Textbook of Angiology

Springer
New York
Berlin
Heidelberg
Barcelona
Hong Kong
London
Milan
Paris
Singapore
Tokyo

Textbook of Angiology

John B. Chang, MD, FACS, FICA

Editor

Associate Editors
Earl R. Olsen, MD, FICA
Kailash Prasad, MD, PhD, FRCP(C), FACC, FICA
Bauer E. Sumpio, MD, PhD, FICA

With 984 Figures

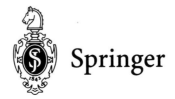 Springer

John B. Chang, MD, FACS, FICA
Chairman, Board of Directors
International College of Angiology, Inc.
    and
Director
Long Island Vascular Center
1050 Northern Boulevard
Roslyn, NY 11576
USA

Earl R. Olsen, MD, FICA
Treasurer and Member,
    Board of Directors
International College of Angiology, Inc.

Kailash Prasad, MD, PhD, FRCP(C), FACC, FICA
Member, Board of Directors
International College of Angiology, Inc.
    and
Associate Member
Department of Medicine
University of Saskatchewan College of Medicine
Saskatoon, Saskatchewan
Canada

Bauer E. Sumpio, MD, PhD, FICA
Vice President, Scientific Council
International College of Angiology, Inc.
    and
Division of Vascular Surgery
Department of Surgery
Yale University School of Medicine
New Haven, CT 06510
USA

Library of Congress Cataloging-in-Publication Data

Chang, John B.
    Textbook of angiology / John B. Chang, Kailash Prasad, Earl R.
Olsen, Bauer E. Sumpio
        p.   cm.
    Includes bibliographical references and index.
    ISBN 0-387-98449-6 (hardcover : alk. paper)
    1. Blood-vessels—Diseases.   I. Prasad, Kailash.   II. Olsen, Earl
R.   III. Sumpio, Bauer E.   IV. Title.
    [DNLM: 1. Cardiovascular Diseases.   2. Blood Vessels—physiology.
3. Blood Vessels—physiopathology.   WG 120 C456t 1998]
    RC691.C518   1998
    616.1′3—dc21
    DNLM/DLC
    for Library of Congress   98-17068

Printed on acid-free paper.

Production coordinated by Impressions Book and Journal Services, Inc. and managed by Terry Kornak;
manufacturing supervised by Jacqui Ashri.
Typeset by Impressions Book and Journal Services, Inc., Madison, WI.
Printed and bound by Maple-Vail Book Manufacturing Group, York, PA.
Printed in the United States of America.

9 8 7 6 5 4 3 2 1

ISBN 0-387-98449-6   Springer-Verlag   New York   Berlin   Heidelberg   SPIN 10660022

This book is dedicated to all the devoted men and women who work so diligently in the field of angiology.

John B. Chang, MD, FACS, FICA
Editor

Preface

Cardiovascular disease is the greatest killer of people in the industrialized nations. With the advances in science during the past decade, our understanding of the disease has increased much more than anticipated. Yet no matter how many goals have been realized and what progress has been made, we are still appalled by the increase in the incidence of cardiovascular disease, its inexorable progression in those afflicted, and the high morbidity and mortality rates. In some areas our understanding of essential basic issues still remains incomplete, imprecise, and clouded by equivocal evidence. It is these problems that dictate the nature of our pursuits for understanding the disease processes and enhancing the capabilities of diagnosis, prevention, and treatment of vascular diseases be it medical or surgical. Although major achievements have been made, they are only minuscule compared with what remains to be achieved.

We have made the most ambitious and formidable undertaking of compiling this book in an attempt to summarize our present knowledge of the understanding of the pathophysiology of vascular diseases, diagnostic modalities, preventive measures, and treatment by medical and surgical means. Information on all aspects of vascular disease has become vast. Thus a single book can no longer adequately cover every aspect of the subject. We have, therefore, selected topics that focus on the important advances in cardiovascular disease that have occurred during the past decade.

We have made an effort to ignore the classical disciplinary boundaries of the medical sciences because they are felt to be irrelevant for the organization of this book. Angiology is a unique discipline that covers all diseases related to blood vessels, including coronary artery disease, hypertension, atherosclerosis, stroke, and peripheral vascular disease. The field of angiology brings together basic scientists and clinicians to enhance our understanding of cardiovascular disease and to improve health care delivery. The interdisciplinary exchange of information and opinions is important because vascular diseases comprise multiple pathophysiological disorders, which are expressed as basic disturbances in the integrative physiology and biochemistry of organ systems. We have attempted to consolidate the knowledge from all disciplines to amplify our understanding of the mechanisms of vascular disease and improve the diagnosis and treatment of these diseases.

This book covers the basic physiological principles of angiology, the pathophysiology and mechanism of disease processes, diagnostic principles, and the prevailing treatments. Topics encompass the integrative control mechanisms, the role of oxygen free radicals in peripheral vascular disease, the mechanism of atherosclerosis, thrombotic and embolic arterial occlusive diseases of the extracranial carotid artery, the aortoiliac segment and visceral arteries, deep vein thrombosis and pulmonary embolism, arterial-venous malformations, aneurysmal diseases of the aorta and peripheral arteries, and the essentials of anesthesia for cardiovascular procedures. Specifically, we have included topics on valvular heart disease, Lyme disease, hypertension, coronary artery disease and bypass surgery, thromboangiitis obliterans, coarctation of the aorta, dissecting aortic aneurysms, the subclavian steal syndrome, thoracic outlet syndrome, popliteal artery entrapment syndrome, vasculitis, diabetic vascular disease, endoluminal grafting, Behçet's disease, renovascular disease, Marfan's syndrome, Budd-Chiari's syndrome, vascular trauma, venous diseases of the upper extremity, occlusive vascular disease in cancer, lymphadenopathy, and phlebology.

The chapters have been organized to provide an overview of the disease in the introduction, the description of the pathophysiology, a characterization of the clinical features, a discussion of the diagnostic modalities, and an assessment of current treatments. We hope that this format will be conducive for facilitating the management of patients.

The contributors of the chapters in this book have provided a comprehensive and authoritative text on the latest concepts in our basic understanding of the pathophysiology of the disease, and for diagnosis and treatment. This book not only examines the mechanism of the disease, application of modern invasive and noninvasive diagnostic techniques, and the management of patients, but also stresses the rationale, techniques, and indications of vascular and cardiac surgery. Particular consideration has been placed on what is considered the cutting-edge of concepts for understanding the pathophysiology of the disease, and for diagnosis and treatment. Where concepts are still ambiguous, multiple authorship has contributed to diverse opinions on some topics. We believe that this book embraces the state of the art for practicing physicians and surgeons, the cutting edge of knowledge in the understanding of vascular disease, and the latest developments concerning the pathophysiology of the disease.

This is the first written in English book on angiology that encompasses every discipline related to blood vessels. Thus, this book should be of value for physicians, surgeons, basic scientists, medical students, residents, interns, and related health care professionals. Health professionals in the field of angiology should find this book very useful in their practice. We hope to continue with further editions of this book to update the changing advances in angiology.

We wish to express our sincere thanks to the contributors, whose names and affiliations are listed elsewhere, for giving their time and effort in making this book possible. The close relationship among the authors contributes to the strengths of this book. We also wish to express our appreciation to our many associates and colleagues who, being experts in their fields, reviewed the chapters and have helped us with their constructive criticism and helpful suggestions.

Editor and Associate Editors

Acknowledgments

A book of this magnitude and scope could not have been written without the assistance and forbearance of numerous individuals. All contributors, reviewers, and the people behind the scenes truly deserve my sincere thanks and appreciation for their roles in the realization of this dream. I extend my profound gratitude to the associate editors and chapter coordinators for their painstaking work that made it possible to undertake and successfully complete this book. I would like to congratulate Springer-Verlag for their outstanding job in producing this book. I thank Ms. Denise M. Rossignol, Executive Director of the International College of Angiology, for her valuable assistance in establishing prompt and timely communications between contributors and the editor. I would also like to thank my associate, Theodore Stein, PhD, for his editorial assistance. Finally, I take this opportunity to express my eternal gratitude and love to Lucy J. Chang, MD, my dear wife and lifetime partner, for her endless support, unwitting sacrifices, and understanding.

John B. Chang, MD, FACS, FICA
Editor

Contents

Editor

John B. Chang, MD, FACS, FICA, Past-President, International College of Angiology, Inc.; Chairman, Board of Directors, International College of Angiology, Inc.; Past-President, The Phlebology Society of America; Chairman, Board of Directors, The Phlebology Society of America; Founding Chairman and Member, Board of Directors, Asian Vascular Society; Editor-in-Chief, *International Journal of Angiology;* Director, Long Island Vascular Center, Roslyn, New York

Associate Editors

Earl R. Olsen, MD, FICA, Past-President, International College of Angiology, Inc.; Treasurer and Member, Board of Directors, International College of Angiology, Inc.; Senior Editor, *International Journal of Angiology;* San Francisco, California

Kailash Prasad, MD, PhD, FRCP(C), FACC, FICA, Past-President, International College of Angiology, Inc.; Member, Board of Directors, International College of Angiology, Inc.; Chairman, Scientific Committee, International College of Angiology, Inc.; Senior Editor, *International Journal of Angiology;* Associate Member, Department of Medicine, University of Saskatchewan College of Medicine, Saskatoon, Saskatchewan, Canada

Bauer E. Sumpio, MD, PhD, FICA, Vice President, Scientific Council, International College of Angiology, Inc.; Co-Chairman, Scientific Committee, International College of Angiology, Inc.; Senior Editor, *International Journal of Angiology;* Division of Vascular Surgery; Department of Surgery; Yale University School of Medicine, New Haven, Connecticut

Chapter Coordinators

Jose Alemany, MD, FICA, President-Elect and Member, Board of Directors, International College of Angiology, Inc.; Editor, *International Journal of Angiology;* Head, Department of Surgery, Knappschafts-Krankenhaus, Bottrop, Germany

John D. Corson, MB, ChB, FICA, Professor of Surgery; Vice President, Scientific Council, International College of Angiology, Inc.; Co-Chairman, Scientific Committee, International College of Angiology, Inc.; Editor, *International Journal of Angiology;* Chief, Department of Vascular Surgery, University of Iowa Hospitals and Clinics, Iowa City, Iowa

John A. Elefteriades, MD, FICA, Professor of Surgery; Co-Chairman, Scientific Committee, International College of Angiology, Inc.; Editor, *International Journal of Angiology;* Chief, Department of Cardiothoracic Surgery, Yale University School of Medicine, New Haven, Connecticut

Robert Gasser, MD, PhD, FICA, Professor of Internal Medicine and Cardiology; Vice President, International College of Angiology, Inc.; Co-Chairman, Scientific Committee, International College of Angiology, Inc.; Editor, *International Journal of Angiology;* Department of Medicine, Division of Cardiology, University of Graz, Graz, Austria

Shunichi Hoshino, MD, PhD, FICA, Professor of Surgery; Editor, *International Journal of Angiology;* Department of Cardiovascular Surgery, Fukushima University School of Medicine, Fukushima, Japan

Anthony Imparato, MD, Professor of Surgery; Editor, *International Journal of Angiology;* Division of Vascular Surgery, New York University Medical Center, New York, New York

Fritz Kaindl, MD, FICA, Professor of Cardiology; Honorary Fellow, International College of Angiology, Inc.; Founding Member, International College of Angiology, Inc.; Member, Board of Directors, International College of Angiology, Inc.; Member, Advisory Council, International College of Angiology, Inc.; Past-President, International College of Angiology, Inc.; Senior Editor, *International Journal of Angiology;* Vienna, Austria

Tatsuki Katsumura, MD, FICA, Professor of Surgery; President and Member, Board of Directors, International College of Angiology, Inc.; Editor, *International Journal of Angiology;* Dean, Kawasaki Medical School, Kurashiki City, Okayama, Japan

Yoshihiko Kubo, MD, FICA, Professor of Surgery; Vice President, Scientific Council, International College of Angiology, Inc.; Co-Chairman, Membership Committee, International College of Angiology, Inc.; Editor, *International Journal of Angiology;* First Department of Surgery, Asahikawa Medical College, Asahikawa, Japan

Dirk A. Loose, MD, FICA, Editor, *International Journal of Angiology;* Center for Circulatory Disturbances and Vascular Defects, Hamburg, Germany

Elmo Mannarino, MD, Department of Clinical Medicine, Pathology, and Pharmacology, Università Degli Studi di Perugia, Perugia, Italy

Michael Martin, MD, FICA, Professor of Medicine; Editor, *International Journal of Angiology;* Personalhaus I der Städtischen Kliniken, Duisburg, Germany

Maurice W. Nicholson, MD, FICA, Editor, *International Journal of Angiology;* Neurological Surgery, Queens Medical Center, Honolulu, Hawaii

Travis J. Phifer, MD, FICA, Associate Professor of Surgery; Member, Board of Directors, The Phlebology Society of America; Past-President, The Phlebology Society of America; Editor, *International Journal of Angiology;* Chief, Division of Vascular Surgery, Louisiana State University Medical Center, Shreveport, Louisiana

Peter Polterauer, MD, Professor of Surgery; Chairman and Director, Vascular Surgery, University of Vienna Medical School, Vienna, Austria

Kailash Prasad, MD, PhD, FRCP(C), FACC, FICA, Professor Emeritus; Past-President, International College of Angiology, Inc.; Member, Board of Directors, International College of Angiology, Inc.; Chairman, Scientific Committee, International College of Angiology, Inc.; Senior Editor, *International Journal of Angiology;* Associate Member, Department of Medicine, University of Saskatchewan College of Medicine, Saskatoon, Saskatchewan, Canada

John H. Scurr, FRCS, FICA, Editor, *International Journal of Angiology;* Senior Lecturer and Consultant Surgeon, Middlesex and University College Hospital, The Lister Hospital, London, England

Vikrom S. Sottiurai, MD, PhD, FICA, Professor of Clinical Surgery; Vice President, Scientific Council, International College of Angiology, Inc.; Co-Chairman, Scientific Committee, International College of Angiology, Inc.; President and Member, Board of Directors, The Phlebology Society of America; Editor, *International Journal of Angiology;* Louisiana State University School of Medicine in New Orleans, New Orleans, Louisiana

Bauer E. Sumpio, MD, PhD, FICA, Professor and Vice Chairman of Surgery; Vice President, Scientific Council, International College of Angiology, Inc.; Co-Chairman, Scientific Committee, International College of Angiology, Inc.; Senior Editor, *International Journal of Angiology;* Chief, Division of Vascular Surgery; Department of Surgery; Yale University School of Medicine, New Haven, Connecticut

Francis Vella, MD, MA (OXON), PhD, DSc (Hon. Causo), Acting General Secretary, The International Union of Biochemistry and Molecular Biology, Department of Biochemistry, College of Medicine, University of Saskatchewan, Saskatoon, Saskatchewan, Canada

Keishu Yasuda, MD, PhD, FICA, Professor of Surgery; Vice President, Scientific Council, International College of Angiology, Inc.; Editor, *International Journal of Angiology;* Chairman, Department of Cardiovascular Surgery, Hokkaido University School of Medicine, Sapporo, Japan

Section 1
Basic Physiologic Principles
in Angiology

1

Structure and Function
of Various Vascular Beds

Kailash Prasad

Blood leaving the left ventricle of the heart is distributed to the tissues through the aorta, arteries (large and small), arterioles, and capillaries. Blood is collected from the capillaries via venules, which join repeatedly to form increasingly large veins that finally reach the heart (Figure 1.1). The systemic circulation includes the blood vessels originating from the left ventricle (aorta) and terminating at the right atrium. Pulmonary circulation constitutes the vessels lying between the right ventricle and the left atrium. Vessels are classified according to function: distribution, resistance, exchange, and capacitance or storage. Shunt vessels provide channels that bypass capillary beds. The resistance vessels include small arteries, arterioles, and precapillary sphincters. Capacitance vessels include small and large veins. Capacitance vessels have great capacity to distend. For a similar rise in pressure, capacitance vessels may accommodate 20 times more blood than resistance vessels. Exchange vessels include the capillaries.

Structure

Structurally, after leaving the aorta, the arterial branches become narrower and their walls become thinner and change histologically as they progress to the periphery. The normal large arterial wall consists of three layers: tunica intima, tunica media, and adventitia (Figure 1.2). The tunica intima consists of endothelial cells and an internal elastic lamina. Endothelial cells line the lumen of all the arteries. They form a continuous single-cell layer. The subendothelial tissue between the internal elastic lamina and endothelial cell layer comprises collagen, elastin fibers, nonstriated myocytes, and macrophages. Endothelial cells not only form a barrier that controls the entry of substances from blood into the arterial wall, but also secrete a variety of substances that regulate the lumen of the blood vessels and affect coagulation. The

tunica media, a fibromuscular structure, extends from the internal to the external elastic lamina. It consists of smooth muscle cells (single or multiple laminae) surrounded by small amounts of collagen and elastic fibers. Smooth muscle cells produce collagen, elastic fibers, and proteoglycans. The tunica adventitia is the outermost layer of the artery, lying outside the external elastic lamina. It consists of a mixture of collagen and elastic fibers and fibroblasts. This layer also contains the vasa vasorum and nerves.

As one moves from aorta to capillaries the branches become narrower and their walls thinner and histologically different (Figure 1.3). Moving from capillaries to the venous system, the changes occur in reverse order. Larger arteries have a large proportion of elastic fibers and collagen and fewer smooth muscle cells. These elastic elements permit the proximal aorta and large arteries to be readily stretched during systole to accommodate the blood. As one goes from the aorta to the arterioles, the elastin and collagen content decreases and the smooth muscle cell component increases, becoming proportionately larger in the arterioles. Capillaries consist of a single layer of endothelial cells permitting rapid exchange of water and solutes with tissue. Capillaries do not have elastic tissue or smooth muscle cells. As one moves from the capillaries to the large veins, elastin and smooth muscle cells begin to appear.

Blood and Nerve Supply of Arteries

Larger arteries are supplied by the vasa vasorum, which may be branches of the artery itself or of a vessel at some distance from their distribution. They supply the tunica adventitia and outer part of the tunica media. The remainder of the wall is supplied by diffusion of blood

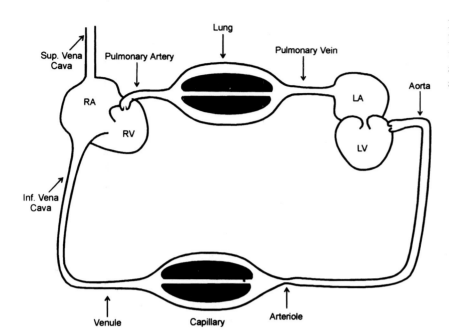

FIGURE 1.1. Schematic diagram of the circulatory system showing the heart and systemic and pulmonary circulation. RA, right atrium; RV, right ventricle; LA, left atrium; and LV, left ventricle.

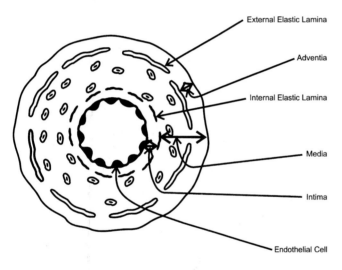

FIGURE 1.2. Diagram showing the principal components of the arterial wall.

from these vessels or from the vascular lumen. Arteries and veins are richly supplied by sympathetic fibers that elicit vasoconstriction via activation of α-adrenergic receptors. Some arterioles also respond to sympathetic stimulation by vasodilation via β₂-adrenergic receptors. Arterioles are richly supplied with sympathetic fibers and act as a stopcock mechanism regulating both arterial pressure and blood flow to the organs.

Capillaries (Exchange Vessels)

The capillary network is schematically shown in Figure 1.4. Arterioles give rise directly to capillaries or metarterioles, which in turn give rise to capillaries. Metarterioles

are a high resistance pathway and sometimes connect directly to venules, without giving rise to capillaries. This constitutes an arteriovenous (A–V) shunt. Capillaries are composed of a single thin layer of endothelial cells with a thin basement membrane to provide support. Numerous capillaries arise from single arterioles or metarterioles. They branch and anastomose repeatedly. Average length of a capillary varies from 0.5 to 1 mm. At the point of origin from the arterioles, capillaries have a smooth muscle coat called the precapillary sphincter. The precapillary sphincter and arterioles regulate blood flow in the capillaries. Constriction of these structures decreases and relaxation increases the flow through capillaries. Capillaries ultimately terminate in venules. Capillary density varies from tissue to tissue, and is greatest

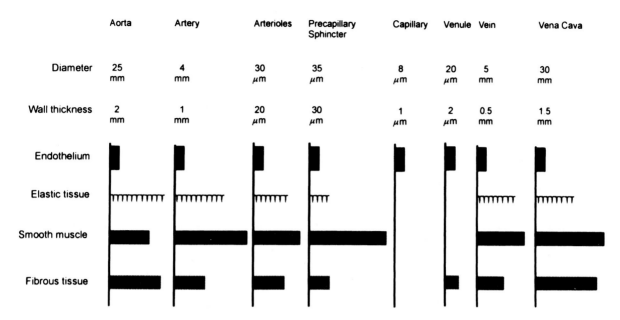

	Aorta	Artery	Arterioles	Precapillary Sphincter	Capillary	Venule	Vein	Vena Cava
Diameter	25 mm	4 mm	30 μm	35 μm	8 μm	20 μm	5 mm	30 mm
Wall thickness	2 mm	1 mm	20 μm	30 μm	1 μm	2 μm	0.5 mm	1.5 mm
Endothelium								
Elastic tissue								
Smooth muscle								
Fibrous tissue								

FIGURE 1.3. Diagram showing the principal components, diameter, and thickness at the various levels of vasculature.

in active tissue. Blood flow in capillaries is not uniform. The average velocity of blood flow is about 1 mm/s; however this can vary from zero to several millimeters per second within a short period in the same vessel. Precapillary vessels show a rhythmic behavior caused by alternate contraction and relaxation (vasomotion). This may be due to an intrinsic contractile behavior of vascular smooth muscle cells or to changes in the transmural pressure. At any one time only 5% to 20% of capillaries are open. If all the capillaries were open at one time,

most of the blood would accumulate in them and cardiac output would decrease dramatically, as occurs in the terminal stage of hemorrhagic shock. When the mast cell lining adjacent to a closed capillary becomes slightly anoxic, it secretes histamine, which causes the capillary to open. Histamine is destroyed quickly in the blood and does not circulate. When mast cells are oxygenated, they stop histamine secretion and the capillary closes. As a result, capillaries open in turn.

Mechanism of Vascular Contraction

Vascular muscle cells contain three types of filaments: thick, thin, and intermediate (Figure 1.5). The function of intermediate filaments is not known. Thin filaments are composed of contractile protein, actin, and the modulatory protein tropomyosin. Troponin complex, which is present in cardiac cells, is absent in vascular smooth muscle cells. The exact role of tropomyosin in vascular contraction is not known. Thick filaments are composed of myosin, which consists of a tail and a head. The head contains the active sites for interaction with actin filaments and contains two parts consisting of heavy chains and two pairs of low molecular weight light chains. Myosin ATPase activity in the head region hydrolyzes adenosine triphosphate (ATP). One pair of light chains is capable of being phosphorylated in a calcium-dependent manner and is called P-light chains. Myosin light-chain kinase is present in myosin heads in inactive form. Its activity is dependent upon calcium and calmodulin. Myosin light-chain phosphatase in the myosin head cat-

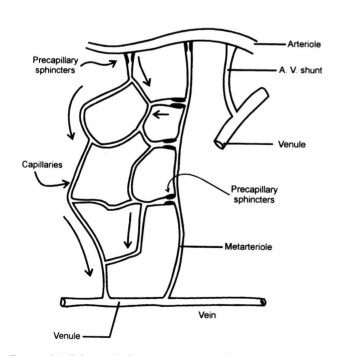

FIGURE 1.4. Schematic diagram of the capillary network.

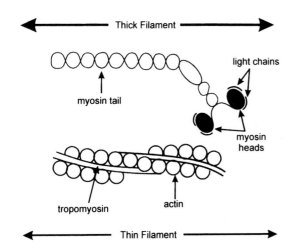

FIGURE 1.5. Ultrastructure of the vascular smooth muscle.

alyzes dephosphorylation of P-light chains and of myosin light-chain kinase (MLCK).

The mechanism of vascular contraction and relaxation is schematically presented in Figure 1.6. Four calcium ions bind to four metal binding sites on calmodulin to form a calcium–calmodulin complex, which then binds to inactive MLCK to form active MLCK. MLCK catalyzes phosphorylation of the myosin P-light chain through activation of Mg-ATPase (transfer of phosphate from Mg^{2+}-ATP to myosin P-light chain). Phosphorylated myosin P-light chain activates actomyosin ATPase activity, resulting in interaction of actin and myosin filaments

and contraction via a sliding mechanism. Myosin light-chain phosphatase dephosphorylates the myosin P-light chain, resulting in relaxation.

Calcium Fluxes in Vascular Smooth Muscle

Calcium (Ca^{2+}) enters the cell through three mechanisms (Figure 1.7): potential-dependent channels (PDC), receptor-operated channels (ROC), and passive leak. Potential-dependent channels open by depolarization (electrical stimulation and potassium). Receptor-operated channels are stimulated by drugs such as norepinephrine. When muscle is in the resting state, potential-dependent channels and receptor-operated channels are closed but the membrane is still permeable to calcium. This passive leak is insensitive to calcium-channel blockers. Potential-dependent channels are more sensitive than receptor-operated channels to calcium-channel blockers. Receptors in receptor-operated channels are activated by agonists and activate phospholipase C in a reaction coupled to guanine nucleotide–binding G proteins. Phospholipase C hydrolyzes phosphatidylinositol bisphosphate in the membrane to yield diacylglycerol and inositol triphosphate. Inositol triphosphate releases Ca^{2+} from the sarcoplasmic reticulum. Calcium entering through receptor-operated channels directly releases Ca^{2+} from the sarcoplasmic reticulum. For relaxation, Ca^{2+} is taken up by the sarcoplasmic reticulum. This uptake is active and energy dependent (ATP and Ca^{2+}-ATPase). Ca^{2+} is extruded from the cell by a calcium pump that is ATP dependent, by sodium–calcium exchange, by a sodium–potassium pump, and by sodium–hydrogen exchange.

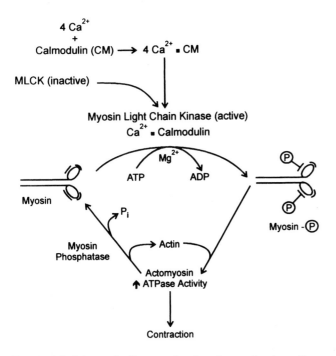

FIGURE 1.6. Schematic diagram showing the mechanism of contraction and relaxation of the vascular smooth muscle. Myosin-P, phosphorylated myosin.

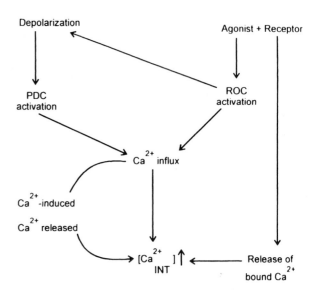

FIGURE 1.7. Mechanism of calcium influx and release of calcium bound to calcium store (sarcoplasmic reticulum).

Calcium Pump

There are two types of calcium pumps: plasmalemmal (sarcolemmal) and sarcoplasmic reticular. The sarcolemmal calcium pump is ATP dependent, pumps Ca^{2+} outward, and is regulated by calcium–calmodulin complex. The sarcoplasmic calcium pump is ATP dependent and transports calcium from the cytosol to the sarcoplasmic reticulum during relaxation. It is stimulated by a phosphorylation reaction catalyzed by protein kinase A. Phospholamban, a regulatory protein, inhibits the sarcoplasmic reticular Ca^{2+} pump. This inhibitory effect of phospholamban is reversed when it is phosphorylated by protein kinase A.

Sodium–Calcium Exchange

Three sodium ions are exchanged for one calcium ion, generating an electrical current with a gain of intracellular positive charge. There is a direct relationship between $[Ca^{2+}]_o/[Na^+]_o$ for this exchange. This exchanger carries sodium or calcium in either direction across the sarcolemma. The amounts of either ion carried are determined by their relative concentrations on either side of the membrane. The driving force for calcium efflux via sodium–calcium exchange is the sodium gradient $[Na^+]_i/[Na^+]_o$. The efflux of Ca^{2+} is about 30 times higher through this exchange mechanism than through the calcium pump. Increasing intracellular sodium increases intracellular calcium through this mechanism.

Sodium–Potassium Pump

The sodium–potassium pump (Mg^{2+}-dependent Na^+-K^+-ATPase) pumps sodium out of the cell and potassium into the cell against their concentration gradient. This pump is activated by internal sodium and external potassium and requires ATP to function. Three sodium ions are transported out of the cell in exchange for two potassium ions that enter the cell; hence, this pump is electrogenic. Because of this, it is also called the electrogenic sodium pump. Drugs that inhibit the sodium–potassium pump increase intracellular sodium, which then increases intracellular calcium through the Na^+-Ca^{2+} exchange mechanism. Increasing Ca^{2+} increases vascular tone. Cardiac glycosides and vanadium inhibit this pump and therefore increase cardiac contractility and vascular tone.

Sodium–Hydrogen Exchange

The exchange of Na^+ for H^+ plays a role in regulating intracellular Na^+ and H^+. During ischemia when intracellular pH decreases due to anaerobic glycolysis, this exchange mechanism removes excess H^+. The amount of Na^+ that enters the cell then increases intracellular Ca^{2+} through the Na^+-Ca^{2+} exchange mechanism.

Role of Endothelium

Endothelium serves several functions besides that of a passive filter that permits passage of water and small molecules across the vessel wall and retains blood cells and large molecules within the vascular compartments. Other functions of endothelium are modulation of vascular tone, coagulation, vascular wall remodeling, and mediation of inflammatory and immunologic responses. Endothelial cell function is described in detail in another chapter in this book.

Modulation of Vascular Tone

Vasodilators

Vascular endothelium synthesizes and releases both vasodilator and vasoconstrictor agents. Vasodilators (relaxant factors) include endothelium-derived relaxing factor (EDRF), endothelium-derived hyperpolarizing factor (EDHF), prostaglandin (PG) I_2, PGE_2, adenosine, ammonia, oxygen radicals, and 11,12,15-hydroxyeicosatetraenoic acid. Contractile factors include endothelin, thromboxane A_2 (TXA_2), angiotensin II, $PGF_{2\alpha}$, serotonin, and oxygen radicals.

Endothelium-Derived Relaxing Factor

Endothelium-derived relaxing factor is actually nitric oxide (NO). Its synthesis pathway is shown schematically in Figure 1.8. NO is synthesized by conversion of L-arginine to L-citrulline by an enzyme, nitric oxide synthetase. NO increases the activity of guanylate cyclase, which acts on guanosine triphosphate (GTP) to form cyclic guanosine monophosphate (cGMP), which is associated with vascular relaxation. NO-induced relaxation could be due to

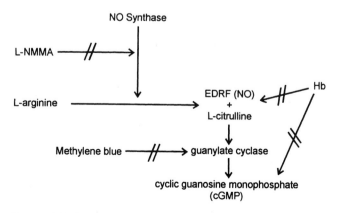

FIGURE 1.8. Synthesis of NO and cGMP and their inhibitors.

formation of a hydroxyl radical (·OH), which also activates guanylate cyclase. Various agents (Figure 1.8) affect the formation and amount of NO. L-*N*-monomethyl arginine (L-NMMA) is a false precursor amino acid that competes with L-arginine for the enzyme nitric oxide synthetase and is the most specific inhibitor of NO formation. Hemoglobin binds NO and thus reduces formation of cGMP. Methylene blue and to some extent also hemoglobin inhibit guanylate cyclase.

Superoxide anion reacts with NO to generate peroxynitrite, which is then converted to peroxynitrous acid at physiological pH. This acid is very unstable and decomposes to form the hydroxyl radical ·OH, which is a vasodilator. Factors such as acetylcholine, ATP, thrombin, bradykinin, histamine, serotonin, substance P, shear stress, hypoxia, flow, and mechanical stretching are able to release EDRF from endothelium. EDRF (NO) has numerous functions: (1) it is a vasodilator; (2) it inhibits platelet aggregation and adhesion; (3) it disaggregates platelets already aggregated; (4) it inhibits smooth muscle proliferation; (5) it modulates vascular tone by suppressing expression of endothelial vasoconstrictor and platelet-derived growth factor B, a potent mitogen with some vasoconstrictor property; (6) it causes depression of myocardial contractility; (7) it inhibits leukocyte adhesion to endothelium and leukocyte aggregation.

The clinical implications of EDRF are numerous. EDRF levels are lower than normal in smokers, children with hypercholesterolemia, and people with atherosclerosis, hypertension, diabetes mellitus, or acute renal failure.

Endothelium-Derived Hyperpolarizing Factor

EDHF depolarizes the membrane by opening ATP-sensitive potassium channels or by activating the sodium–potassium pump. Hyperpolarization inactivates voltage-sensitive calcium channels, reduces the sensitivity of contractile proteins to increases in intracellular calcium, and inhibits activation of phospholipase C and the mobilization of intracellular calcium. The actual chemical nature of EDHF is not known.

Prostaglandins

Endothelial cells synthesize and release PGI_2. Formation of prostaglandins from arachidonic acid are schematically shown in Figure 1.9. Phospholipase A_2 releases arachidonic acid from membrane phospholipid. Arachidonic acid is converted to PGG_2 by cyclooxygenase. Prostaglandin hydroperoxidase converts PGG_2 to PGH_2, which is then converted into PGE_2, PGD_2, PGI_2, and TXA_2 in different organs by the respective prostaglandin synthetases. PGI_2 is a vasodilator that inhibits platelet aggregation and adhesion. Synthesis and release of PGI_2 are increased by acetylcholine, ATP, thrombin, brady-

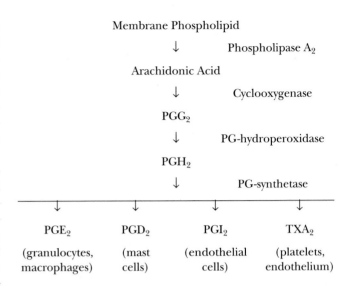

FIGURE 1.9. Formation of various prostaglandins from arachidonic acid metabolism in various tissues.

kinin, histamine, PDGF, high-density lipoprotein cholesterol, leukotrienes, TXA_2, hypoxia, shear stress, serotonin, interleukin 1, vitamins C and E, estradiol, insulin, calcium antagonists, angiotensin-converting enzyme inhibitors nitrates, streptokinase, dipyridamole, and diuretic agents. Synthesis is inhibited by cyclooxygenase inhibitors such as indomethacin, aspirin, nonsteroidal antiinflammatory drugs, and nicotine. PGI_2 synthesis is inhibited by low-density lipoprotein cholesterol, glucocorticoids, and superoxide anion. Glucocorticoids inhibit synthesis by stimulating formation of lipocortin, which inhibits phospholipase A_2 activity.

Oxygen Radicals

Oxygen radicals in endothelial cells are produced mainly by the xanthine–xanthine oxidase pathway and during synthesis of prostaglandins. Low levels of oxygen radicals stimulate cyclooxygenation of arachidonic acid. Increased concentrations inactivate NO and inhibit PGG_2, PGH_2, and PGI_2 synthetases. Oxygen radicals have varying effects on vascular smooth muscle. Superoxide anion produces contraction, hydrogen peroxide produces transient relaxation followed by contraction, and hydroxyl radicals produce only relaxation.

Vasoconstrictors

Endothelium synthesizes and releases numerous vasoconstrictors including endothelin, TXA_2, $PGF_{2\alpha}$, angiotensin II, serotonin, and oxygen radicals.

Endothelin

There are three families of endothelin (ET): ET-1, ET-2, and ET-3. Endothelial cells produce ET-1 only. Endothelins are formed by the conversion of "big" endothelin to endothelin by one or two endothelin-converting enzymes. There are two classes of endothelin receptors, ET_A and ET_B. Both are G protein linked. ET_B has two subtypes. ET_A is found on vascular smooth muscle cells and is responsible for vasoconstriction. Endothelin-induced vasoconstriction is mediated through activation of calcium channels and phospholipase C and A_2. Many substances (including thrombin, epinephrine, and calcium ionophore) cause slow release of ET-1. The usual stimulus for release is damage to the endothelium. Endothelin is a potent vasoconstrictor (10 times more than angiotensin II). It has a mitogenic effect on vascular smooth muscle cells, fibroblasts, and mesangial cells.

Thromboxane A_2

The synthesis pathway of TXA_2 is shown in Figure 1.9. TXA_2 is synthesized not only in the platelets but also in endothelium. Synthesis is inhibited by cyclooxygenase inhibitors, as pointed out in the previous section. Aspirin inhibits cyclooxygenase irreversibly by acetylation of a serine residue at its active site. Since nonnucleated platelets can not produce cyclooxygenase, thromboxane synthesis can occur only with newly formed platelets. The life span of platelets is about 8 to 10 days. Therefore the effect of aspirin has long duration. The formation of PGI_2 is unopposed because cyclooxygenase in endothelial cells recovers within a few hours. Dazoxiben interferes with synthesis of TXA_2 by inhibiting thromboxane synthase. TXA_2 is a vasoconstrictor and helps in aggregation and adhesion of platelets. Its action is just opposite to that of PGI_2.

Angiotensin

Angiotensin II has already been discussed in detail. It should be noted that tissue can also produce angiotensin II. The cells contain rennin, angiotensin-converting enzyme, and angiotensinogen. Angiotensin I is formed in the cell and is then converted to angiotensin II, which has autocrine and paracrine effects. Autocrine effects occur in the same cells where angiotensin II is produced. Paracrine effects occur in other cells. Angiotensin II opens calcium channels and releases Ca^{2+} from the sarcoplasmic reticulum.

Serotonin and Oxygen Radicals

Serotonin will be described later in the section titled "Endothelial Modulation of Vascular Tone." Oxygen radicals have been described earlier in this chapter.

Coagulation

Endothelium regulates intravascular coagulation by participation in and separation of procoagulant pathways, inhibition of procoagulant protein, regulation of fibrinolysis, and production of thromboregulating compounds.

Participation in and Separation of Procoagulant Pathways

Endothelium produces several factors (high molecular weight kininogen, factor V, factor VIII, and tissue factor) involved in coagulation. Also there are binding sites for high molecular weight kininogen and factors VIII, IX, IXa, X, and Xa on endothelial cells, which provide an additional mechanism for procoagulant activity. Endothelium separates intravascular coagulation factor (VIIa) from subendothelial tissue factor and prevents platelets from being exposed to subendothelial proaggregating factors such as collagen and von Willebrand factor. Endothelial cells produce the proteoglycan heparin sulfate, which increases the activity of antithrombin III.

Inhibition of Procoagulant Proteins

Endothelial cells inhibit procoagulant proteins (protein C, protein S, and thrombomodulin). Activated protein C inactivates factors Va and VIIIa. Thrombomodulin and protein S enhance the activity of protein C.

Regulation of Fibrinolysis

Endothelium synthesizes plasminogen activators (PA), urokinase (uPA), and tissue (tPA) type. They activate plasminogen bound to endothelial cells to plasmin, which is fibrinolytic. Normal endothelial cells express only tPA. When stimulated by cytokines, endothelial cells synthesize uPA preferentially. Endothelial cells also synthesize and secrete the plasminogen inhibitors PAI-1 and PAI-2.

Vascular Wall Remodeling

Endothelial cells produce both growth-promoting and growth-inhibitory factors.

Growth-Promoting Factors

Endothelial cells synthesize platelet-derived growth factor (PDGF), basic fibroblast growth factor, thrombospondin, and insulinlike growth factor (IGF-1). PDGF is a potent mitogen for vascular smooth muscle cells. IGF-1 and thrombospondin are required to stimulate smooth muscle cell proliferation. PDGF is known to induce expression of thrombospondin and IGF-1 in endothelial cells. IGF-1 acts on connective tissue to increase cell growth and to enhance organization and maturation of collagen fibers. Other factors derived from endothelium (angiotensin II, endothelin, oxygen radicals) have been shown to be mitogenic.

Growth-Inhibiting Factors

NO and PGI$_2$ (prostacyclin) are antimitogenic. In addition, the endothelial cells produce glycoprotein, glycosaminoglycans, and transforming growth factor β (TGF-β). Although TGF-β alone stimulates proliferation of fibroblast lines, it is capable of blocking PDGF-dependent growth.

Inflammatory and Immunologic Responses

Inflammatory and immunologic responses by endothelium involve cell adherence, cell activation, and cell migration. These processes are linked to an interplay between the expression of adhesion molecules by endothelial cells, leukocyte activation, and local cytokines. Three types of adhesion molecules (selectins, immunoglobulins, and integrins) are involved in interaction between endothelial cells and leukocytes. Interleukin 1 (IL-1), tumor necrosis factor α (TNF-α), TGF-β, and bacterial endotoxin stimulate endothelial cells to produce IL-1, IL-6, and IL-8. IL-8 regulates transendothelial migration of polymorphonuclear leukocytes.

When stimulated by cytokines or thrombin, endothelial cells express endothelial cell leukocyte adhesion molecule 1 (ELAM-1), and intercellular adhesion molecule 1 (ICAM-1). Platelet-activating factor modulates expression of adhesion molecules. The selectin (ELAM-1) is expressed within hours. Immunoglobulin (intercellular adhesion molecule 1) expression facilitates adhesion of both polymorphonuclear leukocytes and lymphocytes. Intercellular adhesion molecule 2 (immunoglobulin family) mediates binding of T and B lymphocytes to the endothelial cells. Vascular cell adhesion molecule 1 (VCAM-1) of the immunoglobulin series binds lymphocytes and monocytes to endothelial cells.

Clinical Implications

Healthy endothelial cells are essential to ward off vascular diseases. Dysfunctional or damaged endothelial cells lead to various vascular diseases including atherosclerosis, hypertension, diabetes mellitus, coronary and vascular spasm, ischemia–reperfusion injury, intimal hyperplasia, and restenosis.

Acknowledgments
The excellent secretarial assistance provided by Ms. Gloria Schneider is gratefully acknowledged. The author is also grateful to Mr. R. Hutchinson for drawings.

Bibliography

Anderson KL. The cardiovascular system in exercise. In: Falls HB, ed. *Exercise Physiology.* New York, NY: Academic Press; 1968:79–128.

Bharadwaj L, Prasad K. Mediation of H$_2$O$_2$-induced vascular relaxation by endothelium-derived relaxing factor. *Mol Cell Biochem.* 1995;149/150:267–270.

———. Mechanism of hydroxyl radical–induced modulation of vascular tone. *Free Radic Biol Med.* 1997;22:381–390.

Cliff WJ. *Blood Vessels.* Cambridge, England: Cambridge University Press; 1976.

Davies MG, Hagen PO. The vascular endothelium. A new horizon. *Ann Surg.* 1993;218:593–609.

Dobrin PB. Mechanical properties of arteries. *Physiol Rev.* 1978;58:397–460.

Folkow B, Neil B. *Circulation.* New York, NY: Oxford University Press; 1971.

Hardaway RM. *Clinical Management of Shock.* Springfield, Ill: Charles C Thomas Publisher; 1968.

Krogh A. *The Anatomy and Physiology of Capillaries.* New York, NY: Hafner Co; 1959.

Loscalzo J, Welch G. Nitric oxide and its role in the cardiovascular system. *Prog Cardiovasc Dis.* 1995;38:87–104.

Milnor WR. *Hemodynamics.* Baltimore, Md: Williams & Wilkins; 1982.

Moncada S, Palmer RMJ, Higgs EA. Nitric oxide: physiology, pathophysiology and pharmacology. *Pharmacol Rev.* 1991;43: 109–142.

Prasad K, Bharadwaj L. Hydroxyl radical—a mediator of acetylcholine-induced vascular relaxation. *J Mol Cell Cardiol.* 1996;28:2033–2041.

Prasad K, Lee P, Kalra J. Influence of endothelin on cardiovascular function, oxygen free radicals and blood biochemistry. *Am Heart J.* 1991;121:178–187.

Somlyo AV, Somlyo AP. Electrochemical and pharmacomechanical coupling in vascular smooth muscle. *J Pharmacol Exp Ther.* 1968;159:129–145.

Somlyo A. Ultrastructure of vascular smooth muscle. In: Bohr DF, Somlyo A, Sparks HV Jr, eds. *The Cardiovascular System.* Vol 2. Bethesda, Md: American Physiological Society; 1980;33–67. *Handbook of Physiology.*

Vane JR, Anggard EE, Botting RM. Regulatory functions of the vascular endothelium. *N Engl J Med.* 1990;323:27–36.

Vanhoutte PM, Mombouli JV. Vascular endothelium: vasoactive mediators. *Prog Cardiovasc Dis.* 1996;39:229–238.

2

Endothelial Modulation of Vascular Tone

Johan Van de Voorde and Bert Vanheel

The vascular endothelium forms a monolayer lining the luminal surface throughout the cardiovascular system. For a long time endothelium was considered a passive physical barrier whose only function was to provide vessels a smooth surface that prevented clotting and turbulence of the blood flow. The development of new research techniques such as culture of endothelial cells has revolutionized ideas about the function of the endothelium and revealed that it has many fascinating features. With its strategic anatomical position at the border of circulating blood and tissue, it is now considered to be a very active metabolic and endocrine organ with multiple functions. It forms a barrier with well-developed mechanisms for exchanging molecules between the lumen and the subendothelial space; it is the first barrier to circulating antigens and actively participates in defense reactions. Endothelium is also important for angiogenesis. It also synthesizes factors that promote or inhibit the coagulation of blood (platelet adhesion and aggregation), the growth of vascular smooth muscle cells, and the synthesis of extracellular matrix. These processes are dynamically influenced by many different factors, including a pivotal role of endothelium in their regulation.[1,2]

Endothelium also has an important function as regulator of the vascular tone, either by changing plasma concentrations of circulating vasoactive substances or by producing and releasing vasoactive substances. Endothelial enzymes affect circulating vasoactive substances by biotransformation. Circulating norepinephrine and serotonin are actively taken up by endothelial cells and metabolized by monoamine oxidase (MAO). One endothelial membrane enzyme catalyzes the conversion of inactive angiotensin I to the potent vasopressor angiotensin II and also catalyzes the inactivation of bradykinin. These mechanisms are not discussed further in this chapter.

Endothelium is also the site of production and release of some very potent vasoactive substances that have a crucial role in physiological and pathophysiological regulation of vascular tone. The extent to which these substances contribute to cardiovascular control became increasingly apparent in the 1980s. In this chapter we focus on these factors.

Endothelial Relaxing Factors

Nitric Oxide

Historical Notes

That endothelium mediates relaxation in response to certain vasoactive substances was first described in 1980 by Furchgott and Zawadzki.[3] Furchgott and Zawadzki were fascinated by the apparently conflicting observation that acetylcholine elicited contraction of isolated spirally cut strips of rabbit aorta, but when ring segments from the same artery were studied relaxation was the response to acetylcholine. In an effort to explain this discrepancy, they found that ring segments had an intact endothelium, whereas the endothelium of spirally cut strips was disrupted by manipulation during preparation. The different responses may have been related to the state of the endothelium, either intact and functioning or disrupted and nonfunctioning, and this was established experimentally by showing that ring segments also contracted in response to acetylcholine when the endothelium was intentionally disrupted by rubbing the ring segments' intimal surfaces. These experiments gave an acceptable explanation for the long-standing enigma that acetylcholine elicits vasodilation effects in vivo but very often shows contractile effects on isolated preparations.

This observation showing an impressively different response to acetylcholine in preparations with and without endothelium has led to an explosive growth of vascular science. Numerous studies were designed to explore the potential influence of endothelium on the vascular effects of many kinds of vasoactive substances. It became clear that endothelium not only modulates the vascular effect of acetylcholine but also that of many other physiologically important vasoactive substances (Figure 2.1). In Table 2.1 a list of stimuli with an established endothelium-dependent effect is presented. It has been documented that endothelium-dependent relaxation is elicited by substances as varying as neurotransmitters, hormones, autacoids, and some released by aggregating platelets (adenosine diphosphate, serotonin) and by physical forces such as the shear stress exerted on the endothelial cell surface by circulating blood.[4]

Since then endothelium-mediated relaxation has been described in all types of blood vessels, from conduit arteries and resistance arteries to veins, and in many species, including humans. Except for acetylcholine, which elicits endothelium-dependent relaxation on almost all blood vessels, most substances show an impor-

TABLE 2.1. Stimuli that elicit endothelial-dependent relaxation of isolated blood vessels.

Acetylcholine	Insulin
Adenosine diphosphate	Leukotrienes
Adenosine triphosphate	Norepinephrine
Arachidonic acid	Oxytocin
Bradykinin	Serotonin
Calcitonin gene-related peptide	Shear stress
Cholecystokinin	Substance P
Ergometrin	Thrombin
Flow	Vasoactive intestinal peptide
Histamine	Vasopressin

tant interspecies and regional heterogeneity in the role of endothelium in the vascular effects.[4,6]

In their original publication, Furchgott and Zawadzki already showed that the endothelium-dependent relaxation was mediated by a humoral factor released from endothelium.[3] This factor was named *endothelium-derived*

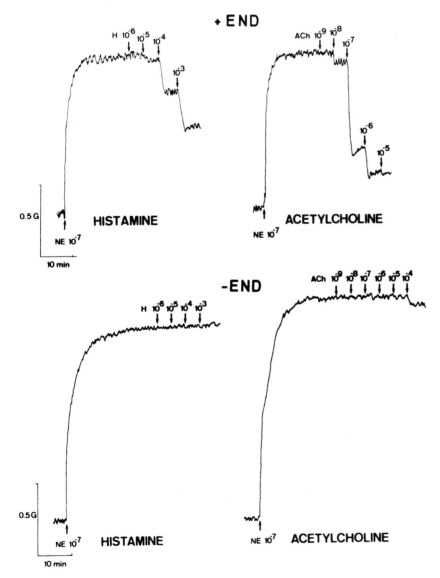

FIGURE 2.1. Original recording of an experiment on isolated rat thoracic aorta with and without endothelium (END). Addition of increasing molar concentrations of histamine (H) or acetylcholine (ACh) to preparations precontracted with norepinephrine (NE; 10^{-7} M) elicits relaxation only if endothelium is present (from Van de Voorde and Leusen[5] with kind permission from Elsevier Science NL, Saraburgeihartstreet 25, 1055 KV Amsterdam, The Netherlands).

relaxing factor, or EDRF. From bioassay experiments it soon became clear that EDRF was a very labile substance. A half-life of 6 seconds was reported.[7] This extreme lability hampered the chemical identification of EDRF. However, it was soon found that EDRF-induced relaxation of the smooth muscle was due to activation of soluble guanylyl cyclase and increased cytosolic cyclic guanosine monophosphate (GMP) levels[8] (Figure 2.2). This mechanism of action was already known to be responsible for the relaxing action of the nitrovasodilators (nitroglyc-

erin, isosorbide dinitrate). These drugs, after being metabolized to nitric oxide (NO), relax vascular smooth muscle cells by activation of guanylyl cyclase.[9] This led to the hypothesis that EDRF might be NO. Comparative studies showing that NO and EDRF displayed analogous biological and biochemical characteristics provided strong evidence in support of this hypothesis.[10,11] The ultimate chemical identification of EDRF as NO was reported in 1987 by Palmer et al.[12] Although it is accepted that NO is the biologically active component of EDRF, there is still some controversy as to whether EDRF is NO or an NO-containing compound (e.g., a nitrosothiol).

Identification of EDRF as NO raised the question of what the biological precursor might be of this simple, very labile, but obviously very potent endothelial relaxing substance. Once again, Palmer et al. provided very convincing evidence that NO was derived from the amino acid L-arginine.[13,14] The strict structural and stereoisomeric specificity of the biological precursor suggested involvement of an enzymatic reaction. The enzyme was called NO synthase (NOS). Enzymatic conversion of L-arginine to NO could be blocked by certain analogs of L-arginine, including NG-monomethyl-L-arginine (L-NMMA), NG-nitro-L-arginine (L-NNA) and NG-nitro-L-arginine methyl ester (L-NAME). These analogs compete with L-arginine and act as stereospecific inhibitors of NOS. They proved to be specific blockers of endothelium-dependent relaxation and provided excellent tools for exploring the physiological importance of NO in the cardiovascular system.[15] It became more and more clear that NO plays an important role in the regulation of cardiovascular homeostasis (besides its roles in many other physiological and pathophysiological processes).

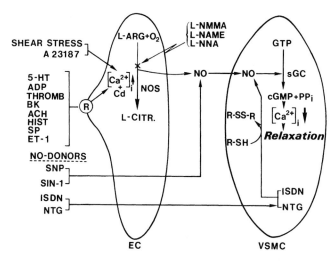

FIGURE 2.2. Schematic representation of the L-arginine–NO–cyclic guanosine monophosphate (GMP) pathway in vasculature and its relation to NO donors. NO is formed during conversion of L-arginine (L-ARG) to L-citrulline (L-CITR) in endothelial cells (EC) by NO synthase (NOS). The enzyme is activated through nonreceptor (e.g., shear stress, calcium ionophore A23187) and receptor (R)-mediated mechanisms (e.g., serotonin [5-HT], adenosine diphosphate [ADP], thrombin [THROMB], bradykinin [BK], acetylcholine [ACh], histamine [HIST], substance P [SP], and endothelin 1 [ET-1]). These stimuli increase endothelial intracellular calcium concentration. Calcium, in the presence of calmodulin (Cd), activates NOS. NOS activity is inhibited by substrate analogs of L-arginine (e.g., NG-monomethyl-L-arginine [L-NMMA], NG-nitro-L-arginine-methyl ester [L-NAME], and NG-nitro-L-arginine [L-NNA]). NO diffuses to the vascular smooth muscle cells (VSMC), where it activates soluble guanylyl cyclase (sGC) to enhance formation of cyclic GMP from guanosine triphosphate (GTP). Cyclic GMP activates cyclic GMP-dependent protein kinases, activating mechanisms that ultimately lead to a decrease in cytosolic calcium concentration and result in relaxation. NO donors have a similar mechanism of action but do not need endothelium for NO formation. NO is formed spontaneously from the NO donor molecule (e.g., sodium nitroprusside [SNP] and the active metabolite of molsidomine [SIN-1]) or after metabolism in smooth muscle cell (e.g., isosorbide dinitrate [ISDN] and nitroglycerin [NTG]). This metabolism requires the presence of reduced thiol groups (R-SH).

Synthesis of NO

Palmer et al.[13,14] very elegantly demonstrated that NO is derived from L-arginine. They found that endothelial cells, cultured in a medium without L-arginine, released a minimal amount of EDRF after stimulation with bradykinin. Only after adding the amino acid to the medium did cells start to release EDRF.

Using radiolabeled L-arginine, Palmer and colleagues[13,14] showed that NO originated from the terminal guanidino group of L-arginine. NO production involves stepwise N-oxidation of the guanidino atoms of L-arginine via formation of NG-hydroxy-L-arginine to L-citrulline. NO is generated in the latter conversion. Incorporation of molecular oxygen into NO and citrulline is mediated by NOS.[16] NOS from human endothelial cells has been isolated, characterized, and cloned.[17] It belongs to the family of P-450 cytochrome oxidoreductases. NOS activity is not restricted to endothelial cells but is also present in platelets, vascular smooth muscle cells, macrophages, hepatocytes, and neuronal tissue.

NO formed by these tissues may have important functions.[18,19] Three isozymes of NOS are produced from three distinct gene loci.

Endothelial NOS isozyme requires the cofactors tetrahydrobiopterin (BH_4), flavin adenine dinucleotide (FAD), flavin mononucleotide (FMN), and reduced nicotinamide adenine dinucleotide phosphate (NADPH). Activation of NOS in endothelial cells is initiated by an increase in cytosolic calcium and requires calmodulin. NO is formed within seconds. Thus NO can be involved in rapid regulatory mechanisms. Expression and activity of NOS in endothelial cells is the rate-limiting factor in formation of NO. Under physiological conditions the supply of L-arginine does not appear to be rate limiting for NO synthesis.[20]

Coupling Endothelial Excitation and NO Secretion

The importance of calcium in endothelium-dependent relaxation was established very early in EDRF research.[21] In the absence of extracellular calcium, EDRF release was much depressed yet still present. Measurement of intracellular calcium activity in endothelial cells showed a biphasic increase upon stimulation with various agonists. An initial sharp rise, due to release of calcium from intracellular stores, is followed by a partial recovery to a calcium level still higher than in absence of an agonist. This plateau depends on a maintained influx of calcium from the extracellular medium.[22]

The initial increase in endothelial cell calcium is mediated by the phosphatidylinositol pathway. Following stimulation by appropriate agonists, phospholipase C activation generates inositol trisphosphate and diacylglycerol. Inositol trisphosphate then mobilizes intracellular calcium from the endoplasmic reticulum while diacylglycerol activates protein kinase C and enhances the influx of extracellular calcium.

Although the importance of extracellular calcium in the full expression of endothelium-dependent relaxation is well-defined, the route of its entry in the endothelial cells is less clear. These cells are generally believed to lack voltage-operated calcium channels, but the following have been proposed as likely participants in the maintained phase of calcium influx: receptor-operated calcium channels, calcium leak channels, stretch-activated calcium channels, and sodium–calcium exchange. Whatever the route of entry, the extent of calcium increase is modified by the membrane potential of the endothelial cells, because the transmembrane potential determines the electrochemical gradient and provides the driving force for calcium influx. Therefore, given the lack of voltage-activated (depolarization-activated) calcium channels, opening of potassium channels with hyperpolarization of the endothelial cells facilitates calcium entry and thus synthesis of NO.[23]

Coupling NO and Vascular Smooth Muscle Relaxation

NO is very labile and reactive and thus has a short action radius. Its half-life in solution is only a few seconds. NO has a great affinity for heme groups. After release at the luminal side of the endothelial cell, NO enters the circulation and binds with hemoglobin. It is then oxidized to nitrite and nitrate, and ultimately both are excreted in urine. There is some evidence that NO may also bind to other plasma constituents including thiols, albumin, and other proteins.[24] Some of these substances prolong its half-life and may act as NO carriers in the circulation.

When NO is released at the abluminal side of the endothelium, it diffuses into the cytosol of adjacent smooth muscle cells and rapidly causes relaxation. NO does not require a cell surface receptor to mediate its action. Being a very small and lipophilic compound, it traverses cell membranes very rapidly. When NO enters the cytosol of smooth muscle, it binds to the heme moiety of soluble guanylyl cyclase. This binding results in a conformational change that activates the enzyme. Enzyme activation promotes conversion of guanosine triphosphate to cyclic GMP. This mechanism of action is similar to that of nitrovasodilators because their active principle is NO, generated either spontaneously (e.g., nitroprusside, molsidomine) or via interaction with tissue components (e.g., nitroglycerin, isosorbide dinitrate). Elevation of cyclic GMP activates cyclic GMP–dependent protein kinases and activates mechanisms that lead to relaxation of vascular smooth muscle cells[25] (Figure 2.2).

Physiological Role of NO on Vascular Tone

It is unlikely that NO acts as a humoral vasoregulator. When it enters the bloodstream, circulating hemoglobin rapidly binds and inactivates it. NO released from the endothelium must thus be considered as a locally active hormone and effective only in the immediate vicinity of the cell that releases it. Luminally released NO helps to provide endothelial cells with an antithrombogenic surface because it prevents platelet aggregation and adhesion. In this respect NO acts in synergy with prostacyclin.[26,27]

Abluminally released NO, acting on smooth muscle cells, is a major physiological regulator of vascular smooth muscle tone. This has become apparent when L-arginine analogs became available as tools for selective and reversible knock out of the L-arginine–NO–cyclic GMP pathway.

Basal Release of NO

When an isolated donor blood vessel with intact endothelium is perfused with physiological salt solution, the effluent induces relaxation in a vessel mounted for detecting the presence of vasoactive substances. No relaxation is seen with the effluent of a vessel segment without endothelium. Thus, the early bioassay experiments provided evidence for release of NO under basal conditions.[28]

In vessels contracted with various agonists, preparations with endothelium often showed an attenuated contraction as compared with those that lacked endothelium. The basal release of EDRF thus influenced the response of isolated vessels. NO was indicated as this factor because addition of arginine analogs that specifically blocked NO formation induced tension increases in noncontracted and contracted isolated vascular rings with endothelium but not in rings without endothelium (Figure 2.3A).

Basal release of NO is important in determining the tone of not only great conduit arteries but also of resistance arteries. This role is substantiated by the many studies showing that blockade of NOS results in increased resistance in several perfused vascular beds from various species, including humans. For example, infusion of the L-arginine analog L-NMMA in the brachial artery reduces forearm blood flow by 40%[29] (Figure 2.3B).

In 1989 Rees et al.[30] found that intravenous injection of the L-arginine analog L-NMMA (but not of D-NMMA, illustrating the stereoselectivity of this agent) induced a rapid and strong increase in blood pressure in rabbits. This increase was rapidly normalized by injection of an excess of L-arginine but not of D-arginine. The conclusion that the increase in blood pressure was due to an increase in total peripheral resistance and not to an increase in cardiac output is supported by the observation that both heart rate and stroke volume were diminished after administration of the arginine analog. The increase in peripheral resistance seen in vivo is likely related to a blockade of basal NO release. This is supported by the finding that blockers of angiotensin-converting enzyme (ACE) do not prevent the increase in blood pressure, excluding possible involvement of the renin–angiotensin–aldosterone mechanism. Also, prazosin, phentolamine, or denervation of baroreceptors have no influence, excluding involvement of an increased sympathetic influence.[31,32]

Blood pressure increase after blockade of NOS has been shown in different species, including humans. L-NMMA increased mean arterial pressure by 10% and total peripheral resistance by 46% in healthy humans.[33] The data have led to the conviction that basal NO exerts a continuous dilatory influence on vascular tone in the organism, counterbalancing the sympathetic contractile influence. This dilatory influence is of major physiological importance because NOS inhibitors elicit drastic effects on vascular tone. In comparison, inhibitors of ACE or of endogenous mediators of vasorelaxation other than NO have only minimal effects on basal blood pressure. It is likely that NO-dependent vasodilator tone is entirely regulated locally and, as such, is probably one of the simplest and yet most fundamental adaptive mechanisms in the cardiovascular system.

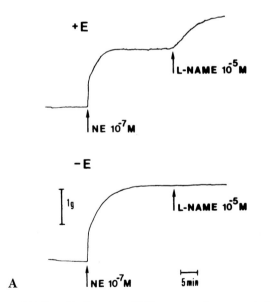
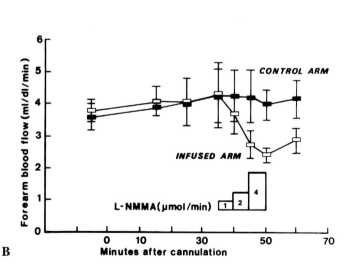

FIGURE 2.3. Basal influence of NO on vascular tone. **A,** Inhibition of NOS with L-NAME (10^{-5} M) further contracts an isolated rat aorta, which was induced to a certain level of tone by norepinephrine (NE; 10^{-7} M), if endothelium is intact ($+$E), but not if endothelium is removed ($-$E) (personal observation). **B,** Influence of infusion of NOS inhibitor L-NMMA into brachial artery on forearm blood flow. Blockade of basal influence of NO diminishes blood flow in the infused arm due to a local effect since blood flow in the control arm is not affected (from Vallance, Collier, and Moncada[29] with kind permission of The Lancet Ltd.).

Flow-Mediated NO Release

Flow-induced relaxation of large arteries is a well-known phenomenon. When blood flow increases, shear stress exerted by blood elements on the luminal surface of the vascular wall also increases. This increased shear force is thought to activate mechanoreceptors on the surface of the endothelium, which promotes NOS activity and results in relaxation. This adaptive mechanism helps to ensure sufficient blood flow to the distal vascular beds when they dilate because of increased metabolic needs.

For many years it was believed that this large vessel dilation was due to a retrograde signal from smaller downstream vessels. The importance of endothelium in mediating this vascular response has been repeatedly demonstrated in vivo and in vitro by showing that flow-induced dilation disappears after removal of endothelium.[34] It is noteworthy that flow-mediated dilation has been demonstrated in human coronary circulation in situ.[35,36]

Coupling between blood flow and release of NO probably occurs through shear stress–sensitive ion channels. A shear stress–gated potassium channel has been identified in endothelial cell membranes, and the channel opening may hyperpolarize the endothelial cell, increase the electrical gradient, and facilitate the calcium entry required to synthesize NO.[37] In addition, a nonselective cation channel has been identified that exhibits an increased frequency of opening induced by pressure and/or stretch.[38] Opening of a nonselective channel is also likely to increase intracellular calcium activity, either directly (through calcium influx) or via sodium–calcium exchange (sodium influx).

NO in Cerebral Vasculature

In the cerebral circulation, besides a basal influence, NO also mediates the vasodilation in response to local neuronal activation. Thus NO may act as a coupler of cerebral blood flow to metabolism. Brain blood vessels are very sensitive to carbon dioxide, and hypercapnia is one of the most potent stimulators of cerebral blood flow. Several studies suggest that cerebral vasodilation during moderate hypercapnia is dependent on formation of NO because hypercapnia-associated increases in cerebral blood flow are attenuated by inhibitors of NOS in several species. This reduction is not coupled to reduced cerebral metabolism. Inhibition of NOS also inhibits increases in cerebral blood flow in response to extracellular acidosis, suggesting it is not carbon dioxide but rather the hypercapnia-induced acidosis that triggers hypercapnic NO-dependent vasodilation.[39]

Role of NO in Renal Vasculature

NO probably has the most prominent influence in renal circulation. Inhibitors of NO synthesis decrease renal blood flow in doses that produce no systemic effects. Both the glomerular and medullary microcirculations appear to be regulated by endogenous NO. The source of NO may not be restricted to the endothelium. Indeed, NOS has been identified in macula densa. NO inhibits renin release from juxtaglomerular cells and thus may have indirect effects on intrarenal vascular tone by decreasing the generation of angiotensin II. Tubuloglomerular feedback, which is regulated by the macula densa, appears to be mediated in part by NO. The ability of NO to regulate arteriolar diameter in the kidney may thus be a key determinant of renin release and the homeostasis of intravascular volume and pressure.[40]

NO and Veins

Endothelium-dependent relaxation is much more pronounced in arterial than in venous blood vessels. On the other hand, veins are more sensitive to nitrovasodilators, suggesting that veins produce less NO. This difference in NO production between arteries and veins has been suggested as a determinant in the higher patency rate of arterial grafts compared with venous grafts.[41] Inhibitors of NOS did not cause an increase in basal tone in a variety of venous preparations from animals or humans.[42] Local administration of L-NMMA into a dorsal hand vein of healthy volunteers did not cause vasoconstriction, providing evidence that there is little if any basal release of NO in veins.[43] This finding is consistent with the observation that L-arginine analogs have no influence on central venous pressure.

Pathophysiological Role of NO

The importance of endothelial NO in lowering vascular tone inevitably suggests that dysfunction of this mechanism may contribute to the pathogenesis of a variety of human vascular diseases. Impairment of the protective relaxing influence of endothelial NO tends to increase resistance and to diminish tissue perfusion. It may tip the balance of vessel tone toward contraction and lead to paradoxical effects in response to certain stimuli. Aggregating platelets release substances (serotonin, adenosine diphosphate, thrombin) that normally stimulate release of NO from endothelium and thus induce relaxation; it may also elicit a vasospastic reaction in vessels with endothelial dysfunction because the released substances exert only their direct contractile effect on smooth muscle cells.

Hypertension

Basal NO has a role in lowering vascular resistance, and any decrease in NO generation or vascular response to NO may thus have a substantial effect on tissue blood flow and blood pressure. A decrease in NO generation, action, or both may provide an acceptable mechanism for the increased vascular resistance in hypertension. Indeed, many studies have shown that relaxation responses to endothelium-mediated substances are impaired in large conduit arteries and resistance arteries of hypertensive rats[44–46] (Figure 2.4). Endothelium-independent vasodilation is not modified, illustrating that the capacity of vascular smooth muscle to relax is not affected. The mechanisms involved are not settled. An endothelial contractile substance is formed in some vessels from spontaneously hypertensive rats.[45] However, this mechanism could not be established in all vessels from hypertensive animals. Impairment of endothelium-dependent relaxation is related to the pressure as such and not to a more generalized neuronal or humoral regulatory mechanism. This is clearly illustrated in experiments on preparations from rats with experimental coarctation of the aorta that showed impairment of endothelium-dependent relaxation in the high-pressure zone proximal to the stenosis; the endothelium-dependent relaxation is not influenced in the normal pressure zone distal to the stenosis.[47,48] Loss of endothelial relaxation seems to be secondary to elevation in blood pressure. Regimens that lower pressure may lead to a restoration of the impaired endothelial dilating influence.[48,49]

In patients with essential hypertension, both basal NO release (assessed as a decrease in blood flow after NOS inhibition) and stimulated NO release (assessed as an increase in blood flow with acetylcholine) are impaired in

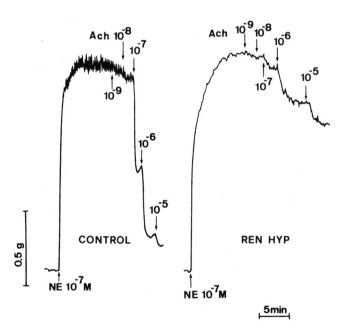

FIGURE 2.4. Original recording of an experiment showing that the relaxation effects of increasing concentrations (molar) of acetylcholine (ACh) on a contracted (norepinephrine [NE], 10^{-7} M) aorta preparation of a renal hypertensive (REN HYP) rat are impaired compared with the effects on preparations of a control normotensive rat (from Van de Voorde and Leusen[46] with kind permission of American Physiological Society).

forearm vasculature.[50–52] The degree of functional attenuation of the NO system increases as blood pressure increases. There is also a strong association between hypertension and impaired coronary relaxation in response to acetylcholine.[53] Exogenous L-arginine, the substrate of NOS, decreased blood pressure in salt-sensitive rats but not in spontaneously hypertensive rats.[54] Administration of L-arginine did not lower blood pressure in patients with essential hypertension and did not improve the impaired vasodilation response to acetylcholine in the forearm vasculature of hypertensive patients.[55] In the latter, the forearm response to acetylcholine remained abnormal even when blood pressure was controlled.[56]

In hypertension due to renal failure, an additional endothelium-related mechanism may be involved. Endogenous inhibitors of NO synthesis accumulate in renal failure. One of these inhibitors, asymmetric dimethyl arginine, approaches plasma concentrations that may influence blood pressure. Those concentrations have indeed been shown to increase vascular tone in rat aortic rings, to increase blood pressure in anesthetized guinea pigs, and to increase forearm vascular resistance in healthy humans.[57]

Enhanced generation of endogenous NO may be involved in the decrease of vascular resistance in the maternal vascular system during pregnancy.[58] Lack of this adaptive response could account for pregnancy-induced hypertension and preeclampsia.[59] Many studies have shown signs of endothelial dysfunction (e.g., decreased formation of prostacyclin, enhanced formation of endothelin) in patients with preeclampsia. The decreased relaxation in response to acetylcholine in isolated human subcutaneous arteries from patients with preeclampsia suggests that the L-arginine–NO–cyclic GMP pathway is impaired.[60] This decreased relaxation response may, however, be related to altered receptor function. In umbilical arteries from patients with preeclampsia, the release of NO is diminished in response to histamine and bradykinin but not to the receptor-independent calcium ionophore (A 23187). Basal release of NO from umbilical vessels is even enhanced in preeclampsia.[61]

Atherosclerosis

That atherosclerosis is associated with a defective endothelial NO mechanism is substantiated by many experimental data.[62] Endothelium-dependent relaxations are severely decreased in blood vessel rings isolated from animals with atherosclerotic lesions.[63] Also, in isolated atherosclerotic human coronary arteries, endothelium-mediated relaxation is impaired.[64]

Although the endothelium remains intact in early stages of atherogenesis, pronounced functional alterations already occur. Oxidized low-density lipoproteins may have an important role in these phenomena. It has been shown that oxidized low-density lipoproteins decrease endothelium-dependent relaxation.[65] Interestingly, in hyperlipidemic rabbits, infusion of L-arginine improved the impaired endothelium-dependent relaxation. Chronic treatment with oral L-arginine even reduced atherosclerotic lesions and endothelial dysfunction.[66,67] At least in regards to normal endothelial function, this finding is not very evident because substrate availability is not primarily rate limiting for formation of NO. It could suggest that NOS kinetics are changed in hyperlipidemia.

Besides administration of L-arginine, dietary adaptation can restore impaired endothelium-dependent responses in atherosclerosis. Monkeys fed an atherogenic diet for 18 months developed severe arterial atherosclerotic lesions, and endothelium-dependent vasodilation was markedly diminished. Other monkeys, fed the atherogenic diet for 18 months followed by normal diet for another 18 months, displayed almost complete regression of the atherosclerotic lesions and intact endothelium-dependent vasodilation.[68] This indicates that endothelial dysfunction in atherosclerosis is reversible if fat consumption is decreased. The lack of endothelial relaxing influence in hypercholesterolemia may be related to the generation of large quantities of superoxide anions that inactivate NO. This is suggested by the observation that treatment with polyethylene-glycolated superoxide dismutase markedly enhanced endothelium-dependent relaxation in isolated vessels from rabbits fed cholesterol.[69]

The clinical relevance of these findings was highlighted in a series of studies in patients with coronary heart disease undergoing routine cardiac catheterization. In these patients, the epicardial coronary artery segments that appeared irregular or stenotic in coronary angiograms displayed severely diminished vasodilation or even moderate constriction in response to challenge with acetylcholine, leg exercise, or an increase in flow, cold exposure, or mental stress.[35,70–73] At the same time, angiographically smooth coronary segments dilated in response to these stimuli. Interestingly, stenotic and irregular arterial segments did not differ from smooth segments in their response to nitroglycerin. Hence, endothelium-dependent vasodilation was impaired, but endothelium-independent vasodilation was maintained. Similar observations were made on coronary resistance vessels.[74]

Endothelial dysfunction does not require manifest atherosclerotic lesions to materialize. Even when no visible lesions are present and coronary arteries look normal on angiography, significant differences in response to intracoronary acetylcholine are obtained between patients with and without functional coronary artery disease.[75] Hence, the response to acetylcholine is already impaired

before lesions are detectable with conventional angiography, so that it has been suggested that intracoronary injection of acetylcholine might be useful for early diagnosis of coronary artery disease. Patients with familial hypercholesterolemia have signs of endothelial dysfunction that can be detected as early as in childhood.[76] Long-time smoking, a major risk factor for development of atherosclerosis, is associated with diminished NO-dependent basal vascular tone and impaired endothelium-dependent vasodilator response in otherwise clinically healthy subjects.[77] The beneficial effects of L-arginine have also been documented in humans with hyperlipidemia. Infusion of L-arginine into the coronary artery or the forearm circulation normalizes the impaired endothelium-dependent vasodilation to acetylcholine[74,78] (Figure 2.5). The clinical relevance of these results requires further substantiation. Because reduced plasma levels of the amino acid are found in hypercholesterolemic patients, improvement may be related to a deficiency of L-arginine.[79] The supply of L-arginine may

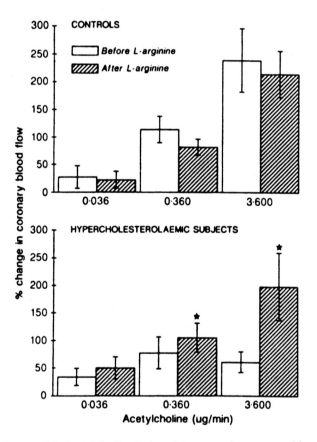

FIGURE 2.5. Acetylcholine-induced increases in coronary blood flow before and after L-arginine administration in control subjects (upper) and hypercholesterolemic subjects (lower). Whereas L-arginine has no influence in control subjects, it restores the impaired coronary dilator response to acetylcholine in hypercholesterolemic subjects (from Drexler et al.[74] with kind permission of The Lancet Ltd.).

thus become rate limiting for NO synthesis in this situation.

A study of patients with coronary heart disease showed that lowering plasma lipids might reverse endothelial dysfunction in atherosclerosis.[80] Endothelium-dependent and endothelium-independent dilation of coronary epicardial arteries was measured before and 6 months following a lipid-lowering regimen, consisting of dietary restrictions and oral treatment with a cholesterol synthesis inhibitor. A decrease in plasma cholesterol of about 30% was achieved. Before treatment, coronary infusion of acetylcholine elicited vasoconstriction in epicardial arteries, whereas at follow-up a moderate vasodilation was observed. It thus appears that lowering of plasma lipids may reverse endothelial dysfunction and thereby also improve myocardial perfusion.

Microvascular Angina: Syndrome X

Patients with microvascular angina, or syndrome X, show anginalike chest pain and pathologic exercise electrocardiogram in the presence of a normal coronary angiogram. These patients show normal epicardial endothelium-dependent vasodilation. The endothelial function of the coronary resistance vessels, assessed as the increase in blood flow in response to acetylcholine, is lower in these patients than in matched control subjects.[81,82] It is thus possible that endothelial dysfunction may be limited to specific zones of the systemic vascular tree.

Diabetes

Although no consistent results have been reported, several studies on different models of diabetic animals report that endothelium-dependent vasodilation is impaired in the blood vessels of diabetic animals.[83] Defective endothelial NO function may be involved in diabetic microangiopathy. Pretreatment with L-arginine potentiated endothelium-dependent relaxation in the aorta from diabetic rats but not in the aorta from control rats. A defect in utilization of L-arginine by NOS may thus play a role.[84] Free radical scavengers restore endothelial dysfunction in mesenteric resistance arteries of diabetic rats,[85] suggesting that increased destruction or inactivation of NO may also be involved.

Isolated blood vessels from patients with insulin-dependent diabetes mellitus show diminished relaxation to acetylcholine.[86] Basal NO influence in the human forearm arterial bed is impaired in patients with insulin-dependent diabetes mellitus.[87] In patients with insulin-independent diabetes, endothelial and smooth muscle function is impaired. Interestingly, it appears that endothelium-dependent vascular responses may be improved in these patients by dietary treatment with polyunsaturated fatty acids from fish oil.[88]

Ischemia and Reperfusion

Ischemia followed by reperfusion reduced endothelial NO-mediated relaxation in several vascular beds in vivo and in vitro.[89] Of particular interest is the fact that the endothelial dysfunction persists for up to 3 months after reperfusion.[90] NO is a highly reactive species that is inactivated by free radicals. The diminished NO-induced relaxation may therefore be due to the rapid inactivation of NO by free radicals produced by injured endothelial cells and adhering leukocytes. This hypothesis is supported by the observation that ischemia followed by reperfusion produces impaired endothelium-dependent responses of cerebral arterioles, which can be restored to normal with scavengers of oxygen radicals. Thus, formation of oxygen radicals impairs endothelial function in cerebral arterioles after ischemia. It could be argued, therefore, that stimulation of NO formation (e.g., by administration of L-arginine) could be protective against ischemia–reperfusion injury. However, this may result in a deleterious effect. When NO scavenges superoxide anions, the reaction product (peroxynitrite) can decompose, forming even more tissue-damaging agents such as hydroxyl radicals. This may explain why, in animals with postischemic endothelial damage, administration of NO or L-arginine provides no, or only a modest, improvement in tissue perfusion.[91]

Cerebral Vasospasm

Endothelium-dependent relaxation of cerebral vessels is reduced after subarachnoid hemorrhage in experimental animals and humans. Hemoglobin, which may play an important role in producing vasospasm after subarachnoid hemorrhage, may constrict cerebral vessels by inhibition of the basal influence of NO. In intact cerebral vessels, hemoglobin decreases basal levels of cyclic GMP to levels similar to those produced by either NOS inhibition or removal of the endothelium. This inhibition has been attributed either to a defect in endothelial cells or to the presence of hemoglobin in cerebrospinal fluid that binds and inactivates NO.[92]

Heart Failure

Systemic vasoconstriction is a hallmark of severe chronic congestive heart failure. In experimental heart failure, endothelial dysfunction has been described in both cardiac and systemic circulations. Patients with congestive heart failure also have impaired receptor-mediated release of endothelial NO.[93] On the other hand, the decrease in blood flow induced by NOS inhibition is enhanced in cardiac failure, indicating increased basal NO release. Also, the plasma levels of nitrate are higher in patients with heart failure than in healthy individuals. The increase in NO-mediated vasodilator tone probably represents a counterregulatory mechanism attempting to compensate for the vasoconstrictor effect of neurohumoral adaptation to heart failure.[94]

Endotoxic Shock

Besides the NOS that is always present in the endothelial cells (constitutive NOS [cNOS]), an inducible form of NOS(iNOS) may become active in endothelial cells and smooth muscle cells after stimulation with cytokines such as bacterial lipopolysaccharide (endotoxin), tumor necrosis factor α, and interleukin-1β. As a consequence, massive amounts of NO are produced, causing profound vasodilation and hypotension. It is believed that this mechanism may be responsible for the severe hypotension, resistant to vasoconstrictors and volume repletion, seen in patients with endotoxic shock.[95] Therefore, inhibitors of NOS have been thought to be potentially beneficial in the treatment of septic shock. L-NMMA is indeed able to reverse tumor necrosis factor– and lipopolysaccharide-induced hypotension in animals. L-NMMA has been administered to humans with life-threatening hypotension due to sepsis and was found to increase their blood pressure.[96] Since the classic arginine analogs inhibit not only iNOS but also cNOS their administration leads to severe disruption of cardiovascular control, tissue hypoperfusion, and even death.[97] The development of selective iNOS inhibitors may lead to drugs useful in treating septic shock.

Pharmacological Implications

NO is involved in many aspects of the physiological and pathophysiological control of vascular tone. It is therefore inevitable that new drugs based on the L-arginine–NO pathway will emerge.

Although NO is a very toxic gas that induces pulmonary inflammation, it can be used in low doses in the treatment of several forms of pulmonary hypertension. Inhaled NO, acting as a selective pulmonary vasodilator without systemic effects (since it is inactivated when it reaches the systemic circulation), improves oxygenation and decreases pulmonary hypertension in patients with adult respiratory distress syndrome.[98] Inhaled NO has also been used successfully for treatment of pulmonary hypertension of the newborn,[99,100] pulmonary hypertension of congenital heart disease,[101] idiopathic pulmonary hypertension,[102] and severe airway disease.[103]

Nitrovasodilators such as nitroglycerin, acting through the generation of NO, have been used for more than 100 years, mainly as treatment for angina but also for other cardiovascular pathologies. The observation that NO-mediated effects are diminished in a variety of human vascular disorders has led to the idea that the NO donors may be regarded as substitution therapy for a failing physiological mechanism.

Research on endothelium-dependent effects has revealed an additional beneficial influence of ACE inhibitors. Bradykinin is an endogenous circulating peptide that causes endothelium-dependent relaxation through stimulation of a bradykinin B_2 receptor. Bradykinin is inactivated by ACE that also converts angiotensin I to angiotensin II. It has been suggested that the prevention of degradation of endogenous bradykinin significantly contributes in the hypotensive effect of ACE inhibitors. There is indeed evidence that ACE inhibitors enhance basal synthesis of NO from endothelial cells and potentiate its release upon stimulation by bradykinin.[104] The cardioprotective influence of ACE inhibitors after an ischemic insult in isolated guinea pig hearts was shown to result from NO release under the influence of endogenous bradykinin.[105]

NO is rapidly destroyed by superoxide anions that are formed under several pathological conditions. Superoxide anion scavengers have been shown to protect endothelium-dependent relaxation in vessels from hypercholesterolemic rabbits.[69] Interest in substances that inactivate superoxide anions such as superoxide dismutase analogs can therefore be expected.

The potential role of L-arginine administration to increase NO synthesis is not clear. Although under normal physiological conditions the availability of L-arginine is not rate limiting for the production of NO, administration of L-arginine to increase NO levels may have both beneficial and detrimental effects. Beneficial effects of NO include maintenance of blood flow and inhibition of aggregation and adherence of platelets. Detrimental effects of NO are possible because high concentrations of NO are cytotoxic after combination with superoxide to form peroxynitrite. This is especially important considering the fact that superoxide anion concentrations are increased in several vascular pathologies, especially after ischemia. In atherosclerosis there is evidence for a beneficial effect of L-arginine on endothelial relaxing function, but the clinical relevance of this effect remains to be established.[62,106]

Hyperpolarizing Factor

In 1988 evidence became available that endothelium-dependent relaxation elicited by different agonists (including acetylcholine, histamine, bradykinin, and substance P) was accompanied by an endothelium-dependent hyperpolarization of smooth muscle cell membranes.[107,108] Although NO can induce some hyperpolarization, it soon became clear that the endothelium-dependent hyperpolarization was not mediated by NO because it was not (or was only partially) inhibited by hemoglobin (which binds and inactivates NO) or by the arginine analogs that efficiently inhibit formation of NO.[109] Some bioassay experiments proved that endothelium-dependent hyperpolarization is mediated by an extremely labile diffusable endothelial factor,[110] and was termed the *endothelium-derived hyperpolarization factor* (EDHF). However, the release of EDHF is difficult to demonstrate,[111] which agrees with the proposed abluminal secretion of the factor.[112] The nature of this EDHF is not yet established, although there is evidence that it may be a metabolite of arachidonic acid formed though a cytochrome P-450 epoxygenase pathway.[112] Like the release of NO, release of EDHF depends on endothelial intracellular calcium.

The change in smooth muscle cell membrane potential induced by EDHF is due to an increase in membrane conductance for potassium. As a result, potassium moves out of the cell, driven by its transmembrane electrochemical gradient. The loss of positive charges hyperpolarizes the cell membrane. This hyperpolarization inhibits calcium entry by closing the voltage-dependent calcium channels of the vascular smooth muscle cells and results in relaxation. The potassium channels activated by EDHF are not definitively characterized, but with the exception of cerebrovascular smooth muscle, endothelium-dependent hyperpolarization in most vascular beds is resistant to blockers of adenosine triphosphate–sensitive potassium channels.[108] Tetrabutylammonium or charybdotoxin, blockers of calcium-dependent potassium channels, block the EDHF-mediated relaxation in some vessels.

The functional significance of EDHF is not clear. Its rapid and mostly transient character suggests that it may be mainly important in initiation of relaxation. Its functional role is probably more prominent in small arterioles than in large arteries, because smooth muscle contraction in small arterioles appears to be more dependent on extracellular calcium influx. Indeed, a much larger component of the endothelium-dependent relaxation is NO independent in more peripheral and smaller vessels.[113] Because endothelial cells are electrically coupled, hyperpolarization with resulting release of EDHF does not have to be limited to the site of stimulation but can eventually spread, even in "upstream" direction, to the feeding arterioles.[114]

Interestingly, endothelium-mediated hyperpolarization is strongly depressed in hypertension. When EDHF proves to have an important role in regulating vascular tone in smaller resistance vessels, the finding may help to explain the increased vascular resistance of hypertension.[115]

Prostacyclin

Prostacyclin was discovered in 1976 and is a major product of the metabolism of arachidonic acid, through the cyclooxygenase pathway, in vascular tissue.[116] Its formation occurs primarily in endothelium but also in media and adventitia. It is a powerful vasodilator, and its formation is stimulated by pulsatile pressure, a number of endogenous mediators, and some drugs. Prostacyclin may partially participate in endothelium-mediated relaxation elicited by several endogenous substances.

From a physiological point of view, prostacyclin is a local rather than a circulating hormone because plasma levels are too low to have systemic effects. The role of prostacyclin as an endogenous regulator of vascular tone is questionable because inhibition of its synthesis does not result in substantial effects on either systemic arterial blood pressure or blood flow in many organs.[117]

Endothelial Contracting Factors

Endothelin

Historical Notes

In 1985 Hickey et al.[118] discovered that the addition of a culture medium of bovine aortic endothelial cells to vascular smooth muscle cells elicited a slowly developing and long-lasting contraction of muscle cells. In an attempt to characterize the triggering mechanism, they demonstrated that the contraction was mediated by a peptide, but they could not find a relation to any known peptidergic vasoconstrictor. This endothelial peptidergic contractile factor was isolated, purified, sequenced, and cloned by Yanagisawa et al.,[119] who named it endothelin (ET). Its structure is related to that of the highly toxic group of snake venoms, the sarafotoxins.

Three structurally and pharmacologically separate isotypes of ET have been discovered. The human genome contains three distinct genes that encode for the three different ET peptides: ET-1, ET-2, and ET-3.[120] The potent biological effects, rapid commercial availability, and relatively low cost of ETs have led to explosive research activity on the ET family. ETs were found to be produced not only by endothelium but also by a wide variety of other cells and were found to be widely distributed in the organism (e.g., in the spleen, kidney, lung, gastrointestinal tract, and central nervous system). Hence, the name *endothelins* is actually a misnomer. ETs are not simply a curiosity from an obscure phylogenic past. Much evidence suggests that they are important biological mediators in many physiological and pathophysiological processes.[121] In this chapter, we focus on ETs only in their relation to vascular smooth muscle tone.

Structure and Synthesis of Endothelin 1

All members of the ET family are closely related peptides consisting of 21 amino acids, with a compact globular conformation. Four cysteine residues form two disulfide bridges that hold the C-terminal region close to the N-terminal region of the molecule.[122] Endothelial cells appear to produce ET-1 exclusively. Its structure is shown in Figure 2.6.

ET-1 is synthesized with a considerable time lag between stimulus and secretion, since different consecutive steps are involved in its formation (Figure 2.7). Translation of mRNA generates a 212-residue polypeptide named preproendothelin 1. This is enzymatically processed to a 38-residue propeptide termed *big endothelin* (big ET-1). Some big ET-1 is secreted by endothelial cells, as it could be found in plasma.[123] The binding affinity and contractile potency of big ET-1, however, are much less than those of ET-1 itself.[124] Further processing of big ET-1 is required for full expression of its biological activity. Big ET-1 is cleaved to the very potent 21-residue ET-1 by endothelin-converting enzyme,[125] which is a membrane-bound neutral metalloprotease inhibited by phosphoramidon. By reference to ACE, endothelin-converting enzyme may prove to be an important target in controlling the release of ET-1. This may be of therapeutic interest considering the potential role of increased ET-1 activity in several important pathologies (see the following).

ET-1 is continuously released from the endothelium. Once synthesized, it is secreted via a constitutive pathway without further regulation at the level of exocytosis. Its release is modulated by different stimuli. ET-1 release is inhibited by NO, nitrovasodilators, and atrial natriuretic peptide, all substances that increase cyclic GMP levels. On the other hand, ET-1 release is increased by thrombin, the calcium-ionophore A23187, arginine vasopressin (AVP), angiotensin II, oxyhemoglobin, decrease in shear stress, tumor necrosis factor α, transforming growth factor β, cyclosporin, and oxidized low-density lipoprotein. This stimulation occurs at the transcriptional level.[126,127]

Kinetics of ET-1

In several species significant quantities of ET-1 are detected in circulating plasma using specific radioimmunoassay methods. Circulating plasma concentrations of immunoreactive ET-1 are in the low picomolar range

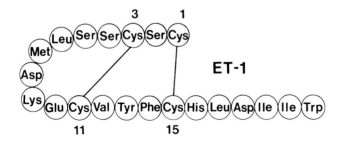

FIGURE 2.6. The primary amino acid sequence of endothelin 1 showing the position of the disulfide bridges.

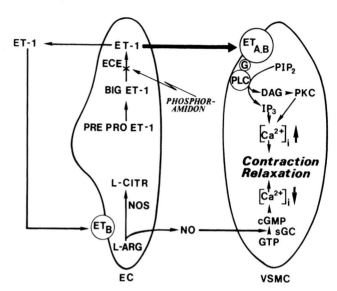

FIGURE 2.7. Schematic representation of the mechanisms of formation and action of endothelin 1 (ET-1) on vascular smooth muscle tone. Translation of mRNA generates in the endothelial cell (EC) preproendothelin 1 (212 amino acids), which is cleaved to proendothelin 1 or big endothelin 1 (38 amino acids). This peptide is further cleaved by endothelin-converting enzyme (ECE) to ET-1 (21 amino acids). This last conversion is blocked by phosphoramidon. ET-1 acts on both ET_A and ET_B receptors on the vascular smooth muscle cell (VSMC). These receptors are coupled to phospholipase C (PLC) via G proteins. This activates the conversion of phosphatidylinositol 4,5-bisphosphate (PIP_2) to diacylglycerol (DAG), thus activating protein kinase C (PKC) and inositol trisphosphate (IP_3), which directly increases intracellular calcium, ultimately leading to contraction. ET-1 released in the vascular lumen may also stimulate endothelial ET_B receptors, leading to NOS activation, enhancing the conversion of L-arginine (L-ARG) to L-citrulline (L-CITR) and NO. NO diffuses to the smooth muscle cell, where it activates soluble guanylyl cyclase (sGC). This results in an enhanced conversion of guanosine triphosphate (GTP) to cyclic GMP (cGMP), activating cyclic GMP–dependent protein kinases that decrease intracellular calcium concentration and ultimately lead to relaxation. The importance of this endothelium-mediated relaxing influence of ET-1 varies from blood vessel to blood vessel.

in healthy humans but are elevated in several pathological conditions (see later section).

Plasma concentrations of ET-1 are stable. However, the plasma half-life of intravenously injected ETs is very short. Approximately 60% of intravenously injected ET-1 is removed from the circulation within the first minute.[128] The quick clearance of ET-1 from the circulation is mainly due to the 50% first-pass elimination by the lung.[129] The kidney (and to a smaller extent the liver) also contributes to elimination of the peptide from the circulation. The concentrations of ET-1 in human urine samples were found to be higher than those in plasma.[130]

ET-1 is inactivated when it is cleaved by a neutral met-alloendopeptidase. Inhibition of this enzyme elevates plasma and urine concentrations of endogenous and exogenous ET-1, illustrating the significant contribution of this enzyme in the elimination of the peptide from the circulation in vivo.[131]

Notwithstanding their short half-life, circulating ETs elicit long-lasting functional effects. This apparent discrepancy is explained by the extremely slow rate of dissociation of receptor–ligand complexes.[132]

Interaction of ET-1 With Vascular Smooth Muscle

ET-1 Receptors

Like most other peptides, ETs exert their effects through interaction with a receptor located on the cell surface. The receptor is proposed to consist of an extracellular NH_2-terminal region, seven transmembrane helices separated by three extracellular and three cytoplasmic loops, and a cytoplasmic COOH-terminal region.[121]

The effects of ETs are mediated by several receptor subtypes. The existence of ET_A and ET_B receptors is generally accepted. On the ET_A receptor, the potency order is ET-1 = ET-2 > ET-3. On the ET_B receptor all three ET isoforms are equipotent. ET-1 elicits contraction of vascular smooth muscle cells through interaction with ET_A and/or ET_B receptors.[133,134] The possible existence of subtypes of these receptors has been suggested.[135] Selective agonists and antagonists for these receptor subtypes are available. In diseases associated with increased ET levels (see following section), ET receptors may be an important therapeutic target. As already noted, there is a particularly strong interaction between ET-1 and its receptors, which may account for the prolonged nature of responses to ET-1. On the other hand, ET receptors, like many other peptide cell surface receptors, are subject to long-lasting (up to 18 hours) ligand-induced down-regulation.[132]

Signal Transduction

ET-1–induced contraction of isolated blood vessels is more slowly developing, maintained for a longer time, and more resistant to agonist removal than is contraction evoked by most other vasoconstrictor agents. This suggests that the peptide is involved in long-term changes rather than in acute responses to certain stimuli. Several signal transduction mechanisms for ET-1–induced vascular contraction have been suggested.[136] They are coupled to the ET receptor through G proteins.[137]

Numerous studies give evidence that ET-1 induces contraction by activating phospholipase C, catalyzing phosphatidylinositol 4,5-bisphosphate breakdown, and resulting in the formation of inositol trisphosphate and diacylglycerol. Inositol triphosphate stimulates release of calcium from sarcoplasmic reticulum. Diacylglycerol mediates contraction through activation of protein kinase C.

Vascular contraction in response to ET-1 is accompanied by an increase in cytosolic calcium concentration; it consists of two components: a rapid initial transient phase, due to mobilization of calcium from intracellular (sarcoplasmic reticulum) stores by inositol triphosphate, followed by a sustained increase in cytosolic calcium, resulting from transmembrane calcium influx. Although it was originally proposed that ET is an endogenous direct ligand of L-type calcium channels,[119] it is now believed that the observed activation of calcium entry via L-type voltage-operated channels is the consequence of indirect gating of the channels by ET-1.[138] Activation of voltage-operated channels may be secondary to ET-1–induced membrane depolarization seen in a variety of vascular smooth muscle cells.[139] Considerable evidence also exists that ET-1 stimulates calcium influx into vascular smooth muscle cells through other calcium channels than L-type voltage-operated channels.[140]

ET has also been reported to activate phospholipase A_2 in some tissues, leading to release of arachidonic acid. Activation of the calcium-sensitive phospholipase A_2 may occur directly or indirectly through an increase in intracellular calcium concentration. Arachidonic acid is then further metabolized to prostaglandins, thromboxanes, and leukotrienes. This suggests the possibility that eicosanoid metabolites may have a role as second messengers in mediating some of the biological effects of ETs.

Effects of ET-1 on Vascular Tone

Influence on Isolated Blood Vessels

ET-1 is one of the most potent vasoactive endogenous substances known and induces contraction of isolated blood vessels. Arterial preparations of various anatomical origins, isolated from a variety of animal species including humans, show slowly developing and long-lasting contractions. This contraction is elicited by binding of ET-1 to the ET_A receptors on vascular smooth muscle cells. In some vascular preparations, including human blood vessels, vasoconstriction can also be mediated by the ET_B receptor.[133,134]

ET-1 also contracts isolated veins. ET-1 is 3-fold to 10-fold more potent in veins than in arteries.[141] However, in the pulmonary circulation, arteries are more sensitive than veins. This greater sensitivity might be due to the difference in oxygen tension.

ET-1 is also a potent constrictor of resistance arteries. This is evidenced by many studies performed on isolated microvessels in vitro and on microcirculation in situ.[142]

Considering the low plasma concentrations, it is important to mention that ET-1, besides its direct vasoconstricting effect, also potentiates, at threshold or subthreshold concentrations, the contractile response of other vasocontracting substances such as norepinephrine and serotonin. This potentiation is reciprocal because small amounts of these substances also potentiate the effect of ET-1. In that way, even small amounts of locally produced ET-1 can exert a profound regulatory influence on vascular tone.

Endothelial Modulation

In spite of its potent contractile effect, ET can in some blood vessels induce relaxation effects that depend on the presence of intact endothelium. This relaxation is mediated by endothelial ET_B receptors that trigger the release of NO. In addition, ETs stimulate release of prostacyclin from endothelial cells.[121] Release of NO and prostacyclin are thought to be responsible for the transient hypotensive effects elicited by ET-1 in vivo.

Hemodynamic Effects of ET-1

Intravenous infusion of ET-1 causes a rapid and transient hypotension followed by a profound and long-lasting increase in blood pressure. The hypotension is probably due to release of endothelial relaxing factors (prostacyclin, NO), and the pressor response is due to direct activation of vascular smooth muscle cells. Although ETs have positive chronotropic and inotropic effects on the heart, blood pressure increase may occur without changes in heart rate or cardiac output, indicating that ETs increase total peripheral resistance. Renal and mesenteric vascular beds seem to be most sensitive to ET.[143]

Indirect Influence of ET-1 on Vascular Tone

Besides its direct influence on vascular smooth muscle cells, ET-1 may also influence smooth muscle tone through interference with endocrine and nervous mechanisms (Figure 2.8).

Via Endocrine Systems

ET-1 may increase vascular tone through activation of the renin–angiotensin–aldosterone system. Interactions with ET-1 have been described at different levels of this system. In vivo and in vitro studies suggest that ET-1 modulates renin secretion from the juxtaglomerular cells. However, the studies provided divergent results: ET-1 suppressed renin secretion in vitro,[144] whereas injection of ET-1 in vivo had no effect or increased plasma renin activity.[145,146] In healthy human volunteers no change in plasma renin activity was found after infusion of ET-1 in a concentration that increased diastolic blood pressure, reduced heart rate and renal plasma flow, increased renal vascular resistance, and elevated the plasma ET-1 level to that found in several pathological conditions.[147,148]

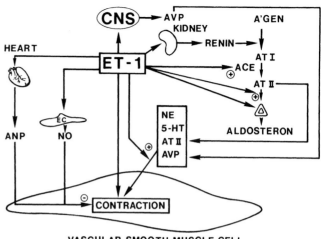

FIGURE 2.8. Schematic representation of the direct and indirect influences of endothelin 1 (ET-1) on vascular smooth muscle tone. The direct effect on smooth muscle is contraction. In vivo ET-1 can also induce contraction in indirect ways. It stimulates the release of arginine vasopressin (AVP) from the central nervous system (CNS) and stimulates the kidney to release renin, leading to an enhanced formation of angiotensin I (AT I) from circulating angiotensinogen (A'GEN). Angiotensin I is further processed to angiotensin II (AT II) by the angiotensin-converting enzyme (ACE). Angiotensin II stimulates the release of aldosterone from the adrenals. The latter two processes are potentiated by ET-1. The contractile effects of angiotensin II, AVP, serotonin (5-HT; released from aggregated platelets), and norepinephrine (NE; released from adrenergic nerve terminals) are also potentiated by ET-1. These contractile effects of ET-1 are to a certain degree counterbalanced by a relaxing influence through indirect mechanisms. ET-1 increases the release of atrial natriuretic peptide (ANP) from the heart, which besides its natriuretic influence on the kidney also has a relaxing influence on the vascular smooth muscle cells. In addition, circulating ET-1 also stimulates the endothelial cells to release NO.

ET-1 also stimulates conversion of angiotensin I to angiotensin II by ACE.[149] Angiotensin II is one of the most potent stimulators of ET-1 synthesis and release,[150] and angiotensin II and ET-1 act synergistically to induce vasoconstriction.

ET-1 also interacts with aldosterone secretion. Specific ET binding sites are present in the aldosterone-producing zona glomerulosa of the adrenal cortex. ET-1 stimulates aldosterone secretion in vitro and in vivo. In secretion of aldosterone from the adrenal cortex, angiotensin II and ET-1 act synergistically.[151]

There is a reciprocal interaction between ET-1 and AVP. ET-1 synthesis is stimulated by AVP.[152] On the other hand, ET-1 administered systemically or centrally stimulates AVP secretion from the neurohypophysis and elevates plasma levels of AVP.[153] The reciprocal influence at the level of the effector organs is not universal; whereas

ET-1 and AVP act synergistically as vasoconstrictors,[154] ET appears to inhibit AVP-induced water reabsorption in renal collecting tubules.[155]

ET-1 also interacts with atrial natriuretic peptide. ET-1 stimulates the release of atrial natriuretic peptide from atrial myocytes.[156] Elevated circulating plasma levels of atrial natriuretic peptide are found after injection of ET-1 with a dose that does not enhance blood pressure and/or right atrial pressure.[157] On the other hand, atrial natriuretic peptide effectively reduces ET-1 production in endothelial cells.[158,159] In several biological systems, ETs and atrial natriuretic peptide show functional antagonism. Atrial natriuretic peptide is a potent vasodilator and reduces plasma volume and osmolarity through its natriuretic influence. These actions are effectively antagonized by the biological actions of ET-1: vasoconstriction, reduction in renal plasma flow and glomerular filtration rate, and consequently reduced natriuresis and diuresis.

Via the Nervous System

ET-1 may interfere with the activity of the peripheral nervous system. Most experimental evidence in vitro indicates that ET-1 inhibits norepinephrine release from the sympathetic nerve terminals but potentiates the biological effects of norepinephrine on postjunctional vascular smooth muscle cells.[160,161] Studies in healthy human volunteers showed, however, that intraarterial infusion of ET-1 had no effect on sympathetically mediated or exogenously induced vasoconstriction in the forearm.[162]

ET-1 also interferes with the central nervous system. Intracerebroventricular injection of ET-1 in rats produces profound pressor responses.[163] The pressor effect of centrally administered ET-1 results from activation of both the sympathoadrenal and the AVP systems.[164–166]

The baroreflex is one of the most important mechanisms in blood pressure homeostasis. Activation of baroreflex stimulates release of ET into plasma.[167] This may contribute to the baroreflex-mediated cardiovascular homeostasis. On the other hand, topical administration of ET-1 to the carotid sinus desensitizes the reflex[168] and could promote hypertension. Systemic administration of ET-1 has no or a desensitizing influence on baroreflex.[157,169] Administration of ET-1 into the cerebrospinal fluid significantly increases baroreceptor sensitivity by affecting the vagal but not the sympathetic component of the baroreflex.[170]

Physiological Significance of ET-1 in the Cardiovascular System

In spite of the tremendous research efforts since 1988, the physiological role of ETs is not yet clearly established. The concentration of ET-1 in blood or tissues is less than the pharmacological concentration necessary to elicit functional responses. However, due to the short half-life and the long-lasting binding to the receptors, ET concentrations near the receptor may be much higher than those found in blood. Blood levels may only represent an overspill of a local paracrine secretion of the peptides. This suggestion fits with the observation that the release of ET occurs preferentially at the abluminal side of the endothelial cells.[171] Some hypotheses of its role in cardiovascular homeostasis have been proposed but need to be further substantiated.

Maintenance of Basal Vascular Tone

ET-1 is continuously released in small amounts by endothelial cells. It is not stored, and release results from continuous de novo synthesis. Because of its high vasoconstrictor potency and long-lasting action, the continuous release of small amounts of ET could contribute to maintenance of vascular tone. It may induce a direct contraction of vascular smooth muscle cells. But it may also have a role in continuous control of basal vascular tone and resistance by indirect mechanisms, including interference with baroreflex, modulation of noradrenaline release from sympathetic nerve terminals, potentiation of postsynaptic effects of norepinephrine, modulation of the synthesis and/or release of angiotensin II, and endothelial relaxing factors (NO, prostacyclin; see previous section, "Endothelial Relaxing Factors"). Haynes and Webb reported that endogenously generated ET-1 probably exerts a continuous influence on the human cardiovascular system. They found that local inhibition of ET-1 generation or of ET-1 action on ET_A receptors causes vasodilation of the forearm in healthy human volunteers[172] (Figure 2.9). These observations need to be further confirmed before ET-1's importance in determining basal vascular tone can be accepted without question.

Contribution to Hemostasis

When a blood vessel is injured, local vasoconstriction prevents blood loss and promotes primary hemostasis by diminishing perfusion pressure at the place of injury. Serotonin released from the aggregating platelets has an important role in the local vasoconstriction. Blood vessel injury also initiates the coagulation cascade that results in the formation of thrombin. Thrombin potently stimulates ET release from the endothelium.[127] The consequent long-lasting vasoconstriction triggered by the peptide may help prevent blood loss and promote local hemostasis. In addition, it may potentiate the vasocontraction induced by serotonin released from activated platelets. This mechanism may be especially effective in the case of endothelial dysfunction, because thrombin and serotonin are potent stimulators of NO release.

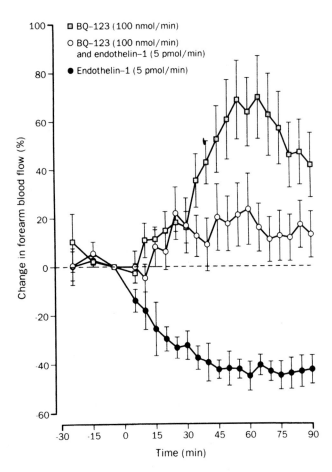

FIGURE 2.9. Intraarterial infusion of endothelin 1 (ET-1) and the ET$_A$ receptor antagonist BQ-123 on human forearm blood flow. Vasoconstriction to intraarterial ET-1 is abolished by BQ-123. Blockade of endogenous ET-1 by infusion of BQ-123 alone causes progressive forearm vasodilatation, suggesting that endogenous ET-1 contributes to basal vascular tone (from Haynes and Webb[172] with kind permission of The Lancet Ltd.).

Contribution to Systemic Blood Pressure Homeostasis

It is likely that ET-1 helps to ensure perfusion pressure when vascular volume decreases. Under these conditions systemic sympathetic activity and the renin–angiotensin–aldosterone system are activated. Angiotensin II stimulates ET release. As noted earlier, small amounts of ET potentiate the contractile effects of norepinephrine and angiotensin II. Additionally, ET-induced venoconstriction would increase cardiac preload and thus also increase cardiac output.

The effects of ET-1 on renal vasculature also protect against volume depletion.[173] ET-1 is the most potent agent known to increase renal vascular resistance.[174,175] In addition, ET-1 reduces glomerular filtration rate due to contraction of mesangial cells, reducing the filtering surface area and filtration coefficient.[176,177] These actions of ET-1 enhance fluid retention. All of these ac-

tions of ET-1 may contribute to blood pressure homeostasis and the preservation of perfusion pressure when vascular volume decreases.

Pathophysiological Significance of ET-1 in the Cardiovascular System

Although the physiological role of ET-1 in the vascular system still needs to be firmly established, its contribution to several pathological events is more generally assumed.

Hypertension

Considering the very potent direct vasocontractile effects of ET-1 and the many indirect actions causing elevation of peripheral resistance, the hypothesis that ET-1 may be involved in the pathophysiology of hypertension and its complications was self-evident. Many studies have focused on this hypothesis, but the pathogenic role of ET-1 in hypertension remains unclear.

Systemic Hypertension

Increased plasma levels of ET-1 would be a strong argument favoring a role for ET-1 in hypertension. In rats with various forms of experimental hypertension, no significant differences were found in circulating plasma levels of ET-1.[178] Plasma ET-1 levels were even significantly lower in genetically hypertensive rats.[179,180] Increased levels were found only in malignant forms of hypertension.[181] Also, in patients with essential hypertension, no or only moderately elevated plasma ET levels were observed.[182–185] Elevated ET levels were convincingly demonstrated in severe forms of hypertension with end-organ complications, such as advanced atherosclerosis or renal failure.[186] Because ET is a sensitive marker of endothelial injury, these elevated levels may simply reflect diffuse endothelial injury. It is also interesting to note that elevated ET-1 levels were found in cerebrospinal fluid of patients with hypertension. Central ET-1–mediated effects may thus also play a role in hypertension.[187]

In the absence of increased ET-1 plasma levels, an increased responsiveness to ET-1 could also lead to hypertension. However, the question of whether the responsiveness of blood vessels to ET-1 is altered in hypertension is unsettled. In spontaneously hypertensive rats, the pressor responses to ET have been reported to be elevated, reduced, or unaltered.[188,189] Divergent results were also obtained on isolated vessels from hypertensive animals. The sensitivity to ETs was reported to be enhanced, reduced, or unchanged.[190–192] Renal arteries isolated from spontaneously hypertensive rats show increased reactivity to ETs.[179] Based on the importance of renal vasculature in blood pressure regulation, alteration of ET responsiveness in this vascular bed may be important in long-term elevation of systemic blood pressure. In patients with essential hypertension, ET-1–induced constriction of the dorsal hand vein is significantly greater than in normotensive subjects. In addition, sympathetically mediated venoconstriction is substantially potentiated by ET-1 in hypertensive but not normotensive subjects.[193] ET-1 may thus contribute to the reduction of venous capacity occurring in the early stages of essential hypertension.

If ET-1 contributes to the increased vascular resistance in hypertension, one would expect a drop in blood pressure after blockade of ET synthesis or ET receptors. In spontaneously hypertensive rats, inhibition of ET-1 production was reported to decrease blood pressure,[194] but anti-ET antibody had no effect.[195] Administration of the selective ET_A receptor antagonist BQ-123 significantly decreased blood pressure in stroke-prone but not in normal spontaneously hypertensive rats,[196] suggesting that ET_A receptors may be involved in the elevated blood pressure in this severe form of hypertension.

The possible pathophysiological role for ET-1 in hypertension is further supported by findings on patients with hemangioendothelioma, a malignant tumor associated with hypertension and a 15-fold to 20-fold increase in plasma ET-1 levels. After surgical excision of the tumor, normal blood pressure and plasma ET-1 concentration are restored. Recurrence of the hemangiothelioma was associated with redevelopment of hypertension and elevated circulating ET levels.[197]

ET-1 thus seems to have a role in certain severe forms of hypertension. However, no convincing evidence exists for the involvement of ET-1 in mild and moderate forms of arterial hypertension.

Pulmonary Hypertension

Pulmonary hypertension is associated with elevated circulatory ET-1 levels.[198] Increased production of ET-1 occurs in the lungs of rats and patients with primary pulmonary hypertension.[199–201] In patients with secondary pulmonary hypertension due to valvular heart disease, the circulating plasma ET-1 level is also significantly elevated. The ET-1 level normalizes after surgical correction of valvular disease.[202] The increased ET-1 available and the observation that constrictor sensitivity to ET-1 increases after prolonged exposure to hypoxia[203] suggest that ET-1 may be involved in sustaining chronic hypoxic pulmonary hypertension.

Preeclampsia

Many studies report elevations of plasma ET-1 levels in pregnancy-induced hypertension.[204–208] On the other hand, in some studies no change of circulating ET-1 level was found in the maternal plasma during preeclampsia.[209,210] Magnesium infusions that reduce blood pressure in these patients also reduce plasma ET-1 levels. Magnesium had no effect in normal pregnant women.[205] Within 48 hours following cesarean section, elevated plasma ET-1 levels return to control values and show good correlation with the time course of blood pressure reduction.[208] Although several studies have shown a good correlation between symptoms of preeclampsia and circulating plasma ET-1 levels, the causal relationship remains to be established.[205,208]

Ischemia

The possible role of ETs in the pathophysiology of ischemic injury is supported by several lines of evidence. Under ischemic conditions, the vasoactive effects of ET-1 are enhanced. Hypoxia increases both ET production and its efficacy.

Cerebral Ischemia

The possible involvement of ET-1 in the pathophysiology of cerebral ischemia is supported by several findings. ET-1 potently constricts cerebral arteries.[211–213] Intravenous, intraarterial, or intracisternal injection of ET-1 causes cerebral vasoconstriction, electroencephalographic signs of cerebral ischemia, and reduction of cerebrospinal fluid production via sustained vasoconstriction in the choroid plexus.[214] Experimental cerebral ischemia followed by reperfusion has been shown to increase ET-1 levels.[215,216] The potential clinical relevance of all these experimental findings can be deduced from the work of Ziv et al.[217] They demonstrated that plasma ET-1 levels in patients with nonhemorrhagic cerebral infarction is fourfold higher than in healthy volunteers. These authors postulated that the excessive production of ET-1 may cause vasoconstriction in the collateral circulation, thereby enlarging the area of infarct size.

Myocardial Ischemia

Significant elevated circulating plasma ET-1 levels are found in patients with acute myocardial infarction. Plasma ET-1 level elevation is probably an early sign of acute myocardial infarction.[218] Plasma ET-1 levels correlate well with the severity of the infarction.[219] Especially high plasma ET-1 levels are found in patients with hemodynamic complications.[220] No change in ET-1 plasma level occurs in patients with stable angina pectoris (i.e., myocardial ischemia but no infarction).[219,221] In patients following percutaneous transluminal coronary angioplasty, significantly increased ET-1 levels are detected in the coronary sinus but not in systemic circulation.[222]

Animal studies point to the fact that these elevated levels may have important consequences. Administration of

ET-1 constricts large and small coronary arteries, leading to signs of myocardial ischemia.[223–226] Coronary artery occlusion followed by reperfusion causes significant facilitation of ET-1–induced coronary vasoconstriction.[227–231] In addition, increased binding of ET-1 to cardiac membranes has been shown following ischemia and reperfusion.[232] ET-1 synthesis/release from the heart is also increased.[227,233,234] Convincing evidence for the role of ET-1 in myocardial ischemia and infarction is provided by the observations that inhibition of ET-1 biosynthesis[235] and treatment with the monoclonal antibody against ET-1[234] significantly reduced the infarct size in anesthetized rats after ischemia.

Renal Ischemia

Renal vasculature is one of the most sensitive to the constrictor action of ET-1. Systemic injection of subpressor doses of ET-1 reduces renal blood flow in dogs[236] and human volunteers.[148]

Reversible renal ischemia augments ET-1 mRNA in the kidney[237] and results in an elevation of plasma and urine levels of ET-1 in rats.[238,239] Administration of exogenous ET-1 mimics the syndrome of acute renal failure, with the following effects: vasoconstriction, reduction in renal plasma flow, reduction in glomerular filtration rate, and reduction of tubular function.[239–241] Also, nephrotoxic substances increase the levels of ET-1. This has been shown with amphotericin B,[242] x-ray contrast medium,[243] endotoxin,[244] and cyclosporin A.[245,246]

Very often renal vasoconstriction after ischemia or nephrotoxic substances could be prevented with anti–ET-1 monoclonal antibodies.[238,240,246] The use of ET antagonists has been shown to protect against ischemia-induced renal damage[247] and cyclosporin A–induced contraction of afferent arterioles.[248] The increase in plasma ET-1 found in patients with acute renal failure[249] suggests that these findings might be of clinical relevance.

Vasospasm

Cerebral Vasospasm

Cerebral vasospasm is a major sequela of subarachnoid hemorrhage. ET-1 may be an important mediator in this effect. Injection of exogenous ET-1 mimics cerebral vasospasm.[250,251] ET-1 is a potent vasoconstrictor of basilar arteries (a common site of vasospasm) isolated from several animal species and humans. After subarachnoid hemorrhage, the reactivity of the cerebral blood vessels to ET-1 is potentiated.[250,252–254] It is also known that hemoglobin stimulates the release of ET-1 from cultured endothelial cells.[255]

Elevated ET-1 levels in plasma and cerebrospinal fluid have been demonstrated in patients with subarachnoid hemorrhage.[256–259] Plasma levels are higher in patients in whom subarachnoid hemorrhage is followed by cerebral vasospasm. No change in ET-1 level in cerebrospinal fluid was observed in the first 3 days following hemorrhage, but the ET-1 level increased significantly on days 5 and 7 after hemorrhage, coinciding with the onset of cerebral vasospasm.[259] No change in ET-1 level in cerebrospinal fluid was observed in subarachnoid hemorrhage patients without vasospasm. Studies have provided convincing evidence for an important role of ET-1 in cerebral vasospasm by inhibiting the influence of endogenous ET-1 through the following means: inhibition of ET-1 biosynthesis,[260] administration of monoclonal antibodies against ET-1,[261] and administration of the selective ET_A receptor antagonist BQ-123[262]; each means of ET-1 inhibition significantly reduced or prevented vasospasm following subarachnoid hemorrhage in dogs. These data support the idea that ET-1 is an important mediator of cerebral vasospasm after subarachnoid hemorrhage.

Coronary Vasospasm

Several arguments support the view that ET-1 may have a role in coronary vasospasm. Animal studies have shown that the contractile effect of ET-1 is augmented in coronary arteries with endothelial denudation or dysfunction due to ischemia and reperfusion.[229–231] ET-1 causes long-lasting coronary contractions, and subthreshold concentrations of ET-1 potentiate the coronary vasoconstrictor action of other contractile agents (e.g., serotonin and norepinephrine in isolated human coronary arteries).[263,264] This increased sensitivity toward serotonin in the presence of ET-1 may perhaps contribute to vasospasm induced by aggregating platelets. ET-1 plasma levels in patients are elevated in the coronary circulation during vasospastic episodes (angina). This might occur without significant changes in ET-1 levels in systemic circulation.[265,266] Wieczorek et al.[267] reported higher plasma ET levels in patients with unstable angina at rest or non–Q-wave myocardial infarction than in healthy control subjects. Interestingly, compared with the patients who had an uneventful course in the 9 weeks after presentation, patients with subsequent events had significantly higher plasma ET levels at presentation and 9 weeks later.

Raynaud's Disease

Some data support the involvement of ET-1 in the excessive spasm of finger arteries on exposure to cold. ET-1 levels were found to be elevated in patients with Raynaud's disease.[268,269] Cooling of the hands caused a moderate elevation of plasma ET-1 levels in healthy subjects but a more pronounced increase in patients with Raynaud's disease.[269] Elevated ET levels were also found in the cutaneous vasculature of patients with Raynaud's disease.[270] Recovery after cold challenge–induced vasoconstriction is abnormally prolonged in these patients, which may be related to the long-lasting constriction induced by ET-1.

Hypercholesterolemia and Atherosclerosis

Patients with hypercholesterolemia[271] and those with coronary artery atherosclerosis[272] show elevated plasma ET-1 levels. This elevation probably develops because oxidized low-density lipoproteins and several cytokines (tumor necrosis factor α, interleukin-1β) that are involved in the vascular injury process of atherosclerosis stimulate the production of ET-1 by the endothelium.[273,274] The enhanced levels of ET-1 might have an important role in the pathophysiology of atherosclerotic disease and its complications. This role is further confirmed by the observations that contractions to ET-1 are potentiated in vessels with atherosclerotic lesions[263] and that ET-1 also induces smooth muscle proliferation.[275] This trophic effect could account for the vascular wall hypertrophy in atherosclerosis.

Congestive Heart Failure

Elevated circulating plasma ET-1 levels are found in humans with heart failure.[276,277] This increase in ET-1 may be secondary to the increased levels of angiotensin II and vasopressin, substances known to stimulate the production of ET-1.[153] It could also be due to a decrease in clearance of ET from the circulation in congestive heart failure.[278] In a dog model of chronic heart failure, systemic blood pressure and resistance were reduced by a selective ET$_A$ antagonist, suggesting that elevated endogenous ET contributes to the increase of systemic vascular resistance in severe congestive heart failure.[279]

Shock

Elevated circulating plasma ET-1 levels were reported in patients with hemorrhagic, cardiogenic, or septic shock.[280,281] From in vitro studies it is known that endotoxin, lipopolysaccharide, and tumor necrosis factor (substances mediating the syndrome of septic shock) stimulate the release of ET-1 from endothelial cells.[282,283] Considering the great sensitivity of the renal circulation to ET-1, it is possible that increased local and systemic production of ET-1 may contribute significantly to the renal failure associated with septic shock.

Hepatorenal Syndrome

ET-1 may also be involved in the hepatorenal syndrome. Circulating ET-1 levels are significantly elevated in patients with liver cirrhosis.[284,285] Because the renal vascular bed is the most sensitive to ET-1, the plasma levels may be sufficient to induce renal insufficiency in cir-

rhotic patients (hepatorenal syndrome). Evidence for this hypothesis is provided by studies showing that renal dysfunction was most prominent in cirrhotic patients with the highest levels of ET-1.[285,286]

Other Endothelial Contracting Factors

There is evidence that endothelial cells, especially in veins, can release other contractile factors under certain conditions. Their formation is inhibited by cyclooxygenase inhibitors. Arachidonic acid induces, in some vessels, endothelium-dependent contraction that is blocked by cyclooxygenase blockers. These endothelial contractile factors thus are probably metabolites of the cyclooxygenase pathway of arachidonic acid metabolism. The involvement of the endoperoxide PGH$_2$ is suggested.[287] Furthermore, the cyclooxygenase pathway is a source of superoxide anions that can mediate endothelium-dependent contraction either by breakdown of NO or by direct effects on vascular smooth muscle cells.[288]

Stretch of canine basilar arteries results in endothelium-dependent contraction, a mechanism that may be involved in autoregulation of cerebral blood flow.[289] Hypoxia elicits prostanoid-induced endothelium-mediated contraction.[290] Also, the aorta from spontaneously hypertensive and from diabetic rats releases, in response to acetylcholine, an endothelial contractile factor that is sensitive to cyclooxygenase blockers.[45,291] Whether these endothelial contractile factors have a functional significance is not established.

Conclusion

Vascular tone is partially regulated by the endothelial cells. These cells release relaxing and contracting factors under basal conditions, and the release is modulated by many different physiological stimuli. The physiological role of ET is diametrically opposed to that of NO. A yin and yang relationship exists between these two very different endothelium-derived mediators. The position of the endothelium, between circulating blood and vascular smooth muscle cells, makes it an ideal signal transduction interface for changes in the environment but also makes it a target for vascular diseases such as atherosclerosis, hypertension, vasospasm, and diabetes. It appears that functional changes of the endothelium are a common hallmark of several forms of cardiovascular disease and therefore a primary candidate to serve as mediator of these disease states and their complications. Reduced release of endothelium-derived relaxant factors and enhanced liberation of endothelial-derived contraction factors are common under these conditions. The understanding of the role of endothelial vasoregulatory factors in health and disease will likely emerge in new pharmacological tools with great value in medicine and in new approaches for successful treatment of cardiovascular diseases.

References

1. Fajardo LF. The complexity of endothelial cells. *Am J Clin Pathol.* 1989;92:241–250.

2. Shepro D, D'amore PA. Physiology and biochemistry of the vascular wall endothelium. In: Renkin EM, Michel CC, Geiger SR, eds. *Microcirculation. Handbook of Physiology.* Section II, vol 4. Bethesda, Md: American Physiological Society; 1984;103–164.

3. Furchgott RF, Zawadzki JV. The obligatory role of endothelial cells in the relaxation of arterial smooth muscle by acetylcholine. *Nature.* 1980;288:373–376.

4. Furchgott RF, Vanhoutte PM. Endothelium-derived relaxing and contracting factors. *FASED J.* 1989;3:2007–2018.

5. Van de Voorde J, Leusen I. Role of the endothelium in the vasodilator response of rat thoracic aorta on histamine. *Eur J Pharmacol.* 1983;87:113–120.

6. Van de Voorde J, Leusen I. Effect of histamine on aorta preparations of different species. *Arch Int Pharmacodyn Ther.* 1984; 268:95–105.

7. Förstermann U, Trogisch G, Busse R. Species-dependent differences in the nature of endothelium-derived vascular relaxing factor. *Eur J Pharmacol.* 1985;106:639–643.

8. Holzmann S. Endothelium-induced relaxation by acetylcholine associated with larger rises in cyclic GMP in coronary arterial strips. *J Cyclic Nucleotide Res.* 1982;8:409–419.

9. Ignarro LJ, Lippton H, Edwards JC, et al. Mechanism of vascular smooth muscle relaxation by organic nitrates, nitrites, nitroprusside, and nitric oxide: evidence for the involvement of S-nitrosothiols as active intermediates. *J Pharmacol Exp Ther.* 1981;218:739–749.

10. Furchgott RF. Studies on relaxation of rabbit aorta by sodium nitrite: the basis for the proposal that the acid-activatable inhibitory factor from bovine retractor penis is inorganic nitrite and the endothelium-derived relaxing factor is nitric oxide. In: Vanhoutte PM, ed. *Vasodilatation: Vascular Smooth Muscle, Peptides, Autonomic Nerves, and Endothelium.* New York, NY: Raven Press; 1988:401–414.

11. Ignarro LJ, Byrns RE, Wood KS. Biochemical and pharmacological properties of endothelium-derived relaxing factor and its similarity to nitric oxide radical. In: Vanhoutte PM, ed. *Vasodilatation: Vascular Smooth Muscle, Peptides, Autonomic Nerves, and Endothelium.* New York, NY: Raven Press; 1988:427–435.

12. Palmer RMJ, Ferrige AG, Moncada S. Nitric oxide release accounts for the biological activity of endothelium-derived relaxing factor. *Nature.* 1987;327:524–526.

13. Palmer RMJ, Ashton DS, Moncada S. Vascular endothelial cells synthesize nitric oxide from L-arginine. *Nature.* 1988;333:664–666.

14. Palmer RMJ, Rees DD, Ashton DS, Moncada S. L-Arginine is the physiological precursor for the formation of nitric oxide in endothelium-dependent relaxation. *Biochem Biophys Res Commun.* 1988;153:1251–1256.

15. Rees DD, Palmer RMJ, Schulz R, Hodson HF, Moncada S. Characterization of three inhibitors of endothelial nitric oxide synthase in vitro and in vivo. *Br J Pharmacol.* 1990; 101:746–752.

16. Leone AM, Palmer RMJ, Knowles RG, Francis PL, Ashton DS, Moncada S. Constitutive and inducible nitric oxide synthases incorporate molecular oxygen into both nitric oxide and citrulline. *J Biol Chem.* 1991;266:23790–23795.

17. Marsden PA, Schappen KT, Chen HS, et al. Molecular cloning and characterization of human endothelial nitric oxide synthase. *FEBS Lett.* 1992;307:287–293.

18. Gibaldi M. What is nitric oxide and why are so many people studying it? *J Clin Pharmacol.* 1993;33:488–496.

19. Moncada S, Palmer RMJ, Higgs EA. Nitric oxide: physiology, pathophysiology, and pharmacology. *Pharmacol Rev.* 1991;43:109–141.

20. Nathan C. Nitric oxide as a secretory product of mammalian cells. *FASEB J.* 1992;6:3051–3064.

21. Singer HA, Peach MJ. Calcium- and endothelial-mediated vascular smooth muscle relaxation in rabbit aorta. *Hypertension.* 1982;4(suppl):II19–II25.

22. Schilling WP, Ritchie AK, Navarro LT, Eskin SG. Bradykinin-stimulated calcium influx in cultured aortic endothelial cells. *Am J Physiol.* 1988;255:H219–H227.

23. Pearson PJ, Vanhoutte PM. Vasodilator and vasoconstrictor substances produced by the endothelium. *Rev Physiol Biochem Pharmacol.* 1993;122:1–67.

24. Stamler JS, Jaraki O, Osbourne J, et al. S-nitrosylation of protein with nitric oxide: synthesis and characterization of biologically active compounds. *Proc Natl Acad Sci U S A.* 1992;89:444–448.

25. Ignarro LJ. Signal transduction mechanisms involving nitric oxide. *Biochem Pharmacol.* 1991;41:485–490.

26. Radomski WM, Palmer RMJ, Moncada S. Comparative pharmacology of endothelium-derived relaxing factor nitric oxide and prostacyclin in platelets. *Br J Pharmacol.* 1987;92:181–187.

27. Radomski MW, Palmer RMJ, Moncada S. Endogenous nitric oxide inhibits human platelet adhesion to vascular endothelium. *Lancet.* 1987;2:1057–1058.

28. Griffith TM, Edwards DH, Lewis MJ, Newby AC, Henderson AH. The nature of endothelium-derived vascular relaxant factor. *Nature.* 1984;308:645–647.

29. Vallance P, Collier J, Moncada S. Effects of endothelium-derived nitric oxide on peripheral arteriolar tone in man. *Lancet.* 1989;2:997–1000.

30. Rees DD, Palmer RMJ, Moncada S. Role of endothelium-derived nitric oxide in the regulation of blood pressure. *Proc Natl Acad Sci U S A.* 1989;86:3375–3378.

31. Aisaka K, Gross SS, Griffith OW, Levi R. N^G-methylarginine an inhibitor of endothelium-derived nitric oxide synthesis is a potent pressor agent in the guinea pig: does nitric oxide regulate blood pressure in vivo? *Biochem Biophys Res Commun.* 1989;160:881–886.

32. Dusting GJ, Dubbin PN, Woodman OL, Zambetis M. Mechanism of hypertension induced by N^G-nitro-L-arginine in rats and rabbits. *Arch Int Pharmacodyn Ther.* 1990; 305:242.

33. Haynes WG, Noon JP, Walker BR, Webb DJ. Inhibition of nitric oxide synthesis increases blood pressure in healthy humans. *J Hypertens.* 1993;11:1375–1380.

34. Pohl U, Holtz J, Busse R, Bassenge E. Crucial role of endothelium in the vasodilator response to increased flow in vivo. *Hypertension.* 1986;8:37–44.

35. Cox DA, Vita JA, Treasure CB, et al. Atherosclerosis impairs flow-mediated dilation of coronary arteries in humans. *Circulation.* 1989;80:458–465.

36. Drexler H, Zeiher AM, Wollschläger H, Meinertz T, Just H, Bonzel T. Flow-dependent coronary artery dilatation in humans. *Circulation.* 1989;80:466–474.

37. Olesen SP, Clapham DE, Davies PF. Haemodynamic shear stress activates a K^+ current in vascular endothelial cells. *Nature.* 1988;331:168–170.

38. Lansman JB, Hallman TJ, Rink TJ. Single stretch-activated ion channels in vascular endothelial cells as mechanotransducers? *Nature.* 1987;325:811–813.

39. Faraci FM, Brian JE. Nitric oxide and the cerebral circulation. *Stroke.* 1994;25:692–703.

40. Raij L. Nitric oxide and the kidney. *Circulation.* 1993;87 (suppl 5):V26–V29.

41. Lüscher TF, Diederich D, Siebenmann R, et al. Difference between endothelium-dependent relaxation in arterial and in venous coronary bypass grafts. *N Engl J Med.* 1988; 319:462–467.

42. Yang Z, Von Segesser L, Bauer E, Stulz P, Turina M, Lüscher TF. Different activation of the endothelial L-arginine and cyclooxygenase pathway in the human internal mammary artery and saphenous vein. *Circ Res.* 1991; 68:52–60.

43. Vallance P, Collier J, Moncada S. Nitric oxide synthesised from L-arginine mediates endothelium dependent dilatation in human veins in vivo. *Cardiovasc Res.* 1989;23: 1053–1057.

44. Diederich D, Yang Z, Bühler FR, Lüscher TF. Impaired endothelium-dependent relaxations in hypertensive resistance arteries involve cyclooxygenase pathway. *Am J Physiol.* 1990;258:H445–H451.

45. Lüscher TF, Vanhoutte PM. Endothelium-dependent contractions to acetylcholine in the aorta of the spontaneously hypertensive rat. *Hypertension.* 1986;8:344–348.

46. Van de Voorde J, Leusen I. Endothelium-dependent and independent relaxation of aortic rings from hypertensive rats. *Am J Physiol.* 1986;250:H711–H717.

47. Lockette W, Otsuka Y, Carretero O. The loss of endothelium-dependent vascular relaxation in hypertension. *Hypertension.* 1986:8(suppl 2):II61–II66.

48. Van de Voorde J, Vanheel B, Leusen I. Depressed endothelium-dependent relaxation in hypertension: relation to increased blood pressure and reversibility. *Pflügers Arch Eur J Physiol.* 1988;411:500–504.

49. Lüscher TF, Vanhoutte PM, Raij L. Antihypertensive therapy normalizes endothelium-dependent relaxations in salt-induced hypertension of the rat. *Hypertension.* 1987; 9(suppl 3):193–197.

50. Calver AL, Collier JG, Moncada S, Vallance PJT. Effect of local intra-arterial N^G-monomethyl-L-arginine in patients with hypertension: the nitric oxide dilator mechanism appears abnormal. *J Hypertens.* 1992;10:1025–1031.

51. Linder L, Kiowski W, Bühler FR, Lüscher TF. Indirect evidence for release of endothelium-derived relaxing factor in human forearm circulation in vivo: blunted response in essential hypertension. *Circulation.* 1990;81:1762–1767.

52. Panza JA, Quyyumi AA, Brush JE, Epstein SE. Abnormal endothelium-dependent vascular relaxation in patients with essential hypertension. *N Engl J Med.* 1990;323:22–27.

53. Treasure CB, Manoukian SV, Klein JL, et al. Epicardial coronary artery responses to acetylcholine are impaired in hypertensive patients. *Circ Res.* 1992;71:776–781.

54. Chen PY, Sanders PW. L-Arginine abrogates salt-sensitive hypertension in Dahl/Rapp rats. *J Clin Invest.* 1991; 88: 1559–1567.

55. Panza JA, Casino PR, Badar DM, Quyyumi AA. Effect of increased availability of endothelium-derived nitric oxide precursor on endothelium-dependent vascular relaxation in normals and in patients with essential hypertension. *Circulation.* 1993;87:1475–1481.

56. Creager MA, Roddy M, Coleman SM, Dzau VJ. The effect of ACE inhibition on endothelium-dependent vasodilation in hypertension. *J Vasc Res.* 1992;29:97–98.

57. Vallance P, Leone A, Calver A, Collier J, Moncada S. Accumulation of an endogenous inhibitor of nitric oxide synthesis in chronic renal failure. *Lancet.* 1992;339:572–575.

58. Weiner C, Martinez E, Zhu LK, Ghodsi A, Chestnut D. In vitro release of endothelium-derived relaxing factor by acetylcholine is increased during the guinea pig pregnancy. *Am J Obstet Gynecol.* 1989;161:1599–1605.

59. Yallampalli C, Garfield RE. Inhibition of nitric oxide synthesis in rats during pregnancy produces signs similar to those of preeclampsia. *Am J Obstet Gynecol.* 1993;169: 1316–1320.

60. McCarthy AL, Woolfson RG, Raju SK, Poston L. Abnormal endothelial cell function of resistance arteries from women with preeclampsia. *Am J Obstet Gynecol.* 1993;168: 323–1330.

61. Akar F, Ark M, Uydes BS, et al. Nitric oxide production by human umbilical vessels in severe pre-eclampsia. *J Hypertens.* 1994;12:1235–1241.

62. Harrison DG. Endothelial dysfunction in atherosclerosis. *Cardiovasc Res.* 1994;27(suppl 1):87–102.

63. Verbeuren TJ, Jordaens FH, Zonnekeyn LL, Van Hove CE, Coene MC, Herman AG. I: Endothelium-dependent and endothelium-independent contractions and relaxations in isolated arteries of control and hypercholesterolemic rabbits. *Circ Res.* 1986;58:552–564.

64. Förstermann U, Mügge A, Alheid U, Haverich A, Frölich JC. Selective attenuation of endothelium-mediated vasodilation in atherosclerotic human coronary arteries. *Circ Res.* 1988;62:185–190.

65. Kugiyama K, Kerns SA, Morrisett JD, Roberts R, Henry PD. Impairment of endothelium-dependent arterial relaxation by lysolecithin in modified low-density lipoproteins. *Nature.* 1990;344:160–162.

66. Cooke JP, Singer AH, Tsao P, Zera P, Rowan RA, Billingham ME. Antiatherogenic effects of L-arginine in the hypercholesterolemic rabbit. *J Clin Invest.* 1992;90: 1168–1172.

67. Girerd XJ, Hirsch AT, Cooke JP, Dzau VJ, Creager MA. L-Arginine augments endothelium-dependent vasodilation in cholesterol-fed rabbits. *Circ Res.* 1990;67:1301–1308.

68. Harrison DG, Armstrong ML, Freiman PC, Heistad DD. Restoration of endothelium-dependent relaxation by dietary treatment of atherosclerosis. *J Clin Invest.* 1987; 80:1808–1811.

69. Mügge A, Elwell JH, Peterson TE, Hofmeyer TG, Heistad DD, Harrison DG. Chronic treatment with polyethylene glycolated superoxide dismutase partially restores en-

dothelium-dependent vascular relaxations in cholesterol-fed rabbits. *Circ Res.* 1991;69:1293–1300.

70. Gordon JB, Ganz P, Nabel EG, et al. Atherosclerosis influences the vasomotor response of epicardial coronary arteries to exercise. *J Clin Invest.* 1989;83:1946–1952.

71. Ludmer PL, Selwyn AP, Shook TL, et al. Paradoxical vasoconstriction induced by acetylcholine in atherosclerotic coronary arteries. *N Engl J Med.* 1986;315:1046–1051.

72. Nabel EG, Ganz P, Gordon JB, Alexander RW, Selwyn AP. Dilation of normal and constriction of atherosclerotic coronary arteries caused by the cold pressor test. *Circulation.* 1988;77:43–52.

73. Yeung AC, Vekshtein VI, Krantz DS, et al. The effect of atherosclerosis on the vasomotor response of coronary arteries to mental stress. *N Engl J Med.* 1991;325:1551–1556.

74. Drexler H, Zeiher AM, Meinzer K, Just H. Correction of endothelial dysfunction in coronary microcirculation of hypercholesterolaemic patients by L-arginine. *Lancet.* 1991;338:1546–1550.

75. Werns SW, Walton JA, Hsia HH, Nabel EG, Sanz ML, Pitt B. Evidence of endothelial dysfunction in angiographically normal coronary arteries of patients with coronary artery disease. *Circulation.* 1989;79:287–291.

76. Celermajer DS, Sorensen KE, Gooch VM, et al. Non-invasive detection of endothelial dysfunction in children and adults at risk of atherosclerosis. *Lancet.* 1992;340:1111–1115.

77. Kiowski W, Linder L, Stoschitzky K, et al. Diminished vascular response to inhibition of endothelium-derived nitric oxide and enhanced vasoconstriction to exogenously administered endothelin-1 in clinically healthy smokers. *Circulation.* 1994;90:27–34.

78. Creager MA, Gallagher SJ, Girerd XJ, Coleman SM, Dzau VJ, Cooke JP. L-Arginine improves endothelium-dependent vasodilation in hypercholesterolemic humans. *J Clin Invest.* 1992;90:1248–1253.

79. Jeserich M, Münzel T, Just H, Drexler H. Reduced plasma L-arginine in hypercholesterolaemia. *Lancet.* 1992;339:561.

80. Leung WH, Lau CP, Wong CK. Beneficial effect of cholesterol-lowering therapy on coronary endothelium-dependent relaxation in hypercholesterolaemic patients. *Lancet.* 1993;341:1496–1500.

81. Egashira K, Inoue T, Hirooka Y, Yamada A, Urabe Y, Takeshita A. Evidence of impaired endothelium-dependent coronary vasodilation in patients with angina pectoris and normal coronary angiograms. *N Engl J Med.* 1993;328:1659–1664.

82. Motz W, Vogt M, Rabenau O, Scheler S, Lückhoff A, Strauer BE. Evidence of endothelial dysfunction in coronary resistance vessels in patients with angina pectoris and normal coronary angiograms. *Am J Cardiol.* 1991;68:996–1003.

83. Durante W, Sen AK, Sunahara FA. Impairment of endothelium-dependent relaxation in aortae from spontaneously diabetic rats. *Br J Pharmacol.* 1988;94:463–468.

84. Pieper GM, Peltier BA. Amelioration by L-arginine of a dysfunctional arginine/nitric oxide pathway in diabetic endothelium. *J Cardiovasc Pharmacol.* 1995;25:397–403.

85. Diederich D, Skopec J, Diederich A, Dai FX. Endothelial dysfunction in mesenteric resistance arteries of diabetic rats: role of free radicals. *Am J Physiol.* 1994;266:H1153–H1161.

86. Saenz de Tajeda I, Goldstein I, Azadzoi K, Krane RJ, Cohen RA. Impaired neurogenic and endothelium-mediated relaxation of penile smooth muscle from diabetic men with impotence. *N Engl J Med.* 1989;320:1025–1030.

87. Calver AL, Collier JG, Vallance PJT. Inhibition and stimulation of nitric oxide synthesis in the human forearm arterial bed of patients with insulin-dependent diabetes. *J Clin Invest.* 1992;90:2548–2554.

88. McVeigh GR, Brennan GM, Johnston GD, et al. Dietary fish oil augments nitric oxide production or release in patients with type 2 (non-insulin-dependent) diabetes mellitus. *Diabetologia.* 1993;36:33–38.

89. Mehta JL, Nichols WW, Donnelly WM, et al. Impaired canine responses to acetylcholine and bradykinin after occlusion-reperfusion. *Circ Res.* 1989;64:43–54.

90. Pearson PJ, Schaff HV, Vanhoutte PM. Long-term impairment of endothelium-dependent relaxations to aggregating platelets after reperfusion injury in canine coronary arteries. *Circulation.* 1990;81:1921–1927.

91. Weyrich AS, Ma XL, Lefer AM. The role of L-arginine in ameliorating reperfusion injury after myocardial ischemia in the cat. *Circulation.* 1992;86:279–288.

92. Macdonald RL, Weir BKA. A review of hemoglobin and the pathogenesis of cerebral vasospasm. *Stroke.* 1991;22:971–982.

93. Drexler H, Hayoz D, Münzel T, Just H, Zelis R, Brunner HR. Endothelial function in congestive heart failure. *Am Heart J.* 1993;126:761–764.

94. Habib F, Dutka D, Crossman D, Oakley CM, Cleland JGF. Enhanced basal nitric oxide production in heart failure: another failed counter-regulatory vasodilator mechanism? *Lancet.* 1994;344:371–373.

95. Stoclet JC, Fleming I, Gray G, et al. Nitric oxide and endotoxemia. *Circulation.* 1993;87 (suppl 5):V77–V80.

96. Petros A, Bennett D, Vallance P. Effect of nitric oxide synthase inhibitors on hypotension in patients with septic shock. *Lancet.* 1991;338:1557–1558.

97. Wright CD, Rees DD, Moncada S. Protective and pathological roles of nitric oxide in endotoxin shock. *Cardiovasc Res.* 1992;26:48–57.

98. Rossaint R, Falke KJ, Lopez F, et al. Inhaled nitric oxide for the adult respiratory distress syndrome. *N Engl J Med.* 1993;328:399–405.

99. Kinsella JP, Neish SR, Shaffer E, Abman SH. Low-dose inhalational nitric oxide in persistent pulmonary hypertension of the newborn. *Lancet.* 1992;340:819–820.

100. Roberts JD, Polaner DM, Lang P, Zapol WM. Inhaled nitric oxide in persistent pulmonary hypertension of the newborn. *Lancet.* 1992;340:818–819.

101. Roberts JD, Lang P, Bigatello LM, Vlahakes GJ, Zapol WM. Inhaled nitric oxide in congenital heart disease. *Circulation.* 1993;87:447–453.

102. Pepke-Zaba J, Higenbottam TW, Dinh-Xuan AT, Stone D, Wallwork J. Inhaled nitric oxide as a cause of selective pulmonary vasodilatation in pulmonary hypertension. *Lancet.* 1991;338:1173–1174.

103. Adatia I, Thompson J, Landzberg M, Wessel DL. Inhaled nitric oxide in chronic obstructive lung disease. *Lancet.* 1993;341:307-308.

104. Wiemer G, Scholkens BA, Becker RH, Busse R. Ramiprilat enhances endothelial autocoid formation by inhibiting breakdown of endothelial derived bradykinin. *Hypertension.* 1991;18:558–563.

105. Massoudy P, Becker BF, Gerlach E. Nitric oxide accounts for postischemic cardioprotection resulting from angiotensin-converting enzyme inhibition: indirect evidence for a radical scavenger effect in isolated guinea pig heart. *J Cardiovasc Pharmacol.* 1995;25:440–447.

106. Lüscher TF, Haefeli WE. L-Arginine in the clinical area: tool or remedy? [Editorial Comment]. *Circulation.* 1993; 87:1746–1748.

107. Chen G, Suzuki H, Weston AH. Acetylcholine releases endothelium-derived hyperpolarizing factor and EDRF from rat blood vessels. *Br J Pharmacol.* 1988;95:1165–1174.

108. Taylor SG, Southerton JS, Weston AH, Baker JRJ. Endothelium-dependent effects of acetylcholine in rat aorta: a comparison with sodium nitroprusside and cromakalim. *Br J Pharmacol.* 1988;94:853–863.

109. Vanheel B, Van de Voorde J, Leusen I. Contribution of nitric oxide to the endothelium-dependent hyperpolarization in rat aorta. *J Physiol (Lond).* 1994;475:277–284.

110. Kauser K, Stekiel WJ, Rubanyi G, Harder DR. Mechanism of action of EDRF on pressurized arteries: effect on K^+ conductance. *Circ Res.* 1989;65:199–204.

111. Kauser K, Rubanyi GM. Bradykinin-induced, N^ω-nitro-L-arginine-insensitive endothelium-dependent relaxation of porcine coronary arteries is not mediated by bioassayable relaxing substances. *J Cardiovasc Pharmacol.* 1992;20(suppl 12):S101–S104.

112. Hecker M, Bara AT, Bauersachs J, Busse R. Characterization of endothelium-derived hyperpolarizing factor as a cytochrome P450-derived arachidonic acid metabolite in mammals. *J Physiol (Lond).* 1994;481:407–414.

113. Garland CJ, Plane F, Kemp BK, Cocks TM. Endothelium-dependent hyperpolarization: a role in the control of vascular tone. *Trends Pharmacol Sci.* 1995;16:23–30.

114. Daut J, Standen NB, Nelson MT. The role of the membrane potential of endothelial and smooth muscle cells in the regulation of coronary blood flow. *J Cardiovasc Electrophysiol.* 1994;5:154–181.

115. Van de Voorde J, Vanheel B, Leusen I. Endothelium-dependent relaxation and hyperpolarization in aorta from control and renal hypertensive rats. *Circ Res.* 1992;70:1–8.

116. Moncada S, Gryglewski R, Bunting S, Vane JR. An enzyme isolated from arteries transforms prostaglandin endoperoxides to an unstable substance that inhibits platelet aggregation. *Nature.* 1976;263:663–665.

117. Moncada S, Vane JR. Pharmacology and endogenous roles of prostaglandin endoperoxides thromboxane A_2 and prostacyclin. *Pharmacol Rev.* 1978;30:293–331.

118. Hickey KA, Rubanyi GM, Paul RJ, Highsmith RF. Characterization of a coronary vasoconstrictor produced by cultured endothelial cells. *Am J Physiol.* 1985;248: C550–C556.

119. Yanagisawa M, Kurihara H, Kimura S, et al. A novel potent vasoconstrictor peptide produced by vascular endothelial cells. *Nature.* 1988;332:411–415.

120. Inoue A, Yanagisawa M, Kimura S, Kasuya Y, et al. The human endothelin family: three structurally and pharmacologically distinct isopeptides predicted by three separate genes. *Proc Natl Acad Sci U S A.* 1989;86:2863–2867.

121. Rubanyi GM, Polokoff MA. Endothelins: molecular biology, biochemistry, pharmacology, physiology, and pathophysiology. *Pharmacol Rev.* 1994;46:325–415.

122. Riddihough G. A twist in the tail of human endothelin. *Nature.* 1994;369:84.

123. Miyauchi T, Yanagisawa M, Tomizawa T, et al. Increased plasma concentrations of endothelin 1 and big endothelin 1 in acute myocardial infarction. *Lancet.* 1989;2: 53–54.

124. Hirata Y, Kanno K, Watanabe TX, et al. Receptor binding and vasoconstrictor activity of big endothelin. *Eur J Pharmacol.* 1990;176:225–228.

125. Opgenorth TJ, Wu Wong JR, Shiosaki K. Endothelin converting enzymes. *FASEB J* 1992;6:2653–2659.

126. Huggins JP, Pelton JT, Miller RC. The structure and specificity of endothelin receptors: their importance in physiology and medicine. *Pharmacol Ther.* 1993;59:55–123.

127. Miller RC, Pelton JT, Huggins JP. Endothelins: from receptor to medecine. *Trends Pharmacol Sci.* 1993;14:54–60.

128. Anggard E, Galton D, Rae G, et al. The fate of radioiodinated endothelin 1 and endothelin 3 in the rat. *J Cardiovasc Pharmacol.* 1989;13(suppl 5):S46–S49.

129. De Nucci G, Thomas R, D'Orleans-Juste P, et al. Pressor effects of circulating endothelin are limited by its removal in the pulmonary circulation and by the release of prostacyclin and endothelium derived relaxing factor. *Proc Natl Acad Sci U S A.* 1988;85:9797–9800.

130. Berbinschi A, Ketelslegers JM. Endothelin in urine. *Lancet.* 1989;2:46.

131. Abassi Z, Golomb E, Keiser HR. Neutral endopeptidase inhibition increases the urinary excretion and plasma levels of endothelin. *Metabolism.* 1992;41:683–685.

132. Hirata Y, Yoshimi H, Takaichi S, Yanagisawa M, Masaki T. Binding and receptor down regulation of a novel vasoconstrictor endothelin in cultured rat vascular smooth muscle cells. *FEBS Lett.* 1988;239:13–17.

133. Davenport AP, Maguire JJ. Is endothelin-induced vasoconstriction mediated only by ET_A receptors in humans? *Trends Pharmacol Sci.* 1994;15:9–11.

134. Seo B, Oemar BS, Siebenmann R, von Segesser L, Lüscher TF. Both ET_A and ET_B receptors mediate contraction to endothelin-1 in human blood vessels. *Circulation.* 1994;89:1203–1208.

135. Bax WA, Saxena PR. The current endothelin receptor classification: time for reconsideration. *Trends Pharmacol Sci.* 1994;15:379–386.

136. Sokolovsky M. Endothelins and sarafotoxins: physiological regulation, receptor subtypes and transmembrane signaling. *Pharmacol Ther.* 1992;54:129–149.

137. Kasuya Y, Takuwa Y, Yanagisawa M, Masaki T, Goto K. A pertussis toxin sensitive mechanism of endothelin action in porcine coronary artery smooth muscle. *Br J Pharmacol.* 1992;107:456–462.

138. Silberberg SD, Poder TC, Lacerda AE. Endothelin increases single channel calcium currents in coronary arterial smooth muscle cells. *FEBS Lett.* 1989;247:68–72.

139. Nakao K, Inoue Y, Oike M, Kitamura K, Kuriyama H. Mechanisms of endothelin induced augmentation of the electrical and mechanical activity in rat portal vein. *Pflügers Arch Eur J Physiol.* 1990;415:526–532.

140. Inoue Y, Oike M, Nakao K, Kitamura K, Kuriyama H. Endothelin augments unitary calcium channel currents on the smooth muscle cell membrane of guinea pig portal vein. *J Physiol (Lond).* 1990;423:171–191.

141. Cocks TM, Faulkner NL, Sudhir K, Angus J. Reactivity of endothelin 1 on human and canine large veins compared with large arteries in vitro. *Eur J Pharmacol.* 1989;171: 17–24.

142. Randall MD. Vascular activities of the endothelins. *Pharmacol Ther.* 1991;50:73–93.

143. Gardiner SM, Compton AM, Bennett T. Regional haemodynamic effects of endothelin-1 and endothelin-3 in conscious Long Evans and Brattleboro rats. *Br J Pharmacol.* 1990;99:107–112.

144. Moe O, Tejedor A, Campbell WB, Alpern RJ, Henrich WL. Effects of endothelin on in vitro renin secretion. *Am J Physiol.* 1991;260:E521–E525.

145. Madeddu P, Troffa C, Glorioso N, et al. Effect of endothelin on regional hemodynamics and renal function in awake normotensive rats. *J Cardiovasc Pharmacol.* 1989;14: 818–825.

146. Nakamoto H, Suzuki H, Murakami M, et al. Effects of endothelin on systemic and renal haemodynamics and neuroendocrine hormones in conscious dogs. *Clin Sci.* 1989; 77:567–572.

147. Gasic S, Wagner OF, Vierhapper H, Nowotny P, Waldhausl W. Regional hemodynamic effects and clearance of endothelin 1 in humans: renal and peripheral tissues may contribute to the overall disposal of the peptide. *J Cardiovasc Pharmacol.* 1992;19:176–180.

148. Vierhapper H, Wagner O, Nowotny P, Waldhausl W. Effect of endothelin 1 in man. *Circulation.* 1990;81: 1415–1418.

149. Kawaguchi H, Sawa H, Yasuda H. Endothelin stimulates angiotensin I to angiotensin II conversion in cultured pulmonary artery endothelial cells. *J Mol Cell Cardiol.* 1990;22:839–842.

150. Scott-Burden T, Resink TJ, Hahn AW, Vanhoutte PM. Induction of endothelin secretion by angiotensin II: effects on growth and synthetic activity of vascular smooth muscle cells. *J Cardiovasc Pharmacol.* 1991;17(suppl 7): S96–S100.

151. Cozza EN, Chiou S, Gomez-Sanchez CE. Endothelin 1 potentiation of angiotensin, II: stimulation of aldosterone production. *Am J Physiol.* 1992;262:R85–R89.

152. Emori T, Hirata Y, Ohta K, et al. Cellular mechanism of endothelin 1 release by angiotensin and vasopressin. *Hypertension.* 1991;18:165–170.

153. Wall KM, Ferguson AV. Endothelin acts at the subfornical organ to influence the activity of putative vasopressin and oxytocin secreting neurons. *Brain Res.* 1992;586:111–116.

154. Wong-Dusting HK, La M, Rand MJ. Endothelin 1 enhances vasoconstrictor responses to sympathetic nerve stimulation and noradrenaline in the rabbit ear artery. *Clin Exp Pharmacol Physiol.* 1991;18:131–136.

155. Tomita K, Nonoguchi H, Marumo F. Effect of endothelin on peptide dependent cyclic adenosine monophosphate accumulation along the nephron segments of the rat. *J Clin Invest.* 1990;85:2014–2018.

156. Fozard JR, Part ML. No major role for atrial natriuretic peptide in the vasodilator response to endothelin 1 in the spontaneously hypertensive rat. *Eur J Pharmacol.* 1990; 180:153–159.

157. Nakamoto H, Suzuki H, Murakami M, et al. Different effects of low and high doses of endothelin on haemodynamics and hormones in the normotensive conscious dog. *J Hypertens.* 1991;9:337–344.

158. Hu RM, Levin ER, Pedram A, Frank HJ. Atrial natriuretic peptide inhibits the production and secretion of endothelin from cultured endothelial cells. Mediation through the C receptor. *J Biol Chem.* 1992;267: 17384–17389.

159. Kohno M, Yasunari K, Yokokawa K, Murakawa K, Horio T, Takeda T. Inhibition by atrial and brain natriuretic peptides of endothelin 1 secretion after stimulation with angiotensin II and thrombin of cultured human endothelial cells. *J Clin Invest.* 1991;87:1999–2004.

160. Wiklund NP, Ohlen A, Cederquist B. Adrenergic neuromodulation by endothelin in guinea pig pulmonary artery. *Neurosci Lett.* 1989;101:269–273.

161. Wong-Dusting HK, La M, Rand MJ. Mechanisms of the effects of endothelin on responses to noradrenaline and sympathetic nerve stimulation. *Clin Exp Pharmacol Physiol.* 1990;17:263–273.

162. Crockcroft JR, Clarke JG, Webb DJ. The effect of intraarterial endothelin on resting blood flow and sympathetically mediated vasoconstriction in the forearm of man. *Br J Clin Pharmacol.* 1991;31:521–524.

163. Siren AL, Feurerstein G. Hemodynamic effects of endothelin after systemic and central nervous system administration in the conscious rat. *Neuropeptides.* 1989;14: 231–236.

164. Kawano Y, Yoshida K, Yoshimi H, Kuramochi M, Omae T. The cardiovascular effect of intracerebroventricular endothelin in rats. *J Hypertens.* 1989(suppl);7:S22–S23.

165. Matsumura K, Abe I, Tsuchihashi T, Tominaga M, Kobayashi K, Fujishima M. Central effect of endothelin on neurohormonal responses in conscious rabbits. *Hypertension.* 1991;17:1192–1196.

166. Yamamoto T, Kimura T, Ota K, et al. Central effects of endothelin 1 on vasopressin and atrial natriuretic peptide release and cardiovascular and renal function in conscious rats. *J Cardiovasc Pharmacol.* 1991;17(suppl 7): S316–S318.

167. Kaufmann H, Oribe E, Oliver JA. Plasma endothelin during upright tilt: relevance for orthostatic hypotension? *Lancet.* 1991;338:1542–1545.

168. Chapleau MW, Hajduczok G, Abboud FM. Suppression of baroreceptor discharge by endothelin at high carotid sinus pressure. *Am J Physiol.* 1992;263:R103–R108.

169. Knuepfer MM, Han SP, Trapani AJ, Fok KF, Westfall TC. Regional hemodynamic and baroreflex effects of endothelin in rats. *Am J Physiol.* 1989;257:H918–H926.

170. Itoh S, Van Den Buuse M. Sensitization of baroreceptor reflex by central endothelin in conscious rats. *Am J Physiol.* 1991;260:H1106–H1112.

171. Wagner O, Christ G, Wojta J, et al. Polar secretion of endothelin-1 by cultured endothelial cells. *J Biomed Chem.* 1992;267:16066–16068.

172. Haynes WG, Webb DJ. Contribution of endogenous generation of endothelin-1 to basal vascular tone. *Lancet.* 1994;344:852–854.

173. Reid JJ. Endothelin-1 may be a physiologic modulator of vasoconstriction in rat kidney. *J Cardiovasc Pharmacol.* 1993;22(suppl 8):S267–S270.

174. Cairns HS, Rogerson ME, Fairbanks LD, Neild GH, Westwick J. Endothelin induces an increase in renal vascular resistance and a fall in glomerular filtration rate in the rabbit isolated perfused kidney. *Br J Pharmacol.* 1989;98:155–160.

175. Ferrario RG, Foulkes R, Salvati P, Patrono C. Hemodynamic and tubular effects of endothelin and thromboxane in the isolated perfused rat kidney. *Eur J Pharmacol.* 1989;171:127–134.

176. Badr KF, Murray JJ, Breyer MD, Takahashi K, Inagami T, Harris RC. Mesangial cell glomerular and renal vascular responses to endothelin in the rat kidney. Elucidation of signal transduction pathways. *J Clin Invest.* 1989;83:336–342.

177. Simonson MS, Dunn MJ. Endothelin 1 stimulates contraction of rat glomerular mesangial cells and potentiates beta adrenergic mediated cyclic adenosine monophosphate accumulation. *J Clin Invest.* 1990;85:790–797.

178. Suzuki N, Miyauchi T, Tomobe Y, et al. Plasma concentrations of endothelin-1 in spontaneously hypertensive rats and DOCA-salt hypertensive rats. *Biochem Biophys Res Commun.* 1990;159:1304–1308.

179. Tomobe Y, Miyauchi T, Saito A, et al. Effects of endothelin on the renal artery from spontaneously hypertensive and Wistar Kyoto rats. *Eur J Pharmacol.* 1988;152:373–374.

180. Vemulapalli S, Chiu PJ, Rivelli M, Foster CJ, Sybertz EJ. Modulation of circulating endothelin levels in hypertension and endotoxemia in rats. *J Cardiovasc Pharmacol.* 1991;18:895–903.

181. Kohno M, Murakawa K, Horio T, et al. Plasma immunoreactive endothelin 1 in experimental malignant hypertension. *Hypertension.* 1991;18:93–100.

182. Haak T, Jungmann E, Felber A, Hillmann U, Usadel KH. Increased plasma levels of endothelin in diabetic patients with hypertension. *Am J Hypertens.* 1992;5:161–166.

183. Lerman A, Click RL, Narr BJ, et al. Elevation of plasma endothelin associated with systemic hypertension in humans following orthotopic liver transplantation. *Transplantation (Baltimore).* 1991;51:646–650.

184. Schiffrin EL, Thibault G. Plasma endothelin in human essential hypertension. *Am J Hypertens.* 1991;4:303–308.

185. Shichiri M, Hirata Y, Ando K, et al. Postural change and volume expansion affect plasma endothelin levels. *JAMA.* 1990;263:661.

186. Widimsky J Jr, Horky K, Dvorakova J. Plasma endothelin 1,2 levels in mild and severe hypertension. *J Hypertens.* 1991;9(suppl):S194–S195.

187. Nakajima M, Morimoto S, Takamoto S, et al. Endothelin-1 in cerebrospinal fluid in elderly patients with hypertension and dementia. *Hypertension.* 1994;24: 97–100.

188. Hirata Y, Matsuoka H, Kimura K, et al. Renal vasoconstriction by the endothelial cell derived peptide endothelin in spontaneously hypertensive rats. *Circ Res.* 1989;65:1370–1379.

189. Winquist RJ, Bunting PB, Garsky VM, Lumma PK, Schofield TL. Prominent depressor response to endothelin in spontaneously hypertensive rats. *Eur J Pharmacol.* 1989;163:199–203.

190. Clozel M. Endothelin sensitivity and receptor binding in the aorta of spontaneously hypertensive rats. *J Hypertens.* 1989;7:913–917.

191. Criscione L, Nellis P, Riniker B, Thomann H, Burdet R. Reactivity and sensitivity of mesenteric vascular beds and aortic rings of spontaneously hypertensive rats to endothelin: effects of calcium entry blockers. *Br J Pharmacol.* 1990;100:31–36.

192. Dohi Y, Lüscher TF. Endothelin in hypertensive resistance arteries: intraluminal and extraluminal dysfunction. *Hypertension.* 1991;18:543–549.

193. Haynes WG, Hand MF, Johnstone HA, Padfield PL, Webb DJ. Direct and sympathetically mediated venoconstriction in essential hypertension: enhanced responses to endothelin-1. *J Clin Invest.* 1994;94:1359–1364.

194. McMahon EG, Palomo MA, Moore WM. Phosphoramidon blocks the pressor activity of big endothelin (1–39) and lowers blood pressure in spontaneously hypertensive rats. *J Cardiovasc Pharmacol.* 1991;17(suppl 7):S29–S33.

195. Takagi Y, Fukase M, Takata S, et al. Role of endogenous endothelin in the development of hypertension in rats. *Am J Hypertens.* 1991;4:389–391.

196. Nishikibe M, Tsuchida S, Okada M, et al. Antihypertensive effect of a newly synthesized endothelin antagonist, BQ 123, in a genetic hypertensive model. *Life Sci.* 1993;52:717–724.

197. Yokokawa K, Tahara H, Kohno M, et al. Hypertension associated with endothelin secreting malignant hemangioendothelioma. *Ann Intern Med.* 1991;114:213–215.

198. Stewart DJ, Levy RD, Cernacek P, Langleben D. Increased plasma endothelin 1 in pulmonary hypertension: marker or mediator of disease? *Ann Intern Med.* 1991;114:464–469.

199. Giaid A, Yanagisawa M, Langleben D, et al. Expression of endothelin 1 in the lungs of patients with pulmonary hypertension. *N Engl J Med.* 1993;328:1732–1739.

200. Shirakami G, Nakao K, Saito Y, et al. Acute pulmonary alveolar hypoxia increases lung and plasma endothelin 1 levels in conscious rats. *Life Sci.* 1991;48:969–976.

201. Stelzner TJ, O'Brien RF, Yanagisawa M, et al. Increased lung endothelin 1 production in rats with idiopathic pulmonary hypertension. *Am J Physiol.* 1992;262:614–620.

202. Chang H, Wu GJ, Wang SM, Hung CR. Plasma endothelin levels and surgically correctable pulmonary hypertension. *Ann Thorac Surg.* 1993;55:450–458.

203. Eddahibi S, Raffestin B, Braquet P, Chabrier PE, Adnot S. Pulmonary vascular reactivity to endothelin 1 in normal and chronically pulmonary hypertensive rats. *J Cardiovasc Pharmacol.* 1991;17(suppl 7):S358–S361.

204. Clark BA, Halvorson L, Sachs B, Epstein FH. Plasma endothelin levels in preeclampsia: elevation and correlation with uric acid levels and renal impairment. *Am J Obstet Gynecol.* 1992;166:962–968.

205. Mastrogiannis DS, Kalter CS, O'Brien WF, Krammer J, Benoit R. Effect of magnesium sulfate on plasma endothelin 1 levels in normal and preeclamptic pregnancies. *Am J Obstet Gynecol.* 1992;167:1554–1559.

206. Nova A, Sibai BM, Barton JR, Mercer BM, Mitchell MD. Maternal plasma level of endothelin is increased in preeclampsia. *Am J Obstet Gynecol.* 1991;165:724–727.

207. Schiff E, Ben Baruch G, Peleg E, et al. Immunoreactive circulating endothelin 1 in normal and hypertensive pregnancies. *Am J Obstet Gynecol.* 1992;166:624–628.

208. Taylor RN, Varma M, Teng NN, Roberts JM. Women with preeclampsia have higher plasma endothelin levels than women with normal pregnancies. *J Clin Endocrinol Metab.* 1990;71:1675–1677.

209. Benigni A, Orisio D, Gaspari F, Frusca T, Amuso G, Remuzzi G. Evidence against a pathogenetic role for endothelin in preeclampsia. *Br J Obstet Gynaecol.* 1992;99: 798–802.

210. Lumme R, Laatikainen T, Vuolteenaho O, Leppaluoto J. Plasma endothelin, atrial natriuretic peptide (ANP), and uterine and umbilical artery flow velocity waveforms in hypertensive pregnancies. *Br J Obstet Gynaecol.* 1992; 99:761–764.

211. Fuxe K, Kurosawa N, Cintra A, et al. Involvement of local ischemia in endothelin 1 induced lesions of the neostriatum of the anaesthetized rat. *Exp Brain Res.* 1992;88: 131–139.

212. Macrae I, Robinson M, McAuley M, Reid J, McCulloch J. Effects of intracisternal endothelin 1 injection on blood flow to the lower brain stem. *Eur J Pharmacol.* 1991;203: 85–91.

213. Mima T, Yanagisawa M, Shigeno T, et al. Endothelin acts in feline and canine cerebral arteries from the adventitial side. *Stroke.* 1989;20:1553–1556.

214. Schalk KA, Faraci FM, Heistad DD. Effect of endothelin on production of cerebrospinal fluid in rabbits. *Stroke.* 1992;23:560–563.

215. Willette RN, Ohlstein EH, Pullen M, Sauermelch CF, Cohen A, Nambi P. Transient forebrain ischemia alters acutely endothelin receptor density and immunoreactivity in gerbil brain. *Life Sci.* 1993;52:35–40.

216. Yamashita J, Kataoka Y, Niwa M, et al. Increased production of endothelins in the hippocampus of stroke prone spontaneously hypertensive rats following transient forebrain ischemia: histochemical evidence. *Cell Mol Neurobiol.* 1993;13:15–23.

217. Ziv I, Fleminger G, Djaldetti R, Achiron A, Melamed E, Sokolovsky M. Increased plasma endothelin 1 in acute ischemic stroke. *Stroke.* 1992;23:1014–1016.

218. Stewart DJ, Kubac G, Costello KB, Cernacek P. Increased plasma endothelin 1 in the early hours of acute myocardial infarction. *J Am Coll Cardiol.* 1991;18:38–43.

219. Yasuda M, Kohno M, Tahara A, et al. Circulating immunoreactive endothelin in ischemic heart disease. *Am Heart J.* 1990;119:801–806.

220. Tomoda H. Plasma endothelin 1 in acute myocardial infarction with heart failure. *Am Heart J.* 1993;125:667–672.

221. Stewart JT, Nisbet JA, Davies MJ. Plasma endothelin in coronary venous blood from patients with either stable or unstable angina. *Brit Heart J.* 1991;66:7–9.

222. Tahara A, Kohno M, Yanagi S, et al. Circulating immunoreactive endothelin in patients undergoing percutaneous transluminal coronary angioplasty. *Metabolism.* 1991;40:1235–1237.

223. Ezra D, Goldstein RE, Czaja JF, Feuerstein GZ. Lethal ischemia due to intracoronary endothelin in pigs. *Am J Physiol.* 1989;257:H339–H343.

224. Hom GJ, Touhey B, Rubanyi GM. Effects of intracoronary administration of endothelin in anesthetized dogs: comparison with Bay k 8644 and U 46619. *J Cardiovasc Pharmacol.* 1992;19:194–200.

225. Kurihara H, Yamaoki K, Nagai R, et al. Endothelin: a potent vasoconstrictor associated with coronary vasospasm. *Life Sci.* 1989;44:1937–1943.

226. Muramatsu K, Tomoike H, Ohara Y, Egashra S, Nakamura M. Effects of endothelin 1 on epicardial coronary tone, coronary blood flow, ECG, ST change, and regional wall motion in anesthetized dogs. *Heart Vessels.* 1991;6: 191–196.

227. Brunner F, Du Toit EF, Opie LH. Endothelin release during ischaemia and reperfusion of isolated perfused rat hearts. *J Mol Cell Cardiol.* 1992;24:1291–1305.

228. Clozel JP, Sprecher U. Influence of a low perfusion pressure on effect of endothelin on coronary vascular bed. *Am J Physiol.* 1991;260:H893–H901.

229. Neubauer S, Zimmermann S, Hirsch A, et al. Effects of endothelin 1 in the isolated heart in ischemia/reperfusion and hypoxia/reoxygenation injury. *J Mol Cell Cardiol.* 1991;23:1397–1409.

230. Saito T, Fuchimi E, Abe T, et al. Augmented contractile response to endothelin and blunted endothelium dependent relaxation in post ischemic reperfused coronary arteries. *Jpn Circ J.* 1992;56:657–670.

231. Watts JA, Chapat S, Johnson DE, Janis RA. Effects of nisoldipine upon vasoconstrictor responses and binding of endothelin 1 in ischemic and reperfused rat hearts. *J Cardiovasc Pharmacol.* 1992;19:929–936.

232. Liu J, Chen R, Casley DJ, Nayler WG. Ischemia and reperfusion increase ^{125}I-labeled endothelin 1 binding in rat cardiac membranes. *Am J Physiol.* 1990;258:H829–H835.

233. Tsuji S, Sawamura A, Watanabe H, Takihara K, Park SE, Azuma J. Plasma endothelin levels during myocardial ischemia and reperfusion. *Life Sci.* 1991;48:1745–1749.

234. Watanabe T, Suzuki N, Shimamoto N, Fujino M, Imada A. Contribution of endogenous endothelin to the extension of myocardial infarct size in rats. *Circ Res.* 1991;69: 370–377.

235. Grover GJ, Sleph PG, Fox M, Trippodo NC. Role of endothelin 1 and big endothelin 1 in modulating coronary vascular tone contractile function and severity of ischemia in rat hearts. *J Pharmacol Exp Ther.* 1992;263: 1074–1082.

236. Lerman A, Hildebrand FL Jr, Aarhus LL, Burnett JC Jr. Endothelin has biological actions at pathophysiological concentrations. *Circulation.* 1991;83:1808–1814.

237. Firth JD, Ratcliffe PJ. Organ distribution of the three rat endothelin messenger RNAs and the effects of ischemia on renal gene expression. *J Clin Invest.* 1992;90: 1023–1031.

238. Lopez-Farre A, Gomez Garre D, Bernabeu F, Lopez Novoa JM. A role for endothelin in the maintenance of

post ischemic renal failure in the rat. *J Physiol (Lond)*. 1991;444:513–522.

239. Shibouta Y, Suzuki N, Shino A, et al. Pathophysiological role of endothelin in acute renal failure. *Life Sci*. 1990; 46:1611–1618.

240. Firth JD, Ratcliffe PJ, Raine AE, Ledingham JG. Endothelin: an important factor in acute renal failure? *Lancet*. 1988;2:1179–1182.

241. Kon V, Yoshioka T, Fogo A, Ichikawa I. Glomerular actions of endothelin in vivo. *J Clin Invest*. 1989;83: 1762–1767.

242. Heyman SN, Clark BA, Kaiser N, et al. In vivo and in vitro studies on the effect of amphotericin B on endothelin release. *J Antimicrob Chemother*. 1992;29:69–77.

243. Margulies KB, Hildebrand FL, Heublein DM, Burnett JC. Radiocontrast increases plasma and urinary endothelin. *J Am Soc Nephrol*. 1991;2:1041–1045.

244. Morel DR, Lacroix JS, Hemsen A, Steinig DA, Pittet JF, Lundberg JM. Increased plasma and pulmonary lymph levels of endothelin during endotoxin shock. *Eur J Pharmacol*. 1989;167:427–428.

245. Kon V, Awazu M. Endothelin and cyclosporine nephrotoxicity. *Renal Failure*. 1992;14:345–350.

246. Perico N, Dadan J, Remuzzi G. Endothelin mediates the renal vasoconstriction induced by cyclosporine in the rat. *J Am Soc Nephrol*. 1990;1:76–83.

247. Mino N, Kobayashi M, Nakajima A, et al. Protective effect of a selective endothelin receptor antagonist BQ 123 in ischemic acute renal failure in rats. *Eur J Pharmacol*. 1992;221:77–83.

248. Lanese DM, Conger JD. Effects of endothelin receptor antagonist on cyclosporine induced vasoconstriction in isolated rat renal arterioles. *J Clin Invest*. 1993;91: 2144–2149.

249. Tomita K, Ujiie K, Nakanishi T, et al. Plasma endothelin levels in patients with acute renal failure. *N Engl J Med*. 1989;321:1127.

250. Asano T, Ikegaki I, Satoh S, et al. Endothelin: a potential modulator of cerebral vasospasm. *Eur J Pharmacol*. 1990; 190:365–372.

251. Ide K, Yamakawa K, Nakagomi T, et al. The role of endothelin in the pathogenesis of vasospasm following subarachnoid haemorrhage. *Neurol Res*. 1989;11:101–104.

252. Alafaci C, Jansen I, Arab MA, Shiokawa Y, Svendgaard NA, Edvinsson L. Enhanced vasoconstrictor effect of endothelin in cerebral arteries from rats with subarachnoid haemorrhage. *Acta Physiol Scand*. 1990;138:317–319.

253. Papadopoulos SM, Gilbert LL, Webb RC, D'Amato CJ. Characterization of contractile responses to endothelin in human cerebral arteries: implication for cerebral vasospasm. *Neurosurgery*. 1990;26:810–815.

254. Willette RN, Sauermelch C, Ezekiel M, Feuerstein G, Ohlstein EH. Effect of endothelin on cortical microvascular perfusion in rats. *Stroke*. 1990;21:451–458.

255. Ohlstein EH, Storer BL. Oxyhemoglobin stimulation of endothelin production in cultured endothelial cells. *J Neurosurg*. 1992;77:274–278.

256. Kraus GE, Bucholz RD, Yoon KW, et al. Cerebrospinal fluid endothelin 1 and endothelin 3 levels in normal and neurosurgical patients: a clinical study and literature review. *Surg Neurol*. 1991;35:20–29.

257. Levesque H, Sevrain L, Freger P, Tadie M, Courtois H, Creissard P. Raised plasma endothelin in aneurysmal subarachnoid haemorrhage. *Lancet*. 1990;335:290.

258. Suzuki H, Sato S, Suzuki Y, et al. Endothelin immunoreactivity in cerebrospinal fluid of patients with subarachnoid haemorrhage. *Ann Med*. 1990;22:233–236.

259. Suzuki R, Masaoka H, Hirata Y, Marumo F, Isotani E, Hirakawa K. The role of endothelin 1 in the origin of cerebral vasospasm in patients with aneurysmal subarachnoid hemorrhage. *J Neurosurg*. 1992;77:96–100.

260. Matsumura Y, Ikegawa R, Suzuki Y, et al. Phosphoramidon prevents cerebral vasospasm following subarachnoid hemorrhage in dogs: the relationship to endothelin 1 levels in the cerebrospinal fluid. *Life Sci*. 1991;49:841–848.

261. Yamaura I, Tani E, Maeda Y, Minami N, Shindo H. Endothelin 1 of canine basilar artery in vasospasm. *J Neurosurg*. 1992;76:99–105.

262. Clozel M, Watanabe H. BQ 123, a peptidic endothelin ET_A receptor antagonist, prevents the early cerebral vasospasm following subarachnoid hemorrhage after intracisternal but not intravenous injection. *Life Sci*. 1993;52:825–834.

263. Chester AH, O'Neil GS, Allen SP, Luu TN, Tadjkarimi S, Yacoub MH. Effect of endothelin on normal and diseased human coronary arteries. *Eur J Clin Invest*. 1992;22: 210–213.

264. Yang ZH, Richard V, Von Segesser L, et al. Threshold concentrations of endothelin 1 potentiate contractions to norepinephrine and serotonin in human arteries: a new mechanism of vasospasm? *Circulation*. 1990;82:188–195.

265. Matsuyama K, Yasue H, Okumura K, et al. Increased plasma level of endothelin 1 like immunoreactivity during coronary spasm in patients with coronary spastic angina. *Am J Cardiol*. 1991;68:991–995.

266. Toyo-oka T, Aizawa T, Suzuki N, et al. Increased plasma level of endothelin 1 and coronary spasm induction in patients with vasospastic angina pectoris. *Circulation*. 1991; 83:476–483.

267. Wieczorek I, Haynes WG, Webb DJ, Ludlam CA, Fox KA. Raised plasma endothelin in unstable angina and non-Q wave myocardial infarction: relation to cardiovascular outcome. *Br Heart J*. 1994;72:436–441.

268. Biondi M, Marasini B, Bassani C, Agastoni A. Increased plasma endothelin levels in patients with Raynaud's phenomenon. *N Engl J Med*. 1991;324:1139–1140.

269. Zamora MR, O'Brien RF, Rutherford RB, Weil JV. Serum endothelin 1 concentrations and cold provocation in primary Raynaud's phenomenon. *Lancet*. 1990;336:1144–1147.

270. Dowd PM, Bunker CB, Bull HA, et al. Raynaud's phenomenon, calcitonin gene related peptide, endothelin, and cutaneous vasculature [letter]. *Lancet*. 1990;336:1014.

271. Bath PM, Martin JF. Serum platelet derived growth factor and endothelin concentrations in human hypercholesterolaemia. *J Intern Med*. 1991;230:313–317.

272. Lerman A, Edwards BS, Hallett JW, Heublein DM, Sandberg SM, Burnett JC Jr. Circulating and tissue endothelin immunoreactivity in advanced atherosclerosis. *N Engl J Med*. 1991;325:997–1001.

273. Boulanger CM, Tanner FC, Bea ML, Hahn AW, Werner A, Lüscher TF. Oxidized low density lipoproteins induce

mRNA expression and release of endothelin from human and porcine endothelium. *Circ Res.* 1992;70:1191–1197.

274. Martin Nizard F, Houssaini HS, Lestavel Delattre S, Duriez P, Fruchart JC. Modified low density lipoproteins activate human macrophages to secrete immunoreactive endothelin. *FEBS Lett.* 1991;293:127–130.

275. Komuro I, Kurihara H, Sugiyama T, Yoshizumi M, Takaku F, Yazaki Y. Endothelin stimulates c fos and c myc expression and proliferation of vascular smooth muscle cells. *FEBS Lett.* 1988;238:249–252.

276. Lerman A, Kubo SH, Tschumperlin LK, Burnett JC Jr. Plasma endothelin concentrations in humans with end stage heart failure and after heart transplantation. *J Am Coll Cardiol.* 1992;20:849–853.

277. Stewart TJ, Cernacek P, Costello KB, Rouleau JL. Elevated endothelin 1 in heart failure and loss of normal response to postural change. *Circulation.* 1992;85:510–517.

278. Cavero PG, Miller WL, Heublein DM, Margulies KB, Burnett JC Jr. Endothelin in experimental congestive heart failure in the anesthetized dog. *Am J Physiol.* 1990; 259: F312–F317.

279. Clavell AL, Wright RS, Thomas MR, Brandt RR, Opgenorth TJ, Burnett JC. Elevated endogenous endothelin mediates systemic vasoconstriction in experimental chronic congestive heart failure. *J Am Coll Cardiol.* 1994;23:172A.

280. Cernacek P, Stewart DJ. Immunoreactive endothelin in human plasma: marked elevations in patients in cardiogenic shock. *Biochem Biophys Res Commun.* 1989;161: 562–567.

281. Weitzberg E, Lundberg JM, Rudehill A. Elevated plasma levels of endothelin in patients with sepsis syndrome. *Circ Shock.* 1991;33:222–227.

282. Nakamura T, Kasai K, Sekiguchi Y, et al. Elevation of plasma endothelin concentrations during endotoxin shock in dogs. *Eur J Pharmacol.* 1991;205:277–282.

283. Voerman HJ, Stehouwer CD, Van Kamp GJ, et al. Plasma endothelin levels are increased during septic shock. *Crit Care Med.* 1992;20:1097–1101.

284. Kraus T, Mehrabi A, Klar E, et al. Peri and postoperative plasma kinetics of big endothelin and endothelin 1/2 after liver transplantation. *Transplant Proc.* 1992;24: 2569–2571.

285. Moore K, Wendon J, Frazer M, Karani J, Williams R, Badr K. Plasma endothelin immunoreactivity in liver disease and the hepatorenal syndrome. *N Engl J Med.* 1992;327: 1774–1778.

286. Uchihara M, Izumi N, Sato C, Marumo F. Clinical significance of elevated plasma endothelin concentration in patients with cirrhosis. *Hepatology.* 1992;16:95–99.

287. Kato T, Iwama Y, Okumura K, Hashimoto H, Ito T, Satake T. Prostaglandin H_2 may be the endothelium-derived contracting factor released by acetylcholine in the aorta of the rat. *Hypertension.* 1990;15:475–481.

288. Lin PJ, Pearson PJ, Cartier HV, Schaff HV. Superoxide anion mediates the endothelium-dependent contractions to serotonin by regenerated endothelium. *J Thorac Cardiovasc Surg.* 1991;102:378–385.

289. Katusic ZS, Shepherd JT, Vanhoutte PM. Endothelium-dependent contractions to stretch in canine basilar arteries. *Am J Physiol.* 1987;252:H671–H673.

290. Lin PJ, Pearson PJ, Schaff HV. Hypoxia releases a vasoconstrictor substance from the endothelium of the human internal mammary artery. *Surg Forum.* 1990;41: 311–312.

291. Tesfamariam B, Brown ML, Deykin D, Cohen RA. Elevated glucose promotes generation of endothelium-derived vasoconstrictor prostanoids in rabbit aorta. *J Clin Invest.* 1990;85:929–932.

3

Peripheral Circulation and Its Control Mechanism

Kailash Prasad

The peripheral circulation is concerned with the transport of blood, blood flow distribution, exchange between blood and tissue, and storage of blood (venous system). It comprises the systemic circulation, which supplies blood to all parts of the body except the lungs, and the pulmonary circulation, which supplies blood to the lungs. Its function is to alter the blood distribution to meet the needs of the different tissues. The aorta is mainly an elastic structure. Peripheral arteries become more and more muscular until the arterioles, where the muscular layer predominates (as described in Chapter 1).

A few features are characteristic of the peripheral vascular system: (1) The pressure in the aorta is almost similar to that in the large arteries, but drops gradually from large arteries to capillaries. The pressure drop is significant in arterioles but greatest in the venular end of capillaries, where the pressure is approximately 15 mm Hg, as compared with 110 mm Hg in the aorta. (2) The aorta has very little resistance as compared with the arterioles, where the resistance is maximal. (3) Pulsatile flow becomes steady flow as blood moves from arteries to capillaries. (4) Cross-sectional area of the vessels increases from the aorta to the capillaries, where it is maximal. (5) Velocity of flow is inversely related to the cross-sectional area; hence it is maximal in aorta and arteries and decreases drastically to a minimum in capillaries (1 mm/s). It increases again from venules to large veins because of a decrease in total cross-sectional area. (6) Sixty-seven percent of the total blood volume resides in the venous side of the systemic circulation. Of the total blood volume, about 5% is in capillaries, 11% in the aorta, arteries, and arterioles, 12% in pulmonary circulation, and 5% in the heart.

There are two types of blood vessels: resistance and capacitance. Resistance vessels include the arterioles and small arteries, whereas the capacitance vessels comprise the venules and veins, which serve as collecting channels and storage areas.

Factors That Affect Blood Flow

Blood flow through the vascular system is affected by both the vascular system and blood. Under normal conditions blood flow is streamlined.

Flow–Velocity Relationship

Velocity of flow is directly proportional to flow and inversely proportional to cross-sectional area of the vessels. This is represented as $V = Q/A$, where V is velocity (distance per unit time), Q is flow (volume per unit time), and A is cross-sectional area of the vessels. In other words, flow is the product of velocity and cross-sectional area. A combination of velocity and cross-sectional area is used to determine flow, using an electromagnetic flowmeter. This relationship also explains why the velocity of flow in the capillaries is very small. From the aorta to the capillaries, the total cross-sectional area increases markedly.

Pressure–Flow Relationship

When there is a steady laminar flow of Newtonian fluid, the flow (1) varies directly as the pressure difference between inflow and outflow pressure, (2) varies directly as the fourth power of the radius of the blood vessels, (3) is inversely proportional to the length of the tube, and (4) is inversely proportional to viscosity of the blood. These relationships were first described by the French physician Jean Poiseuille; hence this relationship is called the Poiseuille law and is stated as $Q = \pi \Delta P r^4 / 8 l n$, where Q is flow, ΔP is the pressure difference, r is the radius of the tube, l is the length of the tube, n is the viscosity of the fluid; and $\pi/8$ is a constant of proportionality.

Flow–Resistance Relationship

Resistance in an electrical circuit is defined as the ratio of voltage drop to current flow. By analogy, resistance (R) in the circulatory system is defined as $\Delta P/Q$, where ΔP is the pressure difference (drop), and Q is the flow.

$$R = \Delta P/Q$$

Substituting Q from the equation in the previous section in this equation, we obtain the following:

$$R = \Delta P/(\pi\Delta P r^4/8ln) = 8ln\Delta P/\pi\Delta P r^4 = 8ln/\pi r^4$$

Because the length of the tube (l) and viscosity (n) do not change much and $8/\pi$ is constant, the resistance depends mainly on the caliber of the blood vessels. Total resistance of the tubes in series equals the sum of the resistance in individual tubes. Also, the reciprocal of the total resistance of tubes in parallel equals the sum of the reciprocals of the resistance in individual tubes.

In hemodynamics, resistance is expressed in hybrid resistance units (HRU) or absolute resistance units (ARU).

HRU (millimeters of mercury per liter) equals mean driving pressure (millimeters of mercury) per mean flow, where mean flow is in liters per minute.

ARU (dynes $\times$ seconds $\times$ centimeters^{-5}) equals mean driving pressure (dynes per square centimeter) divided by mean flow, which is in cubic centimeters per second.

1 mm Hg = 1333 dynes/cm^2

ARU = HRU $\times$ 80

Following are formulas for these commonly used resistances:

TSVR = $(SA_m - RA_m)/CO$, where TSVR is total systemic vascular resistance, SA_m is mean systemic arterial pressure (millimeters of mercury), RA_m is mean right atrial pressure (millimeters of mercury), and CO is cardiac output (liters per minute).

$TPR = PA_m/CO$, where TPR is total pulmonary resistance, and PA_m is mean pulmonary arterial pressure (millimeters of mercury).

$PAR = (PA_m - LA_m)/CO$, where PAR is pulmonary arteriolar resistance, PA_m is mean pulmonary arterial pressure (millimeters of mercury), and LA_m is mean left atrial pressure (millimeters of mercury).

Viscosity

Viscosity is the ratio of shear stress to the shear rate of the fluid. This affects resistance within the vessels. Viscosity is affected by various factors:

1. *Hematocrit.* At normal or low hematocrit the viscosity rises progressively with the rise in hematocrit. A rise in hematocrit above the normal level of 45% produces proportionately greater changes in the viscosity. This

TABLE 3.1. Distribution of cardiac output (blood flow in milliliters per minute).

Organs	Rest	Exercise		
		Light	Moderate	Severe
Brain	750	750	750	750
Heart	250	350	750	1000
Kidney	1100	900	600	250
Skeletal muscle	1200	4500	12,500	22,000
Splanchnic tissue	1400	1100	600	300
Skin	500	1500	1900	600
Other (skeleton, fat, connective tissue)	600	400	500	100

explains why the peripheral resistance is increased in polycythemia.

2. *Flow.* The viscosity of blood increases with a decrease in blood flow. This explains the contribution of viscosity in increased resistance during cardiovascular shock.

3. *Vessel diameter.* The apparent viscosity of blood increases with increase in diameter of the tube up to a diameter of 0.3 mm, above which it stays unchanged. The change in viscosity is less when measured in living tissue.

Distribution of Cardiac Output (Blood Flow)

Blood flow to the organs is dependent upon metabolic need. The blood flow (milliliters per minute) in different organs during rest and exercise is shown in Table 3.1.

Microcirculation

Microcirculation consists of capillaries that are ideally designed for exchange of fluids, gases, or solutes (Figure 3.1). The density of the capillaries varies according to the tissue in which they are located. They are numerous in metabolically active tissues such as heart, skeletal muscle, and glands. Capillary density is low in less-active tissue, such as subcutaneous tissue and cartilage. Following are the characteristic features of capillaries:

1. They have a single layer of endothelial cells and do not have smooth muscle cells; hence, they cannot regulate their own luminal caliber. Blood flow in capillaries is dependent upon the precapillary sphincter and the pressure in the arterioles.

2. Capillary diameter varies.

3. Blood flow in the capillaries is very slow (1 mm/s).

4. Capillaries can withstand high internal pressure without bursting because of their narrow lumen.

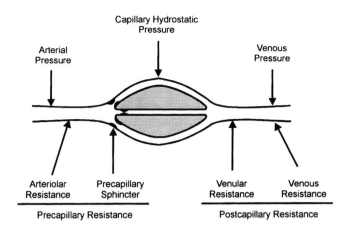

FIGURE 3.1. Schematic diagram showing the precapillary and postcapillary resistance and capillaries.

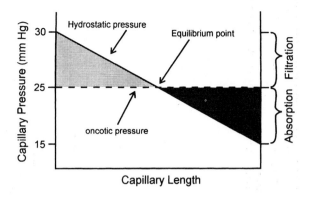

FIGURE 3.2. Diagram showing the changes in the hydrostatic pressure (30 to 15 mm Hg) and oncotic pressure (25 mm Hg) from the arteriolar to the venular end of the capillary. Equilibrium point is the point of intersection of hydrostatic and oncotic pressure where there is neither filtration nor absorption.

In nutritional flow, the blood flows through capillaries, whereas in nonnutritional flow it bypasses the capillaries and goes directly from the arterial to venous side. It is so defined because capillaries are the site for exchange of water and nutrients. Nutritional flow takes place in the active tissues. Nonnutritional flow is primarily found in the fingertips, palms of the hand, toes, soles of the feet, ears, nose, and lips.

Movement of water and nutrients through the capillaries occurs by diffusion, filtration, and pinocytosis.

Diffusion

Diffusion results from random motion of particles due to their thermal energy. Under normal conditions approximately 300 mL of water/100 g of tissue per minute crosses back and forth across the capillary wall by diffusion. Plasma concentrations of sodium chloride, urea, and glucose exchange 120, 100, and 40 times a minute, respectively, with an equal volume of extracellular volume. Diffusion of water is 40 times greater than the rate it is brought by blood flow in tissues; hence exchange of small lipid-insoluble molecules is flow limited. Diffusion is slow with large molecules. Molecules larger than 60,000 kDa do not cross the capillaries. Lipid-soluble substances such as oxygen and carbon dioxide pass directly through the endothelial cells.

Filtration

Under normal conditions 0.06 mL of water/100 g of tissue per minute crosses back and forth across the capillary wall by filtration. The flux (the direction and magnitude of movement) of water across the capillary wall is dependent upon the algebraic sum of the hydrostatic and oncotic (colloid osmotic) pressure across the capillary wall (Figure 3.2). An increase in the effective hydrostatic pressure (difference between the intracapillary hydrostatic pressure and the interstitial pressure) forces fluid from capillary to interstitial space.

On the other hand, an increase in the effective oncotic pressure (difference between the intracapillary and interstitial oncotic pressure) in a capillary favors movement of fluid into it from interstitial space. The forces responsible for capillary filtration were first formulated in 1896 by Ernest Starling in what is called Starling's hypothesis. This hypothesis states that

$$\text{fluid movement} = K[(P_c + p_i) - (P_i + p_p)]$$

where P_c is capillary hydrostatic pressure, P_i is interstitial hydrostatic pressure, p_p is plasma oncotic pressure, p_i is interstitial oncotic pressure, and K is the filtration constant for capillary membrane. A positive algebraic sum favors filtration, whereas a negative one favors absorption.

Hydrostatic Pressure

Capillary hydrostatic pressure is variable from tissue to tissue but averages 32 mm Hg at the arteriolar end of capillaries and 15 mm Hg at the venular end. Capillary hydrostatic pressure is affected more by change in the venous pressure than by a similar change in arterial pressure. Eighty percent of the increase in venous pressure is transmitted back to the capillaries. The interstitial hydrostatic pressure outside capillaries varies from −1 to −10 mm Hg and is probably due to protein or to the physical–chemical characteristics of the interstitial gel-like extracellular matrix.

Oncotic Pressure

Oncotic pressure is the osmotic pressure exerted by protein. The total osmotic pressure of plasma is approximately 6000 mm Hg and is dependent on its electrolyte content. Electrolyte content of plasma and interstitial fluid is similar, and therefore osmotic pressure is similar in the intravascular and interstitial spaces. Osmotic pressure due to electrolytes, therefore, does not have a role in movement of water across the capillaries. Oncotic pressure is only 25 to 28 mm Hg but plays an important role in filtration. As discussed earlier, oncotic pressure is created by proteins that are primarily confined to the intravascular space. Plasma protein (7.3 g/dL) consists of albumin (4.5 g/dL), globulins (2.5 g/dL), and fibrinogen (0.3 g/dL). The oncotic pressures exerted by albumin, globulins, and fibrinogen are approximately 21.8, 6.0, and 0.2 mm Hg, respectively. About 75% to 78% of the oncotic pressure is exerted by albumin and 15% to 21% by globulins. Fibrinogen exerts very little oncotic pressure (0.7%). Albumin has a molecular weight of 69,000 and is about one-half the size of an average globulin molecule (molecular weight is 150,000). Albumin exerts high oncotic pressure not just because it has a small molecular weight and is present in large quantities as compared with globulin, but also for other reasons.

At normal blood pH, albumin is negatively charged and attracts and retains cations, mainly sodium chloride, in the intravascular compartment. Albumin also binds to a small number of chloride ions, which increases the negative charge, increasing the ability of the capillary to retain more sodium. Interstitial oncotic pressure depends upon the amount of albumin escaping from capillaries. The concentration of protein in the interstitial space varies depending on the integrity of the vascular endothelium. Protein content of interstitial fluid of liver and muscle is about 25% and 10% that of plasma, respectively. Interstitial oncotic pressure is approximately 0.1 to 5 mm Hg. Plasma oncotic pressure is about 25 to 28 mm Hg. Capillary filtration in an ideal capillary is shown in Figure 3.2.

The point of intersection of hydrostatic pressure and oncotic pressure is the equilibrium point at which there is no flux of water. To the left of the equilibrium point there is filtration, whereas to the right of the equilibrium point there is absorption. Kidney capillaries show filtration, whereas intestinal mucosa capillaries show absorption throughout their entire length. Only 2% of the plasma flowing through the vascular system is filtered. Eighty-five percent of filtered plasma is reabsorbed into capillaries and venules. The remaining 20% is returned to the vascular system through the lymphatic system.

Edema develops when a large amount of fluid accumulates in the interstitial space as a result of increased filtration. Normally, edema does not develop because fluid is returned to the vascular system through lymphatic vessels. Edema generally develops in the dependent part of the body where the hydrostatic pressure is greatest, for example, in the loose tissue around the eyes and scrotum. Edema formation may be caused by the following reasons:

1. *Increased capillary hydrostatic pressure.* Increased hydrostatic pressure may result from elevated venous pressure, as in thrombophlebitis of a deep vein and congestive heart failure. In these conditions the equilibrium point is shifted to the right, so that filtration is greater and absorption is less.
2. *Low plasma protein concentration.* A decrease in plasma protein concentration decreases plasma oncotic pressure. This shifts the equilibrium point to the right (toward venous side), resulting in increased filtration and decreased absorption. Nephrosis is one pathological condition in which plasma protein concentration is decreased.

Conservation of fluid through capillaries may result from the following:

1. *Decreased hydrostatic pressure.* A decrease in hydrostatic pressure, as occurs in hemorrhagic shock, moves the equilibrium point to the left (toward the arteriolar side), resulting in increased absorption and decreased filtration surface.
2. *Increased oncotic pressure.* Plasma protein concentration is increased in dehydration (prolonged sweating, severe vomiting, diarrhea, and water deprivation), which moves the equilibrium point to the left, resulting in decreased filtration and increased absorption.

Pinocytosis

A very small amount of substance (large, lipid-insoluble molecules) leaves capillaries by pinocytosis. In this process the substance attaches to the endothelial cell surface; this portion of the cell membrane invaginates into the interior of the cell until it is completely pinched off and a vesicle is formed containing the substance. These vesicles move to the other side of the capillary wall to deliver the substance.

Peripheral Vascular Control Mechanism

We now turn to the control of blood flow to the vascular beds of the organs throughout the body. Arterioles, the resistance vessels, are involved in regulating blood flow through their cognate capillaries. These vessels are also important in regulating arterial blood pressure. When arterioles are dilated, organ perfusion (blood flow) is increased and the arterial pressure falls (Figure 3.1). The reverse occurs when arterioles are constricted. There are two control mechanisms that regulate tissue blood flow: the intrinsic (local) and extrinsic.

Intrinsic Control

Smooth muscle of resistance vessels is normally in a state of partial contraction and therefore exhibits resting tone. Intrinsic control is dependent upon the caliber of resistance vessels, as modified by various factors based on the needs of the tissue.

Increased perfusion pressure at constant tissue metabolism increases vascular resistance to maintain constant flow. Decreased perfusion pressure at constant tissue metabolism, however, decreases vascular resistance to maintain constant flow (Figure 3.3). This mechanism is called autoregulation of blood flow. As depicted in Figure 3.3, when the pressure is raised suddenly from 100 mm Hg, there is a sudden increase in flow, which is followed within 30 to 60 seconds by a return of the flow to the base level. On the other hand, when perfusion pressure is lowered below 100 mm Hg, there is a sudden decrease in flow, followed within 30 to 60 seconds by the return of

the flow to the base level. The exact mechanism is not known. Various possible mechanisms are discussed next.

Myogenic Mechanism

The myogenic mechanism postulates that the vascular smooth muscle contracts in response to an increase in intramural pressure (wall tension) and relaxes in response to a decrease in wall tension. Thus, an increase in microvascular flow and the concomitant increase in arteriolar diameter due to elevation in perfusion pressure are countered by increased vascular tone and an increase in vascular resistance. The initial flow increase as a result of increased perfusion pressure is caused by passive stretching of arterioles.

Metabolic Mechanism

As already stated, blood flow is regulated by the metabolic needs of the organs. According to the metabolic hypothesis, an oxygen supply inadequate for tissue requirements results in production of metabolites that are vasodilators. Inadequate oxygen supply could be due to either decreased oxygen delivery or increased oxygen demand as a result of increased metabolic activity.

Vasodilator metabolites locally dilate the resistance vessels. Various metabolites (including low PO_2, high PCO_2, low pH, lactic acid, potassium, phosphate, and adenosine) have been implicated in local vasodilation; however, each has a deficiency. It is known that an increase in PO_2 produces contraction, whereas a decrease produces relaxation. However, in the normal range of PO_2 (11 to 343 mm Hg), there is no correlation between PO_2 tension and arteriolar diameter. Also the reactive hyperemia cannot be explained on the basis of PO_2. Induction of vasodilation by lactic acid, low pH, or high PCO_2 is inadequate when compared with the observed vasodilation during increased metabolic activity. Potassium and phosphate cause active hyperemia (increased blood flow from enhanced tissue activity). Potassium release occurs initially but is not sustained during contraction of muscle. However, the vasodilation is sustained. Adenosine is a potent vasodilator and is involved in the regulation of coronary blood flow. It may also be involved in regulation of blood flow in other organs.

Reactive hyperemia, which occurs in organs if the blood supply is momentarily interrupted, can be explained by the metabolites that are released during decreased O_2 supply. On the release of vascular occlusion, tissue blood flow is increased above the resting level and remains elevated until metabolic conditions have returned to normal. Within limits, peak flow and duration of reactive hyperemia are proportional to duration of occlusion. Occlusion of blood vessels increases the concentration of vasodilator metabolites, and, when the occlusion is removed, these metabolites dilate the blood

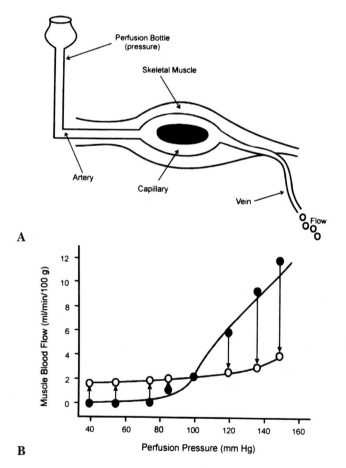

FIGURE 3.3. **A,** Skeletal muscle is perfused at different pressure head, and blood flow is measured. **B,** Diagram showing the relationship between perfusion pressure and blood flow in skeletal muscle. Open circles represent the steady flow, and closed circles represent the initial momentary change in flow when the perfusion pressure is changed.

vessels to increase the blood flow above resting levels. The increased flow acts to close the feedback control loop by increasing the oxygen supply to the tissue and washing out vasodilator metabolites. There are numerous candidates for metabolic vasodilation. Many of them may be found in any vascular bed, and different metabolites are important for different tissues.

Endothelial-Mediated Mechanism

Endothelial cells synthesize and release various vasodilators and constrictors. These agents can regulate vascular tone locally. They are discussed in detail in Chapter 1.

Extrinsic Control

Extrinsic control involves the autonomic nervous system. The autonomic nervous system, vasomotor center, and the reflex vascular control mechanism of vascular tone are discussed in detail in Chapter 4. Here they are discussed in brief. The vasomotor center regulates the activity of the autonomic nervous system. Norepinephrine released at the postganglionic sympathetic nerve endings constricts arterioles to decrease blood flow to the organ and increases arterial pressure. The parasympathetic system has very little control over arterioles compared with the sympathetic system. At postganglionic nerve endings of the parasympathetic system, acetylcholine is released, which dilates the arterioles, resulting in an increase in local blood flow and a decrease in blood pressure. The vasomotor center is under the influence of neurogenic impulses that arise from baroreceptors, chemoreceptors, the ischemic central nervous system, cortex, hypothalamus, skin, and viscera.

Arterial Baroreceptor Reflex

When baroreceptors in the carotid sinus and aortic arch are stimulated by a rise in arterial pressure, an increased number of impulses is generated by the receptors, which ultimately suppresses the vasoconstrictor area and stimulates the vasodepressor area and dorsal motor nucleus of the vagus nerve. These changes produce a decrease in sympathetic activity and an increase in parasympathetic activity and result in arteriolar dilation and, hence, increased local blood flow. The reverse occurs when arterial pressure falls suddenly.

Cardiopulmonary Baroreceptors

Cardiopulmonary baroreceptors are located in the low-pressure part of the cardiovascular system, for example, the cardiac chambers and pulmonary artery. Stimulation of receptors with a rise in pressure reflexively inhibits the vasoconstrictor area in the vasomotor center. Besides this reflex mechanism, atria also synthesize and release atrial natriuretic peptide, which is a vasodilator.

Chemoreceptor Reflex

When stimulated by a fall in blood pressure (as a result of a decrease in PO_2), chemoreceptors in the carotid and aortic bodies reflexively stimulate the vasoconstrictor area to increase arteriolar resistance, which results in a decrease in local blood flow.

Central Nervous System Ischemic Response

Increases in PCO_2 and hydrogen ion concentration stimulate the vasoconstrictor area to increase sympathetic activity and, hence, arteriolar tone and vascular resistance.

Hypothalamus

The hypothalamus regulates blood pressure and flow through (1) stimulation of the anterior hypothalamus, producing a decrease in the arterial pressure and bradycardia; and (2) stimulation of the posterolateral region, producing an increase in arterial pressure and tachycardia. It also regulates pressure through the temperature regulating center. Cooling constricts, whereas warmth dilates cutaneous vessels.

Cerebrum

Stimulation of the motor and premotor areas of the cerebral cortex elicits vasoconstriction. Emotional stimuli elicit a vasodepressor response, as observed in blushing.

Skin and Viscera

Painful stimuli produce vasoconstriction. Distension of the abdominal viscera elicits vasodilation.

Organ-Specific Peripheral Vascular Control Mechanisms

The existence of extrinsic and intrinsic control of blood flow allows the body to direct blood to the organ with greatest need and to divert it away from organs with less immediate need. Intrinsic mechanisms are dominant in heart and brain, which have no tolerance for ischemia. Skin, renal, and splanchnic blood vessels have predominantly extrinsic control. Both intrinsic and extrinsic mechanisms play a role in vascular control in skeletal muscle. In resting skeletal muscle, extrinsic control is dominant. The intrinsic mechanism assumes control in exercising muscle and overrides extrinsic control.

Acknowledgments
The excellent secretarial assistance of Ms. Gloria Schneider is gratefully acknowledged. The author is also grateful to Mr. R. Hutchinson for drawings.

Bibliography

Airkland K, Nicoloysen G. Interstitial fluid volume. Local regulatory mechanism. *Physiol Rev.* 1981;61:556–643.

Anderson KL. Cardiovascular system in exercise. In: Falls HB, ed. *Exercise Physiology.* New York, NY: Academic Press; 1968: 79–128.

Bharadwaj L, Prasad K. Mechanism of hydroxyl radical-induced modulation of vascular tone. *Free Radic Biol Med.* 1996; 22:381–390.

———. Mediation of H_2O_2-induced vascular relaxation by endothelium-derived relaxing factor. *Mol Cell Biochem.* 1995;149/150:267–270.

Braunwald E. *Heart Disease: A Textbook of Cardiovascular Medicine.* Philadelphia, Pa: WB Saunders Co; 1992.

Cohn PF, Brown EJ, Vlay SC. *Clinical Cardiovascular Physiology.* Philadelphia, Pa: WB Saunders Co; 1985.

Eyzaguirre C, Fitzgerald RS, Lahiri S, Zapata P. Arterial chemoreceptors. In: Shepherd JT, Abboud FM, Geiger SR, eds. *The Cardiovascular System—Peripheral Circulation and Organ Blood Flow.* Vol 3. Bethesda, Md: American Physiological Society; 1983:557–621.

Furchgott RF, Vanhoutte PM. Endothelium-derived relaxing and contracting factors. *FASEB J* 1989;3:2007–2018.

Folkow B. Description of myogenic hypothesis. *Circ Res.* 1964;15(suppl I):279–287.

Folkow B, Neil E. *Circulation.* New York, NY: Oxford University Press; 1971.

Guyton AC. Peripheral circulation. *Annu Rev Physiol.* 1959;21: 239–270.

Guyton AC, Granger HJ, Taylor AE. Interstitial fluid pressure. *Physiol Rev.* 1971;51:527–563.

Johnson PC. Local regulatory mechanism in the microcirculation. *Federation Proceedings.* 1975; 34:2005–2037.

Johnson PC, Henrick HA. Metabolic and myogenic factors in local regulation of the microcirculation. *Federation Proceedings.* 1975;34:2020–2024.

Kapoor R, Prasad K. Role of polymorphonuclear leukocytes in cardiovascular depression and cellular injury in hemorrhagic shock and reinfusion. *Free Radic Biol Med.* 1996;21: 609–618.

Katz AM. *Physiology of the Heart.* New York, NY: Raven Press; 1992.

Krogh A. *The Anatomy and Physiology of Capillaries.* New York, NY: Hafner; 1959.

Lee RT, Kamm RD. Vascular mechanics for cardiologists. *J Am Coll Cardiol.* 1994;23:1289–1295.

Little RC, Ginsburg JM. The physiological basis for clinical edema. *Arch Intern Med.* 1984;144:1661–1664.

Mancia G, Mark AL. Arterial baroreflexes in humans. In: Shepherd JT, Abboud FM, eds. *The Cardiovascular System—Peripheral Circulation and Organ Blood Flow.* Vol. 3. Bethesda, Md: American Physiological Society; 1983:755–793.

Mellander S. Systemic circulation: local control. *Annu Rev Physiol.* 1970;32:313–344.

Michel CC. Fluid movement through capillary wall. In: Renkin EM, Michel CC, eds. *The Cardiovascular System—Microcirculation.* Vol. 4. Bethesda, Md: American Physiological Society; 1984:375–409.

Prasad K, Bharadwaj L. Hydroxyl radical: a mediator of acetylcholine-induced vascular relaxation. *J Mol Cell Cardiol.* 1996;28:2033–2041.

Rosell S. Neuronal control of microvessels. *Annu Rev Physiol.* 1980;42:359–371.

Smith JJ, Kampine JP. *Circulatory Physiology: The Essentials.* Baltimore, Md: Williams & Wilkins; 1990.

Sparks HV Jr. Effect of local metabolic factors on vascular smooth muscle. In: Bohr DF, Somylo AP, Sparks HV Jr, eds. *The Cardiovascular System—Vascular Smooth Muscle.* Vol. 2. Bethesda, Md: American Physiological Society; 1980: 475–513.

Taylor AE. Capillary fluid filtration. Starling forces and lymph flow. *Circ Res.* 1981;49:557–575.

Yang SS, Bentivoglio LG, Maranhao V, Goldberg H. *From Cardiac Catheterization Data to Hemodynamic Parameters.* Philadelphia, Pa: FA Davis Company; 1972.

Zucker IH, Gilmore JP. *Reflex Control of Circulation.* Boca Raton, Fla: CRC Press; 1991.

Zweifach BW, Lipowsky HH. Pressure–flow relations in blood and lymph microcirculation. In: Renkin EM, Michel CC, eds. *The Cardiovascular System—Microcirculation.* Vol. 4. Bethesda, Md: American Physiological Society; 1984:251.

4

Blood Pressure and Its Control Mechanism

Kailash Prasad

Arterial blood pressure is the lateral pressure exerted by the column of blood against the arterial walls. During the cardiac cycle the highest pressure attained is the systolic pressure and the lowest pressure is the diastolic pressure. The mean blood pressure (MBP) is the geometric mean, and calculation of MBP requires integration of pressure pulse. However, a crude estimate of MBP is given by the following formulas:

1. MBP = [systolic pressure + 2(diastolic pressure)]/3.
2. MBP = diastolic pressure + (pulse pressure)/3. Pulse pressure is the difference between the systolic and diastolic pressures.

The MBP (in millimeters of mercury) is the product of cardiac output (liters per minute) and total peripheral resistance (millimeters of mercury per liter per minute).

Determinants of Systolic Pressure and Diastolic Pressure

Systolic pressure depends on stroke volume, peak-systolic cardiac ejection rate, and arterial compliance (distensibility). For example, systolic pressure increases with increased stroke volume, peak-systolic ejection rate, and decreased arterial compliance and decreases with the relations reversed. Arterial compliance decreases with age as a consequence of arteriosclerosis and hence pressure increases with volume; therefore the extent of the increase in pressure is directly related to age. Diastolic pressure is determined by total peripheral resistance, heart rate, systolic pressure, and arterial elastic recoil (i.e., increases or decreases in these parameters increase or decrease, respectively, the diastolic pressure). Loss of elastic recoil in the arterial wall that occurs with aging decreases the diastolic pressure. Pulse pressure is approximately one-half of the diastolic pressure and is affected in various clinical situations as outlined in Table 4.1.

Normal Arterial Pressure

The arterial pressure on the first day after birth is approximately 70/50 mm Hg and increases gradually during the next several months to about 90/60 mm Hg. During the subsequent years the rise is very slow until the adult pressure of 115/70 mm Hg is attained at adolescence. The normal blood pressure for adults is 110 to 140 mm Hg systolic and 60 to 90 mm Hg diastolic. There may be great variations in blood pressure within a few minutes because of excitement, apprehension, and various other factors. Eating, smoking, and exercise may raise blood pressure. Strenuous exercise may raise the pressure as high as 200/100 mm Hg. During sleep, the systolic pressure may fall by 15 to 30 mm Hg. There is a progressive increase in the pressure with age in the average population. The systolic pressure rises approximately 1 mm Hg/y from 110 mm Hg at the age of 15 years. This probably reflects progressive reduction in arterial compliance, especially beyond the age of 60 years. Diastolic pressure increases about 0.4 mm Hg/y from 70 mm Hg at the age of 15 years. This rise probably reflects an increase in total peripheral resistance. The progressive increase in pressure with age also results from the effects of aging on the long-term blood pressure control mechanism. Although the average pressure of a population rises with age, some people never experience a rise in pressure with age. Therefore, the mean for a population is composed of a group of normotensive individuals whose blood pressure does not change with time and of hypertensive individuals whose pressure increases with age. Because there is no dividing line between normal and high blood pressure, arbitrary levels have been established to define those who have increased risk of developing morbid cardiovascular events and/or clearly benefit from medical therapy. The logic is to define hypertension at levels where treatment can provide benefits that outweigh risks. Life expectancy is inversely pro-

TABLE 4.1. Clinical conditions that affect pulse pressure.

Increased	Decreased
1. Decreased total peripheral resistance	1. Mechanical obstruction
• Anxiety	• Aortic stenosis
• Exercise	• Mitral stenosis
• Fever	• Mitral regurgitation
• Hyperthyroidism	
• Anemia	
• Paget's disease of bone	
• A–V fistula	
2. Decreased arterial compliance	2. Decreased stroke volume
• Atherosclerosis	• Heart Failure
• Hypertension	• Shock
	• Tachycardia
	• Cardiac temponade
3. Increased stroke volume	
• Bradycardia	
• Complete heart block	
• Aortic regurgitation	

portional to arterial pressure (systolic, diastolic, MBP). There is no desirable blood pressure level. All pressure is somewhat damaging. A systolic pressure of 140 mm Hg or lower and a diastolic pressure of 90 mm Hg or lower is considered normal blood pressure for all ages. Males with normal diastolic pressure but elevated systolic pressure (>158 mm Hg) have a 2½-fold increase in cardiovascular mortality rates when compared to individuals with similar diastolic pressure but normal systolic pressure. The blood pressure is slightly higher in the right arm than in the left arm. Simultaneous recording of blood pressure in both arms shows a difference of 10 mm Hg (both systolic and diastolic) in about 3% of normotensive and 6% of hypertensive individuals. When pressure is taken at different times (not simultaneously) in alternate arms, a difference of 10 mm Hg or more in systolic pressure is present in about 20% of normotensive and 30% of hypertensive individuals, and a difference in diastolic pressure of 10 mm Hg or more is observed in about 10% of normotensive and 15% of hypertensive individuals. Systolic pressure in the thigh is about 10 to 40 mm Hg higher than in the arms, but diastolic pressure is similar in the arms and thighs.

Factors That Affect Blood Pressure

Blood pressure varies throughout the day and with various activities.

Diurnal Variation

Blood pressure changes are closely related to the levels of arousal. Following the onset of sleep, blood pressure falls gradually and reaches the lowest level (decrease of 15%–20%) after 2 hours. Blood pressure rises immediately on waking and tends to be highest in the morning with a gradual decrease over the course of the day. The increase during the early hours of the morning could contribute to the high incidence of cerebral hemorrhage and myocardial infarction in these hours. Diurnal variation may be due to morning diurnal peaks in total blood volume, central blood volume, sympathetic activity, and plasma renin activity.

Physical Activity

Blood pressure increases with physical activity. Intense physical activity can lead to a rise of pressure to a level of 240 mm Hg in patients with mild hypertension. The type of activity determines the amount of rise in blood pressure. Talking is also a potent pressor stimulus.

Meals

There is an increase in the heart rate, a decrease in the diastolic pressure, and little change in systolic pressure for 3 hours after a meal. In older individuals, there may be a marked fall in both systolic and diastolic pressure following a meal.

Mental Activity

Mental activity raises blood pressure.

Seasonal Variation

In temperate climates, blood pressure is about 5 mm Hg higher in winter than in summer. This appears to be related to the effect of the cold in winter on the vasoconstrictor area. Also, warmer climates are vasodilative. Systemic vasoconstriction is due to a reflex response to cold exposure.

Sex

Under the age of 40 to 50 years, systolic and diastolic pressure are lower in women than in men and are higher in women than in men after the age of 50 years. This change may be due to hormonal changes in women that take place at menopause.

Weight

Systolic and diastolic pressure are directly related to the weight of the subject.

Posture

Cardiac output and thoracic arterial pressure decrease in the erect position due to a decrease in venous return.

Compensatory increases in heart rate and systemic vascular resistance cause an increase in both systolic and diastolic pressure, the increase being greater in the latter.

Race and Socioeconomic Status

Blood pressure levels are higher in blacks than in whites, across all ages and for both sexes. Genetic and environmental factors, particularly socioeconomic, may be responsible for this difference.

Pain

Headache and other types of chronic pain raise arterial pressure.

Hypoglycemia

A sudden decrease in blood glucose raises blood pressure through increased sympathetic activity.

Arterial Pressure Control Mechanisms

Arterial pressure has numerous functions: (1) It moves blood throughout the body to provide nutrients to the tissue. This requires hydrostatic pressure to overcome the colloid osmotic pressure. (2) It overcomes gravity and opposes intracranial pressure and the resistance generated by contracting muscles. (3) It enables regulation of blood flow under varying conditions, such as exercise and rest. Arterial pressure is regulated to maintain tissue perfusion during various pathophysiologic conditions. Three mechanisms regulate arterial pressure: (1) a rapidly acting pressure control mechanism, (2) an intermediate time-period pressure control mechanism, and (3) a long-term pressure control mechanism.

Neural Control of Arterial Pressure

I will review briefly the autonomic neural control of the cardiovascular system before discussing the pressure control mechanisms. The organization of the autonomic nervous system is shown in simplified form in Figure 4.1. The vasomotor center is located bilaterally in the medulla and lower third of the pons. It comprises three areas: vasoconstrictor, vasodilator, and sensory (nucleus tractus solitarius [NTS]). The vasoconstrictor area is situated in the anterolateral part of the medulla. Fibers from the vasoconstrictor area descend and synapse in the intermediolateral gray matter of the spinal cord (T1 to L2 or L3). The fibers (preganglionic) then leave the cord

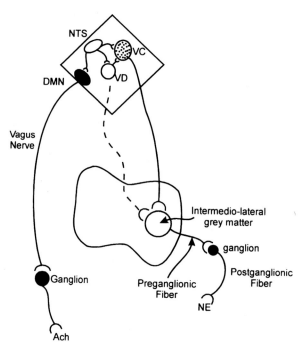

FIGURE 4.1. Organization of the vasomotor center and autonomic nervous system. Diamond-shaped area is medulla of the brain, whereas the near rectangular area is the spinal cord. NTS indicates nucleus tractus of solitarius; VC, vasoconstrictor area; VD, vasodilator area; DMN, dorsal motor nucleus of vagus nerve; Ach, acetylcholine; and NE, norepinephrine.

to join paravertebral sympathetic ganglia. Postganglionic fibers arise from these ganglia and innervate the arteries, veins, and heart. Norepinephrine is released at the postganglionic sympathetic nerve endings and produces vasoconstriction via alpha-adrenergic receptors of the smooth muscle of the blood vessels. Norepinephrine increases the rate, force of contraction, and conduction in the heart. The vasoconstrictor area is tonically active, fires continuously at a rate of one-half to two impulses per second, and maintains a partial tone in the blood vessels. Reflexes or humoral stimuli that enhance this activity produce an increase in the frequency of firing and hence vasoconstriction. Inhibition of the vasoconstrictor area reduces the firing frequency and results in vasodilation. The vasoconstrictor area may show rhythmic changes in tonic activity resulting in oscillations of arterial pressure. Traube-Hering waves occurring at the frequency of respiration are due to increase in sympathetic activity during inspiration. Mayer waves are independent of respiration and are due to oscillation of baroreceptor and chemoreceptor reflexes, and central nervous system (CNS) ischemic response.

The vasodepressor area, which is situated caudal and ventromedial to the vasoconstrictor area, produces a decrease in blood pressure when stimulated. It exerts its effect by direct spinal inhibition and by inhibition of the vasoconstrictor area.

The parasympathetic nervous system has two divisions: cranial division (III, VII, IX, and X nerves) and sacral division (second through fourth sacral nerves). About 75% of all parasympathetic nerve fibers are in the vagus nerve (X). Blood vessels are mainly supplied by the sympathetic nervous system. The parasympathetic system supplies a very small number of blood vessels. Preganglionic parasympathetic fibers originate in the dorsal motor nucleus of the medulla and travel in the vagus nerve. These fibers synapse with ganglia close to the organs. At the postganglionic nerve ending acetylcholine is released. Acetylcholine relaxes blood vessels and decreases the rate and force of contraction of the heart.

Rapidly Acting Pressure Control Mechanism

Rapidly acting pressure control mechanisms are neural. They include baroreceptor, chemoreceptor, and CNS ischemic responses. They become active within seconds.

Baroreceptor (Pressoreceptor) Reflexes

Baroreceptors are located in the carotid sinuses (internal carotid artery at the points of origin from the common carotid artery) and in the aortic arch (Figure 4.2). They are very sensitive to changes in pressure. The impulses from the carotid sinus travel up the sinus nerve to the glossopharyngeal nerve and then to the NTS, the sensory area. Impulses from the aortic arch arrive at the NTS through the aortic nerve via the vagus nerve. Baroreceptors in the carotid sinus and aortic arch are stimulated by the rise in blood pressure and therefore the frequency of firing is increased. These impulses stimulate the NTS. Stimulation of the NTS inhibits the vasoconstrictor area to decrease sympathetic activity and hence blood pressure. Stimulation of the NTS also stimulates the dorsal nucleus of the vagus and vasodepressor areas, contributing to a further fall in blood pressure. Thus baroreceptor stimulation decreases blood pressure by decreasing vasoconstrictor activity and increasing vagal and vasodepressor activity. When there is a rise in blood pressure, the baroreceptor reflex mechanism lowers the blood pressure by (1) decreasing sympathetic activity to produce vasodilation and decrease in cardiac output and (2) increasing parasympathetic activity to produce vasodilation and decrease in cardiac output (Figure 4.3). The reverse occurs when the blood pressure falls (Figure 4.3). As fewer impulses arrive at the NTS, the result is less inhibition of the vasoconstrictor area and an increase in sympathetic activity. Also, there is decreased activity of the vasodepressor area and dorsal nucleus of the vagus that contributes to the rise in blood pressure.

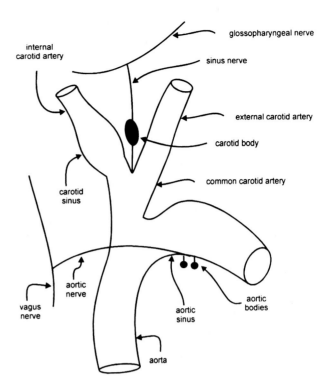

FIGURE 4.2. Schematic diagram showing aortic and carotid sinuses, bodies, and their connections to various efferent nerves.

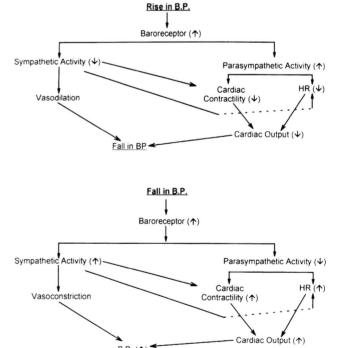

FIGURE 4.3. Diagram showing the baroreceptor mechanism control of blood pressure when the pressure rises or falls. BP indicates blood pressure; HR, heart rate; ↓, decrease; and ↑, increase.

The blood pressure threshold for stimulation of the sinus nerve is about 50 mm Hg and maximum is attained at around 200 mm Hg. Receptors in the carotid sinus are more sensitive than those in the aortic sinus. Baroreceptor sensitivity decreases in hypertension when the carotid sinus becomes stiffer and less deformable. In some individuals carotid sinus receptors are very sensitive. Tight collars or other forms of external pressure over the carotid sinus region in such individuals may result in hypotension and fainting. The baroreceptor reflex mechanism is a potent regulator of arterial pressure when the pressure is in the normal range, but it becomes useless when the pressure falls below 60 to 70 mm Hg. Feedback gain (amount of correction of abnormality divided by the remaining degree of abnormality, i.e., effectiveness of control system) for baroreceptor is less than for the CNS ischemic response but greater than for the chemoreceptor reflex mechanism.

Chemoreceptor Reflex

Chemoreceptors are highly vascular bodies located at the bifurcation of the common carotid artery (carotid body) and the aortic arch (aortic body) (Figure 4.2). They are in close contact with blood, are very sensitive to changes in the Po_2, and are sensitive to changes in the Pco_2 and pH (less so than to changes in Po_2). Low Po_2, high Pco_2, and low pH stimulate the chemoreceptors. Impulses from the chemoreceptors reach the vasoconstrictor area through the glossopharyngeal nerve via the sinus nerve (carotid bodies) and through the vagus nerve via the aortic nerve (aortic bodies) resulting in increased tone in resistance vessels. Whenever blood pressure falls below critical levels, chemoreceptors are stimulated because of decreased blood flow and hence, decreased levels of oxygen, increased Pco_2, and decreased pH. The chemoreceptor reflex mechanism is not a powerful controller of arterial pressure in the normal range because receptors are stimulated strongly only when the arterial pressure falls below 60 to 70 mm Hg. It works until the pressure falls to 40 mm Hg. The response occurs in seconds and the feedback gain is smallest among the nervous control mechanisms.

CNS Ischemic Response

Chemosensitive areas of the vasoconstrictor zone are very sensitive to high Pco_2 and low pH. Ischemia can stimulate the vasoconstrictor area through a rise in Pco_2 and decrease in pH. Po_2 has relatively little effect on the vasoconstrictor area. Moderate reduction in Po_2 stimulates the vasoconstrictor area while severe reduction produces depression of the area. CNS ischemic response is very intense and can raise the arterial pressure to as high as 250 mm Hg. This system works best in the arterial

pressure range of 40 to 20 mm Hg. When the pressure falls below 20 mm Hg, the CNS ischemic response becomes useless. This is called the "last ditch stand" pressure control mechanism. Cushing's response is a type of CNS ischemic response that results from increased intracranial pressure.

Cardiopulmonary Baroreceptors

Atria, ventricles, and pulmonary arteries have baroreceptors (low pressure receptors). Atria have A receptors that are activated during atrial contraction and B receptors that are activated during atrial filling. Stimulation of these receptors decreases sympathetic activity to the kidneys and increases activity to the sinus node. Stimulation of cardiopulmonary receptors also depresses the vasoconstrictor area. Low pressor receptor stimulation inhibits release of angiotensin, aldosterone, and antidiuretic hormone. These hormones increase the blood volume and hence, cardiac output and blood pressure. Overstretch of the atria from excess blood volume results in release of atrial natriuretic peptide from specific cells of the atria. Atrial natriuretic peptide enters the circulation where it inhibits reabsorption of sodium by kidney tubules (collecting ducts) and increases glomerular filtration through vasodilator activity. This results in increased excretion of salt and water, which reduces the blood volume towards control value. A decrease in blood volume decreases arterial pressure. Neither excessive amounts of nor lack of atrial natriuretic peptide cause major changes in blood volume (arterial pressure), because these changes are easily overcome by the small changes in arterial pressure through pressure natriuresis.

Intermediate Time-Period Pressure Control Mechanism

The intermediate mechanism includes renin–angiotensin, stress–relaxation, and capillary fluid shift, and becomes mostly activated within 30 minutes to several hours. The intermediate mechanism is effective for long periods of time (days if necessary) and is important, because by this time the nervous mechanisms are less active.

Renin–Angiotensin-Vasoconstriction Mechanism

When the arterial pressure falls below 100 mm Hg the kidneys synthesize and secrete increased amounts of renin that leads to formation of angiotensin and aldosterone, which in turn raises arterial pressure (Figure 4.4). There are three hypotheses for renin release: (1) The baroreceptor hypothesis postulates that the renal afferent arterioles, which contain juxtaglomerular

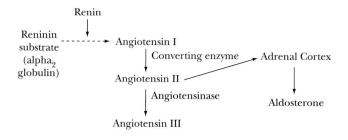

FIGURE 4.4. Renin–Angiotensin–Aldosterone synthesis and release mechanism.

(JG) cells, respond to decreases in stretch as a result of reduced perfusion pressure and renal blood flow by releasing renin. (2) The macula densa hypothesis postulates that as a result of reduction in glomerular filtration due to reduced pressure, the sodium load reaching the distal tubule is reduced. This reduction is sensed by the macula densa, which is in close proximity to JG cells, and possibly through the action of a local hormone that releases renin from JG cells. (3) The adrenergic hypothesis states that when there is a fall in arterial pressure there is an increase in sympathetic activity that results in release of norepinephrine. Juxtaglomerular cells are supplied by the renal sympathetic nerve and are stimulated by norepinephrine to release renin. Elevated plasma levels of norepinephrine during hypotension also stimulate JG cells. The receptor in the JG cells that triggers renin release is β_1-adrenergic receptor. Direct chemical stimuli and inhibitors also affect renin release from JG cells: catecholamines and prostaglandins stimulate whereas angiotensin and potassium inhibit.

Renin is synthesized and stored in an inactive form. It acts on a plasma globulin called renin substrate (angiotensinogen) that is formed in the liver. Renin substrate synthesis is increased by estrogens such as oral contraceptives. Formation of angiotensin II and III from angiotensinogen is shown in Figure 4.4.

Renin acts on angiotensinogen to produce angiotensin I. Renin activity in the blood lasts for 30 to 60 minutes, during which angiotensin I is formed. Angiotensin I is converted into angiotensin II within a few seconds in the lung by converting enzyme present in the endothelium of lung blood vessels. Angiotensin II is then converted into angiotensin III by angiotensinase. Angiotensin III is almost as powerful a vasoconstrictor as angiotensin II. The converting enzyme produces angiotensin II and also destroys the vasodilator bradykinin. This explains why angiotensin-converting enzyme inhibitors are used in the treatment of patients with hypertension. Angiotensin II and III stimulate aldosterone production. Angiotensin II persists in the blood for only 1 or 2 minutes, before it is rapidly inactivated by angiotensinase.

Actions of Angiotensin II

Angiotensin II has various functions:

1. Produces vasoconstriction
2. Increases aldosterone production by the zona glomerulosa of adrenal cortex
3. Increases release of antidiuretic hormone from posterior pituitary
4. Increases thirst by stimulating thirst center
5. Increases vasomotor center activity
6. Releases catecholamines from adrenal medulla and sympathetic nerve endings
7. Increases reabsorption of sodium ions and water in kidney tubules.

Angiotensin II elevates the arterial pressure in two principal ways: (1) by direct vasoconstriction and by the release of norepinephrine through nerve endings and through stimulation of the vasomotor center; and (2) by the increase in blood volume following the increase in sodium reabsorption in the kidneys, increase in thirst, and increase in water reabsorption by antidiuretic hormone. Angiotensin II could possibly increase sodium reabsorption via alteration in peritubular capillary dynamics. Angiotensin II increases arteriolar resistance and, therefore, will produce a decrease in peritubular capillary hydrostatic pressure resulting in an increase in peritubular capillary reabsorption. Peritubular capillary colloid osmotic pressure would increase because of the increased filtration fraction (a result of decreased renal blood flow due to increased arteriolar resistance). The long-term effect of changes in extracellular volume is more powerful than the acute vasoconstrictor effect in returning the arterial pressure to control level. This mechanism of renin–angiotensin–aldosterone works best in the pressure range of 60 to 110 mm Hg and begins acting within a few minutes. Feedback gain is smaller than for the chemoreceptor reflex mechanism.

Stress–Relaxation Mechanism

With the rise in arterial pressure the blood vessels slowly begin to stretch allowing the pressure to fall towards the control value. This is called the stress–relaxation mechanism. Reverse stress–relaxation causes blood vessels to contract around the diminished blood volume. This occurs in hypovolemic shock. Stress–relaxation can serve as an intermediate-term pressure buffer. Feedback gain is better than in the renin–angiotensin mechanism. The stress–relaxation mechanism works at all values of arterial pressure and quickly, within a few minutes of the change in pressure.

Capillary Fluid Shift Mechanism

The capillary fluid shift mechanism works through hydrostatic pressure in capillaries. When the arterial pressure is elevated, capillary hydrostatic pressure is increased leading to transudation of fluid from the capillaries with decreasing blood volume and fall in arterial pressure. Conversely when the arterial pressure falls capillary hydrostatic pressure also falls, fluid is reabsorbed, thus increasing the blood volume and hence, the arterial pressure. This mechanism gets activated within 30 minutes to several hours. The feedback gain is the least of all the mechanisms and it works at all values of arterial pressure.

Aldosterone

There are various mechanisms of release of aldosterone when the arterial pressure falls: (1) Decrease in the arterial pressure releases aldosterone through the renin–angiotensin–aldosterone mechanism (as discussed previously). (2) A change in sodium and potassium concentration also affects aldosterone release. Aldosterone causes renal tubules to reabsorb sodium in large quantities. Increased extracellular sodium also increases release of antidiuretic hormone, which helps in reabsorbing water from kidney tubules. The blood volume increases and leads to an increase in blood pressure toward the control value. The aldosterone mechanism works best in the pressure range of 40 to 150 mm Hg. The feedback gain is not well determined but is similar to that for the stress–relaxation mechanism.

Long-Term Pressure Control Mechanism

Long-term pressure regulation is mainly provided by the renal–body-fluid pressure control mechanism. This involves control of blood volume with consequent effects on arterial pressure. It also partly controls kidney function through renin–angiotensin–aldosterone. The physiologic basis of the renal–body-fluid mechanism for arterial pressure regulation is the direct effect of arterial pressure on output of salt and water from the kidneys. The kidneys excrete sodium and water in proportion to arterial pressure (Figure 4.5).

When the arterial pressure falls to about 50 mm Hg, urinary output falls to zero. However, when arterial pressure rises from the normal value of 100 mm Hg to 200 mm Hg, the output of salt and water increases six- to eightfold (Figure 4.5). The curve in Figure 4.5 is called the renal output curve or renal function curve. A rise in pressure increases sodium output (pressure natriuresis) besides urinary output. The renal–body-fluid mechanism for pressure control depends upon (1) the renal output curve for salt and water, and (2) the net intake of water and salt. The net intake is defined as intake minus the nonrenal output such as through the gut or by sweating. Over a long period of time the net intake equals renal output, and the arterial pressure is determined by

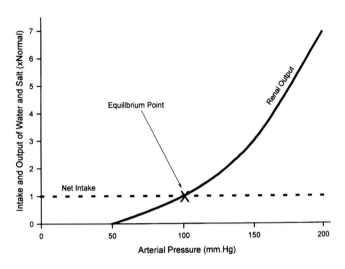

FIGURE 4.5. Diagram showing the renal output with changes in the arterial pressure.

the point that the two curves intersect, at the equilibrium point (100 mm Hg). If arterial pressure rises to 150 mm Hg, urinary output of water and salt increases to about three times normal (urinary output is three times the intake) when the net intake remains unchanged. In such circumstances the body loses fluid, causing a decrease in blood volume, cardiac output, and arterial pressure. The decrease in arterial pressure is also due to a decrease in total peripheral resistance due to autoregulation. When pressure reaches 100 mm Hg, the renal output and net intake become equal again, and the arterial pressure stabilizes at that point. When the arterial pressure falls below the equilibrium point (100 mm Hg pressure) and the net intake of water and salt remains unaltered, renal output decreases. Hence, at low pressure the net intake will be greater than renal output, so that salt and water will accumulate, leading to an increase in blood volume, cardiac output, and arterial pressure, until the pressure returns to the equilibrium point. When the arterial pressure rises (net intake remaining unaltered), renal output of water and salt is greater than net intake. The extracellular volume and cardiac output decrease leads to a decrease in arterial pressure directly and through autoregulation by decreasing total peripheral vascular resistance. The pressure at the equilibrium point can be altered in two ways: (1) shifting the renal output curve for salt and water (degree of shift of renal output curve), and (2) changing the net intake. A new value of the arterial pressure would be attained by changing one or both of these basic determinants of the long-term arterial pressure control mechanism. The feedback gain for the renal–body-fluid mechanism is useless for regulation of arterial pressure over a period of minutes or hours. This mechanism starts later than the other mechanisms, but works until the pressure is back to normal.

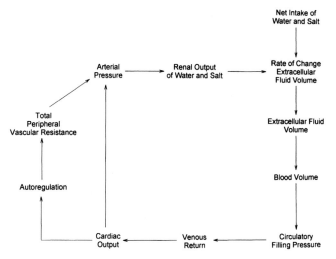

FIGURE 4.6. The feedback control circuit of the renal–body-fluid arterial pressure control mechanism.

Mechanism of Feedback Loop

A detailed outline of the different factors involved in the renal–body-fluid pressure control mechanism is shown in Figure 4.6.

The rate of change of extracellular fluid volume is determined by net intake and renal output of salt and water. A positive rate of change increases extracellular fluid volume while a negative change decreases it. If arterial pressure falls below normal, the sequence of changes outlined in Figure 4.6. will occur provided the net intake remains unchanged. When renal output becomes less than net intake, the extracellular fluid volume increases, and hence blood volume, mean circulatory filling pressure, venous return, and cardiac output are increased. Increase in cardiac output increases arterial pressure in two ways: (1) Cardiac output directly affects blood pressure because this is the product of cardiac output and vascular resistance. (2) Excessive cardiac output causes excessive blood flow to local tissue causing vasoconstriction (autoregulation) and, hence,. increases in vascular resistance (total peripheral resistance). Rise in arterial pressure as a consequence of increased cardiac output is initially due to the direct effect of cardiac output. Autoregulation becomes activated over several days and most of the increase in arterial pressure then is caused by increase in peripheral vascular resistance.

Advantages and Disadvantages of Complex Pressure Regulating Systems

Advantages

1. Cooperation of regulatory systems allows rapid and certain responses to emergencies.

2. Fine tuning capabilities exist.
3. Fail-safe and backup systems enable removal of entire component without loss of control (e.g., adrenalectomy, nephrectomy).
4. Complexity allows local changes to supersede systemic ones in vital organs.

Disadvantages

1. There is a potential danger in having sensors independent of each other. For example, renal ischemia can overdrive the system because local conditions near one sensor may not reflect the status of the body as a whole.
2. The system fails to sense the capacity of the effectors to perform.
3. There is a lack, on the part of regulatory system, to sense the total fluid volume.
4. Absolute level of pressure is not sensed by the regulatory system.

Acknowledgments
Excellent secretarial assistance of Ms. Gloria Schneider is gratefully acknowledged. The author is also grateful to Mr. R. Hutchinson for drawings.

Bibliography

Athanassiadis D, Draper GJ, Honour AJ, Cranston WI. Variability of automatic blood pressure measurements over 24-hour periods. *Clin Sci.* 1969;36:147–156.

Cowley AW Jr, Liard, JF, and Guyton AC. Role of baroreceptor reflex in daily control of arterial blood pressure and other variables in dog. *Circ Res.* 1973;32:564–576.

Davis JO, Freeman RH. Mechanisms regulating renin release. *Physiol Rev.* 1976;56:1–56.

Fagan TC, Conrad KA, Mar HJ, Nelson L. Effects of meals on hemodynamics: implications for antihypertensive drug studies. *Clin Pharmacol Ther.* 1986;39:255–260.

Goodfriend TL. *Hypertension Essentials: Current Concept of Cause and Control.* New York, NY: Grune & Stratton; 1983.

Guyton AC, Coleman TG, Cowley AW Jr, Scheel KW, Manning RD Jr, Norman RA Jr. Arterial pressure regulation. Overriding dominance of the kidneys in long-term regulation and in hypertension. *Am J Med.* 1972;52:584–594.

Guyton AC, Coleman TG, Granger HJ. Circulation: overall regulation. *Annu Rev Physiol.* 1972;34:13–46.

Guyton AC, Hall JE. *Textbook of Physiology.* 9th ed. Philadelphia, Pa: WB Saunders Co; 1996.

Kenner T. Arterial blood pressure and its measurement. *Basic Res Cardiol.* 1988;83:107–121.

Little RC, Little WC. *Physiology of the Heart and Circulation.* 4th ed. Boca Raton, Fla: Year Book Medical Publishing Inc; 1989.

O'Rourke MF. The arterial pulse in health and disease. *Am Heart J.* 1971;82:687–702.

Pascarelli EF, Bertrand CA. Comparison of blood pressure in arms and legs. *N Engl J Med.* 1964;270:693–698.

Peach MJ. Renin-angiotensin system: biochemistry and mechanism of action. *Physiol Rev.* 1977;57:313–370.

Pelletier CL, Shepherd JT. Circulatory reflexes from mechanoreceptors in cardio-aortic area. *Circ Res.* 1973;33: 131–138.

Reid IA, Morris BJ, Ganong WF. The renin-angiotensin system. *Annu Rev Physiol.* 1978;40:377–410.

Richardson DW, Honour AJ, Goodman AC. Changes in arterial pressure during sleep in man. *Hypertens.* 1968;16:62–78.

Rushmer RF. *Cardiovascular Dynamics.* 3rd ed. Philadelphia, Pa: WB Saunders Co; 1970.

Smith OA. Reflex and central mechanisms involved in the control of the heart and circulation. *Annu Rev Physiol.* 1974; 36:93–123.

5

Coronary Vasculature and Endothelium

Rolf Bünger and Patricia A. Gwirtz

Epidemiology of Coronary Heart Disease

General Statistics of Cardiovascular Disease

According to "Heart and Stroke Facts: 1995 Statistical Supplement," published by the American Heart Association,[1] about 59 million Americans—one quarter of the total US population—have one or more forms of cardiovascular disease. Leading forms of cardiovascular disease are hypertension (affecting 50 million people), coronary heart disease (affecting 11.2 million people), stroke (affecting 3.1 million individuals), and rheumatic heart disease (affecting 1.35 million people). One in six men and one in eight woman, age 45 years and older, have had myocardial infarction or stroke. In 1992 cardiovascular diseases claimed 925,000 lives, which amounts to 42.5% of all deaths in the United States. For comparison, in that same year, cancer claimed 521,000 lives, and human immunodeficiency virus (HIV) infection claimed 33,600 lives. Thus cardiovascular disease ranks far ahead of cancer and HIV as a cause of death.

The age-adjusted cardiovascular disease death rates for men and women are 244.9 and 13.4, respectively. The age-adjusted cancer death rates for men and women are 165 and 113, respectively. From 1982 to 1992 death rates from cardiovascular disease declined 24.5%. In 1950 the death rate from cardiovascular disease was 424; in 1991 it had dropped to 186. Medical scientists have made substantial progress in fighting cardiovascular disease. Even so, every 34 seconds a person dies in the United States of cardiovascular disease. Since 1919 more than 42% of all deaths each year have been caused by cardiovascular disease. As the population ages cardiovascular diseases have an even greater human and economic impact. Heart failure is becoming more and more prevalent. If all forms of cardiovascular diseases were eliminated the total life expectancy would increase by almost 10 years; if all forms of cancer were eliminated total life expectancy would increase by 3 years.

Coronary Heart Disease

Coronary heart disease caused 1 of every 4.5 deaths in the United States in 1992, establishing myocardial infarction as the single largest killer of American men and women. It was predicted that about 1.5 million Americans would have myocardial infarction in 1995. More than half of all people with myocardial infarction die within an hour of the onset of symptoms and before they reach the hospital. About 11.2 million people alive today have a history of myocardial infarction, angina pectoris, or both. The least educated have a higher risk of death from myocardial infarction than the most educated. In the decade from 1982 to 1992, the death rate from myocardial infarction declined 31%; between 1950 and 1991 it declined from 226 to 108. It is not clear which portion of these improvements is due to improved and faster ambulance services as compared with advances in medical diagnosis, treatment, and technology in the intensive care unit and operating room of the hospital.

Sex and Ethnic Factors

According to the Framingham Heart Study, 5% of all myocardial infarctions are suffered by people younger than 40 years, and 45% occur in people younger than 65 years. An estimated 57,000 men and 21,000 women under age 65 die of myocardial infarction each year. From ages 35 to 74 years, the death rate from myocardial infarction for black women is about two times that of white women. The average prevalence of coronary heart disease is 7.2% for the general population, 7.5% for whites, 6.9% for blacks, and 5.6% for Mexican Americans. Black men have a 46.8% higher death rate from cardiovascular disease than white men. For black women the rate was 68.9% higher than for white women.

Risk Factors

The danger of myocardial infarction within 8 years is 3.1% and 0.5% in men and women, respectively, in the absence of risk factors. The three major risk factors are cigarette smoking, high levels of blood cholesterol, and high blood pressure. Cigarette smoking alone increases the danger of myocardial infarction for men to 4.6% and for women to 0.9%. If high blood cholesterol is also present the probabilities rise to 6.4% in men and 1.4% in women. If hypertension is added as a risk factor to cigarette smoking and elevated blood cholesterol, the probability of myocardial infarction for men is 9.5% and for women 2.3%. Smoking-related illnesses cost the United States about $50 billion annually in medical care. In 1990 an estimated 417,000 people died of smoking-related diseases, about 38,500 from exposure to environmental tobacco smoke. Smoking in the United States is less common than in the other industrialized Western nations in Europe and Asia. Women who are smokers and use oral contraceptives are up to 39 times more likely to have myocardial infarction than nonsmoking women who do not use birth control pills. Blood cholesterol levels below 200 mg/dL in middle-aged adults seem to indicate a low risk of coronary heart disease. In the United States, it is estimated that almost 95 million adults (52%) have blood cholesterol levels of 200 mg/dL or higher, and about 37 million have levels of 240 mg/dL or above. Women 55 years and older have higher cholesterol levels than men of the same age group. In general blood cholesterol levels rise with age regardless of ethnic background. An estimated 50 million Americans age 60 years or older have high blood pressure (i.e., their systolic aortic pressure is 140 mm Hg or higher and/or their diastolic pressure is 90 mm Hg or higher). Physical inactivity and obesity are additional risk factors. Persons with such sedentary lifestyles have a 30% to 50% higher chance of developing high blood pressure. Coronary heart disease is about twice as likely in physically immobile individuals, regardless of other risk factors. Obesity increased in the United States between 1960 and 1991 by about 27% in all ethnic groups.

Surgical Treatment and Estimated Costs

Coronary bypass surgery was performed on 310,000 people in 1992; 46% were under 65 years of age and 74% were men. Heart transplantations have increased from about 100 in the early 1980s to 2300 in 1993. More than 78% of heart transplant patients are men; 82% of them are white. The 30-day survival rate is 91.6%, the 1-year survival rate is 81.6%, and the 2-year survival rate is 77%. There are about 1100 specialized coronary intensive care units in general hospitals nationwide for myocardial in-farction patients; the coronary intensive care units can reduce in-hospital deaths by about 30%.

The American Heart Association estimated that the cost of cardiovascular disease in 1996 would be about $138 billion. Nearly half of that, $60.5 billion, would be due to coronary heart disease; $18.7 billion would be due to hypertensive heart disease. Of the coronary heart disease costs the greater portion (>65%) is due to hospitalization, followed by those due to physician and nurse services (about 15%). Included in these estimates is lost productivity, which accounts for another 15%. The remaining costs are due to drugs.

Functional Anatomy and Ultrastructure

Arterial Blood Supply

Two arteries, the left and right coronary arteries, originate from the aorta ascendens at the level of the base of the heart (i.e., at the root of the aorta). These vessels and their main branches course over the surface of the heart before penetrating the myocardium.

The right coronary artery supplies the right atrium, a large portion of the right ventricular free wall, the cone of the right ventricle, and small posterior portions of the interventricular septum and of the posterior left ventricular wall. This pattern is found in most human and porcine hearts. In the dog, on the other hand, the right coronary artery does not perfuse significant portions of the left ventricle.[2] The conducting system comprising sinoatrial and atrioventricular nodes, the atrioventricular bundle and its right fasciculus, are usually supplied by the right coronary artery. However, in about 40% of human hearts, the sinoatrial node is supplied by the left coronary artery.

The left coronary artery has two main branches, the left anterior descending branch and the left circumflex branch. The left coronary artery supplies the left atrium, the front of the left ventricular free wall, small portions of the right ventricular free wall, the cardiac apex, the front and lower portions of the interventricular septum, and the posterior lateral wall of the left ventricle. The left fasciculus of the atrioventricular bundle is supplied by both the left and right coronary arteries.

Macroscopic anastomoses between right and left coronary arteries with diameters up to 500 μm are found throughout the ventricular walls; their density in humans is lowest in the epicardium. However, collateral flow has traditionally been considered inadequate to maintain function of the affected ventricle or to reduce infarct size if blood supply to the high-energy-demand myocardium of the left ventricle is acutely impaired. There is now recent evidence for considerable collateral blood flow in patients with chronic coronary artery disease.[3] Thus coronary arteries should no longer be considered "end arteries" without collaterals.

Microscopic anastomoses with diameters less than 90 μm have also been identified in experimental chronically collateral-dependent canine myocardium. Such a system may be of significance in ischemia resulting from small-vessel obstruction.[4] The clinical relevance of such small collaterals is not known.

Arterioles are defined histologically as containing a single smooth muscle cell layer in the media. Physiologically speaking, however, arterioles are the small arterial vessels with diameters less than 100 μm, which makes them a significant but not the sole controller of coronary resistance. The autonomic nervous system directly innervates small arteries and arteriolar smooth muscle. There may be up to one nerve ending per arteriole providing the anatomical substrate for autonomic influence on coronary resistance. Autonomic nerve fibers also run parallel to the large coronary arteries. These nerve fibers form varicosities in the adventitia of the larger vessels and thus innervate only the outer smooth muscle layer. It has also been shown that autonomic fibers form direct contacts with the endothelium. The exact role of these endothelial nerve endings is not clear, but they might be involved in the regulation of capillary flow and/or endothelial permeability.

Vascular smooth muscle cells are spindle-shaped, 5 to 10 mm in diameter in their widest portion, 35 to 100 μm in length, and capable of finely graded but relatively slow contractions. The cell surface area is increased by 25% to 70% by membrane invaginations (caveolae), which are located strikingly close to (within 5 nm of) mitochondria. There is also a close spatial association between mitochondria and the sarcoplasmic reticulum, which actively takes up, stores, and releases calcium required for mechanical activity. Vascular smooth muscle cells probably constitute a nonsyncytial system, which allows for precise local resistance control by minimizing electrical activations across cellular boundaries. Unlike in heart and skeletal myocytes, there is no transverse tubule system that can carry the electrical activation close to the cell center. The vascular smooth muscle cell is approximately 10 times smaller than the skeletal muscle fiber. Diffusion distances for intracellular ions, second messengers, and other solutes are thus relatively small. In the larger-striated (heart, skeletal) myocytes, excitation–contraction coupling is facilitated by the transverse tubule system. This system greatly reduces the distances between membrane calcium channels and the sarcoplasmic reticulum, which effects the calcium-induced calcium release producing contraction (see Rüegg[5] for review). Smooth muscle cells, much like skeletal myocytes, contain up to 2000 mitochondria/cell (1 to 13 mg mitochondrial protein per gram of tissue);

but cardiomyocytes contain many more mitochondria, up to 50 mg mitochondrial protein per gram of tissue. The presence of mitochondria in smooth muscle explains observed couplings between smooth muscle oxygen uptake and developed tension.[6,7] Interestingly, vascular smooth muscle also has the capability to generate more than 15% of its adenosine triphosphate (ATP) demand through anaerobic glycolysis.[6] When this feature is considered in context with the very low energetic cost of smooth muscle tension development (30-fold to 500-fold lower compared with skeletal muscle[7]), it becomes plausible why vascular smooth muscle contraction has conventionally been considered to be virtually independent from local oxygen concentration or tissue P_{O_2}. However, isolated coronary arteries in vitro can relax in response to even mild degrees of hypoxia, but whether this may be mediated by the endothelium is controversial (see section titled "Oxygen" under "Mediators of Metabolic Coronary Flow Regulation").

Capillaries and Endothelium

Capillaries do not contain vascular smooth muscle and adventitia but consist of a single layer of endothelial cells surrounded by a basement membrane. Capillaries are abundant in mammalian hearts (about 300,000 to 500,000 capillaries/cm²). The cells are about 0.2 μm thick except in the region of their nucleus. The mean intercapillary distance in the myocardium, that is, the distance over which nutrients, oxygen, carbon dioxide, and other metabolites, as well as hormones, drugs, and anesthetics must be transported and/or diffuse, is about 18 to 20 μm. The diffusion of molecules is inversely related to their molecular weight or radius but directly proportional to concentration gradient and absolute temperature. Thus, temperature changes in the near-physiologic range have only negligible influence on metabolite transport by diffusion. There is about one capillary for each muscle fiber in both heart and skeletal muscle, and this relation appears to remain constant when the heart hypertrophies (the size of the myocyte increases, not the number of myocytes), which implies that diffusion distances increase and that capillary growth does not normally keep pace with myocyte growth during hypertrophy. In normal heart muscle, capillary density (number of capillaries per centimeter squared) is about 2.5-fold higher than in skeletal muscle. This results from the fact that the skeletal muscle fiber is about 50 μm in diameter compared with about 20 μm in diameter for the heart muscle fiber. For faster solute exchange between blood and interstitium, functional capillary pores of 5 Å have been postulated, but their existence could not be confirmed by electron microscopy.

Endothelial cells extend around the entire inner circumference of small vessels and capillaries. The extremes of these cells often overlap to form apparently long endothelial clefts. These junctions may allow for relatively fast junctional transport or for ultrafiltration of solutes including lipid substances up to the size of plasma proteins. Functional coronary endothelium channels allowing free passage of charged adenine nucleotides in colloid-free perfused hearts have been identified.[8] Besides diffusion and junctional transport, pinocytosis and transport via fused vesicles that can form transiently open channels across the entire endothelial cell are known to occur. In functional terms, the capillaries of the heart have been estimated to be about 15 times more permeable to small molecules than those of skeletal muscle.[9] Nevertheless, cardiac capillaries are continuous and nonfenestrated and thus much less permeable than, for instance, the discontinuous capillaries of liver sinusoids that have large physical gaps of 1 μm or more. For some metabolites such as vasodilator adenosine and other purine nucleosides, the anatomical continuity of cardiac endothelium establishes a physical and metabolic barrier. There is a relative impermeability to 0.2 to 1.0 μM adenosine via intracoronary application. Most likely, one reason for this barrier function of the endothelium is its rich endowment with enzymes of purine nucleoside metabolism,[10] which allows quick degradation of adenosine to inosine, xanthine, and hypoxanthine.[8] The activity of the interconvertible xanthine oxidase, the enzyme that catalyzes the formation of urate from hypoxanthine, is extremely low in human, porcine, and rabbit coronary endothelia in contrast to rat and guinea pig coronary endothelia.[11] Endothelium also contains glycogen, ATP, adenosine diphosphate (ADP), adenosine monophosphate (AMP), creatine phosphate, adenylate kinase plus the full enzyme cascade for adenosine formation (5′-nucleotidase), degradation (adenosine deaminase, purine nucleoside phosphorylase), and rephosphorylation (adenosine kinase).[12] Since endothelium has creatine kinase,[13] free ribosomes, and mitochondria, these cells, much like vascular smooth muscle and striated cardiomyocytes, have at their disposal complete glycolytic and oxidative–phosphorylation outfits for anaerobic and aerobic energy production, respectively. However, endothelium comprises only about 2% to 3% of total myocardial mass.[14] Nevertheless, it is not a metabolically inert cobblestone layer of capillaries or larger vessels. The discovery by Furchgott[15] that it also can elaborate specific vasoactive factor(s) (see section titled "Specific Aspects of Coronary Control Linked to Endothelium") has furthered acceptance of the concept that the endothelium comprises a biologically and metabolically highly active system integrated in and modulating the overall function of the coronary and other vascular beds. Moreover, under pathophysiological conditions there can be direct neutrophil–endothelium interactions facilitated by complement activation in response to myocardial ischemia. The activated neutrophils migrate transvascularly, which is associated with production of cytotoxic oxygen-derived free radicals, short-lived highly reactive oxidizing agents known to contribute to reperfusion injury (see Lucchesi[16] for review).

Venous Drainage

All major veins open into the coronary sinus, which is about 3 cm long and situated in the posterior atrioventricular groove of the heart. The coronary sinus ends in the right atrium between the orifice of the inferior vena cava and the atrioventricular orifice. A semilunar incompetent valve marks the ending of the coronary sinus. The great cardiac vein begins at the cardiac apex and runs parallel to the left anterior descending branch, then curving to the left and reaching the back of the heart to open into the coronary sinus. It receives several tributaries and drains the left atrium and both ventricles. The small cardiac vein runs between the right atrium and the ventricle posteriorly, receiving blood from the right atrium and right ventricle. The oblique vein of the left atrium descends obliquely on the back of the left atrium and ends in the coronary sinus near its ending. All major veins except the oblique vein are provided with valves at their openings into the coronary sinus. Several veins do not end in the coronary sinus: the anterior cardiac veins collecting blood from the anterior wall of the right ventricle open directly into the right atrium; the thebesian veins comprise a number of minute veins within the ventricular walls that open directly into the right atrium and the ventricles. Thebesian flow is small, perhaps about 2% of total coronary flow; the relative magnitude of thebesian flow into the heart chambers depends on the pressure gradients between the veins and the chambers; thus thebesian flow into the left ventricle is smaller than into the right ventricle or right atrium.

Lymphatic Drainage

The myocardium has three lymphatic plexuses: subendocardial, midmyocardial, and subepicardial. Direction of lymph flow is from endocardial to subepicardial plexus from which right and left collecting channels originate. Vessels of the left ventricle converge into a main lymph channel that can be visibly identified at the base of the left atrium and the anterior surface of the pulmonary artery and that then connects to the cardiac lymph node. The rate of cardiac lymph flow is increased with perfusion pressure, inotropic state, and sympathetic nerve stimulation. Basal flow rates are about 2 to 3 mL/h in the dog heart. The ionic composition of lymph is essentially the same as that of plasma, but protein content is reduced by 25% to 50%; also a few thousand red and white blood cells per milliliter can be found in cardiac lymph. Macromolecules such as intracellular enzymes (e.g., creatine kinase, lactate dehydrogenase) have been found in the lymph during or following 15- to 20-minute periods of myocardial ischemia.[17]

Regulation of Coronary Flow

There are seven major factors controlling myocardial perfusion. The two main physical determinants are the driving coronary perfusion pressure and the opposing intramural myocardial compressive forces. A third is the myogenic vascular smooth muscle tone, which is in essence the contractile response of smooth muscle to a quick stretch or a physical stimulus; the mechanism is not known but may include stretch-related calcium influx or increased spontaneous electrical activity of the smooth muscle itself. The other factors are ultimately chemical in nature: (1) the local and humoral factors, (2) the influence of the autonomic nervous system (adrenergic and cholinergic neural control), (3) the metabolically related chemicals and vasodilator factors (metabolic coronary control) elaborated in the working myocardium in response to altered oxygen demand or cardiac oxygenation, and (4) the vasoactive factors of endothelial origin. Other rheological factors such as hematocrit and plasma viscosity become important under clinical conditions of hemodilution or severe hemorrhages; hemodilution and decreased plasma viscosity reduce coronary resistance whereas hemoconcentration and increased plasma viscosity increase coronary resistance.

During the cycle of a single heartbeat coronary flow is characteristically phasic rather than constant, although mean aortic and mean right atrial pressures are normally constant from beat to beat. The phasic nature of this instantaneous coronary flow reflects the interplay of the physical rather than chemical determinants during the cardiac cycle. Myogenic, neural, metabolic, and endothelial factors, on the other hand, exert their influences over several beats or even a longer time base and can minimize changes in coronary flow utilizing the vascular myogenic tone mechanism or adjust flow on a sustained basis due to altered steady-state levels of neural or metabolic vasoactive factors.

Myocardial oxygen extraction is already very high in the heart beating at rest, so myocardial perfusion is characterized by yet another unique feature. Coronary sinus PO_2 is lower than the venous PO_2 in most other vascular beds, 20 to 25 mm Hg. As a result the arteriovenous oxygen concentration difference across the coronary circulation is 10 to 15 vol% larger than the arteriovenous oxygen concentration difference across most other organs (compared with kidney the difference in oxygen extraction is even larger). In adult men the heart's mass is about 0.4% of total body mass, and coronary flow, 0.8 to 1.0 mL/min per gram, is about 4% of resting cardiac output of about 5 to 6 L/min. For comparison, the kidney constitutes 0.5% of the body mass but receives 20% of resting cardiac output. The overperfused kidney can thus significantly increase oxygen consumption by simply increasing the oxygen extraction, whereas the heart, already extracting at rest a relatively large amount of oxygen, meets altered oxygen demand primarily through altered coronary flow (i.e., through adjustments of oxygen delivery).

Coronary Perfusion Pressure

Net coronary driving pressure normally is the aortic root pressure (80 to 120 mm Hg in healthy humans) minus the right atrial pressure (0 to 5 mm Hg). If there is a severe coronary artery stenosis the effective coronary inflow pressure is the pressure distal to the obstruction. During the cardiac cycle ejection of blood can only occur when intraventricular pressures exceed aortic root or pulmonary artery pressures, respectively; these pressure gradients open the one-way semilunar valves, allowing the heart to move blood volume down the pressure gradients into the aortic or pulmonary artery outflow tracts. During early ejection the myocardium continues to increase contractile force (auxotonic ventricular contraction), thus increasing the effective ejection pressure; this results in a further rise in aortic root pressure and hence coronary perfusion pressure. When the ventricles relax at the end of systole, intraventricular pressures rapidly fall below aortic and pulmonary root pressures, resulting in closures of the aortic and pulmonary valves. The aortic valve closure produces the dicrotic aortic notch that marks the beginning of diastole. During ventricular diastole, coronary inflow pressure essentially equals diastolic aortic root pressure, and the intraventricular pressures rapidly fall to values close to zero and then only slightly rise toward the end of diastole (end diastolic pressure) due to ventricular filling. Effective coronary perfusion pressure is thus well maintained during diastole, although the ventricles are relaxed and do not actively generate pressure.

An important aspect of left coronary artery inflow is that it is predominantly diastolic, although the inflow pressures are higher during systole than during diastole. In other vascular beds, tissue perfusion is mainly systolic, but in the normal heart 60% to 80% of left coronary inflow occurs during diastole. This is in part due to the shorter duration of systole compared with diastole; more important are the effects of extravascular coronary resistance caused by compressive forces of the contracting myocardium surrounding intramyocardial coronary arteries. During tachycardia, because of shorter diastoles, as well as during acute myocardial failure, especially when combined with high heart rates, myocardial perfusion during diastole decreases(i.e., there is a relative increase in the systolic portion of myocardial perfusion).

Coronary vascular resistance is not solely regulated at the level of the smallest arterioles; rather, the entire microvasculature, arterioles, capillaries, and venules contribute. Direct pressure measurements at different levels within the microcirculation of the beating cat heart indicate that 95% of the resistance resides in microvessels <300 μm in diameter; more than 50% resides in the precapillary resistance vessels <100 μm in diameter (i.e., the small arterioles[18,19]). Also, microvessels and arterioles <150 μm in diameter are more sensitive to vasodilator adenosine than the large epicardial vessels. Maximal pharmacological coronary dilation shifts a portion of the resistance to the larger arterioles and venules, such that now up to 30% of total resistance resides in the venules that normally account for only about 7% to 10% of the resistance.[18] In dog foreleg, skeletal muscle vasodilators, such as histamine, can reduce the small vessel resistance even below that of the large arteries.[20] Thus, in contrast to traditional views, the small coronary arterioles do not account for nearly the entire coronary resistance, especially not during maximal coronary dilation.

Myocardial Tissue Pressure

Intramyocardial pressure, a major determinant of the extravascular coronary resistance, varies considerably and characteristically during the cardiac cycle. During systole the myocardium compresses the intramural vessels, thus effectively reducing the driving coronary perfusion pressure. In the left ventricle, systolic compression initially produces a precipitous fall of coronary inflow. Sometimes left coronary flow even reverses direction to become a transient, but brief, flow out of the coronary artery. Inflow remains low during systole despite the rising aortic pressure. When intramyocardial pressures are enhanced by aortic outflow tract obstruction or β-adrenergic inotropic stimulation, phasic left coronary flow tracings usually record an early systolic, albeit transient, backflow in dogs. In hypodynamic decompensating ventricles, on the other hand, systolic left circumflex flow constitutes a relatively larger fraction of total coronary inflow (see Olsson et al.[21] for review). In the right coronary artery, the phasic coronary inflow component during systole is about as large as the diastolic flow component. This physiologic difference between right and left coronary artery phasic flows is most probably due to the lower systolic compressive forces in the myocardium of the right ventricle.

Myocardial tissue pressure is not uniform across the ventricular wall. In the endocardial portion intramyocardial pressure approximates left ventricular chamber pressure; consequently it is close to left ventricular end diastolic pressure (LVEDP), about 3 to 6 mm Hg, at the end of diastole in the normal heart. Similarly, systolic in-

tramyocardial pressure is maximal in the inner layer, intermediate in the middle layer, and nearly zero in the outer layer. Systolic compression of intramyocardial arteries is therefore much more effective in the inner than outer layers. One important physiological consequence is that inner myocardial layers receive arterial blood only during diastole.[22,23] Interestingly, this does not appear to limit total flow to the inner layer in the normal dog heart even during strenuous exercise. Feigl[24] reports that flow to the inner layer at rest was even slightly higher (about 10%) than that to the outer layer and remained essentially equal to that of the outer layer during exercise. During isolated left heart failure (e.g., due to severe acute myocarditis, aortic valve stenosis, and subvalvular [muscular] aortic stenosis), LVEDP and hence diastolic tissue pressure, particularly in the inner myocardial layer, can be markedly elevated, especially during exercise. If the right ventricle is functioning normally, diastolic inner layer pressure in the left ventricle will be higher than the coronary sinus outflow pressure in the right atrium. Under such conditions the driving pressure for left coronary inflow is reduced, because it equals the difference between aortic root pressure and intramyocardial pressure rather than the overall arteriovenous pressure gradient. This can lead to subendocardial ischemia, especially during exercise, even in the absence of macroscopic coronary artery abnormalities due to atherosclerosis.

Humoral and Local Factors

Numerous humoral and local factors are potential modulators of coronary vascular resistance. Circulating epinephrine from the adrenal medulla can cause direct mild coronary dilation, whereas circulating norepinephrine causes coronary constriction. Angiotensin II is a powerful arteriolar constrictor peptide, formed via circulating angiotensinogen (the substrate for renin) from angiotensin I, which is cleaved by angiotensin-converting enzyme (ACE), a dipeptidyl-peptidase, to release the biologically active vasoconstrictor angiotensin II. ACE is present in high concentration in the luminal membrane of capillary endothelial cells. Renin, a proteinase highly selective for circulating angiotensinogen, is principally stored by the juxtaglomerular cells of the afferent arteriole of the kidney. This proteinase is released in response to (1) a sustained decrease in renal arterial pressure, (2) an increase in renal sympathetic activity or circulating catecholamines, (3) a decrease in distal tubular sodium due to lowered plasma sodium, and (4) other factors including potassium and prostaglandins.

Renin activity and ACE have also been demonstrated in isolated cardiomyocytes and perfused rat hearts. Cardiac ACE is concentrated in the atria, coronary vasculature, conduction system, and cardiac valves. The cardiac renin–angiotensin system is fully functional, being independent of the circulating system and responsive to chronic sodium loads.[25] Chronic dietary sodium, diuretics, and a chronically elevated sympathetic discharge are therefore clinical complications that could influence the cardiac renin–angiotensin system and thus long-term coronary microvascular or arteriolar tone.

Serotonin (5-hydroxytryptamine) is stored in high concentration in platelets and usually produces coronary constriction upon platelet disintegration. A hypothetical circulating ouabain-like factor remains ill-defined, but it might cause coronary constriction much like ouabain itself, the specific cardiac glycoside that inhibits Na^+, K^+-ATPase and depolarizes the cell membrane, resulting in smooth muscle contraction.

Bradykinins belong to a class of polypeptides generated by proteolysis of α_2-globulins catalyzed by kallikrein, an enzyme present in plasma and tissue fluids. Bradykinins have short half-lives of a few minutes due to inactivation by carboxypeptidase. Kallikrein itself is normally inactive; it becomes activated by nonspecific stimuli such as tissue damage, hemodilution, and blood contact with nonnatural surfaces such as glass or certain plastics. A kallikrein inhibitor of the body fluids deactivates kallikrein. Bradykinins are strong coronary dilators, and they also increase capillary permeability, resulting in edema. Histamine from mast cells and eosinophils is usually released in response to tissue damage. Histamine, much like bradykinin, is a general vasodilator with additional effects on capillary permeability; it plays a role in inflammatory vasodilation, edema formation, and allergic reactions.

Prostaglandins and thromboxanes are formed from arachidonic acid, a cell membrane constituent, in the cyclooxygenase reaction in myocardium and many other tissues. These substances are derived from phospholipids, but they are not stored in cells; instead they are rapidly synthesized and released in response to a variety of physiological and pharmacological stimuli. This class comprises potent vasoconstrictors (e.g., prostaglandin $F_{2\alpha}$), vasodilators (e.g., prostaglandin E_2), and platelet aggregators (thromboxane A_2). Collectively these compounds are referred to as eicosanoids; their synthesis is highly sensitive to aspirin or indomethacin inhibition. Eicosanoids are rapidly degraded in a single pass through the pulmonary circulation. Needleman[26] and others reported that ischemic and hypoxic myocardium, as well as hearts subjected to excessive workloads, release increased amounts of vasodilatory prostaglandins. However, prostaglandin synthesis requires oxygen, indicating that these substances do not cause ischemic or anoxic coronary dilation. In addition, indomethacin has inconsistent effects on coronary autoregulation or reactive hyperemia following a brief period of ischemia or sustained hypoxia. Also, during exercise hyperemia in the heart, prostaglandins appear to be synthesized with a delay only after the metabolically linked coronary dilation is fully established.

Neuropeptides such as substance P (vasodilator), neurotensin (vasoconstrictor in some species), neuropeptide Y (vasoconstrictor of adrenergic nerve endings), and enkephalins (modulators of local release of norepinephrine) have diverse effects on coronary vascular smooth muscle. Also, the roles of two other local neuropeptides, α-neoendorphin and somatostatin (vasoactive peptide of the parasympathetic system), are presently ill-defined. Some of the neuropeptides are mitogens, which raises the possibility that they may be involved in stimulation of coronary collateral growth. It has also been suggested that these or similar agents may be involved in the pathophysiology of coronary spasm.

In general, most if not all of the local and humoral factors mentioned appear to modulate or potentiate, not substitute for, the classical neurotransmitters. Also, it remains difficult to link these factors stoichiometrically to the known strict correlations between coronary flow and acute myocardial energy usage, or the state of cardiomyocyte oxygenation during hypoxia or ischemia. It is this type of problem that continues to raise skepticism that, indeed, at least some of these local and humoral factors may be physiologically crucial controllers of coronary flow. Thus, major revisions about what has been established concerning autonomic, myogenic, metabolic, and endothelial coronary control mechanisms may not be required, at least as far as the regulation of coronary flow under physiological and the major pathological conditions (i.e., hypoxia, ischemia, reactive hyperemia) is concerned.

Myogenic Control

A manifestation of active myogenic coronary smooth muscle tone is the relative constancy of total coronary flow over the aortic pressure range from 60 to 140 mm Hg in blood-perfused hearts. Over this pressure range the coronary flow versus perfusion pressure curve is flatter than above and below this range (i.e., flow changes only slightly despite substantial changes in perfusion pressure). This phenomenon is known as the autoregulation of coronary flow. Coronary flow autoregulation is quite substantial because the flow–pressure curve becomes virtually horizontal (flow totally independent from pressure) when the effects of altered myocardial oxygen consumption (which turns on metabolic controls) caused by altered aortic pressure and hence ventricular afterload are accounted for adequately.[27,28] Efficient flow autoregulation also exists in other major vascular beds (e.g., those of kidney and brain). Coronary flow autoregulation is not dependent on neural or circulating humoral factors, since it is retained in denervated completely isolated heart preparations that are perfused with oxygenated Krebs-Henseleit media, which does not contain plasma factors, platelets, or hemoglobin[27,29,30] (see Figure 5.1). It is also not mediated by metabolically

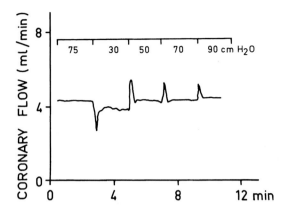

FIGURE 5.1. Dynamic coronary flow–pressure relations in the normoxic completely isolated and denervated nonworking guinea pig heart. To stabilize the heart energetically, it was perfused with 2 mM pyruvate as the main energy-yielding substrate in presence of 95% O_2/5% CO_2.[27,29] To minimize myocardial oxygen demand, the heart was *empty beating*, a term that means it was not generating isovolumic intraventricular pressure, nor was it performing external pressure–volume work. Original tracing displays mean coronary inflow rate monitored with an electromagnetic flow meter. Upper x-axis refers to mean coronary perfusion pressure at the aortic root. A rapid and maintained reduction in perfusion pressure from 75 to 30 cm H_2O was followed by a rapid initial decrease in coronary flow that subsequently increased toward the control value. Conversely, after a sudden increase in perfusion pressure, the flow was initially elevated, but returned within 2 to 3 minutes toward the value measured before the pressure change. Steady-state flow rates before and after pressure changes were almost identical in this heart, if the step changes in pressure were in the range between 50 and 90 cm H_2O. The mean physiological aortic pressure in the guinea pig is about 90 cm H_2O. The pressure steps did not alter spontaneous heart rate, but did alter myocardial oxygen consumption. Between 50 and 90 cm H_2O, coronary flow autoregulation was virtually perfect.[27] The autoregulatory range at subphysiological pressures extends to levels as low as 40 cm H_2O (about 30 mm Hg) in isolated guinea pig hearts. Perfused heart data from R. Bünger. For corresponding data from heart in situ see Olsson et al.[21]

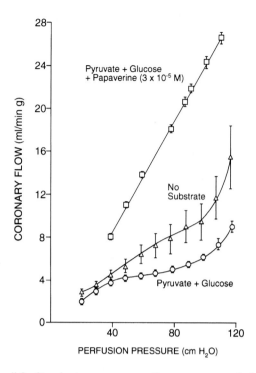

FIGURE 5.2. Steady-state coronary flow–pressure relations in normoxic completely isolated and denervated nonworking guinea pig hearts. Hearts that were energetically stabilized by 95% O_2 and pyruvate plus glucose as substrates almost completely autoregulated coronary flow over the range 50 to 80 cm H_2O. Such hearts were also characterized by low levels of interstitial adenosine (<0.1 μM) as judged by epicardial purine nucleoside levels.[27] When hearts were perfused at constant pressure without metabolic substrates, coronary flow increased steadily over time[29] and autoregulation was markedly impaired; such substrate-free perfused hearts, although normocapnic and normoxic, were deenergized, exhibiting markedly elevated interstitial adenosine levels (up to 0.8 μM,).[27] When a maximal dilatory dose of papaverine was added to the perfusion medium of autoregulating and energetically stable hearts, coronary flow increased twofold to fourfold and became an essentially linear function of perfusion pressure. Thus, pharmacological paralysis of vascular smooth muscle abolishes coronary autoregulation entirely. Perfused heart data from R. Bünger.[29] For corresponding data from heart in situ see Olsson et al.[21]

linked vasoactive chemicals such as adenosine, because interstitial vasodilator adenosine levels increase rather than decrease during autoregulatory increases in coronary resistance in response to rising perfusion pressures.[27]

Not all investigators believe that coronary autoregulatory constriction reflects the intrinsic ability of vascular smooth muscle to contract in response to increased stretch (rising perfusion pressure [Bayliss response]) or to relax in response to decreased stretch (falling perfusion pressure). Direct microvascular pressure measurements have clearly shown, however, that coronary dilation due to decreased pressure predominantly occurs in small vessels with diameters of 100 μm or less (i.e., near or at the level of the small arterioles).[18] Since most known vasoactive chemicals linked to cardiac energy metabolism are coronary vasodilators, these agents would attenuate, not mediate, the flow-minimizing autoregulatory resistance increase during rising aortic pressure, which in turn increases ventricular afterload and thus normally stimulates oxidative myocardial metabolism. Thus, if a vasodilator drug such as papaverine is infused into the coronary arteries, autoregulation is completely abolished, that is, the flow–pressure curve is now linear, with a marked increase in slope; the characteristic relatively flat portion that occurs over the autoregulatory range has been abolished by a coronary dilator substance (Figure 5.2).

Above and below the normal autoregulatory range, coronary flow is strongly dependent on coronary perfusion pressure. The absence of autoregulation at low perfusion pressures is not due to exhaustion of the vasodilator reserve, because coronary blood flow can still be increased pharmacologically at these low pressures. Also, a transmural difference across the ventricular wall in coronary autoregulation has been noted by some investigators: the capacity of the epicardial arteries to autoregulate flow is larger than that of the endocardial vessels[21]; the mechanism of these differences in the autoregulatory capacity is not understood.

Coronary flow–pressure autoregulation minimizes intravascular volume. This may be considered an oxygen sparing effect, since it minimizes myocardial oxygen consumption in response to altered aortic pressure, a feature known as the Gregg or garden hose phenomenon. Besides conserving oxygen, coronary flow autoregulation obviously also protects the microcirculatory structures from sustained hypertension and, importantly, maximizes the delivery of arterial blood to the body.

Neural Control

Coronary artery vessels have a modest adrenergic α-receptor constrictor mechanism and also a powerful β-receptor dilator mechanism (see Feigl[24] for review). Sympathetic α-adrenergic constrictor fibers store and release norepinephrine from their nerve endings. The coronary smooth muscle β-receptors are relatively insensitive to norepinephrine but highly responsive to pharmacological β-adrenergic agonists such as isoproterenol. However, electrical stimulation of cardiac sympathetic nerves of the heart in situ or infusion of norepinephrine into isolated perfused guinea pig hearts produces large increases, not the expected α-adrenergic decreases, in coronary flow. This coronary dilation is one classical example for what is commonly known as *metabolic coronary dilation*, since it is mainly secondary to metabolic cardiomyocyte stimulation in response to the β-adrenergic positive chronotropic and positive inotropic effects of norepinephrine. The norepinephrine stimulation of cardiac function and hence oxidative myocardial metabolism occurs mainly in the working cardiomyocytes. The myocytes, according to the metabolic flow control hypothesis, produce local metabolic vasodilator factors, which in turn prevail over the norepinephrine α-adrenergic vascular constriction. The modest α-adrenergic constrictor component becomes unmasked when the β-adrenergic receptors are blocked with propranolol. According to Holtz and Bassenge[31] and Feigl,[24] basal coronary flow and the metabolic vasodilation during sympathetic activation are both reduced by about 30% due to the primary α-adrenergic constriction; this is a relatively small effect when compared with the coronary dilator reserve of greater than 400%.

The physiologic α-adrenergic constrictor tone probably acts synergistically with the more powerful myogenic constriction in response to stretch. Opposing these adrenergic and myogenic constrictor effects is an apparently tonic vasodilator release due to nitric oxide (NO) from endothelial cells: inhibition of endothelial NO formation by 10 mM N^G-methyl-L-arginine reversibly decreases basal coronary flow in constant pressure–perfused guinea pig hearts by 19%.[21] However, the normal balance between these three factors does not greatly raise basal coronary flow (i.e., the net effect of these mechanisms maintains coronary flow at a markedly low rate despite a very large oxygen extraction).

In the dog a marked parasympathetic coronary vasodilation can be demonstrated when the vagal decrease in heart rate is prevented by electrical pacing. This effect of vagus stimulation can be blocked by the classical muscarinic antagonist atropine and mimicked by acetylcholine (ACh).[24] As Furchgott and Zawadzki[32] discovered, the vasorelaxant effect of ACh, in contrast to that of adenosine, requires an intact endothelium, which releases a factor, the endothelial-derived relaxant factor, that is chemically indistinguishable from NO[32,33] (e.g., see section "Specific Aspects of Coronary Control Linked to Endothelium").

When the carotid sinus baroreceptors are subjected to hypotension they elicit reflex activation of sympathetic cardiac fibers. Again, the reflex tachycardia, increased cardiac work, and contractility produce metabolic vasodilation that is somewhat limited by the direct α-receptor–mediated vasoconstriction. Carotid baroreceptor hypertension, on the other hand, results in inhibition of cardiac sympathetic discharge accompanied by an increase in parasympathetic tone. The resulting change in coronary flow may be minimal, because reduced heart rate and contractility lower coronary flow via reduced metabolic vasodilator mechanisms that act synergistically with the vasodilation due to reduced α-adrenergic tone but oppose active parasympathetic vasodilation.

The carotid body chemoreceptors are stimulated by nicotine; when stimulated by hypoxia or hypercarbia they produce hyperpnea. This appears to inhibit the sympathetic α-receptor coronary constriction, thus resulting in a modest coronary vasodilation (see Feigl[24] for review). Dogs also have a pulmonary hyperinflation reflex, probably mediated by stretch receptors within the lung, that produces a modest vagally mediated increase in coronary flow.

Metabolic Control

Because the myocardial capacity for anaerobic energy production via glycolysis is only 10% to 13% of the energy requirements of a heart performing physiological pressure–volume work,[34,35] hydraulic cardiac work performance strongly depends on mitochondrial oxidative phosphorylation; normal mitochondrial energetic function in turn requires the supply of oxygen and metabolic substrate. In blood-perfused hearts, transcoronary oxygen extraction is about 60% to 70% at rest and can increase to about 90% during maximum exercise, resulting in a fall of coronary sinus P_{O_2} from near 20 mm Hg to below 10 mm Hg. According to Severinghaus[36] such a fall in P_{O_2} corresponds to a decrease in oxyhemoglobin saturation from nearly 27% to 7% in humans, which reaches the limits imposed by the kinetics of oxygen binding to hemoglobin under intravascular conditions. Thus, only minor increases in myocardial oxygen consumption (MVO_2) of about 30% are possible by means of increased oxygen extraction alone. Most physiologic increases in MVO_2 are much larger, twofold to fourfold above resting MVO_2. Such changes in oxygen demand can only be met by increased oxygen delivery (i.e., by increased coronary blood flow). This principle is the basis of the long-established and essentially linear correlation between coronary flow and MVO_2 (for review see Feigl[24]). This nearly obligatory and direct flow–MVO_2 relation also is one of the foundations of the metabolic hypothesis for the control of coronary blood flow.

Metabolic coronary control is independent from neural input, because flow and MVO_2 are also directly related in ex vivo hearts perfused with donor blood. Humoral factors are also not essential, because isolated heart preparations perfused with oxygenated saline media still control coronary flow as a direct essentially linear function of MVO_2. The coronary circulation thus represents a vascular bed wherein blood flow is primarily under the control of mechanisms linked to the energy metabolism of the heart whose mechanically working myocytes are the quantitatively paramount users of oxygen.

Skeletal muscle and brain circulation also show a strong metabolic flow control component. A distinctive feature of a vascular bed under metabolic control is that the basal vascular resistance is high relative to the rate of energy expenditure or ATP turnover. The relatively high but physiological basal coronary resistance does not compromise myocardial energetics or ventricular function; it seems to be mediated by the intrinsic smooth muscle myogenic constrictor tone in combination with the tonic α-adrenergic discharge, both of which are only modestly attenuated by endothelial NO as detailed previously. Efficient metabolic flow control may thus mainly rely on vasoactive metabolites, which are primarily vascular smooth muscle relaxants that modulate or, if necessary, completely override the basal vasconstrictor tone. This concept does not postulate a single vasodilator metabolite uniquely related to all kinds of metabolically induced changes in coronary resistance; it also does not imply that flow control mechanisms based on vasodilatory metabolites may not be redundant. The potential role intramyocardial oxygen (tissue P_{O_2}), which is not a metabolite of myocardial metabolism, may play in the context of metabolic coronary control is covered in the detailed description of individual candidate chemicals for metabolic flow control. Note also that metabolic flow control via vasoconstrictor metabolites may theoretically be possible, but no examples are known.

In contrast to heart, the kidney and lung are examples in which basal vascular resistance is very low. Thus blood flow is high relative to the rate of energy use and is not directly determined by substrate and oxygen demand. Accordingly, the kidney can appreciably change oxygen extraction in addition to blood flow to meet changes in ATP turnover. It is interesting to note that, again, in contrast to heart and skeletal muscle, vasoactive adenosine is an afferent arteriolar constrictor not dilator in the kidney.

Endothelial Factors

The vascular endothelium is a single layer of squamous epithelial cells lining the inner circumference of blood vessels. A number of vasoactive factors produced by the endothelium serve a modulating role in regulating coronary vasomotor tone.[108,109] These factors include the relaxing factors, NO and prostacyclin (PGI_2), and vasoconstrictor factors such as various endothelins. These substances are produced by vascular endothelial cells under basal conditions and when activated by neurotransmitters, autacoids or physical stimuli. They act on the vascular smooth muscle cells in a paracrine (autacoid) fashion. Other important functions served by the endothelium include (1) uptake and metabolism of norepinephrine, serotonin, and purine nucleosides (e.g., adenosine); (2) conversion of angiotensin and bradykinin by ACE and other peptidases; and (3) production of anticoagulant and antiplatelet substances (prostacyclin), fibrinolytic substances (plasminogen activator), procoagulants (von Willebrand factor), and connective tissue macromolecules. Endothelial-dependent modulation of coronary blood flow also interacts with the metabolic, hormonal/humoral, and neural control mechanisms already described.[15]

Myocardial Energy Charge Versus Thermodynamic Phosphorylation Potential

As coronary blood flow adjusts to the acute myocardial energy use, the essence of metabolic coronary control appears to maintain or optimize the energy balance of the cardiomyocytes. The system operates to match energy supply to energy use, thus preventing cellular energy state to fall below physiologically safe limits. The *energy charge*, a complex metabolite ratio relating the *total chemical contents* (designated by curly brackets) of cardiac adenylates, is defined as follows:

$$\text{Energy charge} = (\{ATP\} + 1/2\{ADP\})/ (\{ATP\} + \{ADP\} + \{AMP\})$$

This ratio has originally been used to quantitate cellular energy state.[37] However, cardiac adenylates are strictly compartmented between cytosol and mitochondria and further subcompartmented due to ADP binding to actin and myofilaments and to AMP sequestration in the mitochondria.[38–40,66] It is therefore difficult to attach any thermodynamic meaning to the energy charge ratio. Also, the ratio is not stoichiometrically involved in physiological or metabolic processes. The concentration terms in the expression for the energy charge do not represent those actually occurring at the sites of cellular metabolic reactions.

An index that is thermodynamically meaningful is the phosphorylation or energy state of cytosolic ATP, also termed *phosphorylation potential*, and defined as the following metabolite ratio:

$$\text{Phosphorylation potential (of ATP)} = [ATP]/([ADP] \cdot [P_i])$$

The rectangular brackets designate the free concentrations of the adenylates within one subcellular compartment as distinct from their total myocardial contents that ignore cellular metabolic units such as cytosol and mitochondria. Total tissue metabolite contents comprise cytosolic plus mitochondrial free levels plus those fractions that are bound to, for example, contractile proteins, kinases, and adenosine triphosphatases (ATPases); total metabolite content thus refers to *free content* plus *bound content* plus contents of all subcellular solvent spaces. Only the free adenylates in a given subcellular compartment have biochemical impact on metabolic reactions (i.e., only their concentrations in free solution refer to the thermodynamically relevant amount in that compartment). Adenylates that are bound to cytoplasmic actin or sequestered by mitochondria do not impact the pathways of energy metabolism, ion transport, or phosphate transfer of the cytoplasm.

The $[ATP]/([ADP] \cdot [P_i])$ ratio has real meaning, being the concentration term of the expression that describes the free energy change of ATP hydrolysis in the cytosol or that of ATP synthesis in the mitochondria. Normally mitochondrial oxidative phosphorylation determines the level of $[ATP]/([ADP] \cdot [P_i])$ in the cytosol. Although ATP is the immediate energy source for all major endergonic cellular activities, the actual amount of energy per mol ATP, that is, the free energy change of ATP hydrolysis, termed ΔG_{ATP}, is a function of the energy state of ATP—the $[ATP]/([ADP] \cdot [P_i])$ ratio—not of the ATP concentration per se, according to the following formula:

$$\Delta G_{ATP} = \Delta G°_{ATP} + R \cdot T \cdot \ln([ADP] \cdot [P_i]/[ATP]),$$

where $\Delta G°_{ATP}$, the standard free energy change (-7.73 kcal/mol $= -32.3$ kJ/mol at 38°C, ionic strength $= 0.25$),[50] is nearly constant under most physiologic conditions and many reversible pathological conditions, provided intracellular free magnesium level and intracellular pH are also near normal. R indicates gas constant (1.98 cal/mol $\cdot$ K), T indicates absolute temperature ($273°C + 37°C = 310$ K for normal body temperature), and ln indicates natural logarithm.

ΔG_{ATP} values for ATP hydrolysis/synthesis in the cytosol normally range between -57 and -60 kJ/mol ATP in cardiac muscle. The $[ATP]/([ADP] \cdot [P_i])$ ratio of the heart varies greatly as a function of physiologic or pathologic states, between about 2000/M during extreme stress and ischemic deenergization and 50,000/M to 100,000/M during rest and the absence of hydraulic workloads. ΔG_{ATP} sustains cellular sodium and calcium homeostases and powers the organ-specific cellular functions. In cardiac muscle the obviously most important physiologic functions are contraction, ejection, and relaxation followed by filling. Also physiologically very important to the cells is the sodium homeostasis, which is directly dependent on $[ATP]/([ADP] \cdot [P_i])$[41] in accordance with the $3:2/Na^+:K^+$ stoichiometry of the Na^+,K^+-transport ATPase[42]:

$$3\,Na^+_i + 2\,K^+_o + ATP <\!\!=\!\!=\!\!=\!\!> \\ 3\,Na^+_o + 2\,K^+_i + ADP + P_I$$

$$[ATP]/([ADP] \cdot [P_i]) = K_{eq}. \cdot [Na^+_o]^3 \cdot \\ [K^+_i]^2/([Na^+_i]^3 \cdot [K^+_o]^2)$$

The Na^+ pump catalyzes the active transport of Na^+ ions from the cytoplasm across the cell membrane to the interstitium, utilizing the energy of ATP hydrolysis in the cytosol as the driving force. This process strictly follows the preceding reaction, and its stoichiometry is given by the mass-action equation as indicated. When the Na^+ gradient across the sarcolemma collapses (e.g., during severe ischemic cardiomyocyte deenergization and trauma), the Na^+–Ca^{2+} exchanger of the cell membrane becomes active and mediates increased calcium influx; this can lead to a dangerous intracellular calcium overload. Calcium accumulation can threaten cellular survival because it may cause contracture and stimulate proteases, phospholipases, and endonucleases that, when active on a sustained basis, produce structural cellular and DNA damage and irreversible cellular autolysis and/or programmed cell death (apoptosis).[43,44]

$[ATP]/([ADP] \cdot [P_i])$ also is strictly linked to the chemical reactions of the calcium pumps (Ca^{2+}-ATPases) at sarcoplasmic reticulum and plasma membranes. Thermodynamics dictate that the electrochemical potential of the cellular Na^+ or Ca^{2+} gradients cannot be larger than ΔG_{ATP}. Ca^{2+} reuptake into the sarcoplasmic reticulum can only take place when ΔG_{ATP} is larger than the energy in the Ca^{2+} gradient across the sarcoplasmic reticulum membrane. The extent and direction of the reactions of the ion transport ATPases are governed by mass-action relations and the level of ΔG_{ATP} as well, not by receptor-mediated second messengers. It has been estimated that a ΔG_{ATP} of about -50 kJ/mol ATP is sufficient to drive the major cellular cation pumps.[45] Stability and minimum level of [ATP]/([ADP] $\cdot$ [P_i]) is thus crucial for cellular cation homeostasis. Calcium homeostasis is particularly important because cardiomyocyte relaxation requires cytosolic free calcium near 0.1 μM, a level four orders of magnitude below the concentration of the extracellular or intravesicular sarcoplasmic reticulum calcium. [ATP]/([ADP] $\cdot$ [P_i]) is also stoichiometrically involved in mechanical muscle shortening, providing the energy for cross-bridge cycling and myofilament sliding, and hence for contractile force, hydraulic work output, and the state of contractility. Obviously, the maximum possible hydraulic work is limited by ΔG_{ATP} and also influenced by the energetic efficiency of the contractile apparatus as a whole. Note that unlike receptor-linked second messengers [ATP]/([ADP] $\cdot$ [P_i]) does not directly influence sensitivity (K_M) or the speed (V_{max}) of ATPases or kinases.

Indicators of Phosphorylation Potential

[ATP]/([ADP] $\cdot$ [P_i]) cannot be directly measured because the free concentrations of ADP in the cytosol are below the detection limit of current nuclear magnetic resonance technologies and also below that of microanalytic enzymatic-optic and high-performance liquid chromatography techniques. Since in muscle most ADP is bound to actin, measurements of total heart muscle ADP grossly overestimate the thermodynamically relevant free ADP concentration ([ADP]), which is the term that appears in the denominator of the [ATP]/([ADP] $\cdot$ [P_i]) ratio. However, there are four readily measurable metabolite indicators of [ATP]/([ADP] $\cdot$ [P_i]) that can be used to assess the level and/or directional change of [ATP]/([ADP] $\cdot$ [P_i]). These indicators are illustrated in Figure 5.3 and described in detail in the next section.

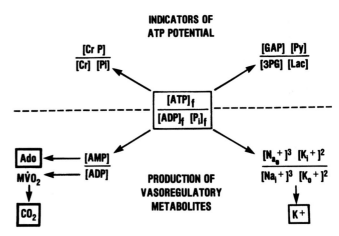

FIGURE 5.3. Proposed relation between myocardial energy state and vasoactive cardiac metabolites. Lower portion of figure: proposed link between the production of vasoregulatory metabolites (adenosine [Ado], carbon dioxide [CO_2], and potassium ion [K^+]) and the cytosolic ATP phosphorylation potential, [ATP]/([ADP] $\cdot$ [P_i]) ratio (as described in text).[66,67] All concentration terms of [ATP]/([ADP] $\cdot$ [P_i]) refer to the free cytosolic concentrations (emphasized by the subscript f) of the reactants in the cardiomyocytes, not to their overall myocardial contents. It is only when this constraint applies that this metabolite ratio is thermodynamically relevant and accordingly has real physical meaning. This stipulation is especially important in heart and skeletal muscle (and probably smooth muscle and brain, too), because here the bulk of extramitochondrial ADP is bound to actomyosin and therefore does not influence [ATP]/([ADP] $\cdot$ [P_i]), the index of the energy state.[21,66] Note that free cytosolic AMP ([AMP]), the immediate precursor of adenosine, is integrated with [ATP]/([ADP] $\cdot$ [P_i]) via the myokinase whose reactants are ATP, ADP, and AMP. Thus, the cytosolic concentration of free AMP, [AMP], is *energy-linked* and so are all AMP degradatives. [ADP], the free cytosolic concentration of ADP, serves as substrate for oxidative phosphorylation and hence is directly related to MVO_2; it also is the precursor of cytosolic AMP, and hence adenosine, and has a number of allosteric effects including stimulation of phosphofructokinases or *endo*-5'-nucleotidase. Upper portion of figure: intracellular indicators of [ATP]/([ADP] $\cdot$ [P_i]) as described in text. CrP, creatine phosphate; Cr, creatine; P_i, orthophosphate; GAP, glyceraldehyde-3-phosphate; 3PG, 3-phosphoglycerate; Py, pyruvate; and Lac, lactate. Subscripts o and i in the $N[K^+_i]^2/(N[Na^+_i]^3 N[K^+_o]^2)$ ratio refer to extracellular and intracellular ion concentrations (strictly speaking to their activities), respectively. (Graph reproduced from Olsson and Bünger.[67])

[CrP]/([Cr] $\cdot$ [P_i]) Ratio

[ATP]/([ADP] $\cdot$ [P_i]) is stoichiometrically linked to the [CrP]/([Cr] $\cdot$ [P_i]) ratio (CrP indicates creatine phoshate; Cr, creatine; and P_i, orthophosphate) via the pH- and Mg^{2+}-dependent creatine kinase. This is true for heart, skeletal muscle, vascular smooth muscle, brain, and also endothelium, and for all cellular systems that contain a creatine kinase/mitochondria system powerful

enough to catalyze a near-equilibrium reaction between ATP-dependent phosphorylation of creatine at mitochondrial sites and creatine phosphate-dependent rephosphorylation of ADP at cytosolic sites. Therefore, in such tissues, free [ATP]/[ADP] and [ATP]/([ADP] $\cdot$ [P_i]) can be assessed by measuring the reactants of creatine kinase (creatine phosphate, creatine, H^+), inorganic phosphate, and intracellular volume.[39] The formal expression that relates these equilibria is[49]

$$[ATP]/([ADP] \cdot [P_i]) = \\ [CrP]/([Cr] \cdot [P_i]) \cdot [H^+]/K_{CK}$$

The pH and Mg^{2+} dependence of the creatine kinase equilibrium constant K_{CK} was investigated by Lawson and Veech.[46] A convenient operational relation linking pH_i and K_{CK} is as follows[8,49]:

$$K_{CK} = [H^+]/antilog_{10}(7.52 + (3.12 \cdot [\text{free cytosolic} \\ Mg^{2+}]^{0.11}) - (0.97 \cdot pH_i))$$

Free Mg^{2+} and pH_i may be estimated using complex indicator metabolite computer routines and/or highly sophisticated ^{31}P-nuclear magnetic resonance (NMR) technologies as adapted by Mallet et al.[8,47] and defined by Radda and Veech,[48] respectively.

$[GAP] \cdot [PYR]/([3PG] \cdot [LAC])$ Ratio

$[ATP]/([ADP] \cdot [P_i])$ is also stoichiometrically linked to glycolysis, at the level of the powerful combined glyceraldehyde-3-phosphate dehydrogenase/phosphoglycerate kinase (GAPDH/PGK) system. Thus, $[ATP]/([ADP] \cdot [P_i])$ can be assessed using the measured $[GAP] \cdot [PYR]/([3PG] \cdot [LAC])$ ratio (GAP indicates glyceraldehyde-3-phosphate; PYR, pyruvate; 3PG, 3-phosphoglycerate; and LAC, lactate),[49,51] provided net metabolic fluxes through glycolysis and lactate dehydrogenase (LDH) are small (<5%–10%) compared with the total activities of GAPDH/PGK and LDH.[49] It is important to note that only under such conditions can these exclusively cytoplasmic enzymes (GAPDH, PGK, LDH) be assumed to catalyze near-equilibrium reactions, a prerequisite to reach acceptable values for $[ATP]/([ADP] \cdot [P_i])$ based on the $[GAP] \cdot [PYR]/([3PG] \cdot [LAC])$ ratio. This condition obtains in heart muscle at low glycolytic rate such as the nonworking Langendorff heart model.[49] The following relation has been found to hold in guinea pig hearts and superfused rat liver cells[49-51]:

$$[ATP]/([ADP] \cdot [P_i]) = [GAP] \cdot [PYR]/([3PG] \cdot \\ [LAC]) \cdot ([H^+]/K_{LDH}) \cdot (K_{G+G}/[H^+])$$

The pH and Mg^{2+} dependence of the $K_{GAPDH} \cdot K_{PGK}$ was investigated by van der Meer and Tager et al.[51]; a computer fit of this exponential relation is published in Bünger et al.[49] Note that the $[GAP] \cdot [PYR]/([3PG] \cdot [LAC])$ ratio is useful in assessments of cytosolic $[ATP]/([ADP] \cdot [P_i])$ in nonmuscle tissues (liver, kidney), which contain little or no creatine kinase, but of course only if near-equilibrium constraints are met. Also, measurements of the $[GAP] \cdot [PYR]/([3PG] \cdot [LAC])$ ratio does not require sophisticated ^{31}P-NMR equipment, knowledge of intracellular water volume or pH_i, or measurements of cytosolic phosphate.

Extracellular Potassium

$[ATP]/([ADP] \cdot [P_i])$ is stoichiometrically linked to the distribution of sodium and potassium ions across the cell membrane, the reaction being catalyzed by the Na^+,K^+-ATPase as described previously. Therefore, a fall in $[ATP]/([ADP] \cdot [P_i])$ will result in an increase in extracellular K^+ concentration,[41] which can be readily measured. Thus, increased myocardial potassium release usually indicates a decrease in $[ATP]/([ADP] \cdot [P_i])$.

Released Adenosine and Other Purines

There are good examples in which changes in $[ATP]/([ADP] \cdot [P_i])$ can be judged, albeit not in quantitative terms, from directionally similar changes in extracellularly released ATP/AMP degradatives.[27,38,39,52,66-69] These compounds are diffusible phosphate-free purine nucleosides (i.e., adenosine, inosine, and hypoxanthine); urate is a degradative of xanthine that appears in coronary venous blood only when cardiac endothelium contains active xanthine oxidase as in rat and guinea pig heart, but not normally in pig, rabbit, and human heart. The relation between adenosine degradatives and myocardial energy state (see Figure 5.8) is derived from the cytosolic $[ATP]/[ADP]$ ratio, which is an integral component of $[ATP]/([ADP] \cdot [P_i])$ while stoichiometrically and obligatorily linked to cytosolic free AMP (via myokinase[39]), whose hydrolytic dephosphorylation (via 5'-nucleotidase) yields adenosine. Thus, increased production and release of purine nucleosides such as adenosine and inosine often signal a fall in the $[ATP]/[ADP]$ ratio, which is often, but not always,[53] the consequence of a fall in $[ATP]/([ADP] \cdot [P_i])$.[55,67] Relatively small increases in intracellular free magnesium can also stimulate adenosine formation because Mg^{2+} is an allosteric activator of cytosolic or *endo*-5'-nucleotidase,[8,54] the enzyme generally considered to catalyze the dephosphorylation of AMP to adenosine (see Figure 5.8). Net adenosine plus degradative releases rise greater than free [AMP] when ATP-dependent purine reutilization by *salvage* pathway enzymes (adenosine kinase, hypoxanthine phosphoribosyltransferase) becomes less intense due to cardiac deenergization during, for example, hypoxia.[52] These relations qualify for inclusion under the concept of *energy-linked* production/reuptake of purine nucleosides[55]because both intracellular free AMP and the capability to rephosphorylate adenosine/hypoxanthine are linked to cytosolic $[ATP]/[ADP]$ and hence $[ATP]/([ADP] \cdot [P_i])$, the index of myocardial energy state.[66]

There is also an energy-independent (extracellular) component of cardiac purine nucleoside release. The extracellular source of cardiac purine nucleosides is based on interstitial AMP rather than cytosolic free AMP as the precursor of released adenosine.[8,55] Because interstitial AMP is located extracellularly, it is physically separated from the free AMP pool of the cytosol. Unlike cytosolic free AMP, interstitial AMP is not integrated in or stoichiometrically coupled to the cytosolic adenylate system. Therefore, the production of vasodilator adenosine based on interstitial AMP is not linked to $[ATP]/([ADP] \cdot [P_i])$. The extracellularly formed adenosine would thus not fall into the category of vasodilator metabolites coupled to myocardial energy metabolism and would therefore not qualify for consideration by the metabolic hypothesis of coronary control. Indeed, at the normally extremely low cytosolic AMP levels of around 100 nM, levels characteristic of the well-oxygenated and highly energized myocardium, the residual adenosine/inosine release is extremely low, about 5 nmol/min per gram dry mass (Figure 5.4), and may be in part due to hydrolysis of interstitial AMP by *ecto*-5′-nucleotidases.[8] This residual rate is about 0.5% of the near-maximum rate observed during cardiomyocyte deenergization by severe low-flow ischemia.[56]

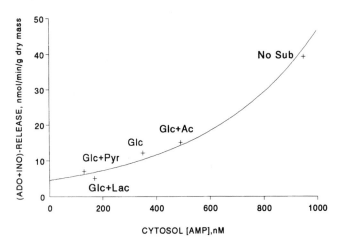

FIGURE 5.4. Observed relation between coronary venous purine nucleoside [adenosine (ADO) and inosine (INO)] release and estimated free cytosolic AMP in isolated perfused heart. Isolated nonworking guinea pig hearts were spontaneously beating at physiological aortic pressure and were normoxic and normocapnic.[27] Myocardial energy state, $[ATP]/([ADP] \cdot [P_i])$ and hence free [AMP], was varied in the absence of hypoxia (perfusion pressure of 87 cm H_2O, Krebs-Henseleit medium oxygenated with 95% O_2/5% CO_2) at normal intracellular pH (pH_i 7.15–7.25) by supplying favorable and unfavorable metabolic substrates according to Bünger et al.[27,29] The fitted smooth curve intersected the ordinate (free [AMP] = 0) at about 3 to 4 nmol/min per gram dry mass. Consequently, this residual rate was unrelated to intracellular free AMP and hence, $[ATP]/([ADP] \cdot [P_i])$. Such purine nucleoside release has been termed *energy-independent*.[55] Likely precursors for this portion of cardiac purine nucleosides are interstitial adenylates and possibly also the intracellular S-adenosylhomocysteine hydrolase (SAH) system, as discussed in text. No sub indicates substrate-free perfusion; Glc, 5 mM glucose; Ac, 5 mM Acetate; Pyr, 5 mM pyruvate; and Lac, 5 mM lactate. Graph based on data from Bünger et al.[55]

Another energy-independent purine nucleoside production mechanism is related to transmethylation pathways, the S-adenosylhomocysteine hydrolase (SAH) system. The hydrolysis of S-adenosylhomocysteine yielding adenosine and homocysteine is a product of S-adenosylmethionine-dependent transmethylation and not linked to cardiac energy metabolism.[57] It seems to account for up to 30% of basal adenosine release from normoxic guinea pig hearts. Not surprisingly, hypoxic perfusion that stimulates adenosine release by nearly two orders of magnitude has no effect on S-adenosylhomocysteine hydrolysis,[58] consistent with the prevalence of the energy-dominated pathways that couple adenosine release and reuptake to $[ATP]/[ADP]$ and cytosolic free AMP. Also, the activities of cardiac, liver, and renal SAH, are minute[58,61] and orders of magnitude smaller than those of powerful systems such as GAPDH, LDH, and creatine kinase.[59] SAH firmly binds over 90% of cardiac and renal adenosine.[60,61] The enzyme can release bound adenosine when intracellular magnesium levels increase.[61] However, the dissociation of the adenosine-SAH complex as assessed in vitro occurs with a half-life of over 2 hours,[60,61] a rate much too low to be of significance for metabolic coronary control.[60] Thus, the SAH concept of coronary flow control is incompatible with the metabolic flow control theory.

Linking Coronary Flow and Myocardial [ATP]/[ADP] or Phosphorylation Potential

Reductions in myocardial $[ATP]/[ADP]$ or $[ATP]/([ADP] \cdot [P_i])$ are associated with decreased coronary resistance under highly diverse experimental conditions. Prolonged metabolic substrate deprivation due to substrate-free perfusion can reduce $[ATP]/([ADP] \cdot [P_i])$ in isolated hearts, which is typically associated with rising interstitial adenosine levels and impaired autoregulatory constriction at increased coronary flow[27,29] (Figure 5.2). Similarly, inhibition of glucose oxidation by aminooxyacetate, a metabolic poison of the malate–aspartate shuttle, can reduce myocardial energy state and decrease coronary resistance, which is accompanied by a severalfold increase in lactate formation due to increased rate of glycolysis.[62] Dinitrophenol uncoupling of oxidative phosphorylation stimulates $\dot{V}O_2$max and cytosolic $[ATP]/([ADP] \cdot [P_i])$ falls while coronary flow rises.[63] Amytal inhibition of mitochondrial electron transport inhibits $\dot{V}O_2$max, $[ATP]/([ADP] \cdot [P_i])$ falls, and again coronary flow rises although, venous PO_2 and lactate production rise severalfold.[64] During maximal norepinephrine stimulation of cardiac function myocardial ATP turnover increases severalfold and myocardial $[ATP]/([ADP] \cdot [P_i])$ decreases in isolated and in situ hearts; this is associated with a large increase in coronary flow (but only a small increase in oxygen extraction) despite the primary α-adrenergic vasoconstrictor effect of norepinephrine (Figure 5.5). Ischemic insults decrease coronary resistance and are usually associated with marked declines in [ATP]/[ADP] and [ATP]/([ADP] · [P_i]), especially if the heart is inotropically stimulated in attempts to maintain cardiac output and aortic pressure.[56] Even during very short ischemic periods of only 2 minutes, [ATP]/([ADP] · [P_i]) decreases 64% in isolated rat hearts; this fall in [ATP]/[ADP] and phosphorylation potential is followed by increased adenosine and purine nucleoside production (inosine, hypoxanthine).[65] Similarly, in normoxic and normocapnic isolated hearts in which myocardial energy state is manipulated by altering metabolic substrate supply, [ATP]/([ADP] · [P_i]) is inversely and free [AMP] is exponentially related to the release of adenosine and its degradatives.[55] Coronary flow increases in substrate-free perfused energy-depleted hearts with low [ATP]/([ADP] · [P_i]) and high free [AMP][27] (Figure 5.6). Taken together these experimental data strongly imply or directly demonstrate a consistent and inverse relation between coronary flow and myocardial [ATP]/[ADP] or [ATP]/([ADP] · [P_i]). Because about 97% of the myocardium is nonendothelial mass, it is the predominant cardiomyocyte compartment whose energy state is monitored by chemical or ^{31}P-NMR assessments of [ATP]/[ADP] or [ATP]/([ADP] · [P_i]) reported in the literature. Consequently, cardiomyocyte [ATP]/[ADP] and [ATP]/([ADP] · [P_i]) and coronary resistance appear to be directly related under many physiological and pathophysiological conditions.

It has been reasoned[66] that it is the persistent, albeit limited, energy deficit actually incurred by the cardiomyocytes, characterized by the difference between acute energy production (ADP rephosphorylation) and actual energy utilization (ATP hydrolysis, ATP-dependent phosphorylations) that is the key to the observed decreases in [ATP]/([ADP] · [P_i]) during metabolic coronary dilation. Deficit-producing stimuli may be physiological in nature but encompass of course pathological, pharmacological, toxic, or traumatic incidents as well. For example, during infusion of norepinephrine into normoxic hearts, work output and hence ATP hydrolysis rise fully within 2 to 5 minutes, but the metabolically linked adjustments of coronary flow, $\dot{V}O_2$max, and substrate oxidation are delayed and require about 6 to 12 minutes for complete adjustment (Figure 5.5). During left ventricular failure caused by enzyme or mitochondrial blockade or due to substrate depletion, ADP rephosphorylation to ATP declines despite adequate oxygen supply. During myocardial ischemia or hypoxia, ADP accumulates in the cytosol and cannot be rephosphorylated primarily because accumulated mitochondrial–reduced nicotinamide-adenine dinucleotide (NADH)

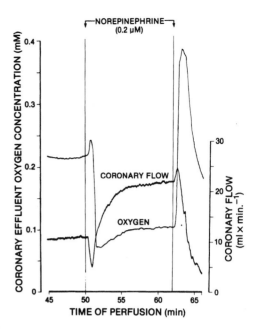

FIGURE 5.5. Time course of metabolic coronary dilation in response to near-maximum norepinephrine stimulation of a completely isolated working guinea pig heart. The heart was perfused with 95% O_2/5% CO_2 Krebs-Henseleit saline (arterial $[O_2]$ = 0.8 mM, P_{O_2} = 630 mm Hg) at constant preload (left atrial filling pressure = 12 cm H_2O) and constant mean aortic pressure of 80 cm H_2O. The oxygen tracing shows that myocardial O_2 extraction was about 79% prior to norepinephrine (NE) rising to 90% during norepinephrine stimulation, a 15% increase. Coronary venous P_{O_2} initially rapidly decreased from about 170 mm Hg to below 80 mm Hg during infusion norepinephrine. The venous P_{O_2} recovered only slightly, but there was a relatively slow, yet large curvilinear increase in coronary flow despite continued strong α-adrenergic constrictor input by norepinephrine. Thus, metabolically linked coronary dilator mechanisms overrode and outcompeted the imposed α-adrenergic constrictor tone. In such hearts, heart rate, intraventricular dP/dt, left ventricular peak pressure, and external pressure–volume work typically reach their new higher performance values in less than 4 minutes, whereas the full recruitment of oxidative phosphorylation and the new metabolic flow adjustment requires about 8 to 12 minutes.[122] Thus, full metabolic coronary adjustment lags behind the fast positive chronotropic and inotropic responses of the ventricles.[123] This is consistent with the notion that, during the norepinephrine transition, the stimulated cardiomyocytes incur a limited, nondamaging energy deficit that would be reflected by an adaptive fall in [ATP]/([ADP] · [P_i]); such a fall in cellular energy state is viewed as physiological, because it occurs at increased cardiac performance; it obviously does not jeopardize functional and energetic stability even at increased or maximum mechanical performance.[39,55,56] Data from R. Bünger. For corresponding data on time courses and an adrenoceptor-limited coronary dilation during severe exercise in dog see Murray and Vatner.[123]

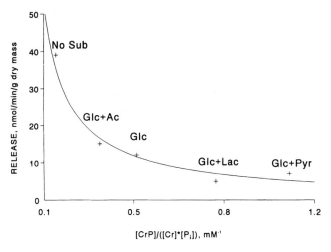

FIGURE 5.6. Reciprocal relation between intracellular $[CrP]/([Cr] \cdot [P_i])$ and coronary venous purine nucleoside release in normoxic, normocapnic myocardium. Hearts (described in Figure 5.4) were freeze clamped and extracted to measure $[CrP]/([Cr] \cdot [P_i])$, an index of cardiomyocyte $[ATP]/([ADP] \cdot [P_i])$. The observed changes in $[CrP]/([Cr] \cdot [P_i])$ occurred in fully oxygenated myocardium at normal intracellular pH. Similar physiological variations of $[CrP]/([Cr] \cdot [P_i])$ in the normoxic myocardium were reported previously.[39] These data demonstrate that $[ATP]/([ADP] \cdot [P_i])$ can vary substantially in the absence of oxygen deficiency, acidosis, or changes in intracellular free Mg^{2+}. Purine nucleoside (adenosine plus inosine) release rates increase when $[ATP]/([ADP] \cdot [P_i])$ decreases, most likely because free ADP and hence free AMP increase, according to the text and Figure 5.4. Thus marked variations in adenosine (plus inosine) release can be induced simply as a consequence of an adaptive, nonhypoxic fall in $[ATP]/([ADP] \cdot [P_i])$ caused, for instance, by switching metabolic substrate from predominantly pyruvate to predominantly acetate or the medium-chain fatty acid octanoic acid.

cannot be oxidized due to lack of oxygen. Thus, a commonality shared by substrate or oxygen deprivation, as well as metabolic poisoning and increased energy demand, is that cytosolic ADP accumulates and $[ATP]/([ADP] \cdot [P_i])$ falls. An important feature of this energy deficit concept is that it allows for ADP-linked AMP accumulation (via myokinase) and hence vasodilator formation (adenosine, potassium) in normoxic, oxygen-deficient, metabolically stressed, and damaged/poisoned hearts, simply as a function of the instantaneous cardiomyocyte energy state.[65–69]

Mediators of Metabolic Coronary Flow Regulation

A quantitative and causal relation to cardiomyocyte energy state, or its rate of ATP turnover, is considered the

key criterion that identifies a mediator of metabolic coronary flow control. Using this relatively broad definition even a compound such as oxygen, although not a metabolic product of mammalian cells, may qualify as a mediator of coronary flow. This is the case because intramyocardial concentration of oxygen (tissue Po_2) reflects the balance between oxygen usage (MVO_2) or ATP turnover by cardiomyocytes and O_2 supply by coronary blood flow. Most studies show that metabolic coronary control is not uniquely linked to a single tissue chemical; instead it appears to reflect the combined influence of several compounds including traditional vasodilator metabolites such as K^+ and adenosine, and possibly also the tissue oxygen concentration. Also, the relative impact of these mediators on coronary vascular tone appears to be affected by the particular conditions prevailing within the myocardium for a given physiological or pathological state. In the following sections, current candidates most plausibly involved in metabolic coronary control are described.

Oxygen

Myocardial ischemia and hypoxia are among the most powerful coronary dilator stimuli. Coronary vasoregulation could thus simply reflect a direct effect of myocardial Po_2 on the coronary microvasculature (independent from the cardiomyocytes' energy metabolism). Such a mechanism could either directly affect the energetics or the membrane potential and hence the function of the vascular smooth muscle or indirectly affect smooth muscle tone via an oxygen-sensitive endothelium that would elaborate vasoactive factors (e.g., prostaglandins). Such an oxygen-control model assumes that the local oxygen concentration (tissue Po_2) rather than coronary flow itself is the controlled variable. The model also assumes a hypothetical oxygen-sensitive resistance that would decrease in response to hypoxia (and conversely increase in response to hyperoxia) and is assumed to reside entirely within the microvasculature or small blood vessels.[70] One problem with this model concerns the unknown nature of the signal(s) from the microvascular sensor, which must be able to program endothelium or smooth muscle to precisely adjust the vessel's resistance to the instantaneous oxygen needs of the working cardiomyocytes. It seems conceivable that the coronary microvasculature might be uniquely engineered such that its potential oxygen sensitivity can preempt or minimize cardiomyocyte energy deficits by maximizing the level and stability of interstitial Po_2. A model of such forward control of coronary resistance by Po_2 could complement, not necessarily contradict, the classical metabolic flow control hypothesis, which is based on the premise that the energetic needs of the working myocytes are the primary mechanisms responsible for the release of vasoactive metabolites.

The basis of the oxygen-sensitive resistance model in cell physiology is speculative. Recent literature appears to implicate the ATP-sensitive potassium channel (K_{ATP}) of vascular smooth muscle. Historically, Noma[71] in 1983 first described a special outward K^+ current in rat cardiomyocytes (not in smooth muscle) that becomes uninhibited in response to extreme depletions of ATP to levels near 0.1 mM (normal cardiac ATP levels are between 5 and 9 mM). This current has been used to explain the hypoxic shortening of the cardiomyocyte action potential and the resulting decline in contractile force. More recently it has also been pointed out that submillimolar levels of free ADP (100–500 μM), known to be attained during moderate to severe myocardial ischemias and hypoxias, can open K_{ATP} channels in cardiac and vascular smooth muscle.[72,73] Thus, opening of the K_{ATP} channel prior to complete exhaustion of the ATP pool seems possible simply in response to a decrease in the free [ATP]/[ADP] ratio. Indeed, large changes in the cellular [ATP]/[ADP] ratio can occur, even without energetic failure, reflecting adaptive responses of the free adenylates to various cellular stimuli and metabolic stressors.[39,41,63,64,66,67,69]

Opening of K_{ATP} channels hyperpolarizes the smooth muscle cell membrane, thereby reducing the probability of open calcium channels; the resulting fall in cytosolic calcium promotes relaxation. Closure of the K_{ATP} channel depolarizes arteriolar coronary muscle from about −60 mV to −40 mV, resulting in increased vessel tone.[74] Daut et al.[75] observed that a 2-mM dose of the K_{ATP} channel blocker glibenclamide nearly completely blunted hypoxic coronary dilation as well as that due to exogenous adenosine in the potassium-arrested guinea pig heart. This raised the possibility that adenosine can act as a K_{ATP}-channel opener in coronary smooth muscle. Belloni et al.[76] used glibenclamide to inhibit adenosine coronary dilation in the normoxic fully energized dog heart in situ; and Olsson et al.[77] reported that glibenclamide caused rightward shifts of the dose-vasodilator–response curves of various synthetic adenosine receptor agonists, but not of adenosine itself, in the normoxic guinea pig heart. Thus adenosine may exert a twofold action on the microvasculature in the absence of smooth muscle deenergization, one of which comprises opening of the K_{ATP} channel and the other the pharmacological profile of an A_2-type vasodilator adenosine receptor agonist (for review see Olsson and Pearson[78]).

A weakness of the hypothesis of a physiologically appropriate oxygen sensitivity of the coronary smooth muscle K_{ATP} channel is that glibenclamide, when used in a nanomolar dose (50 nM) rather than the usual micromolar dose, did not decrease the amplitude of hypoxic coronary dilation but retained full selectivity against pharmacological K_{ATP}-channel openers.[79] This raises concerns regarding the selectivity of the micromolar doses of sulfonylureas usually applied in tests for possible physiological roles of the K_{ATP} channel. Mellemkjaer et al.[80] found involvement of the K_{ATP} channels in hypoxic coronary dilation only under conditions of severe smooth muscle deenergization due to glucose deprivation combined with 2-deoxyglucose inhibition of glycolysis. With glycolysis intact, relaxation of isolated porcine coronary arteries due to hypoxic PO_2s (about 20 mm Hg) were not blocked even by micromolar glibenclamide. During high-flow hypoxic vasodilations in situ, it is unlikely that glycolysis of coronary smooth muscle becomes inhibited at the level of GAPDH[81] because glucose and insulin are always present and the continued washout of lactate plus protons prevents intracellular accumulation of NADH and H^+. High-flow hypoxic or anoxic in situ conditions favor maximum glycolytic flux and anaerobic ATP synthesis, which according to Mellemkjaer[80] could imply that deenergization and K_{ATP} opening via the intrinsic mechanisms of the vascular smooth muscle are only of minor, if any, importance under such conditions. Also, removal of the endothelium only minimally attenuated hypoxic relaxation,[80] which is somewhat unexpected because previous reports by Pohl and Busse et al.[82,83] suggested that hypoxia stimulates the release of endothelial-derived relaxant factor.

It also seems unlikely that in the normoxic physiologically performing myocardium when stimulated, for example by norepinephrine, local PO_2 ever becomes low enough to effect a fall in smooth muscle internal [ATP]/[ADP] sufficient to deinhibit the vascular K_{ATP} channel. As mentioned, vascular smooth muscle generates >15% of total ATP via glycolysis already under aerobic conditions[6] (although glycolysis is highly restrained at the level of the phosphofructokinase) and has an uncommonly low energetic cost of tension development.[7] Obviously, this combination of high mechanical efficiency with substantial glycolytic capacity tends to reduce the dependence of the smooth muscle's [ATP]/[ADP] ratio on local oxygen. Moreover, oxygen demand by tension-developing arteries is at least 20 times lower[6,84,85] than the basal oxygen uptake of 2 to 4 μmol O_2/min per gram wet mass of working hearts,[24,35,39] which argues against the possibility that the [ATP]/[ADP] ratio of the coronary smooth muscle might be more sensitive to hypoxia than the ratio of the working cardiomyocytes.

Despite these arguments it has been established that isolated coronary arteries relax in response to even mild degrees of hypoxia. It might thus be assumed that oxygen-sensitive dilator mechanisms do exist in the vasculature but are independent from the [ATP]/[ADP] ratio of the smooth muscle. In this context, endothelial-derived vasoactive substances have been considered by some investigators and questioned by others.[80] Endothelial mediators under consideration include potent vasodilator prostaglandins (PGI$_2$, PGE$_2$), as well as NO. However, the mechanism by which a decreased ambient Po$_2$ triggers formation and release of nonmyogenic vasodilators in coronary arteries with intact endothelium is not known.[82,83]

The existence of graded hypoxic relaxations of isolated coronary arteries does not prove, but certainly raises the possibility, that Po$_2$-sensitive mechanisms may be available to the intact vessel within the working myocardium. To what extent the microvasculature in situ actually utilizes its intrinsic Po$_2$-responsive mechanisms, totally independent from the energy-linked signals from cardiomyocytes, is unknown. However, the interstitial level of oxygen itself contains metabolic information from the working cardiomyocytes, because the instantaneous tissue Po$_2$ reflects the difference between the rate of oxygen influx (determined by coronary resistance, perfusion pressure, and arterial Po$_2$) and the rate of oxygen uptake (dominated by the mitochondria-rich working cardiomyocytes). The intramyocardial [O$_2$] is thus partly under the influence of the respiration rate of the working cardiomyocytes. Although oxygen acts proximal to cellular energetics, its interstitial concentration could be responsive to the ATP turnover of the cardiomyocytes. Such a design could link the oxygen-control model of the vasculature to the oxidative energy metabolism of the cardiomyocytes (Figure 5.7).

Unlike adenosine, O$_2$ is a substrate for oxidative phosphorylation of ADP, not a vasoactive metabolite of myocardial energy metabolism; O$_2$ is not formed and released in proportion to the ATP turnover rate, or to a fall in the [ATP]/([ADP] · [P$_i$]) ratio in mammalian cells. But if decreased Po$_2$ could stimulate dilator mechanisms within the vasculature itself, the effects would help maximize interstitial O$_2$ concentrations, which in turn would maximize the capability of the cardiomyocytes to maintain [ATP]/([ADP] · [P$_i$]) within physiologic limits. Feigl[24] designated models in which tissue Po$_2$ is the controlled variable as substrate models in distinction to metabolite models in which MVO$_2$ (i.e., the rate of ATP turnover) controls coronary flow. Figure 5.7 indicates that the two models are not mutually exclusive. Also, the relative importance of local control by oxygen may be

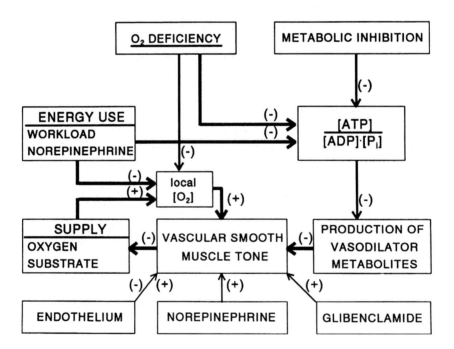

FIGURE 5.7. Integrated model of multifactorial metabolic and endothelial control of coronary tone. The three most important physiological variables are underlined. Proposed are two main elements of the metabolic flow control apparatus: they are the cellular energy state ([ATP]/([ADP] · [P$_i$])), or its major constituent free [ADP], and local Po$_2$ (local [O$_2$]). During normoxia, the system is designed to stabilize cardiomyocyte— [ATP]/([ADP] · [P$_i$])—or prevent adaptive responses beyond physiologically permissible limits. During hypoxia, the system elaborates vasoactive metabolites according to the fall in [ATP]/([ADP] · [P$_i$]), and the reduced local [O$_2$] may act synergistically at the vascular level to maximize relaxation; this would tend to minimize the hypoxic fall of [ATP]/([ADP] · [P$_i$]), thus improving the chances for full recovery from hypoxic injury. The endothelium modulates vascular smooth muscle tone by elaborating vasodilator factors and vasoconstrictor factors. These factors are released in response to a variety of chemical stimuli and also physical factors such as shear stress or cellular deformation. The latter trigger the release of the vasodilator NO.[124,125] The symbols (−) and (+) indicate that a change in one variable causes a reciprocal and parallel change, respectively, in another.

modulated by the energy state of the vascular smooth muscle,[80] while the relative importance of control by vasoactive metabolites appears to be determined by $[ATP]/([ADP] \cdot [P_i])$ of the cardiomyocytes (Figure 5.6). Common to both models is the feature to maximize both level and stability of cardiomyocyte $[ATP]/([ADP] \cdot [P_i])$ for a given increase in MVO_2 or decrease in myocardial O_2 concentration. It seems plausible that during moderate oxygen deficiency the potential intrinsic vascular mechanisms may become dominated by extrinsic signals generated by the cardiomyocytes. If for instance sufficient adenosine is released, it may directly bind to vascular vasodilator receptors and may induce opening of K_{ATP} channels resulting in smooth muscle relaxation even in the absence of vascular deenergization.

Carbon Dioxide/Hydrogen Ion

The preponderantly aerobic metabolism of cardiac muscle generates carbon dioxide (CO_2) continuously and in proportion to MVO_2, which is determined by the respiratory quotient. Being highly diffusible intramyocardial CO_2 has no difficulty reaching coronary resistance vessels. Changes in arterial P_{CO_2} produce consonant changes in coronary flow; therefore, hypercapnia increases and hypocapnia decreases coronary flow. Sorting out whether the coronary effects of CO_2 are due to gaseous CO_2 or to the protons generated consequent to CO_2 hydration is not possible, because CO_2 is rapidly hydrated, both nonenzymatically and by carbonic anhydrase, and the carbonic acid thus formed readily dissociates into HCO_3^- and H^+ at physiologic pH. The central issue here is the question: what is the relation between coronary flow and the concentration of intravascular CO_2 at the microvascular level? Because this relation is not known, the role of CO_2 gas in metabolic coronary control remains poorly defined. Also the mechanism that CO_2 might use to alter the contractile state of vascular smooth muscle is not clear. However, it has been demonstrated that hypercapnia enhances the vasoactivity of cardiac metabolites, such as adenosine,[86] suggesting that CO_2 may play an auxiliary rather than primary role in metabolic vasoregulation.

Potassium

The main source of endogenous K^+ is the beating cardiomyocyte itself, K^+ efflux occurring with each action potential. Net efflux of K^+ changes concordantly with heart rate, contractile force, or state of oxygenation. Fiolet et al.[41] have shown that myocardial ischemia causes a redistribution of Na^+ and K^+ across the sarcolemma in accordance with cytosolic $[ATP]/([ADP] \cdot [P_i])$; it is also predicted because this ratio is stoichiometrically coupled to the Na^+,K^+-ATPase (see section "Myocardial

Energy Charge Versus Thermodynamic Phosphorylation Potential"). Thus, severe myocardial deenergizations obligatorily raise intracellular Na^+ and interstitial K^+ levels. However, to what extent such K^+ redistributions contribute to ischemic coronary dilation is not entirely clear. The intracoronary administration of small amounts of K^+ (up to 12 mmol/L) causes dose-dependent yet transient coronary dilations in isolated guinea pig hearts, a response that can be inhibited by the specific the Na^+, K^+-ATPase blocker ouabain.[87] On the other hand, reactive hyperemias following short periods (up to 1 minute) of cardiac ischemia or coronary dilations in response to moderate hypoxias are only slightly inhibited by ouabain suggesting that K^+ plays only a limited role in this type of metabolic vasoregulation.[87,88] This was further detailed by Murray and Sparks[89] who examined open-chest normoxic dog hearts that were subjected to a step increase in heart rate by 75 beats per minute; this caused the expected sustained increase in MVO_2 and coronary flow. Coronary venous K^+ levels initially rose and reached a peak at 0.5 mmol/L higher than the control K^+ concentration. In six of nine dogs K^+ then declined to control, but coronary resistance did not increase. The three remaining dogs exhibited a sustained increase in coronary sinus K^+ levels. By considering the permeability–surface area product of K^+, the authors argued that interstitial K^+ reached levels that could account for about half the measured change in coronary resistance in these three dogs. In the six dogs wherein venous K^+ was elevated only transiently, other more powerful mechanisms must have been responsible for most, if not all of the sustained hyperemic response. The generally accepted view is therefore that potassium may facilitate the development, but not the maintenance of active coronary hyperemia.

Adenosine

Sixty-eight years ago Drury and Szent-Györgi[90] described the coronary dilator activity of adenosine and two years later Lindner and Rigler[91] proposed that adenosine may be the physiological regulator of coronary flow. Evidence accumulated over the past 30 years and reviewed by R. M. Berne implicates adenosine in blood flow regulation.[92] Adenosine may indeed play such a role (see next section), recently defined as a vasoactive metabolite linked to myocardial energy metabolism and $[ATP]/([ADP] \cdot [P_i])$. It has also become clear that there are at least three sources of adenosine in the myocardium: the major one is coupled to cardiomyocyte energy state, the other two are independent of it. The mechanisms of the latter two alternate pathways of myocardial adenosine formation are the SAH system and the interstitial adenylates, AMP in particular, as described previously.

Two enzymes, adenylate kinase (myokinase) associated with the intermembrane space of the mitochondria (this

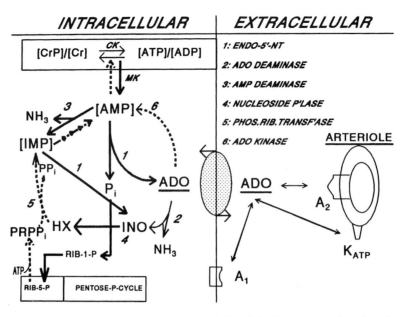

FIGURE 5.8. Simplified model of cardiomyocyte and endothelial adenosine metabolism. Thick solid arrows indicate catabolic pathways, thick dotted arrows synthetic or *salvage* pathways. Free intracellular AMP ([AMP]) is stoichiometrically coupled to the free intracellular [ATP]/[ADP] and hence the [ATP]/([ADP] · [P_i]) ratio via the myokinase reaction (MK). [ATP]/[ADP] is in near-equilibrium with the readily measurable [CrP]/[Cr] and [CrP]/([Cr] · [P_i]) ratios via the powerful creatine kinase (CK). AMP is the precursor of both adenosine (ADO) via the soluble *endo*-5'-nucleotidase (*endo*-5'-NT) and inosine monophosphate (IMP) via adenylate deaminase (AMP deaminase). Possibly, an acid phosphatase could also account for AMP dephosphorylation to adenosine within the cardiomyocytes, especially during extreme intracellular acidosis below pH 6.0. However, at the normal slightly alkaline intracellular pH 7.2, the cardiac acid phosphatase (pH optimum at 5.5) operates far above its pH optimum and is therefore nearly completely inactive[96]; this physiological pH inactivation is intensified by ATP, a powerful allosteric inhibitor ($K_i^{ATP} = 180$ μM) whose physiological concentration is 25-fold to 50-fold its K_i value. Adenosine deaminase (ADO deaminase, $K_M^{ADO} = 40$ μM) and purine nucleoside phosphorylase (nucleoside P'lase, $K_M^{INO} = 30$ μM, $K_M^{Pi} = 1$ μM) are predominantly located in the endothelium.[96] Adenosine inside the endothelium is deaminated to inosine (INO) via ADO deaminase. IMP may also directly contribute to overall myocardial inosine formation via the cardiomyocyte *endo*-5'-NT, or possibly via the Nees phosphatase.[27,96] Inside the endothelium the purine nucleoside phosphorylase reversibly catalyzes inosine interconversion into hypoxanthine (HX) and ribose-1-phosphate (Rib-1-P). HX can be recycled (salvaged) into the IMP pool via the HX phosphoribosyltransferase ($K_M^{HX} = 8$ μM) whose equilibrium is far on the side of IMP; the transferase uses 5-phosphoribose 1-pyrophosphate (PRPP$_i$) as the donor of the ribose-5-phosphate group and pyrophosphate (PP$_i$) is released. PRPP$_i$ is generated after mutation of Rib-1-P to ribose-5-phosphate (Rib-5-P), which in turn becomes pyrophosphorylated at the carbon-1 position by ATP to yield PRPP$_i$ and IMP, an extremely energy-costly process. The other important salvage enzyme is the adenosine kinase (ADO kinase, $K_M^{ADO} < 1$ μM) that readily rephosphorylates adenosine to AMP due to its high affinity; the kinase equilibrium is linked to [ATP]/[ADP] thus responding to myocardial energy state.[52] A hypoxic fall in [ATP]/[ADP] would reduce the ability of the kinase to rephosphorylate adenosine, which would increase the net release of adenosine and degradatives from the myocardium and amplify the effect of free cytosolic AMP on net release of purine nucleosides.[52] Net release of purines is the difference between adenosine purines formed and adenosine purines salvaged. Free intracellular adenosine can reversibly exit into the interstitial space via facilitated diffusion using the nucleoside transporter protein of the cell membrane (represented by dotted oval; $K_M^{ADO} = 35-320$ μM). However, adenosine (as well as other nucleosides) can cross the cell membrane by simple diffusion when the nucleoside transporter is blocked by drugs like dipyridamole. Interstitial adenosine has a number of physiological functions: It can bind to and stimulate the adenosine A_2 vasodilator receptor (stimulating adenyl cyclase) of vascular smooth muscle, the cardioprotective adenosine A_1 receptor (inhibiting stimulated adenyl cyclase) of the cardiomyocytes,[78,126] and perhaps also stimulate K^+ efflux by activating the hyperpolarizing K_{ATP} channel of the microvasculature.[76,77] However, the existence of a receptor for adenosine near or on the K_{ATP} channel of vascular coronary myocytes remains speculative; the number of interstitial binding sites for adenosine is unknown. The endothelium, comprising about 3% of myocardial mass, divides the extracellular compartment into its interstitial and intravascular components. If adenosine is taken up by the endothelium it becomes readily deaminated and further degraded to inosine and hypoxanthine. If however adenosine bypasses the endothelial cytoplasm by diffusing through functional endothelial pores, it crosses the endothelial metabolic barrier intact. Thus coronary sinus concentrations of adenosine and inosine are likely to differ from the interstitial concentrations of adenosine and inosine, especially when cardiac [ATP]/([ADP] · [P_i]) is high and interstitial nucleoside concentrations are low[27]; under such conditions the enzymatic capacity of the endothelium could suffice to quantitatively process the interstitial nucleosides. However, when the [ATP]/([ADP] · [P_i]) ratio decreases substantially due to maximal adrenergic stimulation, metabolic poisoning, anoxia or ischemia, interstitial adenosine concentration rises sharply thereby increasingly saturating the limited transport and metabolic capacities of the endothelium; this will result in increasing equality between interstitial and intravascular adenosine/inosine concentration ratios. Enzyme K_M values from pertinent references cited and Bergmeyer[127], respectively.

intracellular region is metabolically part of the cytosol, not of the mitochondrial matrix), and cytosolic 5′-nucleotidase couple intracellular adenosine production to [ATP]/[ADP] and hence the cellular energy potential (Figure 5.8). The myokinase equilibrium favors ATP formation from 2 molecules of ADP thereby generating AMP according to the following equation:

$$[AMP] = K_{MYK} \cdot [ADP]^2/[ATP] = K_{MYK} \cdot [ADP] \cdot ([ATP]/[ADP])^{-1},$$

where K_{MYK} is the equilibrium constant of the myokinase; K_{MYK} is pH-dependent and Mg^{2+}-dependent, and its value at physiologic temperature, intracellular pH of 7.2, and cytosolic free magnesium near 0.5 mM is about 1.0. Due to the power term $[ADP]^2$ of the myokinase equation, free [AMP] will increase exponentially at constant free magnesium and pH when [ATP]/[ADP] and hence [ATP]/([ADP] · [P_i]) decrease. Thus myokinase can operate as an amplification mechanism, effectively translating changes in cardiac energy state into changes in free cytosolic AMP levels.[67]

5′-Nucleotidase exists in two main forms, membrane-bound and cytosolic (soluble intracellularly). The distribution and regulation of the isoforms were recently reviewed by Newby et al.[93] Histochemically, *ecto*-5′-nucleotidase is located on pericytes in dogs and rabbits, not cardiomyocytes.[94] The enzyme irreversibly hydrolyses AMP to adenosine and orthophosphate (P_i):

$$AMP + H_2O ===> Adenosine + P_i$$

The K_M for AMP of the soluble cytosolic isoform, the *endo*-5′-nucleotidase, is not well-defined except that all published values are in the lower micromolar to millimolar range.[54,93] The rabbit, rat, dog, and pigeon cardiac *endo*-5′-nucleotidases have greater affinity for AMP than for inosine-5′-monophosphate (IMP)[95] (i.e., $K_M^{AMP} < K_M^{IMP}$ with alkaline pH optim). Free cytosolic concentrations of AMP in normoxia and moderate ischemia/hypoxia are likely in the submicromolar to lower micromolar range,[39,49,66–69] which renders the enzyme far from even half-saturated with AMP. It is activated by submillimolar ADP[95] (100–500 µM, which is also K_{ATP} channel-activating); this distinguishes the *endo*-form from the membrane-bound *ecto*-5′-nucleotidase which is inhibited by ADP and hypoxia. It is clear that activator ADP concentrations can rise severalfold from a normoxic level of 30 to 50 µM prior to any significant ATP pool depletion. This can account for normoxic and hypoxic cardiomyocyte adenosine and degradative formation in the absence of measurable declines in myocardial ATP contents. Like cellular kinases the 5′-nucleotidases are Mg^{2+} and pH dependent.[8] Anions like fluoride or metal ions like zinc and nickel are inhibitors. True end product inhibition by adenosine or inosine may occur; end-product inhibition by P_i requires millimolar levels and appears to inhibit more effectively IMP hydrolysis than AMP hydrolysis. In general the kinetics and regulation of the soluble *endo*-5′-nucleotidase appear suitable to maximize changes in adenosine formation in response to changes in [ATP]/([ADP] · [P_i]) at minimal expense to the cytosolic ATP pool, which ensures minimal loss of essential purine moieties during physiological and moderate pathological stresses.

From enzyme studies in highly purified isolated guinea pig cardiomyocytes compared to cardiac endothelium and pericytes, Nees et al.[96] concluded that the cardiomyocytes, which represent about 85% by volume of the ventricle, are virtually devoid of *endo*-5′-nucleotidase. The authors suggested instead that an acid phosphatase that is chiefly present (90%) in the myocytes and characterized by a 150-fold higher affinity for IMP ($K_M^{IMP} = 1.7$ µM) than AMP ($K_M^{AMP} = 250$ µM), would catalyze IMP hydrolysis (inosine formation), not AMP dephosphorylation (adenosine formation) at normal intracellular pH. If the Nees concept would apply to the intact myocardium, adenosine would be eliminated as a candidate for metabolic coronary control in all normoxic flow adaptations and nonacidotic hypoxic hyperemias as well. Skladanowski and Newby[93] have suggested that the Nees phosphatase may actually be a lysosomal 5′-nucleotidase based on K_M^{AMP} and acid pH characteristics. Judged by the V_{max}/K_M ratio, which measures the efficiency of an enzyme, the acid phosphatase is only about 10 times, not 150-fold more catabolically active with IMP than with AMP at pH 7.1.[96] Considering further that, in normal as well as deenergized but normocapnic guinea pig hearts, IMP levels are two orders of magnitude higher than free [AMP],[27] a greater rate of IMP than AMP dephosphorylation is plausible even based on the Nees kinetics of a soluble *endo*-5′-nucleotidase.[54,93] The fact that inosine, not adenosine, is often the main purine nucleoside released from normoxic or hypoxic hearts[27] does not necessarily imply that *endo*-5′-nucleotidase activity is negligible in the cardiomyocytes of the intact myocardium. Also, adenosine-derived inosine is formed when adenosine from deenergized cardiomyocytes is released into the interstitium and diffuses through endothelial cells wherein it will be deaminated by the adenosine deaminase (Figure 5.8). In addition, in normoxic normocapnic guinea pig hearts, interstitial adenosine can rise up to near 0.8 µM in response to substituting pyruvate metabolic substrate for the fatty acid octanoic acid, a maneuver that does not produce acidosis and is unlikely to produce local hypoxia.[27] Substantial normoxic interstitial adenosine levels are difficult to reconcile with the extremely low activity of the Nees acid phosphatase at normal intracellular pH with AMP as substrate. Also, it is interesting to note that during extreme intracellular acidosis (pH 5.5) the V_{max}/K_M ratio of the acid phosphatase with respect to IMP is 60-fold lower, not higher than that with AMP[96]; this implies a more efficient adenosine formation during cardiac ischemia, even if the acid phosphatase solely accounts for intracellular AMP or IMP degradation. Taken together the reported kinetics of the acid phosphatase, much like those of the endo-5′-nucleotidase, predict that adenosine formation during normocapnic normoxias or mild hypoxias is highly restrained, but that it increases strongly during ischemic acidosis, two predictions that have experimental support.

Cytosolic free AMP is the immediate precursor of both adenosine and IMP (Figure 5.8). The origin of most cardiac inosine, much like that of adenosine, is thus free AMP which is closely integrated with [ATP]/[ADP] and hence the $[ATP]/([ADP] \cdot [P_i])$ ratio. Endothelial cells contain the bulk of cardiac adenosine deaminase, and interstitial adenosine taken up by the endothelium is readily deaminated to inosine; thus coronary venous concentration of inosine probably reflects on the interstitial concentration of adenosine. The capacity of the endothelium to process interstitial nucleosides can become saturated, because endothelium comprises only a very small fraction of the myocardium, about 2% to 3%. Therefore the relations between coronary venous concentrations of adenosine or inosine, and interstitial concentrations of adenosine or inosine, respectively, are likely to vary as a function of the instantaneous interstitial nucleoside level. Also, convective transport through endothelial openings (see section titled "Capillaries" under "Functional Anatomy and Ultrastructure of Coronary Vasculature") will influence the coronary venous adenosine and inosine levels. Because of the complexity of these relations, current efforts are directed at the development of comprehensive computer models that can validly predict interstitial adenosine levels in relation to coronary resistance, using readily measurable coronary venous nucleosides, kinetics of myocardial enzymes, and levels of free adenylate.[97]

Many current estimates based on epicardial transudate analysis place the interstitial adenosine concentration in the normoxic heart close to 0.1 μM, a level considered at or below the threshold for coronary smooth muscle relaxation via the adenosine A_2 receptor. Adenosine is therefore considered not to contribute substantially to the control of basal coronary flow. This is consistent with the intrinsic strong myogenic coronary smooth muscle tone, the continuous α-adrenergic constrictor discharge (see section titled "Neural Control" under "Regulation of Coronary Flow"), the well-known inability of adenosine receptor blockers like methylxanthines to decrease basal coronary flow, and finally, also with the apparently tonic NO discharge, a vasodilator stimulus, from the endothelium.[21] As predicted by the metabolic hypothesis implicating free [AMP] and $[ATP]/([ADP] \cdot [P_i])$, adenosine formation and coronary resistance generally

change reciprocally during exercise, high flow myocardial hypoxia, reactive hyperemias, and cellular deenergization due to substrate deprivation (Figure 5.6) or metabolic poisoning.[63,64] Recently it has been shown that hypoxic or reactive hyperemic coronary dilations in the dog can be attenuated (24% or 28%, respectively), but not abolished when the adenosine A_2 receptor antagonist 8-phenyltheophylline is infused.[98] However, in isolated perfused guinea pig hearts, infusion of theophylline in doses that markedly attenuate coronary dilation caused by exogenously administered adenosine, has no appreciable effects on hypoxic or reactive coronary dilation.[88] Nevertheless, intracoronary infusion of adenosine deaminase (to deaminate a portion of interstitial adenosine to vasoinactive inosine) measurably inhibits hypoxic and reactive hyperemic coronary dilation by 20% to 30%.[99] These somewhat disparate and confusing effects of enzymatic adenosine inactivation versus pharmacological adenosine receptor blockade have made it difficult to assign adenosine a clear-cut quantitative role in metabolic coronary control. Nevertheless, the ambiguities resulting from the early adenosine deaminase and methylxanthine studies do not rule out a more definite action of adenosine in the absence of these interventions. These results also do not rule out an adenosine effect completely independent from the vascular A_2 dilator receptor such as opening of the vascular K_{ATP} channel, an adenosine effect that does not require prior deenergization of the coronary smooth muscle.[76,77] Adenosine opening of the K_{ATP} channel is blocked by sulfonylureas, and high doses of glibenclamide, but not methylxanthines, have been shown to blunt anoxic coronary dilation in the guinea pig heart.[75] The only moderate effects of adenosine receptor antagonists and adenosine deaminase on metabolic coronary control responses could perhaps suggest that adenosine is not essential for metabolic flow control in the heart; they certainly imply that multiple metabolically linked vasodilator systems exist that are redundant with the adenosine system.

Dipyridamole, an adenosine transport blocker, can markedly enhance myocardial reactive hyperemic flow possibly as a consequence of enhanced accumulation of interstitial adenosine. Also, adenosine vasodilator receptor blockade by methylxanthines has recently been reported to produce substantial increases in stimulated interstitial or coronary sinus adenosine levels under normoxic and hypoxic conditions.[100–103] Such interstitial adenosine accumulations could well account for the observed blunted-receptor–blocker potencies of methylxanthines during active or reactive/hypoxic myocardial hyperemias.[88,101,103] This is plausible because the interaction between adenosine and methylxanthines is competitive at the level of the vascular receptor.[104] Consequently, accumulated adenosine could outcompete the blocker for receptor binding thus rendering the drugs' inhibitory potencies greatly diminished. This phenomenon has been tentatively termed the *theophylline paradox*[101] and may require reinterpretation of numerous studies of the 1970s and 1980s that employed theophylline or other xanthine derivatives in attempts to quantitate the contribution of endogenous adenosine in metabolic blood flow control.

Specific Aspects of Metabolic Coronary Control Linked to $[ATP]/([ADP] \cdot [P_i])$

Catecholamine Stimulation of Normoxic Adenosine Formation

Depending on the norepinephrine concentration, the changes in cardiac function are typically associated with moderate to severalfold increases in adenosine formation, while intracellular pH only slightly decreases. For example, free cytosolic [AMP] increases during norepinephrine stimulation, provided free intracellular $[Mg^{2+}]$ does not rise; this has been observed in moderate 0.08 μM norepinephrine stimulations.[55] More complicated is the situation during prolonged infusion (>25 min) of high doses of norepinephrine (0.6 μM) where cytosolic ATP, the main physiological Mg^{2+} chelator, decreases by >1 mM from a control of about 8 mM; such net ATP degradation liberates ATP-complexed (bound) Mg^{2+} and estimated free $[Mg^{2+}]$ increases from about 0.4 mM to above 1.0 mM. Under such conditions, the known Mg^{2+}-dependencies of creatine kinase and myokinase[49] predict that estimated free [AMP] does not rise; however measured adenosine release tripled.[55] While this is a clear-cut example of a dissociation between myocardial MVO_2, free AMP and adenosine release,[53] it remains explicable within the theory of free cellular adenylates,[66] as they are linked by pH- and Mg^{2+}-sensitive (creatine and adenylate) kinases and *endo*-5′-nucleotidases. The apparent dissociation paradox may be resolved considering that rising submillimolar levels of free $[Mg^{2+}]$ can effect a severalfold stimulation of the *endo*-5′-nucleotidase.[54] Overall, available evidence supports the concept that cardiomyocyte adenosine formation is under the joint control of free [AMP] as adenosine precursor, free [ATP]/[ADP] as reactants of creatine kinase and precursor of free [AMP] via myokinase, free [ADP] as powerful allosteric activator of *endo*-5′-nucleotidase,[95] and $[P_i]$ as negative feedback inhibitor of the nucleotidase,[55,93] while free $[Mg^{2+}]$[54,55] and pH_i also allosterically shift enzyme activities and optima (see Mallet et al.[8] for detailed discussion). The mechanism of normoxic adenosine formation thus is redundant with respect to AMP, and yet requires cytosolic free [AMP] as the energy-linked immediate precursor of adenosine. Interestingly, metabolic flow control also appears redundant with respect to interstitial adenosine.[67,98]

Microhypoxia Versus Normoxia Model of Adenosine Formation

The classical metabolic flow control hypothesis assumes a microhypoxia stimulus that is responsible for release of vasoactive metabolites from the cardiomyocytes. However, the model implicating $[ATP]/([ADP] \cdot [P_i])$ in metabolic coronary control (Figure 5.7) does not require the microhypoxia stimulus to explain myocardial adenosine formation when oxygen availability is not limiting.[67] Reduced metabolic efficiency (e.g., replacing pyruvate for octanoic acid as energy substrate[27]) or increased metabolic demand due to submaximal norepinephrine produce moderate increases in cytosolic [ADP] during normoxia in isolated perfused hearts.[55,69] The rise in [ADP] accounts for much of the fall in $[ATP]/([ADP] \cdot [P_i])$[39] (Figure 5.6), but this increase in [ADP] is not necessarily evidence of hypoxia, unless it is assumed that low physiological doses of norepinephrine or switching metabolic substrates results in local intramyocardial PO_2s low enough to cause cellular hypoxia. More plausibly, the moderate rise in [ADP] during normoxia is simply an adaptive response to accelerated ATP turnover, elevating [ADP] and $[P_i]$, and is devoid of any implications about myocardial oxygenation or the balance between oxygen supply and demand. In normoxia, the physiological increases in [ADP] always fully support increased mitochondrial respiration ($\dot{V}O_2$max), and also effect amplified changes in free [AMP] as prescribed by the mass-action relation of the myokinase at minor changes of pH_i and free $[Mg^{2+}]$.[39,49,66,67] During anoxia or early ischemia ATP hydrolysis continues and the rate of ADP formation depends on residual contractile function and the energetic drain by the cation pumps, which become stimulated in attempts to maintain intracellular Na^+ and Ca^{2+} homeostasis. Anaerobic glycolysis also becomes stimulated at the level of phosphofructokinase due to rising levels of ADP, AMP, and P_i. Consequently, glycolysis, which responds to increased ADP, can only attenuate but not prevent the increase in [ADP] during anoxia/ischemia.

The instantaneous level of free cytosolic ADP reflects the balance between ATP hydrolysis and net ADP rephosphorylation regardless of the degree of myocardial oxygenation. For example, an ischemic failing myocardium with sufficiently low contractile work output can exhibit near-normoxic levels of ADP or free AMP[66]; conversely, a normoxic myocardium stimulated to perform at maximal contractility and work output may exhibit relatively high [ADP] levels or low [ATP]/[ADP] ratios whose values are near those seen in mild ischemias.[66] Thus, the absolute level of free cytosolic [ADP], not the state of myocardial oxygenation per se, determines the values of [ATP]/[ADP], [ATP]/([ADP] · [P$_i$]) and hence free [AMP] and adenosine formation.

Normoxic Metabolic Flow Control

According to Figure 5.7, when for example, norepinephrine stimulates cardiac energy use, cardiomyocyte [ATP]/([ADP] · [P$_i$]) responds with graded decreases producing graded increases in the release of vasodilatory chemicals (e.g., adenosine, K$^+$) into the interstitium. Then the vasodilators decrease vascular smooth muscle tone, which increases blood flow thus providing increased oxygen and metabolic substrates to the working myocytes. The associated rise in local intramyocardial PO$_2$ could provide, possibly via O$_2$-sensitive mechanisms of the smooth muscle[80] or endothelium,[82,83] a positive feedback that tends to limit vascular smooth muscle relaxation; this mechanism would moderate the dilatory potencies of interstitially accumulated vasodilators. Such an oxygen-sensitive vascular system, acting synergistically with the tonic α-adrenergic constrictor norepinephrine, minimizes normoxic metabolic vasodilation (impeding unrestrained vasorelaxation) and could thus allow for maximum permissible downward flow adjustments that are physiologically safe in terms of the stability of the energy status of the cardiomyocytes. This precision metabolic flow control model effects coronary dilation by graded reversal of a preexisting constraint rather than by activation alone. It is a regulatory principle that also maximizes systemic blood flow output and hence oxygen delivery to the other vital body organs.

Hypoxic Versus Ischemic Metabolic Flow Control

During anoxia or complete ischemia, both [ATP]/([ADP] · [P$_i$]) and local PO$_2$ decrease substantially (Figure 5.7); the resulting collapse of cardiomyocyte [ATP]/([ADP] · [P$_i$]) may cause maximum release of adenosine, K$^+$, and H$^+$ into the interstitium. Simultaneously, the near zero local intramyocardial PO$_2$ provides direct endothelial and/or smooth muscle relaxant stimuli. The changes in interstitial vasoactive chemicals and local vascular [O$_2$] combine to produce unrestrained maximum smooth muscle relaxation. The ischemic/anoxic large accumulation of interstitial adenosine might also directly stimulate the glibenclamide-sensitive K$_{ATP}$ channel in the microvasculature[76,77] producing hyperpolarization and stabilizing relaxation at maximum level. However, the exact dose-response relation between the interstitial concentration of adenosine and opening of the K$_{ATP}$ channel has not been established. Maximum coronary vasodilation would be sustained because local PO$_2$ cannot increase with increased flow, and cardiomyocyte adenosine and H$^+$ production continue to provide vasodilator effectors. During high-flow anoxia the unrestrained maximum coronary blood flow washes out lactate and protons, thus minimizing intracellular acidification and NADH accumulation. This prevents end product inhibition of GAPDH and ensures maximum rate of anaerobic ADP rephosphorylation to ATP via glycolysis. However cardiomyocyte glycolytic capability provides only for about 10% to 13% of the normal myocardial energy requirements.[34,35] During no-flow ischemia, on the other hand, lactate and protons cannot be washed out of the myocardium and accumulate intracellularly; intracellular lactate, acidosis, and accumulated NADH increasingly inhibit GAPDH and hence glycolytic flux, which exacerbates the anaerobic energy deficit, resulting energetic collapse, and intracellular Na$^+$ and Ca^{2+} accumulations. Loss of intracellular calcium control results in cell death, infarct, and apoptosis usually within 20 to 30 minutes. It may be assumed that cardiomyocytes become lethally injured when their [ATP]/([ADP] · [P$_i$]) ratios reach levels too low to support active Na$^+$ extrusion and Ca^{2+} reuptake by the sarcoplasmic reticulum, or active Ca^{2+} export into the extracellular space. Under such circumstances the free energy of ATP hydrolysis in the cytosol is lower than the free energy required to establish cellular Na$^+$ or Ca^{2+} gradients sufficiently high to avert the dangerous loss of Ca^{2+} control.

Specific Aspects of Coronary Control Linked to the Endothelium

Endothelial modulation of coronary vasomotor tone and reactivity is of considerable current interest. A number of diseases and cardiovascular risk factors (arteriosclerotic conditions, hypercholesterolemia, congestive heart failure, hypertension) can damage the endothelium and compromise its function which in turn can cause vascular abnormalities.[105] Vascular endothelium dysfunction can cause disturbances in coronary blood flow, and contribute to the pathophysiology of coronary artery disease and myocardial ischemia.[105-107] For example, impairment of endothelial NO release may lead to increased coronary tone,[107] potentially even vasospasm, platelet aggregation, and thrombosis.

Endothelial-Derived Relaxant Factors

The endothelium synthesizes several vasodilator substances including the classical endothelial-derived relaxant factor (which is thought to be NO), prostacyclin (prostaglandin I$_2$), and endothelial-derived hyperpolarizing factor.

Nitric Oxide

Endothelial-derived relaxant factor, discovered by Furchgott and Zawadski in 1980 and since identified as NO,[15,32] is probably the most important autacoid synthesized in and released from endothelial cells. NO is synthesized from the amino acid L-arginine by NO synthase; its synthesis and hence release can be inhibited by specific L-arginine analogs (e.g., N^G-monomethyl L-arginine and N-nitro-L-arginine). NO stimulates guanylate cyclase, which increases coronary guanosine monophosphate content in vascular smooth muscle, resulting in relaxation. Stimulation of NO synthesis occurs by the majority of known vasoactive agonists, such as ACh from parasympathetic nerves, thrombin, histamine, platelet aggregators [serotonin, ADP], ATP, vasopressin, and catecholamines most likely via α$_2$-adrenergic receptors.[108–110] Thus, for these substances to exert their vasodilator effects, an intact endothelium is obligatorily required. Also, there is continuous, basal release of NO from endothelial cells in the coronary vasculature that is caused by the actions of circulating agonists such as norepinephrine, bradykinin, and thrombin. However, the most important stimuli for NO release appear to be rheological in nature (i.e., laminar shear stress due to blood flow and pulsatile stretching of the intact endothelial lining).[111,112] NO acts on adjacent smooth muscle cells affecting vascular tone and has been shown to contribute to β$_2$-adrenergic receptor mediated coronary vasodilation.[113,114] Only a few vasodilator agonists have been shown to act independently of the vascular endothelium. These include nitroglycerine, nitroprusside, prostacyclin, and adenosine. NO-mediated modulation of vascular tone has been demonstrated in large conductance coronary arteries, but its role in regulation of microvascular resistance vessels is not well established.

Prostenoids

Prostenoids are also released by the vascular endothelium. They stimulate the cell of origin and also adjacent cells, acting as autocrine and paracrine agents, respectively. Of particular interest is prostacyclin (prostaglandin I$_2$ or PGI$_2$), which acts as a coronary vasodilator.[108–110] Prostacyclin is the main product of the vascular cyclooxygenase system. It is synthesized by the endothelium in response to shear stress, hypoxia, pulsatility of flow and intraluminal pressure, and vasoactive mediators including ACh, angiotensin, ATP, bradykinin, histamine, and leukotrienes. The contribution of prostacyclin to endothelial-dependent coronary vascular relaxation, however, is probably negligible. In the porcine coronary artery, prostacyclin stimulates the release of

NO. Its major physiological action appears to be inhibition of platelet aggregation. Other prostaglandins are also synthesized in small amounts in endothelial cells, including PGE$_2$, PGF$_{2\alpha}$, and PGD$_2$, but their role in regulation of coronary blood flow remains to be clarified.

Endothelial-Derived Hyperpolarizing Factor

The endothelium elaborates a hyperpolarizing factor, chemically and physiologically distinct from NO, that may be involved in the coronary relaxation response to ACh.[108–110,115,116] This endothelial-derived hyperpolarizing factor appears to open K$^+_{ATP}$ channels and/or stimulate the Na$^+$, K$^+$-ATPase in vascular smooth muscle, two mechanisms known to cause coronary dilation as described.[74,76,87–89] The hyperpolarization may directly induce endothelial-dependent relaxations or functionally antagonize preexisting or tonic vasoconstrictor stimuli.

Coronary artery tone is the resultant of the balance between competing vasodilator, constrictor factors, and mechanisms. Injury to the vascular endothelium (e.g., due to hypertension, congestive heart failure, coronary artery disease) can disturb this balance; an impaired release of NO, prostacyclin, and/or endothelial-derived hyperpolarizing factor may result in augmented basal vasoconstrictor tone, which functionally antagonizes physiological increases in coronary flow in response to increased cardiac work or contractility. Whether such an endothelial dysfunction materially affects the coronary flow reserve and hence maximum ventricular functional capability has not been established.

Endothelial-Derived Constricting Factors

Endothelial cells of the coronary system also release vasoconstrictor substances, such as endothelin, in response to chemical (hypoxia) and hydraulic (alterations in transmural pressure) stimuli.[108,109,116] Three isoforms of endothelin have been identified (endothelin 1, endothelin 2, and endothelin 3), but vascular endothelial cells appear to produce mainly endothelin 1. Endothelin can produce a strong and long-lasting coronary constrictor response by activating voltage-gated Ca^{2+} channels. However, endothelin is probably insignificant physiologically, because it takes up to 2 hours to synthesize and release it. Also, it is still not established whether a minute basal release of endothelin, if it occurs, could affect vascular mechanical performance. Nevertheless, Yoshizumi et al.[117] demonstrated that shear stress can stimulate secretion of endothelin in endothelial cell cultures. Pathological conditions associated with a damaged endothelium, such as coronary artery disease, congestive heart failure, and hypertension, also may result in increased endothelin release.[106] Under ischemic conditions, endothelin levels are elevated, but whether this exacerbates ischemic damage is not known.

Shear Stress

Blood flow–induced shear stress at the interface between blood and the luminal endothelial surface is probably the most important stimulus among the endothelial-dependent influences on coronary vascular tone.[108,111, 112,124,125] When blood flow through an artery increases, the vessel dilates. This constitutes an endothelial-mediated flow-induced vasodilation that has been demonstrated in conduit arteries, small arteries, and veins. Bassenge, Holtz, and coworkers[109,111] suggested that such flow-induced vasodilation can optimize blood supply to areas where arteriolar resistance has suddenly been reduced (e.g., by exogenous coronary dilators such as dipyridamole), thus counteracting the coronary "steal problem" due to pharmacological vasodilation. Also, flow-induced shear stress appears to functionally antagonize α-adrenergic coronary constriction.[118,119]

Bassenge et al.[108,109] also hypothesized that endothelial cells can actually act as mechanoreceptors; they sense flow-induced shear stress and transduce altered shear stress into biochemical signals that initiate the release of vasoactive substances such as NO. Indeed, there is experimental support for flow-induced, shear-stress–dependent stimulation of NO release from the luminal side of the endothelial lining. In addition, the vasodilator potency of endogenous NO appears to be greatest in large arterioles (i.e., at sites where resistance to flow and shear stress are high). NO release is also known to decrease when the physiologically pulsatile flow becomes completely steady.

In the absence of NO synthesis and/or when endothelial damage occurs endothelial responses to ACh and shear stress are abolished.[106,107] Because exercise is associated with increased shear stress and norepinephrine release, it seems likely that NO release is stimulated by an acute bout of exercise.[120,121] NO not only buffers coronary α-constrictor tone, but also enhances the tonic response to exogenous vasoconstrictors after blockade of NO synthase.[123,124] Thus, NO appears to act as a physiological functional antagonist that inhibits or offsets the tonic vasoconstriction caused by local or systemic prostanoids, angiotensin II, norepinephrine, neuropeptide Y, serotonin, endothelin, and possibly other factors.

Endothelial Dysfunction

The endothelium plays an important role in the pathogenesis of coronary artery disease. Because of its location between circulating blood and vascular smooth muscle, it is a target for vascular injuries, mechanical forces, and cardiovascular risk factors. It is clear that the balance between vasoconstrictor and vasodilator mechanisms for maintaining adequate coronary artery tone is disturbed as the result of aging, arteriosclerosis, myocardial ischemia and/or reperfusion, and hypertension. Aging is an important determinant of coronary artery disease. In humans, the increase in coronary flow induced by ACh declines with aging. This may be due to an increased production of endothelial-derived contracting factors, as well as a decreased production of NO. Mechanical denudation of the coronary artery may occur after percutaneous transluminal coronary angioplasty. This was shown to be associated with endothelial dysfunction and impaired capacity to release NO in porcine coronary arteries, thus favoring vasoconstriction.

Established atherosclerosis in porcine and human coronary arteries has been demonstrated to impair endothelial-dependent relaxation to serotonin, bradykinin, aggregating platelets, and ACh, especially in large epicardial arteries. This endothelial dysfunction may contribute to inappropriate constriction of atherosclerotic coronary stenoses and episodes of ischemic chest pain in patients where epicardial arteries appear normal, but flow in the microcirculation may be impaired. The mechanism mediating this impairment remains unknown.

Endothelial dysfunction occurs early in myocardial ischemia. Brief episodes of ischemia cause loss of endothelial-dependent vasodilation and enhanced coronary artery constrictor responses. Hypoxia can result in endothelial-dependent contractions due to reduced synthesis of NO and release of the vasoconstrictor substance endothelin. After coronary artery occlusion and reperfusion, endothelial-dependent relaxation to thrombin and other agonists is severely impaired in canine and human coronary arteries. Data indicate that ischemia and/or reperfusion result in endothelial damage and vasospastic episodes. In patients with normal coronary arteries (indicated by a vasodilator response to ACh), mental stress causes vasodilation, whereas vasoconstriction is observed in patients with evidence of endothelial dysfunction. Similar constrictor responses are seen in patients with atherosclerotic coronary arteries challenged with a cold pressor test, exercise, and an increase in heart rate. It appears that the loss of NO-mediated dilation in response to increased shear stress or catecholamines in patients with dysfunctional endothelium allows the constrictor effects of catecholamines to act unopposed. Thus, impaired dilator responses of epicardial and resistance vessels may contribute to myocardial ischemia.

Both acute and chronic hypertension are associated with endothelial dysfunction (reduced NO-mediated dilatory responses). Studies indicate that as long as hypertension does not induce left ventricular hypertrophy, the endothelial dysfunction in the coronary vasculature in human patients was confined to large epicardial vessels, which are continuously exposed to high pulsatile pressure and shear stress. The role of endothelin in potentiating the effects of hypertension and mediating a coronary constriction is unclear.

References

1. American Heart Association. Heart and Stroke Facts: 1995 Statistical Supplement.

2. Donald DE, Essex HE. Pressure studies after inactivation of the major portion of the canine right ventricle. *Am J Physiol.* 1954;176:155–161.

3. Sabia PJ, Powers ER, Jayaweera AR, Ragosta A, Kaul S. Functional significance of collateral blood flow in patients with recent acute myocardial infarction. A study using myocardial contrast echocardiography. *Circ Res.* 1992;85:2080–2089.

4. Cicutti N, Rakusan K, Downey HF. Coronary artery occlusion extends perfusion territory boundaries through microvascular collaterals. *Basic Res Cardiol.* 1994;89:427–437.

5. Rüegg JC. *Calcium in muscle activation.* 2nd ed. Berlin, Germany: Springer-Verlag; 1988.

6. Paul RJ, Peterson JW, Caplan SR. Oxygen consumption rate in vascular smooth muscle: relation to isometric tension. *Biochim Biophys Acta.* 1979;306:474–480.

7. Johansson B. Processes involved in vascular smooth muscle contraction and relaxation. *Circ Res.* 1978;43(suppl 1, pt 20):1–14.

8. Mallet RT, Sun J, Fan WL, Kang YH, Bünger R. Magnesium acitvated adenosine formation in intact perfused heart: predominance of ecto-5′-nucleotidase during hypermagnesemia. *Biochim Biophys Acta.* 1996;1290:165–176.

9. Renkin EM. Blood flow and transcapillary exchange in skeletal and cardiac muscle. In: Marchetti G, Taccardi B, eds. *International Symposium on the Coronary Circulation and Energetics of the Myocardium.* New York, NY: S. Karger; 1967.

10. Nees S, Herzog V, Becker BF, Des Rosier C, Gerlach E. The coronary endothelium: a highly active metabolic barrier for adenosine. *Basic Res Cardiol.* 1985;80:515–529.

11. Muxfeldt M, Schaper W. The activity of xanthine oxidase in heart of pigs, guinea pigs, rabbits, rats, and humans. *Basic Res Cardiol.* 1987;82:486–492.

12. Nees S, Gerlach E. Adenine nucleotide and adenosine metabolism in cultured coronary endothelial cells: formation and release of adenine compounds and possible functional implications. In: Berne RM, Rall TW, Rubio R, eds. *Regulatory Function of Adenosine.* Boston, Mass: Martinus Nijhoff Publishers; 1983:347–362.

13. Schrader J, Gruwel M, Decking U, Alves C. Why do endothelial cells require adenosine triphosphate? *Arzneimittelforschung.* 1994;44:436–438.

14. Mall G, Mattfeldt T, Rieger P, Volk B, Frolov VA. Morphometric analysis of the rabbit myocardium after chronic ethanol feeding. Early capillary changes. *Basic Res Cardiol.* 1982;77:57–67.

15. Furchgott RF. The role of endothelium in the responses of vascular smooth muscle. *Circ Res.* 1983;53:557–573.

16. Lucchesi BR. Complement, neutrophils, and free radicals: mediators of reperfusion injury. *Arzneimittelforschung.* 1994;44:420–423.

17. Michael LH. Cardiac lymph: monitor of myocardial membrane and vascular alteration. *Life Sci.* 1981;29:1495–1501.

18. Marcus ML, Chilian WM, Kanatsuka H, Dellsperger KC, Eastham CL, Lamping KG. Understanding the coronary circulation through studies at the microvascular level. *Circulation.* 1990;82:1–7.

19. Chilian WM, Eastham CL, Marcus ML. Microvascular distribution of coronary vascular resistance in beating left ventricle. *Am J Physiol.* 1986;251:H779–H788.

20. Haddy FJ. Effect of histamine on small and large vessel pressures in the dog foreleg. *Am J Physiol.* 1960;198:161–168.

21. Olsson RA, Bünger R, Spaan JAE. Coronary circulation. In: Fozzard HA, Haber E, Jennings RB, Katz AM, Morgan HE, eds. *The Heart and Cardiovascular System. Scientific Foundations.* New York, NY: Raven Press; 1991:1393–1426.

22. Downey JM, Kirk ES. Distribution of the coronary blood flow across the canine heart wall during systole. *Circ Res.* 1974;34:251–257.

23. Hess DS, Bache RJ. Transmural distribution of myocardial blood flow during systole in the awake dog. *Circ Res.* 1976;38:5–15.

24. Feigl EO. Coronary Physiology. *Physiol Rev.* 1983;63:1–205.

25. Dzau VJ, Re RN. Evidence for the existence of renin in the heart. *Circulation.* 1987;73(suppl 1):I134–I136.

26. Needleman E. Triene prostaglandins: prostacyclin and thromboxane biosynthesis and unique biological properties. *Proc Natl Acad Sci U S A.* 1979;76:944–948.

27. Kang YH, Mallet RT, Bünger R. Coronary autoregulation and purine release in normoxic heart at various cytoplasmic phosphorylation potentials: disparate effects of adenosine. *Pflügers Archiv.* 1992;421:188–199.

28. Mosher P, Ross J Jr, McFate PA, Shaw RF. Control of coronary flow by an autoregulatory mechanism. *Circ Res.* 1964;14:250–259.

29. Bünger R, Haddy FJ, Querengässer A, Gerlach E. An isolated guinea pig heart with in vivo like features. *Pflügers Archiv.* 1975;353:317–326.

30. Schrader J, Haddy FJ, Gerlach E. Release of adenosine, inosine, and hypoxanthine from isolated guinea pig heart during hypoxia, flow-autoregulation, and reactive hyperemia. *Pflügers Archiv.* 1977;369:1–6.

31. Holtz J, Saeed M, Sommer O, Bassenge E. Norepinephrine constricts the canine coronary bed via postsynaptic α_2-adrenoreceptors. *Eur J Pharmacol.* 1982;82:199–202.

32. Furchgott RF, Zawadzki JV. The obligatory role of endothelial cells in the relaxation of arterial smooth muscle by acetylcholine. *Nature.* 1980;288:373–376.

33. Kahn MT, Furchgott RF. Additional evidence that endothelium-derived relaxing factor is nitric oxide. In: Rand MJ, Raper C, eds. *Pharmacology.* New York, NY: Elsevier; 1987:341–344.

34. Kobayashi K, Neely JR. Control of maximum rate of glycolysis in rat cardiac muscle. *Circ Res.* 1979;44:166–175.

35. Mallet RT, Hartman DA, Bünger R. Glucose requirement for postischemic recovery of perfused working heart. *Eur J Biochem.* 1990;188:481–493.

36. Severinghaus JW. Blood gas calculator. *J Appl Physiol.* 1966;21:1108–1116.

37. Atkinson DE. The energy charge of the adenylate pool as a regulatory parameter. Interaction with feedback modifiers. *Biochemistry.* 1968;7:4030–4034.

38. Soboll S, Bünger R. Compartmentation of adenine nucleotides in the isolated working guinea pig heart stimulated by noradrenaline. *Zeitschrift für Physiologische Chemie.* 1981;362:125–132.

39. Bünger R, Soboll S. Cytosolic adenylates and adenosine release in perfused working heart. *Eur J Biochem.* 1986; 159:203–213.

40. Schulze K, Becker BF, Shultheiss HP. Autoantibodies to the ADP/ATP carrier, an autoantigen in myocarditis and dilated cardiomyopathy, penetrate into myocardial cells and disturb energy metabolism in vivo. *Circ Res.* 1989; 64:179–192.

41. Fiolet JWT, Baartsheer A, Schumacher CA, et al. The change of the free energy of ATP hydrolysis during global ischemia and anoxia in the rat heart: its possible role in the regulation of transsarcolemmal sodium and potassium gradients. *J Mol Cell Cardiol.* 1984;16:1023–1036.

42. Skou JC. Enzymatic aspects of active linked transport of Na^+ and K^+ through the cell membrane. *Prog Biophys Mol Biol.* 1964;14:133–166.

43. Gottlieb RA, Burlesion KO, Kloner RA, Babior BM, Engler RL. Reperfusion injury induces apoptosis in rabbit cardiomyocytes. *J Clin Invest.* 1994;94:1621–1628.

44. Kroemer G, Petit P, Zamzami N, Vayssiere JL, Mignote B. The biochemistry of programmed cell death. *FASEB J.* 1995;9:1277–1287.

45. Kammermeier H, Schmidt P, Jüngling E. Free energy of ATP hydrolysis: a causal factor of early hypoxic failure of the myocardium? *J Mol Cell Cardiol.* 1982;14:267–277.

46. Lawson JWR, Veech RL. Effects of pH and free Mg^{2+} on the K_{eq} of the creatine kinase reaction and other phosphate hydrolyses and phosphate transfer reactions. *J Biol Chem.* 1979;254:6528–6537.

47. Mallet RT, Kang YH, Mukohara N, Bünger R. Use of cytosolic metabolite patterns to estimate free magnesium in normoxic myocardium. *Biochim Biophys Acta.* 1992;1139: 239–247.

48. Clarke K, Kashiwaya Y, King MT, Gates D, Keon CA, Cross HR, Radda GK, Veech RL. The beta/alpha peak height ratio of ATP. A measure of free $[Mg^{2+}]$ using ^{31}P-NMR. *J Biol Chem.* 1996;271:21142–21150.

49. Bünger R, Mukohara N, Kang YH, Mallet RT. Combined glyceraldehyde-3-phosphate dehydrogenase/phosphoglycerate kinase in catecholamine-stimulated guinea-pig cardiac muscle. Comparison with mass-action ratio of creatine kinase. *Eur J Biochem.* 1991;202:913–921.

50. Veech RL, Lawson JWR, Cornell NW, Krebs HA. Cytosolic phosphorylation potential. *J Biol Chem.* 1979;254: 6538–6547.

51. van der Meer R, Akerboom TPM, Groen AK, Tager JM. Relationship between oxygen uptake of perfused rat-liver cells and the cytosolic phosphorylation state calculated from indicator metabolites and a predetermined equilibrium constant. *Eur J Biochem.* 1978;84:421–428.

52. Decking UK, Schlieper G, Kroll K, Schrader J. Hypoxia-induced inhibition of adenosine kinase potentiates cardiac adenosine release. *Circ Res.* 1997;81:154–164.

53. Decking UK, Arens S, Schlieper G, Schulze K, Schrader J. Dissociation between adenosine release, MVo_2, and en-

ergy status in working guinea pig hearts. *Am J Physiol.* 1997;272:H371–H381.

54. Darvish A, Metting PJ. Purification and regulation of an AMP-specific cytosolic 5'-nucleotidase from dog heart. *Am J Physiol.* 1993;264:H1528–H1534.

55. Bünger R, Mallet RT, Kang YH. Guinea-pig cardiac free, bound, and interstitial adenylates: energy-linked and energy-independent adenosine release. In: Imai S, Nakazawa M, eds. *Role of Adenosine and Adenine Nucleotides in the Biological System.* New York, NY: Elsevier; 1991:337–353.

56. Bünger R, Mallet RT, Hartman DA. Pyruvate-enhanced phosphorylation potential and inotropism in normoxic and postischemic isolated working heart. Near-complete prevention of reperfusion contractile failure. *Eur J Biochem.* 1989;180:221–223.

57. Deussen A, Lloyd HGE, Schrader J. Contribution of S-adenosylhomocysteine to cardiac adenosine formation. *J Mol Cell Cardiol.* 1989;21:773–782.

58. Lloyd HGE, Deussen A, Schrader J. The transmethylation pathway as a source of adenosine in the isolated guinea pig heart. *Biochem J.* 1988;252:489–494.

59. Pette D, Dölken G. Some aspects of regulation of enzyme levels in muscle energy–supplying metabolism. *Adv Enzyme Regul.* 1975;13:355–377.

60. Olsson RA, Saito D, Steinhart CR. Compartmentalization of the adenosine pool of dog and rat hearts. *Circ Res.* 1982;50:617–626.

61. Kloor D, Kurz J, Fuchs S, Faust B, Osswald H. S-adenosyl-homocysteine-hydrolase from bovine kidney: enzymatic binding properties. *Kidney Blood Press Res.* 1996;19: 100–108.

62. Bünger R, Glanert S, Sommer O, Gerlach E. Inhibition by (aminooxy)acetate of the malate aspartate cycle in the isolated working guinea pig heart. *Zeitschrift für Physiologische Chemie.* 1980;361:907–914.

63. Nuutinen EM, Nelson D, Wilson DF, Erecinska M. Regulation of coronary blood flow: effects of 2,4-dinitrophenol and theophylline. *Am J Physiol.* 1983;244:H396–H405.

64. Nuutinen EM, Nishiki K, Erecisnska M, Wilson DF. Role of mitochondrial oxidative phosphorylation in regulation of coronary blood flow. *Am J Physiol.* 1982;243:H159–H169.

65. Bradamante S, Piccine F, Delu C, Janssen M, DeJong JW. NMR evaluation of changes in high energy metabolism produced by short repeated myocardial ischemias. *Biochim Biophys Acta.* 1995;1243:1–8.

66. Bünger R. Thermodynamic state of cytosolic adenylates in guinea pig myocardium. Energy-linked adaptive changes in free adenylates and purine nucleoside release. In: Gerlach E, Becker BF, eds. *Topics and Perspectives in Adenosine Research.* Berlin, Germany: Springer-Verlag; 1987:223–235.

67. Olsson RA, Bünger R. Metabolic control of coronary blood flow. *Prog Cardiovasc Dis.* 1987;29:369–387.

68. Headrick HP, Willis RJ. Adenosine formation and energy metabolism: a ^{31}P NMR study in isolated rat heart. *Am J Physiol.* 1990;258:H617–H624.

69. He MX, Wangler RD, Dillon PF, Romig GD, Sparks HV. Phosphorylation potential and adenosine release during norepinephrine infusion in guinea pig heart. *Am J Physiol.* 1987;253:H1184–H1191.

70. Dankelman J., Spaan JAE, Stassen HG, Vergroesen I. Dynamics of coronary adjustment to a change in heart rate in the anaesthetized goat. *J Physiol (Lond).* 1989;408: 295–312.

71. Noma A. ATP regulated K+ channel in cardiac muscle. *Nature.* 1983;305:147–148.

72. Elliot AC, Smith GL, Allen DG. Simultaneous measurements of action potential duration and intracellular ATP in isolated ferret hearts exposed to cyanide. *Circ Res.* 1989;64:583–591.

73. Beech DJ, Zhang H, Nakoa K, Bolton TB. K+ channel activation by nucleotide diphosphates and its inhibition by glibenclamide in vascular smooth muscle cells. *Br J Pharmacol.* 1993;110:573–582.

74. Klieber HG, Daut J. A glibenclamide sensitive potassium conductance in terminal arterioles isolated from guinea pig heart. *Cardiovasc Res.* 1994;28:823–830.

75. Daut J, Maier-Rudolph W, von Beckerath N, Mehrke G, Günther K, Goedel-Meinen L. Hypoxic dilation of coronary arteries is mediated by ATP-sensitive potassium channels. *Science.* 1990;247:1341–1344.

76. Belloni FL, Hintze TH. Glibenclamide attenuates adenosine-induced bradycardia and coronary vasodilation. *Am J Physiol.* 1991;261:H720–H727.

77. Niiya K, Uchida S, Tsuji T, Olsson RA. Glibenclamide reduces the coronary vasoactivity of adenosine receptor agonists. *J Pharmacol Exp Ther.* 1994;271:14–19.

78. Olsson RA, Pearson JD. Cardiovascular purinoceptors. *Physiol Rev.* 1990;70:761–845.

79. Cyrys S, Daut J. The sensitivity of the coronary vasculature tone to glibenclamide: a study on the isolated perfused guinea pig heart. *Cardiovasc Res.* 1994;28:823–830.

80. Mellemkjaer S, Nielsen-Kudsk JE. Glibenclamide inhibits relaxation of isolated porcine coronary arteries under conditions of impaired glycolysis. *Eur J Pharmacol.* 1994; 270:307–312.

81. Neely JR, Rovetto MJ, Whitmer JT. Rate-limiting steps of carbohydrate and fatty acid metabolism in ischemic hearts. *Acta Med Scand.* 1976;587(suppl):9–15.

82. Busse R, Pohl U, Kellner C, Klemm U. Endothelial cells are involved in the vasodilatory response to hypoxia. *Pflügers Archiv.* 1983;397:78–80.

83. Pohl U, Busse R. Hypoxia stimulates release of endothelium-derived relaxant factor. *Am J Physiol.* 1989;256: H1595–H1600.

84. Howard RO, Richardson DW, Smith MH, Patterson JL. Oxygen consumption of arterioles and venules as studied in the Cartesian diver. *Circ Res.* 1965;16:187–196.

85. Paul RJ, Bauer M, Pease W. Vascular smooth muscle: aerobic glycolysis linked to sodium and potassium transport processes. *Science.* 1979;206:1414–1416.

86. Raberger G, Schütz W, Kraupp O. Coronary reactive hyperemia and coronary dilator action of adenosine during normal respiration and hypercapnic acidoses in the dog. *Clin Exp Pharmacol Physiol.* 1975;2:373–382.

87. Bünger R, Haddy FJ, Querengässer A, Gerlach E. Studies on potassium induced coronary dilation in the isolated guinea pig heart. *Pflügers Archiv.* 1976;363:27–31.

88. Bünger R, Haddy FJ, Querengässer A, Gerlach E. Studies with theophylline and ouabain on the metabolic regulation of coronary flow in the isolated guinea pig heart. *Arzneimittelforschung.* 1977;21(pt 2):1510–1519.

89. Murray PA, Sparks HV. The mechanism of K+ induced vasodilation of the coronary vascular bed of the dog. *Circ Res.* 1978;42:35–42.

90. Drury AN, Szent-Györgi A. The physiological activity of adenine compounds with especial reference to the action upon the mammalian heart. *J Physiol (Lond).* 1929;68: 213–237.

91. Lindner F, Rigler R. Über die Beeinflussung der Weite der Herzkranzgefässe durch Produkte des Zellkernstoffwechsels. *Pflügers Archiv.* 1931;226:697–708.

92. Berne RM, Gidday JM, Hill HE, Curnish RR, Rubio R. Adenosine in the local regulation of blood flow: Some controversies. In: Gerlach E, Becker BF, eds. *Topics and Perspectives in Adenosine Research.* Berlin, Germany: Springer-Verlag; 1987:395–405.

93. Skladanowski AC, Newby AC. 5′-nucleotidase involved in adenosine formation. In: Imai S, Nakazawa M, eds. *Role of Adenosine and Adenine Nucleotides in the Biological System.* Amsterdam: Elsevier; 1991:289–300.

94. Borgers M, Thone F. Species differences in adenosine metabolic sites in the heart. *Histochem J.* 1992;24:445–452.

95. Yamazaki Y, Truong VL, Lowenstein JM. 5′-Nucleotidase I from rabbit heart. *Biochemistry.* 1991;30:1503–1509.

96. Nees S, Dendorfer A. New perspectives in myocardial adenine nucleotide metabolism In: Imai S, Nakazawa M, eds. *Role of Adenosine and Adenine Nucleotides in the Biological System.* Amsterdam: Elsevier; 1991:273–288.

97. Kroll K, Deussen A, Sweet IR. Comprehensive model of transport and metabolism of adenosine and S-adenosylhomocysteine in the guinea pig heart. *Circ Res.* 1992;71: 590–604.

98. Lee S-C, Mallet RT, Shizukada Y, Williams AG Jr, Downey HF. Canine coronary vasodepressor responses to hypoxia are attenuated but not abolished by 8-phenyltheophylline. *Am J Physiol.* 1992;262:H955–H960.

99. Saito D, Steinhart CR, Nixon DG, Olsson RA. Intracoronary adenosine deaminase reduces canine myocardial reactive hyperemia. *Circ Res.* 1981;49:1262–1267.

100. McKenzie JE, Steffen RP, Haddy FJ. Effect of theophylline on adenosine production in canine myocardium. *Am J Physiol.* 1987;252:H204–H210.

101. Mukohara N, Kang YH, Bünger R. Magnesium-induced coronary dilation and adenosine. α,β-methylene adenosine 5′-diphosphate attenuation and theophylline paradox. *Pharmacol Pharm Lett.* 1992;2:12–15.

102. Headrick JP, Ely SW, Matherne GP, Berne RM. Myocardial adenosine, flow, and metabolism during adenosine antagonism and adrenergic stimulation. *Am J Physiol.* 1993;264: H61–H70.

103. Sawmiller DR, Linden J, Berne RM. Effects of xanthine amine congener on hypoxic coronary resistance and venous and epicardial adenosine concentrations. *Cardiovasc Res.* 1994;28:604–609.

104. Bünger R, Haddy FJ, Gerlach E. Coronary responses to dilating substances and competitive inhibition by theophylline in the isolated perfused guinea pig heart. *Pflügers Archiv.* 1975;358:213–224.

105. Vanhoutte PM. Endothelial dysfunction in hypertension. *J Hypertens Suppl.* 1996;15:S83–S93.

106. Lüscher TF, Tanner FC, Tschudi MR, Noll G. Endothelial dysfunction in coronary artery disease. *Annu Rev Med.* 1993;44:395–418.

107. Zeiher A, Drexler H, Saubier B, Just H. Endothelium-mediated coronary blood flow modulation in humans. Effects of age, atherosclerosis, hypercholesterolemia, and hypertension. *J Clin Invest.* 1993;92:652–662.

108. Bassenge E, Busse R. Endothelial modulation of coronary tone. *Prog Cardiovasc Dis.* 1988;30:349–380.

109. Bassenge E. Endothelial regulation of coronary tone. In: Ryan US, Rubanyi GM, eds. *Endothelial Regulation of Vascular Tone.* New York, NY: Marcel Dekker Inc; 1992: 225–264.

110. Shepherd JT, Katuši ZS. Endothelium-derived vasoactive factors, I: endothelium-dependent relaxation. *Hypertension.* 1991;18 (suppl 3):III76–III85.

111. Holtz J, Forstermann U, Pohl U, Giesler M, Bassenge E. Flow-dependent, endothelium-mediated dilation of epicardial coronary arteries in conscious dogs: effects of cyclooxygenase inhibition. *J Cardiovasc Pharmacol.* 1984;6: 1161–1169.

112. Holtz J, Giesler M, Bassenge E. Two dilatory mechanisms of anti-anginal drugs on epicardial coronary arteries in vivo: indirect, flow-dependent, endothelium-mediated dilation and direct smooth muscle relaxation. *Z Kardiol.* 1983;72(suppl 3):98–106.

113. Parent R, Al-Obaidi M, Lavallée M. Nitric oxide formation contributes to β-adrenergic dilation of resistance coronary vessels in conscious dogs. *Circ Res.* 1993;73: 241–251.

114. Van Bibber R, Traub O, Kroll K, Feigl EO. EDRF and norepinephrine-induced vasodilation in the canine coronary circulation. *Am J Physiol.* 1995;268:H1973–H1981.

115. Feletou M, Vanhoutte PM. Endothelium-derived hyperpolarizing factor. *Clin Exp Pharmacol Physiol.* 1996;23: 1082–1090.

116. Katusic ZS, Shepherd JT. Endothelium-derived vasoactive factors, II: endothelium-dependent contraction. *Hypertension.* 1991;18(suppl 3):III86–III92.

117. Yoshizumi M, Kurihara H, Suguyama T, et al. Hemodynamic shear stress stimulates endothelin production by cultured endothelial cells. *Biochem Biophys Res Commun.* 1989;161:859–864.

118. Ishibashi Y, Duncker DJ, Bache RJ. Endogenous nitric oxide masks α_2-adrenergic coronary vasoconstriction during exercise in the ischemic heart. *Circ Res.* 1997;80:196–207.

119. Jones CJH, DeFily DV, Patterson JL, Chilian WM. Endothelium-dependent relaxation competes with α_1- and α_2-adrenergic constriction in the canine epicardial coronary microcirculation. *Circulation.* 1993;87:1264–1274.

120. Berdeaux A, Ghaleh B, Dubois-Randé JL, et al. Role of vascular endothelium in exercise-induced dilation of large epicardial coronary arteries in conscious dogs. *Circulation.* 1994;89:2799–2808.

121. Gwirtz PA, Kim S-J. Intracoronary blockade of nitric oxide synthase limits coronary vasodilation during submaximal exercise. In: Steinacker JM, Ward SA, eds. *Physiology and Pathophysiology of Exercise Tolerance.* New York, NY: Plenum Press; 1996:147–451.

122. Bünger R, Sommer O, Walter G, Stiegler H, Gerlach E. Functional and metabolic features of an isolated perfused guinea pig heart performing pressure-volume work. *Pflügers Archiv.* 1979;380:259–266.

123. Murray PA, Vatner SF. α-Adrenoceptor attenuation of the coronary vascular response to severe exercise in the conscious dog. *Circ Res.* 1979;45:654–660.

124. Pohl U, Herlan K, Huang A, Bassenge E. EDRF-mediated shear-induced dilation opposes myogenic vasoconstriction in small rabbit arteries. *Am J Physiol.* 1991;261: H2016–H2023.

125. Lamontagne D, Pohl U, Busse R. Mechanical deformation of vessel wall and shear stress determine the basal release of endothelium-derived relaxing factor in the intact rabbit coronary vascular bed. *Circ Res.* 1992;70:123–130.

126. Mentzer RM Jr, Bünger R, Lasley RD. Adenosine enhanced preservation of myocardial function and energetics. Possible involvement of the adenosine A_1 receptor system. *Cardiovasc Res.* 1993;27:28–35.

127. Bergmeyer HU, ed. *Methods of Enzymatic Analysis.* 2nd English ed. New York, NY: Academic Press; 1974.

6

Pathophysiology of Atherosclerosis

Kailash Prasad

Atherosclerosis is a disease of large-sized and medium-sized arteries characterized by focal thickening of the inner portion of the arterial wall in association with fatty deposits. Most commonly affected are the aorta and the iliac, femoral, carotid, basilar, vertebral, coronary, and cerebral arteries. Because atherosclerosis can progressively or abruptly interfere with blood flow, particularly through heart and brain, it often causes serious clinical consequences such as heart attack and stroke. Atherosclerosis and its complications, such as myocardial infarction, stroke, and peripheral vascular disease, remain major causes of morbidity and mortality in the Western World. The incidence of disease related to atherosclerosis is as follows: ischemic heart disease, 7 million; peripheral vascular disease, 3 million; and stroke, 0.75 million. Death from ischemic heart disease affects 103/100,000 population and from stroke about 28/100,000 per year. Atherosclerosis is a slowly progressive disease that begins in childhood and does not become manifest until middle age or later. It causes the majority of deaths in the United States, Canada, Europe, and Japan.

In this chapter I describe the pathogenesis and theories of atherosclerosis and its risk factors, with special reference to the role of oxygen free radicals in the initiation and maintenance of hypercholesterolemic atherosclerosis.

Pathogenesis

The pathogenesis of atherosclerosis has been extensively reviewed.[1-3] The intima is the layer predominantly affected by focal lesions of atherosclerosis. Classical types of lesion are referred to as fatty streaks, fibrous plaques, and the so-called complicated lesion according to the stage of progression of atherosclerosis.

Fatty Streaks

Fatty streaks are grossly visible, slightly raised yellow areas that are narrow and longitudinally oriented. They consist of subendothelial aggregates of foam cells that are filled with lipid—mostly cholesterol esters and free cholesterol. Most foam cells are macrophages, but some are smooth muscle cells. T lymphocytes are also present. Fatty streaks stained by the fat-soluble dye oil red O are bright red in color. The lipid is intracellular. The progression of these lesions depends on hemodynamic forces and plasma levels of atherogenic risk factors. Early lesions are considered to be reversible.

Fibrous Plaques

Fibrous plaques are approximately round, raised lesions, usually off-white to white in color. A typical fibrous plaque consists of (1) a fibrous cap composed mostly of smooth muscle cells, a few leukocytes, a relatively dense connective tissue that contains elastin, collagen fibrils, proteoglycans, and a basement membrane; (2) a cellular area beneath and to the side of the cap that consists of a mixture of macrophages, smooth muscle cells, and T lymphocytes; and (3) a deeper necrotic core that contains cellular debris, extracellular lipid droplets, cholesterol crystals, and calcium deposits. The necrotic core often contains large foam cells. The relative content of fibrous tissue and lipid within a plaque is variable, with coronary artery lesions being largely fibrous. The most common site for plaque formation is the lower descending aorta, followed by the coronary arteries, arteries of the lower extremities, descending thoracic aorta, internal carotids, and circle of Willis. Fibrous plaque causes narrowing of the artery.

Complicated Lesions

Complicated lesions are calcified fibrous plaques that have undergone various degrees of necrosis, thrombosis, and ulceration. These lesions predispose vasculature to thrombosis and the intima to rupture, which causes hemorrhage. Progressive weakening of the arterial wall causes aneurysmal dilation. Fragments of plaques can be dislodged into the arterial lumen and cause arterial emboli.

Theories of Atherosclerosis

Of the various theories of atherogenesis, the most accepted one is the *response-to-injury* hypothesis. The concept of atherogenesis must include the following: (1) the mechanism of smooth muscle proliferation, which is the fundamental process in the development of plaque; (2) the presence of lipid in the area of a lesion; (3) the focal nature of the lesions and their general distribution; and (4) the role of major risk factors in development of the atherosclerotic plaque.

Response-to-Injury Hypothesis

In 1956, Virchow pioneered the response-to-injury hypothesis, which was later modified and extended by Ross and Glomset[1] and Ross.[2] It states that some form of injury occurs to the endothelial cells at particular sites in the arterial wall. The injury to endothelium is the key event in this hypothesis. The injury may be manifested in various forms of endothelial dysfunction that need not result in denudation of the endothelial cells. It may simply be a relatively rapid replacement of individual endothelial cells that are lost or an alteration in endothelial permeability or synthesis and release of growth factors and other substances. The injury may be mechanical, chemical, toxicological, viral, or immunological. Dysfunctional endothelial cells lead to exposure of subendothelial tissue to increased concentrations of plasma constituents. This may trigger a sequence of events that include monocyte and platelet adhesion, migration of monocytes into the intima to become macrophages, platelet aggregation and formation of microthrombi, and release of secretory products from platelets and macrophages. Endothelium, platelets, monocytes, macrophages, and lymphocytes are key players in the response-to-injury hypothesis.

The earliest events probably include leakage of plasma constituents into the arterial wall, due to increased permeability of the endothelium and the increased adherence of monocytes and T lymphocytes to the endothelium. The adhesion involves formation of specific sets of adhesion molecules (i.e., endothelium–leukocyte adhesion molecule on both the leukocytes and endothelium). The molecular characterization revealed that the endothelium–leukocyte adhesion molecule in vascular endothelium is vascular cell adhesion molecule 1 (VCAM-1) and in leukocytes very late antigen 4 (VLA-4).[4] This matching endothelium-expressed vascular cell adhesion molecule 1 and monocyte-expressed very late antigen 4 provides a counterreceptor pair for selective adhesion.

In addition to vascular cell adhesion molecule 1 and very late antigen 4 adhesion molecule, there are other endothelium-dependent counterreceptor mechanisms for the recruitment of monocytes. These mechanisms include intercellular adhesion molecule 1, which can interact with the CD11/CD18-integrin complex. The presence of several selectin and integrin classes of molecules leads to increased adherence of monocytes and lymphocytes to the endothelium. Interleukin 1 (IL-1) and tumor necrosis factor (TNF) increase adhesion of leukocytes to endothelium. Hypercholesterolemia or hypercholesterolemic serum lipoproteins promote monocyte adhesion to endothelium. Chemotactic monocyte chemotactic protein-1 (MCP-1) factors generated by endothelium, and perhaps by intimal cells, induce leukocytes to penetrate between endothelial cells, where they localize within the intima.[3,5] Monocytes become active and scavenge oxidized low-density lipoprotein (OX-LDL) to become foam cells.

Various genes expressed in these cells determine the replication of macrophage, smooth muscle migration and replication, T-cell replication, and chemotaxis of additional monocytes. Macrophages generate a host of growth-regulating molecules (platelet-derived growth factor [PDGF], basic fibroblast growth factor [bFGF], heparin-binding epidermal growth factor [HB-EGF], and transforming growth factors [TGF-α and TGF-β]) and cytokines (IL-1, TNF) that affect neighboring cells. Gene expression and transcription in smooth muscle cells could result in the formation of collagen, elastic fiber proteins, and growth-regulating molecules (bFGF, insulinlike growth factor I [IGF-I], HB-EGF, TGF-β) and cytokines (IL-1, TNF-α). Endothelial cells produce growth-promoting molecules (PDGF, bFGF, TGF, IGF-I) and cytokines. T lymphocytes produce TGF-β and cytokines. Smooth muscle cells also produce colony-stimulating factor (macrophage colony-stimulating factor [M-CSF] and granulocyte–monocyte colony-stimulating factor [GM-CSF]). PDGF, bFGF, and IGF-I are critical to the proliferation of smooth muscle cells and possibly of endothelium. Colony-stimulating factor plays a role in macrophage stability and replication. TGF-β is a potent stimulator of synthesis of connective tissue and matrix including collagens, proteoglycans, and elastic fiber proteins; it inhibits the replication of many cells including smooth muscle cells. Cytokines promote smooth muscle cell proliferation. Both PDGF and IGF-I are chemoattractants for smooth muscle cells; fibroblast growth factors and M-CSF are chemoattractants for endothelium and for monocyte-derived macrophages, respectively. Macrophages and smooth muscle cells also generate monocyte chemotactic protein 1 and OX-LDL, which are chemoattractants for monocytes. According to the response-to-injury hypothesis, hyperlipidemia (or some component of hyperlipidemic serum) and other risk factors cause endothelial cell injury, resulting in adhesion of platelets and monocytes and release of various chemoattractants, growth-regulating factors, and cytokines. These mechanisms lead to the proliferation of smooth muscle cells and the migration of monocytes, which results in the development of atherosclerosis.

Lipid Hypothesis

The lipid hypothesis, also called *lipid insudation hypothesis,* is the oldest hypothesis and states that the lipid in the atherosclerotic lesion is derived from lipoproteins in the blood. There is evidence that lipid in the plaques comes from the blood, and good correlation has been found between the severity of atherosclerosis and the levels of hypercholesterolemia. However, the lipid hypothesis does not explain the features of the lesion, which include smooth muscle proliferation and thrombosis, or how hypercholesterolemia initiates atherosclerosis.

Monoclonal Hypothesis

The monoclonal hypothesis states that the cells of any particular plaque arise as a clone from a single progenitor smooth muscle cell. In this process mitogenic or mutagenic factors that might stimulate smooth muscle cell proliferation would act on single cells. The hypothesis is based on the observation that individual plaques of human females' heterozygotes for the X-linked marker glucose-6-phosphate dehydrogenase frequently exhibit one, but not both, of the glucose-6-phosphate dehydrogenase isotypes. At some time, a single cell might be stimulated to enter the growth cycle and undergo several rounds of division, which leads to the atherosclerotic lesion. The mechanism of cell activation for these lesions is not known yet, but similarities proposed by the monoclonal hypothesis are shared with neoplasm. This theory suggests that each lesion is a benign neoplasm derived from cells that have been transformed by agents such as viruses or chemicals. In this case, the lesions might not be affected by the same factors (e.g., platelet factor and plasma lipoproteins) that appear to regulate the proliferation of normal arterial smooth muscle cells. Focal clonal senescence could explain how intrinsic aging processes could lead to atherosclerosis. According to this hypothesis, intimal smooth muscle cells that proliferate to form an atherosclerotic plaque are normally under the feedback control of mitosis inhibitors that are formed by smooth muscle cells in the contiguous media, and this feedback control system tends to decline in activity with advancing age because of death of the cells that control feedback. This hypothesis is supported by the observation that cultured human arterial smooth muscle cells show decline in their ability to replicate as a function of donor age. Many questions concerning the

cellular origin of the lesions are thus raised. Whether the lesions are hyperplastic or neoplastic responses remains to be determined. Any theory that attempts to provide a mechanism for the accumulation of smooth muscle cells in atherosclerotic plaques must take into account this observation of monoclonality.

Endothelium

Endothelium responds to various stimuli by undergoing specific alterations in function, metabolism, and structure. Altered shear stress induces shape changes, whereas turbulent flow increases endothelial replication.[6] Platelets adhere to endothelium treated with chemicals or transformed by simian virus 40 in culture.[7] IL-1 and TNF increase the procoagulant activity of endothelium, adhesion of leukocytes to endothelium, and synthesis of new surface protein molecules. Hypercholesterolemia induces monocyte adhesion to endothelium.[8,9] Both hypertension and hyperlipidemia increase endothelial replication.

Risk Factors

Hyperlipidemia

Hypercholesterolemia is a major risk factor for the development of coronary artery disease (CAD), as evidenced from epidemiological data and clinical trial data[10-13] For every 1% increase in serum cholesterol concentration the risk of CAD increases by 2% to 3%.[14] CAD risk increases as cholesterol concentration increases and climbs steeply from a total blood cholesterol level of 6.7 mmol/L (260 mg/100 mL). Lowering blood cholesterol by 10% reduces CAD risk over 5 years by half for men 40 years of age and by a quarter for men 60 years of age.

Plasma Cholesterol Metabolism

There are two pathways by which cholesterol is transported in the body. A third pathway, called the *reverse cholesterol transport,* involves removal of cholesterol from peripheral tissues to the liver, where it is reused for synthesis of new lipoproteins, excreted into the bile, or converted to bile acids.

In the exogenous pathway, dietary cholesterol is packaged, together with dietary fatty acids, by intestinal epithelial cells into chylomicrons. These triglyceride-rich lipoprotein particles are secreted into the lymph and enter the plasma via the thoracic lymph duct. Lipoprotein lipase in the capillary beds digests the triglyceride (TG) in chylomicrons and releases free fatty acids. The resultant particles (depleted of TG) are called chylomicron remnants and contain dietary cholesterol. Chylomicron remnants are taken up by the liver, where their cholesterol can be used to form very-low-density lipoproteins (VLDLs) or diverted to bile acid production. Chylomicrons are composed mostly of apolipoprotein (apo) B, apo E, and cholesterol.

The endogenous pathway starts in the liver with production of VLDLs whose principal lipid component is TG. These particles also contain significant amounts of cholesterol that are either synthesized in the liver or delivered via the exogenous pathway. Lipoprotein lipase hydrolyzes TG to release free fatty acids, leaving VLDL remnants that are usually called intermediate-density lipoproteins. Intermediate-density lipoproteins may be taken up directly by the liver or may be converted to low-density lipoproteins (LDLs). Categories of TG-rich lipoproteins include chylomicron remnants, VLDL, and several types of VLDL remnants (small VLDLs, intermediate-density lipoproteins, and β-VLDLs). LDL interacts with the LDL receptor and is internalized by endocytosis. In lysosomes, LDL protein is digested and cholesterol is released for tissue use. VLDL is taken to the liver, where about half is converted to LDL by addition of cholesterol esters derived from action on free cholesterol by a lecithin–cholesterol acyltransferase.

High-density lipoproteins (HDLs) appear to originate as nascent particles secreted from intestine, liver, macrophages, and other tissues. HDL has two subclasses: HDL_3 consists of dense and relatively small particles, and HDL_2 consists of less dense and larger particles. It is cleared by a hepatic HDL receptor.

Reverse cholesterol transport involves transport of cholesterol from peripheral tissue to the liver by HDL and thus prevents development of atherosclerosis. HDL also helps create LDL from VLDL via the lecithin–cholesterol acyltransferase reaction and thus may enhance the risk of atherosclerosis. The composition of major lipoproteins is shown in Table 6.1.

Lipoprotein(a), or Lp(a), a lipoprotein particle produced in the liver, has two components: one closely resembling LDL in structure that is partially wrapped by a chainlike apolipoprotein (apo) B-100 and the other a molecule of apolipoprotein (A).

The major apolipoproteins are apo A and apo B. apo A is associated with HDL, and measurement of apo A has been proposed as a better index of atherogenic risk than assay of HDL cholesterol. apo B comprises most of the protein component of LDL. apo B-100 is also the major B apolipoprotein component of VLDL. The normal values for various lipoproteins are shown in Table 6.2.

TABLE 6.2. Normal values for lipids and lipoproteins.

	(mmole Serum/L)	(mg/100 Serum mL)
Triglycerides	2.82	250
Total cholesterol (C)	<5.15	<200
High-density lipoprotein (C)	1.17	45
Low-density lipoprotein (C)	<3.36	130
Lipoprotein (a)		20

Atherogenic Risk

In the absence of at least a moderate increase in total cholesterol concentrations, especially LDL cholesterol, CAD is relatively rare. Populations with high concentrations of cholesterol have a high mortality from CAD. The probability of developing myocardial infarction increases with plasma cholesterol level. Borderline high-risk total cholesterol is from 5.15 to 6.18 mmol/L and high-risk total cholesterol is ≥6.20 mmol/L.

Triglycerides

Using TGs as an indicator of risk for CAD has been very controversial.[11,15] However, several prospective studies suggest that TGs are an important risk factor.[16–18] Hypertriglyceridemia promotes atherogenesis through the metabolic consequences of TG. Presence of high concentrations of VLDL TGs gives rise to other atherogenic abnormalities, including small, dense LDL and low HDL cholesterol concentrations that are atherogenic. High TG levels produce a procoagulant state by increasing factor VII, activated factor VII–phospholipid complexes, inhibitor of tissue plasminogen activator (tPA), amplified factor X, fibrinogen formation, and thrombin generation. A procoagulant state may increase the risk of myocardial infarction. TGs are increased in obesity, severe acute stress, estrogen therapy, alcohol intake, glucocorticoid therapy, high-fat diet, diabetes mellitus, and kidney disease.

LDL Cholesterol

LDLs, especially small, dense LDL particles, are related to increased atherogenicity,[19] probably because smaller particles enter easily into the arterial wall, are more susceptible to oxidation,[20] or both. The desirable LDL cholesterol value is <3.36 mmol/L (<130 mg/100 mL); borderline values are 3.36 to 4.11 mmol/L (130–159 mg/100 mL), and high-risk values are ≥4.14 mmol/L (160 mg/100 mL).

TABLE 6.1. Composition of major lipoproteins (in percentages).

Lipoproteins	Triglycerides	Cholesterol	Phospholipid	Protein
Chylomicrons	85	5	5	2
Very-low-density lipoproteins	60	15	15	10
Low-density lipoproteins	10	45	20	25
High-density lipoproteins	5	15	30	50

HDL Cholesterol

Several studies have suggested that HDL concentration has a strong inverse correlation with risk of atherosclerotic CAD. Low HDL seems to be an independent risk factor. A reduced HDL cholesterol level generally reflects a reduction in the number of HDL particles, particularly HDL_2 and HDL particles containing apo A-I, usually considered protective against CAD.[21,22] High HDL concentrations retard the rate of atherogenesis,[23] whereas HDL reduction accelerates atherogenesis.[24] For every 1 mg/dL decrease in HDL cholesterol concentration, the risk for CAD is increased by 2% to 3%.[25] Several mechanisms may be involved in protecting against atherosclerosis by HDL. HDL is involved in the process of reverse cholesterol transport, which may slow down the progression of atherosclerosis and may interfere with the atherogenic effect of LDL. It may prevent aggregation of LDL within the arterial wall[26] or oxidation of LDL.[27] Low HDL concentrations are observed in cigarette smokers, obese patients, those who do not exercise or have hypothyroidism, and patients who take thiazides, β-blockers, or sympatholytic medications. Hyperthyroidism, alcohol intake, and exercise all elevate HDL concentrations in serum.

Apolipoproteins

apo A is associated with HDL and apo B with VLDL, intermediate-density lipoprotein, LDL and Lp(a). apo B provides a better index of atherosclerotic risk than LDL cholesterol. The relative risk of CAD is suggested by the ratio of apo A-I to apo B, the average being 1.4. A ratio of 1 increases the risk threefold.

Lipoprotein(a)

Several studies suggest that Lp(a) elevation is a very significant independent risk factor for CAD.[28] This genetically determined lipoprotein promotes not only atherosclerosis but also thrombosis by virtue of its homology to plasminogen.[29] Elevation above 30 mg/100 mL serum increases the CAD risk by twofold or more. Lp(a) concentration is increased in patients with familial hypercholesterolemia, chronic renal failure, and postmenopausal decrease in estrogen levels. Lp(a) concentration is decreased in chronic alcoholic patients. Syndrome X (deadly quartet) includes the risk factors of high TG, low HDL, glucose intolerance, and android obesity.

CAD Risk Index

Although the focus has been on the independent role of various lipoproteins, the combined effects of lipids are of greater importance. Various indices have been used for this purpose:

1. Total cholesterol/HDL cholesterol (normal ratio is 5)
2. LDL cholesterol/HDL cholesterol (normal ratio is 3)
3. Lipid tetrad index: total cholesterol × TGs × Lp(a)/HDL cholesterol (all in mg/dL)

An index of <10,000 is considered desirable, from 10,000 to 20,000 borderline, and >20,000 high. An index >100,000 is associated with marked prematurity and severity of CAD.[29]

Oxidative Hypothesis of Atherosclerosis

According to the oxidative hypothesis, LDL is readily modified by oxidation[30] and produces cholesterol deposition in tissue macrophages that leads to foam cell formation characteristic of early atherosclerotic fatty streak lesions. In the early stage of atherogenesis, plasma proteins and LDL accumulate in the subendothelial space and are subjected to oxidative modification by endothelial cells, smooth muscle cells, and resident monocytes/macrophages.[31-35] The proposed mechanism of the oxidative hypothesis of atherosclerosis[35] is shown in Figure 6.1. LDL becomes mildly oxidized and is called *minimally modified LDL* (MMLDL). Smooth muscle cells and endothelial cells exposed to minimally modified LDL produce monocyte chemotactic protein 1, which is involved in monocyte migration. Minimally modified LDL is further oxidized to produce OX-LDL, which can directly augment monocyte recruitment by virtue of its lysolecithin content. Monocytes adhere to the endothelium and then penetrate the subendothelial space. Monocytes/macrophages express the LDL receptor, but the rate of uptake of native LDL is insufficient to produce foam cells. OX-LDL is a ligand for the scavenger re-

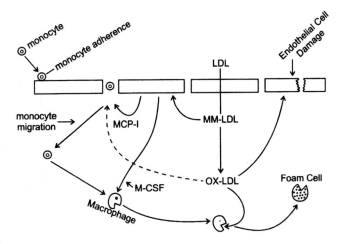

FIGURE 6.1. Mechanism of oxidative hypothesis of atherosclerosis. LDL, low-density lipoprotein; MM-LDL, minimally modified LDL; OX-LDL, oxidized LDL; MCP-1, monocyte chemotactic protein 1; M-CSF, macrophage colony-stimulating factor.

ceptor that is expressed as monocytes differentiate into tissue macrophages. This monocyte/macrophage differentiation is facilitated by release of M-CSF from endothelial cells under the influence of minimally modified LDL. Macrophages have receptors for OX-LDL, which is taken up by the receptors to produce foam cells. The production of foam cells is an early stage of atherosclerosis. Monocyte adhesion involves surface expression of endothelial–leukocyte adhesion molecules (ELAMs) and secretion of a variety of adhesive cytokines, such as IL-1β and M-CSF. Foam cells also produce oxygen radicals. OX-LDL could contribute to atherogenesis in various ways: (1) it is chemotactic for circulating monocytes; (2) it inhibits motility of resident macrophages, thus trapping them at sites of developing lesions; (3) it damages endothelial cells; (4) it stimulates release of monocyte chemotactic protein 1 and M-CSF from endothelial cells; and (5) it favors generation of foam cells.

A modern view of atherogenesis has been presented by Schwartz et al.[33] Consensus is now emerging on the mechanism of atherosclerosis. The factors involved in atherosclerosis include the following:

1. Focal intimal influx and accumulation of plasma lipoproteins
2. Focal intimal monocyte recruitment
3. Generation of oxygen radicals within the intima by endothelial cells, smooth muscle cells, and macrophages
4. Oxidative modification of LDL and Lp(a)
5. Foam cell formation due to uptake of oxidized lipoprotein by macrophages
6. Foam cell necrosis due to the cytotoxic effects of OX-LDL, which gives rise to an extracellular lipid core and is less readily reversible
7. Smooth muscle cell migration to and proliferation in the arterial intima, a process in which PDGF acts as a chemoattractant; fibroblast growth factor likely regulates smooth muscle proliferation
8. Plaque rupture at sites of greatest microphage density; metalloproteases released by macrophages may stimulate plaque rupture, which ultimately leads to mural or occlusive thrombosis
9. Autoimmune inflammation is probably the result of autogenic epitopes of OX-LDL, as reflected by lymphocytic infiltration of adventia

Cell Adhesion Molecules, Atherosclerosis, and Antioxidants

Endothelium, platelets, monocytes, macrophages, lymphocytes, and smooth muscle cells are key players in the response-to-injury hypothesis. Cell adhesion molecules are involved in interaction between circulating blood cells and vascular endothelium.[36] They have a role in atherogenesis.[37,38] Circulating concentrations of P-selectin, E-selectin, intercellular adhesion molecule 1 (ICAM-1), and VCAM-1 are elevated in atherosclerosis.[39] Expression of adhesion molecules by arterial endothelial cells, which mediate monocyte adhesion and their transmigration process, has been demonstrated in tissue cultures and experimental animals to be modulated by free radicals and oxidative stress and suppressed by antioxidants.[40,41] Several studies have demonstrated that antioxidants can reduce or block expression of cell adhesion molecules.[42–44] Antioxidants (vitamin E) reduced the expression of soluble intercellular adhesion molecule 1 (sICAM-1) and other cell adhesion molecules and decreased the adhesion of endothelial cells to monocytes when cells were exposed to LDL or stimulated with IL-1.[40,41,45] Supplemental vitamin E preserves endothelium-dependent vessel relaxation in cholesterol-fed rabbits.[46] Dietary antioxidants may modulate several mechanisms involved in the pathogenesis of atherosclerosis, including production of cytokines and other mediators, expression of adhesion molecules by endothelial cells and immune cells, and monocyte adhesion to endothelium. The interaction and adhesion of monocyte to endothelium have been recognized as important steps in the development and progression of atherosclerosis.[47,48] After their adhesion to the endothelial cell lining of the vessel walls, monocytes transmigrate to the intima, where they are transformed into activated macrophages and accumulate lipids to become foam cells, a major component of fatty streaks.[49]

Possible Sources of Oxygen Radicals in Hypercholesterolemia

Hypercholesterolemia is a major risk factor for the development of atherosclerosis.[2,12,50–52] Endothelial cell injury has been theorized to be the basic mechanism for initiation and maintenance of atherosclerosis. Hypercholesterolemia-induced atherosclerosis may be due to endothelial cell injury produced by cholesterol. Cholesterol may increase the concentration of oxygen free radicals (OFRs), which may damage the endothelial cells. Endothelial and smooth muscle cells, neutrophils, monocytes, and platelets may be sources of OFRs. Possible sources of OFRs have been described in detail by Prasad and Kalra[50] and Prasad et al.[51] Hypercholesterolemia increases the cholesterol content of platelets, polymorphonuclear leukocytes (PMNLs), endothelial cells, smooth muscle cells, and monocytes.[53–55] Cholesterol-rich platelets release substances including thrombin, histamine, and adenosine diphosphate (ADP).[56] Histamine and ADP activate phospholipase A₂,[57] which acts on membrane phospholipids to release arachidonic acid.[58] An increase in phospholipase A₂ activity may also

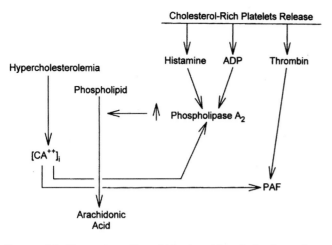

FIGURE 6.2. Formation of arachidonic acid and platelet activating factor in hypercholesterolemia. PAF, platelet activating factor; ADP, adenosine diphosphate.

arise from increases in intracellular Ca^{2+} concentration[58] that accompany hypercholesterolemia.[59] Activated phospholipase A_2 increases the formation of arachidonic acid and hence synthesis of prostaglandins and leukotrienes in various cells. Synthesis and release of platelet activating factor (PAF) depend on thrombin and intracellular Ca^{2+}.[60] The formation of arachidonic acid and PAF is schematically shown in Figure 6.2.

The intermediate steps in the biosynthesis of prostaglandins[61] and leukotrienes[62] from arachidonic acid generate OFRs. The generation of OFRs in hypercholesterolemia is schematically shown in Figure 6.3. Hypercholesterolemia activates complement components C3 and C5 (C3a, C5a).[63] Leukotriene B_4 is formed during metabolism of arachidonic acid by leukocytes. Leukotriene B_4, PAF, C3a, and C5a would activate PMNLs to generate OFRs (superoxide anion, H_2O_2, ·OH and

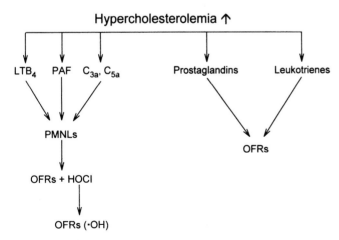

FIGURE 6.3. Generation of oxygen free radicals in hypercholesterolemia. LTB$_4$, leukotriene B$_4$; PAF, platelet activating factor; C3a and C5a, activated complement C3 and C5, respectively; OFRs, oxygen free radicals; HOCl, hypochlorous acid.

hypochlorous acid) during hypercholesterolemia.[64-66] Hypochlorous acid in combination with superoxide anion produces ·OH. OFRs are produced by endothelial cells,[67] smooth cells,[68] monocytes,[69] and PMNLs.[70,71] Hypercholesterolemia increases production of superoxide anion in endothelial cells.[72] OFRs damage endothelial cells. Prasad and Kalra[50] proposed that hypercholesterolemia increases concentrations of OFRs and leads to endothelial cell injury, thus setting the stage for initiation and maintenance of atherosclerosis. This explanation fits with the response-to-injury hypothesis of atherogenesis.[2] According to this hypothesis, endothelial cell injury is a prerequisite for the development of atherosclerosis. OFRs produced through various sources could oxidize the LDL. OX-LDL may also produce atherogenesis, as proposed by Steinberg.[35]

Hypertension

Hypertension is associated with an increased incidence of CAD and other atherosclerotic disease[73]; this association is independent of other risk factors. Diastolic pressure greater than 115 mm Hg is associated with a greater risk of organic complications of atherosclerosis. Other studies show that elevated systolic pressure may be a more potent risk factor.[74] Obesity and alcohol intake cause a significant increase in blood pressure. Effective control of blood pressure reduces morbidity and mortality rates. The mechanism of atherosclerosis in hypertension is poorly understood. However, a few observations may shed some light on the mechanism of atherosclerosis. Both medial smooth muscle hypertrophy and intimal hyperplasia occur with hypertension.[75] The stimulated sympathetic nervous system in hypertension can induce vascular wall growth. Angiotensin II, whose level is elevated in patients with hypertension, can induce smooth muscle hyperplasia. Other vasoactive substances such as serotonin, endothelin, and thrombin can stimulate smooth muscle replication. Both endothelial dysfunction in experimental hypertension with monocyte adhesion and transendothelial migration of adherent cells (similar to hypercholesterolemia) have been reported.[76] Endothelial dysfunction could be due to an elevation of OFR concentration observed in hypertension (discussed in Chapter 34, titled "Oxygen Free Radicals and Peripheral Vascular Disease"). Mechanical stress can injure endothelial cells. Endothelial dysfunction can promote atherogenesis. Hypertension alters endothelial permeability and increases lysosomal enzyme activity.

Diabetes

Diabetes mellitus is associated with an increased risk for atherosclerosis, myocardial infarction, atherothrombotic brain infarction, and intermittent claudication. Diabetes mellitus is an independent risk factor for CAD and cardiovascular death. The incidence of myocardial infarction in patients with diabetes is at least twice that of individuals without diabetes. The mechanism of atherosclerosis is not clear. Platelets from patients with diabetes release more growth factor than those from nondiabetic patients. Platelets release PDGF and IGF-I, and an injured artery expresses increased mRNA for IGF-I. Insulin and IGF-I increase the proliferative effects of growth factor and stimulate uptake of LDL by smooth muscle cells. Glycation, the nonenzymatic binding of glucose to proteins, increases the atherogenic potential of certain plasma constituents including LDL. Advanced glycosylation end products, which accumulate in patients with diabetes, are cytotoxic and may be associated with atherogenesis. Glycation of LDL results in enhanced uptake of LDL by macrophages.[77] Glycoxidation is free radical–mediated oxidation of lipoproteins, and the glycoxidation products are atherogenic. Glycosylation end products are chemotactic for human monocytes and may play a role in atherosclerosis. Uptake of glycosylation end products by macrophages results in an increase in TNF-α and IL-1. Increased glucose concentration stimulates proliferation of cultured arterial smooth muscle cells. Hyperglycemia in diabetes could produce OFRs in various ways as outlined in Chapter 34, titled "Oxygen Free Radicals and Peripheral Vascular Disease." Oxygen radicals produce dysfunctional endothelium, which is a prerequisite for development of atherosclerosis. Patients with diabetes have dysfunctional endothelium.

Cigarette Smoking

Cigarette smoking has a strong and independent link to CAD, atherosclerotic peripheral vascular disease, and cerebrovascular disease.[78,79] Risk of cardiovascular death remains high in patients who smoke. The degree of aortic and coronary atherosclerosis is greater in those who smoke than in those who do not. Risk of having a first-time major coronary event in patients who smoke (one or more packs of cigarettes per day) is 2.5 to 3.2 times greater than that for patients who do not smoke. Men who smoke one pack of cigarettes per day have about a 70% greater death rate and a threefold to fivefold increase in risk of ischemic heart disease compared with those who do not smoke. There is an increase in ischemic heart disease mortality in women over the age of 35 years who take oral contraceptives and smoke cigarettes. Cessation of smoking reduces the incidence of cardiovascular death. Smoking influences the incidence of sudden death by triggering lethal events in those who already have compromised coronary circulation. Patients who smoke and die of causes other than ischemic heart disease have been found at autopsy to have more

TABLE 6.3. Effects of smoking.

 1. Increased platelet aggregation and thrombosis
 2. Hypercoagulability
 3. Increased fibrinogen levels
 4. Decreased fibrinolytic activity
 5. Enhanced platelet thrombus formation
 6. Increased blood viscosity
 7. Constricts blood vessels
 8. Increased heart rate
 9. Increased myocardial oxygen demand
10. Interference with oxygen supply due to formation of carboxyhemoglobin as a result of increased carbon monoxide level in blood
11. Decreased threshold for ventricular fibrillation
12. Decreased plasma concentrations of vitamins B_{12}, E, C, and folic acid
13. Decreased concentrations of serum high-density lipoproteins
14. Increased concentrations of plasma C_{5a}
15. Increased concentrations of oxygen free radicals in blood
16. Increased production of oxygen free radicals by polymorphonuclear leukocytes
17. Increased risk of atherogenicity
18. Cigarette smoke contains reactive peroxy radicals and can damage the endothelium and also have mutagenic effect

Averbook et al.,[220] Kalra et al.[80]

coronary atherosclerosis than those who do not smoke. Cessation of smoking results in a prompt decline in risk, and patients who smoke may reach the risk level of those who do not smoke as early as 1 year after cessation.

The adverse effects of cigarette smoking on atherogenesis are complex. The effects of smoking are summarized in Table 6.3. The cigarette smoke–induced atherosclerosis, to some extent, is due to the effect of smoking on the clotting factor. By-products of smoke such as peroxy radical may injure endothelial cells. Cigarette smoking increases OFR production by PMNLs through various mechanisms.[80] Nicotine in cigarettes enhances PMNL responsiveness to C5a. The concentration of OFRs is elevated in patients who smoke.[80] OFRs can induce endothelial cell injury, then initiate and sustain the development of atherosclerosis. Also, OFRs are mutagenic. Recent studies have shown a direct effect of OFRs on cell proliferation.[81,82] Cigarette smoking may expose the arteries to OFRs, which may stimulate the smooth muscle cells to proliferate. A decrease in serum HDL concentration may increase the susceptibility to atherogenesis.

Alcohol

Moderate alcohol consumption is associated with a decreased incidence of CAD,[83] but there is a positive association between heavy consumption of alcohol and CAD.[84] Moderate consumption increases serum HDL concentration and decreases serum LDL concentration.[85] Alcohol consistently increases plasma TGs. The protective effect of moderate consumption of alcohol may be due to an increase in serum HDL concentration and a decrease in serum LDL concentration. Some studies report an increase in HDL_2 concentration[86] and others report an increase in HDL_3[87] with alcohol consumption. Alcohol and the levels of OFRs are discussed in detail in Chapter 34, titled "Oxygen Free Radicals and Peripheral Vascular Disease." Increased concentrations of TGs and OFRs may induce atherogenesis. The dangers of acute and chronic excessive use of alcohol outweigh theoretical benefits from alcohol-induced elevated HDL or lowered LDL concentrations.

Obesity

Obesity is a risk factor for development of CAD and stroke. It is associated with increased incidence of CAD, particularly angina pectoris and sudden death.[88] Obese persons develop twice as much cardiac failure and brain infarction as persons of normal weight.[88] There is no apparent association between obesity and occlusive peripheral arterial disease. Abdominal obesity (android obesity) is associated with CAD, hypertension, hyperinsulinemia, impaired glucose tolerance, hypertriglyceridemia, hypercholesterolemia, hyperglycemia, reduced HDL cholesterol concentration, and hyperuricemia.[88,89] Most of the risk is mediated through the associated changes in the mentioned parameters. Obesity is an independent risk factor but to a lesser extent. Hypertriglyceridemia, hypercholesterolemia, and reduced HDL concentration may lead to atherogenesis. Insulin may directly affect arterial wall metabolism and lead to increased endogenous lipid synthesis, thus predisposing a patient to atherosclerosis. Insulin stimulates proliferation of arterial smooth muscle, enhances binding of LDL and VLDL to cells, and decreases binding of HDL to cells. These attributes of insulin could induce atherosclerosis. Finally, hyperglycemia and hypercholesterolemia could increase the concentration of OFRs, which could damage endothelial cells and set the stage for atherosclerosis.

Coffee

A retrospective case-control study has shown a relationship between coffee consumption and myocardial infarction.[90] Tea containing comparable amounts of caffeine was not associated with myocardial infarction. Acute effects of caffeine are inconsistent increases in blood pressure and heart rate and coronary dilation. Increased myocardial irritability and a decreased ventricular fibrillation threshold in animals have been suggested as possible causes of sudden death in coffee drinkers.[91] Prospective studies have failed to implicate coffee in atherosclerotic disease.[92] In some recent studies coffee consumption has been associated with an increased risk of coronary heart disease.[93] Coffee-induced atherosclerosis may be due to an increase in the serum cholesterol concentration. Coffee consumption is associated with elevated serum cholesterol and TG concentration.[94] Consumption of boiled coffee (ground coffee beans boiled directly with water) has a hypercholesterolemic effect, but filtered coffee (coffee percolated through a filter) does not increase serum cholesterol concentration.[95,96] The LDL cholesterol–raising effect of boiled coffee is due to the diterpene alcohols cafestol and kahweol, which are removed on filtering.[97,98] Recently Post et al.[99] have shown that a decrease in bile acid synthesis and down-regulation of the LDL receptor may explain the rise in serum cholesterol concentration in humans who consume boiled coffee. They have shown that cafestol suppresses bile acid synthesis, whereas kahweol and isokahweol are less active.

Infection

In recent years, certain viral and bacterial infections have been implicated in the pathogenesis of atherosclerosis. In this section I describe some of the highlights of infection in atherogenesis.

Human coxsackievirus B, human cytomegalovirus, and the genus herpes simplex viruses have been implicated in atherogenesis.[100–103] Viral infection can predispose infected birds to atherosclerosis. Chickens infected with a widespread avian herpes virus develop arterial plaques resembling those of human atherosclerosis.

Dental infections (teeth, gingivae, caries, peridontitis) have been implicated in coronary atherosclerosis.[104] The oropharyngeal flora include *Haemophilus influenzae*, *Streptococcus pneumoniae*, viridans and nonhemolytic streptococci; the *Neisseria* and *Corynebacterium* species and Spirochaetes; and other anaerobic cocci. Dental caries are associated with the presence of *Lactobacillus* species. *Helicobacter pylori* has been implicated in the development of peptic ulcer. It is also a risk factor for CAD.[105]

Chlamydia pneumoniae is one of the strongest contenders in the search for infectious factors in atherogenesis. Numerous papers and reviews discuss the role of *C pneumoniae* in atherogenesis.[106–111] Both serological and histopathological evidence suggests the association of *Chlamydia* infection with atherosclerosis.[111]

Mechanism of Infection-Induced Atherosclerosis

Possible mechanisms of infection-induced atherosclerosis include an immunological response and its effect on thrombogenesis, lipid metabolism, and changes in local turbulence. During sepsis, production of monocyte-derived cytokines (IL-1β, IL-6, IL-8, and TNF) is increased. Both TNF and IL-1 inhibit production of lipoprotein lipase and cause expression of leukocyte adhesion molecules of the macrophage 1 antigen (CD11b/CD18) and leukocyte function–associated antigen 1 family on endothelial cells.[112,113] IL-1 is mitogenic, and TNF, IL-1β and IL-6 increase the procoagulant activity of endothelial cells and activate platelets to release PAF.

Bacterial products (endotoxin and muramyldipeptide) increase synthesis of cholesterol ester. In sepsis, LDL cholesterol is elevated and can be oxidized by OFRs from endothelial cells or monocyte/macrophages. There is endothelial expression of immunoglobulin receptors in infection, with consequent complement activation and release of PAF, which could release mitogenic factors.

Infection with *C pneumoniae* is associated with increased concentrations of serum TGs, total cholesterol, and LDL cholesterol and decreased concentrations of HDL cholesterol.[114,115] Acute microbial infections caused by gram-negative bacteria raise serum TG and lower serum HDL concentrations[116]; these changes are risk factors for atherosclerosis. *C pneumoniae* has lipopolysaccharides with a strongly acidic ketodeoxyoctane–containing immunoreactive hydrophilic residue that may react with LDL cholesterol and then be oxidized. *C pneumoniae* induces production of IL-1, IL-6, and TNF-α in mononuclear leukocytes.[117] Endotoxin from bacteria releases PAF from PMNLs and activates complement components. Bacteria, IL-1, activated complement component, PAF, and TNF activate PMNLs to release OFRs that can damage endothelial cells and set the stage for atherosclerosis. OFRs can also oxidize LDL, and OX-LDL can initiate atherosclerosis. Chronic macrophage infection may contribute to local inflammation and development of atheromatous plaques.

Infection increases blood viscosity by raising the concentrations of plasma fibrinogen, factor VIII, β-thromboglobulin, and thromboxane.[111] Infections also increase platelet aggregation and reduce the concentration of antithrombin III.[118] An increased procoagulant state would increase the risk of coronary thrombosis. Thrombogenesis is intimately related to atherogenesis. Hypercoagulable states predispose one to atherosclerosis. These data support the hypothesis that infections may play a role in pathogenesis of atherosclerosis.

Oxygen Radicals and Hypercholesterolemic Atherosclerosis

Hypercholesterolemia

Some evidence suggests that OFRs are involved in the genesis and maintenance of hypercholesterolemic atherosclerosis. Hypercholesterolemic atherosclerosis is associated with an increase in (1) the production of OFRs by PMNLs[50,119]; (2) the lipid peroxidation product malondialdehyde (MDA), an indirect index of levels of OFRs in blood[50,51,120,121]; (3) the aortic tissue MDA[50,51,121]; and (4) the presence of OX-LDL in the plasma of both patients and New Zealand White Rabbits[122] and in atherosclerotic lesions.[35] Antioxidant reserve in the atherosclerotic tissue is decreased in association with hypercholesterolemic atherosclerosis.[51,120,121] Antioxidant enzyme (superoxide dismutase [SOD], catalase, glutathione peroxidase [GSH-P$_X$]) activity is also affected in hypercholesterolemic atherosclerosis. SOD and GSH-P$_X$ activity decreased, whereas catalase activity increased in the blood.[123] SOD, catalase, and GSH-P$_X$ activity in atherosclerotic aorta increased significantly in rabbits.[121,123,124]

Antioxidants

Vitamin E

Vitamin E is a potent lipid-soluble antioxidant. It protects LDL against oxidative modification and inhibits proliferation of vascular smooth muscle.[125]

In Watanabe heritable hyperlipidemic rabbits, the extent of atherosclerosis, along with serum cholesterol concentration and LDL oxidation, was reduced with dietary vitamin E.[126] Vitamin E significantly reduces the extent of hypercholesterolemic atherosclerosis in rabbits[50,127] and monkeys.[128] Reduction in the extent of atherosclerosis (approximately 75%) with vitamin E is associated with a decrease in serum MDA concentrations[50] and an increase in blood SOD and GSH-P$_X$ activity but without any change in catalase activity.[123] Vitamin E prevents the cholesterol-induced rise in catalase and GSH-P$_X$ activity in the atherosclerotic aorta but does not prevent the rise in SOD activity.[123] Other investigators have observed no beneficial effect of vitamin E on hypercholesterolemic atherosclerosis.[129]

Several small clinical trials of vitamin E in intermittent claudication have been reported, but the results are inconclusive.[130] Vitamin E has been used in patients undergoing percutaneous transluminal coronary angioplasty to determine the incidence of restenosis.[131] The results were inconclusive. In the Health Professional Follow-Up Study involving 39,910 men who were followed for 4 years, Rimm et al.[132] showed that increased dietary intake of vitamin E was associated with a lower risk of CAD. In the Nurses' Health Study involving 87,245 women who were followed for 8 years, Stampfer et al.[133] reported that vitamin E supplementation was associated with a 40% reduction in risk of major CAD. Also, there was a trend toward a greater decrease in risk with higher daily doses of vitamin E. An inverse relationship exists between vitamin E and ischemic heart disease.[134]

Vitamin C

Vitamin C is a water-soluble vitamin that prevents LDL oxidation[135] and lipid peroxidation in LDL and plasma.[136] Vitamin C–deficient guinea pigs on an atherogenic diet develop atherosclerosis, which can be prevented by ascorbic acid supplementation.[137]

Probucol

Probucol is an antioxidant[138] that prevents oxidation of LDL.[35] It is a cholesterol-lowering agent that suppresses the permeability of LDL, uptake of modified LDL by macrophages, and secretion of smooth muscle cell proliferation factor.[139] Kita et al.[140] showed that a reduction in the extent of atherosclerosis in Watanabe heritable hyperlipidemic rabbits by probucol was associated with a decrease in the copper-mediated oxidation of the LDL isolated from these rabbits. In models of cholesterol-fed rabbits[51,141] and monkeys,[142] probucol inhibits the development of atherosclerosis. Prasad et al.[51] showed that the reduction of atherosclerosis by probucol is inversely dependent on the concentrations of cholesterol. Reduction of atherosclerosis was associated with a decrease in the aortic MDA concentration. They also showed that the ineffectiveness of probucol in reducing the extent of atherosclerosis in the 1% cholesterol diet was associated with no effect on MDA and antioxidant reserve. Probucol is ineffective in altering the 0.5% cholesterol diet–induced increase in activity of SOD and catalase in aorta.[124] However, it raised the level of GSH-P$_X$ activity. Probucol is ineffective in altering antioxidant enzymes in aortas of 1% cholesterol-fed rabbits.

In the Probucol Quantitative Regression Swedish Trial the effects of probucol on development of femoral atherosclerosis were measured in hypercholesterolemic individuals.[143] Probucol reduced the total cholesterol level by 17%, LDL cholesterol by 10%, and HDL cholesterol by 31%. It prevented oxidation of LDL and reduced formation of MDA. A decrease in HDL concentration with probucol has also been observed in hypercholesterolemic rabbits.[51] These results suggest that the antioxidant activity of probucol may be responsible for the reduction in the extent of atherosclerosis in hypercholesterolemia. Probucol has recently been found to be effective in reducing the incidence of restenosis following percutaneous transluminal coronary angioplasty.[144]

Estrogen

Estrogen reduces the extent of atherosclerosis in ovariectomized monkeys and baboons on an atherogenic diet[145] and apolipoprotein-deficient mice.[146] It protects LDL against oxidation by copper ions, monocyte, and endothelial cells in vitro.[147,148]

Antioxidant effects of estrogen are due to the presence of a phenolic group in the molecule. Its antioxidant action may occur either directly or indirectly by increasing HDL, which in turn has been shown to prevent oxidation of LDL in vitro.[27] Most of the antioxidant actions of estrogen on LDL oxidation have been shown in vitro.[149] Equine estrogen is a more potent antioxidant than human estrogen.[150] Some studies suggest that estrogens have antioxidant actions in vivo.[149] Estrogen lowers the total plasma cholesterol concentration, especially the LDL and VLDL fractions,[151] and raises both plasma TG[152] and HDL levels.[153] The antiatherogenic activity of estrogen could be due to (1) the decrease in LDL and VLDL and the increase in HDL levels, (2) the antioxidant effect, (3) the inhibition of vascular smooth muscle proliferation, or (4) the inhibition of collagen synthesis and prevention of platelet thrombus.

Garlic

Garlic is a potent antioxidant.[154,155] It is effective in retarding hypercholesterolemic atherosclerosis in rabbits.[121,156] Hypercholesterolemic atherosclerosis was associated with increased levels of MDA and activity of antioxidant enzymes and decreased levels of antioxidant reserve in atherosclerotic aorta.[121] Garlic supplement reduced development of hypercholesterolemic atherosclerosis by 38%. This protection was associated with a decrease in the MDA concentration and activity of catalase and GSH-P$_X$, and an increase in antioxidant reserve in aorta.

Flaxseed and Secoisolariciresinol Diglucoside

Flaxseed reduces the development of hypercholesterolemic atherosclerosis in rabbits by 46%. This protection was associated with a decrease in the OFR producing activity of PMNLs.[119] Serum TGs and total cholesterol concentrations remained unaltered. The protective effect could be due to a decrease in the OFR-producing activity of PMNLs and/or the ω-3 fatty acid content of flaxseed.

The antiatherosclerotic effect of flaxseed could not be due to the ω-3 fatty acid content of flaxseed because a variety of flaxseed (called *Crop Development Center [CDC] flaxseed*), which has a very low content of ω-3 fatty acid, reduces hypercholesterolemic atherosclerosis by 69% in a dose similar to flaxseed.[157] An antiatherosclerotic effect was associated with decreases in serum total cholesterol and LDL cholesterol levels and total cholesterol/HDL cholesterol ratio by approximately 30%. The antiatherosclerotic effect of CDC-flaxseed could be due in part to decreases in the concentrations of total cholesterol and LDL cholesterol produced by it. However, an antiatherosclerotic effect could also be due to the antioxidant activity of flaxseed lignans contained in the flaxseed meal.

Secoisolariciresinol diglucoside isolated from flaxseed meal (devoid of oil) has antioxidant activity.[158] Secoisolariciresinol diglucoside decreases the development of hypercholesterolemic atherosclerosis in rabbits by 73%.[159] Reduction in atherosclerosis was associated with decreases in aortic MDA, serum total cholesterol, and LDL cholesterol levels and an increase in serum HDL cholesterol concentration. Prevention of hypercholesterolemic atherosclerosis by secoisolariciresinol diglucoside could be due to a fall in serum total cholesterol and LDL cholesterol levels, a rise in serum HDL cholesterol concentration, and antioxidant activity.

Hyperhomocysteinemia

Hyperhomocysteinemia is a newly emerging risk factor for atherosclerosis. From 30% to 50% of atherosclerosis is related to hyperhomocysteinemia. Both hereditary and nutritional factors contribute to its occurrence. It is an independent risk factor for CAD.

Synthesis and Metabolism

Homocysteine is a sulfur-containing amino acid derived from methionine metabolism. It is essential for a number of biochemical processes including metabolism of nucleic acids, fats, and high-energy bonds. Synthesis and metabolism of homocysteine are shown in Figure 6.4.

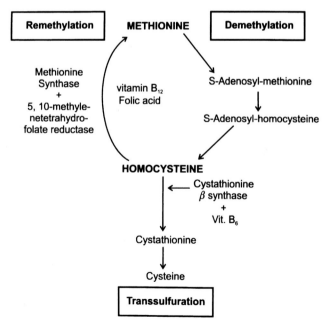

FIGURE 6.4. Synthesis and metabolism of homocysteine.

Demethylation

Demethylation converts methionine to homocysteine through the intermediate metabolites S-adenosylmethionine and S-adenosylhomocysteine.

Transmethylation

In the transmethylation pathway homocysteine is remethylated to methionine in the presence of methionine synthase and 5,10-methylenetetrahydrofolate reductase. This reaction requires folic acid and vitamin B_{12}. In normal metabolism the majority (>50%) of homocysteine is remethylated to methionine.

Transsulfuration

In transsulfuration homocysteine is converted to cystathionine and then cysteine. This process requires cystathionine β-synthase and vitamin B_6 as a cofactor.[160] Cysteine is further broken down into sulfate and excreted through the kidney.

Normal Values

The normal total plasma homocysteine concentration ranges from 5 to 15 μmol/L. About 70% of the plasma homocysteine is bound to serum protein[161] and is in equilibrium with free homocysteine.

Causes of Hyperhomocysteinemia

The plasma concentration of homocysteine rises with age. Causes of hyperhomocysteinemia are shown in Table 6.4. Hyperhomocysteinemia can be due to enzyme deficiencies, vitamin deficiencies, disease states, and drugs; it is caused by a defect in the transsulfuration of

TABLE 6.4. Etiology of hyperhomocysteinemia.

Enzyme deficiency
  Cystathionine β-synthase
  Methionine synthase
  5,10-methylenetetrahydrofolate reductase
Vitamin deficiency
  Vitamin B_{12}
  Folic acid
  Vitamin B_6
Drugs
  Inhibitor of dihydrofolate reductase: methotrexate
  Folic acid antagonist: phenytoin, carbamazepine
  Methionine synthase inhibitor: nitrous oxide
  Vitamin B_6 antagonist: theophylline, 6-azauridine triacetate
Diseases
  Chronic renal failure
  Acute lymphoblastic anemia
  Psoriasis
  Coronary and peripheral atherosclerosis
  Hypertension
  Extracranial carotid artery stenosis

homocysteine to cysteine, because of a defect in the gene for cystathionine or in the genes for the enzymes (methionine synthase or 5,10-methylenetetrahydrofolate reductase) responsible for the remethylation of homocysteine to methionine.[162] Deficiency in vitamin B_6, vitamin B_{12}, and folic acid interferes with both the transsulfuration and remethylation processes, and hence there is an increase in plasma concentration of homocysteine.[163,164]

Effects of Homocysteine

Homocysteine produces thromboembolism, atherosclerosis, and vascular endothelial cell damage. It increases platelet adhesion and aggregation, inhibition of Na^+,K^+–adenosinetriphosphatase activity, and hemolysis of erythrocytes.

Mechanism of Atherosclerosis in Hyperhomocysteinemia

Endothelial cell damage is the prerequisite for development of atherosclerosis according to the response-to-injury hypothesis of atherosclerosis. Homocysteine is toxic to endothelial cells,[165–171] possibly because of generation of OFRs from homocysteine. As such, the sulfhydryl group of homocysteine is believed to act catalytically with ferric or cupric ions in a mixed-function oxidation system to generate hydrogen peroxide, oxygen radicals, and homocysteinyl radicals.[172–174] High concentrations of homocysteine increase intracellular reduced homocysteine, which participates in the transsulfuration pathway and can replace cysteine in the synthesis of glutathione. Reduced homocysteine concentrations in the presence of copper ions in the cell culture medium are directly toxic to the cells. The cell toxicity may be due to the OFRs formed by thiol autooxidation.[175] Superoxide anions are formed during oxidation (by oxygen) of homocysteine to homocysteine.[168]

There is a decrease in the activity of antioxidant enzymes (SOD, catalase, and GSH-P_X) in the plasma of rabbits with methionine-induced atherosclerosis.[176] However antioxidant enzymes of aorta increased with such a diet. In erythrocytes, SOD activity increased, catalase activity remained normal, and GSH-P_X activity decreased. The lipid peroxidation product MDA increased in both plasma and aorta.[176] Homocysteine decreases intracellular glutathione and NAD^+ levels[170] and the ratio between intracellular concentrations of reduced and oxidized glutathione.[174] The toxic effect of homocysteine alone and homocysteine plus Cu^{2+} was associated with an increase in lipid peroxidation that was prevented by catalase and reduced by deferoxamine mesylate.[171] Homocysteine may cause vascular injury by promoting oxidation of LDL cholesterol.[168] Homocysteine, in the presence of a transition metal (iron or copper) causes

oxidation of LDL.[177,178] OX-LDL has been implicated in the development of atherosclerosis.[35] Another mechanism of endothelial cell injury could be the inability to sustain S-NO-homocysteine formation owing to an imbalance between the production of nitric oxide by dysfunctional endothelium and the concentration of homocysteine. It is known that brief exposure of endothelial cells to homocysteine stimulates secretion of nitric oxide, which leads to the formation of S-nitric oxide–homocysteine, a potent antiplatelet agent and vasodilator. It generates H_2O_2 and unlike homocysteine does not undergo conversion to homocysteine thiolactate.[173,179] Homocysteine thiolactate is believed to be cytotoxic. Homocysteine-induced endothelial cell dysfunction eventually leads to atherosclerosis. Vascular smooth muscle cells are adversely affected by homocysteine, which stimulates proliferation of smooth muscle cells in culture.[180]

Hyperhomocysteinemia and CAD

Homocysteine may play a role in the etiology of CAD. Hyperhomocysteinemia is an independent risk factor for CAD.[163,166,181–186] Many studies suggest that hyperhomocysteinemia is associated with an increased risk of CAD.[168,181,187–189] A modest increase in the concentration of homocysteine (>15 to 20 μmol/L) has been reported in patients with CAD, stroke, and peripheral vascular disease.[163,164] Plasma folate and vitamin B_{12} concentrations are inversely associated with homocysteine concentrations.[190,191] Studies have shown that elevated plasma homocysteine concentrations can be normalized by treatment with folate or vitamin B_{12}.[183,191] Patients with CAD and other forms of atherosclerosis have lower plasma concentrations of vitamin B_6 than control subjects.[192,193] Lower plasma concentrations of vitamin B_6 are associated with hyperhomocysteinemia. Treatment with vitamin B_6 reduces LDL cholesterol concentration by 17%.[194] Morrison et al.[195] have reported that persons with lower plasma folate concentrations had a higher 15-year coronary mortality rate.

Stroke and Peripheral Vascular Disease and Homocysteinemia

Homocysteine concentration is elevated in patients with stroke and peripheral vascular disease.[163,164,196] Lower limb atherosclerotic disease is associated with high fasting homocysteine concentrations.[197] An increased concentration of homocysteine is seen in patients with premature CAD, peripheral vascular disease, and cerebrovascular disease.[185,198,199] High plasma homocysteine concentration and low concentrations of folate and vitamin B_6 are associated with an increased risk of extracranial carotid artery stenosis in the elderly.[200,201] Plasma homocysteine concentration is elevated in patients with carotid artery intimal wall thickening.[202] In normotensive subjects a high normal homocysteine concentration is associated with an increased prevalence of carotid artery wall thickening.[203]

Deep Venous Thrombosis and Homocysteinemia

Hyperhomocysteinemia is a common risk factor for recurrent venous thrombosis.[201] Patients with homocystinuria have the most frequent thrombotic complications, such as deep venous thrombosis.[204] Plasma homocysteine concentrations of 25% of patients with recurrent venous thrombosis were high during both fasting and methionine-loading tests.[205]

Renal Disease and Hyperhomocysteinemia

The kidney plays a part in homocysteine metabolism.[206] The incidence of vascular disease is increased in patients with continuous ambulatory peritoneal dialysis[207] and acute dialysis.[208] Patients with renal failure, end-stage renal disease, and chronic uremia have hyperhomocysteinemia and are at risk for atherosclerosis.[209-211]

Organ Transplant and Homocysteine

Homocysteine concentration was elevated (70%) after cardiac transplant and remained elevated for 12 months.[212] Associated with an increase in homocysteine was a decrease in plasma concentrations of vitamin B_{12} and folic acid. Homocysteine concentration is also elevated in patients who have undergone kidney, lung, or liver transplant. The vascular complications in transplant patients may be due to hyperhomocysteinemia, which is atherogenic and thrombogenic.

Type I Diabetes Mellitus and Homocysteine

Homocysteine levels in plasma are lower in patients with type I diabetes than normal subjects.[213] Accelerated atherosclerosis in such patients could be due to factors other than homocysteine.

Experimental Atherosclerosis and Homocysteine

A diet high in methionine content (3% D,L-methionine) increased the plasma concentration of TGs, cholesterol, homocysteine, cysteine, and lipid peroxides and was associated with the development of aortic atherosclerosis.[214] Rabbits on a diet of 0.3% methionine for 6 to 9 months had increased plasma and aortic lipid peroxida-

tion product levels and aortic antioxidant enzyme activity.[176] However, plasma antioxidant activity decreased. In erythrocytes, SOD activity increased, catalase activity remained normal, and GSH-P_X activity decreased. These changes were associated with the development of atherosclerosis in aorta. High doses of methionine in normotensive rats and spontaneous hypertensive rats had variable effects.[169] The methionine diet increased the serum homocysteine concentration and was associated with aortic atherosclerosis. Hyperhomocysteinemia was associated with considerable loss of endothelium, degradation of media cells and degenerating mitochondria, and elevation of cystathione concentration in the aortic wall. Spontaneous hypertensive rats had higher serum homocysteine and cystathione levels than the normotensive rats. Methionine-induced atherosclerotic changes in the aorta were more pronounced and developed earlier in spontaneous hypertensive rats than in normotensive rats.

Therapeutic Regimen for Hyperhomocysteinemia

Folic acid decreases the serum concentration of homocysteine in normal subjects and patients with vascular disease and chronic renal failure.[163,164,209] Chauveau et al.[209] used folic acid (10 mg/d) and vitamin B_6 (70 mg/d) for two 3-month periods in nondialyzed chronic renal failure patients. They concluded that folic acid (but not vitamin B_6) was effective in lowering plasma homocysteine concentrations. Naurath et al.[215] used folic acid (1.1 mg/d), vitamin B_{12} (1 mg/d), and vitamin B_6 (5 mg/d) to normalize elevated homocysteine concentrations. In patients with CAD, folic acid in daily doses of 0.4 mg, 1.0 mg, or 5 mg for 3 months reduced the homocysteine concentration by 30%.[216] High doses of folic acid (15 mg/d or more) are required to reduce homocysteine concentrations in renal failure patients.

Individuals with elevated plasma homocysteine levels are normalized by treatment with folic acid or vitamin B_{12}.[183,217-219] A threshold for increasing homocysteine appears when the folate concentration is less than 12.5 nmol/L and for vitamin B_{12} 225 pmol/L.[191] In the United States the accepted lower limit for normal fasting plasma folate is 6.8 nmol/L, whereas the World Health Organization lower limit is 13.6 nmol/L.

Fish oil has been administered to patients with hyperhomocysteinemia. The results are conflicting. Fish oil (12 g/d) lowers serum homocysteine levels in patients with type IIa or IIb lipoproteinemia or hypertriglyceridemia.[172] However, Holdt et al.[207] reported that fish oil did not lower serum homocysteine concentration in patients on continuous ambulatory peritoneal dialysis.

Acknowledgment

I am very thankful to Ms. Gloria Schneider for her excellent assistance in preparing this manuscript.

References

1. Ross R, Glomset JA. The pathogenesis of atherosclerosis. *N Engl J Med.* 1976;295:369–377, 420–425.

2. Ross R. The pathogenesis of atherosclerosis: an update. *N Engl J Med.* 1986;314:488–500.

3. Ross R. Atherosclerosis: a defense mechanism gone awry [Rous-Whipple Award Lecture]. *Am J Pathol.* 1993;143: 987–1002.

4. Gimbrone MA Jr. Vascular endothelium: an integrator of pathophysiologic stimuli in atherosclerosis. *Am J Cardiol.* 1995;75:67B–70B.

5. Denholm EM, Lewis JC. Monocyte chemoattractants in pigeon aortic atherosclerosis. *Am J Pathol.* 1987;126: 464–475.

6. Davies PF, Remuzzi A, Gordon EJ, Dewey CF, Gimbrone MA Jr. Turbulent fluid shear stress induces vascular endothelial cell turnover in vitro. *Proc Natl Acad Sci U S A.* 1986;83:2114–2117.

7. Duff GL, McMillan GC. Pathology of atherosclerosis. *Am J Med.* 1951;11:92–108.

8. Endemann G, Pronczuk A, Friedman G, Lindsey S, Alderson L, Hayes KC. Monocyte adherence to endothelial cells in vitro is increased by beta-VLDL. *Am J Pathol.* 1987; 126:1–6.

9. Joris T, Nunnari JJ, Krolikowski FJ, Majno G. Studies on the pathogenesis of atherosclerosis, I: adhesion and emigration of mononuclear cells in the aorta of hypercholesterolemic rats. *Am J Pathol.* 1983;113:341–358.

10. Anderson KM, Castelli WP, Levy D. Cholesterol and mortality: 30 years follow-up from Framingham Study. *JAMA.* 1987;257:2176–2180.

11. Castelli WP. The triglyceride issue: a view from Framingham. *Am Heart J.* 1986;112:432–437.

12. Castelli WP. Cholesterol and lipids in the risk of coronary artery disease: the Framingham Heart Study. *Can J Cardiol.* 1988;4(suppl A):5A–10A.

13. Lipid Research Clinic Program. The Lipid Research Clinics coronary primary prevention trial results. *JAMA.* 1954;251:351–374.

14. Davis C, Rifkind B, Brenner H, Gordon D. A single cholesterol measurement underestimates the risk of CHD: an empirical example from the Lipid Research Clinic's mortality followup study. *JAMA.* 1990;264:3044–3046.

15. Austin MA. Plasma triglycerides as a risk factor for coronary artery disease: the epidemiological evidence and beyond. *Am J Epidemiol.* 1989;129:249–259.

16. Fontbonne AM, Eschwege EM. Insulin and cardiovascular disease: Paris Prospective Study. *Diabetes Care.* 1991;14: 461–469.

17. Enas EA, Yusuf S, Mehta JL. Prevalence of coronary artery disease in Asian Indians. *Am J Cardiol.* 1992;70:945–949.

18. Steinberg D, Witztum JL. Lipoproteins and atherogenesis: current concepts. *JAMA.* 1990;264:3047–3052.

19. Austin MA, King MC, Vranizam KM, et al. Atherogenic lipoprotein phenotype: a proposed genetic marker for coronary heart disease risk. *Circulation.* 1990;82:495–506.

20. deGraff J, Hak-Lemmers HLM, Hectors PNM, et al. Enhanced susceptibility to in vitro oxidation of the dense low density lipoprotein subfractions in healthy subjects. *Arteriosc Thromb.* 1991;11:298–306.

21. Anderson DW, Nichols AV, Pan SS, et al. High density lipoprotein distribution: resolution and determination of three major components in normal population sample. *Atherosclerosis.* 1978;29:161–179.

22. Montali A, Vega GL, Grundy SM. Concentrations of apolipoprotein A-1 containing particles in patients with hypoalphalipoproteinemia. *Arteriosc Thromb.* 1994;14: 511–517

23. Rubin EM, Krauss RM, Spangler EA, et al. Inhibition of early atherogenesis in transgenic mice by human apolipoprotein A-1. *Nature.* 1991;353:265–267.

24. Karathanasis SK, Ferris E, Haddad IA. DNA inversion within the apolipoprotein AI/C III/ATV encoding gene cluster of certain patients with premature atherosclerosis. *Proc Natl Acad Sci U S A.* 1987;84:7198–7202.

25. Grundy SM. Atherogenic dyslipidemia: lipoprotein abnormalities and implications for therapy. *Am J Cardiol.* 1995; 75(suppl B):B45–B52.

26. Khoo JC, Miller E, McLoughlin P, et al. Prevention of low density lipoprotein aggregation by high density lipoprotein or apolipoprotein A-1. *J Lipid Res.* 1990;31:645–658.

27. Parthsarathy S, Barnett J, Fong LG. High density lipoprotein inhibits the oxidative modification of low density lipoprotein. *Biochem Biophys Acta.* 1990;1044:275–283.

28. Utermann G. Lipoprotein(a). In: Seriver CK, Beaudet AL, Sly WS, Valle D, eds. *The Metabolic and Molecular Bases of Inherited Disease.* New York, NY: McGraw Hill; 1995: 1887–1912.

29. Enas EA. Rapid angiographic progression of coronary artery disease in patients with elevated lipoprotein (a). *Circulation.* 1995;92:2352–2354.

30. Henriksen T, Mahoney EM, Steinberg D. Enhanced macrophage degradation of low density lipoprotein previously incubated with cultured endothelial cells: recognition by receptor for acetylated low density lipoproteins. *Proc Natl Acad Sci U S A.* 1981;78:6499–6503.

31. Keany JF Jr, Vita JA. Atherosclerosis, oxidative stress, and antioxidant protection in endothelium-derived relaxing factor action. *Prog Cardiovasc Dis.* 1995;38:129–154.

32. Chisolm GM III. Antioxidant and atherosclerosis: a current assessment. *Clin Cardiol.* 1991;14:25–30.

33. Schwartz CJ, Valenta AJ, Sprague EA. A modern view of atherogenesis. *Am J Cardiol.* 1993;71(suppl B):B9–B14.

34. Steinberg D, Parthasarathy S, Carew TE. In vivo inhibition of foam cell development by probucol in Watanabe rabbits. *Am J Cardiol.* 1988;62(suppl B):B6–B12.

35. Steinberg D. Antioxidant and atherosclerosis: a current assessment. *Circulation.* 1991;84:1420–1425.

36. Gimbrone MA Jr. Vascular endothelium: an integrator of pathophysiologic stimuli in atherosclerosis. *Am J Cardiol.* 1995;75:67B–70B.

37. Ridker PM, Hennekens CH, Roitman-Johnson B, Stampfer MJ, Allen J. Plasma concentration of soluble intercellular adhesion molecule and risks of future myocardial infarction in apparently healthy men. *Lancet.* 1998;351:88–92.

38. Holvoet P, Collen D. Thrombosis and atherosclerosis. *Curr Opin Lipidol*. 1997;8:320–328.

39. Gearing AJH, Newman W. Circulating adhesion molecules in disease. *Immunol Today*. 1993;14:506–512.

40. Martin A, Foxall T, Blumberg JB, Meyadani M. Vitamin E inhibits low-density lipoprotein-induced adhesion of monocytes to human aortic endothelial cells in vitro. *Arterioscler Thromb Vasc Biol*. 1997;17:429–436.

41. Faruqi R, de la Motta C, DiCorleto P. Alpha-tocopherol inhibits agonist-induced monocytic cell adhesion to cultured human epithelial cells. *J Clin Invest*. 1994;94:592–600.

42. Chiu JJ, Wung BS, Shyy JY, Hsieh HJ, Wang DL. Reactive oxygen species are involved in shear stress–induced intercellular adhesion molecule-1 expression in endothelial cells. *Arterioscler Thromb Vasc Biol*. 1997;17:3570–3577.

43. Kaneko M, Hayashi J, Saito I, Miyasaka N. Probucol down regulates E-selectin expression in cultured human vascular endothelial cells. *Arterioscler Thromb Vasc Biol*. 1996;16:1047–1051.

44. Xia L, Pan J, Yao L, McEver RP. A protease inhibitor, and antioxidant, or a salicylate, but not glucocorticoid, blocks constitute and cytokine inducible expression of P-selectin in human endothelial cells. *Blood*. 1998;91:1625–1632.

45. Devaraj S, Li D, Jialal I. The effects of alpha tocopherol supplementation on monocyte function: decreased lipid oxidation, interleukin 1β secretion, and monocyte adhesion to endothelium. *J Clin Invest*. 1996;98:756–763.

46. Keaney JF Jr, Gaziano JM, Xu A, Frei B, Curran-Celentano J, Shwaery GT, Loscalzo J, Vita JA. Low-dose α-tocopherol improves and high-dose α-tocopherol worsens endothelial vasodilator function in cholesterol-fed rabbits. *J Clin Invest*. 1994;93:844–851.

47. DiCorleto PE, Chisolm GM. Participation of the endothelium in the development of atherosclerotic plaque. *Prog Lipid Res*. 1986;25:365–374.

48. Libby P, Hansson GK. Biology of disease. Involvement of the immune system in human atherogenesis: current knowledge and unanswered questions. *Lab Invest*. 1991;64:5–15.

49. Ross R. The pathogenesis of atherosclerosis: a prospective for the 1990s. *Nature*. 1993;362:801–809.

50. Prasad K, Kalra J. Oxygen free radicals and hypercholesterolemic atherosclerosis: effect of vitamin E. *Am Heart J*. 1993;125:958–973.

51. Prasad K, Kalra J, Lee P. Oxygen free radicals as a mechanism of hypercholesterolemic atherosclerosis: effects of probucol. *Int J Angiol*. 1994;3:100–112.

52. Gotto AM, Gorry GA, Thompson JR, et al. Relationship between plasma, lipid concentration, and coronary artery disease in 496 patients. *Circulation*. 1977;56:875–883.

53. Görg P, Kakkar VV. Increased uptake of monocyte-treated low density lipoproteins by aortic endothelium in vivo. *Atherosclerosis*. 1987;65:99–107.

54. Prisco D, Rogasi PG, Matucci M, et al. Age related changes in platelet lipid composition. *Thromb Res*. 1986;44:427–437.

55. Stuart MJ, Gerrard JM, White JG. Effect of cholesterol on production of thromboxane B$_2$ by platelets in vitro. *N Engl J Med*. 1980;302:6–10.

56. Henry RL. Platelet function. *Semin Thromb Hemost*. 1977;4:93–122.

57. Ruzicka T, Printz MP. Arachidonic acid metabolism in skin: a review. *Rev Physiol Biochem Pharmacol*. 1984;100:121–160.

58. Vanden Bosch H. Intracellular phospholipases A. *Biochem Biophys Acta*. 1980;604:191–246.

59. Quan-sang KHL, Levenson J, Simon A, et al. Platelet cytosolic free Ca^{++} concentration and plasma cholesterol in untreated hypertensives. *J Hypertens*. 1987;5(suppl 5):S251–S254.

60. Whatley RE, Nelson P, Zimmerman GA, et al. The regulation of platelet-activating factor production in endothelial cells: the role of calcium and protein kinase *Can J Biol Chem*. 1989;264:6325–6333.

61. Egan RW, Paxton J, Kuehl FA Jr. Mechanism for irreversible self-deactivation of prostaglandin synthetase. *J Biol Chem*. 1976;251:7329–7335.

62. Murota SI, Morita I, Suda N. The control of vascular endothelial cell injury. *Ann N Y Acad Sci*. 1990;598:182–187.

63. Vogt W, Von Zabern I, Damerau B, et al. Mechanisms of complement activation by crystalline cholesterol. *Mol Immunol*. 1985;22:101–106.

64. Ford-Hutchinson AW, Bray MA, Doig MV, et al. Leukotriene B$_4$, a potent chemokinetic and aggregating substance released from polymorphonuclear leukocytes. *Nature*. 1980;286:264–267.

65. Hanahan DJ. Platelet-activating factor: a biologically active phosphoglyceride. *Annu Rev Biochem*. 1986;55:483–509.

66. Webster RO, Hong SR, Johnston RB Jr, et al. Biological effects of human complement fragments of C5a and C5a des Arg on neutrophil function. *Immunopharmacology*. 1980;2:201–219.

67. Rosen GM, Freeman BA. Detection of superoxide generated by endothelial cells. *Proc Natl Acad Sci U S A*. 1984;81:7269–7273.

68. Heinecke JW, Baker L, Rosen H, et al. Superoxide mediated modification of low density lipoprotein by human arterial smooth muscle cells in culture. *J Clin Invest*. 1986;77:757–761.

69. Hiramatsu K, Rosen H, Heinecke JW, et al. Superoxide initiates oxidation of low density lipoprotein by human monocytes. *Atherosclerosis*. 1986;7:50–60.

70. Prasad K, Kalra J, Chaudhary AK, Debnath D. Effect of polymorphonuclear leukocyte-derived oxygen free radicals and hypochlorous acid on cardiac function and some biochemical parameters. *Am Heart J*. 1990;119:538–550.

71. Prasad K, Chaudhary AK, Kalra J. Oxygen-derived free radical producing activity and survival of activated polymorphonuclear leukocytes. *Mol Cell Biochem*. 1991;103:51–62.

72. Ohara Y, Peterson TE, Harrison DG. Hypercholesterolemia increases endothelial superoxide anion production: the Framingham Study. *J Clin Invest*. 1993;91:2546–2551.

73. Kannel WB. Role of blood pressure in cardiovascular disease: the Framingham Study. *Angiology*. 1975;26:1–14.

74. Rosenman RH, Sholtz RI, Brand RJ. A study of comparative blood pressure measures in predicting risk of coronary heart disease. *Circulation*. 1976;54:51–58.

75. Owens GK. Control of hypertrophic versus hyperplastic growth of vascular smooth muscle cells. *Am J Physiol.* 1989;257(suppl):H1755–H1765.

76. Chobanian AV. Corcoran lecture: adaptive and maladaptive responses of arterial wall to hypertension. *Hypertension.* 1990;15:666–674.

77. Lyons TJ. Glycation and oxidation: a role in the pathogenesis of atherosclerosis. *Am J Cardiol.* 1993;71:26B–31B.

78. Fielding JE. Smoking: health effects and control (pt 1). *N Engl J Med.* 1985;313:491–498.

79. Friedman GD, Dales LG, Ury HK. Mortality in middle-aged smokers and nonsmokers. *N Engl J Med.* 1979;300: 213–217.

80. Kalra J, Chaudhary AK, Prasad K. Increased production of oxygen free radicals in cigarette smokers. *Int J Exp Pathol.* 1991;72:1–7.

81. Burdon RH, Rice-Evans C. Free radicals and the regulation of mammalian cell proliferation. *Free Radical Res Commun.* 1989;6:345–358.

82. Murrell GAL, Francis MJO, Bromley L. Modulation of fibroblast proliferation by oxygen free radicals. *Biochem J.* 1990;265:659–665.

83. Hennekens CH, Rosner B, Cole DS. Daily alcohol consumption and coronary artery disease. *Am J Epidemiol.* 1978;107:196–200.

84. Schmidt W, deLint J. Causes of death of alcoholics. *Q J Stud Alcohol.* 1972;33:171–185.

85. Castelli WP, Doyle JT, Gordon T, et al. Alcohol and blood lipids: the cooperative lipoprotein phenotyping study. *Lancet.* 1977;2:153–155.

86. Haffner J, Appelbaum-Bowden D, Hoover J, et al. Association of high-density lipoprotein cholesterol 2 and 3 with Querelet, alcohol, and smoking, The Seattle Lipid Research Clinic population. *Cardiovascular Disease Epidemiol Newsl.* 1982;31: 20–22.

87. Haskell WL, Camargo C, Williams PT, et al. The effect of cessation and resumption of moderate alcohol intake on serum high-density lipoprotein subfractions. *N Engl J Med.* 1984;310:805–810.

88. Gordon T, Kannel WB. Obesity and cardiovascular disease: the Framingham Study. *Clin Endocrinol Metab.* 1976;5: 367–375.

89. Ashley FW Jr, Kannel WB. Relation of weight change to changes in atherogenic traits: the Framingham Study. *J Chronic Dis.* 1974;27:103–114.

90. Jick H, Miettinen OS, Neff RK, et al. Coffee and myocardial infarction. *N Engl J Med.* 1973;289:63–67.

91. Bellet S, Horstmann E, Roman LR, et al. Effect of caffeine on the ventricular fibrillation threshold in normal dogs and dogs with acute myocardial infarction. *Am Heart J.* 1972;84:215–227.

92. Kannel WB, Dawber TR. Coffee and coronary disease. *N Engl J Med.* 1973;289:100–101.

93. Tverdal A, Stensvold I, Solvall K, et al. Coffee consumption and death from coronary heart disease in middle aged Norwegian men and women. *BMJ.* 1990;300: 566–569.

94. Thelle DS, Heyden S, Fodor JG. Coffee and cholesterol in epidemiological and experimental studies. *Atherosclerosis.* 1987;67:97–103.

95. Bak AAA, Grobbee DE. The effect on serum cholesterol levels of coffee brewed by filtering or boiling. *N Engl J Med.* 1989;321:1432–1437.

96. Zock PL, Katan MB, Merkus MP, et al. Effect of lipid-rich fraction from boiled coffee on serum cholesterol. *Lancet.* 1990;335:1235–1237.

97. Heckers H, Gobel U, Kleppel U. End of coffee mystery: diterpene alcohol raise serum low-density lipoprotein cholesterol and triglyceride levels. *J Intern Med.* 1994;235: 192–193.

98. Weusten-Vander Wouw MPME, Katan MB, Viani R, et al. Identity of the cholesterol-raising factor from boiled coffee and its effect on liver function enzymes. *J Lipid Res.* 1994;35:721–733.

99. Post SM, deWit ECM, Princen HMG. Cafestol, the cholesterol-raising factor in boiled coffee, suppresses bile acid synthesis by downregulation of cholesterol 7 α-hydroxylase and sterol 27-hydroxylase in rat hepatocytes. *Arterioscler Thromb Vasc Biology.* 1997;17: 3064–3070.

100. Nicholls AC, Thomas M. Coxsackie virus infection in acute myocardial infarction. *Lancet.* 1997;1:883–884.

101. Melnick JL, Adam E, DeBakey ME. Cytomegalovirus and atherosclerosis. *Eur Heart J.* 1993;14(suppl K):30–38.

102. Benditt EP, Barrett T, McDougall JK. Viruses in the etiology of atherosclerosis. *Proc Natl Acad Sci U S A.* 1983; 80:6386–6389.

103. Jacob HS. Newly recognized causes of atherosclerosis: the role of microorganisms. *J Lab Clin Med.* 1994;123: 808–816.

104. Mattila KJ, Valle MS, Nieminen MS, et al. Dental infections and coronary atherosclerosis. *Atherosclerosis.* 1993; 103:205–211.

105. Mendall MA, Goggin PM, Molineaux N, et al. Relation of *Helicobacter pylori* in coronary heart disease. *Br Heart J.* 1994;71:437–439.

106. Saikku P. *Chlamydia pneumoniae* and atherosclerosis: an update. *Scand J Infect Dis Suppl.* 1997;104:53–56.

107. Gupta S, Leatham EW. The relation between chlamydia pneumoniae and atherosclerosis. *Heart.* 1997;77:7–8.

108. Jackson LA, Campbell LA, Schmidt RA, et al. Specificity of detection of *Chlamydia pneumoniae* in vascular atheroma: evaluation of the innocent bystander hypothesis. *Am J Pathol.* 1997;150:1785–1790.

109. Wimmer MLJ, Sandmann-Strupp R, Saikku P, et al. Association of chlamydia infection with cerebrovascular disease. *Stroke.* 1996;27:2207–2210.

110. Moazed TC, Kuo CC, Patton DL, et al. Animal model: experimental rabbit models of *Chlamydia pneumoniae* infection. *Am J Pathol.* 1996;148:667–676.

111. Cook PJ, Lip GYH. Infectious agents and atherosclerotic vascular disease. *Q J Med.* 1996;89:727–735.

112. Gamble JR, Harlan JM, Klebanoff SJ, et al. Stimulation of adherence of neutrophils to umbilical vein endothelium by human recombinant tumor necrosis factor. *Proc Natl Acad Sci U S A.* 1985;82:8667–8671.

113. Bella J, Kolatkar PR, Marlor CW, Greve JM, Rossmann MG. The structure of the two aminoterminal domains of human ICAM-1 suggests how it functions as a rhinovirus

receptor and as an LFA-1 integrin ligand. *Proc Natl Acad Sci U S A*. 1998;95:4140–4145.

114. Laurila A, Bloigu A, Näyhä S, et al. Chronic *Chlamydia pneumoniae* infection is associated with a serum lipid profile known to be a risk factor for atherosclerosis. *Arterioscler Thromb Vasc Biol*. 1997;17:2910–2913.

115. Laurila A, Bloigu A, Näyhä S, et al. *Chlamydia pneumoniae* antibodies and serum lipids in Finnish males. *BMJ*. 1997;14:1456–1457.

116. Gallin JI, Kaye D, O'Leary WM, et al. Serum lipids in infection. *N Engl J Med*. 1969;281:1081–1086.

117. Kaukoranta-Tolvanen SS, Teppo AM, Laitinen K, et al. Growth of *Chlamydia pneumoniae* in cultured peripheral blood mononuclear cells and induction of a cytokine response. *Microb Pathogen*. 1996;21:215–221.

118. Richardson SGN, Mathews KB, Gruikshank JK, et al. Coagulation activity and hyperviscosity in infection. *Br J Haematol*. 1979;42:469–480.

119. Prasad K. Dietary flaxseed in prevention of hypercholesterolemic atherosclerosis. *Atherosclerosis*. 1997;132:69–76.

120. Prasad K, Mantha SV, Kalra J, et al. Purpurogallin in the prevention of hypercholesterolemic atherosclerosis. *Int J Angiol*. 1997;6:157–166.

121. Prasad K, Mantha SV, Kalra J, et al. Prevention of hypercholesterolemic atherosclerosis by garlic, an antioxidant. *J Cardiovasc Pharmacol Ther*. 1997;2:309–320.

122. Palinski W, Rosenfeld ME, Ylä-Herittuala S, et al. Low density lipoprotein undergoes oxidative modification in vivo. *Proc Natl Acad Sci U S A*. 1989;86:1372–1376.

123. Mantha SV, Prasad M, Kalra J, Prasad K. Antioxidant enzymes in hypercholesterolemia and effects of vitamin E in rabbits. *Atherosclerosis*. 1993;101:135–144.

124. Mantha SV, Kalra J, Prasad K. Effects of probucol on hypercholesterolemia-induced changes in antioxidant enzymes. *Life Sci*. 1996;58:503–509.

125. Boscoboinik D, Szewczyk A, Azzi A. α-tocopherol (vitamin E) regulates vascular smooth muscle cell proliferation and protein kinase C activity. *Arch Biochem Biophys*. 1991; 286:264–269.

126. Williams RJ, Motteram JM, Sharp CH, et al. Dietary vitamin E and attenuation of early lesion development in modified Watanabe rabbits. *Atherosclerosis*. 1992;94: 153–159.

127. Bocan TM, Mueller SB, Brown EQ, et al. Antiatherogenic effects of antioxidants are lesion specific when evaluated in hypercholesterolemic New Zealand white rabbits. *Exp Mol Pathol*. 1992;57:70–83.

128. Verlangieri AJ, Bush MJ. Effects of *d*-alpha-tocopherol supplementation on experimentally induced primate atherosclerosis. *J Am Coll Nutr*. 1992;11:131–138.

129. Godfried SL, Combs GF, Saroka JM. Potentiation of atherosclerotic lesions in rabbits by high dietary level of vitamin E. *Br J Nutr*. 1989;61:607–617.

130. Haeger K. Long-time treatment of intermittent claudication with vitamin E. *Am J Clin Nutr*. 1974;27:1179–1181.

131. DeMaio S, King SB III, Lembo NJ, et al. Vitamin E supplementation, plasma lipids, and incidence of restenosis after percutaneous transluminal coronary angioplasty. *J Am Coll Nutr*. 1992;11:68–73.

132. Rimm EB, Stampfer MJ, Ascherio A, et al. Vitamin E consumption and the risk of coronary heart disease in men. *N Engl J Med*. 1993;328:1450–1456.

133. Stampfer MJ, Hennekens CH, Manson JE, et al. Vitamin E consumption and the risk of coronary artery disease in women. *N Engl J Med*. 1993;328:1444–1449.

134. Gey KF. Inverse correlation of vitamin E and ischemic heart disease. *Int J Vitam Nutr Res Suppl*. 1989;30:224–237.

135. Jailal I, Vega GL, Grundy SM. Physiologic levels of ascorbate inhibit oxidative modification of low-density lipoprotein. *Atherosclerosis*. 1990;82:185–191.

136. Kimura H, Yamada Y, Morita Y, et al. Dietary ascorbic acid depresses plasma and low density lipoprotein lipid peroxidation in genetically scorbutic rabbits. *J Nutr*. 1992;122: 1904–1909.

137. Ginter E, Babala J, Cerven J. The effect of chronic hypovitaminosis C on the metabolism of cholesterol and atherogenesis in guinea pigs. *J Atheroscl Res*. 1969;10: 341–352.

138. Bridges AB, Scott NA, Belch JJF. Probucol, a superoxide free radical scavenger in vitro. *Atherosclerosis*. 1991;89: 263–265.

139. Yamamoto A, Hara H, Takaichi S, et al. Effect of probucol on macrophages, leading to regression of xanthomas and atheromatous vascular lesion. *Am J Cardiol*. 1988;62(suppl B):B31–B36.

140. Kita T, Nagano Y, Yokode M, et al. Prevention of atherosclerotic progression in Watanabe rabbits by probucol. *Am J Cardiol*. 1988;62(suppl B):B13–B19.

141. Daugherty A, Zweifel BS, Schonfeld G. Probucol attenuates the development of aortic atherosclerosis in cholesterol-fed rabbits. *Br J Pharmacol*. 1989;98:612–618.

142. Sasahara M, Raines E, Chait A, et al. Inhibition of hypercholesterolemia-induced atherosclerosis in the nonhuman primate by probucol, I: is the extent of atherosclerosis related to resistance of LDL to oxidation? *J Clin Invest*. 1994;94:155–164.

143. Walldius G, Regnström J, Nilsson J, et al. The role of lipids and antioxidative factors for development of atherosclerosis: the Probucol Quantitative Regression Swedish Trial (PQRST). *Am J Cardiol*. 1993;71:15B–19B.

144. Watanabe K, Sekiya M, Ikeda S, et al. Preventive effects of probucol on restenosis after percutaneous transluminal coronary angioplasty. *Am Heart J*. 1996;132:23–29.

145. Adams MR, Kaplan JR, Manuck SB, et al. Inhibition of coronary artery atherosclerosis by 17-beta estradiol in ovariectomized monkeys: lack of an effect of added progesterone. *Arteriosclerosis*. 1990;10:1051–1057.

146. Bourassa PAK, Milso PM, Gaynor BJ, Breslow JL, Aiello RJ. Estrogen reduces atherosclerotic lesion development in apolipoprotein E-deficient mice. *Proc Natl Acad Sci U S A*. 1996;93:10022–10027.

147. Maziere C, Auclair M, Ronveaux MF, et al. Estrogens inhibit copper and cell-mediated modification of low density lipoprotein. *Arteriosclerosis*. 1991;89:175–182.

148. Rifici VA, Kachadurian AK. The inhibition of low-density lipoprotein oxidation by 17-beta estradiol. *Metab Clin Exp*. 1992;41:1110–1114.

149. Nathan L, Chaudhuri G. Estrogens and atherosclerosis. *Annu Rev Pharmacol Toxicol*. 1997;37:477–515.

150. Subbiah MT, Kessel B, Agrawal M, et al. Antioxidant potential of specific estrogens on lipid peroxidation. *J Clin Endocrinol Metab.* 1993;77:1095–1097.

151. Kushwaha RS, Hazzard WR. Exogenous estrogens attenuate dietary hypercholesterolemia and atherosclerosis in the rabbit. *Metabolism.* 1981;30:359–366.

152. Knopp RH, Zhu X, Bonet B. Effects of estrogens on lipoprotein metabolism and cardiovascular disease in women. *Atherosclerosis.* 1994;110:583–591.

153. Bush TL. The epidemiology of cardiovascular disease in postmenopausal women. *Ann N Y Acad Sci.* 1990;592:263–271.

154. Prasad K, Laxdal VA, Yu M, et al. Antioxidant activity of allicin, an active principle in garlic. *Mol Cell Biochem.* 1995;148:183–189.

155. Prasad K, Laxdal VA, Yu M, et al. Evaluation of hydroxyl radical scavenging property of garlic. *Mol Cell Biochem.* 1996;154:55–63.

156. Mirhadi SA, Singh S. Effect of garlic supplementation to cholesterol rich diet on development of atherosclerosis in rabbits. *Indian J Exp Biol.* 1991;29:162–168.

157. Prasad K, Mantha SV, Muir AD, Westcott ND. Reduction of hypercholesterolemic atherosclerosis by CDC-flaxseed with very low alpha-linolenic acid. *Atherosclerosis.* 1998;136:367–375.

158. Prasad K. Hydroxyl radical-scavenging property of secoisolariciresinol diglucoside (SDG) isolated from flaxseed. *Mol Cell Biochem.* 1997;168:117–123.

159. Prasad K. Prevention of hypercholesterolemic atherosclerosis by secoisolariciresinol diglucoside (SDG) isolated from flaxseed [abstract]. *Proceedings of the 4th International Symposium on Multiple Risk Factors in Cardiovascular Disease: Strategies of Prevention of Coronary Heart Disease, Cardiac Failure, and Stroke.* Houston, Tex: Giovanni Lorenzini Medical Foundation; 1997:68.

160. Kang SS, Wong PWK, Norusis M. Homocysteinemia due to folate deficiency. *Metabolism.* 1987;36:458–462.

161. Kang S-S, Wong PWK, Zhou J, et al. Thermolabile methylenetetra-hydrofolate reductase in patients with coronary artery disease. *Metabolism.* 1988;37:611–613.

162. Kang S-S, Zhou J, Wong PWK, et al. Intermediate homocysteinemia: a thermolabile variant of methylenetetrahydrofolate reductase. *Am J Hum Genet.* 1988;43: 414–421.

163. Boushey CJ, Beresford SA, Omenn GS, et al. A quantitative assessment of plasma homocysteine as a risk factor for vascular disease: probable benefits of increasing folic acid intakes. *JAMA.* 1995;274:1049–1057.

164. Mayer EM, Jacobsen DW, Robinson K. Homocysteine and coronary atherosclerosis. *J Am Coll Cardiol.* 1996;27: 517–527.

165. Weimann BJ, Kuhn H, Baumgartner HR. Effect of homocysteine on cultured bovine and human endothelial cells. *Experientia.* 1980;36:762.

166. Starkebaum G, Harlan JM. Endothelial cell injury due to copper-catalyzed hydrogen peroxide generation from homocysteine. *J Clin Invest.* 1986;77:1370–1376.

167. Harker LA, Slichter SJ, Scott CR, et al. Homocystinemia: vascular injury and arterial thrombosis. *N Engl J Med.* 1974;291:537–543.

168. Harker LA, Ross R, Slichter SJ, et al. Homocystine-induced arteriosclerosis: the role of endothelial cell injury and platelet response in its genesis. *J Clin Invest.* 1976; 58:731–741.

169. Mathias D, Becker CH, Riezler R, et al. Homocysteine-induced arteriosclerosis-like alteration of the aorta in normotensive and hypertensive rats following application of high doses of methionine. *Atherosclerosis.* 1996;122: 201–216.

170. Blundell G, Jones BG, Rose FA, et al. Homocysteine mediated endothelial cell toxicity and its amelioration. *Atherosclerosis.* 1996;122:163–172.

171. Jones BG, Rose FA, Tudball N. Lipid peroxidation and homocysteine induced toxicity. *Atherosclerosis.* 1994;105: 165–170.

172. Olszewski AJ, McCully KS. Homocysteine metabolism and the oxidative modification of proteins and lipids. *Free Radical Biol Med.* 1993;14:683–693.

173. Stamler JS, Osborne JA, Jaraki O, et al. Adverse vascular effects of homocysteine are modulated by endothelium-derived relaxing factor and related oxides of nitrogen. *J Clin Invest.* 1993;91:308–318.

174. Welch GN, Upchurch GR, Keaney JF, et al. Homocyst(e)ine decreases cell redox potential in vascular smooth muscle cells [abstract]. *J Am Coll Cardiol.* 1996;27(suppl A):A163.

175. Hultberg B, Andersson A, Isaksson A. Metabolism of homocysteine, its relation to the other cellular thiols, and its mechanism of cell damage in a cell culture line (human histiocytic cell line). *Biochem Biophys Acta.* 1995;1269: 6–12.

176. Toborek M, Kopieczna-Grzebieniak E, Drozdz M, et al. Increased lipid peroxidation as a mechanism of methionine-induced atherosclerosis in rabbits. *Atherosclerosis.* 1995;115:217–224.

177. Heinecke JA, Rosen H, Suzuki LA, et al. Iron and copper promote modification of low density lipoprotein by human arterial smooth muscle cells in culture. *J Clin Invest.* 1984;74:1890–1894.

178. Heinecke JA, Rosen H, Suzuki LA, et al. The role of sulfur-containing amino acids in superoxide production and modification of low density lipoprotein by arterial smooth muscle cells. *J Biol Chem.* 1987;262:98–103.

179. Stamler JS, Loscalzo J. Endothelium-derived relaxing factor modulates the atherothrombogenic effects of homocysteine. *J Cardiovasc Pharmacol.* 1992;20(suppl 12): S202–S204.

180. Tsai JC, Perrella MA, Yoshizumi M, et al. Promotion of vascular smooth muscle cell growth by homocysteine: a link to atherosclerosis. *Proc Natl Acad Sci U S A.* 1994;91: 6369–6373.

181. Clarke R, Daly L, Robinson K, et al. Hyperhomocysteinemia: an independent risk factor for vascular disease. *N Engl J Med.* 1991;324:1149–1155.

182. Coull BM, Malinow MR, Beamer N, et al. Elevated plasma homocyst(e)ine concentration as a possible independent risk factor for stroke. *Stroke.* 1990;21:572–576.

183. Stampfer MJ, Malinow MR, Willett WC, et al. A prospective study of plasma homocyst(e)ine and risk of myocar-

dial infarction in US physicians. *JAMA*. 1992;268:
877–881.

184. Ellis JM, McCully KS. Prevention of myocardial infarction
by vitamin B$_6$. *Res Commun Mol Pathol Pharmacol*. 1995;89:
208–220.

185. Frohlich JJ. Lipoproteins and homocysteine as risk factors
for atherosclerosis: assessment and treatment. *Can J Cardiol*. 1995;1(suppl C):C18–C23.

186. Glueck CJ, Shaw P, Lang JE, et al. Evidence that homocysteine is an independent risk factor for atherosclerosis in
hyperlipidemic patients. *Am J Cardiol*. 1995;75:132–136.

187. Kang S-S, Wong PWK, Cook HY, et al. Protein-bound homocyst(e)ine: a possible risk factor for coronary artery
disease. *J Clin Invest*. 1986;77:1482–1486.

188. Olszewski AJ, Szostak WB. Homocysteine content of
plasma proteins in ischemic heart disease. *Atherosclerosis*.
1988;69:109–113.

189. Israelsson B, Brattström LE, Hultberg BJ. Homocysteine
and myocardial infarction. *Atherosclerosis*. 1988;71:
227–234.

190. Ubbink JB, Vermaak WJ, van der Merwe A, et al. Vitamin
B$_{12}$, vitamin B$_6$, and folate nutritional status in men with
hyperhomocysteinemia. *Am J Clin Nutr*. 1993;57:47–53.

191. Pancharuniti N, Lewis CA, Sauberlich HE, et al. Plasma
homocysteine, folate, and vitamin B$_{12}$ concentrations are
risk for early onset coronary artery disease. *Am J Clin Nutr*.
1994;59:940–948.

192. Robinson K, Mayer EL, Miller DP, et al. Hyperhomocysteinemia and low pyridoxal phosphate: common and independent reversible risk factors for coronary artery disease. *Circulation*. 1995;92:2825–2830.

193. Leklem JJ. Vitamin B$_6$. In: Shils ME, Olson JA, Shike M,
eds. *Modern Nutrition in Health, Disease*. 8th ed. Philadelphia, Pa: Lea & Febiger; 1994:383–394.

194. Brattström L, Stavenow L, Galvard H, et al. Pyridoxine reduces cholesterol and low-density lipoprotein and increases antithrombin III activity in 80-year-old men with
low plasma pyridoxal 5-phosphate. *Scand J Clin Lab Invest*.
1990;50:873–877.

195. Morrison HI, Schaubel D, Desmeules M, et al. Serum folate and risk of fatal coronary heart disease. *JAMA*.
1996;275:1893–1896.

196. Fortin LJ, Genest J Jr. Measurement of homocysteine in
the prediction of arteriosclerosis. *Clin Biochem*. 1995;28:
155–162.

197. Van-den-Berg M, Stehouwer CD, Bierdrager E, et al.
Plasma homocysteine and severity of atherosclerosis in
young patients with lower limb atherosclerotic disease.
Arterioscler Thromb Vasc Biol. 1996;16:165–171.

198. Berwanger CS, Jeremy JY, Stansby G. Homocysteine and
vascular disease. *Br J Surg*. 1995;82:726–731.

199. Malinow MR. Homocysteine and arterial occlusive diseases. *J Intern Med*. 1994;236:603–617.

200. Selhub J, Jacques PF, Bostom AG, et al. Association between plasma homocysteine concentrations and extracranial carotid artery stenosis. *N Engl J Med*. 1995;332:
328–329.

201. Ubbink JB. Homocysteine: an atherogenic and a thrombogenic factor? *Nutr Rev*. 1995;53:323–325.

202. Malinow MR, Nieto FJ, Szklo M, et al. Carotid artery intimal-medial wall thickening and plasma homocysteine in
asymptomatic adults. *Circulation*. 1993;87:1107–1113.

203. Willinek WA, Lennarz M, Dudek M, et al. High normal
serum homocysteine concentrations are associated with
an increased risk for early atherosclerotic carotid artery
wall lesions in normotensive subjects [abstract]. *Proceedings of the 4th Symposium on Multiple Risk Factors in Cardiovascular Disease: Strategies of Prevention of Coronary Heart Disease, Cardiac Failure, and Stroke*. Washington, DC; 1997:39.

204. Mudd SH, Skovby F, Levy HL, et al. The natural history of
homocystinuria due to cystathionine β-synthase deficiency. *Am J Hum Genet*. 1985;37:1–31.

205. den Heijer M, Blom HJ, Gerrits WBJ, et al. Is hyperhomocysteinaemia a risk factor for recurrent venous thrombosis? *Lancet*. 1995;345:882–885.

206. Bostom AG, Brosnan JT, Hall B, et al. Net uptake of
plasma homocysteine by the rat kidney in vivo. *Atherosclerosis*. 1995;116:59–62.

207. Holdt B, Korten G, Knippel M, et al. Increased serum
level of total homocysteine in CAPD patients despite fish
oil therapy. *Perit Dial Int*. 1996;16(suppl 1):S246–S249.

208. Bostom AG, Shemin D, Yoburn D, et al. Lack of effect of
oral *N*-acetylcysteine on acute dialysis-related lowering of
total plasma homocysteine in hemodialysis patients. *Atherosclerosis*. 1996;120:241–244.

209. Chauveau P, Chadefaux B, Conde M, et al. Long-term
folic acid (but not pyridoxine) supplementation lowers
elevated plasma homocysteine level in chronic renal failure. *Miner Electrolyte Metab*. 1996;22:106–109.

210. Chauveau P, Chadefaux B, Conde M, et al. Hyperhomocysteinemia, a risk factor for atherosclerosis in chronic
uremic patients. *Kidney Int Suppl*. 1993;41(suppl):
S72–S77.

211. Robinson K, Gupta A, Dennis V, et al. Hyperhomocysteinemia confers an independent increased risk of atherosclerosis in end-stage renal disease and is closely linked
to plasma folate and pyridoxine concentrations. *Circulation*. 1996;94:2743–2748.

212. Berger PB, Jones JD, Olson LJ, et al. Increase in total
plasma homocysteine concentration after cardiac transplantation. *Mayo Clin Proc*. 1995;70:125–131.

213. Robillon JF, Canivet B, Candito M, et al. Type I diabetes
mellitus and homocysteine. *Diabete Metab*. 1994;20:
494–496.

214. Koyama J. The influence of methionine and its metabolites on the progression of atherosclerosis in rabbits. *Nippon Ika Daigaku Zasshi*. 1995;62:596–604.

215. Naurath HJ, Joosten E, Reizler R, et al. Effects of vitamin
B$_{12}$, folate, and vitamin B$_6$ supplements in elderly people
with normal serum vitamin concentrations. *Lancet*. 1995;
346:85–89.

216. Abou-Gazala T, Lobo A, Alsous F, et al. High plasma homocysteine, in patients with coronary artery disease, can
be reduced by folic acid supplementation [abstract]. *J Am
Coll Cardiol*. 1997;27(suppl 2A):488A.

217. Malinow MR, Kang SS, Taylor LM, et al. Prevalence of hyperhomocyst(e)inemia in patients with peripheral arterial occlusive disease. *Circulation*. 1989;79:1180–1188.

218. Taylor LM, DeFrang RD, Harris EJ, et al. The association of elevated plasma homocyst(e)ine with progression of symptomatic peripheral arterial disease. *J Vasc Surg.* 1991; 13:128–136.

219. Ueland PM, Refsum H. Review article. Plasma homocysteine, a risk factor for vascular disease: plasma levels in health, disease, and drug therapy. *J Lab Clin Med.* 1989; 114:473–501.

220. Averbook A, White GH, Wilson SE. Epidemiology and anatomic distribution of atherosclerosis in man. In: White RA, ed. *Atherosclerosis and Arteriosclerosis: Human Pathology and Experimental Animal Methods and Models.* Boston, Mass: CRC Press; 1990:17–46.

7

Cellular Mechanisms of Myocardial Hibernation, Stunning, and Ischemic Preconditioning

Herwig Köppel, Ernst Pilger, and Robert Gasser

Myocardial hibernation, stunning, and ischemic preconditioning are different pathological entities related to reduced blood supply to the myocardium.

The phenomenon known as hibernation describes an impairment of contractile function in myocardial regions subjected to low coronary flow. This local reduction of myocardial contractility and the subsequent local decrease in oxygen consumption can be seen as a cardioprotective mechanism: in the affected region cardiac metabolism is reduced, whereas in well-perfused areas normal contractile force persists to prevent pump failure. The mechanisms underlying reduced contractile force during myocardial hibernation are still poorly understood. One major finding, however, is a decreased level of Ca^{2+} in the cardiac myocytes. Stunning, on the other hand, refers to decreased contractility following a period of low coronary perfusion. Unlike hibernation, stunning results from Ca^{2+} overload in the cell.

Ischemic preconditioning refers to a short episode of myocardial ischemia that renders the myocardium resistant to severe damage from subsequent longer periods of low myocardial oxygen supply. Although hibernation, stunning, and ischemic preconditioning must be regarded as distinct entities, they may coexist in some clinical conditions such as variable angina. In this chapter we summarize the cellular mechanisms as known so far and stress the different properties of these phenomena and the need for a different therapeutic approach.

Background

The term *myocardial hibernation* was introduced by Rahimtoola in 1984 in a National Heart, Lung, and Blood Institute Workshop on the Treatment of Coronary Artery Disease. He used it to express the persistently impaired left ventricular function due to reduced coronary blood flow. Myocardial function, however, can be partially or completely reversed if the balance between substrate demand and supply is returned to normal. Hence, the impaired ventricular function can be considered as the response of the heart to cope with the reduced oxygen supply to avoid necrosis.[1] Another salient characteristic of hibernation is the absence of pain. Therefore, Marban[2] defines the characteristics of myocardial hibernation as contractile dysfunction during low coronary flow, regardless of duration, in which necrosis is absent, normal phosphorus metabolites are maintained, and the condition is quickly reversible.

The term *myocardial stunning* was coined by Kloner and Braunwald in 1982.[3] In contrast to myocardial hibernation, stunning is a phenomenon that occurs during reperfusion. In both dysfunctions, there is no necrosis, but stunning is only slowly reversible, and the adenosine triphosphate (ATP) levels are significantly decreased (see also Table 7.1). After introduction of the term *myocardial stunning*, impaired ventricular function during ischemic periods was termed *chronic myocardial stunning*. However, it should have been named hibernation, because stunning refers only to reperfusion-induced damage. In 1975 Heyndrickx[4] showed myocardial stunning in the hearts of intact animals with local ischemia. Experiments followed that demonstrated the occurrence of stunning adjacent to necrotic tissue[5] in isolated hearts rendered globally ischemic or anoxic[6] and when a transient imbalance between the supply and demand of myocardial oxygen existed.[7] Myocardial stunning occurs not only under experimental conditions but also in the following clinical circumstances: reperfusion after thrombotic occlusion of a coronary artery, following ischemic arrest in patients undergoing cardiac surgery, and after episodes of unstable angina or Prinzmetal's angina. To date, the underlying cellular mechanisms of stunning have not been elucidated. Ca^{2+} antagonists, neutrophil depletion, and oxygen free radical scavengers have all shown beneficial effects in the treatment of myocardial stunning and thus point at some basic principles of the possible cellular mechanisms.

TABLE 7.1. Main properties of myocardial hibernation and stunning.

Hibernation	Stunning
$CA^{2+} \downarrow$	$Ca^{2+} \uparrow$
No necrosis	No necrosis
Quick recovery	Slow recovery
Coronary flow $\downarrow$	Coronary flow $\uparrow$
Adenosine triphosphate $\uparrow\downarrow$	Adenosine triphosphate $\uparrow$

The mechanisms of ischemic preconditioning are also not well defined. Murray et al.[8] first showed that preconditioning with ischemia caused a delay of lethal cell injury. Subsequent studies have implicated the involvement of adenosine A_1-receptors[9–11] and α_1-adrenoceptors.[12] ATP-sensitive potassium (K_{ATP}) channels (e.g., see Mullane[13] and Van Winkle et al.[14]) may be common targets for the activated receptors. The exact mechanism of the link between the receptors (adenosine A_1-receptors and α_1-adrenoceptors) and the K_{ATP} channel, however, remains unresolved. Proposed mechanisms for the intracellular signal transduction in preconditioning are G_i proteins[15,16] and/or protein kinase C (PKC).[17–19]

Hibernation

Little is known about the cellular factors involved in hibernation, mainly because of the lack of experimental models. Development of animal models with chronic low-flow ischemia is difficult due to occlusion of the coronary stenosis by platelet or fibrin thrombi. Because hibernation is caused by insufficient blood supply, one would expect to observe ATP depletion as a major finding in cardiac myocytes. Marban,[2] however, who used nuclear magnetic resonance spectroscopy, could not detect any evidence of metabolic failure. In isolated perfused hearts he found a significant decrease of intracellular Ca^{2+} but only little change in phosphorus metabolism as gauged by the ^{31}P spectrum, which indicates intracellular ATP levels. Hence, hibernation seems to be an impaired excitation–coupling process due to a decreased availability of Ca^{2+}. Possible explanations include a reduced inward current of Ca^{2+}, reduced intraluminal Ca^{2+} storing capacity of the sarcoplasmic reticulum, and diminished release of Ca^{2+} from the sarcoplasmic reticulum due to raised Mg^{2+} levels.[2] Recent patch clamp studies suggest that inhibition of potential-dependent Ca^{2+} current through L-type calcium channels is responsible for the diminished availability of Ca^{2+}.[20] In the study from Marban,[2] changes in Ca^{2+} availability occurred consistently and in a range that sufficiently explained the attenuated contractile force. The decrease in force was quickly reversible, so that a decreased Ca^{2+} responsiveness of myofilaments seems unlikely. Limitations of

this study are the buffering of Ca^{2+} and the limited time resolution.[21]

Decreased intracellular Ca^{2+} stores as a simple explanation for as complex a phenomenon as hibernation seems, however, unlikely. Ferrari et al.[22] investigated the involvement of heat shock proteins (hsp) in hibernating myocardium. They exposed an isolated heart to 8 minutes of total ischemia, followed by 5 hours of reduced coronary perfusion and 60 minutes of reperfusion. They found that the concentration of hsp 72 (heat shock proteins are named according to their molecular weight; in this case the molecular weight is 72 kd) was statistically elevated in the right and left ventricles, with higher levels in the right than in the left ventricle. Originally considered to be a reaction to hyperthermia, the expression of heat shock proteins seems to be a stereotype reaction of heart cells to stress at the molecular level, because increased expression of hsp 72 can also be detected in hearts with congestive heart failure[22] or other forms of disturbance (see next section). Their role in cardioprotection, however, remains elusive.

Stunning

The basic cellular mechanisms of decreased contractile force that occur during myocardial stunning remain unknown. Hibernation is caused by diminished intracellular Ca^{2+} levels, whereas the opposite seems to be true for stunned myocardium. Hearse et al.[23] described a link between abrupt reoxygenation, or reperfusion, and changes of intracellular Ca^{2+} levels, possibly caused by oxygen radicals. Bolli et al.[24] have related this link of the *oxygen paradox* and the *calcium paradox* with the pathological events of stunned myocardium. Free radical–induced oxidant stress may change the activity of thiol-regulated proteins involved in the regulation of intracellular Ca^{2+} homeostasis.[25] Radicals can cause structural injury to proteins, as well as alter the permeability of the cell or of the intracellular membranes by lipid peroxidation.[25] Thiol-regulated proteins affected by these free radicals are the sodium–calcium exchanger, Na^+, K^+-ATPase, and the calcium pump of the sarcolemma.[26–29] Dysfunction of the sarcolemmal Ca^{2+} release channel (equivalent to the ryanodine receptor) has recently been shown to cause intracellular Ca^{2+} accumulation due to reduced Ca^{2+} extrusion.[30] Further evidence for involvement of oxygen radicals derives from observations in which antioxidant enzymes such as superoxide dismutase and catalase showed beneficial effects in stunned myocardium[31,32]; the major source of free radicals is neutrophils. Chemotactic factors activate neutrophils, which release mediators such as lipid peroxidation products of arachidonic acid or platelet activating factor.[33] Activated neutrophils adhere to the myocytes via interaction between CD18 and intercellular adhesion molecule 1 (ICAM-1); the adherence promotes generation and release of hydrogen peroxide, which leads to contracture of the myocytes.[34] Evidence for involvement of neutrophils is also based on the finding that removal of neutrophils from the blood before it enters the coronary circulation reduced the degree of stunning.[35,36] Due to involvement of intracellular Ca^{2+} overload as a cause for reperfusion-induced disturbances, the beneficial effects of Ca^{2+} antagonists such as verapamil hydrochloride,[37] nifedipine,[38] diltiazem hydrochloride,[39] or amlodipine besylate[40] appear logical. Another property of Ca^{2+} antagonists in the treatment of postischemic damage is to scavenge free radicals.[41,42] It should be noted, however, that observations of beneficial effects of Ca^{2+} antagonists are only of experimental origin. The clinical use of such agents in treatment of postischemic dysfunction after thrombolysis or cardiopulmonary bypass surgery awaits proof.

Factors other than Ca^{2+} overload may also contribute to stunning. Kusuoka et al.[43] and Marban et al.[44] found that the sensitivity of myofibrils decreases with Ca^{2+} overload. Paradoxically, reduced contractility may be overcome by inotropic agents such as dobutamine.[45] Even if sensitivity to Ca^{2+} is reduced, the contractile apparatus can still contract, if provided with enough Ca^{2+}, due to α-adrenergic stimulation. These findings, however, appear surprising in view of the fact that stunning is caused by Ca^{2+} overload, and α-adrenergic stimulation further increases intracellular Ca^{2+} levels.

There is still dispute among scientists as to whether stunning is a real pathological occurrence or is merely an energy down-regulation. Consideration of molecular mechanisms may help to resolve this question. As stated previously, heat shock proteins are synthesized by cells after exposure to hyperthermia or other disturbances. These proteins protect cells against damage that otherwise would have been lethal.[46] In stunned myocardium, Fleischmann et al.[47] detected expression of hsp 70, which indicated the exposure of cells to sublethal damage and that stunning is more than just energy down-regulation. Furthermore, they observed enhanced expression of c-*myc* and c-*fos* transcription factor genes.[47] Such genes code for proteins that bind to specific regions of DNA, thereby regulating the activity of gene transcription. Increased expression of such transcription factor genes can often be noticed in cells after sublethal stress.

Ischemic Preconditioning

Ischemic preconditioning is known as a cardioprotective mechanism in which the heart develops resistance against severe damage caused by a long period of ischemia after exposure to several short episodes of myocardial ischemia. Murray et al.[8] first described the phenomenon of preconditioning with ischemia, and its efficacy has been confirmed in dogs,[10] rabbits,[9] rats,[12] and pigs.[48] Emerging data suggest its occurrence in humans.[49,50] Clinical evidence of ischemic preconditioning comes from percutaneous transluminal coronary angioplasty procedures that indicate ischemic preconditioning provides a strong means of cardioprotection.[50]

Activation of adenosine A_1-receptors has been implicated in ischemic preconditioning.[9–11] Under ischemic circumstances, adenosine is released from cardiac myocytes, which causes dilation of the coronary arteries and is responsible for opening K_{ATP} channels of the myocytes.[10,11] One way of coupling adenosine A_1-receptors to the K_{ATP} channel are G proteins, especially the α-subunit of the pertussis-sensitive inhibitory G protein (G_i).[51] The role of G proteins in preconditioning is unresolved. Some investigators detected abolition of the protective effects by inhibition of G proteins,[15,16] whereas others found no involvement of G proteins.[52,53] Another possible pathway is the activation of PKC via diacylglycerol. Stimulation of adenosine A_1-receptors enhances translocation of PKC in rat ventricular myocytes.[54] The translocated PKC activates K_{ATP} channels, possibly by changing the stoichiometry of ATP binding to the channel.[55]

Activation of another receptor, $α_1$-adrenoceptors, stimulates PKC via diacylglycerol.[12] Whereas activated $α_1$-adrenoceptors are generally thought to increase diacylglycerol through phospholipase C, adenosine rather promotes phospholipase D to increase diacylglycerol.[56] Involvement of agonists of $α_1$-adrenoceptors (such as noradrenaline) in preconditioning would not be surprising, because an episode of myocardial ischemia raises plasma levels of noradrenaline, and stimulation of $α_1$-adrenoceptors could constitute a physiological way of ameliorating cardiac function (see Figure 7.1).

Recently, calcitonin gene–related peptide (CGRP) was found to be involved in ischemic preconditioning. Xiao and coworkers[57] found that cardioprotective effects of preconditioning could be abolished by a specific CGRP receptor antagonist. Li et al.[58] found that CGRP was also effective in protecting the heart against reperfusion-induced injury in rat heart. This finding was confirmed by Feng et al.,[59] who demonstrated reduction and delay in the occurrence of reperfusion-induced arrythmias in rats. CGRP is released from nerves surrounding arteries and causes vasodilation through activation of K_{ATP} channels.[60] Stimulus for the release of CGRP is ischemia/hypoxia of the heart, possibly via prostacyclin.[61] This hypothesis needs further investigation. In cardiac myocytes, however, CGRP enhances activity of PKC,[62] and although not established, activation of a K_{ATP} current is most likely the final effect. Other factors such as

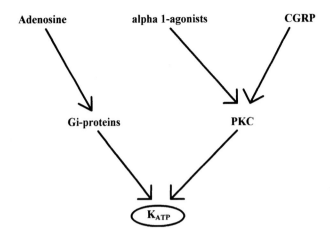

FIGURE 7.1. Adenosine stimulates pertussis-sensitive G protein (G_i) and protein kinase C (PKC). Stimulation of PKC is also produced by α_1-agonists such as noradrenaline and calcitonin gene–related peptide (CGRP). Final effect is opening of the K_{ATP} channel.

bradykinin,[63] peripheral opioid receptors,[64] and β-adrenergic receptors[65] mimic preconditioning like cardioprotection. The precise cellular mechanisms are still a matter of discussion. The so-called delayed preconditioning, also known as the second window of protection, is a phenomenon that exerts cardioprotection 24 to 72 hours after ischemic preconditioning. Heat shock proteins (hsp 70 and hsp 90)[66] and tyrosine kinase inhibitors[67] have been shown to be crucial elements, but many questions remain unresolved.

Conclusions

Myocardial hibernation (an impaired ventricular function during low coronary flow) and myocardial stunning (an essentially postischemic dysfunction) are important complications related to coronary heart disease, which is one of the most widespread diseases of the Western countries. An exact diagnosis can be made only if both coronary flow and contractile function are known. Little is known about the intracellular events during hibernation or stunning, and therapeutic interventions are also still undefined. There is evidence, however, that coronary artery bypass grafting improves left ventricular function and survival rates, whereas pharmacological treatment is without effect.[68] Closely related is ischemic preconditioning, a mechanism that protects the heart after a short period of ischemia against severe damage caused by a subsequent longer episode of myocardial ischemia. In preconditioning, opening of K_{ATP} channels and subsequent shortening of the action potential duration have been found to be crucial; in delayed pre-

conditioning, heat shock proteins and tyrosine kinase inhibitors are involved, but intracellular signal transduction pathways are still not well established. Hence, more experimental work is necessary to clarify the intracellular mechanisms and thus provide effective therapeutic intervention.

References

1. Rahimtoola SH. The hibernating myocardium. *Am Heart J.* 1989;117:211–221.
2. Marban E. Myocardial stunning and hibernation: the physiology behind the colloquialisms. *Circulation.* 1991; 83:681–688.
3. Braunwald E, Kloner RA. The stunned myocardium: prolonged, postischemic ventricular dysfunction. *Circulation.* 1982;66:1146–1149.
4. Heyndrickx GR, Millard RW, McRitchie RJ. Regional myocardial functional and electrophysiological alterations after brief coronary occlusion in conscious dogs. *J Clin Invest.* 1975;56:978–985.
5. Ellis SG, Henschke CI, Sandor T. Time course of functional and biochemical recovery of myocardium salvaged by reperfusion. *J Am Coll Cardiol.* 1983;68(suppl I):8–15.
6. Nayler WG, Elz JS, Buckley DJ. The stunned myocardium: effect of electrical and mechanical arrest and osmolality. *Am J Physiol.* 1988;254(suppl):H60–H69.
7. Thaulow E, Guth BD, Heusch G. Characteristics of regional myocardial stunning after exercise in dogs with left ventricular hypertrophy. *Am J Physiol.* 1989;257(suppl): H113–H119.
8. Murray CE, Jennings RB, Reimer KA. Preconditioning with ischemia: a delay of lethal cell injury in ischemic myocardium. *Circulation.* 1986;74:1124–1136.
9. Liu GS, Thornton J, Van Winkle DM, Stanley AWH, Olsson RA, Downey JM. Protection against infarction afforded by preconditioning is mediated by adenosine A_1-receptors in rabbit heart. *Circulation.* 1991;84:350–356.
10. Auchampach JA, Gross GJ. Adenosine A_1-receptors, K_{ATP} channels, and ischemic preconditioning in dogs. *Am J Physiol.* 1993;264(suppl):H1327–H1336.
11. Grover GJ, Sleph PG, Dzwonczyk BS. Role of myocardial ATP-sensitive potassium channels in mediating preconditioning in the dog heart and their possible interaction with adenosine A_1-receptors. *Circulation.* 1992;86:1310–1316.
12. Hu K, Nattel S. Mechanisms of ischemic preconditioning in rat hearts: involvement of alpha-adrenoceptors, pertussis toxin sensitive G-proteins, and protein kinase C. *Circulation.* 1995;92;2259–2265.
13. Mullane K. Adenosine, ATP-sensitive potassium channels, and myocardial preconditioning. In: Escande D, Standen NB, eds. *K Channels in Cardiovascular Medicine.* Paris: Springer-Verlag; 1993:273–283.
14. Van Winkle DM, Chien GL, Wolff RA, Soifer BE, Kuzume K, Davis RF. Cardioprotection provided by adenosine receptor activation is abolished by blockade of the K_{ATP} channel. *Am J Physiol.* 1994;266:H829–H839.
15. Thornton JD, Liu GS, Downey JM. Pretreatment with pertussis toxin blocks the protective effects of precondition-

ing: evidence for a G-protein mechanism. *J Mol Cell Cardiol.* 1993;25:311–320.

16. Piacentini L, Wainwright CL, Parratt JR. The antiarrhythmic effect of ischemic preconditioning in isolated rat heart involves a pertussis toxin sensitive mechanism. *Cardiovasc Res.* 1993;27:674–680.

17. Liu Y, Dong GW, O'Rourke B, Marban E. Synergistic modulation of ATP-sensitive K currents by protein kinase C and adenosine: implications for ischemic preconditioning. *Circ Res.* 1996;78:443–454.

18. Speechly-Dick ME, Grover GJ, Yellon DM. Does ischemic preconditioning in the human involve protein kinase C and the ATP-dependent K-channel? Studies of contractile function after simulated ischemia in an atrial in vitro model. *Circ Res.* 1995;77:1030–1035.

19. Light PE, Sabir AA, Allen BG, Walsh MP, French RJ. Protein kinase C–induced changes in the stoichiometry of ATP binding activate cardiac ATP-sensitive K channels: a possible mechanistic link to ischemic preconditioning. *Circ Res.* 1996;79:399–406.

20. Alekseev AE, Markevich NI, Korysiova AE, Lankina DA, Kokoz YM. The kinetic characteristics of the L-type calcium channels in cardiocytes of hibernators, I: development of a kinetic model. *Membr Cell Biol.* 1997;11:31–34.

21. Marban E, Kitakaze M, Koretsune Y, Yue DT, Chacko VP, Pike MM. Quantification of $(Ca^{2+})_i$ in perfused hearts: critical evaluation of the 5F-BAPTA and nuclear magnetic resonance method as applied to the study of ischemia and reperfusion. *Circ Res.* 1990;66:1255–1267.

22. Ferrari R, Bongrazio M, Cargnoni A, et al. Heat shock protein changes in hibernation: a similarity with heart failure? *J Mol Cell Cardiol.* 1996;28:2383–2395.

23. Hearse DJ, Humphrey SM, Bullock JR. The oxygen paradox and the calcium paradox: two facets of the same problem? *J Moll Cell Cardiol.* 1978;10:641–668.

24. Bolli R. Oxygen-derived free radicals and postischemic myocardial dysfunction ("stunned myocardium"). *J Am Coll Cardiol.* 1988;12:239–249.

25. Halliwell B, Gutteridge JMC. *Free Radicals in Biology and Medicine.* 2nd ed. Oxford, England: Clarendon Press; 1989.

26. Reeves JP, Bailey C, Hale CC. Redox modification of sodium-calcium exchange activity in cardiac sarcolemmal vesicles. *J Biol Chem.* 1986;561:4948–4955.

27. Abramson JJ, Cronin JR, Salama G. Oxidation induced by phthalocyanine dyes causes rapid calcium release from sarcoplasmatic reticulum. *J Bioenergetics Biomemb.* 1989;21:283–294.

28. Yamada S, Ikemoto N. Distinction of thiols involved in the specific reaction steps of the Ca^{2+}-ATPase of the sarcoplasmatic reticulum. *J Biol Chem.* 1978;253:6801–6807.

29. Shi ZQ, Davison AJ, Tibbits GF: Effects of active oxygen generated by DTT/Fe^{2+} on cardiac Na^+/Ca^{2+} exchange and membrane permeability to Ca^{2+}. *J Mol Cell Cardiol.* 1989;21:1009–1016.

30. Valdivia C, Hegge JO, Lasley RD, Valdivia HH, Mentzer R. Ryanodine dysfunction in porcine stunned myocardium. *Am J Physiol.* 1997;273(suppl):H796–H804.

31. Gross GJ, Faber NE, Hardman HF. Beneficial actions of superoxide dismutase and catalase in stunned myocardium of dogs. *Am J Physiol.* 1986;250(suppl):H372–H377.

32. Przyklenk K, Kloner RA. "Reperfusion injury" by oxygen-derived free radicals? Effects of superoxide dismutase plus catalase, given at the time of reperfusion, on myocardial infarct size, contractile function in the canine model of the "stunned myocardium." *Circ Res.* 1986;58:148–156.

33. Mullane KM, Westlin W, Kraemer R. Activated neutrophils release mediators that may contribute to myocardial injury and dysfunction associated with ischemia and reperfusion. *Ann N Y Acad Sci.* 1988;524:103–121.

34. Entmann ML, Youker K, Shappel SB. Neutrophil adherence to isolated adult canine myocytes: evidence for a CD18 dependent mechanism. *J Clin Invest.* 1990;85: 1497–1506.

35. Engler R, Covell JW. Granulocytes cause reperfusion ventricular dysfunction after 15-minute ischemia in the dog. *Circ Res.* 1987;61:20–28.

36. Westlin W, Mullane KM. Alleviation of myocardial stunning by leukocyte and platelet depletion. *Circulation.* 1989; 80:1828–1836.

37. Przyklenk K, Kloner RA. Effect of verapamil on postischemic "stunned" myocardium: importance of the timing of treatment. *J Am Coll Cardiol.* 1988;11:614–623.

38. Przyklenk K, Ghafari GB, Eitzmann DT. Nifedipine administered postreperfusion ablates systolic contractile dysfunction of postischemic "stunned" myocardium. *J Am Coll Cardiol.* 1989;13:1176–1183.

39. Taylor AL, Golino P, Eckels R. Differential enhancement of postischemic segmental systolic thickening by diltiazem. *J Am Coll Cardiol.* 1990;15:737–747.

40. Dunlap ED, Matlib MA, Millard RW. Protection of regional mechanics and mitochondrial oxidative phosphorylation by amlodipine in transiently ischemic myocardium. *Am J Cardiol.* 1989;64(suppl):I84–I93.

41. Shridi F, Robak J. The influence of Ca-channel blockers on superoxide anions. *Pharmacological Research Communications.* 1988;20:13–21.

42. Koller PT, Bergmann SR. Reduction of lipid peroxidation in reperfused isolated rabbit hearts by diltiazem. *Circ Res.* 1989;65:838–846.

43. Kusuoka H, Koretsune Y, Chacko VP. Excitation-contraction coupling in postischemic myocardium: does failure of activator Ca^{2+} transients underlie stunning? *Circ Res.* 1990;66:1268–1276.

44. Marban E, Litakaze M, Kusuoka H. Intracellular free calcium concentration measured with ^{19}F NMR spectroscopy in intact ferret hearts. *Proc Natl Acad Sci U S A.* 1987; 84:6005–6009.

45. Schulz R, Myazaki S, Miller M. Consequences of regional inotropic stimulation of ischemic myocardium on regional myocardial blood flow and function in anesthetized swine. *Circ Res.* 1989;84:1118–1128.

46. Schlesinger M. Heat shock proteins. *J Biol Chem.* 1990;265: 12111–12114.

47. Fleischmann KE, Brand T, Sharma HS. Gene expression in a preconditioning model [abstract]. *Circulation.* 1990; 82(suppl 3):III464.

48. Schott RJ, Rohrmann S, Braun ER, Schaper W. Ischemic preconditioning reduces infarct size in swine myocardium. *Circ Res.* 1990;66:1133–1142.

49. Yellon DM, Alkhulaifi AM, Pugsley WB. Preconditioning the human myocardium. *Lancet.* 1993;342:276–277

50. Deutsch E, Berge M, Kussmaul WG, Hirshfeld JW, Herrmann HC, Laskey WK. Adaption to ischemia during percutaneous transluminal coronary angioplasty: clinical, hemodynamic, and metabolic features. *Circulation.* 1990;82:2044–2051.

51. Kirsch GE, Codina J, Birnbaumer L, Brown AM. Coupling of ATP-sensitive K-channels to A_1-receptors by G-proteins in rat ventricular myocytes. *Am J Physiol.* 1990;259(suppl):H820–H826.

52. Liu Y, Downey JM. Preconditioning against infarction in the rat heart does not involve a pertussis toxin sensitive G-protein. *Cardiovasc Res.* 1993;27:608–611.

53. Lawson CS, Coltart DJ, Hearse DJ. The antiarrhythmic effect of ischemic preconditioning in rat hearts does not involve functional G-proteins. *Cardiovasc Res.* 1993;27:681–687.

54. Henry P, Demolombe S, Puceat M, Escande D: Adenosine A_1 stimulation activates ∂-protein kinase C in rat ventricular myocytes. *Circ Res.* 1996;78:161–165.

55. Light PE, Sabir AA, Allen BG, Walsh MP, French RJ. Protein kinase induced changes in the stoichiometry of ATP binding activate cardiac ATP-sensitive K channels. *Circ Res.* 1996;79:399–406.

56. Cohen MV, Liu Y, Liu GS, et al. Phospholipase D plays a role in ischemic preconditioning in rabbit heart. *Circulation.* 1996;94:1713–1718.

57. Xiao ZS, Li YJ, Deng HW. Ischemic preconditioning by calcitonin gene related peptide in isolated rat hearts. *Acta Pharmacologica Sinica.* 1996;175:445–448.

58. Li YJ, Xiao ZS, Peng CF, Deng HW. Calcitonin gene related peptide induced preconditioning protects against ischemia-reperfusion injury in isolated rat hearts. *Eur J Pharmacol.* 1996;311:163–167.

59. Feng ZJ, Jin L, Xuan-Zong L, Ming Yue L, Shu-li S, Wan-Jiang W. The effect of calcitonin gene related peptide on ischemic reperfusion-induced arrhythmias in rats. *Int J Cardiol.* 1994;46:33–36.

60. Quayle JM, Bonev AD, Brayden JE, Nelson MT. Calcitonin gene related peptide activates ATP-sensitive K currents in rabbit arterial smooth muscle via protein kinase A. *J Physiol.* 1994;475:9–13.

61. Franco-Cereceda A, Källner G, Lundberg J. Cyclooxygenase products released by low pH have capsaicin-like actions on sensory nerves in the isolated guinea pig heart. *Cardiovasc Res.* 1994:28:365–369.

62. Bell D, Schluter KD, Zhou XJ, McDermott BJ, Piper HM. Hypertrophic effects of CGRP and amylin on adult ventricular cardiomyocytes. *J Mol Cell Cardiol.* 1995;27:2433–2443.

63. Parratt JR, Vegh A, Zeitlin IJ, et al. Bradykinin and endothelial-cardiac myocyte interactions in ischemic preconditioning. *Am J Cardiol.* 1997;80(suppl 3A):124A–131A.

64. Schultz JJ, Hsu Ak, Gross GJ. Ischemic preconditioning is mediated by a peripheral opioid receptor mechanism in the intact rat heart. *J Mol Cell Cardiol.* 1997;29:1355–1362.

65. Nasa Y, Yabe K, Takeo S. Beta-adrenoceptor stimulation-mediated preconditioning-like cardioprotection in perfused rat hearts. *J Cardiovasc Pharmacol.* 1997;29:436–443.

66. Nayeem MA, Hess ML, Qian YZ, Loesser KE, Kukreja RC. Delayed preconditioning of cultured rat cardiac myocytes: role of 70- and 90-kDa heat stress proteins. *Am J Physiol.* 1997;273(suppl):H861–H868.

67. Imagawa J, Baxter GF, Yellon DM. Genistein, a tyrosine kinase inhibitor blocks the "second window of protection" 48h after ischemic preconditioning in the rabbit. *J Mol Cell Cardiol.* 1997;29:1885–1893.

68. Gunning MG, Chua TP, Harrington D, et al. Hibernating myocardium: clinical and functional response to revascularisation. *Eur J Cardiothorac Surg.* 1997;11:1105–1112.

8

Calcium Antagonists and Ischemic Heart Disease

Andrea Obernosterer and Robert Gasser

Calcium antagonists (Ca^{2+} antagonists) have been used for more than two decades in the treatment of ischemic heart disease. Their use was initially promoted for treatment of variant angina but soon expanded to all forms of ischemic heart disease, including stable and unstable angina. Based on promising experimental findings, these drugs have also been used in the treatment of myocardial infarction and secondary prevention but with disappointing results. The basic principle underlying Ca^{2+}-antagonistic therapy of ischemic heart disease is improvement of the myocardial oxygen balance. On the one hand, Ca^{2+} antagonists (in particular, verapamil hydrochloride and diltiazem hydrochloride) reduce myocardial oxygen demand via negative inotropic and chronotropic action; on the other hand, the afterload is reduced by peripheral vasodilatation. In addition, coronary dilation improves oxygen delivery, especially during exercise. Ca^{2+} antagonists inhibit transsarcolemmal Ca^{2+} influx and thus prevent deleterious myocardial Ca^{2+} overload, as seen during ischemia and in atherosclerosis. Recent human studies have shown that calcium channel blockers may prevent atherosclerosis.

The discovery of Ca^{2+} antagonists and their principle of action has revolutionized cardiovascular therapy over the past 20 years. Since their discovery, the therapeutic spectrum of these drugs—which are used to treat arrhythmias, hypertension, and ischemic heart disease—has constantly increased. In this context, important developments have taken place. Ca^{2+} antagonists have been shown to reduce afterload via a decrease in peripheral resistance, lower myocardial oxygen demand, and inhibit Ca^{2+} overload in cardiac and vascular tissue. The drugs may also have an antiatherosclerotic effect, as evidenced by numerous animal experiments and a number of multicenter trials with patients.[1]

Ca^{2+} antagonists can be effectively used in the treatment of the following conditions: stable and unstable angina, hypertensive heart disease, transient ischemia, and myocardial stunning. The specific calcium channel blocker diltiazem hydrochloride has been used effectively in treating acute nontransmural infarction. Other studies, however, suggest that use of Ca^{2+} antagonists during acute myocardial infarction is problematic, especially in patients with left ventricular dysfunction.

Ca^{2+} antagonists have been ineffective in secondary prevention, and it is generally accepted that they should not be used for this purpose. Ca^{2+} antagonists of the dihydropyridine group increase heart rate and can be effectively combined with β-blockers.[2] The use of different types of Ca^{2+} antagonists requires differentiation of patients and substance classes.

Recent research has focused on the development of highly specific and more selective subgroups of Ca^{2+} antagonists; for example, dihydropyridines show little negative effect on inotropy and tend to decrease reactive neurohumoral activation, which is favorable for the treatment of ischemic cardiomyopathy. In this chapter we provide an overview of the various types of Ca^{2+} antagonists and their use in the treatment of ischemic heart disease.

Historical Review

In 1882, after Sydney Ringer had hired a new laboratory assistant, his isolated perfused Langendorff hearts stopped beating. Some time later Ringer found that his former laboratory assistant used the dirty water of the Thames, whereas his new assistant used distilled water, to produce the solutions for the perfusate. The dirty water of the Thames contained enough soluble Ca^{2+} to allow contractility. Our knowledge that Ca^{2+} is needed for electromechanical coupling results from this laboratory accident.[3] Thirty years later, Cow[4] investigated the effect of Ca^{2+} on isolated smooth muscle. Ebashi[5] later described the interdependence of actin, myosin, troponin, and adenosine triphosphate activity, together with Ca^{2+}. Figure 8.1 shows the interdependence of free intracellular Ca^{2+} and contractile force in myocardial tissue.

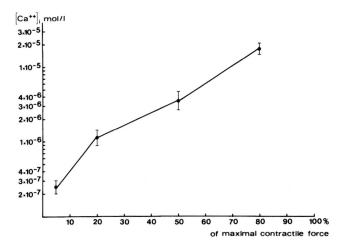

FIGURE 8.1. Correlation between free intracellular Ca^{2+} and percentage of maximal contractile force in a guinea pig papillary muscle. (From Gasser et al.[6])

Ca^{2+} antagonists have long been used to treat ischemic heart disease. More than 3000 years ago, the Chinese began using tea from the Dan Shen plant (which contains a naturally available Ca^{2+} antagonist called *Tanshinone*) to treat angina pectoris.[7] In 1963 Albrecht Fleckenstein was asked to investigate *iproveratril* (later verapamil hydrochloride) and *prenylamin*. Fleckenstein and coworkers found that these substances affected myocardial contractility and smooth muscle tone. The effect was comparable to that of Ca^{2+} withdrawal; when Ca^{2+} was added back to the solution, contractility was recovered.[8] Fleckenstein[9] was the first to postulate the principle of Ca^{2+}-antagonistic action. Only 10 years later, Lewis and coworkers[10] began to use these drugs to treat hypertension. Around the same time, the first dihydropyridine-type Ca^{2+} antagonist was discovered. A substance called *Bay A 1040* had previously been used as a yellow pigment. Fleckenstein and coworkers[11] then showed that the substance has a highly specific vasodilator effect. Nikajima and coworkers[12] found in 1975 that another class of highly specific Ca^{2+} antagonists—diltiazem hydrochloride—was related to benzodiazepines. The blockade of slow calcium channels as a fundamental principle of calcium antagonism had first been postulated by Kohlhart and Fleckenstein in 1972.[13] Their work confirmed the earlier concept of Ca^{2+}-antagonistic action as a slow channel blocker. Livsley and coworkers[14] were the first to introduce Ca^{2+} antagonists for the treatment of angina pectoris. Glossman and associates[15] described receptor binding at the calcium channel for these substances in 1984. Several authors—including Bourdellion, Henry, Clark, and Fleckenstein[16-19]—have since described Ca^{2+}-antagonistic myocardial protection.

Classification of Ca^{2+} Antagonists

The two major groups of Ca^{2+} antagonists are group A (highly specific Ca^{2+} antagonists) and group B (less specific Ca^{2+} antagonists).[18,20]

Group A

Group A Ca^{2+} antagonists consist of three subgroups:

1. Dihydropyridine-type Ca^{2+} antagonists (e.g., nifedipine, nicardipine, nisoldipine, niludipine, isradipine, nitrendipine, amlodipine, flordipine, silvadipine, and darodipine)
2. Verapamil-type Ca^{2+} antagonists (e.g., verapamil, gallopamil, anipamil, romipamil, and tiapamil)
3. Benzodiazepine-type Ca^{2+} antagonists (diltiazem and derivatives)

The one thing Ca^{2+} antagonists have in common is that they inhibit the slow transsarcolemmal Ca^{2+} influx without influencing Na^+ currents. Moreover, these Ca^{2+} antagonists are able to suppress Ca^{2+}-dependent action potentials without influencing Mg^{2+}-dependent membrane phenomena.[18] These substances allow the suppression of Ca^{2+}-dependent electromechanical coupling in ventricular myocardium up to 100% without influencing Na^+ influx in these concentrations. The drugs bind stereospecifically to characteristic receptor subunits of Ca^{2+} transport proteins that act as slow calcium channels.[18]

Class A Ca^{2+} antagonists are subdivided into subgroup 1 (verapamil hydrochloride), subgroup 2 (nifedipine), and subgroup 3 (benzotiazepine) based on the classification of the World Health Organization.[20] Dihydropyridine-type Ca^{2+} antagonists are vasodilators that act mainly on vascular smooth muscle cells. Verapamil-type Ca^{2+} antagonists also tend to dilate vessels but reduce conduction velocity and pacing rate. Hence, they have negative inotropic and chronotropic effects. Dihydropyridine-type Ca^{2+} antagonists may cause tachycardia because of a quick decrease in blood pressure via the baroreceptor reflex. Such a reflective tachycardia may cause an attack of angina pectoris. Another group of Ca^{2+} antagonists—the so-called benzotiazepine Ca^{2+} antagonists and their derivatives—have properties between group 1 and group 2. Diltiazem hydrochloride is not only cardiodepressive but also vasodilative.[21]

Group B

Group B includes the less specific Ca^{2+} antagonists: prenylamine, fendiline, terodiline, caroverine, perhexiline, cinnarizine, flunarizine, and bepridil.[18,21] These substances have a lower affinity to the calcium channels, and the Ca^{2+}-antagonistic activity is less pronounced than in group A. They also affect the fast sodium current. Various authors have shown that this group of Ca^{2+} antagonists is involved in the Mg^{2+}-dependent bioelectrical membrane phenomena. Fleckenstein used this criterion as the second important principle to differentiate between the two groups of Ca^{2+} antagonists.[18,21] Group B Ca^{2+} antagonists are only rarely used in clinical treatment today.

Coronary Artery Disease and Ca^{2+} Antagonists

The therapeutic spectrum of drugs available to treat ischemic heart disease is wide. Interventional cardiology and bypass surgery and pharmacotherapeutic principles are used. The latter entail nitrates, β-blockers, and Ca^{2+} antagonists. The multifaceted genesis of angina pectoris requires different strategies which may imply Ca^{2+} antagonists.

Basic Pathophysiological Principles of Coronary Artery Disease

The basic pathogenic principle of coronary artery disease is an imbalance between oxygen delivery and oxygen demand (Figure 8.2). This imbalance can be related to an increased oxygen demand of the myocardium or occur secondary to a decreased coronary blood supply. In most cases, we find a mixed form in which reduced coronary flow cannot provide the substrate and oxygen needed by the myocardium.[22-25] Decreased coronary delivery can have various causes including vasospasm, concentric and eccentric coronary stenosis, and partial or complete coronary occlusion. The different forms of coronary insufficiency can also be mixed. For most cases, the predominant components remain unclear. Coronary artery disease must thus be treated with a strategy of trial and error combined with the knowledge of certain underlying principles.

Ca^{2+} Antagonists in the Treatment of Coronary Artery Disease

Albrecht Fleckenstein was the first to allude to the possibility of using Ca^{2+} antagonists in the treatment of coronary artery disease.[9] Later work by Maseri and coworkers[26] has consistently implicated coronary spasm as one of the important causes of myocardial ischemia. In this context, Ca^{2+} antagonists have become important tools in treating coronary artery disease.[26] However, the limitations of other coronary treatments (e.g., tolerance development in nitrate therapy) demand therapeutics such as Ca^{2+} antagonists. In particular, Ca^{2+} antagonists with a negative chronotropic and inotropic effect that at the same time enact a vasodilative effect (verapamil hydrochloride) seem to be excellent medications for the treatment of coronary artery disease.[27,28] The combination of dihydropyridines and β-blockers has also been used successfully. The anticalcinotic and antiatherosclerotic effects of Ca^{2+} antagonists have opened a new era of Ca^{2+}-antagonistic therapy for coronary artery disease (Figure 8.3). Numerous animal experiments and a few larger clinical trials have confirmed this effect of Ca^{2+}-antagonistic drugs.[1,11,29-33]

Mechanisms of Action and Indications for Ca^{2+} Antagonists in Patients With Ischemic Heart Disease

A detailed discussion of the mode of action of various Ca^{2+} antagonist subtypes is beyond the scope of this chapter (see Gasser,[1] Fleckenstein,[21] Morad et al.,[34] and Nayler[35]). Following is a brief description:

1. In principle, Ca^{2+} antagonists act via a relaxation of epicardial and intramyocardial coronary arteries, which increases oxygen delivery and inhibits coronary spasm. Oxygen delivery and coronary spasm play important roles in the genesis of angina pectoris.[21,36]
2. Ca^{2+} antagonists also provide for vascular relaxation by acting directly on the smooth muscle cell in the peripheral artery. Peripheral resistance is thus decreased and so is afterload, which reduces myocardial oxygen demand and improves myocardial oxygen bal-

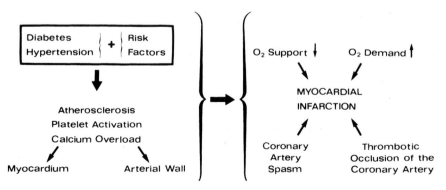

FIGURE 8.2. Various risk factors enhance cellular Ca^{2+} uptake and thus lead to vasospasm, increased myocardial oxygen consumption, and Ca^{2+} overload.

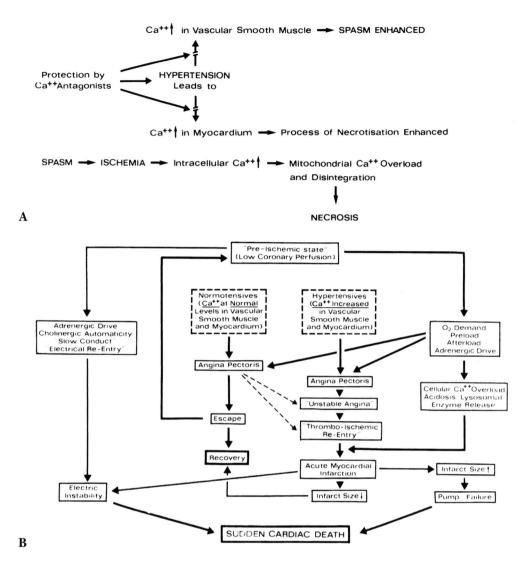

FIGURE 8.3. **A,** Hypertension leads to increased Ca^{2+} influx and thus to enhanced spasm. Ischemia-induced necrosis is also positively influenced by Ca^{2+} channel blockade. **B,** Flow diagram of myocardial ischemia.

ance. The intensity and frequency of angina pectoris attacks are hence decreased.[21,36,37]

3. The blockade of calcium influx in myocytes of the working myocardium decreases adenosine triphosphate consumption, which reduces oxygen and substrate demand. In clinical terms, angina becomes less frequent.[21,36]

4. The prolongation of conduction velocity leads to a negative chronotropicity of Ca^{2+} antagonists, which prolongs the duration of diastole and improves cardiac output because of a more effective Frank–Starling mechanism. In this context, oxygen consumption is decreased as well.[21,38]

The clinical efficacy of Ca^{2+} antagonists in the treatment of ischemic heart disease is evidenced by the following:

1. A subjective decrease in the frequency of angina attacks[25,36,39,40] and use of nitrates[25,36]

2. A decrease in heart rate and blood pressure (heart rate may not be decreased in the presence of dihydropyridines, a phenomenon described and discussed first by Loaldi[32]; this phenomenon is prominent during exercise[25,36–38])

3. An increased exercise tolerance, which improves the patient's quality of life[25,36–40]

4. A reduction in exercise-induced ST depression[39,40]

How, When, and Which Ca^{2+} Antagonist to Use in the Treatment of Coronary Artery Disease

Vasospastic Angina

The importance of vasospasm in the genesis of ischemic heart disease was described in 1959 by Prinzmetal.[41] We continue to see patients with angina pectoris and normal coronary angiograms. In many of these cases, the vasospastic form of angina is the predominant cause. To date, however, the pathophysiology of vasospastic angina has not been completely elucidated. The importance of vasospasm in the context of the development of myocardial infarction has been discussed by numerous authors.[23,26,42-47] Many sudden cardiac deaths occur because myocardial infarction did not result from occlusive thrombosis in any of the coronary arteries.[48,49]

Coronary spasm can be induced by cold, stress, and various unknown factors. Endothelial factors, platelet-borne substances, and neurogenic mechanisms are also likely to play a role in coronary artery spasm.[50-54] Dihydropyridines thwart vasospastic angina. Intravenous nifedipine has vasodilative effects that control coronary spasm.[55] Numerous other authors have confirmed the data, and dihydropyridines are now an established treatment for coronary artery spasm.[56-58] Some data show that verapamil hydrochloride and diltiazem hydrochloride also reduce the incidence of coronary artery spasm.[57] However, other data suggest that nifedipine and diltiazem hydrochloride are more effective than verapamil hydrochloride.[59] Ca^{2+} antagonists, in particular dihydropyridines, are effective in the treatment of vasospastic angina. In serious cases of vasospastic angina, dihydropyridines have been administered intravenously.[60] Figure 8.3 demonstrates the effects of Ca^{2+} overload and Ca^{2+} antagonistic action in coronary spasm and angina pectoris.

The advantage of administering Ca^{2+} antagonists is that tolerance development (as occurs with nitrates) is avoided. Numerous authors (e.g., Hill et al.[56]) have alluded to the superiority of dihydropyridines over nitrates.

Silent Ischemia

The pathophysiology of silent ischemia has not yet been elucidated. The spontaneous occurrence in the presence of physical and psychological stress suggests a vasospastic component. Hence, Ca^{2+} antagonists are highly effective in the treatment of such episodes. β-Blockers, however, have proved superior to Ca^{2+} antagonists in this area. Rizzon and coworkers[61] have shown that silent episodes of ischemia can be managed well with either nifedipine (120 mg/d) or verapamil hydrochloride (480 mg/d); both are superior to nitrates in this application.[61] Repetitive ischemic episodes may lead to myocardial stunning, which can also be treated with Ca^{2+} antagonists.

Stable and Exercise-Induced Angina

Eccentric Coronary Artery Sclerosis

Dihydropyridine-type Ca^{2+} antagonist therapy is appropriate for patients with stable angina and eccentric coronary artery disease. Eccentric atherosclerosis involves contractible sections of the arterial wall that can be dilated when Ca^{2+} antagonists are used. Because use of Ca^{2+} antagonists can lead to only partial vasodilatation, the combination with a negative inotropic or chronotropic substance such as a β-blocker seems prudent and has various advantages. Therefore, the combination of β-blockers and Ca^{2+} antagonists has been recommended. β-blockers prevent an increase in heart rate, secondary to a reduction in blood pressure, while reducing oxygen demand.[62] It has also been shown that a combination of dihydropyridines and β-blockers is superior to a combination of nitrates and β-blockers. However, the nitrate–β-blocker combination exerts a favorable influence on left ventricular function during exercise.[63] Diltiazem hydrochloride has also been used effectively in this context to treat ischemic heart disease. Subramanian[36] has worked extensively in this area.

Concentric Coronary Artery Sclerosis

In the case of concentric coronary artery sclerosis, Ca^{2+} antagonists may have a negative effect.[32,36,37,64] In particular, Ca^{2+} antagonists of the dihydropyridine class may lead to peripheral vasodilatation, an increase in heart rate (via the baroreceptor reflex), and more important to the so-called steal phenomenon. The steal phenomenon involves dilatation of the vascular bed in other sections of the coronary artery not affected by atherosclerosis. As a result, blood is "stolen" from the areas that are situated distally from the concentric atherosclerotic lesion. The vessels of such areas are stiff and cannot be dilated.[65,66] Hence, Ca^{2+} antagonists are less likely to be successful in treating this type of coronary artery disease. However, dihydropyridines and diltiazem hydrochloride can be given successfully in combination with β-blockers in this context.[62,63]

Ca^{2+} antagonists of the benzotiazepine type and verapamil hydrochloride are appropriate treatments for this type of coronary artery disease in patients with stable angina.[36,38-40,67] Gallopamil, verapamil hydrochloride, and diltiazem hydrochloride have been shown to be effective. However, the main effect of the drugs in this particular subtype of coronary artery disease is the decrease in oxygen consumption by the myocardium, because of negative chronotropic and inotropic effects. The combined use of verapamil hydrochloride and propanolol was suggested as a possible treatment.[68,69] However, this combination seems dangerous, because it can lead to atrioventricular block III and asystole.[70,71]

During physical exercise the relative tension of the arterial wall can be increased (possibly a result of increased concentrations of catecholamines).[72] Because of this increased tension, coronary artery dilation via Ca^{2+} antagonists could be even more effective during exercise than during rest.[72,73] Improved oxygen delivery could be the main source of the antianginal effect of nifedipine.[2,74] Another important pathomechanism in ischemic heart disease is increased diastolic stiffness of the myocardium, which is an early manifestation of ischemia.[1,75] Verapamil hydrochloride improves left ventricular filling but does not affect diastolic ventricular function to the same extent.[73,75,76]

Unstable Angina

Unstable angina may be very different from stable angina regarding pathophysiology. Unstable angina entails vasospastic forms of angina and formations of intermittent coronary thrombi[77-79] (Figure 8.4). Clinically, unstable angina appears as angina at rest; affected patients require hospitalization and intravenous therapy to avoid progression into myocardial infarction. Depending on the possibility and the severity of unstable angina, intracoronary and intravenous administration of Ca^{2+} antagonists has proven useful.[55,56] A crossover study has shown that intravenous nifedipine is more effective than intravenous nitroglycerin in controlling ischemic episodes.[80] Previtali and coworkers[81] have treated patients who tend toward spastic angina, as well as those with unstable forms of angina, using oral nifedipine, diltiazem hydrochloride, and verapamil hydrochloride. Nifedipine and diltiazem hydrochloride, and to a lesser extent verapamil hydrochloride, have been shown to be highly effective in the prevention of ischemic attacks.[81] However, verapamil hydrochloride has still shown a better antianginal effect than propanolol.[5] Figure 8.5 depicts therapeutic strategies in the context of the pathophysiology of ischemic heart disease.

Ischemic Cardiomyopathy

Most Ca^{2+} antagonists with negative inotropy should be avoided in treating ischemic cardiomyopathy because the Ca^{2+} antagonists will further decrease the already deficient left ventricular function. The negative humoral effects in dilated cardiomyopathy especially can be po-

tentiated by the short-acting type of Ca^{2+} antagonists: dihydropyridines, benzothiazepines, and verapamil hydrochloride. In this case, nitrates and angiotensin-converting enzyme inhibitors would be preferred. Patients with ischemic cardiomyopathy often suffer from an adrenergic overdrive that leads to tachycardia. β-Blockers have been used effectively to counteract this adrenergic overdrive. This results in improved diastolic filling and thus an improved hemodynamic situation of the heart. Studies are under way that will eventually provide the results of the use of newer generations of Ca^{2+} antagonists. Jusuf and Fuhrberg published a meta-analysis of long-term and short-term investigations of myocardial infarction that showed an increased mortality rate (6%) in patients who had been treated with Ca^{2+} antagonists after myocardial infarction. This analysis shows no favorable effects of Ca^{2+} antagonists in secondary prevention. Because the evidence for positive effects in certain subgroups of Ca^{2+} antagonists is scant, we would not recommend those drugs in the treatment of myocardial infarction.

Primary Prevention

Larger primary prevention studies for Ca^{2+} antagonists are rare. Lichtlen[31] looked at normotensive patients with coronary artery disease after 3 years of treatment with nifedipine and reported some degree of prevention of atherosclerotic plaque development. Several experimental studies alluded to the antiatherosclerotic effect of Ca^{2+} antagonists. The link between arterial wall cholesterol and Ca^{2+} is still missing, however (Figure 8.6). The reduction of cardiovascular events such as myocardial infarction and sudden cardiac death has not been demonstrated in this study; progression of coronary artery disease was also not affected. These results have been supported by a Canadian study that used nicardipine hydrochloride.[82] Klein and coworkers[29] and Kober and coworkers (personal communication) have found some indication that diltiazem hydrochloride and verapamil

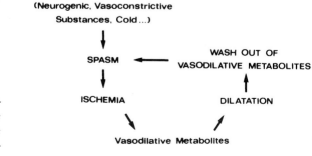

FIGURE 8.4. Unstable angina resulting from vasospasm and repetitive thrombosis. In severe cases, unstable angina results in myocardial necrosis.

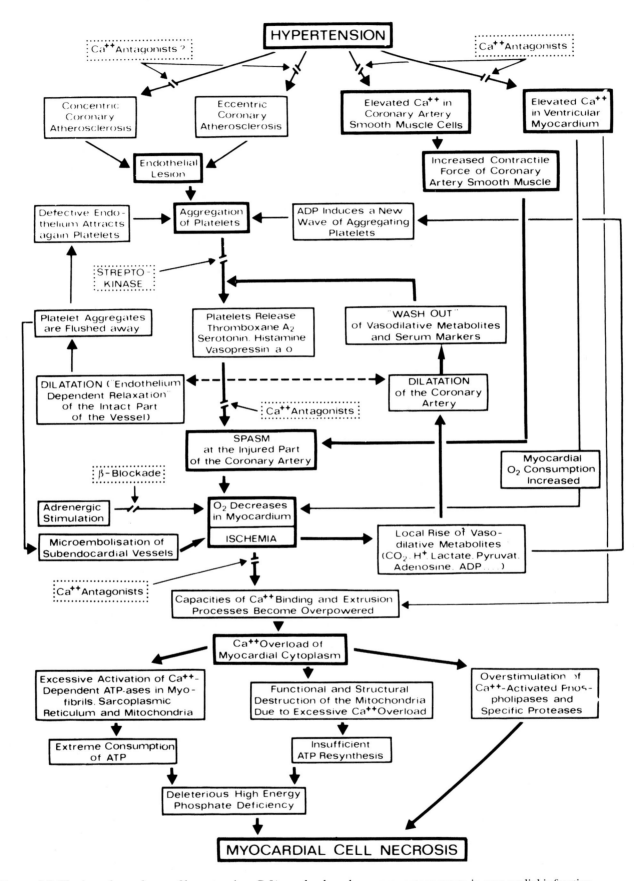

FIGURE 8.5. The interdependence of hypertension, Ca^{2+} overload, and coronary artery spasm in myocardial infarction.

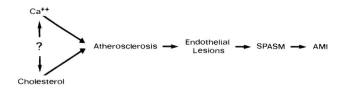

(Ca⁺⁺Antagonists Protect against Experimental Atherosclerosis)

FIGURE 8.6. Missing link between arterial wall cholesterol and Ca^{2+} antagonism.

hydrochloride may cause a regression of atherosclerotic plaques. However, these results were gathered from retrospective analyses.

References

1. Gasser R. Antiarteriosklerotische Wirkung von Calcium-antagonisten und coronare Herzkrankheit. Wien: Fakultas; 1990.
2. Opie LH. Calcium channel antagonists, II: use and comparative properties of the three prototypical calcium antagonists in ischaemic heart disease, including recommendations based on an analysis of 41 trials. In: Opie LH, ed. *Clinical Use of Calcium Channel Antagonist Drugs.* 2nd ed. Boston, Mass: Kluwer Academic Publishers; 1990.
3. Ringer S. A further contribution regarding the influence of different constituents of blood on the contraction of the heart. *J Physiol.* 1883;4: 29–34.
4. Cow D. Some reactions of surviving arteries. *J Physiol.* 1911;42:125–140.
5. Ebashi S. Ca^{2+} and the contractile proteins. *J Mol Cell Cardiol.* 1984;16:129–136.
6. Gasser R, Frey M, Fleckenstein-Grün. Free calcium in rat papillary muscle at contraction assessed with Ca-sensitive micro-electrodes. *Angiology.* 1989;41:736–741.
7. Parodi O, Simonetti I, L'Abbate A, Marei A. Verapamil versus propanolol for angina at rest. *Am J Cardiol.* 1982;50: 923–929.
8. Fleckenstein A, Kammermeier H, Döring HJ, Freund HJ, Grün G, Kienle A. Zum Wirkungsmechanismus neuartiger Coronardilatatoren mit gleichzeitigen sauerstoffeinsparenden Myocardeffekten, Prenylamin und Iproveratil. *Z Kreislaufforsch.* 1967;56:716–839.
9. Fleckenstein A. Specific inhibitors and promoters of calcium action in the excitation-contraction coupling of heart muscle and their role in the prevention of production of myocardial lesions. In: Harris P, Opie LH, eds. *Calcium and the Heart.* London: Academic Press; 1971: 135–142.
10. Lewis GRJ, Morley KD, Lewis BM, Bones PJ. The treatment of hypertension with verapamil. *N Z Med J.* 1978;87: 351–363.
11. Fleckenstein A, Tritthart H, Döring HJ, Byon YK. Bay a 1040-ein hochaktiver Ca-antagonistischer Inhibitor der elektromechanischen Koppelungsprozesse im Warmblüter-myocard. *Arzneim-Forsch/Drug Res.* 1972;22:22–29.
12. Nikajima H, Hoshiyima M, Yamashita K, Kiyomoto A. Effect of diltiazem on electrical and mechanical activity of isolated cardiac ventricular muscle of guinea pig. *Jpn J Pharmacol.* 1975;25:383–392.
13. Kohlhart E, Bauer B, Krause H, Fleckenstein A. Differentiation of the transmembrane Na and Ca channel in mammalian cardiac fibres by use of specific inhibitors. *Pflügers Arch.* 1972;335:309–315.
14. Livesely B, Catley PF, Campbell RC, Oram S. Double blind evaluation of verapamil, propanolol, and isosorbide dinitrate in the treatment of angina pectoris. *BMJ.* 1973;1: 375–378.
15. Glossmann H, Ferry DR, Goll A, Rambush M. Molecular pharmacology of the calcium channel: evidence of subtypes, multiple drug receptor sites, channel subunits, and the development of a radioiodinated, 1,4-dihydropyridine calcium channel label (¹²⁵I Iodipine). *J Cardiovasc Pharmacol.* 1984; 6:608–617.
16. Bourdellion PO, Poole-Wilson PA. Effect of verapamil, K, quiescence, and cardioplegia on calcium exchange and mechanical function in ischaemic rabbit myocardium. *Circ Res.* 1982;50:360–368.
17. Clark RE, Ferguson TB, Marbarger J. The first American trial of nifedipine in cardioplegia. *J Thoracic Cardiovasc Surg.* 1981;82:848–853.
18. Fleckenstein A, Van Breemen C, Groβ R, Hoffmeister F, eds. *Cardiovascular Effects of Dihydropyridine-Type Calcium Antagonists and Agonists.* Berlin: Springer-Verlag; 1985.
19. Henry PD, Schuchleib R, Borda LJ, Roberts R, Williamson JR, Soebel BE. Effects of nifedipine on myocardial perfusion and ischaemic injury in dogs. *Circ Res.* 1978;43: 372–379.
20. Vanhoutte PM, Paoletti R. The WHO classification of calcium antagonists. *Trends Pharmacodyn.* 1987;172:235–241.
21. Fleckenstein A. *Calcium Antagonism in Heart and Smooth Muscle: Experimental Facts and Therapeutic Prospects.* New York, NY: Wiley; 1983.
22. Dienstl F. A mathematical model of the prehospital period in the first 24 hours of myocardial infarction. Paper presented at: Interna Symposium; Baden-Baden, Germany: Witzstock; 1977:128–130.
23. Gasser R. The interdependence of hypertension, calcium overload, and coronary spasm in the development of myocardial infarction. *Angiology.* 1988;39:761–772.
24. Gasser R. Calcium antagonists: pharmacological agents in search of new clinical indications. *Angiology.* 1990;41: 36–41.
25. Klein W, Eber B, Dusleag J, et al. New concepts in ischaemia prevention. *J Cardiovasc Pharmacol.* 1991;18(suppl 9):S7–S14.
26. Maseri A, Abbate AL, Baroldi G. Coronary spasm as a possible cause of myocardial infarction: a conclusion derived from the study of preinfarction angina. *N Engl J Med.* 1978;299:271–274.
27. Gasser R, Kickenweiz E, Brussee H, Klein W. Myokard-und Gef-βprotektion durch Kalziumantagonisten bei koronarer Herzkrankheit. *Therapiew Österr.* 1991;6:480–486.
28. Gibson RS, Boden WE, Theroux P, et al. The diltiazem reinfarction study group. *N Engl J Med.* 1986;315:423–429.
29. Klein W, Lufty A, Schreyer H. Effect of longterm treatment with calcium blockers on human arteriosclerosis. In: Fleckenstein A, Hashimoto K, Hermann M, Schwartz A,

Seipel L, eds. *New Calcium Antagonists: Recent Developments and Prospects.* Stuttgart, Germany: Gustav Fischer; 1983: 183–189.

30. Leaf A, Weber PC. Prevention and noninvasive therapy of atherosclerosis. *Atherosclerosis Reviews.* Vol 21. New York, NY: Raven Press; 1989.

31. Lichtlen PR, Hugenholtz PG, Rafflenbeul W, Hecker H, Jost S, Deckers JW. Retardation of angiographic progression of coronary artery disease by nifedipine. *Lancet.* 1990;335:1109–1113.

32. Loaldi A, Polese A, Montorsi P. Comparison of nifedipine, propanolol, and isosorbide dinitrate on angiographic progression and regression of coronary arterial narrowings in anginal pectoris. *Am J Cardiol.* 1989;64:433–439.

33. Schettler G, Gross R, eds. *Arteriosklerose.* Köln: Deutscher Ärzteverlag; 1985.

34. Morad M, Nayler W, Kazda S, Schramm M, eds. *The Calcium Channel: Structure, Function, and Implications.* Berlin: Springer-Verlag; 1988.

35. Nayler W. *Calcium Antagonists.* London: Academic Press; 1988.

36. Subramanian VB. *Calcium Antagonists in Chronic and Stable Angina Pectoris.* Amsterdam: Excerpta Medica; 1983.

37. Smith T, ed. *DHP Calcium Antagonists: New Possibilities in Angina Pectoris and in Hypertension.* Brussels: Dehapse Publisher; 1987.

38. Zanchetti A, Krokler DM. *Calcium Antagonism in Cardiovascular Therapy. Experience with Verapamil.* Amsterdam: Excerpta Medica; 1981.

39. Chaitman BR, Wagniart P, Pasternac A. Improved exercise tolerance after propanolol, diltiazem, or nifedipine in angina pectoris: comparison at 1, 3, and 8 hours and correlation with plasma drug concentration. *Am J Cardiol.* 1984;53:1–5.

40. Frischman W, Charlap S, Kimmel B. Diltiazem, nifedipine, and their combination in patients with stable angina pectoris: effects on angina, exercise tolerance, and the ambulatory electrocardiographic ST segment. *Circulation.* 1988;77:774–786.

41. Prinzmetal M, Kennamer R, Merliss R, Wada T, Bor N. Angina pectoris, I: a variant form of angina pectoria: preliminary report. *Am J Med.* 1959;27:375–388.

42. Braunwald E. Coronary artery spasm as a cause of myocardial ischaemia. *J Lab Clin Med.* 1981;97:299–307.

43. Gasser R, Dienstl F, Puschendorf B, Hauptlorenz S, Moll M, Dworzak E. New perspectives on the function of coronary artery spasm in acute myocardial infarction: the thrombo-ischemic re-entry mechanism. *Angiology.* 1986;37: 880–887.

44. Gasser R. Spontaneous intermittent reperfusion in early myocardial infarction. *Lancet.* 1988;2:1189.

45. Gasser R, Schafhalter-Zoppoth I, Schwarz T, Eber B, Koppel H, Lechleitner P, Puschendorf B, Dienstl F, Klein W. Cyclic phenomena in early myocardial infarction. *Acta Med Austriaca.* 1995;22:69–72.

46. Oliva PB, Breckinridge JC. Arteriographic evidence of coronary arterial spasm in acute myocardial infarction. *Circulation.* 1977;56:366–372.

47. Prinzmetal M, Kennamer R, Merliss R. A angina pectoris: a variant form of angina pectoris. *Am J Med.* 1959;27: 375–382.

48. Gasser R, Dienstl F, Henn R. Impact of thrombo-ischemic reentry: mechanism on coronary thrombosis and microembolism in acute myocardial infarction. *Angiology.* 1987;38:562–567.

49. Schwartz CJ, Gerrity RG. Anatomical pathology of sudden, unexpected cardiac death. *Circulation.* 1975;51/52 (suppl 2):18–25.

50. Metha J, Metha P, Feldmann RL, Horalek C. Thromboxane release in coronary artery disease. *Am Heart J.* 1984; 107:286–292.

51. Ogasawara K, Aizawa T, Nishimura K, Satoh H, Fujii J, Katoh K. β-Thromboglobulin release within coronary circulation: a potential role of platelets in ergonovine-induced coronary artery spasm. *Int J Cardiol.* 1985;10:15–22.

52. Brum JM, Sufan Q, Lane G, Bove AA. Increased vasoconstrictor activity of proximal coronary arteries with endothelial damage in intact dogs. *Circulation.* 1984; 70:1066–1073.

53. Ganz P, Alexander W. New insights into the cellular mechanisms of vasospasm. *Am J Cardiol.* 1985(suppl);56: 11E–15E.

54. Kazda S, Mayer D. Postischaemic impaired reperfusion and tissue damage: consequences of a calcium-dependent vasospasm? In: Godfraind E, Fleckenstein A, Lichtlen PR, et al., eds. *Calcium Entry Blockers and Tissue Protection.* New York, NY: Raven Press; 1985:129–138.

55. Rafflenbeul W: Adalat intravenös bei Koronarspasmen. In: Meyer J, Erbel R, eds. *Intravenöse und intrakoronare Anwendung von Adalat.* Berlin: Springer-Verlag; 1985:61–64.

56. Hill JA, Feldman RL, Pepine CJ, Conti CR. Randomised double-blind comparison of nifedipine and isosorbide dinitrate in patients with coronary arterial spasm. *Am J Cardiol.* 1982;49:431–441.

57. Johnson SM, Mauritson DR, Willerson JT, Hillis LD. Comparison of verapamil and nifedipine in the treatment of variant angina pectoris: preliminary observations in 10 patients. *Am J Cardiol.* 1981;47:1295–1298.

58. Previtali M, Salerno JA, Tavazzi L. Treatment of angina at rest with nifedipine: a short term controlled study. *Am J Cardiol.* 1980;45:825–832.

59. Kishida H. Application of calcium antagonists in patients with Prinzmetal angina pectoris. In: Fleckenstein A, Rosskamm H, eds. *Calcium Antagonismus.* Berlin: Springer-Verlag; 1980:246–251.

60. Meyer J, Erbel R, eds. *Intravenöse und intrakoronare Anwendung von Adalat.* Berlin: Springer-Verlag; 1985.

61. Rizzon P, Scrutino D, Mangini SG. Randomised placebo-controlled comparative study of nifedipine, verapamil, and isosorbide dinitrate in the treatment of angina at rest. *Eur Heart J.* 1986;7:67–76.

62. Daniel WG, Reil G-H, Schober O, Creuzig H, Lichtlen PR. Effects of combined nifedipine and propanolol treatment on regional myocardial blood flow in coronary patients. In: Lichtlen PR, ed. *6th International Adalat Symposium: New Therapy of Ischaemic Heart Disease and Hypertension.* Amsterdam: Excerpta Medica; 1986:414–421.

63. Nesto R, White H, Ganz P, et al. Nifedipine is superior to nitrates when added to β-blocker therapy in stable angina: analysis by left ventricular performance during exercise. In: Lichtlen PR, ed. *6th International Adalat Symposium: New Therapy of Ischaemic Heart Disease and Hypertension.* Amsterdam: Excerpta Medica; 1986:345–346.

64. Patmore L, Whiting RL. Calcium entry blocking properties of tanshinone 11-A sulphonate, an active principle of an antianginal extract Dan Shen. *Br J Pharmacol.* 1982;75: 149–155.

65. Jariwalla AG, Anderson EG. Side effects of drugs: production of ischaemic cardiac pain by nifedipine. *BMJ.* 1978;1: 1181–1182.

66. Stone PH, Muller JE, Turi ZG. Efficacy of nifedipine therapy in patients with refractory angina pectoris: significance of the presence of coronary vasospasm. *Am Heart J.* 1983;106:644–652.

67. Hossack KF, Pool PE, Steele P. Effect of diltiazem on angina effort: a multicenter trial. *Am J Cardiol.* 1982; 49:567–578.

68. Bassan M. Additive antianginal effect of verapamil in patients receiving propanolol. *BMJ.* 1978;1:1067–1072.

69. Lessem J. Combined administration of verapamil and β-blockers in patients with angina pectoris. In: Zanchetti A, Krikler DM, eds. *Calcium Antagonism in Cardiovascular Therapy: Experience With Verapamil.* Amsterdam: Excerpta Medica; 1981:159–166.

70. Benaim ME. Asystole after verapamil. *BMJ.* 1972;2: 349–354.

71. Denis B, Pellet J, Machecourt J, Martin-Noel P. Verapamil et β-bloquant. Une association therapeutic dangereuse. *Nouv Presse Med (Moscow).* 1977;10:100–109.

72. Heusch G, Guth BD, Seitelberger R. Attenuation of exercise-induced myocardial ischaemia in dogs with recruitment of coronary vasodilator reserve by nifedipine. *Circulation.* 1987;75:482–490.

73. Bonow RO, Leon MB, Rosing DR. Effects of verapamil and propanolol on left ventricular systolic function and diastolic filling in patients with coronary artery disease: radionuclide angiographic studies at rest and during exercise. *Circulation.* 1981;65:1337–1350.

74. Ardissino D, de Servi S, Salerno JA. Efficacy, duration, and mechanism of action of nifedipine in stable exercise-induced angina pectoris. *Eur Heart J.* 1983;4:873–881.

75. Bolognesi R, Cucchini F, Manca C. Effects of verapamil and nifedipine on rate of left ventricular relaxation in coronary artery disease patients with normal systolic function. *N Y Acad Sci Abstract Book;* 1987:66.

76. Apstein CS, Grossman W. Opposite initial effects of supply and demand ischaemia on the left ventricular diastolic compliance: the ischaemia-diastolic paradox. *J Mol Cell Cardiol.* 1987;19:119–128.

77. Gasser R, Dienstl F. Acute myocardial infarction: an episodic event of several coronary spasms followed by dilatation? *Clin Physiol.* 1986;6:397–403.

78. Hacket D, Davies G, Chierchia S, Maseri A. Intermittent coronary occlusion in acute myocardial infarction: value of combined thrombolytic and vasodilator therapy. *N Engl J Med.* 1987;317:1055–1059.

79. Maseri A. Pathogenic mechanisms of angina pectoris: expanding views. *Br Heart J.* 1980;43:431–439.

80. Rafflenbeul W, Bosaller C, Lichtlen PR. Intravenous infusion of nifedipine versus intravenous infusion of nitroglycerin in patients with unstable angina pectoris. In: Lichtlen PR, ed. *6th International Adalat Symposium: New Therapy of Ischaemic Heart Disease and Hypertension.* Amsterdam: Excerpta Medica; 1986:264–268.

81. Previtali M, Salerno JA, Panciroli C, Guast L, Chimienti M, Montemartini C. Short-term effectiveness of nifedipine, diltiazem, and verapamil in Prinzmetal's variant angina: evaluation by Holter monitoring and ergometrine testing. In: Lichtlen PR, ed. *6th International Adalat Symposium: New Therapy of Ischaemic Heart Disease and Hypertension.* Amsterdam: Excerpta Medica; 1986:280–286.

82. Waters D, Lesperance J, Francetich M, et al. A controlled clinical trial to assess the effect of a calcium channel blocker on the progression of coronary atherosclerosis. *Circulation.* 1990;82:1940–1972.

9

Basic Mechanisms of Action of Nitrovasodilators and Development of Tolerance to Organic Nitrates

Johan Van de Voorde and Marc Bogaert

Nitrovasodilators are among the oldest but still most widely used drugs in cardiovascular medicine.[1] As early as 1867, Brunton noted that inhalation of amyl nitrite relieved anginal pain within seconds,[13] and in 1879, Murrell established the use of nitroglycerin for prophylaxis and relief of acute anginal attacks.[64] Even though the beneficial effects of nitrates were recognized more than 100 years ago, their impact on the organism and their cellular mechanism of action were elucidated only in the 1970s and 1980s. Nitrovasodilators were then found to be a peculiar kind of prodrug; they undergo biotransformation to their active form, nitric oxide (NO), at their site of action, mainly the vascular smooth muscle. NO synthesized by vascular endothelial cells has an important role in physiological regulation of vascular smooth muscle tone (see Chapter 2 in this book). Recognition of the physiological role of NO renewed interest in the nitrovasodilators, because they were then seen as a substitute for failing endogenous NO in patients with endothelial dysfunction (e.g., in angina and myocardial infarction).

Based on their capacity to diminish cardiac preload and afterload and to dilate coronary vessels, nitrates reduce the oxygen consumption of myocardium. These drugs have proved to be useful for treatment of angina pectoris and heart failure. A major problem associated with nitrovasodilators is attenuation of their effects with time, which limits their clinical usefulness.[10,24,28,56,77] In this chapter we focus on the basic mechanism of action of nitrovasodilators, the mechanisms thought to be involved in attenuation of their effects in time, and potential strategies to overcome this problem.

Classification of Nitrovasodilators

For insight into the mechanism of action of nitrovasodilators and the development of tolerance to nitrates, a classification of nitrovasodilators is useful (Figure 9.1).

1. *Organic nitrates* are polyalcohol esters of nitric acid (R-O-NO$_2$). They are commonly used in medicine. The prototype is the powerful explosive glyceryl trinitrate, or nitroglycerin, the trinitrate ester of the polyalcohol glycerol. Other members of this group are isosorbide dinitrate, isosorbide-5-mononitrate, erythrityl tetranitrate, and pentaerythritol tetranitrate.

2. *Organic nitrites* also may have vasodilative activity. They are alcohol esters of nitrous acid (R-O-NO), such as amyl nitrite, whose antianginal properties were recognized before those of nitroglycerin. Medical use of amyl nitrite, administered by inhalation, has been abandoned.

3. Other substances with an *NO moiety*, such as sodium nitroprusside and molsidomine, liberate NO in biological fluids. Nitroprusside is a potent vasodilator effective in the treatment of acute hypertension, but its use is limited because of toxicity of its cyanide moiety. Molsidomine (SIN-10), a more recently developed molecule, is a prodrug activated in the liver by enzymatic conversion to SIN-1 (*N*-carboxy-3-morpholinosydnonimine ethylester). SIN-1 is converted in blood to the very labile SIN-1A, which is further metabolized to the inactive SIN-1C. NO is released in the latter conversion.[69] Several other molecules with an NO moiety will probably become available.

4. *NO* itself is a very toxic gas, but inhalation of low concentrations is thought to be useful for the treatment of primary and secondary forms of pulmonary hypertension.[45,79,81]

Cellular Mechanisms of Action of Nitrovasodilators

Leaving aside some data that indicate involvement of prostacyclin[54] or smooth muscle hyperpolarization,[40,100] it is generally accepted that the main mechanism of action of nitrovasodilators is stimulation of guanylyl cy-

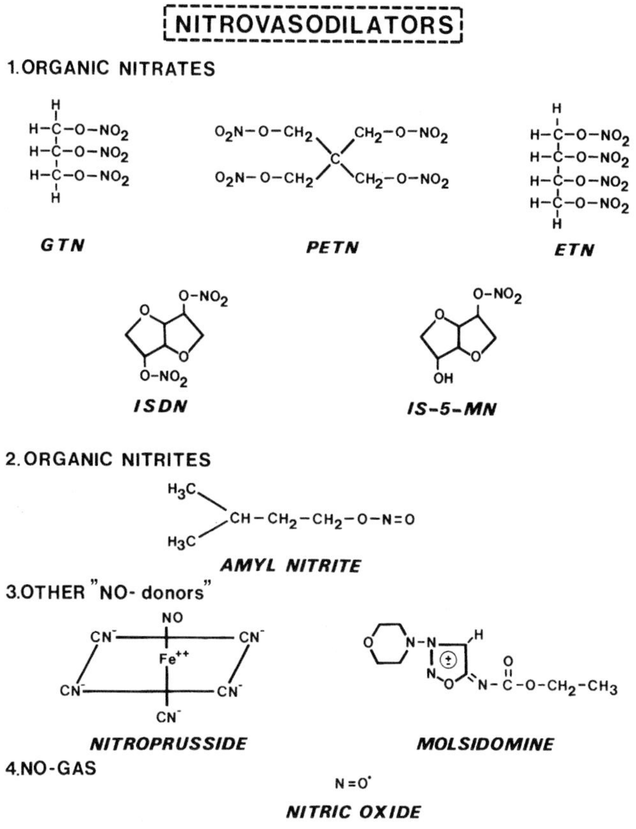

NITROVASODILATORS

1.ORGANIC NITRATES

GTN

PETN

ETN

ISDN

IS-5-MN

2.ORGANIC NITRITES

AMYL NITRITE

3.OTHER "NO- donors"

NITROPRUSSIDE

MOLSIDOMINE

4.NO-GAS

NITRIC OXIDE

FIGURE 9.1. Classification and chemical structure of different types of nitrovasodilators. GTN indicates glyceryl trinitrate, nitroglycerin; PETN, pentaerythritol tetranitrate; ETN, erythrityl tetranitrate; ISDN, isosorbide dinitrate; and IS-5-MN, isosorbide-5-mononitrate.

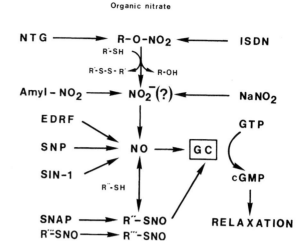

FIGURE 9.2. Schematic representation of mechanisms considered to be involved in the relaxation of vascular smooth muscle cells under the influence of nitrovasodilators. NTG, nitroglycerin; R-O-NO$_2$, organic nitrate; ISDN, isosorbide dinitrate; R'-SH, R''-SH, R'''-SH, different thiol-containing molecules; R'-S-S-R', oxidized thiol; R-OH, denitrated organic nitrate; NO$_2^-$, nitrite; EDRF, endothelial-derived relaxant factor; NO, nitric oxide; SNP, sodium nitroprusside; SNAP, S-nitroso-N-acetylpenicillamine; R''-SNO, R'''-SNO, organic nitrosothiols; and GC, guanylyl cyclase. (Adapted with permission from Van de Voorde.[95])

clase, which results in increased levels of cyclic guanosine monophosphate (cGMP) and leads to relaxation of contractile machinery of the vascular smooth muscle cell.[1,49] Thus, Kukovetz and Holzmann[50] found good correlation between the degree of relaxation and the accumulation of cGMP in bovine coronary arteries in response to nitroglycerin, nitroprusside, and SIN-1 under different conditions.

Although the evidence for the role of cGMP as mediator of smooth muscle relaxation in response to nitrovasodilators is extensive, there are reports that drug-induced relaxation and cGMP elevation are not well correlated.[65] It is thus possible that, besides formation of cGMP, other mechanisms may be involved in the relaxation produced by nitrovasodilators.

How do nitrovasodilators lead to accumulation of cGMP? Measurements of the content of thiol groups in smooth muscle cells by Needleman et al.[67] and the extensive biochemical work by Ignarro et al.[36] have led to the concept that the spasmolytic effect of organic nitrates occurs through a complex cascade of intracellular biochemical events (Figure 9.2) that involve denitration

of the organic nitrates by reaction with a thiol-containing group (most probably cysteine). Liberation of inorganic nitrite, followed by its conversion to NO, stimulates guanylyl cyclase, directly or through formation of a nitrosothiol. Related compounds such as amyl nitrite, sodium nitrite, nitroprusside, SIN-1, endothelium-derived nitric oxide, S-nitrosoacetylpenicillamine, and other nitrosothiols also fit into this scheme but enter the pathway at different levels. NO is the common active principle of the nitrovasodilators, the biotransformation of nitrovasodilators to NO being a prerequisite for vascular relaxation.

The exact mechanism that mediates formation of NO from organic nitrates in vascular smooth muscle is not fully established. Although inorganic nitrite is the predominant nitrogen oxide–containing species formed, its role as intermediate in the formation of an activator of guanylyl cyclase is questionable because it has low vasodilator potency and the endogenous levels of this species are high relative to the amounts that could be formed from pharmacologically relevant concentrations of organic nitrates.[4] There are probably multiple biotransformation systems, with different affinities for the various nitrates and different selectivities for the molecular site of denitration of the nitrates, that contribute to NO formation from organic nitrates. NO formation from relatively high concentrations of nitroglycerin can occur nonenzymatically by interaction with cysteine. Also, glutathione-S-transferases and cytochrome P-450 mediate denitration of nitroglycerin. The relative importance of these biotransformation systems in the formation of NO from organic nitrates has not been established.[1,4]

Attenuation of the Effect of Nitrates

The main disadvantage of organic nitrates is the attenuation of their effects on repeated exposure so that increasing doses are required to achieve the same effect. This phenomenon is known as *tolerance*. However, *nitrate tolerance* is sometimes used in a much more specific and restrictive manner to denote the decreased response of vascular smooth muscle toward a given nitrate concentration. This so-called *vascular tolerance* has mainly been demonstrated in animal studies. Attenuation of the effects of nitrates on chronic administration might, however, also be due to counterregulatory mechanisms.

Tolerance to nitrovasodilators may also develop in blood platelets. Indeed, nitrovasodilators have not only vasodilative effects but also antiplatelet activity.[20,55] Nitroglycerin inhibits platelet aggregation and prevents platelet adhesion to damaged intimal lining.[52] Nitrates may also dissolve formed platelet aggregates. The effects on platelets are also due to increased levels of cGMP. In patients with impaired nitrate-induced vasodilation due to nitrate tolerance, the increase in intracellular formation of cGMP in platelets is diminished.[104]

Before further discussion of nitrate tolerance, the problem of sorption of organic nitrates should be mentioned. Nitroglycerin and isosorbide dinitrate adhere strongly to several materials, especially polyvinylchloride.[1,18,19] This adhesion may result in a marked reduction of the dose administered to the patient by injection or infusion. In case of a lack of effectiveness of nitrates, such adherence should be excluded before concluding that tolerance has developed.

Historical Note

Tolerance to nitrovasodilators was recognized at the end of the nineteenth century by observation of workmen who handled nitroglycerin for production of explosives.[89] When they began working, they suffered from severe headache and syncopal tendency due to exposure to nitrates in the environment. After a few days these symptoms disappeared; that is, the workers became tolerant. During the weekends, they were no longer exposed to nitroglycerin, and tolerance disappeared. After the weekend, on renewed exposure to nitrates, the typical syndrome (known as Monday morning disease) was again seen. Workers soon realized that they could prevent this syndrome by during the weekends applying nitrate paste to their skin or wearing hats with headbands that had been impregnated with nitrate.

Tolerance to the therapeutic effects of nitrovasodilators was also already recognized in the nineteenth century. In 1867, Brunton wrote that with prolonged use of amyl nitrite, the dose had to be increased to maintain beneficial effects.[13] Very soon after introduction of nitroglycerin in clinical practice, Stewart reported the very rapid establishment of tolerance.[86]

Mechanisms of Nitrate Tolerance

Tolerance could theoretically result from *pharmacokinetic changes* such as reduction in absorption, changes in distribution, and enhancement of metabolism or excretion of the administered nitrates or their active metabolites. However, it has been established that tolerance to nitrovasodilators is not due to pharmacokinetic alterations, because plasma drug levels are not decreased when tolerance develops after long-term treatment.[27] It can be added that the poor relationship between plasma concentrations and the therapeutic effects of nitrates limits interest in the pharmacokinetics of these substances.[1,11]

Nitrate tolerance is due to *pharmacodynamic changes,* either a decrease in responsiveness of vascular smooth muscle cells or the development of counterregulatory mechanisms. A large amount of evidence shows that the responsiveness of vascular smooth muscle cells is clearly decreased when animals become tolerant. This vascular tolerance was first demonstrated in 1968.[9] Isolated vessel segments taken from animals treated in vivo for some days with, for example, nitroglycerin show a marked decrease in sensitivity to the effects of this drug (Figure 9.3).[9,66,96] Incubation of isolated blood vessel segments in a physiological solution that contains high concentrations of nitroglycerin for only 1 hour also results in a marked decrease in sensitivity to the effects of the drug.[2,47,68] Such in vitro experiments clearly demonstrate that a decrease in sensitivity to nitrates may occur simply by direct contact of the nitrate with vascular smooth muscle cells.

What could be the mechanism of vascular tolerance? Considering the mechanism of action of nitrovasodilators presented in Figure 9.2, vascular tolerance can be explained by several hypotheses. Tolerance could be due to a decreased effect of cGMP on the relaxation mechanisms. This is not the case, as it has been reported repeatedly that 8-bromo-cyclic GMP, a lipophilic analog of cGMP that readily penetrates cell membranes, elicits similar relaxation in control and in nitroglycerin-tolerant vessels.[42,58] It has also been shown repeatedly that tolerance is associated with impaired elevation of the cGMP level.[2,42,43,47,58] This could be due to an increase in cGMP

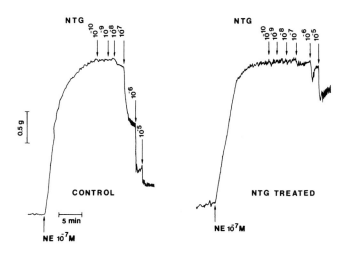

FIGURE 9.3. Original tracings of tension measurements on isolated rat thoracic aorta, showing relaxation effects elicited by increasing concentrations (in molar units) of nitroglycerin (NTG) after precontraction with norepinephrine (NE, 10^{-7} M). **Left,** Preparation taken from a control rat. **Right,** Preparation taken from a rat treated with nitroglycerin (three subcutaneous injections of 100 mg/kg for 2 days).

phosphodiesterase activity, which is responsible for cGMP breakdown. Zaprinast, a phosphodiesterase inhibitor, indeed restores vasoreactivity in nitrate-tolerant vessels.[73] Such an effect could not be confirmed in human volunteers with the phosphodiesterase inhibitor dipyridamole.[90] Decreased cGMP formation as seen in tolerant animals may also be due to enhanced production of vascular superoxide anion. Superoxide anions rapidly inactivate NO, and inactivation of superoxide anions by superoxide dismutase increases responses to nitrate in nitroglycerin-tolerant rabbit aorta.[63] Decreased cGMP levels in tolerant animals may also result from decreased guanylyl cyclase activity in tolerant smooth muscle cells. Thus, enzyme prepared from nitroglycerin-tolerant vessels is less responsive to the effect of certain nitrovasodilators than that prepared from control vessels.[60,103] However, desensitization of guanylyl cyclase in cell-free preparations in vitro may not accurately reflect the situation within intact cells.

If tolerance is due to increased cGMP–phosphodiesterase activity, enhanced production of superoxide anion, or decreased activity of guanylyl cyclase, one would expect nitrate-tolerant vessels to have impaired relaxation in response to all substances that elicit relaxation through NO-induced activation of guanylyl cyclase, including nitroprusside, SIN-1, and endothelial NO. Some studies do indeed show a small decrease of sensitivity to the direct-acting activators of guanylyl cyclase.[33,51,58,80] But the changes in relaxation response to SIN-1, endothelium-derived nitric oxide, or inorganic nitrovasodilators in these studies are much less pronounced than those seen with organic nitrovasodilators. Increased

cGMP–phosphodiesterase activity, enhanced production of superoxide anion, and decreased activity of guanylyl cyclase may thus occur, but their contribution to nitrate tolerance is modest compared with that of a major desensitization mechanism that more specifically involves the organic nitrates.

Many studies report development of tolerance to, and cross-tolerance between, organic nitrates without concomitant desensitization to nitroprusside, nitrosothiols, SIN-1, or endothelium-derived nitric oxide.[5,47,48,61,84, 85,87,92,97] This rather specific desensitization mechanism for organic nitrates is thought to be due to diminished metabolism of these drugs by smooth muscle cells. Basic observations leading to this theory were published by Needleman,[67] who introduced the organic nitrate receptor theory. He found a diminished concentration of thiol groups in tolerant vessels. This has led to the concept that when organic nitrate enters the cell, it reacts with a thiol group, most probably from cysteine, resulting in denitration of the organic nitrate and oxidation of the thiols to disulfides. Because the availability of thiol groups in vascular smooth muscle cells is limited, prolonged exposure to nitrate leads to exhaustion of the thiol pool, and lack of intracellular metabolism of the nitrate leads to tolerance. This hypothesis is strengthened by observations that destruction of thiol groups with alkylating agents reduces the efficacy of nitroglycerin and that tolerance can be reversed by treatment with the disulfide-reducing agent dithiothreitol.[2,67] The observation that hydralazine attenuates tolerance may be due to inhibition of catabolism of methionine and cysteine, enhancing the availability of thiol groups.[3,93] The hypothesis that nitrate tolerance arises from impaired metabolism of the drug is also supported by the diminished production of nitrate metabolites in nitrate-tolerant vessels.[12,14,30,82,83] That nitrate tolerance in vivo is associated with diminished metabolism of nitrate to NO is supported by the reduction of exhaled NO in tolerant animals. Measurement of exhaled NO may even be useful as a marker for organic nitrate tolerance.[35]

An implication of this organic nitrate receptor theory is that tolerance develops toward all substances that require this "nitrate receptor" for metabolism to active product. This can explain the well-established cross-tolerance observed between organic nitrates.[1,68,74,96]

A characteristic of tolerance to nitrates is its very fast disappearance after cessation of nitrate administration. Reversal of tolerance has been found in animal experiments after a nitrate-free interval of less than 1 hour.[74] This reversal could result from regeneration of thiol groups in the vascular smooth muscle cell by cell metabolism.

Although the mechanisms of tolerance presented earlier have gained wide acceptance, they do not explain all experimental findings. The matter is obviously more complicated. Nitrate tolerance in vivo was reported not to be associated with depletion of arterial or venous thiol levels.[7] Incubation of tolerant bovine coronary arteries with cysteine or glutathione in vitro does not significantly reverse tolerance to nitroglycerin-induced cGMP accumulation or relaxation, despite substantial rise in tissue concentration of thiol compounds.[32] It may be that nitrate tolerance is associated with, but not caused by, thiol depletion.[46]

Other mechanisms probably involved in attenuation of the effects of nitrates are *counterregulatory neurohormonal adaptations*. The organism possesses complex regulatory mechanisms that may adapt and counterregulate the long-term effects of nitrovasodilators. The best evidence for the existence of counterregulatory mechanisms is the increase of anginal attacks sometimes observed after withdrawal of nitrates (see section titled "Nitrate Withdrawal Phenomenon").

Factors that could explain counterregulation are orthosympathetic stimulation and activation of the renin–angiotensin–aldosterone system. Activation of this system increases vascular volume, characterized by hemodilution and weight gain. Several data indicate that nitrate therapy is indeed associated with activation of the renin–angiotensin–aldosterone system.[23,59,70,72,76] Activation of the system increases the venous capacity and may be responsible for the attenuation of the effect of nitrates. The beneficial action of nitrates relies at least in part on an increase in venous capacity, which cannot develop as effectively when venous capacity is already substantially increased.

Another mechanism that may explain counterregulation is a diminished influence of the protective, endogenously released NO from the vascular endothelium after prolonged exposure of the vessel to exogenous NO derived from nitrate. A study performed on rat vessels provides evidence that this hypothesis is probably not correct.[98]

Attenuation of Effects of Nitrates in Humans

Attenuation of the effects of nitrates in clinical use is now well established. This is true for different types of molecules (with cross-tolerance) and different routes of administration. Attenuation has been observed in patients with angina pectoris and with congestive heart failure.[24,39,56,71] Despite early recognition of the problem of tolerance, patients continue to receive nitrates uninterrupted, and many physicians doubt that tolerance is clinically relevant. It is clear that tolerance does not necessarily lead to a complete disappearance of the nitrate effect but only to its attenuation. Also, many dosage schemes are accompanied by periods of low nitrate levels that allow for disappearance of the tolerance phenomenon (see "Nitrate-Free Intervals"). Attenuation of nitrate effects has become prominent with the introduction of

preparations that lead to sustained and uninterrupted nitrate levels in the organism. There is no longer any doubt about the clinical relevance of nitrate tolerance.[10,24,28,39,56,77]

It can be questioned whether vascular tolerance (i.e., smooth muscle cell desensitization) has a role in the attenuation of the effects of nitrates seen in patients. Indeed, in both in vitro and animal studies, very high, clinically irrelevant doses are often used. In one study, however, isolated mammary arteries from patients treated therapeutically with nitroglycerin were found to be much less sensitive to the nitrate.[21]

Strategies to Avoid Attenuation of the Effects of Nitrates

Based on the proposed mechanisms involved in nitrate tolerance, several strategies have been designed to prevent or reverse attenuation of the effects of nitrates.[15,24,28,56]

Administration of a Thiol Group Donor

The critical importance of thiol groups in the development of tolerance suggests that tolerance may be prevented or reversed by enhancing thiol group availability. The precursor of cysteine, *N*-acetylcysteine, has often been used for this purpose. Nitrate drugs that contain a cysteine moiety are being developed.[105] Although *N*-acetylcysteine has been successfully applied in some animal experiments and in some clinical settings, most studies have yielded disappointing results.[8,34,57,62,71,78,91,102] Enhanced responsiveness after *N*-acetylcysteine administration could be rather nonspecific, independent of tolerance, and the consequence of *S*-nitrosocysteine formed extracellularly.[29] *N*-acetylcysteine may also alter counterregulation by inhibiting angiotensin-converting enzyme (ACE) activity.[6]

Nitrate-Free Intervals

Another strategy based on the exhaustion of thiol groups is programming a nitrate-free period into the treatment schedule.[15,56] It is established that tolerance to nitrates rapidly disappears when contact with the nitrate is stopped. This is explained by the rapid regeneration of thiol groups in vascular smooth muscle cells by cell metabolism and by the disappearance of counterregulatory responses. Therefore, development of tolerance can be prevented by introduction of a nitrate-free period into the regimen. The aim is to reach low nitrate plasma levels for, for example, 6 to 8 hours by removing the nitroglycerin patch during the night or by not giving the night dose of an oral nitrate. Actually, nitrate-free periods often occur spontaneously because of the preparations used and the poor compliance of patients prescribed oral formulations of nitrates. This may explain why the problem of tolerance has long been underestimated. Poor compliance is not surprising in view of the headache often associated with nitrate treatment.

Nitrate-free periods need to be programmed in harmony with the patient's complaints. A patient who tends to have anginal attacks in the early morning is not advised to have a nitrate-free interval during the night. On the other hand, a nitrate-free interval must be avoided during the daytime in patients who have problems induced by exercise.

A disadvantage of including a nitrate-free interval is that patients are not protected during the nitrate-free period. Therefore, patients need to be protected with another antianginal drug such as a β-blocker or a calcium antagonist. This approach is certainly indicated because some studies have reported a rebound phenomenon, consisting of anginal attacks during the nitrate-free period. This *zero hour effect* has been reported even in patients who did not have anginal attacks before start of treatment.[17,26]

Administration of ACE Inhibitors and Diuretics

Because attenuation of the effects of nitrates may be due to activation of the renin–angiotensin–aldosterone system or other counterregulatory processes, some studies have been performed to investigate whether ACE inhibitors can prevent nitrate tolerance.[41,53,99] It was found that captopril inhibits development of tolerance in an isolated vessel. This beneficial effect is probably related to the presence of a thiol group in the captopril molecule, because an ACE inhibitor that lacked a thiol group was not effective.[53] In clinical settings, ACE inhibitors with or without a thiol group prevented attenuation of the effects of nitrates.[41,99] This can be explained if ACE inhibitors diminish fluid retention and preserve the venodilative effect of nitrates. Not all studies show a beneficial effect of ACE inhibitors.[16,22,76] More detailed studies are required to determine whether ACE inhibitors have a beneficial influence on the development of nitrate tolerance.

Because diminished fluid retention may be beneficial, studies were performed to investigate the influence of a decrease in intravascular volume produced by diuretics. They yielded mixed results.[75,88,101] More study is needed before useful conclusions can be drawn.

Administration of Thiol-Independent NO Donors

Because vascular tolerance is believed to be mainly due to a diminished metabolism to NO, NO donors that do not require metabolism by means of thiol groups may have the same beneficial effects as nitrates without inducing tolerance. Molsidomine is such a thiol-independent NO donor. It is metabolized in liver to SIN-1, which reaches the circulation and then spontaneously releases

NO. At least in vitro, such drugs seem to produce less tolerance and cross-tolerance.[37,96] Whether clinical development of tolerance is avoided remains to be established.[38,44,94] It should be mentioned here that NO inhalation for the treatment of pulmonary hypertension in humans remains effective for up to 53 days, indicating that NO as such does not induce tolerance in pulmonary vessels.[81]

Nitrate Withdrawal Phenomenon

When intermittent nitrate therapy is used, the strong influence of counterregulatory mechanisms after withdrawal of nitrates can result in an overshoot of compensation, or *rebound*, and lead to undesirable effects (e.g., anginal attacks). The rebound phenomenon has been recognized for a long time. Anginal attacks and sudden death after removal from a nitrate-rich environment were described in the nineteenth century in workmen in the explosives industry. For many years the nitrate withdrawal phenomenon in therapeutics received limited attention. The introduction of nitrate patches with sudden nitrate-free periods clearly revealed the risk of a rebound effect. The risk of rebound during nitrate withdrawal can be lessened by avoiding an abrupt decline in blood nitrate concentration or by concomitant administration of additional antianginal drugs.[25]

Concluding Remarks

Nitrates are useful drugs, notwithstanding the attenuation of their effect with time. This attenuation is a complex multifactorial process that involves cellular and systemic mechanisms. The complexity is further illustrated by the differences between arterial and venous circulation. Susceptibility to development of nitrate tolerance in humans is higher in the venous than in the arterial circulation.[31] Nitrate tolerance may also depend on the individual clinical condition of the patient. The most widely accepted mechanism of nitrate tolerance is depletion of thiol groups in vascular smooth muscle cells; thiol groups are necessary to metabolize organic nitrates to the active component, NO. Strategies used to prevent attenuation (such as administration of *N*-acetylcysteine, allowing a nitrate-free period, or the use of drugs that do not require thiol groups for their effect) are all based on this basic mechanism. Besides depletion of thiol groups, neurohumoral counterregulation (e.g., by the renin–angiotensin–aldosterone system) may also contribute to attenuation of the effect of nitrates. Concomitant use of diuretics or ACE inhibitors with nitrates may therefore be useful. However, no adjuvant pharmacological intervention has been conclusively demonstrated to have a beneficial influence on nitrate tolerance.

References

1. Ahlner J, Andersson RGG, Torfgard K, Axelsson KL. Organic nitrate esters: clinical use and mechanisms of actions. *Pharmacol Rev.* 1991;43:351–423.

2. Axelsson KL, Andersson RGG, Wikberg JES. Vascular smooth muscle relaxation by nitro compounds: reduced relaxation and cGMP elevation in tolerant vessels and reversal of tolerance by dithiothreitol. *Acta Pharmacol Toxicol.* 1982;50:350–357.

3. Bauer JA, Fung HL. Concurrent hydralazine administration prevents nitroglycerin-induced hemodynamic tolerance in experimental heart failure. *Circulation.* 1991;84:35–39.

4. Bennett BM, McDonald BJ, Nigam R, Simon WC. Biotransformation of organic nitrates and vascular smooth muscle cell function. *Trends Pharmacol Sci.* 1994;15:245–249.

5. Berkenboom G, Fontaine J, Degré S. Persistence of the response to SIN-1 on isolated coronary arteries rendered tolerant to nitroglycerin in vitro or in vivo. *J Cardiovasc Pharmacol.* 1988;12:345–349.

6. Boesgaard S, Aldershvile J, Poulsen HE, Christensen S, Dige-Petersen H, Giese J. *N*-acetylcysteine inhibits angiotensin converting enzyme in vivo. *J Pharmacol Exp Ther.* 1993;265:1239–1244.

7. Boesgaard S, Aldershvile J, Poulsen HE, Loft S, Anderson ME, Meister A. Nitrate tolerance in vivo is not associated with depletion of arterial or venous thiol levels. *Circ Res.* 1994;74:115–120.

8. Boesgaard S, Iversen HK, Wroblewski H, et al. Altered peripheral vasodilator profile of nitroglycerin during long-term infusion of *N*-acetylcysteine. *J Am Coll Cardiol.* 1994;23:163–169.

9. Bogaert MG. Tolerance towards glyceryltrinitrate (trinitrin) in rabbits. *Arch Int Pharmacodyn Ther.* 1968;172:228–230.

10. Bogaert M. Clinical relevance of tolerance to nitrovasodilators. *J Cardiovasc Pharmacol.* 1991;17(suppl 3):S309–S313.

11. Bogaert MG. Clinical pharmacokinetics of nitrates. *Cardiovasc Drugs Ther.* 1994;8:693–699.

12. Brien JF, McLaughlin BE, Breedon TH, Bennet BM, Nakatsu K, Marks GS. Biotransformation of glyceryl trinitrate occurs concurrently with relaxation of rabbit aorta. *J Pharmacol Exp Ther.* 1986;237:608–614.

13. Brunton TL. On the use of nitrite of amyl in angina pectoris. *Lancet.* 1867;2:97–98.

14. Chung SJ, Fung HL. Relationship between nitroglycerin-induced vascular relaxation and nitric oxide production. Probes with inhibitors and tolerance development. *Biochem Pharmacol.* 1993;45:157–163.

15. Cowan JC. Avoiding nitrate tolerance. *Br J Clin Pharmacol.* 1992;34:96–101.

16. Dakak N, Makhoul N, Frugelman MY, et al. Failure of captopril to prevent nitrate tolerance in congestive heart failure secondary to coronary heart disease. *Am J Cardiol.* 1990;66:608–613.

17. DeMots H, Glasser SP. Intermittent transdermal nitroglycerin therapy in the treatment of chronic stable angina. *J Am Coll Cardiol.* 1989;13:786–795.

18. De Muynck C, Remon JP, Colardyn F. The sorption of isosorbide dinitrate to intravenous delivery systems. *J Pharm Pharmacol.* 1988;40:601–604.

19. De Rudder D, Remon JP, Neyt E. The sorption of nitroglycerin by infusion sets. *J Pharm Pharmacol.* 1987;39:556–558.

20. Diodati J, Theroux P, Latour JG, Lacoste L, Lam JY, Waters D. Effects of nitroglycerin at therapeutic doses on platelet aggregation in unstable angina and acute myocardial infarction. *Am J Cardiol.* 1990;66:683–688.

21. Du ZY, Buxton BF, Woodman OL. Tolerance to glyceryl trinitrate in isolated human internal mammary arteries. *J Thorac Cardiovasc Surg.* 1992;104:1280–1284.

22. Dupuis J, Lalonde G, Bichet D, Rouleau JL. Captopril does not prevent nitroglycerin tolerance in heart failure. *Can J Cardiol.* 1990;6:281–286.

23. Dupuis J, Lalonde G, Lemieux R, Rouleau JL. Tolerance to intravenous nitroglycerin in patients with congestive heart failure: role of increased intravascular volume, neurohumoral activation, and lack of prevention with *N*-acetylcysteine. *J Am Coll Cardiol.* 1990;16:923–931.

24. Elkayam U. Tolerance to organic nitrates: evidence, mechanisms, clinical relevance, and strategies for prevention. *Ann Intern Med.* 1991;114:667–677.

25. Ferratini M. Risk of rebound phenomenon during nitrate withdrawal. *Int J Cardiol.* 1994;45:89–96.

26. Ferratini M, Pirelli S, Merlini P, Silva I, Pollavini G. Intermittent transdermal nitroglycerin monotherapy in stable exercise-induced angina: a comparison with a continuous schedule. *Eur Heart J.* 1989;10:998–1002.

27. Fung H-L. Pharmacokinetics and pharmacodynamics of organic nitrates. *Am J Cardiol.* 1987;60(suppl):4H–9H.

28. Fung H-L, Bauer JA. Mechanisms of nitrate tolerance. *Cardiovasc Drugs Ther.* 1994;8:489–499.

29. Fung H-L, Chong S, Kowaluk E, Hough K, Kakemi M. Mechanisms for the pharmacologic interaction of organic nitrates with thiols. Existence of an extracellular pathway for the reversal of nitrate vascular tolerance by *N*-acetylcysteine. *J Pharmacol Exp Ther.* 1988;245:524–530.

30. Fung H-L, Poliszczuk R. Nitrosothiol and nitrate tolerance. *Z Kardiol.* 1986;75(suppl 3):25–27.

31. Ghio S, Deservi S, Perotti R, Eleuteri E, Montemartini C, Specchia G. Different susceptibility to the development of nitroglycerin tolerance in the arterial and venous circulation in humans: effects of *N*-acetylcysteine administration. *Circulation.* 1992;86:798–802.

32. Gruetter C, Lemke SM. Dissociation of cysteine and glutathione levels from nitroglycerin-induced relaxation. *Eur J Pharmacol.* 1985;111:85–95.

33. Henry PJ, Horowitz JD, Louis WJ. Nitroglycerin-induced tolerance affects multiple sites in the organic nitrate bioconversion cascade. *J Pharmacol Exp Ther.* 1989;248:762–768.

34. Hogan JC, Lewis MJ, Henderson AH. *N*-acetylcysteine fails to attenuate haemodynamic tolerance to glyceryl trinitrate in healthy volunteers. *Br J Clin Pharmacol.* 1989;28:421–426.

35. Husain M, Adrie C, Ichinose F, Kavosi M, Zapol WM. Exhaled nitric oxide as a marker for organic nitrate tolerance. *Circulation.* 1994;89:2498–2502.

36. Ignarro LJ, Lippton H, Edwards JC, et al. Mechanism of vascular smooth muscle relaxation by organic nitrates, nitrites, nitroprusside, and nitric oxide: evidence for the involvement of S-nitrosothiols as active intermediates. *J Pharmacol Exp Ther.* 1981;218:739–749.

37. Isono T, Sato N, Yamamoto T, et al. Tolerance to the vascular effect of a novel nitric oxide-donating vasodilator, FK409. *Eur J Pharmacol.* 1994;260:163–168.

38. Jansen W, Eggeling T, Meyer L, Tauchert M, Hilger HH. Acute and chronic effects of molsidomine on pulmonary artery pressure and work capacity in patients with coronary heart disease. *Eur Heart J.* 1987;8:870–877.

39. Jordan RA, Seth L, Casebolt P, Haynes MJ, Wilen MM, Franciosa J. Rapidly developing tolerance to transdermal nitroglycerin in congestive heart failure. *Ann Intern Med.* 1986;104:295–298.

40. Karashima T. Actions of nitroglycerine on smooth muscles of the guinea-pig and rat portal veins. *Br J Pharmacol.* 1980;71:489–497.

41. Katz RJ, Levy WS, Buff L, Wasserman AG. Prevention of nitrate tolerance with angiotensin converting enzyme inhibitors. *Circulation.* 1991;83:1271–1277.

42. Keith RA, Burkman AM, Sokoloski TD, Fertel RH. Vascular tolerance to nitroglycerin and cyclic GMP generation in rat aortic smooth muscle cells. *J Pharmacol Exp Ther.* 1982;221:525–531.

43. Keith RA, Burkman AM, Sokoloski TD, Fertel RH. Nitroglycerin tolerance and cyclic GMP generation in the longitudinal smooth muscle of the guinea-pig ileum. *J Pharmacol Exp Ther.* 1983;225:29–34.

44. Kinoshita M, Sawamura M, Motomura M, Takayama Y, Kawaguchi Y, Kawakita S. Long-term effects of molsidomine on exercise tolerance in patients with exertional angina pectoris. *Jpn Circ J.* 1983;47:1398–1405.

45. Kinsella JP, Neish SR, Shaffer E, Abman SH. Low-dose inhalational nitric oxide in persistent pulmonary hypertension of the newborn. *Lancet.* 1992;340:819–820.

46. Kojda G, Meyer W, Noack E. Influence of endothelium and nitrovasodilators on free thiols and disulfides in porcine coronary smooth muscle. *Eur J Pharmacol.* 1993;250:385–394.

47. Kowaluk EA, Fung H-L. Dissociation of nitrovasodilator-induced relaxation from cyclic GMP levels during in vitro nitrate tolerance. *Eur J Pharmacol.* 1990;176:91–95.

48. Kühn M, Förstermann U. Endothelium-dependent vasodilatation in human epicardial coronary arteries: effect of prolonged exposure to glyceryl trinitrate or SIN-1. *J Cardiovasc Pharmacol.* 1989;14(suppl 11):S47–S54.

49. Kukovetz WR, Holzmann S. Cyclic GMP as the mediator of molsidomine-induced vasodilatation. *Eur J Pharmacol.* 1986;122:103–109.

50. Kukovetz WR, Holzmann S. Mode of action of nitrates with regard to vasodilatation and tolerance. *Z Kardiol.* 1986;75(suppl 3):8–11.

51. Kukovetz WR, Holzmann S. Tolerance and cross-tolerance between SIN-1 and nitric oxide in bovine coronary arteries. *J Cardiovasc Pharmacol.* 1989;14(suppl 11):S40–S46.

52. Lam JYT, Chesebro JH. Platelets, vasoconstriction, and nitroglycerin during arterial wall injury. *Circulation.* 1988;78:712–716.

53. Lawson DL, Nichols WW, Mehta P, Mehta JL. Captopril-induced reversal of nitroglycerin tolerance: role of sulfhydryl group vs. ACE-inhibitory activity. *J Cardiovasc Pharmacol.* 1991;17:411–418.

54. Levin RI, Jaffe EA, Weksler BB, Tack-Goldman K. Nitroglycerin stimulates synthesis of prostacyclin by cultured human endothelial cells. *J Clin Invest.* 1981;67:762–769.

55. Loscalzo J. Antiplatelet and antithrombotic effects of organic nitrates. *Am J Cardiol.* 1992;70(suppl):18B–22B.

56. Mangione NJ, Glasser SP. Phenomenon of nitrate tolerance. *Am Heart J.* 1994;128:137–146.

57. May DC, Popma JJ, Black WH, et al. In vivo induction and reversal of nitroglycerin tolerance in human coronary arteries. *N Engl J Med.* 1987;317:805–809.

58. Molina CR, Andresen JW, Rapoport RM, Waldman S, Murad F. Effect of in vivo nitroglycerin therapy on endothelium-dependent and independent vascular relaxation and cyclic GMP accumulation in rat aorta. *J Cardiovasc Pharmacol.* 1987;10:371–378.

59. Muiesan ML, Agabiti-Rosei E, Romanelli G, et al. Transdermal nitroglycerin efficacy in patients with chronic stable angina pectoris as related to sympathetic and renin-angiotensin-aldosterone activity. *Eur Heart J.* 1992;13:15–21.

60. Mülsch A, Busse R, Bassenge E. Clinical tolerance to nitroglycerin is due to impaired biotransformation of nitroglycerin and biological counterregulation, not to desensitization of guanylate cyclase. *Z Kardiol.* 1989;78(suppl 2):22–25.

61. Mülsch A, Busse R, Winter I, Bassenge E. Endothelium- and sydnonimine-induced responses of native and cultured aortic smooth muscle cells are not impaired by nitroglycerin tolerance. *Naunyn Schmiedebergs Arch Pharmacol.* 1989;339:568–574.

62. Münzel T, Holtz J, Mülsch A, Stewart DJ, Bassenge E. Nitrate tolerance in epicardial arteries or in the venous system is not reversed by N-acetylcysteine in vivo but tolerance-independent interactions exist. *Circulation.* 1989;79:188–197.

63. Münzel T, Sayegh H, Freeman BA, Tarpey MM, Harrison DG. Evidence for enhanced vascular superoxide anion production in nitrate tolerance. A novel mechanism underlying tolerance and cross-tolerance. *J Clin Invest.* 1995;95:187–194.

64. Murrel W. Nitro-glycerine as a remedy for angina pectoris. *Lancet.* 1879;1:80–81, 113–115, 151–152, 225–227.

65. Nakatsu K, Diamond J. Role of cGMP in relaxation of vascular and other smooth muscle. *Can J Physiol Pharmacol.* 1989;67:251–262.

66. Needleman P. Tolerance to the vascular effects of glyceryl trinitrate. *J Pharmacol Exp Ther.* 1970;171:98–102.

67. Needleman P, Jakschik B, Johnson EM. Sulfhydryl requirement for relaxation of vascular smooth muscle. *J Pharmacol Exp Ther.* 1983;187:324–331.

68. Needleman P, Johnson EM. Mechanism of tolerance development to organic nitrates. *J Pharmacol Exp Ther.* 1973;184:709–715.

69. Noack E, Feelisch M. Molecular aspects underlying the vasodilator action of molsidomine. *J Cardiovasc Pharmacol.* 1989;14(suppl 11):S1–S5.

70. Olivari M, Carlyle P, Levine BS, Cohn J. Hemodynamic and hormonal response to transdermal nitroglycerin in normal subjects and in patients with congestive heart failure. *J Am Coll Cardiol.* 1983;2:872–888.

71. Packer M, Lee WH, Kessler PD, Gottlieb SS, Medina N, Yushak M. Prevention and reversal of nitrate tolerance in patients with congestive heart failure. *N Engl J Med.* 1987;317:799–804.

72. Packer M, Meller J, Medina N, Yushak M, Gorlin R. Determinants of drug responses in severe chronic heart failure. Activation of vasoconstrictor forces during vasodilatory therapy. *Circulation.* 1981;64:506–514.

73. Pagani ED, VanAller GS, O'Connor B, Silver PJ. Reversal of nitroglycerin tolerance in vitro by the cGMP-phosphodiesterase inhibitor zaprinast. *Eur J Pharmacol.* 1993;243: 141–147.

74. Parker JC, Di Carlo FJ, Davidson IWF. Comparative vasodilator effects of nitroglycerin, pentaerythritol trinitrate and biometabolites, and other organic nitrates. *Eur J Pharmacol.* 1975;31:29–37.

75. Parker JD, Farrell B, Fenton T, Parker JO. Effects of diuretic therapy on the development of tolerance during continuous therapy with nitroglycerin. *J Am Coll Cardiol.* 1992;20:616–622.

76. Parker JD, Parker JO. Effect of therapy with an angiotensin-converting enzyme inhibitor on hemodynamic and counterregulatory responses during continuous therapy with nitroglycerin. *J Am Coll Cardiol.* 1993;21: 1445–1453.

77. Parker JO. Update on nitrate tolerance. *Br J Clin Pharmacol.* 1992;34(suppl 1):11S–14S.

78. Parker JO, Farrell B, Lahey KA, Rose BF. Nitrate tolerance: lack of effect of *N*-acetylcysteine. *Circulation.* 1987;76: 572–576.

79. Pepke-Zaba J, Higenbottam TW, Dinh-Xuan AT, Stone D, Wallwork J. Inhaled nitric oxide as a cause of selective pulmonary vasodilatation in pulmonary hypertension. *Lancet.* 1991;338:1173–1174.

80. Rapoport RM, Waldman SA, Ginsburg R, Molina CR, Murad F. Effects of glyceryl trinitrate on endothelium-dependent and -independent relaxation and cyclic GMP levels in rat aorta and human coronary artery. *J Cardiovasc Pharmacol.* 1987;10:82–89.

81. Rossaint R, Falke KJ, Lopez F, Slama K, Pison U, Zapol WM. Inhaled nitric oxide for the adult respiratory distress syndrome. *N Engl J Med.* 1993;328:399–405.

82. Salvemini D, Pistelli A, Vane J. Conversion of glyceryl trinitrate to nitric oxide in tolerant and non-tolerant smooth muscle and endothelial cells. *Br J Pharmacol.* 1993;108: 162–169.

83. Slack CJ, McLaughlin BE, Brien JF, Marks GS, Nakatsu K. Biotransformation of glyceryl trinitrate and isosorbide dinitrate in vascular smooth muscle made tolerant to organic nitrates. *Can J Physiol Pharmacol.* 1989;67:1381–1385.

84. Slack CJ, McLaughlin BE, Nakatsu K, Marks GS, Brien JF. Nitric oxide-induced vasodilation of organic nitrate-tolerant rabbit aorta. *Can J Physiol Pharmacol.* 1988;66: 1344–1346.

85. Smith MP, Humphrey SJ, Kerr SW, Mathews WR. In vitro vasorelaxant and in vivo cardiovascular effects of S-nitrosothiols: comparison to and cross tolerance with standard nitrovasodilators. *Methods Find Exp Clin Pharmacol.* 1994;16:323–335.

86. Stewart DD. Remarkable tolerance to nitroglycerin. *Polyclinic.* 1888;6:171–172.

87. Stewart DJ, Holtz J, Bassenge E. Long-term nitroglycerin treatment: effect on direct and endothelium-mediated large coronary artery dilation in conscious dogs. *Circulation.* 1987;75:847–856.

88. Sussex BA, Campbell NR, Raju MK. Nitrate tolerance is modified by diuretic treatment [abstract]. *Circulation.* 1990;82(suppl 2):200.

89. Swartz AM. The cause, relief, and prevention of headache arising from contact with dynamite. *N Engl J Med.* 1946; 235:241–244.

90. Torfgard KE, Ahlner J. Effect of low dose of dipyridamole on glyceryl trinitrate tolerance in healthy volunteers. *J Cardiovasc Pharmacol.* 1993;21:516–521.

91. Torresi J, Horowitz JD, Dusting GJ. Prevention and reversal of tolerance to nitroglycerin with *N*-acetylcysteine. *J Cardiovasc Pharmacol.* 1985;7:777–783.

92. Unger P, Berkenboom G, Brekine D, Fontaine J. Nitrate tolerance and aging in isolated rat aorta. *Eur J Pharmacol.* 1993;248:145–149.

93. Unger P, Berkenboom G, Fontaine J. Interaction between hydralazine and nitrovasodilators in vascular smooth muscle. *J Cardiovasc Pharmacol.* 1993;21:478–483.

94. Unger P, Vachiery JL, de Canniere D, Staroukine M, Berkenboom G. Comparison of the hemodynamic responses to molsidomine and isosorbide dinitrate in congestive heart failure. *Am Heart J.* 1994;128:557–563.

95. Van de Voorde J. Mechanisms involved in the development of tolerance to nitrovasodilators. *J Cardiovasc Pharmacol.* 1991;17(suppl 3):S304–S307.

96. Van de Voorde J, Claeys M, Leusen I. Relaxations to endothelium-derived relaxing factor and the metabolite of molsidomine, SIN-1, in the aorta and the hindquarters of the rat. *J Cardiovasc Pharmacol.* 1989;14(suppl 11): S55–S61.

97. Van de Voorde J, Vanheel B, Leusen I. Influence of vascular tolerance to nitroglycerin on endothelium-dependent relaxation. *Arch Int Pharmacodyn Ther.* 1987;290:215–221.

98. Van de Voorde J, Vyt S, Vanheel B. The basal endothelial inhibitory influence on vascular tone is not affected in nitroglycerin-tolerant rat aorta. *Can J Physiol Pharmacol.* 1994; 72:1094–1097.

99. Van Gilst WH, de Graeff PA, Scholtens E. Potentiation of isosorbide dinitrate-induced coronary dilatation by captopril. *J Cardiovasc Pharmacol.* 1987;9:254–255.

100. Vanheel B, Van de Voorde J, Leusen I. Contribution of nitric oxide to the endothelium-dependent hyperpolarization in rat aorta. *J Physiol (Lond).* 1994;475:277–284.

101. Varriale P, David WJ, Chryssos BE. Hemodynamic resistance to intravenous nitroglycerin in severe congestive heart failure and restored response after diuresis. *Am J Cardiol.* 1991;68:1400–1402.

102. Vincent J, Kongpatanakul S, Blaschke TF, Hoffman BB. Desensitization of nitrate-induced venodilation-reversal with oral *N*-acetylcysteine in humans. *J Cardiovasc Pharmacol.* 1992;20:907–912.

103. Waldman SA, Rapoport RM, Ginsburg R, Murad F. Desensitization to nitroglycerin in vascular smooth muscle from rat and human. *Biochem Pharmacol.* 1986;35:3525–3531.

104. Watanabe H, Kakihana M, Ohtsuka S, Enomoto T, Yasui K, Sugishita Y. Platelet cyclic GMP: a potentially useful indicator to evaluate the effects of nitroglycerin and nitrate tolerance. *Circulation.* 1993;88:29–36.

105. Zanzinger J, Feelisch M, Bassenge E. Novel organic nitrates are potent dilators of large coronary arteries with reduced development of tolerance during long-term infusion in dogs: role of sulfhydryl moiety. *J Cardiovasc Pharmacol.* 1994;23:772–778.

10

Coronary Microcirculation

M. G. Trivella and G. Pelosi

Microcirculation and the Concept of Coronary Reserve in Coronary Pathophysiology

Although the term *coronary microcirculation* includes all the vessels from small arteries to small veins, it is currently used to define the precapillary vasculature, because common knowledge of coronary physiology localizes the main site of flow regulation at the precapillary level, and there is difficulty in identifying possible dysfunction of capillary or postcapillary vessels in humans.[71]

Coronary flow varies under different conditions, being strictly linked to cardiac metabolic demand. The change in coronary flow from the resting state to maximal vasodilation is defined as *coronary reserve*, which is generally expressed as the ratio of maximal to baseline coronary blood flow. The limit at which maximal coronary flow is attained is not known; in experimental research, physiologic stimuli such as ischemia induce less vasodilation than obtained by pharmacological vasodilators, and the extent of pharmacological vasodilation is affected by the agent employed and the specific experimental setting.[31,65,70]

Major determinants of coronary blood flow are aortic pressure, myocardial extravascular compression, myocardial metabolism, and neural control.[20] The complex interrelations among these variables play a fundamental role in the physiology and pathophysiology of the coronary microcirculation.[8,44]

Coronary Resistance and Coronary Reserve in Experimental Models

Coronary resistance can be considered as the sum of three components: vascular anatomy, vascular tone, and extravascular compression. The anatomical component is the result of the architecture of the coronary vasculature; that is, the diameters and lengths of all vascular segments, branching angles, and total number of vessels at each branching level. This component can be measured only when functional tone is absent, under maximal vasodilation of the coronary circulation. The functional component is due to the vasomotor tone of the resistance vessels, which keeps their diameter smaller than their anatomical size. Vasomotor tone can vary in different physiologic and pathologic conditions, thereby accounting for coronary autoregulation of flow within a wide range (60–140 mm Hg) of perfusion pressures. The extravascular component is due to myocardial compression of the resistance vessels (*intramyocardial pressure*). This compression varies during the cardiac cycle—being greater during systole—and is influenced by intracavitary pressure. This component can be assessed only during maximal coronary vasodilation.[20,28]

The most appropriate method to measure total coronary resistance and its three components is based on the pressure–flow relation. This relation can be derived by different approaches. Pressure–flow curves can be obtained under steady state, when different levels of pressure and flow are maintained for a period sufficient to stabilize systemic and coronary hemodynamics. Diastolic pressure–flow curves are obtained by the spontaneous decrease of perfusion pressure and coronary flow during long diastoles, being affected by coronary capacitance and changes in metabolic autoregulation. Instantaneous pressure–flow relations are obtained by sudden changes of pressure or flow within the time interval (1–7 seconds) when capacitance effects are minimal and autoregulatory tone is not yet modified, and they are more representative of baseline coronary resistance.[28,30]

Resistance of the coronary tree, in contrast to other vascular districts, is given by the ratio of the pressure drop between input artery and intramyocardial pressure to the coronary flow, because intramyocardial pressure is higher than venous pressure (the waterfall theory).[15,32]

Thus, coronary flow stops when perfusion pressure is positive, with a value ranging from 10 to 20 mm Hg under maximal vasodilation to 45 mm Hg during autoregulation, when zero flow pressure is the effect of both extravascular pressure and vascular tone.[15]

When metabolic requirements do not vary, the heart maintains a constant blood flow, despite wide changes in arterial pressure. This phenomenon is called *autoregulation*. To evaluate the autoregulatory state it is necessary to keep metabolic needs constant. In experimental models, by cannulating and perfusing a coronary artery, it is possible to change coronary perfusion pressure without any change in aortic pressure and in left ventricular work and to obtain a pressure–flow relation of the autoregulating coronary circulation at constant myocardial oxygen consumption. In this experimental preparation with intact tone, the flow is almost unchanged over a wide range of perfusion pressures. The curve has a sigmoid shape with a plateau of steady flow. When myocardial oxygen consumption varies, the autoregulation limits vary accordingly. It is then possible to describe a family of different autoregulation curves, determined by changes in the functional component of coronary resistance. These curves are shifted parallel to the baseline relation, with higher or lower flow values at a given perfusion pressure if myocardial oxygen consumption is increased or decreased, respectively (Figure 10.1). In fact, coronary circulation is regulated by a myogenic component (which accounts for the changes in vascular tone that compensate for changes in pressure and ensure a constant myocardial perfusion) and a metabolic component (which makes it possible to match the increased myocardial metabolic requirements by increasing flow supply). This latter component accounts for the parallel shift of the autoregulation curves at different myocardial workloads. These two components of coronary autoregulation, however, can hardly be separated under physiologic conditions.

When vascular tone is abolished by administration of vasodilators, the pressure–flow relation is the only method to selectively assess the vascular anatomical and the extravascular components of coronary resistance (Figure 10.1). Pressure–flow relation under maximal vasodilation can be obtained, in an in situ, working heart preparation, by perfusing a coronary artery at different flow or pressure levels after reaching the maximal vasodilation of the coronary vascular territory, generally by intracoronary adenosine infusion. The mean values of pressure and flow are commonly used. Such pressure–flow curves display an initial (curvilinear) portion between 10 to 20 mm Hg (which is the zero flow–pressure value) and 40 mm Hg. Above this value the relation is almost linear, and coronary flow is the ratio of pressure difference between perfusion pressure and extravascular pressure to the anatomical resistance of the coronary vascula-

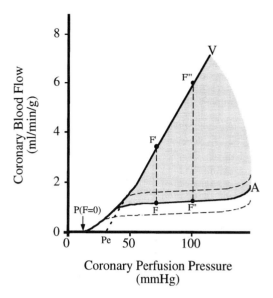

FIGURE 10.1. Pressure–flow relations during autoregulation (curve A) and during maximal vasodilation (curve V) at constant oxygen consumption. The A curve displays similar flow values within a wide range of perfusion pressures; it is shifted upward or downward by higher or lower oxygen consumption, respectively (dashed A curves). The V curve originates from zero flow pressure, $P(F = 0)$; it has a curvilinear initial part (vascular waterfall) and a linear main portion, which intercepts the pressure axis at a value corresponding to the mean extravascular pressure, Pe. Thus, coronary flow F is given by the formula $F = (P - Pe)/Rv$, where P is the coronary perfusion pressure, Pe is the mean extravascular pressure, and Rv is the vascular resistance, which corresponds to the F/P slope of the linear part of the V curve. The dark area between the A and V curves represents the coronary reserve: the simple ratio of resting to maximal flow, which does not take into account the pressure level, can lead to gross errors, as evidenced by the marked difference between the flow ratios F/F' and F''/F''' (dashed lines).

ture. The slope of this linear part of the curve indicates the actual vascular anatomical resistance, whereas the intercept of this line to the pressure axis is the mean extravascular pressure, and the zero flow–pressure value is the minimal extravascular pressure.[28,32]

The pressure–flow relations during maximal vasodilation and during autoregulation enclose an area that represents the reserve of coronary flow (*coronary reserve*), which adapts myocardial perfusion to metabolic requirements under different pathophysiologic conditions. The more common definition of coronary reserve as the ratio of baseline to maximal coronary flow clearly appears inappropriate, because it does not take into account the level of perfusion pressure where coronary reserve is measured. The flow ratio can vary by three to six times for relatively small differences in perfusion pressure level (Figure 10.1). In experimental models, coronary reserve has been assessed after transient ischemic periods by using the peak hyperemic flow values. Hyperemic vasodilation is due to an early myogenic component and release of endogenous vasodilators, especially adenosine.[46,58] Steady-state pressure–flow curves have also been obtained during intracoronary exogenous adenosine infusion. In these conditions, coronary flow, at a perfusion pressure of 70 mm Hg, can increase by seven to eight times above the baseline value, whereas reactive hyperemia elicits only a fourfold increase.[70] Therefore, vasodilation of different magnitudes can be elicited by different stimuli, and the magnitude of coronary reserve may change according to different vasodilators or experimental procedures.

The limit beyond which coronary vascular reserve is completely exhausted is not yet known. Physiologic stimuli, such as ischemia, elicit a lower reserve than that evidenced by pharmacological vasodilation, the magnitude of which is affected both by the agent employed and, possibly, by the experimental design. Knowledge of the upper limit of vasodilation achievable in the coronary vascular system is not of purely physiologic interest. In the absence of coronary atherosclerosis, it is possible that abnormalities in myocardial perfusion, such as described in cardiomyopathies or syndrome X, could be the consequence of reduced maximal vasodilation capacity.

The maximal coronary vasodilation that can be elicited by an intracoronary infusion of adenosine—the most powerful coronary vasodilator available—may also be significantly different in different experimental preparations, as demonstrated by the marked variability in flow values (ranging from 4 to 9 mL/min per gram) obtained at comparable and physiologic levels of perfusion pressure (80–100 mm Hg) that are reported in the literature.[12,13,17,65] Moreover, even in the same experiment, significant changes in adenosine-induced vasodilation can be noted, a biphasic pattern of vasodilation having been observed with a greater (approximately 50%) increase in flow after 20 minutes' infusion.[31] Therefore, differences in experimental preparations and methodological procedures employed in the same experiment may affect the maximal value of coronary reserve.

Regional Coronary Resistance

Under normal hemodynamic conditions, coronary flow is evenly distributed within the left ventricular wall, with a slight predominance in the subendocardial layer. This general uniformity can be modified by several factors. In many experimental studies of the maximally dilated coronary system, the anatomical resistance of the subendocardial vasculature has been the lowest.[32] This can be interpreted as a compensatory mechanism for the greater extravascular compression of the subendocardial

vasculature. The opposite transmural gradients of vascular resistance and extravascular compression help to maintain a uniform myocardial perfusion within the ventricular wall, even in the absence of coronary autoregulation, provided there is a normal range of perfusion pressures. Beyond this anatomical compensation, coronary autoregulation can minimize the effects of extravascular pressure on myocardial perfusion by modifying microvascular pressure through changes in arteriolar diameter.

Complete distension of subendocardial vasculature can be attained in the maximally vasodilated circulation at high-perfusion pressure after blockage of myocardial contractility. In these particular conditions, subendocardial flow becomes two or three times greater than subepicardial flow.[28,33] On the other hand, when significant coronary stenosis is present, the low post-stenotic perfusion pressure is unable to compensate for extravascular compression of the vasodilated subendocardial microcirculation, leading to preferential subendocardial underperfusion.[22,23] A different experimental model of myocardial ischemia, by distal rather than proximal obstruction, is coronary microembolization. In this model, the progressive occlusion of an equal number of arterioles 15 to 25 μm in diameter in the inner and outer layers of the ventricular wall leads to preferential underperfusion of the subepicardium because of the lower arteriolar density of this layer.[53,54]

Regional coronary resistance of left ventricular layers can be assessed by regional steady-state pressure–flow curves using radioactive microspheres for measurement of specific flow per gram of tissue.[75] During vasodilation, a lower subendocardial flow has been observed in the beating heart, in contrast with a higher subendocardial flow in the arrested heart.[28] In particular, in the arrested heart the subendocardial pressure–flow curve indicates lower vascular and extravascular resistances, whereas in the beating heart the slopes have an almost equal value (similar vascular resistance), but the intercept on the subendocardial pressure axis is greater, suggesting a greater extravascular pressure. Such findings seem to exclude the possibility of a uniform transmural myocardial flow within the left ventricular wall at maximal vasodilation. Other studies, however, have demonstrated that the subendocardial pressure–flow relation has a greater pressure-axis intercept but a lower vascular resistance than the subepicardial pressure–flow relation. This finding can be explained by a greater total vascular cross section of the subendocardium, which has a lower anatomical vascular resistance, whereas the extravascular compression is greater than that in the subepicardium.[32]

When autoregulation is absent, coronary flow is dependent not only on perfusion pressure but also on several hemodynamic variables such as heart rate, myocardial contractility, and left ventricular pressure, all of which can modify extravascular pressure and its distribution.

An increase in left ventricular diastolic pressure leads to an increase in subendocardial extravascular pressure and to consequent reduction of flow in this layer. Also, an increase in left ventricular systolic pressure can reduce subendocardial flow.[34] Under physiologic conditions, however, the effects of systolic left ventricular pressure on transmural flow distribution are practically absent because of parallel changes in aortic, and thus coronary, perfusion pressure. It has also been documented that it is, in particular, the ratio of coronary diastolic pressure to left ventricular systolic pressure that influences subendocardial perfusion.[27] This can be due either to selective perfusion of the subepicardium during systole or to the time interval between end of systole and start of diastolic subendocardial perfusion; in fact, this time interval depends on extravascular compression (systolic occlusion) of coronary vessels during the previous systole. The vessels that are more compressed during systole would thus be perfused for a shorter time during the subsequent diastole.[20,28]

The effect of myocardial contractility itself, independent of ventricular pressure, has been experimentally evaluated by selectively abolishing or increasing the contractility of limited regions of the left ventricle. Reduction of contractility favors subendocardial perfusion, whereas increase of contractility reduces subendocardial flow.[20,28,33,37]

The role of ventricular pressure and volume, wall thickness, and myocardial contractility in modifying extravascular pressure and its distribution is especially crucial in determining the onset and severity of ischemia. When the microcirculation is vasodilated downstream of a fixed severe coronary stenosis, which markedly lowers perfusion pressure, myocardial perfusion becomes directly dependent on extravascular pressure.[43]

Heart rate influences the duration of diastole, myocardial oxygen consumption, and therefore myocardial perfusion. Under maximal vasodilation, the effect of heart rate on coronary resistance is more evident, mainly because of changes in extravascular pressure and its distribution. Although total coronary resistance is increased by only 10% to 15% after a heart rate increase of 100 beats per minute, its transmural distribution is markedly changed. In the anesthetized dog, the ratio of subendocardial to subepicardial flow decreases from 1.0 to 0.5–0.4 when the heart rate increases from 100 to 210–250 beats per minute. When the heart is arrested (heart rate = 0) the subendocardial-to-subepicardial ratio value is 1.4 to 1.6.[20,74] When autoregulation is present, the heart rate has no effect on myocardial blood flow distribution, because changes in functional subendocardial resistance can compensate for the shorter diastolic time and greater extravascular compression. On the other hand, when maximal vasodilation is present and the coronary reserve is fully elicited, the extravascular component of coronary resistance increases in the subendocardium in proportion to heart rate.

Microcirculatory Function and Coronary Reserve in Humans

Small artery control of coronary resistance can be altered by endothelial damage, smooth muscle hyperreactivity to vasoconstrictor stimuli, reduced response to vasodilators, and structural abnormalities of the vascular wall. Abnormalities of the extravascular components (e.g., cellular and matrix alterations) can impair vasodilation. Each of these abnormalities requires an adequate diagnostic and therapeutic approach.

It is well known that epicardial arteries and small resistance vessels display an opposite response to nitrates (marked dilation of epicardial arteries with little increase in coronary flow) and to dipyridamole or adenosine (marked increase in flow but little coronary dilation).[10,73] Different agents are likely to elicit different responses at different levels of the microcirculation by inducing complex responses due to selective activation of different receptors, neural pathways, and metabolic changes. In experimental research with different models, it has been possible to evaluate such mechanisms individually.[21,29,64,69]

The individual mechanisms that act on microcirculation, and the different vascular components of total coronary resistance, cannot be adequately identified and studied in humans. The estimate of total coronary resistance as the ratio of mean aortic pressure to mean coronary flow provides a global measurement that is the sum of all vascular (anatomical and functional) and extravascular components of coronary resistance. In addition, lack of high-resolution techniques for assessment of transmural coronary flow makes it impossible to evaluate the subepicardial and subendocardial resistance.

Assessment of total coronary resistance can be useful only when no heterogeneity in resistance distribution is present; moreover, the global estimate of coronary resistance includes extravascular factors that are unrelated to microcirculatory dysfunction.

Study of coronary microcirculation in humans is based on indirect evaluation of the vasomotor response to different and specific stimuli (vasoconstrictors or vasodilators), assessed by measurement of coronary flow and arterial pressure.[38] Methods that are validated and currently employed to measure coronary flow in humans provide the following information:

1. Mean flow per gram of myocardium
2. Total flow of the coronary sinus or of a large coronary artery

3. Regional flow within the myocardium per gram of tissue with a spatial resolution of a few cubic centimeters

Mean flow per gram of tissue can be assessed by diffusible indicator techniques that apply the Fick principle, thus measuring the arteriovenous difference of inert gases such as hydrogen, argon, or helium. This technique requires blood sampling from the coronary sinus in the absence of hemodynamic changes.[38,41] The thermodilution technique measures flow in the coronary sinus relative to the coronary sinus segment where the catheter is positioned and refers to the portion of the heart draining in that particular venous site. This technique underestimates high flows and so is inaccurate in evaluating coronary vasodilation. Its major limit, however, is the time required for the measurement itself, which makes difficult the evaluation of transient effects such as the responses of coronary flow to vasoconstricting or vasodilating stimuli. Rapid changes in flow, on the other hand, can be evaluated by Doppler catheters that measure flow velocity in a large coronary artery. If the diameter of the artery is known, the mean flow velocity can be converted into mean flow. However, this measurement cannot be expressed per unit mass, because the extent of the perfused region is unknown and varies according to the position of the catheter. Also, measurement of flow velocity depends on the position and direction of the catheter. Irregularities in vessel diameter and branching sites can also affect the measured values. Therefore, this technique is more accurate for assessment of flow changes than for absolute flow values and is unrelated to myocardial mass.[38,57]

Regional myocardial blood flow can be evaluated by positron emission tomography (PET), whose only intrinsic limits are the spatial resolution of the scanner and its cost.[52] Furthermore, each measurement requires 2 to 5 minutes of a stationary hemodynamic state, which is the limit of the temporal resolution of this technique.

All these methods have an intrinsic error of about 20% of measured values. In particular, the indicator dilution technique is unable to identify heterogeneities in regional myocardial flow; thermodilution and Doppler catheter techniques are unrelated to myocardial mass, thus making it impossible to estimate whether a reduced coronary reserve is the consequence of high resting flow or of reduced maximal flow; and use of PET for regional flow measurement is limited by its spatial and temporal resolution. Therefore, all the currently available techniques for assessment of coronary blood flow in humans are often inadequate to identify microcirculatory dysfunction unless flow impairment is marked, homogeneous, and extensive. In spite of these methodological limitations, coronary reserve is still measured in humans by these techniques, the most common being Doppler catheters for absolute flow and PET for regional myocardial perfusion assessment.

Because of the difficulty of obtaining a pressure–flow relation in clinical studies by evaluation of coronary flow during autoregulation and during maximal vasodilation over a wide range of perfusion pressures, coronary reserve in humans is commonly estimated by the ratio of resting to maximal flow, an approach that leads to gross errors. Furthermore, most of the pharmacological and physical interventions that modify perfusion pressure by changing aortic pressure are likely to vary myocardial oxygen consumption and/or vasomotor tone and also lead to errors in the estimate of maximal coronary reserve. Another difficulty in patients is determining whether maximal flow has actually been achieved. It is well known from experimental studies that reactive hyperemic flow after a transient coronary occlusion is lower than that elicited by vasodilators such as adenosine, dipyridamole, and papaverine.[25,26,70] Transient occlusions during surgery have indeed been used to evaluate coronary reserve in people, as well as hyperosmolar radiopaque contrast agents,[2] pacing, maximal exercise, and infusion of several vasodilators. Flows 2 to 2.5 times the control value have been obtained by pacing, intracoronary injection of contrast media, or infusion of isoproterenol.[35] Greater increases are obtained by maximal exercise (two to four times the control values). Vasodilators such as papaverine, adenosine, and dipyridamole produce maximal vasodilation in humans (up to four to five times the control values), as well as 20-second transient occlusion in anesthetized patients at surgery (fivefold to sixfold increase in peak flow velocity).[36] Dobutamine and other inotropic agents that dilate the coronary microcirculation by increasing cardiac work have also been employed to assess vasodilatory capability in patients with dilated cardiomyopathy.[16,42] However, dobutamine and other inotropic agents elicit a vasodilation smaller than the fourfold increase in flow produced by other direct vasodilators.

Pathophysiology of the Coronary Microcirculation

Functional or structural abnormalities in the coronary precapillary microcirculation have been suggested in several heart diseases when impaired vasodilation of resistance vessels is ascertained in the absence of coronary stenoses at angiography.[9] In syndrome X, ischemic heart disease that follows successful coronary angioplasty, dilated and hypertrophic cardiomyopathy, and hypertension, microcirculatory abnormalities have been reported, and a pathogenetic role of microcirculatory dysfunction has been suggested.

Syndrome X

Pathology of small coronary resistance vessels has been suggested in patients with angina and normal epicardial arteries, who display ST-segment depression on exercise, without the changes in cardiac contractility and cardiac metabolism typical of coronary heart disease.[19,56] However, no specific microvascular abnormalities have been documented by cardiac biopsy.[48] An abnormal vasodilatory response to pacing and to some vasodilator agents has been demonstrated in some patients.[19] Presence of a real impairment of coronary reserve in syndrome X is still debated, and conflicting results have been reported.[11,40,48]

Recently, direct measurement of regional myocardial blood flow by PET has revealed a uniform perfusion of the left ventricular myocardium both in autoregulation and during vasodilation (dipyridamole). Moreover, the vasodilatory response in subjects given dipyridamole is not significantly different from that of a control group of subjects. An increased adrenergic tone of coronary arterioles has been hypothesized on the basis of marked increase in flow after administration of α-blocking agents.[5]

Ischemic Heart Disease

In patients with early-stage coronary atherosclerotic lesions, microvascular disease has been documented[76] in association with the hydraulic obstacle caused by stenosis. Angiographic evidence of vasoconstriction of small arteries distal to severe stenosis in the absence of coronary spasm after an ergonovine test is indirect evidence that the increase in microcirculatory resistance contributes to modulation of coronary flow in ischemic heart disease.[39,67] In patients with complete occlusion of a coronary branch, the presence of resting myocardial ischemia has been attributed to increased microvascular tone, as suggested by the disappearance of the collateral circulation as shown on angiography.[55] Finally, some PET studies have documented, in patients with single-vessel disease, reduction in resting perfusion and in coronary reserve and impaired response to atrial pacing in the remote territory supplied by a normal coronary artery.[59,60,68] In addition, parallel to experimental evidence of microvascular disease in hypercholesterolemic animals, PET studies in asymptomatic subjects with hyperlipidemia have demonstrated reduced vasodilatory response to adenosine, which was normalized by lowering the plasma cholesterol level.[14,24]

Coronary Reperfusion

After successful coronary angioplasty of a stenosed coronary artery, either electively or during acute myocardial infarction, ischemia can still be detected in the distal territory by scintigraphy and echo stress test or by angiography (which shows diffuse vasoconstriction of distal vessels).[66] In addition, after coronary angioplasty in patients with unstable angina and intracoronary thrombus, ischemia associated with low runoff of contrast medium has been described. A microvascular constric-

tion by agents derived from thrombus fragmentation has been hypothesized.[18,72] All these findings cannot be attributed to a dynamic stenosis (the ergonovine test is negative) but are considered to be the consequences of microvascular damage in the reperfused myocardium. This hypothesis is supported by direct evidence, obtained by intracoronary Doppler and PET measurements, of reduced coronary reserve early after coronary angioplasty, which returns to normal levels in all patients after 6 months.[66] Therefore, an altered microvascular vasomotor response can be a component of chronic ischemic heart disease and a mechanism of the modulation of residual coronary reserve after successful percutaneous coronary angioplasty.

Dilated Cardiomyopathy

Several abnormalities of the coronary microcirculation have been described in dilated cardiomyopathy, though unrelated to specific structural alterations at cardiac biopsy or autopsy.[47] Some studies have reported reduction in resting flow[50] and in vasodilatory capability.[6,47,63] Severe impairment of ventricular function could greatly affect myocardial perfusion by modifying extravascular components of coronary resistance; elevated left ventricular end-diastolic pressure, increased ventricular volume, and wall tension can all contribute to reduced myocardial flow. In the early stage of the disease, alterations in myocardial perfusion were found both in resting conditions and during application of vasodilating stimuli (atrial pacing and dipyridamole).[45] These findings indicate that basal perfusion and coronary reserve are markedly affected even before clinical evidence of ventricular insufficiency. A primary role of microcirculatory dysfunction in reducing myocardial perfusion in the early stages of dilated cardiomyopathy is therefore likely, though its influence in the evolution toward ventricular insufficiency is still unclear.

Hypertrophic Cardiomyopathy

Myocardial ischemia with normal coronary arteries is a common feature of hypertrophic cardiomyopathy. Abnormalities of the structure of intramyocardial arterioles at autopsy and a reduced vasodilatory capacity have been documented in patients.[1,7]

In spite of a normal basal perfusion, patients with hypertrophic cardiomyopathy display reduced vasodilation (with dipyridamole infusion) even in regions of the left ventricular wall that are not hypertrophic.[4] This finding suggests that coronary microcirculatory alterations are independent of myocardial hypertrophy. The possibility that both myocardial fibers and vascular smooth muscle cells could be morphologically altered has been proposed.[1]

Recent PET studies have documented a preferential subendocardial ischemia during dipyridamole infusion, a finding that can be explained by the contribution of mechanical determinants of coronary blood flow distribution to the impairment of coronary reserve. In particular, increase in the extravascular component of coronary resistance, due to increased intramyocardial pressure, a higher ventricular stiffness, and a higher intraventricular pressure, accounts for the preferential subendocardial ischemia in these patients, independent of microcirculatory changes.[3,7]

Hypertension

Hypertension induces microcirculatory damage not only in the renal and cerebral blood vessels but also in the coronary circulation. In hypertension, coronary reserve is reduced by both hemodynamic factors and structural changes of the small coronary arteries; these mechanisms can potentially provoke ischemia in hypertensive patients. Cardiac hypertrophy, with a greater intramyocardial pressure or left ventricular dilation, can increase the extravascular component of coronary resistance, whereas the structural abnormalities of coronary microvessels can increase the vascular anatomical resistance.[62] Experimental models of hypertension have documented a higher myocardial oxygen demand (caused by a greater afterload and left ventricular dilation) and morphofunctional changes of coronary microvessels.

Although hypertensive patients display a normal basal flow, the hyperemia following an increase in metabolic demand is reduced. The coronary reserve elicited by vasodilatory agents (e.g., dipyridamole and papaverine) is also reduced.[49] Recently, a reduced resting flow and an impaired vasodilation with pacing and dipyridamole infusion have been documented by PET studies in both hypertrophic and nonhypertrophic regions of the left ventricle.[51]

The microcirculatory changes in hypertension are both functional and morphological. Some studies[49] have documented a reduced response of coronary microcirculation to vasodilators such as dipyridamole, in the absence of anatomical changes (histological and ultrastructural) of microvessels in cardiac biopsy specimens.

Morphological changes have been described in animal models of long-lasting hypertension. Capillary angiogenesis, vascular remodeling, and hyperplasia of the arteriolar media have been described. In endomyocardial biopsy specimens, an abnormally high media-to-lumen ratio of coronary microvessels and an increased perivascular fibrosis have been reported.[61] The clinical relevance of such findings is still debated, and most studies emphasize functional rather than morphological abnormalities of coronary microcirculation in hypertension.

References

1. Baroldi G, Camerini F, Goodwin JF. *Advances in Cardiomyopathies*. Berlin: Springer-Verlag; 1990:7–175.

2. Bassan M, Ganz W, Marcus HS, Swan HJC. The effect of intracoronary injection of contrast medium upon coronary blood flow. *Circulation.* 1975;51:442–445.

3. Camici PG, Cecchi F, Gistri R, et al. Dipyridamole-induced subendocardial underperfusion in hypertrophic cardiomyopathy assessed by positron emission tomography. *Coron Artery Dis.* 1991;2:837–841.

4. Camici PG, Chiriatti G, Lorenzoni R, et al. Coronary vasodilation is impaired both in hypertrophied and nonhypertrophied myocardium of patients with hypertrophic cardiomyopathy: a study with ^{13}N-ammonia and positron emission tomography. *J Am Coll Cardiol.* 1991;17:879–886.

5. Camici PG, Marraccini P, Gistri R, Salvadori PA, Sorace O, L'Abbate A. Adrenergically-mediated coronary vasodilation in patients with syndrome X. *Cardiovasc Drugs Ther.* 1994;8:221–226.

6. Cannon RO, Cannon RE, Parrillo JE, et al. Dynamic limitation of coronary vasodilator reserve in patients with dilated cardiomyopathy and chest pain. *J Am Coll Cardiol.* 1987;10:1190–1200.

7. Cannon RO, Rosing DR, Maron BJ, et al. Myocardial ischemia in patients with hypertrophic cardiomyopathy: contribution of inadequate vasodilator reserve and elevated left ventricular filling pressures. *Circulation.* 1985; 71:234–243.

8. Chilian MW. Coronary microcirculation in health and disease. *Circulation.* 1997;95:522–528.

9. Cianflone D, Lanza GA, Maseri A. Microvascular angina in patients with normal coronary arteries and with other ischaemic syndromes. *Eur Heart J.* 1995;16(suppl 1):96–103.

10. Cohen MV, Kirk ES. Differential response of large and small coronary arteries to nitroglycerin and angiotensin: autoregulation and tachyphylaxis. *Circ Res.* 1973;33: 445–453.

11. Crake T, Canepa-Anson R, Shapiro LM, Poole-Wilson PA. Continuous recording of coronary sinus oxygen saturation during atrial pacing in patients with coronary artery disease and with syndrome X. *Br Heart J.* 1988;89:31–38.

12. Crystal GJ, Downey HF, Bashour FA. Small vessel and total coronary blood volume during intracoronary adenosine. *Am J Physiol.* 1981;241:H194–H201.

13. Crystal GJ, Downey HF, Bashour FA. Persistent coronary vasodilation during long-term, supramaximal doses of adenosine. *Am J Physiol.* 1984;247:H869–H873.

14. Dayanikli F, Grambow D, Muzik O, Mosca L, Rubenfire M, Schwaiger M. Early detection of abnormal coronary flow reserve in asymptomatic men at high risk for coronary artery disease using positron emission tomography. *Circulation.* 1994;90:808–817.

15. Downey JM, Kirk ES. Inhibition of coronary blood flow by a vascular waterfall mechanism. *Circ Res.* 1975;36:753–760.

16. Dubois-Randé JL, Marlet P, Duval-Moulin AM, et al. Coronary vasodilating action of dobutamine in patients with idiopatic dilated cardiomyopathy. *Am Heart J.* 1993;125: 1329–1336.

17. Eliasen P, Amtorp O. Effect of intracoronary adenosine upon regional blood flow, microvascular blood volume and hematocrit in canine myocardium. *Int J Microcirc Clin Exp.* 1984;3:3–12.

18. El-Tamimi H, Davies GJ, Crea F, Sritara P, Hackett D,

Maseri A. Inappropriate constriction of small coronary vessels as a possible cause of a positive exercise test soon after successful coronary angioplasty. *Circulation.* 1991;84: 2307–2312.

19. Epstein SE, Cannon RO III. Site of increased resistance to coronary flow in patients with angina pectoris and normal epicardial coronary arteries. *J Am Coll Cardiol.* 1986;8: 459–461.

20. Feigl EO. Coronary physiology. *Physiol Rev.* 1983;63:1–205.

21. Feigl EO, Buffington CW, Nathan HJ. Adrenergic coronary vasoconstriction during myocardial underperfusion. *Circulation.* 1987;75(suppl I):1–I5.

22. Gallagher KP, Folts JD, Shebuski RJ, Rankin JHG, Rowe GG. Subepicardial vasodilator reserve in the presence of critical coronary stenosis in dogs. *Am J Cardiol.* 1980;46: 67–73.

23. Gould KL, Lipscomb K, Hamilton GW. Physiologic basis for assessing critical coronary stenosis. Instantaneous flow response and regional distribution during coronary hyperemia as measures of coronary flow reserve. *Am J Cardiol.* 1974;33:87–94.

24. Gould KL, Martucci JP, Goldberg DI, et al. Short-term cholesterol lowering decreases size and severity of perfusion abnormalities by positron emission tomography after dipyridamole in patients with coronary artery disease. A potential noninvasive marker of healing coronary endothelium. *Circulation.* 1994;89:1530–1538.

25. Gould KL, Westcott RJ, Albro PC, Hamilton GW. Noninvasive assessment of coronary stenoses by myocardial imaging during pharmacologic coronary vasodilatation. II. Clinical methodology and feasibility. *Am J Cardiol.* 1978; 41:279–287.

26. Hoffman JIE. Maximal coronary flow and the concept of coronary vascular reserve. *Circulation.* 1984;70:153–159.

27. Hoffman JIE, Buckberg GD. The myocardial supply : demand ratio. A critical review. *Am J Cardiol.* 1978;41: 327–331.

28. Hoffman JIE, Spaan JAE. Pressure–flow relations in coronary circulation. *Physiol Rev.* 1990;70:331–390.

29. Huang AH, Feigl EO. Adrenergic coronary vasoconstriction helps maintain uniform transmural blood flow distribution during exercise.*Circ Res.* 1988;62:286–298.

30. Klocke FJ, Mates RE, Canty JM, Ellis AK. Coronary pressure–flow relationships: controversial issues and probable implications. *Circ Res.* 1985;56:310–323.

31. L'Abbate A, Camici P, Trivella MG, et al. Time dependent response of coronary flow to prolonged adenosine infusion: doubling of peak reactive hyperaemic flow. *Cardiovasc Res.* 1981;15:282–286.

32. L'Abbate A, Marzilli M, Ballestra AM, et al. Opposite transmural gradients of coronary resistance and extravascular pressure in the working dog's heart. *Cardiovasc Res.* 1980;14:21–29.

33. L'Abbate A, Marzilli M, Ballestra AM, Camici P. Myocardial contraction: an additional determinant of transmural flow distribution. In: Maseri A, Klassen G, Lesch M, eds. *Primary and Secondary Angina Pectoris.* New York: Grune & Stratton; 1978:21.

34. L'Abbate A, Trivella MG, Camici P, Ballestra AM, Pelosi G, Taddei Le Davies GJ. Beneficial effect on subendocardial perfusion of lowering left ventricular afterload in the absence of coronary reserve. In: Mason DT, Neri Serneri GG, Oliver MF, eds. *Florence International Meeting on Myocardial Infarction.* Amsterdam: Excerpta Medica; 1979:560.

35. MacLeod CA, Bahler RC, Davies B. Pacing-induced changes in cardiac venous blood flow in normal subjects and patients with coronary artery disease. *Am J Cardiol.* 1973;32:686–692.

36. Marcus M, Wright C, Doty D, et al. Measurements of coronary velocity and reactive hyperemia in the coronary circulation of humans. *Circ Res.* 1981; 49:877–891.

37. Marzilli M, Goldstein S, Sabbah HN, Lee T, Stein PD. Modulating effect of regional myocardial performance on local myocardial perfusion in the dog. *Circ Res.* 1979;45: 634–641.

38. Maseri A, ed. *Myocardial Blood Flow in Man. Methods and Significance in Coronary Disease.* Torino, Italy: Minerva Medica; 1972.

39. Maseri A, Crea F, Cianflone D. Myocardial ischemia caused by distal coronary vasoconstriction. *Am J Cardiol.* 1992;79:1602–1605.

40. Maseri A, Crea F, Kaski JC, Crake T. Mechanisms of angina pectoris in syndrome X. *J Am Coll Cardiol.* 1991;17: 499–506.

41. Maseri A, L'Abbate A, Michelassi C, et al. Possibilities, limitations, and technique for the study of regional myocardial perfusion in man by xenon-133. *Cardiovasc Res.* 1977;11:277–290.

42. Mason Jr, Palac RT,Freeman ML, et al. Thallium scintigraphy during dobutamine infusion: non-exercise dependent screening test for coronary disease. *Am Heart J.* 1984;107: 481–485.

43. McGinn AL, White CW, Wilson RF. Interstudy variability of coronary flow reserve: influence of heart rate, arterial pressure and ventricular preload. *Circulation.* 1990;81: 1319–1330.

44. Muller JM, Davis MJ, Chilian WM. Integrated regulation of pressure and flow in coronary microcirculation. *Cardiovasc Res.* 1996;32:668–678.

45. Neglia D, Parodi O, Gallopin M, et al. Myocardial blood flow response to pacing tachycardia and to dipyridamole infusion in patients with dilated cardiomyopathy without overt heart failure. A quantitative assessment by positron emission tomography. *Circulation.* 1995;92:796–804.

46. Olsson R.A., Patterson RE. Adenosine as a physiological regulator of coronary blood flow. In: Hahn FE, ed. *Progress in Molecular and Subcellular Biology.* New York: Springer-Verlag; 1976:227.

47. Opherk D, Schwartz F, Mall G, Manthey J, Baller D, Kubler W. Coronary dilatory capacity in idiopathic dilated cardiomyopathy: analysis of 16 patients. *Am J Cardiol.* 1983; 51:1657–1662.

48. Opherk D, Zede H, Weihe E, et al. Reduced coronary dilatory capacity and ultrastructural changes of the myocardium in patients with angina pectoris but normal coronary arteries. *Circulation.* 1981;63:817–825.

49. Opherk G, Mall G, Zede H, et al. Reduction of coronary reserve: a mechanism for angina pectoris in patients with arterial hypertension and normal coronary arteries. *Circulation.* 1984;69:1–7.

50. Parodi O, De Maria R, Oltrona I, et al. Myocardial blood flow distribution in patients with ischemic heart disease or dilated cardiomyopathy undergoing heart transplantation. *Circulation.* 1993;88:509–522.

51. Parodi O, Neglia D, Palombo C, et al. Regional myocardial blood flow response to pacing tachycardia and dipyridamole in arterial hypertension: a quantitative study by positron emission tomography [abstract]. *Circulation.* 1990;82(suppl 2):478.

52. Parodi O, Sambuceti G. The role of coronary microvascular dysfuction in the genesis of cardiovascular diseases. *J Nucl Med.* 1996;40:9–16.

53. Pelosi G, L'Abbate A, Trivella MG, et al. Persistence of subendocardial perfusion after subtotal coronary embolisation. *Cardiovasc Res.* 1988;22:113–121.

54. Pelosi G, Saviozzi G, Trivella MG, L'Abbate A. Transmural redistribution of coronary resistance during embolization: a clue to intramyocardial small artery architecture. *Microvasc Res.* 1990;39:322–340.

55. Pupita G, Maseri A, Kaski JC, Galassi AR, Gavrielides S, Dacies G, Crea F. Myocardial ischemia caused by distal coronary constriction in stable angina pectoris. *N Engl J Med.* 1990;323:514–520.

56. Rosano GMC, Lindsay DC, Pool-Wilson PA. Syndrome X: an hypothesis for cardiac pain without ischaemia. *Cardiologia.* 1991;36:885–895.

57. Rossen JD, Oskarsson H, Stenberg RG, Braun P, Talman CL, Winniford MD. Simultaneous measurement of coronary flow reserve by left anterior descending coronary artery Doppler and great cardiac vein thermodilution methods. *J Am Coll Cardiol.* 1992;20:402–407.

58. Rubio R, Berne RM. Regulation of coronary blood flow. *Prog Cardiovasc Dis.* 1975;18:105–122.

59. Sambuceti G, Marzullo P, Giorgetti A, et al. Global alteration in perfusion response to increasing oxygen consumption in patients with single vessel coronary artery disease. *Circulation.* 1994;90:1696–1705.

60. Sambuceti G, Parodi O, Marcassa C, et al. Alteration in regulation of myocardial blood flow in one vessel coronary artery disease determined by positron emission tomography. *Am J Cardiol.* 1993;72:538–543.

61. Schwartzkopff B, Motz W, Frenzel H, Vogt M, Knauer S, Strauer BE. Structural and functional alterations of the intramyocardial coronary arterioles in patients with arterial hypertension. *Circulation.* 1993;88:993–1003.

62. Tomanek RJ, Palmer PJ, Pfeiffer GL, Schreiber KL, Eastham CL, Maecus ML. Morphometry of canine coronary arteries, arterioles and capillaries during hypertension and left ventricular hypertrophy. *Circ Res.* 1986;58:38–46.

63. Treasure CB, Vita JA, Cox DA, et al. Endothelium dependent dilation of the coronary microvasculature is impaired in dilated cardiomyopathy. *Circulation.* 1990;81:772–779.

64. Trivella MG, Broten TP, Feigl EO. β-Receptor subtypes in the canine coronary circulation. *Am J Physiol.* 1990;259: H1575-H1585.

65. Trivella MG, Pelosi G, Nevola E, et al. Functional components and adenosine vasodilation: complex behavior of minimal coronary resistance [abstract]. *Clin Res.* 1992; 40(2)AFCR:257A.

66. Uren N, Crake T, Lefroy DC, De Silva R, Davies GJ, Maseri A. Delayed recovery of coronary resistive vessel function after coronary angioplasty. *J Am Coll Cardiol.* 1993;21: 612–621.

67. Uren N, Crake T, Lefroy DC, De Silva R, Davies GJ, Maseri A. Reduced coronary vasodilator response in infarcted and normal myocardium after infarction. *N Engl J Med.* 1994;331:222–227.

68. Uren NG, Marraccini P, Gistri R, De Silva R, Camici PG. Altered coronary vasodilator reserve and metabolism in myocardium subtended by normal arteries in patients with coronary artery disease elsewhere. *J Am Coll Cardiol.* 1993;22:650–658.

69. Van Winkle DM, Feigl EO. Acetylcholine causes coronary vasodilation in dogs and baboons. *Circ Res.* 1989;65: 1580–1593.

70. Warltier DC, Gross GJ, Brooks HL. Pharmacologic- vs. ischemia-induced coronary artery vasodilation. *Am J Physiol.* 1981;240:H767–H774.

71. Wiedeman MP, Tuma RF, Mayrovitz HN. *An Introduction to Microcirculation.* New York: Academic Press; 1981:30.

72. Wilson RF, Lesser JF, Laxson DD, White CW. Intense microvascular constriction after angioplasty of acute thrombotic arterial lesions. *Lancet.* 1989;1:807–811.

73. Winbury MM, Howe BB, Hefner MA. Effect of nitrates and other coronary dilators on large and small coronary vessels: hypothesis for the mechanism of action of nitrates. *J Pharmacol Exp Ther.* 1969;168:70–95.

74. Wusten B, Buss DD, Deist H, Schaper W. Dilatory capacity of the coronary circulation and its correlation to the arterial vasculature in the canine left ventricle. *Basic Res Cardiol.* 1977;72:636–650.

75. Yipintsoi T, Dobbs WA Jr, Scanlon PD, Knopp TJ, Bassingthwaighte JB. Regional distribution of diffusible tracers and carbonized microspheres in the left ventricle of isolated dog hearts. *Circ Res.* 1973;33:573–587.

76. Zeiher AM, Drexler H, Wollschlaeger, Just H. Endothelial dysfunction of coronary microvasculature is associated with impaired flow regulation in patients with early atherosclerosis. *Circulation.* 1991;84:1984–1992.

11

Occupational Cardiovascular Risk Factors

Francesco Tomei, Tiziana Paola Baccolo, Arianna Izzo, Bruno Papaleo,
Benedetta Persechino, Enrico Tomao, and Maria Valeria Rosati

Occupational Cardiovascular Diseases

Despite much progress in recent years, only a few studies have looked into the relations between occupational factors and cardiovascular pathology. Rosenmann[141] estimated that the traditional cardiovascular risk factors explained not more than 50% of cardiac ischemic pathology. Olsen and Kristensen[119] maintained that 16% of premature cardiovascular mortality among men and 22% among women could be avoided by taking preventive measures in the workplace.

Hypertension, disorders of carbohydrate and lipid metabolism, cigarette smoking, and obesity are all known vascular risk factors, but there are others, often misunderstood, underestimated, and classified as minor. Chemical and physical agents, once found only in the workplace, are becoming more important because they are increasingly encountered in all walks of life. Psychosocial factors are also largely acknowledged as co-causative agents in various pathological conditions.

All too frequently the term *essential hypertension*—a condition of primary importance in the pathogenesis of vascular disease—is used as a handy label behind which to hide limited knowledge of the underlying etiologic and physiopathogenic factors. Clarifying the influence of vascular factors other than the traditional ones may cast useful light on the pathogenesis of vascular diseases and help define more clearly the rather vague clinical condition referred to as essential hypertension.

Besides exposure to chemicals, psychosocial–occupational factors such as stress and shift work and physical factors such as vibration, ionizing radiation, and noise are all important in relation to cardiovascular diseases.

Chemicals

The harmful effects on the vascular system of high doses of metals and other chemicals have long been known, although they tend to be overlooked when disturbances are being diagnosed. Much more complex is the relation between vascular damage and exposure to the low doses of toxic substances likely to be encountered in the everyday environment. For many years this was purely a question of occupational medicine, since these toxic substances were mostly limited to the workplace (Table 11.1). Now that many of them are spreading throughout the environment, however, the issue has become of more general interest.

The chemicals most likely to cause vascular damage are lead, cadmium, mercury, arsenic, carbon monoxide, carbon disulfide, nitroderivatives, halogenated hydrocarbons, and vinyl chloride (Table 11.2).

Lead

Numerous epidemiological, biochemical, and clinical studies have investigated how lead is related to the development of vascular pathology. Observations on saturnism and the association of nephropathy and hypertension arising from massive, long-term absorption of lead are part of medical history. The effects of prolonged exposure to low doses of lead are worth considering in view of their implications in the pathogenesis of hypertension. The question is all the more important considering that much of the population may be affected by this type of exposure and that lead is frequently found in the environment, in food, and in drinking water.

Lead is an extremely frequent atmospheric contaminant. The amount estimated to enter the atmosphere every year is 18,000 tons of natural origin and no less than 440,000 tons resulting from human activities, approximately 400,000 of this amount coming from vehicle emissions. The use of lead-free gasoline should help reduce the levels of lead in the air. Blood levels of lead in the United States were reduced by 37% between 1976 and 1980, mainly as a result of hygienic measures on foods and the elimination of lead from gasoline. Pirkle et al.[130] have hypothesized that this reduction may lower

TABLE 11.1. The main cardiovascular toxins and their occupational uses.

Lead
Smelting and recovery, manufacturing accumulators, polyvinyl articles, rifle ammunition, pewter work, preparation of enamels, and tile enameling

Cadmium
Treatment of metal serfaces, accumulators, paints, and glass

Mercury
Mining, thermometers, electrical and scientific equipment, and amalgams

Arsenic
Mining and processing, production of paints and enamels, drugs, and vulcanization of rubber

Carbon monoxide
Industrial treatment of carbon monoxide, mining, coke works, blast furnaces, glassworks, gas and arc welding, engine testing, and fire fighting

Carbon disulfide
Rayon and flock manufacture, extraction of oil from seed husks, cellulose solvent, cold vulcanization of rubber, and pesticides

Nitroderivatives
Production of explosives and drugs

Hydrocarbons
Production of explosives, perfumes and perfumed soaps, chemicals, and pharmaceuticals

Vinyl chloride monomer
Production of polyvinyl chloride (PVC) and use of PVC in manufacturing plastic

TABLE 11.2. Vascular pathologies caused by chemicals: clinical and epidemiological data.

Lead
High blood concentrations of lead in hypertensives, high incidence of hypertension in areas with high lead content in water, high lead concentrations in atheromatous plaques, and increased mortality from vascular pathologies among subjects exposed to lead

Cadmium
High blood and urinary cadmium concentrations in hypertensive patients

Mercury
Hypertension among exposed subjects and potentiation of the atherogenic effect of cholesterol

Arsenic
Cardiac lesions with subepicardial hemorrhage and alterations in repolarization

Carbon monoxide
Increased atheromatous processes and increased thrombaxane concentrations with platelet hyperaggregability

Carbon disulfide
Cerebral and renal vascular disease and hypertension among exposed subjects

Nitroderivatives
Monday morning syndrome, peripheral vasodilatation, and Raynaud's syndrome

Hydrocarbons
Alterations to lipid metabolism, rhythm disturbances, dilatory cardiomyopathy, and stroke

Vinyl chloride monomer
Alterations to microcirculation in the limbs, rhythm disturbances, Raynaud's syndrome, and cerebrovascular pathologies

the incidence of myocardial infarction by 4.7% and stroke by 6.7% over the next 10 years. They also showed that for blood lead levels between 7 and 34 μg/dL it was impossible to establish a threshold below which they were not correlated with blood pressure (BP). The dose–response curve showed that at relatively low blood lead concentrations BP tended to rise considerably, whereas at higher concentrations it plateaued out.[130]

Most lead in food comes from milk (pastures treated with lead salts or those close to main roads), from vegetables (land contaminated with the metal as a result of lead arsenate treatment or storage in pottery crocks treated with lead-based varnish), from wine (storage in enameled metal containers or tiled vats, exposure to grouting for tiling, etc.), from cigarette smoke, and from water (lead carbonate encrusting pipes and dissolved by the action of chlorine) (Table 11.3). The lead content in the water has been found to be higher in areas where the incidence of hypertension is high,[187] and hypertensive patients have been reported to have significantly higher blood lead levels than normotensive subjects. Concentrations of lead were high in the arterial walls and atheromatous plaques of patients who died from coronary disease.[186]

Epidemiological, clinical, and toxicological studies of the relation between exposure to low doses of lead and high BP have indicated that even low doses may raise BP and thus also the risk of cardiovascular disease.[50,90,140, 141,154,186] Although no firm conclusions can be drawn, there are many reports of a high incidence of cardiovascular and cerebrovascular diseases among workers occupationally exposed to high levels of lead.[36,39,41,72,108,147, 148,152] The association between hypertension and lead has been demonstrated for low-dose exposure also (serum lead concentrations of 2 to 15 μg/dL).[151,157–159,186] The evaluation of both systolic and diastolic cardiac functions by Doppler echocardiography in workers exposed to lead showed an increase of systolic cardiac function, a decrease of diastolic cardiac function, and an increase of the MB isoenzyme of creatine phosphokinase (CPK-

TABLE 11.3. Daily lead intake.

Food	150–500 μg
Water	20 μg
Air	4–40 μg
Cigarette smoke	1–15 μg

MB). The increase of CPK-MB was correlated with lead burden.[188]

Experimental data on the relations between lead intake and the vascular system have provided new topics for research (Table 11.4), indicating the main mechanisms of action of the metal: its renal effects linked to action on the renin–angiotensin system and effects resulting from changes in calcium-mediated control of vascular smooth muscle.[80,82] Studies in animals made hypertensive by exposure from birth to 500 ppm of lead have revealed elevated plasma renin concentrations; if lead dosing was started in utero (5 to 500 ppm) hypertension was already detectable 1 month after birth.[177,180,181] When the animals were exposed to the metal for another 4 to 5 months, however, renin levels dropped. In all cases rats exposed to lead had reduced renin secretion in response to specific stimuli, and those exposed to the highest concentrations showed angiotensin-converting enzyme (ACE) inhibition also.[177]

Workers exposed to lead presented a dose-related decrease in urinary excretion of kallikrein; plasma renin activity was below normal in elderly people with chronic lead intoxication and rose in workers exposed to low doses for weeks or months.[105] The decreases in kallikrein and angiotensin II appear to be correlated to lead's inhibitory effect on ACE, the enzyme responsible for converting angiotensin I to angiotensin II. In light of these findings, the relation between lead-induced hypertension and the activity of the renin–angiotensin system appears to merit further investigation. Boscolo et al.[23] suggested there may also be a relation between changes in the copper and zinc metabolism and lead's effects on the cardiovascular system.

Lead causes spasm of gastrointestinal smooth muscle; if it also produces spasm in vascular smooth muscle, its hypertensive effects may be explained. Studies using caudal arterial preparations from rats exposed to low-dose lead revealed an increased contractile response of the smooth muscle fiber cells to adrenergic agonists, noradrenaline (NA), and electrical stimulation.[181] Rats exposed to lead present different cardiovascular effects, including potentiation of the cardiovascular responses resulting from activation of α_2-, β_1-, and β_2-adrenergic receptors and cardiac and vascular dopaminergic receptors, hyporeactivity of the afferent baroreflex pathways,

changes in plasma renin activity and/or in the activity of ACE, increased central sympathetic tonic activity associated with a diminution of vagal tone, and interference with cyclic AMP-dependent contractile processes in the vascular and cardiac muscle cells.[20-22,53] Lead, by activating adrenergic and dopaminergic receptors, may affect the availability of intracellular free calcium, though it does not appear to have much effect on the passage of calcium ions through the plasma membrane slow channels. The final prohypertensive effect of lead is certainly the sum of a combination or combinations of its multiple effects—some of which may be antagonistic—on catecholaminergic receptors and on the autonomic nervous system.

Cadmium

Cadmium is a nonessential element with no biological functions. It is highly toxic for mammals. It is ubiquitous and found in air, earth, and water. It enters the food chain, and the body picks it up daily in its water and food, as well as from cigarette smoke. Cadmium is virtually undetectable in newborns, except for a trace—about 1 μg—derived from the mother, through the placenta. Cadmium accumulates mainly in kidneys and liver, with a very long biological half-life (10 to 30 years). Accumulation peaks around the age of 50 years, when levels reach 15 to 20 mg.

Cadmium's role in the pathogenesis of hypertension is widely studied. High doses have well-known vascular effects, but current research focuses mainly on the effects of exposure to low doses of the metal. Studies in experimental animals (Table 11.5) suggest it has some prohypertensive effect, but epidemiological studies provide no firm conclusions. In hypertensive patients, however, high cadmium concentrations in serum and urine and accumulation in the kidneys have been reported.[106,146,187] A relation has even been found between atmospheric levels of cadmium and an increase in mortality from vascular pathology.[101]

Low doses of cadmium in genetically susceptible rats may induce persistent hypertension. The mechanism of this cadmium-dependent rise in BP appears to involve increases in cardiac inotropism and peripheral vascular resistance. The latter rises in relation to various factors such as the reduced activity of the kallikrein–kinin system, action on the renin–angiotensin system, and increased NA release from peripheral adrenergic neurons.

TABLE 11.4. Vascular toxicity due to lead: experimental data.

- Increased systemic blood pressure and cardiac inotropism
- Enhanced α_2-, β_1-, and β_2-adrenergic responses
- Enhanced dopaminergic responses
- Reduced baroceptor reflexes
- Action on the renin–angiotensin system
- Enhanced central tonic–sympathetic activity
- Reduction of vagal tonus
- Action on cyclic adenosine monophosphate–dependent contractile processes

TABLE 11.5. Vascular toxicity due to cadmium: experimental data.

- Increased systemic blood pressure and cardiac inotropism
- Enhanced peripheral vascular responses
- Reduced kallikrein–kinin system activity
- Action on the renin–angiotensin system
- Increased peripheral noradrenaline release

Other factors important in the onset of experimental cadmium-induced hypertension include interference with the metabolism of Ca^{2+} ions and other bivalent cations (Zn, Cu, Mg, Co, Fe) required as cofactors by enzymes that inactivate hypertensive substances; when these enzymes are inhibited the road is clear to hypertension. Cadmium also probably induces hypertension through other mechanisms such as a reduction in prostacyclin synthesis and an increase in adrenal catecholamine release.[23,158] Some authors indicated that cadmium-mediated modifications in atrial natriuretic peptide receptor density and affinity may be involved in BP rise.[55,56] The mechanism of such an effect may be attributed to a cadmium-induced peroxidative damage of the cell membrane.[113,121] Extrapolating the animal data to humans, it would appear that the dose that induces hypertension in the rat—5 µg/kg per day—corresponds to 175 to 350 µg/d in humans. In most Western countries, daily dietary intake of cadmium is 50 to 70 µg, although foods such as oysters, liver, rice, and wheat—all rich in this element—may raise this figure considerably (Table 11.6). Water provides about 5 µg/L, and cigarette smoking (average 20 cigarettes) adds 1 to 2 µg/d; at least 20% to 50% of this amount is absorbed. The amount of cadmium inhaled with air varies much more than that ingested with food (Table 11.6). Overall daily cadmium intake may therefore reach the equivalent of the hypertensive dose in the rat. From these figures we cannot state with certainty that cadmium has no role in the pathogenesis of hypertension and cardiovascular pathology.[90]

Mercury

Mercury is a protoplasmic toxin that denatures cell proteins and thus damages cell integrity. It comes mainly from food, although there are numerous other possible sources in everyday life—it is used in antiseptics, paints, floor waxes, furniture polish, fabric softeners, and air-conditioning filters, to name a few. From 20% to 25% of the population, not exposed to mercury in their work, nevertheless have appreciable concentrations of the metal in their body fluids. Daily intake of mercury with food is 5 to 20 µg; water provides about 0.1 µg/d, and cigarette smoking results in inhalation of 0.1 to 0.5 µg/d.

Mercury poisoning can cause hypertension, with left ventricular hypertrophy and myocardiosclerosis. The presumed mechanism involves early generalized athero-

TABLE 11.6. Daily cadmium intake.

Food	50–70 µg
Water	5 µg
Cigarette smoke	1–2 µg
Air at rural sites	0.005–0.215 µg
Air at industrial sites	0.01–3.5 µg
Air close to the source	0.05–25 µg

TABLE 11.7. Vascular toxicity due to mercury: experimental data.

- Increased systemic blood pressure and cardiac inotropism
- Increased peripheral noradrenaline release
- Reduced baroceptor reflexes
- Action on cyclic nucleotide system
- Action on verapamil-sensitive calcium channels

sclerosis, resulting from mercury's enhancement of the atherogenic action of cholesterol.

Other pathogenic theories have been proposed, based on experimental data (Table 11.7). In the rat low doses of mercury increase cardiac inotropism and raise BP. These effects appear to be linked to increased NA release from peripheral adrenergic neurons through action on the presynaptic membrane. The afferent component of the baroreflex arc is also reduced, and response to stimulation of β_1- and β_2-adrenergic receptors is increased. Mercury interferes with the cyclic nucleotide system and with verapamil-sensitive calcium channels.[23] The combined and contrasting effects on neurons and receptors may give rise to hypertension.

The prevalence of hypertension in organisms chronically exposed to mercury is significantly higher than in the general population.[102,187] Investigation of symptoms related to autonomic dysfunction in subjects exposed to low levels of mercury vapors for an average of 16 years revealed a tendency to reduced cardiovascular reflexes and a slight increase in subjective symptoms.[129] Among workers without hypertension or renal pathologies who were exposed to mercury, there was a significant rise in urinary transferrin, an early marker of renal pathological modification.[61] There are also reports of increased urinary excretion of intestinal alkaline phosphatase (IAP), which is a sensitive and specific marker of alterations in the S3 proximal tubular segment, preferential site of action for various nephrotoxins.[118]

Arsenic

Acute or chronic arsenic poisoning causes myocardial damage whose histological findings are typical subepicardial hemorrhages. It also commonly alters repolarization, sometimes leading to serious ventricular arrhythmias. Not all epidemiological data on the relation between chronic arsenic intake and vascular pathology are concordant, although most do agree that the relation is likely.[91,166,187]

Experimentally, arsenic given to rats at a concentration of 50 µg/mL water for from 320 days to 18 months did not affect BP or cardiac inotropism. Longer treatments, however, raised peripheral vascular resistance and reduced cardiac output. Arsenic's vascular effects appear to be linked to an action on β_1- and β_2-adrenergic responses and to rises in central sympathetic and vagal tone.[23]

Carbon Monoxide

Carbon monoxide (CO) is formed in incomplete combustion, whenever there is not enough oxygen for carbon to be converted to carbon dioxide. Gas water heaters, liquid-gas room heaters, and other such combustion devices may be dangerous if used in inadequately oxygenated premises. CO is one of the ingredients of city gas, except when pure methane is supplied.

The relation between CO and cardiovascular disease has been amply dealt with in the literature. There is no question about the consequences of high, acute exposure to CO, but the possible effects of exposure to this gas in the development of atherosclerosis are still debated. Some investigators conclude that CO raises the risk of cardiovascular disease, whereas others take a more prudent stance.[63,89,187]

Exposure to CO interferes with the eicosanoid balance, causing a quantitative or functional increase in thromboxane, with concomitant platelet hyperaggregability.[163] When cardiovascular homeostatic mechanisms are working properly, this situation does not necessarily lead to overt pathology, but its pathogenic potential is always latent. Significant increases in plasma fibrinogen level and blood viscosity and reduced red cell deformability have been found.[163] The general population is exposed to CO through environmental pollution from vehicle emissions and through cigarette smoke, thus creating a situation of potential vascular risk.[57,90,131,139]

The association between chronic exposure to CO and atherosclerosis is greatly debated. On the one hand are the conflicting data from experimental animal studies; on the other hand are the perplexities arising from observations on groups of smokers with different levels of carboxyhemoglobin and occupational categories of exposed workers such as firefighters and foundry workers.[90,159,187] However, the presence of carboxyhemoglobin, known to be correlated with cardiovascular risk, may simply be a marker of absorption of other components of tobacco smoke or other toxic compounds encountered in the workplace. Kosekela[81] investigated long-term effects of CO exposure on foundry workers' morbidity and mortality from cardiovascular diseases and found that exposure to CO increases the risk of both cardiovascular morbidity and mortality.

Carbon Disulfide

Carbon disulfide's effects on the vascular system have long been known. It mainly affects the brain and kidneys and less frequently the heart and circulatory system. Some studies on exposed workers have found an increase in retinal arterial pressure and retinal angiospasm.[187] Early alterations to ocular microcirculation are very important in the diagnosis of subclinical poisoning.

Current knowledge suggests that the relation between hypertension and exposure to carbon disulfide is based on the toxin's atherogenic action. Peripheral vascular disturbances have also been reported in patients with carbon disulfide poisoning who presented a clear picture of intermittent claudication but frequently also had peripheral vascular alterations detectable by oscillography and plethysmography.[66,83,84] Those who had been most exposed had significantly higher mortality rates than those less exposed from all causes of death, but particularly from ischemic heart disease. The increase in mortality from this latter disease was directly correlated to the degree of exposure. There is widespread agreement that cardiovascular mortality diminishes when exposure stops, which contrasts with the proposed atherogenic action of carbon disulfide.[49] This finding suggests that carbon disulfide's effect is at least partially reversible and that in fact discontinuation results in cessation of some direct cardiotoxic or thrombotic action.[162]

Chronic morbidity has been examined in young people exposed occupationally to carbon disulfide. They presented a higher prevalence of hypertension than subjects of the same age who were not exposed to the gas.[92]

Carbon disulfide pathology is not often observed today, but the poisoning is still being studied. The mechanisms of action of the gas and the pathogenesis of the intoxication must be clarified, and the causal relations between vascular pathology and exposure must be investigated to establish the nontoxic level. Among exposed subjects there is an excess of mortality due to ischemic heart disease attributable to the toxin, but it is difficult to specify the exact roles of biochemical and functional parameters such as BP and lipid and carbohydrate metabolism that, if altered, constitute known risk factors for atherosclerosis.

Although it has been suggested that carbon disulfide concentrations below 30 to 35 mg/m³ (10 ppm) do not constitute a cardiovascular risk factor, the toxin can interfere with many of the body's structures and functions and is potentially toxic to different organs and systems. It therefore remains a risk factor and may act in synergy with other such factors, possibly facilitating the onset, or aggravating the course, of the pathology.[42,49]

Nitroderivatives

Nitroderivatives are used in dynamite factories to prepare explosive mixtures and lower the freezing point of dynamite and in the pharmaceutical industry. They enter the body mainly through the lungs and skin. The most serious pathology likely to result from their intake is the cardiac electrical withdrawal syndrome, also known as Monday morning syndrome, which may cause sudden death. Asymptomatic cardiac electrical disturbances have been reported.[187] Overload and impregnation syndromes mainly cause headache, peripheral vasodilation, and Raynaud's syndrome.[178] An association has been reported between occupational exposure to nitroderivatives and cardiac morbidity and mortality.[48]

From studies of the relations between environmental nitroglycerin and nitroglycol levels and cardiac alterations, a theory has been proposed to explain the causes of sudden death after exposure. The theory suggests that the withdrawal hazard does not result from cessation of the vasodilator effect of the nitroderivatives but is a rebound stimulation in response to the effect of inhalation of these substances on the production of endothelial prostaglandins, and especially on endothelial-derived relaxant factor. Stopping inhalation of the nitroderivatives would, according to this theory, remove a vascular and coronary protection mechanism in the case of generic cardiovascular toxins.[10,48,164]

Halogenated Hydrocarbons

Inhalation of halogenated hydrocarbons can cause poisoning not only among those exposed occupationally but also among "sniffers" and people using curative products in sprays or for domestic spot removal and the like. Their effect on the vascular system appears to be the result of their ability to sensitize the heart to the effects of endogenous and exogenous adrenaline, giving rise to rhythm disturbances and even sudden death.

Alterations of lipid metabolism have been observed after exposure to or inhalation of organic compounds generally referred to as solvents, such as amyl acetate, gasoline, liquid paraffin, monoiodoacetate, methylstyrene, 1,3-butadiene, and trichloroethylene.[89] Whether these compounds actually have an atherogenic effect, however, remains to be proved.

The possibility of long-term effects, arrhythmias, and dilative cardiomyopathies is based exclusively on sporadic reports on sniffers[187] and in a retrospective study on exposed workers.[47] There are even sporadic reports of stroke among young sniffers: the proposed pathogenic mechanism involves vasospasm secondary to inhalation of the substances as a result of receptor sensitization to circulating catecholamines.[27]

Epidemiological studies have found that many solvents (e.g., methylene hydrochloride, trichloroethane, fluorocarbons, phenol, and dinitrotoluene) can cause vascular disease. Methylene hydrochloride, for example, through its metabolism to CO, facilitates and can precipitate myocardial infarct. Other solvents cause cardiac sensitization, inducing fatal arrhythmias in subjects exposed to high doses. Epidemiological evidence suggests that more moderate doses of the fluorocarbon dichlorodifluoromethane cause vascular toxicity.[185] Among normotensive workers without renal pathology who are exposed to solvents, a significant rise was reported in the urinary superoxide dismutase, considered to be an early marker of pathological renal modification.[61]

Vinyl Chloride Monomer

Vinyl chloride monomer is a systemic toxin with particular vascular tropism. The endothelium is its target organ, so it acts on the tiny vessels of the extremities and the skin in the systemic circulation and the hepatic and splenic parenchymas. Vinyl chloride monomer poisoning affects various organs. Generally the clinical picture is of a syndrome of the extremities, in which Raynaud's phenomenon is associated with acro-osteohalisteresis and pseudoscleroderma. Poisoning often causes symptoms of central and peripheral nervous system impairment, hepatopathy, and pulmonary failure. Vinyl chloride monomer poisoning has an uncertain prognosis and responds poorly to therapy. Cessation of exposure leads to spontaneous regression of only some of the symptoms. The toxin is metabolized by hepatic microsomes, forming alkylating compounds that bind to biological structures and altering their antigenic properties. When the metabolites bind to plasma proteins the immune complexes formed can promote typical vascular lesions with perivasal inflammatory infiltrates.[90,187] Cutaneous, skeletal, pulmonary, and soft-tissue alterations are thus the outcome of repeated vascular occlusion. Some reports describe a high incidence of alterations to the vascular system, particularly hypertension, electrocardiographic (ECG) abnormalities (extrasystoles; altered atrioventricular or intraventricular conduction; P wave morphological anomalies; and signs of myocardial infarction, repolarization disturbances, and ECG anomalies indicating right heart involvement).[90,94,140,141]

Pesticides

In investigations of the relation between agricultural work and cardiovascular pathologies, much attention has been paid to the chemical risk in agriculture. Many studies in animals and humans have investigated the effects of acute exposure to pesticides. Cardiovascular effects have been reported after exposure to organophosphorus compounds (e.g., altered repolarization, arrhythmias, acute vascular insufficiency, and myocardiopathies),[15,82] to organochlorides (e.g., myocardial hyperexcitability, atherosclerosis, and ECG anomalies),[90,187] to carbamates (atherosclerosis),[90,187] to paraquat (heart failure),[90,187] and to dioxins (coronary disease and atherosclerosis).[90,93,187]

The cardiovascular effects of pesticides are highly complex and derive from an indirect mechanism resulting because many of these substances inhibit acetylcholinesterase, causing muscarinic and nicotinic effects, with consequent changes in cardiac activity (mainly a brief sympathetic discharge and persistent parasympathetic hypertonus).[73,138] Pesticides have direct cardiotoxicity through peroxidation of the cell membrane or action on the enzymes of oxidative phosphorylation.[187] It has been suggested that the organophosphorus compounds modify heart rhythm through effects on calcium ions.[11] Brezenoff [26] suggested their effect may also be linked to stimulation of the central muscarinic receptors. Koyama et al. showed that iminoctadine, a fungicide used widely in fruit culture, causes circulatory failure in humans and acute oral poisoning and vasodilatation in rats due mostly to its α_1-adrenoceptor antagonizing action and partly to endothelial-dependent mechanisms.[82,83,87]

Psychosocial–Occupational Factors

Stress

The roles of emotional factors, personality, psychosocial stress, and stressful events of life have been widely studied in the last 30 years in relation to the pathogenesis of vascular disease. Increasing attention is being paid now, as a result, to the possibility of psychosocial–occupational factors being involved in the etiology of vascular diseases, particularly coronary disease, and especially because several large-scale epidemiological studies[7,31,34,35, 44,67,71,104,114,165] have produced significant results. These factors may contribute to causing cardiovascular diseases through either a direct mechanism, whereby stress activates the adrenergic and hypothalamic–pituitary–adrenal systems, or an indirect mechanism, by aggravating the impact of conventional risk factors.

In the 1930s Selye defined *stress* as the organism's nonspecific response to demands on it.[150] Stimuli that induce this type of response, known as stressors, take numerous forms. Selye underlined that the response to stress was completely aspecific and stereotyped and served as a defense for the organism, as part of a general adaptation syndrome. This syndrome develops in three steps: the first is alarm, involving biochemical modifications; the second is resistance, in which the body organizes its defenses. In the third phase, exhaustion, the defenses fail and the ability to further adapt to the stressors is completely lost. Subsequent research showed that adaptation to stress can be triggered by emotional activation, depending on the nature and intensity of the stressors.[125,137] The response to different stressors requires activation of the hypothalamic–pituitary–adrenal system, the adrenal medullary catecholaminergic system, and the autonomic nervous system. This complex neuroendocrine mobilization ensures biological defense and provides the energy the body needs.[137] Stress is therefore not a pathological response but a physiologically useful one, enabling the organism to adapt to a wide variety of conditions. It can however become pathogenic if the stressor is not eliminated, and its persistence and intensity may cause the body's defenses to fail and thus enter the exhaustion phase. Circulating levels of corticos-

TABLE 11.8. Metabolic changes during stress.

Change		Mechanism	
Glucose	↑	Adrenaline	↑
		Thyroxine	↑
		17-hydroxycorticosteroid	↑
		Growth hormone	↑
		Insulin	↓
Nonesterified fatty acids	↑	Catecholamines	↑
Cholesterol	↑	17-hydroxycorticosteroid	
Triglycerides	↑ ↔	Catecholamines	↑
Platelet aggregation	↑	Nonesterified fatty acids	↑
		Catecholamines	↑
		Nonesterified fatty acids	↑

teroids and catecholamines rise, leading—in a series of metabolic steps—to increased concentrations of glucose and fatty acids; these high-energy compounds enable the body to cope with changes in its environment (Table 11.8). The neuroendocrine response to acute stress exhausts itself in a short time, especially when it is possible to control or eliminate the stressor through an appropriate behavioral response. In chronic stress situations, however, the final aim of removal of the stressor cannot be achieved or is inadequate; the biological activation then persists, leading to a tonic state that can exhaust the body's defense resources and eventually give rise to pathology.

Four main conditions are now known to involve a risk of vascular pathology: socioeconomic difficulties, chronic or hard-to-solve problems at work, lasting emotional disturbances, and type A behavioral modalities (see later section).[45] There are innumerable potential sources of stress at work: physical factors such as heat or noise, chemicals (e.g., direct cardiotoxins such as lead), and all the psychological or psychosocial stimuli that may bother an individual. The overall causes of stress at work can be classified under six main headings (Table 11.9).[68] Some factors arising routinely in certain working conditions may act as stressors: examples are too much or too little work, excessively rigid definition of tasks or the opposite, exasperation due to role conflicts, the absence or excess of responsibility, and the combination of high performance expectations and low decisional profile. The way work is organized may constitute a cause of stress: repetitive, monotonous jobs; monotony combined with the need for high levels of alertness; heavy psychophysical load; and heavy responsibility for others.[17,25,110]

TABLE 11.9. Causes of occupational stress.

- Factors intrinsic to the work
- Factors depending on relations with the outside world
- Retirement
- Career development and prospects
- Organizational climate and structure
- Relational factors within the work environment

One of the ways through which the organization of work and life in our technologically advanced society can contribute to aggravating cardiovascular disease risk is by selecting and motivating type A behavior, predisposing people to cardiovascular risk factors.[45] In daily clinical practice it has long been suspected that certain emotional features of vascular disease patients were somehow linked to the onset of the disease.[30] For instance, such patients have a tendency to get too involved emotionally in their work or to respond to life's different situations with a constant form of repressed aggression.

In the 1960s Rosenmann et al.[142] found a statistically significant association between coronary disease and the complex of personality and behavioral traits they defined as type A behavior pattern, subsequently referred to briefly as type A personality. Type A personality is defined as a particular behavioral–emotional pattern shown or possessed by an individual fighting chronically and excessively to obtain an unlimited number of things from his or her environment in the shortest possible time, despite the efforts and resistance of the persons and situations around the individual.[143] The characteristics of this type of personality have been defined operatively, distinguishing type A—predisposed to coronary disease—from its opposite, type B—at low risk of coronary disease. Type A people are usually fiercely competitive, constantly aggressive but controlled, impatient, and intolerant with people who work at a different rhythm; they feel the need to exercise constant, total control over their environments and are always in a hurry, trying constantly to pack a vast number of tasks into a limited time.

These emotional–behavioral traits are chronic or subchronic in all our daily activities but tend to become much more evident in jobs in which they are associated with high levels of achievement and yield. Thus type A individuals receive continual reinforcement from their environment to carry on with the same type of behavior. In work involving a high level of competition, those with the greatest productivity and best performance are recompensed not only economically but also socially. Type A individuals, therefore, are potentially predisposed to this type of behavior but certainly manifest it more or less openly depending on the social interactions around them. Type A individuals tend to make lifestyle choices, such as cigarette smoking, alcohol drinking, taking drugs and medicines, and limiting physical activity, that put them at risk for cardiovascular pathologies. Those with type A personalities live in a condition of chronic stress, in a continual "state of emergency" that ends up changing their blood chemistry and physical constants so that in the long run they become susceptible to coronary diseases. The predictive value of type A behavior in relation to cardiovascular disease has been confirmed.[33,45] This finding mainly reflects the fact that type A individuals do not have a one-dimensional personality and behavioral construct.[46] The personality and behavioral traits linked to hostility and aggressivity are now believed to be more significantly correlated to the predictivity for myocardial infarct than type A behavior as a whole.[29,45,46,68,69,114]

Shift Work

The term *shift work* is used in general to refer to any work schedule that interrupts the biological daily rhythm and/or social rhythms and thus refers not only to night shifts but also to rotating weekly shifts and the like. Shifts and night work are increasingly used to fully exploit technically advanced factories and make the most of their productive capacities. About 7% to 15% of the working population in the industrialized countries works night shifts, either regularly or occasionally. Numerous studies have found a correlation between shift work and coronary disease and/or the onset of hypertension.[3,4,8,16,24,62,75,76,89,116,122,124,161,165,189,190,191] Andersen[12] reported that the higher mortality from cardiovascular diseases in those in certain occupations—cooks, bakers, factory workers, domestic staff, emergency service drivers, hotel and restaurant personnel, and taxi drivers—may be linked to shift work. The greater risk of cardiovascular disease may persist in former shift workers even after changing schedules.[13,76,78,79,191] The combination of shift work and monotonous tasks or noise at work may raise the risk of myocardial infarction.[7,12]

Physical Agents

Ionizing radiation, vibration, and noise are among the particularly topical physical agents suspected of being cardiovascular risk factors.

Ionizing Radiation

The harmful effects of ionizing radiation on the vascular system have been well studied in patients receiving radiation therapy for tumors. Vascular alterations can usually be seen in the irradiated areas. These alterations are dose related and affect not only the large vessels but particularly the small ones, whose endothelia specifically show small-cell infiltrate, impairment of the internal lamina elastica (which presents hyalinosis and fragmentation), and alterations of the vasa vasorum.[19,58,107,120,123] The large vessels affected by radiation present marked, early atherosclerosis, with circumscribed calcifications in the arteries, necrosis of the aortic wall, fibrous hyperplasia of the intima, and parietal thrombosis (aortic arch syndrome). These findings are confirmed in experimental animals that develop early atherosclerosis of the large vessels after exposure to high-dose radiation.[43,149]

The alterations to microcirculation caused by high-dose ionizing radiation are well known, but the effects of lower doses have not been investigated much and are less clear-cut.[54,65,86–88] Chronic ionizing irradiation on the skin is a particular problem for health workers dealing with radioactive substances. The skin of the hands is the most frequent site of lesions, which may become disabling. Even moderate doses of ionizing radiation (less than 5 rem/y) may cause capillary occlusion through a process of hyperplasia/hypertrophy of the endothelial cells, visible with the capillaroscope.[171] The damage can be seen early in the skin microcirculation, the small vessels at the end of the terminal arterioles, and just above the terminal venules, with a caliber less than 30 μm. Chronic manifestations may follow either an acute radiodermatitis or repeated exposure to low doses, not enough on their own to induce clinical symptoms. The first clinical signs of chronic radiodermatitis are lesions mainly on the dorsal surface of the hands, especially on the extensor surfaces of the second and third phalanges, with frequent early involvement of the nail bed.[115,128]

Vibration

The vascular alterations caused by vibration have been widely investigated; they mainly involve angioneurotic signs and produce a picture of Raynaud's phenomenon, particularly for frequencies between 25 and 250 Hz. The causal relation between angioneurosis and the use of vibrating tools has long been established, and the condition is considered an occupational disease in most of the socially advanced countries.[176,179] The main cardiovascular symptoms include bradycardia, hypertension, and hypocoagulation.[52,89,141,187]

Recently Koiwa et al.[77] investigated whether the left ventricular relaxation rate could be modulated by phase-controlled mechanical vibration applied to the patient's anterior chest wall and whether there are some quantitative differences in the response of normal, hypertrophied, and failing ventricles. The study showed that phase-controlled, small-amplitude vibration on the chest wall can directly modulate left ventricular relaxation rate, especially in subjects with hypertrophy or failing ventricle.

Al Nashash et al.[8] recently described in subjects exposed for 15 minutes to vertical vibrations in the frequency range 5 to 30 Hz either depression or elevation of the ST segment of the ECG, indicating heart muscle fatigue.

Much less is known about the effects of generalized vibrations and the cerebrovascular system, but on the whole biomechanical effects appear to prevail over the strictly physiological ones.

Cardiovascular Effects of Noise

The question of pathology caused by noise is extremely important as industrial technology continues to develop, traffic grows, and the sources of sound pollution increase. Research is thus stimulated, with a view to preventing noise-induced damage on the human body (auditory and extraauditory effects) and on the economy, deriving from the high cost of industrial noise in terms of absenteeism for illness and reduced performance due to stress.

People have grown so used to noise that it is no longer possible to establish a threshold of tolerance. Noise may already cause harm to the hearing system at levels likely to be encountered in a routine traffic jam—90 dB. Clearly numerous types of work and industrial activities cause considerable auditory stress. Equally risky are habitual or emerging social habits involving large parts of the population, such as rifle shooting and the use of stereo earphones to listen to music at high volume. In most discotheques the threshold of 90 dB is largely exceeded, and in fact the sound level that causes extraauditory effects is probably lower.

Questions are now beginning to be asked about the emotional effects and effects on the central nervous system of various types of music such as rock and night music, with its strong symmetrical melodies and almost complete lack of high tones. The basic features of rock music are repetition and the use of low notes to arouse alarm reactions similar to those induced by certain natural rhythms and sounds. Rock music appears to overstimulate the brain, making it responsive only to the stimuli exceeding a certain threshold, which itself has risen as a result of exposure to this type of sound. Night music has the opposite effect of rock music, in that it combines repetition, echoes, and dissonance with natural, relaxing sounds such as those of the waves of the sea, the wind, or a waterfall. It is evocative and relaxing when it reduces muscle tension and induces regular breathing. However, it may have extremely exciting and disinhibiting effects when it presents low, repetitive sounds in crescendo, such as drum solos.

It would be useful to investigate neuronal reactions in the reticular formation of the brain stem and deep nuclei of the brain in relation to ECG recordings taken with the subject listening to these different types of music. Music as a form of communication has a topographic organization in the cerebral cortex fairly similar to verbal communication. The temporal and frontal areas of the left hemisphere decodify and shape all kinds of logical communication. These areas thus recognize the underlying structure of a piece of music and are employed in its composition. The right hemisphere, on the other hand, is involved in the emotional aspects of musical communication, as in verbal communication. Lesions to the right hemisphere can block the emotional understanding of music, just as they cause defects in grasping certain aspects of verbal communication. The emotional connotations of a piece of music, however, do not depend solely on the effects of the notes on the cerebral cortex but also call into play the ability to produce alarm reactions involving the subcortical and limbic centers.

There are innumerable reports of increases in various pathologies connected with noise. Nevertheless, a clear etiopathogenic and nosological definition is still lacking. Difficulties arise mainly from the fact that existing data are conflicting, the effects are not specific, and establishing a definite relation between the various physical characteristics of noise and their effects has never proved possible.

It can be presumed that extraauditory effects involve a series of nervous circuits acting on the cardiovascular, gastrointestinal, and neuroendocrine systems and on the mind and central nervous system; they may also use the autonomic nervous system as an efferent pathway. The autonomic connections between the auditory pathways and the reticular formation may explain the effects of noise on cortical arousal, pain, and sleep. The auditory apparatus can be viewed as a warning system that works by sending signals to the higher centers and, through the autonomic nervous system, prepares the individual to respond, using heart rate, vessels, muscles, and the adrenals as target systems (Table 11.10).

Exposure to noise has different effects on humans depending on the physical characteristics of the noise, the time and modality of exposure to it, and the individual's specific responsiveness. The duration of the noise and individual sensitivity are factors weighing in the balance of acoustic and general well-being. The most widely studied form of noise-induced damage is that involving the hearing apparatus. Pathologies of various types increase in relation to exposure to noise, the harm growing with exposure time, though not in direct proportion. The

lack of subjective sensations, or their scarcity, is not real proof of habituation to the noise.

The type of response varies in relation to the type of stimulus: sudden and intense or chronic and expected. Multiple factors may influence the effects of noise, the most important being the sound pressure, exposure time, and frequency. There are various strata of harmfulness, different methods of emission, with the presence of impulsive components and masking effects, the latter influencing mental fatigue, performance at work, and the rate of accidents at work. The spectral characteristics, presence of tonal components, infrasonic and ultrasonic waves, and recovery time must all be considered. Further factors are individual sensitivity, the "surprise" effect, semantic content, and identifiability of the sound source. Considering all these points allows us to draw some conclusions to help interpret the numerous, often discordant reports of the effects of noise on the body.

There are numerous responses to noise, but the central and peripheral nervous system responses are important, as are those of the respiratory apparatus and the endocrine, gastrointestinal, visual, reproductive, immune, and cardiovascular systems. The central and autonomic nervous systems respond in a wide variety of ways to noise, depending on the interactions between cortical structures, the limbic system, and reticular formation (Table 11.11). These different effects at different levels depend largely on the anatomical connections between the auditory pathways and the reticular substance, as

TABLE 11.10. Probable pathophysiological mechanisms of the extra-auditory effects of noise.

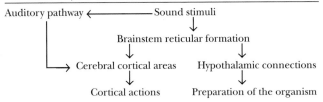

Prompt response: exhausts itself if the stimulus is repetitive
- Increased heart rate
- Increased blood pressure
- Increased respiratory frequency
- Increased gastric secretion and motility
- Increased adrenal hormone secretion
- Peripheral vasoconstriction

Delayed response
- May appear in response to expected stimuli
- Persists as long as the stimulus lasts
- Strength of response depends on sound level

TABLE 11.11. Summary of effects of noise on the central nervous system and mind.

Insomnia, tiredness, headache, speech difficulties, and muscle tension
Increased intracranial pressure
Increased motor nerve excitability
Electroencephalographic changes
Irritability, anxiety, depression, and aggressivity
Changes in output

Andrén L. *Acta Med Scand.* 1982;657:1. Aparicio-Ramon DV et al. *J Environ Pathol Toxicol Oncol.* 1993;12:237. Bach V et al. *Eur J Appl Physiol.* 1911;63:330. Belojevic G et al. *Int Arch Occup Environ Health.* 1992;64:293. Berglund B et al. *J Acoust Soc Am.* 1996;99:2985. Breschi MC et al. *Int J Neurosci.* 1994;75:73. Cetinguc M. *Aviat Space Environ Med.* 1992;63:905. Guignard JC, King PF. AGARD Conference Proceeding No 151. Washington DC: NATO, 1972. Hodge B, Thompson JF. *Lancet.* 1990;335:891. Ickes W, Espil J. *J Speech Hear Res.* 1979;22:334. Kryter KD. *Psychol Med.* 1990;20:1022. Levy-Le Boyer C. *Work Stress.* 1989;3:315. Lowry S. *BMJ.* 1990;13:211. Lyxell B et al. *Scand Audiol.* 1993;22:67. Melamed S et al. *Psychosom Med.* 1993;55:185. Nakamura H. *Eur J Appl Physiol.* 1994;68:62. Nakamura M et al. *Epilepsy Res.* 1994;17:249. Picano JJ. *Aviat Space Environ Med.* 1990;61:356. Smith A, Miles C. *Int Arch Occup Environ Health.* 1987;59:83. Smith AP. *Int Arch Occup Environ Health.*1988;60:307. Smith AP. *Int Arch Occup Environ Health.* 1990; 62:1. Sparrow D et al. *Circulation.* 1984;70:533. Stansfeld SA. *Psychol Med Monogr Suppl.* 1992;22:1. Wu TN et al. *Int Arch Occup Environ Health.* 1986; 60:99. Wu TN et al. *Am J Ind Med.* 1987;12:431. Wu TN et al. *Int Arch Occup Environ Health.* 1988;60:99.

well as between the hypothalamus and cortical centers. A main function of the hypothalamus is control of the autonomic nervous system. The posterior and lateral nuclei that control the sympathetic system induce responses linked to its activation: systemic hypertension, midriasis, piloerection, sweating, and NA and adrenaline release, with electroencephalographic and behavioral signs of arousal. The hypothalamus processes behavioral engrams and autonomic responses activated by natural conditions of satisfaction of instincts. Stimulation of the anterior hypothalamus may induce parasympathetic responses. The connections between the cortex and the tractus solitarius nucleus, between the cortex and limbic system, and between the cortex and hypothalamus appear to influence sympathetic output. The frontal cortex plays a major role: one of the main output pathways of the frontal cortex crosses the dorsal subthalamic and hypothalamic regions, influencing the activity of the visceral nuclei and thus controlling visceral responses and cardiac vulnerability. If exposure to noise is sufficiently protracted it may lead to pathology in the target organs.

An unexpected acoustic stimulus causes an orientation reaction; this alarm triggers activation of the sympathetic nervous system, with subsequent synaptic catecholamine release, and stimulates adrenal medullary output. If the stimulus continues the body moves into the adaptation step, with increased pituitary output of the adrenocorticotropic hormone; this increased secretion leads to stimulation of the adrenal cortex, which in turn releases and produces corticosteroids.

The impact of sound on the body is through a mechanism very similar to that of stress. The organism responds to frequent repeated stimuli with a series of adaptation reactions, each one stronger than the previous one, until the effector system is exhausted, at which point the risk arises of somatization of the damage. Insomnia—difficulty in falling asleep, waking early, and influence on the duration and quality of sleep—is a frequent effect of exposure to noise. Other effects are tiredness, headache, speech difficulty, and irritability. Exposure to loud noise may raise intracranial pressure and increase the excitability of motor nerves, reducing their chronaxy. Noise louder than 80 dB can cause electroencephalographic changes that vary in relation to the strength and duration of the stimulus. Predisposed subjects may suffer convulsions on exposure to noise. Low levels of noise in places where the work is monotonous may increase workers' performance, whereas exposure to the same levels of sound during work requiring concentration may reduce output.

The psychological effects of exposure to noise vary widely, depending on individual responses; these responses are mediated by emotional activation and cognitive assessment of the stimulus, taking the form of irritability, anxiety, arousal of conflict states, depression, and aggression, all of which affect a worker's efficiency and performance on the job. The effects of noise on the central nervous and neuroendocrine systems must be considered together (Table 11.12). Sound acts on the diencephalon and pituitary, activating the hypothalamus and pituitary and peripheral endocrine glands, raising the blood concentrations of glycocorticoids and mineralocorticoids and other hormones, while also increasing output of sympathomimetic amines through activation of the sympathetic system. These hormonal changes are followed by metabolic and hemodynamic changes.

Like the stress reaction chain, this phase of endocrine hyperfunction may be followed by a second phase of inhibition and/or adaptation; functional activity may eventually be restored—with a tendency to hyperactivity—during rest, until the organism's capacity to respond to a persistent stimulus is exhausted. It has been suggested that once they reach the central auditory nucleus, impulses travel across the reticular formation, reaching the hypothalamic nuclei, from which they reach the pituitary, with neuroendocrine effects, thus closing the auditory–hypothalamus–pituitary–endocrine system loop.

The hypothalamus plays a pivotal role in the interactions between the central nervous and endocrine systems. It serves as the control panel for the signals traveling to and from the superior nerve centers and the periphery. The hypothalamus sends the chemical messages to the pituitary, to control its secretory activity and circadian rhythm, and also to the brain areas responsible for behavioral output, such as the limbic cortex, which sends it important nerve fiber message patterns.

TABLE 11.12. Summary of effects of noise on the gastrointestinal and endocrine systems.

Gastrointentinal system
Increase or decrease in gastric motility
Changes in gastric secretion
Dyspepsia
Peptic and duodenal ulcers
    Bergmann JF et al. *Agressologie.* 1991;32:127. Gue M. *Digestive Diseases and Sciences.* 1987;32:1411. Pellegrini A et al. *Boll Soc Ital Biol Sper.* 1991;67: 111. Sonnenberg A et al. *Scand J Gastroenterol.* 1984;89:45. Sparrow D et al. *Circulation.* 1984;70:533. Tomei F et al. *Am J Ind Med.* 1994;26:367.

Endocrine system
Hyperactivity of the pituitary, thyroid, and adrenals
    Axelsson A, Lindgren F. *Acta Otolaryngol.* 1985;100:379. Colletti V. *Acta Otolaryngol.* 1987;104:217. Colletti et al. NATO Advanced Study Workshop, 1985. Dengerink HA et al. NATO Advanced Study Workshop, 1985. Duncan RC. *Environ Int.* 1993;19:359. Gamallo A. *Physiol Behav.* 1992;51:1201. Gue M. *Digestive Diseases and Sciences,* 1987;32:1411. Mallion JM et al. *Nouv Presse Med.* 1974;3:2003. Manninen O. *Int Arch Occup Environ Health.* 1988;60:249. Smookler HH, Buckey, JP. *Int J Neuropharmacol.* 1969;8:33. Softowa A. *Zantralb Allg Pathol.* 1983;127:85. Theorell T. *Scand J Work Environ Health.* 1990;16:74. Van Dijk FJH. *Int Arch Occup Environ Health.* 1986;58:321.

Acute exposure to noise immediately activates adaptation mechanisms, whether behavioral, endocrine, or autonomic, which work to reestablish the body's homeostasis by biological activation, the endocrine and autonomic systems providing the somatic backing the body needs to adapt, and by behavioral activation aimed at removing the stimulus. If the stimulus does in fact cease, the behavioral and biological mechanisms are rapidly disactivated and the body restores its normal balance.

As long as the response mechanisms can reestablish homeostasis the process can be considered normal. However, reestablishing homeostasis becomes gradually more difficult as the stimulus becomes chronic and behavioral activation can do nothing about it. The constant behavioral, endocrine, and autonomic activation needed, interacting with each individual's biological, psychological, and psychodynamic characteristics, can lead eventually to somatic or psychiatric pathology.

How exposure to noise affects the gastrointestinal system has been amply examined; increases or decreases in both gastric motility and secretion ulcers have been reported in relation to noise levels (Table 11.12). Dyspepsia due to gallbladder dyskinesia has also been reported in response to noise, spasm, and a significantly elevated incidence of peptic and duodenal ulcers[18,121,155,156] (Table 11.12). Our own studies have shown that these contrasting effects on gastric secretion may depend on differences in baseline secretion in the noise-exposed subjects.[172]

Exposure to noise may increase the respiratory rate and reduce vital capacity, with the extent varying by individual.[51] It has been reported that noise may even cause laryngeal disorders arising from the loss of audiophonic control because of the masking effect on verbal communications and vasomotor-congestive rhinopathies[37] (Table 11.13).

Effects on vision (important for drivers, pilots, etc.) have been described, with loss of visual acuity and color vision, narrowing of the visual field, midriasis, and accommodation problems. These disturbances appear to be due to interference with the nerve fibers connecting the diencephalic and cortical visual centers.[37,70,96,99] Recently a decrease in visual reaction time has been described in workers exposed to sound levels of between 90 and 113 dBA.[144] Effects on the reproductive system—reduced fertility, loss of libido, and influence on fetal development—have also been reported[2,74] (Table 11.13). In the immune system, noise may even affect the proliferative ability of lymphocytes[50,153,183] (Table 11.13).

The serious effects of noise on hearing are well known, but it has only recently been questioned whether noise may cause hypertension and cardiovascular disease. Noise appears to have a particularly marked effect, either direct or indirect, on the cardiovascular system. Investigations have been conducted in humans and animals exposed to acute and chronic noise, continuous or intermittent, industrial (e.g., metalworking, mechanical, textile, chemical, and other processes), town traffic, and white noise, with intensity up to 115 dBA. Most studies have considered the effects of noise louder than 85 dBA. Most investigators have concluded that noise, taken as a decisive etiological factor, raises heart rate (Table 11.14) and BP (Table 11.15), peripheral vascular resistances (Table 11.16), blood and urinary concentrations of NA, and often blood and urinary concentrations of adrenaline as well (Table 11.17).

The relations between auditory damage and hypertension have also been investigated, but few results have so

TABLE 11.13. Summary of effects of noise on the respiratory, reproductive, and immune systems.

Respiratory System
Increased respiratory frequency
Decreased vital capacity
    Berglund B et al. *J Acoust Soc Am.* 1996;99:2985. Cosa H, Nicoli M. Edizioni Scientifiche associate, Roma 1989. ESA, Roma, 1989. Fruhstorfer B, Hensel H. *J Appl Physiol Respirat Environ Exer Physiol.* 1980;49:985.

Reproductive system
Reduced fertility, loss of libido, and influence on fetal growth
    Agnew J et al. *Am J Ind Med.* 1991;19:433. Kisilevsky BS et al. *Obstet Gynecol.* 1989;73:971. Zhang J. *Am J Ind Med.* 1992;21:397.

Immune system
Influence on lymphocyte and monocyte proliferative capacity and on phagocytosis
    Freire-Garabal M et al. *Res Immunol.* 1993;122:311. Silve MJ. *Mut Res.* 1996;369:113. Weisse CS et al. *Brain Behav Immun.* 1990;4:339.

TABLE 11.14. Summary of effects of noise on heart rate.

Heart Rate
Increase
    Colletti V. *Acta Otolaryngol.* 1987;104:217. Duclos JC, Khaurand A. *Arch Mal Prof.* 1987;48:151. Fruhstorfer B. *J Appl Physiol Health.* 1980; 12:476. Green MS et al. *J Occup Med.* 1991;33:879. Gue M. *Digestive Diseases and Sciences.* 1987;32:1411. Kirby DA et al. *Physiol Behav.* 1984;32:779. Linden W et al. *Int J Psychophisiol.* 1985;3:67. Ortiz GA et al. *Hormone Res.*1974;5:57. Parrot J. *Int Arch Occup Environ Health.* 1992;63:477. Petiot JC et al. *Int Arch Occup Environ Health.* 1992;63:485. Ray RL et al. *Int J Psychophysiol.* 1984;1:335. Reinharez D. *Phlébologie.* 1989;42:215. Sanden A, Axellsson A. *Acta Otolaryngol.* 1981;92:75. Verdun di Cantohno L et al. *Acta Otolaryngol.* 1976;339:55. Wu TN et al. *Int Arch Occup Environ Health.* 1993;65:119.
Decrease
    Casazza F et al. *G Ital Cardiol.* 1977;7:829. Froelich GR. AGARD Conference Proceedings No 151 Washington DC: NATO, 1975.
No change
    Andrén L et al. *Acta Med Scand.* 1983;213:31. Baker CF. *Crit Care Nurs Q.* 1993;16:831. Cartwright LB, Thompson RH. *Am Ind Hyg Assoc J.* 1975;36:653. Franco G et al. *Med Lav.* 1976;67:511. Gold S et al. *J Occup Med.* 1989;31:933. Ising H et al. *Int Arch Occup Environ Health.* 1980;47:179. Kriter KD, Poza F. *J Acoust Soc Am.* 1980;67:2036. Peterson EA et al. *Science.* 1981;211:1450. Sonnenberg A et al. *Scand J Gastroenterol.* 1984;Suppl 89:45.

TABLE 11.15. Summary of effects of noise on blood pressure.

Blood pressure
Increase

Andrén L et al. *Acta Med Scand.* 1980;207:493. Andrén L et al. *Clin Sci.* 1981;61:89. Andrén L. *Acta Med Scand.* 1982;657:1. Andrén L et al. *Clin Sci.* 1982;62:137. Babish W et al. *Arch Environ Health.* 1988;43:407. Bartsch R et al. *Int Arch Occup Environ Health.* 1986;58:217. Belli S et al. *Am J Ind Med.* 1984;6:59. Cohen S et al. *Am Sci.* 1981;69:528. Colletti V et al. NATO Advanced Study Workshop, 1985. Ducan RC. *Environ Int.* 1993;19:359. Eggertsen R. *Acta Med Scand.* 1984;221:159. Eggertsen R et al. *Acta Med Scand.* 1987;221:159. Gamallo A et al. *Hormone Metab Res.* 1988;20:336. Gamallo A. *Physiol Behav.* 1992;51:1201. Green R. *Public Health Res.* 1991;19:277. Idzior-Walus B. *Eur Heart J.* 1987;8:1040. Ising H et al. *Int Arch Occup Environ Health.* 1980;47:179. Ising H. *Int Arch Occup Environ Health.* 1990;62:357. Jagaden D et al. *Arch Mal Prof.* 1986;47:15. Knipschild P, Salle H. *Int Arch Occup Environ Health.* 1979;44:55. Lahoz-Zamarro MT et al. *Acta Otorinolaringol Esp.* 1993;44:11. Lang T et al. *Int Arch Occup Environ Health.* 1992;63:369. Ledesert B. *Eur J Epidemiol.* 1994;10:609. Manninen O, Aro S. *Int Arch Occup Environ Health.* 1979;42:251. Manninen O. *Int Arch Occup Environ Health.* 1985;56: 251–274. Mazzuero G. *G Ital Cardiol.* 1989;19:1028. Michalak R. *Int Arch Occup Environ Health.* 1989;62:365. Milkovic-Kraus S. *Int Arch Occup Environ Health.* 1990;62:259. Nowak S. *Pol Merkuriusz Lek.* 1996;1:389. Ortiz GA et al. *Hormone Res.* 1974;5:57. Parvizpoor D. *J Occup Med.* 1976;18:730. Ray RL et al. *Int J Psychophysiol.* 1984;1:335. Rosenman KD. *Arch Environ Health.* 1984;39:218. Saha S et al. *Indian J Physiol Pharmacol.* 1996;40:35. Sokas RK. *Am J Ind Med.* 1997;31:188. Sonnenberg A et al. *Scand J Gastroenterol.* 1984;89:45. Talbott EO et al. *J Occup Med.* 1990;32: 685. Theorell T. *Scand J Work Environ Health.* 1990;16:74. Tomei F et al. *Int J Cardiol.* 1991;33:393. Tomei F et al. *Angiology.* 1992;43:904. Tomei F et al. *Int J Angiology.* 1995;4:117. Tomei F et al. *Med Lav.* 1996;87:394. Vacheron A. *Bull Acad Natl Med.* 1992;176:387. Van Dijk FJH et al. *Int Arch Occup Environ Health.* 1986;58:325. Van Dijk FJH et al. *Int Arch Occup Environ Health.* 1987;59:55. Verbeek JHAM et al. *Int Arch Occup Environ Health.* 1987;59:51. Verdun di Cantogno L et al. *Acta Otolaryngol.* 1976;339:55. Von Eiff AW et al. *Munch J Med Wochenscher.* 1981;123:420. Wright JW et al. *Hear Res.* 1985;17:41. Wu TN et al. *Int Arch Occup Environ Health.* 1988:60:99. Wu TN et al. *Int Arch Occup Environ Health.* 1993;65: 119–123. Zhao Y et al. *Br J Ind Med.* 1991;48:179.

Reduced diastolic BP

Bartsch R et al. *Int Arch Occup Environ Med.* 1986;58:217. Reinharez D. *Phlébologie.* 1989;42:215.

No change

Cartwright LB, Thompson RN. *Am Ind Hyg Assoc J.* 1975;36:653. Colletti V. *Acta Otolaryngol.* 1987;104:17. Garcia AM, Garcia A. *Med Clin Barc.* 1992;98:5. Hedstrand H et al. *Lancet.* 1977;2:1291. Hessel PA et al. *Arch Environ Health.* 1994;49:128. Hirai A et al. *J Hypertens.* 1991;9:1069. Lees REM, Roberts JH. *Can Med Assoc J.* 1979;120:1082. Lercher P et al. *Int Arch Occup Environ Health.* 1993;65:23. Malchaire JB, Mullier M. *Ann Occup Hyg.* 1979;22:63. Petiot JC et al. *Int Arch Occup Environ Health.* 1992;63:485. Sanden A, Axelsson A. *Acta Otolaryngol.* 1981;92:75. Santana VS, Barberino JR. *Rev Saude Publ.* 1995;29:478. Takala J et al. *Lancet.* 1977;2:974. Talbott E et al. *Am J Epidemiol.* 1985;121:501. Van Dijk FJH et al. *Int Arch Occup Environ Health.* 1987;59:55. Verbeek JHAM et al. *Int Arch Occup Environ Health.* 1987;59:51. Wu TN. *Int J Epidemiol.* 1996;25:791.

TABLE 11.16. Summary of effects of noise on the coronary disturbances and peripheral vascular resistances.

Coronary disturbances

Capellini A, Moroni M. *Med Lav.* 1974;65:297. Garcia AM, Garcia A. *Schriftenr Ver Wasser Boden Lufthyg.* 1993;88:212. Green MS et al. *Public Health Res.* 1992;19: 277. Idzior-Walus B, Walus B. *Eur Heart J.* 1987;4:1040. McHenry P et al. *Circulation.* 1984;70:547. Olsen O, Kristensen TS. *Epidemiol Community Health.* 1994;45:4. Tomei F et al. *Int J Cardiol.* 1991;33:393. Tomei F et al. *Angiology.* 1992;43:904. Tomei F et al. *Int J Angiology.* 1995;6:117. Vacheron A. *Bull Acad Natl Med.* 1992;176:387. Verdun di Cantogno L et al. *Acta Otolaryngol.* 1976;339(suppl):55.

Peripheral vascular resistances

Andrén L et al. *Acta Med Scand.* 1980;207:493. Andrén L et al. *Clin Sci.* 1981;61:89. Andrén L. *Acta Med Scand.* 1982;657:1. Bach V et al. *Eur J Appl Physiol.* 1991;63:330. Borg E. *Acta Otolaryngol.* 1978;83:153. Eggertsen R. *Acta Med Scand.* 1984;689:1. Eggertsen R et al. *Acta Med Scand.* 1987;221:159. Fruhstorfer B, Hensel H. *J Appl Physiol Respirat Environ Exer Physiol.* 1980;49:985. Ickes W, Espili J. *J Speech Res.* 1979;22:334. Kryter KD, Poza F. *J Acoust Soc Am.* 1980;67:2036. Millar K, Steels MJ. *Aviat Space Environ Med.* 1990;61:695. Neus H et al. *Int Arch Occup Environ Health.* 1980;47:9. Ortiz GA et al. *Hormone Res.* 1974;5:57. Petiot JC et al. *Int Arch Occup Environ Health.* 1992;63:485. Ray RL et al. *Int J Psychophysiol.* 1984;1:335. Tomei F et al. *Int J Cardiol.* 1991;33:393. Tomei F et al. *Angiology.* 1992;43:904. Tomei F et al. *Int J Angiology.* 1992;176:387. Vacheron A. *Bull Acad Natl Med.* 1992;176:387.

TABLE 11.17. Summary of effects of noise on biochemical and humoral indexes and myocardiac contractility and anatomy and histology of the myocardium and vessels.

Biochemical and humoral indexes

Altura BM. *Schriftenr Ver Wasser Boden Lufthyg.* 1993;88:65. Andrén L et al. *Clin Sci.* 1982;62:137. Babish W et al. *Arch Environ Health.* 1988;43:407. Borg E. *Acta Otolaryngol.* 1981;92:1. Friedman M et al. *Am J Physiol.* 1967;212:1174. Gamallo A. *Physiol Behav.* 1992;51:1201. Garcia AM, Garcia A. *Schriftenr Ver Wasser Boden Lufthyg.* 1993;88:212. Iwamoto M. *J Sound Vibrat.* 1988;127:431. Lercher P et al. *Int Arch Occup Environ Health.* 1993;65:23. Melamed S. *J Occup Environ Med.* 1996;38:252. Ortiz GA et al. *Hormone Res.* 1974;5:57–64. Rai RM et al. *Int Arch Occup Environ Health.* 1981;48:331. Reinharez D. *Phlébologie.* 1989;42:215. Rosenman KD. *Arch Environ Health.* 1984;39:218. Saha S et al. *Indian J Physiol Pharmacol.* 1996;40:35. Sanden A, Axelsson A. *Acta Otolaryngol.* 1981;92: 75. Schmid AP et al. *Biomed Biochem Acta.* 1989;48:453. Sudo A et al. *Ind Health.* 1996;34:279. Turkkan JS et al. *Physiol Behav.* 1984;33:21. Yamamura K, Aoshima K. *Eur J Physiol.* 1980;44:9.

*Myocardiac contractility and anatomy and
histology of the myocardium and vessels*
Reduced cardiac output

Lehmann G. *Intern Z Angew Physiol.* 1956;16:217. Taccola A, Franco G. *Lavoro Umano.* 1963;15:571.

Morphological changes to the myocardium and atheromatous lesions in the aorta and medium-caliber arteries.

Friedman M et al. *Am J Physiol.* 1967;212:1174. Pellegrini A. *Submicrosc Cytol Pathol.* 1996;28:507. Scano A. *Minerva Aerospaziale.* 1989;1:20. Softowa A. *Zentralb Allg Pathol.* 1983;127:85.

far been reported, and they tend to be too contradictory to permit any firm conclusions. In our studies we started from the assumption that noise, depending on its intensity and duration, the type, and individual susceptibility, may have effects at different thresholds for different systems (cardiovascular and auditory) and cause different types and degrees of damage: hearing deficits, hypertension, or both.

Although coronary disorders have been investigated less than the other variables, it does seem widely acknowledged that exposure to noise may induce them, especially in people who have already had coronary disease (Table 11.17). Noise appears to cause direct and indirect changes in cardiovascular dynamics and in the myocardial and vascular structure and histology[126] (Table 11.17).

We still do not understand the pathophysiological mechanism by which these cardiovascular and humoral changes arise. The most widely accepted theory is that they are due to stimulation of the adrenergic system, with repercussions on the pituitary–adrenal axis as well.[111,144,145,161]

In light of this theory, much work has been done to investigate blood and urinary concentrations of NA and adrenaline and—less extensively—corticosteroids and adrenocorticotropic hormone in blood and urinary 17-OH corticosteroids. Pharmacological block of adrenergic receptors has provided interesting information: the rise in BP is not prevented by blocking α-receptors and β-receptors, although pressure is lower than with placebo in the same experimental conditions.

β-Blockade helps protect people with coronary disease from the effects of noise. Peripheral vascular resistances appear to be elevated in noise-exposed hypertensive patients treated with β-blockers, whereas blocking α-receptors has no such effect. In our own studies we worked on the hypothesis that the postural drop in BP is a more sensitive sign of cardiovascular effects, responding to lower noise levels than hypertension and ECG anomalies.[173–175]

It has still not been clarified—or even widely investigated—how chronic noise affects the cardiovascular system. Our theory was that baroceptor sensitivity may be altered as a consequence of chronic sympathetic activation in response to chronic noise. This activation would result in exposure to high catecholamine levels, with consequent catecholamine depletion and/or reduced catecholamine response, partly due to β-receptor desensitization, which is reversible for only a certain time. Initially the mechanism serves to protect against arrhythmias and toxic effects on the myocardium.

The different effects on the cardiovascular apparatus may therefore depend on whether the clinical or experimental investigation is done in the early, intermediate, or chronic phases of noise exposure. Studies are also needed to check whether low-frequency noise has greater or more specific hypertensive action on the cardiovascular system.

Occupational Venous Diseases

Venous disease constitutes a large and still rising category of social pathology. The importance and role of venous disorders in the world of work are amply documented because these pathologies, which may afflict from 10% to 40% of a population, create considerable demand for medical care and hospital admissions and cause long- or short-term absence from work and disability.[9,14,38,95,100,117,167,187] Clinical and epidemiological studies of the topic are not numerous but highlight the importance of varicose disease.[28,32,40,60,64,97,98,103,109,112, 169,170,182]

Varicose veins in the legs hold seventh place among chronic ailments in the United States, and 17% of the population suffers in the United Kingdom. In France an average of 65,000 saphenectomies are performed every year; it is the fifth most frequent type of surgery in the nation, and third as regards costs for only one type of operation. Recent statistics indicate that about 10% of the Italian population over 40 years of age has varicose veins, including 1 out of 5 women and 1 out of 15 men.[32,38,59]

The social cost is heavy. It has been estimated that venous pathology of the legs caused a mean loss of 22 working days per person per year.[32,168] One third of the people who suffer venous diseases eventually become either partially or totally disabled, 16% have to change their jobs, and 10% are left total invalids.[59] Besides the medical costs actually related to them, varicose veins tend to become disabling and give rise to a high incidence of complications, sometimes serious. A study of patients admitted to hospitals in Piedmont for vascular diseases between 1976 and 1987 found that varicose veins of the legs reached the highest rate of hospital admissions, with 4794 cases per year, rising to 6980 if complications such as thrombophlebitis and pulmonary embolism were included.[132,133]

The critical review by Alexander[5] showed that varices were common in industrial societies but infrequent in primitive ones. Many of the factors associated with the higher incidences could be excluded as main causes but may well serve to accelerate the process, acting on veins that were already more susceptible because of the mainly sedentary Western lifestyle.

It does appear that venous pathology is often either totally or partially caused by occupational factors. Few reports have been published on the relationships between venous disease and work, and they provide incomplete and discordant data.[28,40] This result reflects the variety of methods adopted and the almost universal lack of any real analysis of the workers' jobs (only broad occupational categories rather than specific tasks are usually used) and place of work.

With specific reference to work, it is widely believed that the workers who most commonly suffer varicose veins are cooks, ironing staff, foundry workers, surgeons, dentists, assembly line workers, retail sales staff, hairdressers, housewives, waiters, textile workers, teachers, and bank clerks. Such workers' hydrodynamic factors are altered by long periods of standing or by too little movement.[98] One of the most important occupational factors that influences venous pathology is in fact the body posture at work, although there is disagreement as to the relative weights of standing, walking, and sitting.[60,98,100]

An identifiable risk factor that we believe has probably the greatest weight is having to stand for long periods. Data regarding walking and sitting seem less important because walking around during work is usually limited to small movements and working in a sitting position certainly is less important than standing. A significantly higher prevalence of varicose veins was found among workers of both sexes who spent a lot of time standing compared with those who walked around or worked seated.[1,32,85,109,136,160] There is also a considerably higher prevalence of venous thromboembolism among subjects who spend a lot of time on their feet compared with other categories of workers.[135] The duration of standing is also important: standing for more than 8 hours a day is particularly related to varicose veins.[134,170] Prolonged standing combined with limited physical activity facilitates the onset of varices; this may explain the different frequencies of the disease among industrial workers (especially the textile and metal-mechanical sectors)—1160 out of 100,000 insured—and workers in commerce (679 out of 100,000 insured) and agriculture (627 out of 100,000 insured).[14] Furthermore, the incidence of admissions to hospitals seems to be higher during the years of work (particularly for blue-collar workers rather than for pensioners, housewives, and students).[134]

Marshall[103] underlined the considerable medical and socioeconomic impact of chronic venous diseases, which often appear during a person's working life. In Germany such diseases cause 2500 cases of pensionable disability every year. However, chronic venous pathology has not been recognized by sickness insurance organizations and social medicine, so it is often difficult to obtain treatment and rehabilitation at work for people suffering from varices. Although Marshall maintains that it is difficult to show that venous diseases are occupational diseases, they must be borne in mind in the field of occupational medicine because jobs that require standing cause appreciable fatigue in the peripheral venous system. Heavy work and venous system trauma are other potential causes of thrombosis. There appear to be various connections between the treatment of venous pathology

and work. The effectiveness of compression bandages, for example, is negatively influenced by sedentary work.

An unequivocal influence on the frequency of varicose veins was also attributed to lifting weights during work[32] and to heavy work.[14] Another risk factor is the possible role of the microclimate in the workplace, because the prevalence of varices was higher among people exposed to high temperatures.[32,98]

Our group[169] studied 150 workers with venous disease. We recorded their types of occupation, family histories, social classes, ages, and sexes. Subjects who spent long periods standing at work presented ectasia and insufficiency of the internal saphenous vein and often had superficial dermohypodermatitis and ulcers, which tended not to heal because of the poor blood flow to the lower perforator veins. Workers who moved around more during their work presented a lower prevalence of venous disease and dermatitis and fewer ulcers. In a subsequent investigation[170] we studied 447 men from three different occupational categories: 151 industrial workers, 159 construction workers, and 137 office employees. They completed a targeted questionnaire regarding occupational and extraoccupational risk factors for venous diseases, focusing on the time spent standing, walking, and sitting at work. Each subject received a general clinical examination and a venous check-up, both lying down and standing. The three groups of workers were comparable regarding age, family history, and conventional risk factors for venous disease. The findings indicated that the industrial workers were at high risk of venous disease (38.4%), compared with the construction workers (25.1%) and office employees (22.6%). The main risk factor in this case list was standing for half or more of the working day.

It thus appears that venous diseases are often related to occupational causes, which frequently become decisive on their own or in combination with other factors. These pathologies often lead to temporary or permanent disability of some degree and even severe complications (pulmonary embolism). Occupational medicine should therefore pay more attention to venous diseases and their relationship with the patient's job, aiming at prevention and early hygienic–therapeutic measures rather than viewing the question simply as a matter of suitability for a job. The future development of relations between occupation and onset of venous diseases will require establishment of preventive measures and treatments applicable on the job. Preventive measures will involve better organization of work (alternating tasks and introducing active breaks when workers can move around); measures will have to be taken to identify subjects at risk when hiring them; and periodic checkups must be planned to detect early signs of venous problems and therapy recommended, such as elastic hosiery. Such measures would not only reduce or at least delay the onset of this pathology but also avoid its complications and the risk of permanent disability.

References

1. Abramson JH, Hopp C, Epsein LM. The epidemiology of varicose veins. A survey in western Jerusalem. *J Epidemiol Community Health.* 1981;35:213.

2. Agnew J, McDiarmid MA, Lees PS, Duffy R. Reproductive hazards of fire fighting, I: Non-chemical hazards. *Am J Ind Med.* 1991;19:433–445.

3. Akerstedt T, Knutsson A, Alfredsson L, Theorell T. Shift work and cardiovascular disease. *Scand J Work Environ Health.* 1984;10:409.

4. Akerstedt T, Knutsson A. Cardiovascular disease and shift work. *Scand J Work Environ Health.* 1997;23:241.

5. Alexander CJ. The epidemiology of varicose veins. *Med J Aust.* 1972;1:215.

6. Alfredsson L, Karasek R, Theorell T. Myocardial infarction risk and psychosocial work environment: an analysis of the male Swedish working force. *Soc Sci Med.* 1982;16:463.

7. Alfredsson L, Spetz CL, Theorell T. Type of occupation and near-future hospitalization for myocardial infarction and some other diagnoses. *Int J Epidemiol.* 1985;14:378.

8. Al Nashash H, Qassem W, Zabin A, Othman M. ECG response of the human body subjected to vibrations. *J Med Eng Technol.* 1996;20:2.

9. Alos J, Carreno P. Coexistencia en nuestro medio de los factores de riesgo en los pacientes con sindromo varicoso. *Angiologia.* 1992;13:17.

10. Amnon BD. Cardiac arrest in an explosives factory worker due to withdrawal from nitroglycerin exposure. *Am J Ind Med.* 1989;15:719.

11. Anand M, Gulati A, Gopal K, Khanna RN, Ray PK. Changes in cardiac rhythm and calcium levels in guinea pigs treated chronically with Fenitrothion. *Toxicol Environ Chem.* 1989;24:199.

12. Andersen O. *Mortality and Occupation 1970–1980.* Copenaghen: Danmarks Statistik; 1985.

13. Angersbach D, Knauth P, Loskant H, Karvonen MJ, Undeutsch K, Rutenfranz J. A retrospective cohort study comparing complaints and diseases in day and shift workers. *Int Arch Occup Environ Health.* 1980;45:127.

14. Bartolo M. Socioeconomic impact of venous diseases in Italy. *Phlébologie.* 1992;45:423.

15. Bataillard A, Sannajust F, Yoccoz D, Blauchet G, Sentenoc-Roumanous IT, Savarol J. Cardiovascular consequences of organophosphorus poisoning and of antidotes in conscious unrestrained rats. *Pharmacol Toxicol.* 1990;67:27.

16. Baumgart P, Walger P, Fuchs G, v. Eiff M, Vetter H, Rahn KH. Diurnal variations of blood pressure in shift workers during day and night shifts. *Int Arch Occup Environ Health.* 1989;61:463.

17. Beilin LJ. Stress, coping, lifestyle, and hypertension: a paradigm for research, prevention, and non pharmacological management of hypertension. *Clin Exp Hypertens.* 1997; 19:739.

18. Bergmann JF, Caulin C, Geneve J, Simoneau G, Segrestaa JM. Effect of psychological stress on gastric potential difference in man. *Agressologie.* 1991;32:127.

19. Boivin J, Hutchison GB. Coronary heart disease mortality after irradiation for Hodgkin's disease. *Cancer.* 1982;49: 2470.

20. Boscolo P, Carmignani M, Carelli G, Finelli VN, Giuliano G. Zinc and copper in tissues of rats with blood hypertension induced by long-term lead exposure. *Toxicol Lett.* 1992;63:135.

21. Boscolo P, Carmignani M, Preziosi P, Giuliano G. Regolazione della funzione vascolare e cardiaca nella esposizione cronica sperimentale a metalli tossici. *Atti 51° Congresso Nazionale Società Italiana Medicina Lavoro Igiene Industriale.* 1988;1:337.

22. Boscolo P, Carmignani M, Preziosi P, Giuliano G, Luongo F. Esposizione cronica a piombo e ipertensione arteriosa. Meccanismi di azione del tossico sul sistema di regolazione pressoria. *Min Angiol.* 1990;15:405.

23. Boscolo P, Carmignani M, Preziosi P, Giuliano G. Meccanismi di tossicità dell'esposizione cronica a piombo sul sistema che regola la pressione arteriosa. *Atti 53° Congresso Nazionale Società Italiana Medicina Lavoro Igiene Industriale.* 1990;2:1007.

24. Boucsein W, Oltmann W. Psychophysiological stress effects from the combination of night shift-work and noise. *Biol Psychol.* 1996;42:301.

25. Bourbonnais P, Brisson C, Moisan J, Vezina M. Job strain and psychological distress in white collar workers. *Scand J Work Environ Health.* 1996;22:139.

26. Brezenoff HE, Giuliano R. Cardiovascular control by cholinergic mechanism in the central nervous system. *Ann Rev Pharmacol Toxicol.* 1982;22:341.

27. Brust JCM. Stroke and drugs. In: Vinken PJ, Bruyn GW, Klawans HL, eds. *Handbook of Clinical Neurology: Vascular Diseases.* Vol 55. Part III. Amsterdam: Elsevier; 1986:517.

28. Callam MJ. Epidemiology of varicose veins. *Br J Surg.* 1994; 81:167.

29. Caprara GV, Pastorelli C. Toward a reorientation of research on aggression. *Europ J Personal.* 1989;3:121.

30. Carasso R, Yehuda S, Ben-Uriah Y. Personality type, life events, and sudden cardiovascular attack. *Int J Neurosci.* 1981;14:223.

31. Cas LD, Metra M, Nodari S, Nardi M, Giubbini R, Visioli O. Stress and ischemic heart disease. *Cardiologia.* 1993; 38(suppl 1):415.

32. Catilina P, Domont A, Dreyfus JP, et al. Chronic venous insufficiency in the workplace today. *Proceedings of the 24th International Congress on Occupational Health.* Nice; 1993: 2–13.

33. Cesana GC, Ferrario M, Sega R, Duzioni F, Zanettini R, Grieco A. Nuovi problemi in medicina del lavoro: indagine sul rischio di coronaropatia nel terziario. *Med Lav.* 1989;80:192.

34. Cesana GC, Poncato E, Tenconi MT, et al. Indagine psicometrica delle misure dei comportamenti predisponenti alla coronaropatia (Tipo A) in popolazioni lavorative, I: La scala di Bortner. *Med Lav.* 1988;79:110.

35. Chapman A, Mandryk JA, Frommer MS, Edye BV, Fergu-

son DA. Chronic perceived work stress and blood pressure among Australian government employees. *Scand J Work Environ Health.* 1990;16:258.

36. Cooper WC, Wong O, Kheifets L. Mortality among employees of lead battery plants and lead producing plants 1947–1980. *Scand J Work Environ Health.* 1985;11:331.

37. Cosa M, Nicoli M. *Valutazione e controllo del rumore e delle vibrazioni.* Roma: Edizioni Scientifiche Associate; 1989.

38. Cottenot F, Carton FX, Tessler L. Incidences èconomiques du mode de traitement des ulcères de jambe. *Phlébologie.* 1979;32:333.

39. Davies JM. Long term mortality studies of chromate pigment workers who suffered lead poisoning. *Br J Ind Med.* 1984;41:170.

40. De Backer G. Epidemiology of chronic venous insufficiency. *Angiology.* 1997;48:569.

41. Dingwall-Fordyce I, Lane RE. A follow-up study of lead workers. *Br J Ind Med.* 1963;20:313.

42. Drexler H, Uhm K, Hubmann M, et al. Carbon disulphide, III: Risk factors for coronary heart diseases in workers in the viscose industry. *Int Arch Occup Environ Health.* 1995; 67:243.

43. Dudchenko NN, Okladnikova ND. Ischemic heart disease in workers of radiochemical industry chronically exposed to radiation dosage less than MPEL. *Med Tr Prom Ekol.* 1995;6:7.

44. Emdad R, Belkic K, Theorell T. Cardiovascular dysfunction related to threat, avoidance, and vigilant work: application of event-related potential and critique. *Integr Physiol Behav Sci.* 1997;32:202.

45. Eysenck HJ. Personality as a risk factor in coronary heart disease. *Europ J Personal.* 1991;5:81.

46. Eysenck HJ. Type A behaviour and coronary heart disease: the third stage. *J Soc Behav Personal.* 1990;5:25.

47. Flesch-Janys D, Berger J, Gurn P, et al. Exposure to polychlorinated dioxius and furans (PCDD/F) and mortality in a cohort of workers from a herbicide producing plant in Hamburg, Federal Republic of Germany. *Am J Epidemiol.* 1995;142:1165.

48. Forman SA, Helmkamp JC, Bone CM. Cardiac morbidity and mortality associated with occupational exposure to 1,2 propylene glycole dinitrate. *JOM.* 1987;29:445.

49. Franco G, Candura F. Aspetti vascolari della tossicità da solfuro di carbonio: epidemiologia, meccanismi d'azione e ipotesi patogenetiche. *Atti 51° Congresso Nazionale Società Italiana Medicina del Lavoro Igiene Industriale.* 1988;1:167.

50. Freire-Garabal M, Nunez MJ, Fernandez-Rial JC, Couceiro J, Garcia-Vallejo L, Rey-Mendez M. Phagocytic activity in stressed mice: effects of alprazolam. *Res Immunol.* 1993; 144:311.

51. Fruhstorfer B, Hensel H. Extra-auditory responses to long-term intermittent noise stimulation in humans. *J Appl Physiol Respirat Environ Exer Physiol.* 1980;49:985.

52. Gasakure E, Massin N. Revue bibliographique des principaux facteurs étiologiques des maladies cardio-vasculaires "professionelles." *Arch Mal Prof.* 1991;57:477.

53. Gatagonova TM. Functional state of the cardiovascular system in workers employed in lead production. *Med Tr Prom Ekol.* 1995;1:15.

54. Gelas M, Giraud M, Righi E, Tobajas L. Medical surveillance of workers exposed to ionizing radiations. *Med Lav.* 1994;85:193.

55. Giridhar J, Isom GE. Alteration of atrial natriuretic peptide levels by short term cadmium treatment. *Toxicology.* 1991;70:185.

56. Giridhar J, Rathinavelu A, Isom GE. Interaction of cadmium with atrial natriuretic peptide receptors: implication for toxicity. *Toxicology.* 1992;75:133.

57. Glueck CJ, Kelley W, Wang P, Gartside PS, Black D, Tracy T. Risk factors of coronary heart disease among firefighters in Cincinnati. *Am J Ind Med.* 1996;30:331.

58. Gomory JM, Levy P, Weshler Z. Radiation induced aneurysm of the basilar artery: a case report. *J Vasc Dis.* 1987;3:147.

59. Gorin JP, Nossin F, Radier P. Quelques aspects èconomiques de la chirurgie des varices. Pladoyer pour un traitement ambulatoire. *Phlébologie.* 1979;32:325.

60. Griton PH, Escalie R, Imbert M, Cuffit A. La maladie variques: étude épidémiologique, à propos de 1600 cas. *Phlébologie.* 1987;40:923.

61. Gruener N. Early detection of changes in kidney function in workers exposed to solvents and heavy metals. *Isr J Med Sci.* 1992;28:605–607.

62. Hakola T, Harma MI, Laitinen JT. Circadian adjustment of men and women to night work. *Scand J Work Environ Health.* 1996;22:133.

63. Hinderliter AL, Kirkwood FA, Price CJ, Herbst MC, Koch G, Sheps DS. Effects of low-level carbon monoxide exposure on resting and exercise-induced ventricular arrhythmias in patients with coronary artery disease and no baseline ectopy. *Arch Environ Health.* 1989;44:89.

64. Hopewell JW, Calvo W, Jaenke R, Reinhold HS, Robbins MEC, Whitehouse EM. Microvasculature and radiation damage. Recent Results. *Cancer Res.* 1993;130:1.

65. Hopkins PN, Williams RR. A survey of 246 suggested coronary risk factors. *Atherosclerosis.* 1981;40:1.

66. Horowitz SF, Fischbein A, Matza D, et al. Evaluation of right and left ventricular function in hard metal workers. *Br J Ind Med.* 1988;45:742.

67. Hurrel JJ, Murphy LR. Occupational stress intervention. *Am J Ind Med.* 1996;29:338.

68. Jaffe MP, Smolmsky MH, Wun CC. Sleep quality and physical and social well being in North American petrochemical shiftworkers. *South Med J.* 1996;89:305.

69. Hobson J. Venous insufficiency at work. *Angiology.* 1997; 48:577–582.

70. Jansen G. Noise as a cause of disease. *Dtsch Med Wochenschr.* 1967;92:2325.

71. Jenkins CD. Psychosocial risk factors for coronary heart disease. *Acta Med Scand.* 1982;660(suppl):123.

72. Kaye WE, Novotny T, Tucker M. New ceramics-related industry implicated in elevated blood lead levels in children. *Arch Environ Health.* 1987;42:161.

73. Khosla SN, Nitya N, Kumar P. Cardiovascular complications of aluminium phosphide poisoning. *Angiology.* 1988; 355:359.

74. Kisilevsky BS, Muir DW, Low JA. Human fetal responses to sound as a function of stimulus intensity. *Obstet Gynecol.* 1989;73:971.

75. Knutsson A, Akerstedt T, Jonsson BG. Prevalence of risk factors for coronary artery disease among day and shift workers. *Scand J Work Environ Health.* 1988;14:317.

76. Knutsson A. Shift work and coronary heart disease. *Scand J Soc Med.* 1989;17:1.

77. Koiwa Y, Honda H, Takagi T, Kikuchi J, Itoshi N, Takashima T. Modification of human left ventricules relaxation by small amplitude, phase-controlled mechanical vibration on the chest wall. *Circulation.* 1997;95:156.

78. Koller M, Kundi M, Cervinka R. Field studies of shift work at an Austrian oil refinery, I: health and psychosocial well being of workers who drop out of shift-work. *Ergonomics.* 1978;21:835.

79. Koller M. Health risks related to shift work. *Int Arch Environ Health.* 1983;53:59.

80. Kopp SJ, Barron JT, Tow JP. Cardiovascular actions of lead and relationship to hypertension: a review. *Environ Health Prospect.* 1988;78:91.

81. Koskela RS. Cardiovascular diseases among foundry workers exposed to carbon monoxide. *Scand J Work Environ Health.* 1994;20:286.

82. Koyama K, Goto K, Yamashita M. Circulatory failure caused by a fungicide containing iminoctadine and a surfactant: a pharmacological analysis in rats. *Toxicol Appl Pharmacol.* 1994;126:197.

83. Koyama K, Yamashita M, Miyauchi T, Goto K. A fungicide containing iminoctadine causes circulatory failure in acute oral poisoning. *Vet Hum Toxicol.* 1993;35:512.

84. Koyama K, Yamashita M, Miyauchi T, Goto K. Mechanisms of hypotension in iminoctadine poisoning: pharmacological analysis in rats. *Eur J Pharmacol.* 1994;270:151.

85. Krijnen RM, de Boer EM, Ader HJ, Bruynzeel DP. Venous insufficiency in male workers with a standing profession, I: epidemiology. *Dermatology.* 1997;194:111.

86. Krishnan EC, Krishnan L, Botteron GW, Dean RD, Jewell WR. Effect of irradiation on microvasculature: a quantitative study. *Cancer Detect Prev.* 1987;10:121.

87. Krishnan EC, Krishnan L, Jewell B, Bhatia P, Jewell WR. Dose dependent radiation effect on microvasculature and repair. *J Natl Cancer Inst.* 1987;79:1321.

88. Krishnan L, Krishnan EC, Jewell WR. Immediate effect of radiation on microvasculature. *Int J Radiat Oncol Biol Phys.* 1988;15:47.

89. Kristensen TS. Cardiovascular diseases and the work environment: a critical review of the epidemiologic literature on nonchemical factors. *Scand J Work Environ Health.* 1989;15:165.

90. Kristensen TS. Cardiovascular diseases and the work environment: a critical review of the epidemiologic literature on chemical factors. *Scand J Work Environ Health.* 1989; 15:245.

91. Krstev S, Mitic V, Farkic B. Evaluation of health status among workers exposed to carbon disulphide. *Arh Hig Rada Tksikol.* 1989;40:221.

92. Krstev S, Perunicic B. Some epidemiological characteristics of hypertension related to occupation. *Med Lav.* 1986;67:90.

93. Kurppa K, Hietanen E, Klockars M. Chemical exposures at work and cardiovascular morbidity: atherosclerosis, ischemic heart disease, hypertension, cardiomyopathy, and arrhythmias. *Scand J Work Environ Health.* 1984;10:381.

94. Laplanche A, Clavel F, Contassot JC, Lanouziere C. Exposure to vinyl chloride monomer: report on a cohort study. *Br J Ind Med.* 1987;44:711.

95. Laurikka J, Sisto T, Auvinen O, Tarkka M, Läärä M, Hakama M. Varicose veins in Finnish population aged 40–60. *J Epidemiol Community Health.* 1993;47:355.

96. Leturneau JE. The effect of noise on vision. *Eye, Ear, Nose Thr Monthly.* 1972;51:441.

97. Lorenzi G, Bavera P, Cipolat L, Carlesi R. The prevalence of primary varicose veins among workers of a metal and steel factory. In: Davy A, Stemmer R, eds. *Plebology '85.* Paris: John Libbey Eurotext; 1986:163–165.

98. Lorenzi G. General and occupational risk factors in the etiology of varicose veins. In: Davy A, Stemmer R, eds. *Phlebology '89.* Paris: John Libbey Eurotext; 1989:315–318.

99. Loth MD. Rapport initial sur les recherches effectuées sur le thème: Bruit- Santé. Ministère Environnement, Collect. Recherche Environn; 1983.

100. Maffei FH, Magaldi C, Pinho SZ, et al. Varicose veins and chronic venous insufficiency in Brazil: prevalence among 1755 inhabitants of a country town. *Int J Epidemiol.* 1986; 15:210.

101. Magnavita N, Sacco A. Effetti nefrotossici e cardiovascolari dei metalli pesanti cadmio e piombo. *Archivio Scienze Lavoro.* 1989;5:187.

102. Marek K, Zajac Nezola M, Rala E, Wocka Maiek T, Languarer Lewowicka H, Witecki K. Examination of health effects after exposure to metallic mercury vapors in workers engaged in production of chlorine and acetic aldehyde, I: evaluation of general health status. *Med Pr.* 1995;46:101.

103. Marshall M. Chronic venopathies in occupational and social medicine. *Arbeitsmed Sozialmed Praventivmed.* 1988; 23:3.

104. Martin JK, Blun TC, Beach SR, Roman PM. Subclinical depression and performance at work. *Soc Psychatry Psychiatr Epidemiol.* 1996;31:3.

105. Mason H, Somervaille L, Wright A, Chettle D, Scott M. The renin-angiotensin axis and urinary kallikrein excretion in lead exposed workers. *Proceedings of the 7th International Conference: Heavy Metals in the Environment.* Vol 2. Geneva; 1989:254.

106. Mazzella Di Bosco M, Esposito Iacenna V, Giuliano G. Cadmio ed ipertensione arteriosa. *Archivio Scienze Lavoro.* 1989;5:73.

107. McCready RA, Hide GL, Bivings BA, Mattingly S, Griffen WO. Radiation-induced arterial injuries. *Surgery.* 1983;93: 306.

108. McMichel AJ, Johnson HM. Long term mortality profile of heavily exposed lead smelter workers. *JOM.* 1982;24: 375.

109. Mekky S, Schilling RSF, Walford J. Varicose veins in women cotton workers: an epidemiological study in England and Egypt. *BMJ.* 1969;2:591.

110. Melamed S, Ben Avi I, Luz J, Green MS. Repetitive work, work underload, and coronary heart disease risk factors among blue-collar workers: the CORDIS study. Cardiovascolar Occupational Risk Factors Determination in Israel. *J Psychosom Res.* 1995;39:19.

111. Melamed S, Bruhis S. The effects of chronic industrial noise exposure on urinary cortisol, fatigue, and irritabil-

ity: a controlled field experiment. *J Occup Environ Med.* 1996;38:252.

112. Merlen JF. Le médecin du travail devant l'insuffisance veineuse chronique. *Arch Mal Prof.* 1979;40:939.

113. Mikhaleva LM, Zhavoronkov AA, Cherniacev AL, Koshelev WB. Morphofunctional characteristics of cadmium induced arterial hypertension. *Biull Eksp Biol Med.* 1991;11:420.

114. Mincheva L, Hadjiolova I, Deyanov C. Cardiovascular changes at work: relation with some individual risk factors. *Rev Environ Health.* 1994;10:57.

115. Mole B. Radiodermatitis. *Presse Med.* 1987;16:1802–1805.

116. Naitoh P, Kelly TL, Englund C. Health effects of deprivation. *Occup Med.* 1990;5:209–238.

117. Norgren L. Quelques aspects de la phlébologie en suede. *Phlébologie.* 1992;45:444.

118. Nuyts GD, Roels HA, Verpooten GF, Bernard AM, Lauwerys RR, De Broe ME. Intestinal-type alkaline phosphatase in urine as an indicator of mercury induced effects on the S3 segment of the proximal tubule. *Nephrol Dial Transplant.* 1992;7:225.

119. Olsen O, Kristensen TS. Impact of work environment on cardiovascular diseases in Denmark. *J Epidemiol Community Health.* 1991;45:4.

120. Om A, Samer E, Vetrovec GW. Radiation induced coronary artery disease. *Am Heart J.* 1992;124:1598.

121. Oner G. Role of cadmium-induced lipid peroxidation in the kidney response to atrial natriuretic hormone. *Nephron.* 1996;72:257.

122. Orth-Gomer K, Knutsson A, Freden K, Akerstedt T. Direct and indirect evidence of ischemic heart disease in shift workers. *Med Lav.* 1986;77:90.

123. Orzan F, Brusca A. Radiation-induced constrictive pericarditis: associated cardiac lesions, treatment, and follow up. *G Ital Cardiol.* 1994;24:817.

124. Ottmann W, Karvonen MJ, Schmidt KH, Knauth P, Ruterfranz J. Subjective health status of day- and shift-working policemen. *Ergonomics.* 1989;32:847.

125. Pancheri P. Psiconeuroendocrinologia. In: Pancheri P, ed. *Trattato di Medicina Psicosomatica.* Vol 1. Firenze: USES; 1984:179–223.

126. Pellegrini A, Soldani P, Gesi M, Lenzi P, Paparelli A. The action of diazepam on noise-induced alterations in rat atrial tissue: an ultrastructural study. *J Submicrosc Cytol Pathol.* 1996;28:507.

127. Pellegrini A, Soldani P, Ricciardi MP, Paparelli A. Morpho-histochemical observations on the liver parenchyma of adult albino rats subjected to acute acoustic stress. *Boll Soc Ital Biol Sper.* 1991;67:111.

128. Petruzzellis V, Lospallutti M, Scardigno A. Correlazioni capillaroscopiche e cliniche nelle radiodermiti croniche professionali. *G Ital Med Lav.* 1985;7:231–235.

129. Piikivi L. Cardiovascular reflexes and low long-term exposure to mercury vapour. *Intern Arch Occup Environ Health.* 1989;61:391.

130. Pirkle JL, Schwartz J, Landis JR, Harlan WR. The relationship between blood lead levels and blood pressure and its cardiovascular risk implications. *Am J Epidemiol.* 1985; 121:246.

131. Pribyl CR, Racca J. Toxic gas exposure in ice arenas. *Clin J Sport Med.* 1996;6:232.

132. Raso AM, Castagno PL, Muncinelli M, Sisto G, Puleo V. Conseguenze socio-economiche dei ricoveri per vasculopatie in Piemonte (periodo 1976–1987) e studio pilota sul reinserimento socio-lavorativo dei soggetti sottoposti ad interventi di chirurgia arteriosa. *Min Angiol.* 1990; 15:59.

133. Raso AM, Castagno PL. Epidemiologia delle flebopatie. *Min Angiol.* 1992;17:75.

134. Raso AM, Levis P, Rispoli P, Durando R, Carlin R. Studio clinico-epidemiologico sui pazienti affetti da patologie flebolinfatiche ricoverati negli Ospedali della Regione Piemonte nel periodo 1976–1979. *Min Med.* 1983;74: 1479.

135. Raso AM, Sisto G, Castagno PL, Muncinelli M. Studio della trombosi venosa profonda nella regione piemonte durante il periodo 1976–85. *Min Angiol.* 1991;16:533.

136. Recoules-Achè J. Importance du sedentarisme debout dans l'evolution et les complicationes des varices: etude statistique. *Angeiologie.* 1965;17:17.

137. Rees WL. Stress, distress, and disease. *Br J Psychol.* 1976; 28:3.

138. Robineau P, Guittin P. Effects of an organophosphorus compound on cardiac rhythm and haemodynamics in anesthetized and conscious beagle dogs. *Toxicol Lett.* 1987;37:95.

139. Ronneberg A. Mortality and cancer morbidity in workers from an aluminium smelter with prebacked carbon anodes, III: mortality from circulatory and respiratory diseases. *Occup Environ Med.* 1995;52:255.

140. Rosenman KD. Cardiovascular disease and workplace exposures. *Arch Environ Health.* 1984;39:218.

141. Rosenman KD. Cardiovascular disease. In: Levy BS, Wegmen DH, eds. *Occupational Health: Recognizing and Preventing Work-Related Diseases.* Boston, Mass: Little, Brown; 1983:331–340.

142. Rosenman RH, Friedman M, Strauss R. A predictive study of coronary heart disease. *JAMA* 1964;189:103.

143. Rosenman RH, Friedman M. Relationship of type A behaviour pattern to coronary heart disease. In: Selye H, ed. *Selye's Guide to Stress Research.* New York, NY: Van Nostrand Reinhold; 1983:250–261.

144. Saha S, Gandhi A, Das S, Kaur P, Singh SH. Effects of noise stress on some cardiovascular parameters and audiovisual reaction time. *Indian J Physiol Pharmacol.* 1996; 40:35.

145. Santana VS, Barberino JL. Occupational noise exposure and hypertension. *Rev Saude Publica.* 1995;29:478.

146. Schroeder HA. Cadmium, chromium, and cardiovascular disease. *Circulation.* 1967;35:570.

147. Selevan SG, Landrigan PJ, Stern FB, Jones JH. Lead and hypertension in a mortality study of lead smelter workers. *Environ Health Perspect.* 1988;78:65.

148. Selevan SG, Landrigan PJ, Stern FB, Jones JH. Mortality of lead smelter workers. *Am J Epidemiol.* 1985;122:673.

149. Selwyn AP. The cardiovascular system and radiation. *Lancet.* 1983;2:152.

150. Seyle H. A syndrome produced by diverse nocuous agents. *Nature.* 1936;138:32.

151. Sharp DS, Becker CE, Smith AH. Chronic low-level lead exposure: its role in the pathogenesis of hypertension. *Med Toxicol.* 1987;2:210.

152. Sharp DS, Osterhol J, Becker CE, et al. Blood pressure and blood lead concentration in bus drivers. *Environ Health Perspect.* 1989;78:131.

153. Silve MJ, Corathers A, Castelbianco N, Dias A, Boavida MG. Sister chromatidid exchange analysis in workers exposed to noise and vibration. *Mutat Res.* 1996;369:113.

154. Sokas RK, Simmens S, Sophar K, Welch LS, Liziewski T. Lead levels in Maryland construction workers. *Am J Ind Med.* 1997;31:188.

155. Sonnenberg A, Donga M, Erckenbrecht JF, Wienbeck M. The effect of mental stress induced by noise on gastric acid secretion and mucosal blood flow. *Scand J Gastroenterol.* 1984;89:45.

156. Sparrow D, Tifft CP, Rosner B, Weiss ST. Postural changes in diastolic blood pressure and the risk of myocardial infarction: the normative aging study. *Circulation.* 1984; 70:533–537.

157. Staessen J, Yeoman WB, Fletcher AE, et al. Blood lead concentration, renal function, and blood pressure in London civil servants. *Br J Ind Med.* 1990;47:442.

158. Staessen JA, Buchet JP, Ginucchio G, et al. Public health implication of environmental exposure to cadmium and lead: an overview of epidemiological studies in Belgium. *J Cardiovasc Risk.* 1996;3:26.

159. Stern FB, Halperin WE, Hornung RW, Ringerburg VL, McCammon CS. Heart disease mortality among bridge and tunnel officers exposed to carbon monoxide. *Am J Epidemiol.* 1988;128:1276.

160. Stvirtinova V, Kolesar J, Wimmer G. Prevalence of varicose veins of the lower limbs in the women working at a department store. *Int Angiol.* 1991;10:2.

161. Sudo A, Nguyen AL, Jonai H, et al. Effects of earplugs on catecholamine and cortisol excretion in noise-exposed texile workers. *Ind Health.* 1996;34:279.

162. Sweetnam PM, Taylor SWC, Elwood PC. Exposure to carbon disulphide and ischaemic heart disease in a viscose rayon factory. *Br J Ind Med.* 1987;44:220.

163. Taccola A, Pisati P, Imbriani M, Gotti GB, Di Maio D, Carenzio G. Sul meccanismo patogenetico delle alterazioni cardiovascolari nell'ossicarbonismo. *Med Lav.* 1988;79:444.

164. Taccola A, Zaliani A, Di Maio D, Gobba F. Rilievi cardiocircolatori in un gruppo di lavoratori esposti a nitroderivati. Una ipotesi patogenetica del "Withdrawal Hazard." *G Ital Med Lav.* 1987;9:153.

165. Tenkanen L, Sjoblom T, Kalimo R, Alikoski T, Harma M. Shift work, occupation, and coronary heart disease over 6 years of follow-up inthe Helsinki Heart Study. *Scand J Work Environ Health.* 1997;23:257.

166. Theorell T. Family history of hypertension: an individual trait interacting with spontaneously occurring job stressors. *Scand J Work Environ Health.* 1989;16:74.

167. Tollenstrup K, Daling JR, Allard J. Mortality in a cohort of orchard workers exposed to lead argenate pesticide spray. *Arch Environ Health.* 1995;50:221.

168. Tomei F, Bartolo M. La sindrome post-flebitica. Valutazione clinica e schemi di trattamento. *Sett Osp.* 1977;19: 135.

169. Tomei F, Baccolo TP, Papaleo B, Tomao E. Flebopatie professionali. *Arch Scienze Lav.* 1991;7:105.

170. Tomei F, Tomao E, Baccolo TP, Papaleo B. Venous diseases and occupation. *16th World Congress of the International Union of Angiology.* Paris: International Union of Angiology; 1992:373.

171. Tomei F, Baccolo TP, Papaleo B, Rosati MV, et al. Flebopatie professionali nell'industria, nell'edilizia, e nel terziario. *Prevenzione Oggi.* 1995;1:123–155.

172. Tomei F, Papaleo B, Iavicoli S, Fantini S, Rosati MV. Vascular effects of occupational exposure to low-dose ionizing radiation. *Am J Ind Med.* 1996;30:72–77.

173. Tomei F, Papaleo B, Baccolo TP, Persechino B, Spanò G, Rosati MV. Noise and gastric secretion. *Am J Ind Med.* 1994;26:367.

174. Tomei F, Papaleo B, Baccolo TP, Tomao E, Alfi P, Fantini S. Chronic noise exposure and the cardiovascular system in aircraft pilots. *Med Lav.* 1996;87:394.

175. Tomei F, Rosati MV, D'Anna M, et al. Rischio di patologia cardiovascolare in agricoltura. *Prevenzione Oggi.* 1996;1: 53–75.

176. Tomei F, Tomao E, Papaleo B, Baccolo TP, Cirio AM, Alfi P. Epidemiological and clinical study of subjects occupationally exposed to noise. *Int J Angiology.* 1995;4:117.

177. Tzvetkov D. Effect of vibrations on the organism possibilities for development of non-specific diseases and their prognostication. *Cent Eur J Public Health.* 1993;1:10.

178. Vander AJ. Chronic effects of lead on the renin-angiotensin system. *Environ Health Perspect.* 1988;78:78.

179. Vandevoir D, Gournay M. Pathologie coronarienne et vasculaire des travailleurs des dynamiteries. *Phlébologie.* 1989; 42:223.

180. Vergnano P, Serra A, Talamo R, Coscia GC, Castagno L. Indagini vascolari in esposti a vibrazioni agli arti inferiori. *Atti 54° Congresso Società Nazionale Medicina del Lavoro Igiene Industriale.* 1991;2:819.

181. Victery W. Evidence for effects of chronic lead exposure on blood pressure in experimental animals: an overview. *Environ Health Perspect.* 1988;78:71.

182. Webb RC, Winquist RJ, Victery W, Vander AJ. In vivo and in vitro effects of lead on vascular reactivity in rats. *Am J Physiol.* 1981;241:211.

183. Weddel JM. Varicose veins pilot survey, 1966. *Br J Prev Soc Med.* 1969;23:179.

184. Weisse CS, Pato CN, McAllister CG, Littman R, Breier A, Paul SM. Differential effects of controllable and uncontrollable acute stress on lymphocyte proliferation and leukocyte percentages in humans. *Brain Behav Immun.* 1990;4:339.

185. Widmer LK, Wandeler JM. Leg complaints and peripheral venous disorders. In: Widmer LK, ed. *Peripheral Venous Disorders.* Bern, Switzerland: Hans Huber; 1978: 58–63.

186. Wilcosky TC, Simonsen NR. Solvent exposure and cardiovascular disease. *Am J Ind Med.* 1991;19:569.

187. Wu TN, Shen CY, Ko KN, et al. Occupational lead exposure and blood pressure. *Int J Epidemiol.* 1996;25:791.

188. Zanettini R, Pavlova Kotzeva K, Agostoni O, Cesana G. Esposizione professionale ad agenti chimico-fisici e malattie cardiovascolari. *Archivio di Scienze del Lavoro.* 1989;5:347.

189. Zou HJ, Ding Y, Huang KL, et al. Effects of lead on systolic and diastolic cardiac functions. *Biomed Environ Sci.* 1995;8:281.

190. Zwingenberger W, Schneider R, Faulhaber HD. Observa-tions on the development of borderline-hypertension in ore miners under different work loads. *Z Gesamte Hyg Ihre Grenzgeb.* 1990;36:176.

191. Zwingerberger W, Nestler K, Faulhaber HD, Schneider R. Blood pressure response in shift workers with hyperten-sion level. *Z Gesamte Hyg Ihre Grenzgeb.* 1989;35:552.

12

Pathophysiological Basis of the Acute Coronary Syndromes

Kurt Huber and Fritz Kaindl

Background

In typical chronic stable angina, pain is related to an increase in myocardial oxygen demand, most commonly induced by physical activity and/or emotion. Underlying fixed coronary artery obstruction is usually present and responsible for a fixed limited oxygen supply. Accordingly, factors that lead to increased activity of the heart and to increased oxygen demand (e.g., exercise, emotional stress, fever, and tachycardias from other causes) precipitate ischemia and angina. There is also increasing evidence that angina may be caused by transient reduction of oxygen supply as a consequence of coronary vasoconstriction.[1] In patients with severe fixed obstruction to coronary flow, only a minor increase in dynamic vasoconstriction is necessary for blood flow to fall below a critical level and cause myocardial ischemia.

Acute coronary syndromes are caused in most patients by acute thrombotic coronary artery obstruction and are mainly precipitated by reduction in myocardial oxygen supply. However, acute unstable angina and myocardial infarction, as one might expect, are not necessarily a consequence of an already preexistent fixed high-grade coronary stenosis: data from angiographic studies over the past decade have clearly shown that the lesions most likely to precipitate an infarct-provoking thrombosis often have not been highly stenotic before the acute event.[2-5] Acute thrombus formation is a consequence of plaque disruption of a vulnerable plaque, but not all disruptions of atherosclerotic plaque lead to acute clinical symptoms.[6,7] Subclinical episodes of plaque fissuring with accompanying hemodynamically inactive thrombus formation and subsequent organization of thrombotic material seem to represent an important pathway for plaque progression[7] and may in part also explain silent angina (intermittent ischemic electrocardiographic alterations without chest pain). Recent studies on possible plaque regression by use of lipid-lowering drugs have demonstrated that only minimal effects on angiographi-

cally established stenotic lesions were accompanied by a significant decrease in acute coronary events.[8] Taken together, these data indicate the greater importance of plaque composition for development of acute coronary syndromes than the grade of luminal narrowing.

Vulnerable Plaque and Triggers of Plaque Rupture

Several studies have shown that coronary occlusions evolve most frequently from mild to moderate stenoses, which are more lipid rich and vulnerable and by far outnumber severely obstructive plaques.[2-5,9,10] The risk of plaque disruption is related to intrinsic properties of individual plaques (*vulnerability*) and extrinsic forces acting on plaques (*trigger mechanisms of rupture*) (Table 12.1). The former predispose plaques to rupture, whereas the latter may precipitate disruption if vulnerable plaques are present.

Vulnerability of Atherosclerotic Plaques

Plaque disruption occurs most frequently where the fibrous cap is thinnest and most heavily infiltrated by macrophage/foam cells (e.g., at the junction between plaque and adjacent less-diseased vessel wall, or shoulder region).[11] The vulnerability of atherosclerotic plaques depends on (1) the size and consistency of the atheromatous core, (2) the thickness and collagen content of the fibrous cap, (3) the local inflammation within the plaque and fibrous cap, and (4) the "fatigue" of the cap due to long-term cyclic stresses acting on it[12] (Table 12.1).

Atheromatous Core

Compared with stable plaques, which are composed mainly of collagen-rich sclerotic tissue and a relatively small lipid-rich core in the central portion of the eccen-

TABLE 12.1. Properties and triggers of plaque disruption.

Intrinsic properties
    Size and consistency of the atheromatous core
    Thickness and collagen content of the fibrous cap
    Local inflammation
    Fatigue of the fibrous cap

Extrinsic forces
    Cap tension
    Plaque compression
    Circumferential bending
    Longitudinal flexion
    Shear stress

External triggers
    Circadian variation of contributing factors
    Seasonal variation of contributing factors
    Emotional stress
    Physical stress (vigorous exercise)

trically thickened intima, a vulnerable plaque has a much bigger atheromatous (soft, lipid-rich) component[12] that destabilizes it, makes it prone to rupture, and is highly thrombogenic.[13,14]

Cap Thickness

The thickness and collagen content of the fibrous cap overlying this lipid-rich core fundamentally determine the stability of an atherosclerotic plaque. Rupture-prone plaques tend to have thin, friable fibrous caps.[11,15] Stable plaques have thicker fibrous caps that are more resistant to circumferential stress and other mechanical forces.[16] Interstitial collagen, elastin, and proteoglycans are synthesized by smooth muscle cells, which are important constituents of the cap region. In vulnerable plaques, collagen synthesis is impaired by mechanisms such as focal chronic inflammation and immune stimulation (e.g., by action of the cytokine interferon-γ, which is produced by chronically activated T cells).[17,18] Interferon-γ also inhibits smooth muscle cell proliferation[19] and can contribute to activation of apoptosis,[20] both of which may reduce the content of smooth muscle cells in the fibrous cap.

Inflammation

Disrupted fibrous caps are usually heavily infiltrated by activated macrophage/foam cells, indicating ongoing inflammation at the site of plaque rupture.[17] In addition, foam cell infiltration and inflammation occur preferably at the shoulder region of the plaque,[11] thereby reducing tensile strength and easing rupture at this site.[21,22] Activated macrophages are capable of degrading extracellular matrix by phagocytosis or secretion of proteolytic enzymes such as plasminogen activators (tissue type and urokinase type[23]) and metalloproteinases (collagenases,

gelatinases, and stromelysins[24-26]) that weaken the fibrous cap.

Increased fibrinolytic activity has been reported in extracts of intima of coronary atheromas[27] and is mainly mediated by urokinase-type plasminogen activator localized in macrophage-rich areas of advanced lesions.[23] Receptor-bound urokinase-type plasminogen activator and plasmin are the key enzymes of extracellular proteolysis regulation.[28] Plasmin may activate metalloproteinases released in latent form by macrophages, with subsequent degradation of collagen, elastin, and proteoglycans of the fibrous cap.[26]

As already mentioned, activated macrophage/foam cells are the main source of tissue factor responsible for rapid thrombus formation and luminal occlusion after plaque rupture and exposure of subendothelial structures to the blood stream.[14,29]

Other cells involved in inflammatory processes of the shoulder region of advanced plaques are activated mast cells, which can produce and secrete powerful proteolytic enzymes (e.g., tryptase and chymase, which can activate zymogen precursors of metalloproteinases[30]) and neutrophils.[31]

Recently, Liuzzo et al.[32] demonstrated elevated levels of C-reactive protein and serum amyloid A in unstable patients with unfavorable outcome, indirectly indicating the importance of the extent of local inflammatory processes in acute coronary syndromes. Thompson et al.[33] also found a positive relationship between increased incidence of angina and plasma levels of C-reactive protein. These results have led to the measurement of C-reactive protein and serum amyloid as prognostic markers in unstable coronary artery disease.[34]

Cap "Fatigue"

Repetitive chronic stress caused by cyclic stretching, compression, bending, flexion, shear, and pressure fluctuations may lead to sudden spontaneous fracture of the tissue due to fatigue.[35] Differences between stable and "vulnerable" plaques are summarized in Table 12.2.

Trigger Mechanisms of Plaque Rupture

Stresses imposed on plaques are usually concentrated at weak points where the fibrous cap is thinnest. External forces that stress the plaque are (1) cap tension, (2) plaque compression, (3) bending (circumferential), (4) flexion (longitudinal), and (5) shear stress[12] (Table 12.1).

Cap Tension

The higher the blood pressure and the larger the luminal diameter, the more tension stress develops in the vessel wall (Laplace's law)[36] and concentrates at critical

TABLE 12.2. Differences between stable and vulnerable plaques.

	Stable Plaque	Vulnerable plaque
Fibrous cap	Thick	Thin
	High content of SMCs, elastin, collagen, and proteoglycans	Low content of SMCs, elastin, collagen, and proteoglycans
		Infiltration with macrophages/foam cells
Composition	High content of SMCs, elastin, collagen, and proteoglycans	Low content of SMCs, elastin, collagen, and proteoglycans
	Lipid poor	Lipid rich
	Calcification present	
Inflammation	Absent	Present
Thrombogenicity	Low	High (tissue factor)

SMC, smooth muscle cell.

points.[11,37] Thus, tension stress is highest where the fibrous capsule is thinnest and/or where focal macrophage activities and low resistance to plaque fissuring can be found.[11,37] According to Laplace's law, the tension created in fibrous caps of mildly or moderately stenotic lesions (with a bigger vessel lumen) is greater than that in caps of severely stenotic plaques (with smaller lumen) with the same cap thickness and exposed to the same blood pressure. This explains why mildly or moderately stenotic plaques have a higher potential to rupture.

Plaque Compression

Plaque compression is theoretically caused by high blood pressure and vasospasm. However, blood pressure is mainly responsible for tension as compared with compression,[36] and vasospasm seems to be rather a consequence than a cause of plaque rupture.[38,39]

Circumferential Bending

The propagating pulse wave and changes in vascular tone cause changes in lumen size and shape; concentric plaques thus change less than eccentric plaques due to deformation and bending. Bending stress involves especially the junctions between stiff plaque and the more compliant plaque-free vessel wall and may therefore contribute to plaque rupture at these sites[12] from acute circumferential bending stress or chronic fatigue.

Longitudinal Flexion

Like circumferential bending, a sudden accentuated longitudinal flexion may trigger acute plaque disruption, whereas long-term cyclic flexion may contribute to plaque fatigue.[40]

Shear Stress

Low and/or oscillatory chronic shear stress is a trigger of atherogenesis and plaque development at predisposed sites of the coronary vessel tree.[41] In highly stenotic lesions blood velocity can be extremely high and may shear the endothelium away. However, high shear forces alone do not seem to be sufficient to cause plaque rupture but may be a contributing factor in the presence of other triggers.[42]

Pathophysiological Triad of the Acute Coronary Syndromes

The most important contributors to the pathophysiological mechanism of acute coronary syndromes are plaque rupture, acute thrombus formation, and vasoconstriction (Figure 12.1).

External Triggers of Plaque Rupture

Most plaque ruptures and subsequent acute coronary syndromes are caused by external triggers or conditions.[43–45] Unstable angina and acute myocardial infarction occur at increased frequency in morning hours,[44, 46–48] on Mondays,[46,49] during the cold season,[50] during times of emotional stress,[51,52] and during vigorous exercise[53–55] (Table 12.1).

The pattern of onset of acute coronary syndromes in morning hours may be explained by the temporary coincidence of several factors: (1) early morning activation of sympathetic activity leading to a sudden increase in

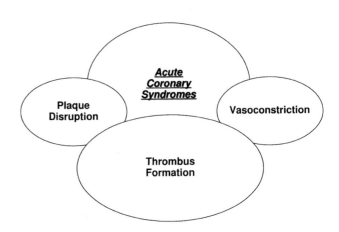

FIGURE 12.1 Acute coronary syndromes: pathophysiological triad.

pulse rate, blood pressure, ventricular contraction, and coronary blood flow[53]; (2) a diurnal systemic prothrombotic state due to platelet hyperaggregability[56,57] and impaired endogenous fibrinolysis[47,58–61] that may aggravate and accelerate occlusive thrombus formation in case of plaque disruption; and (3) an increased tendency toward vasoconstriction of epicardial vessels in the morning.[62]

Acute Thrombus Formation After Plaque Disruption

Acute thrombus formation with rapid alteration of the atherosclerotic plaque and high-grade narrowing or occlusion of the vessel lumen is probably the most important consequence of plaque rupture.[63] Exposure of a subendothelial atheromatous core to blood leads immediately to platelet activation and aggregation and thrombin formation mainly caused by induction of the very potent tissue factor pathway.[14] Several local and systemic factors present at the time of plaque rupture may influence the degree and duration of thrombus deposition and account for various pathological and clinical manifestations[63] (Table 12.3).

Local Factors

Local factors that contribute to thrombus formation are (1) degree of plaque fissuring, (2) degree and geometry of stenosis, (3) composition of disrupted plaque, and (4) surface of residual thrombus.

Degree of Plaque Fissuring

In patients with unstable angina, complex coronary artery lesions suggestive of deep fissuring or ulceration of a plaque are markers of a more persistent coronary occlusion.[64,65]

Degree and Geometry of Stenosis

The acute thrombotic response depends in part on the sudden geometric changes or the degree of stenosis that follows the plaque fissuring and is due to increased platelet deposition and shear-induced platelet activation.[66] Platelet-rich thrombi tend to be less amenable to fibrinolytic therapy than thrombin-rich thrombi.

Composition of Disrupted Plaque

The rough surface after plaque disruption stimulates development of an occlusive thrombus,[13] as does the exposure of atheromatous gruel. The latter may function by tissue factor–mediated procoagulant activity[14] and/or release of platelet activators from macrophages.[22,67]

Surface of Residual Thrombus

Spontaneous endogenous lysis of acutely developed thrombi is an important physiological mechanism in acute coronary syndromes.[68,69] Compared with a deeply injured vessel wall, the residual thrombus after spontaneous or therapeutic thrombolysis is very thrombogenic, possibly due to high local thrombin activity on the surface of the partially lysed thrombus.[70] As a consequence, enhanced platelet and thrombin activation occur and contribute to rethrombosis.[71] Residual thrombin acts as a very potent vasoconstrictor[38] and is therefore a main trigger of thrombus-related focal vasospasm.

Systemic Thrombogenic Risk Factors

Several systemic factors can account for a hypercoagulable, prothrombotic, or antifibrinolytic state and therefore favor focal thrombosis after plaque disruption. These factors include (1) high plasma levels of catecholamines, (2) alterations of the renin–angiotensin system, (3) lipid disorders and other metabolic states, (4) hypercoagulation, and (5) a reduced endogenous fibrinolytic system (Table 12.2).

Catecholamines

Activation of platelets and thrombin is catecholamine dependent.[72,73] Catecholamines are the mediators of the onset of acute coronary syndromes[57] and represent the

TABLE 12.3. Plaque disruption: local and systemic thrombogenic risk factors.

Local risk factors	Systemic risk factors
Degree of plaque disruption	Catecholamines
Degree of stenosis	stress, smoking, diurnal variation
change in geometry	Renin–angiotensin system
Plaque composition	DD genotype, impairment of fibrinolysis
lipids, macrophages, tissue factor, plasminogen	Lipoprotein (a)
activators, metalloproteinases	Insulin resistance, hyperinsulinemia, and diabetes mellitus
Residual thrombus	Hypercoagulation
	fibrinogen, clotting factor VII, fibrinopeptide A, prothrombin fragments,
	von Willebrand's factor
	Impaired fibrinolysis
	plasminogen activator–inhibitor type 1, tissue plasminogen activator

link between emotional stress,[74] severe exercise,[54] smoking,[75] cocaine use,[76] and atherothrombotic events.

Renin–Angiotensin System

An activated renin–angiotensin system may be related to increased risk for myocardial infarction in the presence of the angiotensin-converting enzyme-DD genotype.[77,78] It is postulated that in patients with this phenotype, angiotensin II is capable of increasing the plasma concentration of plasminogen activator–inhibitor type 1, thus impairing the endogenous fibrinolytic potential.[79,80]

Lipoprotein(a)

Elevation of plasma lipoprotein(a) concentration is an important and independent coronary risk factor.[81] Apolipoprotein(a) is known for its close structural homology with plasminogen[82] and may therefore be capable of interfering with plasminogen-binding sites on the fibrin molecule, on endothelial cells, and on monocytes, thus preventing plasmin formation from plasminogen[83] and reducing the fibrinolytic response to thrombus formation. Lipoprotein(a) also increases plasminogen activator–inhibitor type 1 and reduces synthesis of tissue plasminogen activator in endothelial cells.[84,85] Several isoforms of lipoprotein(a) have been described, and only the low molecular weight isoforms compete with plasminogen for the respective binding sites.[86]

Insulin Resistance, Hyperinsulinemia, and Diabetes Mellitus

Hyperinsulinemia, an independent coronary risk factor, is often related to increased plasma levels of fibrinogen[87,88] and/or plasminogen activator–inhibitor type 1[87,88] and is therefore accompanied by an increased tendency to thrombus formation (see later section). The prothrombotic state in patients with manifest diabetes mellitus is caused by increased platelet activity, hypercoagulation, and impaired fibrinolysis.[89]

Fibrinogen

Fibrinogen is an independent coronary risk factor,[90,91] being especially related to onset of unstable angina,[92] acute myocardial infarction,[93] and sudden cardiac death.[94] Increased fibrinogen levels are also predictors of future acute coronary syndromes.[33] Fibrinogen levels increase with smoking, age, obesity, diabetes, and emotional stress.[95,96]

Factor VII

Elevated plasma levels of clotting factor VII are associated with unstable coronary syndromes.[91] Factor VII levels can be elevated by increasing dietary fat[97] and are found to be increased in postmenopausal women.[98]

Fibrinopeptide A and Prothrombin Fragments (F_{1+2})

The plasma markers of thrombin activity fibrinopeptide A and prothrombin fragments (F_{1+2}) are elevated in patients with unstable angina and acute myocardial infarction for longer than the duration of the acute clinical phase.[99] Fibrinopeptide A and prothrombin fragments may be triggers of rethrombosis, recurrent instability, and reinfarction.[99]

von Willebrand's Factor

von Willebrand's factor is important in early adhesion of platelets to a defective endothelium. Elevations can be provoked systemically by cigarette smoking[100] and focally by mediators of inflammation (interleukins and tumor necrosis factor)[101]; elevations are associated with diabetes and an increase in body weight–index and plasma triglyceride levels.[102] Elevated von Willebrand's factor levels are positively correlated with acute fatal coronary events.[103]

Impaired Endogenous Fibrinolysis

A defect of the endogenous fibrinolytic system can be attributed mainly to elevated plasma levels of plasminogen activator–inhibitor type 1, which rapidly impairs the action of tissue plasminogen activator. Elevated plasminogen activator–inhibitor type 1 levels are associated with an increased incidence of acute coronary syndromes[104–111] and reinfarction[112] and have been considered to represent an important coronary risk factor.[113] Interestingly, elevation of tissue plasminogen activator antigen levels are an even stronger predictor of future acute coronary events.[33,114,115] This paradoxical finding may be explained by (1) the way elevated tissue-type plasminogen activator antigen levels parallel increased inhibitor levels due to reactive chronic production and secretion triggered by the inhibitor-induced prothrombotic state and (2) by the tissue–plasminogen activator antigen (as determined by enzyme-linked immunosorbent assay systems) being complexed with the inhibitor and therefore not completely active.[116]

Vasoconstriction

Abnormal constriction of epicardial coronary arteries contributes to the pathogenesis of acute coronary syndromes.[117–119] The augmented vasoconstrictor responsiveness associated with atherosclerosis can in large part be attributed to an impairment in endothelial-dependent relaxation due to the disability of the atherosclerotic endothelium to produce and release endothelial-derived relaxant factor,[120] thereby favoring the action of endothelin 1, which is the most important endothelial vasoconstrictor.[121] As a consequence transient vasoconstriction is frequently present after plaque disruption and thrombus formation[38,117] and is mainly thrombin dependent[122] and platelet dependent (mediated by serotonin and thromboxane A_2).[38,122,123] Vasoconstriction as a response to endothelial dysfunction may occur near the culprit lesion or be a response to deep arterial damage or plaque disruption of the culprit lesion itself.[38] However, vasoconstriction as the causal pathomechanism of plaque disruption, or as primary initiator of acute coronary syndromes without plaque fissuring, seems to be extremely rare.

References

1. Ganz P, Abben RP, Barry WH. Dynamic variations in resistance of coronary arterial narrowings in angina pectoris at rest. *Am J Cardiol.* 1987;59:66–74.

2. Alderman EL, Corley SD, Fisher LD, et al., and CASS Participating Investigators and Staff. Five-year angiographic follow-up of factors associated with progression of coronary artery disease in the Coronary Artery Surgery Study (CASS). *J Am Coll Cardiol.* 1993;22:1141–1154.

3. Ambrose J, Tannenbaum M, Alexopoulos D, et al. Angiographic progression of coronary artery disease and the development of myocardial infarction. *J Am Coll Cardiol.* 1988; 12:56–62.

4. Hackett D, Davies G, Maseri A. Pre-existing coronary stenoses in patients with first myocardial infarction are not necessarily severe. *Am Heart J.* 1988;9:1317–1323.

5. Nobuyoshi M, Tanaka M, Mosaka H, et al. Progression of coronary atherosclerosis: is coronary spasm related to progression? *J Am Coll Cardiol.* 1991;18:904–910.

6. Davies MJ, Thomas AC. Plaque fissuring: the cause of acute myocardial infarction, sudden ischemic death, and crescendo angina. *Br Heart J.* 1985;53:363–373.

7. Fuster V, Lewis A. Conner Memorial Lecture. Mechanisms leading to myocardial infarction: insights from studies of vascular biology. *Circulation.* 1994;90:2126–2146.

8. Blankenhorn DH, Hodis HN. Arterial imaging and atherosclerosis reversal. *Arterioscler Thromb.* 1994;14:177–192.

9. Giroud D, Li JM, Urban P, Meier B, Rutishauer W. Relation of the site of myocardial infarction to the most severe coronary arterial stenosis at prior angiography. *Am J Cardiol.* 1992;69:729–732.

10. Little WC, Constantinescu M, Applegate RJ, et al. Can coronary angiography predict the site of subsequent myocardial infarction in patients with mild-to-moderate coronary artery disease? *Circulation.* 1988;78:1157–1166.

11. Richardson RD, Davies MJ, Born GVR. Influence of plaque configuration and stress distribution on fissuring of coronary atherosclerotic plaques. *Lancet.* 1989;2:941–944.

12. Falk E, Shah PK, Fuster V. Coronary plaque disruption. *Circulation.* 1995;92:657–671.

13. Fernandez-Ortiz A, Badimon JJ, Falk E, et al. Characterization of relative thrombogenicity of atherosclerotic plaque components: implications for consequences of plaque rupture. *J Am Coll Cardiol.* 1994;23:1564–1569.

14. Wilcox JN. Thrombotic mechanisms in atherosclerosis. *Coron Artery Dis.* 1994;5:223–229.

15. Loree HM, Kamm RD, Stringfellow RG, Lee RT. Effect of fibrous cap thickness on peak circumferential stress in model atherosclerotic vessels. *Circ Res.* 1992;71:850–858.

16. Burleigh MC, Briggs AD, Lendon CL, Davies MJ, Born GV, Richardson PD. Collagen types I and III, collagen content, GAGs, and mechanical strength of human atherosclerotic plaque caps: span-wise variations. *Atherosclerosis.* 1992; 96:71–81.

17. Van der Wal AC, Becker AE, Van der Loos CM, Das PK. Site of intimal rupture or erosion of thrombosed coronary atherosclerotic plaques is characterized by an inflammation process irrespective of the dominant plaque morphology. *Circulation.* 1994;89:36–44.

18. Warner SJC, Freidman GB, Libby P. Regulation of major histocompatibility gene expression in cultured human vascular smooth muscle cells. *Arteriosclerosis.* 1989;9:279–288.

19. Hansson GK, Jonasson L, Holm J, Clowes MK, Clowes A. Gamma interferon regulates vascular smooth muscle proliferation and Ia expression in vivo and in vitro. *Circ Res.* 1988;63:712–719.

20. Majno G, Joris I. Apoptosis, oncosis, and necrosis: an overview of cell death. *Am J Pathol.* 1995;146:3–15.

21. Lendon CL, Davies MJ, Born GVR, Richardson PD. Atherosclerotic plaque caps are locally weakened when macrophage density is increased. *Atherosclerosis.* 1991;87:87–90.

22. Moreno PR, Falk E, Palacios IF, Newell JB, Fuster V, Fallon JT. Macrophage infiltration in acute coronary syndromes: implications for plaque rupture. *Circulation.* 1994;90:775–778.

23. Lupu F, Heim DA, Bachmann F, Hurni M, Kakkar VV, Kruithof EKO. Plasminogen activator expression in human atherosclerotic lesions. *Arterioscler Thromb Vasc Biol.* 1995;15:1444–1455.

24. Brown DL, Hibbs MS, Kearney M, Loushin C, Isner JM. Identification of 92-kD gelatinase in human coronary atherosclerotic lesions: association of active enzyme synthesis with unstable angina. *Circulation.* 1995;91:2125–2131.

25. Galis ZS, Sukhova GK, Lark MW, Libby P. Increased expression of matrix-metalloproteinases and matrix degrading activity in vulnerable regions of human atherosclerotic plaques. *J Clin Invest.* 1994;94:2493–2503.

26. Henney AM, Wakeley PR, Davies MJ, et al. Localization of stromelysin gene expression in atherosclerotic plaques by in situ hybridization. *Proc Natl Acad Sci U S A.* 1991;88:8154–8158.

27. Underwood MJ, de Bono DP. Increased fibrinolytic activity in the intima of atheromatous coronary arteries: protection at a price. *Cardiovasc Res.* 1993;27:882–885.

28. Ellis V, Behrendt N, Dano K. Cellular receptor for urokinase-type plasminogen activator: function in cell-surface proteolysis. *Methods Enzymol.* 1993;223:223–233.

29. Leatham EW, Bath PMW, Tooze JA, Camm AJ. Increased monocyte tissue factor expression in coronary disease. *Br Heart J.* 1995;73:10–13.

30. Kaartinen M, Penttilä A, Kovanen PT. Accumulation of activated mast cells in the shoulder region of human coronary atheroma, the predilection site of atheromatous rupture. *Circulation.* 1994;90:1669–1678.

31. Weiss SJ. Tissue destruction by neutrophils. *N Engl J Med.* 1989;320:365–376.

32. Liuzzo G, Biasucci LM, Gallimore JR, et al. The prognostic value of C-reactive protein and serum amyloid A protein in severe unstable angina. *N Engl J Med.* 1994;331:417–424.

33. Thompson SG, Kienast J, Pyke SDM, Haverkate F, van de Loo JCW, for the European Concerted Action on Thrombosis and Disabilities Angina Pectoris Study Group. Hemostatic factors and the risk of myocardial infarction or sudden death in patients with angina pectoris. *N Engl J Med.* 1995;332:635–641.

34. Alexander RW. Inflammation and coronary artery disease. *N Engl J Med.* 1995;332:468–469.

35. MacIsaac AI, Thomas DJ, Topol EJ. Toward the quiescent coronary plaque. *J Am Coll Cardiol.* 1993;22:1228–1241.

36. Lee RT, Grodzinsky AJ, Frank EH, Kamm RD, Schoen FJ. Structure-dependent dynamic mechanical behaviour of fibrous caps from human atherosclerotic plaques. *Circulation.* 1991;83:1764–1770.

37. Cheng GC, Loree HM, Kamm RD, Fishbein MC, Lee RT. Distribution of circumferential stress in ruptured and stable atherosclerotic lesions: a structural analysis with histopathological correlation. *Circulation.* 1993;87: 1179–1187.

38. Bogaty P, Hackett D, Davies G, Maseri A. Vasoreactivity of the culprit lesion in unstable angina. *Circulation.* 1994; 90:5–11.

39. Zeiher AM, Schächinger V, Weitzel SH, Wollschläger H, Just H. Intracoronary thrombus formation causes focal vasoconstriction of epicardial arteries in patients with coronary artery disease. *Circulation.* 1991;83:1519–1525.

40. Stein PD, Hamid MS, Shivkumar K, Davis TP, Khaja F, Henry JW. Effects of cyclic flexion of coronary arteries on progression of atherosclerosis. *Am J Cardiol.* 1994;73: 431–437.

41. Gibson CM, Diaz L, Kandarpa K, et al. Relation of vessel wall shear stress to atherosclerosis progression in human coronary arteries. *Arterioscler Thromb.* 1993;13:310–315.

42. Gertz SD, Roberts WC. Hemodynamic shear force in rupture of coronary arterial atherosclerotic plaques. *Am J Cardiol.* 1990;66:1368–1372.

43. Muller JE, Abela GS, Nesto RW, Tofler GH. Triggers, acute risk factors, and vulnerable plaques: the lexicon of a new frontier. *J Am Coll Cardiol.* 1994;23:809–813.

44. Muller JE, Tofler GH, Stone PH. Circadian variation and triggers of onset of acute cardiovascular disease. *Circulation.* 1989;79:733–743.

45. Willich SN, Maclure M, Mittleman M, Arntz H-R, Muller JE. Sudden cardiac death: support for a role of triggering in causation. *Circulation.* 1993;87:1442–1450.

46. Gnecchi-Ruscone T, Piccaluga E, Guzzetti S, Contini M, Montano N, Nicolis E. Morning and Monday: critical periods for the onset of acute myocardial infarction: the GISSI 2 Study experience. *Eur Heart J.* 1994;15:882–887.

47. Huber K, Resch I, Rosc D, Schuster E, Glogar D, Binder BR. Circadian variation of plasminogen activator inhibitor and tissue plasminogen activator levels in plasma of patients with unstable coronary artery disease and acute myocardial infarction. *Thromb Haemost.* 1988;60:372–376.

48. Willich SN, Collins R, Peto R, Linderer T, Sleight P, Schröder R. ISIS-2 (Second International Study of Infarct Survival) Collaborative Group. Morning peak in the incidence of myocardial infarction: experience in the ISIS-2 trial. *Eur Heart J.* 1992;13:594–598.

49. Willich SN, Löwel H, Lewis M, Hörmann A, Arntz H, Keil U. Weekly variation of acute myocardial infarction: increased Monday risk in the working population. *Circulation.* 1994;90:87–93.

50. Ornato JP, Siegel L, Craren EJ, Nelson N. Increased incidence of cardiac death attributed to acute myocardial infarction during winter. *Coron Artery Dis.* 1990;1:199–203.

51. Gelernt MD, Hochman JS. Acute myocardial infarction triggered by emotional stress. *Am J Cardiol.* 1992;69: 1512–1513.

52. Meisel SR, Kutz I, Dayan KI, et al. Effect of Iraqui missile war on incidence of acute myocardial infarction and sudden death in Israeli civilians. *Lancet.* 1991;338:660–661.

53. Curfman GD. Is exercise beneficial—or hazardous—to your heart? *N Engl J Med.* 1993;329:1730–1731.

54. Mittleman MA, Maclure M, Tofler GH, Sherwood JB, Goldberg RJ, Muller JE. Triggering of acute myocardial infarction by heavy physical exertion: protection against triggering by regular exertion. *N Engl J Med.* 1993;329: 1677–1683.

55. Willich SN, Lewis M, Löwel H, Arntz H-R, Schubert F, Schröder R. Physical exertion as a trigger of acute myocardial infarction. *N Engl J Med.* 1993;329:1684–1690.

56. Grignani G, Soffiantino F, Zucchella M, et al. Platelet activation by emotional stress in patients with coronary artery disease. *Circulation.* 1991;83(suppl 2):II128–II136.

57. Tofler GH, Brezinski D, Schafer AI, et al. Concurrent morning increase in platelet aggregability and the risk of myocardial infarction and sudden cardiac death. *N Engl J Med.* 1987;316:1514–1518.

58. Andreotti F, Davies GJ, Hackett DR, et al. Major circadian fluctuations in fibrinolytic factors and possible relevance to time of onset of myocardial infarction, sudden cardiac death, and stroke. *Am J Cardiol.* 1988;62:635–637.

59. Angleton P, Chandler WL, Schmer G. Diurnal variation of tissue-type plasminogen activator and its rapid inhibitor (PAI-1). *Circulation.* 1989;79:101–106.

60. Bridges AB, McLaren M, Scott NA, Pringle TH, McNeill GP, Belch JJ. Circadian variation of tissue plasminogen activator and its inhibitor, von Willebrand factor antigen, and prostacyclin stimulating factor in men with ischemic heart disease. *Br Heart J.* 1993;69:121–124.

61. Huber K, Beckmann R, Lang I, Schuster E, Binder BR. Circadian fluctuations in plasma levels of tissue plasminogen activator antigen and plasminogen activator inhibitor activity. *Fibrinolysis.* 1989;3:41–43.

62. Quyyumi AA, Panza JA, Diodati JG, Lakatos E, Epstein SE. Circadian variation in ischemic threshold: a mechanism underlying the circadian variation in ischemic events. *Circulation.* 1992;86:22–28.

63. Fuster V, Badimon L, Badimon JJ, Chesebro JH. The pathogenesis of coronary artery disease and the acute coronary syndromes (pt 2). *N Engl J Med.* 1992;326: 310–318.

64. Davies SW, Marchant B, Lyons JP, Timmis AD. Irregular coronary lesion morphology after thrombolysis predicts clinical instability. *J Am Coll Cardiol.* 1991;18:669–674.

65. Pozzati A, Bugiardini R, Borghi A, et al. Transient ischemia refractory to conventional medical treatment in unstable angina: angiographic correlates and prognostic implications. *Eur Heart J*. 1992;13:360–365.

66. Badimon L, Badimon JJ. Mechanism of arterial thrombosis in nonparallel streamlines: platelet thrombi grow at the apex of stenotic severely injured vessel wall: experimental study in a pig model. *J Clin Invest*. 1989;84:1134–1144.

67. Serneri GGN, Sensini GF, Possesi L, et al. The role of extraplatelet thromboxane A$_2$ in unstable angina investigated with a dual thromboxane A$_2$ inhibitor: importance of activated monocytes. *Coron Artery Dis*. 1994;5:137–145.

68. Rentrop KP, Felt F, Blanke H, Sherman W, Thornton JC. Serial angiographic assessment of coronary artery obstruction and collateral flow in acute myocardial infarction. *Circulation*. 1989;80:1166–1175.

69. Van Lierde J, DeGeest H, Verstraeet M, Van de Werf F. Angiographic assessment of the infarct-related residual coronary stenosis after spontaneous or therapeutic thrombolysis. *J Am Coll Cardiol*. 1990;16:1545–1549.

70. Meyer BJ, Badimon JJ, Mailhac A, et al. Inhibition of growth of thrombus on fresh mural thrombus: targeting optimal therapy. *Circulation*. 1994;90:2432–2438.

71. Fitzgerald DJ, Fitzgerald GA. Role of thrombin and thromboxane A$_2$ in reocclusion following coronary thrombolysis with tissue-type plasminogen activator. *Proc Natl Acad Sci U S A*. 1989;86:7585–7589.

72. Kimura S, Nishinaga M, Ozawa T, Shimada K. Thrombin generation as an acute effect of cigarette smoking. *Am Heart J*. 1994;128:7–11.

73. Larsson PT, Wallen NH, Hjemdahl P. Norepinephrine-induced human platelet activation in vivo is only partly counteracted by aspirin. *Circulation*. 1994;89:1951–1957.

74. Yeung AC, Vekshtein VI, Krantz DS, et al. The effect of atherosclerosis on the vasomotor response of coronary arteries to mental stress. *N Engl J Med*. 1991;325:1551–1556.

75. Winniford MD, Wheeland KR, Kremers MS, et al. Smoking-induced coronary vasoconstriction in patients with atherosclerotic coronary artery disease: evidence for adrenergically mediated alterations in coronary artery tone. *Circulation*. 1986;73:662–667.

76. Moliterno DJ, Willard JF, Lange RA, et al. Coronary-artery vasoconstriction induced by cocaine, cigarette smoking, or both. *N Engl J Med*. 1994;330:454–459.

77. Cambien F, Poirier O, Lecerp L, et al. Deletion polymorphism in the gene for angiotensin-converting enzyme is a potent risk factor for myocardial infarction. *Nature*. 1992;359:641–644.

78. Tiret L, Kee F, Poirier O, et al. Deletion polymorphism in angiotensin-converting enzyme gene associated with parental history of myocardial infarction. *Lancet*. 1993; 341:991–992.

79. Ridker PM, Gaboury CL, Conlin PR, Seely EW, Williams GH, Vaughan DE. Stimulation of plasminogen activator inhibitor in vivo by infusion of angiotensin II: evidence of a potential interaction between the renin-angiotensin system and fibrinolytic function. *Circulation*. 1993;87: 1969–1973.

80. van Leeuwen RTJ, Kol A, Andreotti F, Kluft C, Maseri A, Sperti G. Angiotensin II increases plasminogen activator inhibitor type I and tissue-type plasminogen activator messenger RNA in cultured rat aortic smooth muscle cells. *Circulation*. 1994;90:362–368.

81. Ridker PM, Hennekens CH, Stampfer MJ. A prospective study of lipoprotein(a) and the risk of myocardial infarction. *JAMA*. 1993;270:2195–2199.

82. McLean JW, Tomlinson JE, Kuang WJ, et al. cDNA sequence of human apolipoprotein(a) is homologous to plasminogen. *Nature*. 1987;30:132–137.

83. Loscalzo J. Lipoprotein(a): a unique risk factor for atherothrombotic disease. *Arteriosclerosis*. 1990;10: 672–679.

84. Etingin O, Hajjar D, Hajjar K, Harpel P, Nachman R. Lipoprotein(a) regulates plasminogen activator inhibitor-1 expression in endothelial cells. *J Biol Chem*. 1991;266: 2459–2465.

85. Levin EG, Miles LA, Fless GM. Lipoproteins inhibit the secretion of tissue plasminogen activator from human endothelial cells. *Arterioscler Thromb*. 1994;14:438–442.

86. Angles-Cano E, Hervio L, Loyau S. Relevance of lipoprotein(a) in cardiovascular disease: methododical approaches. *Fibrinolysis*. 1993;7:66–68.

87. Juhan-Vague I, Thompson SG, Jespersen J, for the ECAT Angina Pectoris Study Group. Involvement of the hemostatic system in the insulin resistance syndrome. A study of 1500 patients with angina pectoris. *Arterioscler Thromb*. 1993;13:1865–1873.

88. Landin K, Tengborn L, Smith U. Elevated fibrinogen and plasminogen activator inhibitor (PAI-1) in hypertension are related to metabolic risk factors for cardiovascular disease. *J Intern Med*. 1990;227:273–278.

89. Schneider DJ, Sobel BE. Effect of diabetes on the coagulation and fibrinolytic systems and its implications for atherogenesis. *Coron Artery Dis*. 1992;3:26–32.

90. Folsom AR, Wu KK, Shahar E, Davis CE, for the Atherosclerosis Risk in Communities (ARIC) Study Investigators. Association of hemostatic variables with prevalent cardiovascular disease and asymptomatic carotid artery atherosclerosis. *Arterioscler Thromb*. 1993;13:1829–1836.

91. Meade TW, Ruddock V, Stirling Y, Chakrabarti R, Miller GJ. Fibrinolytic activity, clotting factors, and long-term incidence of ischemic heart disease in the Northwick Park Heart Study. *Lancet*. 1993;342:1076–1079.

92. Al-Nozha M, Gader AMA, Al-Momen AK, Noah MS, Jawaid M, Arafa M. Hemostatic variables in patients with unstable angina. *Int J Cardiol*. 1992;43:269–277.

93. Kannel WB, Wolf PA, Castelli WP, D'Agostino RB. Fibrinogen and risk of cardiovascular disease: the Framingham study. *JAMA*. 1987;258:1183–1186.

94. Lauribe P, Benchimol D, Dartigues J-F, et al. Biological risk factors for sudden death in patients with coronary artery disease and without heart failure. *Int J Cardiol*. 1992;34: 307–318.

95. Green D, Ruth KJ, Folsom AR, Liu K. Hemostatic factors in the coronary artery risk development in young adults (CARDIA) study. *Arterioscler Thromb*. 1994;14:686–693.

96. Rosengren A, Wilhelmsen L, Welin L, Tsipogianni A, Teger-Nilsson AC, Wedel H. Social influences and cardiovascular risk factors as determinants of plasma fibrinogen concentration in a general population sample of middle aged men. *BMJ*. 1990;330:634–638.

97. Conelly JB, Roderick PJ, Cooper JA, Meade TW, Miller GJ. Positive association between self-reported fatty food consumption and factor VII coagulant activity, a risk factor for coronary heart disease. *Thromb Haemost.* 1993;70: 250–252.

98. Scarabin PY, Bonothon-Kopp C, Bara L, Maljema A, Guize L, Samama M. Factor VII activation and menopausal status. *Thromb Res.* 1990;57:227–234.

99. Merlini PA, Bauer KA, Oltrona L, et al. Persistent activation of coagulation mechanisms in unstable angina and myocardial infarction. *Circulation.* 1994;90:61–68.

100. Blann AD, McCollum CN. Adverse influence of cigarette smoking on the endothelium. *Thromb Haemost.* 1993;70: 707–711.

101. van der Poll T, van Deventer SJH, Pasterkamp G, van Mourik JA, Büller HR, ten Cate JW. Tumor necrosis factor induces von Willebrand factor release in healthy humans. *Thromb Haemost.* 1992;67:623–626.

102. Conlan MG, Folsom AR, Finch A. Associations of factor VIII and von Willebrand factor with age, race, sex, and risk factors for atherosclerosis. The atherosclerosis risk in communities (ARIC) study. *Thromb Haemost.* 1993;70: 380–385.

103. Jansson J-H, Nilsson TK, Johnson O. von Willebrand factor in plasma: a novel risk factor for recurrent myocardial infarction and death. *Br Heart J.* 1991;66:351–355.

104. Geppert A, Beckmann R, Graf S, et al. Tissue-type plasminogen activator and type-1 plasminogen activator inhibitor in patients with coronary artery disease—relations to clinical variables and cardiovascular risk factors. *Fibrinolysis.* 1995;9:109–113.

105. Hamsten A, Wiman B, De Faire U, Blombaeck M. Increased levels of a rapid inhibitor of tissue plasminogen activator in young survivors of myocardial infarction. *N Engl J Med.* 1985;313:1557–1563.

106. Huber K, Resch I, Stefenelli T, et al. Plasminogen activator inhibitor-1 levels in patients with chronic angina pectoris with or without angiographic evidence of coronary sclerosis. *Thromb Haemost.* 1990;63:336–339.

107. Juhan-Vague I, Alessi MC. Plasminogen activator inhibitor-1 and atherothrombosis. *Thromb Haemost.* 1993;70: 138–143.

108. Olofsson BO, Dahlen G, Nilsson TK. Evidence for increased levels of plasminogen activator inhibitor and tissue plasminogen activator in plasma of patients with angiographically verified coronary artery disease. *Eur Heart J.* 1989;10:77–82.

109. Paramo JA, Colucci M, Collen D. Plasminogen activator inhibitor in blood of patients with coronary artery disease. *Br Med J.* 1985;291:573–574.

110. Rocha E, Paramo JA. The relationship between impaired fibrinolysis and coronary heart disease. *Fibrinolysis.* 1994; 8:294–303.

111. Salomaa V, Stinson V, Kark JD, Folsom AR, Davis CE, Wu KK. Association of fibrinolytic parameters with early atherosclerosis. The ARIC study. *Circulation.* 1995;91: 284–290.

112. Hamsten A, DeFaire U, Walldius G, et al. Plasminogen activator inhibitor in plasma: risk factor for recurrent myocardial infarction. *Lancet.* 1987;2:3–9.

113. Dawson S, Henney A. The status of PAI-1 as a risk factor for arterial and thrombotic disease. *Atherosclerosis.* 1992; 95:105–117.

114. Jansson JH, Olofsson BO, Nilsson TK. Predictive value of tissue plasminogen activator mass concentration on long term mortality in patients with coronary artery disease. A 7-year follow up. *Circulation.* 1993;88:2030–2034.

115. Wieczorek I, Ludlam CA, Fox KAA. Tissue-type plasminogen activator and plasminogen activator inhibitor activities as predictors of adverse events in unstable angina. *Am J Cardiol.* 1994;4:424–429.

116. Huber K, Hornykewycz S, Angles-Cano E. Risikoprädiktion und Sekundärprävention bei Angina pectoris und nach Herzinfarkt. *Der Internist.* 1995;36:883–890.

117. Berk BC, Alexander W, Brock TA, Gimbrone MAJ, Webb RC. Vasoconstriction: a new activity for platelet-derived growth factor. *Science.* 1986;232:87–89.

118. Hackett D, Davies G, Chierchia S, Maseri A. Intermittent coronary occlusion in acute myocardial infarction: value of combined thrombolytic and vasodilator therapy. *N Engl J Med.* 1987;317:1055–1059.

119. Vanhoutte PM, Houston DS. Platelets, endothelium, and vasospasm. *Circulation.* 1985;72:728–734.

120. Meredith IT, Yeung AC, Weidinger FF, et al. Role of impaired endothelium-dependent vasodilation in ischemic manifestations of coronary artery disease. *Circulation.* 1993;87(suppl. 5):V56–V66.

121. Yanagisawa M, Kurihara H, Kimura S, et al. A novel potent vasoconstrictor peptide produced by vascular endothelial cells. *Nature.* 1988;332:411–415.

122. Vanhoutte PM, Shimkova H. Endothelium-derived relaxing factor and coronary vasospasm. *Circulation.* 1989; 80:1–9.

123. Willerson JT, Golino P, Eidt J, Campbell WB, Buja LM. Specific platelet mediators and unstable coronary artery lesions: experimental evidence and potential clinical implications. *Circulation.* 1989;80:198–205.

13

Clinical Subsets

Otmar Pachinger and Fritz Kaindl

Angina pectoris is the leading symptom of coronary artery disease; determining the type of angina pectoris is important in selecting the proper management for affected patients. The term *angina pectoris* was coined by William Heberden when he described sufferers from "a disorder of the breast. . . . The seat of it and sense of strangling and anxiety with which it is attended may make it not improper to be called Angina Pectoris."[1] Heberden therefore gave a description rather than a definition and described a symptom rather than a disease.

Definition

Angina pectoris is the traditional term for intermittent chest pain, usually of short duration, not associated with acute myocardial infarction. The most common form of it is provoked by exercise or excitement and relieved by rest.

Longer attacks occurring without apparent excitation factors have been designated by various names (e.g., *coronary insufficiency, coronary failure, angina decubitus,* etc.), none of which has been widely accepted. The present terminology divides angina pectoris into two subsets: (1) stable angina pectoris and (2) unstable angina pectoris.

Anginal pain is not the only manifestation of reversible ischemia; it may be present in patients who exhibit the following:

- No symptoms at all
- Anginal pain
- Anginal equivalents (dyspnea, dizziness, and apprehension)
- Arrhythmias

The diagnosis of angina pectoris is enabled by a thorough history and the analysis of the patient's symptoms. Various characteristics of pain description have to be considered:

- Quality of symptoms
- Localization of symptoms
- Duration of symptoms
- Triggering factors
- Factors relieving the symptoms
- Behavior of the patient

The symptom complex leading to the diagnosis of angina is invariably important even if the intensity of the discomfort described by the patient appears slight. Pain seldom occurs only in the left precordial area, and a discomfort lasting continuously over several hours is unlikely to be cardiac ischemia unless it is caused by myocardial infarction or uncorrected cardiac rhythm disturbance. Patients with angina usually prefer to rest, sit, or stop walking during attacks.[2,3]

It is not clear why some patients with clear-cut evidence of ischemic heart disease experience no chest discomfort; diabetics appear to have a higher frequency of silent ischemia, perhaps because of autonomic denervation. The fact that the discomfort of angina is not uniform and that other entities can mimic it often makes the differential diagnosis of chest pain difficult.

A host of disorders, including esophageal disorders, biliary colic, costosternal syndrome, cervical radiculitis, and cardiovascular disorders (e.g., pulmonary hypertension, pulmonary embolism, acute pericarditis, and acute myocardial infarction), can cause chest discomfort (Table 13.1).

Patients with stable angina require selective evaluation. Obviously, the sequential use of all available diagnostic techniques is not indicated in all cases. The overall goal of the diagnostic approach to coronary artery disease includes the analysis of pain (i.e., whether it is cardiac or noncardiac in origin), the detection of coronary artery disease with atypical features, and the evaluation of myocardial function

The *clinical history* is the fundamental part of the diagnostic approach; on the basis of a history a definitive di-

TABLE 13.1. Cardiovascular disorders that can lead to angina pectoris.

Aortic valve disease
Hypertrophic obstructive cardiomyopathy
Mitral stenosis
Hypertension
Primary pulmonary hypertension
Pulmonary stenosis
Shunt (left to right)
Hyperthyroidism, obesity, anemia

agnosis can be established. The characteristic features of anginal pain are illustrated in Table 13.2.

The *physical examination* is important diagnostically during an attack of angina pectoris. A patient with angina, during a spontaneous or provoked attack, prefers to stand still or sit. A patient's immobility and distracted and often anxious expression are characteristic of an attack of angina pectoris. The face is often pale; only in severe attacks is a gray tint or even sweating present. There is often dyspnea, and there may be eructation. Examination of the patient's heart is frequently unremarkable. An S_4 gallop sound is often detected, yet this finding has low specificity.

Findings that may support the diagnosis of angina include development of (1) an S_3 gallop sound during pain, (2) an apical systolic murmur, (3) an abnormal systolic precordial pulsation, and (4) arrhythmias. Additional information obtained during examination includes the detection of possible risk factors (hypertension and evidence of hyperlipidemia) and, in later stages of the disease, signs of cardiac failure and other cardiac complications.[4]

Electrocardiography represents an important diagnostic tool in ischemic heart disease; however, in the stage of

TABLE 13.2. Some features differentiating cardiac from noncardiac chest pain.

Favoring ischemic origin	Against ischemic origin
	Character of pain
Constricting	Dull ache
Squeeziing	Knifelike, sharp, stabbing
Burning	Jabs aggravated by respiration
Heaviness, Heavy feeling	
	Location of pain
Substernal	Left submammary area
Across midthorax	Left hemithorax
Both arms, shoulders	
Neck, cheeks, teeth	
Forearms, fingers	
Interscapular region	
	Factors provoking pain
Exercise	Completion of exercise
Excitement	Specific body motion
Other forms of stress	
Cold weather	
After meals	

stable or unstable angina pectoris, the electrocardiogram is frequently normal or may show nondiagnostic abnormalities. The principal value of the electrocardiogram lies in the following:

- Identification of a previous myocardial infarction
- Demonstration of ischemia in tracings taken during an attack of pain
- Demonstration of ischemia during stress tests

Clinical Manifestations of Coronary Artery Disease

The various stages of ischemic heart disease are illustrated in Table 13.3.

Asymptomatic Stage

The asymptomatic stage of angina pectoris can best be defined as a state in which some clinical manifestations of ischemic heart disease can be established in patients who do not have (or do not admit) symptoms. Such manifestations include past myocardial infarction, past angina pectoris with complete remission, and definite evidence of painless ischemia as shown by electrocardiography or scintigraphy. Asymptomatic ischemic heart disease thus consists of two populations: patients with past evidence of the disease, and those with active ischemia but absence of pain or its equivalent.

The problem of painless, or silent, ischemia has never been completely clarified. The obvious explanation of a faulty pain mechanism signaling ischemia appears to apply only to some patients (Table 13.4).

Patients who have anatomic evidence of coronary artery disease without active symptoms fall into two categories: those with a fully compensated state and ade-

TABLE 13.3. Clinical spectrum of coronary artery disease.

Asymptomatic stage
Coronary artery disease with reversible ischemia
Stable subsets
Stable angina
Positive exercise tests
Angina equivalents
Silent myocardial ischemia
Unstable subsets
Unstable angina and equivalents
Post–myocardial infarction angina pectoris
Prinzmetal's angina pectoris
Silent ischemia
Myocardial infarction
Cardiac arrhythmias
Sudden death
Syncope
Coronary artery disease in combination with other conditions

TABLE 13.4. Reasons for lack of symptoms.

Poor history taking by physician
Limiting of physical activity
Sedentary existence of patient
Denial syndrome of patient
Diabetes or transplanted heart
Ischemia and infarction during anesthesia or coma
True silent ischemia

quate perfusion and those with asymptomatic ischemia; the proportion in each category is not known.

Stage of Stable Angina

Stable angina pectoris is defined as recurrent attacks of pain appearing in response to an obvious provocation that increases myocardial oxygen demands. Attacks usually show consistency in circumstances provoking them. Effort angina represents the most common clinical manifestation of coronary artery disease. Less common factors include emotional stress, excitement, attacks of tachycardia, and so forth. Nocturnal attacks do not automatically place a patient in the stage of unstable angina if the attacks are related to exciting dreams, nightmares, or paroxysmal arrhythmias. Cold weather, wind, and post-prandial state often reduce the threshold of pain.

Changes in effort tolerance, if very slow and gradual, do not justify reclassification of patients into unstable angina. Many changes may be related to factors such as changes in body weight, effects of treatment, intercurrent illnesses, and so on. Patients who respond well to treatment by cessation of anginal attacks, or those who reduce activities below anginal threshold, should still be considered as having stable angina, even though they are asymptomatic.[5,6]

The extent of functional impairment can best be evaluated by an objective stress test. Clinical history can classify the stage of the disease according to the scheme of the Canadian Cardiovascular Society[7]:

I. No angina during daily activity
II. Modest angina during daily activity
III. Moderate to severe impairment of daily activity
IV. No activity without symptoms

Atypical Angina (Chest Pain)

Patients' symptoms are termed atypical if the physician is convinced that the patient has coronary artery disease but one or several features do not qualify for cardiac or anginal origin (e.g., pain localization, radiation, or its response to nitroglycerin).

The prevalence of these syndromes is increased in the female population at around 50 years of age. In many of these disorders angina pectoris can be excluded by a careful history and physical examination. It must be emphasized, however, that ischemic heart disease can and frequently does coexist with many of these conditions.

Chest Pain With Normal Coronary Arteriogram

The syndrome of angina pectoris with a normal coronary arteriogram is an important clinical entity.[8–14] In this condition, sometimes referred to as *syndrome X*, the prognosis is usually excellent and its recognition is important. The cause of the syndrome is unknown; many mechanisms (e.g., inadequate vasodilator reserve, abnormality affecting the small resistance vessels, etc.) are postulated, but true myocardial ischemia is present in only a small fraction of these patients.

Unstable Angina

The definition of unstable angina is generally broad, including all forms of angina that do not fall under the definition of stable angina. Unstable angina ranges from rapidly progressing effort angina to prolonged attacks of pain, formerly referred to as coronary insufficiency, coronary failure, intermediate syndrome, and preinfarction angina. A controversial pattern of unstable angina is de novo angina, or angina developing for the first time.[15–22] In 1994 the American Heart Association defined unstable angina in its guidelines as rest angina, new-onset severe exertional angina, or recent acceleration of stable angina.

Unstable angina is a clinical syndrome with different pathophysiological mechanisms in different clinical subsets. These subsets differ in prognosis and therefore management approach (Table 13.5). The identification of high-risk subsets is of utmost importance for proper therapeutic management.

Unstable angina is by definition a transient state. It can resolve into acute myocardial infarction or sudden death, regress into stable angina, or even change into an asymptomatic state. Even severe attacks at rest may respond to hospitalization and intensive medical therapy and subsequently resolve completely.

Some attacks, unresponsive to medical therapy, may require emergency surgery or acute revascularization procedures such as percutaneous transluminal coronary

TABLE 13.5. Subsets in clinical practice.

Documented coronary artery disease without myocardial infarction
Prior myocardial infarction
Variant angina
Post–myocardial infarction
Post–percutaneous transluminal coronary angioplasty
Post–coronary artery bypass graft
Noncardiac chest pain

| | Clinical circumstances | | |
Severity	A. Develops in presence of extracardiac condition that intensifies myocardial ischemia (secondary UA)	B. Develops in absence of extracardiac condition (primary UA)	C. Develops within 2 weeks of AMI (postinfarction UA)
I. New onset of severe angina or accelerated angina (no rest pain)	IA	IB	IC
II. Angina at rest within past month but not within preceding 48 h (angina at rest, subacute)	IIA	IIB	IIC
III. Angina at rest within 48 h (angina at rest, acute)	IIIA	IIIB	IIIC

FIGURE 13.1. Braunwald classification of unstable angina.

angioplasty. The ischemic episodes of unstable angina are not related to obvious precipitating factors, such as anemia, infection, thyrotoxicosis, or cardiac arrhythmias.

Clinical Findings

The chest discomfort in unstable angina is similar in quality to that of exercise-induced angina, although it is usually more intense and of longer duration (up to 20 to 30 minutes). Clues that alert the physician that a patient may be experiencing unstable angina include (1) change in anginal pattern; (2) abrupt and persistent reduction of anginal threshold; (3) increase in frequency, severity, and duration of pain; and (4) new features associated with the pain (e.g., diaphoresis, nausea, and palpitations).

High-risk subsets include patients with (1) pain that continues even after prolonged rest, (2) ST-T changes during the attacks, (3) recent histories of myocardial infarction, and (4) angina associated with hemodynamic compromise (e.g., hypotension, pulmonary edema, murmur during attack, etc.).

It is now widely recognized that patients with unstable angina have a high incidence of ischemic electrocardiographic changes and that these findings have a high prognostic power. Increased levels of troponin also have an adverse prognostic implication.[23,24]

In 1989 Braunwald introduced a new classification of unstable angina to separate patients into a manageable number of meaningful and easily understood subgroups (Figure 13.1).[25,26] A group of Dutch investigators found in a subsequent clinical study that survival without infarction was 80% to 91%, with the best prognosis in

Braunwald's classes I, II, and B and the worst prognosis in classes III and C.[27]

The classification proposed by Braunwald can be used easily in clinical practice; the pain-free period is a better risk indicator than the distinction between accelerated angina and angina at rest. The probability of developing new chest pain decreased to <20% and <10% after 48 hours and 3 days, respectively. In the recent GUSTO trial the investigators were able to stratify the patients according to their electrocardiographic and enzyme changes (Figure 13.2).[28]

Prinzmetal's Variant Angina

In 1959 Prinzmetal described an unusual syndrome of cardiac pain that occurs almost exclusively in patients at rest, usually is not precipitated by physical exertion or emotional stress, and is associated with ST-segment elevations on the electrocardiogram.

This syndrome may be associated with acute myocardial infarction, severe cardiac arrhythmias (including malignant ventricular arrhythmias), and sudden death. Variant angina has been demonstrated to be due to coronary spasm. It is defined as a transient, abrupt, and marked reduction in the diameter of an epicardial artery resulting in myocardial ischemia in the absence of any preceding increases in myocardial oxygen demand.[29–34]

The history differs from that of typical angina: the principal finding is angina at rest. Exercise capacity is usually well preserved; the anginal discomfort may be extremely severe and accompanied by syncope. Occasionally, patients with vasospastic angina have little or no

| | Non-ST group | | ST Elevation group | |
Outcomes	TROP-T neg $N = 201$	TROP-T pos $N = 123$	TROP-T neg $N = 324$	TROP-T pos $N = 176$
Death	1%	9%	5%	12%
Shock	2%	6%	3%	9%
MI	6%	11%	5%	7%
CHF	7%	16%	10%	15%

Gusto IIa Investigators, 1995.

FIGURE 13.2 Risk stratification in acute coronary syndromes.

pain with their ischemia; such patients may present with episodic arrhythmias or syncope as the sole manifestation. These findings suggest that some proportion of patients with sudden cardiac death may have undiagnosed vasospastic angina.[35,36]

The prognosis in these patients is variable. Those with normal or minimally atherosclerotic coronary arteries appear to do well, although a few patients develop infarction or sudden death.[37,38] Patients with severe atherosclerotic changes appear to have a higher incidence of infarction, and revascularization procedures are often necessary.

The most important factor in prognosis is a change in the patient's symptoms. When a patient with stable angina pectoris has a change in symptoms or a patient with asymptomatic coronary artery disease develops complaints, the prognosis worsens for the next 3 to 6 months, the unstable phase. Clinical recognition and prompt attention to evaluation and therapy are of critical importance in patients with new-onset angina or change in symptoms because the incidence of sudden cardiac death and myocardial infarction in the 3 to 6 months following onset of an unstable syndrome is higher than in stable patients.

Sudden Death

Sudden death is the initial and final event in nearly one third of patients with coronary artery disease. Sudden death is defined as unexpected cardiac death in a patient with or without pre-existing disease within 1 hour of having been free of symptoms .

Most patients with ischemic heart disease who suffer sudden death have extensive coronary artery disease, frequently associated with ventricular scarring. They usually do not experience prodromal symptoms, and most patients are affected outside of the hospital. Attempts to improve our ability to predict which patients might suffer cardiac death, particularly as the first manifestation, have resulted in the hypothesis that the risk factors for sudden death are the same as those for other manifestations of coronary artery disease.

References

1. Heberden W. Some account of a disorder of the breast. *Med Trans.* 1772;2:59.
2. Kannel WB, Feinleib M. Natural history of angina pectoris in the Framingham study. *Am J Cardiol.* 1972;29:154–163.
3. Reeves TJ, Oberman A, Jones WB, Sheffield LT. Natural history of angina pectoris. *J Cardiol.* 1974;33:423–430.
4. Vlodaver Z, Neufeld HN, Edwards JE. Pathology of angina pectoris. *Circulation.* 1972;46:1048–1064.
5. Douglas JS, Hurst JW. Limitations of symptoms in the recognition of coronary atherosclerotic heart disease. In: Hurst JW, ed. *The Heart.* New York, NY: McGraw-Hill; 1979: 3–12.
6. Epstein SE, Richmond DR, Goldstein RE. Angina pectoris: pathophysiology, evaluation, and treatment. *Ann Intern Med.* 1971;75:263.
7. Campeau L. Grading of angina pectoris. *Circulation.* 1976; 54:522–523.
8. Bemiller CR, Pepine CJ, Rogers AK. Long-term observation in patients with angina and normal coronary arteriograms. *Circulation.* 1973;47:36–43.
9. Dwyer EM, Weiner L, Cox JW. Angina pectoris in patients with normal and abnormal coronary arteriograms: hemodynamic and clinical aspects. *Am J Cardiol.* 1969;23:639–649.
10. Kemp HG, Elliott WC, Gorlin R. The anginal syndrome with normal coronary arteriography. *Trans Assoc Am Physiol.* 1967;80:59–70.
11. Kemp HG, Vokonas PS, Cohn PF, Gorlin R. The anginal syndrome associated with normal coronary arteriograms: report of six year experience. *Am J Med.* 1973;54:735–742.
12. Ockene JS, Shay MJ, Alpert JS, Weiner BH, Dulen JE. Unexplained chest pains in patients with normal coronary arteriograms. *N Engl J Med.* 1980;303:1249–1252.
13. Opherk D, Zebe H, Weihe E, et al. Reduced coronary dilatory capacity and ultrastructural changes of the myocardium in patients with angina pectoris and normal coronary arteriograms. *Circulation.* 1981;63:817–895.
14. Waxler EB, Kimbiris D, Dreifus LS. The fate of women with normal coronary arteriograms and chest pain resembling angina pectoris. *Am J Cardiol.* 1971;28:25–32.
15. Chahine RA. Unstable angina: the problem of definition. *Br Heart J.* 1975;37:1246–1249.
16. Fahri J-I, Cohen M, Fuster V. The broad spectrum of unstable angina pectoris and its implications for future controlled trials. *Am J Cardiol.* 1986;58:547–550.
17. Fulton M, Duncan B, Lutz W. Natural history of unstable angina. *Lancet.* 1972;1(7762):1244.
18. Gazes PC, Mobley EM, Faris HM, Duncam RC, Humphries GB. Preinfarctional (unstable) angina: a prospective study. Ten year follow-up. *Circulation.* 1973;48:331–337.
19. Gorlin R, Fuster V, Ambrose JA. Anatomic-physiologic links between acute coronary syndromes. *Circulation.* 1986; 74:6–9.
20. Heng MK, Norris RM, Singh BN, Partridge JB. Prognosis in unstable angina. *Br Heart J.* 1976;38:921–925.
21. Krauss KR, Hutter AM, DeSanctis RW. Acute coronary insufficiency: course and follow-up. *Arch Intern Med.* 1972; 129:808–813.
22. Mulcahy R, Daly L, Graham I, et al. Unstable angina: natural history and determinants of prognosis. *Am J Cardiol.* 1981;48:525–528.
23. Vakil RJ. Preinfarction syndrome: management and follow-up. *Am J Cardiol.* 1964;14:55–63.
24. Wilcox I, Freedman B, McCredie RJ, Carter GS, Kelly DT, Harris PJ. Risk of adverse outcome in patients admitted to the coronary care unit with suspected unstable angina pectoris. *Am J Cardiol.* 1989;64:845–848.
25. Braunwald E. Unstable angina: a classification. *Circulation.* 1989;80:410–414.
26. Braunwald E, Mark DB, Jones RH, et al. *Clinical Practice Guideline Number 10: Unstable Angina: Diagnosis and Man-*

agement. Rockville, Md: US Department of Health and Human Services, Agency for Health Care Policy and Research; 1994. AHCPR publication 94-0602.

27. van Miltenburg-van Zijl AJM, Simoons ML, Veerhoek RJ. Incidence and follow-up of Braunwald subgroups in unstable angina pectoris. *J Am Coll Cardiol.* 1995;25:1286–1292.

28. The GUSTO Angiographic Investigators. The comparative effect of tissue plasminogen activator, streptokinase, or both on coronary artery patency, ventricular function, and survival after acute myocardial infarction. *N Engl J Med.* 1993;329:1615–1622.

29. Cheng TO, Bashour T, Kelser GA, Weiss L, Bacos J. Variant angina of Prinzmetal with normal coronary arteriograms. *Circulation.* 1973;47:476–485.

30. Conti CR, Curry RC. Coronary artery spasm and myocardial ischemia. *Mod Concepts Cardiovasc Dis.* 1980;49:1–6.

31. Conti CR, Pepine CJ, Curry JC. Coronary artery spasm: an important mechanism in the pathophysiology of ischemic heart disease. *Curr Probl Cardiol.* 1979;4:1–70.

32. Graves EJ. Detailed diagnosis and procedures. National Hospital Discharge Survey, 1992. National Center for Health Statistics. Vital Health Statistics. 13,1994;118:1–281.

33. Maseri A, Severi S, DesNes M, et al. "Variant" angina: one aspect of a continuous spectrum of vasospastic myocardial ischemia. *Am J Cardiol.* 1978;42:1019–1035.

34. Prinzmetal M, Kennamer R, Merliss R. Angina pectoris, I: a variant form of angina pectoris. *Am J Med.* 1959;27:375.

35. Selzer A, Langston M, Ruggeroli C. Clinical syndrome of variant angina with normal coronary arteriogram. *N Engl J Med.* 1976;295:1343–1347.

36. Severi S, Michelassi C, Orsini E, Marraccini P, L'Abbate A. Long-term prognosis of transient acute ischemia at rest. *Am J Cardiol.* 1989;64:889–895.

37. Theroux P. A pathophysiologic basis for the clinical classification and management of unstable angina pectoris. *Circulation.* 1987;75(suppl 5):V103–V109.

38. Whiting RB, Klei MD, Vanderveer J, Lown B. Variant angina pectoris. *N Engl J Med.* 1970;282:709–715.

14

Echocardiography in Coronary Artery Disease

S. Globits, A. Hassan, M. Zehetgruber, and D. H. Glogar

Over the past three decades, there have been many innovations in echocardiography, including the development of transducer technology, the improvement in image acquisition and display, and the discovery of new clinical applications. Although other noninvasive cardiac imaging techniques, such as magnetic resonance imaging, computerized tomography, nuclear cardiology, and positron emission tomography, are also undergoing technical improvement, echocardiography is still the most widely used imaging modality in clinical cardiology.

In the 1970s, M-mode and two-dimensional echocardiography became available for the study of cardiac anatomy and function. In the early 1980s, introduction of pulsed-wave, continuous-wave, and color flow Doppler imaging allowed evaluation of intracardiac blood flow and accurate estimates of pressure gradients, shunt fractions, valvular areas, and severity of regurgitant lesions. In the late 1980s, transesophageal echocardiography became an established clinical technique. With the introduction of single-plane, then biplane, and recently multiplane transesophageal echocardiography transducers, it became possible to acquire unlimited tomographic views of the heart and the great vessels. This technique has proved to be very valuable in the evaluation of ventricular and valvular function in critically ill patients. In addition, transesophageal echocardiography has been shown to provide important diagnostic information in patients undergoing cardiac surgery, which allows for modification of the surgical plan. Most postoperative surgical complications can be diagnosed quickly with this bedside technique. In this chapter we provide an overview of the rapidly growing field of echocardiography in coronary artery disease (CAD) including various aspects of recent developments in this evolving diagnostic field.

Imaging Techniques in CAD

M-Mode

Quantitative M-mode echocardiographic assessment of cardiac chamber size, wall thickness, and valve excursion is widely performed in clinical practice. The excellent temporal resolution of M-mode echocardiography allows various measurements of diameters of left and right ventricular chambers, septal and posterior left ventricular walls, aortic root, left atrium, and aortic and mitral valve openings in respect to the electrocardiogram. Mean values of healthy subjects for these parameters are shown in Table 14.1. The so-called mitral-septal separation, the perpendicular distance between the E point (most anterior deflection of the tip of the anterior leaflet of the mitral valve in early diastole) and a tangent drawn to the most posterior point reached by the interventricular septum within the same cycle, is a simple and useful indicator of left ventricular function.[1] In the absence of significant aortic regurgitation, a measured value for mitral-septal separation exceeding 10 mm reliably indicates significant global left ventricular systolic dysfunction with an ejection fraction below 40%. Another M-mode echocardiographic index of left ventricular systolic function is the shortening fraction of the left ventricular minor axis, which indicates the fractional distance that the left ventricle moves from its maximum end-diastolic to its minimum end-systolic dimension. End diastole can be marked at the peak of the R wave of the electrocardiogram, immediately after mitral valve closure. End systole can be marked at the end of the T wave or the video frame with maximum systolic myocardial contraction immediately before the mitral valve opening. M-mode echocardiographic measurements are

TABLE 14.1 Normal M-mode measurements of the heart.

Parameter	Range
Right ventricular end-diastolic diameter (mm)	9–26
Left ventricular end-diastolic diameter (mm)	35–56
Left ventricular end-diastolic index (mm/m2)	< 33
Left ventricular end-systolic diameter (mm)	27–37
Fractional shortening (%)	> 30
Posterior left ventricular wall thickness (mm)	6–11
Ventricular septal wall thickness (mm)	6–11
Left atrial dimension (mm)	19–40
Aortic root dimension (mm)	20–37
Aortic cusp separation (mm)	15–26

simple, rapid, and highly reproducible; numerous published results are available for both healthy persons and cardiac patients. M-mode quantitation can be performed frequently, allowing long-term evaluation of progression of cardiac disease or therapeutic interventions. A possible disadvantage of M-mode measurement is that it does not reflect variations in regional cardiac function and size, which are demonstrated on two-dimensional echocardiographic images. For example, a patient who has CAD with an apical aneurysm or a lateral wall motion abnormality might have normal M-mode values for left ventricular diameter and shortening fraction, because these parameters are measured near the cardiac base in an anteroposterior direction.

Two-Dimensional Echocardiography

In two-dimensional images, the contracting heart appears similar to a left ventricular cineangiogram. Consequently, left ventricular ejection fraction, volume, and mass can be determined by two-dimensional echocardiography showing a close correlation with simultaneously performed cineangiographic techniques, radionuclide methods, and autopsy data.[2–4] Although echocardiography tends to underestimate left ventricular volume determined by angiography, which is due to the exclusion of trabecular volume, this effect has been minimized by improvements in ultrasonic beam width, tracing methods, transducer position, and scan plane orientation within the ventricle.

Two-dimensional echocardiography has become the procedure of choice to study cardiac morphology in patients with CAD. However, although two-dimensional echocardiography provides better anatomic imaging with a more accurate and comprehensive assessment of left ventricular geometry, the M-mode technique is more suitable for highly reproducible measurements.

In two-dimensional echocardiography, left ventricular volumes are measured using an application of the biplane Simpson's rule.[2,5] Left ventricular volume and ejection fraction are calculated from the apical two- and four-chamber views. End-diastolic volumes are traced at the peak of the R wave of the electrocardiogram; end-

systolic volumes are traced at the frame preceding mitral valve opening. For assessment of left ventricular mass, the truncated ellipsoid formula can be used to determine epicardial and endocardial end-diastolic volume. The difference between the volumes yields the myocardial volume, which is then multiplied by the density of myocardium (1.05 g/mL). This technique has been validated in animal and human studies.[6,7] The biplane Simpson's rule method for left ventricular volume has been shown to be superior to M-mode single-plane area length and biplane area length methods by correlation with angiography.[8] Most studies show that two-dimensional echocardiographic tracing techniques show the same variation of reproducibility (between 3% and 15%) for left ventricular volume as angiographic studies or radionuclide studies and a beat-to-beat variation between 10% and 37% on sequential ventriculograms. Using the interobserver variability and 95% confidence limits for a given laboratory, a significant change in two-dimensional echocardiographic morphology for a given patient can be determined. In previous studies, an interobserver variability of 23% for left ventricular end-diastolic volume, 33% to 62% for end-systolic volume, and 12% to 45% for ejection fraction was demonstrated.[2,4] Using grouped data, it has been shown that mean population changes of 2% for end-diastolic volume and 5% for end-systolic volume can be considered to be significant. Current development of computer-assisted endocardial edge detection may improve the reproducibility of volume measurements. However, errors due to quantitative planimetry tend to exceed those due to image acquisition, especially in technically suboptimal studies. Ejection fraction, left ventricular mass, and average wall thickness tend to be the most reproducible two-dimensional echocardiographic measurements, whereas volume measurements show the most variability.

Application of Echocardiography in CAD

Wall Motion Abnormalities

Two-dimensional echocardiography permits real-time assessment of left ventricular wall motion and wall thickening, which is useful in the diagnosis of myocardial infarction and ischemia. The area of wall motion abnormality correlates with the vascular distribution of the coronary arteries (Figure 14.1). Transmural or Q-wave myocardial infarctions are usually associated with left ventricular regional wall motion abnormalities, thinning of myocardium, and increased signal intensity of the respective area. Wall motion abnormalities include hyperkinetic, akinetic, or dyskinetic wall segments confined to the area of coronary artery occlusion. Occlusion of the sep-

FIGURE 14.1. Schematic representation of left ventricular wall segments on two-dimensional echocardiogram in relation to coronary artery distribution. LAX, parasternal long-axis view; 4-C, four-chamber view; 2-C, two-chamber view; SAX MV, parasternal short-axis view at mitral valve level; SAX PM, parasternal short-axis view at papillary muscle level; SAX AP, parasternal short-axis view at apical level; sept, septal; ant, anterior; lat, lateral; post, posterior; inf, inferior. (Reproduced, with permission, from Siostrzonek P, Mundigler G, Hassan A, Zehetgruber M. Echocardiographic diagnosis of segmental wall motion abnormalities. *Acta Anaesthesiologica Scandinavica.* 1997;111 [suppl]: 271.)

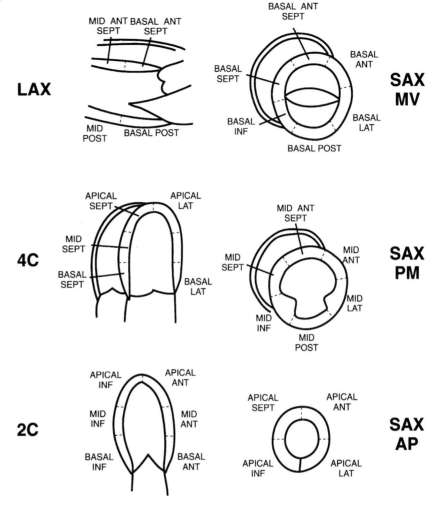

tal branches generally leads to septal asynergy, whereas occlusion of the diagonal branches leads to anterolateral or lateral wall asynergy. The interventricular septum can be visualized in multiple views, including parasternal short- and long-axis, apical four-chamber, and subcostal views. The anterior wall of the left ventricle is best displayed in the parasternal short-axis and apical two-chamber views (Figure 14.1).

Transmural inferior myocardial infarction (due to acute occlusion of the right or circumflex coronary artery) is demonstrated by wall motion abnormalities of the inferior or posterior wall segments. These segments are best imaged in the parasternal short-axis and apical two-chamber views. Lateral wall infarctions seem to be less common on echocardiography than anterior or inferior infarctions and are secondary to acute occlusion in the distribution of the circumflex artery or diagonal branches of the left anterior descending coronary artery. The lateral wall can be demonstrated in the parasternal short-axis and apical four-chamber views, although visualization of the lateral wall is usually hampered by a re-

duced image quality due to limited lateral resolution of the ultrasonic beam.

Diagnosis of Acute Myocardial Infarction

Two-dimensional echocardiography is very useful in the emergency room or coronary care unit setting for diagnosing acute myocardial infarction.[9] In patients with acute chest pain in whom thrombolytic therapy is being considered, this technique may be helpful in differentiating acute coronary occlusion from pericarditis or pulmonary embolism. In this context, echocardiography is most useful in detecting and localizing a patient's first transmural myocardial infarction. The efficacy of this technique decreases in patients with previous myocardial infarctions. In patients with acute myocardial infarction, in whom adequate image quality can be achieved, asynergy with preserved wall thickness and normal gray-scale intensity can be demonstrated. In contrast, chronic infarctions tend to show focal myocardial thinning and high gray-scale intensity, consistent with the presence of scar tissue. However, diagnosis of asynergy may be difficult in patients with bundle branch block, pacemaker, or severe ischemic cardiomyopathy with dilated left ventricle.

In patients with peripheral coronary occlusions, the base of the heart shows normal wall motion, whereas middle or apical segments of the ventricle can demonstrate asynergy. Therefore, global left ventricular function cannot be assessed from a parasternal short-axis view, and quantitative assessment of systolic contractility from M-mode tracing at the base of the heart is not representative for the total left ventricular ejection fraction.

Complications of Myocardial Infarction

Echocardiography, in conjunction with Doppler sonography, can be considered to be the leading diagnostic tool for detection or confirmation of complications of myocardial infarction (Table 14.2). As a readily available bedside diagnostic noninvasive test, it yields instantaneous information in patients with infarction-associated hypotension, new systolic murmurs, and pulmonary edema. For example, in a patient with acute anterior myocardial infarction, a prominent decrease in blood pressure may be secondary to hypervolemia, cardiogenic shock, cardiac rupture with tamponade, papillary muscle dysfunction, or right ventricular infarction. Echocardiography allows complete evaluation of the size and contractility of both ventricles, presence or absence of pericardial effusion, respiratory behavior of the inferior vena cava, and presence or degree of mitral regurgitation.

Systolic Murmur

In a patient with acute infarction and a new systolic murmur, two-dimensional echocardiography in conjunction with Doppler sonography can differentiate ventricular septal rupture from acute mitral regurgitation. In patients with ischemic ventricular septal defect, the defect can often be directly visualized and a shunt flow can be confirmed by detection of high-velocity turbulent blood flow by color-coded Doppler.[10]

In patients with acute myocardial infarction, mitral regurgitation is due to either dilatation of the left ventri-

cle, ischemia or infarction of the papillary muscle, or rupture of chordae tendinae. The regurgitant jet is readily depicted on color-coded Doppler images, which also allow a semiquantitative assessment of severity.

Aneurysm Formation

Two-dimensional echocardiography is very helpful in detecting and distinguishing between aneurysm and pseudoaneurysm.[11–13] A true aneurysm comprises all layers of the myocardial wall (endocardium, myocardium, epicardium, and pericardium) and is characterized by dyskinetic wall motion, a wide neck, and a low risk of cardiac rupture. In contrast, a pseudoaneurysm is due to myocardial rupture, with formation of a saccular structure with a narrow neck often located at the inferior wall and a relatively high risk of rupture.

Thrombus Formation

Left ventricular thrombus formation complicates about 30% to 40% of anterior myocardial infarctions and less than 5% of inferior infarctions.[14–16] Two-dimensional echocardiography is the leading modality for the diagnosis and follow-up of these lesions. Although anticoagulation appears to provide protection against embolic events, resolution of left ventricular thrombi does not always occur with this therapy.[16] Thrombi usually appear as apical structures that have an echogeneity similar to the liver and must be distinguished from left ventricular trabeculae, false chordae, and chest wall artifacts. To appreciate the full size of an apical thrombus, anterior and posterior angulation of the transducer may be helpful. Furthermore, alternative sonographic windows such as the epigastric view may facilitate visualization of apical thrombi. Echocardiographic features that are associated with increased risk of thrombus formation after myocardial infarction include left ventricular aneurysm, spontaneous contrast indicating slow flow in the ventricle, and reverse or circular diastolic flow in the cardiac apex as documented by pulsed-wave Doppler.[17] Two-dimensional echocardiography is ideally suited for serial studies, especially in patients with protruding or freely mobile thrombi.

Pericardial Effusion

Pericardial effusion can occur either early in the infarct period (peri-infarct pericarditis) or late in the course of recovery (Dressler's syndrome). In rare cases, echocardiography can be helpful in acute cardiac rupture associated with cardiac tamponade because it leads to subsequent successful repair of the lesion.

Right Ventricular Infarction

Right ventricular infarction complicates approximately one third of inferior myocardial infarctions and can be

TABLE 14.2 Complications of acute myocardial infarction.

New systolic murmur	Ventricular septal defect
	Mitral regurgitation
Aneurysm formation	
Thrombus formation	
Pericardial effusion	Peri-infarct pericarditis
	Dressler's syndrome
	Cardiac rupture
Right ventricular infarction	
Cardiogenic shock	

diagnosed by echocardiography as right ventricular free wall asynergy on a parasternal, apical, or subcostal view. However, the presence of right ventricular free wall motion abnormalities does not correlate with the hemodynamic importance of a right ventricular infarction. Blunted respiratory response of the inferior vena cava indicates elevated right atrial pressure, whereas poor movement of the right ventricular base indicates a decreased right ventricular contractile state.[18]

Quantification of Ischemic Muscle

The current approach recommended by the American Society of Echocardiography is to use a wall motion score index based on the 16-segment approach.[19] Each segment is judged as to whether it is normal or abnormal based on the following scheme: 1, normal; 2, hypokinetic; 3, akinetic; 4, dyskinetic; and 5, aneurysmal segment. The left ventricular score index is then derived by summing up the scores and dividing them by the number of segments evaluated. If a segment cannot be visualized it is not scored and is not included in the denominator. Consequently, with increasing numbers of segments not visualized, the score index becomes more and more unreliable. This wall scoring index has been modified so that the segments are assigned to different coronary artery distributions. Two overlap areas, the apical septum and the apical lateral wall, are assigned to their appropriate arteries, depending on whether there are also wall motion changes in corresponding segments. For example, an abnormal apical inferior segment is assigned to the left anterior descending artery (LAD) if the apical septum is also abnormal. If, however, the apical septum is normal and the basal inferior wall is abnormal, then the apical inferior wall is assigned to the right coronary artery. Many other schemes have been used for evaluating regional dysfunction with two-dimensional echocardiography, but most are too tedious for routine clinical use.[20,21]

The most preferred method for quantitative evaluation of regional wall function is the so-called center line technique developed in angiographic laboratories.[22,23] On two-dimensional images, endocardial borders are traced in diastole and systole. The computer then calculates the center line between the two contours and generates the deviation from the center line of each of 100 segments. Since echocardiography can also trace the epicardium, a modification of this technique can be used to display wall thickness and endocardial excursion. However, this technique is very tedious and requires high-quality images for accurate measurements.

Stress Echocardiography for Assessment of Viable Myocardium

Since the first report that showed the clinical utility of exercise echocardiography for detection of CAD more than 15 years ago,[24] stress echocardiography has entered the clinical area as a cost-effective alternative to nuclear cardiology. One major advantage of this technique in a clinical setting is its ability to provide instantaneous and on-line results for clinical decision making.

Early limitations were primarily overcome with the introduction of a new generation of two-dimensional scanners and development of digital acquisition systems in combination with quad-screen format and display of preexercise and postexercise images side by side in a continuous cineloop format. Recent studies show that exercise and dobutamine stress echocardiography have comparable sensitivities and specificities to those of exercise and dipyridamole stress thallium perfusion imaging for diagnosis of CAD[25-29] (Table 14.3). This method is clearly superior to analysis of only symptoms and electrocardiographic responses for diagnosis of CAD. Obviously, the levels of accuracy reported in the literature depend on the skill and expertise of experienced, dedicated investigators. Recently, issues of patient prognosis and clinical decision making have been addressed. In particular the prognosis after normal findings on stress echocardiography, prognosis after myocardial infarction without treatment, and risk assessment before noncardiac surgical procedures have been investigated. Stress echocardiography can be performed with the use of either exercise-related or pharmacologically induced stress. Pacing is less commonly used.

TABLE 14.3 Diagnosis of coronary artery disease: myocardial perfusion imaging (MPI) versus stress echocardiography.

Study	Type of stress	No.	Sensitivity		Specificity	
			MPI	Echocardiography	MPI	Echocardiography
Galanti et al.[25]	Exercise	53	27/27 (100%)	25/27 (93%)	24/26 (92%)	25/26 (96%)
Pozzoli et al.[26]	Exercise	75	41/49 (84%)	35/49 (71%)	23/26 (88%)	25/26 (96%)
Quinones et al.[27]	Exercise	112	65/86 (76%)	64/86 (74%)	21/26 (81%)	23/26 (88%)
	Exercise	30	23/30 (77%)	20/30 (67%)	—	—
	Exercise	50	37/42 (88%)	40/50 (80%)	—	—
Forster et al.[28]	Dobutamine	21	10/12 (83%)	9/12 (75%)	8/9 (89%)	8/9 (89%)
Marwick et al.[29]	Dobutamine	217	108/142 (76%)	102/142 (72%)	50/75 (67%)	62/75 (83%)
Total			311/388 (80%)	295/396 (74%)	126/162 (78%)	143/162 (88%)

Exercise Echocardiography

A normal response to exercise is an increase in left ventricular contractility. In the presence of coronary artery stenosis, stress-induced myocardial ischemia results in a decrease of contractility in myocardial regions supplied by stenosed vessels.[30] This alteration of contractility can be detected echocardiographically as an area of hypokinesia, akinesia, or dyskinesia.[31-33] Experimental studies have shown that exercise-induced regional myocardial dysfunction appears earlier and persists longer than ischemic electrocardiographic changes.[34]

Early validation studies on exercise echocardiography used bicycle ergometry with imaging during exercise.[24,35] Exercise echocardiography is usually performed with supine ergometry on a tilting exercise table, with a table tilted to 30 degrees of the left lateral decubitus position. Exercise is started with a workload of 20 W and increased by 20 W every 3 minutes. Other working groups use upright bicycle exercise and imaging before, during, and after exercise.[36,37] With this sequential approach, the sensitivity for detecting CAD can be increased by 10% to 30% in comparison with imaging after bicycle exercise alone.

Since several studies have shown that regional wall motion abnormalities persist up to 30 minutes after a treadmill exercise test,[24,38] this technique can also be used for detection of CAD. Although it has been found satisfactory for the assessment of CAD, this technique is associated with certain technical difficulties. Most importantly, images have to be acquired during the critical postexercise period of 1 minute to maximize the diagnostic accuracy.

Data Acquisition

Before exercise, resting echocardiographic images are obtained from parasternal and apical windows. The subcostal approach can also be used, but this approach is limited by respiratory motion postexercise. The study is recorded on a videotape, and a representative cardiac cycle is acquired, digitized, and stored on a floppy disk for each of the views. Postexercise imaging acquisition is challenging because of lung and motion artifacts and the limited time window after exercise. With the currently available imaging equipment, it is possible to capture several consecutive cardiac cycles, the best being selected for comparison with the resting images. The digitized images are displayed side by side for comparison with the resting images in a continuous cineloop.[39]

Image interpretation is performed by using the 16-segment model recommended by the American Society of Echocardiography.[40] Each segment is analyzed individually and scored on the basis of its motion and systolic wall thickening: 1, normal; 2, hypokinetic; 3, akinetic; 4, dyskinetic; and 5, aneurysmal. By dividing the sum of the scores by the total number of segments analyzed, a global left ventricular wall motion score index at rest and after exercise can be generated. The normal response to exercise is an increasing contractility. Myocardial ischemia is diagnosed when the postexercise echocardiographic images document a new regional wall motion abnormality or when no hyperdynamic motion develops despite good exercise performance. In the presence of regional wall motion abnormality at rest, the postexercise images may display worsening of the resting abnormality. This worsening may be due to additional ischemia that occurs in a prior infarction[41] or may be related to hibernating myocardium, which means profound ischemia in association with persisting tissue viability. Most importantly, these wall segments can show recovery function after successful angioplasty or surgical revascularization.[42] A wall motion abnormality that remains fixed after exercise is often related to a previous myocardial infarction. The possibility of hibernating myocardium has to be considered in this situation, especially if the involved wall segments show normal or near normal wall thickness or the patient has no history or electrocardiographic evidence of prior infarction.

The 16 anatomic segments are classified into three coronary artery distributions (anterior, inferior, and lateral). However, it has to be kept in mind that possible individual variations related to coronary dominance and varying vascular supply of the apex exist. In addition, global left ventricular response to stress is analyzed. Normally, ejection fraction increases with exercise and end-systolic volume decreases with exercise.

Studies have suggested that the feasibility of this technique ranges between 90% and 99% for treadmill exercise echocardiography.[43-46] However, these data were acquired in well-established laboratories with experienced sonographers and the published data pertain to only a small number of patients. The diagnostic accuracy of exercise echocardiography has been reported with a sensitivity of 84% and a specificity of 87%. However, in patients with single vessel disease and normal left ventricular function the sensitivity may be lower (approximately 75%). For application of these results to clinical practice, it has to be emphasized that for most published data the visual interpretation of the coronary angiography was used with its limitations relative to the prediction of the physiological significance of a stenosis.[47] Limited data suggest that quantitative indexes of severity of coronary artery stenosis correlate better with exercise echocardiographic results than qualitative angiographic interpretation.[48]

Pharmacological Stress Echocardiography

Compared with exercise testing, pharmacological tests may have several advantages, such as better image quality, feasibility in patients unable to exercise, and high specificity and sensitivity for the diagnosis of CAD.[49–53] Two classes of drugs have been used: (1) coronary vasodilators such as dipyridamole and adenosine, which induce subendocardial ischemia through a coronary steal phenomenon, and (2) sympathomimetic agents such as dobutamine, which increases the myocardial oxygen demand by increasing heart rate and contractility.

Dipyridamole-Stress Echocardiography

Dipyridamole-stress echocardiography is performed at a total dose of 0.84 mg/kg body weight over 10 minutes.[52] In radionuclide studies dipyridamole has been shown to induce blood flow heterogeneity in patients with CAD. However, not all blood flow heterogeneity indicates true myocardial ischemia; this form of stress, which results in a rather low sensitivity (average 65%, range 48%–82%), is thus not ideal in diagnosing CAD.

Adenosine-Stress Test

Adenosine increases resting coronary blood flow more than fourfold in normal subjects. However, it has not been widely used. Data published so far indicate a sensitivity of around 85%.[54] The high cost of the drug and frequent side effects may limit its use.

Dobutamine-Stress Echocardiography

Dobutamine increases myocardial contraction at low doses (5–20 µg/kg per minute) and increases heart rate at high doses (30–50 µg/kg per minute). The dobutamine test usually begins with an infusion rate of 5 µg, with subsequent increases every 3 minutes to 10, 20, 30, and 40 µg/kg per minute. During each state of infusion, echocardiographic images are acquired for assessment of global and segmental left ventricular function. The blood pressure response varies during administration of dobutamine but usually increases by 10 to 30 mm Hg. The heart rate increases gradually. In patients in whom the target heart rate is not achieved, atropine has been used.[55] The safety of this test has been well established; the incidence of arrhythmias is approximately 10% to 15%. Less than 2% of patients experience nonsustained ventricular tachycardia. During the infusion of dobutamine, progressive reduction in end-diastolic and end-systolic volumes is observed; myocardial wall thickening also increases progressively. In areas of ischemia the percentage of myocardial thickening may reach only 30% to 40%; these areas are then identified as relatively hypokinetic. Severe ischemia can be seen as akinesis or dyskinesis. The sensitivity of this method ranges from 72% to 95% (mean 85%), with a specificity between 66% and 93% (mean 81%).[56] Various studies have shown that dobutamine-stress echocardiography compares favorably with radionuclide techniques.[52,55–57]

Assessment of Myocardial Viability With Dobutamine Echocardiography

Since patients with poor left ventricular function and significant CAD often show an improvement in contractile function after revascularization,[58] methods of assessing myocardial viability are necessary to determine which patients will benefit most from coronary angioplasty or bypass surgery. Dysfunctional myocardium can be classified as either stunned (severe but transient decrease in coronary blood flow) or hibernating (severe chronic reduction of coronary blood flow). Dysfunctional myocardium can be differentiated from myocardial scar by the induction of contractile (inotropic) reserve during use of low-dose dobutamine infusion. The presence of contractile reserve during low-dose dobutamine infusion in patients with chronic ventricular dysfunction has been shown to predict improved survival and functional improvement after revascularization.[59] Low-dose dobutamine stress echocardiography predicts recovery of function in 75% to 85% of myocardial segments after revascularization.[60]

Comparison of Different Pharmacological Stress Tests

A recent study by Dagianti[61] showed a feasibility for pharmacological tests of 100% but only 95% for exercise testing, mainly due to inadequate image acquisition during exercise. For detection of CAD on the basis of wall motion abnormalities, exercise-stress echocardiography showed an overall sensitivity of 76%, dipyridamole-stress echocardiography showed 52%, and dobutamine-stress echocardiography showed 72%. Specificity data for exercise were 94%, for dipyridamole 97%, and for dobutamine 97%, yielding a diagnostic accuracy of 87% for exercise, 78% for dipyridamole, and 87% for dobutamine. For prediction of the extent of significant CAD, exercise showed a 40% accuracy rate compared with 17% by dipyridamole and 46% by dobutamine. This study suggests that exercise and dobutamine echocardiography demonstrate a higher sensitivity when compared with dipyridamole echocardiography for diagnosis of CAD. However, other investigators found a significantly higher sensitivity for exercise (89%) than for dipyridamole (43%).[62] Dipyridamole echocardiography also appears to be less sensitive in patients with multivessel disease.[63]

Transesophageal Stress Echocardiography

In obese patients or patients with obstructive lung disease and chest wall deformities, transthoracic echocardiographic image quality is not good enough to allow accurate delineation of endocardial borders. In these patients the transesophageal approach can overcome these limitations with improved visualization of epicardial and endocardial borders.

A recent report[64] has shown that transesophageal dobutamine-stress echocardiography is feasible and safe, with sensitivity and specificity of 82% and 93%, respectively. However, this method also has potential limitations. Approximately 4% of the studies had to be terminated because of patient discomfort. The total transesophageal probe insertion time was 15 minutes. In 8% of patients pure echocardiographic images related to the presence of hiatal hernia or gastroesophageal disease were present.

The limited data on transesophageal stress echocardiography show similar results with dipyridamole[65] and atrial pacing.[66] Segar et al.[57] showed that detection of stenosis in individual coronary arteries is improved in lesions with a minimal lumen diameter of <1 mm (sensitivity 86%), indicating that these stenoses are more likely to be physiologically significant.

A potential limitation of the transesophageal approach is that ischemia confined to the apex may be missed. However, use of a biplane transducer with a longitudinal imaging plane can improve visualization of wall motion abnormalities in these segments.

Prognostic Implications of Stress Echocardiographic Studies

The most powerful predictor of cardiac events is the presence and extent of jeopardized viable myocardium on myocardial perfusion imaging. The cardiac event rate appears to be substantially higher among patients with negative stress echocardiography (more than 12% per year) compared with myocardial perfusion imaging (4% per year).[67,68] This difference is greatest when prevalence of underlying CAD is high. Therefore normal stress echocardiography does not appear to reliably identify a low-risk group, especially in patients with known CAD.[69,70]

Assessment of Left Ventricular Diastolic Function

Symptoms of congestive heart failure are usually attributed to left ventricular systolic dysfunction. Within the last decade it has become apparent that left ventricular diastolic dysfunction may also account for dyspnea on exertion or pulmonary edema. Patients with diabetes, hypertension, aortic stenosis, and other forms of pathological left ventricular hypertrophy often demonstrate noncompliant left ventricular pressure to volume relationships such that small increases in left ventricular volume lead to marked increases in filling pressure. A notable exception is the physiological left ventricular hypertrophy acquired by highly trained athletes who usually have normal compliance characteristics.

Several echocardiographic parameters correlate well with invasively determined criteria for left ventricular diastolic dysfunction. M-mode markers include abnormal posterior aortic root motion and mitral valve motion. Motion of the posterior aortic root mirrors changes in left atrial volume.[71] In the normal compliant left ventricle, the aortic root moves rapidly posteriorly in early diastole, reflecting vigorous passive filling. In noncompliant hearts, early posterior diastolic motion occurs slowly, but late diastolic motion is more prominent, reflecting dependence of left ventricular filling on atrial kick. M-mode tracings of mitral valve motion also demonstrate an exaggerated atrial filling wave in patients with stiff ventricles. In addition, abnormal diastolic function is reflected by flattened mitral E/F slope, abnormal diastolic left ventricular posterior wall motion, and enlarged left atrium despite sinus rhythm.

Currently, the most commonly used echocardiographic technique to evaluate left ventricular diastolic function is the Doppler analysis of mitral inflow.[72,73] The healthy young adult in sinus rhythm has a dominant or large early mitral peak flow velocity (E wave) and a smaller late mitral peak flow velocity (A wave), representing atrial contraction, as well as a short E-wave deceleration time. In patients with left ventricular diastolic dysfunction, a reversal of this pattern occurs, with a small E wave, a large A wave, an E-to-A ratio less than 1, and an increased E-wave deceleration time. In patients with hypertension, serial studies have shown that development of this Doppler criterion occurs early and precedes echocardiographic evidence of left ventricular hypertrophy.[74] However, several important limitations in the application of Doppler sonography for diagnosis of diastolic dysfunction have to be mentioned. First, the normal heart shows an increasing tendency to display an inversed E-to-A ratio with age. In addition, parameters of mitral inflow depend on many factors such as heart rate, loading conditions, ventricular contractility, and presence or absence of mitral regurgitation.

Evaluation of Coronary Blood Flow by Echocardiographic Techniques

Transesophageal Doppler Echocardiography

The simple anatomical evaluation of severity of coronary artery stenosis is of limited value because coronary flow reserve, the real indicator of functional importance of a stenosis, only modestly correlates with anatomical severity.[75] Therefore, growing interest exists in methods that can assess coronary blood flow reserve by measuring flow before and after drug-induced increases in flow.[76,77] Besides invasive, catheter-guided methods (see later section), transesophageal echocardiography has emerged

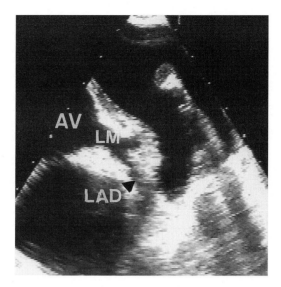

FIGURE 14.2. Transesophageal echocardiographic image visualizing the aortic root slightly above the aortic valve (AV), left main coronary artery (LM), and left anterior descending artery (LAD).

cation. Transducer adjustments include up and down movements, right and left movements, and retroflexion. Because of cyclic cardiac movement, the LAD does not always lie in the same position throughout the entire cardiac cycle. However, during diastole the position of LAD is stable, thus making ultrasound exploration feasible by placing a Doppler sample volume in the vascular lumen.

Coronary blood flow velocity in LAD has a biphasic pattern, with a greater diastolic component and a smaller systolic component. Usually, the following parameters are measured: maximal systolic velocity, maximal diastolic velocity, mean systolic velocity, and mean diastolic velocity. Coronary blood flow reserve is then calculated as the ratio of stress to rest maximal diastolic velocity. Interobserver and intraobserver variability of this method is around 3%, with a reproducibility rate of 2%.[81] Peak diastolic velocities in a normal LAD range from 12 to 50 cm/s (mean 35 cm/s) at baseline and from 63 to 139 cm/s (mean 109 cm/s) during dipyridamole infusion. In patients with severe coronary artery stenosis, defined as more than 75% decrease of lumen in angiography, the dipyridamole response is significantly blunted, with a maximum diastolic velocity during dipyridamole of 53 to 104 cm/s (mean 75 cm/s) (Figure 14.3A,B). As shown recently,[81] blood flow measurements can be adequately recorded in about 70% of patients, and short-term reproducibility of this method is good. In patients without CAD, blood flow velocity increases significantly with pharmacological interventions (Figure 14.4A,B).

Similar to measurements of transesophageal flow velocity in the proximal LAD, coronary sinus flow velocity before and after dipyridamole administration also allows assessment of coronary flow reserve. A modified four-chamber view with dorsal angulation of the transducer is used to visualize the ostium of the coronary sinus (Figure 14.5). Coronary sinus flow velocity recordings are

as a semi-invasive method with high-quality images that provide visualization of proximal parts of the LAD.[78,79] Furthermore, pulsed-wave Doppler can be used to measure coronary blood flow velocity in the LAD directly before and after pharmacological intervention.[80]

Transesophageal echocardiography is usually performed with the patient in the left lateral decubitus position. The LAD is visualized by placing the transducer at a level just above the aortic valve leaflets. LAD, arising from the corresponding sinus, is seen as an echo-free space (Figure 14.2). Small adjustments in transducer orientation are usually necessary to visualize the vessel along its full length from aortic root to its y-shaped bifur-

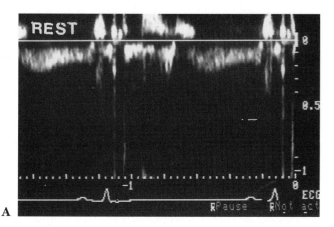

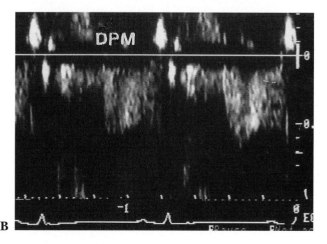

FIGURE 14.3. **A,** Typical coronary blood flow velocity pattern of the left anterior descending artery (LAD) in a patient with severe proximal LAD stenosis at rest. **B,** After dipyridamole (DPM) administration, flow velocity increases only moderately, resulting in a coronary flow reserve of 1.9.

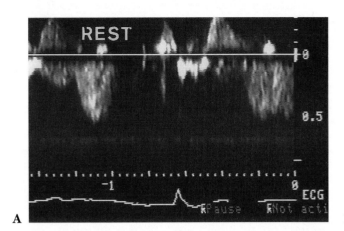

A   B

FIGURE 14.4. **A,** Coronary blood flow velocity pattern of the left anterior descending artery (LAD) in a patient without coronary artery disease at rest. **B,** After dipyridamole (DPM) ad-

ministration, a marked increase in flow velocity occurs, resulting in a coronary flow reserve of 3.0.

performed with the Doppler sample placed in the coronary sinus within a distance up to 10 mm from its ostium. Typically, a biphasic anterograde flow pattern and short mid-diastolic or end-diastolic periods of retrograde flow are observed. Recent studies demonstrate the feasibility of this technique for the assessment of coronary flow reserve in patients with dilated cardiomyopathy, severe LAD disease, and syndrome X.[82,83] Figure 14.6A,B demonstrates a significant increase in coronary sinus flow velocity after dipyridamole in a patient without CAD. In contrast, only a minor change in coronary sinus

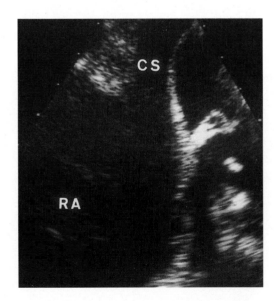

FIGURE 14.5. Modified transesophageal four-chamber view visualizing the coronary sinus (CS) draining into the right atrium (RA).

flow velocity occurs in a patient with syndrome X (Figure 14.7A,B).

Limitations of Transesophageal Doppler Echocardiography

Following are limitations of transesophageal Doppler echocardiography:

1. Transesophageal echocardiography cannot be considered as a noninvasive technique. However, it is definitely safer than cardiac catheterization.
2. The feasibility of transesophageal Doppler evaluation of coronary blood flow is around 70% using the LAD technique and around 90% using the coronary sinus technique. However, invasive methods also have some technical difficulties and limitations.
3. Due to the angle between the exploring ultrasound beam and the direction of blood flow velocities, measured values can be lower then the real velocities. However, since flow reserve (the ratio between baseline and stress values) is calculated, the effect of the angle between blood flow direction and ultrasound beam is eliminated.
4. Doppler techniques measure velocities but not blood flow volume. To calculate blood flow volume, one needs to know the cross-sectional area of the vessel. Since dipyridamole increases the area of the vessel only modestly, changes in coronary blood flow velocities induced by dipyridamole closely reflect changes in coronary blood flow.
5. Transesophageal LAD and coronary sinus techniques are limited to flow reserve calculations within the territory of the left coronary artery. Regional coronary flow reserve cannot be determined by the coronary sinus technique.

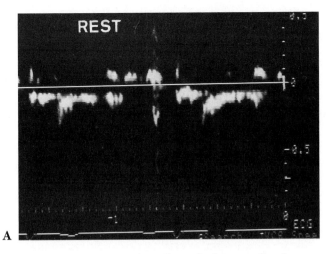

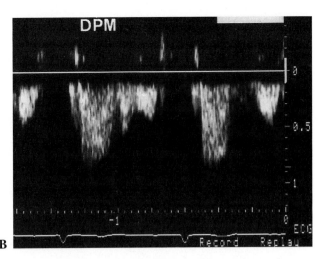

FIGURE 14.6. **A,** Coronary sinus flow velocity recording in a patient without coronary artery disease with normal coronary flow reserve at rest. **B,** After dipyridamole (DPM) administration, a marked increase in flow velocity occurs.

Clinical Implications of Transesophageal Doppler Echocardiography

Transesophageal Doppler evaluation of coronary blood flow reserve appears to be particularly useful for physiopathological studies requiring serial evaluation of coronary flow reserve, such as assessment of effects of pharmacological interventions on coronary blood flow velocity and evaluation of coronary blood flow reserve in cardiac diseases. Another possible clinical implication could be the measurement of effects of angioplasty on LAD. In cardiac disease with diffuse reduction of coronary flow reserve, as in patients with syndrome X, evaluation of global flow reserve by the coronary sinus technique seems particularly sensitive.

Invasive Measurements of Coronary Flow Reserve

Invasive methods of measuring coronary flow reserve include thermodilution techniques, Doppler catheters, and digital coronary angiograms at baseline conditions and during maximal vasodilation induced pharmacologically.[76,77]

Doppler Methods

Until recently, all intracoronary Doppler measurements were made using either intracoronary Doppler catheters or modified Judkins catheters with a caudally mounted piezoelectric crystal.[84] This generation of catheters was

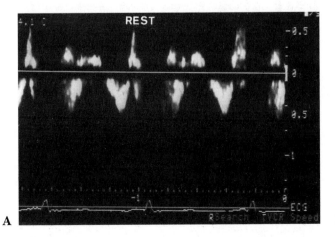

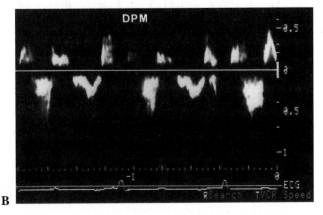

FIGURE 14.7. **A,** Coronary sinus flow velocity recording in a patient with syndrome X at rest. **B,** After dipyridamole (DPM) administration, the flow velocity pattern is not altered.

constructed with either end-mounted or side-mounted Doppler crystals and was generally 3 F in size. Due to the relatively large size of these catheters, Doppler measurements were limited to the proximal portions of large epicardial vessels. These limitations have been overcome by development of a Doppler-tipped guide wire including a 12- and 15-MHz piezoelectric ultrasound transducer. The forward-directed ultrasound beam diverges at a 27-degree angle from the Doppler transducer. The signal from the piezoelectric transducer is processed by a real-time spectral analyzer using on-line fast Fourier transformation.[85] The Doppler guide wire is steerable and can be used during interventional procedures. Due to its small size, this guide wire does not create much turbulence and can therefore assess flow velocities in large portions of the epicardial vessels.

Measurement of Normal Coronary Blood Flow

In the normal coronary circulation, blood flow velocity signals have a characteristic diastolic predominant flow pattern, which is secondary to systolic filling of epicardial capacitance vessels followed by diastolic runoff into intramyocardial vessels. Integrating the area under the systolic and diastolic flow velocity curves to generate velocity integrals demonstrates a diastolic to systolic flow velocity integral ratio of more than 1.5 in normal coronary arteries.[86] The right coronary artery usually has a less marked diastolic predominant flow velocity pattern, resulting in a lower diastolic to systolic flow velocity integral ratio. Mean velocities in the LAD equal 31 ± 15 cm/s, in the circumflex 25 ± 8 cm/s, and in the right coronary artery 26 ± 7 cm/s. Using the Doppler catheter, the ratio of maximal hyperemic coronary blood flow to baseline blood flow can be calculated and is known as coronary flow reserve. As mentioned previously, the coronary flow reserve in normal patients has been demonstrated to be three to six times greater than resting flow values.[87]

Assessment of Severity of Coronary Stenosis

Translesional pressure gradients, absolute and normalized for aortic pressure, have been used to define the resting hemodynamic significance of coronary stenosis.[88] More recently, peak hyperemic translesional gradients and distal coronary artery pressures during hyperemia have been used as an advancement of the hemodynamic assessment of functional characteristics of stenosis.[89] Measurement of coronary flow reserve as an effective method for assessing physiological characteristics of a stenosis was established by Goldstein et al.[90] In contrast to animal studies, in humans the hyperemic coronary flow has demonstrated variable results in predicting the functional significance of angiographically defined coronary stenosis.[75,91] The variable results are due mainly

to the proximal measurements of flow reserve being summations of the flow reserve in the index epicardial artery and proximal branches. Doppler guide wire technology has overcome this problem by measuring flow reserve distal to stenosis. Three major markers of altered coronary flow velocity characterize physiologically significant coronary stenosis:

1. Translesional flow velocity.
2. Phasic coronary velocity ratio: animal and human studies have found a reduction of diastolic flow velocity with an unchanged systolic flow velocity distal to significant stenosis, resulting in a lowered diastolic to systolic velocity ratio.[89,92]
3. Distal coronary flow reserve: coronary reserves of 2.0 or less are strongly correlated with the presence of a reversible perfusion defect on technetium Sestamibi single photon emission computed tomography scintigraphic imaging.[93] The 89% correlation rate between perfusion imaging and distal coronary flow reserves was superior to that with proximal to distal flow velocity integral ratios or quantitative angiography.

Limitation of Intracoronary Doppler Technique

Doppler measurements may be affected by three-dimensional geometry of stenosis; intracoronary velocity profile, especially in diffusely diseased vessels; and interrogation angle between the piezoelectric crystal and major flow vector of blood. Doppler guide wires have a very small sample volume and may not measure maximal blood flow velocity, especially in large arteries. Extrapolation from Doppler velocity measurements to volumetric blood flow calculations may also be difficult.

Intravascular Ultrasound

Intravascular ultrasound (IVUS) uses miniature transducers at the tip of the catheter to provide cross-sectional images of small and large arteries. For IVUS imaging, 20- to 50-MHz transducers (with 2.9- to 4.3-F catheters) are used. Catheters are of mechanical or solid-state (phased array) design. The advantage of the solid-state multielement system is the lack of a drive shaft for rotating the ultrasound element, thus allowing the central lumen to be used as a guide wire. In addition, absence of a rotating component prevents potential distortion resulting from nonuniform rotational velocity in mechanical systems. However, the lateral resolution of solid-state designs is presently slightly inferior to the resolution of mechanical systems. A limitation common to all of these instruments is the lack of forward-viewing capability. However, a prototype catheter that allows visualization beyond the catheter tip has recently been developed.[94]

Major complications with IVUS are rare and occur only during interventional procedures. Minor complications, predominantly spasm reversed by nitroglycerin, may occur during diagnostic cases but are very uncommon (0.8%–8%).

With IVUS imaging, normal muscular arteries have a three-layered appearance. By using microdissection, the media have been shown to be responsible for the echolucent middle zone in normal adult human arteries. This zone is often thinner or absent at arterosclerotic sites when mechanical systems are used.[95] It has also been shown that reflectivity of the inner echogenic layer of a plaque is greater in regions with more calcium and proteoglycan and less lipid. An increase in collagen in the media results in echogenicity and reflectivity similar to that of the intima. Therefore, in a diseased coronary artery with a three-layered appearance, the inner echogenic layer may represent both the intima and part of the media. Since it is usually difficult to delineate the intimal surface, Hausman et al.[96] have shown that the boundary between arterial wall and blood can be enhanced by use of contrast agents.

Correlations between IVUS and angiographic measurements are very good in normal segments ($r = 0.92$) but very weak after coronary angioplasty ($r = 0.28$).[97] Other studies have shown that the extent and severity of CAD are significantly underestimated by angiography.[98–100] This underestimation is due to possible disease of the reference segment and compensatory enlargement (arterial remodeling) of the diseased segment.

IVUS has been extremely useful in elucidating mechanisms of various interventions. Arterial expansion and dissection are the principal mechanisms responsible for improved lumen dimensions after balloon angioplasty.[101] IVUS allows for the assessment of calcification within the target lesion, which can help in choosing the right device. Clinical experiments have shown that IVUS influences catheter-based therapy in 48% of cases including upsizing of a device, placement of a perfusion catheter, change in device selection, and alteration in the orientation of a atherectomy device. IVUS can also be used to assess results after coronary stenting[102] (Table 14.4).

Intracardiac Echocardiography

Intracardiac echocardiography is another catheter-based ultrasound modality allowing visualization of intracardiac structures. Compared with IVUS, for intracardiac echocardiography lower-frequency (10- to 20-MHz) catheters are mandatory. Catheter size varies from 6 to 10 F. Larger sizes are required for lower-frequency catheters. With this method cardiac anatomy can be defined easily, and valvular abnormalities, ventricular dysfunction, cardiac masses, and pericardial effusions can be identified (Table 14.5). However, this type of catheter does not allow reliable visualization of left heart structures from the right side of the heart in adults.

TABLE 14.4 Applications of intravascular ultrasound.

Assessment of the extent of atherosclerosis and other arterial diseases
Better understanding of arterial remodeling and disease of the reference segment
Use in studies on regression of atherosclerosis
Assessment of left main coronary artery disease
Diagnosis of aortic dissection
Assessment of coronary involvement in Kawasaki's syndrome

Assessment of dynamic abnormalities
Use in studies of vasomotor and endothelial function
Characterization of different coronary syndromes, such as vasospasm bridging, and syndrome X

Use during interventions
Selection of type and size of device in coronary and peripheral arteries
Monitoring during balloon angioplasty and atherectomy
Use in coronary artery stenting
Monitoring in children (closure of patent ductus arteriosus and balloon dilation of coarctation)

TABLE 14.5 Potential applications of intracardiac echocardiography.

Electrophysiology laboratory
Use during transseptal catheterization
Positioning of tip of ablation catheter
Optimization of tissue electrode contact
Monitoring during energy application
Visualization of ablation lesions
Rapid identification of complications
Decrease in fluoroscopy time

Catheterization laboratory
Assessment of regional and global systolic function
Assessment of the viability of a ventricular segment
Assessment of the functional significance of coronary stenosis
Assessment of collateral flow to specific territory in combination with contrast echocardiography
Use during transseptal catheterization
Wire and balloon positioning during valvuloplasty
Monitoring during catheter closure of atrial septal defect
Rapid identification of complications

Coronary care unit and operating room
Monitoring of ventricular function
Early detection of myocardial ischemia

Contrast Echocardiography

Myocardial contrast echocardiography (MCE) uses introduction of microbubbles of air into the coronary circulation during concurrent two-dimensional echocardiographic imaging. The subsequent increased myocardial contrast can be quantified in a spatial and temporal fashion. MCE is a pure intravascular tracer technique. Since initial use of the technique,[103] attention has focused on characterization of regional distribution of coronary blood flow and measurements of myocardial perfusion.

The magnitude of contrast enhancement is proportional to the sixth power of the bubble radius.[104] Therefore, an ideal microbubble must be sufficiently large to produce myocardial opacification yet suitably small to move freely through the capillaries. An ideal microbubble can be created with a recently developed method using sonication of liquid media containing air or other gases.[105] However, sonicated noniodinated and iodinated radio-opaque dyes produce transient effects on systemic hemodynamics and left ventricular function. In contrast, sonicated 5% human albumin produces myocardial opacification without affecting coronary blood flow, systemic hemodynamics, or left ventricular function (Albunex, Molecular Biosystems, Inc, San Diego, CA, USA).[106] This contrast medium shows a favorable safety profile and has been approved by the US Food and Drug Administration. After intravenous injection of Albunex one can see opacification of the left ventricular cavity, followed by the opacification of the left ventricular myocardium. Time–activity and time–intensity curves can be obtained. Alternatively, palmitic acids encapsulated in polysaccharides have been developed, which can be produced in reproducible sizes of 3 to 6 μm. After injection into the central venous system, the microbubbles pass through the lungs and are stable for four to five heart cycles (Laevovist, Schering, Berlin, Germany).

Clinical Application

Because of the no- or low-reflow abnormalities in microvascular reserve, an intravascular tracer can be used to distinguish infarct from viable tissue during postischemic reperfusion.[107] No-reflow abnormalities refer to failure of tissue perfusion despite re-establishment of epicardial coronary artery patency after sustained coronary artery occlusion.[108] This phenomenon corresponds pathologically to microvascular obstruction and necrosis, occurs exclusively in necrotic tissue, and is proportional to the extent of myocardial infarction. As a result of the no-reflow phenomenon, MCE perfusion defects correlate directly with the size of myocardial infarction.[107] Coronary hyperemia occurs immediately after reflow, and therefore the perfusion defect tends to underestimate the size of the infarct. Despite the presence of resting hyperemia, however, microvascular reserve within infarct tissue is impaired.[109] Therefore, when a coronary vasodilator is administered exogenously, no further increase in flow occurs within the infarct zone, whereas normal tissue demonstrates a marked increase in flow. Therefore, infarcted tissue shows less perfusion during coronary vasodilation despite resting hyperemia.[107] Repeat MCE studies after 1 month of angiographically documented patency of the infarct-related artery showed that recovery of regional ventricular function was less in no-reflow regions compared with those with successful tissue perfusion.[110]

Assessment of Collateral Blood Flow

Since MCE microbubbles are smaller than 10 μm, assessment of collateral blood flow appears to be superior to coronary arteriography, which can only detect collaterals greater than 100 μm in diameter. Therefore, MCE is able to demonstrate collateral blood flow within an infarct bed despite the presence of a persistently occluded infarct-related artery. The spatial extent of collateral perfusion within the infarct bed is associated with improved regional systolic function after antegrade blood flow is restored to the infarct zone, even when achieved late after acute infarction.[111]

Assessment of Coronary Blood Flow Reserve

MCE can reveal the presence of a reduced vascular reserve in the perfusion bed of a stenotic artery by use of pharmacological vasodilation.[112] It may also be possible to measure the relative myocardial blood flow using MCE.[113] When microbubbles are injected as a rapid bolus directly into a coronary artery, the wash-in and wash-out characteristics of the contrast medium are manifested as a rise and fall in video intensity over time. The width of the time–intensity curve is related to the rate of transit of the microbubbles through the myocardium, which is proportional to the ratio of blood flow to intravascular blood volume of the myocardial region supplied by the artery. However, when microbubbles are not delivered directly into the coronary artery as a tight bolus, the input function is dispersed over multiple cardiac cycles and is longer than the transit time of the tracer through the myocardium. Nonetheless, the peak intensity of contrast in the myocardium can be used as a measure of myocardial blood volume (i.e., the volume of blood within myocardial arterioles, capillaries, and venules).[113]

In summary, MCE is a clinically useful technique for assessment of myocardial perfusion in patients with CAD. Its application is limited by the necessity of injecting microbubbles directly into the arterial circulation. Newer contrast agents, capable of producing myocardial opacification from a venous injection, are likely to broaden significantly the application of this technique. Development of new ultrasound systems capable of demonstrating the linear relationship between tissue concentration of microbubbles and video intensity will make this method a truly quantitative one.

Two-Dimensional Tissue Doppler Imaging Technique

The advent of a tissue Doppler imaging technique has permitted two-dimensional measurement of tissue motion velocity in real time.[114–116] Myocardial thickening is an important indicator of regional left ventricular contraction.[117-119] In a normally contracting heart the endocardium moves faster than the epicardium during myocardial contraction, reflecting the rate of increase in wall thickness. Therefore, the velocity gradient between the endocardium and epicardium in systole is an indicator of regional myocardial contraction, as shown recently.[120]

With tissue Doppler technique, color flow Doppler images are used to depict velocities within the myocardium for quantitative assessment of regional left ventricular contraction. For a conventional color Doppler scanner the frame rate is usually limited to 10 to 20 frames/s. However, to analyze wall motion, a rate at least comparable to that of conventional two-dimensional echocardiography (30 frames/s) is necessary to obtain a spatially undistorted velocity image using tissue Doppler imaging.[120] Other problems in clinical application of this method include detection of the sum of the velocities associated with regional wall motion in combination with the parallel motion of the whole heart and the dependence of velocity measurements on the Doppler angle of incidence. Therefore, two-dimensional myocardial velocity gradients have been used by setting a hypothetical center of contraction in a left ventricular short-axis view to overcome these problems. In a recent study of 11 normal volunteers,[120] myocardial velocity gradients derived from M-mode tissue Doppler measurements in the left ventricular posterior wall reflected the rate of changing wall thickness. A serious limitation is still the lack of spatial orientation.

References

1. Massie BM, Schiller NB, Ratshin RA, Parmley WM. Mitral-septal separation: new echocardiographic index of left ventricular function. *Am J Cardiol.* 1977;39:1008–1016.

2. Schiller NB, Acquatella H, Ports TA, et al. Left ventricular volume from paired biplane two-dimensional echocardiographs. *Circulation.* 1979;60:547–555.

3. Reichek N, Helak J, Plappert T, et al. Anatomic validation of left ventricular mass estimates from clinical two-dimensional echocardiography: initial results. *Circulation.* 1983; 67:348–352.

4. Ren JF, Dotler MN, DePace NL, et al. Comparison of left ventricular ejection fraction and volumes by two-dimensional echocardiography, radionuclide angiography, and cineangiography. *J Cardiol Ultrason.* 1983;2:213–218.

5. Cohn PF, Levine JA, Bergeron FA, Gorlin R. Reproducibility of the angiographic left ventricular ejection fraction in patients with coronary artery disease. *Am Heart J.* 1974;88: 713–720.

6. Schiller NB, Skiodebrand C, Schiller E, et al. In vivo assessment of left ventricular mass by two dimensional echocardiography. *Circulation.* 1983;68:210–216.

7. Byrd BF III, Wahr DW, Wang YS, Bouchard A, Schiller NB. Left ventricular mass and volume/mass ratio determined by two-dimensional echocardiography in normal adults. *J Am Coll Cardiol.* 1985;6:1021–1025.

8. Silverman NH, Ports TA, Snider AR, Schiller NB, Carlsson E, Heilbron DC. Determination of left ventricular volume in children: echocardiographic and angiographic comparison. *Circulation.* 1987;62:548–556.

9. Horowitz RS, Morganroth J, Parrotto C, Chen CC, Soffer J, Pauletto FJ. Immediate diagnosis of acute myocardial infarction by two-dimensional echocardiography. *Circulation.* 1982;65:323–329.

10. Farcot JC, Boisante L, Rigaud M, Bardet J, Bourdarias JP. Two-dimensional echocardiographic visualization of ventricular septal rupture after acute anterior myocardial infarction. *Am J Cardiol.* 1980;45:370–377.

11. Erlebacher JA, Weiss JL, Eaton LW, Kallman C, Weisdfeldt ML, Bulkley BH. Late effects of acute infarct dilation of heart size: a two-dimensional echocardiographic study. *Am J Cardiol.* 1982;49:1120–1126.

12. Weyman AE, Peskoe SM, Williams ES, Dillon JC, Feigenbaum H. Detection of left ventricular aneurysms by cross-sectional echocardiography. *Circulation.* 1976;54:936–944.

13. Davidson KH, Parisi AF, Harrington JJ, Barsamian EM, Fishbein MC. Pseudoaneurysm of the left ventricle: an unusual echocardiographic presentation. *Ann Intern Med.* 1977;86:430–433.

14. Asinger RW, Mikell FL, Elsperger J, Hodges M. Incidence of left-ventricular thrombosis after acute transmural myocardial infarction. *N Engl J Med.* 1981;305:297–302.

15. Keating EC, Gross SA, Schlamowitz RA, et al. Mural thrombi in myocardial infarctions: prospective evaluation by two-dimensional echocardiography. *Am J Med.* 1983;74: 989–995.

16. Weinreich DJ, Burke JF, Pauletto FJ. Left ventricular mural thrombi complicating acute myocardial infarction: long-term follow-up with serial echocardiography. *Ann Intern Med.* 1984;100:789–799.

17. Maze SS, Kotler MN, Parry WR. Flow characteristics in the dilated left ventricle with thrombus: qualitative and quantitative Doppler analysis. *J Am Coll Cardiol.* 1989;13: 873–881.

18. Goldberger JJ, Himelman RB, Wolfe CL, Schiller NB. Right ventricular infarction: recognition and hemodynamic significance by two-dimensional echocardiography. *J Am Soc Echocardiogr.* 1991;4:140–146.

19. Bourdillon PDV, Broderick TM, Sawada SG, et al. Regional wall motion index for infarct and noninfarct regions after reperfusion in acute myocardial infarction: comparison with global wall motion index. *J Am Soc Echocardiogr.* 1989; 2:398–406.

20. Guyer DE, Goale RA, Gillam LD, Wilkins GT, Guerrero JL, Weyman AE. An echocardiographic technique for quantifying and displaying the extent of regional left ventricular dyssynergy. *J Am Coll Cardiol.* 1986;8:830–835.

21. Gillam LD, Franklin TD, Foale RA, et al. The natural history of regional wall motion in the acutely infarcted canine ventricle. *J Am Coll Cardiol.* 1986;7:1325–1334.

22. McGillem MJ, Mancini J, DeBoe SF, Buda AJ. Modification of the centerline method for assessment of echocardiographic wall thickening and motion: a comparison with areas of risk. *J Am Coll Cardiol.* 1988;11:861–866.

23. Sheehan FH, Bolson EL, Dodge HT, Mathey DG, Schofer J, Woo HW. Advantages and applications of the centerline method for characterizing regional ventricular function. *Circulation.* 1986;74:293–305.

24. Wann LS, Faris JV, Childress RH, Dillon JC, Weyman AE, Feigenbaum H. Exercise cross-sectional echocardiography in ischemic heart disease. *Circulation.* 1979;60:1300–1308.

25. Galanti G, Sciagra R, Comeglio M, et al. Diagnostic accuracy of peak exercise echocardiography in coronary artery disease: comparison with thallium-201 myocardial scintigraphy. *Am Heart J.* 1991;122:1609–1616.

26. Pozzoli MA, Fioretti PM, Salustri A, Reijs AEM, Roelandt JRTC. Exercise echocardiography and technetium-99m MIBI single-photon emission computed tomography in the detection of coronary artery disease. *Am J Cardiol.* 1991;67:350–355.

27. Quinones MA, Verani MS, Haichin RM, Mahmarian JJ, Suarez J, Zoghbi WA. Exercise echocardiography versus 201-Tl single-photon emission computed tomography in evaluation of coronary artery disease, analysis of 292 patients. *Circulation.* 1992;85:1026–1031.

28. Forster T, McNeill AJ, Salustri A, et al. Simultaneous dobutamine stress echocardiography and technetium 99-m isonitrile single photon emission computed tomography in patients with suspected coronary artery disease. *J Am Coll Cardiol.* 1993;21:1591–1596.

29. Marwick T, D'Hondt A, Baudhuin T, et al. Optimal use of dobutamine stress for the detection and evaluation of coronary artery disease: combination with echocardiography or scintigraphy, or both? *J Am Coll Cardiol.* 1993;22:159–165.

30. Tennant R, Wiggers CJ. Effect of coronary occlusion on myocardial contraction. *Am J Physiol.* 1935;112:351.

31. Ross J Jr. Assessment of ischemic regional myocardial dysfunction and its reversibility. *Circulation.* 1986;74:1186–1190.

32. Tomoike H, Franklin D, McKown D, Kemper WS, Guberek M, Ross J Jr. Regional myocardial dysfunction and hemodynamic abnormalities during strenuous exercise in dogs with limited coronary flow. *Circ Res.* 1978;42:487–496.

33. Ross J Jr. Mechanisms of regional ischemia and antianginal drug action during exercise. *Prog Cardiovasc Dis.* 1989;31:455–466.

34. Grover-McKay M, Matsuzaki M, Ross J Jr. Dissociation between regional myocardial dysfunction and subendocardial ST segment elevation during and after exercise-induced ischemia in dogs. *J Am Coll Cardiol.* 1987;10:1105–1112.

35. Mason SJ, Weiss JL, Weisfeldt ML, Garrison JB, Fortuin NJ. Exercise echocardiography: detection of wall motion abnormalities during ischemia. *Circulation.* 1979;59:50–59.

36. Presti CF, Armstrong WF, Feigenbaum H. Comparison of echocardiography at peak exercise and after bicycle exercise in evaluation of patients with known or suspected coronary artery disease. *J Am Soc Echocardiogr.* 1988;1:119–126.

37. Ryan T, Segar DS, Sawada SG, et al. Detection of coronary artery disease with upright bicycle exercise echocardiography. *J Am Soc Echocardiogr.* 1993;6:186–197.

38. Kloner RA, Allen J, Cox TA, Zheng Y, Ruiz CE. Stunned left ventricular myocardium after exercise treadmill testing in coronary artery disease. *Am J Cardiol.* 1991;68:329–334.

39. Feigenbaum H. Exercise echocardiography. *J Am Soc Echocardiogr.* 1988;1:161–166.

40. Schiller NB, Shah PM, Crawford M, DeMaria A, Devereux R, Feigenbaum H. Recommendations for quantification of the left ventricle by two-dimensional echocardiography. *J Am Soc Echocardiogr.* 1989;2:358–362.

41. Ryan T, Armstrong WF, O'Donnell JA, Feigenbaum H. Risk stratification after acute myocardial infarction by means of exercise two-dimensional echocardiography. *Am Heart J.* 1987;114:1305–1316.

42. Broderick T, Sawada S, Armstrong WF, et al. Improvement in rest and exercise-induced wall motion abnormalities after coronary angioplasty: an exercise echocardiography study. *J Am Coll Cardiol.* 1990;15:591–599.

43. Limacher MC, Quinones MA, Poliner LR, Nelson JG, Winters WL Jr, Waggoner AD. Detection of coronary artery disease with exercise two-dimensional echocardiography: description of a clinically applicable method and comparison with radionuclide ventriculography. *Circulation.* 1983;67:1211–1218.

44. Robertson WS, Feigenbaum H, Armstrong WF, Dillon JC, O'Donnell J, McHenry PW. Exercise-echocardiography: a clinically practical addition in the evaluation of coronary artery disease. *J Am Coll Cardiol.* 1983;2:1085–1091.

45. Quinones MA, Verani MS, Haichin RM, Mahmarian JJ, Suarez J, Zoghbi WA. Exercise echocardiography versus 201-Tl single photon emission computed tomography in evaluation of coronary artery disease: analysis of 292 patients. *Circulation.* 1992;85:1026–1031.

46. Labovitz AJ, Lewen M, Kern MJ, et al. The effects of successful PTCA on left ventricular function: assessment by exercise echocardiography. *Am Heart J.* 1989;117:1003–1008.

47. White CW, Wright CB, Doty DB, et al. Does visual interpretation of the coronary arteriogram predict the physiologic importance of a coronary stenosis? *N Engl J Med.* 1984;310:819–824.

48. Sheikh KH, Bengtson JR, Helmy S, et al. Relation of quantitative coronary lesion measurements of the development of exercise-induced ischemia assessed by exercise echocardiography. *J Am Coll Cardiol.* 1990;15:1043–1051.

49. Sawada SG, Segar DS, Ryan T, et al. Echocardiography detection of coronary artery disease during dobutamine infusion. *Circulation.* 1991;83:1605–1614.

50. Previtali M, Lanzarini L, Ferrario M, Tortorici M, Mussini A, Montemartini C. Dobutamine versus dipyridamole echocardiography in coronary artery disease. *Circulation.* 1991;83(suppl 3):III27–III31.

51. Mazeika PK, Nadazdin A, Oakley CM. Dobutamine stress echocardiography for detection and assessment of coronary artery disease. *J Am Coll Cardiol.* 1992;19:1203–1211.

52. Martin TW, Seaworth JF, Johns JP, Pupa LE, Condos WR. Comparison of adenosine, dipyridamole, and dobutamine in stress echocardiography. *Ann Intern Med.* 1992;116:190–196.

53. Salustri A, Fioretti PM, McNeill AJ, Pozzoli MMA, Roelandt JRTC. Pharmacological stress echocardiography in the diagnosis of coronary artery disease and myocardial ischemia: a comparison between dobutamine and dipyridamole. *Eur Heart J.* 1992;13:1356–1362.

54. Zoghbi WA, Cheirif J, Kleiman NS, Verani MS, Trakhtenbroit A. Diagnosis of ischemic heart disease with adenosine echocardiography. *J Am Coll Cardiol.* 1991;18: 1271–1279.

55. McNeill AJ, Fioretti PM, el-Said SM, Salustri A, Forster T, Roelandt JR. Enhanced sensitivity for detection of coronary artery disease by addition of atropine to dobutamine stress echocardiography. *Am J Cardiol.* 1992;70:41–46.

56. Marvick T, D'Hondt AM, Baudhuin T, Willemart B, Wijns W, Detry JM. Optimal use of dobutamine stress for the detection and evaluation of coronary artery disease: combination with echocardiography or scintigraphy, or both? *J Am Coll Cardiol.* 1993;22:159–166.

57. Segar DS, Brown SE, Sawada SG, Ryan T, Feigenbaum H. Dobutamine stress echocardiography: correlation with coronary lesion severity as determined by quantitative angiography. *J Am Coll Cardiol.* 1992;19:1197–1202.

58. Alderman EL, Fisher LD, Litwin P, Kaiser GC, Myers WO, Maynard C. Results of coronary artery surgery in patients with poor left ventricular function. *Circulation.* 1983;68: 785–795.

59. Nesto RW, Cohn LH, Collins JJ Jr, Wynne J, Holman L, Cohn PF. Inotropic contractile reserve: a useful predictor of increased 5-year survival and improved postoperative left ventricular function in patients with coronary artery disease and reduced ejection fraction. *Am J Cardiol.* 1982; 50:39–44.

60. Cigarroa CG, deFilippi CR, Brickner ME, Alvarez LG, Wait MA, Grayburn PA. Dobutamine stress echocardiography identifies hibernating myocardium and predicts recovery of left ventricular function after coronary revascularization. *Circulation.* 1993;88:430–436.

61. Dagianti A, Penco M, Agati L, et al. Stress echocardiography: comparison of exercise, dipyridamole and dobutamine in detecting and predicting the extent of coronary artery disease. *J Am Coll Cardiol.* 1995;26:18–25.

62. Marangelli V, Iliceto S, Piccinni G, De Martino G, Sorgente L, Rizzon P. Detection of coronary artery disease by digital stress echocardiography: comparison of exercise, transesophageal atrial pacing, and dipyridamole echocardiography. *J Am Coll Cardiol.* 1994;24:117–124.

63. Mazeika P, Nihoyannopoulos P, Joshi J, Oakley CM. Uses and limitations of high-dose dipyridamole stress echocardiography for evaluation of coronary artery disease. *Br Heart J.* 1992;67:144–149.

64. Frohwein S, Klein L, Lane A, Taylor R. Transesophageal dobutamine stress echocardiography in the evaluation of coronary artery disease. *J Am Coll Cardiol.* 1995;25: 823–829.

65. Agati L, Renzi M, Sciomer S, et al. Transesophageal dipyridamole echocardiography for diagnosis of coronary artery disease. *J Am Coll Cardiol.* 1992;19:765–770.

66. Lambertz H, Kreis A, Trumper H, Hanrath P. Simultaneous transesophageal atrial pacing and transesophageal

two-dimensional echocardiography: a new method of stress echocardiography. *J Am Coll Cardiol.* 1990;16: 1143–1153.

67. Krivokapich J, Child JS, Gerber RS, Lem V, Moser D. Prognostic usefulness of positive or negative exercise stress echocardiography for predicting coronary events in ensuing twelve months. *Am J Cardiol.* 1993;71:646–651.

68. Brown KA, Rowen M. Extent of jeopardized viable myocardium determined by myocardial perfusion imaging best predicts perioperative cardiac events in patients undergoing noncardiac surgery. *J Am Coll Cardiol.* 1993;21: 325–330.

69. Sawada SG, Ryan T, Conley MJ, Corya BC, Feigenbaum H, Armstrong WF. Prognostic value of a normal exercise echocardiogram. *Am Heart J.* 1990;120:49–55.

70. Bateman TM, O'Keel J, Barnhart C, Handlin LR, Ligon RW. Clinical comparison of cardiac events during follow-up after a non-ischemic exercise test suggests superiority of SPECT Tl-201 over echocardiography [abstract]. *J Am Coll Cardiol.* 1993;21:67A.

71. Strunk BL, Fitzgerald JW, Lipton M, Popp RL, Barry WH. The posterior aortic wall echocardiogram: its relationship to left atrial volume change. *Circulation.* 1976;54:744–750.

72. Danford DA, Huhta JC, Murphy DJ. Doppler echocardiographic approaches to ventricular diastolic function. *Echocardiography.* 1986;3:33–41.

73. Spirito P, Maron BJ, Bonow RO. Noninvasive assessment of left ventricular diastolic function: comparative analysis of Doppler echocardiographic and radionuclide angiographic techniques. *J Am Coll Cardiol.* 1986;7:518–526.

74. Phillips RA, Coplan NL, Krakoff LR, et al. Doppler echocardiographic analysis of left ventricular filling in treated hypertensive patients. *J Am Coll Cardiol.* 1987;9:317–322.

75. White CW, Wright CB, Doty DB, Hiratza LF, Eastham CC, Harrison DG. Does visual interpretation of the coronary angiogram predict the physiologic importance of a coronary stenosis? *N Engl J Med.* 1984;310:819–824.

76. Marcus ML, Wilson RF, White CW. Methods of measurement of myocardial blood flow in patients: a critical review. *Circulation.* 1987;76:245–253.

77. Ganz W, Tamura K, Marcus HS, Donoso R, Yoshida S, Swan HJC. Measurement of coronary sinus blood flow by continuous thermodilution in man. *Circulation.* 1971;44: 181–195.

78. Iliceto S, Memmola C, DeMartino G, Piccinni G, Rizzon P. Visualization of the coronary artery using transesophageal echocardiography. In: Erbel R, Khandheria BK, Brennecke R, Meyer J, Seward JB, Tajik AJ, eds. *Transesophageal Echocardiography: A New Window to the Heart.* Berlin: Springer-Verlag; 1989:86.

79. Taams MA, Gussenhoven EJ, Cornel JH, et al. Detection of left coronary stenosis by transesophageal echocardiography. *Eur Heart J.* 1988;9:1162–1166.

80. Yamagishi M, Miyatake K, Beppu S, et al. Assessment of coronary blood flow by transesophageal two-dimensional pulsed Doppler echocardiography. *Am J Cardiol.* 1988;62: 641–644.

81. Iliceto S, Marangelli V, Memmola C, DeMartino G, Rizzon P. Transesophageal Doppler echocardiography evaluation

of coronary blood flow velocity in baseline conditions and during dipyridamole-induced coronary vasodilation. *Circulation*. 1991;83:61–69.

82. Siostrzonek P, Kranz A, Heinz G, et al. Non-invasive estimation of coronary flow reserve by transesophageal Doppler sonographic measurement of coronary sinus flow. *Am J Cardiol*. 1993;72:1334–1337.

83. Zehetgruber M, Mundigler G, Christ G, et al. Estimation of coronary flow reserve by transesophageal coronary sinus Doppler measurements in patients with syndrome X and patients with significant left coronary artery disease. *J Am Coll Cardiol*. 1995;25:1039–1045.

84. Kern MJ. A simplified method to measure coronary blood flow velocity in patients: validation and application of a new Judkins-style Doppler-tipped angiographic catheter. *Am Heart J*. 1990;1202–1212.

85. Doucette JW, Corl PD, Payne HM, et al. Validation of a Doppler guidewire for intravascular measurement of coronary flow velocity. *Circulation*. 1992;85:1899–1911.

86. Ofili EO, Kern MJ, Labovitz AJ, St. Vrain JA, Egal J, Aguirre F. Analysis of coronary artery blood flow velocity dynamics in angiographically normal and stenosed arteries before and after endolumen enlargement by angioplasty. *J Am Coll Cardiol*. 1993;21:308–316.

87. Bach RG, Al-Joundi B, Kern MJ, et al. High-dose dipyridamole compared with standard infusion fail to further augment coronary hyperemia in patients. *J Am Coll Cardiol*. 1994;127A:736.

88. Wijns W, Serruys PW, Reiber JHC, et al. Quantitative angiography of the left anterior descending coronary artery: correlations with pressure gradient and results of exercise thallium scintigraphy. *Circulation*. 1985;71:273–279.

89. Gould KL, Lipscomb K, Hamilton GW. Physiologic basis for assessing critical coronary stenosis: instantaneous flow responses and regional distribution during coronary hyperemia as measures of coronary flow reserve. *Am J Cardiol*. 1974;33:87–94.

90. Goldstein RA, Kirkeeide RL, Demer LL, et al. Relation between geometric dimensions of coronary artery stenoses and myocardial perfusion reserve in man. *J Clin Invest*. 1987;79:1473–1478.

91. Zijlstra F, van Ommeren J, Reiber JHC, Serruys PW. Does the quantitative assessment of coronary artery dimensions predict the physiologic significance of a coronary stenosis? *Circulation*. 1987;75:1154–1161.

92. Kajiya F, Tsujioka K, Ogasawara Y, et al. Analysis of flow characteristics in post-stenotic regions of the human coronary artery during bypass graft surgery. *Circulation*. 1987;76:1092–1100.

93. Miller DD, Donohue TJ, Younis LT, et al. Correlation of pharmacologic 99m-Sestamibi myocardial perfusion imaging with post-stenotic coronary flow reserve in patients with angiographically immediately documented coronary artery stenoses. *Circulation*. 1994;89:2150–2160.

94. Evans JL, Ng KH, Vonesh MJ, Kramer BL, et al. Arterial imaging with a new forward-viewing intravascular ultrasound catheter, I: initial studies. *Circulation*. 1994;89:712–717.

95. Siegel RJ, Chae JS, Maurer G, Berlin M, Fishbein MC. Histopathologic correlation of the three-layered intravascular ultrasound appearance of normal adult human muscular arteries. *Am Heart J*. 1993;126:872–878.

96. Hausmann D, Sudhir K, Mullen WL, Fitzgerald PJ, Ports TA, Daniel WG. Contrast-enhanced intravascular ultrasound: validation of a new technique for delineation of the vessel wall boundary. *J Am Coll Cardiol*. 1994;23:981–987.

97. De Scheerder I, De Man F, Herregods MC, et al. Intravascular ultrasound versus angiography for measurement of luminal diameters in normal and diseased coronary arteries. *Am Heart J*. 1994;127:243–251.

98. Alfonso F, Macaya C, Goicolea J, et al. Intravascular ultrasound imaging of angiographically normal coronary segments in patients with coronary artery disease. *Am Heart J*. 1994;127:536–544.

99. Porter TR, Sears T, Xie F, et al. Intravascular ultrasound study of angiographically mildly diseased coronary arteries. *J Am Coll Cardiol*. 1993;22:1858–1865.

100. Gerber TC, Erbel R, Gorge G, Ge J, Rupprecht HJ, Meyer J. Extent of atherosclerosis and remodeling of the left main coronary artery determined by intravascular ultrasound. *Am J Cardiol*. 1994;73:666–670.

101. Tenaglia AN, Buller CE, Kisslo KB, Stack RS, Davidson CJ. Mechanisms of balloon angioplasty and directional coronary atherectomy as assessed by intracoronary ultrasound. *J Am Coll Cardiol*. 1992;20:685–691.

102. Laskey WK, Brady ST, Kussmaul WG, Waxler AR, Krol J, Herrman HC. Intravascular ultrasonographic assessment of the results of coronary artery stenting. *Am Heart J*. 1993;125:1576–1583.

103. DeMaria AN, Bommer WJ, Rigg SK, et al. Echocardiographic visualization of myocardial perfusion by left heart and intracoronary injection of echo contrast agents [abstract]. *Circulation*. 1980;62(suppl 3):III143.

104. Albers VM. *Underwater Acoustic Handbook*. State College: Pennsylvania State University Press; 1960.

105. Feinstein SB, Ten Cate FJ, Zwehl W, et al. Two-dimensional contrast echocardiography, I: in-vitro development and quantitative analysis of echo contrast agents. *J Am Coll Cardiol*. 1984;3:14–20.

106. Keller MW, Glasheen W, Gear A, Kaul S. Myocardial contrast echocardiography without significant hemodynamic effects or reactive hyperemia: a major advantage in the imaging of myocardial perfusion. *J Am Coll Cardiol*. 1988;12:1039–1047.

107. Villanueva FS, Glasheen WD, Sklenar J, Kaul S. Assessment of risk area during coronary occlusion and infarct size after reperfusion with myocardial contrast echocardiography using left and right atrial injections of contrast. *Circulation*. 1993;88:596–604.

108. Kloner RA, Ganote CE, Jennings RB. The 'no-reflow' phenomenon after temporary coronary occlusion in the dog. *J Clin Invest*. 1974;54:1496–1508.

109. Johnson WB, Malone SA, Pantely G, Anselone CG, Bristow JD. No reflow and extent of infarction during maximal vasodilation in the porcine heart. *Circulation*. 1988;78:462–472.

110. Ito H, Tomooka T, Sakai N, et al. Lack of myocardial perfusion immediately after successful thrombolysis: a predictor of poor recovery of left ventricular function in

anterior myocardial infarction. *Circulation.* 1992;85: 1699–1705.

111. Sabia PJ, Powers ER, Ragosta M, Sarembock IJ, Burwell LR, Kaul S. An association between collateral blood flow and myocardial viability in patients with recent myocardial infarction. *N Engl J Med.* 1992;327:1825–1831.

112. Keller MW, Smucker ML, Burwell L, Glasheen WP, Watson DD, Kaul S. Myocardial contrast echocardiography in humans, II: assessment of coronary blood flow reserve. *J Am Coll Cardiol.* 1988;12:925–934.

113. Skyba DM, Jayaweera AR, Goodman NC, Ismail S, Camarano G, Kaul S. Quantification of myocardial perfusion with myocardial contrast echocardiography during left atrial injection of contrast: implication for venous injection. *Circulation.* 1994;90:1513–1521.

114. McDicken WN, Sutherland GR, Moran CM, Gordon LN. Colour Doppler velocity imaging of the myocardium. *Ultrasound Med Biol.* 1992;18:651–654.

115. Miyatake K, Yamagishi M, Tanaka N. A new method for evaluation of left ventricular wall motion by color-coded tissue Doppler echocardiography: in vitro and in vivo studies [abstract]. *Circulation.* 1993;88(suppl):I48.

116. Sutherland GR, Stewart MJ, Groundstroem KWE, et al. Color Doppler myocardial imaging: a new technique for the assessment of myocardial function. *J Am Soc Echocardiogr.* 1994;7:441–458.

117. Miyatake K, Yamagishi M, Tanaka N. A new method for the evaluation of left ventricular wall motion by color-coded tissue Doppler imaging: in vitro and in vivo studies. *J Am Coll Cardiol.* 1995;25:717–724.

118. Heusch G, Guth BD, Widman T, Peterson KL, Ross J Jr. Ischemic myocardial dysfunction assessed by temporal Fourier transform of regional myocardial wall thickening. *Am Heart J.* 1987;113:116–124.

119. Guth BD, Schulz R, Heusch G. Time course and mechanisms of contractile dysfunction during acute myocardial ischemia. *Circulation.* 1993;87(suppl 4):IV35–IV42.

120. Uematsu M, Miyatake K, Tanaka N, et al. Myocardial velocity gradient as a new indicator of regional left ventricular contraction: detection by a two-dimensional tissue Doppler imaging technique. *J Am Coll Cardiol.* 1995;26: 217–223.

15

Intravascular Ultrasound

Franz F. Weidinger, Paul Yang, and Ali Hassan

Intravascular ultrasound (IVUS) is an invasive diagnostic technique that has evolved rapidly over the past 10 years and is now widely used as an adjunct to conventional angiography in interventional catheterization laboratories. With its capability to provide high-resolution cross-sectional images, it has become possible to obtain detailed information on the structure of the vessel wall and to provide a histologylike view of the artery in vivo.[1-3] Thus, incremental information on the anatomy of the arterial wall that is not available from radiography's longitudinal contour images of the vessel lumen can be gained. These capabilities have challenged selective coronary angiography as the gold standard for diagnosis of coronary artery disease. IVUS has emerged as a more sensitive method to detect diffuse atherosclerosis and to identify plaque morphology along with a cross-sectional view of the stenosis. Recent advances in IVUS technology include further miniaturization of ultrasound catheters, three-dimensional reconstruction of images, combined imaging and therapeutic devices, and backscatter analysis for tissue characterization.

Limitations of Angiography

Although angiography has been accepted as the gold standard for the diagnosis of obstructive vascular disease, several limitations have been recognized for many years.[4-7] First, visual interpretation of the angiogram is subjective and results in considerable intraobserver and interobserver variability.[5,7] Several studies have compared angiographic assessment of the severity of coronary stenoses with postmortem histological examination.[4,6] Observed discrepancies between angiographic and histological assessment have been attributed to the fact that diffuse atherosclerosis is often undetected by angiography.[8,9] Assessment of percent diameter stenosis compares the stenotic segment with an adjacent "normal" reference segment, which histologically may ex-

hibit diffuse atherosclerotic changes, thereby leading to an underestimation of lesion severity. Second, remodeling of the artery may lead to compensatory enlargement of the entire vessel, a process that accommodates the growing plaque and, in the early stage of atherosclerosis, prevents significant narrowing of the lumen.[10] Detection of this phenomenon depends on visualization of the entire vessel wall as provided by IVUS. The discrepancy between angiographic and histological evaluation of lesion severity has been further supported by in vivo studies that compare angiographic percent diameter stenosis with the physiological effects of the lesions, which have shown poor correlation.[11,12]

Advantages of IVUS

The tomographic view of the entire circumference of the vessel lumen and the vessel wall provided by IVUS has major advantages over the longitudinal view of the lumen provided by angiography.[13] First, lumen area and lumen diameter can be measured directly, even in the presence of irregular lumen shape or eccentric plaque configuration.[14,15] With angiographic assessment, only vessel diameter can be measured directly, and considerable inaccuracy can occur at sites with eccentric stenoses, even with the use of multiple projections. Second, vessel wall morphology can be visualized directly by IVUS, such that tissue quality and the configuration of the atherosclerotic plaque can be assessed in vivo.[16] This qualitative information provided by IVUS may have prognostic importance, because there is increasing evidence that conversion of stable to unstable coronary syndromes is due to changes of plaque composition rather than gradual increases in stenosis severity.[17,18] In addition, information on plaque morphology may be useful for the choice of catheter-based interventions and for the control of preventive measures such as lipid-lowering therapy.[19,20]

Technical Aspects

Currently available IVUS systems are based on two different transducer designs: *mechanically rotated* and *electronic phased-array* catheters.

The mechanical system uses a single-element transducer connected to an external motor drive, operating at about 1800 rpm, and incorporated in an acoustically transparent housing. In another design, the transducer is fixed and a rotating mirror located in front of the transducer reflects the acoustic beam. In the most recently developed catheter systems, the transducer core is moved inside a transparent, fluid-filled sheath, which is itself introduced into the artery over a 0.014-in guide wire beyond the region of interest, thus avoiding direct contact of the moving parts with the vessel wall. The mechanical systems have the advantage of a large effective aperture of the single-element transducer, which offers maximum delivery of acoustic power and high image quality. The size of the catheters ranges from 2.9 to 3.5 F (0.96–1.17 mm). The disadvantage of mechanical systems is the use of a rotating drive shaft, which limits flexibility and may lead to image artifacts due to nonuniform rotational speed of the transducer, particularly in small or tortuous vessels.

Electronic systems consist of multiple-transducer elements (32 or 64 elements) arranged in a circular fashion at the tip of the catheter. The device relies on the synthetic aperture principle for image generation. A high-speed array processor reconstructs each picture element by integrating signals obtained from a variable number of transducer elements. The absence of moving parts results in catheters with good flexibility and guide wire tracking. However, currently available devices provide suboptimal image quality due to the small size of the individual transducer elements, which limits the acoustic power, and the requirement for a complex image reconstruction computer, which limits the temporal resolution to 10 frames/s (as compared with 30 frames/s with mechanical systems). Both mechanical and electronic systems use ultrasound frequencies ranging from 20 to 30 MHz, which provides high spatial resolution at a depth of 3 to 5 mm.

Validation Studies

In vitro and in vivo studies that compare IVUS measurements with histological preparations or angiography have generally shown close correlations for the assessment of lumen diameter, cross-sectional area, and plaque dimensions (Table 15.1). For IVUS and quantitative angiographic measurements of lumen diameter and lumen area, correlations were close for normal arteries and concentric atherosclerotic lesions but less close or very poor for eccentric lesions[14] and sites with previous balloon angioplasty,[16] presumably due to the complex lumen shape that results from these interventions.

TABLE 15.1. Validation studies comparing intravascular ultrasound with histological or angiographic measurements.

Author	Study design	Vessel	Reference method	Parameters, correlation coefficient
Tobis [15]	In vitro	Human peripheral arteries	Histology	Lumen cross-sectional area $r = .88$
Mallery[21]	In vitro	Human peripheral arteries	Histology	Intimal thickness $r = 0.92$
				Wall thickness, $r = -0.87$
				Medical thickness, $r = 0.83$
Gussenhoven[22]	In vitro	Human peripheral arteries	Histology	Plaque thickness, $r = 0.84$
				Lumen area, $r = 0.85$
Nishimura[23]	In vitro	Phantom	Phantom	Lumen area, $r = 0.99$
		Peripheral arteries	Histology	Lumen area $r = 0.98$
Potkin[24]	In vitro	Human coronary arteries	Histology	Lumen area, $r = 0.85$
				Total vessel area, $r = 0.94$
				Plaque plus medial area, $r = 0.92$
Pandian[25]	In vivo	Canine pulmonary arteries	Histology	Lumen area, $r = 0.99$
				Lumen diameter, $r = 0.92$
				Wall thickness, $r = 0.85$
Nissen[26]	In vivo	Canine peripheral arteries	Angiography	Lumen area, $r = 0.96$
				Lumen diameter, $r = 0.98$
Tobis[16]	In vivo	Human coronary arteries	Angiography	Lumen area at normal sites, $r = 0.26$
				Lumen area after percutaneous transluminal coronary angioplasty $r = 0.12$
Nissen[14]	In vivo	Human coronary arteries	Angiography	Lumen diameter
				Normal segments, $r = 0.92$
				Concentric lesions, $r = 0.93$
				Eccentric lesions, $r = 0.77$

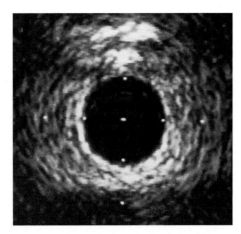

FIGURE 15.1. Normal coronary morphology by intracoronary ultrasound demonstrating a single-layered wall in a cardiac transplant recipient.

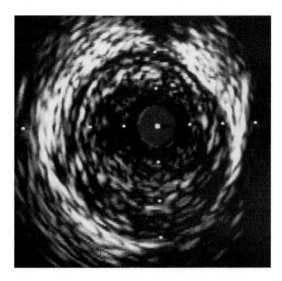

FIGURE 15.2. Ultrasound image showing a soft atheroma with lower echodensity than the surrounding adventitia. The lesion is rather concentric and causes severe lumen narrowing.

Normal and Pathological Vascular Morphology

Normal Morphology

Initial studies examined the ultrasound appearance of normal and abnormal vessel wall structures in isolated arterial preparations in vitro.[22–24] These studies have shown that the normal muscular artery has a three-layered wall, with a thin echogenic intimal layer, an echolucent medial zone, and an echogenic adventitia. In contrast, elastic arteries showed a single-layered echogenic wall. These findings have been contradicted in part by later in vivo studies performed in young hearts of cardiac transplant recipients that showed that normal coronary arteries may reveal a single-layered wall (Figure 15.1). In 10 of 25 patients with angiographically normal coronary arteries, studied within 1 month of cardiac transplantation, the vessel wall had a single-layer appear-

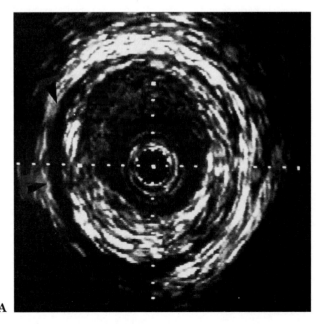

A

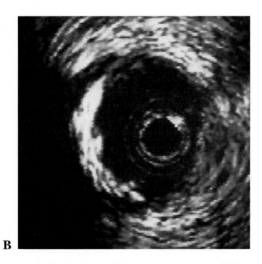

B

FIGURE 15.3. Two examples of echogenic lesions. **A,** The lesion is mildly eccentric and reveals the echolucent medial zone (arrows). **B,** The bright plaque (position between 6 and 11 o'clock) causes acoustic shadowing of deeper structures, which suggests calcification.

ance, whereas the remaining 15 patients showed three-layered vessel walls.[27] The mean donor age of the single-layered group was 20 years and of the three-layered group 32 years. It is assumed that the thickness of the "normal" intima lies below the axial resolution of the most frequently used 30-MHz ultrasound transducer. In vitro studies supported this theory by showing that the three-layered appearance is present only when the intima exceeds 148 μm in thickness.[28]

Atherosclerotic Plaque Morphology

The appearance of ultrasound images depends on the acoustic properties of the tissue (i.e., on the relative differences in acoustic impedance between tissue components). Histological studies have shown that atherosclerotic lesions can be classified according to their echodensity.[22–24] *Soft plaques,* appearing less echogenic than the adventitia, contain lipids or have a predominantly cellular (fibromuscular) component (Figure 15.2). These lesions may be homogeneous in appearance or contain areas of different echodensity when compared with the bright adventitia on the one side or with the echolucent lumen on the other. The latter may exhibit echogenic elements in small or stenotic vessels where the IVUS catheter may cause near obstruction and thus blood stasis; in such cases it may become difficult to distinguish soft plaque from lumen. *Bright echogenic lesions* (Figure 15.3) contain increased amounts of fibrotic tissue and are thought to represent more advanced, stable forms of atherosclerotic plaque. Highly echogenic lesions with attenuation of structures behind them, a phenomenon known as acoustic shadowing, represent *calcified plaques* (Figure 15.3). Although acoustic shadowing may limit the diagnostic information on deeper structures, it enhances the sensitivity for the detection of cal-

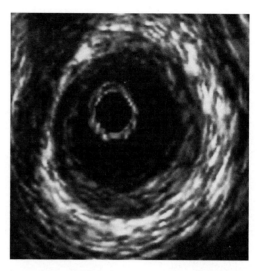

FIGURE 15.5. Example of mild concentric intimal thickening without lumen encroachment in a cardiac transplant recipient.

cium, where IVUS has been shown to be superior to angiography.[29] Atherosclerotic lesions can be further classified according to their shape and extent within the circumference of the vessel wall. Early changes appear as intimal thickening not protruding into the lumen and often with a crescent shape. These *eccentric* lesions (Figure 15.4) can be distinguished from the normal part of the circumference. *Concentric* lesions can appear as mild intimal thickening (Figure 15.5) or, in more advanced stages, as massive atheromas causing luminal encroachment (Figure 15.2). *Complex atheromas* (Figure 15.6) are characterized by irregular luminal borders and inhomogeneous echogenic (fibrous and/or calcified) and echolucent (lipoid/necrotic or fibrocellular) tissue components.

Clinical Applications

Clinical applications of IVUS include the diagnosis of vessel wall morphology and the guidance of catheter-based interventions (Table 15.2).

Diagnostic IVUS

Diagnosis of Diffuse Atherosclerosis and Borderline Lesions

Diffuse atherosclerosis can frequently be detected by IVUS in angiographically normal coronary segments[13,27] (Figure 15.7), which may have important implications for the assessment of stenosis severity. In particular, a stenosis of borderline angiographic significance (e.g., 50%–70% diameter stenosis) may be underestimated in the presence of diffuse atherosclerosis in the proximal

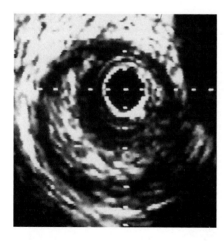

FIGURE 15.4. Ultrasound image of an eccentric, crescent-shaped atheroma (position between 3 and 11 o'clock). The plaque exhibits similar echodensity compared with the adventitia, which suggests fibrous tissue.

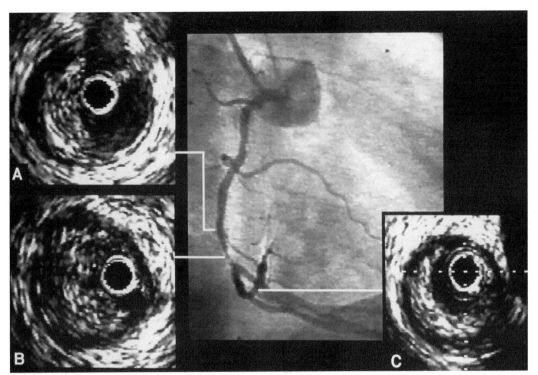

FIGURE 15.6. Complex lesion morphology as revealed by intracoronary ultrasound. **A,** Intravascular ultrasound findings at a proximal reference site. **B,** Massive eccentric atheroma with irregular surface and mixed components (cellular, fibrous, and lipid) at the site of severe angiographic narrowing. **C,** Intravascular ultrasound findings at a distal reference site. Despite a normal angiographic appearance, ultrasound reveals significant amounts of plaque extending into the reference sites.

and/or distal reference segments because a normal lumen size is no longer present and not measurable on the arteriogram.[11,13] On the other hand, reference segments associated with ectatic atherosclerosis and more distant segments showing a narrower lumen but normal or less diseased wall morphology may lead to overestimation of percent diameter stenosis.

Predilection sites for early atherosclerosis, such as the left main coronary artery,[30] branch points, and tortuous segments, can be clearly identified with IVUS, which may be considered in the case of a symptomatic patient in whom angiography yields ambiguous or negative findings.

Diagnosis of the true plaque burden is desirable when alternative interventional devices such as directional or rotational atherectomy are considered. The extent and thickness of plaque may be underestimated by angiography in severely eccentric lesions or in segments showing

TABLE 15.2. Clinical applications of intravascular ultrasound.

Detection of diffuse atherosclerosis
Assessment of plaque morphology and composition
Guidance of catheter-based interventions
    Detection of reference segment disease
    Detection of target lesion calcification
    Assessment of the acute result
    Diagnosis of dissection
    Optimization of stent deployment
    Control of plaque removal by directional atherectomy
Detection of cardiac allograft vasculopathy

remodeling (compensatory enlargement) (Figure 15.8) adjacent to, or extending into, the target lesion site.[31] Detection of severe plaque burden in a remodeled segment with a preserved or moderately stenosed lumen may be clinically important if it shows low echogenicity, which suggests high lipid content or soft, potentially vulnerable plaque, more often seen in culprit lesions of patients with unstable angina.[32]

Transplant Coronary Vasculopathy

Transplant coronary vasculopathy, an accelerated form of atherosclerosis, is distinct from native coronary disease in that it usually affects the entire coronary artery and involves diffuse concentric intimal thickening rather than localized narrowing.[33] The incidence of graft atherosclerosis may be as high as 50% at 5 years after transplant, and it represents the major cause of death and retransplantation in patients who survive more than 1 year after transplantation.[34] Because angiography has a low sensitivity in the diagnosis of the early stage of this disease,[35] IVUS has been tested as an adjunctive diagnostic modality during routine (usually annual) follow-up angiography.[36,37] Of 80 patients studied 2 weeks to 13 years after cardiac transplantation, 60 patients showed at least minimal intimal thickening on IVUS. Of these 60 patients, 42 (70%) had angiographically normal coronary arteries, 21 (50%) of whom had moderate or severe intimal thickening.[37] The same group of investigators has shown that serial ultrasound imaging of the same vessel sites is feasible, with 39% of the patients showing pro-

FIGURE 15.7. Intra-
coronary ultrasound
findings (A, B, and
C) at angiographi-
cally normal sites
(D). **A,** Intracoro-
nary ultrasound re-
veals a concentric le-
sion in the left main
coronary artery. **B,**
Crescent-shaped inti-
mal thickening in
the proximal portion
of the left anterior
descending coronary
artery. **C,** Crescent-
shaped intimal thick-
ening in the midpor-
tion of the left
anterior descending
coronary artery.

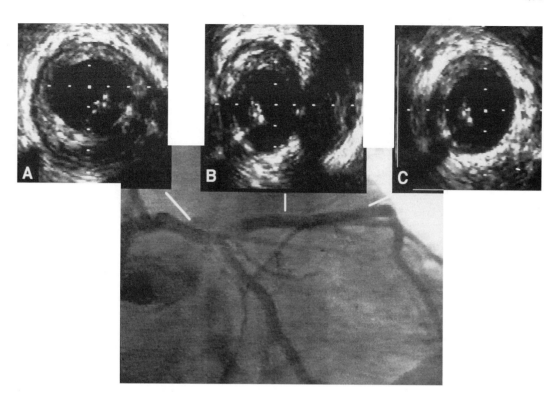

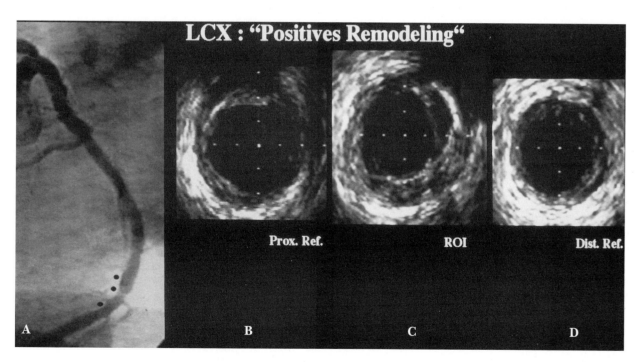

FIGURE 15.8. Example of arterial remodeling. **A,** The angiographic appearance of a stenosis in the distal portion of the left
circumflex artery (dots indicating the location of the ultrasound probe; center of stenosis—middle, proximal, and distal
reference sites—upper and distal, respectively). **B, C, D,** Ultrasound evidence of compensatory vessel enlargement. In the region of interest (ROI), the artery exhibits a soft eccentric
plaque with an increase of the total vessel circumference in
comparison with the proximal and distal reference sites.

gression of intimal thickening from one year to the next, with a mean time after transplantation of 3 years in the initial study.[36] Therefore, IVUS may be particularly useful in this setting due to its high sensitivity for angiographically silent intimal thickening. Although effective therapy is lacking, the early detection of transplant vasculopathy will undoubtedly provide new insights into its natural history and will hopefully help to identify subsets of patients at higher risk of rapid progression and to develop preventive or therapeutic strategies.

IVUS in Interventional Cardiology

Coronary Angioplasty

The most valuable role for intracoronary ultrasound is in the control and guidance of catheter-based therapeutic interventions. In the setting of balloon angioplasty, ultrasound imaging provides complementary information to angiographic assessment in several ways:

1. *Detection of diffuse atherosclerosis involving the reference segments:* as mentioned earlier, the tomographic orientation of ultrasound imaging enables the diagnosis of angiographically undetected reference segment disease (Figure 15.6). Studies have shown that a minority of angiographically normal reference segments are normal by IVUS and that atherosclerosis may reduce luminal diameter by more than 50% in these segments.[32,38] Ultrasound findings in reference segments may reveal diffuse or ectatic disease. Because adequate sizing of balloon or other interventional devices largely depends on correct assessment of the reference segment, IVUS may provide useful information for preprocedural decision making.

2. *Assessment of the predominant plaque component:* detection of calcification within the target lesion has important implications for the immediate success of balloon angioplasty and for the choice of alternative interventions. Large amounts of calcium limit the success of balloon angioplasty because the resistance of the lesion will require high inflation pressures. With more localized calcium deposits, the risk of dissection may be increased at the border of these and adjacent softer plaque materials due to high shear forces at these sites.[39,40] IVUS is more sensitive than angiography in the detection of calcium.[29] Also, the localization and assessment of the extent of calcification may be important components of lesion evaluation when alternative devices such as directional and rotational atherectomy are considered.[41]

3. *Immediate result and mechanism of balloon angioplasty:* lumen enlargement by angioplasty is often associated with or even dependent on tears or dissections (Figure 15.10). These acute sequelae of angioplasty may not be apparent angiographically or merely cause a "haziness" of the lumen. Dissections may contribute in large part to the therapeutic effect of lumen enlargement by creating new blood channels[42] but may also be the cause of rapid deterioration and acute closure. The tomographic view of the complex lumen shape after angioplasty provided by IVUS may help to assess the severity and depth of dissections and to decide whether additional intervention is necessary. In addition, IVUS can reveal the predominant mechanism of the initial lumen gain in angiographically ambiguous situations. These mechanisms include stretching of the vessel wall, occurring particularly in eccentric stenoses, which is often followed by elastic recoil, a cause of early lumen loss; other mechanisms include plaque compression, plaque fracture, and variable degrees of plaque dissection.

4. *Mechanism and prediction of restenosis:* the late outcome of angioplasty and other catheter-based revascularization procedures remains limited by a persistently high rate of restenosis, despite multiple efforts to reduce this occurrence.[43,44] Although the predominant mechanism of restenosis has been attributed to proliferation of smooth muscle cells and matrix formation,[45] recent IVUS studies have shown that shrinkage or negative remodeling of the arterial wall (Figure 15.9) in the dilated segment accounts for more than 50% of the late lumen loss and that the proliferative component of restenosis may have been overemphasized.[46–48] Studies are under way to examine whether ultrasound variables of lumen and plaque dimensions before and immediately following balloon angioplasty and other catheter interventions are able to predict the later occurrence of restenosis. Preliminary follow-up data of two studies suggest that residual percent cross-sectional plaque burden, defined as the area of plaque plus media divided by the area encompassed by the external elastic membrane (also termed *percent cross-sectional narrowing*), and the luminal cross-sectional area after intervention are strong independent predictors of restenosis and/or late recurrence of symptoms.[49,50]

Stenting

The use of intracoronary stents has rapidly increased since two randomized trials comparing stents and balloon angioplasty for elective treatment of de novo coronary lesions reported a significant reduction in the restenosis rate in the stented patients.[51,52] In the early phase of stenting, major limitations of this new device included a high incidence of stent thrombosis and bleeding complications due to the aggressive anticoagulation regimen used. IVUS studies have contributed to an improved understanding of the mechanism of coronary

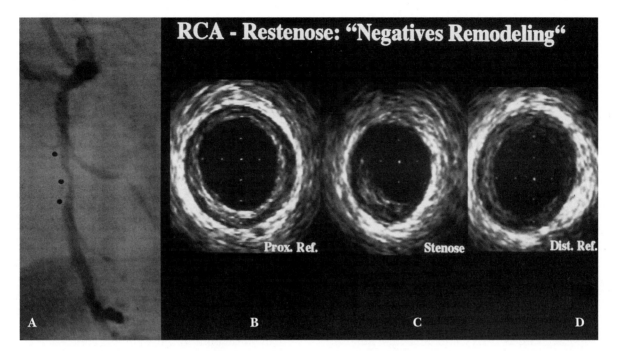

FIGURE 15.9. Example of negative remodeling. **A,** A tubular stenosis in the midportion of the right coronary artery (dots indicating the location of the ultrasound probe; center of stenosis—middle, proximal, and distal reference sites—upper and distal, respectively). **B, C, D,** Ultrasound images reveal an eccentric plaque with a marked decrease of the total vessel circumference in the center of the stenosis in comparison with the proximal and distal reference sites. The amount of plaque, however, is nearly equal in all three segments.

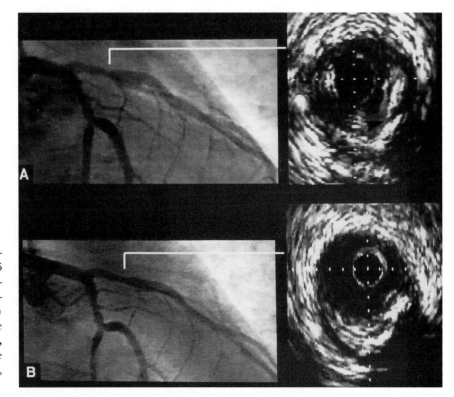

FIGURE 15.10. Angiographic and ultrasound images immediately (A) and 6 months (B) following balloon angioplasty of a proximal left anterior descending artery. **A,** A fracture (arrow) within a calcified plaque as a possible mechanism of lumen enlargement. **B,** After 6 months, ultrasound of the same site no longer reveals plaque fracture, suggesting that healing has occurred.

stenting. These studies have revealed that residual lumen narrowing, incomplete stent expansion, and apposition of the struts against the vessel wall are still present despite an acceptable angiographic result in more than 80% of patients.[53] Based on these findings obtained with ultrasound guidance, gradual modifications in the strategy used for stent deployment have been developed and are now widely accepted. These modifications include additional balloon dilation inside the stent with high-pressure balloons to achieve optimal stent expansion and proper strut apposition and the placement of additional stents to cover residual lumen narrowing in adjacent segments.[53,54] Several IVUS criteria regarding optimal stent deployment have been proposed. The criteria being evaluated prospectively in randomized trials include (1) complete apposition of the stent struts against the vessel wall over the entire length of the stent and (2) minimal in-stent cross-sectional area >80% of the average reference lumen cross-sectional area or minimal in-stent cross-sectional area equal to or greater than the distal reference lumen cross-sectional area.[53] Reference sites are defined as less diseased vessel segments (proximal and distal) adjacent to but at least 0.5 mm from the target lesion.

With the consistent use of high-pressure dilation and increased operator experience, a gradual reduction in the incidence of stent thrombosis to less than 1% has been observed, and the aggressive anticoagulation regimen has been replaced by a combined antiplatelet therapy with ticlopidine and aspirin. Large-scale multicenter registries that have examined the safety and efficacy of this regimen confirmed a reduction of the rate of subacute thrombosis, the rate of bleeding complications, and the length of hospitalization.[55]

Other Devices

Directional atherectomy is another catheter-based procedure that has the advantage of plaque removal (debulking) and lumen dilation. The initial expectation that this method could reduce restenosis was tempered by the results of the Coronary Angioplasty Versus Excisional

Atherectomy Trial,[56] which showed a restenosis rate of 50% after directional atherectomy as compared with 57% after angioplasty. One reason for these disappointing findings could be that plaque removal was not sufficiently aggressive. Indeed, IVUS studies revealed a high residual plaque burden despite satisfactory acute angiographic results.[57] This finding has been attributed to the inability of angiography to distinguish between the cutting and mechanical effects of balloon dilation. Ultrasound guidance in this setting is particularly useful because ultrasound can permit visualization of atherectomy cuts and residual plaque distribution (Figure 15.11); more aggressive plaque debulking may lead to better long-term results.[58] Conversely, overly aggressive plaque removal by multiple cuts increases the risk of deep vessel wall injury; in addition, IVUS may reveal highly complex or irregular lumen shapes in this setting, which may explain the relatively high incidence of acute adverse events after directional atherectomy.[56] In an attempt to guide the alignment of the atherectomy device directly in relation to the plaque, a combined imaging–atherectomy catheter that may contribute to a more controlled removal of plaque tissue and minimization of deep vessel wall injury has been developed.

Demonstration and localization of lesion calcium is important for preprocedural decision making, because larger amounts of calcium may prevent the atherectomy device from cutting effectively and thus limit the initial success.[41] In the presence of extensive calcium, as well as in diffuse lesions, *rotational atherectomy (rotablation)* has been shown to be the interventional method of choice. Ultrasound examination after rotablation may help to assess the size and shape of the neolumen and to decide whether further intervention using either larger burrs, directional atherectomy, or balloon is needed.[59,60]

Limitations

Even with the highly miniaturized ultrasound catheters now available, several limitations remain, especially re-

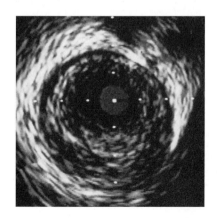 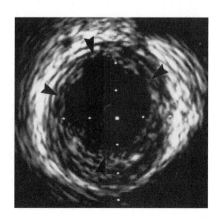

FIGURE 15.11. Intracoronary ultrasound before (left panel) and immediately after (right panel) directional coronary atherectomy. **Left panel,** Soft, rather concentric lesion (see Figure 15.2). **Right panel,** Acute result of atherectomy, with the sites of plaque removal and residual plaque in positions between 3 and 9 o'clock.

garding application in the coronary system. Limited catheter flexibility may lead to a noncoaxial or eccentric position of the ultrasound probe, causing image artifacts or partial loss of signal (echo dropouts). Such positioning may preclude quantification of lumen dimensions, particularly in small or tortuous vessel segments. Spatial orientation and correlation with the angiogram is difficult, the latter being dependent on anatomical landmarks such as side branches. Further current limitations include invasiveness, with the small but inherent risk of vessel wall trauma or transient ischemia due to lumen obstruction, and cost-effectiveness.

Future Developments

Further reduction in the size of IVUS catheters remains an important goal. An imaging probe with the dimensions of a guide wire, which would allow simultaneous imaging during any catheter-based intervention, is under development.

Feasibility of three-dimensional reconstruction has been demonstrated by several investigators[61] (Figure 15.12), but major limitations (mainly arising from motion and other artifacts) remain unresolved. Current areas of investigation include improvement of automated contour detection, electrocardiographic-gated signal acquisition, and motorized pullback of the ultrasound catheter. On-line three-dimensional reconstruction should enable a more comprehensive assessment of lesion characteristics including length, plaque volume, and site of maximal lumen narrowing during interventional procedures. Combination devices currently under preliminary investigation include an imaging-balloon and an imaging-atherectomy catheter. Finally, improved tissue characterization using backscatter analysis could contribute to the identification of vulnerable, rupture-prone plaques, an area undergoing intensive investigation.

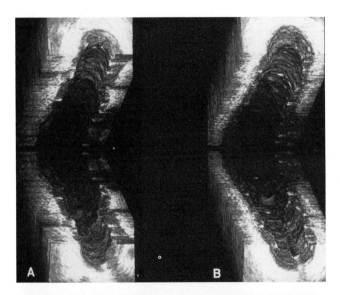

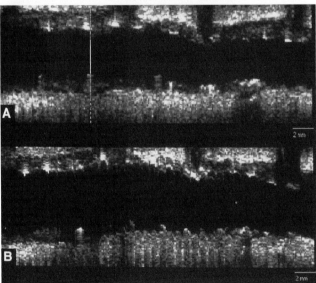

FIGURE 15.12. Three-dimensional reconstruction of serial intracoronary ultrasound images from a patient who has undergone stent implantation. The upper panel shows an open cylindrical presentation allowing a view of the intimal surface of the artery. The lower panel represents the longitudinal reconstruction of the same segment showing lumen diameter and strut apposition over the entire length of the stented artery segment. In this example the result of final high-pressure balloon dilation (B) is compared with the immediate result of stent implantation (A).

References

1. Pandian NG, Kreis A, Brockway B, et al. Ultrasound angioscopy: real-time, two-dimensional, intraluminal ultrasound imaging of blood vessels. *Am J Cardiol.* 1988;62: 493–494.
2. Roelandt J, Serruys PW. Intraluminal real-time ultrasonic imaging: clinical perspectives. *Int J Card Imaging.* 1989;4: 89–97.
3. Yock PG, Linker DT, Angelsen BA. Two-dimensional intravascular ultrasound: technical development and initial clinical experience. *J Am Soc Echocardiogr.* 1989;2:296–304.
4. Arnett EN, Isner JM, Redwood DR, et al. Coronary artery narrowing in coronary heart disease: comparison of cineangiographic and necropsy findings. *Ann Intern Med.* 1979;91:350–356.
5. Galbraith JE, Murphy ML, de Soyza N. Coronary angiogram interpretation: interobserver variability. *JAMA.* 1978;240:2053–2056.
6. Vlodaver Z, Frech R, Van-Tassel RA, Edwards JE. Correlation of the antemortem coronary arteriogram and the postmortem specimen. *Circulation.* 1973;47:162–169.
7. Zir LM, Miller SW, Dinsmore RE, Gilbert JP, Harthorne JW. Interobserver variability in coronary angiography. *Circulation.* 1976;53:627–632.
8. Marcus ML, Harrison DG, White CW, McPherson DD, Wilson RF, Kerber RE. Assessing the physiologic significance of coronary obstructions in patients: importance of diffuse

undetected atherosclerosis. *Prog Cardiovasc Dis.* 1988;31: 39–56.

9. Topol EJ, Nissen SE. Our preoccupation with coronary luminology: the dissociation between clinical and angiographic findings in ischemic heart disease. *Circulation.* 1995;92:2333–2342.

10. Glagov S, Weisenberg E, Zarins CK, Stankunavicius R, Kolettis GJ. Compensatory enlargement of human atherosclerotic coronary arteries. *N Engl J Med.* 1987;316: 1371–1375.

11. Marcus ML, Skorton DJ, Johnson MR, Collins SM, Harrison DG, Kerber RE. Visual estimates of percent diameter coronary stenosis: "a battered gold standard." *J Am Coll Cardiol.* 1988;11:882–885.

12. White CW, Wright CB, Doty DB, et al. Does visual interpretation of the coronary arteriogram predict the physiologic importance of a coronary stenosis? *N Engl J Med.* 1984; 310:819–824.

13. Waller BF, Pinkerton CA, Slack JD. Intravascular ultrasound: a histological study of vessels during life. The new 'gold standard' for vascular imaging. *Circulation.* 1992; 85:2305–2310.

14. Nissen SE, Gurley JC, Grines CL, et al. Intravascular ultrasound assessment of lumen size and wall morphology in normal subjects and patients with coronary artery disease. *Circulation.* 1991;84:1087–1099.

15. Tobis JM, Mallery JA, Gessert J, et al. Intravascular ultrasound cross-sectional arterial imaging before and after balloon angioplasty in vitro. *Circulation.* 1989;80:873–882.

16. Tobis JM, Mallery J, Mahon D, et al. Intravascular ultrasound imaging of human coronary arteries in vivo. Analysis of tissue characterizations with comparison to in vitro histological specimens. *Circulation.* 1991;83:913–926.

17. Falk E, Shah PK, Fuster V. Coronary plaque disruption. *Circulation.* 1995;92:657–671.

18. Fuster V. Lewis A. Conner Memorial Lecture. Mechanisms leading to myocardial infarction: insights from studies of vascular biology. *Circulation.* 1994;90:2126–2146.

19. Brown BG, Zhao XQ, Sacco DE, Albers JJ. Lipid lowering and plaque regression: new insights into prevention of plaque disruption and clinical events in coronary disease. *Circulation.* 1993;87:1781–1791.

20. MacIsaac AI, Thomas JD, Topol EJ. Toward the quiescent coronary plaque. *J Am Coll Cardiol.* 1993;22:1228–1241.

21. Mallery JA, Tobis JM, Griffith J, et al. Assessment of normal and atherosclerotic arterial wall thickness with an intravascular ultrasound imaging catheter. *Am Heart J.* 1990;119:1392–1400.

22. Gussenhoven EJ, Essed CE, Lancee CT, et al. Arterial wall characteristics determined by intravascular ultrasound imaging: an in vitro study. *J Am Coll Cardiol.* 1989;14: 947–952.

23. Nishimura RA, Edwards WD, Warnes CA, et al. Intravascular ultrasound imaging: in vitro validation and pathologic correlation. *J Am Coll Cardiol.* 1990;16:145–154.

24. Potkin BN, Bartorelli AL, Gessert JM, et al. Coronary artery imaging with intravascular high-frequency ultrasound. *Circulation.* 1990;81:1575–1585.

25. Pandian NG, Weintraub A, Kreis A, Schwartz SL, Konstam MA, Salem DN. Intracardiac, intravascular, two-dimensional,

high-frequency ultrasound imaging of pulmonary artery and its branches in humans and animals. *Circulation.* 1990;81:2007–2012.

26. Nissen SE, Grines CL, Gurley JC, et al. Application of a new phased-array ultrasound imaging catheter in the assessment of vascular dimensions: in vivo comparison to cineangiography. *Circulation.* 1990;81:660–666.

27. St. Goar FG, Pinto FJ, Alderman EL, et al. Detection of coronary atherosclerosis in young adult hearts using intravascular ultrasound. *Circulation.* 1992;86:756–763.

28. Fitzgerald PJ, St. Goar FG, Connolly AJ, et al. Intravascular ultrasound imaging of coronary arteries. Is three layers the norm? *Circulation.* 1992;86:154–158.

29. Mintz GS, Popma JJ, Pichard AD, et al. Patterns of calcification in coronary artery disease: a statistical analysis of intravascular ultrasound and coronary angiography in 1155 lesions. *Circulation.* 1995;91:1959–1965.

30. Gerber TC, Erbel R, Gorge G, Ge J, Rupprecht HJ, Meyer J. Extent of atherosclerosis and remodeling of the left main coronary artery determined by intravascular ultrasound. *Am J Cardiol.* 1994;73:666–671.

31. Losordo DW, Rosenfield K, Kaufman J, Pieczek A, Isner JM. Focal compensatory enlargement of human arteries in response to progressive atherosclerosis: in vivo documentation using intravascular ultrasound. *Circulation.* 1994; 89:2570–2577.

32. Hodgson JM, Reddy KG, Suneja R, Nair RN, Lesnefsky EJ, Sheehan HM. Intracoronary ultrasound imaging: correlation of plaque morphology with angiography, clinical syndrome, and procedural results in patients undergoing coronary angioplasty. *J Am Coll Cardiol.* 1993;21:35–44.

33. Billingham ME. Cardiac transplant atherosclerosis. *Transplant Proc.* 1987;19:19–25.

34. Uretsky BF, Murali S, Reddy PS, et al. Development of coronary artery disease in cardiac transplant patients receiving immunosuppressive therapy with cyclosporine and prednisone. *Circulation.* 1987;76:827–834.

35. Gao SZ, Alderman EL, Schroeder JS, Silverman JF, Hunt SA. Accelerated coronary vascular disease in the heart transplant patient: coronary arteriographic findings. *J Am Coll Cardiol.* 1988;12:334–340.

36. Pinto FJ, Chenzbraun A, Botas J, et al. Feasibility of serial intracoronary ultrasound imaging for assessment of progression of intimal proliferation in cardiac transplant recipients. *Circulation.* 1994;90:2348–2355.

37. St. Goar FG, Pinto FJ, Alderman EL, et al. Intracoronary ultrasound in cardiac transplant recipients: in vivo evidence of "angiographically silent" intimal thickening. *Circulation.* 1992;85:979–987.

38. Mintz GS, Painter JA, Pichard AD, et al. Atherosclerosis in angiographically "normal" coronary artery reference segments: an intravascular ultrasound study with clinical correlations. *J Am Coll Cardiol.* 1995;25:1479–1485.

39. Fitzgerald PJ, Ports TA, Yock PG. Contribution of localized calcium deposits to dissection after angioplasty. An observational study using intravascular ultrasound. *Circulation.* 1992;6:64–70.

40. Potkin BN, Keren G, Mintz GS, et al. Arterial responses to balloon coronary angioplasty: an intravascular ultrasound study. *J Am Coll Cardiol.* 1992;20:942–951.

41. Matar FA, Mintz GS, Pinnow E, et al. Multivariate predictors of intravascular ultrasound end points after directional coronary atherectomy. *J Am Coll Cardiol.* 1995; 25:318–324.

42. Losordo DW, Rosenfield K, Pieczek A, Baker K, Harding M, Isner JM. How does angioplasty work? Serial analysis of human iliac arteries using intravascular ultrasound. *Circulation.* 1992;86:1845–1858.

43. Franklin SM, Faxon DP. Pharmacologic prevention of restenosis after coronary angioplasty: review of the randomized clinical trials. *Coron Artery Dis.* 1993;4:232–242.

44. Holmes D Jr, Vlietstra RE, Smith HC, et al. Restenosis after percutaneous transluminal coronary angioplasty (PTCA): a report from the PTCA Registry of the National Heart, Lung, and Blood Institute. *Am J Cardiol.* 1984;53:18–20.

45. Liu MW, Roubin GS, King SB III. Restenosis after coronary angioplasty: potential biologic determinants and role of intimal hyperplasia. *Circulation.* 1989;79:1374–1387.

46. Currier JW, Faxon DP. Restenosis after percutaneous transluminal coronary angioplasty: have we been aiming at the wrong target? *J Am Coll Cardiol.* 1995;25:516–520.

47. Di Mario C, Gil R, Camenzind E, et al. Quantitative assessment with intracoronary ultrasound of the mechanisms of restenosis after percutaneous transluminal coronary angioplasty and directional coronary atherectomy. *Am J Cardiol.* 1995;75:772–777.

48. Mintz GS, Pichard AD, Kent KM, Satler LF, Popma JJ, Leon MB. Intravascular ultrasound comparison of restenotic and de novo coronary artery narrowings. *Am J Cardiol.* 1994;74:1278–1280.

49. Mintz G, Chuang Y, Popma J, et al. The final % cross-sectional narrowing (residual plaque burden) is the strongest intravascular ultrasound predictor of angiographic restenosis. *J Am Coll Cardiol.* 1995;35A:701–702.

50. The GUIDE Trial Investigators. IVUS-determined predictors of restenosis in PTCA and DCA: an interim report from the GUIDE trial, phase II. *Circulation.* 1994;90(pt II): I–23.

51. Fischman DL, Leon MB, Baim DS, et al. for the Stent Restenosis Study Investigators. A randomized comparison of coronary-stent placement and balloon angioplasty in the treatment of coronary artery disease. *N Engl J Med.* 1994;331:496–501.

52. Serruys PW, de-Jaegere P, Kiemeneij F, et al. for the Benestent Study Group. A comparison of balloon-expandable-stent implantation with balloon angioplasty in patients with coronary artery disease. *N Engl J Med.* 1994;331: 489–495.

53. Colombo A, Hall P, Nakamura S, et al. Intracoronary stenting without anticoagulation accomplished with intravascular ultrasound guidance. *Circulation.* 1995;91:1676–1688.

54. Gorge G, Haude M, Ge J, et al. Intravascular ultrasound after low and high inflation pressure coronary artery stent implantation. *J Am Coll Cardiol.* 1995;26:725–730.

55. Morice MC, Zemour G, Benveniste E, et al. Intracoronary stenting without coumadin: one month results of a French multicenter study. *Cathet Cardiovasc Diagn.* 1995;35:1–7.

56. Topol EJ, Leya F, Pinkerton CA, et al. A comparison of directional atherectomy with coronary angioplasty in patients with coronary artery disease. The CAVEAT Study Group. *N Engl J Med.* 1993;329:221–227.

57. Suarez de Lezo J, Romero M, Medina A, et al. Intracoronary ultrasound assessment of directional coronary atherectomy: immediate and follow-up findings. *J Am Coll Cardiol.* 1993;21:298–307.

58. Umans VA, Keane D, Foley D, Boersma E, Melkert R, Serruys PW. Optimal use of directional coronary atherectomy is required to ensure long-term angiographic benefit: a study with matched procedural outcome after atherectomy and angioplasty. *J Am Coll Cardiol.* 1994;24: 1652–1659.

59. Kovach JA, Mintz GS, Pichard AD, et al. Sequential intravascular ultrasound characterization of the mechanisms of rotational atherectomy and adjunct balloon angioplasty. *J Am Coll Cardiol.* 1993;22:1024–1032.

60. Mintz GS, Potkin BN, Keren G, et al. Intravascular ultrasound evaluation of the effect of rotational atherectomy in obstructive atherosclerotic coronary artery disease. *Circulation.* 1992;86:1383–1393.

61. Roelandt JR, di Mario C, Pandian NG, et al. Three-dimensional reconstruction of intracoronary ultrasound images: rationale, approaches, problems, and directions. *Circulation.* 1994;90:1044–1055.

16

Magnetic Resonance Imaging in Cardiovascular Disease

Herbert Frank and Sebastian Globits

Magnetic resonance imaging (MRI) is a noninvasive testing method that in the last decade has become more and more important in evaluation of the heart and cardiovascular system. MRI with electrocardiographic (ECG) gating can provide information about cardiovascular anatomy and function, myocardial tissue characterization, and myocardial metabolism. The combination of inherent contrast between blood flow and chamber wall, high spatial resolution, and lack of ionizing radiation makes MRI an important tool in noninvasive diagnosis of a number of cardiovascular diseases.

Initially, cardiac images were acquired by use of ECG-gated spin-echo (SE) pulse sequences, which produced contrast between the high signal intensity from myocardium and the lack of signal from flowing blood. Cine MRI was developed to permit sequential image acquisition at a single level through the cardiac cycle, which allowed the assessment of cardiac function. Recent developments in the area of fast-imaging techniques are rapidly increasing the utility of MRI for the study of the heart and vascular system.

MRI Techniques

Basic Principles

Magnetic Protons

A strong magnetic field provides the environment for the MRI process. The field magnetizes the tissue and resonates it at a specific radio frequency. For MRI, only protons have been used. In absence of a magnetic field, protons have no preferred orientation. Because of their random orientation, their magnetic properties cancel such that the tissue has no net magnetism. However, when the body is placed in a strong magnetic field, many protons will align with and against the field. Because of differences in energy between the two alignments, there is a slight excess of protons in the lower energy state.

Longitudinal and Transverse Magnetization

When radio-frequency energy at the appropriate frequency (Larmor frequency) is applied, protons reverse their direction and align with the higher energy state, from which they relax back to their original alignment at a rate determined by T_1 and T_2 relaxation times.

Tissue that is magnetized in the same direction as the magnetic field is described as longitudinally magnetized. If tissue is abruptly placed in a magnetic field, protons begin to align and longitudinal magnetization grows exponentially until it reaches a stable maximum value. This growth process is generally referred to as longitudinal relaxation and is characterized in a specific tissue by the T_1 value. Tissue magnetization can be flipped from the longitudinal to the transverse direction by applying a 90 degree pulse. Transverse magnetization is an unstable condition that begins to decay as soon as it is created. It decays in an exponential manner, the rate being determined by the T_2 value of the tissue. T_2 image contrast is created during the decay phase of transverse magnetization. T_1 and T_2 relaxation times depend in a complex way on the physical and chemical characteristics of the tissue.

T_1 and T_2 Contrast

The time required for relaxation, which is the basic characteristic of longitudinal magnetization, is the tissue's T_1 characteristic. The difference in magnetization of two different tissues represents the T_1 contrast between these two tissues. The time required for a tissue to dissipate its transversal magnetization is its T_2 characteristic. If tissues have different T_2 values, their magnetization decays at different rates, and T_2 contrast will be created. The repetition time (TR)—the time between the initiation of the pulse sequence and the beginning of the next sequence—influences T_1 and T_2 contrast. T_1-weighted images usually employ a TR of 0.5 to 1.0 seconds, whereas T_2 contrast is enhanced by a TR of about 2.0 seconds.

Pulse Sequences

The tissue contrast displayed with MRI depends on T_1 and T_2 relaxation times and on the density of protons in the tissue being imaged. By selecting appropriate radio-frequency pulse sequences, the contribution of each parameter can be emphasized, and the relative intensity of different tissue in the image altered accordingly. The most widely used radio-frequency pulse sequence is the spin-echo (SE) pulse sequence, which consists of a 90 degree pulse at the end of the magnetization and a following 180 degree pulse, which inverts the magnetization. There is a variable delay between the initial pulse and receipt of the signal or echo, called *echo time* (TE). TE is the time interval between the 90 degree pulse and the echo event. The primary significance of TE is that it determines the amount of T_2 contrast. If the objective is to create an image with T_2 contrast, then a relatively long TE value is selected. If the image is to be T_1-weighted, T_2 contrast should be reduced by selecting a relatively short TE value.

Formation of Image Contrast

In the process of relaxation, protons produce the magnetic resonance signal in a radio antenna, the body coil that surrounds the patient. Alternatively, specialized small radio antennae, called *surface* or *local coils,* may be used to optimize the image quality over localized regions of the body. Under the influence of the main magnetic field, all spins precess at the same frequency. Applying a magnetic gradient field on the main magnetic field imposes a range of frequencies along the direction of the gradient. Three magnetic gradient systems are incorporated into each scanner, one for each of the three spatial axes (x, y, and z). The three magnetic gradients are separately adjustable and are generated by three electromagnetic coils housed inside the main magnet. Slice selection requires application of a magnetic gradient in a direction orthogonal to the desired slice, and simultaneous application of a radio-frequency field at a frequency designed to coincide with the slice's position. In the same manner, application of a magnetic gradient orthogonal to the selected slice defines planes of spins with distinct frequencies. A gradient applied after slice selection imposes a range of frequencies on the signal originating from the slice. The data thus acquired can be processed into an image by application of a two-dimensional Fourier transformation.

Cardiovascular MRI Techniques

Successful MRI of the cardiovascular system requires ECG gating because of two important factors: (1) ungated images of the heart produce unacceptable degrees of motion artifacts and (2) most of the cardiovascular MRI studies require imaging or data acquisition during a certain cardiac cycle. The trigger delay time is the time between the R-wave seen in the electrocardiogram and the image selection during the heart cycle. Due to the selected trigger delay time in a single-slice imaging mode, either a systolic or diastolic image can be acquired. For volume quantification and assessment of ventricular function, multislice, multiphase pulse sequences in four-chamber (oblique axial or oblique coronal) equivalent projections are required and allow appropriate measurements of the ventricle volumes during an end-systolic and end-diastolic phase. Because MRI is a three-dimensional imaging procedure, it is expected to be more accurate than angiography or two-dimensional echocardiography for quantification of right and left ventricular volumes and stroke volume.[1] Good correlations have been found between MRI and two-dimensional echocardiography measurements of left ventricular volume. MRI can also provide exact measurements of right ventricular volume and yields nearly equivalent values for stroke volume of right and left ventricles in normal subjects.[2]

Two imaging approaches have been widely used in cardiovascular MRI: the spin-echo (SE) sequence for depiction of cardiac and vascular morphology, and the gradient-echo (GRE) sequence for assessment of flow and cardiac function. Using the SE technique, good spatial resolution and the excellent contrast between flowing blood and myocardium facilitate the delineation of the endocardial border. This technique also enables the assessment of ventricular volumes by calculating the areas of each slice and multiplying them by slice thickness and interslice gap.

The GRE technique uses low flip angles, short TR, and gradient-refocused echos for demonstration of blood-flow phenomena.[3] Areas of high velocity and turbulent flow appear as a typical signal void within the regurgitant chamber. By this imaging technique, it is possible to visualize the regurgitant jet in all patients, although the area of signal loss may not always correspond with the extent of the regurgitant jet and therefore may not prove useful for quantitative assessment of the severity of regurgitation.[3] Technologic developments have enabled the quantification of intracardiac blood flow using velocity-encoded cine GRE (VEC) imaging.[4] From the VEC data set, the velocity can be measured for each pixel or within a region of interest encircling the entire vessel cross-sectional area. The product of area and spatial mean velocity yields instantaneous flow volume for a specific time frame in the cardiac cycle. Integration of all instantaneous flow volumes throughout the cardiac cycle gives the volume flow per heartbeat. This technique has been validated in vitro against flow phantoms, and in vivo in healthy subjects by comparing flow measurements in the aorta and pulmonary artery with left and right stroke volume by cine GRE imaging.[5]

Although progress in reducing scan times has been made by implementation of GRE techniques, the echo-planar imaging method, which completes images after a single excitation, is of particular note in cardiology where organ perfusion and functional motion, wall thickness, and the degree of contraction and expansion must be taken in account. Echo-planar techniques acquire all the data necessary to complete an image in as little as 30 ms.[6] This and other fast imaging techniques are suitable to image myocardial perfusion and coronary vasculature and assess myocardial viability.

Congenital Heart Disease

As a tomographic method with a good spatial resolution, MRI allows identification of visceral atrial situs, type of ventricular loop, and relationship of the great vessels.[7] From a comparison with angiographic and two-dimensional echocardiographic images, MRI provides accurate anatomic diagnosis in complex congenital heart diseases. In some instances, MRI can replace the need for invasive cardiac catheterization or reduce the number of catheterizations required in management of patients with complex congenital heart disease. MRI of complex congental heart diseases is necessary for preoperative assessment in adults and infants and influences surgical planning through increased knowledge of the anatomic topography of the vascular malformation and its relation to the bronchial system.

Atrial Septal Defect

Visualization of atrial septal defects (ASDs) by MRI with the SE technique is well established, as is use of dynamic imaging with the GRE technique to visualize ASD shunt flow.[8] The SE technique allows delineation of the atrial septum in two orthogonal views (short axis and four chamber) perpendicular to the plane of the septum. Large atrial septal defects can be identified easily as the absence of, or a large deficit in, the interatrial septum. MRI has high sensitivity and specificity in the diagnosis of primum, secundum, and sinus venosus ASDs.[7] False positive diagnoses of ASDs can occur due to the low signal intensity of the atrial septum in the region of the fossa ovalis. The differentiation between signal dropout in the area of the fossa ovalis and a true secundum atrial defect is especially difficult in images of suboptimal quality.[7] Thus, SE imaging can give erroneously large measurements of secundum ASD size. Ostium primum and sinus venosus ASDs are located primarily in thicker parts of the septum, so these lesions are defined more reliably by septal discontinuity in SE images.[9]

Dynamic imaging with the GRE technique can visualize an ASD shunt jet (Figure 16.1), especially when in-

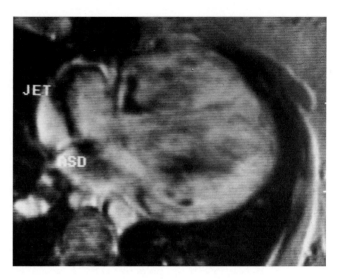

FIGURE 16.1. GRE image in a four-chamber view visualizing the ASD shunt jet (JET) as a signal void into the right atrium.

creased interatrial pressure gradients are present. However, when the interatrial pressure gradient is low, this technique may be inadequate if the jet velocity is low.[9] In such cases, shunt flow can be missed entirely. In studies using VEC imaging of the cross section of the shunt stream at the orifice, researchers were able to identify and assess ASD size that was not apparent in the magnitude image. This technique can yield ASD dimensions and shape with sufficient accuracy to identify patients who require surgical repair versus those who may benefit from nonsurgical ASD closure by catheterization techniques.[9] VEC imaging is also an accurate and reproducible method for measuring Q_p/Q_s. Use of VEC imaging to demonstrate unequal levels of pulmonary and systemic flows in a few patients with various forms of congenital heart disease has already be reported.[10] Studies have demonstrated that VEC imaging can quantify Q_p/Q_s in patients with a left-to-right shunt and that these results correlate closely with oximetric data obtained at cardiac catheterization.[11]

Ventricular Septal Defect

Ventricular septal defects (VSD) can be diagnosed by either SE pulse sequences using transverse or coronal planes, or by the GRE technique. Despite the reported accuracy with SE imaging, small VSDs will be missed and muscular defects not identified. GRE imaging, however, has resulted in improved detectability of VSD because the actual shunt flow is identified. The overall sensitivity of MRI in diagnosis of VSDs was calculated to be 100% at the 95% specificity level.[7] Defects in the trabecular portion of the septum can be identified very easily by MRI. These defects penetrate the muscular septum, are sur-

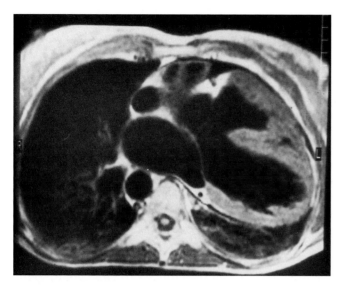

FIGURE 16.2. Large conoventricular septum defect on a transverse SE sequence with right descending aorta.

rounded entirely by muscle, and are not related to the aortic or atrioventricular valve. Conoventricular defects, characteristically with one border formed by the mitral, tricuspid, and aortic fibrous continuity, are often seen on transverse SE images (Figure 16.2). The morphology of this defect and its relationship to the septal leaflet of the tricuspid valve are particularly important because some of these defects are partially covered by the valvular structure, making the defect appear relatively small. Also important is the relationship of this defect to the aortic valve.[12] In these cases, selection of small slice thickness (5 mm) is very important for accurate diagnosis. Supracristal defects are usually related to the pulmonary and aortic valves and are clearly demonstrated by contiguous transverse sections upward to the plane of the pulmonary valve (Figure 16.3).

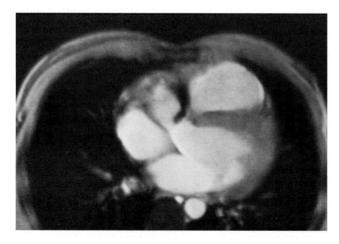

FIGURE 16.3. Small supracristal VSD on a transverse GRE image. The signal void in the right ventricular outflow tract visualizes the left-to-right shunt flow.

Patent Ductus Arteriosus

An important application of MRI is in visualization of a patent ductus arteriosus. Compared to other noninvasive imaging techniques, MRI allows detection and measurement of the extent of a patent ductus arteriosus. The best demonstration is by transverse sections at the level of the great arteries and by coronal sections. The left anterior oblique plane in the SE and GRE techniques is very helpful in visualizing the ductus and verifying blood flow between the aorta and pulmonary artery (Figure 16.4). Best results are achieved if a slice thickness between 3 and 5 mm is selected. However, the accuracy of MRI for diagnosis of a patent ductus arteriosus is still uncertain.[12]

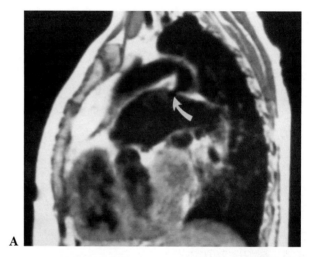

A

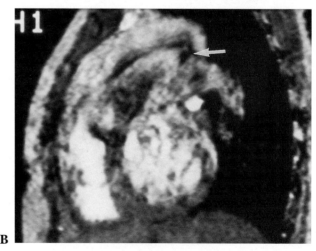

B

FIGURE 16.4. Left anterior oblique plane of a patient with a patent ductus arteriosus (SE and GRE techniques). **A,** The patent ductus arteriosus is visible on this oblique plane (arrow), and the extent of the ductus can be measured. **B,** GRE pulse sequence demonstrating the signal void of the shunt jet into the pulmonary artery (arrow).

Anomalous Venous Connection

Although echocardiography is superior to MRI for detection of valvular abnormalities, MRI is better for showing anomalies of pulmonary venous connection.[13] Visualization of pulmonary veins and diagnosis of an anomalous venous connection requires performing the MRI study with this intention. Partial anomalous pulmonary venous connection is identified from the course of the pulmonary veins to their point of drainage, and by demonstration of lack of communication to the left atrium on one side, and the route of the anomalous connection on the other. The pulmonary veins may be connected to various sites, commonly classified as supracardiac, cardiac, infracardiac, and mixed. Supracardiac connection is to the right superior vena cava or to the innominate vein. Cardiac connection may be to the coronary sinus or directly to the right atrium. Infracardiac connection is through a vertical vein to the inferior vena cava. Transverse SE sections at the level of the left atrium and at the anomalous connection identify the anomaly. Sections of the lung at different levels, and the inferior vena cava on transverse and coronal sections can also delineate anomalous drainage of the pulmonary veins (Figure 16.5).

Tetralogy of Fallot

Tetralogy of Fallot is a complex lesion with VSD, aortic override of the defect, right ventricular outflow obstruction, and right ventricular hypertrophy. A frequent associated anomaly is a right-sided aortic arch. The association of tetralogy of Fallot and absence of pulmonary valve leads to enlarged pulmonary arteries, which may cause bronchial obstruction.

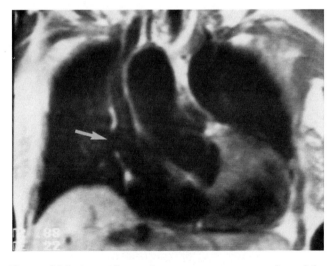

FIGURE 16.5. Anomalous pulmonary venous connection of the supracardiac type on a coronal SE plane image showing drainage of the pulmonary vein to the right superior vena cava (arrow).

Magnetic resonance tomograms in the transverse, sagittal, and coronal planes demonstrate all characteristic lesions of tetralogy of Fallot. The dimensional difference between aorta and pulmonary artery is revealed on transverse images. Sequential transverse and sagittal images can be used to demonstrate pulmonary stenosis. Sagittal images are helpful in the assessment of right ventricular wall thickness.[14] Pulmonary and bronchial arteries can be distinguished on transverse planes at the level of the carina. The origin of bronchial arteries from the descending aorta can be visualized on transverse and coronal images. Cine MRI has been used to demonstrate the right ventricular outflow tract and identify pulmonary regurgitation.[15] Pulmonary regurgitation occurs especially when a transannular patch is used for relief of the outflow tract obstruction of the right ventricle. In the case of residual pulmonary regurgitation, right ventricular overload may predispose to development of ventricular arrhythmia, a risk factor for sudden death. Several studies suggest that postoperative pulmonary regurgitation may be partly responsible for abnormal right ventricular hemodynamics or limited exercise capacity in otherwise asymptomatic patients with tetralogy of Fallot.[16,17] Attempts have been made to estimate severity of pulmonary regurgitation using Doppler echocardiography, contrast ventriculography, or videodensitometry. VEC imaging provides measurement of volumetric flow and is an accurate and noninvasive method for volumetric quantitation of pulmonary regurgitation in patients after surgical repair of tetralogy of Fallot.[18] In addition, the ability of MRI to measure right ventricular volumes tomographically allows a more comprehensive study of pulmonary regurgitation in postoperative tetralogy of Fallot.

MRI provides good visualization of vessel morphology and mediastinal structures and is superior to echocardiography in detection of additional vessel abnormalities such as left brachiocephalic truncus and dextropositioned aorta. In tetralogy of Fallot associated with absence of the pulmonary valve, MRI makes imaging of the bronchial system possible and enables diagnosis of airway obstruction. Neither ultrasonic nor radiographic examinations allow accurate assessment of bronchus anatomy or malstructure. This additional information in tetralogy of Fallot, and in complex congenital heart disease in general, is necessary for preoperative assessment and planning of surgery.[19]

Complete Transposition

In D transposition of great arteries, the aorta arises anteriorly from the right ventricle, whereas the pulmonary artery arises posteriorly from the left ventricle. In L transposition, the morphologic left ventricle lies to the right, the morphologic right ventricle to the left (Figure

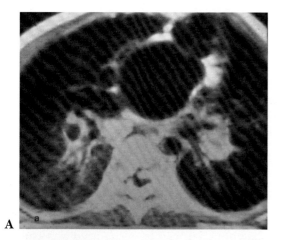

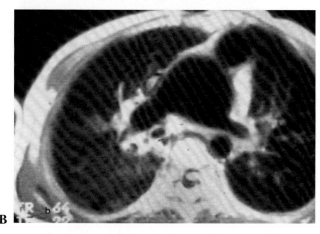

FIGURE 16.6. L transposition of the great arteries on a transverse image plane. **A,** The aorta is visualized anterior and to the left of the pulmonary artery, which is easier to identify by its bifurcation on a cranial plane, **B.**

16.6). In this congenitally corrected aortopulmonary transposition, there is an atrioventricular and ventriculoarterial discordance.

Transverse and coronal scans of the base of the heart reveal the origin of pulmonary artery and aorta. The anatomic right ventricle is recognized by the moderator band. In complete D transposition, sequential transverse images show the anatomic right ventricle with an originating right-sided aorta. Right atrium and right ventricle are normally connected. In transverse magnetic resonance tomograms, the aorta is anteriorly positioned and to the right of the pulmonary artery. In congenitally corrected L transposition, the aorta is visualized anterior and to the left of the pulmonary artery. Additional planes are needed to distinguish the aorta and pulmonary artery unequivocally. The pulmonary artery may be recognized by following transverse images cranially to the pulmonary arterial bifurcation, whereas the ascending aorta is characterized by the aortic arch and brachiocephalic vessels.

The advantage of MRI in congenital heart disease is that additional malformations can be visualized because of the greater field of view. Several other congenital heart anomalies are associated with L transposition and can be detected by MRI. The most frequent additional malformations are VSD, valvular and subvalvular pulmonic stenosis, and Ebstein´s anomaly of the left-sided atrioventricular valve.

Truncus Arteriosus

Truncus arteriosus is a common vessel that overrides both ventricles and the large VSD. Coronary arteries and systemic and pulmonary vessels arise from this common vessel. The branching pattern into pulmonary and aortic circulations allows classification of the different forms of truncus arteriosus.[20] In type I truncus, there is a common pulmonary artery arising from the truncus, whereas the branch pulmonary arteries arise separately in type II truncus. In type III truncus, one of the branch pulmonary arteries is absent and one pulmonary artery is fed from a persistent patent ductus arteriosus. Type IV truncus represents coincidence of a type I truncus with aortic arch interruption, where the ascending aorta is small and the descending aorta is perfused through a widely patent ductus arteriosus. Transverse SE sequences are recommended for visualization and classification of the different forms of truncus arteriosus (Figure 16.7). The site of origin of the pulmonary arteries can be discerned using thin slices (5 mm) on transverse or coronal tomograms. MRI can reliably classify truncus arteriosus by assessing pulmonary artery anatomy. The size of the pulmonary artery and its branches can be measured on transverse, coronal, and sagittal planes. For assessment of pulmonary arteries, a slice thickness of 3 to 5 mm is recommended.

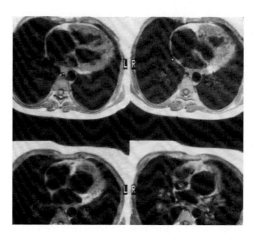

FIGURE 16.7. Four different planes of transverse images of a truncus arteriosus. Magnetic resonance images show the common vessel overriding both ventricles.

Pulmonary Hypertension

MRI is useful in establishing a diagnosis of pulmonary hypertension and can be used to determine the cause of pulmonary hypertension in patients with congenital heart disease, mitral valve disease, dilative cardiomyopathy, and pulmonary fibrosis. However, MRI cannot distinguish between primary pulmonary hypertension and chronic pulmonary embolism. Pulmonary artery pressure can be estimated by assessing the right ventricular free wall and systolic pulmonary flow. Systolic slow-flow phenomenon in the pulmonary artery is evidence that mean pressure in the pulmonary artery is greater than 70 mm Hg. In healthy patients, rapid flow of blood during systole is manifested as a signal void on images that are gated to the systolic phase of the cardiac cycle.[21] An intralumenal signal due to slowly flowing blood can be found only on images gated to end-diastole. Systolic slow-flow phenomena were observed in patients with chronic pulmonary hypertension and a mean pulmonary pressure greater than 70 mm Hg (Figure 16.8). Several authors have reported a correlation between this slow-flow phenomenon and systolic pressure.[22,23] Others found a relationship between pulmonary vascular resistance and intensity of the intravascular signal during systole.[24] This decrease in flow caused by deterioration of cardiac output subsequent to increased pulmonary pressure causes a slow-flow phenomenon during systole.[25]

Of the quantitative parameters, the right ventricular wall thickness correlated best with pulmonary mean pressure ($r = 0.83$, $P = .0001$).[2] For patients with chronic pulmonary hypertension who require many fol-

low-up studies, thickness of the right ventricular wall and systolic slow-flow phenomena are significant parameters for pressure changes.

Valvular Disease

Assessment of Valvular Stenosis

Usually, the severity of a valvular stenosis is described either by the pressure gradient or calculated valve area by means of Doppler echocardiography or cardiac catheterization. Early experience with blood flow–sensitive gradient echo techniques indicated that high-velocity turbulent flow of stenotic jets can be recognized as a typical signal void.[26] With use of velocity-encoded cine MRI it is now possible to gain flow-velocity profiles across all cardiac valves and to accurately measure flow velocities across valvular stenoses.[27]

Quantification of Valvular Stenosis Using Cine GRE Imaging

Cine GRE imaging can be used in a semiquantitative fashion to define mitral stenosis and aortic stenosis. Casolo et al.[28] used cine MRI to characterize mitral leaflet morphology, diastolic transmitral flow, and leaflet separation in 20 patients with various degrees of mitral stenosis. They found a significant correlation between maximum leaflet separation measured by MRI and mitral valve area as calculated from Doppler echocardiography using the pressure half-time method. De Roos and coworkers[29] found that, in 17 patients with aortic stenosis, the following features appear to correlate with severity of aortic stenosis compared with Doppler echocardiography: identification of a narrow, high-velocity transvalvular jet; extensive propagation of turbulence in the ascending aorta; and presence of a prestenotic acceleration flow void. Eichenberger et al.[30] found no correlation between area of signal loss in the proximal ascending aorta and the pressure gradient measured during catheterization in patients with aortic stenosis. This the signal void seems to be mainly related to turbulence and not to high-velocity flow.[31] However, the phenomenon of signal loss is useful in demonstrating the site of stenosis in the subvalvular, valvular, or supravalvular region.

Quantification of Valvular Stenosis Using Velocity-Encoded Cine MRI

With velocity-encoded cine MRI, the phase shifts of protons within various voxels of the image are displayed in the gray level, corresponding to the degree of phase shift. The major factor causing such phase shift is motion, and the phase shift is directly proportional to motion over time and, hence, velocity. On the displayed

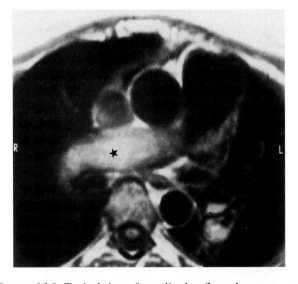

FIGURE 16.8. Typical sign of systolic slow-flow phenomenon in the pulmonary artery (*) in a patient with primary pulmonary hypertension. Due to increased pulmonary resistance, blood is flowing slowly during systole and causes an intralumenal signal increase.

phase images of a velocity-encoded cine MRI sequence, a region of interest can be drawn around the jet to display the ensemble of velocities in the jet during peak systole. From the measured peak velocity across the stenotic lesion, the pressure gradient is determined using the simplified Bernoulli equation (peak gradient = 4 × peak velocity[2]). Possible advantages of MRI over continuous-wave Doppler include freedom of access to jets at any location and in any direction, and reliable depiction of the anatomic location of jets. However, measurement of velocity across the stenotic valve is complicated by the presence of high-velocity turbulent flow, causing loss of signal beyond the valve. Whereas the signal void seen with cine MRI caused by turbulence permits recognition of stenosis and regurgitation, signal loss can vitiate measures of velocity at such sites. Using flow phantom experiments, the mean jet velocity measured by MRI showed an excellent correlation ($r = 0.99$) with that measured by Doppler echocardiography.[27] These authors have shown that a reduction in echo time minimizes the problem of signal loss from high-velocity turbulent jets. Another study demonstrated that velocity-encoded cine MRI can be used to accurately measure velocities up to 700 cm/s in flow phantoms[32] and in patients with valvular stenosis.[33] Eichenberger et al.[30] examined 19 subjects with a wide range of aortic gradients varying from 3 to 148 mm Hg using short-axis velocity-encoded cine MRI perpendicular to the jet and found a close correlation for the pressure gradients compared with Doppler echocardiography ($r = 0.96$) or catheterization ($r = 0.97$). In contrast, Kilner and coworkers[27] found it generally easier to interpret velocity maps parallel rather than perpendicular to the jet, as the former shows the length of the jet in relation to prestenotic and poststenotic flow.

A potential limitation of MRI is that misalignment between the motion–velocity vector and flow-encoding gradient may result in image artifacts due to flow–velocity components within the acquisition plane, the so called in-plane flow. The resulting image artifact is in the direction of the frequency-encoding readout gradient, leading to a distortion of the velocity profile. Despite having the imaging plane perpendicular to flow at time of maximal jet velocity, movement of the aortic valve throughout systole does not allow precise alignment with a fixed imaging plane.[34]

Blood flow across the mitral valve has also been measured by using phase-shift gradient echo techniques.[35] The normal biphasic pattern, can be reproduced in normal volunteers and is altered in patients with severe mitral stenosis.[36] In a study[37] of 16 patients with various degrees of mitral stenosis, significant correlations were shown between Doppler measurements and velocity-encoded cine MRI for the mean pressure gradient ($r = 0.95$) and velocity time integral ($r = 0.89$) (Figure 16.9). The severity of mitral stenosis has also been assessed by

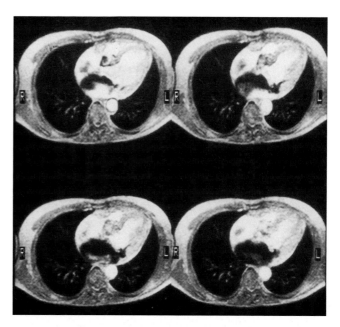

FIGURE 16.9. Transverse GRE single-slice multiphase image in a patient with severe mitral regurgitation. The signal void seen on the images visualizes the eccentric jet of the mitral regurgitation.

measuring pulmonary vein flow, which becomes reversed during systole in severe cases.[38]

Assessment of Regurgitant Lesions

The volume of blood that regurgitates across an incompetent valve is determined by the cross-sectional area of the regurgitant orifice, regurgitant time, total left ventricle (LV) stroke volume, and pressure difference across the valve. Quantification of regurgitant lesions by use of MRI can focus on the description of the characteristics and size of the regurgitant jet or on measurement of regurgitant volume expressed as an absolute value or relative to the forward cardiac output as described by the regurgitant fraction.

Quantification of Regurgitation Using Cine GRE Imaging

Because the signal intensity of blood flow is altered by abnormal flow characteristics,[39,40] cine GRE imaging is sensitive in detection of regurgitant jets. Several studies have demonstrated use of features of the signal void for grading of aortic regurgitation (AR) and mitral regurgitation (MR).[41,42] Aurigemma et al.[43,44] reported that in AR the ratio of maximal area of flow void to the left ventricular area, and in MR the ratio of area of flow void to the left atrial area correlated well with the severity estimated by Doppler echocardiography. Nishimura et al.[45] found that cine MRI correctly classified the degree of

AR in 93% of 30 patients as compared wtih angiographic grading. The best correlation between the two methods was demonstrated for the ratio of the flow void to the left ventricular area. As emphasized in this study, a problem may arise in patients with both AR and mitral stenosis or severe MR (including relative mitral stenosis), because these conditions induce an area of low signal intensity in the left ventricle during diastole and thus cause difficulty in evaluation of aortic regurgitant area in the left ventricular outflow tract.

The cine GRE studies in 62 patients with either AR or MR, and 20 normal subjects were retrospectively reviewed in a blinded fashion by three independent observers.[46] In all patients, MRI results were compared with Doppler and/or angiographic findings, yielding a sensitivity of 0.98, a specificity of 0.95, and a diagnostic accuracy of 0.97 for identification of AR or MR.

The imaging plane can influence considerably the apparent volume of signal void. Maximal size of the flow void for aortic lesions is observed in the coronal plane and for mitral and tricuspid lesions in the horizontal long-axis plane.[41] Size of the flow void may be influenced by several parameters such as field strength of the gradient, flip angle, echo time, imaging plane, and hemodynamic parameters such as preload and afterload, pressure gradient between the two chambers, and orifice size of the regurgitant lesion.[47] Nevertheless, a possible advantage of cine MRI a compared with Doppler echocardiography and angiography is the ability to show regurgitant flow at several levels of the heart and to provide a three-dimensional depiction of the regurgitant jet.

The total volume of the regurgitant jet clearly separates mild, moderate, and severe lesions, with good correlations with Doppler echocardiography and/or angiography.[48,49] These studies showed good reproducibility for measurement of flow void with an intraobserver correlation of 0.98 and an interobserver correlation of 0.94. In 23 patients with pure MR, and in 21 patients with pure AR, regurgitant volume determined by the volume of the signal void and by difference between left and right ventricular stroke volume correlated well ($r = 0.84$) for both lesions.

Cine GRE provides precise and reproducible quantification of ventricular volumes. Good correlations have been shown with other imaging techniques and phantom models.[50–55] In absence of regurgitation, the stroke volumes of the left and right ventricles are nearly equal.[56] In patients with MR or AR, the stroke volume of the left ventricle exceeds that of the right ventricle by the regurgitant volume. Consequently, the regurgitant fraction can be calculated as the regurgitant volume divided by the stroke volume of the regurgitant ventricle in patients with isolated valvular lesions.[3]

Another possible application of MRI in quantification of valvular regurgitation is the assessment of the so-called proximal convergence zone. As flow accelerates proximal to the regurgitant orifice, a flow void is produced in cine GRE images. Several recent MRI and Doppler studies suggest that measurements of this proximal convergence zone may offer a more precise method of determining regurgitant flow.[57] Yoshida et al.[58] found that the size and persistence of the proximal convergence zone on cine GRE imaging can be used to discriminate among several grades of aortic regurgitation with better success than the size of the regurgitant jet. This notion is supported by other authors.[59]

Quantification of Regurgitation Using Velocity-Encoded Cine MRI

Phase-mapping methods are accurate in measuring flow over a wide range of velocities in flow models and in patients.[60,61] By using VEC-MRI, the stroke volume ejected by the left or right ventricle can be determined from time-integrated measurements of flow volume in the ascending aorta or pulmonary artery. Kondo et al.[5] demonstrated that left and right ventricular stroke volumes measured by VEC-MRI were equal and comparable to left ventricular stroke volumes determined by cine MRI in 12 healthy volunteers. However, one major limitation of VEC-MRI is that it does not measure blood-flow changes on a beat-to-beat basis as does Doppler echocardiography. The data for flow measurements are acquired over 128 to 256 heartbeats and represent an average value. Nevertheless, blood flow can be presented in a phasic fashion for an average cardiac cycle by plotting flow for each of the multiple images corresponding to an average cardiac cycle.

In patients with isolated MR or AR, the regurgitant volume has been measured in several ways. Regurgitant volume can be determined in two ways (1) The regurgitant volume can be calculated from the difference between the left ventricular stroke volume measured in the ascending aorta, and the right ventricular stroke volume measured in main pulmonary artery. (2) In AR, net antegrade and retrograde flow can be measured directly from aortic flow phase data, where retrograde flow over one cardiac cycle is a direct measure of regurgitant volume even in presence of additional valvular diseases. By using this direct flow measurement in the ascending aorta in 10 patients with AR, Dulce et al.[62] demonstrated a close correlation for regurgitant volume and fraction data derived from VEC-MRI as compared with volumetric measurements from cine MR studies ($r = 0.97$). The interstudy reproducibility for VEC-MRI is high ($r = 0.97$), and the interstudy variability is low, making this technique an ideal tool for serial follow-up studies and for monitoring pharmacological intervention.

Sondergaard et al.[63] showed that, in 10 patients with isolated AR, there is a high correlation ($r = 0.97$) between stroke volume calculated from left ventricular end-diastolic and end-systolic volumes using cine magnetic resonance images, and the stroke volume quantified by VEC-MRI. They also found a significant correlation between left ventricular end-diastolic volume and regurgitant volume by VEC-MRI ($r = 0.80$) and between regurgitant volume by MRI and the angiographic grading ($r = 0.80$), respectively. The wide variation in regurgitant volumes within one angiographic grade was partially related to shortcomings of angiography because rapid dilution of the contrast medium entering a dilated chamber may cause subjective underestimation of the regurgitant volume.[64,65]

Using VEC-MRI, regurgitant volume and fraction can also be assessed with MRI using the difference between ventricular outflow as measured in the ascending aorta, and ventricular inflow as measured at the mitral valve annulus. Fujita et al.[66] compared MRI results with Doppler echocardiography in 19 patients with MR and showed significantly different regurgitant volumes among groups with mild, moderate, and severe MR. Regurgitant fraction also correlated well with Doppler echocardiography grading ($r = 0.87$).

Evaluation of Prosthetic Heart Valves

Although image artifacts and flow-masking effects caused by cardiac prostheses interfere with the diagnostic accuracy of transthoracic and transesophageal echocardiography, the value of this method has been well established in assessment of artificial valves.[67] Nevertheless, cardiac catheterization has remained the reference standard in evaluation of such patients despite the fact that signs and symptoms of prosthetic dysfunction are often too subtle or nonspecific to justify exposing the patient to a costly invasive procedure that does not allow repeated or longitudinal studies.[68]

Previous in vitro and in vivo studies have shown that patients with artificial heart valves can be safely examined with high-field magnets.[69-71] The diagnostic value of cine MRI in detecting regurgitation in artificial valves was compared with that of transesophageal color Doppler echocardiography in a study conducted by Deutsch et al.[49] They examined 47 patients with a total of 55 prostheses (32 aortic, 22 mitral, and 1 tricuspid) of various types and found 96% agreement between both methods in distinguishing physiologic from pathologic regurgitation across prosthetic valves. When the degree of regurgitation was graded according to the area covered by the regurgitant jet, results were identical in 75% of valve prostheses. Quantification of jet length and area showed good correlation ($r = 0.85$ and $r = 0.91$, respectively) between the two methods.[49]

Measurement of Blood Flow

Several techniques have been developed for measuring blood flow. One is called the *time-of-flight* technique, in which protons are tagged at one anatomical level and imaged at another level further downstream within the blood vessel. Because the time between measurement and tagging of the protons within flowing blood and the distance between the two sites is known, it is possible to calculate the velocity of blood flow. Another technique measures the change in phase of protons that are in motion relative to nonmobile protons, which maintain the same phase during the MRI sequence. It is based on the proportionality of phase change to velocity of motion of spins that flow along a magnetic gradient during the imaging sequence. This technique, referred to as the velocity-encoded cine MRI (VEC-MRI) technique, is perhaps the most effective one for measuring blood flow (Figure 16.10).[52,57] With this technique, it is possible to measure peak blood flow, blood flow at any site across the lumen of the vessel, and mean blood flow in the vessel. The technique provides a magnitude image on which the cross-sectional area of the vessel is measured, and a phase image on which flow velocity is measured for any voxel in the lumen.

The quantitative phase technique has been verified in flow phantom and in patient studies. In an experimental setting, measurements have been found to correlate precisely over a flow range of 10 to 600 cm/s for a TE value of 7 ms with a 1.5-T magnet.[57] In vivo validation has been achieved by comparison of measurement of left ventricular stroke volume defined by the quantitative phase tech-

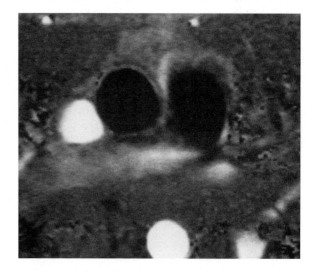

FIGURE 16.10. On VEC-MR images, superior-to-inferior flow (superior vena cava, descending aorta, and internal mammary arteries [IMAs]) is considered positive and is represented as a white area, whereas inferior-to-superior flow (ascending aorta, main pulmonary artery, and internal mammary veins) is considered negative and is thus represented as a black area.

nique, with left ventricular stroke volume measured by volume calculations from a stack of cine magnetic resonance images.[57] Correlation between these measurements has been excellent ($r = 0.95$), with a low standard error of the estimate (4.8 mm/s). VEC-MRI has also been compared to Doppler echocardiography measurements in the pulmonary artery, and there is good agreement between the methods. As expected, the values for peak velocity were nearly identical, but those for the mean blood flow rate by VEC-MRI and Doppler echocardiography were not the same, due to the difference in temporal resolution between methods.

VEC-MRI has been used to measure blood flow separately in right and left pulmonary arteries. The precision of this technique is indicated by the finding that the sum of the blood flow within right and left pulmonary arteries correlated nearly precisely with the measurement of blood flow in the main pulmonary artery. The technique can also be used to demonstrate the difference in pulmonary blood-flow pattern in normal individuals and in patients with pulmonary arterial hypertension. Whereas the flow pattern in the normal pulmonary artery showed almost no retrograde flow during diastole or during systole, in pulmonary arterial hypertension, the peak velocity of blood flow is reached earlier during the systolic period, and there is retrograde flow during portions of systole and diastole. Additionally, direction of blood flow in the pulmonary artery during systole was antegrade in some regions and retrograde in other regions in patients with pulmonary arterial hypertension.

There are numerous applications for blood-flow measurements in cardiovascular diagnosis, including measurement of right and left ventricular stroke volume and calculation of cardiac output. The technique can be used to compare right and left ventricular stroke volumes to quantitate volumes of intracardiac shunts or singular regurgitant valve lesions. Further indications include measurement of pressure gradients across stenotic heart valves, assessment of systolic pulmonary artery pressure from tricuspid regurgitant jet velocity, and quantitation of filling properties of both ventricles. One of the most exciting applications is the quantitative assessment of blood flow in native coronary arteries and bypass grafts.

Cardiac Masses

The goals of imaging cardiac and paracardiac masses by MRI include clear definition of cardiac anatomy, localization, and determination of mass size, configuration, mobility, and hemodynamic relevance. The major advantages are the ability to noninvasively assess extension of the mass and its relation to the adjacent mediastinal structures and to differentiate the mass tissue.

Primary heart tumors are very rare, with an incidence between 0.0017% and 0.19% in unselected patients at autopsy. Most are benign cardiac tumors, and of these, myxomas and lipomas are the most common. Primary malignant cardiac tumors (e.g., angiosarcoma, rhabdomyosarcoma, fibrosarcoma, and malignant lymphoma) are found less frequently. Secondary metastatic tumors are 20 to 40 times more common than primary tumors. The most frequent diagnosis of an intracardial mass is intracardial thrombus.

Technical Considerations

The routine magnetic resonance diagnostic procedures of cardial and paracardial masses make use of SE and GRE pulse sequences. Use of paramagnetic contrast agents can be very helpful for tissue characterization. Pulse sequences should include multislice SE sequences in at least two orientations. Some artifacts may lead to decreased image quality. Susceptibility effects from pulmonary air, motion-induced artifacts from respiratory and cardiovascular motion, and flow phenomena may affect diagnostic accuracy.[72] Flow phenomena may lead to difficulties in differentiation between slow blood flow and laminated structures. To minimize these artifacts, an alternating flow-related signal, which creates black blood with spatial presaturation and white blood with gradient moment nulling, is required.[73]

Another method to improve image quality is slice acquisition during systole in the caudocranial direction. This may lead to better visualization especially in the lower mediastinum for evaluation of the pericardium at the level of cardiac chambers and myocardium, and the ability to see intracavitary structures such as papillary muscles, moderator bands, and atrioventricular valves.[72] Magnetic resonance tomography also has the potential for use in quantitative tissue characterization by allowing the comparison of the T_1 and T_2 values of different tissues to a reference tissue.

Benign Masses

Myxoma

As mentioned earlier, primary tumors of the heart are very rare, with an incidence between 0.0017% and 0.19% in unselected patients at autopsy. Three quarters of tumors are benign and nearly half are myxomas. About 75% of myxomas originate in the left atrium, and 15% to 20% originate in the right atrium. They usually develop from the interatrial septum at the border of the fossa ovalis. Few myxomas are located in the ventricles. Myxomas are neoplasms of endocardial origin and contain multipotential mesenchymal cells. They are generally polyploid, often pedunculated, round or oval with a smooth surface, and often covered with thrombi. Tumor diameters range from 1 to 15 cm, with an average of 5 to 6 cm. Their histologic structure shows a myxoid matrix, large blood vessels at the base, and often cysts and areas of hemorrhage. Clinical symptoms appear as embolism, intracardiac obstruction, and constitutional problems and are determined by size, location, and mobility of the tumor. Embolism is reported in 30% to 40% of patients with myxomas. Left atrial location of the tumor is frequently followed by systemic embolism, and cerebral and peripheral embolism may occur.

Two-dimensional echocardiography is the technique of choice in evaluating atrial myxomas. Because the sensitivity and specificity of two-dimensional echocardiography is not 100% reliable, additional methods are required.[74] In MRI, myxoma is mainly diagnosed by its typical pedunculated, prolapsing appearance and the intensity characteristics in combination with clinical data (Figures 16.11 and 16.12).[75] Cine display should be obtained to show the degree of mobility of the tumor; a larger field of view allows better assessment of the presence of secondary valvular obstruction and cardiac chamber dilation, when these are present.[76] Cardiac myxomas are of variable signal intensity. Most frequently the intensity is similar to that of myocardium, but this usually does not interfere with the diagnosis.[77] Some myxomas may contain calcified areas and hemorrhage. Calcification is consistent with areas of low signal intensity in SE sequences, whereas subacute and chronic hemorrhage is characterized by high signal intensity on short

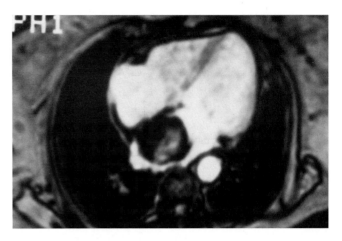

FIGURE 16.12. GRE image of a myxoma in the left atrium with internal hemorrhage (signal increase).

and long echo times.[78] MRI gives important additional anatomic information regarding the relationship of the tumor to normal intracardiac structures and its extension to adjacent vascular and mediastinal structures.[79] In addition, MRI is also helpful in differentiating extracardiac structures (eg., hiatal hernia, a tortuous descending aorta, or a bronchogenic cyst) with external compression of the atrium simulating an intracardiac mass.[80]

Lipoma

Intracardiac lipomas are the second most frequent intracardiac benign tumors They are commonly located in the right atrium. There are several special forms, of which the most frequent is lipomatous hypertrophy of the interatrial septum. Extended epicardial fat tissue with variable extracardiac location is rarely visible. MRI in these cases is indicated to differentiate the benign condition of lipomatous hypertrophy from myxoma, thrombus, and other tumors. Lipomatous hypertrophy of the atrial septum is histologically characterized by infiltration of lipomatous cells between atrial muscle fibers, and unlike true lipomas, they are unencapsulated and contain lipoblasts and mature fat cells.[81] Classically, lipomas occur in older, overweight patients who frequently have atrial fibrillation.[82] Normally on MRI, the atrial septum is a thin structure with a signal intensity similar to that of myocardium. In lipomatous hypertrophy a bilobed atrial septum thickening with a signal intensity comparable to subcutaneous fat on T_1- and T_2-weighted images can be visualized. Signal intensity is about twice that of cardiac muscle.[83,84] Subcutaneous fat appears brightest because muscle has relatively low signal intensity in T_1-weighted images. In T_2-weighted images, fat has a medium signal intensity. To differentiate lipomatous hypertrophy of the interatrial septum from thrombus, myxoma, and the very rare liposarcoma of the

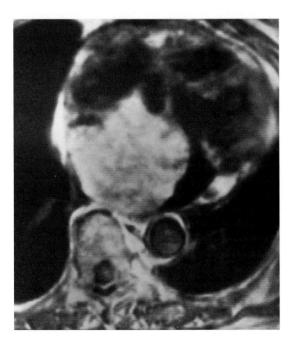

FIGURE 16.11. T_2-weighted image of a myxoma in the left atrium. The myxoma takes up almost the whole atrium and shows a typical signal increase on T_2.

heart, one should note the prolonged relaxation time and the lower signal intensity of these lesions.

Fibroma

Fibroma occurs mostly in young patients. An intramyocardial location in the anterior wall of the left chamber or in the ventricular septum is typical. MRI shows a decrease in signal intensity relative to myocardium from the first to the second echo, depending on the short T_2 time of fibrous tissue.[85,86] Another problem that concerns fibrous tissue is that fibromuscular structures can exist in the normal right atrium and lead to misdiagnosis. In a small population, the incidence of nodular soft-tissue structures (mean diameter 6 mm) along the posterior right atrial wall was reported to be 90%; These may

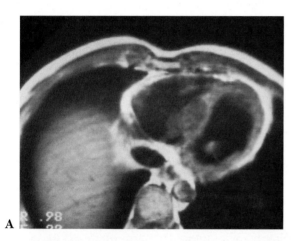

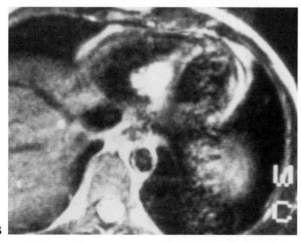

FIGURE 16.13. T_1-weighted (**A**) and T_2-weighted (**B**) image of an intramural echinococcus cyst in the interventricular septum. Cysts are rare lesions and appear on MRI images as structures with long T_1 and T_2 values and flow void, indicating fluid-filled structures. They have low signal intensity on T_1-weighted and increased signal intensity on T_2-weighted images. After the administration of gadolinium-DTPA, intracystic septae can be observed. The significant advantage of MRI is its ability to differentiate these lesions from solid masses and avoid explorative surgery to determine the diagnosis.

simulate the appearence of an atrial tumor or mass.[87] Histologically, this region of nodular thickening consists of myocyte hypertrophy and fibrosis and correlates anatomically with the crista terminalis and the Chiari network. Other authors deny the real danger of misdiagnosing pseudomasses.[88] Cine MRI and phase-contrast techniques can be used to exclude suggested intra-atrial masses (Figure 16.13).

Malignant Masses

Nearly a quarter of all cardiac tumors are malignant. Metastases are 20 to 40 times more common than primary malignant tumors and appear in 6% of postmortem autopsies in malignant diseases. They occur within the cardiac chambers or are present as nodules on the epicardial surface. Some neoplasms tend to grow intralumenally into the right atrium and arise from the vena cava system. Because of the good soft-tissue contrast available with MRI, it became an ideal tool for imaging even small tumors.

Using T_1 and T_2 pulse sequences and gadolinium DTPA (Gd-DTPA), differentiation between benign and malignant lesions may be possible. But because fewer cardiac malignancies have been examined, sensitivity rates for tissue differentiation of cardiac malignancies are not available.

Angiosarcoma is the most frequent primary malignant cardiac tumor. It is usually located in the right atrium and inserts from the interatrial septum. Typically it has a polymorphic configuration with a central region of hyperintensity, and moderate signal intensity in peripheral regions in T_1- and T_2-weighted magnetic resonance images. Until 1979 only 120 cases of a primary leiomyosarcoma of the large arteries and veins had been reported. Some 75% arise from the inferior vena cava. Lupetin et al.[89] reported a case of superior vena cava origin. The neoplasm demonstrated a signal intensity slightly higher than the liver parenchyma, but not as intense as adjacent mediastinal fat. The advantage of MRI is clearly the ability to assess tumor extension into the vena cava superior and heart chambers, where computed tomography may have failed. Garrigue et al.[90] reported two cases of pericardial liposarcoma in which echocardiography showed pericardial effusion, but no mass was detected. With MRI, a heterogeneous pericardial lipomatous mass was detected. Explorative open heart surgery showed a histologically proven liposarcoma.

Metastatic Tumors

Secondary metastasis into the heart is not uncommon and is 20 to 40 times more frequent than primary cardiac tumors. There are three types of metastic implantation into cardiac tissue. The first is direct mediastinal infiltration of heart tissue due to lung cancer, breast cancer, and mediastinal lymphomas. The second is metastasis by systemic tumors such as malignant melanoma, lymphoma, leukemia, and sarcoma. The third is the possibility of transvenous spread. T_1 and T_2 pulse sequences and the signal behavior after administration of Gd-DTPA make MRI diagnosis of metastatic tumors possible. Comparison of gated studies with two-dimensional echocardiography has indicated that MRI more clearly demonstrates the presence, location, and extent of intracardiac masses. The large field of view, capability for imaging noncardiac mediastinal structures, and definition of the limits of cardiac walls are decided advantages of MRI.

Intracardiac Thrombi

Intracardiac thrombi are the most common cardiac masses. They are located in the atrium or left ventricle and caused by atrial fibrillation or blood stasis in myocardial aneurysms or in dilative cardiomyopathy.

For MRI diagnosis of intracardiac thrombi, initial imaging with gated T_1 SE in transverse planes is suggested through the entire heart, with parallel saturation above and below the heart. In addition, multislice cine GRE images are important to delineate intracardiac thrombi. In comparison to intracardiac tumors, no signal enhancement can be found in thrombi after administration of an intravenous contrast agent (Gd-DTPA).

Aortic Diseases

Because MRI provides definite, noninvasive evaluation of the entire thoracic aorta, the technique should be useful for diagnosis of congenital and acquired aortic anomalies. SE pulse sequences in transverse and oblique planes through the aortic arch allow excellent evaluation of aortic morphology. Diameters of the thoracic aortas, arch anomalies, and dissection membranes can be visualized by SE or GRE techniques. Knowledge of the aortic anatomy and the right choice of slice orientation and thickness are prerequisites for reliable evaluation of aortic diseases.

Congenital Aortic Diseases

Marfan's Syndrome

The classic findings of aortic involvement in Marfan's syndrome include disproportionate annular dilation with pre-arch sparing (Figure 16.14). This finding is unusual in other diseases. The diameter of the aortic root can be precisely measured and compared with that of the descending aorta. This ratio is expected to be a use-

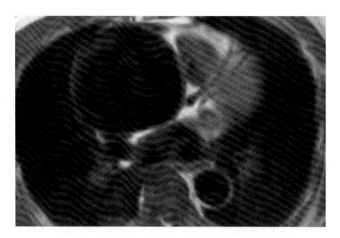

FIGURE 16.14. Classic finding in a patient with Marfan's syndrome. T_1-weighted transverse image shows dilation of the aortic root.

ful indicator of progressive aortic root involvement in the long-term follow-up of patients with Marfan's syndrome.[91] Because patients with Marfan's syndrome have a high incidence of aortic dissection, serial MRI follow-up is recommended, and surgical repair is advocated when the size of the ascending aorta approaches 60 mm.

Aortic Arch Anomalies

Anomalies of the aortic arch and its major branches may be associated with severe congenital heart disease or present as incidental findings in otherwise asymptomatic patients. Studies have indicated the utility of MRI for demonstration of aortic anomalies.[92] Anomalies of the aortic arch may present as a double arch or as a single arch, with variations in course and branching pattern. Kersting-Sommerhoff et al.[93] have shown that MRI can reliably define the various types of aortic arch anomalies. A left aortic arch with aberrant right subclavian artery, the most common aortic arch anomaly, is usually found incidentally in asymptomatic patients. Aortic arch anomalies that lead to clinical symptoms are vascular rings, which may cause tracheal or esophageal compression. Right aortic arches with a left ductus arteriosus or with an aberrant left subclavian artery may form a vascular ring. The most common cause of a symptomatic vascular ring is a double arch, which is seldom associated with other malformations. In two thirds of cases, the right arch is larger than the usually obliterated or atretic left arch. MRI is able to identify the narrower arch and aberrant vessels that form vascular rings.

Coarctation

Coarctation of the aorta is a relatively common congenital lesion that can occur in isolation or in association with other congenital lesions. Occasionally the lesion is not immediately treated by surgery during childhood, and follow-up studies in young adults become essential. With MRI the oblique-sagittal SE images are the most informative, providing high contrast between moving blood (which is black), and tissue, allowing excellent depiction of myocardial or vascular structures. These images permit accurate localization and quantitation of the coarctation diameter and a reliable assessment of the prestenotic and poststenotic segments. Comparison between MRI and angiography in measuring aortic diameters has shown a correlation coefficient of 0.97.[94] MRI was more efficient than echocardiography in diagnosing coarctation.[91,95] The better diagnosis of coarctation by MRI is not suprising because the isthmus is the least accessible portion of the thoracic aorta to ultrasound investigation (Figure 16.15). Even after surgical repair, MRI is better than cross-sectional echocardiography for imaging the aortic arch and measuring its diameter.[94] Prolongation of anterograde blood flow during diastole, measured by VEC-cine MRI in the descending aorta, always indicates a morphological abnormality—an important restenosis or aneurysmal dilatation.[94,96]

Peak coarctation jet velocity measured by VEC-MRI was comparable to that obtained by continuous-wave Doppler echocardiography. Mohiaddin et al.[97] found good correlation between the results of MRI and Doppler echocardiography ($r = 0.95$). MRI velocity mapping is useful if the echo window is limited or alignment of the ultrasound beam is inadequate, because there is no limitation on velocity mapping for site or direction of acquisition data.

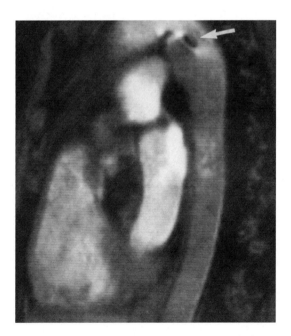

FIGURE 16.15. Oblique-sagittal GRE image provides information about the flow void of the stenotic jet in coarctation (arrow). Please note the poststenotic dilation of the aorta.

Depending on the degree of severity of the coarctation, a variable collateral supply develops to provide blood flow to the descending aorta via the subclavian and intercostal arteries. VEC-MRI provides measurements of blood flow at any site in the cardiovascular system. Steffens et al.[95] have shown in their study, that MRI was able to provide the data needed to calculate the amount of flow change from the proximal to the distal part of the descending aorta and thereby to quantify the volume of collateral flow into the distal descending aorta.

Acquired Aortic Disease

Aortic Aneurysm

Aneurysms of the thoracic aorta enlarge progressively and are often clinically silent until they become life threatening. Early management consists of serial observations for development of symptoms or signs that may indicate the need for surgery, such as a size of 60 mm or more. MRI is an ideal diagnostic imaging method; it is sensitive, accurate, complete, and noninvasive, allowing safe and frequent follow-up examinations. Dinsmore et al.[92] examined the sensitivity of several imaging techniques in detection of aortic aneurysms. MRI was superior to computed tomography and echocardiography, especially in diagnosing small saccular aneurysms and in the evaluation of the aortic wall.

Aortic Dissection

Acute dissection of the thoracic aorta is a life-threatening disorder. Detection and localization of a dissecting membrane and a proximal entry is crucial because patients with a type A dissection of the ascending aorta require surgical correction, whereas a type B dissection of the descending aorta does not need immediate intervention (Figure 16.16). Electrocardiogram-gated SE and GRE images in transverse, coronal, and oblique sagittal planes provide an excellent assessment of the entire thoracic aorta and of the extent of the dissection. MRI allows localization of the entry site, accurate differentiation of true and false lumen, and assessment of thrombus formation (Figure 16.17). Several studies have shown an excellent sensitivity for dissection of the thoracic aorta for MRI and transesophageal echocardiography, in contrast to other imaging modalities.[92,98,99] However, the specificity of TEE was inferior to that of MRI in the ascending aorta.[100] computed tomography was not useful in identifying an entry site, and conventional transthoracic echocardiography was not helpful in detecting communication within the descending aorta. Both echocardiographic techniques were less sensitive for thrombus formation in the ascending aorta and in the arch.[100] Even aortography does not always show con-

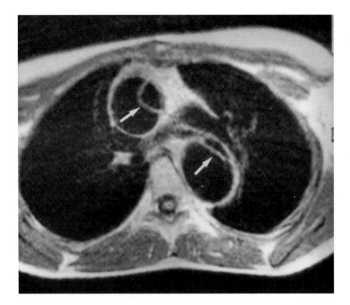

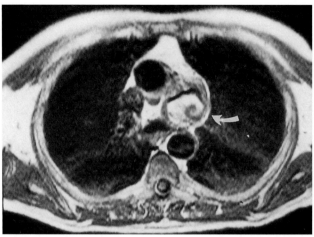

FIGURE 16.16. Transverse SE image demonstrating a type A aneurysm with associated dissection in the entire thoracic aorta (arrow). True and false lumen can accurately be assessed by transverse SE or GRE images.

FIGURE 16.17. Saccular aneurysm of the aortic arch with dissection membrane, mural thrombus formation, and slow-flow phenomenon on a transverse T_1-weighted SE image (curved arrow).

clusive evidence of dissection. Flow of contrast material into the false lumen may temporarily stop at the time of examination, the separated intima may not be imaged tangentially, and the thickened portion of the aortic wall containing the dissecting hematoma may be concealed by adjacent normal and abnormal densities.[100,101] A major advantage of MRI is the reliable visualization of the aortic wall. Aortic wall thickness and intramural hemorrhage can be assessed by SE and GRE images, and the resulting information may be helpful in guiding urgent surgical therapy. In addition, MRI allows identification of aortic insufficiency and pericardial effusion, which are associated findings in type A dissections. In a large group of patients with type A dissection, aortic insufficiency was found in 50% and pericardial effusion in 25%.[100]

White et al.[102] investigated the use of MRI in assessing the aorta after surgery for aortic dissection. Several anatomic features of postoperative aortic dissection could be detected by MRI studies. They included patency of the residual false lumen, aneurysmal dilation of the aorta distal to the graft, slow blood flow and thrombus within the false lumen, and origin of the visceral vessels to vital organs from the false lumen in the dissected abdominal aorta. Differentiation among aortic dissection with slow blood flow, thrombus within its false lumen, and aneurysm with adherent mural thrombus is a well-recognized limitation of both aortography and computed tomography (Figure 16.18).[103] This distinction is important at the time of postoperative follow-up evaluation of aortic dissections, during which confirmation of the presence or absence of recurrence or progression of

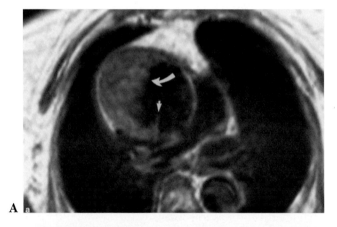

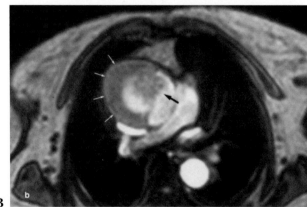

FIGURE 16.18. **A,** Transverse SE image of a type A dissection with a proximal entry and thrombus formation in the false lumen (curved arrow). The small arrow indicates the dissection membrane. **B,** GRE image in the same plane position visualizing mural thrombus (arrows) and turbulent flow through the entry into the false lumen (arrow)

dissection, of aneurysmal dilation of the aorta, or of thrombus within the false lumen may be sought.[102] Also the identification of blood flow within a false lumen in patients after surgery for aortic dissection is important for postsurgical follow-up evaluation. MRI is very sensitive for documenting the presence of at least minimal blood flow within the false lumen, which indicates patency of the residual false lumen.

Pericardial Diseases

The normal pericardium is 1 to 3 mm in thickness. The adjacent visceral and parietal layers are surrounded externally by pericardial fat and internally by subepicardial fat. A pericardial line of low intensity is readily visualized on SE images. The normal pericardial line may also consist of adherent normal pericardial fluid.[104] The pericardium covers the heart and extends to nearly the middle of the ascending aorta and on to the pulmonary artery to the bifurcation. Fluid in the superior pericardial recess is observed in some normal subjects and in patients with even small pericardial effusions.

Pericardial Effusion

Fluid in the superior pericardial recess is observed in many normal subjects and can be demonstrated by MRI.[104] The technique is very sensitive for identifying generalized or loculated pericardial effusions. The wide field of view of MRI renders it effective for defining and depicting the size of loculated effusions.

A hemorrhagic effusion is characterized by high signal intensity on T_1-weighted SE images and low signal intensity on GRE images. On the other hand, a nonhemorrhagic effusion has low intensity on T_1-weighted SE images and high intensity on T_2-weighted images and GRE images.

Pericarditis

In acute pericarditis, MRI shows pericardial effusion and sometimes thickened pericardium. Inflammatory adhesions between the visceral and parietal pericardium may be observed in the presence of intense inflammation from, for example, uremic pericarditis.

In constrictive pericarditis the pericardium is directly visualized on magnetic resonance images. Consequently, MRI is an ideal technique for diagnosis of constrictive pericarditis.[105,106] Normal pericardial thickness is less than 4 mm. A thickness of 4 mm or greater indicates pericardial thickening and, in the proper clinical setting, is a diagnostic finding in constrictive pericarditis. Pericardial thickening can be observed in absence of constrictive pericarditis. The pericardium can be thickened for weeks or months after cardiac surgery, which is con-

sistent with the postpericardiotomy syndrome (Dressler's syndrome). It is also thickened during inflammation by, for example, acute bacterial, viral, or uremic pericarditis. The central cardiovascular structures have a characteristic appearance in constrictive pericarditis; the inferior vena cava, hepatic veins, and right atrium are substantially dilated, while the right ventricle has normal or reduced volume. An elongated, narrow-shaped right ventricle and a sigmoid-shaped ventricular septum are sometimes observed in this disease.[107]

Constriction is sometimes localized to the right side of the heart or even to just the right atrioventricular groove. In many circumstances, pericardial thickening is observed only over the right atrium and right ventricle. Transverse MRI images has displayed pericardial thickening of the right atrioventricular groove, causing narrowing of the tricuspid valve orifice. In 29 patients referred for MRI to establish the diagnosis of constrictive pericarditis, MRI had a diagnostic accuracy of 93%.[108]

MRI can also be employed to distinguish between constrictive pericarditis and restrictive cardiomyopathy. Both diseases cause dilated atria and nearly normal volumes of the ventricles. However, the recognition of pericardial thickening indicates the presence of constrictive pericarditis.

Pericardial Cysts and Tumors

Due to the wide field of view, MRI has been effective for demonstrating pericardial tumors and pericardial cysts.[86,109] The latter, in typical form, are recognized by low signal intensity on a T_1-weighted image and homogeneous high signal intensity on T_2-weighted images (Figures 16.19 and 16.20). With prolongation of the TE in-

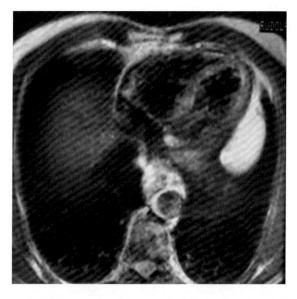

FIGURE 16.19. T_2-weighted image of a left-sided pericardial cyst with typical bright signal intensity.

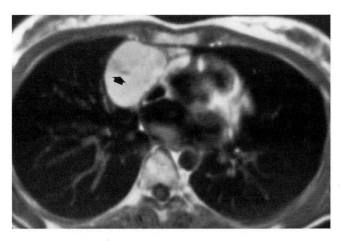

FIGURE 16.20. Right-sided pericardial cyst on a transverse T_2-weighted image with internal septum (arrow).

terval there is generally a progressive increase in signal intensity of fluid within the pericardial cyst. This is typically located in the right cardiophrenic angle but may be located anywhere within the pericardium. When situated in an unusual location, a pericardial cyst may be indistinguishable from a bronchogenic or a thymic cyst. Any cyst containing simple fluid (low protein concentration and nonhemorrhagic) has low intensity on T_1-weighted images and high, homogeneous intensity on T_2-weighted images. However, some pericardial and bronchogenic cysts contain highly proteinaceous fluid, which causes the signal to be high on electrocardiogram-gated T_1-weighted images.

Pericardial tumors generally occur by extension from mediastinal or lung tumors or by metastasis. Pericardial tumors are much more frequently secondary rather than

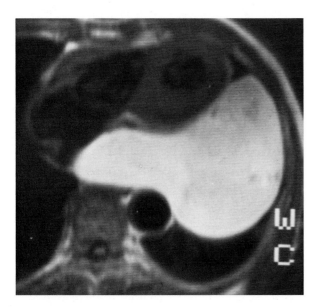

FIGURE 16.21. Pericardial lipoma on a T_1-weighted image with homogeneous fat signal.

primary. A tumor extending to but not through the pericardium can be recognized by the presence of an intact pericardial line. However, tumors that have extended through the pericardium may be recognized by focal obliteration of the pericardial line and presence of a pericardial effusion. Many tumors metastatic to the heart or extending through the pericardium induce a hemorrhagic pericardial effusion. Because of the high signal intensity of the blood within the pericardial sac on SE images, it may not be possible to recognize the tumor itself as separate from the high signal intensity of blood within the pericardial sac.

The most frequent paracardiac masses are pericardial cyst and pseudocysts, enlarged pericardial fat pad, pericardial lipoma (Figure 16.21), lymphoma, teratoma, diaphragmatic eventration and hernia, bronchogenic and metastatic carcinoma, and inferior extension of anterior thoracic tumors (thymoma and teratoma). An intrapericardial pheochromocytoma is an unusual extra-adrenal site for this tumor.

Ischemic Heart Disease

Acute Myocardial Infarction

Within 7 to 10 days after onset of acute myocardial infarction, MRI studies reveal high signal intensity from the infarcted region, which is due to myocardial edema.[110] This can be demonstrated within the first 24 hours from onset of symptoms.[111] Studies by MRI in dogs have demonstrated ischemically injured myocardium with a significant prolongation of T_2 relaxation time as early as 4 hours after coronary occlusion.[112] Differential contrast between infarcted and normal myocardium is improved with greater T_2-weighting of the images. MRI has also shown considerable accuracy in determining the size of acute myocardial infarction in dogs.[113]

On SE images, signal from blood in the left ventricle observed during systole in patients with acute infarcts suggests regional left ventricular dysfunction. It is important to distinguish between the intense signal arising from blood lying stagnant along the ventricular walls and signal from a subendocardial acute infarction. Such distinction can be achieved by using a long TE value on a single-echo sequence. Pitfalls in regard to the recognition of high signal intensity within regions of the left ventricular myocardium include motion artifacts,[114] displacement of high-intensity flow signal into the ventricular wall as a result of the difference in time between application of phase-encoding and readout gradients, and partial volume effects from epicardial fat in the diaphragmatic wall.

To improve depiction of acute myocardial infarction in man, contrast-enhanced MRI has been used with Gd-DTPA.[115,116] Although depiction of acute myocardial infarction is possible on noncontrast T_2-weighted images, image quality is superior on the short-TE contrast-enhanced images due to a better signal-to-noise ratio.[117,118] However, chronic myocardial infarctions have not shown enhancement by contrast media, presumably because the injured myocardium is replaced by scar tissue.

Complications of Acute Myocardial Infarction

Left ventricular mural thrombus is demonstrated on SE images as a mass adherent to the ventricular wall or a mass filling a left ventricular aneurysm.[119] Signal intensity of the thrombus is variable, depending on its age. A subacute thrombus usually has medium to high signal intensity on T_1-weighted images, and bright signal intensity on T_2-weighted images. However, a chronic organized thrombus may have low signal intensity both on T_1- and T_2- weighted SE images.

Left ventricular aneurysms have been recognized on MRI as wall thinning of less than 2 mm and diastolic bulging of the left ventricular wall.[120] MRI can clearly localize the site of aneurysm in various segments of the left ventricle: most true aneurysms are situated in the anterolateral region or apical region of the left ventricle. Less frequently, true aneurysms involve the diaphragmatic or posterior region of the left ventricle. False aneurysms can also be readily identified on gated magnetic resonance images. A false aneurysm is characterized by a larger size than the average true aneurysm, a location on the posterior or diaphragmatic region of the left ventricle, and a relatively small ostium connecting to the aneurysm. When the ostium is less than one half of the diameter of the widest point of the aneurysm, this suggests the presence of a pseudoaneurysm.

Myocardial Function in Ischemic Heart Disease

Cine MRI and multiphasic SE imaging have been used to demonstrate the extent of wall thickening during the cardiac cycle. The normal range for the percent wall thickening and the absolute extent of wall thickening during systole in the various regions of the left ventricle have been defined by MRI.[121-124] Wall thickening is generally about 60%, and absolute wall thickening is greater than 6 mm in normal myocardium. A decrease in percent wall thickening and the absolute extent of wall thickening has been observed at sites of prior myocardial infarctions. Using the uptake of ^{99m}Tc-methoxyisobutyl-isonitrile on single proton emission tomography as a reference for residual viability at sites of myocardial ischemic injury, Sechtem and coworkers[125,126] found that a regional end diastolic wall thickness of less than 6 mm and systolic wall thickening of less than 1 mm on cine MRI are indications of nonviable transmural infarctions.

Another method for measuring wall thickening, wall motion, and wall deformation has been achieved by myocardial tagging using spatial presaturation of the myocardium.[127,128] This method provides precise tracing of the normal and abnormal in-plane rotation and through-plane displacement of the ventricle. Therefore measurements of wall motion and wall thickening can be corrected for in-plane and through-plane movement and can supply precise information about these parameters in ischemic heart disease. The myocardial tagging method has been shown to be a unique method for assessing abnormal motion of the peri-infarction zone of myocardium.[129]

GRE imaging (cine MRI) provides accurate and highly reproducible measurements of left ventricular volumes, ejection fraction, and myocardial mass.[130] Such images, when encompassing the entire heart, provide a three-dimensional data set at multiple phases of the cardiac cycle, including end-diastole and end-systole. Consequently, measurements of volumes and mass are not dependent on assumption of geometrical models, as is required for such measurements obtained by echocardiography and x-ray ventriculography. Because of asymmetry of the ventricle caused by regional infarction and remodeling of the left ventricle, formulas for calculating volumes and mass based on geometrical models have questionable validity, whereas MRI has been accurate for measuring LV mass in the abnormally shaped ventricle after transmural infarction.[131]

Cine MRI can also be performed during pharmacologic stress testing using the administration of dipyridamole[132-134] or dobutamine.[135-137] In patients with known coronary artery disease but normal LV function at rest, cine MRI has been performed to visualize wall motion or wall thickening abnormalities in the potentially ischemic myocardium induced by use of pharmacologic agents that either increase myocardial oxygen requirement or induce disparity of blood flow or both. Dipyridamole-induced wall motion abnormalities shown by cine MRI correlate closely with results of myocardial stress scintigraphy.[134] The sensitivity of dipyridamole-MRI for localization of hemodynamically significant stenoses of major coronary arteries is 84%, and specificity reaches 89% when compared with coronary arteriography. With the use of dobutamine for inducing pharmacologic stress during MRI, a sensitivity of 91% and a specificity of 100% for detection of significant coronary artery disease can be reached.[137]

Myocardial Perfusion

With development of fast imaging techniques, such as fast GRE or echo planar imaging, it is possible to estimate regional myocardial perfusion by monitoring first-pass kinetics of distribution of various types of magnetic

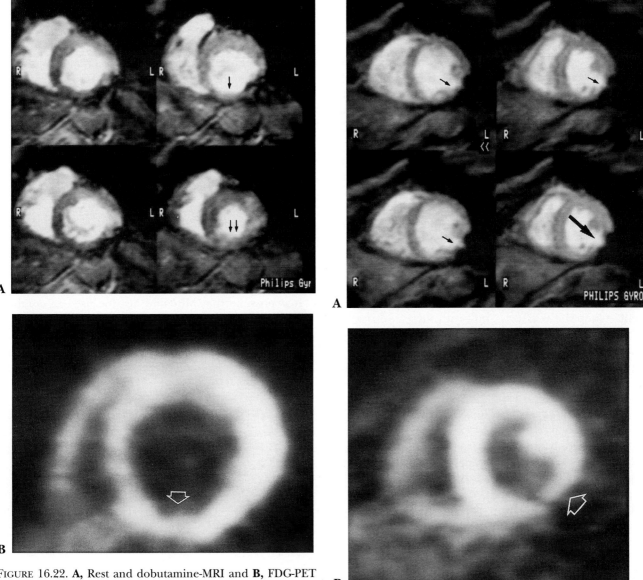

FIGURE 16.22. **A,** Rest and dobutamine-MRI and **B,** FDG-PET basal short-axis tomogram of a patient with inferior myocardial infarction. At rest (upper left panel) the end-diastolic thickness of the inferior wall appears slightly reduced, but the same region shows a lack of wall thickening (arrow) at end-systole (upper right panel). During dobutamine infusion, significant systolic wall thickening (lower right panel) of the basally akinetic inferior wall (arrows) could be induced, which is in agreement with the preserved FDG uptake (arrow) of the inferior wall demonstrated in the corresponding PET short-axis tomogram. With permission from Baer et al.[138]

FIGURE 16.23. **A,** Rest and dobutamine-MRI and **B,** FDG-PET midventricular short-axis tomograms of a patient with inferolateral myocardial infarction. The end-diastolic phase shows reduced wall thickness at rest (upper left panel) and during dobutamine infusion (lower left panel) in the lateral wall (arrow). At end-systole the rest–contraction pattern (upper right panel) demonstrates normal wall thickening of the anterolateral wall but lack of wall thickening in the lateral region (arrow). During dobutamine infusion (lower right panel) the lateral wall remains akinetic (thick arrow), which corresponds to the lateral region, with markedly reduced FDG uptake (arrow) in the corresponding PET short-axis tomogram. With permission from Baer et al.[138]

resonance contrast media (Figures 16.22 and 16.23). In general, MRI contrast media consist of paramagnetic ions such as gadolinium (Gd), manganese (Mn), or dysprosium (Dy) complexed to larger molecules such as DTPA.[139] The distribution space of an MRI contrast agent (i.e., intravascular or extravascular; intracellular or extracellular) depends on the nature of the ligand utilized to form the complex.

Differentiation of normal from ischemic myocardium using MRI has been accomplished by demonstrating the differential distribution of two different types of contrast media.[140–144] The first type consists of T_1-enhancing and magnetic susceptibility agents and T_1-enhancing agents such as Gd-DTPA. They shorten the T_1 relaxation time of myocardial tissue, thus increasing signal intensity on T_1-weighted images. This contrast-producing effect of the agent depends on delivery by myocardial perfusion and tissue water content. Following contrast agent infusion, normally perfused myocardial regions experience the T_1-shortening effect of the delivered contrast molecules, and signal intensity is increased. Delivery of contrast medium to hypoperfused myocardium is reduced, so these zones appear hypointense compared with enhanced normal myocardium (a cold spot). The second type consists of magnetic susceptibility agents that cause shortening of the T_2 relaxation time, which results in decreased signal intensity in areas to which they are distributed. Visualized image signal intensity depends on delivery by perfusion and compartmentalization of the contrast agent. With compartmentalization, contrast molecules are prevented from entering myocardial cells by the intact cell membrane, and this causes the magnetic susceptibility effect. Thus, with these contrast media, normally perfused myocardial regions (which compartmentalize the contrast molecules) are depleted of signal intensity, whereas zones of attenuated perfusion do not lose signal and appear hyperintense (a hot spot).

In order to enhance the difference between normal and hypoperfused myocardium, the vasodilator dipyridamole has been used in several studies.[145–147] However, although there is some experience with use of magnetic resonance contrast media in patients with ischemic heart disease,[148–150] most information has been obtained in experimental animal models.[145,146,151–156]

Contrast-enhanced first-pass magnetic resonance perfusion imaging cannot only detect but can also quantify myocardial ischemia.[157,158] Fast GRE sequences were used to follow the first pass of Gd-DTPA in dogs with varying grades of stenosis of the left anterior descending coronary artery. Imaging performed before and after application of dipyridamole showed that magnetic resonance perfusion imaging can define different levels of myocardial perfusion. In comparisons of absolute myocardial blood flow with signal intensity versus time curves obtained from magnetic resonance images, the inverse mean transit time of the contrast agent had a linear correlation with absolute blood flow in the myocardium. These results suggest that quantification of myocardial blood flow may be feasible using first-pass magnetic resonance perfusion imaging.[159]

Another potential application of MRI could be the determination of successful reperfusion after thrombolytic therapy and assessment of irreversibly injured myocardial tissue within jeopardized regions; this application would yield information similar to that obtained by studies with myocardial contrast echocardiography.[160–161] In animal experiments, contrast-enhanced MRI with a T_1-enhancing agent was effective in differentiating occlusive from reperfused myocardial infarction. Irreversibly injured myocardium is enhanced significantly more than reperfused, reversibly injured, or normal myocardium. Occlusive infarcts have a complicated enhancement pattern consisting of multiple zones. After contrast administration epicardial and endocardial margins of the infarcts enhance immediately and homogeneously, whereas central zones are initially hypointense, gradually increasing in intensity during the following 60 minutes following contrast administration (Figure 16.24).[141] Enhanced occlusive infarct margins have been referred to as the *peri-infarction zone*.[142] Unfortunately, clinical circumstances in patients frequently do not involve purely occlusive or reperfused myocardial infarcts, but rather a heterogeneous myocardial injury with components of both. Consequently, it has been more difficult to determine the effectiveness of contrast-enhanced MRI for the differentiation of these two conditions in humans.[115,162]

It is possible that MRI may also be used to combine functional and perfusion imaging in one study for patients with ischemic heart disease. In patients with perfusion deficits previously demonstrated by thallium scintigraphy, breath-hold cine MRI has been used to display the

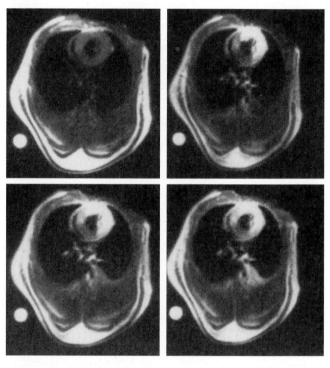

FIGURE 16.24. Magnetic resonance image of irreversible injury obtained before (top left) and 15 (top right), 30 (bottom left), and 60 (bottom right) minutes after the administration of manganese chelate of N,N′-bis(pyridoxal-5-phosphate) ethylene diamine N,N′ diacetic acid (Mn-DPDP) (400 mmol/kg). Increase in signal intensity with Mn-DPDP administration is demonstrated. With permission from Saeed et al.[164]

extent of the deficit in wall thickening, whereas inversion recovery–prepared fast-gradient echo imaging during the first pass of gadodiamide injection has been used to demonstrate the perfusion deficit. Concordance has been shown between thallium deficit and functional and perfusion deficits, as defined by MRI.[163]

Assessment of Coronary Arteries and Bypass Grafts

Visualization of coronary arteries by MRI has been limited by prolonged imaging times, cardiac and respiratory motion, and the small diameter, tortuosity, and mobility of these vessels.[165,166] Ultrafast breath-hold GRE sequences with k-space segmentation, which depict laminar blood flow as bright and turbulent flow as a signal void, have been successfully used to demonstrate vessels similar in size to coronary arteries, such as intracranial or renal vessels.[167,168] Burstein showed the feasibility of this technique in demonstrating coronary arteries in isolated hearts and in animals.[169] Meyer et al. were able to visualize up to 80 mm of the right coronary artery in normal subject by using fat-suppressed fast GRE imaging and k-space segmentation.[170] Utilizing the same technique, Manning et al.[171] examined 19 healthy volunteers and 6 patients with known coronary artery disease. On

overlapping transverse images, the left main coronary artery was visualized in 96% of patients, with a mean diameter of 4.8 mm and a mean length of 10 mm. The left anterior descending artery was seen in 100% of subjects, with a mean length of 44 mm, and the circumflex artery in 76% of patients, with an average length of 25 mm. For examination of the right coronary artery, multiple oblique images were used, leading to identification of the vessel in 100% of patients, with an average length of 58 mm (Figure 16.25). Comparison with quantitative angiography of the proximal segments revealed a good correlation, with MRI-determined lumen diameters of $r = 0.86$ ($P < .002$). A study of healthy volunteers by Sakuma et al.[172] indicated visibility of the left anterior descending artery for a mean length of 62 mm and of the right coronary artery for 65 mm. The imaging protocol included interleaved transaxial images, single oblique images along the heart axis, multiangle oblique images tangential to the epicardial surface for the left coronary artery, and interleaved oblique coronal images for the right coronary artery.

MRI slightly overestimates angiographically determined lumen diameter, probably due to a combination of partial volume averaging related to the reduced magnetic resonance spatial resolution and movement of the vessel during the imaging period. On MRI, occluded ves-

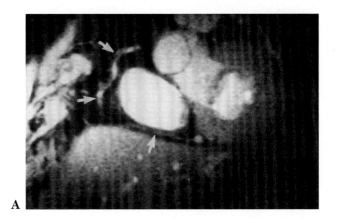

A

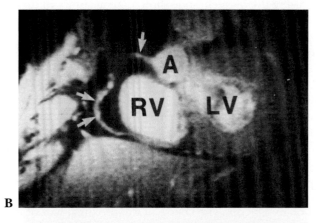

B

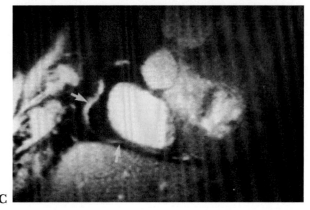

C

FIGURE 16.25. Sequential oblique magnetic resonance scans of the right coronary artery without substantial stenoses. LV indicates left ventricle; RV, right ventricle; A, aortic root. With permission from Manning et al.[182]

sels display a signal void distal to the occlusion, whereas vessels with significant angiographic stenoses demonstrate signal loss at the area of stenosis, with visualization of the vessel more distally. Minor lumenal irregularities may also lead to significant local turbulence with subsequent signal loss in absence of significant stenosis in angiography. Although partial volume effects and signal dropout caused by turbulence preclude the use of quantitative magnetic resonance coronary angiography to measure the diameter of stenoses, use of shorter echo times may minimize signal loss, and use of specially designed small surface coils will enhance the signal-to-noise ratio and permit increased spatial resolution.

Besides evaluation of morphologic aspects of coronary artery disease, assessment of blood flow has become possible by using velocity-encoded cine MRI. Edelman et al.[173] used flow-sensitive, segmented fast GRE sequences in normal subjects to quantify flow in the right and left coronary artery. Morover, this technique allowed demonstration of a significant increase in coronary blood flow after application of adenosine, a potent vasodilator.

Coronary artery bypass grafts are typically much larger than native vessels and show less respiratory and cardiac motion. Herfkens et al.[174] were first to report the MRI appearance of a coronary artery bypass graft on transaxial MRI of the chest. Since then, MRI has been used to assess the patency of coronary artery bypass grafts. Studies using the SE technique showed an accuracy in detection of patent grafts of 90% to 92%, and of 72% to 85% in detection of occluded grafts.[175-177] The application of cine MRI did not significantly improve these results,[178,179] with an overall sensitivity of 88% to 93%, and a specificity of 86% to 100%. However, patency alone does not exclude the presence of a significant stenosis, nor does it obviate invasive catheterization in a symptomatic patient. Underwood et al. used velocity-encoded cine MRI in the quantification of coronary bypass graft flow.[180]Debatin et al.[181] showed the feasibility of this method in measuring blood flow in native and grafted internal mammary arteries, with successful evaluation in 14 of 15 patients. The course of the proximal half of the IMA bypass graft parallel to the chest wall makes it particularly suitable for evaluation with VEC cine MRI. Limiting factors include metallic surgical devices that obscure the graft vessel, and postoperative residual mediastinal hematoma, because the surrounding hemosiderin causes dephasing artifacts.[181]

References

1. Mogelvang J, Stubgaard M, Thomsen C, et al. Evaluation of right ventricular volumes measured by magnetic resonance imaging. *Eur Heart J.* 1988;9:529–533.
2. Frank H, Globits S, Glogar D, et al. Detection and quan-

tification of pulmonary artery hypertension with MR imaging: results in 23 patients. *AJR.* 1993;161:27–31.
3. Sechtem U, Pflugfelder P, Cassidy M, et al. Mitral or aortic regurgitation: quantification of regurgitant volumes with CINE MR imaging. *Radiology.* 1988;167:425–430.
4. Mostbeck G, Caputo G, Higgins C. MR measurement of blood flow in the cardiovascular system. *AJR.* 1992;159:453–461.
5. Kondo C, Caputo G, Semelka R, et al. Right and left ventricular stroke volume measurements with velocity-encoded cine MR imaging: in vitro and in vivo validation. *AJR.* 1991;157:9–16.
6. Cohen M, Fordham J. Developments in magnetic resonance imaging. *Invest Radiol.* 1993;28(suppl 4):S32–S37.
7. Kersting-Sommerhoff B, Diethelm L, Teitel D, et al. Magnetic resonance imaging of congenital heart disease: sensitivity and specificity using receiver operating characteristic curve analysis. *Am Heart J.* 1989;118(1):155–161.
8. Theissen P, Sechtem U, Mennicken U, et al. Noninvasive diagnosis of atrial septal defects and anomalous pulmonary venous return by magnetic resonance imaging. *Nuklear Medizin.* 1989;28:172–180.
9. Holmvang G, Palacios I, Vlahakes G, et al. Imaging and sizing of atrial septal defects by magnetic resonance. *Circulation.* 1995;92:3473–3480.
10. Rees S, Firmin D, Mohiaddin R, et al. Application of flow measurements by magnetic resonance velocity mapping to congenital heart disease. *Am J Cardiol.* 1989;64:953–956.
11. Brenner L, Caputo G, Mostbeck G, et al. Quantification of left to right atrial shunts with velocity-encoded cine nuclear magnetic resonance imaging. *J Am Coll Cardiol.* 1992;20(5):1246–1250.
12. Soto B, Cranney G, Blackwell G. Congenital heart disease in adult. In: Blackwell G, Cranney G, Pohost G, eds. *MRI: Cardiovascular System.* New York, NY: Gower Medical; 1992:50–58.
13. Fellows K, Weinberg P, Baffa J, et al. Evaluation of congenital heart disease with MR imaging: current and coming attractions. *AJR.* 1992;159:925–931.
14. Higgins C, Caputo G. Role of MR imaging in acquired and congenital cardiovascular disease. *AJR.* 1993;161:13–22.
15. Chung K, Simpson I, Newman R, et al. Cine magnetic resonance imaging for evaluation of congenital heart disease: role in pediatric cardiology compared with echocardiography and angiography. *J Pediatr.* 1988;113:1028–1035.
16. Bove E, Byrum C, Thomas F, et al. The influence of pulmonary insufficiency on ventricular function following repair of tetralogy of Fallot. *J Thorac Cardiovasc Surg.* 1983;85:691–696.
17. Horneffer P, Zahka K, Rowe S, et al. Long-term results of total repair of tetralogy of Fallot in childhood. *Ann Thorac Surg.* 1990;50:179–185.
18. Rebergen S, Chin J, Ottenkamp J, et al. Pulmonary regurgitation in the late postoperative follow-up of tetralogy of Fallot: volumetric quantitation by nuclear magnetic resonance velocity mapping. *Circulation.* 1993;88(1):2257–2266.
19. Frank H, Salzer U, Popow C, et al. Magnetic resonance imaging of absent pulmonary valve syndrome. *Pediatr Cardiol.* 1996;17:35–39.

20. Calder L, Van Praagh R, Van Praagh S, et al. Truncus arteriosus communis. Clinical, angiocardiographic and pathologic findings in 100 patients. *Am Heart J.* 1976;92:23–38.

21. Mazer M, Carroll F, Falke T. Practical aspect of gated magnetic resonance imaging of the pulmonary artery. *Journal Thoracic Imaging.* 1988;3(3):73–84.

22. Schulthess G, Fisher M, Higgins C. Pathologic blood flow in pulmonary vascular disease as shown by gated magnetic resonance imaging. *Ann Intern Med.* 1985;103:317–323.

23. Bouchard A, Higgins C, Byrd BI, et al. Magnetic resonance imaging in pulmonary arterial hypertension. *Am J Cardiol.* 1985;56:938–942.

24. Didier D, Higgins C. Estimation of pulmonary vascular resistance by MRI in patients with congenital cardiovascular shunt lesions. *AJR.* 1986;146:919–924.

25. Conces D, Tarver R, Augustyn G. Nonangiographic imaging of the pulmonary arteries: CT and MR. *Critical Reviews in Diagnostic Imaging.* 1987;27(3):237–269.

26. Sechtem U, Pflugfelder P, White P, et al. Cine MRI: potential for the evaluation of cardiovascular function. *AJR.* 1987;148:239–246.

27. Kilner P, Firmin D, Rees R, et al. Valve and great vessel stenosis: assessment with MR jet velocity mapping. *Radiology.* 1991;178:229–235.

28. Casolo G, Zampa V, Rega L, et al. Evaluation of mitral stenosis by cine magnetic resonance imaging. *Am Heart J.* 1992;123:1252–1260.

29. De Roos A, Reichek N, Axel L, et al. Cine MR imaging in aortic stenosis. *J Comput Assist Tomogr.* 1989;13:421–425.

30. Eichenberger A, Jenni R, von Schulthess G. Aortic valve pressure gradients in patients with aortic valve stenosis: quantification with velocity-encoded cine MR imaging. *AJR.* 1993;160:971–977.

31. Tarnawski M, Porter D, Graves M, et al. Flow determination in small vessels by magnetic resonance imaging [abstract]. In: *Book of Abstracts: Society of Magnetic Resonance in Medicine.* Berkeley, CA: Society of Magnetic Resonance in Medicine; 1989:869.

32. Mostbeck G, Caputo G, Madlumdar S, et al. Assessment of vascular stenoses with MR jet phase velocity mapping at 1.5 T: in vitro validation [abstract]. *Radiology.* 1991;181: 264.

33. Caputo G, Duerinckx A, Hartiala J, et al. Assessment of aortic valve pressure gradients with phase contrast MRI [abstract]. *Circulation.* 1992;86(suppl I):163.

34. Yoganathan A, Cape E, Sung H, et al. Review of hydrodynamic principles for the cardiologist: applications to study blood flow and jets by imaging techniques. *J Am Coll Cardiol.* 1988;12:1344–1353.

35. Sondergaard L, Thomsen C, Stahlberg F, et al. Mitral and aortic valvular flow: quantification with MR phase mapping. *J Magn Reson Imaging.* 1992;2:295–302.

36. Kilner P, Mancara C, Mohiaddin R, et al. Magnetic resonance jet velocity mapping in mitral and aortic valve stenosis. *Circulation.* 1993;87:1239–1248.

37. Heidenreich P, Steffens J, Fujita N, et al. The evaluation of mitral stenosis with velocity-encoded cine MRI. *Am J Cardiol.* 1995;75:365–369.

38. Mohiaddin R, Amanuma M, Kilner P, et al. MR phase-shift velocity mapping of mitral and pulmonary venous flow. *J Comput Assist Tomogr.* 1991;15:237–243.

39. Evans A, Hedlund L, Herfkens R, et al. Evaluation of steady and pulsatile flow with dynamic MRI using limited flip angles and gradient refocused echoes. *Magn Reson Imaging.* 1987;5:475–482.

40. Evans A, Blinder R, Herfkens R, et al. Effects of turbulence in signal intensity in gradient echo images. *Invest Radiol.* 1988;23:512–518.

41. Ohnishi S, Fukui S, Kusuoka H, et al. Assessment of valvular regurgitation using cine MRI coupled with phase compensating technique: comparison with Doppler color flow mapping. *Angiology.* 1992;43:913–924.

42. Higgins C, Wagner S, Kondo C, et al. Evaluation of valvular heart disease with cine gradient echo MRI. *Circulation.* 1991;84 (suppl I):198–207.

43. Aurigemma G, Reichek N, Schiebler M, et al. Evaluation of aortic regurgitation by cardiac cine magnetic resonance imaging: planar analysis and comparison to Doppler echocardiography. *Cardiology.* 1991;78:340–347.

44. Aurigemma G, Reichek N, Schiebler M, et al. Evaluation of mitral regurgitation by cine MRI. *Am J Cardiol.* 1990;66: 621–625.

45. Nishimura F. Oblique cine MRI for the evaluation of aortic regurgitation: comparison with cineangiography. *Clin Cardiol.* 1992;15:73–78.

46. Wagner S, Auffermann W, Buser P, et al. Diagnostic accuracy and estimation of the severity of valvular regurgitation from the signal void on cine magnetic resonance images. *Am Heart J.* 1989;118:760–767.

47. Suzuki J, Caputo G, Kondo C, et al. Cine MR Imaging of valvular heart disease: Display and imaging parameters affect the size of the signal void caused by valvular regurgitation. *AJR.* 1990;155:723–727.

48. Pflugfelder P, Landzberg J, Cassidy M, et al. Comparison of cine MR imaging with Doppler echocardiography for the evaluation of aortic regurgitation. *AJR.* 1989;152: 729–735.

49. Pflugfelder P, Sechtem U, White R, et al. Noninvasive evaluation of mitral regurgitation by analysis of left atrial signal loss in cine magnetic resonance. *Am Heart J.* 1989;117: 1113–1119.

50. Rehr R, Malloy C, Filipchuk N, et al. Left ventricular volumes measured by MR imaging. *Radiology.* 1985;156: 717–719.

51. Markiewicz W, Sechtem U, Kirby R, et al. Measurement of ventricular volumes in the dog by nuclear magnetic resonance imaging. *J Am Coll Cardiol.* 1987;10:170–177.

52. Dilworth L, Aisen A, John-Mancini G, et al. Determination of left ventricular volumes and ejection fraction by magnetic resonance imaging. *Am Heart J.* 1987;113:24–32.

53. Longmoore D, Underwood S, Bland C, et al. Dimensional accuracy of magnetic resonance in studies of the heart. *Lancet.* 1985;1:1360–1362.

54. Underwood S, Gill C, Klipstein R, et al. Left ventricular volume measured rapidly by oblique magnetic resonance imaging. *Br Heart J.* 1988;60:188–195.

55. Cranney G, Lotan C, Dean L, et al. Left ventricular volume measurement using cardiac axis nuclear magnetic resonance imaging validation by calibrated ventricular angiography. *Circulation.* 1990;82:154–163.

56. Sechtem U, Pflugfelder P, Gould R, et al. Measurement of

right and left ventricular volumes in healthy individuals with cine MR imaging. *Radiology.* 1987;163:697–702.

57. Bargiggia G, Tronconi L, Sahn D, et al. A new method for quantification of mitral regurgitation based on color flow Doppler imaging of the flow convergence proximal to regurgitant orifice. *Circulation.* 1991;84:1481–1489.

58. Yoshida K, Yoshikawa J, Hozumi T, et al. Assessment of aortic regurgitation by the acceleration flow signal void proximal to the leaking orifice in cinemagnetic resonance imaging. *Circulation.* 1991;83:1951–1955.

59. Cranney G, Benjelloun H, Perry G, et al. Rapid assessment of aortic regurgitation and left ventricular function using cine nuclear magnetic resonance imaging and the proximal convergence zone. *Am J Cardiol.* 1993;71:1074–1081.

60. Meier D, Maier S, Boesiger P. Quantitative flow measurements on phantoms and on blood vessels with MR. *Magn Reson Med.* 1988;8:25–34.

61. Duerk J, Pattany P. In-plane flow velocity quantification along the phase encoding axis in MRI. *Magn Reson Imaging.* 1988;6:321–333.

62. Dulce M, Mostbeck G, O'Sullivan M, et al. Severity of aortic regurgitation: Interstudy reproducibility of measurements with velocity-encoded cine MR imaging. *Radiology.* 1992;185:235–240.

63. Sondergaard L, Lindvig K, Hildebrandt P, et al. Quantification of aortic regurgitation by magnetic resonance velocity mapping. *Am Heart J.* 1993;125:1081–1090.

64. Hunt D, Baxley W, Kennedy J, et al. Quantitative evaluation of cineaortography in the assessment of aortic regurgitation. *Am J Cardiol.* 1973;31:696–700.

65. Fujita N, Chazouilleres A, Hartiala J, et al. Quantification of mitral regurgitation by velocity encoded cine nuclear magnetic resonance imaging. *J Am Coll Cardiol.* 1994;23:951–958.

66. Sprecher D, Adamick R, Adams D, et al. In vitro color flow, pulsed and continuous wave Doppler ultrasound masking of flow by prosthetic valves. *J Am Coll Cardiol.* 1987;9:1306–1310.

67. Labovitz A. Assessment of prosthetic heart valve function by Doppler echocardiography. A decade of experience. *Circulation.* 1989;80:707–709.

68. Soulen R, Budinger T, Higgins C. Magnetic resonance imaging of prosthetic heart valves. *Radiology.* 1985;154:705–707.

69. Randall P, Kohman L, Scalzetti E, et al. Magnetic resonance imaging of prosthetic cardiac valves in vitro and in vivo. *Am J Cardiol.* 1988;62:973–976.

70. Frank H, Buxbaum P, Huber L, et al. In-vitro behaviour of mechanical heart valves in a 1.5 Tesla superconducting magnet. *Eur Radiol.* 1992;2:555–558.

71. Deutsch H, Bachmann R, Sechtem U, et al. Regurgitant flow in cardiac valve prostheses: diagnostic value of gradient echo nuclear magnetic resonance imaging in reference to transesophageal two-dimensional color Doppler echocardiography. *J Am Coll Cardiol.* 1992;19:1500–1507.

72. Chako A, Tempany C, Zerhouni E. Effect of slice Acquisition Direction on Image Quality in Thoracic MRI. *J Comput Assist Tomogr.* 1995;19(6):936–940.

73. Schulthess G, Higgins C. Blood flow imaging with MR: spin-phase phenomena. *Radiology.* 1985;157:687–695.

74. Green S, Joynt L, Fitzgerald P, et al. In vivo ultrasonic tissue characterization of human intracardiac masses. *Am J Cardiol.* 1983;51:231–236.

75. Lund J, Ehman R, Julsrud P, et al. Cardiac masses: assessment by MR imaging. *AJR.* 1989;152:469–473.

76. Go R, O'Donnell J, Underwood D, et al. Comparison of gated cardiac MRI and 2D Echo of intracardiac neoplasms. *Am J Rad.* 1985;145:21–25.

77. Gomes A, Lois J, Child J, et al. Cardiac tumors and thrombus: evaluation with MR imaging. *A J Rad.* 1987;149: 895–899.

78. Roos A, Weijers E, Duinen S, et al. Calcified right atrial myxoma demonstrated by MRI. *Chest.* 1989;95:478–79.

79. Freedberg R, Kronzon I, Rumancik W, et al. The contribution of MRI to the evaluation of intracardiac tumors diagnosed by echocardiography. *Circulation.* 1988;77:96–103.

80. Menegus M, Greenberg M, Spindola-Franco H, et al. MRI of suspected atrial tumors. *Am Heart J.* 1992;123:1260–1268.

81. Kluge W. Lipomatous hypertrophy of the interatrial septum. *Northwest Med.* 1969;68:25–30.

82. Hutter AJ, Page D. Atrial arrhythmias and lipomatous hypertrophy of the cardiac interatrial septum. *Am Heart J.* 1971;82:16–21.

83. Levine R, Weyman A, Dinsmore R, et al. Noninvasive tissue characterization: diagnosis of lipomatous hypertrophy of the atrial septum by nuclear magnetic resonance imaging. *J Am Coll Cardiol.* 1986;7:688–692.

84. Applegate P, Tajik A, Ehman R, et al. Two-dimensional echocardiographic and magnetic resonance imaging observations in massive lipomatous hypertrophy of the atrial septum. *Am J Cardiol.* 1987;59:489–491.

85. Winkler M, Higgins C. Suspected intracardiac masses: evaluation with MR imaging. *Radiology.* 1987;165:117–122.

86. Amparo E, Higgins C, Farmer K, et al. Gated magnetic resonance imaging (MRI) of cardiac and paracardiac masses. *Am Heart J.* 1984;143:1151–1156.

87. Mirowitz S, Gutierrez F. Fibromuscular elements of the right atrium: pseudomass at MR imaging. *Radiology.* 1992;182:231–233.

88. Meier R, Hartnell G. MRI of right atrial pseudomass: it is really a diagnostic problem. *J Comput Assist Tomogr.* 1994;18:398–401.

89. Lupetin A, Dash N, Beckman I. Leiomyosarcoma of the superior vena cava: diagnosis by cardiac gated MR. *Cardiovasc Intervent Radiol.* 1986;9:103–105.

90. Garrigue S, Robert F, Roudaut R, et al. Assessment of noninvasive imaging techniques in the diagnosis of heart liposarcoma. *Eur Heart J.* 1995;16:139–141.

91. Fletcher B, Jacobstein M. MRI of congenital abnormalities of the great arteries. *AJR.* 1986;146:941–948.

92. Dinsmore R, Liberthson R, Wismer G, et al. Magnetic resonance imaging of thoracic aortic aneurysms: comparison with other imaging methods. *AJR.* 1986;146:309–314.

93. Kersting-Sommerhoff B, Sechtem U, Fisher M, et al. MR imaging of congenital anomalies of the aortic arch. *AJR.* 1987;149:9–13.

94. Mühler E, Neuerburg J, Rüben A, et al. Evaluation of aortic coarctation after surgical repair: role of magnetic resonance imaging and Doppler ultrasound. *Br Heart J.* 1993;70:285–290.

95. Steffens J, Bourne M, Sakuma H, et al. Quantification of collateral blood flow in coarctation of the aorta by velocity encoded cine magnetic resonance imaging. *Circulation.* 1994;90(2):937–943.

96. Didier D, Ratib O, Friedli B, et al. Cine gradient echo MR imaging in the evaluation of cardiovascular diseases. *Radiographics.* 1993;13:561–573.

97. Mohiaddin R, Kilner P, Rees S, et al. Magnetic resonance volume flow and jet velocity mapping in aortic coarctation. *J Am Coll Cardiol.* 1993;22:1515–1521.

98. Nienaber C, von Kodolitsch Y, Nicolas V, et al. The diagnosis of thoracic aortic dissection by noninvasive imaging procedures. *N Engl J Med.* 1993;328:1–9.

99. Deutsch H, Sechtem U, Meyer H, et al. Chronic aortic dissection: comparison of MR imaging and transesophageal echocardiography. *Radiology.* 1994;192:645–650.

100. Nienaber C, Spielmann R, Kodolitsch Y, et al. Diagnosis of thoracic aortic dissection: magnetic resonance imaging versus transesophageal echocardiography. *Circulation.* 1992;85:434–447.

101. Paulin S. Imaging of suspected aortic dissection. *AJR.* 1993;161:494–495.

102. White R, Ullyot D, Higgins C. MR imaging of the aorta after surgery for aortic dissection. *AJR..* 1988;150:87–92.

103. White R, Lipton M, Higgins C, et al. Noninvasive evaluation of suspected thoracic aortic disease by contrast-enhanced computer tomography. *Am J Cardiol.* 1986;57:282–290.

104. Sechtem U, Tscholakoff D, Higgins C. MRI of the normal pericardium. *AJR.* 1986;147:239–244.

105. Sechtem U, Tscholakoff D, Higgins C. MRI of the abnormal pericardium. *AJR.* 1986;147:245–256.

106. Soulen R, Stark D, Higgins C. Magnetic resonance imaging of constrictive pericardial heart disease. *Am J Cardiol.* 1985;55:480–484.

107. Mueller C, Globits S, Glogar D, et al. Constrictive pericarditis without significant hemodynamic changes as a cause of oedema formation due to protein-losing enteropathy. *Eur Heart J.* 1991;12:1140–1143.

108. Masui T, Finck S, Higgins C. Constrictive pericarditis and restrictive cardiomyopathy: evaluation with MR imaging. *Radiology.* 1992;182:369–373.

109. Barakos J, Brown J, Higgins C. Magnetic resonance imaging of secondary cardiac and paracardiac masses. Pictorial essay. *AJR.* 1989;153:47–50.

110. McNamara M, Higgins C, Schechtmann N, et al. Detection and characterization of acute myocardial infarctions in man with use of gated magnetic resonance imaging. *Circulation.* 1985;71:717–724.

111. Johnson D, Mulvagh S, Cashion R, et al. NMR imaging of acute myocardial infarction within 24 hours of chest pain onset. *Am J Cardiol.* 1989;64:172–179.

112. Tscholakoff D, Higgins C, McNamara M, et al. Early phase myocardial infarction: Evaluation by magnetic resonance imaging. *Radiology.* 1986;159:667–672.

113. Caputo G, Sechtem U, Tscholakoff D, et al. Measurement of myocardial infarct size at early and late time intervals using MR Imaging: an experimental study in dogs. *AJR.* 1987;149:237–243.

114. Filipchuk W, Peshock R, Malloy C, et al. Detection and lo-

calization of recent myocardial infarction by MRI. *Am J Cardiol.* 1986;58:214–219.

115. De Roos A, van Rossum A, van der Wall E, et al. Reperfused and nonreperfused myocardial infarction: diagnostic potential of Gd-DTPA-enhanced MR imaging. *Radiology.* 1989;172:717–720.

116. Nishimura T, Kobayashi H, Ohara Y, et al. Serial assessment of myocardial infarction by using gated MRI and Gd-DTPA. *AJR.* 1990;153:715–720.

117. De Roos A, Doornbos J, van der Wall E, et al. MR imaging of acute myocardial infarction: value of Gd-DTPA. *AJR.* 1988;150:531–534.

118. Matheijsen N, de Roos A, van der Wall E, et al. Acute myocardial infarction:comparison of T_2-weighted and T_1-weighted gadolinium-DTPA enhanced MR imaging. *Magn Reson Med.* 1991;17:460–469.

119. Dooms G, Higgins C. MR imaging of cardiac thrombi. *J Comput Assist Tomogr.* 1986;10:415–420.

120. McNamara M, Higgins C. Magnetic resonance imaging of chronic myocardial infarcts in man. *AJR.* 1986;146:315–320.

121. Peschock R, Rokey R, Malloy G, et al. Assessment of myocardial systolic wall thickening using nuclear magnetic resonance imaging. *J Am Coll Cardiol.* 1989;14:653–659.

122. Sechtem U, Sommerhoff B, Markiewicz W, et al. Regional left ventricular wall thickening by magnetic resonance imaging: evaluation in normal persons and patients with global and regional dysfunction. *Am J Cardiol.* 1987;59:145–151.

123. McDonald K, Parrish T, Wennberg P, et al. Rapid accurate and simultaneous noninvasive assessment of right and left ventricular mass with nuclear magnetic resonance imaging using the snapshot gradient method. *J Am Coll Cardiol.* 1992;19:1601–1607.

124. Underwood S, Rees R, Savage P, et al. Assessment of regional left ventricular function by magnetic resonance. *Br Heart J.* 1986;56:334–339.

125. Baer F, Smolarz K, Jungehuelsing M, et al. Chronic myocardial infarction: assessment of morphology, function and perfusion by gradient-echo magnetic resonance imaging and 99mTc-methoxyisobutyl-isonitrile-SSPECT. *Am Heart J.* 1992;123:636–645.

126. Sechtem U, Voth E, Schneider C, et al. Assessment of residual viability in patients with myocardial infarction using magnetic resonance imaging. *Int J Card Imaging.* 1993;9:931–940.

127. Zerhouni E, Parish D, Rogers W, et al. Human heart: tagging with MR imaging—a method for noninvasive assessment of myocardial motion. *Radiology.* 1988;169:59–63.

128. Clark N, Reichek N, Bergey P, et al. Circumferential myocardial shortening in the abnormal human left ventricle. Assessment by magnetic resonance imaging using spatial modulation of magnetization. *Circulation.* 1991;84:67–74.

129. Kramer C, Lima J, Reichek N, et al. Regional differences in function within noninfarcted myocardium during left ventricular remodeling. *Circulation.* 1993;88:1279–1288.

130. Wagner S, Auffermann W, Buser P, et al. Functional description of the left ventricle in patients with volume overload, pressure overload, and myocardial disease using

cine magnetic resonance imaging. *Am J Cardiac Imag.* 1991;5:87–97.

131. Shapiro E, Rogers W, Beyar R, et al. Determination of left ventricular mass by magnetic resonance imaging in hearts deformed by acute infarction. *Circulation.* 1989;79: 706–711.

132. Pennell D, Underwood S, Longmore D. Detection of coronary artery disease using MR imaging with dipyridamol infusion. *J Comput Assist Tomogr.* 1990;14:167–170.

133. Baer F, Smolarz K, Jungehulsing M, et al. Feasibility of high-dose dipyridamole-magnetic resonance imaging for the detection of coronary artery disease and comparison with coronary angiography. *Am J Cardiol.* 1992;69:51–56.

134. Baer F, Smolarz K, Theissen P, et al. Identification of hemodynamically significant coronary artery stenoses by dipyridamole-magnetic resonance imaging and 99m Tc-methoxyisobutyl-isonitrile-SPECT. *Int J Cardiac Imag.* 1993;9:133–145.

135. Pennell D, Underwood S, Manzara C, et al. Magnetic resonance imaging during dobutamine stress in coronary artery disease. *Am J Cardiol.* 1992;70:34–40.

136. Baer F, Voth P, Theissen P, et al. Dobutamine-MRI in comparison to simultaneously assess 99m Tc-MIBI-SPECT for the localization of hemodynamically significant artery stenoses [abstract]. In: *Book of Abstracts: Society of Magnetic Resonance in Medicine.* Berkeley, CA: Society of Magnetic Resonance in Medicine; 1993:224.

137. Van Rugge F, van der Wall E, de Roos A, et al. Dobutamine stress magnetic resonance imaging for detection of coronary artery disease. *J Am Coll Cardiol.* 1993;22: 431–439.

138. Baer FM, Voth E, Schneider CA, et al. Comparison of low-dose dobutamine-gradient-echo magnetic resonance imaging and positron emission tomography with (18F) fluorodeoxyglucose in patients with chronic coronary artery disease: a functional and morphological approach to the detection of residual myocardial viability. *Circulation.* 1995;91:1006–1015.

139. Higgins C, Saeed M, Wendland M, et al. Contrast media for cardiothoracic MR imaging. *J Magn Reson Imaging* 1993;3:265–276.

140. Rosen B, Belliveau J, Vevea J, et al. Perfusion imaging with NMR contrast agents. *Magn Reson Med.* 1990;14:249–265.

141. Saeed M, Wagner S, Wendland M, et al. Occlusive and reperfused myocardial infarcts: Differentiation with Mn-DPDP-enhanced MR Imaging. *Radiology.* 1989;172:59–64.

142. Masui T, Saeed M, Wendland M, et al. Occlusive and reperfused myocardial infarcts: MR imaging differentiation with nonionic Gd-DTPA-BMA. *Radiology.* 1991;181: 77–83.

143. Saeed M, Wendland M, Higgins C. Characterization of reperfused myocardial infarctions with T_1-enhancing and magnetic susceptibility—enhancing contrast media. *Invest Radiol.* 1991;26:239–241.

144. Saeed M, Wendland M, Yu K, et al. Identification of myocardial reperfusion with echo planar magnetic resonance imaging: discrimination between occlusive and reperfused infarctions. *Circulation.* 1994;90:1492–1501.

145. Miller D, Holmvang G, Gill J, et al. MRI detection of myocardial perfusion changes by gadolinium-DTPA infusion during dipyridamole hyperemia. *Magn Reson Med.* 1989; 10:246–255.

146. Schaefer S, Lange R, Gutekunst D, et al. Contrast-enhanced magnetic resonance imaging of hypoperfused myocardium. *Invest Radiol.* 1991;26:551–556.

147. Gould K. Noninvasive assessment of coronary stenosis by myocardial perfusion imaging during pharmacologic coronary vasodilatation, I: physiologic basis and experimental validation. *Am J Cardiol.* 1978;41:267–278.

148. Manning W, Atkinson D, Grossman W, et al. First-pass nuclear magnetic resonance imaging studies using gadolinium-DTPA in patients with coronary artery disease. *J Am Coll Cardiol.* 1991;18:959–965.

149. Schaefer S, van Tyen R, Saloner D. Evaluation of myocardial perfusion abnormalities with gadolinium-enhanced snapshot MR imaging in humans. *Radiology* 1992;185: 795–801.

150. Van Rugge F, Boreel J, van der Wall E, et al. Cardiac first-pass and myocardial perfusion in normal subjects assessed by subsecond Gd-DTPA enhanced MR imaging. *J Comput Assist Tomogr.* 1991;15:959–965.

151. Atkinson J, Burstein D, Edelman R. First pass cardiac perfusion: evaluation with ultrafast MR imaging. *Radiology.* 1990;174:757–762.

152. Saeed M, Wendland M, Sakuma H, et al. Detection of myocardial ischemia using first pass contrast-enhanced inversion recovery and driven equilibrium fasr GRE imaging [abstract]. In: *Book of Abstracts: Society of Magnetic Resonance in Medicine.* Berkeley, CA: Society of Magnetic Resonace in Medicine; 1993:536.

153. Saeed M, Wendland M, Sakuma H, et al. MR-enhanced myocardial perfusion imaging: identification of hemodynamically significant coronary ertery stenosis in dogs [abstract]. In: *Book of Abstracts: Society of Magnetic Resonance in Medicine.* Berkeley, CA: Society of Magnetic Resonance in Medicine; 1994:745.

154. Schmiedl U, Ogan M, Paajanen H, et al. Albumin labeled with Gd-DTPA as an intravascular, blood-pool enhancing agent for MR imaging: biodistribution and imaging studies. *Radiology.* 1987;162:205–210.

155. Wilke N, Engels G, Koroneos A, et al. First pass myocardial perfusion imaging with ultrafast gadolinium-enhanced MR imaging at rest and during dipyridamole administration [abstract]. *Radiology.* 1992;185:33.

156. Wendland M, Saeed M, Masui T, et al. Echo-planar MR imaging of normal and ischemic myocardium with gadodiamide injection. *Radiology.* 1993;186:535–542.

157. Wilke N, Simm C, Zhang J, et al. Contrast enhanced first pass myocardial perfusion imaging: correlation between myocardial blood flow in dogs at rest and during hyperemia. *Magn Reson Med.* 1993;29:485–497.

158. Wendland M, Saeed M, Masui T, et al. First pass of an MR susceptibility contrast agent through normal and ischemic heart: gradient-recalled echo-planar imaging. *J Magn Reson Imaging.* 1993;3:755–760.

159. Sakuma H, O´Sullivan M, Lucas J, et al. Effect of magnetic susceptibility contrast medium on myocardial signal intensity with fast gradient-recalled echo and spin-echo MR imaging: initial experience in humans. *Radiology.* 1994;190:161–166.

160. Ito H, Tomooka T, Sakai N, et al. Lack of myocardial perfusion after successful thrombolysis: a predictor of poor recovery of left ventricular function in anterior myocardial infarction. *Circulation.* 1992;85:1699–1705.

161. Saeed M, Wendland M, Takehara Y, et al. Reversible and irreversible injury in the reperfused myocardium: differentiation with contrast material-enhanced MR imaging. *Radiology.* 1990;175:633–637.

162. De Roos A, Matheijssen N, Doornbos J, et al. Myocardial infarct size after reperfusion therapy: Assessment with Gd-DTPA-enhanced MR imaging. *Radiology.* 1990;176:517–521.

163. Bourne M, Numerow L, Amidon L, et al. The assessment of the extent of myocardial functional and perfusion abnormality with fast gradient echo (FGRE) magnetic resonance imaging in patients with chronic myocardial infarction: comparison with thallium 201 SPECT [abstract]. In: *Book of Abstracts: Society of Magnetic Resonance in Medicine.* Berkeley, CA: Society of Magnetic Resonance in Medicine; 1994:1014.

164. Saeed M, Wendland MF, Takehara Y, Higgins CB. Reversible and irreversible injury in the reperfused myocardium: differentiation with contrast-enhanced MR imaging. *Radiology.* 1990;175:633–637.

165. Paulin S, Schulthess G, Fossel E, et al. MR imaging of the aortic root and proximal coronary arteries. *AJR.* 1987;148:665–670.

166. Alfidi R, Masaryk T, Haacke E, et al. MR angiography of peripheral, carotid and coronary arteries. *AJR.* 1987;149:1097–1109.

167. Ruggieri P, Laub G, Masaryk T, et al. Intracranial circulation: pulse-sequence considerations in three-dimensional (volume) MR angiography. *Radiology.* 1989;171:785–791.

168. Kent K, Edelman R, Kim D, et al. Agnetic resonance imaging: a reliable test for the evaluation of proximal atherosclerotic renal arterial stenosis. *J Vasc Surg.* 1991;13:311–318.

169. Burstein D. MR imaging of coronary artery flow in isolated and in-vivo hearts. *J Magn Reson Imaging.* 1991;1:337–346.

170. Meyer C, Hu B, Nishimura D, et al. Fast spiral coronary artery imaging. *Magn Reson Med.* 1992;28:202–213.

171. Manning W, Li W, Boyle N, et al. Fat suppressed breath-hold magnetic resonance coronary angiography. *Circulation.* 1993;87:94–104.

172. Sakuma H, Caputo G, Steffens J, et al. Breath-hold MR angiography of coronary arteries using optimal double-oblique imaging planes [abstract]. In: *Book of Abstracts: Society of magnetic Resonance in Medicine.* Berkeley, CA: Society of Magnetic Resonance in Medicine; 1994:221.

173. Edelman R, Manning W, Gervino E, et al. Flow velocity quantification in human coronary arteries with fast breathhold MR angiography. *J Magn Reson Imaging.* 1993;3:699–703.

174. Herfkens R, Higgins C, Hricak H, et al. Nuclear magnetic resonance imaging of the cardiovascular system: normal and pathologic findings. *Radiology.* 1983;147:749–759.

175. Gomes A, Lois J, Drinkwater D, et al. Coronary artery bypass grafts: visualization with MR imaging. *Radiology.* 1987;162:175–179.

176. White R, Caputo G, Mark A, et al. Coronary artery bypass graft patency: noninvasive evaluation with MR imaging. *Radiology.* 1987;164:681–686.

177. Rubinstein R, Askenase A, Thickman D, et al. Magnetic resonance imaging to evaluate patency of aortocoronary bypass grafts. *Circulation.* 1987;76:786–791.

178. White R, Pflugfelder P, Lipton M, et al. Coronary artery bypass graft: evaluation of patency with cine MR imaging. *AJR.* 1988;150:1271–1274.

179. Aurigemma G, Reichek N, Axel L, et al. Noninvasive determination of coronary artery bypass graft patency by cine magnetic resonance imaging. *Circulation.* 1989;80:1595–1602.

180. Underwood S, Firmin D, Klipstein R, et al. The assessment of coronary artery bypass grafts using magnetic resonance imaging with velocity mapping. *Br Heart J.* 1987;57:93–99.

181. Debatin J, Strong J, Sostman H, et al. MR characterization of blood flow in native and grafted internal mammary arteries. *J Magn Reson Imaging.* 1993;3:443–450.

182. Manning WJ, Li W, Edelman RR. A preliminary report comparing magnetic resonance coronary angiography with conventional angiography. *N Engl J Med.* 1993;328:823–832.

17

Nuclear Cardiology

Hans Martin Hoffmeister

Nuclear cardiology is a discipline that involves cardiology and nuclear medicine. It developed as a new field in the 1970s with the introduction of several radiopharmaceutical agents for cardiac imaging and with ongoing progress in the development of camera systems and dedicated computers. The scope of the procedures includes not only diagnostic approaches to identify patients with coronary heart disease, but more dedicated tools to characterize regional perfusion and metabolic and functional status of the left ventricular myocardium in order to optimize the diagnostic and therapeutic strategies in patients with cardiac diseases. The techniques are also used to obtain information on prognosis and are recommended for risk stratification in various patient groups. In this chapter, radiopharmaceuticals and camera systems are introduced first, followed by a description of imaging modalities. Clinical applications of the methods are described thereafter.

Conventional Nuclear Cardiology (Single Photon Emission Scintigraphy)

Radiopharmaceutical Agents and Camera Systems

Imaging Agents

Compounds labeled with thallium 201 (Tl 201) and technetium 99m (Tc 99m) are at present the agents used for studying myocardial perfusion with gamma camera systems. Several Tc 99m–labeled compounds have been developed for myocardial imaging. Most frequently used is Tc 99m hexakis-2-methoxy-2-isobutyl isonitrile (sestaMIBI or Tc 99m MIBI). Additional Tc 99m–labeled radiopharmaceutical compounds are Tc 99m teboroxime and tetrofosmin. Other agents are under development, but Tl 201, Tc 99m MIBI, Tc 99m tetrofosmin, and Tc 99m teboroxime are the most frequently used perfusion markers. Use of these compounds may vary in different countries, depending on their approval for clinical indications.

Thallium-201

Tl-201 is a cyclotron-derived product emitting mainly (88%) x-rays at 69 to 83 keV and gamma rays between 135 and 167 keV. These characteristics make it less favorable for standard gamma camera systems. Tl-201 has a relatively long physical half-life of about 74 hours and an unfavorable biological half-life of the same length. Therefore only small amounts of Tl 201 can be administered. Depending on the camera system used, amounts of 2.0 to 3.5 mCi are injected. Initially Tl 201 is accumulated in the left ventricular myocardium in relation to myocardial blood flow with a high extraction rate (> 80%).[1,2] Thereafter a transmembranous exchange of Tl 201 occurs. The uptake of Tl 201 is in part an active process dependent on the Na^+,K^+-ATPase system. The behavior of thallium is similar to that of potassium, but experimental analyses confirmed that distinct differences between the handling of thallium and potassium exist. Therefore, Tl 201 is not only a pure perfusion marker but is also dependent on metabolic processes. Several technical features of this imaging agent are listed in Table 17.1.

Due to its relatively high emission of radiation, only small amounts of Tl 201 can be administered. This is a disadvantage especially when the unfavorable radiation profile for gamma camera systems is taken into account. Tl 201 also has very interesting advantages. There is an ongoing exchange between myocytes and the blood pool after the first accumulation. Thus, exercise-induced perfusion defects on poststress Tl 201 scans can fill in (relative uptake in postischemic regions versus wash-out in normal regions) during reperfusion following the acute ischemia.[3] This so-called redistribution is used in conventional Tl 201 perfusion protocols, with

TABLE 17.1. Comparsion of some properties of Tl 201 and Tc 99m MIBI, the most frequently used agents to examine myocardial perfusion using gamma camera systems.

	Tl 201	Tc 99m MIBI
Half-life (physical/biological)	74/58 h	6.6 h
Heart half-life	3–4 h	6 h
Emissions	69–83, 135, 165, 167 keV	140 keV
Dose	2.5–3.5 mCi	30 mCi
Myocardial extraction fraction	80%–90%	60%–70%
Whole body radiation dose	0.21 rad/mCi	0.02 rad/mCi

delayed imaging either 2 to 4 hours or even up to 24 hours after the stress test in order to discriminate myocardial ischemia from irreversibly damaged myocardium, which persists as a regional defect. Thus, standard thallium protocols consist of a first study (within 5 to 10 minutes) after the injection at the maximum of an exercise- or pharmacologically induced perfusion disorder to detect the flow-dependent initial myocardial accumulation of the tracer. Then a second study, after redistribution, is obtained for information about the extent of viable myocardium. With this protocol, reversible (ischemia-like) and irreversible (persistent) defects can be distinguished. A rare observation is the "reverse redistribution." This means either enlargement or occurrence of a defect on the delayed images, whereas the defect on the initial study was smaller or even absent. This phenomenon was observed after thrombolytic therapy in myocardial infarction,[4] but was critically discussed with respect to technical and kinetic problems.[5,6] Reverse redistribution can disappear after reinjection.[7] In recent years this type of standard protocol was improved either by adding very delayed images (up to 24 hours) or by additional reinjection of smaller amounts of Tl 201 at rest conditions on top of the previous thallium injection, or by a combination of the two. Using such advanced protocols, accuracy of Tl 201 imaging to identify viable myocardium was significantly improved.[8–12] Despite its unfavorable physical characteristics, Tl 201 is the most frequently used tracer to detect myocardial viability with gamma camera systems.

Technetium-99m–Labeled Myocardial Imaging Agents

Tc 99m MIBI

Tc-99m has a favorable gamma emission spectrum with a photo peak at 140 keV suitable for standard camera equipment. With physical and biological half-lives of about 6 hours, the absorbed radiation dose is less than with Tl 201. From the point of dosimetry, the target for Tc 99m MIBI is the upper gastrointestinal tract, whereas the most critical organs for Tl 201 are the kidneys and the urinary bladder.[13] Tc-99m MIBI is excreted by the hepatobiliary system, its uptake by the lung is not critical for imaging modalities. Tc 99m MIBI has several advantages over Tl 201, such as the radiation spectrum, which

is much better suited for gamma camera systems (Tc 99 is the "work horse" isotope for imaging in nuclear medicine), the much more favorable radiation profile with a shorter half-life (allowing larger doses to be administered), and easier technical handling (not cyclotron dependent, and "fixed" in the myocardium after injection, resulting in the possibility of uncoupling of the strict timing between injection and imaging). Its favorable imaging characteristics make feasible an assessment of regional and global function after electrocardiogram (ECG) gating of the perfusion study. Myocardial distribution of Tc 99m MIBI is proportional to myocardial blood flow at least at normal flow rates, but at higher flow rates the relation becomes inaccurate.[3,14,15] The extraction fraction is less than that of thallium, the most likely main entry into myocytes being passive diffusion. Inside the myocyte, Tc 99m MIBI is bound to mitochondria, and further uptake occurs during recirculation.[16] Redistribution of Tc 99m MIBI is relatively low compared with thallium. Several studies examined its use to characterize viability.[17–23] Tc 99m MIBI results in "frozen" perfusion images without the delayed additional filling-in in initially existing defects, as occurs on delayed thallium images (depending on the pathophysiological state of the initial perfusion defect). For practical purposes, imaging should be delayed by more than 1 hour after injection and the patient should have a meal after injection of the agent so as to make sure the liver is cleared before imaging of the myocardium is initiated. Protocols with Tc 99m MIBI for detection of myocardial ischemia include two separate injections, one at maximum coronary flow maldistribution (e.g., peak exercise) and one at rest in absence of myocardial ischemia.

Tc 99m Teboroxime and Tc 99m Tetrofosmin

Tc-99m teboroxime is a perfusion-imaging agent with an extraction fraction greater than that of thallium, and with a flow-related uptake.[24,25] Tc 99m teboroxime also has a high liver uptake with slow wash-out kinetics. Lung uptake is higher than with Tc 99m MIBI. The most marked difference is the myocardial wash-out, which is flow dependent and fast for Tc 99m teboroxime, with a clearance of most of the accumulated Tc 99 teboroxime within minutes during the rapid first phase of the washout.[26] Fast wash-out is followed by a slow wash-out phase with a half-life of clearance of 3 to 4 hours. Because the clearance is flow dependent, myocardial segments with reduced coronary flow are cleared more slowly and result in a redistribution effect if serial images are performed. The fast kinetics of Tc 99m teboroxime demand imaging during the first minutes after injection. Since actual silent ischemia may influence defect size at rest, nitrate pretreatment is recommended.[27]

Technetium-99m tetrofosmin is a perfusion agent that does not have as rapid wash-out as teboroxime, so that myocardial perfusion imaging within the first minutes after injection is not mandatory. Results with this agent correlate very well with thallium and coronary angiography findings.[28,29]

Other Pharmaceutical Agents

Besides Tl 201 and Tc 99m MIBI, several other compounds are used in nuclear cardiology. A number of imaging agents are coupled with Tc 99m. The majority of infarct-avid imaging studies today are performed with Tc 99m pyrophosphate. Another agent is indium 111 antimyosin. Although imaging with Tc 99m has the abovementioned advantages, indium 111 (In 111) causes a certain background activity by dissociation from the antibody. Additionally it also has a long half-life of about 72 hours, thus limiting the maximum dose. Furthermore, depending on local circumstances, In 111 is not always available and needs to be delivered. Other agents for assessment of myocardial viability are coupled with iodine 123 (I 123).[30]

Other pharmaceutic agents include labeled fatty acids for single-photon metabolic imaging, the majority of them being labeled with I 123. For study of cardiac sympathetic innervation, metaiodobenzylguanidine (MIBG–I 123) is used. Other compounds include lymphocytes and platelets labeled with In 111 and labeled low-density lipoproteins. Newer tracers for cardiac hypoxia are currently under investigation.

For radionuclide angiography, Tc 99m is used in several modes of application, as described in the section on radionuclide angiography.

Imaging Systems

Systems for imaging consist of a radiation detector equipped with a collimator (gamma camera) and a dedicated computer system (using a 64 × 64 or 128 ×128 matrix) for acquisition and processing of data. The standard gamma camera has a single crystal; multicrystal cameras with higher sensitivity but lower spatial resolution are preferable for first-pass studies. The gamma camera for planar imaging has a detector that is 10 to15 inches in diameter (the latter is called a *large field-of-view camera*). The standard detector is circular, but an increas-

ing number of newer camera heads are rectangular. In most cases of imaging with Tl 201, an all-purpose parallel-hole collimator is used, whereas for technetium-labeled compounds a high-resolution parallel-hole collimator is preferable. The camera system should be optimized for linearity and field homogeneity. The resolution, which is usually given as "full width at half maximum, is inversely related to sensitivity. For the complete gamma camera system including collimator, resolution is typically in the range of 10 to 15 mm.

The energy range of the gamma camera can be preselected for the compound used. For Tl 201, a double window set at 80 and 167 keV is used, whereas for Tc 99m, a 20% window at the 140 keV peak is adequate.

In general, conventional planar imaging has to be differentiated from tomographic imaging, known as emission computed tomography (ECT). In planar imaging, three to four projections are chosen with the patient lying supine or turned to the right (anterior, left anterior oblique, and left lateral [60 to 80 degrees]). Imaging time is adjusted to obtain a sufficient number of counts in the field of view.

For tomographic studies, the gamma camera has a gantry that allows rotation of the camera head around the patient who is in a supine position. An alternative to this supine position, to avoid or modify attenuation artifacts by the left hemidiaphragm or by the tomographic table, is the right lateral decubitus position or a prone position.[31–35] The camera head rotates either in a circle or in a pre-set orbit for 180 degrees, with 32 stops of 20 to 60 seconds.[36] Alternatively a 360 degree arc is possible.[37] Newer developments in ECT systems resulted in double- or triple-head cameras with reduced acquisition times. After acquisition, the data have to be processed using filtered back-projection or iterative reconstruction. Then several heart-axis–oriented short- and long-axis slices are displayed. To condense this information, the left ventricular myocardium can be displayed in a polar map fashion. If a dedicated ECT camera system is not available, a planar gamma camera can be equipped with a seven-pinhole–collimator to obtain some three-dimensional information.[38,39] However, this technique has several limitations and has not been shown to be superior to advanced ECT systems.

Myocardial Scintigraphy

Myocardial Perfusion Imaging

The aim of perfusion imaging is to describe myocardial blood flow on a regional basis to detect local disturbances of coronary flow. The tracer should be fixed in the myocardium in a sufficiently proportional relation to coronary flow in an extended range of blood flow, but this goal is not perfectly fullfilled, especially in the upper flow range, with the currently available tracers.[15,40] A limitation of perfusion imaging with standard gamma camera equipment is the impossibility of quantitative determination of flow per gram of myocardium. The gamma camera studies provide information only about the relative distribution of flow in the left ventricular myocardium, and information is displayed normalized to the "hottest" pixel. Therefore, coronary stenoses with a balanced limitation of coronary flow (e.g., when stenosis of the left main and right coronary artery are of equal importance) may cause a homogeneous reduction in left ventricular myocardial blood flow and result in a homogeneous tracer distribution without evidence for severe coronary heart disease. However, in the overwhelming majority of patients with coronary artery disease, the reduction in coronary blood flow is not homogeneous, especially if wash-out kinetics are taken into account,[41-43] and therefore the perfusion disturbances are detectable.

Several methods are used to provide distribution disturbances of coronary flow as a diagnostic indicator for coronary artery disease. The most common way is an exercise test resulting in a stress-induced myocardial ischemia, with tracer injection at peak exercise. If a patient is unable to exercise, a pharmacologic stress test (e.g., dobutamine) can be performed.[44] An alternative method is the induction of coronary blood flow inhomogeneities using intravenous adenosine or dipyridamole (indirect action via adenosine) [45-56]; further stress modalities are "handgrip" or "cold pressor" stress. An extensive summary of the pharmacologic techniques indicates the overall low incidence of severe side effects,[3] but for application in patients who are able to exercise adequately, there is no striking advantage of either catecholamine stress or vasodilation (adenosine or dipyridamole) for general use.

There are several variations on images of normally perfused left ventricles that must be taken into account during interpretation. The apical region often appears to be thinner, especially in hypertrophied and dilated left ventricles.[57(p291)] The valve plane (mitral and aortic valve) and the membraneous part of the septum show variation that results in some difficulty in judging the end of the posterior wall or septum versus defects due to minor infarctions. The posterolateral region usually appears with a higher count rate compared with the septal wall. Other artifacts may result from a "partial volume" effect, if the target source is markedly smaller compared with the pixel size. Additional evaluation of local function using gated studies and a Tc 99m tracer[58] may be helpful in solving this problem.

Quantitative data on coronary blood flow cannot be obtained with gamma camera imaging, therefore, in most cases, perfusion studies are judged qualitatively for the presence of perfusion defects. Quantitative approaches, which in some studies resulted in slightly higher test ac-

curacy, do not provide quantitative data on myocardial blood flow but refer to normal ranges of relative activities and wash-out in various left ventricular regions.[59,60] Qualitatively, the extent and severity of perfusion defects can be classified using scoring systems.[61] Further useful information from perfusion studies includes the assessment of transient or persistent pathological enlargement of the left ventricles,[62,63] enforced visualization of the right ventricle (indicating pulmonary hypertension), and increased lung activity (on unprocessed planar Tl 201 scans).[64,65]

The most frequently used tracer for myocardial-perfusion imaging is Tl 201. In the majority of studies, Tl 201 is injected at maximum point of an exercise stress test. Because Tl 201 is initially distributed in relation to myocardial blood flow, this first image mainly represents a pure perfusion image of the left ventricular myocardium during stress. Tl 201 has quantitatively important redistribution effects, and imaging should be started soon after the stress test to avoid a decrease in sensitivity. On the other hand, within the first few minutes after maximum exercise, a slight relative movement of the heart after the patient is positioned in the supine position influences the images (the so-called upward creep effect[66]). This artifact can be avoided by a delayed start of the imaging procedure. Starting at the end of the stress test, the redistribution process in the left ventricular myocardium results in filling in of the viable regions, which were less perfused during stress (Figure 17.1). Therefore, the standard images obtained 2 to 4 hours poststress are not pure perfusion images but represent the result of the stress-induced perfusion inhomogeneity, redistribution effects, the relative coronary flow during the poststress period, and metabolic effects. If zones of the left ventricular myocardium with exercise-induced ischemia are filled in after 3 to 4 hours of redistribution (reversible defect), absence of myocardial infarction is indicated. In contrast, from an incomplete or absent fill-in (fixed indicates persistent or irreversible defect), the presence of irreversibly damaged myocardial tissue cannot be conclusively inferred. Several studies have shown that such regions may also consist of viable myocardium with severe but reversible injury. To cope with this problem, several improvements have been proposed for thallium-imaging protocols[8-12]. Prolongation of reperfusion time results in a longer time span for filling in of an initially present perfusion defect but is limited by the impairment of count statistics (especially on 24-hour delayed studies). The decrease in the total count rate results in longer acquisition times with increased statistical problems and less clearly delineated left ventricular myocardium because the target-to-background ratio is also impaired. Another proposed protocol modification is the "reinjection" of a smaller amount of Tl 201 during the redistribution pe-

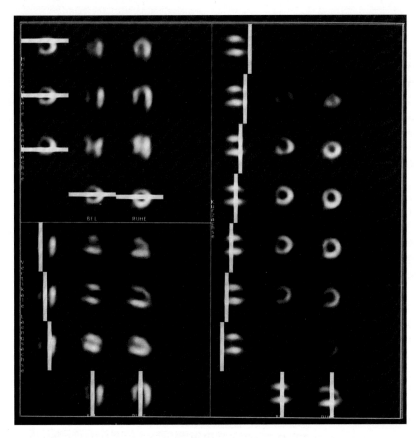

FIGURE 17.1. Tl 201 stress and 3-hour redistribution myocardial perfusion scintigraphy. Exercise-induced ischemia in the anterolateral, apical, and septal segments in a patient with single-vessel coronary artery disease (proximal 90% stenosis of the left anterior descending coronary artery). On the upper left panel, horizontal long-axis tomograms (apex on the top, septum on the left, and lateral wall on the right side); on the left bottom, vertical long-axis tomograms (anterior wall on top, inferior wall at the bottom, apex on the right side); on the right panel, short-axis tomograms (septum on the left, lateral wall on the right, anterior wall on the upper side, inferior wall on the bottom of each slice). All tomograms are displayed in a top-to-bottom format, starting with the anterior wall for the horizontal slices, with the septal wall for the vertical long-axis slices, and with the apical region for the short-axis slices. Parallel display of the stress images (on the left) and redistribution images (on the right) for direct comparison. A larger anterolateral-septal-apical perfusion defect is displayed on the stress images, which is completely reversible on the redistribution images.

riod to push the filling in of initial perfusion defects, which consist of still-viable myocardium (Figure 17.2). Several modifications of these approaches have been proposed. Since some protocols are rather time consuming, shorter versions with early reinjection after the stress image acquisition[67,68] (done only if a stress-induced defect is present) with half of the initial Tl 201 dose, and imaging after one to several hours of redistribution are being examined for feasibility. If only the perfusion at rest is of interest, tracer injection can also be performed without initial exercise and results in a resting coronary flow image. If the exact extent of viable myocardium is of interest, any actual myocardial ischemia at the time of injection should be avoided (e.g.,

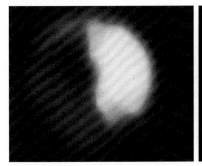 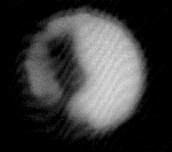 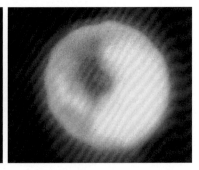

FIGURE 17.2. Tl 201 myocardial perfusion scintigraphy of a patient with multivessel coronary artery disease and severely reduced left ventricular function. The images are displayed as polar maps (condensed information of all short-axis slices. with the septum on the left, the lateral wall on the right, the anterior wall on the top, and the inferior wall on the bottom of each polar map. From left to right: stress scan, 3-hour redistribution scan, and reinjection scan (1 mCi after the 3-hour redistribution scan, imaging after redistribution). There is an extended perfusion defect including several left ventricular regions on the stress scan. Some redistribution is visible on the 3-hour poststress image, with additional redistribution after reinjection. The reinjection–redistribution scan results were identical to those of an F 18 FDG study performed later for exact delineation of viable myocardium.

administration of nitrates). For the most exact delineation of viable myocardium, rest-redistribution or rest-reinjection studies have been performed with Tl 201.[69-71]

With Tc 99m MIBI no considerable redistribution occurs. This results in a "frozen" image of myocardial blood flow at the time of injection. For detection of exercise-induced ischemia, it is recommended that exercise be continued for up to 120 seconds postinjection. The acquisition time after injection is not critical as with thallium but should be delayed to profit from liver and gall bladder clearance. In contrast to studies with Tl 201, a second study with injection of Tc 99m MIBI during resting conditions (with pretreatment to avoid myocardial ischemia[72]) is necessary to compare flow distribution during stress and during rest in order to identify stress-induced myocardial ischemia. One- and 2-day protocols give essentially the same results.[73,74] Also dual isotope protocols have been proposed. Because Tc 99m MIBI is a perfusion marker without clinically important redistribution effects, its main advantage is exact characterization of relative distribution of myocardial blood flow and not the quantitative delineation of viable myocardium (defects on Tc 99m MIBI scans done at rest are often larger compared with those assessed by reinjection–redistribution Tl 201 scans[75]). Detection of viability using Tc 99m MIBI can be improved by nitroglycerin administration.[72]

For other technetium compounds, different approaches and protocols are under investigation, depending on the specific perfusion agent. Tc 99m teboroxime especially requires data acquisition within minutes after injection[48,76] Tc 99m tetrofosmin is clinically similar to Tc 99m MIBI.[28,29]

Infarct Imaging

With respect to imaging strategy, acute myocardial infarctions have to be distinguished from chronic myocardial infarctions. Imaging techniques for the latter group are described in the section on coronary heart disease.

In acute myocardial infarction, either positive or negative infarction imaging can be performed. For negative myocardial infarction imaging, the perfusion tracers can be used to delineate a perfusion defect at the site of the acute myocardial infarction.[77] Tl-201 is not perfect in this situation because several redistribution effects may occur; rapid imaging after injection is necessary if the area of risk is to be determined. Furthermore, follow-up studies with respect to reperfusion therapy are not possible. With Tc 99m MIBI, the perfusion defect at the time of injection is "frozen" for several hours and therefore makes judgement of the management (e.g., thrombolytic therapy) of the patients easier.[78-82] However, because in more than about 10% to 20% of patients spontaneous thrombolysis occurs, perfusion images delayed after the onset of the acute chest pain may miss the correct diagnosis. An additional disadvantage is the non-

specificity of perfusion imaging in the differentiation between acute and chronically persistent perfusion defects (chronic myocardial infarctions) and also the differentiation between perfusion defects that result in reversible versus irreversible tissue damage.

In contrast to imaging of infarcts as defects, positive imaging (with infarct-avid agents) can be performed. The standard tracer is Tc 99m pyrophosphate, and it is used in patients within the first days after acute myocardial infarction without diagnostic ECG, and in patients early after coronary artery bypass grafting.[83-86] This agent has medium sensitivity and specificity for diagnosing acute myocardial infarction.[87,88] There are several reasons for false-positive results such as intracardiac calcifications and recent myocardial infarctions. On the other hand, if the study is performed too early (<24 hours) or too late (1 week) after the onset of infarction, false-negative results may be observed, and smaller infarcts may be not diagnosed due to the use of planar imaging.[89] For improving infarct-avid scintigraphy, an antibody (antimyosin) labelled with In 111 was proposed,[90,91] but this technique resulted in sensitivities similar to those of infarct scintigraphy with Tc 99m pyrophosphate. Disadvantages of the In 111 scintigraphy are the low total dose that can be administered (due to the long half-life), slow blood clearance, and dissociation from the antibody. Therefore, imaging can be started about 24 hours after injection and repeated at 48 hours after injection. The best time for injection is similar to that for Tc 99m pyrophosphate, that is, after 48 hours from onset of the acute infarction. Because In 111 images taken early after the injection are difficult to read due to the substantial blood pool activity, dual-isotope–scintigraphy (similar to the use of Tl 201 and Tc 99m pyrophosphate[92,93]) with Tl 201 and In 111 antimyosin has been proposed for easier reconstruction and orientation.[94]

The infarct-avid imaging agents available may be indicated in certain circumstances, but for the majority of patients with acute myocardial infarction the profile of imaging modalities and the time delay after the acute onset of the chest pain do not make these agents a first-line diagnostic tool for general purposes.

Prognosis after acute myocardial infarction is related to the quantity of myocardial tissue damaged. A further prognostic aspect is related to Tc 99m pyrophosphate scintigraphy in patients with unstable angina pectoris. Patients with unstable angina pectoris and positive pyrophosphate scan have a worse prognosis than patients with negative test results.[95]

Results with a similar prognostic impact have been observed in comparable patient groups with Tc 99m MIBI scans and with plasma markers of myocardial necrosis such as troponin T, demonstrating a possible future indication of perfusion scans for patients with chest pain and nondiagnostic ECG results.[96-99]

Fatty Acid Analogue Imaging

In single-photon imaging, labeled fatty acid analogues have been used as myocardial imaging agents.[100-103] Several different fatty acids have been labeled with iodine isotopes. I 123 hexadecanoic acid scans were compared with Tl 201 scintigraphy and both tracers were described as equally potent for detection of areas of myocardial infarction.[104] Redistribution of another analogue (*p*-phenylpentadecanoic acid) has also been extensively explored.[105-109] Because images obtained with *p*-phenylpentadecanoic acid are influenced by myocardial flow, dual imaging was proposed to relate fatty acid uptake to myocardial flow.[110] Imaging with iodine-labeled fatty acid analogues is a promising approach for assessment of myocardial metabolism with SPECT, but the contribution of coronary flow and metabolism to the images is still not resolved, and clinical usefulness has to be investigated with special attention to the competitiveness of PET metabolic imaging.

Additional Imaging Modalities

Myocardial neurone scintigraphy can be performed using metaiodobenzylguanidine (MIBG) labeled with I 123 as a marker of adrenergic neurones. This compound allows imaging of the sympathetic nerve endings in the left ventricular myocardium. Dae and coworkers[111] studied coronary flow and MIBG uptake in dogs. Comparing MIBG distribution to that of Tl 201, it was shown that in some regions MIBG uptake was negative but thallium uptake was positive, indicating regional denervation. MIBG defects were also demonstrated in human myocardial infarction.[112,113] In several studies[114-116] MIBG was studied in patients with dilated cardiomyopathy. The results indicate some inverse relationship of the cardiac uptake of MIBG to the level of circulating catecholamines,[117] and also an influence of fibrosis. Pathological findings were also reported in patients with diabetes mellitus.[118] MIBG scintigraphy was used to study patients with ventricular tachycardia.[113,119,120] In general, MIBG studies of regional denervation need thallium imaging to assess perfusion defects. Denervation is diagnosed from the mismatch between the magnitude of the (larger) MIBG-defined defects and the persistent thallium-defined defect.[111,113] It was also suggested that MIBG be used as a diagnostic tool in patients with long-QT syndrome. However, the clinical value of this imaging modality has not yet been settled.

Platelets can be labeled with In 111; this makes imaging of thrombi in different locations of the body with a gamma camera system feasible. Using this technique, thrombi in the left ventricular cavity and other cardiac chambers[121-128] and in arteries[129-132] have been observed; however, thrombi in the coronary arteries in particular are often too small for the resolution power of the standard camera systems and may be missed.

Lymphocytes can also be labeled with In 111. This has been proposed for detection of cardiac rejection after transplantation.[133,134]

An interesting approach is the labeling of low-density lipoprotein (LDL) with Tc 99m[135] and In 111.[136,137] The advantage of In 111 over technetium is the better stability of the labeling of the LDL and the more favorable half-life of LDL. The technique is hampered by the lack of uptake of tracer into old plaques, whereas soft, new lesions are more easily labeled with marked LDL. Quantitative evaluation is further limited by blood pool activity.

Radionuclide Angiography

Two different approaches can be used to assess cardiac performance using radio-pharmaceutical agents. One approach, which is less frequently performed, is the first-pass technique. More frequently, the equilibrium ECG-gated technique is used. A critical summary of the methods and the clinical data of both techniques have recently been published.[3]

The most important information obtained with both radionuclide ventriculography techniques concerns global ventricular function (Table 17.2). Quantitative data with good test accuracy for left ventricular function can be derived, especially in patients not suited for quantitative echocardiography examination for various reasons. For information about certain coronary stenosis (severity, restenosis, etc.), advanced perfusion scintigraphy techniques are more suitable, as has been pointed out in an ACC/AHA statement.[138]

First-Pass Radionuclide Angiography

This technique detects activity of a radioactive bolus passing through the right and then the left heart during a few heart beats. Several technical prerequisites are necessary. The tracer (usually a bolus of Tc 99m pertechnetate) should be administered as an optimal bolus by an injection via the cubital vein. The camera system should be capable of detecting with good sensitivity the high

TABLE 17.2. Information available from radionuclide ventriculography.

Left ventricle	Right ventricle
Ejection fraction	Ejection fraction
End-systolic and end-diastolic volumes	End-systolic and end-diastolic volumes
Diastolic function	Regional wall motion
Cardiac output	Intracardiac shunts
Mean pulmonary transit time	Regurgitation fraction
Regional wall motion	Localization of some rhythm abnormalities
Intracardiac shunts	
Regurgitation fraction	
Localization of some rhythm abnormalities	

level of radioactivity within a short time. Major dead-time losses result in inaccurate results. Also, linearity at high count rates and a dedicated computer system are necessary. Within the few beats used for analysis no arrhythmias should be present.[139] To meet these technical problems, multicrystal camera systems have been used. At present, new digitized camera systems may also be appropriate. Compared with the equilibrium technique, the spatial resolution of the first-past technique is lower due to the enhanced sensitivity of the systems (due to the need for more sensitive collimators). The availability of newer technetium-labeled perfusion agents may lead to an increase of first-pass scans after bolus injection of the tracer, before the myocardial perfusion studies are performed, to obtain more comprehensive information about the left ventricle.[140,141]

The data of first-pass studies are usually processed in frame mode in dedicated computer systems. Because the bolus passes through the right ventricle first, the first-pass imaging modality is the tool of choice to assess right ventricular function. Other tracers used for this purpose include, for example, gold-195m.[142,143] Further applications of first-pass studies are the detection and quantification of intracardiac shunts.[144] A reference region over the lung is used for this purpose. For detection of stress-induced functional disturbances of the left or right ventricle, separate studies during stress and at rest have to be performed with the first-pass technique, but only one camera view can be studied.

ECG-Gated Equilibrium Blood Pool Radionuclide Angiography

For this technique the blood pool must be labeled either by in vivo or in vitro techniques. To label erythrocytes, Tc 99m (standard dose 20 mCi) is used, and unlabeled stannous pyrophosphate facilitates its reaction in vivo. Also feasible is preparation with Tc 99m pertechnetate, after the patients own blood is collected for the in vitro preparation. With these techniques data acquisition can be performed over a span of some hours, enabling stress and rest examinations, studies from different camera views, and the short-term control of interventions. Data acquisition is performed using ECG gating in a frame mode (data processed and then stored) list mode (data stored and processed later), or hybrid mode (intermediate list mode acquisition of one actual cycle with subsequent decision on acceptance and storage in frame mode). Several hundred heart cycles are summed to obtain a sufficient target-to-background ratio.[145] To avoid artifacts, the patient must remain in one position during the time of data acquisition (up to 10 minutes per view). Arrhythmias can disturb the data collection, but dedicated correction systems can exclude such cardiac cycles. A further limitation of equilibrium radionuclide ven-

triculography is the background activity. In a state of equilibrium, radioactivity is present in all chambers of the heart and in the great vessels and pulmonary vessels. Compared with imaging that uses a bolus, as in first-pass ventriculography, the overlap of these activities is a limitation of the equilibrium technique. This is especially true for evaluation of the right ventricle.[146,147] At rest, acquisition of several views of the left ventricle allows improved diagnosis of regional dysfunction with the equilibrium technique, the count statistics are better with the equilibrium approach, and the regional spatial resolution is also higher due to the need for a less-sensitive camera.

The standard orientation for gated blood pool ventriculography is the 35 to 45 degree left anterior oblique orientation. With this orientation and a slight caudal tilt for the contribution of the left atria, a clear separation of the right and left ventricle is obtained, otherwise the degree of obliqueness should be optimized (best septal view). Using this orientation, global left ventricular function is examined and stress studies are performed. Anterior and lateral views are added thereafter to obtain information about respective areas of the left ventricle. Regarding regional information, it must be stressed that the spatial resolution of radionuclide ventriculography techniques is poor compared with contrast cine ventriculography, echocardiography, and MRI techniques.[148–151] However, radionuclide ventriculography not only provides a contour of the left ventricle with moderate resolution but also gives information in a third dimension because of the count statistics, an advantage not given by any of the methods that rely on contours. This advantage is used for calculation of the ejection fraction and for determination of ventricular volumes with equilibrium radionuclide ventriculography. Blood sampling for calibration standards is necessary for the determination of ventricular volumes; also, attenuation for radiation must be taken into account.[152–154]

After some data processing, the left ventricular curve can be used to determine the ejection fraction and left ventricular (rapid) filling properties. For regional analysis, the contour method can be used with a cine loop, or multiple frames from the representative heart cycle or a center-line method for quantitative evaluation can be applied.[155–157] Another approach to the assessment of regional function is the phase analysis of contraction with display of the data on parametric images (Figure 17.3). With parametric Fourier analysis–based evaluation on a pixel base, both the amplitude of contraction and its timing within the left ventricle of each region can be assessed. This technique was pioneered by Adam and coworkers.[158,159] It can easily be used to identify left ventricular aneurysms or zones of hypokinesia or akinesia.[160] The overlap in this technique requires that several views be taken so that abnormalities of regional wall mo-

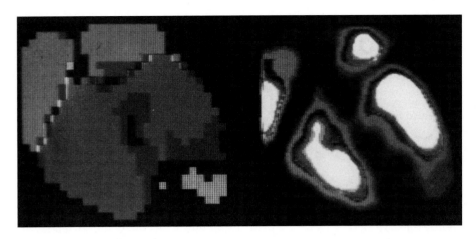

FIGURE 17.3. Tc 99m equilibrium ECG-gated ventriculography of a patient with a large apicoanterior aneurysm. Display of parametric images from a 40 degree LAO view, with phase images on the left and amplitude images on the right side. Both ventricles and both atria are clearly separated. On the phase images, a phase shift characterizing an aneurysm is visible in the apical and anteroseptal region. Correspondingly, an apical and anteroseptal amplitude defect is present on the amplitude image.

tion are not missed. In preliminary reports this technique was used for analysis of arrhythmias and their impact on cardiac function. The parametric approach has the advantage of not being contour derived and therefore not being so dependent on the low resolution of the radionuclide ventriculography, but it gives all the information provided by the equilibrium contour technique.

Newer techniques include SPECT-gating techniques[161–164] and combination of a first-pass acquisition followed by a perfusion study.[165]

Using the equilibrium approach, a nonimaging probe for long-term evaluation of left ventricular function was developed (called a *nuclear stethoscope*).[166] Ambulant monitoring systems that use a similar approach are under development to provide data on left ventricular function over the long-term.[167]

Clinical Application

Coronary Heart Disease

Detection of Chronic Ischemic Heart Disease

Myocardial ischemia occurs in patients with coronary heart disease when the ratio of supply to demand is disturbed. It results in a relative hypoperfusion of left ventricular myocardial regions. Radiolabeled perfusion markers have been used extensively since the 1970s to identify the presence of coronary heart disease and to enable risk stratification of patients. Because the identification of a relative hypoperfusion is dependent on the presence of ischemia at the time of tracer injection, coronary heart disease can be identified only at rest in the presence of either an acute or old myocardial infarction, or unstable angina pectoris with actual ischemia.

To detect exercise-induced myocardial ischemia in patients with possible stable chronic coronary heart disease, it is necessary to perform a stress test to induce relative regional hypoperfusion. Also, patients with sus-

pected silent ischemia can be examined with perfusion scintigraphy.[168–170] The most commonly used test is exercise stress, with Tl 201 administered by intravenous injection at peak exercise and the patient exercising for a further 40 to 60 seconds. Thereafter the stress image is obtained. If a patient is unable to exercise, pharmacologic stress (e.g., dobutamine) or pharmacologically induced vasodilation using dipyridamole or adenosine with consecutive relative hypoperfusion in poststenotic myocardial areas can be performed, with comparable test accuracy and safety.[52,171–174] The most frequently used marker for these tests is Tl 201, but the newer Tc 99m–labeled agents have the same diagnostic accuracy (Figure 17.4).[13,74,141,175–179] For imaging in these cases, either planar or SPECT camera systems may be used, with a slightly higher diagnostic accuracy reported for the SPECT technique, especially for localization of hypoperfused areas and for prediction of the number of vessels involved.[39,180,181] With the planar technique the accuracy (mainly sensitivity) for the circumflex artery is low, whereas the best results are obtained in the left anterior descending artery region.[182–184] The test accuracy for detection of chronic coronary artery disease was evaluated in the 1970s and 1980s; sensitivity and specificity values were found to be in the mid 80% range with qualitative visual image analysis.[151,185–188] Quantitative evaluation of the images results in a slight increase of accuracy.[60,185,189–194] The results of testing by different evaluation modalities have recently been summarized extensively.[3] Increase in diagnostic accuracy by quantitative methods is mainly due to an increase in sensitivity, whereas specificity is not improved. However, the number of stenoses is more accurately assessed.[195,196] Several reports described a higher detection frequency for coronary heart disease with SPECT systems.[182,194,197–199] Using a quantitative approach to SPECT, Tl 201 polar maps can be constructed and compared with normalized data. Polar mapping or bull's-eye plotting for diagnosing stable coronary heart disease increases the sensitivity up to

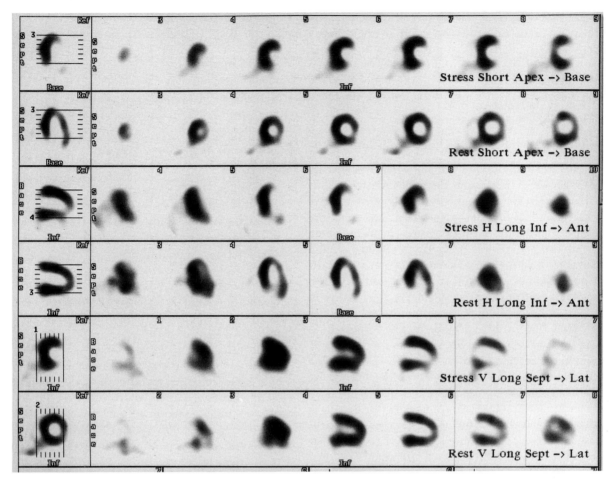

FIGURE 17.4. Tc 99 tetrofosmin stress and rest myocardial reperfusion scintigraphy with exercise-induced ischemia in the apical, posterolateral, and diaphragmal segment in a patient with multivessel coronary artery disease. From top to bottom: stress and rest short-axis slices, stress and rest horizontal long-axis slices, and stress and rest vertical long-axis slices.

90% with a specificity of about 70%.[182] It has been recently discussed whether the reduced specificity in those studies may be due to a bias caused by a selection factor, because many patients with consecutive normal SPECT study results would not have coronary angiography. To compensate for such a referral bias a normalcy rate instead of specificity was proposed, which is the fraction of negative studies in clinically normal patients. This normalcy rate for quantitative Tl 201 SPECT is about 89%.[138] With respect to the extent of severe coronary heart disease (multivessel or left main), there is a very high probability for an abnormal perfusion scan,[60,183,192, 196,200,201] but in a certain percentage, only one perfusion defect is found in multivessel disease (probably the culprit lesion). The accuracy of different tests in the identification of a coronary stenosis depends on the location of the stenosis.

The vast majority of studies on use of perfusion tracers to detect coronary heart disease were performed with Tl 201, but some recent reports summarize experience with Tc 99m MIBI and Tc 99m tetrofosmin and conclude that both tracers have about the same accuracy.[28,29,178,179] In general, comparison of data for sensitivity and specificity among different studies has to take into account not only differences in the camera systems or tracers used, but also the patient populations investigated. For comparison it is of utmost importance to know whether patients were referred to a specialized cardiology unit after previous diagnostic testing or whether the scintigraphic tests were performed in a less homogeneous population.

Several conditions may influence the accuracy of a perfusion test to diagnose coronary heart disease. From a pathophysiological point of view myocardial ischemia is a prerequisite for identification of a relative hypoperfusion. All pharmacological treatments that decrease the extent or prohibit the occurrence of ischemia during a stress test reduce the probability of detecting of coronary heart disease; but, on the other hand, the stress test can be used to document therapeutical success. This limitation includes all anti-ischemic drugs. Radionuclide-perfusion imaging with a stress test may nevertheless be more sensitive in drug-treated patients compared with exercise ECG, because a smaller extent of ischemia in treated patients may be still detectable by quantitative scintigraphy. In patients with premedication that cannot be discontinued for an appropriate time before the exercise test, pharmacological induction of relative regional hypoperfusion by dipyridamole or adenosine may be a helpful alternative.[52,202,203]

Left Bundle Branch Block and Other Limitations

In patients with left bundle branch block, exercise-induced myocardial perfusion defects have frequently been observed in spite of angiographically normal coronary arteries.[204-207] In some cases, pharmacologically induced stress modalities seem to be superior for imaging this condition,[203,208-211] but no large comparative studies are available. It cannot be predicted whether such a defect is present only in the stress study or also in the at-rest perfusion study. Conclusively, only a negative test result in patients with left bundle brunch block can be considered normal. In contrast, a positive finding (especially in the septal/anterior region) does not have a high specificity for the presence of coronary heart disease, and a defect located only in this region does not exclude ischemic heart disease.

Further limitations of perfusion imaging for detection of coronary heart disease include attenuation artifacts. Because perfusion markers give the relative regional perfusion of the left ventricle, regional attenuation artifacts may cause false-positive results. There are two main reasons for such artifacts: attenuation in obese patients and breast attenuation, especially of anterior wall activity in women.[212,213] Even if Tl 201 scans are obtained with additional attenuation correction, such artifacts cannot be excluded. Tc-99m MIBI, which is not so dependent on attenuation because of its physical properties, could be superior in this situation. Another approach to compensate for attenuation artifacts is to position the patient in both a supine and prone position.[31,33] Ongoing studies are examining the clinical impact of compensation for attenuation by using new dedicated software and digital cameras.[214]

Several other conditions may also cause inaccuracy in perfusion stress tests with respect to the diagnosis of coronary heart disease. False-negative results are sometimes obtained if the stress test was not adequate to induce myocardial ischemia or if the patient had anti-ischemic treatment.[215] Other reasons may be a too-delayed start of the scanning (redistribution has already abolished the ischemic defect), interpretation problems, or rare conditions such as balanced hypoperfusion or nonlimiting collateral supply. On the other hand, several conditions such as hypertension, diabetes mellitus, various cardiomyopathies (but not mitral valve prolapse[216p473]), coronary vasospasm, syndrome X, and others may result in false-positive test results.[217-224] The term *false-positive*

for these patients remains a semantic point because many of these patients have disturbances of coronary flow, especially in the small vessels, and a reduced coronary flow reserve, even if an angiographycally detectable coronary heart disease is excluded. The number of such patients in a study population can influence the sensitivity and specificity considerably.

Radionuclide Ventriculography for Detection of Coronary Heart Disease

Radionuclide ventriculography as a first-pass (studies at rest and during exercise) technique and as an equilibrium ECG-gated technique can be performed for detection of coronary heart disease but provide only indirect (functional) assessment of perfusion abnormalities. The exercise ejection fraction is expected to be about 5% higher than the ejection fraction at rest but is affected by several influences.[225-228] Reduction of the ejection fraction during exercise or (depending on the laboratory standard) a failure of the ejection fraction to increase significantly are the main global parameters. Occurrence of exercise-induced local wall motion abnormalities are the regional markers for exercise-induced ischemia. Persistent regional dysfunction during stress and rest studies are indicative of myocardial infarction; however, other pathophysiological circumstances such as hibernation cannot be ruled out with this technique. The numbers for overall sensitivity and specificity for detection of coronary heart disease have been at the lower range of those reported for perfusion agents.[3,151] With the improved, newer perfusion-imaging techniques, the indirect method of radionuclide ventriculography for detection of coronary heart disease has become less important for establishing the diagnosis of ischemic heart disease. Radionuclide ventriculography is—especially with the equilibrium technique, which allows better regional detection of abnormalities—limited by motion artifacts caused by exercise during the relatively long acquisition period for gated studies. Inadequate exercise (because severe ischemia is not tolerated by most patients for a prolonged period of data acquisition) and the performance of exercise in only one view decreases the sensitivity for detection of ischemia in regions that are not directly visualized. Nevertheless, this indirect method for the identification of coronary heart disease has a great prognostic implication because the ejection fraction is strongly correlated with the prognosis.

Radionuclide Tests for Diagnosis of Coronary Heart Disease

As already mentioned, sensitivity and specificity also depend on the prevalence of the disease in the patient population. Test accuracy is better with radionuclide techniques than with a stress ECG test but is not 100%.

Therefore, the applicability of these tests should be critically considered for each individual patient. According to Bayes' theorem, the use of such a test system in a patient with relatively low or relatively high pretest probability for the presence of coronary heart disease would not result in improved post-test information. That means that in a young patient with very little evidence for coronary heart disease a positive test has only a limited predictive value, and a negative test in a patient with very high pre-test probability for coronary heart disease decreases the post-test probability by only a small percentage.[229-234] Thus, such a test is useful only in patients with a medium-range probability for coronary heart disease, in whom the post-test probability can be expected to differ markedly from the pretest probability and have an important impact on the further diagnostic and therapeutic strategy. Aside from the purely diagnostic aspect, a Tl 201 study nevertheless adds further prognostic information because even patients with angiographically proved coronary heart disease and a normal Tl 201 scan or low-risk (small single defect) results after maximum exercise have very good prognosis.[235-239] Thus, quantitative aspects of the Tl 201 study add information beyond the probability of the presence of coronary heart disease. The perfusion scans are additionally valuable for prognostic purposes and the prediction of clinical events besides other clinical diagnostic tests.[233,240-245]

Detection of Myocardial Ischemia in Patients With Known Coronary Artery Disease

The determination of severity and localization of myocardial ischemia in patients with proved coronary artery disease gain increasing importance over testing to establish diagnosis of ischemic heart disease. Nuclear cardiology techniques are used (1) to investigate the hemodynamic relevance of a given stenosis that appears angiographically borderline in the presence of nontypical chest pain or a nondiagnostic exercise ECG test;[182,246,247] (2) for the identification of the "culprit" lesion in patients with multivessel disease, especially if patients have several high-degree stenoses and previous myocardial infarctions; (3) to document effects of therapeutic procedures and reexamine symptomatic patients or patients with pathological stress ECG test results after revascularization.[248-250]

For such problems, SPECT-perfusion scintigraphy is obviously preferable to planar imaging. SPECT studies have an improved segmental resolution (not hampered by overlap of left ventricular regions). A certain stenosis can thus be related to a region of ischemia found in the SPECT scintigraphy, especially if the findings from the coronary angiography are taken into consideration. Putting together the information obtained from the coronary angiography and from the stress-perfusion study, the "target" stenosis for interventions and the he-modynamic relevance of a given stenosis can be identified. A limitation, however, is the dependence of scintigraphy on the presence of ischemia during the stress test. If the stress test has to be terminated due to the occurrence of severe angina pectoris or ST-segment alterations on a low-stress level caused by the most severe coronary artery stenosis of the patient, other stenoses in multivessel disease, which are relevant only at higher levels of exercise, may be missed. It could be asked whether quantitative evaluation of the scintigrams or pharmacological flow maldistribution by adenosine may be more sensitive, but conclusive information from large studies on this problem is not available. As long as gamma camera systems with single-photon imaging tracers with the currently available technologies are used, no quantification of regional myocardial flow (only relative information on the tracer distribution over the left ventricular myocardium) will be obtained. The functional significance of a given coronary stenosis is not very important in patients undergoing coronary bypass grafting (if in these patients all angiographycally significant suitable vessels will be grafted), but it is important in percutaneous transluminal coronary angioplasty that aims to improve patients' symptoms by dilating the ischemia-provoking "culprit" stenosis. Results differ about the suitability of thallium perfusion scintigraphy after percutaneous transluminal coronary angioplasty, but 4 to 10 weeks after coronary angioplasty, the functional outcome of the intervention can be assessed with high accuracy.[251-255] Tc 99m MIBI was also shown to be useful after percutaneous transluminal coronary angioplasty.[256] Similarly, the exercise ejection fraction should be increased after a successful revascularization procedure if the ejection fraction was limited either by exercise-induced ischemia or by hibernating myocardium.[257,258] Perfusion scintigraphy seems to be especially useful in patients after intervention if postrevascularization atypical chest pain is present or develops during follow-up, and the stress ECG results are not diagnostic due to pre-existing ST-T alterations. In those patients, a perfusion stress test may be helpful in guiding further diagnostic and therapeutic strategies.

Myocardial Viability

With the increasing number of revascularization procedures in patients with coronary heart disease and reduced left ventricular function, accurate assessment of myocardial viability is of great interest. In the first decade of perfusion imaging with Tl 201, a rest scintigram performed up to 4 hours after the initial poststress study was regarded as diagnostic for irreversibly injured myocardium (persistent perfusion defect in a delayed study considered as myocardial infarction). With increasing knowledge of the pathophysiology of ischemic heart disease it became obvious that dysfunctional myocardium diagnosed by, for example, contrast ventriculography is not identical with irreversibly injured tissue but may represent entities such as stunned myocardium (postischemic reversibly injured dysfunctional myocardium[259]) and hibernating myocardium (hypoperfused, downregulated, but viable myocardium with the capability to regain contraction upon revascularization[260]). Regions affected, particularly by the latter condition, profit from revascularization; left ventricular function then improves. In hearts with multivessel coronary artery disease and a history of myocardial infarction, exact characterization of the pathophysiological conditions (including the peri-infarct border zone, recurrent ischemia, severity of given stenoses versus collateral supply, and eventually silent periods of ischemia) complicate the assessment of the status of certain left ventricular myocardial segments and demand more information than is required to define only local dysfunction (e.g., contrast cine ventriculography). Measurement of the residual Tl 201 activity provides some information about viability and questions the use of a sharp cut-off between viable and nonviable regions on the Tl 201 scans.[261] The observation of late filling-in on thallium studies delayed up to 24 hours or after reinjection of a smaller amount (usually 1 mCi Tl 201) of the tracer,[9,71,262-264] challenged the concept that the 2- to 4-hour redistribution study correctly identifies the extent of myocardial scarring. Further evidence against the usefulness of early (2- to 4-hour) post-stress Tl 201 scans for correct quantitative identification of myocardial infarction stems from the observation that late filling-in correlates, in selected patient groups, with functional improvement after reperfusion, and with the observation of viable myocardium by metabolic PET imaging in such regions with "fixed" thallium defect.[8]

For correct identification of viable myocardium, different scintigraphic protocols have been examined.[8-12, 70,71,265] With a gamma camera system, Tl 201 is the most suitable viability marker because it has redistribution properties as well as initial distribution in the left ventricular myocardium in relation to the blood flow. For optimal identification of viable myocardium this tracer should be injected at rest in patients who are free of ischemia, and a second redistribution or reinjection/redistribution study several hours later should be performed. In contrast, with Tc 99m MIBI (which, clinically, has no relevant redistribution properties), a possible ischemia at the time of injection may be fixed, or viable myocardial regions with low flow perfusion may not be sufficiently visualized. Thus the feasibility of this agent for delineating viable myocardium is controversial.[18,23, 266,267] Experimental data suggested some redistribution effects after Tc 99m MIBI administration,[22] but their clinical importance is not settled. Use of Tc 99m–based perfusion agents for detection of viability is still considered to be investigational.[138]

Protocols that combine detection of ischemia and identification of viable myocardium usually consist of an initial Tl 201 stress scan followed by a series of either delayed thallium scans (up to 24 hours) or reinjection of about half of the initial dose relatively early, if a substantial defect is present in the first series of images. The majority of Tl 201–positive segments identified with this technique respond to positive inotropic stimulation, indicating viability.[268] Even after reinjection, however, a certain time for redistribution is necessary to obtain optimal results for identification of the extent of viable myocardium.[75]

Radionuclide Tests and Prognosis

Much information regarding the prognosis for patients can be derived from thallium or Tc 99m MIBI studies.[233,240-245,269-273] The size of myocardial infarction is related to prognosis.[274] By visualizing viable and nonviable myocardium, an assessment of infarct size is possible.[275,276] The relation to prognosis was shown for perfusion defect size[277] and for increased Tl 201 lung uptake or occurrence of right ventricular visualization in patients with myocardial infarction.[176,278,279] Similar information has been obtained with radionuclide ventriculography after acute myocardial infarction; it is known that global left ventricular function is correlated to prognosis,[201,275,280-286] especially the ejection fraction during exercise.[284,287] Overall, the extent and severity of ischemia on Tl 201 stress images are related to the extent of coronary heart disease and therefore are also linked to prognosis.[280,288-293] Patients with larger defects imaged by Tl 201 scans have a higher risk for subsequent cardiac events.[290,291,294-296] A similar relation was found for patients at discharge after myocardial infarction.[42,297,298] These findings are in accordance with large comparative studies on sensitivity of thallium perfusion scintigraphy that indicate that patients, in whom the diagnosis of coronary heart disease was missed, had single-vessel disease (whereas a higher sensitivity for ischemia and subsequent diagnosis of coronary heart disease was found in multivessel disease[191,196,299-301]). In contrast, after sufficient stress, a normal Tl 201 study is related to a low rate of cardiac events even if the presence of coronary artery disease is proven angiographically.[237-239,292]

These prognostic aspects make Tl 201 imaging suitable for examination of patients who are undergoing major noncardiac surgery.[47,54,233,302,303] In patient subgroups with increased risk for perioperative cardiac events, especially in patients undergoing operations for diseases of the noncardiac greater vessels, identification of high-risk individuals is of great importance. In the majority of reports,[304-307] but not in all,[308] patients with large defects on Tl 201 scans or with other scintigraphic markers of significant myocardial ischemia had a higher risk compared with those with no or only a small perfusion defect. In patients who are being considered for major noncardiac vascular surgery, an exercise test is often not possible. These patients are typical candidates for a pharmacologic stress test.[257,309,310] Using radionuclide ventriculography, the absolute value of the ejection fraction and of failure of ejection fraction to increase during exercise can also be used as markers for prognosis.[280,287,311]

Nonischemic Myocardial Diseases

Radionuclide techniques can also be used to assess nonischemic cardiac disease. If ventricular systolic or diastolic performance may be involved, radionuclide ventriculography with or without exercise testing provides quantitative information. Perfusion-imaging agents, on the other hand, primarily detect only perfusion defects, which in some ventricular diseases may be associated with increased connective tissue content or circumscribed scarring. Information derived from perfusion markers is, thus, mainly indirect (e.g., enlarged left ventricle), and differentiation between dilated cardiomyopathy and coronary heart disease as the cause for left ventricular dilation by radionuclide techniques is difficult.[257,312–314]

Cardiomyopathy

Cardiomyopathy may be a primary disease or secondary to other causes. If no improvement as a result of reversible transient diseases can be expected, prognosis is mainly related to global left ventricular function.[83,312] Inhomogeneous left ventricular thallium distribution or spotty persisting defects are relatively specific indicators for dilated cardiomyopathy.[218,315] Larger perfusion defects are more common after extended myocardial infarction and, in general, are indicative of so-called ischemic cardiomyopathy.[316] Extensive perfusion defects are also observed in dilated cardiomyopathy, as are reversible defects after a stress study (even if coronary artery disease is angiographically excluded). Such defects are moderately closely related to regional function[317,318] and may be related to an increased connective tissue content.[319] There is some relation between the extent of defects and prognosis in dilated cardiomyopathy.[320,321] In patients with dilated cardiomyopathy, the existence of additional coronary heart disease can be excluded only in the absence of perfusion defects, however, the presence of defects does not provide sufficient further information about the status of the individual coronary arteries. In patients with suspected dilated cardiomyopathy, Tc 99m pyrophosphate, gallium 97 citrate, and In 111 antimyosin scintigraphy have been performed particularly to attempt detection of inflammatory processes, but the results have added little diagnostic information so far.

In patients with active myocarditis, however, In 111 antimyosin scintigraphy was reported to have good specificity combined with low sensitivity.[322] Other myocardial markers have been disappointing in the assessment of myocarditis. Improvement of reduced left ventricular function over time detected by radionuclide ventriculography may also be a strong indicator for a reversible process, as in myocarditis (versus dilated cardiomyopathy).

In secondary cardiomyopathies, for example, in dose-dependent cardiomyopathy after treatment with toxic antineoplastic agents, radionuclide ventriculography is an established tool to monitor the development of cardiotoxicity.[323–325]

In hypertrophic cardiomyopathy, using a Tl 201 test to detect reversible perfusion defects may provide some prognostic information,[221,222,326] but the specificity for coronary heart disease is reduced. Abnormalities in fatty acid metabolism have also been described in these patients.[327,328]

In other diseases that affect the left ventricular myocardium (e.g., systemic sclerosis, amyloidosis, sarcoidosis, and tumors), persistent defects seen with Tl 201 or Tc 99m MIBI scans,[329,330] as well as pathological uptake of Tc 99 pyrophosphate and gallium, can be observed.[331–334] However, the clinical value of radionuclide tests in these conditions has not yet been determined.

Valvular Heart Disease

Radionuclide ventriculography can be used in patients with insufficiency of cardiac valves to quantify the regurgitant fraction. However, this approach is limited if insufficiency of several valves is present. Left ventricular global function and volumes can be determined at rest and during exercise. The usefulness for timing of valve replacement in aortic valve insufficiency has been discussed[335] but not proved in larger studies. However, most of this information can also be obtained by echocardiography. Quantitative data on regurgitation (obtained from the comparison of right and left ventricular stroke counts) is limited by the overlap of heart chambers in diseases with enlargement either of ventricles or atria secondary to valve insufficiency. Tl 201 scintigraphy has been used in patients with valvular heart disease to diagnose concomitant coronary artery disease. Because reversible or persistent defects have been described in patients with valvular heart disease even in the absence of significant coronary artery disease,[336–338] only a negative Tl 201 scan provides information about the absence of significant coronary artery disease. A reversible or fixed defect may also be found in patients without coronary heart disease.[339] However, contradictory results were reported for adenosine–Tl 201 scintigraphy[340] and for dipyridamole–Tc 99m MIBI tests.[341] Studies in patients with decreased left ventricular function and aortic valve insufficiency revealed a spotty defect pattern, as in dilated cardiomyopathy, with Tl 201 SPECT testing.[339]

Other Diseases

Diabetes mellitus and hypertensive heart disease are conditions with an increased risk for coronary heart disease. In these diseases disturbances of myocardial blood flow on the level of the microvasculature are present,[219] and therefore the value of myocardial perfusion scintigraphy to diagnose coronary heart disease positively is limited.[217,224] A negative perfusion scan, however, has a high accuracy in excluding significant coronary heart disease. Radionuclide ventriculography can provide important prognostic information about systolic left ventricular function. Diastolic dysfunction, as frequently present in hypertrophied left ventricles, can be diagnosed[342,343] by abnormal filling indices (peak filling rate and time to peak filling). However, disturbed diastolic filling properties are not specific for hypertrophy but may also be found in restrictive cardiomyopathies and coronary heart disease.[344]

Posttransplantation

In posttransplant hearts, radionuclide ventriculography can be used for determination of left and right ventricular function to detect posttransplant deterioration of left ventricular function. In 111 antimyosin has been proposed as a tool to detect rejection.[345] There was good overall correlation with biopsy findings.[346] As a quantitative marker, the heart-to-lung ratio is useful after transplantation.[345,347,348] For other imaging techniques, such as gallium 67 or In 111–labeled lymphocytes, only preliminary results have been published.[349,350]

Positron Emission Tomography

Radiopharmaceutical Agents and Camera Systems

A large number of tracers have been proposed for clinical PET studies. The most frequently used is fluorine 18 fluorodeoxyglucose (F 18 FDG) to determine myocardial glucose metabolism.[8,351–358] It has the advantage of the relatively long half-life of fluorine 18 (near 2 hours), so it may be transported to PET centers that lack a cyclotron. Other markers for metabolism include fatty acids labeled with carbon 11 (C 11),[359] and C 11 acetate (for assessment of oxidative metabolism[360–362]). Both markers are hampered by the relatively short half-life of 20 minutes for C 11. These tracers therefore can only be used by centers equipped with a cyclotron. Myocardial

perfusion can be measured with oxygen 15 (O 15) water and nitrogen 13 (N 13) ammonia.[363] O 15 water has the advantage of being metabolically inert,[364] whereas trapping of N 13 ammonia may be influenced by metabolic abnormalities.[365] O 15 and N 13 have a half-life of 2 and 10 minutes, respectively, and need a stand-by cyclotron. In contrast rubidium 82 (Rb 82) (half-life of 75 seconds),which can also be used to determine myocardial perfusion, can be delivered from a small on-site generator without a cyclotron. Besides its use in flow imaging, Rb 82 was also examined for use in identification of myocardial viability, compared with Tl 201. In this comparison the smaller defects were observed with PET scans.[366] For research purposes, labeling of receptor ligands and monoclonal antibodies is a promising new technique in PET.

PET equipment has a fixed ring of detectors. The long-axis section window of newer generation scanners is 15 cm wide, allowing imaging of the left ventricle within a single acquisition section. With PET scanners, both simultaneously emitted photons can be detected. This approach has the advantage of coincidence detection of scatter. PET also provides a higher spatial resolution compared with SPECT and a true tissue photon attenuation correction. Therefore, quantification of activity, which can be translated by dedicated computer programs into quantitative measurement of physiological and metabolic processes, is feasible with PET. Unfortunately, costs of a PET center are significantly higher than those of dedicated SPECT systems, but cost-effectiveness with respect to the higher accuracy of PET imaging must also be taken into account.[233] Therefore, many studies are being performed to examine whether the higher costs of PET imaging have a significantly greater impact on diagnostic and therapeutic strategies compared with SPECT imaging. Independent of the cost-related issues, PET imaging is considered to be an advanced and powerful research tool for studies of human physiology and pathophysiology.[367]

Myocardial PET Imaging

Perfusion Imaging

Perfusion imaging with PET to detect coronary heart disease is feasible using dipyridamole as a coronary vasodilator and Rb 82, N 13 ammonia, and O 15 water as perfusion markers. The sensitivity and specificity are slightly higher than with SPECT, being up to 97% and 100%, respectively.[368–371] There are few studies that directly compare Tl 201 SPECT and Rb 82 as perfusion markers for detection of coronary heart disease, but the results have been discussed critically.[139] Because PET is a relatively expensive tool for diagnosis of coronary heart disease,[233] the possible slight improvement in diagnostic accuracy does not justify its use as a primary tool for this purpose. Depending on the local situation, conventional radionuclide studies are also performed less frequently to diagnose coronary heart disease than they are to answer more sophisticated questions such as identification of target lesions and myocardial viability. Measurement of coronary flow reserve can be performed with PET.[372–374] After a standard dose of dipyridamole (0.56 mg/kg intravenously over 4 minutes), a 2.5- to 4-fold increase in coronary flow was reported in volunteers.[365,375] Using Rb 82, a decreased flow reserve was found in hypertrophied myocardium.[376] In patients without angiographic coronary heart disease but typical chest pain, a reduction of the flow reserve with dipyridamole was reported using O 15–labeled water.[377] Similarly a reduction of flow reserve was observed in coronary heart disease.[378] The testing of flow reserve was used for the assessment of the impact of several risk factors for coronary heart disease and for follow-up studies.[379–383]

Tracers of Myocardial Metabolism

F 18 FDG (Figure 17.5) is the most widely used tracer for determination of exogenous glucose utilization, but the uptake is linearly related for utilization only during steady-state conditions and depends on the glucose transporter.[384] Some prerequisites are important to obtain such standard conditions.[16,385–387] Positive F 18 FDG uptake in regions of the left ventricle with severe hypoperfusion diagnosed by perfusion markers is termed *flow-metabolism mismatch,* indicating severely ischemic or hibernating myocardium that is still viable.[388] This mismatch identifies viable dysfunctional myocardium with preserved ability for functional recovery after reperfusion.[357,374,388–391] In contrast, in dysfunctional regions with reduced flow and F 18 FDG uptake (termed *flow-metabolism match*), no functional improvement after revascularization is to be expected. Imaging with F 18 FDG was recently found to be feasible using gamma cameras.[392–394] Examination of myocardial viability has a great impact on therapeutic options and prognosis in patients with coronary heart disease and poor left ventricular function.[395] Further markers for myocardial metabolism are C 11 acetate for oxidative metabolism[396,397] and C 11 palmitate, which were also proposed to identify dysfunctional but viable left ventricular segments.

Additional Tracers

Using other tracers to mark β-adrenergic receptors, to detect hypoxia, and to diagnose other signaling and metabolic pathway defects[398–402] is considered investigational at present.

Left Ventricular Function Evaluation

Using ECG gating and a dedicated computer system, several attempts have been undertaken to determine left ventricular function using PET. A new approach, using a special Fourier-based smoothing and reconstruction, provided promising results in detection of local left ventricular wall motion. With this technique, regional metabolism of F 18 FDG and regional wall motion could be identified in a single set of data. This avoids any transfer problems between different functional and metabolic imaging modalities (e.g., tomography versus left contrast cine ventriculography or echocardiography)[403–405] and makes feasible an assessment of metabolism and function on a segmental level.

Clinical Application

Because PET is not readily available, it is not considered the method of choice for acute coronary syndromes. As discussed, it is a tool for diagnosis of coronary heart disease using pharmacologic vasodilation (or other stress modalities). Most important clinically is the use of PET studies for detection of myocardial viability.[353,356,395, 406–409] The finding that Tl 201–negative and F-18 FDG–positive left ventricular severely dysfunctional regions may regain contractile function upon coronary revascularization and therefore prognosis may be improved challenged the conventional strategies of thallium imaging for diagnosing myocardial scars.[371,410,411] The development of sophisticated Tl 201 protocols has

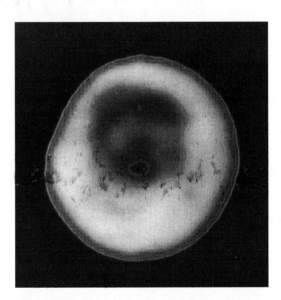

FIGURE 17.5. Polar plot of an F 18 FDG PET scan of a patient with severely compromised left ventricular function and multivessel coronary heart disease. A large central, anteroseptal, and anterolateral zone without tracer uptake is visible, indicating absence of viable myocardium in this left ventricular region (anterobasal is at the top, posterobasal at the bottom, septal at the left, and lateral at the right side of the plot.

improved accurate detection of viable myocardium by using reinjection or rest–redistribution techniques.[8,391,412] Thus, results of PET studies enforced the development of more advanced Tl 201 SPECT protocols to detect myocardial viability accurately. Whether PET F 18 FDG studies can add significantly more clinical information to the results of the more advanced Tl 201 viability studies is still under investigation. Data for other metabolic markers and their diagnostic and prognostic impact are not available from larger prospective studies. Important limitations of the concept of diagnosing viability by radionuclides include the following: (1) the limited spatial resolution does not allow to differentiation of transmural extension and (2) there is a lack of standardization of criteria for determining the transition from "viability" to "nonviability" on the images. Therefore, whether a segment will be considered viable depends on the degree of transmurality of the overall content of scar. Thus a sharp quantitative cut-off is always arbitrary and hampered by false judgements with regard to functional recovery upon reperfusion. Functional recovery is also often incomplete. One reason may be nontransmural or disseminated scarring. Other reasons are related to the "gold standard" of functional recovery: some early restenosis or graft occlusion may occur before severely injured but histologically viable myocardium[413] has regained normal function (or, vice versa, the postrevascularization test is performed prior to recovery of function). The number of periprocedural (smaller or larger) myocardial infarctions (which are not always easy to diagnose), even if the vessel is patent, and the methodological and data transfer problems at the subsegment level between tomographic multislice tracer studies and biplane cine ventriculography limit the value of the "gold standard." These points may provide some biological and methodological explanations for why 100% predictive accuracy of functional recovery as proof of viability cannot be expected. New techniques, which make subsegmental functional examination from the F 18 FDG data set itself feasible, will in the near future reduce some of these problems.[403,405]

Because of its physical properties, PET has advantages over SPECT in all patients in whom attenuation problems may play a role, especially if breast attenuation artifacts or attenuation artifacts in the posterior wall are presumed in the study of a patient. This problem is of importance especially in patients with dilated left ventricles and severe dysfunction. In such patients PET may be clinically preferable for the accurate diagnosis of left ventricular perfusion and myocardial viability.

PET is today a rapidly developing field in nuclear cardiology. With each generation of cameras the spatial resolution increases. With dedicated and standardized computer programs able to quantify regional flow and metabolism, especially if information on regional func-

tion can be added, a comprehensive set of data is provided, which in future may strengthen the impact of PET in the routine clinical diagnostic and therapeutic strategies in ischemic and nonischemic heart disease. Most applications of PET are still investigational but provide stimulating insights into ischemic heart disease and into metabolic and receptor-related disorders in several cardiac diseases.

Acknowledgment

The author wishes to thank Prof. Dr. Bares, Prof. Dr. Feine, and Prof. Dr. Müller-Schauenburg (Department of Nuclear Medicine) for their excellent cooperation and especially for their critical advice and the provision of figures for this chapter.

References

1. Nielson AP, Morritz KG, Murdock R, et al. Linear relationship between the distribution of thallium-201 and blood flow in ischemic and nonischemic myocardium during exercise. *Circulation*. 1980;61:769–772.
2. Weich HF, Strauss HW, Pitt B. The extraction of thallium-201 by the myocardium. *Circulation*. 1977;56:188–191.
3. Iskandrian AD, Verani MS. *Nuclear Cardiac Imaging: Principles and Applications*. Philadelphia, Pa: FA Davis; 1996.
4. Weiss AT, Maddahi J, Lew AS, et al. Reverse redistribution of thallium-201. A sign of nontransmural myocardial infarction with patency of the infarct-related coronary artery. *J Am Coll Cardiol*. 1986;7:61–67.
5. Leppo JA, O'Brien J, Rothendler JA, Getchell JD, Lee VW. Dipyridamole-thallium-201 scintigraphy in the prediction of future cardiac events after acute myocardial infarction. *N Engl J Med*. 1984;310:1014–1018.
6. Liu P, Burns RJ. Easy come, easy go: time to pause and put thallium reverse redistribution in perspective. *J Nucl Med*. 1993;34:1692–1694.
7. Marin-Neto JA, Dilsizian V, Arrighi JA, et al. Thallium reinjection demonstrates viable myocardium in regions with reverse redistribution. *Circulation*. 1993;88:1736–1745.
8. Bonow RO, Dilsizian V, Cuocolo A, Bacharach SI. Identification of viable myocardium in patients with chronic coronary artery disease and left ventricular dysfunction: comparison of thallium scintigraphy with reinjection and PET imaging with F-18 fluorodeoxyglucose. *Circulation*. 1991; 83:26–37.
9. Dilsizian V, Rocco TP, Freedman NMT, Leon MB, Bonow RO. Enhanced detection of ischemic but viable myocardium by the reinjection of thallium after stress-redistribution imaging.*N Engl J Med*. 1990;323:141–146.
10. Dilsizian V, Smeltzer WR, Freedman NT, Dextras R, Bonow RO. Thallium reinjection after stress-redistribution imaging: does 24-hour delayed imaging following reinjection enhance detection of viable myocardium? *Circulation*. 1991;83:1247–1255.
11. Dilsizian V, Bonow RO. Differential uptake and apparent Tl-201 washout after thallium reinjection: options regard-

ing early redistribution imaging before reinjection or late redistribution imaging after reinjection. *Circulation.* 1992; 85:1032–1038.

12. Dilsizan V, Freedman NT, Bacharach SL Perrone-Filardi P, Bonow RO. Regional thallium uptake in irreversible defects: magnitude of change in thallium activity after reinjection distinguishes viable from nonviable myocardium. *Circulation.* 1992;85:627–634.

13. Wackers FJT, Berman DS, Maddahi J, et al. Technetium-99m hexakis 2-methoxyisobutyl isonitrile: human biodistribution, dosimetry, safety, and preliminary comparison of thallium-201 for myocardial perfusion imaging. J *Nucl Med.* 1989;30:301–311.

14. Glover DK, Ruiz M, Edwards NC, et al. Comparison between thallium-201 and Tc-99m sestamibi uptake during adenosine-induced vasodilation as a function of coronary stenosis severity. *Circulation.* 1995;91:813–820.

15. Melon PG, Beanlands RS, Degrado TR, Nguyen N, Petry NA, Schwaiger M. Comparison of technetium-99m sestamibi and thallium-201 retention characteristics in canine myocardium. *J Am Coll Cardiol.* 1992;20:1277–1283.

16. Marshall RC, Leidholdt EM, Zhang DY, Barnett CA. Technetium-99m hexakis 2-methoxy-2-isobutyl isonitrile and thallium-201 extraction, washout, and retention at varying coronary flow rates in rabbit heart. *Circulation.* 1990; 82:998–1007.

17. Chua T, Kiat H, Germano G, et al. Gated technetium-99m sestamibi for simultaneous assessment of stress myocardial perfusion, postexercise regional ventricular function and myocardial viability. *J Am Coll Cardiol.* 1994;23:1107–1114.

18. Dilsizian V, Arrighi JA, Diodati JG, et al. Myocardial viability in patients with chronic coronary artery disease. *Circulation.* 1994;89:578–587.

19. Kauffman GJ, Boyne TS, Watson DD, Smith WH, Beller GA. Comparison of rest thallium-201 imaging and rest technetium-99m sestamibi imaging for assessment of myocardial viability in patients with coronary artery disease and severe left ventricular dysfunction. *J Am Coll Cardiol.* 1996;27:1592–1597.

20. Marzullo P, Sambuceti G, Parodi O. The role of sestamibi scintigraphy in the radioisotopic assessment of myocardial viability. *J Nucl Med.* 1992;33:1925–1930.

21. Maurea S, Cuocolo A, Pace L, et al. Left ventricular dysfunction in coronary artery disease: comparison between rest-redistribution thallium-201 and resting technetium 99m methoxyisobutyl isonitrile cardiac imaging. *J Nucl Cardiol.* 1994;1:165.

22. Sinusas AJ, Bergin JD, Edwards NC, et al. Redistribution of Tc-99m sestamibi and Tl-201 in the presence of a severe coronary artery stenosis. *Circulation.* 1994;89:2332–2341.

23. Udelson JE, Coleman PS, Metherall J, et al. Predicting recovery of severe regional ventricular dysfunction. *Circulation.* 1994;89:2552–2561.

24. DiRocco RJ, Rumsey WL, Kuczynski BL, et al. Measurement of myocardial blood flow using a co-injection technique for technetium-99m teboroxime, technetium-96-sestamibi and thallium-201. *J Nucl Med.* 1992;33:1152–1159.

25. Stewart RE, Heyl B, O'Rourke RA, Blumhardt R, Miller DD. Demonstration of differential post-stenotic myocardial technetium-99m teboroxime clearance kinetics after experimental ischemia and hyperemia stress. *J Nucl Med.* 1991;32:2000–2008.

26. Seldin DW, Johnson LL, Blood D, et al. Myocardial perfusion imaging with technetium-99m SQ30217: comparison with thallium-201 and coronary anatomy. *J Nucl Med.* 1989;30:312–319.

27. Bisi G, Sciargrà R, Santoro GM, Zerauschek F, Fazzini PF. Sublingual isosorbide dinitrate to improve technetium-99m teboroxime perfusion defect reversibility. *J Nucl Med.* 1994;35:1274–1278.

28. Rigo P, Leclercq B, Itti R, Lakini A, Braat S. Technetium-99m-tetrofosmin myocardial imaging: a comparison with thallium-201 and angiography. *J Nucl Med.* 1994;35: 587–593.

29. Zaret BL, Rigo P, Wackers FJT, et al. Myocardial perfusion imaging with Tc-99m tetrofosmin. *Circulation.* 1995;91: 313–319.

30. Marie PY, Angioi M, Danchin N, et al. Assessment of myocardial viability in patients with previous myocardial infarction by using single-photon emission computed tomography with a new metabolic tracer [123]I-16-iodo-3-Methylhexadecanoic acid (MIHA). *J Am Coll Cardiol.* 1997; 30:1241–1248.

31. Esquerre JP, Coca FJ, Martinez SJ, Guiraud RF. Prone decubitus: a solution to inferior wall attenuation in thallium-201 myocardial tomography. *J Nucl Med.* 1989;30:398–401.

32. O'Connor MK, Bothun ED. Effects of tomographic table attenuation on prone and supine cardiac imaging. *J Nucl Med.* 1995;36:1102–1106.

33. Segal GM, Davis MJ. Prone versus supine thallium myocardial SPECT: a method to decrease artifactual inferior wall defects. *J Nucl Med.* 1989;30:548–555.

34. Suzuki A, Muto S, Oshima M, et al. A new scanning method for thallium-201 myocardial SPECT: semi-decubital position method. *Clin Nucl Med.* 1989;14:736–741.

35. Nohara R, Kambara H, Suzuki Y. Stress scintigraphy using single-photon emission computed tomography in the evaluation of coronary artery disease. *Am J Cardiol.* 1984;53: 1250–1254.

36. Gottschalk SC, Salem D, Lim CB, Wake RH. SPECT resolution and uniformity improvements by noncircular orbit. *J Nucl Med.* 1983;24:822–828.

37. Coleman RE, Jaszczak RJ, Cobb FR. Comparison of 180 degree and 360 degree data collection in thallium-201 imaging using single-photon emission computerized tomography (SPECT): concise communication. *J Nucl Med.* 1982; 23:655–660.

38. Bateman T, Garcia E, Maddahi J, et al. Clinical evaluation of sevenpinhole tomography for the detection and localization of coronary artery disease: comparison with planar imaging using quantitative analysis of myocardial thallium-201 distribution and washout after exercise. *Am Heart J.* 1983;106:263–271.

39. Massie BM, Wisneski JA, Hollenberg M, Gertz EW, Henderson S. Quantitative analysis of seven-pinhole tomographic thallium-201 scintigrams: improved sensitivity and estimation of the extent of coronary involvement by evaluation of radiotracer uptake and clearance. *J Am Coll Cardiol.* 1984;3:1178–1186.

40. Dahlberg ST, Leppo JA. Physiologic properties of myocardial perfusion tracers. *Cardiol Clin.* 1994;12:169–185.

41. Bateman TM, Maddahi J, Gray RJ, et al. Diffuse slow washout of myocardial thallium-201: a new scintigraphic indicator of extensive coronary artery disease. *J Am Coll Cardiol.* 1984;4:55–64.

42. Gerwitz H, Paladino W, Sullivan M, Most AS. Value and limitations of myocardial thallium washout rate in the noninvasive diagnosis of patients with triple-vessel coronary artery disease. *Am Heart J.* 1983;106:681–686.

43. Sklar J, Kirch D, Johnson T, Hasegawa B, Peck S, Steele P. Slow late myocardial clearance of thallium: a characteristic phenomenon in coronary artery disease. *Circulation.* 1982;65:1504–1510.

44. Vaduganathan P, He ZX, Raghavan C, Mahmarian JJ, Verani MS. Detection of left anterior descending coronary artery stenosis in patients with left bundle branch block: exercise, adenosine or dobutamine imaging. *J Am Coll Cardiol.* 1996;28:543–550.

45. Albro PC, Gould KL, Westcott RJ, Hamilton GW, Ritchie JL, Williams DL. Noninvasive assessment of coronary stenoses by myocardial imaging during pharmacologic coronary vasodilation, III: clinical trial. *Am J Cardiol.* 1978;42:751–760.

46. Coyne EB, Belvedere DA, Vande Streek PR, Weiland FL, Evans RB, Spaccavento LJ. Thallium-201 scintigraphy after intravenous infusion of adenosine compared with exercise thallium testing in the diagnosis of coronary artery disease. *J Am Coll Cardiol.* 1991;17:1289–1294.

47. Emlein G, Villegas B, Dahlberg S, Leppo J. Left ventricular cavity size determined by preoperative dipyridamole thallium scintigraphy as a predictor of late cardiac events in vascular surgery patients. *Am Heart J.* 1996;131:907–914.

48. Glover DK, Ruiz M, Bergmann EE, et al. Myocardial technetium-99m-teboroxime uptake during adenosine-induced hyperemia in dogs with either a critical or mild coronary stenosis: comparison to thallium-201 and regional blood flow. *J Nucl Med.* 1995;36:476–483.

49. Gould KL. Noninvasive assessment of coronary stenoses by myocardial perfusion imaging during pharmacologic coronary vasodilatation: physiologic basis and experimental validation. *Am J Cardiol.* 1978;41:267–278.

50. Gould KL, Westcott RJ, Albro PC, Hamilton GW. Noninvasive assessment of coronary stenosis by myocardial imaging during pharmacologic coronary vasodilatation, II: clinical methodology and feasibility. *Am J Cardiol.* 1978; 41:279–287.

51. Kumar EB, Steel SA, Howey S, Caplin JL, Aber CP. Dipyridamole is superior to dobutamine for thallium stress imaging: a randomised crossover study. *British Heart Journal.* 1994;71:129–134.

52. Marwick T, Willemart B, D'Hondt AMD, et al. Selection of the optimal nonexercise stress for the evaluation of ischemic regional myocardial dysfunction and malperfusion. *Circulation.* 1982;87:345–354.

53. Nguyen T, Heo J, Ogilby JD, Iskandrian AS. Single-photon emission computed tomography with thallium-201 during adenosine-induced coronary hyperemia: correlation with coronary arteriography, exercise thallium imaging and two-dimensional echocardiography. *J Am Coll Cardiol.* 1990;16:1375–1383.

54. Stratmann HG, Younis LT, Wittry MD, Amato M, Miller DD. Dipyridamole technetium-99m sestamibi myocardial tomography in patients evaluated for elective vascular surgery: prognostic value for perioperative and late cardiac event. *Am Heart J.* 1996;31:923–929.

55. Verani MS, Mahmarian JJ, Hixson JB, Boyce TM, Staudacher RA. Diagnosis of coronary artery disease by controlled coronary vasodilation with adenosine and thallium-201 scintigraphy in patients unable to exercise. *Circulation.* 1990;82:80–87.

56. Nishimura S, Mahmarian JJ, Boyce TM, Verani MS. Quantitative thallium-201 single-photon emission computed tomography during maximal pharmacologic coronary vasodilation with adenosine for assessing coronary artery disease. *J Am Coll Cardiol.* 1991;18:736–745.

57. Wackers FJT. Myocardial perfusion imaging. In: Gottschalk A, Hoffer PB, Potchen EJ, eds. *Diagnostic Nuclear Medicine.* 2nd ed. Baltimore, Md: Williams & Wilkins; 1988.

58. Nallamothu N, Araujo L, Russell J, Geo J, Iskandrian AE. Prognostic value of simultaneous perfusion and function assessment using Tc-99m sestamibi. *Am J Cardiol.* 1996; 78:562–563.

59. Garcia E, Maddahi J, Berman DS, Waxman A. Space/time quantitation of thallium-201 myocardial scintigraphy. *J Nucl Med.* 1981;22:309–317.

60. Wackers FJ, Fetterman RC, Mattera JA, Clements JP. Quantitative planar thallium-201 stress scintigraphy: a critical evaluation of the method. *Semin Nucl Med.* 1985;15:46–66.

61. Reisman S, Maddahi J, van Train K, Garcia E, Berman D. Quantitation of extent, depth, and severity of planar thallium defects in patients undergoing exercise thallium-201 scintigraphy. *J Nucl Med.* 1986;27:1273–1281.

62. Akinboboye OO, Haines FA, Atkins HL, Oster ZH, Brown EJ. Assessment of left ventricular enlargement from planar thallium-201 images. *Am Heart J.* 1994;127:148-151.

63. Weiss AT, Berman DS, Lew AS, et al. Transient ischemic dilation of the left ventricle on stress thallium-201 scintigraphy: a marker of severe and extensive coronary artery disease. *J Am Coll Cardiol.* 1987;9:752–759.

64. Boucher CA, Zir LM, Beller GA, et al. Increased lung uptake of thallium-201 during exercise myocardial imaging: clinical, hemodynamic and angiographic implications in patients with coronary artery disease. *Am J Cardiol.* 1980; 46:189–196.

65. Nishimura S, Mahmarian JJ, Verani MS. Significance of increased lung thallium uptake during adenosine thallium-201 scintigraphy. *J Nucl Med.* 1992;33:1600–1607.

66. Friedman J, Van Train K, Maddahi J, et al. "Upward creep" of the heart: a frequent source of false-positive reversible defects during thallium-201 stress-distribution SPECT. *J Nucl Med.* 1989;30:1718-1722.

67. Galli M, Marcassa C. Thallium-201 redistribution after early reinjection in patients with severe stress perfusion defects and ventricular dysfunction. *Am Heart J.* 1994; 128:41–52.

68. Van Eck-Smit BLF, Van Der Wall EE, Zwinderman AH, Pauwels EK. Clinical value of immediate thallium-201 reinjection imaging for the detection of ischaemic heart disease. *Eur Heart J.* 1995;16:410–420.

69. Charney R, Schwinger ME, Chun J, et al. Dobutamine echocardiography and resting-redistribution thallium-201 scintigraphy predicts recovery of hibernating myocardium after coronary revascularization. *Am Heart J.* 1994;128: 864–869.

70. Dilsizian V, Perrone-Filardi P, Arrighi JA, et al. Concordance and discordance between stress-redistribution-reinjection and rest-redistribution thallium imaging for assessing viable myocardium. *Circulation.* 1993;88:941–952.

71. Rocco TP, Dilsizian V, McKusick KA, Fischman AJ, Boucher CA, Strauss HW. Comparison of thallium redistribution with rest "reinjection" imaging for the detection of viable myocardium. *Am J Cardiol.* 1990;66:158–163.

72. Galli M, Marcassa C, Imparato A, Campini R, Orrego PS, Giannuzzi P. Effects of nitroglycerin by technetium-99m sestamibi tomoscintigraphy on resting regional myocardial hypoperfusion in stable patients with healed myocardium infarction. *Am J Cardiol.* 1994;74:843–848.

73. Berman DS, Kiat HS, Van Train KF, Germano G, Maddahi J, Friedman JD. Myocardial perfusion imaging with technetium-99m sestamibi: comparative analysis of available imaging protocols. *J Nucl Med.* 1994;35:681–688.

74. Taillefer R, Laflamme L, Durpas G, Picard M, Phaneuf DC, Leveille J. Myocardial perfusion imaging with Tc-99m methoxy-isobutyl-isonitrile (MIBI): comparison of short and long time intervals between rest and stress injections. *Eur J Nucl Med.* 1988;13:515–522.

75. Helber U, Fenchel G, Müller-Schauenburg W, Hoffmeister HM. Effect of the redistribution time after reinjection on quantification of viable myocardium in multi-vessel coronary disease: comparison with post-revascularization defect size [abstract]. *Circulation.* 1994;90:1961.

76. Johnson LL. Myocardial perfusion imaging of a flow tracer: clinical experience with teboroxime. In: Zaret BL, Beller GA, eds. *Nuclear Cardiology–State of the Art and Future Directions.* St Louis, Mo: CV Mosby, 1993:209–215.

77. ACC/AHA Task Force. Guidelines for the early management of patients with acute myocardial infarction. *J Am Coll Cardiol.* 1996;28:1328–1428.

78. Gibson RJ, Verani MS, Behrenbeck T, et al. Feasibility of tomographic Tc-99m hexakis-2-methoxy-2-methylpropyl-isonitrile imaging for the assessment of myocardial area at risk and the effect of treatment in acute myocardial infarction. *Circulation.* 1989;80:1277–1286.

79. Santoro GM, Bisi G, Sciaga R, Leoncini M, Fazzini PF, Meldolesi U. Single photon emission computed tomography with technetium-99m hexakis 2-methoxy isobutyl isonitrile in acute myocardial infarction before and after thrombolytic treatment: assessment of salvaged myocardium and prediction of late functional recovery. *J Am Coll Cardiol.* 1990;15:301–314.

80. Sinusas AJ, Trautmann KA, Bergin JD, et al. Quantification of area at risk during coronary occlusion and degree of myocardial salvage after reperfusion with technetium-99m methoxyisobutyl isonitrile. *Circulation.* 1990;82: 1424–1437.

81. Verani MS, Jeroudi MO, Mahmarian JJ, et al. Quantification of myocardial infarction during coronary occlusion and myocardial salvage after reperfusion using cardiac imaging with technetium-99m hexakis-2-methoxyisobutyl isonitrile. *J Am Coll Cardiol.* 1988;12:1573–1581.

82. Wackers FJT, Gibbons RJ, Verani MS, et al. Serial quantitative planar technetium-99m isonitrile imaging in acute myocardial infarction: efficacy for noninvasive assessment of thrombolytic therapy. *J Am Coll Cardiol.* 1989;14:861–873.

83. Burdine JA, DePuey G, Orzan F, Mathur VS, Hay RJ. Scintigraphic, electrocardiographic, and enzymatic diagnosis of perioperative myocardial infarction in patients undergoing myocardial revascularization. *J Nucl Med.* 1979;20: 711–714.

84. Klausner SC, Botvinick EH, Shames D, et al. The application of radionuclide infarct scintigraphy to diagnose perioperative myocardial infarction following revascularization. *Circulation.* 1977;56:173–181.

85. Righetti A, Crawford MH, O'Rourke RA, et al. Detection of perioperative myocardial damage after coronary artery bypass graft surgery. *Circulation.* 1977;55:173–178.

86. Rude RE, Parkey RW, Bonte FJ, et al. Clinical implications of the technetium-99m stannous pyrophosphate myocardial scintigraphic "doughnut" pattern in patients with acute myocardial infarcts. *Circulation.* 1979;59:721–730.

87. Coleman RE, Klein MS, Roberts R, Sobel BE. Improved detection of myocardial infarction with technetium-99m stannous pyrophosphate and serum MB creatine phosphokinase. *Am J Cardiol.* 1976;37:732–735.

88. Corbett JR, Lewis M, Willerson JT, et al. 99m-Tc-pyrophosphate imaging in patients with acute myocardial infarction: comparison of planar imaging with single-photon tomography with and without blood pool overlay. *Circulation.* 1984;69:1120–1128.

89. Massie BM, Botvinick EH, Werner JA, Chatterjee K, Parmley WW. Myocardial scintigraphy with technetium-99m stannous pyrophosphate: an insensitive test for nontransmural myocardial infarction. *Am J Cardiol.* 1979;43: 186–192.

90. Johnson LL, Seldin DW, Becker LC, et al. Antimyosin imaging in acute transmural myocardial infarction: results of a multicenter clinical trial. *J Am Coll Cardiol.* 1989;13: 27–35.

91. Ouzan J, Metz D, Jolly D, Liehn JC, Elaerts J. What factors determine indium-111 antimyosin monoclonal antibody uptake in patients with myocardial infarction. *Int J Cardiol.* 1993;40:257–263.

92. Asano H, Sone T, Tsuboi H, et al. Diagnosis of right ventricular infarction by overlap images of simultaneous dual emission computed tomography using technetium-99m pyrophosphate and thallium-201. *Am J Cardiol.* 1993;71: 902–908.

93. Schofer J, Spielman RP, Brömel T, Bleifeld W, Mathey DG. Thallium-201/technetium-99m pyrophosphate overlap in patients with acute myocardial infarction after thrombolysis: prediction of depressed wall motion despite thallium uptake. *Am Heart J.* 1986;112:291–295.

94. Johnson LL, Seldin DW, Keller AM, et al. Dual isotope thallium and indium antimyosin SPECT imaging to identify acute infarct patients at further ischemic risk. *Circulation.* 1990;81:37–45.

95. Olson HG, Lyons KP, Aronow WS, Stinson PJ, Kuperus J,

Waters HJ. The high-risk angina patient: identification by clinical features, hospital course, electrocardiography and technetium-99m stannous pyrophosphate scintigraphy. *Circulation.* 1981;64:674–684.

96. Goldman L, Cook EF, Johnson PA, Brand DA, Ronan GW, Lee TH. Prediction of the need for intensive care in patients who come to emergency departments with acute chest pain. *N Engl J Med.* 1996;334:1498–1504.

97. Hilton TC, Thompson RC, Williams HJ, et al. Technetium-989-sestamibi myocardial perfusion imaging in the emergency room evaluation of chest pain. *J Am Coll Cardiol.* 1994;23:1016–1022.

98. Ohman EM, Armstrong PW, Christenson RH, et al. Cardiac troponin T levels for risk stratification in acute myocardial ischemia. *N Engl J Med.* 1996;335:1333–1341.

99. Varetto T, Cantalupi D, Altiero A, Orlandi C. Emergency room technetium-99m-sestamibi imaging to rule out acute myocardial ischemic events in patients with nondiagnostic electrocardiograms. *J Am Coll Cardiol.* 1993;22:1804–1808.

100. Hansen CI, Corbett JR, Pippin JJ, et al. Iodine-123-phenylpentadecanoic acid and single photon emission computed tomography in identifying left ventricular regional metabolic abnormalities in patients with coronary heart disease: Comparison with thallium-201 tomography. *J Am Coll Cardiol.* 1988;12:78–87.

101. Kahn JK, Pippin JJ, Akers MS, Corbett JR. Estimation of jeopardized left ventricular myocardium in symptomatic and silent ischemia as determined by iodine-123 phenylpentadecanoic acid rotational tomography. *Am J Cardiol.* 1989;63:540–544.

102. Kennedy PL, Corbett JR, Kulkarni PV, et al. Iodine-123 phenylpentadecanoic acid myocardial scintigraphy. Usefulness in the identification of myocardial ischemia. *Circulation.* 1986;74:1007–1015.

103. Walamies M, Turjanmaa V, Koskinen M, Uusitalo A. Diagnostic value of I-123 phenylpentadecanoic acid (IPPA) metabolic and thallium-201 perfusion imaging in stable coronary artery disease. *Eur Heart J.* 1993;14:1079–1087.

104. Van der Wall EE, Heidendal GA, den Hollander W, Westera G, Roos JP. I-123 labeled hexadecanoic acid in comparison with thallium-201 for myocardial imaging in coronary heart disease. *Eur J Nucl Med.* 1980;5:401–405.

105. Machulla HJ, Marsmann M, Dutschka K. I-131-(phenyl)-pentadecanoic acid, a highly promising radioiodinated fatty acid for myocardial studies, I: development of synthesis and radiopharmaceutical quality. *Radioactive Isotope in Klinik und Forschung.* Vienna, Austria: H Engerman. 1980;14:363–368.

106. Machulla HJ, Marsmann M, Dutschka K. Biochemical concept and synthesis of radioiodinated phenyl fatty acid for in vivo metabolic studies of myocardium. *Eur J Nucl Med.* 1980;5:171.

107. Machulla HJ, Marsmann M, Dutschka K. Radiopharmaceuticals: synthesis of radioiodinated phenyl fatty acids for studying myocardial metabolism. *Journal of Radioanalytical Chemistry.* 1980;56:253–261.

108. Machulla HJ, Knust EJ, Vyska K. Radioiodinated fatty acids for cardiological diagnosis. *International Journal of Radiation Applications and Instrumentation.* 1986;37:777–788.

109. Reske SN, Sauer W, Machulla HJ, Winkler C. 15(p-[I-123] iodophenyl) pentadecanoic acid as a tracer of lipid metabolism: comparison with [14-C] palmitic acid in murine tissues. *J Nucl Med.* 1984;25:1335–1342.

110. Vyska K, Machulla HJ, Stremmel W, et al. Regional myocardial free fatty acid extraction in normal and ischemic myocardium. *Circulation.* 1988;78:1218–1233.

111. Dae MW, O'Connell JW, Botvinick EH, et al. Scintigraphic assessment of regional cardiac adrenergic innervation. *Circulation.* 1989;79:634–644.

112. McGhie AI, Corbett JR, Akers MS, et al. Regional cardiac adrenergic function using I-123 meta-iodobenzylguanidine tomographic imaging after acute myocardial infarction. *Am J Cardiol.* 1991;67:236–242.

113. Stanton MS, Tuli MM, Radtke NL, et al. Regional sympathetic denervation after myocardial infarction in human detected noninvasively using I-123-metaiodobenzylguanidine. *J Am Coll Cardiol.* 1989;14:1519–1526.

114. Glowniak JV, Turner FE, Gray LL, Palace RT, Lagunas-Solar MC, Woodward WR. Iodine-123 metaiodobenzylguanidine imaging of the heart in idiopathy congestive cardiomyopathy and cardiac transplants. *J Nucl Med.* 1989;30:1182–1191.

115. Henderson EB, Kahn JK, Corbett JR, et al. Abnormal I-123 metaiodobenzylguanidine myocardial washout and distribution may reflect myocardial adrenergic derangement in patients with congestive cardiomyopathy. *Circulation.* 1988;78:1192–1199.

116. Schofer J, Spielman, R, Schuchert A, Weber K, Schlüter M. Iodine-123 metaiodobenzylguanidine scintigraphy: a noninvasive method to demonstrate myocardial adrenergic nervous system distegrity in patients with idiopathic dilated cardiomyopathy. *J Am Coll Cardiol.* 1988;12:1252–1258.

117. Nakajo M, Shapiro B, Glowniak J, Sisson JC, Beierwaltes WH. Inverse relationship between cardiac accumulation of METAP [I-131] iodobenzylguanidine (I-131 MIBG) and circulating catecholamines in suspected pheochromocytomas. *J Nucl Med.* 1983;24:1127–1134.

118. Kreiner G, Wolzt M, Fasching P, et al. Myocardial I-123m iodobenzylguanidine scintigraphy for the assessment of adrenergic cardiac innervation in patients with IDDM. *Diabetes.* 1995;44:543–549.

119. Mitrani RD, Klein LS, Miles WM, Hackett FK, Burt RW, Wellman HN. Regional cardiac sympathetic denervation in patients with ventricular tachycardia in the absence of coronary artery disease. *J Am Coll Cardiol.* 1993;22:1344–1353.

120. Wichter T, Hindricks G, Lerch H, et al. Regional myocardial sympathetic dysinnervation in arrhythmogenic right ventricular cardiomyopathy. *Circulation.* 1994;89:667–683.

121. Ezekowitz MD, Leonard JC, Smith ED, Allen EW, Taylor FB. Identification of left ventricular thrombi in man using indium-111 labeled autologous platelets. *Circulation.* 1981;63:803–810.

122. Ezekowitz MD, Wilson DA, Smith EO, et al. Comparison of indium-111 platelet scintigraphy and two-dimensional echocardiography in diagnosis of left ventricular thrombi. *N Engl J Med.* 1982;306:1509–1513.

123. Ezekowitz MD, Burow RD, Heath PW, Streitz T, Smith EO, Parker DE. Diagnostic accuracy of indium-111 platelet scintigraphy in identifying left ventricular thrombi. *Am J Cardiol.* 1983;51:1712–1716.

124. Ezekowitz MD, Smith EO, Rankin R, Harrison LH, Krous HF. Left atrial mass: diagnostic value of transesophgageal two-dimensional echocardiography and indium-111 platelet scintigraphy. *Am J Cardiol.* 1983;51:1563–1564.

125. Ezekowitz MD, Kellerman DJ, Smith EO, Streitz TM. Detection of active left ventricular thrombosis during acute myocardial infarction using indium-111 platelet scintigraphy. *Chest.* 1984;86:35–39.

126. Nishimura T, Misawa T, Park YD, Ühara T, Hayashida K, Hayasti M. Visualization of right atrial thrombus associated with constrictive pericarditis by indium-111 oxine platelet imaging. *J Nucl Med.* 1987;28:1344.

127. Stratton JR, Ritchie JL. In-111 platelet imaging of left ventricular thrombi: predictive value for systemic emboli. *Circualtion.* 1990;81:1182–1189.

128. Vandenberg BF, Deabold JE, Conrad GR, et al. In-111 labeled platelet scintigraphy and two dimensional echocardiography for detection of left atrial appendage thrombi: studies in a new canine model. *Circulation.* 1988;78:1040–1046.

129. Bergmann SR, Lerch RA, Mathias CJ, Sobel BE, Welch MJ. Noninvasive detection of coronary thrombi in In-111 platelets: concise communication. *J Nucl Med.* 1983;24:130–135

130. Fox KAA, Bergmann SR, Mathias CJ, et al. Scintigraphic detection of coronary artery thrombi in patients with acute myocardial infarction. *J Am Coll Cardiol.* 1984;4:975–986.

131. Pope CF, Ezekowitz MD, Smith EO, et al. Detection of platelet deposition at the site of peripheral balloon angioplasty using indium-111 platelet scintigraphy. *Am J Cardiol.* 1985;55:495–497.

132. Riba AL, Thakur ML, Gottschalk A, Zaret BL. Imaging experimental coronary artery thrombosis with indium-111 platelets. *Circulation.* 1979;60:767–775.

133. Bergmann SR, Lerch RA, Carlson EM, Saffitz JE, Sobel BE. Detection of cardiac transplant rejection with radiolabeled lymphocytes. *Circulation.* 1982;65:591–595.

134. McKillop JH, Wallwork J, Reitz BA, et al. The use of In-111-labeled lymphocyte imaging to evaluate graft rejection following cardiac transplantation in dogs. *Eur J Nucl Med.* 1982;7:162–165.

135. Lees AM, Lees RS, Schön FJ. Imaging human atherosclerosis with Tc-99m labeled low-density lipoprotein in human subjects. *Arteriosclerosis.* 1988;8:461–470.

136. Rosen JM, Butler SP, Meinken GE, et al. Indium-111-labelled LDL: a potential agent for imaging atherosclerotic disease and lipoprotein disease and lipoprotein biodistribution. *J Nucl Med.* 1990;31:343–350.

137. Sinzinger H, Virgolini I. Nuclear medicine and atherosclerosis. *Eur J Nucl Med.* 1990;17:160–178.

138. ACC/AHA Task Force Report. Guidelines for clinical use of cardiac radionuclide imaging. *Circulation.* 1995:91:1278–1303.

139. Dymond DS, Elliot A, Stone D, Hendrix G, Spurrell R. Factors that affect the reproducibility of measurments of left ventricular function from first-pass radionuclide ventriculograms. *Circulation.* 1982;65:311–322.

140. Baillet G, Mena IG, Kuperus JH, Robertson JM, French WJ. Simultaneous technetium-99m MIBI angiography and myocardial perfusion imaging. *J Nucl Med.* 1989;30:38–44.

141. Iskandrian AS, Heo J, Kong HJ, Lyons E, Marsch S. Use of technetium-99m isonitrile (RP-30A) in assessing left ventricular perfusion and function at rest and during exercise in coronary artery disease and comparison with coronary arteriography and exercise thallium-201 SPECT imaging. *Am J Cardiol.* 1989;64:270–275.

142. Cheng C, Trevis S, Samuel A, Treves S, Davis MA. A new osmium-191-iridium-191m generator. *J Nucl Med.* 1980;21:1169–1176.

143. Wackers FJ, Stein R, Pytlik L, et al. Gold-195m for serial first pass radionuclide angiocardiography during upright exercise in patients with coronary artery disease. *J Am Coll Cardiol.* 1983;2:497–505.

144. Gelfand MJ, Hannon DW. Pediatric Nuclear Cardiology. In: Gerson MC, ed. *Cardiac Nuclear Medicine.* 1st ed. New York, NY: McGraw-Hill; 1987:437.

145. Imaging guidelines for nuclear cardiology procedures. *J Nucl Cardiol.* 1996;3:G1–G46.

146. Hooper W, Horn M, Moser K, et al. Right ventricular size and function: the discrepancy between cardiac blood pool imaging techniques. *Cathet Cardiovasc Diagn.* 1982;8:597–606.

147. Rezai K, Weiss R, Stanford W, Preslar J, Marcus M, Kirchner P. Relative accuracy of three scintigraphic methods for determination of right ventricular ejection fraction: a correlative study with ultrafast computed tomography. *J Nucl Med.* 1991;32:429–435.

148. Bodenheimer MM, Banka VS, Fooshee CM, Hermann GA, Helfant RH. Quantitative radionuclide angiography in the right anterior oblique view: comparison with contrast ventriculography. *Am J Cardiol.* 1978;41:718–723.

149. Brady TJ, Thrall JH, Keyes GW, Brymer JF, Walton JA, Pitt B. Segmental wall-motion analysis in the right anterior oblique projection: comparison of exercise equilibrium radionuclide ventriculography and exercise contrast ventriculography. *J Nucl Med.* 1980;21:617–621.

150. Freeman MR, Berman DS, Staniloff HM, et al. Improved assessment of inferior segmental wall motion by the addition of a 70-degree left anterior oblique view in multiple gated equilibrium scintigraphy. *Am Heart J.* 1981;101:169–173.

151. Hoffmeister HM, Hanke H, Unterberg R, Voelker W, Müller-Schauenburg W, Karsch KR. Ischämieerkennung mit Thallium-201-Single-Photon-Emissionscomputer-tomographie (SPECT) und Radionuklidventrikulographie im Vergleich zur Belastungscineventrikulographie. *Z Kardiol.* 1988;77:115–119.

152. Fearnow EC, Stanfield JA, Jaszczak RJ, Harris CC, Coleman RE. Factors affecting ventricular volume as determined by a count-based equilibrium method. *J Nucl Med.* 1985;26:1042–1047.

153. Links JM, Becker LC, Shindledecker JG, et al. Measurements of absolute left ventricular volume from gated blood pool studies. *Circulation.* 1982;65:82–91.

154. Verani MS, Gaeta J, LeBlanc AD, et al. Validation of left ventricular volume measurements by radionuclide angiography. *J Nucl Med*. 1985;26:1394.

155. Duncan JS, Fetterman R, Greene R, et al. Quantification of left ventricular wall motion from multiple view equilibrium angiocardiography (ERNA). *Automedica*. 1988;10:1–3.

156. Wackers FJ, Terrin ML, Kayden DS, et al. Quantitative radionuclide assessment of regional ventricular function after thrombolytic therapy for acute myocardial infarction: results of phase I thrombolysis in myocardial infarction (TIMI) trial. *J Am Coll Cardiol*. 1989;13:998–1005.

157. Zaret BL, Wackers FJ. Radionuclide methods for evaluating the results of thrombolytic therapy. *Circulation*. 1987;76(suppl II):8–17.

158. Adam WE, Tarkowska A. Evaluation of myocardial function using gated blood pool procedures. In: Pabst HW, Adam WE, Ell P, Gör G, Kriegel H, eds. *Handbook of Nuclear Medicine*. Stuttgart, Germany: Fischer; 1992.

159. Sigel H, Adam WE, Geffers H, Bitter F, Stauch M. Radionuklid-Ventrikulographie, III: klinische Ergebnisse: Parameter der regionalen Wandbewegung. *Nuklear Medizin*. 1978;17:216–220.

160. Brateman L, Buckley K, Keim SG, Wargovich TJ, Williams CM. Left ventricular regional wall motion assessment by radionuclide ventriculography: a comparison of cine display with fourier imaging. *J Nucl Med*. 1991;32:777–782.

161. Boonyaprapa S, Ekmahachai M, Thanachaikun N, Jaiprasert W, Sukthomya V, Poramatikul N. Measurement of left ventricular ejection fracton from gated technetium-99m sestamibi myocardial images. *Eur J Nucl Med*. 1994;22:528–531.

162. Cerqueira MD, Harp GD, Richie JL. Quantitative gated blood pool tomographic assessment of regional ejection fraction: definition of normal limits. *J Am Coll Cardiol*. 1992;20:934–941.

163. Faber TL, Stokely EM, Templeton GH, Akers MS, Parkey RW, Corbett JR. Quantification of three-dimensional left ventricular segmental wall motion and volumes from gated tomographic radionuclide ventriculograms. *J Nucl Med*. 1989;30:638–649.

164. Moore HL, Murphy PH, Burdine JA, et al. ECG-gated emission computed tomography of the cardiac blood pool. *Radiology*. 1980;134:233–235.

165. Borges-Neto S, Coleman RE, Jones RH. Perfusion and function at rest and treadmill exercise using technetium-99m stestamibi: comparison of one- and two-day protocols in normal volunteers. *J Nucl Med*. 1990;31:1128–1132.

166. Wagner HN, Wake R, Nickoloff E, Natarajan TK. The nuclear stethoscope: a simple device for generation of left ventricular volume curves. *Am J Cardiol*. 1976;38:747–750.

167. Tamaki N, Yasuda T, Moore R, et al. Continuous monitoring of left ventricular function by an ambulatory radionuclide detector in patients with coronary artery disease. *J Am Coll Cardiol*. 1988;12:669–679.

168. Hecht HS, Shaw RE, Bruce T, Myler RK. Silent ischemia: evaluation by exercise and redistribution tomographic thallium-201 myocardial imaging. *J Am Coll Cardiol*. 1989; 14:895–900.

169. Hecht HS, Shaw RE, Chin HL, Ryan C, Stertzer SH, Myler RK. Silent ischemia after coronary angioplasty: evaluation of restenosis and extent of ischemia in asymptomatic patients by tomographic thallium-201 exercise imaging and comparison with symptomatic patients. *J Am Coll Cardiol*. 1991;17:670–677.

170. Mahmarian JJ, Pratt CM, Cocanougher MK, Verani MS. Altered myocardial perfusion in patients with angina pectoris or silent ischemia during exercise as assessed by quantitative thallium-201 single-photon emission computed tomography. *Circulation*. 1990;82:1305–1315.

171. Abreu A, Mahmarian JJ, Nishimura S, Boyce TM, Verani MS. Tolerance and safety of pharmacologic coronary vasodilation with adenosine in association with thallium-201 scintigraphy in patients with suspected coronary artery disease. *J Am Coll Cardiol*. 1991;18:730–735.

172. Leppo JA. Thallium washout analysis: fact or fiction [editorial]? *J Nucl Med*. 1987;28:1058.

173. Mason JR, Palace RT, Freeman ML, et al. Thallium scintigraphy during dobutamine infusion: nonexercise-dependent screening test for coronary disease. *Am Heart J*. 1984;107:481–485.

174. Pennell DJ, Underwood SR, Swanton RH, Walker JM, Ell PJ. Dobutamine thallium myocardial perfusion tomography. *J Am Coll Cardiol*. 1991;18:1471–1479.

175. Kahn JK, McGhie I, Akers MS, et al. Quantitative rotational tomography with Tl-201 and Tc-99m 2-methoxy-isobutyl-isonitrile: a direct comparison in normal individuals and patients with coronary artery disease. *Circulation*. 1989;79:1282–1293.

176. Kiat H, Berman DS, Maddahi J. Comparison of planar and tomographic exercise thallium-201 imaging methods for the evaluation of coronary artery disease. *J Am Coll Cardiol*. 1989;13:613–616.

177. Maddahi J, Kiat H, Van Train KF, et al. Myocardial perfusion imaging with technetium-99m sestamibi SPECT in the evaluation of coronary artery disease. *Am J Cardiol*. 1990;66:55E–62E.

178. Maddahi J, Kiat H, Friedman JD, Berman DS, Van Train KK, Garcia EV. Technetium-99m-sestamibi myocardial perfusion imaging for evaluation of coronary artery disease. In: Zaret BL, Beller GA, eds. *Nuclear Cardiology: State of the Art and Future Directions*. St Louis, Mo: Mosby; 1993: 191–200.

179. Verani MS. Thallium-201 and technetium-99m perfusion agents: where we are in 1992. In: Zaret BL, Beller GA, eds. *Nuclear Cardiology: State of the Art and Future Directions*. St Louis, Mo: Mosby; 1993:216–224.

180. Fintel DJ, Links JM, Brinker JA, Frank TL, Parker M, Becker LC. Improved diagnostic performance of exercise thallium-201 single photon emission computed tomography over planar imaging in the diagnosis of coronary artery disease: a receiver operating characteristic analysis. *J Am Coll Cardiol*. 1989;13:600–612.

181. Mahmarian JJ, Boyce TM, Goldberg RK, Cocanouger MK, Roberts R, Verani MS. Quantitative exercise thallium-201 single-photon emission computed tomography for the enhanced diagnosis of ischemic heart disease. *J Am Coll Cardiol*. 1990;15:318–329.

182. Mahmarian JJ, Verani MS. Exercise thallium-201 perfusion scintigraphy in the assessment of coronary artery disease. *Am J Cardiol*. 1991;67:2D–11D.

183. Massie BM, Botvinick EH, Brundage BH. Correlation of thallium-201 scintigrams with coronary anatomy. Factors affecting region by region sensitivity. *Am J Cardiol.* 1979; 45:616–622.

184. Rigo P, Bailey IK, Griffith LS, et al. Value and limitations of segmental analysis of stress thallium myocardial imaging for localization of coronary artery disease. *Circulation.* 1980;61:973–981.

185. Detrano R, Janosi A, Lyons KP, Marcondes G, Abbassi N, Froelicher VF. Factors affecting sensitivity and specificity of a diagnostic test: the exercise thallium scintigram. *Am J Med.* 1988;84:699–710.

186. Gibson RS, Beller GA. Should exercise electrocardiographic testing be replaced by radioisotope methods? In: Rahimtoola SH, Brest AN, eds. *Controversies in Coronary Artery Disease.* Philadelphia, Pa: FA Davis Co; 1981:1–31.

187. Okada RD, Boucher CA, Strauss HW, Pohost GM. Exercise radionuclide imaging approaches to coronary artery disease. *Am J Cardiol.* 1980;46:1188–1204.

188. Verani MS, Marcus ML, Razzak MA, Ehrhardt JC. Sensitivity and specificity of thallium-201 perfusion scintigrams under exercise in the diagnosis of coronary artery disease. *J Nucl Med.* 1978;19:773–782.

189. Hoffmeister HM, Kaiser W, Hanke H, et al. Erkennung, Quantifizierung und Lokalisation von Myokardinfarkten: Vergleich der Thallium-Single-Photon-Emissions-Computertomographie mit biplaner Angiographie. *Z Kardiol.* 1985;74:625–632.

190. Hoffmeister HM, Hanke H, Unterberg R, Voelker W, Müller-Schauenburg W, KarschKR. Quantification of myocardial ischemia and infarction with single photon emission computed tomography. *Eur J Nucl Med.* 1989;15:26–31

191. Kaul S, Boucher CA, Newell JB, et al. Determination of the quantitative thallium imaging variables that optimize detection of coronary artery disease. *J Am Coll Cardiol.* 1986;7:527–537.

192. Kaul S, Chesler DA, Okada RD, Boucher CA. Computer versus visual analysis of exercise thallium-201 images: a critical appraisal in 325 patients with chest pain. *Am Heart J.* 1987;114:1129–1137.

193. Maddahi J, Garcia EV, Berman DS, Waxman A, Swan HJC, Forrester J. Improved noninvasive assessment of coronary artery disease by quantitative analysis of regional stress myocardial distribution and washout of thallium-201. *Circulation.* 1981;64:924–935.

194. Zaret BL, Wackers FJT, Soufer R. Nuclear cardiology. In: Braunwald E, ed. *Heart Disease.* Philadelphia, Pa: WB Saunders; 1992:276–311.

195. Iskandrian AS, Heo J, Lemlek J, Ogilby JD. Identification of high risk patients with left main and three-vessel coronary artery disease using stepwise discriminant analysis of clinical exercise and tomographic thallium data. *Am Heart J.* 1993;125:221–225.

196. Maddahi J, Abdulla A, Garcia EV, Swan HJC, Berman DS. Noninvasive identification of left main and triple vessel coronary artery disease: improved accuracy using quantitative analysis of regional myocardial stress distribution and washout of thallium-201. *J Am Coll Cardiol.* 1986; 7:53–60.

197. Gerson MC, Thomas SR, Van Heertum RL. Tomographic myocardial perfusion imaging. In: Gerson MC, ed. *Cardiac Nuclear Medicine.* 2d ed. New York, NY: McGraw-Hill Inc; 1991:25–52.

198. Tamaki N, Yonekura Y, Mukai T, et al. Segmental analysis of stress thallium myocardial emission tomography for localization of coronary artery disease. *Eur J Nucl Med.* 1984; 9:99–105.

199. Tamaki N, Yonekura Y, Mukai T, et al. Stress thallium-201 transaxial emission computed tomography: quantitative versus qualitative analysis for evaluation of coronary artery disease. *J Am Coll Cardiol.* 1984;4:1213–1221.

200. Chae SC, Heo J. Identification of extensive coronary artery disease in women by exercise single-photon emission computed tomographic (SPECT) thallium imaging. *J Am Coll Cardiol.* 1993;21:1305–1311.

201. The Multicenter Post-Infarction Research Group. Risk stratification and survival after myocardial infarction. *N Engl J Med.* 1983;309:331–336.

202. Esquivel L, Pollock SG, Beller GA, Gibson RS, Watson DD, Kaul S. Effect of the degree of effort on the sensitivity of the exercise thallium-201 stress test in symptomatic coronary artery disease. *Am J Cardiol.* 1989;63:160–165.

203. O'Keefe JH Jr, Bateman TM, Silvestri R, Barnhart C. Safety and diagnostic accuracy of adenosine thallium-201 scintigraphy in patients unable to exercise and those with left bundle branch block. *Am Heart J.* 1992;124:614–621.

204. Braat SH, Brugaeda P, Bar FW, Gorgels APM, Wellens HJJ. Thallium-201 exercise scintigraphy and left bundle branch block. *Am J Cardiol.* 1985;55:224–226.

205. DePuey EG, Guertler-Krawczynska E, Robbins WL. Thallium-201 SPECT in coronary artery disease patients with left bundle branch block. *J Nucl Med.* 1988;29:1479-1485.

206. Hirzel HO, Senn M, Nuesch K, et al. Thallium-201 scintigraphy in complete left bundle branch block. *Am J Cardiol.* 1984;53:764–769.

207. McGowan RL, Welch TG, Zaret BL, Bryson AL, Martin ND, Flamm MD. Noninvasive myocardial imaging with potassium-43 and rubidium-81 in patients with left bundle branch block. *Am J Cardiol* 1976;38:422–428.

208. Burns RJ, Galligan L, Wright LM, Lawand S, Burke RJ, Gladstone PJ. Improved specificity of myocardial thallium-201 single-photon emission computed tomography in patients with left bundle branch block by dipyridamole. *Am J Cardiol.* 1991;68:504–508.

209. Jukema JW, Van der Wall EE, Van der VisMeesen MJ, Kruyswijk HH, Bruschke AVG. Dipyridamole thallium-201 scintigraphy for improved detection of left anterior descending coronary artery stenosis in patients with left bundle branch block. *Eur Heart J.* 1993;14:53–56.

210. O'Keefe JH, Bateman TM, Barnhart CS. Adenosine thallium-201 is superior to exercise thallium-201 for detection coronary artery disease in patients with left bundle branch block. *J Am Coll Cardiol.* 1993;21:1332–1338.

211. Rocett JF, Wood WC, Moinuddin M, Loveless V, Parrish B. Intravenous dipyridamole thallium-201 SPECT imaging in patients with left bundle branch block. *Clin Nucl Med.* 1990;15:401–407.

212. Friedman TD, Greene AC, Iskandrian AS, Hakki AH, Kane SA, Segal BL. Exercise thallium-201 myocardial

scintigraphy in women: correlation with coronary arteriography. *Am J Cardiol.* 1982;49:1632–1637.

213. Johnstone DE, Wackers FJ, Berger HJ, et al. Effect of patients positioning of left lateral thallium-201 myocardial images. *J Nucl Med.* 1979;20:183–188.

214. Ficaro EP, Fessler JA, Shreve PD, Kritzman JN, Rose PA, Corbett JR. Simultaneous transmission/emission myocardial perfusion tomography: diagnostic accuracy of attenuation-corrected 99m Tc-sestamibi single photon emission computed tomography. *Circulation.* 1996;93:463–473.

215. McLaughlin PR, Martin RP, Doherty P, et al. Reproducibility of thallium-201 myocardial imaging. *Circulation.* 1977;55:497–503.

216. Iskandrian AS, Gerson M. Valvular heart disease. In: Gerson MC, ed. *Cardiac Nuclear Medicine.* 2d ed. New York, NY: McGraw-Hill; 1991.

217. Genda A, Mizuno S, Nunoda S, et al. Clinical studies on diabetic myocardial disease using exercise testing with myocardial scintigraphy and endomyocardial biopsy. *Clin Cardiol.* 1986;9:375–382.

218. Hoffmeister HM, Riesner C, M,ller-Schauenburg W, Karsch KR. Myocardial pattern of thallium-201 distribution in patients with dilated cardiomyopathy. *American Journal of Noninvasive Cardiology.* 1991;5:235–239.

219. Houghton JL, Frank MJ, Carr AA, Dohlen TW, Prisant M. Relations among impaired flow reserve, left ventricular hypertrophy and thallium perfusion defects in hypertensive patients without obstructive coronary artery disease. *J Am Coll Cardiol.* 1990;15:43–51.

220. Maseri A, Parodi O, Severi S, Pesola A. Transient transmural reduction of myocardial blood flow, demonstrated by thallium-201 scintigraphy, as a cause of variant angina. *Circulation.* 1976;54:280–288.

221. O'Gara PJ, Bonow RO, Maron BJ, et al. Myocardial perfusion abnormalities in patients with a hypertrophic cardiomyopathy: assessment with thallium-201 emission computed tomography. *Circulation.* 1987;76:1214–1223.

222. Pitcher D, Wainright R, Maisey M, et al. Assessment of chest pain in hypertrophic cardiomyopathy using exercise thallium-201 myocardial scintigraphy. *British Heart Journal.* 44:650–656.

223. Ricci DR, Orlick AE, Doherty PW, Cipriano PR, Harrison DC. Reduction of coronary blood flow during coronary artery spasm occuring spontaneously and after provocation by ergonovine maleate. *Circulation.* 1978;57:392–395.

224. Tubau JF, Szachcic J, Hollenberg M, Massie BM. Usefulness of thallium-201 scintigraphy in predicting the development of angina pectoris in hypertensive patients with left ventricular hypertrophy. *Am J Cardiol.* 1989;64:45–49.

225. Hakki AH, Iskandrian AS. Effect of gender on left ventricular function during exercise in patients with coronary artery disease. *Am Heart J.* 1986;111:543–546.

226. Hanley PC, Zinmeister AR, Clements IP, Bove AA, Brown ML, Gibbons RJ. Gender-related differences in cardiac response to supine exercise assessed by radionuclide angiography. *J Am Coll Cardiol.* 1989;13:624–629.

227. Kuo L, Bolli R, Thornby J, Roberts R, Verani MS. Effects of exercise tolerance, age, and gender on the specificity of radionuclide angiography and sequential ejection fraction analyis during multistage exercise. *Am Heart J.* 1987;113:1180–1189.

228. Port S, Cobb FR, Coleman RE, Jones RH. Effect of age on the response of the left ventricular ejection fraction to exercise. *N Engl J Med.* 1980;303:1133–1137.

229. Diamond GA, Forrester JS. Analysis of probability as an aid to the clinical diagnosis of coronary artery disease. *N Engl J Med.* 1979;300:1350–1358.

230. Epstein SE. Implications of probability analysis on the strategy used for noninvasive detection of coronary artery disease. *Am J Cardiol.* 1980;46:491–499.

231. Patterson RE, Horrowitz SF, Eng C, et al. Can exercise electorcardiography and thallium-201 myocardial imaging exclude the diagnosis of coronary artery disease? *Am J Cardiol.* 1982;49:1127–1135.

232. Patterson RE, Eng C, Horowitz SF. Pratical diagnosis of coronary artery disease: a Bayes' theorem nomogram to correlate clinical data with noninvasive exercise test. *Am J Cardiol.* 1984;53:252–256.

233. Patterson RE, Eisner RL, Horowitz SF. Comparison of cost-effectivness and utility of exercise ECG, single photon emission computed tomography, positron emission tomography, and coronary angiography for diagnosis of coronary artery disease. *Circulation.* 1995;91:54–65.

234. Weintraub WS, Madeira SW, Bodenheimer MM, et al. Critical analysis of the application of Bayes' theorem to sequential testing in the noninvasive diagnosis of coronary artery disease. *Am J Cardiol.* 1984;54:43–49.

235. Fleg JL, Girstenblith G, Zonderman AB, et al. Prevalence and prognostic significance of exercise-induced silent myocardial ischemia detected by thallium scintigraphy and electrocardiography in asymptomatic volunteers. *Circulation.* 1990;81:428–436.

236. Heo J, Thompson WO, Iskandrian AS. Prognostic implications of normal exercise thallium images. *American Journal of Noninvasive Cardiology.* 1987;1:209–212.

237. Pamelia FX, Gibson RS, Watson DD, Craddock GB, Sirowatka J, Beller GA. Prognosis with chest pain and normal thallium-201 exercise scintigrams. *Am J Cardiol.* 1983;55:920–926.

238. Wackers FJT, Russo DJ, Russo D, Clements JP. Prognostic significance of normal quantitative planar thallium-201 stress scintigraphy in patients with chest pain. *J Am Coll Cardiol.* 1985;6:27–30.

239. Wahl J, Hakki AH, Iskandrian AS. Prognostic implications of normal exercise thallium-201 images. *Arch Intern Med.* 1985;145:253–256.

240. Blumenthal RS, Becker DM, Moy TF, Coresh J, Wilder LB, Becker LC. Exercise thallium tomographypredicts future clinically manifest coronary heart disease in a high-risk asymptomatic population. *Circulation.* 1996;93:915–923.

241. Califf RM, Armstrong PW, Carver JR, D'Agostino RB, Strauss WE. Task force stratification of patients into high, medium and low-risk subgroups for purpose of risk factor management. *J Am Coll Cardiol.* 1996;27:964–1047.

242. Marie PY, Danchin N, Durand JF, et al. Long-term prediction of major ischemic events by exercise thallium-201 single photon emission computed tomography: Incre-

mental prognostic value compared with clinical exercise testing, catheterization and radionuclide angiographic data. *J Am Coll Cardiol*. 1995;26:879–886.

243. Mazzotta G, Pace L, Bonow RO. Risk stratification of patients with coronary artery disease and left ventricular dysfunction by exercise radionuclide angiography and exercise electrocardiography. *J Nucl Cardiol*. 1994;1:529–539.

244. Nallamothu N, Ghods M, Heo J, Iskandrian AS. Comparison of thallium-201 single photon emission computed tomography and electrocardiographic response during exercise in patients with normal rest electrocardiographic results. *J Am Coll Cardiol*. 1995;25:830–836.

245. Pancholy SB, Fattah AA, Kamal AA, et al. Independent and incremental prognostic value of exercise single-photon emission computed tomographic imaging in women. *J Nucl Cardiol*. 1995;2:110–116.

246. Marcus ML, Skorton DJ, Johnson MR, Collins SM, Harrison DG, Kerber RE. Visual estimates of percent diameter coronary stenosis: a battered gold standard. *J Am Coll Cardiol*. 1988;11:882–885.

247. White CW, Wright CB, Doty DB, et al. Does visual interpretation of the coronary arteriogram predict the physiologic importance of a coronary stenosis? *N Engl J Med*. 1984;310:819–824.

248. Lakkis NM, Mahmarian JJ, Verani MS. Exercise thallium-201 single photon emission computed tomography for evaluation of coronary artery bypass graft patency. *Am J Cardiol*. 1995;76:107–111.

249. Ritchie JL, Narahara KA, Trobaugh GB, Williams DL, Hamilton GW. Thallium-201 myocardial imaging before and after coronary revascularization: assessment of regional myocardial blood flow and graft patency. *Circulation*. 1977;56:830–836.

250. Verani MS, Marcus ML, Spoto G, Rossi NP, Ehrhardt JC, Razzak MA. Thallium-201 myocardial perfusion scintigrams in the evaluation of aorto-coronary venous bypass surgery. *J Nucl Med*. 1978;19:765–772.

251. Hecht HS, Shaw RE, Bruce RT, Ryan C, Stertzer SH, Myler RK. Usefulness of tomographic thallium-201 imaging for detection of restenosis after percutaneous transluminal coronary angioplasty. *Am J Cardiol*. 1990;66:1314–1318.

252. Hirzel HO, Neusch K, Gruentzig AR, Luetolf UM. Short and long-term changes in myocardial perfusion after percutaneous transluminal coronary angioplasty assessed by thallium-201 exercise scintigraphy. *Circulation*. 1981;63:1001–1007.

253. Hoffmeister HM, Kaiser W, Hanke H, Müller-Schauenburg W, Karsch KR, Seipel L. Myocardial perfusion and left ventricular function early after successful PTCA in 1-vessel coronary artery disease. *Nuclear Medicine*. 1994;33: 68–72.

254. Miller DD, Verani MS. Current status of myocardial perfusion imaging after percutaneous transluminal coronary angioplasty. *J Am Coll Cardiol*. 1994;24:260.

255. Verani MS, Tadros S, Raizner AE, et al. Quantitative analysis of thallium-201 uptake and washout before and after transluminal coronary angioplasty. *Int J Cardiol*. 1986;13: 109–124.

256. Avery PG, Hudson NM, Hubner PJB. Assessment of myocardial perfusion and function using gated methoxy-isobutyl-isonitrile scintigraphy to detect restenosis after coronary angioplasty. *Coron Artery Dis*. 1993;4:1097–1102.

257. Iskandrian AS. Single-photon emission computed tomographic thallium imaging with adenosine, dipyridamole, and exercise. *Am Heart J*. 1991;122:279–284.

258. Kent KM, Bonow RO, Rosing DR, et al. Improved myocardial function during exercise after successful percutaneous transluminal coronary angioplasty. *N Engl J Med*. 1982;306:441–446.

259. Braunwald EB, Kloner RA. The stunned myocardium: prolonged, postischemic ventricular dysfunction. *Circulation*. 1982;66:146–1149.

260. Rahimtoola SH. The hibernating myocardium. *Am Heart J*. 1989;117:211–221.

261. Zimmermann R, Mall G, Rauch B,et al. Residual Tl-201 activity in irreversible defects as a marker of myocardial viability. *Circulation*. 1995;91:1016–1021.

262. Cloninger KG, DePuey EG, Garcia EV, et al. Incomplete redistribution of delayed thallium-201 single photon emission computed tomographic (SPECT) images: an overestimation of myocardial scarring. *J Am Coll Cardiol*. 1988;12:955–963.

263. Cuocolo A, Pace L, Maurea S, et al. Enhanced thallium-201 uptake after reinjection relation to regional ventricular function myocardial perfusion and coronary anatomy. *J Nucl Biol Med*. 1994;38:6–13.

264. Kiat H, Berman DS, Maddahi J, et al. Late reversibility of tomographic myocardial thallium-201 defects: an accurate marker of myocardial viability. *J Am Coll Cardiol*. 1988;12:1456–1463.

265. Mahmarian JJ, Pratt CM, Boyce T, Verani MS. The variable extent of jeopardized myocardium in patients with single vessel coronary artery disease. Quantification of thallium-201 single-photon emission computed tomography. *J Am Coll Cardiol*. 1991;17:355–362.

266. Rocco TP, Dilsizian V, Strauss HW, Boucher CA. Technetium-99m isonitrile myocardial uptake at rest. Its relation to clinical markers of potential viability. *J Am Coll Cardiol*. 1989;14:1678–1684.

267. Sawada SG, Allman KC, Muzik O, et al. Positron emission tomography detects evidence of viability in rest technetium-99m sestamibi defects. *J Am Coll Cardiol*. 1994;23: 92–98.

268. Panza JA, Dilsizian V, Laurienzo JM, Curiel RV, Katsiyiannis PT. Relation between thallium uptake and contractile response to dobutamine. *Circulation*. 1995;91:990-998.

269. Beller GA. Myocardial perfusion imaging with thallium-201. *J Nucl Med*. 1994;35:674–680.

270. Brown KA. Prognostic value of thallium-201 myocardial perfusion imaging. *Circulation*. 1991;83:363–381.

271. Heller GV, Brown KA. Prognosis of acute and chronic coronary artery disease by myocardial perfusion imaging. *Cardiol Clin*. 1994;12:271–287.

272. Koss JH, Kobren S, Grunwald AW, Bodenheimer MM. Role of exercise thallium-201 myocardial perfusion scintigraphy in predicting prognosis in suspected coronary artery disease. *Am J Cardiol*. 1987;59:531–534.

273. Gibson RS, Watson DD, Craddock GB, et al. Prediction of cardiac events after uncomplicated myocardial infarction: a prospective study comparing predischarge exercise

thallium-201 scintigraphy and coronary angiography. *Circulation*. 1983;68:321–336.

274. Machecourt J, Longeère P, Farget D, et al. Prognostic value of thallium-201 single-photon emission computed tomographic myocardial perfusion imaging according to extent of myocardial defect. *J Am Coll Cardiol*. 1994; 23:1096–1106.

275. Cerqueira MD, Maynard C, Ritchie JL, Davis KB, Kennedy JW. Long-term survival in 618 patients from the Western Washington streptokinase in myocardial infarction trials. *J Am Coll Cardiol*. 1992;20:1452–1459.

276. Hakki AH, Bestico PF, Heo J, Unwala AA, Iskandrian AS. Relative prognostic value of rest thallium-201 imaging, radionuclide ventriculography and 24-hour ambulatory electrocardiographic monitoring after acute myocardial infarction. J Am Coll Cardiol. 1987;10:25–32.

277. Braunwald EB, Mark DB, Jones RH, et al. *Clinical Practice Guidelines: Unstable Angina: Diagnosis and Managment*. Rockville, Md: US Dept of Health and Human Servies, Agency for Health Care Policy and Research; 1994. AHCPR publication 94-0602.

278. Gill JB, Ruddy TR, Newell JB, Finkelstein DM, Strauss HW, Boucher CA. Prognostic importance of thallium uptake by the lungs during exercise in coronary artery disease. *N Engl J Med*. 1987;317:1486–1489.

279. Iskandrian AS, Heo J, Nguyen T, Lyons E, Paugh E. Left ventricular dilatation and pulmonary thallium uptake after single-photon-emission computer tomography using thallium-201 during adenosine-induced coronary hyperemia. *Am J Cardiol*. 1990;66:807–811.

280. Bonow RO, Kent KM, Rosing DR, et al. Exercise-induced ischemia in mildly symptomatic patients with coronary artery disease and preserved left ventricular function: identification of subgroups at risk of death during medical therapy. *N Engl J Med*. 1984;311:1339–1345.

281. Christian TF, Behrenbeck T, Pellikka PA, Huber KC, Chesebro JH, Gibbons RJ. Mismatch of left ventricular function and infarct size demonstrated by technetium-99m isonitrile imaging after reperfusion therapy for acute myocardial infarction: identification of myocardial stunning and hyperkinesia. *J Am Coll Cardiol*. 1990;16: 1632–1638.

282. Corbett JR, Dehmer GJ, Lewis SE, et al. The prognostic value of submaximal exercise testing with radionuclide ventriculography before hospital discharge in patients with recent myocardial infarction. *Circulation*. 1981;64: 535–544.

283. Harris PJ, Harrell FE Jr, Lee KL, Behar VS, Rosati RA. Survival in medically treated coronary artery disease. *Circulation*. 1979;60:1259–1269.

284. Lee KL, Pryor DB, Pieper KS, et al. Prognostic value of radionuclide angiography in medically treated patients with coronary artery disease: a comparsion with clinical and catheterization variables. *Circulation*. 1990;82:1705–1717.

285. Mock MB, Ringqvist I, Fisher LD, et al. Survival of medically treated patients in the coronary artery surgery study (CASS) registry. *Circulation*. 1982;66:562–568.

286. Simoons ML, Vos J, Tijssen JGP, et al. Long-term benefit of early thrombolytic therapy in patients with acute myocardial infarction: 5 year follow-up of a trial conducted by the Interuniversity Cardiology Institute of the Netherlands. *J Am Coll Cardiol*. 1989;14:1609–1615.

287. Pryor DB, Harrell FE, Lee KI, et al. Prognostic indicators from radionuclide angiography in medically treated patients with coronary artery disease. *Am J Cardiol*. 1984; 53:18–22.

288. Hendel RC, Layden JJ, Leppo JA. Prognostic value of dipyridamole thallium scintigraphy for evaluation of ischemic heart disease. *J Am Coll Cardiol*. 1990;15:109–116.

289. Iskandrian AS, Heo J, Decoskey D, Askenase A, Segal BL. Use of exercise thallium-201 imaging for risk stratification of elderly patients with coronary disease. *Am J Cardiol*. 1988;61:269–272.

290. Kaul S, Lilly DR, Gasho JA, et al. Prognostic utility of the exercise thallium-201 test in ambulatory patients with chest pain: comparison with cardiac catheterization. *Circulation*. 1988;77:745–758.

291. Landenheim ML, Pollock BH, Rozanski A, et al. Extent and severity of myocardial hypoperfusion as predictors of prognosis in patients with suspected coronary artery disease. *J Am Coll Cardiol*. 1986;7:464–471.

292. Staniloff HM, Forrester JS, Berman DS, Swan HJC. Prediction of death, myocardial infarction, and worsening chest pain using thallium scintigraphy and exercise electrocardiography. *J Nucl Med*. 1986;27:1842–1848.

293. Stratmann HG, Mark AL, Walter KE, Williams GA. Prognostic value of atrial pacing and thallium-201 scintigraphy in patients with stable chest pain. *Am J Cardiol*. 1989;64: 985–900.

294. Abraham RD, Freedman SB, Dunn RF, et al. Prediction of multivessel coronary artery disease and prognosis early after acute myocardial infarction by exercise electrocardiography and thallium-201 myocardial perfusion scanning. *Am J Cardiol*. 1986;58:423–427.

295. Bairey CN, Rozanski A, Maddahi J, Resser KJ, Berman DS. Exercise thallium-201 scintigraphy and prognosis in typical angina pectorix and negative exercise electrocardiography. *Am J Cardiol*. 1989;64:282–287.

296. Brown KA, Boucher CA, Okada RD, et al. Prognostic value of exercise thallium-201 imaging in patients presenting for evaluation of chest pain. *J Am Coll Cardiol*. 1983;1:994–1001.

297. Heller LI, Tresgallo M, Sciacca RR, Blood DK, Seldin DW, Johnson LL. Prognostic significance of silent myocardial ischemia on a thallium stress test. *Am J Cardiol*. 1990;65: 718–721.

298. Leppo JA. Dipyridamole-thallium imaging: the lazy man's stress test. *J Nucl Med*. 1989;30:281–287.

299. Christian TF, Miller TD, Bailey KR, Gibbons RJ. Noninvasive identification of severe coronary artery disease using exercise tomographic thallium-201 imaging. *Am J Cardiol*. 1992;70:14–20.

300. Nygaard TW, Gibson RS, Ryan JN, Gascho JA, Watson DD, Beller GA. Prevalence of high-risk thallium-201 scintigraphic findings in left main coronary artery stenosis: comparison with patients with multiple- and single-vessel coronary artery disease. *Am J Cardiol*. 1984;53:462–469.

301. Rehn T, Griffith LS, Achuff SC, et al. Exercise thallium-201 myocardial imaging in left main coronary artery disease: sensitive but not specific. *Am J Cardiol*. 1981;48: 217–223.

302. ACC/AHA Task Force. Guidelines for preoperative cardiovascular evaluation of noncardiac surgery. *Circulation.* 1996;93:1280–1317.

303. Mangano DT, Goldman L. Preoperative assessment of patients with known or suspected coronary disease. *N Engl J Med.* 1995;333:1750–1756.

304. Lette J, Lapointe J, Waters D, Cerino M, Picard M, Gagnon A. Transient left ventricular cavitary dilation during dipyridamole-thallium imaging as an indicator of severe coronary artery disease. *Am J Cardiol.* 1990;66: 1163–1170.

305. Levinson JR, Boucher CA, Coley GM, Guiney TE, Strauss W, Eagle KA. Usefulness of semiquantitative analysis of dipyridamole-thallium-201 redistribution for improving risk stratification before vascular surgery. *Am J Cardiol.* 1990;66:406–410.

306. Shaw L, Miller DD, Kong BA, et al. Determination of perioperative cardiac risk by adenosine thallium-201 myocardial imaging. *Am Heart J.* 1992;124:861–869.

307. Wong T, Detsky AS. Preoperative cardiac risk assessment for patients having peripheral vascular surgery. *Ann Intern Med.* 1992;116:743–753.

308. Baron JF, Mundler O, Bertrand M, et al. Dipyridamole-thallium scintigraphy and gated radionuclide angiography to assess cardiac risk before abdominal aortic surgery. *N Engl J Med.* 1994;330:663–669.

309. Elliott BM, Robison JG, Zellner JL, Hendrix GH. Dobutamine Tl-201 imaging. *Circulation.* 1991;84(suppl III): III54–III60.

310. Zellner JL, Elliot BM, Robison JG, Hendrix GH, Spicer KM. Preoperative evaluation of cardiac risk using dobutamine-thallium imaging in vascular surgery. *Ann Vasc Surg.* 1990; 4:238–243.

311. Morris KG, Palmeri ST, Califf RM, et al. Value of radionuclide angiography in predicting specific cardiac events after acute myocardial infarction. *Am J Cardiol.* 1985;55: 318–324.

312. Bulkley BH, Hutchins GM, Bailey I, Strauss HW, Pitt B. Thallium-201 imaging and gated blood pool scans in patients with ischemic and idiopathic congestive cardiomyopathy: a clinical and pathologic study. *Circulation.* 1977; 55:753–760.

313. Eichhorn EJ, Kosinski EJ, Lewis SM, Hill TC, Emond EH, Leland OS. Usefulness of dipyridamole-thallium-201 perfusion scanning for distinguishing ischemic from nonischemic cardiomyopathy. *Am J Cardiol.* 1988;62:945–951.

314. Greenberg JM, Murphy JH, Okada RD, Pohost GM, Strauss WH, Boucher CA. Value and limitations of radionuclide angiography in determining the cause of reduced left ventricular ejection fraction: comparison of idiopathic dilated cardiomyopathy and coronary artery disease. *Am J Cardiol.* 1985;55:541–544.

315. Dunn R, Uren R, Sadick N, et al. Comparison of thallium-201 scanning in idiopathic dilated cardiomyopathy and severe coronary artery disease. *Circulation.* 1982;66: 804–810.

316. Tauberg SG, Orie JE, Bartlett BE, Cottington EM, Flores AR. Usefulness of thallium-201 for distinction of ischemic from idopathic dilated cardiomyopathy. *Am J Cardiol.* 1993;71:674–680.

317. Jullière Y, Mariet PY, Danchin N, et al. Radionuclide assessment of regional differences in left ventricular wall motion and myocardial perfusion in idiopathic dilated cardiomyopathy. *Eur Heart J.* 193;14:1163–1169.

318. Yamaguchi S, Tsuiki K, Hayasaka M, Yasui S. Segmental wall motion abnormalities in dilated cardiomyopathy: hemodynamic characteristics and comparison with thallium-201 myocardial scintigraphy. *Am Heart J.* 1987;113: 1123–1128.

319. Schwarz F, Mall G, Zebe H, et al. Quantitative morphological findings of the myocardium in idiopathic dilated cardiomyopathy. *Am J Cardiol.* 1983;51:501–506.

320. Suzuki Y, Kadota K, Nohara R, et al. Dilated cardiomyopathy: evaluation by thallium-201 emission computed tomography [abstract]. *Circulation.* 1983;68(suppl III).

321. Yoshinori LD, Chikamori T, Takata J, et al. Prognostic value of thallium-201 perfusion defects in idiopathic dilated cardiomyopathy. *Am J Cardiol.* 1991;67:188–193.

322. Dec GW, Palacios I, Yasuda T, et al. Antimyosin antibody cardiac imaging: its role in the diagnosis of myocarditis. *J Am Coll Cardiol.* 1990;16:97–104.

323. Alexander J, Dainiak N, Berger HJ, et al. Serial assessment of doxorubicin cardiotoxicity with quantitative radionuclide angiocardiography. *N Engl J Med.* 1979;300: 278–283.

324. Palmeri ST, Bonow RO, Myers CE, et al. Prospective evaluation of doxorubicin cardiotoxicity by rest and exercise radionuclide angiography. *Am J Cardiol.* 1986;58:607–613.

325. Schwartz RG, McKenzie WB, Alexander J, et al. Congestive heart failure and left ventricular dysfunction complicating doxorubicin therapy: seven-year experience using serial radionuclide angiocardiography. *Am J Med.* 1987;82: 1109–1118.

326. Dilsizian V, Bonow RO, Epstein SE, Fananapazir L. Myocardial ischemia is a frequent cause of cardiac arrest and syncope in young patients with hypertrophic cardiomyopathy. *J Am Coll Cardiol.* 1993;22:796–804.

327. Ohtsuki K, Sugihara H, Umamoto I, Nakamura T, Nakagawa T, Nakagawa M. Clinical evaluation of hypertrophic cardiomyopathy by myocardial scintigraphy using I-123 labelled 15-(*p*-iodophenyl)-3-R, S-methylpentadecanoic acid (I-123 BMIPP). *Nucl Med Commun.* 1994;15:441–447.

328. Shimonagata T, Nishimura T, Uehara T, et al. Discrepancies between myocardial perfusion and free fatty acid metabolism in patients with hypertrophic cardiomyopathy. *Nucl Med Commun.* 1993;14:1005–1013.

329. Kinney EL, Jackson GL, Reeves WC, Zelis R, Beers E. Thallium-scan myocardial defects and echocardiographic abnormalities in patients with sarcoidosis without clinical cardiac dysfunction. *Am J Med.* 1980;68:497–503.

330. Le Guludec D, Menad F, Faraggi M, Weinmann P, Battesti JP, Valeyre D. Myocardial sarcoidosis: clinical value of technetium-99 sestamibi tomoscintigraphy. *Chest.* 1994; 106:1675–1682.

331. Follansbee WP, Curtis EJ, Medsger TA Jr, et al. Physiologic abnormalities of cardiac function in progressive systemic sclerosis with diffuse scleroderma. *N Engl J Med.* 1984; 310:142–148.

332. Forman MB, Sandler MP, Sacks GA, Kronenberg MW, Powers TA. Radionuclide imaging in myocardial sarcoido-

sis: demonstration of myocardial uptake of technetium pyrophosphate-99m and gallium. *Chest.* 1983;83:570–580.

333. Fournier C, Grimon G, Rinaldi JP, et al. Usefulness of technetium-99m pyrophosphate myocardial scintigraphy in amyloid polyneuropathy and correlation with echocardiography. *Am J Cardiol.* 1993;72:854–857.

334. Tawarahara K, Kurata C, Okayama K, Kobayashi A, Yamazaki N. Thallium-201 and gallium-67 single photon emission computed tomographic imaging in cardiac sarcoidosis. *Am Heart J.* 1992;124:1383–1384.

335. Borer JS, Bacharach SL, Green MV, et al. Exercise-induced left ventricular dysfunction in symptomatic and asymptomatic patients with aortic regurgitation: assessment by radionuclide cineangiography. *Am J Cardiol.* 1978;42:351–356.

336. Bailey IK, Come PC, Kelly DT, et al. Thallium-201 perfusion imaging in aortic valve stenosis. *Am J Cardiol.* 1977;40:889–899.

337. Dunn RF, Wolff L, Wagner S, Botvinick EH. The inconsistent pattern of thallium defects: a clue to false positive perfusion scintigram. *Am J Cardiol.* 1981;48:224-232.

338. Pfisterer M, Müller-Brand J, Brundler H, Cueni T. Prevalence and significance of reversible radionuclide ischemic perfusion defects in symptomatic aortic valve disease patients with and without concomitant coronary disease. *Am Heart J.* 1982;103:92–96.

339. Nies R, Hanke H, Helber U, Müller-Schauenburg W, Hoffmeister HM. Untersuchungen zur Perfusion des linksventrikulären Myokards bei Patienten mit Aortenklappenvitien mittels Single-Photon-Emisssions-Computertomographie. *Z Kardiol.* 1994;83:864–869.

340. Samuels B, Kiat H, Friedman JD, Berman DS. Adenosine pharmacologic stress myocardial perfusion tomographic imaging in patients with significant aortic stenosis. *J Am Coll Cardiol.* 1995;25:99–106.

341. Kettunen R, Huikuri HV, Heikkilä J, Takkunen JT. Preoperative diagnosis of coronary artery disease in patients with valvular heart disease using technetium-99m isonitrile tomographic imaging together with high dose dipyridamole and handgrip exercise. *Am J Cardiol.* 1992;69:1442–1445.

342. Fouad FM, Slomindki JM, Tarazi RC. Left ventricular diastolic function in hypertension: relation to left ventricular mass and function. *J Am Coll Cardiol.* 1984;3:1500-1506.

343. Iskandrian AS, Hakki A. Age-related changes in left ventricular diastolic performance. *Am Heart J.* 1986;112:75–78.

344. Bonow RO, Kent KM, Rosing DR, et al. Improved left ventricular diastolic filling in patients with coronary artery disease after percutaneous transluminal coronary angioplasty. *Circulation.* 1982;66:1159-1163.

345. Carrio I, Berna L, Ballester M, et al. Indium-111 antimyosin scintigraphy to assess myocardial damage in patients with suspected myocarditis and cardiac rejection. *J Nucl Med.* 1988;29:1893–1900.

346. Frist W, Yasuda T, Segall G, et al. Noninvasive detection of human cardiac transplant reinjection with indium-111 antimyosin (Fab) imaging. *Circulation.* 1987;76(suppl V):V81–V85.

347. Ballester M, Obrador D, Carrio I, et al. Indium-111-mono-

clonal antimyosin antibody studies after the first year of heart transplantation: identification of risk groups for developing rejection during long-term follow-up and clinical implications. *Circulation.* 1990;82:2100–2108.

348. De Nardo D, Scibilia G, Macchiarelli AG, et al. The role of indium-111 antimyosin (Fab) imaging as a noninvasive surveillance method of human heart transplant rejection. *Journal of Heart Transplantation.* 1989;8:407–412.

349. Addonizio LJ. Detection of cardiac allograft rejection using radionuclide techniques. *Prog Cardiovasc Dis.* 1990;33:73–83.

350. Meneguetti JC, Camargo EE, Soares J, et al. Gallium-67 imaging in human heart transplantation: correlation with endomyocardial biopsy. *Journal of Heart Transplantation.* 1987;6:171–176.

351. Berry JJ, Pieper S, Hanson MW, Hoffmean JM, Coleman RE. The effect of metabolic milieu on cardiac PET imaging with fluorine-18 doxyglucose and nitrogen-13 ammonia in normal volunteers. *J Nucl Med.* 1991;32:1518–1525.

352. Camici P, Araujo LI, Spinks T, et al. Increased uptake of F-18 fluorodeoxyglucose in post-ischemic myocardium of patients with exercise-induced angina. *Circulation.* 1986;74:81–88.

353. Czernin J, Porenta G, Brunken R, et al. Regional blood flow, oxidative metabolism, and glucose utilization in patients with recent myocardial infarction. *Circulation.* 1990;88:884–895.

354. Gropler RJ, Siegal BA, Lee KJ, et al. Nonuniformity in myocardial accumulation of F-18 fluorodeoxyglucose in normal fasted humans. *J Nucl Med.* 1990;31:1749–1756.

355. Marshall RC, Tillisch JH, Phelps ME, et al. Identification and differentiation of resting myocardial ischemia and infarction in man with positron computed tomography, F-18 labeled fluorodeoxyglucose and N-13 ammonia. *Circulation.* 1981;64:766–778.

356. Perrone-Filardi P, Bacharach SL, Dilsizian V, Maurea S, Frank JA, Bonow RO. Regional left ventricular wall thickening. Relation to regional uptake of F-18 fluorodeoxyglucose and Tl-201 in patients with chronic coronary artery disease and left ventircular dysfunction. *Circulation.* 1992;86: 125–1137.

357. Tamaki N, Yonekura Y, Yamashita K, et al. Positron emission tomography using fluorine-18 deoxyglucose in evaluation of coronary artery bypass grafting. *Am J Cardiol.* 1989;64:860–865.

358. Van der Wall EE, Blanksma PK, Niemeyer MG, Paans AMJ. *Cardiac Positron Emission Tomography: Viability, Perfusion, Receptors and Cardiomyopathy.* Dordrecht, Germany: Kluwer Academic Publisher; 1995.

359. Schelbert HR, Henze E, Keen R, et al. C-11 palmitate acid for the noninvasive evaluation of regional myocardial fatty acid metabolism with positron computed tomography, IV: in vivo demonstration of impaired fatty acid oxidation in acute myocardial ischemia. *Am Heart J.* 1983;106:736–750.

360. Armbrecht JJ, Buxton DB, Schelbert HR. Validation of [1–11C] acetate as a tracer for noninvasive assessment of oxidative metabolism with positron emission tomography in normal, ischemic, postischemic, and hyperemic canine myocardium. *Circulation.* 1990;81:1594–1605.

361. Buxton DB, Schwaiger M, Nguyen A, Phelps ME, Schelbert HR. Radiolabeled acetate as a tracer of myocardial tricarboxylic acid cycle flux. *Circ Res.* 1988;63:628–634.

362. Walsh MN, Geltman EM, Brown MA, et al. Noninvasive estimation of regional myocardial oxygen consumption by positron emission tomography with carbon-111 acetate in patients with myocardial infarction. *J Nucl Med.* 1989; 30:1798–1808.

363. Kuhle WG, Porenta G, Huang SC, et al. Quantification of regional myocardial blood flow using N-13 ammonia and reoriented dynamic positron emission tomographic imaging. *Circulation.* 1992;86:1004–1017.

364. Iida H, Kanno I, Takahashi A, et al. Measurement of absolute myocardial blood flow with H2-15O and dynamic positron emission tomography: strategy for quantification in relation to the partial-volume effect. *Circualtion.* 1989; 78:104–115.

365. Bergmann SR, Hack S, Tweson T, Welch MJ, Sobel BE. The dependence of accumulation of NH3–13 by myocardium on metabolic factors and its implications for the quantitative assessment of perfusion. *Circulation.* 1980; 61:34–43.

366. Stewart RE, Popma J, Gacioch GM, et al. Comparison of thallium-201 SPECT redistribution patterns and rubidium-82 PET rest-stress myocardial blood flow imaging. *International Journal of Cardiac Imaging.* 1994; 10: 15–23.

367. Schelbert HR, Bonow RO, Geltman EN, et al. Clinical use of cardiac positron emission tomography: Positron statement of the Cardiovascular Council of the Society of Nuclear Medicine. *J Nucl Med.* 1993;34:1385–1388.

368. Demer LL, Gould KL, Goldstein RA, et al. Assessment of coronary artery disease severity by positron emission tomography: comparison with quantitative arteriography in 193 patients. *Circulation.* 1989;79:825–835.

369. Go RT, Marwick TH, MacIntyre WJ, et al. A prospective comparison of rubidium-82 PET and thallium-201 SPECT myocardial perfusion imaging utilizing a single dipyridamole stress in the diagnosis of coronary artery disease. *J Nucl Med.* 1990;31:1899–1905.

370. Grover-McKay M, Ratib O, Schwaiger M. Detection of coronary artery disease with positron emission tomography and thallium-201 SPECT imaging for detection of coronary artery disease. *Am J Cardiol.* 1992;67:1303–1310.

371. Tamaki N, Yonekura Y, Yamashita K, et al. Relation of left ventricular perfusion and wall motion with metabolic activity in persistent defects on thallium-201 tomography in healed myocardial infarction. *Am J Cardiol.* 1988;62: 202–208.

372. Beanlands RS, Muzik O, Melon P, et al. Noninvasive quantification of regional myocardial flow reserve in patients with coronary atherosclerosis using nitrogen-13 ammonia positron emission tomography. *J Am Coll Cardiol.* 1995;26: 1465–1475.

373. DeSilva R, Camici PG. Role of positron emission tomography in the investigation of human coronary circulation. *Cardiovasc Res.* 1994;28:1595–1612.

374. Di Carli MF, Davidson M, Little R, et al. Value of metabolic imaging with positron emission tomography for evaluating prognosis in patients with coronary artery diease and left ventricular dysfunction. *Am J Cardiol.* 1994;73:527–533.

375. Di Carli M, Czernin J, Hoh CK, et al. Relation among stenosis severity, myocardial blood flow, and flow reserve in patients with coronary artery disease. *Circulation.* 1995; 91:1944–1951.

376. Goldstein RA, Haynie M. Limited myocardial perfusion reserve in patients with left ventricular hypertrophy. *J Nucl Med.* 1990;31:255–258.

377. Geltman E, Henes C, Senneff M, Sobel BE, Bergmann SR. Increased myocardial perfusion at rest and diminished perfusion reserve in patients with angina and angiographically normal coronary arteries. *J Am Coll Cardiol.* 1990;16:586–595.

378. Uren NG, Melin JA, De Bruyne B, Wijns W, Baudhuin T, Camici PG. Relation between myocardial flow and the severity of coronary artery stenosis. *N Engl J Med.* 1994; 330: 1782–1788.

379. Czernin J, Sun K, Brunken R, Bottcher M, Phelps M, Schelbert H. Effect of acute and long-term smoking on myocardial blood flow and flow reserve. *Circulation.* 1995; 91:2891–2997.

380. Czernin J, Barnard RJ, Sun KT, et al. Effect of short-term cardiovascular conditioning and low-fat diet on myocardial blood flow and flow reserve. *Circulation.* 1995;92: 197–204.

381. Gould KL, Martucci JP, Goldberger DI, et al. Short-term cholesterol lowering decreases size and severity of perfusion abnormalities by positron emission tomography after dipyridamole in patients with coronary artery disease: a potential noninvasive marker of healing coronary endothelium. *Ciculation.* 1994;89:1530–1538.

382. Gould KL, Ornish D, Scherwitz L, et al. Changes in myocardial perfusion abnormalities by positron emission tomography after long-term intense risk factor modification. *JAMA.* 1995;274:894–901.

383. Superko HR, Drauss RM. Coronary artery disease regression: convincing evidence for the benefit of aggressive lipoprotein management. *Circulation.* 1994;90:1056-1069.

384. Hariharan R, Bray M, Ganim R, Doenst T, Goodwin GW, Taegtmeyer H. Fundamental limitations of F-18 2-dioxy-2-fluoro-D-glucose for assessing myocardial glucose uptake. *Circulation.* 1995;91:2435–2444.

385. Knuuti MJ, Nuutila P, Ruotsalainen U, et al. Euglycemic hyperinsulinemic clamp and oral glucose load in stimulating myocardial glucose utilization during positron emission tomography. *J Nucl Med.* 1992;33:1255–1262.

386. Locher JT, Frey LD, Seybold K, Jenzer H. Myocardial F18-FDG-PET: experiences with euglycemic hyperinsulinemic clamp technique. *Angiology.* 1995;46:313-320.

387. Tamaki N, Yonekura Y, Konishi J. Myocardial FDG studies with the fasting oral glucose-loading or insulin clamp methods [editorial]. *J Nucl Med.* 1992;33:1263–1268.

388. Tillisch J, Brunken R, Marshall R, et al. Reversibility of cardiac wall-motion abnormalities predicted by positron tomography. *N Engl J Med.* 1986;314:884–888.

389. Eitzman D, Al-Aouar Z, Kanter HL, et al. Clinical outcome of patients with advanced coronary artery disease after viability studies with positron emission tomography. *J Am Coll Cardiol.* 1992;20:559–565.

390. Nienaber CA, Brunken RC, Sherman CT, et al. Metabolic and functional recovery of ischemic human myocardium after coronary angioplasty. *J Am Coll Cardiol.* 1991;18:966–978.

391. Tamaki N, Ohtani H, Yamashita K, et al. Metabolic activity in the areas of new fill-in after thallium-201 reinjection: comparison with positron emission tomograpy using fluorine-18-deoxyglucose. *J Nucl Med.* 1991;32:673–678.

392. Bax JJ, Visser FC, van Lingen A, et al. Feasibility of assessing regional myocardial uptake of F-18 fluorodeoxyglucose using single photon emission computed tomography. *Eur Heart J.* 1993;14:1675–1682.

393. Bax JJ, Visser FC, van Lingen A, et al. Relation between myocardial uptake of thallium-201 chloride and F-18 fluorodeoxyglucose imaged with SPECT in normal volunteers. *Eur J Nucl Med.* 1995;22:56–60.

394. Huitnik JM, Visser FC, van Lingen A, et al. Feasibility of planar fluorine-18-FDG imaging after recent myocardial infarction to assess myocardial viability. *J Nucl Med.* 1995;36:975–981.

395. Maddahi J, Schelber H, Brunken R, DiCarli M. Role of thallium-201 and PET imaging in evaluation of myocardial viability and management of patients with coronary artery disease and left ventricular dysfunction. *J Nucl Med.* 1994;35:707–715.

396. Armbrecht JJ, Buxton DB, Brunken RC, Phelps ME, Schelbert HR. Regional myocardial oxygen consumption determined noninvasively in humans with [1–11C] acetate and dynamic positron tomography. *Circulation.* 1989;80:863–872.

397. Gropler RJ, Geltman EM, Sampathkumaran K, et al. Functional recovery after coronary revascularization for chronic coronary artery disease is dependent on maintenance of oxidative metabolism. *J Am Coll Cardiol.* 1992;20:569–577.

398. Caldwell JH, Revenaugh JR, Martin GV, Johnson PM, Rasey JS, Krohn KA. Comparison of fluorine-18-fluorodeoxyglucose and tritiated fluoromisonidazole u take during low-flow ischemia. *J Nucl Med.* 1995;36:1633–1638.

399. Calkins H, Lehmann MH, Allman K, Wieland D, Schwaiger M. Scintigraphic pattern of regional cardiac sympathetic innervation in patients with familial long QT syndrome using positron emission tomography. *Circulation.* 1993;87:1616–1621.

400. Delforge J, Syrota A, Lancon JL, et al. Cardiac fl-adrenergic receptor density measured in vivo using PET, CGP12177, and a new graphical method. *J Nucl Med.* 1991;32:739–748.

401. Syrota A. Positron emission tomography: evaluation of cardiac receptors. In: Marcus ML, Schelbert HR, Skorton DJ, Wolf GL, eds. *Cardiac Imaging: A Companion to Braunwald's Heart Disease.* Philadelphia, Pa: WB Saunders Company; 1991:1256–1270.

402. Ziegler SI, Frey AW, Überfuhr P, et al. Assessment of myocardial reinnervation in cardiac transplants by positron emission tomography: functional significance tested by heart rate variability. *Clin Sci (Colch).* 1996;91:126–128.

403. Hoffmeister HM, Müller-Schauenburg W, Helber U, Feine U, Seipel L. EKG-getriggerte FDG-Positron-Emissions-Computertomographie zur Identifikation von vitalem Myokard [abstract]. *Z Kardiol.* 1995;84(suppl 1):3.

404. Hoffmeister HM, Müller-Schauenburg W, Helber U, Machulla HJ, Feine U, Bares R. LV segmental metabolism and function in multi-vessel coronary heart disease detected with ECG-gated PET and dobutamine stress [abstract]. *Circulation.* 1997;96(suppl 1):68.

405. Müller-Schauenburg W, Hoffmeister HM, Helber U, Litzenmayer U, Feine U. Gated cardiac FDG PET improved by Fourier analysis in comparison with cine ventriculography [abstract]. *J Nucl Med.* 1995;36:141.

406. Perrone-Filardi P, Bacharach SL, Dilsizian V, et al. Clinical significance of reduced regional myocardial glucose uptake in regions with normal blood flow in patients with chronic coronary artery disease. *J Am Coll Cardiol.* 1994;23:608–616.

407. Soufer R, Dey HM, Ng CK, Zaret BL. Comparison of sestamibi single-photon emission computed tomography with positron emission tomography for estimating left ventricular myocardial viability. *Am J Cardiol.* 1995;75:1214–1219.

408. Tamaki N, Kawamoto M, Tadamura E, et al. Prediction of reversible ischemia after revascularization. *Circulation.* 1995;91:1697–1705.

409. vom Dahl J, Muzik O, Wolfe E, Allman C, Hutchins G, Schwaiger M. Myocardial rubidium-82 tissue kinetics assessed by dynamic positron emission tomography as a marker of myocardial cell membrane integrity and viability. *Circulation.* 1996;93:238–245.

410. Brunken RC, Kottou S, Nienaber CA, et al. PET detection of viable tissue in myocardial segments with persistent defects at Tl-201 SPECT. *Radiology.* 1989;65:65–73.

411. Haas F, Hähnel C, Sebening F, Meisner H, Schwaiger M. Effect of preoperative PET viability on peri- and postoperative risk [abstract]. *J Am Coll Cardiol.* 1996;27:300A.

412. Brunken RC, Mody FV, Hawkins RA, Nienaber C, Phelps ME, Schelbert HR. Positron emission tomography detects metabolic viability in myocardium with persistent 24 hours single-photon emission computed tomography Tl-201 defects. *Circulation.* 1992;86:1357–1369.

413. Flameng W, Suy R, Schwarz F, et al. Ultrastructural correlates of left ventricular contraction abnormalities in patients with chronic ischemic heart disease: determinants of reversible segmental asynergy. *Am Heart J.* 1981;102:846–857.

18

Medical Treatment of Coronary Artery Disease

Ming K. Heng

Coronary Artery Disease Syndromes

Current medical treatment of coronary artery disease (CAD) consists of interventions to increase coronary artery flow, reduce myocardial oxygen demand, prevent coronary artery thrombosis, and lyse existing coronary artery thrombi. The strategies used depend on the patient's ischemic syndromes. Patients with CAD may present to the physician with stable angina, unstable angina, myocardial infarction, or silent ischemia. To a physician seeing a CAD patient for the first time, the disease may manifest itself in any one of the mentioned syndromes. Over a period of time, most patients will experience a change from one syndrome to another. Although the physician cannot eliminate CAD in a patient, the goal of therapy is to keep the patient in a stable state consistent with the best quality of life and the lowest risk from either myocardial infarction or death. Patients are at lowest risk when they are free from ischemia, whether symptomatic or silent, or are in a state of stable angina with symptoms that are infrequent and brought on only by moderate to severe exertion.

Stable Angina

Angina pectoris, the pain brought on by myocardial ischemia, occurs whenever myocardial oxygen demand exceeds oxygen supply. In the majority of patients with angina, the underlying pathophysiology is reduced blood flow (i.e., reduced oxygen supply), because of luminal obstruction from CAD or coronary artery vasospasm. Hence in most patients presenting with anginalike chest pain, the diagnosis is usually CAD, particularly if there are associated risk factors for CAD. Coronary artery vasospasm without pre-existing CAD is an uncommon cause of angina but should be suspected in younger patients who take cocaine or present with Prinzmetal's angina. In addition, angina may be associated with conditions involving decreased oxygen supply without diminished blood flow, as in anemia. Even in these clinical circumstances, however, chest pain in patients with preexisting CAD is most likely due to angina.

Angina may also occur because of abnormally increased oxygen demands in conditions associated with increased myocardial mass—that is, left ventricular hypertrophy from either pressure overload (e.g., left or right ventricular hypertension or aortic or pulmonary valve stenosis) or volume overload (e.g., aortic or pulmonary regurgitation or mitral or tricuspid regurgitation). Most patients with angina involving increased oxygen demand have increased left ventricular mass, with angina originating from the left ventricular structural abnormality. Rarely, angina from this mechanism occurs from right ventricular pathology. Patients with severe pulmonary hypertension, for example, often have angina in the absence of CAD or left ventricular hypertrophy.

Another possible mechanism for angina in patients who have increased myocardial mass may be decreased coronary artery reserve, a condition in which the coronary arteries have a limited ability to dilate and increase myocardial blood flow to meet myocardial oxygen demand. Coronary artery flow reserve is the relative increase in blood flow during conditions of vasodilatation expressed as a percentage of the blood flow at rest. Patients with conditions associated with left ventricular pressure overload (e.g., hypertension, valvular aortic stenosis, and hypertrophic subaortic stenosis) may be particularly prone to decreased coronary artery reserve. Many older patients with these conditions also have underlying CAD, and angina may be present largely due to a combination of luminal obstruction and diminished coronary artery reserve

Angina pectoris is characterized by left precordial pain, tightness, or pressure, often radiating to the neck, jaw, or inner side of the left arm. The discomfort increases in severity over several minutes and dissipates over another few minutes. It is unusual for angina to be constant and present for hours. Angina is usually brought on or aggravated by physical exercise, large meals, cold exposure, and emotional stress and is relieved when these precipitating conditions disappear. Angina is usually relieved within 1 to 5 minutes of taking sublingual nitroglycerin. When all these elements are present, the patient has typical angina. Atypical angina is present when one or more of these elements are absent. Patients with only one or none of these elements are experiencing noncardiac chest pain. Ascertaining whether the symptom is typical angina, atypical angina, or noncardiac chest pain is helpful in determining CAD probability. In middle-age adults, the incidence of CAD is 90% in those with typical angina, 50% in those with atypical angina, 16% in those with noncardiac chest pain, and 3% to 4% in those without symptoms.[1]

Treatment of Stable Angina

General measures that should be applied in all patients with CAD must be incorporated into the treatment of those with stable angina. Although these measures may not relieve acute episodes of chest pain, in the long term they may be helpful in improving both longevity and quality of life, including reducing angina symptoms. General therapeutic measures for stable angina are directed toward correction of all classical risk factors for CAD, including control of hypertension, smoking cessation, optimum treatment of diabetes and hyperlipidemia, weight reduction if indicated, and institution of an exercise program. All patients with CAD must be repeatedly reminded of the importance of reducing risk factors because significant and permanent changes in lifestyle, which cannot be achieved without patient collaboration, are necessary. All patients with CAD should take aspirin (80–325 mg/d) unless its use is contraindicated. The routine use of aspirin for such patients has been shown to be associated with a reduction in cardiac events.[2–5]

Current drug therapy for stable angina is based on the principle of improving the myocardial oxygen supply and demand balance, with either drugs or one or more of the revascularization procedures. The latter include surgical bypass or one of the angioplasty procedures, discussed in greater detail elsewhere in this book. Some an-

tianginal drugs reduce myocardial oxygen demand by reducing heart rate, blood pressure, and contractility; others increase coronary blood flow. The major classes of antianginal medications currently in use have pharmacological properties that address one or more of these physiological goals. For example, the major effect of β-adrenergic blockers in angina is to reduce myocardial oxygen demand, whereas calcium channel blockers and nitrates increase coronary blood flow.

Nitrates

Nitrates relieve angina by two physiological actions:

1. Vasodilatation of normal and stenotic epicardial coronary arteries (i.e., medium to large conductance vessels), producing an increase in myocardial blood flow[6]
2. Vasodilatation of systemic veins, decrease in venous return, and fall in volume and pressure of all cardiac chambers,[7] which have the net effect of reducing myocardial oxygen demand

Although the endothelium is now known to be extremely active with regard to the production of chemical mediators that regulate vasomotion, the vasodilatory actions of nitrates are believed to be independent of endothelium function.[8] Nitrates increased intracellular nitric oxide formation directly, leading to an increase in cellular guanylate cyclase activity and corresponding increase in cyclic guanosine monophosphate. The increase in cyclic guanosine monophosphate produces vascular relaxation and vasodilation. Formation of nitric oxide and guanylate cyclase activity depends on the availability of sulfhydryl groups.[9] The development of nitrate tolerance to long-acting oral nitrates or transdermal patches is believed to be due to depletion of sulfhydryl groups with uninterrupted nitrate administration. Consequently, nitrates should be prescribed so that there is a 10- to 12-hour nitrate-free interval to decrease the likelihood of nitrate tolerance. To ensure sufficient nitrate-free intervals, nitrate patches should be applied for no longer than 14 hours at a time, and long-acting nitrate preparations should be given no more than two to three times daily, with one nitrate-free interval of at least 10 hours between dosages.

TABLE 18.1. Commonly used nitrate preparations.

Preparation	Dosage	Duration of action	Frequency
Sublingual NTG	0.3–0.5 mg	15–20 min	As required
Aerosol NTG	0.4 mg	15–20 min	As required
NTG ointment	2–4 CM (1–2 in)	4–6 h	Every 6 hr
NTG patches	0.1–0.6 mg/h	Continuous	Every 12–24 h
Oral ISDN	5–30 mg	3–6 h	Every 2–3 h
Oral ISDN (SR)	40–80 mg	6–8 h	Every 8–12 h
Oral ISMN	10–40 mg	30 min	Every 6–8 h
Oral ISMN (SR)	40–100 mg	30 min	Every 12 h

NTG, nitroglycerin; ISDN, isosorbide dinitrate; SR, sustained release; ISMN, isosorbide mononitrate.

Table 18.1 lists the most common nitrate preparations in clinical use for the treatment of angina. They may be divided into the very-short-acting preparations used to immediately relieve angina and the longer-acting preparations used to prevent recurrence of angina.

Sublingual Nitroglycerin

Sublingual preparations are the preferred treatment for acute episodes of angina occurring during either exercise or rest. A dose of 0.3 to 0.6 mg relieves angina within 1 to 5 minutes. Doses can be repeated every 5 minutes if needed, to a maximum of 1.2 mg in 15 to 20 minutes. Angina not relieved after this period requires the patient to seek medical assistance for either unstable angina or acute myocardial infarction. Sublingual nitroglycerin is also indicated before activities known to provoke angina in a particular patient. Taken prophylactically in this way, the medication can prevent episodes of angina for the duration of its serum half-life (i.e., 30 minutes). Tolerance does not usually develop from sublingual nitrate administration, presumably because this route does not produce persistence of nitrate blood levels for prolonged periods.

Aerosol Nitroglycerin

Aerosol nitroglycerin is used in much the same way as sublingual nitroglycerin; it contains oral nitroglycerin in a canister that delivers metered doses of 0.4 mg of aerosolized medication into the mouth. Aerosol nitroglycerin was developed to prolong the shelf life of sublingual nitroglycerin, which deteriorates on exposure to light. Side effects, indications, and contraindications for this preparation are similar to those of sublingual nitroglycerin.

Topical Nitroglycerin

Nitroglycerin can be administered through the skin in either an ointment or a patch. The ointment (about 15 mg/2 cm) is usually applied on the front of the chest in dosages of 1 to 4 cm (0.5–2 in) every 4 to 6 hours and covered with water-resistant plastic or paper adhesive. Because the ointment may stain clothing, it is usually not recommended for ambulatory patients. However, this preparation is extremely useful in hospitalized patients who have to remain in bed because of unstable angina or acute myocardial infarction. To avoid nitrate tolerance, the ointment should be removed to allow nitrate-free intervals of about 10 hours every 24 hours.

Nitroglycerin transdermal patches contain nitroglycerin in a matrix that allows continuous and predictable absorption through the skin. The patch can be applied anywhere on the skin of the body but is usually placed on the upper arm or front of the chest. The patch dosage varies from 0.1 to 0.6 mg/h (Table 18.1). Patients should be started on the lower doses and moved to higher doses if indicated. Like all nitrate preparations given continuously, the patch should be administered in a manner that allows a nitrate-free interval of 10 to 12 hours every 24 hours to prevent the development of nitrate tolerance.

Long-Acting Oral Nitrate Preparations

Isosorbide dinitrate is a long-acting nitrate preparation given to prevent angina by providing therapeutic blood levels on a prolonged basis. It is administered by either swallowing or chewing. The oral preparation has a longer onset and duration of action than the chewable form (Table 18.1). The oral preparation is therefore more suitable for prolonged protection from angina, whereas the chewable form may be given for either treatment of established angina or prophylaxis during activities that are known to provoke angina (e.g., physical activity or emotional stress). Isosorbide dinitrate is metabolized rapidly by the liver, but blood levels after oral administration vary considerably among patients. Accordingly, isosorbide dinitrate is usually given in increasing doses until the desired clinical effects are obtained. To prevent nitrate tolerance, isosorbide dinitrate is usually given two to three times daily in eccentric schedules to allow 10-hour or longer nitrate-free intervals. For example, a two-times-daily schedule may be at 8:00 AM and 5:00 PM, and a three-times-daily schedule may be at 8:00 AM, 1:00 PM, and 5:00 or 6:00 PM. For patients who have angina at night, the schedule should be readjusted to cover the night hours with a different nitrate-free interval or the use of a long-acting β-blocker or calcium channel blocker timed to ensure adequate drug levels at night.

Isosorbide dinitrate has a major metabolite—isosorbide 5-mononitrate—that is pharmacologically active, with a long half-life. Isosorbide 5-mononitrate is available commercially and has the advantage over its parent compound of a longer duration of action, requiring no more than twice-daily dosing (e.g., at 8:00 AM and 2:00 PM).

Nitrates are generally well tolerated by patients; the most troublesome side effects are headache and flushing. These side effects occur mainly in patients taking the drugs for the first time or at high doses. The side effects usually subside after a few days with continuation of therapy or reduction in dose. Headaches can usually be alleviated with nonsteroidal analgesic, which usually need to be given no longer than a few days.

β-Adrenergic Blocking Drugs

β-Adrenergic blockers (β-blockers) are major antianginal drugs that relieve angina by reducing myocardial oxygen demand by decreasing the heart rate, myocardial contractility, and blood pressure. As the name suggests, β-blockers block signal transduction of β-adrenergic receptors by catecholamines. This blockade results in a decrease in intracellular cyclic adenosine monophosphate formation and cyclic adenosine monophosphate–dependent protein kinase activity.[10] Because the latter mediates the physiological processes that occur secondary to increased catecholamine levels, the end result of β-blockade is a physiological state in which sympathetic drive is below normal (i.e., low heart rate, decreased contractility, and reduced blood pressure).

The two subtypes of β-adrenergic receptors, β_1 and β_2, have different physiological actions.[10,11] Stimulation of β_1-adrenergic receptors results mainly in an increase in myocardial contractility and heart rate, whereas stimulation of β_2-adrenergic receptors produces bronchial and peripheral vasodilation. As shown in Table 18.2, β-blockers' different affinity for blocking the two β-adrenergic receptors determine their clinical use.[12] Thus certain β-blockers (e.g., atenolol and metoprolol) that have greater affinity for the β_1-adrenergic receptors are regarded as cardioselective β-blockers, whereas others (e.g., propranolol and timolol) that do not possess this property are regarded as noncardioselective β-blockers. The β-blocker action that makes this class of drugs particularly useful in treating angina (i.e., reduced myocardial oxygen demand) can be achieved with most β-blockers. However, in patients who have peripheral vascular disease, asthma, and chronic obstructive pulmonary disease, it is more appropriate to use a cardioselective preparation if a β-blocker is indicated. It should be emphasized, however, that this cardioselectivity is relative and that at higher doses cardioselective β-blockers may significantly block β_2-adrenergic receptors, which results in bronchospasm or claudication. In patients who have peripheral vascular disease or a tendency for bronchospasm, cardioselective β-blockers should be started at

TABLE 18.2. Commonly used β-adrenergic blockers.

	Nonselective	Selective	ISA	α-Blocking
Acebutolol		+	+	
Atenolol		+		
Betaxoplol		+		
Bucindolol	+			+
Carvedilol	+			+
Esmolol		+		
Labetalol	+		+	+
Metoprolol		+		
Nadolol	+			
Pindolol	+		+	
Propranolol	+			
Sotalol	+			
Timolol	+			

ISA, intrinsic sympathomimetic activity; + pharmacological activity present.

the lowest possible dose and monitored closely for any adverse effects before the dose is increased.

Other pharmacological properties of some β-blockers are of uncertain significance in their use for angina. Thus the β-blocker labetol has an α-adrenergic receptor blocking property that produces peripheral vasodilation in addition to its β-blocking effects. Although peripheral vasodilation may have some theoretical advantages in use of the drug for hypertension, it is unclear whether it is better than other β-blockers in treating angina. Some β-blockers (e.g., pindolol) have intrinsic sympathomimetic activity that results in an interesting combination of both β-adrenergic inhibitory and stimulatory properties. Although the drugs with intrinsic sympathomimetic activity may have theoretical advantages in terms of less myocardial depression, bronchospasm, and so forth, it is still unclear whether these β-blockers are clinically better for treating angina than those without intrinsic sympathomimetic activity.

The side effects of β-blockers are predictable from their pharmacological actions. Side effects include aggravation of heart failure associated with low ejection fraction, bronchospasm, sinus bradycardia, bradycardia associated with atrioventricular conduction block, impotence, and aggravation of peripheral vascular disease. In addition, β-blockers may mask hypoglycemic attacks due to insulin overdose in diabetic patients. Many patients also complain of fatigue and lethargy; however, these side effects often improve after 1 to 2 weeks of β-blocker use.

Calcium Channel Blockers

Calcium channel blockers, another major class of antianginal medication, are highly effective in the treatment of angina. The movement of calcium ions across calcium channels is responsible, in large part, for myocardial contraction, spontaneous cardiac electrical activity, and maintenance of vascular smooth muscle tone. Using drugs to block calcium channels results in less forceful cardiac contractions (i.e., negative inotropism), slowed pacemaker function of both atrioventricular and sinus nodes (negative chronotropism), and decreased smooth muscle tone (decreased systemic vascular resistance). Commonly used calcium channel blockers are listed in Table 18.3.

Drugs shown to have calcium channel blocking properties are heterogeneous with respect to their chemical structures and pharmacological actions.[13,14] These drugs, based on their pharmacological action, are usually considered as belonging to the following groups largely based on their pharmacologic action: the dihydropyridines, diltiazem, verapamil, and bepridil. The group that is derived from dihydropyridines include nifedipine, nicardipine, amodipine, isradipine, felodipine, and nimodipine. Diltiazem is derived from benzodiazepine, verapamil has a chemical structure that resem-

TABLE 18.3. Commonly used calcium channel blockers.

	Heart rate	AV node conduction	Peripheral resistance	Myocardial contractility	Cardiac output
Amlodipine	↑	–	↓↓	↓	↑–
Felodipine	↑	–	↓↓	–	↑–
Nifedipine	↑	–	↓↓	↓	↑–
Nicardipine	↑	–	↓↓	–	↑–
Nimodipine	↑	–	↑↓	–	↑–
Diltiazem	↓	↓↓	↑↓	↓	↑↓
Verapamil	↑↓	↓↓	↓	↓↓	↑↓
Bepridil	↓	↓↓	–	↑↓	↑↓

AV, atrioventricular; ↑, increase; ↓, decrease; ↑↓, variable, may increase or decrease in individual patients; –, no change.

bles papaverine, and bepridil has a unique chemical structure unrelated to any currently used cardiac drug.

Calcium blocking drugs vary in their effect on myocardial contraction, spontaneous cardiac electrical activity, and maintenance of vascular smooth muscle tone. All calcium channel blockers depress myocardial contractility and produce coronary arterial vasodilation by smooth muscle relaxation.[15] The dihydropyridine derivatives are much more potent peripheral vasodilators than the other groups but have little effect on nodal conduction.[16,17] Use of the dihydropyridine derivatives, in general, results in an increase in coronary blood flow, a decrease in blood pressure, either no change or an increase in heart rate, and a decrease in myocardial contractility. The negative inotropic effects of this group of drugs may be offset by a fall in peripheral resistance, so that deterioration of ejection fraction and systolic heart failure may not occur. The main cardiac side effects of these drugs are reflex tachycardia and hypotension.

Diltiazem significantly slows both sinus and atrioventricular nodal conduction but only moderately reduces cardiac contractility and peripheral resistance. The common cardiac side effects of diltiazem therapy are sinus bradycardia (especially in older patients with preexisting sick sinus syndrome), atrioventricular nodal block, and aggravation of systolic heart failure.

Verapamil has potent negative inotropic action, significantly slows nodal conduction (particularly of the atrioventricular node), and moderately reduces peripheral resistance. The latter action is usually not sufficient to overcome verapamil's negative inotropic effects. Because of these actions, important cardiac side effects of verapamil therapy are atrioventricular nodal block and aggravation of systolic heart failure.

Bepridil, in addition to being a calcium channel blocker, has sodium channel blocking actions that give the drug quinidine-like effects. Consequently, bepridil may lengthen the QT interval and prolong the effective refractive periods of the atria and ventricles. Because of these actions, bepridil may induce new arrhythmias, particularly new premature ventricular contractions, ventricular tachycardia, and ventricular fibrillation. Because

of QT-interval prolongation, bepridil use may, on rare occasions, cause torsade de pointes–type ventricular tachycardia, particularly in patients with low serum potassium levels. Bepridil also significantly blocks sinus and atrioventricular nodal conduction but has less effect on cardiac contractility and peripheral resistance. The major concern with bepridil therapy is the development of ventricular arrhythmias. Accordingly, use of bepridil as an antianginal medication should be limited to patients with chronic stable angina who have failed to respond adequately to other antianginal medications.

It is clear that the different drugs in the family of calcium channel blockers have varying effects on different organs. This variation occurs partly because drugs belonging to different groups of the family exert qualitatively similar but quantitatively different effects on the same organ system and partly because the effects on one organ system may be offset by those on another system. Knowledge of the different effects of each member of the calcium channel blocker family can be used to the patient's advantage by selecting the drug that best fits the patient's clinical profile. For example, a dihydropyridine derivative, especially amlodipine, is better suited for treatment of angina in patients with coexisting systolic heart failure. Similarly, diltiazem and verapamil are more suitable drugs for the treatment of angina in patients with coexisting atrial arrhythmias because these medications also assist in controlling ventricular rate by slowing atrioventricular nodal conduction.

Use of Combinations of Antianginal Medications

The different classes of antianginal medications provide considerable options for optimizing therapy in patients with angina. Depending on the severity of symptoms, physicians have the choice of using one, two, or all three classes of antianginal drugs. In general, physicians should avoid prescribing combinations of two drugs in the same class (e.g., two β-blockers or two long-acting nitrate preparations). However, because calcium channel blockers have diverse effects, physicians may prescribe two concurrently. Such combinations are used only rarely when combination therapy is needed in a patient who is unable to tolerate either nitrates or β-blockers. Before prescribing two calcium channel blockers, the physician should fully understand the drugs and ensure that their adverse effects are not potentiated by each other.

Patients at low risk for serious cardiac events (e.g., those with single-vessel disease or normal left ventricular function) and with mild symptoms can be treated with sublingual nitrates either with or without a long-acting nitrate preparation. Patients with moderate symptoms require combinations of two or more drugs, generally nitrates with a β-blocker or calcium channel blocker. Because there is good evidence that the long-term use of β-blockers is associated with a reduction in mortality rate after myocardial infarction,[18] the combination of a β-blocker and a nitrate should be considered first. However, this combination may not be suitable for patients in whom the side effects of β-blockers may be particularly problematic. Such patients include men who may develop impotence and those with heart failure secondary to low ejection fraction, atrioventricular block, and bronchospastic lung disease. In these patients, a nitrate–calcium channel blocker combination may be more appropriate.

If combination therapy with nitrate–calcium channel blockers is used, it is important to remember that both nitrates and the dihydropyridine group of drugs produce reflex tachycardia. A combination of these drugs may thus result in an excessive increase in heart rate, an undesirable side effect in patients with CAD. A nitrate–calcium channel blocker combination should begin with a nitrate–diltiazem or nitrate–verapamil combination.

Antilipid Therapy

The concept of cholesterol-lowering therapy as an integral part of the management of CAD is now the subject of much interest and discussion. Cholesterol-lowering therapy refers to the practice of (1) aggressively treating elevated cholesterol levels with the goal of CAD regression or delayed progression and (2) administering cholesterol-lowering drugs even when the cholesterol level is not elevated to the range conventionally regarded as requiring therapy (i.e., drug treatment is offered regardless of the initial cholesterol levels). As reviewed by Brown,[19] the importance of cholesterol-lowering therapy has arisen because of studies on the effects of cholesterol lowering with the goal of CAD regression. In these studies, although the anatomical changes in CAD with respect to regression or delay in progression have been extremely small, the reduction in clinical cardiac events has been much more impressive. The general trend in most of these reports is a reduction of the rate of CAD progression, usually measured by the minimum obstruction diameter or mean segmental diameter of the affected coronary arteries, on the order of 0.05 to 0.1 mm between treated and untreated patients. Yet despite these relatively small anatomical changes, clinical events in the treated groups may be about 20% to 40% less compared with those of the untreated groups. The reduction in clinical events include cardiac deaths, myocardial infarctions (fatal and nonfatal), angioplasty, coronary artery bypass, unstable angina, transient ischemic episodes, and strokes.

The probable mechanism for the small anatomical changes and the larger reduction in clinical events is plaque stabilization. Despite the seemingly small changes in lumen diameter, treated patients may have atherosclerotic lesions that are much less prone to rupture compared with those in untreated patients. Another possible mechanism may be less coronary artery vasomotor lability in treated patients because of lower cholesterol levels. Hyperlipidemia has been shown to cause loss or attenuation of endothelial-dependent vasodilation.[20] The combination of plaque stability and improved coronary vasodilatory function probably accounts for much of the improvement in clinical outcome despite unimpressive anatomical changes.

The extent of lipid lowering needed to reduce cardiovascular events with antilipid therapy is not known at present. Moreover, it is also unknown whether the extent of lowering of lipid levels for reduction of CAD events is different from that of CAD regression. Because the relationship between the risk of cardiovascular events and lipid levels appears continuous, any reduction in lipid levels is beneficial. In terms of a target level for the purpose of therapy, it appears reasonable to adopt the US National Cholesterol Education Program recommendation for patients with CAD (i.e., total cholesterol < 200 mg/dL and LDL cholesterol < 100 mg/dL).[21]

Antiplatelet and Anticoagulation Therapy

In patients with CAD, the potential usefulness of platelet inhibition (e.g., aspirin) and anticoagulation (e.g., coumadin and heparin) therapy has been recognized for a long time. Only in recently, however, have trials clarified whether such therapy produces clinical benefits in terms of reduction in mortality or morbidity rates.

The atherosclerotic process is associated with endothelial injury and dysfunction, including loss of the anticoagulant activity that allows normal endothelium to maintain a smooth and thrombus-free surface.[22] Loss of this function, particularly when associated with disruption of the endothelial layer and exposure of subendothelial material such as lipids and collagen to blood, results in platelet activation and aggregation at the site of atherosclerotic lesions. Platelet aggregation causes mechanical obstruction of luminal blood flow, release of cytokines that mediate further platelet aggregation, vasoconstriction, and intimal hyperplasia. Aspirin inhibits platelet cyclo-oxygenase, leading to a reduction of thromboxane A_2 and prostacyclin formation.[23] Low doses of aspirin (85–325 mg/d) probably reduce thromboxane A_2 production more than prostacyclin production.[24] Because thromboxane A_2 produces vasoconstriction and platelet aggregation, whereas prostacyclin has the opposite effect, the result of the relatively greater inhibition of thromboxane A_2 is prevention of periodic intense vasoconstriction and acute ischemic syndromes.

Several large studies have shown that aspirin in low doses reduces the risk of myocardial infarction when given either for primary prevention in patients at high risk for CAD or for secondary prevention in patients with known disease.[25] When the results of trials for secondary prevention in CAD are pooled, aspirin appears to reduce the mortality rate by about 15% and repeat myocardial infarction by 30%.

The issue of the appropriate dose of aspirin has been debated at length for many years. The doses of aspirin used in the studies cited earlier ranged from 300 to 1500 mg/d; some investigators studied aspirin in combination with dipyridamole. Because aspirin is most useful when its therapeutic action is directed mainly toward thromboxane A_2 rather than prostacyclin inhibition, it has been increasingly recognized in recent years that this goal is best achieved with low rather than high doses of the drug. The currently recommended dose for long-term primary or secondary prevention is between 80 and 325 mg/d. Side effects are uncommon at this dose range but when present are mainly gastrointestinal, including gastritis, gastric or duodenal ulceration, and gastrointestinal bleeding. In patients who have gastrointestinal irritation without frank bleeding or ulceration, aspirin therapy can be continued with enteric-coated preparations. Aspirin therapy is contraindicated in patients with known hypersensitivity to the drug and should be used with caution in patients with impaired renal function.

Other known antiplatelet agents currently available include dipyridamole and ticlopidine. Even though dipyridamole has been investigated in combination with aspirin in some trials, no clear-cut data support the use of dipyridamole as a platelet inhibitor to prevent cardiac events in patients with CAD.[26] Similarly, the role of the newer antiplatelet agent ticlopidine in patients with CAD and chronic angina is not yet known.

The therapeutic value of long-term oral anticoagulation administration in patients with CAD has long been the subject of controversy. The concept that coronary thrombosis is a major cause of myocardial infarction was recognized several decades ago, and a number of trials of oral anticoagulation were conducted between 1950 and 1970 in patients who had experienced myocardial infarction.[27] The results of these trials were inconclusive because of small sample sizes, poor study design, and inadequate control of the anticoagulation level. The routine use of long-term anticoagulation therapy in patients with CAD was largely abandoned by most physicians for a number of years.

In the 1980s, however, a number of larger and more carefully designed studies reopened the question of the therapeutic efficacy of chronic anticoagulation therapy after myocardial infarction.[28-30] These studies showed that long-term oral anticoagulation therapy significantly reduces the incidence of recurrent myocardial infarction (30%–50%) and cerebrovascular events (40%–55%) but has equivocal effects on mortality rates. Oral anticoagulation therapy was associated with an increase in bleeding and cerebral hemorrhage. In comparing the results of aspirin and oral anticoagulation therapies in trials that studied each agent separately, the two therapies appeared to have similar effects for patients at low risk for future cardiac events (i.e., patients without heart failure, cardiomegaly, atrial fibrillation, or known intracardiac thrombus). Currently, aspirin is the preferred treatment for such low-risk patients because it has fewer side effects than oral anticoagulation therapy. In contrast, patients with one or more of the mentioned clinical features may benefit more from oral anticoagulation medications, provided they understand that there is a small but significant risk of bleeding. Studies are currently under way to directly compare the relative benefits of aspirin and oral anticoagulation medications by randomizing patients into one of the two groups. Until the results of such studies are available, it is prudent to use aspirin mainly for patients with uncomplicated CAD and oral anticoagulation preparations for higher-risk patients with heart failure or risk of embolic events. The issue of whether combinations of the two forms of therapy are better than either alone awaits further study.

Antioxidant Therapy

The potential role of antioxidants in the long-term treatment of CAD has recently been the subject of much interest and debate. The concept that antioxidants may be beneficial for patients with CAD is based on the results of many experimental studies that indicate that an important mechanism of atherogenesis is oxidation injury. Low-density lipoproteins (LDLs) in arterial walls undergo oxidation by oxygen free radicals produced by many cells within atherosclerotic lesions.[31] Oxidized LDLs have been clearly shown to be cytotoxic and may be critical in the onset of atherogenesis.[32,33] Because oxidized LDL is taken up by scavenger receptors of macrophages, accumulations of oxidized LDL in the macrophage population within arterial lesions are postulated to constitute an important cause of arterial wall injury and atherosclerosis. The hypothesis that arterial wall injury by oxidized LDL is one mechanism of atherogenesis has led to studies that attempted to determine whether antioxidant therapy may either retard or stop the progression of CAD. Investigations have focused on probucol, a lipid-lowering drug, and vitamins A, C, and E, which are naturally occurring antioxidants found in many food sources.

Probucol, a cholesterol-lowering drug that has been available for many years, lowers both low-density and high-density lipoprotein levels by mechanisms that are still unknown. The drug prevents the oxidation of LDL by oxygen free radicals, possibly through its ability to function as a scavenger for peroxyl and lipid radicals.[34] Some studies with animals suggest that probucol is antiatherogenic because it retards atherosclerosis in animals with high-lipid diets.[35] A recent clinical study appears to indicate that endothelial function, as measured by vasodilation in response to acetylcholine, may be restored by a year of probucol therapy.[36] However, no long-term clinical study has suggested that CAD morbidity or mortality rates are significantly lowered by the drug. The combination of these findings supported the hypothesis that antioxidants may prevent or retard CAD and stimulated the recent interest in vitamins A, C, and E as potentially therapeutic antioxidants.

Most reports of the relationship between the intake of naturally occurring antioxidant vitamins and the risk of CAD are observational epidemiological studies. Several epidemiological studies have examined the relationship between dietary intake of vitamin E and risk of CAD; these studies suggest that high intake of the agent is related to a reduced risk of CAD.[37-39] The major foods considered by these studies to be high in vitamin E were nuts and seeds. Because the studies relied on the patients' memories of specific foods consumed, the relationship between vitamin E intake and CAD is presumed and imprecise. In contrast, attempts to provide more precise validation to the hypothesis by intake of known dosages of vitamin E supplements in a study population have not shown a definite inverse relationship between vitamin supplements and CAD.[39]

Epidemiological data suggest that high dietary intake of fruits and vegetables containing beta carotene is associated with a lowered risk of CAD.[40] However, this result was not confirmed in a recent large report on another observational epidemiological study in postmenopausal women.[39] Increased intake of beta carotene by supplementation has not been shown to have a definite inverse relationship with risk of CAD. On the contrary, results from two large randomized prospective trials suggest that beta carotene supplementation may be associated with a higher incidence of lung cancer and increased total and cardiovascular mortality rates, particular among smokers.[41,42] The data with vitamin C intake and CAD risk are related solely to observational studies and do not show definitively that vitamin C intake lowers CAD risk.[39]

The balance of evidence at this time suggests that increased dietary intake of vitamin E, and possibly beta carotene, reduces the risk of CAD. It does not indicate that vitamin C also has this effect or that supplementation with any antioxidant vitamin or drug will unequivocally reduce CAD risks in humans. Furthermore, there is no clear evidence that any antioxidant will retard the rapid progression of atherosclerosis seen after vascular angioplasty. The discrepancy between the epidemiological studies of dietary intake and prospective studies of vitamin supplementation, especially of vitamin E and beta carotene, may be due to the fact that dietary intake of the vitamins is associated with other nutrients not contained in the form of pure supplements. Patients concerned about CAD should be encouraged to eat a varied diet that contains moderate to large amounts of fruit and vegetable products rich in vitamin E and beta carotene. Because no evidence indicates that probucol has antioxidant effects in humans at clinical doses, use of probucol should not extend beyond its anticholesterol role.

Unstable Angina

Definition of Unstable Angina

Unstable angina is a condition in which a recent pattern of angina is increasing in severity or frequency. Unstable angina, part of the spectrum of clinical manifestations of CAD, is intermediate in clinical severity and prognosis between stable angina at one end and acute myocardial infarction at the other. In recognition of this, and the observation that acute myocardial infarction is often preceded by unstable angina, previous terms for the syndrome have included *preinfarction angina, impending myocardial infarction, accelerated angina, crescendo angina,* and *intermediate coronary syndrome.* Although the risk of acute myocardial infarction is increased in patients with unstable angina compared with stable angina, it is apparent that the risk is not as high as previously thought. Consequently, the term *unstable angina* has become accepted over other terms that carry more serious implications.

Because of previous confusion regarding the definition of unstable angina, which in turn affected clarification of the natural history and optimum treatment of the syndrome, Braunwald proposed a definition of unstable angina that also permitted a classification based on severity of angina, possible etiology, and underlying treatment.[43] From a purely functional viewpoint, however, the syndrome of unstable angina is present[44] when any one of the following clinical presentations is occurring: rest angina lasting more than 20 minutes and occurring within 1 week of presentation, new onset of angina within the last 2 months with a severity of Canadian Cardiovascular Society Classification III, or a pattern of increasing angina within 2 months so that the angina severity is increased by at least one class to current Canadian Cardiovascular Society Classification III severity (Table 18.4).

It is important to emphasize that, irrespective of how one chooses to define the condition, unstable angina is essentially a clinical diagnosis. The value of making the diagnosis is to draw attention to a syndrome that, in the presence of underlying CAD, is much more likely than stable angina to lead to serious cardiac events (i.e., myocardial infarction and death) but is also highly treatable. Moreover, clinicians must remember that the con-

TABLE 18.4. Definition and presentation of unstable angina.

Rest angina	Angina at rest, >20 min in duration, occurring within 1 wk of presentation
New-onset angina	Angina of at least CCSC III severity, occurring within 2 mo of presentation
Increasing angina	Angina that is increasing in frequency, longer in duration, or lower in threshold, to at least CCSC III severity; or an increase of CCSC level by at least one class over last 2 mo

CCSC, Canadian Cardiovascular Society Classification (of angina functional status).

dition is a syndrome that requires therapy before laboratory confirmation of either underlying CAD or evolving myocardial infarction. Thus, a number of patients with the clinical diagnosis of unstable angina will turn out, after appropriate investigation, to have either acute myocardial infarction or chest pain due to noncardiac causes. To ensure that the diagnosis of unstable angina is appropriate, particular care should be paid to obtaining a history that would suggest either the presence or an increased likelihood of CAD (e.g., previous myocardial infarction, history of angina, presence of known CAD by laboratory criteria, acute electrocardiographic [ECG] abnormalities, and presence of multiple major risk factors).

In most cases of unstable angina, the pathophysiology is a decrease in coronary artery flow; less frequently, unstable angina is due to an increase in myocardial oxygen demand. Most patients with unstable angina, particularly those presenting with more dramatic acute ischemic syndromes, probably have plaque disruption of established atherosclerotic lesions, which leads to a rapid fall in coronary artery blood flow because of mechanical obstruction and thrombosis.[45] Plaque disruption may decrease the luminal diameter independent of thrombosis if blood enters the fissure and expands the lesion or if an intimal flap that reduces the luminal cross-sectional area is produced. Very commonly, however, plaque disruption leads to thrombus formation because the contact of blood with subendothelial elements (e.g., lipids or collagen) initiates the process of thrombosis. Coronary artery vasoconstriction is likely to be another important mechanism in the pathogenesis of unstable angina.[46] Although coronary artery vasoconstriction may occur in the absence of atherosclerotic disease, it is more commonly seen in patients with known CAD. Atherosclerosis leads to endothelium dysfunction, including loss of control of vasomotor tone from diminished production of nitric oxide by the affected endothelium. The coronary arteries are thus less able to vasodilate, allowing unopposed action of vasoconstrictive substances such as endothelin. The pathophysiological result may be intense coronary vasospasm in focal parts of the coronary arterial circulation, leading to acute coronary ischemic syndromes.

Treatment of Unstable Angina

Treatment of unstable angina is based on present concepts of the pathophysiology of the condition. Thus, major emphasis is placed on therapies directed toward reversing the thrombotic process with anticoagulation or antiplatelet agents and improving the myocardial supply—demand balance with coronary arterial vasodilators and β-blockers.

All patients with unstable angina considered to have intermediate to high risks for an acute cardiac event should be admitted to the hospital in a monitored setting. These include patients with prolonged angina of more than 20 minutes, rest or nocturnal chest pain, recent chest pain brought on by mild or minimal exertion, ECG ST-segment elevation or depression during chest pain, ECG that is different from previous record even in the absence of ongoing pain, and clinical signs of hemodynamic instability (e.g., evidence of hypotension and signs of heart failure as shown by tachycardia, tachypnea, S_3, rales, new or worsening mitral regurgitation, and left ventricular failure on chest x-ray). Patients without these features have a lower risk of acute cardiac events and can be managed as outpatients with aspirin and antianginal medications. They should return as outpatients for reevaluation within 3 to 4 days, when plans should be made for longer-term management.

Antiplatelet Agents

Antiplatelet agents that have been shown to be particularly useful in unstable angina include aspirin and ticlopidine. Because most cases of unstable angina appear to be caused by plaque disruption, the pharmacological actions of antiplatelet agents are particularly important in managing the condition. By preventing thrombin formation and release of cytokines, which mediates vasoconstriction, these drugs assist in maintaining coronary flow in affected arteries.

In recent years several large randomized trials of aspirin in patients with unstable angina have shown a significant reduction in cardiac events with aspirin therapy.[47–50] The results are especially remarkable because the trend is consistent despite differences in drug dosages, duration of follow-up, and definition of unstable angina. Aspirin therapy should be started immediately on diagnosis of unstable angina except if contraindicated. The recommended initial dosage of aspirin need not exceed 325 mg/d for 2 to 3 days, after which daily doses of 80 to 325 mg are recommended for maintenance therapy. Patients already following an aspirin regimen probably do not require higher doses of the drug.

Ticlopidine has a different mechanism of platelet inhibition than aspirin but has also been shown to reduce cardiac events in patients with unstable angina. Ticlopidine probably acts by interfering with platelet activation mechanisms that are adenosine diphosphate dependent and with the platelet glycoprotein IIb/IIIa receptor. Nonfatal myocardial infarction and deaths were reduced by about 40% with this drug.[51] Ticlopidine is given in a dose of 250 mg twice daily. The drug should be prescribed only for patients who are unable to use aspirin; it is far more expensive than aspirin, and there is small (1%–2%) but potentially serious risk of developing neutropenia and agranulocytosis.

Heparin and Other Antithrombin Therapy

Use of heparin is supported by the rationale that prevention of clot formation by inhibiting thrombin formation secondary to plaque rupture maintains coronary flow in the affected artery. Because heparin therapy requires close monitoring of clotting time, the studies are not as extensive as those with aspirin. Heparin is recommended for patients with unstable angina who continue to have angina despite a regimen of aspirin and optimum dosages of antianginal medication, including nitrates and either calcium channel or β-adrenergic blockers. Some evidence suggests that heparin with aspirin is more effective in reducing cardiac events than either agent alone.[50,52]

Heparin is given as a continuous infusion to maintain an activated partial thromboplastin time (aPTT) between 45 and 70 seconds, or 1.5 to 2.5 times control; the aPTT should be measured 6 hours after dosage initiation or change and daily once therapeutic dosages of heparin are reached. Intermittent boluses of heparin may be associated with increased risk of bleeding compared to the continuous infusion. Although the duration of heparin therapy for unstable angina is unknown, 2 to 4 days of heparin therapy are adequate to control acute ischemic symptoms in most patients. The dose of heparin should be continuously reassessed during this period; failure to control angina may be due to inadequate dosages of heparin and antianginal medications rather than to failure of medical therapy.

The major adverse effect of heparin is bleeding from an excessive increase in aPTT; this is prevented by careful monitoring of aPTT with every dose change. A small percentage of patients may develop thrombocytopenia secondary to a hypersensitivity reaction associated with platelet antibodies. Accordingly, platelet counts should be taken daily for 3 to 5 days after initiation of heparin therapy; platelet counts below 100,000 indicate that heparin therapy should be stopped.

Thrombolytic therapy has no defined role in unstable angina at present. A large randomized study of thrombolytic therapy in patients with acute ischemic syndromes not associated with acute ST-segment elevation in the ECG (i.e., unstable angina and non–Q-wave myocardial infarction) has not shown reduction of cardiac events or mortality rates.[53] It should be emphasized, however, that some patients with angina may present with ST-segment elevation without subsequent enzyme changes. These patients should be treated with thrombolysis because the strategy of using the therapy in this setting has been shown to reduce cardiac mortality, as discussed later in the treatment of acute myocardial infarction. Current evidence, however, does not support the use of thrombolysis in patients who present with acute ischemic syndromes associated with ST-segment depression.

Antianginal Therapy

Antianginal therapy with combinations of nitrates, β-blockers, and calcium channel blockers is essential for managing unstable angina. The goal of antianginal therapy is to render the patient asymptomatic and hemodynamically stable without heart failure while maintaining heart rate and blood pressure within physiological ranges. The use of antianginal therapy in patients with unstable angina is based on the rationale that patients with persistent chest pain or hemodynamic instability are more likely to experience acute cardiac events. However, it should be emphasized that there is no definite evidence from randomized clinical trials that antianginal therapy, whether given as a single drug or in a combination of drugs, significantly reduces mortality rates in patients with unstable angina.

Nitrates

All patients with unstable angina should take some form of nitrates. Outpatients can use oral (e.g., isosorbide dinitrate) or topical (e.g., nitroglycerin patches or ointment) nitrates. For inpatients, the choice of oral, topical, or intravenous nitrates is usually based on clinical evaluation; patients who are significantly symptomatic are usually treated with intravenous nitroglycerin. Intravenous nitroglycerin can be started at 5 μg/min, increasing the rate by 5 μ/min every 5 to 10 minutes until the heart rate has increased by 5 to 10 beats per minute, the blood pressure has fallen by 10 mm Hg, or the patient complains of severe headaches. Once started, intravenous nitroglycerin is usually continued for 1 to 3 days without interruption because nitrate-free intervals are not necessary with this parental use of the drug. However, oral and topical nitrates, whether given at the start of unstable angina or after cessation of intravenous nitrate administration, should be given to allow an 8- to 10-hour nitrate-free interval to reduce nitrate tolerance.

β-Adrenergic Blockers

β-Adrenergic blockers in combination with nitrates are considered by many clinicians to be standard therapy for patients with unstable angina, especially those admitted to the hospital for the condition. The combination of the two drugs is physiologically rational and clinically highly effective in reducing anginal symptoms in other settings. The use of β-blockers in patients with unstable angina has not been subjected to the extensive trials undertaken with these agents in relation to acute myocardial infarction. In smaller studies, β-blockers have been shown to reduce chest pain and reduce the incidence of acute myocardial infarction.[54]

The choice of a specific β-blocker is not important, because they all appear to reduce sympathetic tone in the acute ischemic syndromes. However, β-blockers with intrinsic sympathetic activity (e.g., pindolol) should be avoided. β-Blockers should be given in doses that reduce the heart rate to 50 to 60 beats per minute while maintaining a relatively normal blood pressure. These drugs may be particularly useful in patients with high adrenergic tone who have high heart rates and blood pressure at the time of presentation; many of these patients are younger than average CAD patients. β-Blocker therapy can also be started using intravenous preparations (e.g., esmolol, metoprolol, or atenolol); once the desired levels of heart rate and blood pressure are achieved, the patients can be switched to oral β-blockers.

Patients who are already taking β-blockers should continue with their medication but with the dose titrated to maintain heart rate and blood pressure to the levels indicated earlier. For patients who are not taking β-blockers, β-blocker therapy should be initiated only after a careful review of potential contraindications because the development of adverse effects (e.g., bronchospastic disease, heart failure associated with low ejection fraction, and coronary vasospasm) may be especially problematic during ongoing acute coronary ischemia. Patients with heart failure associated with high ejection fractions (i.e., diastolic heart failure) can be treated with β-blockers.

Calcium Channel Blockers

In unstable angina, calcium channel blockers should be regarded as therapy to help reduce chest pain after nitrates and β-blockers have not completely controlled symptoms. Clinical studies of the use of several first-generation calcium channel blockers (e.g., nifedipine, diltiazem, and verapamil) in unstable angina without β-blockers have shown that calcium channel blockers are effective in reducing chest pain but appear to have no salutary effect on cardiac mortality or myocardial infarction.[55] Indeed, short-acting nifedipine as sole therapy may be associated with more nonfatal myocardial infarctions than metoprolol or a combination of both drugs.[56] However, the combination of calcium channel blockers and β-blockers appears to be more effective than either agent alone in reducing chest pain. In view of the studies showing that calcium channel blockers have no definite

survival benefit in patients with unstable angina,[55,56] these agents should be used as an adjunct to an existing regimen of β-blockers and nitrates for better control of chest pain. In patients in whom β-blockers are contraindicated, calcium channel blockers can be used with nitrates. In this case, a calcium channel blocker that does not cause reflex tachycardia (e.g., diltiazem rather than nifedipine) should be used.

In summary, medical treatment of unstable angina consists of routine administration of aspirin, heparin, and generally two or more antianginal medications for each patient (except those in whom aspirin or heparin is contraindicated). Most patients should receive nitrates with β-blockers to initiate antianginal treatment; patients who fail to respond to optimum doses of these agents should have calcium channel blockers added. Patients who improve on this therapy should be scheduled for further workups to assess their risk for future cardiac events, generally starting with noninvasive diagnostic procedures (i.e., some form of stress test). Those who display clinical evidence of high risk for cardiac events during their initial presentation (e.g., ST-segment changes during pain or heart failure) may undergo immediate angiography to define their anatomy for revascularization.

Other Treatment Modalities

Other treatment options for patients with unstable angina include intraaortic balloon counterpulsation and revascularization with surgery and some form of coronary angioplasty. These procedures are discussed in more detail elsewhere in this book.

Aortic counterpulsation is effective in controlling chest pain and hemodynamics in severely symptomatic or unstable patients. It must be used only as a precursor to either surgery or angioplasty. Coronary angioplasty and coronary bypass surgery are indicated in patients who are symptomatic and hemodynamically unstable, despite optimum medical therapy, and those considered at high risk for future cardiac events (e.g., patients with significant ST-segment changes during angina). The choice of angioplasty or surgery in an individual patient depends on coronary anatomy, left ventricular function, and other coexisting conditions that affect the risk for the procedure. At this time, there is no evidence that a strategy of routine revascularization with either angioplasty or surgery in all patients with unstable angina increases survival. A large randomized study (TIMI IIIb) comparing the outcome of early revascularization versus conservative therapy did not show any difference in survival rate.[57] Two randomized studies also failed to show that a strategy of routine bypass surgery was more effective than medical treatment for unstable angina.[58,59]

In general, patients with one or two coronary artery lesions should be considered for angioplasty, and those with left main or three-vessel disease with low ejection fraction are surgical candidates. If possible, angioplasty should be performed after symptoms of the acute ischemic syndrome have been brought under control; angioplasty in the first few days of unstable angina generally carries much higher risk of cardiac events compared with that done later. For reasons discussed earlier, coronary angiography is not routinely indicated in all patients with unstable angina but rather in patients who may need revascularization (i.e., those who fail to respond to medical therapy) or are at high risk for future cardiac events. Patients at high risk for future events include those with unstable angina soon after an acute myocardial infarction (postinfarction angina), significant ischemia on noninvasive stress testing, heart failure, low ejection on echocardiogram or radionuclide studies, and possibly previous angioplasty or bypass surgery.

Prognosis for Patients With Unstable Angina

Because of different definitions of unstable angina, the prognosis varies among studies. Unpublished data from the Duke Cardiovascular Databank show that the mortality rate for patients with unstable angina is highest (about 5%) in the acute stage and falls to baseline levels for the CAD age group in about 2 months.[60] The decline is exponential, so that the greatest drop occurs in the first month; afterward, the rate of decline slows substantially, to reach baseline levels at 2 months. It is mainly because of these data that the current definition of unstable angina uses the time element of 2 months. The risk of myocardial infarction is about 10% in the acute stage and 15% at 3 to 6 months. The definition of unstable angina proposed by Braunwald[43] has some prognostic implications in that patients with angina at rest, having unstable symptoms that cannot be attributed to a secondary cause (e.g., anemia) and despite optimum medical therapy, are very likely to be at high risk for cardiac events and should be candidates for more aggressive management.

Acute Myocardial Infarction

A detailed discussion of acute myocardial infarction is outside the scope of this chapter, and readers are encouraged to consult standard textbooks of cardiology as needed for reference. With regard to etiology, the overwhelming cause of myocardial infarction is CAD. Less frequent causes include coronary artery spasm, embolism, aortic dissection, congenital coronary artery anomalies, vasculitides, and chest trauma. In CAD, most cases of myocardial infarction occur secondary to coronary artery obstruction from thrombus formation following plaque fissuring or rupture.[61] Accordingly, the current therapy for acute myocardial infarction is directed toward lysis of the occluding thrombus with thrombolytic therapy, prevention of further clot formation and propagation with antiplatelet and anticoagulation therapy, improvement of myocardial oxygen supply–demand balance with antianginal medications, improvement of myocardial pump function with agents that reduce left ventricular afterload and increase contractility, and revascularization interventions to improve survival rates and symptoms.

General Measures in the Treatment of Acute Myocardial Infarction

All patients suspected or found to have an acute myocardial infarction must be admitted to an institution equipped to treat the condition. Because 40% to 60% of deaths occur within an hour of acute myocardial infarction, and a window of 6 to 12 hours exists to reduce the extent of ischemic damage in survivors, it is imperative that therapies for acute myocardial infarction be initiated as early as possible. On arrival at the hospital, all patients should undergo continuous ECG monitoring and be administered oxygen at a rate of 2 to 4 L/min and nitroglycerin. Nitroglycerin is usually given as an ointment on an area of 2 to 4 cm (1–2 in) or as intravenous infusion starting at 5 mg/min, increasing by 5 mg/min every 10 minutes until pain decreases, blood pressure falls by 10%, or heart rate increases by 10%. Pain not controlled with nitroglycerin requires intravenous morphine at doses of 2 to 4 mg repeated every 20 to 30 minutes if necessary. Patients who are unusually anxious should be given a mild sedative. These general measures are provided as part of good supportive treatment; there is no evidence that these measures improve mortality rates after acute myocardial infarction.

Aspirin

The use of aspirin in treating acute myocardial infarction has been shown to reduce mortality rates and recurrent infarctions.[62] These effects are similar to those of aspirin in patients with unstable and stable chronic angina. The mechanism for the remarkable consistency of the benefits of aspirin in all forms of CAD manifestation is almost certainly inhibition of platelet function and specifically of thromoxane A_2 production, which prevents platelet aggregation, propagation of the thrombus, and vasoconstriction of the affected coronary artery.

Unless contraindicated because of aspirin hypersensitivity or potential bleeding, all patients with acute myocardial infarction should be given aspirin as soon as possible. The dose of aspirin for patients experiencing acute myocardial infarction has been the subject of debate, much of which was probably unnecessary. In a trial (ISIS-2) that unequivocally showed reduction of cardiac events in myocardial infarction with aspirin, the dose used was 160 mg.[62] As mentioned earlier, the mechanism for the benefit of aspirin in CAD is mainly related to its inhibition of thromboxane A_2 production, which appears to be achieved with doses between 40 and 325 mg/d. This dose of aspirin (either chewed or swallowed whole) can be given for acute myocardial infarction; patients with a history of peptic ulcer disease can be given aspirin in an enteric-coated form. In the absence of adverse effects, all patients with CAD should continue aspirin therapy indefinitely.

β-Adrenergic Blockers

Extensive trials have shown that β-blockers reduce both mortality and recurrent infarction after acute myocardial infarction.[63] The mechanisms of the benefit of β-blockade in this condition are not clear but are probably related to reduction in one or more of the following: ischemic injury, arrhythmias, and the propensity for plaque rupture. After an acute myocardial infarction, β-blockers have been shown to decrease infarct size, reduce arrhythmias, and increase the threshold to ventricular fibrillation.[64–66] Because β-blockade reduces blood pressure and myocardial contractile force, it is possible that the tendency for plaque rupture may be reduced in the same way that these agents help prevent aortic dissection.[67]

β-Blockers (either metoprolol or atenolol) can be given intravenously in the acute myocardial infarction phase.[68–70] Metoprolol is given at a dosage of 5 mg as a slow intravenous bolus and repeated every 5 to 10 minutes to a total dose of 15 mg; oral metoprolol is given at a dosage of 50 mg twice daily on the second day and then at 100 mg twice daily on the third and subsequent days. Atenolol can be initiated at 5 mg as a slow intravenous bolus and repeated in 10 to 15 minutes to a total dose of 10 mg; oral atenolol can be given at a dosage of 50 mg on the second day and 100 mg on the third and subsequent days. β-Blockers (e.g., metoprolol, timolol, and propranolol) can also be given as oral therapy on diagnosis.[63]

Randomized trials of these agents suggest that the reduction of cardiac events after myocardial infarction is due to β-adrenergic blockade as a class action and may be obtained with all drugs possessing significant β-blockade activity. However, β-blockers that also possess significant intrinsic sympathomimetic activity (e.g., pindolol and oxprenolol) may be deleterious in acute myocardial infarction and should be avoided. Although the randomized trials with β-blockers have varied with regard to the timing of β-blocker initiation after an acute myocardial infarction, it is reasonable to start β-blockers once acute myocardial infarction is diagnosed. At the latest, the drug should be given before discharge from the hospital. In general, patients at low risk for future cardiac events after myocardial infarction probably do not benefit as much from long-term β-blocker therapy as those at higher risk. Low-risk patients include those with uncomplicated myocardial infarction, good ejection fraction, and a postinfarction low-level stress test that shows good exercise tolerance and no ischemia. Whether a low-risk patient should be given β-blockers over the long term after myocardial infarction is an issue of individual physician preference.

β-Blockers are contraindicated in patients with a history of bronchospasm, second- and third-degree atrioventricular heart block, bradycardia with heart rates <50 beats per minute, and moderate to severe heart failure with ejection fractions <40% to 45%. Most patients with milder forms of heart failure are usually able to take β-blockers.

Thrombolytic Therapy

Thrombolytic therapy is a major advance in the management of acute myocardial infarction and should be administered to all patients who meet the criteria for treatment. Thrombolytic agents approved for treating acute myocardial infarction act by converting plasminogen to plasmin, the enzyme that breaks down fibrin in clots and produces clot lysis. The action of tissue plasminogen activator (tPA) is relatively specific toward plasminogen contained in the plasminogen–fibrin complex in existing clots. Anistreplase (APSAC) and streptokinase act on circulating and clot-bound plasminogen. In theory, the latter two agents may lead to more bleeding because of the breakdown of circulating fibrinogen and fibrin in clots. As discussed later, bleeding complications are more frequent with tPA use because of the need to use systemic anticoagulation agents.

Several clinical trials have shown that thrombolytic therapy reduces mortality rates after acute myocardial infarction by about 30% more than placebo.[61,71,72] The clinical benefits observed after thrombolysis in acute myocardial infarction are due mainly to lysis of the thrombus in the affected artery. In this regard, an infarction due to a totally closed artery is more likely to respond favorably to thrombolytic therapy than one in which the coronary artery is still partially patent. Thus, a myocardial infarction associated with ECG Q-wave and ST-segment elevation responds favorably to thrombolytic therapy because 80% of such infarctions are associated with a closed coronary artery.[73] In contrast, those with ECG ST-segment depression do not benefit from thrombolytic therapy, presumably because more than 50% of affected arteries in this condition are partially patent.[57]

The indications and contraindications for thrombolytic therapy are given in Table 18.5. In brief, all patients with cardiac chest pain , ST-segment elevation in the ECG consistent with an acute infarction, and no contraindications to thrombolytic therapy should be considered for treatment with one of the agents proven to reduce cardiac mortality after myocardial infarction.

TABLE 18.5. Indications and contraindications for thrombolytic therapy.

Indications
Prolonged ischemic chest pain >20 min and ST-segment elevation ≥ 1 mm in two or more contiguous leads
Prolonged ischemic chest pain >20 min and left bundle branch block

Contraindications
Active bleeding from any internal site
Recent major trauma or surgery in last 6 wk
Known history of bleeding, neoplasm, aneurysm, or arteriovenous malformation in central nervous system (intracranial or spinal cord)
Stroke in last 6 mo
Significant gastrointestinal bleeding in last 6 wk
Recent traumatic cardiopulmonary resuscitation
Severe uncontrolled hypertension (systolic >200 mm Hg, diastolic >120 mm Hg) despite therapy
Significant bleeding diathesis
Pregnancy or 1 mo post-partum
Known allergy to thrombolytic drug or history of streptokinase and anistreplase use between 4 and 5 d and 12 mo

TABLE 18.6. Thrombolytic agents in current use.

Streptokinase
Dosage	1.5 million units over 30–60 min
Side effects	Bleeding, hypotension, and allergic reactions

Tissue plasminogen activator (t-PA)
Dosage	Standard regimen: 100 mg over 3 h (10 mg bolus, 50 mg first hour, and 20 mg over each of the following 2 h)
	Accelerated regimen: ≤100 mg over 1.5 h (15 mg bolus, 0.75 mg/kg but <50 mg over 30 min, and 0.5 mg/kg but <35 mg over 60 min)
	Intravenous heparin should be given with t-PA for 2 d to maintain activated partial thromboplastin time at 60–85 s
Side effects	Bleeding

Anistreplase (APSAC)
Dosage	30 units over 5 min
Side effects	Bleeding, hypotension, and allergic reactions

Patients with prolonged angina (i.e., >20 minutes) and left bundle branch block in the ECG are also candidates for thrombolytic therapy. Although the presence of left bundle branch block obscures the ECG diagnosis of acute myocardial infarction, analysis of patients with this ECG finding in randomized trials shows that the trend to reduced mortality with thrombolytic therapy also applies to this group.[74] It should be emphasized, however, that acute myocardial infarction associated with ST segment depression is not an indication for thrombolytic therapy. Most patients who present with an acute ischemic syndrome associated with ST-segment depression have either non–Q-wave myocardial infarction or unstable angina; randomized studies have shown that thrombolytic therapy does not significantly decrease cardiac events in patients with either condition.[57]

The thrombolytic agents that have been shown to reduce mortality rates in patients following acute myocardial infarction and the recommended regimens for their use are listed in Table 18.6. The issue of the best agent to use in acute myocardial infarction has been extensively debated and investigated. Three large studies—GISSI-2, ISIS-3, and GUSTO—compared the relative efficacy of tPA and streptokinase.[75–77] The first two studies, which used subcutaneous heparin to prevent reocclusion of the affected artery after thrombolysis, failed to show a significant difference in mortality rates between tPA and streptokinase therapies. These two studies also showed a slightly increased incidence of cerebral bleeding with tPA. In contrast, GUSTO, in which a study arm tested intravenous heparin with thrombolysis (to maintain an aPTT of 60–85 seconds for 2 days), showed a small but significant reduction in mortality rates with tPA compared to streptokinase (6.3% versus 7.4%). The same study showed a small but significant increase in cerebral

bleeding between streptokinase with subcutaneous heparin and tPA with intravenous heparin (0.54% versus 0.72%, respectively). However, the difference between the combined end points of death and nonfatal cerebral bleeding was slightly but significantly lower in the tPA group (6.6% versus 7.5%).

In choosing from the thrombolytic agents available, the physician should consider cost and clinical parameters. Currently, the least expensive thrombolytic agent is streptokinase; compared with this agent, APSAC is about 7 to 8 times more expensive and tPA is about 10 times more expensive. Streptokinase and APSAC produce allergic reactions with repeated use, and a second administration should be avoided in the interval between 4 to 5 days and 1 year after the initial dose. These two agents also tend to produce hypotension during infusion and may not be suitable for patients who have low blood pressure. Thus, patients who have been treated with streptokinase or APSAC within the period referred to earlier or who have systolic blood pressures below 90 to 100 mm Hg should not be given either agent. The choice of agents in other patients is based on physician judgment. Patients given tPA should always receive intravenous heparin for about 2 days to maintain aPTT at 60 to 85 seconds; heparin is not indicated in patients given streptokinase or APSAC.

Because of varying selection criteria and results in the major trials of thrombolysis, whether certain groups of patients with acute myocardial infarction are eligible for thrombolytic therapy has been greatly debated. The debate centers on the factors of advanced age, infarct location, and time of presentation. First, review and analysis of the many studies on thrombolytic therapy indicate that age by itself is not a contraindication to thrombolysis. Second, the site of infarction does not affect benefit from thrombolytic therapy; patients with anterior myocardial infarction may benefit more than those with inferior infarction but only because anterior infarctions are associated with a significantly higher mortality rate. Third, there is a strong likelihood that thrombolytic treatment may produce benefits up to 12 hours after the onset of acute myocardial infarction.

Angiotensin-Converting Enzyme Inhibitors

Angiotensin-converting enzyme inhibitor (ACEI) agents have been shown conclusively to be beneficial in patients with subnormal ejection fractions; whether they should be given routinely to all patients with myocardial infarctions is less clear. ACEI agents inhibit the enzyme that converts angiotensin I to angiotensin II (angiotensin-converting enzyme) and also the activity of bradykinin. Inhibiting formation of angiotensin II results in vasodilation, decreased preload and afterload, and reduced aldosterone activity. Inhibition of bradykinin degradation results in dilatation of the efferent glomerular arteriole, fall in hydrostatic pressure across the glomerulus, and some decline in renal function. The beneficial effects of ACEI after an acute infarction are probably related to two mechanisms—prevention of ventricular dilatation and reduction in recurrent ischemic events.

Therapy with ACEI has been shown to reduce mortality rates in patients with heart failure and low ejection fractions.[78,79] Similarly, ACEI decreases mortality and morbidity rates in patients with acute infarctions associated with low ejection fractions, with or without symptoms of heart failure.[80] Unless contraindicated by significant renal failure, all patients with systolic heart failure after a myocardial infarction, with or without symptoms, should be started on an ACEI regimen. The choice of agent does not appear important because the salutary effect of ACEI in systolic heart failure appears to be related to its class action. Current agents available include captopril, enalapril, lisinopril, quinapril, benazapril, and ramapril. The specific benefits of ACEI in patients with myocardial infarction and systolic heart failure have been attributed to improved myocardial remodeling such that in the long term the left ventricle is not as dilated and has more contractile function. This benefit may be seen particularly with use of ACEI after a large anterior myocardial infarction.[81,82]

The issue of whether ACEI agents are also beneficial when given routinely to all patients with myocardial infarction, irrespective of ejection fraction, is less clear-cut. Several large studies examining this question have not been unanimous. However, the two largest and most recent studies, GISSI-3 and ISIS-4, showed small but significant mortality rate reductions of 12% and 7%, respectively, about a month after the infarction.[83,84] Furthermore, meta-analysis of all the studies to date showed a significant reduction of 6.5% in short-term mortality rates with the routine use of ACEI agents after an acute infarction.[85] However, it should be emphasized that these studies included patients who had low ejection fractions; whether the results would be unequivocally favorable in patients who have normal cardiac function is still questionable.

The mechanism involved in the beneficial results seen in patients with myocardial infarction but normal ejection fractions may be related to the effects of ACEI agents on endothelial function. These medications may be antiatherogenic because of their vasodilatory and antimitogenic effects on the endothelium. Previous studies of these drugs on patients with heart failure have shown that the observed reduction in mortality rates is partly due to a lower incidence of myocardial infarction during long-term follow-up.[79,80]

ACEI agents are relatively free from adverse side effects compared with most other cardiac medications. The major problem is decreased renal function, the frequency of which increases with the severity of the heart failure. A decline in renal function occurs mainly in patients who have significant heart failure. Decreasing the dose of the diuretic, ACEI agent, or both usually produces improved renal function. The other side effects include cough, hypotension, rash, and angioneurotic edema.

Other Medications

Despite considerable interest and research in the use of calcium channel blockers, antiarrhythmic drugs, and magnesium in patients with acute myocardial infarction, the balance of evidence at present does not favor a routine role for these medications in this setting. Calcium channel blockers may be given for symptomatic treatment of angina in patients who continue to have chest pain after myocardial infarction despite administration of nitrates and β-blockers.[86] In these patients, it is preferable to use diltiazem or verapamil rather than a dihydropyridine derivative because of studies showing potential adverse effects of short-acting dihydropyridines.[87]

Of the four classes of antiarrhythmic drugs, the roles of class II (β-blocker) and class IV (calcium channel blocker) drugs have already been discussed. Current evidence indicates that there is no benefit from the routine use of class I antiarrhythmic drugs (e.g., lidocaine) after acute myocardial infarctions. On the contrary, both prospective studies and meta-analysis show that routine use of many class I drugs was related to excess mortality rates in treated patients.[88] The role of class III antiarrhythmic drugs (e.g., amiodarone and sotalol) in acute myocardial infarction remains to be defined. The use of antiarrhythmic drugs should therefore be limited to patients who have significant arrhythmias after acute myocardial infarction.

Magnesium was initially used in patients after acute myocardial infarction based on the rationale that the agent may have antiarrhythmic actions. Although several earlier studies have suggested that routine use of Mg^{++} may reduce deaths after acute myocardial infarction, this hypothesis was not confirmed in a subsequent large study.[84] At present, the balance of evidence does not favor the routine use of Mg^{++} in patients after acute myocardial infarction[89] but limits its use to certain groups of patients. Patients who may benefit from Mg^{++} administration include those with recalcitrant arrhythmias and those suspected of having low Mg^{++} levels (e.g., those undergoing chronic diuretic therapy, alcoholic patients, and those with chronic malnutrition). However, the benefits of Mg^{++} therapy in these settings have not been defined.

Silent Ischemia

Definition and Mechanism

In addition to stable angina, unstable angina, and myocardial infarction, CAD may manifest as myocardial ischemia without symptoms. The syndrome of silent ischemia is present when there is objective evidence of ischemia (detected by abnormalities of left ventricular perfusion, metabolism, contractile function, or ECG activity) without angina or equivalent symptoms. Silent ischemia is often classified into two subsets: type 1 occurs in completely asymptomatic patients who may or may not have underlying CAD, and type 2, which is much more common, occurs in patients who manifest angina in some form. In patients with both symptomatic and silent ischemia (type 2), episodes of silent ischemia are actually more frequent than episodes of symptomatic ischemia.

The mechanism of silent ischemia is currently unknown, especially in patients with type 2 silent ischemia who have some episodes of myocardial ischemia associated with chest pain and many others that are silent. One possible mechanism includes a difference in pain threshold between patients with and without silent ischemia.[90,91] Other studies suggest that this diminished pain response may be related to endorphin release[92,93] or neuropathy.[94] Still others have suggested that silent ischemia may indicate less-severe episodes of myocardial ischemia.[95]

Diagnosis

In the clinical setting, silent ischemia is noted commonly during exercise stress testing and ambulatory ECG (Holter) monitoring when there is ECG ST-segment depression without chest pain. That many patients have ST-segment depression during the exercise stress test without chest pain has been observed for years. In a population with a high prevalence for CAD, this test detects CAD (and therefore silent ischemia when chest pain is not present during the test) with well-defined sensitivity and specificity. In more recent years, continuous ambulatory ECG (Holter) monitoring has been studied and used for the diagnosis of silent ischemia. It is important to emphasize that although Holter monitoring has been found to be useful for the detection of silent ischemia in patients with known CAD or high probability for CAD, the technique, unlike the exercise stress test, is not helpful in the diagnosis of CAD. Extensive experience with this technique indicates that, unlike with the exercise stress test, the mere presence of ST-segment depression on the Holter monitor has low specificity and predictive value for CAD, particularly because many patients without confirmed CAD may show this finding. However, limiting the definition of ischemia to the presence of ST-segment depression of at least 1 mm, measured 80 ms after the J point and lasting for at least 30 seconds, significantly increases the specificity of the Holter monitor for silent ischemia.[96]

Prognosis

Many studies indicate that the presence of silent ischemia, on either exercise testing or Holter monitoring, has the same unfavorable prognosis as symptomatic myocardial ischemia in patients with known CAD. Good representative studies of this trend are seen in the reports by Deedwania for chronic angina[97] and the Coronary Artery Surgery Study registry for the postinfarction patient.[98] In unstable angina, patients with silent ischemia have more severe CAD and are more likely to experience cardiac events.[99,100] In this syndrome, the total duration of ischemia (sum of silent and symptomatic ischemic episodes) predicted cardiac mortality and morbidity rates better than either silent or symptomatic ischemia.[101] It is now widely accepted that therapy should correlate with the extent of the disease as assessed by the total number of both symptomatic and silent myocardial ischemic episodes (total ischemic burden) rather than by the symptomatic episodes alone.

In asymptomatic patients, the prognostic significance of ST-segment depression on the Holter or exercise stress test is more problematic. In those with risk factors for CAD, there is a definite but small risk of having occult CAD when such ECG abnormalities are noted even in the absence of angina. However, no data at present provide any information on the prognostic value of these ECG findings in any quantifiable way for this group of asymptomatic CAD patients. In asymptomatic patients who have no risk factors for CAD, the probability of underlying CAD is very low, even if ST-segment abnormality is present, and the overall prognosis is good.

Treatment

Although it is generally agreed that silent ischemia in patients with CAD is associated with an unfavorable prognosis, there is less agreement on therapy. To a large degree, this disagreement results from uncertainty about the end points of treatment and the prognostic implication of treatment.

With symptomatic episodes of ischemia, reduction in the severity and frequency of angina is in itself an important goal of treatment; with silent ischemia, this is not a measurable end point. Accordingly, many workers have used reduction in the ischemic burden and improvement in exercise time before onset of ECG ST-segment depression as end points of therapy. These end points can be achieved with all modalities of treatment traditionally used for angina, including administration of nitrates, β-blockers, and calcium channel blockers and revascularization with percutaneous angioplasty or surgery.[102] Thus, the medical treatment of silent ischemia is similar to that of symptomatic angina with regard to choice of drugs, dosages, and regimens.

As with all patients with CAD, the prognosis of those with silent ischemia is improved by coronary artery bypass surgery if such patients have specific findings on coronary angiography (e.g., left main coronary artery disease or three-vessel disease with low ejection fraction). However, it is not clear at this time whether medical therapy or revascularization improves prognosis for those experiencing silent ischemia. Some preliminary studies suggest that reduction of silent ischemic episodes is associated with better survival rates.[103,104]

References

1. Diamond GA, Forester JS. Analysis of probability as an aid in the clinical diagnosis of coronary artery disease. *N Engl J Med.* 1979;300:1350–1358.
2. Physicians Health Study Research Group. Fiscal report on the aspirin components of the ongoing Physicians' Heath Study. *N Engl J Med.* 1989;321:129–135.
3. Mansm JE, Grobbee DE, Stampfer MJ, et al. Aspirin in the primary prevention of angina pectoris in a randomized trial of United States physicians. *Am J Med.* 1990;89:772–776.
4. Ridker PM, Mansom JE, Gaziahom M, Barihg JE, Hennekens CH. Low-dose aspirin therapy for chronic stable angina. *Ann Intern Med.* 1991;114:835–839.
5. Juul-Moller S, Edvardsson N, Jahnmatz B, et al., for the Sweden Angina Pectoris Aspirin Trial (SAPAT) Group. Double-blind trial of aspirin in primary prevention of myocardial infarction in patients with stable angina pectoris. *Lancet.* 1992;340:1421–1425.
6. Brown BG, Bolson E, Petersen RB, Pierce CD, Dodge HT. The mechanisms of nitroglycerin actin: stenosis vasodilation as a major component of the drug response. *Circulation.* 1981;64:1089–1097.
7. Wilkins RW, Hayes FW, Weiss S. The role of the venous system in the circulatory collapse induced by sodium nitrite. *J Clin Invest.* 1937;85:85–91.
8. Horowitz JD, Antman EM, Lovell BG, et al. Potentiation of the cardiovascular effects of nitroglycerin by N-acetylcysteine. *Circulation.* 1983;68:1247–1253.
9. Murad F. Cyclic guanosine monophosphate as a mediator of vasodilation. *J Clin Invest.* 1986;78:1–5.
10. Behovic JL, Bouvier M, Caron MG, Lefkowitz RJ. Regulation of adenylcyclase-coupled beta-adrenergic receptors. *Annu Rev Cell Biol.* 1988;4:405–428.
11. Lefkowitz RJ, Caron MG. Adrenergic receptors: models for the study of receptors coupled to guananine nucleotide regulatory proteins. *J Biol Chem.* 1988;263:4993–4996.
12. Cruickshank JM. The clinical importance of cardioselectivity and lipophilicity in beta blockers. *Am Heart J.* 1980;100:160–178.
13. Braunwald E. Calcium-channel blockers: pharmacologic considerations. *Am Heart J.* 1982;104:665–671.
14. Schwartz A, Matlib A, Balwierezak J, Lathrop DA. Pharmacology of calcium antagonists. *Am J Cardiol.* 1985;55:3c–7c.
15. Flekenstein A. Specific pharmacology of calcium myocardium, cardiac pacemakers, and vascular smooth muscles. *Annu Rev Pharmacol Toxicol.* 1977;17:149–166.
16. Ellrodt G, Chew CYC, Singh BN. Therapeutic implications of slow-channel blockade in cardiocirculatory disorders. *Circulation.* 1980;62:669–679.
17. Singh BN, Nademanee K, Baky S. Calcium antagonist. *Drugs.* 1983;25:125–153.
18. Yusef S, Peto R, Lewis J, Collins R, Sleight P. β-blockade during and after myocardial infarction: an overview of the randomized trials. *Prog Cardiovasc Dis.* 1985;27:335–371.
19. Brown BG, Fuster V. Impact of management of stabilization of coronary disease. In: Fuster V, Ross R, Topol EJ, eds. *Atherosclerosis and Coronary Artery Disease.* Philadelphia, Pa: Lippincott-Raven; 1996:191–205.
20. Chin JH, Azhar S, Hoffman BB. Inactivation of endothelial derived relaxing factor by oxidized lipoproteins. *J Clin Invest.* 1992;89:10–18.
21. National Cholesterol Education Program. Second report of the Expert Panel on Detection, Evaluation, and Treatment of High Blood Cholesterol in Adults (Adult Treatment Panel II). *Circulation.* 1994;89:1329–1445.
22. Ross R. The pathogenesis of atherosclerosis: a perspective for the 1990's. *Nature.* 1993;362:801–809.
23. Kyrle Pa, Eicler HG, Jager U, Lechner K. Inhibition of prostacyclin and thromboxane A_2 generation by low-dose aspirin at the site of plug formation in man and in vivo. *Circulation.* 1987;75:1025–1029.
24. Patrignani P, Pilabozzi P, Patrono C. Selective cumulative inhibition of platelet thromboxane production by low dose aspirin in healthy subjects. *J Clin Invest.* 1982;69:1366–1372.
25. Steering Committee of the Physicians' Health Study Research Group. Final report on the aspirin component of the ongoing Physicians' Health Study. *N Engl J Med.* 1989;321:129–135.
26. Fitzgerald GA. Dipyridamole. *N Engl J Med.* 1983;316:1247–1257.
27. International Anticoagulant Review Group. Collaborative analysis of long-term anticoagulant administration after acute myocardial infarction. *Lancet.* 1970;1:203–209.
28. Sixty-Plus Reinfarction Study Research Group. A double-blind trial to assess long-term oral anticoagulant therapy

in elderly patients after myocardial infarction. *Lancet.* 1980;2:989–994.

29. Smith P, Arnesen H, Holme I. The effect of warfarin on mortality and reinfarction. *N Engl J Med.* 1990;323: 147–152.

30. Anticoagulants in the Secondary Prevention of Events in Coronary Thrombosis (ASPECT) Research Group. Effect of long-term oral anti-coagulant treatment on mortality and cardiovascular morbidity after myocardial infarction. *Lancet.* 1994;343:499–503.

31. Morel DW, DiCorleto PE, Chisolm GM. Endothelial and smooth muscle cells alter low density lipoprotein in vitro by free radical oxidation. *Arteriosclerosis.* 1984;4:357–364.

32. Steinberg D, Parthasarathy S, Carew TE, Khoo JC, Witztum JL. Beyond cholesterol: modifications of low-density lipoproteins that increase its atherogenicity. *N Engl J Med.* 1989;320:915–924.

33. Aviram M. Modified form of low density lipo-protein and atherosclerosis. *Atherosclerosis.* 1993;98:1–9.

34. Parthasarathy S, Young SG, Witztum JL, Pittman RC, Steinberg D. Probucol inhibits oxidative modification of low density lipoprotein. *J Clin Invest.* 1986;77:641–644.

35. Daugherty A, Zweifel BS, Schofeld G. Probucol attenuates the development of aortic atherosclerosis in cholesterol-fed rabbits. *Br J Pharmacol.* 1989;98:612–618.

36. Anderson TJ, Meredith IT, Charbonneau F, et al. Endothelium-dependent coronary vasomotion relates to the susceptibility of LDL to oxidation in humans. *Circulation.* 1996;93:1647–1650.

37. Stampfer MJ, Hennekens CH, Manson JE, Colditz GA, Rosner B, Willete WC. Vitamin E consumption and the risk of coronary artery disease in women. *N Engl J Med.* 1993;328:1444–1449.

38. Rimm EB, Stampfer MJ, Ascherio A, Giovannucci E, Coldiz GA, Willete WC. Vitamin E consumption and the risk of coronary disease in men. *N Engl J Med.* 1993;328: 1450–1456.

39. Kushi LH, Folsom AR, Prineas RJ, Mink PJ, Wu Y, Bostick RM. Dietary antioxidant vitamins and death from coronary heart disease in postmenopausal women. *N Engl J Med.* 1996;334:1156–1162.

40. Gaziano JM, Manson JE, Buring JE, Hennekens CH. Dietary antioxidants and cardiovascular disease. *Ann N Y Acad Sci.* 1992; 669:249–259.

41. Henneken CH, Buring JE, Manson JE, et al. Lack of effect of long-term supplementation with beta-carotene on incidence of malignant neoplasms and cardiovascular disease. *N Engl J Med.* 1996;334:1145–1149.

42. The Alpha-Tacopherol, Beta Carotene Cancer Prevention Study Group. The effect of vitamin E and beta carotene on the incidence of lung cancer and other cancers in male smokers. *N Engl J Med.* 1994;330:1029–1035.

43. Braunwald E. Unstable angina: a classification. *Circulation.* 1989;80:410–414.

44. *Clinical Practice Guideline Number 10: Unstable Angina: Diagnosis and Management.* Rockville, Md: US Department of Health and Human Services, Agency for Health Care Policy and Research and the National Heart, Lung, and Blood Institute; 1994. AHCPR publication 94-0602.

45. Sherman CT, Litvack F, Grundfest W, et al. Coronary angioscopy in patients with unstable angina pectoris. *N Engl J Med.* 1986;315:913–919.

46. Maseri A, L'Abbate A, Baroldi G, et al. Coronary vasospasm as a possible cause of myocardial infarction: a conclusion derived from the study of "preinfarction" angina. *N Engl J Med.* 1978;299:1271–1277.

47. Lewis HD Jr, Davis JW, Archibald DG, et al. Protective effects of aspirin against acute myocardial infarction and death in men with unstable angina. *N Engl J Med.* 1983; 309:396–403.

48. Cairns JA, Gent M, Singer J, et al. Aspirin, sulfinpyrazone, or both in unstable angina. *N Engl J Med.* 1985;313: 1369–1375.

49. Theroux P, Qiumet H, McCans J, et al. Aspirin, heparin, or both to treat acute unstable angina. *N Engl J Med.* 1988; 319:1105–1111.

50. RISC Group. Risk of myocardial infarction and death during treatment with low dose aspirin and intravenous heparin in men with unstable coronary artery disease. *Lancet.* 1990;336:827–830.

51. Balsano F, Rizzon P, Violi F, et al. Antiplatelet treatment with ticlopidine: a controlled multicenter clinical trial. *Circulation.* 1990;82:17–26.

52. Theroux P, Waters D, Qui S, McCans J, De Guise P, Juneau M. Aspirin vs heparin to prevent myocardial infarction during the acute phase of unstable angina. *Circulation.* 1993;88(pt 1):2045–2048.

53. TIMI IIIA Investigators. Early effects of tissue-type plasminogen activator added to conventional therapy on the culprit coronary lesion in patients presenting with ischemic cardiac pain at rest. *Circulation.* 1993;87:38–52.

54. Yusuf S, Wittes J, Friedman L. Overview of results of randomized clinical trials in heart disease, II: unstable angina, heart failure, primary prevention with aspirin, and risk factor modification. *JAMA.* 1988;260:2088–2093.

55. Held PH, Yusuf S, Furberg CD. Calcium channel blockers in acute myocardial infarction and unstable angina: an overview. *BMJ.* 1989;299:1187–1192.

56. Lubsen J, Tijssen JG. Efficacy of nifedipine and metoprolol in the early treatment of unstable angina in the coronary care unit: findings from the Holland Interuniversity Nifedipine/Metoprolol Trial (HINT). *Am J Cardiol.* 1987; 60:18A–25A.

57. TIMI IIIB Investigators. Effects of tissue plasminogen activator and a comparison of early invasive and conservative strategies in unstable angina and non–Q wave myocardial infarction: results of the TIMI IIIB Trial. *Circulation.* 1994; 89:1545–1556.

58. Luchi RJ, Scott SM, Deupree RH, Principal Investigators, and Their Associates of Veterans Administration Cooperative Study No. 28. Comparison of medical and surgical treatment for unstable angina pectoris. *N Engl J Med.* 1987;316:977–984.

59. Russell RO, Moraski RE, Kouchokos N, et al. Unstable angina pectoris: National Cooperative Study Group to compare surgical and medical therapy, II: in-hospital experience and initial followup results in patients with one, two, and three vessel disease. *Am J Cardiol.* 1978;42: 839–848.

60. Mark DB, Brauwald E. Medical treatment of unstable angina. In: Fuster V, Ross R, Topol EJ, eds. *Atherosclerosis and Coronary Artery Disease*. Philadelphia, Pa: Lippincott-Raven; 1996:1315–1326.

61. Davis M, Thomas A. Plaque fissuring: the cause of acute myocardial infarction, sudden ischemic death, and crescendo angina. *Br Heart J*. 1985;53:363–373.

62. ISIS-2 (Second International Study of Infarct Survival) Collaborative Group. Randomized trial of intravenous streptokinase, oral aspirin, both, or neither among 17,187 cases of suspected myocardial infarctions: ISIS-2. *Lancet*. 1988;2:349–360.

63. Yusuf S, Lewis J, Collins R, Sleight P. Beta-blockade during and after acute myocardial infarction: an overview of the randomized trials. *Prog Cardiovasc Dis*. 1985;27:335–371.

64. Peter T, Norris RM, Clarke ED, et al. Reduction of enzyme release after myocardial infarction in patients by propronolol. *Circulation*. 1978;57:1091–1095.

65. Yusuf S, Sleight P, Rossi PRF, et al. Reduction in infarct size, arrhythmias, chest pain, and morbidity by early intravenous blockade in suspected acute myocardial infarction. *Circulation*. 1983;67(pt 2):32–41.

66. Norris RM, Barnaby PF, Brown MA, et al. Prevention of ventricular fibrillation during acute myocardial infarction by intravenous propranolol. *Lancet*. 1984;2:883–886.

67. Frishman WH, Lazar EJ. Reduction of mortality, sudden death, and non-fatal infarction with beta-adrenergic blockers in survivors of acute myocardial infarction: a new hypothesis regarding the cardioprotective action of beta-adrenergic blockade. *Am J Cardiol*. 1990;65:66G̃70G.

68. ISIS-1 (First International Study of Infarct Survival) Collaborative Group. Randomised trial of intravenous atenonol among 16027 cases of suspected myocardial infarction: ISIS-1. *Lancet*. 1988;2:57–66.

69. MIAMI Trial Research Group. Metoprolol in acute myocardial infarction (MIAMI): a randomized placebo controlled international trial. *Eur Heart J*. 1985;6:199–226.

70. Hjalmarson A, Elmfeldt D, Herlitz J, et al. Effect on mortality of metoprolol an acute myocardial infarction: a randomized trial. *Lancet*. 1981;2:823–827.

71. Gruppo Italiano per lo Studio della streptochinasi nell'Infarcto Miocardico (GISSI). Effectiveness of intravenous thrombolytic therapy in acute myocardial infarction. *Lancet*. 1986;1:397–401.

72. AIMS Trial Study Group. Effect of intravenous APSAC on mortality after acute myocardial infarction: preliminary report of a placebo-controlled clinical trial. *Lancet*. 1988;1:545–549.

73. DeWood MA, Spores J, Notske R, et al. Prevalence of total coronary occlusion during the early hours of transmural myocardial infarction. *N Engl J Med*. 1980;303:897–902.

74. Fibrinolytic Therapy Trialist (FTT) Collaborative Group. Indications for fibrinolytic therapy in suspected acute myocardial infarction: collaborative overview of early mortality and major morbidity results from all randomized trials of more than 1000 patients. *Lancet*. 1994;343:311–322.

75. Gruppo Italiano per lo Studio dell Sopravvivenza nell'Infarcto Miocardico GISSI-2. A factorial randomized trial of alteplase versus streptokinase and heparin versus no hep-

arin among 12,490 patients with acute myocardial infarction. *Lancet*. 1990;336:65–71.

76. ISIS-3 (Third International Study of Infarct Survival) Collaborative Group. ISIS-3: a randomized comparison of streptokinase vs tissue plasminogen activator vs anistreplase and of aspirin plus heparin vs aspirin alone among 41,229 cases of suspected acute myocardial infarction. *Lancet*. 1992;339:753–770.

77. GUSTO Investigators. An international randomized trial comparing 4 thrombolytic agents for acute myocardial infarction. *N Engl J Med*. 1993;329:673–682.

78. CONSENSUS Trial Study Group. Effects of enalapril on mortality on severe congestive heart failure: results of the Cooperative North Scandinavian Enalapril Survival Study (CONSENSUS). *N Engl J Med*. 1987;316:1429–1435.

79. SOLVD Investigators. Effect of enalapril on survival in patients with reduced left ventricular ejection fraction and congestive heart failure. *N Engl J Med*. 1991;325:293–302.

80. Pfeffer MA, Braunwald E, Moye LA, et al. Effect of captopril on mortality and morbidity in patients with left ventricular dysfunction after acute myocardial infarction. *N Engl J Med*. 1992;327:669–677.

81. Sharpe N, Murphy J, Smith H, Hannan S. Treatment of patients with symptomless left ventricular dysfunction after myocardial infarction. *Lancet*. 1988;1:255–259.

82. Pfeffer MA, Lamas GA, Vaughan GE, Parisi AF, Braunwald E. Effect of captopril on progressive left ventricular dilatation after anterior myocardial infarction. *N Engl J Med*. 1988;319:80–86.

83. Gruppo Italiano per lo Studio della Sopravvivenza Nell'Infarcto Miocardio. GISSIS-3: effects of lisinopril and transdermal glyceryl trinitrate singly and together on 6-week mortality and ventricular function. *Lancet*. 1994;343:1155–1121.

84. ISIS-4 (Fourth International Study of Infarct Survival) Collaborative Group. ISIS-4: a randomised factorial trial assessing early oral captopril, oral mononitrate, and intravenous magnesium sulphate in 58,050 patients with suspected acute myocardial infarction. *Lancet*. 1995;345:669–685.

85. Flather MD, Avezum A, Yusuf S. General approach to management of acute myocardial infarction. In: Fuster V, Ross R, Topol EJ, eds. *Atherosclerosis and Coronary Artery Disease*. Philadelphia, Pa: Lippincott-Raven; 1996:939–954.

86. Held P, Yusuf S. Effects of beta-blockers and calcium channel blockers in acute myocardial infarction. *Eur Heart J*. 1993;14(suppl F):18–25.

87. Furberg CD, Psaty BM, Meyer JV. Nifedipine: dose-related increase in mortality in patients with coronary artery disease. *Circulation*. 1995;92:1326–1331.

88. Teo KK, Yusuf S, Furberg CD. Effects of prophylactic antiarrhythmia drug therapy in acute myocardial infarction. *JAMA*. 1993;270:1589–1595.

89. Yusuf S, Flather M. Magnesium in acute myocardial infarction. *BMJ*. 1995;310:1669–1670.

90. Glazier JJ, Chierchia S, Brown M, et al. Importance of generalized defective perception of painful stimuli as a cause of silent ischemia in chronic stable angina pectoris. *Am J Cardiol*. 1986;58:667–672.

91. Falcone C, Sconnochia R, Guasita L, et al. Dental pain threshold and angina pectoris in patients with coronary artery disease. *J Am Coll Cardiol.* 1988;12:348–352.

92. Sheps DS, Adams KF, Hinderliter A, et al. Endorphins are related to pain perception in coronary artery disease. *Am J Cardiol.* 1987;59:523–527.

93. Falcone C, Guasita L, Ochan M, et al. Beta-endorphins during coronary angioplasty in patients with silent or symptomatic myocardial ischemia. *J Am Coll Cardiol.* 1993; 22:1614–1620.

94. Marchant B, Umachandran V, Stevenson R, Kopelman PG, Timmis AD. Silent myocardial ischemia: role of subclinical neuropathy in patients with and without diabetes. *J Am Coll Cardiol.* 1993;22:1433–1437.

95. Chierchia S, Lazzari M, Freedman B, et al. Impairment of myocardial perfusion and function during painless myocardial ischemia. *J Am Coll Cardiol.* 1983;1:924–930.

96. Deanfield JE, Ribiero P, Oakley K, et al. Analysis of ST-segment changes in normal subjects: implications for ambulatory monitoring in angina pectoris. *Am J Cardiol.* 1984;53: 1321–1325

97. Deedwania PC, Carbajal EV. Silent ischemia during daily life is an independent predictor of mortality in stable angina. *Circulation.* 1990;81:748–756.

98. Weiner DA, Ryan TJ, McCabe CH, et al. Significance of myocardial ischemia during exercise testing in patients with coronary artery disease. *Am J Cardiol.* 1987;59: 725–729.

99. Gottlieb S, Weisfeldt ML, Ouyang P, Mellitis D, Gerstenblith G. Silent ischemia as a marker for early unfavorable outcome in patients with unstable angina. *N Engl J Med.* 1986;314:1214–1219.

100. Nademanee K, Intarachot V, Josephson MA, Rieders D, Mody FV, Singh BN. Prognostic significance of silent myocardial ischemia in patients with unstable angina. *J Am Coll Cardiol.* 1987;10:1–9.

101. Romeo F, Rosano GMC, Martuscelli E, Valente A, Reale A. Unstable angina: role of silent ischemia and total ischemic time (silent plus painful episodes), a 6 year followup. *J Am Coll Cardiol.* 1992;19:1173–1179.

102. Cohn PF. Silent ischemia. In: Fuster V, Ross R, Topol EJ, eds. *Atherosclerosis and Coronary Artery Disease.* Philadelphia, Pa: Lippincott-Raven; 1996:1561–1576.

103. Lim R, Dyke L, Dymond DS. Effect on prognosis of abolition of exercise-induced painless myocardial ischemia by medical therapy. *Am J Cardiol.* 1992;69:733–735.

104. Pepine CJ, Cohn PF, Deedwania PC, et al., for the ASIT Study Group. Effects of treatment on outcome in mildly symptomatic patients with ischemia during life: the Atenolol Silent Ischemia Study (ASIT). *Circulation.* 1994; 90:762–768.

19

Cardiovascular Manifestations of Lyme Disease

Peter Lercher, Renate Schöllnast, and Robert Gasser

Borrelia burgdorferi, discovered more than a decade ago, has been identified as a causal agent of numerous disorders and symptoms.[1] Table 19.1 lists the different clinical manifestations of Lyme disease. Cardiovascular symptoms sometimes occur in the context of this systemic disorder. Adequate antibiotic treatment is needed to thwart cardiovascular Lyme disease. Cardiac manifestations in the United States are seen in 8% to 10% of all cases. Our own group has observed cardiovascular manifestations in 15% of 294 studied patients. In this chapter we expand current views on cardiovascular manifestations of Lyme disease. We mention only briefly other manifestations, diagnostic questions, and therapeutic problems but provide references to important publications in the field.

Pathophysiology

Practically all cardiovascular manifestations of Lyme disease relate to *Borrelia*-induced inflammation. Little is known about the histomorphological changes seen in myocardial *Borrelia* infection, because biopsies of the right ventricle are only rarely performed. Cardiovascular Lyme borreliosis manifests as perimyocarditis, epimyocarditis, and endomyocarditis; transmural myocarditis is characterized by interstitial inflammation. Furthermore, vasculitis, showing infiltration of lymphocytes, plasma cells, macrophages, and neutrophils, has been described.[2]

In histomorphological investigations using silver stain, spirochetes are seen only rarely in the affected myocardium. Myocardial necrosis cannot usually be observed in patients with Lyme borreliosis, and pathological serum enzyme levels are within the normal range. This is in contrast to infections caused by *B. recurrentis*, in which myocardial necrosis is the predominant manifestation.

Experimental infection of rats, mice, hamsters, rabbits, and dogs reveals a similar picture: *Borrelia burgdorferi* shows a pronounced tropism for mesenchymal structures. Myocardial cells are only rarely affected. Local edema, inflammation, and microvasculitis cause trophic disturbances, which, in turn, lead to destruction of myocardial cells. Experimental models show a distinct association between the microorganism and interstitial structures, particularly areas of the heart rich in mesenchymal structures such as the area around the valves, the aorta itself, the wall of the coronary arteries, and the adventitia.[2] Histologically, the typical course of the disease has been demonstrated in animal experiments as follows: 6 to 10 days after the primary infection, spirochetes are found for the first time in myocardial tissue. Then, for a period of 10 to 15 days, the number of spirochetes increases and signs of inflammation in the myocardium become more pronounced.[2] The number of spirochetes present in the myocardium subsequently decreases, as do signs of inflammation. However, as demonstrated with silver staining and culture techniques, spirochetes can exist for more than 90 days in the myocardium.[3] Note that *B. burgdorferi* has been cultivated from myocardial biopsies of patients, including those with very-long-standing dilated cardiomyopathy and *Borrelia* infection.

Although different hypotheses have been put forward to answer the question, we do not know why some patients develop cardiac symptoms and signs of inflammation and others do not. Some authors have shown that genetics play a significant role in this context. Some strains of mice show complete resistance against *B. burgdorferi* infection whereas others do not.[4,5] The different strains of *Borrelia* cause different types of infection, tropisms, and effects on the heart, joints, and nervous system.[4,5]

Another possible mechanism by which *B. burgdorferi* affects the myocardial tissue is the release of cardiotoxic

TABLE 19.1. Incidence of cardiovascular manifestations according to reference 1 and observations from our own group of subjective symptoms.

Cardiovascular manifestations	Incidence (%)*
Palpitations	69
Conduction disturbances	19
Myocarditis	10
Dilated cardiomyopathy	5
Pericarditis	2

Subjective symptoms as reported by patients with cardiovascular manifestations
Palpitations
Increased heart rate
Arrhythmias
Angina pectoris
Shortness of breath
Slow heart rate
Irregular heart beat
Dizziness
Syncope

Total of cardiovascular manifestations of Lyme disease seen in 294 patients consecutively admitted to our Lyme disease outpatient care unit
Atrioventricular block, third degree
Bundle branch block
Ventricular tachycardia
Supraventricular tachycardia
Ventricular fibrillation
Ectopic atrial beats
Ectopic ventricular beats, all Lown classifications
Myocarditis
Dilated cardiomyopathy
Coronary vasculitis
Coronary aneurysm
Pericarditis

*From Ciesielsky et al.[1]

substances by the microorganism. This hypothesis is based on the following observations:

1. Successful antibiotic therapy induces bacteriolysis and causes the typical Herxheimer–Jarisch reaction. The latter is dominated by cardiovascular symptoms such as tachycardia. Cardioactive toxins may be liberated in the course of bacteriolysis.
2. The causal agent, *B. burgdorferi*, is only rarely seen in myocardial tissue, even though myocardial tissue is greatly affected by the agent. However, further evidence is needed to understand the mechanisms of *Borrelia*-associated cardiovascular disease. Immunological reactions and activation of autoimmune processes also play a role in the pathophysiology of cardiovascular Lyme disease. Molecular mimicry and persistence of immunological reactions may contribute to late manifestations of Lyme disease. A recent paper by Chiao, Pavia, and Riley[6] reported that *B. burgdorferi* itself exerts an immunosuppressive effect on cellular immunity. This effect is mediated by a specific trypsin-sensitive protein of 62 to 100 kd.

Cardiovascular Symptoms as Reported by Patients

Of the 294 patients admitted to our outpatient clinic for *B. burgdorferi*–associated disorders, 43% suffered from cardiovascular symptoms. The symptoms reported have been described as palpitations, tachycardia, arrhythmias, angina pectoris–like symptoms, and shortness of breath. We have noticed that shortness of breath in patients with Lyme disease can also be a result of neuritis of the phrenic nerve. Despite the fact that 43% of the patients reported symptoms, only 15% had objective evidence of cardiovascular manifestations of Lyme disease. Symptoms have been reported as regularly occurring, episodic in nature, and alternating in character. Only a few published works have alluded to the subjective symptoms of patients. Ciesielski et al.[1] reported data that could be compared with ours. They showed that 69% of 84 patients reported cardiovascular symptoms (Table 19.1). The discrepancy between objective symptoms and clinically verified organic manifestation can be explained by the transient nature of cardiovascular *Borrelia* infection.[7] Somatized depression and memory impairment may also play a role in some cases.

Clinical Manifestations of Cardiovascular Lyme Borreliosis

Arrhythmias

The most common manifestation of cardiovascular Lyme borreliosis is atrioventricular (AV) block of various degrees. In particular, AV block III° in patients with Lyme disease has been reported by several authors.[7,8] Ciesielski et al.[1] reported that 19% of their patients presented with AV block III°. Dufty[7] reported a prevalence of 87% of AV block III° in 52 published cases. However, this high prevalence may be due to preselection of cases. Some authors have pointed out that a PR interval of more than 300 ms could be a risk factor for the development of more serious AV block. Figure 19.1 shows the electrocardiogram of a patient with bradycardia and AV dissociation with acute Lyme carditis. Symptoms reported in the context of AV block are palpitations, shortness of breath, dizziness, and syncope. The pathophysiology underlying AV block in patients with Lyme carditis is likely based on inflammatory edema within the cardiovascular conduction system. Most cases of AV block can be completely reversed with antibiotic treatment.[7,8] When AV block persists, which is rare, implantation of a permanent pacemaker may be required.

Electrophysiological investigations of two patients with AV block III° and small QRS complexes have shown

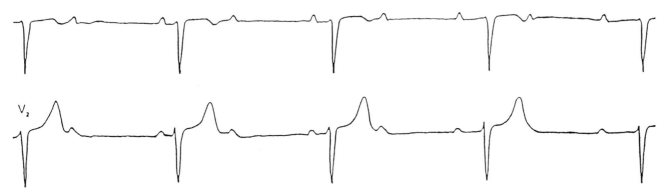

FIGURE 19.1. Electrocardiogram of a patient suffering from acute Lyme carditis revealing bradycardia and atrioventricular dissociation.

suprahisarian block.[9] Further investigations have pointed out that most cases of AV block are suprahisarian or located directly within the AV node.[10] Infrahisarian blocks have been reported only very rarely.

Bundle branch blocks[7-9] are seen in late stages of Lyme carditis, mostly in dilated cardiomyopathy secondary to Lyme carditis. Left anterior hemiblock, incomplete left bundle branch block, left bundle branch block, and bifascicular blocks are commonly seen in late *Borrelia* infection. However, bundle branch blocks in early stages of Lyme carditis have been reported.

Ventricular and supraventricular tachycardia, described only rarely in the literature, are both reversible with antibiotic treatment.[1] We have seen a case of a male colleague, 43 years of age, who reported dizziness, palpitations, and shortness of breath. He showed recurrent nonsustained ventricular tachycardia that improved with antiarrhythmic therapy and did not reoccur after administration of antibiotic therapy. Figure 19.2 shows an electrocardiogram of a male patient, 53 years of age, with *B. burgdorferi*–associated ventricular tachycardia (the tachycardia had to be terminated by electric cardioversion). One of our patients with dilated *Borrelia* cardiomyopathy suffered from recurrent ventricular fibrillation and needed an automatic implantable cardioverter-defibrillator pacemaker.

The palpitations reported by patients could be verified as supraventricular ectopic contractions in most cases. Ventricular premature beats show all Lown classifications, but Lown IVa and IVb are not very common.

Myocarditis

As shown in experiments, 100% of infected animals produce myocardial manifestations. It is very likely that, in humans, myocarditis and myocardial infection are as prominent as in the animal models, but they are clinically silent.[9] Chronic and subchronic forms of myocarditis may lead to dilated cardiomyopathy.

Echocardiographic findings are quite variable in patients with Lyme carditis and may range from normal left ventricular function to global and regional dysfunction. Regional disturbances in left ventricular wall motion have been attributed to coronary vasculitis. Pericardial effusions have only rarely been reported in patients with Lyme disease.[7-10] Ventricular dysfunction is reversible with antibiotic treatment when started early enough.[11] Figure 19.3 shows left ventricular dysfunction of a young female patient with Lyme carditis. Using radioactive markers for leukocytes (gallium 67) and radioactive antimyosin antibodies, it has been shown that both cellular

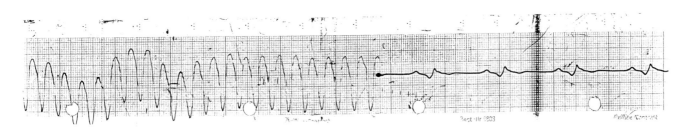

FIGURE 19.2. Electrocardiogram of a male patient, 53 years of age, with *Borrelia*-associated ventricular tachycardia before and after cardioversion.

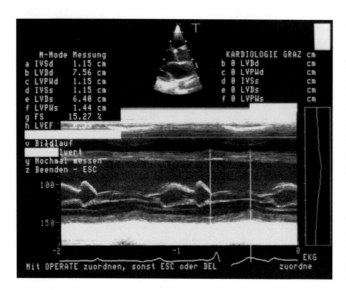

FIGURE 19.3. Left ventricular dysfunction (septum and apex) of a young female patient with Lyme carditis.

infiltration and myocardial cell death occur in humans with Lyme carditis.[12]

Histological investigations of right ventricular biopsies showed diffuse infiltration (predominantly interstitial infiltration) with lymphocytes and plasma cells.[13] The histology of the inflammatory process is not typical or pathognomonic. To confirm Lyme carditis, *Borrelia* must be cultivated from biopsy material or histologically verified using silver stain. However, it is very difficult to demonstrate *Borrelia* infection of myocardial tissue, especially in late stages of the disease. Some authors describe distinct bands of lymphocellular–plasmacellular infiltrates along the endocardium as being typical of *Borrelia* infection. Only rarely can one see disseminated necrosis in the surrounding area of mononuclear infiltrates. Occasionally, signs of fibrinous pericarditis and a rarefication of intramyocardial vessels suspicious for chronic vasculitis) can be found. Angiographically, this type of rarefication of intramyocardial vessels is seen as a "burned tree" angiogram. Few histological or post-mortem studies of the conduction system have been undertaken, and these studies are derived from only a small number of case reports.

Dilated Cardiomyopathy

The etiology of dilated cardiomyopathy is generally unclear and fairly hypothetical. In many cases we can find an inflammatory component early in the development of dilated cardiomyopathy. Several authors have clearly shown that a considerable percentage of cases of dilated cardiomyopathy (up to 25% in certain areas) may be sequelae of Lyme carditis. Although Lyme carditis has been described as transient in nature, convincing evi-

dence has been presented for the association of *B. burgdorferi* infection with dilated cardiomyopathy. Gasser and coworkers[14] found a prevalence of *B. burgdorferi* antibodies in 33% of 54 patients with dilated cardiomyopathy. In contrast, we see a prevalence of 8% in the normal population of this area. Stanek and coworkers have shown that *B. burgdorferi* could be repetitively cultivated from myocardial biopsies of patients with dilated cardiomyopathy.[15] Experimental studies have been performed on Syrian hamsters showing the persistence of *B. burgdorferi* in the dilated myocardial tissue.

In our own study,[14] 11 of 46 patients with dilated cardiomyopathy showed positive serology results and typical case histories for Lyme borreliosis infection. These patients received intravenous standard infusion with ceftriaxone (2 g given twice daily) over 14 days. Of the 46 patients, 55% showed complete recovery of left ventricular ejection fraction, 27% showed a marked improvement, and only 18% had no change in left ventricular ejection fraction. In other words, 82% of all patients showed improvement or complete recovery of left ventricular ejection fraction, whereas only 26% of patients with dilated cardiomyopathy but without *Borrelia* infection showed improvement or recovery. We also noticed a strong correlation between the duration of cardiac symptoms before the onset of treatment and the percentage of improvement of left ventricular ejection fraction. In particular, patients who showed left ventricular dysfunction for more than 6 months rarely recovered with antibiotic therapy.[10] Similar results have been found by other authors who did not find improvement of left ventricular ejection fraction in patients with *B. burgdorferi*–associated dilated cardiomyopathy when symptoms lasted longer than 6 months. Fruhwald and coworkers[16] saw complete recovery of left ventricular ejection fraction in a patient treated with roxithromycin. *Borrelia burgdorferi*–associated left ventricular dysfunction should always be treated as early as possible with adequate antibiotic therapy.

Coronary Artery Disease

Reports concerning coronary artery disease in the context of Lyme borreliosis are rare, but *Borrelia*-associated vasculitis has been reported as a rare cause of stroke. Grisold and coworkers[17] reported on a patient with infarction-like syndrome associated with *B. burgdorferi* infection Inflammatory coronary artery disease in the context of *Borrelia* vasculitis causes rarefication of intramyocardial vessels, which can be clearly seen in *Borrelia*-associated long-standing myocarditis ("burned tree" image shown on coronary angiogram). We reported on cases of *Borrelia*-associated coronary aneurysms of the left coronary artery, but the presence of *B. burgdorferi* in the aneurysmatic artery wall could not be confirmed.[18]

Aortic Aneurysm and Dilation

Late stages of other spirochete infections are often characterized by chronic or subchronic aortitis. The latter has not been described in the literature for *B. burgdorferi* infection. Despite the huge number of cases (100 to 200 per year) of late Lyme disease in our specialized outpatient clinic for *B. burgdorferi*–associated disorders, we have not seen any *Borrelia*-associated aortic dilation or aneurysm or aortic valve incompetence so far. We also looked into the possibility of serological screening of patients with aortic regurgitation or dilation but could not see a higher prevalence of *B. burgdorferi* antibodies in pa-

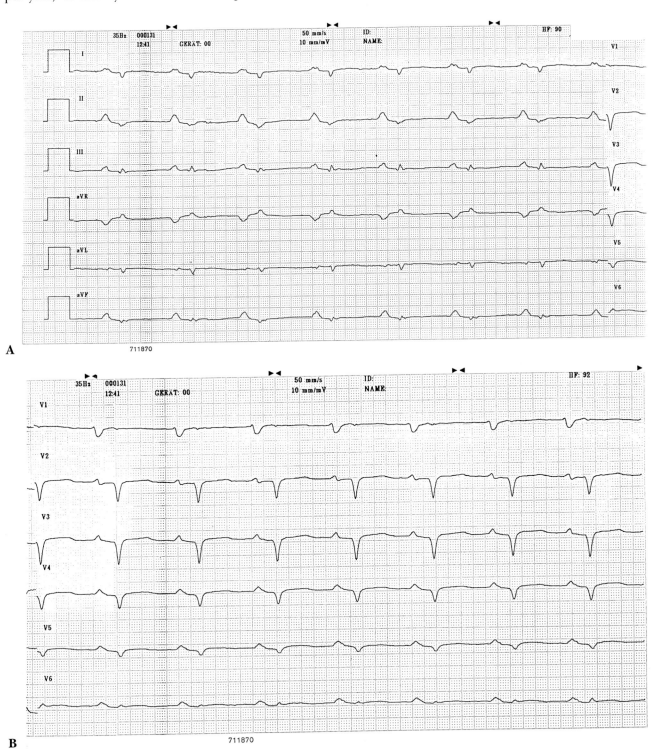

FIGURE 19.4. Electrocardiogram of a 36-year-old patient with exudative *Borrelia*-associated pericarditis showing decreased voltage of the R waves in all leads.

tients with aortic regurgitation compared with the normal population.

Pericarditis

Various authors have described *Borrelia*-associated exudative pericarditis in animal experiments and in humans. Most reports are anecdotal in character, and systematic investigations are absent. *Borrelia burgdorferi*–associated pericarditis has not shown any special characteristics, and its treatment largely depends on its clinical appearance. Steroids, however, are not desirable treatments for *Borrelia*-associated exudative pericarditis. Figure 19.4 shows the electrocardiogram of a 36-year-old patient with exudative *Borrelia*-associated pericarditis.

Summary

Borrelia burgdorferi infection does not often involve the cardiovascular system. However, cardiovascular manifestations still constitute the major source of death in patients with Lyme disease. The predominant manifestations are palpitations, AV block, myocarditis, dilated cardiomyopathy, and pericarditis. General cardiovascular manifestations are transient in nature. However, longlasting chronic myocarditis may lead to dilated cardiomyopathy. If treated early enough, response to antibiotic treatment is good, and left ventricular ejection fraction can be fully restored.

References

1. Ciesielsky CA, Markowitz LE, Horsley R. Lyme disease surveillance in the United States: 1983–1986. *Rev Infect Dis.* 1989;11(suppl 6):1425–1441.
2. Duray PH. Histopathology of clinical phases of human Lyme disease. *Rheum Dis Clin North Am.* 1989;15:691–710.
3. Barthold SW, Beck DS, Hansen GM, Terwilliger GA, Moody KD. Experimental Lyme borreliosis in selected strains and ages in laboratory mice. *J Infect Dis.* 1990;162:133–138.
4. Moody KD, Barthold SW, Terwilliger GA. Lyme borreliosis in laboratory animals: effect of host species and in vitro passage level of *Borrelia burgdorferi. Am J Trop Med Hyg.* 1990;43:87–92.
5. Blizard DA, Welty R. Cardiac activity in the mouse: strain differences. *J Comp Physiol Psychol.* 1971;77:337–344.
6. Chiao JW, Pavia C, Riley M, et al. Antigen of Lyme disease of spirochaete *Borellia burgdorferi* inhibits antigen- or mitogen-induced lymphocyte proliferation. *FEMS Immunol Med Microbiol* 1994;8:151–155.
7. Dufty J. Cardiac manifestations of Lyme disease. *J Musculoskel Med.* September 1992:17–28.
8. Cox J, Krajden M. Cardiovascular manifestations of Lyme disease. *Am Heart J.* 1991;122:1449–1455.
9. Steere AC, Batsford WP, Weinberg M, et al. Lyme carditis: cardiac abnormalities of Lyme disease. *Ann Intern Med.* 1980;92:8–16.
10. Van der Linde MR, Crijns BM, de Koning J, et al. Range of atrioventricular conduction disturbances in Lyme borreliosis: a report of four cases and review of other published reports. *Br Heart J.* 1990;163:162–168.
11. Gasser R, Dusleag J, Fruhwald F, Klein W, Reisinger EC. Early antimicrobial treatment of dilated cardiomyopathy associated with *Borrelia burgdorferi. Lancet.* 1992;340:982.
12. Jacobs JC, Rosen JM, Szer IS. Lyme myocarditis diagnosed by gallium scan. *J Pediatr.* 1984;105:950–952.
13. Reznick JW, Braunstein DB, Walsh RL, et al. Lyme carditis: electrophysiological and histopathological study. *Am J Med.* 1986;81:923–927.
14. Gasser R, Dusleag J, Reisinger EC, et al. Reversal by ceftriaxone of dilated cardiomyopathy in *Borrelia burgdorferi* infection. *Lancet.* 1992;339:1174–1175.
15. Stanek G, Klein J, Bittner R, Glogar D. Isolation of *Borrelia burgdorferi* from the myocardium of a patient with longstanding cardiomyopathy. *N Engl J Med.* 1990;322:249–252.
16. Fruhwald F, Dusleag J, Klein W, et al. Reversibility of dilated cardiomyopathy by low dose oral roxithromycin in a patient with chronic Lyme borreliosis. *Int J Angiol.* 1994;3:126–127.
17. Grisold M, Gasser R, Dusleag J, et al. Infarct like syndrome in acute Lyme borreliosis: a form of coronary vasculitis? Paper presented at: 5th International Conference on Lyme Borreliosis; May 1992; Arlington, Mass.
18. Gasser R, Fruhwald F, Watzinger N, Luha O, Eber B, Klein W. Coronary aneurysms in two patients with longstanding Lyme disease. *Lancet.* 1994;344:1300–1301.

20

Minimally Invasive Direct Coronary Artery Bypass or Limited Access Myocardial Revascularization

Vardhan J. Reddy and Denton A. Cooley

Minimally invasive direct coronary bypass (MIDCAB) through a limited anterior thoracotomy is gaining increasing acceptance.[1-9] This technique retains the internal mammary artery as the conduit of choice, as well as the operative principles of conventional coronary artery bypass grafting (CABG), which have had favorable long-term results. MIDCAB is less invasive and therefore has the benefit of other less invasive techniques, such as percutaneous transluminal coronary angioplasty, while retaining the more favorable long-term outcomes and lower costs of CABG. Percutaneous transluminal coronary angioplasty is often used in patients with proximal coronary stenosis. In 1996, in the United States alone, 482,000 patients (323,000 men and 155,000 women; 234,000 people over the age of 65) underwent percutaneous transluminal coronary angioplasty.[10] After angioplasty, however, the restenosis rate is very high. Although intraluminal stents have recently been used to reduce restenosis after coronary angioplasty, many patients might nonetheless receive long-term benefit from CABG.[1]

Because there is less surgical trauma in MIDCAB than in conventional CABG, MIDCAB avoids the complications related to median sternotomy, cardiopulmonary bypass, and cardiac arrest. Ultimately, lower perioperative morbidity and mortality rates, lower hospital costs, and an increasing public awareness of the benefits of this procedure will encourage surgeons to use MIDCAB more frequently.[1,2]

In MIDCAB, the internal mammary artery undergoes limited mobilization and is directly anastomosed to the left anterior descending coronary artery through a small anterior thoracotomy incision. Other coronary arteries, including the right, diagonal, and circumflex arteries, can also be recanalized via this procedure. The radial artery, saphenous vein, and right gastroepiploic artery are used as alternate grafts in limited myocardial revascularization.[1,9]

Three other minimally invasive cardiac surgical procedures are currently being developed.[3-9] In one procedure, the internal mammary artery is mobilized via thoracoscopy[8] up to the first intercostal space and direct internal mammary coronary anastomosis is accomplished thorough a small anterior thoracotomy, as in MIDCAB. In another procedure—port-access coronary artery bypass grafting[6,7]—percutaneous cardiopulmonary bypass through a triple-lumen catheter is introduced via the femoral artery to occlude the aorta and deliver cardioplegia for cardiac arrest; the internal mammary artery is then anastomosed to the coronary vessel via thoracoscopy. In the third procedure, a small laparotomy is followed by coronary revascularization with right gastroepiploic artery.[1,11]

Of the four minimally invasive coronary revascularization procedures, MIDCAB is used most frequently: an estimated 600 MIDCAB procedures had been performed worldwide by mid-1996.[1,5,9] On the basis of our principle to "modify, simplify, and apply," we believe that the MIDCAB procedure is the most promising of the four. Although greater surgical skill is required in the MIDCAB technique than in the other minimally invasive surgical techniques, technological improvements in optical loops and fiber-optic illumination are continuing to make microvascular surgery less difficult.[1]

Incidence

Cardiovascular disease is a major international health problem.[10] In 1990, in developed countries, 5.3 million (of a total 10.9 million) deaths were attributed to cardiovascular disease, primarily heart disease and stroke. However, the mortality rate from cardiovascular disease fell by more than 60% in men in Japan and by 50% in men in Australia, Canada, France, and the United States. The mortality rate from cardiovascular disease declined less impressively in the Scandinavian countries and in Ireland, Portugal, and Spain and rose by 40% in Hungary, 60% in Poland, and 80% in Bulgaria. In Africa, Western Asia, and Southeast Asia, 15% to 20% of an estimated 20 million deaths are due to cardiovascular disease. In China and India (which contain approximately half of the total population of the developing world), 4.5 to 5 million deaths are attributed to cardiovascular disease. Cardiovascular disease is a growing problem in developing countries, largely due to increases in socioeconomic status and Westernization of diet and culture.

In the United States the estimated annual economic cost of cardiovascular disease is $286.5 billion, and in every year since 1900 (with the exception of 1918) cardiovascular disease has been the principal cause of death.

History

CABG remains one of the most commonly used techniques for myocardial revascularization.[10] In 1993, 485,000 CABG operations were performed in the United States alone, including 176,000 repeat operations. The concept of coronary revascularization was first introduced in 1910 when Alexis Carrel described coronary artery bypass in dogs. In 1946 Vineberg described a technique in which the internal mammary artery was implanted into the myocardium, and in 1952 Demikhov directly anastomosed the internal mammary artery to a coronary vessel in dogs. Not until 1964, however, did Kolessov[12] perform the first sutured anastomosis of the internal mammary artery to a coronary artery in a 44-year-old patient. Since then, many clinical studies from around the world have established the long-term patency of the internal mammary coronary bypass in the treatment of cardiovascular disease. Today, the internal mammary artery graft remains the gold standard for coronary revascularization.

Evolution of MIDCAB

Modern coronary artery bypass employs a median sternotomy, wide exposure of the heart, temporary cardiopulmonary bypass, and cardiac arrest. The major disadvantage of CABG is its invasiveness. After a sternotomy, major infection occurs in 0.4% to 5% of patients, in whom the mortality rate ranges between 7% and 80%.[13-15] The significant risk factors are the interval between hospital admission and surgery, the hospital environment, reoperation, blood transfusion requirements, early chest reexploration, and sternal rewiring. Internal mammary artery harvesting increases the incidence of sternal infection. Diabetes and double mammary mobilization multiply the risk of sternal infection by 13.9. The sequelae in patients who survive a sternal infection can be long lasting and difficult, and hospital charges for such patients are 2.8 times greater than for patients whose postoperative course is uncomplicated.

A sternotomy also increases postoperative pain and delays recovery; 2 to 4 months are generally required for complete rehabilitation after a CABG procedure. In the United States in 1996, the estimated lost output from disability after CABG procedures was $9.6 billion.[10] Patients who have diabetes or severe respiratory disease and those who are obese or are undergoing a reoperation would benefit from avoiding sternotomy procedures. Further, patients who do not undergo sternotomies appear to be at less risk if they require cardiac operation in the future.

Cardiopulmonary bypass also has adverse effects for the CABG patient, including systemic microembolization, activation of complement and neutrophils, abnormal septal wall motion with some diminution in global left ventricular function, arrhythmias, diminished oxygen delivery, and impaired hemostasis. Additional deleterious effects may occur in high-risk patients such as older patients and those with renal failure, respiratory problems, cerebrovascular disease, and acute myocardial infarction. Patients who undergo CABG without cardiopulmonary bypass have a reduced mortality rate (1% versus 4%), a lower incidence of cerebrovascular accidents (0.5% versus 2.3%), a lower blood transfusion rate (19% versus 66%), and a shorter hospital stay. In addition, women, hypertensive patients, and patients with depressed left ventricular function benefit from CABG without cardiopulmonary bypass.

The MIDCAB procedure arose in response to pressure for better outcomes, both fiscal and surgical. The procedure was developed to avoid the complications of median sternotomy, cardiopulmonary bypass, and cardiac arrest and to retain the beneficial outcome from the long-term patency of internal mammary artery grafting. Thus far, postoperative morbidity has been reduced, the mortality rate is acceptable, and both surgical and fiscal outcomes have improved.

Patient Selection

Patients eligible for the MIDCAB procedure are those who exhibit any of the following characteristics.[1,5,9]

1. They have left main or left anterior descending coronary artery disease, and percutaneous transluminal coronary angioplasty is not advisable (because of proximal or complex stenoses), not possible (because of an occluded left anterior descending coronary artery), or has not been successful.

2. They have left anterior descending coronary artery disease and a second occluded vessel (right coronary or circumflex arteries) that has been recanalized, with

mild stenosis or with stenosis that could be dilated.

3. They have left anterior descending coronary artery disease, disease of two other vessels, and a combination of the aforementioned conditions.
4. They have multiple-vessel disease and an unacceptably high risk of morbidity from cardiopulmonary bypass (patients with depressed left ventricular function, cancer, severe renal failure, diffuse cerebrovascular disease, diffuse peripheral vasculopathy, severe respiratory insufficiency, or who are older than 80 years).
5. They have single right coronary artery disease.
6. They are undergoing a repeat CABG and are at high risk for complications of sternotomy, cardiopulmonary bypass, and massive transfusions.
7. They are Jehovah's Witnesses with any of the aforementioned conditions.
8. They do not want a sternotomy, choose a limited-access myocardial revascularization, and have any of the aforementioned conditions.
9. They have severe diabetes mellitus with left anterior descending and right coronary artery disease that requires bilateral mammary arteries and have a subsequent high risk of sternal infection.

Contraindications

Contraindications for the MIDCAB procedure include the presence of any of the following:

1. A calcified distal left anterior descending coronary artery smaller than 1.5 mm in diameter
2. Intramyocardial coronary vessels (often detected by angiography)
3. An internal mammary artery less than 2 mm in diameter at the level of the fourth intercostal space (documented by either a preoperative Doppler echocardiographic study or angiography)
4. Proximal subclavian stenosis, stenosis of the origin of the internal mammary artery, abnormal origin of the internal mammary artery, or anomalous origin of the thyrocervical trunk or the transverse cervical artery from the internal mammary artery (patients with subclavian stenosis greater than 50% may undergo preoperative angioplasty before coronary revascularization)

Previous use of the internal mammary artery is a relative contraindication. The saphenous vein, radial artery, and gastroepiploic artery can be used as alternative conduits, and the subclavian artery can be the site for proximal anastomosis. This technique may be considered when the internal mammary artery is occluded (Figure 20.1A). After the subclavian artery is exposed, the saphenous vein graft is anastomosed proximally (Figure 20.1B) and then distally to the left anterior descending coronary artery (Figure 20.1C,D).

Internal Mammary Artery[16–24]

Thorough knowledge of the anatomy of the internal mammary artery will enable careful planning of the limited myocardial revascularization procedure. The internal mammary artery generally arises from the lower and anterior part of the first part of the subclavian artery opposite the origin of the thyrocervical trunk, although it may arise from the second or third part of the subclavian artery.[16] In 20% of the population, the internal mammary artery has a common origin with other major branches. It arises with the thyrocervical trunk (10%), suprascapular artery (10%), and transverse cervical artery (1%). The average external diameter of the internal mammary artery in cadavers is 3.6 mm, whereas the external diameter of the superior epigastric artery is 1.6 mm and the musculophrenic artery 1.8 mm.[19] In vivo these diameters are smaller: preoperative duplex studies reveal a diameter of 2.4 mm for the left internal mammary artery and 2.6 mm for the right internal mammary artery; angiography reveals a 2.6-mm left internal mammary artery and a 2.8-mm right internal mammary artery; and digital subtraction angiography reveals a 2.7-mm left internal mammary artery and a 2.8-mm right internal mammary artery. The right internal mammary artery is larger than the left, probably because of the predominant right-handedness in the population. The right internal mammary artery is 1.03 cm from the right lateral edge of sternum; the left internal mammary artery is 0.98 cm from the left lateral edge of the sternum.

Various names have been given to the major side branch of the internal mammary artery, including lateral costal artery, high intercostal artery, first intercostal artery, lateral intercostal artery, and lateral internal mammary artery.[23] Lateral costal artery, the preferred term, adequately describes its origin and course. The lateral costal artery, first described by Heister in 1730, is present only on the right side in 8.9% of the population, only on the left side in 13.4%, and on both sides in 5.3%. When present, the lateral costal artery arises about 1 cm below the origin of the internal mammary artery, at or above the first costal cartilage, and runs laterally and obliquely along the anterior axillary line. The caliber of the artery is directly proportional to its length and number of branches. When the lateral costal artery extends beyond the sixth intercostal space, its diameter is more than two thirds the diameter of the internal mammary artery; however, a lateral costal of this size occurs in only 4.5% of the overall population.

The other branches of the internal mammary artery are of a small caliber. Among them are (1) the pericardiophrenic artery, a long slender branch that accompanies the phrenic nerve; (2) the mediastinal arteries, the small vessels distributed to the areolar tissue of the mediastinum; (3) the thymic arteries, which supply the remains of the thymus; (4) the sternal branches, which

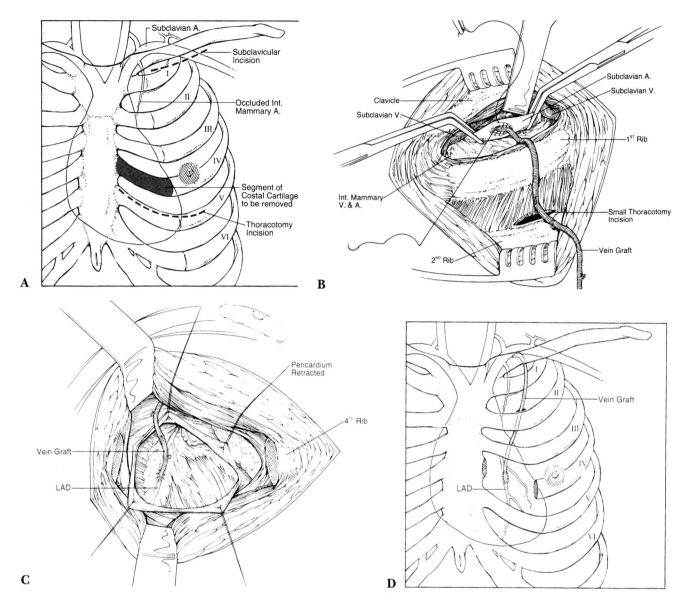

FIGURE 20.1. Anastomosis of the saphenous vein graft to the subclavian artery proximally and the left anterior descending coronary artery distally.

supply the transverse thoracic muscle and become part of the subpleural plexus supplying the sternum; (5) the anterior intercostal arteries (one [in 46% of the population] or two [in 54%]) in the first five or six intercostal spaces; (6) the perforators (one in each of the first six intercostal spaces); (7) the musculophrenic artery, one of the two terminal branches of the internal mammary artery, which runs along the costal cartilage of the false ribs and ends at the last intercostal space; and (8) the superior epigastric artery, the other terminal branch, which runs under the rectus abdominis and connects to the inferior epigastric artery.

Preoperative Preparation for MIDCAB

In addition to the routine preoperative preparation of a patient for a conventional CABG, preoperative assessment of the internal mammary artery is essential in patients undergoing MIDCAB. Coronary subclavian steal is a recognizable and correctable cause of postoperative myocardial ischemia. Subclavian stenosis, which occurs in 0.5% to 2.0% of the patients who require coronary bypass grafts, causes coronary subclavian steal by reverting the flow from coronary to mammary during active use of the upper limb. Unrecognized subclavian stenosis[25-28] is a rare but possible cause of postoperative angina secondary to coronary steal. Consequently, routine subclavian angiography is recommended during cardiac catheterization in patients who have (1) symptoms and signs of upper extremity or cerebrovascular ischemia, (2) the presence of cervical or supraclavicular bruit, or (3) an upper extremity blood pressure differential greater than or equal to 20 mm Hg. The traditional approach to this problem is a carotid–subclavian bypass, but there have been recent successful reports of both preoperative and postoperative angioplasty of subclavian artery stenosis.

Routine subclavian angiography can also reveal stenosis of the origin of the internal mammary artery, which is a very rare contraindication for limited myocardial revascularization.[29] Anomalous origin of major branches of the internal mammary artery, such as the thyrocervical trunk or the transverse cervical artery, is also a contraindication for limited myocardial revascularization.[20] Although the incidence of this anomaly is unknown, it can be detected through arm exercise testing and a duplex sonographic study of flow in the internal mammary artery. (Arm exercise reduces flow in the internal mammary artery.)

Routine angiography of the internal mammary artery is not without complications.[21,22] An ostial intimal tear of the artery that leads to further dissection occurs in 10% to 15% of patients whose internal mammary artery is intubated for either diagnosis or angioplasty of arterial lesions. The internal mammary artery is also subject to intense spasm after selective intubation. Other difficulties, including vascular tortuosity, congenital anomaly, anatomical difficulty, or proximal subclavian stenosis, limit the success of selectively intubating the internal mammary artery to 78% to 80%.

Because of these complications, a noninvasive preoperative procedure such as duplex sonographic evaluation is advisable. Such an evaluation can indicate the size of the internal mammary artery, the presence of large side branches, blood flow, velocity, pulsatility index, and anatomical variability. For use in MIDCAB, an internal mammary artery greater than 2 mm in diameter at the level of the fourth intercostal space is preferable.

As in other systemic arteries,[9] blood flow in the internal mammary artery is triphasic and systolic-dominant; mean blood flow velocity is 21.2 cm/s. After anastomosis of the internal mammary artery to a coronary artery, the flow in the distal part of the internal mammary artery changes to biphasic and diastolic-dominant, whereas flow in the proximal part of the internal mammary artery remains triphasic and systolic-dominant. This finding is similar to those in which the internal mammary artery is

reported to be an active and live conduit that adapts to the demands of the distal coronary vascular bed.

Postoperative demonstration of the change in flow pattern from triphasic and systolic-dominant to biphasic and diastolic-dominant indicates the "patency" of the internal mammary coronary graft and obviates the need for interventional procedures. Duplex sonographic evaluation of the internal mammary artery both preoperatively and postoperatively provides objective physiological evidence of flow and the patency of the vessel.

Surgical Technique

The patient is placed in the supine position on the operating table.[1] The left side of the chest is elevated about 10 degrees with a rolled blanket. The left upper limb is tucked at the side of the patient; special care must be given to protect pressure points with eggshell sponges. The right upper limb is abducted and elevated at the shoulder with a wedge to reduce tension on the brachial plexus. An arterial line, Foley catheter, and jugular triple-lumen catheter are inserted. A Swan-Ganz catheter is used only rarely. Anesthesia is induced with fentanyl and sodium thiopental and maintained with fentanyl and droperidol. Muscular relaxation is obtained with pancuronium bromide. Early in our experience with MIDCAB, we used a double-lumen endotracheal tube to avoid left lung ventilation if necessary, but we no longer do so. In the final part of the operation, a mixture of N_2O and O_2 is used to enable the patient to awaken more rapidly. A perfusion team is available if needed.

A 4-cm curved transverse incision is made over the fourth rib anteriorly with a medial curve parallel to the sternum (Figure 20.2A). The costal cartilage is divided at its junction with the rib end. As the cartilage is retracted forward, it will fracture at the junction with the sternum. This maneuver both protects and exposes the underlying internal mammary artery and vein and allows adequate access for the surgeon to mobilize and prepare the vessel for bypass. Early in our experience, we resected 2 to 3 cm of the third costal cartilage (Figure 20.2B). This resection, however, may predispose the patient to a cosmetic defect and lung herniation. Now, for more flexibility, we divide and retract the third costal cartilage to facilitate the proximal mobilization of an adequate length of the internal mammary artery. The mammary artery is then dissected distally under the fifth costal cartilage and proximally under the third costal cartilage to the level of the second intercostal space (Figure 20.2C). The branches are clipped (with small gold-colored clips) on the mammary side and cauterized on the chest side.

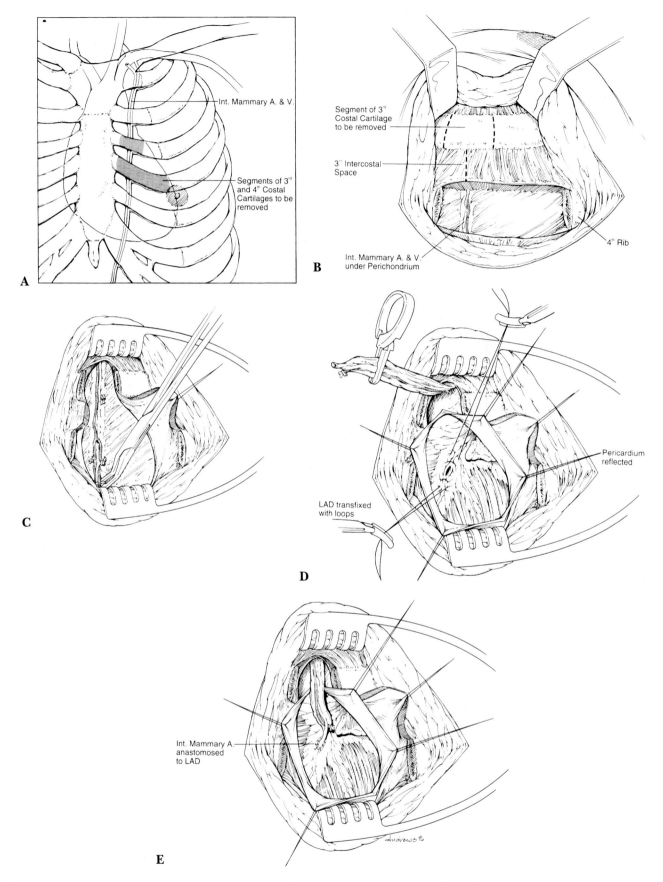

FIGURE 20.2. Surgical technique for minimally invasive direct coronary artery bypass. The left internal mammary artery is anastomosed to the left anterior descending coronary artery. LAD, left anterior descending.

Before the artery is divided, the pericardium is incised parallel to the sternum, the left anterior descending coronary artery is exposed, and its suitability for bypass is assessed. An intramyocardial, severely calcified, very small left anterior descending artery makes anastomosis impossible. Pericardial traction sutures are applied to retract the heart forward and to prevent the insufflated lung from obscuring the surgeon's view (Figure 20.2D). In the MIDCAB procedure, the heart is actually closer to the chest wall than in conventional CABG, because mediastinal ligaments keep the heart well suspended in the pericardial sac close to the anterior chest wall. This phenomenon reduces the length of internal mammary artery required for the bypass operation. The left anterior descending artery is then dissected. If it is suitable for bypass, traction-snare sutures (2-O polypropylene passed around the artery twice) are used to occlude the artery during anastomosis. These sutures also provide regional immobility of the myocardium, which decreases the difficulty of operating on a beating heart. Extra stay sutures passed around the left anterior descending artery may be used to stabilize the myocardium locally. Various innovative measures, such as the "octopus" suction device with 19 to 20 suction domes, have been developed to immobilize the cardiac wall.

An esmolol drip[30] is begun by the anesthesiologist, and the cardiac rate is reduced to between 40 and 60 beats per minute. Heparin, usually 50 mg or less, is injected intravenously. The mammary artery is then divided distally and checked for free flow. The distal part of the mammary artery is skeletonized. If needed, papaverine (1 mg/mL of saline solution) may be injected locally to control spasm.

The traction sutures on the coronary artery are gently retracted and attached to the surgical drapes. A longitudinal incision is made in the artery, and the anastomosis is completed with a 7-O polypropylene suture using a standard, continuous-suture technique starting at the heel and finishing at the toe of the anastomosis (Figure 20.2E). Some centers use an interrupted anastomosis with 7-O polypropylene in the "parachute" technique. We use saline irrigation to visualize the anastomotic site; some centers use CO_2 insufflation for the same purpose.

Although the heart continues to contract, a satisfactory anastomosis can be accomplished with meticulous surgical technique. Our anastomotic time is 3 to 5 minutes, and the left anterior descending artery is occluded for less than 10 minutes. The left internal mammary artery and the left anterior descending coronary artery are unclamped, and hemostasis is carefully checked. Heparin may then be reversed with protamine sulfate. The divided third costal cartilage is sutured back. An intercostal nerve block of 0.5% bupivacaine and 1% lidocaine injected one space above and below the thoracotomy

can increase postoperative comfort levels. In some centers, a small catheter is left in the pleural cavity for the continuous infusion of an analgesic drug (bupivacaine). Insertion of a small chest tube is optional. The surgical incision is closed without pericostal sutures.

Postoperative Course

All patients are admitted to the intensive care unit, where central venous pressure, blood pressure, and urine output are monitored. Patients are remarkably hemodynamically stable because the procedure is much less invasive than conventional CABG and cardiopulmonary bypass is avoided. Patients have minimal blood loss during the operation and postoperatively require smaller quantities of blood products. To date, our patients have not needed pharmacological support to maintain blood pressure.

Most of the patients are extubated 4 to 6 hours after the operation. Even patients with chronic lung disease are extubated early, because there has been less pulmonary intervention intraoperatively. Because patients generally have less postoperative discomfort, we routinely use a single-lumen rather than a double-lumen endotracheal tube. Clear liquid fluids are allowed orally immediately after extubation; fluids are advanced as tolerated.

Obviously, because they have not undergone median sternotomy, most patients have less postoperative pain than they would after conventional CABG. Most patients can sit up and dangle their feet within 12 hours of their operation. Patients seem pleasantly surprised by the relatively lower level of pain. Patients also require less postoperative sedation.

The chest tube, central line, and Foley catheter are removed the day after the operation, and the patient is transferred to floor care with a peripheral intravenous line. Wound dressings are removed, and patients are encouraged to ambulate as they are able. Patients are also encouraged to use incentive spirometry.

A postoperative duplex evaluation of the internal mammary artery may yield valuable information. Because the internal mammary artery remains in its natural position in the first two or three intercostal spaces, the flow pattern is easily detectable. Also, because there is no median sternotomy, the first two to three intercostal spaces are free of edema from surgical trauma. As described earlier, the change in the left internal mammary artery flow from triphasic and systolic-dominant to biphasic and diastolic-dominant demonstrates the patency of the graft. This flow pattern can be compared with that in the right internal mammary artery. Most patients are discharged on the second postoperative day.

Results

Currently, we have only short-term results: the mortality rate is zero, and no patients have required a repeat operation or blood transfusion or have had arrhythmias; all patients are currently asymptomatic. One patient had ST changes immediately after the operation, but these reverted to normal within 2 hours. The ST changes probably occurred as the result of spasm in the internal mammary artery. The patient was discharged uneventfully.

Early graft patency rates in various centers are between 95% and 98%. Follow-up with color duplex sonography is desirable, because it is noninvasive and inexpensive. Color duplex sonography is also easier in MIDCAB patients than in conventional CABG patients because the proximal internal mammary artery remains in its natural position after MIDCAB.

Although early graft failure can result from occlusion of the distal left internal mammary artery at the anastomosis, kinking of the artery against the sternum, or acute angling of the artery, meticulous surgical technique can usually prevent these complications. An intraoperative thermal imaging camera may be helpful in detecting blood flow through the anastomosis. Spasm of the artery can be reduced by perivascular injection of papaverine solution. Special attention should be given to attaining good hemostasis from the intercostal branches of the internal mammary artery.

Lung herniation has been reported when two or more cartilages are divided. We excise the fourth costal cartilage and divide and suture the third costal cartilage, which also provides a good cosmetic result. The wound heals well, and we have not had any wound infections.

Cardiac Rehabilitation

We begin rehabilitation education in the preoperative period and continue it during recovery. In our experience, patients who have undergone the MIDCAB procedure follow postoperative rehabilitation instructions more closely, probably because there is less pain. Postoperative ambulation and incentive spirometry are begun on the day of the operation, and the levels of each are increased until the patient returns to work. Generally, patients may return to daily activities, including desk work, within 2 weeks. Postoperative paresthesia of the anterior chest wall, commonly seen in patients who have undergone conventional CABG, occurs less frequently in patients who have undergone MIDCAB, probably because of the limited mobilization of the internal mammary artery. In addition, patient acceptability of MIDCAB is greater because of the smaller surgical scar.

Comment

MIDCAB leaves the pericardium intact, which provides three-dimensional support to the heart. Further, the pericardium, with intact anterior and posterior ligaments, suspends the heart more closely to the anterior chest wall. As a result, a shorter length of internal mammary artery is required for anastomosis than in conventional CABG, and the internal mammary artery need not be mobilized beyond the second intercostal space. Also, in the MIDCAB procedure, the anterior and posterior movement of the heart during the cardiac cycle is preserved. In conventional CABG, the lateral pericardium and the lungs are displaced, especially on the left side after mobilization of the left internal mammary artery. The heart then falls back and rotates during each cardiac cycle, which requires a greater length of the left internal mammary artery.

Limited Mobilization of the Internal Mammary Artery[11,23,24,31–40]

Limited mobilization maintains the proximal part of the artery in its natural position, with complete innervation, and prevents the occasional complication of rotation of the artery and graft failure that can occur in conventional CABG.[41] With limited mobilization, there is also the issue of whether the proximal branches cause a steal phenomenon. The hemodynamic importance of this anatomical condition is controversial, but increasing evidence from physiological flow studies of the internal mammary artery shows that the collaterals are of no significance.

As discussed earlier, the flow in the distal internal mammary artery is biphasic and diastolic-dominant (with a diastolic-to-systolic velocity ratio of 1.4), whereas the flow in the proximal internal mammary artery is triphasic and systolic-dominant (diastolic-to-systolic velocity ratio = 0.6), and the flow in the proximal collaterals is triphasic and systolic-dominant (diastolic-to-systolic velocity ratio = 0.5). There is no competition between the two flows because they occur in different phases of the cardiac cycle.

After adenosine stimulation, the diastolic flow increase in the left internal mammary artery is 103 mL/min; 70% of this flow goes to the coronary circulation and is not affected by diversion to the side branches. Flow in the internal mammary artery is rarely a limiting factor in the augmentation of myocardial perfusion.

As in any blood vessel, flow in the internal mammary artery depends on distal vascular bed resistance. In the internal mammary artery, most of the resistance is provided by the coronary vessels. When the internal mammary artery diameter is larger than 2 mm, resistance is

negligible; resistance begins to rise when the diameter is less than 2 mm. Many clinical studies have shown that the internal mammary artery has sufficient recruitable physiological flow reserve to supply more than one coronary vascular territory. Most of the T grafts coming from the internal mammary artery remain patent for long periods. The gastroepiploic artery graft provides another example in which larger, proximal, undivided branches before coronary anastomosis do not affect long-term patency. We believe angiographic demonstration of the presence of proximal branches of the internal mammary artery has no hemodynamic or clinical significance and is only a marker for increased coronary vascular resistance due to advancing coronary disease.

Limited mobilization of the internal mammary artery through a MIDCAB incision also prevents phrenic nerve injury.[42-44] Phrenic nerve dysfunction is a significant source of morbidity but a rare cause of mortality. Most injury to the phrenic nerve during cardiac surgery results from ice slush, which is avoided in the MIDCAB procedure. Phrenic nerve dysfunction also occurs after injury to the pericardiophrenic artery during more proximal mobilization of the left internal mammary artery, which is also generally avoided in MIDCAB surgery. Limited mobilization of the internal mammary artery can also prevent rare complications, such as stretch injury of the brachial plexus during sternotomy,[45] left recurrent nerve injury,[46] and chylothorax.[47,48]

Occlusion of the Left Anterior Descending Coronary Artery

In our experience, occlusion of the left anterior descending artery does not cause hemodynamic changes or rhythm disturbances. Ischemic preconditioning of the artery (intermittent or continuous occlusion) may detect myocardial ischemic sensitivity and may increase myocardial ischemic tolerance. Myocardial sensitivity depends on the degree and longevity of the stenosis of the left anterior descending artery and the dominance and collaterals of the coronary vascular system, as well as the myocardial mass. We must emphasize that MIDCAB does not enable rapid cannulation of the patient.

Economics

The economic costs of cardiovascular disease are high.[10] In 1999, the estimated economic cost of cardiovascular disease in the United States will be $286.5 billion, and the cost of heart disease alone will be $183.1 billion. Related estimated costs for 1999 include hospitals and nursing homes, $124.3 billion; services of physicians and nurses, $26.8 billion; and lost work output resulting from disability, $26.5 billion. Because the MIDCAB procedure results in a shorter stay in intensive care, a shorter total

length of stay in the hospital, a shorter recovery period, a quicker rehabilitation, and an earlier return to work, many of the aforementioned costs can be greatly reduced. These savings are particularly beneficial in this period of changing health care delivery. In addition, the MIDCAB procedure may be especially useful in developing countries with limited resources.

Conclusions

Before MIDCAB can become a standard procedure, surgeons will need additional experience to evaluate the efficacy of this new technique. Although MIDCAB demands great surgical expertise, our experience demonstrates that coronary bypass operations can be successfully performed for selected lesions in an operating field that is neither quiet nor bloodless. Ultimately, wider use of the MIDCAB procedure may result in better patient outcomes and lower costs.

References

1. Cooley DA. Limited access myocardial revascularization: a preliminary report. *Tex Heart Inst J*. 1996;23:81–84.
2. Lytle BW. Minimally invasive cardiac surgery [editorial]. *J Thorac Cardiovasc Surg*. 1996;111:554–555.
3. Acuff TE, Landreneau RJ, Griffith BP, Mack MJ. Minimally invasive coronary artery bypass grafting. *Ann Thorac Surg*. 1996;61:135–137.
4. Robinson MC, Gross DR, Zeman W, Stedje-Larsen E. Minimally invasive coronary artery bypass grafting: a new method using an anterior mediastinotomy. *J Card Surg*. 1995;10:529–536.
5. Subramanian VA, Sani G, Bennetti FJ, Calafiore AM. Minimally invasive coronary artery bypass surgery: a multi-center report of preliminary clinical experience [abstract]. *Circulation*. 1995;92(suppl 1):I645.
6. Stevens JH, Burdon TA, Peters WS, et al. Port-access coronary artery bypass grafting: a proposed surgical method. *J Thorac Cardiovasc Surg*. 1996;111:567–573.
7. Schwartz DS, Ribakove GH, Grossi EA, et al. Minimally invasive cardiopulmonary bypass with cardioplegic arrest: a closed chest technique with equivalent myocardial protection. *J Thorac Cardiovasc Surg*. 1996;111:556–566.
8. Benetti FJ, Ballester C. Use of thoracoscopy and a minimal thoracotomy, in mammary-coronary bypass to left anterior descending artery, without extracorporeal circulation: experience in 2 cases. *J Cardiovasc Surg*. 1995;36:159–161.
9. Calafiore AM, Di Giammarco G, Teodori G, et al. Left anterior descending coronary artery grafting via left anterior small thoracotomy without cardiopulmonary bypass. *Ann Thorac Surg*. 1996;61:1658–1665.
10. American Heart Association. *Heart and Stroke Facts: 1996 Statistical Supplement*. Dallas, Tex: American Heart Association; 1996.
11. Suma H, Wanibuchi Y, Terada Y, Fukuda S, Takayama T, Furuta S. The right gastroepiploic artery graft: clinical and

angiographic midterm results in 200 patients. *J Thorac Cardiovasc Surg.* 1993;105:615–623.

12. Olearchyk AS. Vasilii I Kolesov: a pioneer of coronary revascularization by internal mammary-coronary artery grafting. *J Thorac Cardiovasc Surg.* 1988;96:13–18.

13. Ottino G, De Paulis R, Pansini S, et al. Major sternal wound infection after open-heart surgery: a multivariate analysis of risk factors in 2,579 consecutive operative procedures. *Ann Thorac Surg.* 1987;44:173–179.

14. Grossi EA, Esposito R, Harris LJ, et al. Sternal wound infections and use of internal mammary artery grafts. *J Thorac Cardiovasc Surg.* 1991;102:342–347.

15. Loop FD, Lytle BW, Cosgrove DM, et al. J. Maxwell Chamberlain memorial paper. Sternal wound complications after isolated coronary artery bypass grafting: early and late mortality, morbidity, and cost of care. *Ann Thorac Surg.* 1990;49:179–187.

16. Bean RB. A composite study of the subclavian artery in man. *Am J Anat.* 1905;4:303–328.

17. Sabiston DC Jr, Blalock A. Experimental ligation of the internal mammary artery and its effect on coronary occlusion. *Surgery.* 1958;43:906–912.

18. Finci L, Meier B, Steffenino G, Doriot PA, Rutishauser W. Nonselective preoperative digital subtraction angiography of internal mammary arteries. *Cathet Cardiovasc Diagn.* 1990;19:13–16.

19. Sons HJ, Marx R, Godehardt E, Losse B, Kunert J, Bircks W. Duplex sonography of the internal thoracic artery: preoperative assessment. *J Thorac Cardiovasc Surg.* 1994;108:549–555.

20. Bauer EP, Bino MC, von Segesser LK, Laske A, Turina MI. Internal mammary artery anomalies. *Thorac Cardiovasc Surg.* 1990;38:312–315.

21. Kunz RE, Baim DS. Internal mammary angiography: a review of technical issues and newer methods. *Cathet Cardiovasc Diagn.* 1990;20:10–16.

22. Feit A, Reddy CV, Cowley C, Ibrahim B, Zisbrod Z. Internal mammary artery angiography should be a routine component of diagnostic coronary angiography. *Cathet Cardiovasc Diagn.* 1992;25:85–90.

23. Kropp BN. The lateral costal branch of the internal mammary artery. *J Thorac Surg.* 1951;21:421–425.

24. Schmid C, Heublein B, Reichelt S, Borst HG. Steal phenomenon caused by a parallel branch of the internal mammary artery. *Ann Thorac Surg.* 1990;50:463–464.

25. Tyras DH, Barner HB. Coronary-subclavian steal. *Arch Surg.* 1977;112:1125–1127.

26. Marshall WG Jr, Miller EC, Kouchoukos NT. The coronary-subclavian steal syndrome: report of a case and recommendations for prevention and management. *Ann Thorac Surg.* 1988;46:93–96.

27. Laub GW, Muralidharan S, Naidech H, Fernandez J, Adkins M, McGrath LB. Percutaneous transluminal subclavian angioplasty in a patient with postoperative angina. *Ann Thorac Surg.* 1991;52:850–851.

28. Belz M, Marshall JJ, Cowley MJ, Vetrovec GW. Subclavian balloon angioplasty in the management of the coronary-subclavian steal syndrome. *Cathet Cardiovasc Diagn.* 1992;25:161–163.

29. Stullman WS, Hilliard GK. Unrecognized internal mammary artery stenosis treated by percutaneous angioplasty after coronary bypass surgery. *Am Heart J.* 1987;113(pt 1):393–395.

30. Labovitz AJ, Barth C, Castello R, Ojile M, Kern MJ. Attenuation of myocardial ischemia during coronary occlusion by ultrashort-acting beta adrenergic blockade. *Am Heart J.* 1991;121:1347–1352.

31. Ayres RW, Lu CT, Benzuly KH, Hill GA, Rossen JD. Transcatheter embolization of an internal mammary artery bypass graft sidebranch causing coronary steal syndrome. *Cathet Cardiovasc Diagn.* 1994;31:301–303.

32. Singh RN, Sosa JA. Internal mammary artery-coronary artery anastomosis: influence of the side branches on surgical result. *J Thorac Cardiovasc Surg.* 1981;82:909–914.

33. Tartini R, Steinbrunn W, Kappenberger L, Goebel N, Turina M. Anomalous origin of the left thyrocervical trunk as a cause of residual pain after myocardial revascularization with internal mammary artery. *Ann Thorac Surg.* 1985;40:302–304.

34. Pelias AJ, DelRossi AJ, Tacy L, Wolpowitz A. A case of postoperative internal mammary steal [letter]. *J Thorac Cardiovasc Surg.* 1985;90:794–795.

35. Ivert T, Huttunen K, Landou C, Bjork VO. Angiographic studies of internal mammary artery grafts 11 years after coronary artery bypass grafting. *J Thorac Cardiovasc Surg.* 1988;96:1–12.

36. Kuttler H, Hauenstein KH, Kameda T, Wenz W, Schlosser V. Significance of early angiographic follow-up after internal thoracic artery anastomosis in coronary surgery. *Thorac Cardiovasc Surg.* 1988;36:96–99.

37. Kern MJ, Bach RG, Donohue TJ, Caracciolo EA, Wolford T, Aguirre FV. Interventional physiology, XIII: role of large pectoralis branch artery in flow through a patent left internal mammary artery conduit. *Cathet Cardiovasc Diagn.* 1995;34:240–244.

38. Louagie YA, Haxhe JP, Jamart J, Gurne O, Buche M, Schoevaerdts JC. Preoperative hemodynamic study of left internal mammary artery grafts. *Thorac Cardiovasc Surg.* 1995;43:27–34.

39. Barner HB, Naunheim KS, Willman VL, Fiore AC. Revascularization with bilateral internal thoracic artery grafts in patients with left main coronary stenosis. *Eur J Cardiothorac Surg.* 1992;6:66–71.

40. Habbab MA, Amro AA. Nonsurgical (embolization) treatment of the coronary-internal mammary flow diversion phenomenon. *Am Heart J.* 1993;126:456–458.

41. Brown RP. Effect on blood flow of rotation and position of the internal mammary artery pedicle. *Ann Thorac Surg.* 1995;59:416–418.

42. O'Brien JW, Johnson SH, VanSteyn SJ, et al. Effects of internal mammary artery dissection on phrenic nerve perfusion and function. *Ann Thorac Surg.* 1991;52:182–188.

43. Owens WA, Gladstone DJ, Heylings DJ. Surgical anatomy of the phrenic nerve and internal mammary artery. *Ann Thorac Surg.* 1994;58:843–844.

44. Setina M, Cerny S, Grim M, Pirk J. Anatomical interrelation between the phrenic nerve and the internal mam-

mary artery as seen by the surgeon. *J Cardiovasc Surg.* 1993; 34:499–502.

45. Vander Salm TJ, Cereda JM, Cutler BS. Brachial plexus injury following median sternotomy. *J Thorac Cardiovasc Surg.* 1980;80:447–452.

46. Phillips TG, Green GE. Left recurrent laryngeal nerve injury following internal mammary artery bypass. *Ann Thorac Surg.* 1987;43:440.

47. Di Lello F, Werner PH, Kleinman LH, Mullen DC, Flemma RJ. Life-threatening chylothorax after left internal mammary artery dissection: therapeutic considerations. *Ann Thorac Surg.* 1987;44:660–661.

48. Weber DO, Mastro PD, Yarnoz MD. Chylothorax after myocardial revascularization with internal mammary artery graft. *Ann Thorac Surg.* 1981;32:499–502.

21

Aortic Insufficiency

Jacquelyn A. Quin and John A. Elefteriades

Historical Background

Descriptions of aortic valve function and aortic regurgitation date back as far as the ancient Greeks, who performed experiments on valvular competence using columns of water. Other early investigators in Vaslef and Roberts'[1] narrative on the history of aortic valvular function include Galen (AD 130–200) and Leonardo da Vinci (1452–1519), both of whom recognized that the aortic valve prevented flow reversal to the heart. One of the earliest descriptions of the insufficient aortic valve was given in 1706 by William Cowper, a London surgeon. He noted that the semilunar valves of the aorta were thickened, less pliable, and did not approximate well, thus causing blood to "recoil" back into the heart. In 1715 Raymond Vieussens, a Montpellier physician, described the pronounced apical impulse and bounding pulses he found in a 35-year-old man with aortic insufficiency. He predicted the patient's demise; when the patient died, Vieussens went on, at necropsy, to describe the calcified, retracted aortic valves he found.

One of the first successful operations for aortic insufficiency was performed in 1952 by Hufnagel, who implanted an artificial valve in the descending aorta (Figure 21.1).[2] In a subsequent series of 23 patients, reported in 1954, this operation was found successful in 17 patients. These patients postoperatively demonstrated improved exercise tolerance and decreased evidence of heart failure on chest roentgenogram. Six deaths occurred: five of cardiac causes and one from an acute exacerbation of rheumatic fever.[3] There were no reported complications of valve dysfunction or thrombosis. The Hufnagel valve was devised using a free-floating hollow methacrylate ball; after the first several patients, the ball was changed to a nylon core covered with a layer of silicone.[4] After the development of cardiopulmonary bypass, the first successful aortic valve replacement in the anatomical subcoronary position was performed by Harken in 1960.[5]

Other surgical procedures that attempted to ameliorate insufficiency included polliwog and Neuman valves, which were ball valves designed to fall back on and cover the central portion of the aortic valve during diastole (Figure 21.2). A constricting sash of nylon wound around the dilated aortic annulus to provide external support was also used. These procedures met with less success than valve replacement.[7] As such, much of the work in the early years of aortic valve replacement focused on development of an ideal valve prosthesis. The problems encountered included thrombosis, embolization, valve degeneration, and primary valve dysfunction.[8-10] Despite introduction of bioprosthetic valves and homografts and advancement in the design of mechanical valves, problems of graft durability and anticoagulation persist; the perfect valve remains an elusive goal. The pendulum has swung back again, and, once more, current surgical investigations for aortic insufficiency involve the development of methods to repair and preserve the native valve.

Etiology

The multiple causes of aortic insufficiency may be grouped into the broad categories of congenital, inflammatory, infectious, traumatic, and degenerative conditions.[11] In the past, rheumatic fever was responsible for most cases of insufficiency; however, in a recent Mayo Clinic study, the most common cause of isolated aortic insufficiency was dilation of the aortic root.[12] The time course is also important in determining the cause of insufficiency. Acute regurgitation is seen most often resulting from bacterial endocarditis, aortic dissection, and trauma.[13]

Isolated congenital aortic regurgitation is rare.[14] More often, coexisting pathology such as ventricular septal defect (VSD)[15-17] or Marfan's syndrome is found.[18,19] Of the congenital valvular anomalies causing aortic regurgi-

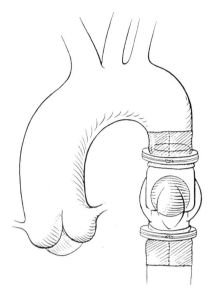

FIGURE 21.1. The Hufnagal ball valve, as shown in the descending aorta, was housed in a unit made of Plexiglas. The ball itself, made of silicone rubber surrounding a hollow nylon core, was of critical weight to respond to minimal changes in aortic pressure. (Reprinted with permission from Hufnagel et al.[6])

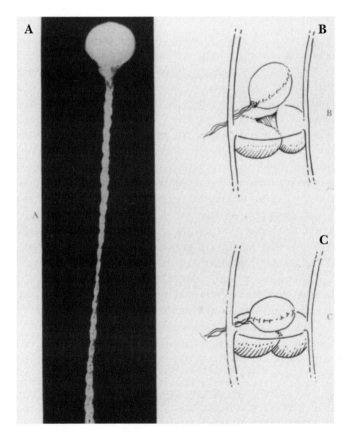

FIGURE 21.2. The polliwog valve was designed to cover the central portion of the aortic valve during diastole. (Reprinted with permission from Bailey and Likoff.[7])

tation, bicuspid valve, estimated to affect 1% to 2% of the general population, is the most common.[20,21] The bicuspid aortic valve becomes calcified and thickened secondary to abnormal hemodynamic stresses across the valve during diastole. Although the initial presentation may be aortic stenosis, insufficiency results over time as the valve leaflets shorten and contract and the edges become unable to coapt during diastole.

A characteristic morphology of the regurgitant bicuspid valve has been elucidated. Sadee et al.,[22] who studied 148 patients with regurgitant bicuspid valves, found that valve cusps were conjoined, with a distinct central indentation on the free edge of the cusp. These patients manifested a relative risk for regurgitation four times greater than patients with bicuspid valves without this indentation. Bicuspid valve is associated with other aortic pathology that may contribute or predispose patients to valvular incompetency, including coarctation,[23,24] aortic dissection,[25,26] and aortic root dilatation.[27,28] In addition, the abnormal bicuspid valve is susceptible to infectious endocarditis, with possible subsequent valve destruction. Aortic insufficiency from spontaneous rupture of a bicuspid aortic valve has also been described.[29]

Aortic root degeneration and dilatation that cause regurgitation are seen in patients with Marfan's syndrome, an autosomal dominant inherited connective tissue disorder related to the gene for fibrillin. In Marfan's syndrome and other connective tissue disorders of the media, the connective tissue of the aorta weakens, causing progressive dilation of the aortic root.[30] As the cross-sectional area of the aorta increases, each valve leaflet must cover a greater area and is required to withstand greater pressures during diastole. As the ability of the valve cusps to coapt progressively deteriorates, insufficiency results. This process may progress at a rapid rate without accompanying symptoms, and severe dilatation can be seen in patients as young as 20 years old.[31] *Annuloaortic ectasia* is the term used to describe the condition of adults with aortic root dilatation who lack the typical Marfanoid body habitus.[32] Although most have associated aortic insufficiency, of greater concern is the high incidence in these patients of accompanying aortic dissection. Despite surgery, the overall prognosis is worse in these patients than those presenting with isolated insufficiency.[33] Patients with the connective tissue disorder Ehlers–Danlos syndrome have also been reported to develop aortic insufficiency. The mechanism of degeneration is thought to involve abnormal collagen fibrils, which cause asymmetric dilation of the sinuses of Valsalva and predispose the aorta to regurgitation.[34]

Rheumatic fever is probably the most common of the inflammatory causes of insufficiency, which develops as a result of valvulitis. The first episode of such an inflammation may be fatal. Patients who survive several attacks develop severe scarring of the aortic valve and distortion of the aortic annulus. The mitral valve is almost invariably affected as well.[35] Insufficiency may result from juvenile rheumatoid arthritis by a mechanism similar to that of rheumatic fever in which progressive weakening and dilation of the aortic valves occur secondary to repeated valvulitis. Although aortic insufficiency is the most common valvular manifestation of this disease, it is nonetheless rare in comparison to rheumatoid pericarditis.[36,37] Other inflammatory and autoimmune diseases that rarely cause aortic insufficiency include Whipple's disease,[38] systemic lupus,[39,40] ankylosing spondylitis,[41,42] Reiter's syndrome,[43] Takayasu's disease,[44,45] Behçet's syndrome,[46,47] and idiopathic or giant cell aortitis.[48,49]

Insufficiency from endocarditis is usually bacterial in nature. The most common responsible organism is *Streptococcus viridans;* however, *Streptococcus fecalis, Staphylococcus* gram-negative bacteria, and fungi are increasing in frequency.[50] Aortic insufficiency complicating disseminated gonorrhea has been described and may be fatal.[51,52] Not surprisingly, preexisting conditions, including rheumatic heart disease, bicuspid valve, and calcific aortic disease, predispose patients to infection. Infectious endocarditis as a complication of hypertrophic cardiomyopathy requires valve replacement.[53] Syphilis, though often described, is now a rare cause of aortic insufficiency. Infiltration of the aortic root by the spirochete causes intense inflammation; perivascular infiltration of lymphocytes and obliteration of the vessels of the vasa vasorum are the earliest findings. Dilation of the aortic root and consequent distortion of the aortic valve occur. Widening of the valvular commissures is the most common finding and often occurs with the development of hyaline plaque. The free margin of the cusp thickens with eversion, rolling, and retraction.[54]

Aortic valvular injury and regurgitation from blunt trauma are uncommon. Injury and regurgitation are usually associated with rapid deceleration in high-speed motor vehicle accidents[55,56] and may occur despite the protective deployment of automobile airbags.[57] It is thought that blood within the ascending aorta continues to have forward inertia after blunt trauma and exerts pressure against the ascending aorta and valve that causes rupture. In this theory, rupture of the valve is more likely during diastole, when the left ventricular pressure is low and provides no counterpressure against the column of blood in the aortic root. During systole, counterpressure within the left ventricle may protect the valve. Although the diagnosis is usually immediately evident after severe blunt trauma, presentations after months[58] and even years[59] have been reported.

When occurring secondary to hypertension and fulminating ascending aortic dissection, valvular insufficiency is usually acute and may be fatal because of left ventricular failure. In the absence of dissection, the insufficiency associated with hypertension is usually mild; however, severe regurgitation that requires valve replacement has been described. The mechanism by which severe hypertension causes aortic insufficiency, however, is unclear.[60]

Other reports of aortic regurgitation are largely anecdotal and include its diagnosis in patients with Turner's syndrome,[61] Down syndrome,[62] polycystic kidney disease,[63] chronic renal insufficiency,[64] and mucopolysaccharide disease.[65] Aortic regurgitation has been described in isolated myxomatous degeneration without associated Marfan's syndrome.[66] Insufficiency as a complication of mediastinal radiation has been reported.[67] Spontaneous aortic valve rupture with no antecedent history of trauma or with hypertension has been described.[68,69] Although artherosclerosis has been suggested as an etiology of aortic insufficiency, evidence of its association is lacking.

Pathophysiology

In aortic insufficiency, the heart must not only accommodate an increased volume but also eject the volume into the high-pressure arterial circuit.[70] Thus, the heart must perform not only increased volume work but also increased pressure work. Aortic insufficiency is distinguished in this way from situations of left ventricular volume overload only, especially mitral regurgitation, in which this excess volume is directed to a low-pressure circuit. Over a prolonged period of aortic insufficiency, the ventricular wall dilates to accommodate the increased volume and hypertrophies to maintain ejection fraction against a normal or increased afterload. This proportionate increase in both thickness and chamber size is termed *eccentric hypertrophy* and is distinguished from settings in which the heart develops hypertrophy only. The latter, termed *concentric hypertrophy,* occurs when the heart compensates for increased pressure only. Concentric hypertrophy would occur with aortic stenosis, in which the left ventricular wall hypertrophies to maintain stroke volume against increased afterload without handling an actual increase in volume.

The volume of regurgitant flow is determined by three factors: the cross-sectional area of incompetence, the pressure gradient between the left ventricle and aorta during diastole, and the time interval of exposure for the pressure difference (i.e., the length of diastole). An increase in any of these three factors increases aortic insufficiency.[71] In severe cases, the regurgitated volume may be twice or three times the forward cardiac output. If the insufficiency progresses slowly, the heart is able to compensate and the patient may remain asymptomatic.[72,73] However, left ventricular systolic function eventually deteriorates and the patient develops symptoms of left ventricular failure and low cardiac output including pulmonary edema and fatigue. If not corrected, pulmonary hypertension and right ventricular failure ensue, with signs and symptoms of systemic congestion progressing to end-stage disease.

Experimental models have demonstrated that the left ventricular hypertrophy of aortic insufficiency results from increased myofibrillar protein synthesis. This increase is most marked in the initial week of regurgitation and gradually slows to reach a steady state after 2 to 3 months. Hypertrophy is maintained as a result of decreased protein degradation.[74] With myocyte hypertrophy in the initial stages of the disease, the heart is able to compensate for the regurgitant volume, placing increased preload pressure on the ventricle as in the well-known Frank–Starling relationship. Over time, however, myocyte hypertrophy can no longer compensate; the Frank–Starling curve is exceeded, and cardiac output begins to fall. Left ventricular end-diastolic pressure increases, and left ventricular compliance decreases. Myocardial oxygen consumption increases from myocardial hypertrophy and increased stroke volume; oxygen delivery, however, is decreased because of decreased diastolic pressure and worsening systolic function. The myocyte hypertrophy and increased interstitial fibrosis that occur with prolonged regurgitation may be irreversible if correction of the regurgitatant valve is delayed beyond the optimal time for repair.[75]

Acute regurgitation presents a much more abrupt picture, because excess volume is presented suddenly to an essentially normal heart that has not yet had time to hypertrophy and dilate. The heart is unable to accommodate the increase in volume, which results in a marked rise in end-diastolic pressure. In severe regurgitation, the increase in end-diastolic pressure may be as high as 50 to 60 mm Hg.[76] If left ventricular pressure exceeds left atrial pressure, premature closure of the mitral valve will result; the heart is then unable to maintain an effective forward stroke volume and cardiac output falls. Severe pulmonary congestion occurs. The decrease in cardiac output evokes sympathetic discharge, which increases myocardial contractility and systemic resistance. However, the increase in myocardial contractility is insufficient to accommodate the volume overload and increased systemic resistance, and acute left ventricular failure may occur.[77,78]

In both chronic and acute insufficiency, the natural history of the disease is one of death from ventricular failure. Saving the patient who presents with acute severe insufficiency requires prompt surgical attention; patients with mild to moderate degrees of acute insufficiency have a natural history that parallels that of chronic insufficiency, albeit with a shorter time course. Although death may be imminent without valve replacement or repair, sudden death due to arrhythmia is rare in patients with isolated aortic insufficiency.[79]

Clinical Features

Patients with acute insufficiency usually present with dramatic complaints of severe breathlessness. The history often reveals the cause for the sudden cardiac decompensation, such as aortic dissection or endocarditis. Patients with chronic insufficiency, however, may remain asymptomatic for decades. Angina due to inadequate diastolic pressure and diastolic coronary flow is uncommon in patients with isolated insufficiency. Its occurrence usually points to concomitant disease such as aortic stenosis or coronary atherosclerosis.[80] Patients who present with peripheral edema and signs of hepatic engorgement, including ascites, most often have right-sided ventricular failure as well.

Early asymptomatic regurgitation is suspected when an aortic diastolic murmur is detected on physical examination. The intensity and duration of the murmur on auscultation may correlate with the severity of the regurgitant flow[81]; however, the murmur itself is easily missed on examination. It is best heard along the left side of the sternum in the third to fourth interspace during expiration and may be accentuated by having the patient lean forward in an upright position. The Austin Flint murmur, an apical diastolic rumbling, was originally described in two patients with aortic regurgitation without associated mitral disease. The etiology of the murmur is controversial; however, recent color flow Doppler echocardiography studies relate the murmur to the regurgitant jet of aortic flow during diastole as it strikes the left ventricular endocardial wall.[82,83] A gallop is heard during cardiac examination of patients with acute insufficiency who lack the diastolic murmur characteristic of chronic insufficiency.[84]

The arterial pulse in aortic insufficiency is characterized by a strong, quick upstroke and an abnormally quick downstroke that is almost collapsing in nature. This water-hammer pulse is termed Corrigan's sign. Arterial pulsations are actually visible, and many signs have been characterized. Musset's sign, described by Delpeuch[85] and named after the French poet with syphilitic aortic disease, refers to the nodding of the head in synchrony with the heart beat. Quincke's pulses, as described by Heinrich Quincke, are visible blanchings in the fingernail beds that correspond to the marked diastolic drop in blood pressure. Pulsations of the uvula are termed Müller's sign. Duroziez's sign describes a to-and-fro double murmur heard over the femoral artery during compression; Traube's sign is a double sound heard over the femoral artery without compression. Normally, there is a slightly higher systolic pressure in the femoral artery than in the brachial artery; Hill's sign refers to an exaggeration of this difference that may be as high as 20 mm Hg in aortic regurgitation.

Progressive heart failure is reflected in the electrocardiogram and chest roentgenogram. The P wave on the electrocardiogram broadens and becomes diphasic, reflecting left atrial hypertrophy. The PR interval is prolonged in severe cases. Left axis deviation and left ventricular hypertrophy are seen. Subtle changes, including an altered QRS complex showing a delayed R peak occurring after the S peak instead of before, may occur early in the course of aortic regurgitation before symptoms develop.[86,87] The chest x-ray shows left atrial and ventricular enlargement. In cases of acute regurgitation, these findings are largely absent. The electrocardiogram is relatively normal acutely, although tachycardia may be an isolated finding. Similarly, on chest x-ray in patients with aortic insufficiency, the cardiac silhouette and aorta are often unremarkable; the only finding may be pulmonary edema.[88]

Because optimal timing of operative intervention is based not only on the presence of symptoms but also on the severity of left ventricular dysfunction, an accurate assessment of the degree of regurgitation is necessary. Although contrast angiography is traditionally used, several alternative diagnostic methods exist to qualitatively and quantitatively assess the severity of aortic insufficiency; most are based on Doppler echocardiography. Klein et al.[89] have reviewed various advances in quantifying aortic insufficiency through Doppler imaging, many of which are discussed below. Advantages of Doppler echocardiographic assessment over angiography include comparable quantitation of regurgitant flow[90] without an invasive procedure or need for ionizing radiation.[91] Although Doppler echocardiography may be overly sensitive in detecting (physiologic) regurgitation in the pulmonic, tricuspid, and mitral valves, it does not appear to have this characteristic in the aortic valve.[92]

Two-dimensional and M-mode echocardiography provide the most basic evaluation of aortic regurgitation; information about the severity of valvular regurgitation is obtained indirectly based on the degree of left ventricular chamber dilatation and dysfunction or on abnormalities of the aortic valve leaflets themselves. Both pulsed-wave and continuous wave Doppler echocardiography provide information on direction and velocity of blood flow; the estimation of regurgitation, however, is considered qualitative only.[93] Pulsed-wave Doppler mapping allows for more accurate assessment of regurgitant flow by measuring flow velocities within the left ventricle and along the left ventricular outflow tract. Although still not considered quantitative, a more accurate estimation of regurgitant flow is obtained based on the area of the left ventricle and the outflow tract occupied by the regurgitant flow (Figure 21.3). Minimal regurgitation involves only the area just below the aortic valve, whereas severe regurgitation involves the entire left ventricle. Involvement of less than 25% of the left ventricular outflow

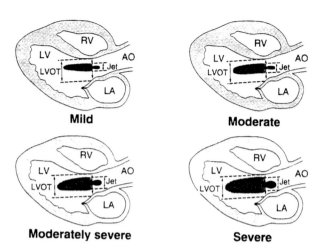

FIGURE 21.3. Aortic regurgitation (parasternal long-axis view) is graded by comparing the height of the regurgitant jet with the height of the left ventricular outflow tract (LVOT). Regurgitation is shown in mild, moderate, moderately severe, and severe degrees. AO, aorta; LA, left atrium; LV, left ventricle; RV, right ventricle. (Reprinted with permission from Klein et al.[89])

tract by the regurgitant jet distinguishes mild (angiographic grade 1+), from moderate (angiographic grade 2+) regurgitation; occupation of more than 40% of the left ventricular outflow tract by the regurgitant jet correlates with severe regurgitation (angiographic grades 3 to 4+).[94] Doppler color flow mapping provides additional information by sampling several points within the left ventricle and outflow tract simultaneously and assigning different rates of flow velocities different colors, which allows for faster and easier visualization of the regurgitant jet. As a method of determining flow, Doppler color flow mapping is still considered semiquantitative. The continuous-wave Doppler pressure half-time index calculates the degree of regurgitation based on the time needed for the pressure gradient between the aorta and the left ventricle during diastole to fall to 29% of the original difference. This interval is inversely proportional to the amount of regurgitation, albeit in a nonlinear fashion that limits exact quantitation.

To determine regurgitant fraction quantitatively, Doppler is used to calculate left ventricular stroke volume based on the flow velocity out of the left ventricular outflow tract. If the volume of flow into the left ventricle is calculated in a similar manner, then, based on the Fick principle, the volume of regurgitant flow is taken simply as the difference between these two volume measurements. This volume, divided by the left ventricular stroke volume, gives a fraction of regurgitation. Provided that no mitral regurgitation or flow abnormalities exist, Doppler-derived estimates of aortic regurgitation compare favorably with angiography estimates.

Transesophageal echocardiography is an alternative Doppler option for assessment of aortic regurgitation. Theoretical advantages over transthoracic echocardiography include better visualization of the heart by virtue of the close proximity and lack of interfering structures of the chest, especially in patients with poor acoustic windows secondary to underlying pulmonary disease or chest wall deformity. It also provides a higher-quality image than the transthoracic approach in aortic insufficiency with associated disease states such as VSD[95] or Marfan's syndrome,[96] and in regurgitation secondary to trauma or endocarditis.[97] It is most useful in cases in which transthoracic imaging is suboptimal.[98] Although it has been suggested that transesophageal echocardiography may be useful in assessing regurgitation based on the depth of penetration of the regurgitant jet into the left ventricle, our study with Rafferty of 30 patients[99] as well as other studies[100] have not supported this claim. We did demonstrate, however, that transesophageal echocardiography for assessment of aortic insufficiency was feasible and correlated with angiography satisfactorily when the regurgitant jet proximal width and area ratios were used.

Magnetic resonance imaging (MRI), a relatively new modality for assessing regurgitation, provides a noninvasive means to diagnose aortic regurgitation; its use is not limited in patients with poor acoustic windows. MRI is able to image the heart in several planes, thus deriving a three-dimensional image, with excellent resolution between moving blood and myocardium. Disadvantages of MRI include the cost and time-consuming nature of the examination.[101] MRI may be used in several ways to evaluate regurgitation. Cine MRI provides a semiquantitative assessment of regurgitation based on the direction and area of the regurgitant jet. This method of determination is similar to the method used in pulsed-wave Doppler or color Doppler mapping and yields similar results.[102] MRI may also be used to calculate left and right ventricular stroke volumes; as in Doppler echocardiography, the regurgitant fraction is based on the difference between the two volumes using the Fick principle. Using this method, Globits demonstrated excellent correlation between MRI and angiography in his study of 30 patients with aortic insufficiency. MRI velocity mapping senses motion through an imaging plane, through which a velocity profile is obtained. Because the MRI is able to measure the cross-sectional area of interest in the imaging plane, flow rates can be calculated. Using this method in a limited number of patients with aortic insufficiency, Søndergaard et al. demonstrated good agreement between MRI mapping and subsequent angiography.[103] Ambrosi et al. described a method of assessing the presence of aortic regurgitation based on diastolic retrograde blood flow of a saturation band positioned across the thoracic aorta. This method requires an imaging time of less than 20 minutes and provides qualitative assessment of regurgitation.[104]

Medical Management

Patients who do not have an indication for surgery should be closely followed and managed medically. With administration of oral arterial vasodilators, left ventricular end-diastolic volume is decreased, with a subsequent improvement in the ejection fraction.[105] Previously, long-term management included administration of hydralazine; however, severe side effects limit its use.[106] Currently, most patients are treated with nifedipine. Because of potent arterial vasodilatation, stroke volume is increased and the regurgitatant fraction is reduced, despite the negative inotropic effect of nifedipine; however, these effects cannot be extrapolated to include other calcium channel blockers or vasodilators.[107,108] Scognamiglio et al.[109] have shown that use of nifedipine can alleviate symptoms of heart failure while protecting left ventricular function and prolonging the time before surgery without adversely affecting the chance for ventricular recovery after correction.

Timing of Operation

The management of severe aortic insufficiency is operative. In the acute setting, surgical intervention may be urgent, because the left ventricle has no compensatory mechanism for the increase in end-diastolic volume. Medical management in preparation for surgery is directed toward reduction of systemic vascular resistance and is usually accomplished with vasodilators such as nitroprusside. Operative risk for these patients is higher than for those with chronic regurgitation; the inciting pathology, such as traumatic dissection or infective endocarditis, poses additional considerations over the patient who presents with isolated chronic regurgitation. In infectious endocarditis, the surgeon must weigh the risks of prosthetic infection against worsening, intractable failure, which usually results in death.

The timing of surgical intervention in chronic aortic insufficiency is controversial. Patients who are symptomatic, despite normal left ventricular function, should undergo repair. Because the development of symptoms is an unreliable indicator of worsening left ventricular function, asymptomatic patients must be followed closely. Repair must be carried out before such dysfunction becomes irreversible. However, because valve replacement is not without risk, surgical correction for the asymptomatic patient must be timed to balance the risks of surgery and possible need for lifetime anticoagulation therapy against the risk of irreversible left ventricular

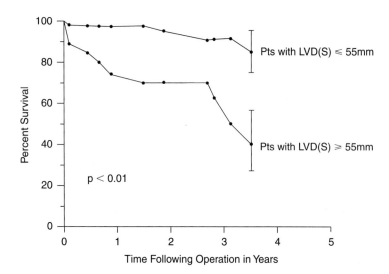

FIGURE 21.4. The influence of preoperative left ventricular end-systolic dimension, LVD(S), on postoperative survival at 3 years. (Reprinted with permission from Bonow et al.[110])

dysfunction. Of the parameters indicating irreversible left ventricular failure, an end-systolic dimension of 55 mm is often used. Patients with end-systolic dimensions of >55 mm showed only a 40% postoperative survival rate at 3-year follow-up; patients with end-diastolic dimensions <55 mm showed a >90% survival rate (Figure 21.4).[110] Patients with extreme left ventricular dilatation (diastolic dimension >80 mm, systolic dimension >55 mm) are at risk for sudden death. These patients, as well as those with any degree of left ventricular contractile dysfunction at rest, should undergo valve replacement surgery.[111] Long-term follow-up of asymptomatic patients reveals an annual mortality rate of less than 5%, with less than 4% per year requiring aortic valve replacement for either development of symptoms or onset of left ventricular dysfunction or dilatation.

Ejection fraction is also used to identify patients needing surgery. Postoperative recovery of left ventricular systolic function generally occurs in patients with an

ejection fraction greater than 40% to 60% but may not be realized in patients with a depressed ejection fraction below 30%. Therefore, repair is recommended when the resting ejection fraction falls below 50% (Figure 21.5).[112,113] Other parameters proposed for operative repair include wall stress of greater than 600 mm Hg[114] and a shortening fraction of less than 30% as visualized with echocardiography.[115] Aortic distensibility, which reflects the change in aortic diameter between systole and diastole, has also been used to predict worsening left ventricular function and the need for valve replacement. Older patients manifested less aortic distensibility, which correlated with the need for subsequent valve replacement.[116]

Technique of Operation

The standard median sternotomy provides excellent exposure for aortic valve replacement. Alternate smaller incisions are currently being explored in this era of "mini" surgery. Venous cannulation may be carried out using two venous cannulae or a single large two-stage venous cannula. If mitral replacement is also considered, a two-cannulae technique is preferred. Aortic cannulation is standard. In patients with aortic insufficiency, it may be necessary to immediately cross-clamp the aorta to prevent acute ventricular fibrillation and left ventricular distention from the sudden infusion of cold priming solution from the pump. Although the operation may be performed without a vent, exposure is facilitated by placing a vent across the left atrium into the ventricle. Antegrade or antegrade–retrograde cardioplegia is given with the initial aortotomy (directly intracoronary in the case of severe insufficiency) and approximately every 30 minutes thereafter. The patient is systemically cooled to 25 to 28°C and topical hypothermia is applied to the heart.

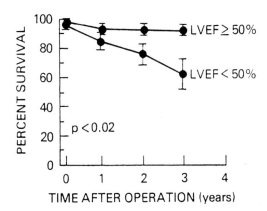

FIGURE 21.5. The influence of preoperative left ventricular ejection fraction (LVEF) on postoperative survival in patients undergoing surgery for aortic regurgitation. (Reprinted with permission from Forman et al.[117])

Precise placement of the aortotomy is crucial and depends on the type of valvular repair.[118] The incision should provide optimal surgical exposure and account for the possible need for aortic root enlargement, type of graft placement (allograft, pulmonary autograft, or prosthesis), and security of closure. The surgeon must be cognizant of the right coronary artery to avoid inadvertent injury to the artery itself or its osteum. The aortotomy is made relatively high on the anterior ascending aorta (1 to 2 cm above the right coronary osteum)[119] in an area free of calcification where the slight increase in wall thickness may allow for better hemostasis and control of the incision at closure. The valve is then inspected and a decision made about the optimal type of valve replacement.

Unless the valve is noncalcified, a moist gauze should be placed within the left ventricle to ensure that no loose fragments of calcium (which may cause complications from embolization) are left behind during valve excision. The tip of the suction catheter is removed to facilitate immediate retrieval of any such calcium fragments. As much of the valve should be removed as possible with the initial incision. However, care must be taken to avoid damaging the ventricular septum, aortic wall, or conduction system. The heavily calcified valve may distort the annulus, and caution must be exercised to avoid damaging the anterior leaflet of the mitral valve when removing the aortic valve noncoronary leaflet. After valve removal, additional cannular débridement is performed with either a small rongeur or a no. 15 blade. The left ventricular gauze packing is removed, and the area is examined for any remaining calcium fragments.

In sizing the valve, the aortic obturator should just engage the annulus without slipping into the ventricle. The type of suture employed in replacement varies according to the surgeon; we have used Teflon-backed mattress sutures of no. 2-O Tycron with success and a perivalvular leak rate of <1%. Three sutures may be placed initially at the commissures to serve as traction for the remaining sutures. The sutures are placed at the juncture of the remaining valve leaflet and the aortic wall. During valve placement, the commissure of the noncoronary and right coronary leaflets is identified. The membranous septum just deep to this area carries the bundle of His; injudicious placement of suture(s) in this area may result in heart block. After carefully seating the valve, sutures are tied in the order of placement, with five to six knots per suture. The aorta is sutured in two layers: first with running horizontal mattress sutures followed by simple running sutures. The patient is placed into a deep Trendelenberg position while the aorta is unclamped to allow for the evacuation of air, which is carried out by venting the anterior ascending aorta and the apex of the left ventricle with a needle. The left ventricle vent is turned off and the patient given a few breaths to expel any air that may have entered into the pulmonary veins.

The choice of graft for replacement, whether pulmonary autograft, cryopreserved allograft (isolated or as a cylinder), or mechanical or bioprosthetic valve, depends on the clinical situation. Although review of the optimal replacement valve is beyond the scope of this chapter, there are general considerations to follow. Placement of an allograft gives very good results and is the valve of choice in replacement for endocarditis or in young female patients for whom pregnancy is a consideration. Allografts should not be used in patients with dilated aortic root (diameter >30 mm at the level of the leaflet commissures). Use of bioprosthetic valves is appropriate in elderly patients because lifelong anticoagulation therapy can be avoided and the valves have satisfactory longevity in this age group. Bioprosthetic valves are not appropriate for young patients (under 45 years of age) or those with aortic roots less than 21 mm in diameter unless aortic root enlargement is undertaken concurrently. They are not used in patients with renal failure and high calcium turnover. A mechanical or bioprosthetic graft is acceptable in an enlarged and thin ascending aorta. Mechanical valves perform well even in patients with small aortic annuli; placement in such patients may sometimes be facilitated by tilting the prosthesis approximately 15 to 20 degrees. Otherwise, the annulus should be enlarged either posteriorly[120,121] or anteriorly.[122] Mechanical prosthetic valves are not generally used in patients who cannot undergo lifelong anticoagulation therapy, including those with potential sources of bleeding (e.g., peptic ulcer disease or colitis) or the potentially gravid patient.

In the patient with an associated ascending aortic aneurysm or annuloaortic ectasia, the aortic valve and ascending aorta are replaced. This procedure is also considered in patients with aortic insufficiency and chronic dissection in which the distal anastamosis may be technically difficult. David and Feindel[123] reported on a number of patients who have undergone aortic valve–sparing replacement of the aortic root for insufficiency with associated annuloaortic ectasia. The aneurysmal portion of the ascending aorta and sinuses of Valsalva are excised, leaving behind the aortic valve itself with part of the aortic wall. The valve is resuspended within a collagen-impregnated Dacron graft with reimplantation of the coronary arteries. This procedure is currently under clinical investigation.[124]

The young patient with aortic insufficiency remains a management challenge for lack of an ideal replacement valve. Although patients with bioprosthetic valves need not undertake lifelong anticoagulation therapy, the longevity of the prosthetic is inadequate for the patient's anticipated life expectancy. An alternative option is the aortic allograft, which offers long-term durability and avoids the need for anticoagulation therapy.[125] The allograft procedure is reported to have a higher rate of freedom from complication after 10 years than the porcine bioprosthetic valve (92% versus 75%).[126] Aortic valve repair is being performed on an experimental basis. Kumar and colleagues[127] reported on 149 consecutive patients, aged 35 years and younger, with aortic regurgitation. Of these, 88 underwent repair; 2 died postoperatively, and 12 required reoperation for aortic (8) or mitral (4) valve dysfunction.[127] Cosgrove et al.[128] reported on an initial series of 28 consecutive patients (age 46.8 ± 14.4 years) who underwent aortic valvuloplasty for insufficiency from leaflet prolapse. Their technique involved plication of the annulus at the commissures (Figure 21.6) and triangular resection of the free edge of the prolapsing cusp (Figure 21.7). The severity of aortic insufficiency, graded from 0 to 4 by color flow Doppler echocardiography, improved significantly from 3.4 ± 0.7 preoperatively to 0.6 ± 0.5 intraoperatively, immediately after repair. In patients with insufficient bicuspid valves, the repair includes resection of the raphe, when present (Figure 21.8). A series of 72 consecutive patients with insufficient bicuspid valves (mean age 39 ± 11 years) underwent such repair; late postoperative echocardiograms, available for 58 patients (mean 16 ± 13 months), revealed an improvement in mean aortic insufficiency from 3.6 ± 0.6 preoperatively to 0.9 ± 0.8 postoperatively.[129]

Aortic valvuloplasty is performed in young patients with insufficiency and an associated VSD. In Trusler's[130] series of 70 patients aged 36 years or younger (mean age 10 years) undergoing such repair, survival and freedom from operation at 10 years were 96% and 85%, respectively. Valvuloplasty success at 10 years was 76%. Hisatomi et al.[131] reported a success rate of 79.6% at 10 years for 11 patients (mean age 7.2 years). None of the patients required reoperation. Correction of insufficiency may also be undertaken using a pulmonary autograft (Ross proce-

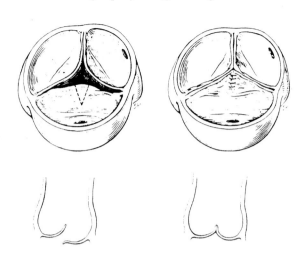

FIGURE 21.7. Triangular resection of the free edge of the prolapsed cusp is performed to restore leaflet size and coaptation. (Reprinted with permission from Cosgrove et al.[128])

dure).[132] The autologous pulmonary valve is implanted as an aortic root replacement with coronary reimplantation. Advantages of the pulmonary autograft include the potential for growth, long-term durability, and freedom from anticoagulation therapy.[133] Al-Halees et al.[134] reported on its use in 78 patients (mean age 18.6 ± 7.4 years); 60 of these patients had aortic insufficiency as the primary diagnosis. Two late deaths occurred from noncardiac causes. Four patients required reoperation for autograft failure. Postoperative progressive aortic regurgitation from recurrent rheumatic activity was seen in 12 patients at follow-up of 2 months or greater and required reoperation in 4 patients.

As emphasized earlier, surgical outcome is favorably influenced if aortic valve replacement or correction is

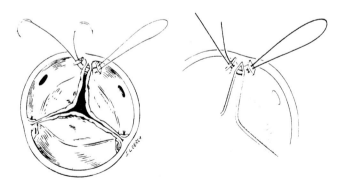

FIGURE 21.6. Horizontal mattress sutures buttressed with Teflon are placed at the commissures in the aortic valvuloplasty for insufficiency. Contact with the leaflet is avoided. (Reprinted with permission from Cosgrove et al.[128])

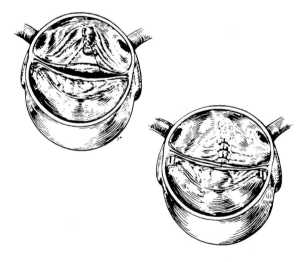

FIGURE 21.8. Repair of bicuspid valve included resection of raphe if present, annuloplasty, and resection of the prolapsing leaflet. (Reprinted with permission from Cosgrove et al.[128])

carried out before the onset of irreversible left ventricular failure. Reversal of left ventricular dilation and improvement in left ventricular systolic performance is usually seen within 6 to 8 months of surgery and is reflected by decreased left ventricular end-diastolic dimension and an improvement in the ejection fraction (Figure 21.9). If an initial increase in the ejection fraction is seen during this early postoperative period, additional long-term improvement may also be anticipated; however, if the ejection fraction fails to increase during this period, subsequent improvement is unlikely.[135] The ratio of left ventricular peak systolic pressure to end-systolic volume has been used for predicting postoperative function. Patients with a ratio of >1.72 preoperatively had improved postoperative recovery compared with those who had a ratio of <1.72.[136] A left ventricular contractility score has

been devised by DiBasi et al.[137] to predict postoperative outcome based on wall kinesis of the left ventricle in 20 subsegments. Patients with a higher score (indicative of worse preoperative contractility) had worse postoperative function and survival rates.[137]

An early improvement in the ejection fraction may increase survival rates. In a Mayo Clinic study of 1012 consecutive patients undergoing aortic valve replacement, 167 patients had a preoperative ejection fraction of less than 45%. Of these 167 patients, the 5-year survival rate was significantly greater in patients who had an initial postoperative increase in ejection fraction of 0.10 or greater.[139]

Although older patients have a relatively higher risk, surgery can be carried out safely. Likewise, although surgery is undertaken with higher risk in patients with severe left ventricular dysfunction, it is nonetheless recommended because the natural history of untreated aortic insufficiency is one of progressively worsening heart failure. Surgery to correct aortic insufficiency is indicated despite advanced left ventricular failure. Valve replacement offers improved cardiac function in some of these patients. In our investigation of 20 consecutive patients with an ejection fraction of ≤35% who underwent aortic valve replacement for insufficiency, a significant increase in ejection fraction was seen postoperatively from 29% to 45% (Figure 21.10). At 1-, 3-, and 4-year follow-up examinations, survival rates were 95%, 87%, and 80%, respectively (unpublished data). At the lowest

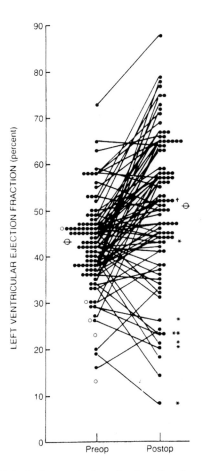

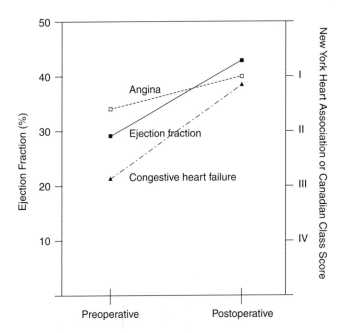

FIGURE 21.9. Left ventricular ejection fraction at rest by radionuclide angiography before and after aortic valve replacement in 93 consecutive patients with chronic aortic insufficiency. An increase in the ejection fraction was seen in the majority of patients postoperatively. Open circles indicate patients who died before 6 months' follow-up; asterisks indicate patients who died of congestive heart failure. One patient (†) died suddenly after the 6-month study. (Reprinted with permission from Bonow.[138] © 1991, American Heart Association.)

FIGURE 21.10. An improvement is seen in the mean ejection fraction of 20 patients with severely depressed ejection fraction (<35%) after valve replacement. Of note, improvement in symptoms of congestive heart failure and angina are also seen. (From JA Elefteriades, unpublished data.)

range of ejection fraction, the question arises as to whether cardiac transplantation should supersede valve replacement. We have recommended that, in general, valve replacement be attempted first. Patients who fail to improve are still candidates for cardiac transplantation provided other selection criteria are met.[139]

References

1. Vaslef S, Roberts WC. Early descriptions of aortic regurgitation. *Am Heart J.* 1993;125:1475–1483.

2. Hufnagel CA, Harvey WP. The surgical correction of aortic regurgitation: preliminary report. *Bull Georgetown Univ Med Center.* 1953;6:60–61.

3. Hufnagel CA, Harvey WP, Rabil PJ, McDermott TF. Surgical correction of aortic insufficiency. *Surgery.* 1954;35:673–683.

4. Hufnagel CA. In the beginning. *Ann Thorac Surg.* 1989;47:475–476.

5. Harken DE, Soroff HS, Taylor JW, et al. Partial and complete prosthesis in aortic insufficiency. *J Thorac Cardiovasc Surg.* 1960;40:744–762.

6. Hufnagel CA, Villegas PD, Nahas H. Experiences with new types of aortic valvular prostheses. *Surgery.* 1958;147:636–645.

7. Bailey CP, Likoff W. The surgical treatment of aortic insufficiency. *Ann Intern Med.* 1955;42:388–406.

8. Kay EB, Suzuki A. Evolution of aortic valvular prostheses. *J Thorac Cardiovasc Surg.* 1963;45:372–381.

9. Kay EB. Early years in artificial valve development. *Ann Thorac Surg.* 1989;48:S24–S25.

10. Harken DE, Taylor WJ, Lefemine AA. Aortic valve replacement with a caged ball valve. *Am J Cardiol.* 1962;9:292–299.

11. Benotti JR, Dalen JE. Aortic valvular regurgitation: natural history and medical treatment in aortic regurgitation. In: Cohn LH, DiSesa VJ, eds. *Aortic Regurgitation: Medical and Surgical Management.* New York, NY: Marcel Dekker; 1986:1–53.

12. Dare AJ, Veinot JP, Edwards WD, Tazelaar HD, Schaff HV. New observations on the etiology of aortic valve disease: a surgical pathologic study of 236 cases from 1990. *Human Pathol.* 1993;24:1330–1338.

13. Morganroth J, Perloff JK, Zeldis SM, Dunkman WB. Acute severe aortic regurgitation: pathophysiology, clinical recognition, and management. *Ann Intern Med.* 1977;87:223–232.

14. Donofrio MT, Allen Engle M, O'Loughlin JE. Congenital aortic regurgitation: natural history and management. *J Am Coll Cardiol.* 1992;20:366–372.

15. Halloran KH, Talmer NS, Browne MJ. A study of ventricular septal defect associated with aortic insufficiency. *Am Heart J.* 1965;69:320–326.

16. Dimich I, Steinfeld L, Litwak RS, et al. Subpulmonic ventricular septal defect associated with aortic insufficiency. *Am J Cardiol.* 1973;32:325–328.

17. Ishikawa S, Morishita Y, Sato Y, et al. Frequency and operative correction of aortic insufficiency associated with ventricular septal defect. *Ann Thorac Surg.* 1994;57:996–998.

18. McKusick V. The cardiovascular aspects of Marfan's syndrome: a heritable disorder of connective tissue. *Circulation.* 1955;11:321–342.

19. Goyette EM, Palmer DW. Cardiovascular lesions in arachnodactyly. *Circulation.* 1953;7:373–379.

20. Edwards WD. Surgical pathology of the aortic valve. In: Waller BF, ed. *Pathology of the Heart and Great Vessels.* New York, NY: Churchill Livingstone; 1980:43–100.

21. Roberts WC. Congenitally bicuspid aortic valve: a study of 85 autopsy cases. *Am J Cardiol.* 1970;26:72–83.

22. Sadee AS, Becker AE, Verhuel HA, et al. Aortic regurgitation and the congenitally bicuspid aortic valve: a clinicopathological correlation. *Br Heart J.* 1992;67:439–441.

23. Fenoglio JJ, McAllister HA, Decastro CM, et al. Congenital bicuspid aortic valve after age 20. *Am J Cardiol.* 1977;39:164–169.

24. Becker AE, Becker MJ, Edwards JE. Anomalies associated with coarctation of the aorta. *Circulation.* 1970;41:1067–1076.

25. Edwards WD, Leaf DS, Edwards JE. Dissecting aortic aneurysm associated with congenital bicuspid aortic valve. *Circulation.* 1978;57:1022–1025.

26. Gore I. Dissecting aneurysm of the aorta in persons under forty years of age. *Arch Pathol.* 1953;55:1–13.

27. Olson LJ, Subramanian R, Edwards WD. Surgical pathology of pure aortic insufficiency: a study of 225 cases. *Mayo Clin Proc.* 1984;59:835–841.

28. Guiney TE, Davies MJ, Parker DJ, et al. The aetiology and course of isolated severe aortic regurgitation: a clinical, pathological, and echocardiographic study. *Br Heart J.* 1987;58:358–368.

29. Becker AE, Dureu DR. Spontaneous rupture of bicuspid aortic valve: an unusual cause of aortic insufficiency. *Chest.* 1977;72:361–362.

30. Roberts WC, Honig HS. The spectrum of cardiovascular disease in the Marfan syndrome: a clinicopathologic study of 18 necropsy patients and comparison to 151 previously reported patients. *Am Heart J.* 1982;104:115–135.

31. Hwa J, Richards JG, Huang H, et al. The natural history of aortic dilatation in Marfan syndrome. *Med J Aust.* 1993;158:558–562.

32. Ellis PR, Cooley DA, DeBakey ME. Clinical consideration and surgical treatment of annulo-aortic ectasia. *J Thorac Cardiovasc Surg.* 1961;42:363–370.

33. Lemon DK, White CV. Annuloaortic ectasia: angiographic hemodynamic and clinical comparison with aortic valve insufficiency. *Am J Cardiol.* 1978;41:482–486.

34. Takahashi T, Kiode T, Yamaguchi H. Ehler-Danlos syndrome with aortic regurgitation, dilation of the sinuses of Valsalva, and abnormal dermal collagen fibrils. *Am Heart J.* 1992;123:1709–1712.

35. Gross L, Silverman G. The aortic commissural lesion in rheumatic fever. *Am J Pathol.* 1937;13:389–404.

36. Özer S, Alehan D, Özme S, et al. Mitral and aortic insufficiency in polyarticular juvenile rheumatoid arthritis. *Pediatr Cardiol.* 1994;15:151–153.

37. Leak AM, Millar-Craig MW, Ansell BA. Aortic regurgitation in seropositive juvenile arthritis. *Ann Rheum Dis.* 1981;40:229–234.

38. Wright CB, Hiratzka LF, Crosslands S, et al. Aortic insufficiency requiring valve replacement in Whipple's disease. *Ann Thorac Surg.* 1978;25:466–469.

39. Demircin M, Dogan R, Peker O, et al. Aortic insufficiency and enterococcal endocarditis complicating systemic lupus erythematosus. *Thorac Cardiovasc Surg.* 1955;43:302–304.

40. Olearchyk AS. Aortic regurgitation in systemic lupus erythematosus. *J Thorac Cardiol Surg.* 1992;103:1026.

41. Simpson J, Borzy MS, Silberbach GM. Aortic regurgitation at diagnosis of HLA-B27 associated spondyloarthropathy. *J Rheumatol.* 1995;22:332–334.

42. O'Neill TW, Bresnihan B. The heart in ankylosing spondylitis. *Ann Rheum Dis.* 1992;51:705–706.

43. Misukiewicz P, Carlson RW, Rowan L. Acute aortic insufficiency in a patient with presumed Reiter's syndrome. *Ann Rheum Dis.* 1992;51:686–687.

44. Trazzera S, Colasacco J, Ong L. Takayasu's arteritis with unstable angina and aortic insufficiency. *Am Heart J.* 1995;130:1122–1124.

45. Satoh T, Chino M, Takahashi M, Suzuki K. Aortitis syndrome with fatal acute aortic regurgitation due to aortic dilatation and aortic valve perforation: a case report. *Angiology.* 1992;42:869–872.

46. Huong DL, Wechsler B, Piette J, et al. Aortic insufficiency and recurrent valve prosthesis dehiscence in MAGIC syndrome. *J Rheumatol.* 1993;20:397–398.

47. González T, Hernádez-Beriain JA, Rodríguez-Lozano B, Martín-Herrera A. Severe aortic regurgitation in Behçet's disease. *J Rheumatol.* 1993;20:1807–1808.

48. Honig HS, Weintraub AM, Gomes MN, et al. Severe aortic regurgitation secondary to idiopathic aortitis. *Am J Med.* 1977;63:623–633.

49. Sooral AS, McKeowen F, Cleland J. Aortic valve replacement for severe aortic regurgitation caused by idiopathic giant cell aortitis. *Thorax.* 1980;35:60–63.

50. Hall RJC, Julian DG. Infective endocarditis. In:, *Diseases of the Cardiac Valves.* New York, NY: Churchill Livingstone; 1989:321–338.

51. Willerson JT, Buja LM. A 17 year old woman with a history of sexually transmitted disease and productive cough who developed cardiogenic shock. *Circulation.* 1993;88(pt 1):1945–1951.

52. Lim YT, Lim MC, Choo MH, et al. Severe aortic regurgitation due to Neisseria mucosal endocarditis. *Singapore Med J.* 1994;35:650–652.

53. Roberts WC, Kishel JC, McIntosh CL, et al. Severe mitral or aortic valve regurgitation, or both, requiring valve replacement of infective endocarditis complicating hypertrophic cardiomyopathy. *J Am Coll Cardiol.* 1992;19:365–371.

54. Saphir O, Scott RW. Observations on the 107 cases of syphilitic aortic insufficiency with special reference to the aortic valve area, the myocardium, and branches of the aorta. *Am Heart J.* 1930;6:56–58.

55. Prêtre R, Faidutti B. Surgical management of aortic valve injury after nonpenetrating trauma. *Ann Thorac Surg.* 1993;56:1426–1431.

56. Paone RT, Kidd JN, Dobrin DJ, DiDonna GJ. Traumatic aortic incompetence associated with transection of the thoracic aorta. *Chest.* 1996;109:1118–1119.

57. Reiland-Smith J, Weintraub RM, Selke FW. Traumatic aortic valve injury sustained despite the deployment of an automobile air bag. *Chest.* 1993;103:1603.

58. Miralles A, Farinola T, Quiroga J, et al. Valvuloplasty in traumatic aortic insufficiency due to subtotal tear of the intima. *Ann Thorac Surg.* 1995;60:1098–1100.

59. Murray EG, Minami K, Körtke H, et al. Traumatic sinus of Valsalva fistula and aortic valve rupture. *Ann Thorac Surg.* 1993;55:760–761.

60. Waller BF, Zoltick JM, Rosen JH. Severe aortic regurgitation from systemic hypertension (without aortic dissection) requiring aortic valve replacement. *Am J Cardiol.* 1982;49:473–477.

61. Oohara K, Yamazaki T, Sakaguchi K, Nakayama M, Kobayashi A. Acute aortic dissection, aortic insufficiency, and a single coronary artery in a patient with Turner's syndrome. *J Card Surg.* 1995;36:273–275.

62. Weinhouse E, Riggs TW, Aughton DJ. Isolated bicuspid aortic valve in a newborn with Down syndrome. *Clin Pediatr.* 1995;34:116–117.

63. Mavromatidis K, Sombolos K, Zoumbaridis N, Natse T, Panidou-Kiriakidou I, Hagekostas G. Retinitis pigmentosa and aortic regurgitation in a patient with adult polycystic kidney disease. *Nephron.* 1992;60:114–115.

64. Storstein O, Örjavik O. Aortic insufficiency in chronic renal failure. *Acta Med Scand.* 1978;203:175–180.

65. Wippermann CF, Beck M, Schranz D, et al. Mitral and aortic regurgitation in 84 patients with mucopolysaccharidoses. *Eur J Pediatr.* 1995;154:98–101.

66. Olinger GN, Korns ME, Bonchek LI. Acute aortic valvular insufficiency due to isolated myxomatous degeneration. *Ann Intern Med.* 1978;88:807–808.

67. Chenu PC, Schroeder E, Buche M, Marchandise B. Bilateral coronary ostial stenosis and aortic valvular disease after radiotherapy. *Eur Heart J.* 1994;151:150–151.

68. Aoyagi S, Fukunga S, Oishi K. Aortic regurgitation due to non-traumatic rupture of the aortic valve commissures: report of two cases. *J Heart Valve Dis.* 1995;4:99–102.

69. Sainani GS, Szatkowski J. Rupture of normal aortic valve after physical strain. *Br Heart J.* 1969;31:653–655.

70. Carabello B. The changing unnatural history of valvular regurgitation. *Ann Thorac Surg.* 1992;53:191–199.

71. Alpert JS. Chronic aortic regurgitation. In: Dalen JE, Alpert JS, eds. *Valvular Heart Disease.* Boston, Mass: Little, Brown; 1987:283–317.

72. Spagnulo M, Koth H, Taranta A, et al. Natural history of rheumatic aortic regurgitation: criteria predictive of death, congestive heart failure, and angina in young patients. *Circulation.* 1978;44:368–380.

73. Goldschlager N, Pfeifer J, Cohn K, et al. The natural history of aortic regurgitation: a clinical and hemodynamic study. *Am J Med.* 1973;54:577–588.

74. Magid NM, Wallerson DC, Borer JS. Myofibrillar protein turnover in cardiac hypertrophy due to aortic regurgitation. *Cardiology.* 1993;82:20–29.

75. Donaldson RM, Floria R, Frickards A, et al. Irreversible

morphological changes contributing to depressed cardiac function after surgery for chronic aortic regurgitation. *Br Heart J.* 1982;118:589–597.

76. Wigle ED, Labrosse CJ. Sudden severe aortic insufficiency. *Circulation.* 1965;32:708–720.

77. Morganroth J, Perloff JK, Zeldis SM, et al. Acute severe aortic regurgitation. *Ann Intern Med.* 1977;87:223–232.

78. Cipriano PR, Griepp RB. Acute retrograde dissection of the ascending thoracic aorta. *Am J Cardiol.* 1978;43:520–528.

79. Von Olshausen K. Arrhythmias in aortic regurgitation: incidence, consequences, and treatment. *Acta Cardiologica.* 1992;47:141–143.

80. Hall RJC, Julian DG. Aortic regurgitation. In: *Diseases of the Cardiac Valves.* New York, NY: Churchill Livingstone; 1989:120–141.

81. Desjardins VA, Enriquez-Sareno M, Tajik J, et al. Intensity of murmurs correlates with severity of valvular regurgitation. *Am J Med.* 1995;100:149–156.

82. Landzberg JS, Pflugfelder PW, Cassidy MM. Etiology of the Austin Flint murmur. *J Am Coll Cardiol.* 1992;20:408–413.

83. Emi S, Nobuo F, Takashi O, et al. Genesis of the Austin Flint murmur: relation to mitral inflow and aortic regurgitant flow dynamics. *J Am Coll Cardiol.* 1993;21:1399–1405.

84. Folland ED, Kriegel BJ, Henderson WG. Implications of third heart sound in patients with valvular heart disease. *N Engl J Med.* 1992;327:458–462.

85. Delpeuch A. Le signe de musset: secousses rhythmées de la tete chez les aortiques. *Presse Méd.* 199;8:237–238.

86. Cantor AA, Gilutz H, Barlow JB. Value of the electrocardiogram in detecting left ventricular dysfunction in asymptomatic patients with aortic regurgitation. *Am J Cardiol.* 1994;74:72–74.

87. Recke SH, Marienhagen J, Feistel H. Electrocardiographic characteristics indicating a risk of irreversibly impaired myocardial function in chronic aortic regurgitation. *Int J Cardiol.* 1993;42:129–138.

88. Rahimtoola SH. Recognition and management of acute aortic regurgitation. *Heart Dis Stoke.* 1993;2:217–221.

89. Klein AL, Davison MB, Vonk G, Tajil AJ. Doppler echocardiographic assessment of aortic regurgitation: uses and limitations. *Cleveland Clinic J Med.* 1992;59:359–368.

90. Wilkenshoff UM, Druck K, Gast D, Schröder R. Validity of continuous wave Doppler and colour Doppler in the assessment of aortic regurgitation. *Eur Heart J.* 1994;15:1227–1234.

91. Xie G, Berk MR, Smith MD, DeMaria AN. A simplified method for determining regurgitant fraction by Doppler echocardiography in patients with aortic regurgitation. *J Am Coll Cardiol.* 1994;24:1041–1045.

92. Jobic Y, Slama M, Tribouilloy C, et al. Doppler echocardiographic evaluation of valve regurgitation in healthy volunteers. *Br Heart J.* 1992;69:109–113.

93. Simpson IA, de Belder MA, Kenny A, et al. How to quantitate valve regurgitation by echo Doppler techniques. *Br Heart J.* 1995;73(suppl 2):1–9.

94. Dolan MS, Castello R, St. Vrain JA, Aguire F, Labovitz AJ. Quantitation of aortic regurgitation by Doppler echocardiography: a practical approach. *Am Heart J.* 1995;129:1014–1020.

95. Leung MP, Chau K, Chiu C, Yung T, Mok C. Intraoperative TEE assessment of ventricular septal defect with aortic regurgitation. *Ann Thorac Surg.* 1996;61:854–860.

96. Simpson IA, deBelder MA, Treasure T, Camm AJ, Pumphrey CW. Cardiovascular manifestations of Marfan's syndrome: improved evaluation by transesophageal echocardiography. *Br Heart J.* 1993;69:104–108.

97. Habre WN, vanGessel EF, Mamie C, Cantieni R, Suter PM. Traumatic or septic aortic regurgitation: diagnosis by esophageal echocardiography. *Acta Anaesthesiol Scand.* 1994;38:612–614.

98. Karalis DG, Ross JJ Jr, Brown, F, Chandrasekaran K. Transesophageal echocardiography in valvular heart disease. In: Frankl WS, Brest AN, eds. *Valvular Heart Disease: Comprehensive Evaluation and Treatment. Cardiovasc Clinics.* 1993;23: 105–123.

99. Rafferty TT, Durkin MA, Sittig D, et al. Transesophageal color flow Doppler imaging for aortic insufficiency in patients having cardiac operations. *J Thorac Cardiovasc Surg.* 1992;104:521–525.

100. Perry GJ, Helmcke F, Nanda NC, Byard C, Soto B. Evaluation of aortic insufficiency by Doppler color flow mapping. *J Am Coll Cardiol.* 1987;9:952–959.

101. Globits S, Frank H, Mayr H, Heuhold A, Glogar D. Quantitative assessment of aortic regurgitation by magnetic resonance imaging. *Eur Heart J.* 1992;13:78–83.

102. Tamai T, Konishi T, Okamoto S, Sakuma H, Takeda K, Nakano T. Evaluation of aortic regurgitation using cine magnetic resonance imaging. *Jpn Heart J.* 1993;34:741–748.

103. Søndergaard L, Lindvig K, Hildebrandt P, et al. Quantification of aortic regurgitation by magnetic resonance velocity mapping. *Am Heart J.* 1993;125:1081–1090.

104. Ambrosi P, Faugère G, Desfossez L, et al. Assessment of aortic regurgitation severity by magnetic resonance imaging of the thoracic aorta. *Eur Heart J.* 1995;16:406–409.

105. Bolen JA, Aldennan EL. Hemodynamic consequences of afterload reduction in patients with chronic aortic regurgitation. *Circulation.* 1976;53:879–883.

106. Grenberg B, Massie B, Bristow JD, et al. Long term vasodilator therapy of chronic aortic insufficiency: a randomized double-blinded placebo-controlled clinical trial. *Circulation.* 1988;78:92–103.

107. Gentile F, Ornaghi M, Esposti D, Triulzi MO. Hemodynamic effects of nifedipine in patients with asymptomatic aortic regurgitation: evaluation by Doppler echocardiography. *Acta Cardiologica.* 1993;48:495–506.

108. Röthlisberger C, Sareli P, Wisenbaugh T. Comparison of single-dose nifedipine and captopril for chronic severe aortic regurgitation. *Am J Cardiol.* 1993;71:799–804.

109. Scognamiglio R, Rahimtoola SH, Fasoli G, Nistri S, Dalla Volta S. Nifedipine in asymptomatic patients with severe aortic regurgitation and normal left ventricular function. *N Engl J Med.* 1994;331:689–694.

110. Bonow RO, Rosing DR, Kent KM, Epstein SE. Timing of operation for chronic aortic regurgitation. *Am J Cardiol.* 1982;50:325–336.

111. Bonow RO. Asymptomatic aortic regurgitation: indications for operation. *J Card Surg.* 1994;9(suppl):170–173.

112. Tornos MP, Olona M, Permanyer-Miralda G. Clinical out-

come of severe asymptomatic chronic aortic regurgitation: a long-term prospective follow-up study. *Am Heart J.* 1995;130:333–339.

113. Gray RJ, Helfant RH. Timing of surgery for valvular heart disease. In: Frankl WS, Breast AN, eds. *Valvular Heart Disease: Comprehensive Evaluation and Treatment.* Philadelphia, Pa: FA Davis; 1993:209–231.

114. Gaash WH, Carroll JD, Levine HJ, Criscitiello MG. Chronic aortic regurgitation: prognostic value of left ventricular end-systolic dimension and end-diastolic radius/thickness ratio. *J Am Coll Cardiol.* 1983;1:775–782.

115. Henry WL, Bonow RO, Rousing DR, Epstein SE. Observations on the optimal timing for operative intervention for aortic regurgitation: serial echocardiographic evaluation of asymptomatic patients. *Circulation.* 1980;61:484–492.

116. Wilson RA, McDonald RW, Bristow JD, et al. Correlates of aortic distensibility in chronic aortic regurgitation and relation to progression to surgery. *J Am Coll Cardiol.* 1992; 19:733–738.

117. Forman R, Firth BF, Barnard MS. Prognostic significance of preoperative left ventricular ejection fraction and valve lesion in patients with aortic valve replacement. *Am J Cardiol.* 1980;45:1120–1125.

118. Kirkland JW, Barratt-Boyes BG, eds. *Cardiac Surgery.* 2nd ed. New York, NY: Churchchill Livingstone; 1993.

119. Agathos EA, Starr A. Aortic valve replacement. *Curr Probl Surg.* 1993;30:601–710.

120. Blank RH, Pupello DF, Besson LN, et al. Method of managing the small aortic annulus during valve replacement. *Ann Thorac Surg.* 1976;22:356–361.

121. Manouguian S, Seybold-Epting W. Patch enlargement of the aortic valve by extending the aortic incision to the anterior mitral leaflet: new operative technique. *J Thorac Cardiovasc Surg.* 1979;78:402–412.

122. Rastan H, Koncz J. Aortoventriculoplasty: a new technique for the treatment of left ventricular outflow obstructions. *J Thorac Cardiovasc Surg.* 1976;71:920–927.

123. David TE, Feindel CM. An aortic valve-sparing operation for patients with aortic incompetence and aneurysm of the ascending aorta. *J Thorac Cardiovasc Surg.* 1992;103: 617–622.

124. David TE, Feindel CM, Bos J. Repair of the aortic valve in patients with aortic insufficiency and aortic root aneurysm. *J Thorac Cardiovasc Surg.* 1995;109:345–352.

125. Keeley SB, Brewer PL, Burdette FM. Homograft root replacement for juvenile rheumatoid aortic valve incompetence. *Ann Thorac Surg.* 1992;53:330–331.

126. Jones EL. Aortic valve replacement in the young. *J Card Surg.* 1994;9(suppl):188–191.

127. Kumar N, Gometza B, Al Halees Z, Duran C. Surgery for aortic regurgitation in the young: repair vs replacement. *J Cardiovasc Surg.* 1992;33:7–13.

128. Cosgrove DM, Rosenkranz ER, Hendren WG, Bartlett JC, Stewart WJ. Valvuloplasty for aortic insufficiency. *J Thorac Cardiovasc Surg.* 1991;102:571–577.

129. Fraser CD, Wang N, Mee RB, et al. Repair of insufficient bicuspid aortic valves. *Ann Thorac Surg.* 1994;58:386–390.

130. Trusler GA, Williams WG, Smallhorn JF, Freedom RM. Late results after repair of aortic insufficiency associated with ventricular septal defect. *J Thorac Cardiovasc Surg.* 1992;103:276–281.

131. Hisatomi K, Isomura T, Sato T, et al. Aortoplasty for aortic regurgitation with ventricular septal defect. *J Thorac Cardiovasc Surg.* 1994;108:396–397.

132. Schoof PH, Hazekamp MG, Huysmans HA. Pulmonary autograft in ventricular septal defect–aortic insufficiency complex. *Ann Thorac Surg.* 1996;61:1005–1006.

133. Reddy VM, Rajasinghe HA, McElhinney DB, et al. Extending the limits of the Ross procedure. *Ann Thorac Surg.* 1993;60(suppl 6):S600–S603.

134. Al-Halees Z, Kumar N, Gallo R, Gometza B, Duran CMG. Pulmonary autograft for aortic valve replacement in rheumatic disease: a caveat. *Ann Thorac Surg.* 1995;60: S172–S176.

135. Bonow RO, Dodd JT, Maron BJ. Long-term serial changes in left ventricular function and reversal of ventricular dilatation after valve replacement for chronic aortic regurgitation. *Circulation.* 1988;78:1108–1112.

136. Pirwitz MJ, Lange RA, Willard JE, Landau C, Glamann DB, Hillis LD. Use of the left ventricular peak systolic pressure/end-systolic volume ratio to predict symptomatic improvement with valve replacement in patients with aortic regurgitation and enlarged end-systolic volume. *J Am Coll Cardiol.* 1994;24:1672–1677.

137. DiBasi P, Pajé A, Salati M, et al. Surgical timing in aortic regurgitation: left ventricular analysis by contractility score. *Ann Thorac Surg.* 1994;58:509–515.

138. Bonow RO. Radionuclide angiography in the management of aortic regurgitation. *Circulation.* 1991;84(suppl 1):I292–I302.

139. Bonow RO, Nikas D, Elefteriades JA. Valve replacement for regurgitant lesions of the aortic or mitral valve in advanced left ventricular dysfunction. *Cardiol Clin.* 1995; 13:73–83.

22

Valvular Heart Disease: Mitral Stenosis

David W. Drucker and John F. Setaro

Incidence and Etiology

Mitral stenosis is recognized when a pathologic process causes obstruction of flow through the mitral valvular orifice. Typically such stenosis is secondary to restriction of valve leaflet movement that arises from severe scarring. Whatever the etiology, mitral stenosis causes a characteristic symptom complex that must be followed closely and treated aggressively. In this chapter we survey the clinical, radiographic imaging, and hemodynamic findings of mitral valvular stenosis.

The most common cause of mitral stenosis remains rheumatic carditis.[1-3] The prevalence of this disorder is decreasing in the industrialized world but rising in Latin America, Asia, Africa, and the Middle East.[2] More than half of affected patients do not recollect a clinical syndrome of acute rheumatic fever. Two thirds of patients with rheumatic heart disease are female, and 25% exhibit pure mitral stenosis as a solitary finding. More commonly, a combination of stenosis and regurgitation is witnessed.[4] Occasionally amyloid deposits accumulate on rheumatic mitral leaflets and may worsen the obstructive syndrome.[3] Severe mitral stenosis requires a minimum of 2 years for full development, and most patients are asymptomatic for 10 or more years. Symptoms are most frequently encountered in the third or fourth decade of life.[5]

Other causes of mitral stenosis are listed in Table 22.1. When mitral stenosis appears in association with an atrial septal defect, the resulting entity is known as Lutembacher's syndrome.[5] In the following we focus on the rheumatic form of the disease, but most management principles are similarly applicable.

Complications of mitral stenosis include atrial fibrillation in 50% of patients and systemic emboli arising from intracardiac thrombi in 20%.[6] Though unusual, bacterial endocarditis should be entertained as a diagnosis in any patient with a consistent history. The prognosis of patients with mitral stenosis who do not receive treat-

TABLE 22.1. Causes of mitral valvular stenosis.

Rheumatic fever

Complication of another systemic disorder
Carcinoid
Lupus erythematosis
Rheumatoid arthritis
Hunter–Hurley type mucopolysaccharidosis
Infective endocarditis
Thrombus formation

Methysergide therapy

Congenital

Leaflet or annular calcification

Conditions that may simulate mitral stenosis
Left atrial myxoma
Cor triatriatum
Parachute mitral valve deformity
Pulmonary veno-occlusive disease
Obstructing mediastinal granulomata
Obstructing metastatic neoplasms

ment with contemporary medical and surgical modalities depends on symptom severity and stage of disease. Asymptomatic patients demonstrate a 10-year survival rate of >60% whereas those evincing New York Heart Association functional class IV characteristics have a 5-year survival rate of 15%.[7]

Pathology and Pathophysiology

A normal mitral valve possesses two cusps and an orifice with a cross-sectional area of 4 to 6 cm^2. Rheumatic fever can induce one or all types of valvular fusion: commisural, cuspal, or chordal.[8] Fusion tends to occur at the edges of the cusps, and additional chordal inflammation produces short, thickened chordae tendineae. The resultant mitral valve is stenotic and has a funnel-shaped orifice that has been described as resembling a button-

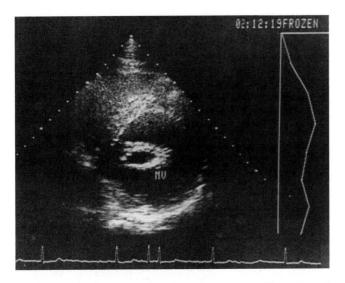

FIGURE 22.1. Echocardiographic evaluation (two-dimensional) of mitral stenosis showing characteristic buttonhole or fish mouth deformity. Calibration dots are 1 cm apart. (Reprinted with permission from Yang et al.[10])

hole or fish mouth (Figure 22.1). Left atrial and pulmonary venous congestion develop later, predisposing the patient to atrial fibrillation, systemic thromboembolization, left and right heart congestive failure, and reactive pulmonary arterial hypertension.[9]

Symptomatology and Natural History

History

The classic presenting symptom of mitral valvular stenosis is dyspnea. This symptom can be precipitated by any condition that swiftly increases left atrial pressure and cardiac output. Frequent provoking factors include exercise, fever, pregnancy, and emotional stress.[4] The onset of atrial fibrillation, with its resultant loss of atrial contraction and often rapid ventricular response, produces dyspnea along with palpitations and fatigue.

Elevation of right-sided pressures can produce hemoptysis,[11] pulmonary hypertension, right heart failure, or ischemic symptoms arising from the right ventricle under strain.[12] Other symptoms include hoarseness (secondary to left atrial compression of the recurrent laryngeal nerve) and neurological impairment due to stroke (left atrial thromboembolization).

Physical Examination

Findings in patients with mitral valvular stenosis may include atrial fibrillation and borderline low systemic blood pressure due to impaired forward cardiac output. On auscultation, the examiner may note an accentuated first heart sound, a low-frequency diastolic rumble best heard at the cardiac apex, and an opening snap. Of these, the opening snap is viewed as the most important. It is produced during maximal excursion of the anterior leaflet of the mitral valve and is usually detected at the cardiac apex.[13] Typically the snap is heard between 0.03 and 0.14 seconds after the second heart sound, with more severe stenosis (and higher left atrial pressures) shortening the interval between aortic closure and the opening snap.[14] Yet the opening snap is not diagnostic of mitral stenosis in that it may also be found in patients with other disorders such as atrial or ventricular septal defect.

In the early stages of mitral stenosis, the diastolic murmur may be heard only with the patient placed in the left lateral decubitus position soon after exercise. The murmur tends to be low pitched and best auscultated with the bell of the stethoscope. The intensity of the murmur does not correlate well with the degree of stenosis and may decrease or even vanish as cardiac output declines in the very late stages of mitral stenosis.

In its advanced stages, mitral stenosis causes pulmonary hypertension, which in turn produces a palpable right ventricular heave along the left sternal border.[15] The diastolic rumble and the first heart sound may also be palpable at the cardiac apex.[16] The intensity of the first heart sound is decreased by valve leaflet immobility or regurgitation and increased by any intervention that shortens the PR interval.[17] With advanced disease, patients may manifest elevated neck veins, systolic pulsation of the jugular veins (caused by functional tricuspid valvular regurgitation), or mitral facies (malar flush with peripheral cyanosis).[18]

Diagnostic Tests

Electrocardiography

Of patients who have mitral stenosis, 25% disclose electrocardiographic evidence of left atrial enlargement. Findings are notable for a broad, notched P wave best appreciated in lead II, with a negative terminal deflection in lead VI.[19] Atrial fibrillation is usually evident, and when pulmonary hypertension supervenes electrocardiographic criteria for right ventricular hypertrophy may be present (rightward deviation of the mean QRS vector).

Roentgenography

The most frequently encountered radiologic findings in mitral stenosis are caused by left atrial enlargement.

These manifestations include straightening of the left cardiac border on a posteroanterior chest film, elevation of the left main stem bronchus, and posterior deviation of the esophagus on a barium swallow study.[20] Elevated left atrial pressure results in prominence of the pulmonary arteries and right ventricular enlargement. Acute increases in left atrial pressure cause roentgenographic findings of pulmonary edema, whereas chronically high pressures produce radiographically visible redistribution of blood flow to the apexes and Kerley's B lines.[21]

Echocardiography

As with many cardiovascular disorders, echocardiography has become extremely useful in the detection and longitudinal evaluation and follow-up of mitral stenosis.[6] Initial M-mode data reveal dense echoes that suggest calcification and restricted leaflet excursion. Currently, two-dimensional images provide the clearest portrait of mitral stenosis (Figure 22.1). These techniques document restricted leaflet movement, left atrial enlargement, valve calcification, and a typical diastolic doming pattern of the valve. Valve area can be calculated by using planimetry (Figure 22.1) or by employing Doppler flow velocity methods to determine a pressure half-time ($T_{1/2}$) (Figure 22.2). Mitral valve area is approximately equal to $220/T_{1/2}$.[10,22] Other significant data made available by two-dimensional echocardiography include left and right ventricular size and function and potential findings that support nonrheumatic etiologies for mitral stenosis.

Transesophageal echocardiography allows for detailed inspection of the mitral valve and subvalvular apparatus without the limitations imposed by the thoracic cavity. Such a degree of detail can be particularly useful when contemplating balloon valvuloplasty or surgical valve repair in favor of valve replacement. In addition, transesophageal echocardiography is especially sensitive for the evaluation of intracardiac thrombi and valvular vegetations. Mitral valve area derived by transesophageal techniques is calculated in a fashion identical to that of a transthoracic study.

Hemodynamic Findings at Right and Left Heart Catheterization

Physiologic pulmonary capillary wedge pressure at 10 to 14 mm Hg reflects left atrial pressure, and no gradient normally exists between left atrial and left ventricular end-diastolic pressure. In mitral stenosis, pulmonary capillary wedge pressure is elevated and a gradient is measurable between pulmonary capillary wedge pressure and left ventricular end-diastolic pressure (Figure 22.3). With increasing degrees of stenosis, greater atrio-

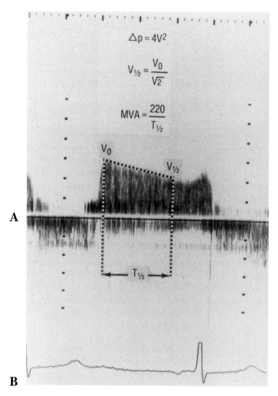

FIGURE 22.2. Mitral valve gradient (A) and area (B) can be estimated using Doppler echocardiography. **A,** Employing the square of the Doppler-derived mitral flow velocity multiplied by four gives the instantaneous mitral valve pressure gradient. **B,** Velocity at half-time ($V_{1/2}$) is calculated by dividing initial flow velocity (V_0) by the square root of 2. Then the $V_{1/2}$ point on the velocity curve is identified, and the time interval (or pressure gradient half-time $T_{1/2}$ in ms) between V_0 and $V_{1/2}$ is measured. The mitral valve area (MVA) is derived by dividing 220 into $T_{1/2}$. (Reprinted with permission from Yang et al.[10])

ventricular pressure differences are required to maintain normal cardiac output. For example, in critical mitral stenosis (<1.0 cm^2 valve area), a transmitral gradient of 20 mm Hg is needed to preserve cardiac output. Atrial contraction contributes to this requirement by augmenting the presystolic transmitral pressure gradient by 30%. The onset of atrial fibrillation therefore represents a significant mechanical disadvantage.

Symptomatic patients usually have either a resting- or exercise-induced elevation of pulmonary capillary wedge pressure. Additional information obtained during catheterization includes quality of ventricular function, presence of coexisting disease in other valves, pressure evaluation of the pulmonary circuit, and assessment for obstructive coronary artery atherosclerotic disease.[10] A pressure gradient of 5 mm Hg or greater between the pulmonary artery end-diastolic pressure and the pulmonary capillary wedge pressure usually indicates the presence of pulmonary hypertension. Depression of left ventricular function in pure mitral valvular stenosis is

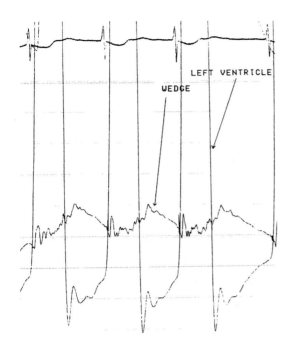

FIGURE 22.3. Hemodynamic findings of mitral stenosis in an 80-year-old patient with a history of rheumatic heart disease. Of note is a gradient in diastole between pulmonary capillary wedge and left ventricle pressure. Valve area was 1.0 cm². Scale is 0 to 40 mm Hg. (Reprinted courtesy of Jerome E. Williams, Jr, MD, and Joseph J. Brennan, Jr, MD, Cardiac Catheterization Laboratory, Yale University School of Medicine.)

rare, although regional wall motion abnormalities may be observed.[6]

A mitral valve area can be calculated once baseline hemodynamic data are obtained using the Gorlin formula, which relates area to flow and gradient,[10] as follows: MVA = (CO/DFP × HR/K √MVG, where MVA = mitral valve area (cm²), CO = cardiac output (mL/min), DFP = diastolic filling period (seconds), HR = heart rate, K = 38 (Gorlin's mitral valve constant), and MVG = mitral valve gradient (typically averaged over 10 contractions).

Medical management of mitral stenosis consists of preventing recurrent bouts of rheumatic fever, preventing and treating bacterial endocarditis, protecting against stroke through anticoagulation therapy, and treating symptoms with appropriate control of intravascular volume and heart rhythm and rate. These medical modalities and catheter-based and surgical therapies are discussed more fully in later chapters.

References

1. Olson LJ, Subramanian R, Ackerman DM. Surgical pathology of the mitral valve: a study of 712 cases spanning 21 years. *Mayo Clin Proc.* 1987;62:22–28.
2. Kumar A, Sinha M, Sinha DNP. Chronic rheumatic heart diseases in Ranchi (India). *Angiology.* 1982;33:141–143.
3. Ladefoged C, Rohr N. Amyloid deposits in aortic and mitral valves. *Virchow's Arch (A).* 1984;404:301–304.
4. Bowe JC, Bland F, Sprague HB, White PD. Course of mitral stenosis without surgery: ten and twenty year perspectives. *Ann Intern Med.* 1960;52:741–746.
5. Gaasch WH, O'Rourke RA, Cohn LH, Rackley CE. Mitral valve disease. In: Hurst JW, Schlant RC, Rackley CE, Sonnenblick EH, Wenger NK, eds. *Hurst's: The Heart.* 8th ed. New York: McGraw-Hill; 1994:1483–1491.
6. Lutas EM. Echocardiographic analysis of mitral stenosis: a critical appraisal of its clinical value in detection of severe stenosis and valvular calcification. *J Cardiovasc Ultrasonog.* 1983;2:131–136.
7. Gaasch WH, Folland ED. Left ventricular function in rheumatic mitral stenosis. *Eur Heart J.* 1991;12(suppl B): 66–69.
8. Abernathy WS, Willis PW. Thromboembolic complications of rheumatic heart disease. *Cardiovasc Clin.* 1973;5: 131–138.
9. Setaro JF, Cleman MW, Remetz MS. The right ventricle in disorders causing pulmonary venous hypertension. *Cardiol Clin.* 1992;10:165–183.
10. Yang SS, Bentivoglio LG, Maranhao V, et al. Assessment of ventricular inflow and outflow obstruction. In: Yang SS, Bentivoglio LG, Maranhao V, Goldberg H, eds. *Cardiac Catheterization Data to Hemodynamic Parameters.* 3rd ed. Philadelphia, Pa: FA Davis; 1988:122–151.
11. Waller BF. Rheumatic and non-rheumatic conditions producing valvular heart disease. In: Frankl WS, Brest AN, eds. *Cardiovascular Clinics Valvular Heart Disease: Comprehensive Evaluation and Management.* Philadelphia, Pa: FA Davis; 1986:3–104.
12. Selzer A, Cohn KE. Natural history of mitral stenosis: a review. *Circulation.* 1972;45:878.
13. Wood P. An appreciation of mitral stenosis. *BMJ.* 1954; 1:1051–1062.
14. Mounsey JP. The opening snap of mitral stenosis. *Br Heart J.* 1953;15:135–138.
15. Ross RS. Right ventricular hypertension as a cause of precordial pain. *Am Heart J.* 1961;61:134–136.
16. Schwartz R, Meyerson RM, Lawrence LT, et al. Mitral stenosis, massive pulmonary hemorrhage, and emergency valve replacement. *N Engl J Med.* 1966;272:755–759.
17. Mounsey JP. Inspection and palpation of the cardiac impulse. *Prog Cardiovasc Dis.* 1967;10:187–196.
18. Dack S, Bleifer S, Grishman A, et al. Mitral stenosis: auscultatory and phonocardiographic findings. *Am J Cardiol.* 1960;5:815–819.
19. Gooch AS, Calatayud JB, Gorman PA, et al. Leftward shift of the terminal P forces in the electrocardiogram associated with left atrial enlargement. *Am Heart J.* 1966;71: 727–729.
20. Chen JT, Behar VS, Morris JJ, et al. Correlation of roentgen findings with hemodynamic data in pure mitral stenosis. *Am J Roentgenol Radium Ther Nucl Med.* 1968;102: 280–292.
21. Meszaros WT. Lung changes in left heart failure. *Circulation.* 1973;47:859–863.
22. Yang SS, Goldberg H. Simplified Doppler estimate of mitral valve area. *Am J Cardiol.* 1985;56:488–492.

23

Valvular Heart Disease: Mitral Regurgitation

Habib Samady and John F. Setaro

Incidence and Etiology

The functional mitral valve apparatus comprises the mitral annulus, the mitral leaflets, the chordae tendineae, the papillary muscles, and the adjacent atrial and ventricular myocardium. Abnormalities in one or more of these structures can lead to mitral regurgitation (MR) (Figure 23.1). *Mitral regurgitation* can be defined as retrograde flow of blood from the left ventricle to the left atrium as a consequence of inadequate closure of the mitral leaflets. The incidence of chronic MR is difficult to ascertain accurately because the condition frequently remains asymptomatic until late in its course. It is often detected on routine physical examination. In the United States, mitral valve prolapse and coronary artery disease account for the majority of cases of MR.

Mitral valve prolapse, the most common form of valvular heart disease, occurs in 5% to 10% of the population.[2] MR frequently occurs as a result of mitral valve prolapse at some stage in the clinical syndrome. Mitral valve prolapse is discussed at length elsewhere in this chapter.

Papillary muscle dysfunction arising from myocardial ischemia can result in MR. The posteromedial papillary muscle, which is supplied by the right coronary artery, is involved more commonly than the anterolateral papillary muscle, which frequently receives blood from both the left anterior descending and circumflex coronary arteries. Among 206 patients with myocardial infarction who entered the Thrombolysis in Myocardial Infarction phase I trial, MR was present in 13%.[3] Transient MR was found in up to 50% to 60% of patients. Acute MR may result from injury or rupture of a papillary muscle due to acute myocardial infarction (Figure 23.2). Acute MR commonly results in severe hemodynamic compromise.

Another important cause of MR is dilatation of the left ventricle, which alters the geometry and function of the mitral apparatus. In particular, with progressive dilatation of the left ventricle, a transition from ovoid to spherical shape of the left ventricle has been correlated with onset of MR.

For many years rheumatic fever, in which MR is often seen in combination with mitral stenosis, was considered to be the most common etiology for MR in the United States. Although rheumatic fever continues to be the most common cause of MR in many parts of the world, its incidence has declined in the United States.

Less commonly MR can be caused by endocarditis, mitral annular calcification, hypertrophic cardiomyopathy, connective tissue diseases such as Ehlers–Danlos syndrome, infiltrative disorders, inflammatory disorders, and congenital disorders. Bacterial endocarditis and myxomatous degeneration with spontaneous or traumatic rupture of the chordae[5,6] can also result in acute MR.

Pathology and Pathophysiology

MR can result from a gradual though relentless process or an abrupt disruption of the valvular apparatus. Although acute MR can become chronic, important differences exist in the pathophysiology of these two states. In acute MR the major burden falls on the pulmonary circulation, whereas in chronic MR the left ventricle sustains the major load.

Sudden development of MR due to disruption of the mitral valve apparatus results in an acute volume overload in the left ventricle. The ventricle, via the Frank–Starling mechanism, accommodates this preload reserve by increasing its stroke volume. In systole, part of the stroke volume flows retrograde into the low-pressure left atrium (regurgitant fraction) and the remainder flows forward through the left ventricular outflow tract (forward output). The small, undiseased left atrium dilates in response to the rapid rise in volume and pressure. These events in turn lead to pulmonary venous congestion and pulmonary edema.

FIGURE 23.1. Transesophageal echocardiographic view of mitral regurgitation (MR) by color flow Doppler technique. LA, left atrium; MV, mitral valve; LV, left ventricle; RA, right atrium; RV, right ventricle; TV, tricuspid valve. (Reprinted with permission from Rafferty et al.[1])

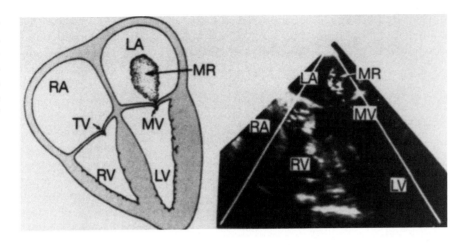

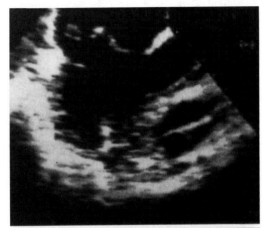

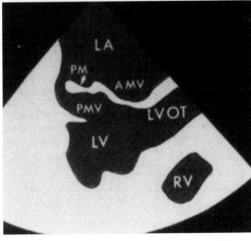

FIGURE 23.2. Transesophageal echocardiogram shows ruptured papillary muscle as a free structure connected to the mitral valve yet appearing in the left atrium. LA, left atrium; LV, left ventricle; LVOT, left ventricular outflow tract; RV, right ventricle; PM, posterior papillary muscle; PMV, posterior mitral valve leaflet; AMV, anterior mitral valve leaflet. (Reprinted with permission from Zotz et al.[4])

Elevated pulmonary artery pressures may produce intimal proliferation and medial hypertrophy of the pulmonary arteries and subsequent right ventricular hypertrophy. When regurgitation is severe the forward stroke volume cannot be maintained and cardiac output falls.

The evolution from acute to chronic MR is attended by a series of compensatory myocardial and circulatory adjustments[7] that culminate in enlargement of the left ventricle. The increased preload results in addition of new sarcomeres, rearrangement of myocardial fibers, and eccentric hypertrophy of the left ventricle. Thus preload at the sarcomere level returns toward normal, and the enhanced stroke volume is mediated through myocyte hyperplasia and hypertrophy. The hyperkinetic small ventricle of acute MR is converted into a large compliant chamber that is well suited to accept and propel a large stroke volume. The left atrium enlarges, becomes more compliant, and accommodates the regurgitant volume from the left ventricle with only a small increase in pressure. In compensated chronic MR the left ventricular mass, end-diastolic volume, and stroke volume are increased without a substantial increase in the left ventricular end-diastolic pressure or pulmonary capillary wedge pressure. As a result, patients may remain asymptomatic for years during the compensated phase of chronic MR.

The sequence of events leading to decompensation in chronic MR has not yet been fully characterized. According to one hypothesis, the left atrium and ventricle progressively enlarge to the point at which mitral annular dilatation further impairs mitral leaflet coaptation, thereby worsening the degree of regurgitation. Atrial fibrillation and subsequent systemic embolization may result from dilatation and stasis in the left atrium. Decompensated MR is characterized by progressive left ventricular enlargement, elevation of left ventricular end-diastolic pressures, and increase in systolic wall stress. These events culminate in a declining ejection fraction, progressive atrial enlargement, atrial arrhythmias, and pulmonary hypertension. Symptoms frequently develop during the transition from the compensated to the decompensated state. Without surgical intervention, the outcome is lethal.

Symptomatology and Natural History

History

The severity of symptoms in chronic MR is a function of the extent of regurgitation, the level of pulmonary artery pressure, and the presence of associated valvular, myocardial, or coronary disease. Patients with mild MR may remain asymptomatic for some time. Early symptoms, which include fatigue and dyspnea, usually signify incipient decompensation of the left ventricle. By the time orthopnea, paroxysmal nocturnal dyspnea, and hepatic and peripheral edema develop, severe and often irreversible left ventricular dysfunction may ensue. Physical exhaustion and light-headedness as a result of low cardiac output are late features of MR.

Palpitations, light-headedness, and systemic embolization can result from the atrial fibrillation that frequently complicates chronic MR. Left atrial appendage thrombi occur less frequently in MR than in mitral stenosis. The large, high-pressure retrograde bolus of blood projected into the left atrium is thought to "wash" the left atrial appendage and thus discourage stasis and thrombus formation.

Acute pulmonary edema also occurs less commonly in patients with MR than in those with mitral stenosis. This lower incidence may be due to the increased compliance of the left atrium, which absorbs the systolic regurgitant load.

Physical Examination

In patients presenting with dyspnea and a systolic murmur, palpation of the carotid arterial pulse may be helpful in distinguishing MR from aortic stenosis. In contrast to the delayed carotid arterial upstroke of aortic stenosis, in MR the carotid upstroke is often brisk and hyperdynamic. This characteristic results from the early ejection of the forward left ventricular output into the aorta before MR occurs. Palpation of the carotid pulse may also alert the observer to the etiology of MR in hypertrophic cardiomyopathy when a characteristic peak-and-dome pattern is found.

Jugular venous distention results from pulmonary hypertension in acute severe MR or in the late stages of decompensated chronic MR. Prominent *a* waves may accompany significant pulmonary hypertension. *v* waves can be seen with associated tricuspid regurgitation.

Precordial palpation reveals lateral displacement of the apical impulse with diffuse hyperdynamic motion that reflects left ventricular enlargement in chronic decompensated MR. A heave in the lower left sternal border may be due to right ventricular enlargement or left atrial expansion. Additionally, a systolic thrill may be palpable in association with loud regurgitant murmurs.

In severe chronic MR, the intensity of the first heart sound is often diminished. The second heart sound may be widely split as a result of shortening of the left ventricular ejection phase and an earlier A_2. When pulmonary hypertension is present, P_2 will be louder than A_2. The increased flow across the mitral valve during the rapid early phase of ventricular filling is associated with an S_3. This finding excludes significant mitral stenosis, unless another cause for an S_3 is present. An S_4 may be present in acute severe MR in conjunction with myocardial ischemia.

The characteristic murmur of MR is a holosystolic murmur beginning with the first heart sound and extending beyond closure of the aortic valve. It is of blowing, high-pitched quality and typically radiates to the axilla and left infrascapular area. When posterior leaflet prolapse occurs, the murmur radiates toward the base, corresponding to the anterior superior regurgitant jet in the left atrium.

Although the intensity of the systolic murmur of MR does not correlate with the severity of the regurgitation, its timing may indicate severity. Indeed, severe MR, which occurs as soon as isovolumic contraction of the left ventricle begins, generates a holosystolic murmur. In contrast, mild MR may not occur until late in systole when enough intraventricular pressure is generated to cause retrograde blood flow across a partially functional mitral apparatus. Examples of the latter include mitral valve prolapse and papillary muscle dysfunction.

The differential diagnosis of systolic murmurs includes MR of various etiologies, mitral valve prolapse, aortic stenosis, tricuspid regurgitation, ventricular septal defect, and hypertrophic cardiomyopathy. Physical examination and physiologic and pharmacological maneuvers are used to ascertain the clinical diagnosis. Aortic stenosis tends to produce a crescendo–decrescendo murmur, heard loudest in the second right intercostal space and radiating to the carotid region. Ventricular septal defects create loud, harsh holosystolic murmurs heard best at the left lower sternal border, often associated with a thrill. The tricuspid regurgitation murmur is also a holosystolic murmur heard best at the left sternal border, but it radiates to the right sternal border and usually increases in intensity with inspiration.

Valsalva's maneuver, standing, exercise, and amyl nitrite all tend to increase the murmurs of mitral valve prolapse and hypertrophic cardiomyopathy and decrease systolic murmurs of other etiologies. Gripping the hand or squatting decreases murmurs of mitral prolapse and hypertrophic cardiomyopathy and increases systolic murmurs of other etiologies. Valsalva's maneuver consists of forced exhalation against a closed glottis. Its diagnostic utility is limited by the complex physiologic response to this maneuver. The strain phase of Valsalva's maneuver results in decreased venous return and subsequent reduction in right and left ventricular chamber sizes (this effect may be achieved more simply by rapid standing). As a result, in hypertrophic cardiomyopathy the decrease in left ventricular size results in an increased gradient across the left ventricular outflow tract, which enhances the dynamic systolic murmur. In mitral valve prolapse, the reduction of left ventricular size causes earlier elevation of left ventricular end-diastolic pressure, which results in the earlier appearance of the click and systolic murmur.

Both gripping and squatting exercises increase afterload and thus decrease the murmur of hypertrophic cardiomyopathy and delay the murmur and click of mitral valve prolapse. Squatting, by increasing venous return to the heart, also augments the left ventricular end-diastolic dimension, further contributing to the lessening of the hypertrophic cardiomyopathy outflow murmur and the later appearance of the mitral valve prolapse murmur and click.

Natural History

Patients with mild asymptomatic MR who receive appropriate endocarditis prophylaxis may remain stable for many years.[8] Severe MR occasionally follows a bout of endocarditis or rupture of a chord. Regurgitation tends to progress. In the presurgical era, the 5-year survival rate of an unselected group of medically treated patients with MR was 80% and the 10-year survival rate was 60%.[9] Patients with combined mitral stenosis and MR had a poorer prognosis, with only 67% surviving for 5 years and only 30% surviving beyond 10 years. In a cohort of patients with more severe MR treated medically,[10] the 5-year survival rate was found to be 44%. The development of effective surgical techniques has had a favorable impact on the natural history of MR.

Diagnostic Tests

Electrocardiography

The major findings of MR with electrocardiography include left atrial enlargement and atrial fibrillation.[11,12] Evidence of left ventricular enlargement and hypertrophy is seen in about 30% of patients with severe MR; right ventricular hypertrophy, reflecting pulmonary hypertension, is seen in about 15% of patients with severe

MR. Although ST-segment changes have been attributed to papillary muscle dysfunction,[13] they are nonspecific changes and may be secondary to left ventricular hypertrophy, digitalis use, or conduction defects.

Roentgenography

Radiographic findings of left atrial enlargement such as elevation of the left main stem bronchus, straightening of the left heart border, and a double shadow of the right heart border may be seen in patients with chronic MR. Left ventricular enlargement and prominent pulmonary vasculature reflect late decompensation of chronic MR. Mitral valve calcification may be seen on fluoroscopy. Acute MR frequently results in pulmonary edema, which is evident on radiography.

Echocardiography

Echocardiography has emerged as the mainstay of the investigation of MR and plays a central role in the diagnosis, determination of etiology, and hemodynamic consequences of MR. It has also proved useful in the follow-up of patients with chronic MR by assessing the severity of MR and demonstrating ventricular dilatation. Transesophageal echocardiography has been used for detailed visualization of the mitral valve apparatus, assessment of prosthetic valve regurgitation, and intraoperative assessment of valvular function.

Left atrial and ventricular enlargement are well visualized by echocardiography. Ruptured chordae,[14] flail leaflets,[15] wall motion abnormalities involving the papillary muscles, mitral annular calcification, and vegetations associated with endocarditis can often suggest the etiology of MR. Color flow and pulsed-wave Doppler techniques can estimate the severity of MR and correlate well with angiographic techniques.[16,17] Tricuspid regurgitation associated with pulmonary hypertension provides an estimate of pulmonary artery systolic pressures.

Right Heart Catheterization

Although the effective (forward) cardiac output is usually depressed in patients with significant MR, the combined left ventricular output (regurgitant fraction and forward flow) is generally elevated until the left ventricle decompensates. The *a* wave of the left atrial pressure tracing is not as prominent in patients with MR as in those with mitral stenosis.[18] The *v* wave, however, is often large, particularly in patients with acute MR in which the left atrium is unaccustomed to the sudden increase in load (Figure 23.3). A *v* wave may also be appreciated in the pulmonary artery tracing. In pure MR, the *y* descent of the left atrial tracing is rapid, whereas when MR is combined with mitral stenosis, because the left atrium is slower to empty, the *y* descent may be more gradual.

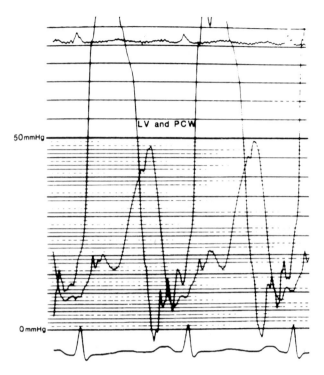

FIGURE 23.3. Large *v* wave visible to 50 mm Hg in a case of severe acute mitral regurgitation. PCW, pulmonary capillary wedge; LV, left ventricle. (Reprinted with permission from Hirshfield.[19])

Angiography

Contrast left ventriculography shows systolic opacification of the left atrium. This opacification can be graded angiographically depending on the extent of left atrial opacification (Figure 23.4). The ejection and regurgitant fractions can be calculated by planimetry.

Equilibrium radionuclide angiography or first-pass angiography calculates an end-diastolic volume as well as the right and left ventricular ejection fraction. The ratio of the left to right ventricular ejection fraction gives an estimate of the regurgitant fraction. These studies may be particularly helpful for interval follow-up of chronic MR.

References

1. Rafferty T, Edwards B, Judd J, et al. An integrated software system for quality assurance–related kappa coefficient analysis of intra-operative transesophageal echocardiography interpretive skills. *Clin Cardiol.* 1993;16:745–752.
2. Savage DD, Garrison RJ, Devereux RB, et al. Mitral valve prolapse in the general population, I: epidemiologic features: the Framingham Study. *Am Heart J.* 1983;106: 571–577.
3. Lehmann KG, Francis CK, Dodge HT, et al. Mitral regurgitation in early myocardial infarction: incidence, clinical detection, and prognostic implications. *Ann Intern Med.* 1992;117:10–17.
4. Zotz RJ, Dohmen G, Genth S, et al. Diagnosis of papillary muscle rupture after acute myocardial infarction by transthoracic and transesophageal echocardiography. *Clin Cardiol.* 1993;19:665–670.
5. Selzer A, Kelly JJ Jr, Vannitamby M, et al. The syndrome of mitral insufficiency due to isolated rupture of the chordae tendineae. *Am J Med.* 1967;43:822–836.

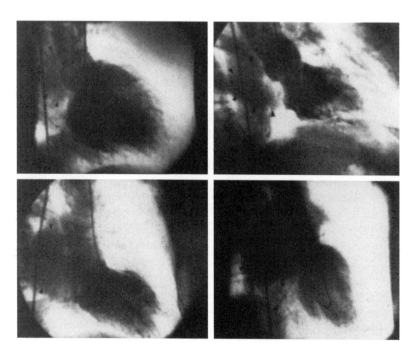

FIGURE 23.4. Angiographic grading (1+, least severe, upper left panel, to 4+, most severe, lower right panel). Arrows identify degree of opacification of left atrium during contrast ventriculography. (Reprinted with permission from Yang et al.[20])

6. Sanders CA, Armstrong PW, Williams JT, et al. Etiology and differential diagnosis of mitral regurgitation. *Prog Cardiovasc Dis.* 1971;14:129–152.

7. Gaasch WH, John RM, Aurgemma GP. Managing asymptomatic patients with mitral regurgitation. *Chest.* 1995;108:842–847.

8. Cohn LS, Mason DT, Braunwald E. Significance of an atrial gallop sound in mitral regurgitation: a clue to the diagnosis of ruptured chordae tendineae. *Circulation.* 1966;35:112–115.

9. Rappaport E. Natural history of aortic and mitral valve disease. *Am J Cardiol.* 1975;35:221–227.

10. Munoz S, Gallardo J, Diaz-Gorrin JR, et al. Influence of surgery on natural history of rheumatic mitral and aortic valve disease. *Am J Cardiol.* 1975;35:234–242.

11. Cooksey JD, Dunn M, Massie E. *Clinical Vectorcardiography and Electrocardiography.* 2nd ed. Chicago, Ill: Chicago Year Book Medical Publishers; 1977.

12. Barlow JB. *Mitral Regurgitation: Perspectives on the Mitral Valve.* Philadelphia, Pa: FA Davis; 1987.

13. Burch GI, Depasquale NP, Phillips JH. The syndrome of papillary muscle dysfunction. *Am Heart J.* 1968;75:399–415.

14. Sweatman T, Selzer A, Kamageki M, et al. Echocardiographic diagnosis of mitral regurgitation due to ruptured chordae tendineae. *Circulation.* 1972;46:580–589.

15. Himelman RB, Kusumoto F, Oken K, et al. The flail mitral leaflet: echocardiographic findings by precordial and transesophageal imaging and Doppler color flow mapping. *J Am Coll Cardiol.* 1991;17:272–279.

16. Blumlein S, Bouchard A, Shiller NB. Quantitation of mitral regurgitation by Doppler echocardiography. *Circulation.* 1986;74:306–314.

17. Dang TY, Gardin JM, Clark S. Redefining the criteria for pulsed Doppler diagnosis of mitral regurgitation by comparison with left ventricular angiography. *Am J Cardiol.* 1987;60:663–666.

18. Braunwald E, Turi ZG. Pathophysiology of mitral valve disease. In: Ionescu MJ, Cohn LH, eds. *Mitral Valve Disease: Diagnosis and Treatment.* London: Butterworths; 1985:3–10.

19. Hirshfield JW. Valve function: stenosis and regurgitation. In: Pepine CJ, ed. *Diagnostic and Therapeutic Cardiac Catheterization.* Baltimore, Md: Williams & Wilkins; 1989: 407.

20. Yang SS, Bentivoglio LG, Maranhao V, Goldberg H. Assessment of valvular regurgitation. In: Yang SS Bentivoglio LG, Maranhao V, Goldberg H, eds. *Cardiac Catheterization Data to Hemodynamic Parameters.* 3rd ed. Philadelphia, Pa: FA Davis; 1988:152–165.

24

Mitral Valve Prolapse

Lynda E. Rosenfeld

Mitral valve prolapse (MVP) is a very common condition, with a prevalence of approximately 5% in the general population.[1] Although it has been associated with a "syndrome" of associated symptoms (and, in a minority of patients, serious complications including significant mitral regurgitation, infective endocarditis, cerebral ischemia, and sudden death), it is overwhelmingly a benign condition. The definition and identification of MVP are very much tied to the development of echocardiography, which along with physical examination is the gold standard by which the diagnosis is made.

The hallmark physical findings of MVP, a midsystolic click or clicks and systolic murmur, were identified by Gallavardin early in the twentieth century. However, they were initially felt to have an extracardiac origin. It was not until the 1960s, when Reid and then Barlow associated late systolic murmurs with the angiographic identification of "billowing" of the mitral valve leaflets into the atrium, that an intracardiac origin was proposed.[2] Beginning in the 1970s with the development of M-mode and then two-dimensional echocardiography, diagnostic criteria for this condition were defined. However, the frequency with which MVP is diagnosed in asymptomatic individuals has raised concern about whether the diagnostic criteria applied in some series have been too lenient or if it may represent a normal variant in some people.

Incidence

The incidence of MVP has ranged from 5% to 15% in various studies and depends on the population examined, the diagnostic criteria used, and to a certain extent the hemodynamic status of the patient at the time of the examination.[3] In the population-based Framingham Study, the overall prevalence, based on echocardiographic criteria, was 5% but ranged from 7% in younger subjects to 3% in older members of the population.[1] There was a decline in prevalence from 17% among women in their 20s to 1% in those over age 80.

Pathophysiology

Appropriate function of the mitral valve requires the interaction of the valve leaflets themselves and the left atrium, valve annulus, chordae tendineae, papillary muscles, and left ventricular muscle. Many theories exist about the cause of MVP.[4,5] The exact etiology may vary in certain subsets of patients, which may explain differences in prognosis. Much attention has focused on the valve leaflets, which are often "hooded," thickened, and enlarged. Pathologically, such valves may contain increased amounts of acid mucopolysaccharides and myxomatous tissue, and there may be disruption of elastic tissue.[6] The association of MVP with Marfan's syndrome and other connective tissue diseases supports structural abnormalities of connective tissue as an etiologic factor. In an echocardiographic study, Weissman et al.[7] found the annuli of MVP patients to be enlarged even in the absence of mitral regurgitation. Hutchins et al.,[8] in a study of MVP pathology, identified disjunction of the mitral annulus in patients with MVP and postulated that hypermobility of the valve apparatus played a role in this condition.

Rupture of chordae tendineae or a papillary muscle may lead to one of the catastrophic complications of MVP, severe mitral regurgitation. Whether this is a primary problem, due to morphological abnormalities of these structures, or secondary to the stresses of supporting an abnormal valve is debated.[4] Liedtke et al.,[9] using angiographic techniques, identified localized inferior contraction abnormalities in patients with MVP and proposed that an inability of the inferior papillary muscle to shorten or sustain shortening leads to lack of support of the posterior leaflet of the mitral valve. Not all patients with mitral valve prolapse have regional contraction abnormalities, and the importance of this component is uncertain.

Devereux et al.[10] have supported a genetic basis for MVP. Based on a study of 45 probands with echocardiographically diagnosed MVP and their first-degree relatives, they proposed an autosomal dominant pattern of inheritance with age- and sex-dependent expression. They did not specifically examine body habitus as a contributing factor to the manifestation of MVP.

Physical Findings

Although echocardiographically documented prolapse of the mitral valve may be "silent," the physical findings associated with this condition are unique and distinctive and have led to one of its synonyms, the click-murmur syndrome. MVP is dynamic and depends on the loading conditions of the left ventricle. Thus, the physical findings associated with this condition respond in a characteristic and diagnostic manner to postural and pharmacological maneuvers.[4]

Patients typically have one or multiple midsystolic clicks that may be snapping in quality and variable in timing. Such clicks may be followed by a mid- to late-systolic murmur (perhaps with a honking quality) best heard at the apex. Occasionally patients may describe hearing honking sounds in certain positions. In the minority of patients with significant mitral regurgitation, the murmur may become holosystolic and obscure the click.

A decrease in left ventricular volume tends to move the click earlier (it may merge with the first heart sound) and prolongs the murmur. In some patients the characteristic auscultatory findings may become apparent only in the standing position. Conditions that increase left ventricular pressure tend to make the murmur more prominent and may increase its honking quality. Thus, standing moves the click forward and tends to lengthen and soften the murmur, whereas sudden squatting moves the click toward the second heart sound, shortening and accentuating the murmur. Typically Valsalva's maneuver and the initial effects of amyl nitrite will move the click forward and lengthen the murmur, which may also become less prominent. The physical findings of MVP may diminish or disappear during pregnancy, when intravascular volume is increased.

MVP has also been associated with an asthenic body habitus and a variety of skeletal abnormalities including pectus excavatum, a narrow chest, loss of the normal lordotic curvature of the lumbar spine (the straight back syndrome),[11] and hypomastia.[12]

Diagnostic Studies

Echocardiography has been critical to defining and diagnosing MVP. The M-mode finding of posterior systolic motion of continuous mitral leaflet interfaces behind the line connecting the valve's opening and closing points (by at least 2 mm for late systolic prolapse and 3 mm for holosystolic prolapse) has been the diagnostic standard since the early 1970s[15] (Figure 24.1). On the two-dimensional parasternal long-axis view, billowing of one or both of the mitral leaflets across the annular plane into the atrium has also been shown to be sensitive and specific in a variety of studies (Figure 24.2). Such motion may also be documented on the four chamber view, which, however, may be overly sensitive. Thickening of one or both mitral leaflets may also be seen, and Doppler studies may identify mitral regurgitation. In all cases, technically excellent studies are necessary, and care must be taken to avoid angulated views that may suggest false prolapse. A lack of caution in ascribing significance to minor degrees of prolapse has led to inflated estimates of the prevalence of MVP and has created unnecessary anxiety and concern among patients.

Angiographic criteria for the diagnosis of MVP are less rigorous than the echocardiographic standards, and there has been concern that clinically insignificant degrees of prolapse have been diagnosed at the time of cardiac catheterization. Generally, scalloping of the mitral valve leaflets and billowing of the leaflets beyond the line connecting the anterior and posterior fornices of the mitral valve as viewed in the right anterior oblique projection have been taken as evidence of prolapse.[4]

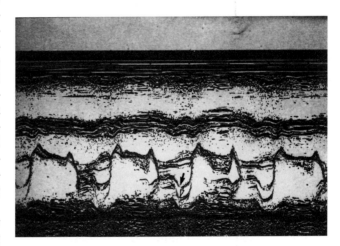

FIGURE 24.1. M-mode echocardiogram demonstrating prolapse of the anterior (solid arrow) and posterior (open arrow) leaflets of the mitral valve.

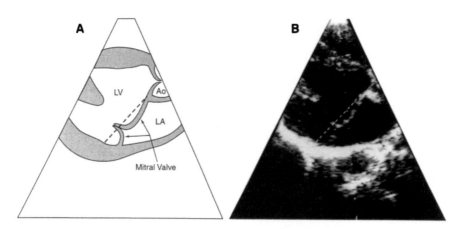

FIGURE 24.2. Diagram (A) and photograph (B) of a two-dimensional echocardiogram demonstrating a parasternal long-axis view of the mitral valve. Both the anterior and posterior leaflets billow beyond the valve plane (dotted line) into the left atrium. Ao, aorta; LA, left atrium; LV, left ventricle.

Natural History

The prognosis of the majority of individuals with MVP is overwhelmingly benign. This is reflected in the recommendations of the American Academy of Pediatrics' Committee on Sports Medicine and Fitness that asymptomatic patients with MVP be allowed to participate in all activities unless they have significant mitral regurgitation or a family history of MVP associated with sudden death.[13]

In Bisset and coworkers'[14] study of 118 children who were referred for evaluation because of a click or murmur and followed for 7 years, no patient died suddenly or developed progressive mitral insufficiency. One patient developed endocarditis, and one had a cerebrovascular accident.

Nishimura et al.[15] found a similarly low (4.2%) rate of complications in an older population identified echocardiographically and followed for 6 years. Several other studies[16,17] have documented a very low risk of complications in individuals identified as having only MVP without other abnormalities of the valve such as thickening or significant mitral regurgitation. Even these low complication rates may be overestimates, because all but one of these studies[16] included only patients specifically referred for evaluation or echocardiography and many asymptomatic patients may not come to medical attention.

Risk factors for the development of serious complications related to MVP have included male sex, age (an increased risk of complications is associated with more advanced age), a holosystolic murmur and enlargement of left-sided chambers (both reflecting the presence of significant mitral regurgitation), and thickening of the mitral valve.[16–18] In contrast to the other studies, Duren et al.[19] described serious complications in 100 of 300 patients, although this was a selected, largely symptomatic population referred to a cardiology center for evaluation.

Mitral Valve Prolapse Syndrome

Many patients with MVP have been identified because of complaints of dyspnea, fatigue, chest pain that is atypical for ischemia, and an awareness of their heartbeat even in the absence of documented arrhythmias. They often have nonspecific electrocardiographic changes, especially in the inferior distribution,[20] thoracic bony abnormalities, and sometimes symptoms of anxiety or panic attacks. These patients have been said to have the MVP syndrome, and their symptoms may be responsive to β-blocker therapy. Whether these symptoms represent a true syndrome or several common conditions occurring in the same patient remains uncertain. Devereux et al.[21] compared patients with echocardiographically documented MVP to their relatives and spouses without echocardiographic abnormalities and found MVP to be associated with thoracic bony abnormalities, low body weight, palpitations, and low blood pressure but not with nonischemic chest pain, dyspnea, panic attacks, or electrocardiographic abnormalities.

Significant Mitral Regurgitation

The development of symptomatic mitral regurgitation that requires mitral valve repair or replacement is one of the most important complications associated with MVP.[1,5,21] In Duren and coworkers' study,[19] 10% of patients developed asymptomatic mitral regurgitation during an average of 6 years, and 7% required mitral valve surgery for progressive mitral insufficiency not due to infective endocarditis. Wilcken et al.[22] calculated that approximately 4% of men and 1.5% of women with MVP will require mitral valve surgery by age 70. The risk of surgery was negligible before the age of 50, however, and was minimal in women. Fukuda et al.[23] have identified the presence of a holosystolic murmur, posterior leaflet prolapse, and thickening of the mitral valve as additional risk factors for the development of severe mitral regurgitation. Despite the low overall incidence of severe mitral regurgitation in patients with MVP, myxomatous degeneration of the valve is now the most common indication for mitral valve repair or replacement among patients with isolated mitral regurgitation.[24]

Although these characteristics may be useful in predicting who will develop severe mitral regurgitation, our ability to identify early on which patients are at high risk remains poor. It has been suggested[25] that the provocation of mitral regurgitation during exercise is predictive in patients without this finding at rest. However, the usefulness of these data as isolated screening tests, independent of the mentioned risk factors, has been criticized.

The mechanisms by which progressive valvular regurgitation develops may vary. Infective endocarditis causes only a minority of cases. In a study of excised pathologic specimens of myxomatous mitral valves, Roberts et al.[26] identified dilatation of the mitral annulus and rupture of chordae tendineae as the primary mechanisms; 58% of the valves exhibited both features. Among patients who undergo valve replacement, the presence of excessive valvular tissue may make them candidates for mitral valve repair, providing an impetus for close follow-up and earlier operative intervention.

Infective Endocarditis

Infective endocarditis may result in significant morbidity, including the need for valve replacement, and mortality in individuals with MVP. In their retrospective review, Nishimura et al.[15] identified a 1.3% incidence of endocarditis, whereas 6% of Duren and coworkers' prospectively followed patients developed this complication.[19] Clemens et al.,[27] using a case-control design, calculated an odds ratio of 8.2 for the development of endocarditis when hospitalized MVP patients referred for echocardiography were compared with other patients without risk factors for endocarditis who also underwent this procedure. However, subsequent studies have suggested a lower risk for this complication.

The risk for endocarditis is clearly low among individuals without significant valvular deformity or mitral regurgitation. At present, the American Heart Association does not recommend antibiotic prophylaxis for patients without mitral regurgitation.[28] Cost-benefit calculations are probably favorable for the treatment of patients with mitral regurgitation.[29]

Cerebral Ischemia

An association between cerebral ischemic events and MVP received attention in the early 1980s.[30,31] These events have been attributed to the embolization of fibrin–platelet thrombi[30] that may be adherent to such valves and are believed to account for an excess of young patients lacking risk factors other than MVP who present with symptoms of cerebral ischemia. Infective endocarditis and atrial fibrillation due to progressive mitral regurgitation represent other well-defined risk factors for cerebral ischemia. Nevertheless, long-term follow-up of two cohorts of patients with MVP has identified an overall risk of cerebral ischemic events of 1% to 4%.[15,19] More recent population-based studies, albeit of an older population, have failed to identify an increased risk for initial[32] or recurrent[33] cerebral ischemia or stroke in patients with MVP.

Atrial and Ventricular Arrhythmias

Palpitations, even in the absence of documented arrhythmias, may be a component of the MVP syndrome. These symptoms lead to the clinical investigation of many patients. Ambulatory electrocardiographic monitoring and exercise testing have documented the presence of atrial and ventricular ectopy of varying complexity in some of these patients.[34] Despite this finding, the majority of individuals with MVP remain free of dangerous arrhythmias.[34]

An association between the Wolff-Parkinson-White syndrome, specifically left-sided accessory connections, and MVP has been suggested but not proven and may be an artifact of the frequency of MVP in the young adults who present with this syndrome.[34] There is no evidence that MVP is a mechanical consequence of the abnormal ventricular activation associated with preexcitation, and, if present, MVP will persist even after ablation of the accessory connection and normalization of contraction.

Sudden death is a rare complication of MVP recognized in 2.5% of Nishimura and coworkers' patients[15] and 1% of Duren and coworkers' study group.[19] In several studies of the pathology of sudden death victims, the incidence of MVP was not different from that of the general population. Yet, there may be a small group of patients, often young women, sometimes with QT prolongation and a family history of sudden death, who do carry an increased risk.[35] Further, the development of hemodynamically significant mitral regurgitation and ventricular dysfunction carries with it a risk for atrial fibrillation and life-threatening ventricular arrhythmias.

Patients with syncope and ventricular dysfunction and those resuscitated from sustained ventricular arrhythmias merit careful evaluation. Although electrophysiology studies may be helpful in managing these patients, their sensitivity and specificity in the larger group with milder symptoms and preserved ventricular function are uncertain.[36] Generally, in this latter group, atrial and ventricular ectopy, even if frequent, does not require suppressive antiarrhythmic therapy, and some of the deaths associated with MVP may actually be the consequence of such treatment. If therapy is felt to be necessary, β-blockade is safe and may be very effective. In contrast, patients with serious ventricular arrhythmias may require treatment with amiodarone or the protection of a defibrillator.

Other Associations

Morphologically abnormal, prolapsing mitral valves are a component of several inherited connective tissue diseases, including Marfan's syndrome, Ehlers–Danlos syndrome, and perhaps pseudoxanthoma elasticum.[37] Most individuals with isolated MVP are not believed to have a form of these conditions, however.

At one time some believed MVP to be a sequela of rheumatic fever. This does not appear to be the case.[38] Associations with autoimmune diseases such as systemic lupus erythematosus,[39] thyroid disease,[40] ophthalmoplegia,[41] abnormal cardiovascular regulation, and a variety of psychiatric syndromes, including panic attacks and anxiety neuroses,[42] have been suggested but not proven.

Summary

MVP is a very common morphological condition defined by physical examination and echocardiographic criteria. Often asymptomatic, it may be associated with a relatively benign but often troublesome syndrome characterized by fatigue, chest pain, and palpitations. Much less commonly, serious complications such as hemodynamically significant mitral regurgitation, infective endocarditis, life-threatening arrhythmias, and stroke may develop.

References

1. Savage DD, Garrison RJ, Devereux RB, et al. Mitral valve prolapse in the general population, I: epidemiologic features: the Framingham Study. *Am Heart J.* 1983;106: 571–576.
2. Barlow JB, Pocock WA. The problem of nonejection systolic clicks and associated mitral systolic murmurs: emphasis on the billowing mitral leaflet syndrome. *Am Heart J.* 1975; 90:636–655.
3. Aufderheide S, Lax D, Goldberg SJ. Gender differences in dehydration-induced mitral valve prolapse. *Am Heart J.* 1994;129:83–86.
4. Devereux RB, Perloff JK, Reichek N, Josephson ME. Mitral valve prolapse. *Circulation.* 1976;54:3–14.
5. Devereux RB, Kramer-Fox R, Kligfield P. Mitral valve pro-

6. Tamura K, Fukuda Y, Ishizaki M, Masuda Y, Yamanaka N, Ferrans VJ. Abnormalities in elastic fibers and other connective-tissue components of floppy mitral valve. *Am Heart J.* 1995;129:1149–1158.
7. Weissman NJ, Pini R, Roman MJ, et al. In vivo mitral valve morphology and motion in mitral valve prolapse. *Am J Cardiol.* 1994;73:1080–1088.
8. Hutchins GM, Moore GW, Skoog DK. The association of floppy mitral valve with disjunction of the mitral annulus fibrosis. *N Engl J Med.* 1986;314:535–540.
9. Liedtke AJ, Gault JH, Leaman DM, Blumenthal MS. Geometry of left ventricular contraction in the systolic click syndrome. *Circulation.* 1973;47:27–35.
10. Devereux RB, Brown WT, Kramer-Fox R, Sachs I. Inheritance of mitral valve prolapse: effect of age and sex on gene expression. *Ann Intern Med.* 1982;97:826–832.
11. Udoshi MB, Shah A, Fisher VJ, Dolgin M. Incidence of mitral valve prolapse in subjects with thoracic skeletal abnormalities: a prospective study. *Am Heart J.* 1979;97:303–311.
12. Rosenberg CA, Derman GH, Grabb WC, Buda AJ. Hypomastia and mitral-valve prolapse. *N Engl J Med.* 1983;309: 1230–1232.
13. Committee on Sports Medicine and Fitness. Mitral valve prolapse and athletic participation in children and adolescents. *Pediatrics.* 1995;95:789–790.
14. Bisset GS III, Schwartz DC, Meyer RA, James FW, Kaplan S. Clinical spectrum and long-term follow-up of isolated mitral valve prolapse in 119 children. *Circulation.* 1980;62: 423–429.
15. Nishimura RA, McGoon MD, Shub C, Miller FA Jr, Ilstrup DM, Tajik AJ. Echocardiographically documented mitral-valve prolapse. *N Engl J Med.* 1985;313:1305–1309.
16. Zuppiroli A, Rinaldi M, Kramer-Fox R, Favilli S, Roman MJ, Devereux RB. Natural history of mitral valve prolapse. *Am J Cardiol.* 1995;75:1028–1032.
17. Marks AR, Choong CY, Sanfilippo AJ, Ferre M, Weyman AE. Identification of high-risk and low-risk subgroups of patients with mitral-valve prolapse. *N Engl J Med.* 1989;320: 1031–1036.
18. Devereux RB, Kramer-Fox R, Shear MK, Kligfield P, Pini R, Savage DD. Diagnosis and classification of severity of mitral valve prolapse: methodologic, biologic, and prognostic considerations. *Am Heart J.* 1987;113:1265–1280.
19. Duren DR, Becker AE, Dunning AJ. Long-term follow-up of idiopathic mitral valve prolapse in 300 patients: a prospective study. *J Am Coll Cardiol.* 1988;11:42–47.
20. Lobstein HP, Horwitz LD, Curry GC, Mullins CB. Electrocardiographic abnormalities and coronary arteriograms in the mitral click-murmur syndrome. *N Engl J Med.* 1973; 289: 127–131.
21. Devereux RB, Kramer-Fox R, Brown WT, et al. Relation between clinical features of the mitral prolapse syndrome and echo-cardiographically documented mitral valve prolapse. *J Am Coll Cardiol.* 1986;8:763–772.
22. Wilcken DEL, Hickey AJ. Lifetime risk for patients with mitral valve prolapse of developing severe valve regurgitation requiring surgery. *Circulation.* 1988;78:10–14.

lapse: causes, clinical manifestations, and management. *Ann Intern Med.* 1989;111:305–317.

23. Fukuda N, Oki T, Iuchi A, et al. Predisposing factors for severe mitral regurgitation in idiopathic mitral valve prolapse. *Am J Cardiol.* 1995;76:503–507.

24. Rosen SE, Borer JS, Hochreiter C, et al. Natural history of the asymptomatic/minimally symptomatic patient with severe mitral regurgitation secondary to mitral valve prolapse and normal right and left ventricular performance. *Am J Cardiol.* 1994;74:374–380.

25. Stoddard MF, Prince CR, Dillon S, Longaker RA, Morris GT, Liddell NE. Exercise-induced mitral regurgitation is a predictor of morbid events in subjects with mitral valve prolapse. *J Am Coll Cardiol.* 1995;25:693–699.

26. Roberts WC, McIntosh CL, Wallace RB. Mechanisms of severe mitral regurgitation in mitral valve prolapse determined from analysis of operatively excised valve. *Am Heart J.* 1987;113:1316–1323.

27. Clemens JD, Horwitz RI, Jaffe CC, Feinstein AR, Stanton BF. A controlled evaluation of the risk of bacterial endocarditis in persons with mitral-valve prolapse. *N Engl J Med.* 1982;307:776–781.

28. Dajani AS, Bisno AL, Chung KJ, et al. Prevention of bacterial endocarditis. *JAMA.* 1990;264:2919–2922.

29. Devereux RB, Frary CJ, Kramer-Fox R, Roberts RB, Ruchlin HS. Cost-effectiveness of infective endocarditis prophylaxis for mitral valve prolapse with or without a mitral regurgitant murmur. *Am J Cardiol.* 1994;74:1024–1029.

30. Hanson MR, Conomy JP, Hodgman JR. Brain events associated with mitral valve prolapse. *Stroke.* 1980;11:499–505.

31. Barnett HJM, Boughner DR, Taylor DW, Cooper PE, Kostuk WJ, Nichol PM. Further evidence relating mitral-valve prolapse to cerebral ischemic events. *N Engl J Med.* 1980; 302:139–144.

32. Orencia AJ, Petty GW, Khandheria BK, et al. Risk of stroke with mitral valve prolapse in population-based cohort study. *Stroke.* 1995;26:7–13.

33. Orencia AJ, Petty GW, Khandheria BK, O'Fallon WM, Whisnant JP. Mitral valve prolapse and the risk of stroke after initial cerebral ischemia. *Neurology.* 1995;45: 1083–1086.

34. Levy S. Arrhythmias in the mitral valve prolapse syndrome: clinical significance and management. *PACE.* 1992;15: 1080–1088.

35. Dollar AL, Roberts WC. Morphologic comparison of patients with mitral valve prolapse who died suddenly with patients who died from severe valvular dysfunction or other conditions. *J Am Coll Cardiol.* 1991;17:921–931.

36. Babuty D, Cosnay P, Breuillac JC, et al. Ventricular arrhythmia factors in mitral valve prolapse. *PACE.* 1994;17: 1090–1099.

37. Lebwohl MG, Distefano D, Prioleau PG, Uram M, Yannuzzi LA, Fleischmajer R. Pseudoxanthoma elasticum and mitral-valve prolapse. *N Engl J Med.* 1982;307:228–231.

38. Zuppiroli A, Roman MJ, O'Grady M, Devereux RB. Lack of association between mitral valve prolapse and history of rheumatic fever. *Am Heart J.* 1996;131:525–529.

39. Comens SM, Alpert MA, Sharp GC, et al. Frequency of mitral valve prolapse in systemic lupus erythematosus, progressive systemic sclerosis, and mixed connective tissue disease. *Am J Cardiol.* 1989;63:369–372.

40. Channick BJ, Adlin EV, Marks AD, et al. Hyperthyroidism and mitral-valve prolapse. *N Engl J Med.* 1981;305:497–500.

41. Darsee JR, Miklozek CL, Heymsfield SB, Hopkins LC Jr, Wenger NK. Mitral valve prolapse and ophthalmoplegia: a progressive, cardioneurologic syndrome. *Ann Intern Med.* 1980;92:735–741.

42. Stringer JC, Obeid A, O'Shea E. Mitral valve prolapse and addictions. *Am J Cardiol.* 1985;56:808–809.

25

Treatment of Mitral Valve Disease

John A. Elefteriades and John Setaro

For the purposes of this chapter, treatment of mitral valve disease is divided into medical management, catheter valvuloplasty, and surgical techniques. Treatments are divided into those for mitral stenosis and those for mitral regurgitation. Specific attention is paid at the conclusion of this chapter to the issues of the results of mitral valve surgery (especially as regards ventricular function and patient outlook), the complications of mitral valve surgery, the controversies of repair versus replacement, and chordal division versus preservation, and the issue of mitral valve surgery in the "bad" ventricle.

Medical Management

Mitral Stenosis

Although the mechanical lesion of valvular obstruction cannot be influenced by medical treatment, complications associated with mitral stenosis can be avoided or ameliorated by appropriate pharmacologic therapies. Thus, prevention of recurrent rheumatic fever, antibiotic prophylaxis and treatment for infective endocarditis, control of heart rate and rhythm, regulation of intravascular volume, and anticoagulation for heart failure or atrial fibrillation represent the foundations of medical treatment for mitral valvular stenosis.

Secondary prophylaxis for patients who have experienced an initial attack of rheumatic fever and are considered at risk for recurrence can avert recurrent episodes and protect against further deterioration in valvular function.[1] The American Heart Association has recommended a secondary prevention program consisting of 1.2 million units of intramuscular benzathine penicillin G monthly, or oral penicillin V at a dose of 250 mg daily; sulfadiazine at a dose of 1 g daily serves as an accepted alternative for patients allergic to penicillin.[2] In low-risk patients, treatment for 5 years or until age 18 has been suggested; lifetime prophylaxis is advocated for higher-risk individuals. Standard infective endocarditis prophylaxis directed against potential local microbial pathogens should be administered in the setting of dental, gynecologic, gastrointestinal, or surgical procedures in which bacterial contamination of the bloodstream may occur.[3] When clinical suspicion exists, a diligent search for the presence, source, and bacteriologic identity of infective endocarditis should be undertaken in patients with mitral stenosis. A full discussion of the diagnosis and treatment of infective endocarditis is beyond the scope of this section and is available elsewhere in this textbook.

Mitral stenosis results in abnormal left ventricular filling and therefore merits careful management of intravascular volume status as well as regulation of heart rate to permit adequate time for filling in diastole. Oral or intravenous diuretics and reduction in sodium intake are useful therapies when symptoms of pulmonary congestion are present. Conditions that result in increased heart rate and cardiovascular demand, such as infection, fever, anemia, and strenuous exercise, may require additional medical adjustments. β-Adrenergic blockers may assist in alleviating symptoms and enhancing exercise capacity for patients who are either in sinus rhythm or in atrial fibrillation. Additional rate control may be achieved by the concomitant use of digitalis glycosides or atrioventricular nodal–blocking calcium channel antagonists such as verapamil or diltiazem. Antiarrhythmic agents can be used to effect conversion to sinus rhythm or to assist in maintaining sinus rhythm following electrical cardioversion. A 3-week program of full anticoagulation prior to elective chemical or electrical cardioversion is desirable so that restoration of sinus rhythm is not complicated by systemic thromboembolization. The prognosis for successful conversion and maintenance of sinus rhythm in mitral stenosis patients with atrial fibrillation is inversely proportional to the duration of the abnormal rhythm and the size of the left atrium. If hemodynamic instability exists with new-onset rapid atrial fibrillation, emergency electrical cardioversion should be considered.

Apart from preparation for cardioversion, full systemic anticoagulation should be administered for stroke prophylaxis to all patients with mitral stenosis and atrial fibrillation, as well as those who exhibit congestive heart failure with a history of a venous thrombotic event. It is not clear that anticoagulation has any beneficial role in the patient with mitral valvular stenosis who is still in normal sinus rhythm.

Mitral Regurgitation

The medical therapy of chronic mitral valvular regurgitation is based on regulation of volume state, left ventricular afterload reduction, and prevention of infective endocarditis.[3] Sodium restriction, administration of oral or intravenous diuretics, anticoagulation in the presence of atrial fibrillation or heart failure and prior venous thrombotic events, and treatment with digitalis glycosides in the context of congestive heart failure or atrial fibrillation constitute the mainstays of medical management. Issues relating to elective or emergent cardioversion from atrial fibrillation in the setting of mitral regurgitation parallel those already listed for patients with mitral stenosis.

Afterload reduction therapy with vasodilating agents is of particular importance in mitral valvular regurgitation of both chronic and acute types. In either case, decreased impedance to left ventricular ejection favors forward physiologic blood flow into the aorta versus retrograde flow across the regurgitant mitral valve into the left atrium. The degree of mitral regurgitation may also be improved by the reduction in left ventricular size and mitral annular diameter achievable with afterload reduction therapy. Hydralazine and angiotensin-converting enzyme inhibitors have been shown to produce clinical improvement, although randomized controlled trials showing that afterload reduction therapy can delay the need for surgical intervention have not been reported for mitral regurgitation. Encouraging reports favoring such therapies for the left ventricular volume overload lesion of aortic valvular regurgitation suggest the need for further study in mitral regurgitation.[4,5]

In acute mitral valvular regurgitation such as that arising from ischemic papillary muscle rupture, torn chordae tendineae, or severe infective endocarditis, afterload reduction using an intravenous vasodilator such as sodium nitroprusside serves to enhance antegrade blood flow and can abolish the V wave observed in the pulmonary capillary wedge tracing (Figure 25.1). When myocardial ischemia or injury is a factor, intravenous nitroglycerin serves as a valuable pharmacologic adjunct. In the acute setting, control of intravascular volume may create only modest benefit, and mechanical ventilation is often indicated. Intra-aortic balloon counterpulsation

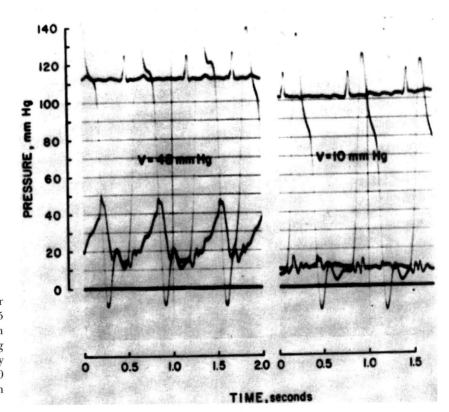

FIGURE 25.1. Severe acute mitral valvular regurgitation with V waves visible to 45 mm Hg (left) prior to the administration of the intravenous afterload-reducing agent nitroprusside. Following therapy (right) the V waves have declined to 10 mm Hg. Reprinted with permission from Harshaw CW, et al.[6]

is frequently helpful because the systolic unloading effect promotes antegrade blood flow into the systemic circuit. Such measures serve as a prelude to surgical intervention, which is the optimal treatment for patients with acute hemodynamically intolerable mitral regurgitation.

Catheter Valvuloplasty

Advances in catheter-based technologies, in the context of the long-standing favorable experiences with closed surgical mitral commissurotomy, have permitted the development of transcatheter methods for treatment of rheumatic mitral valvular stenosis. As in the operative procedure, balloon mitral valvuloplasty achieves its results through the separation of fused commissures upon balloon inflation. Valve area typically is increased by at least 1 cm[2]. Early as well as long-term hemodynamic and clinical results in relation to valve function parallel those of surgical techniques,[7,8,9] and similar benefits are available in relation to pulmonary vascular pressures and right heart function as well.[10,11] A recent report has documented improvement in left ventricular systolic function through preload augmentation following successful balloon valvuloplasty of the stenotic mitral valve.[12]

To determine which patients are appropriate candidates for mitral balloon valvuloplasty, an echocardiographic scoring system has been devised based on four possible findings graded on a scale of 0 to 4 (favorable to unfavorable). These criteria include leaflet rigidity, valvular thickening, subvalvular thickening, and calcification.[13] A score of 8 or less has been linked with favorable early as well as late results in several series. The optimal candidate for balloon mitral valvuloplasty is a young patient with mitral disease of rheumatic origin who has no significant valvular calcification or regurgitation, and no sign of atrial thrombus. Patients who are not ideally

suited for surgical valve replacement for reasons of pregnancy, childbearing potential, or critical comorbid illness may serve as acceptable candidates for a balloon procedure as well.[14] In addition, the balloon technique has proved ideal in international settings where resources are limited and rheumatic heart disease is prevalent in younger patients.

The mitral valve is typically approached via the transinteratrial septal route. Valvuloplasty employs either a system of one or two cylindrical balloons or a single (Inoue) nylon–rubber balloon that possesses a waist that allows it to position itself securely across the valve (Figure 2). The creation of an interatrial septal defect by device passage across the transseptal puncture site is often noted yet is usually of no lasting clinical significance. Infrequent complications include leaflet tears, chordal or papillary rupture leading to mitral regurgitation, cerebral embolic events, cardiac tamponade related to transseptal puncture, and cardiac perforation (witnessed less often with the use of the Inoue device).[14]

Both open surgical commissurotomy and balloon mitral valvuloplasty performed by experienced operators are associated with favorable early and long-term outcomes. A direct comparison of the two methods in patients who were excellent candidates for either (echocardiographic mean score 6.7) showed good early hemodynamic results, with 72% of the balloon valvuloplasty group enjoying New York Heart Association class I status at 3 years; 57% of the surgical group were in class I.[15] Repeat catheterization at the 3-year point showed a significant difference in mitral valve area favoring the balloon-treated group (2.4 versus 1.8 cm[2]). No data is yet available for the comparison of transcatheter and surgical techniques in patients whose mitral valves disclose evidence of more advanced disease. In sum, for patients with flexible noncalcified valves, mitral balloon valvuloplasty should be viewed as an acceptable alternative to surgery.

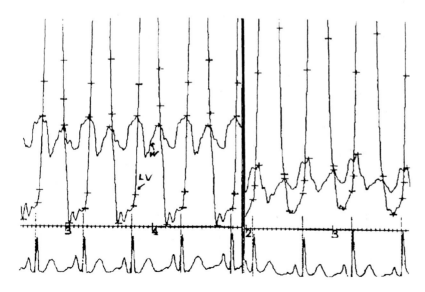

FIGURE 25.2. Hemodynamic study before (left) and after (right) transcatheter treatment of mitral valve stenosis using a single-balloon (Inoue) technique. Note reduction in end-diastolic pulmonary capillary wedge (W) versus left ventricular (LV) gradient from 21.1 to 7.6 mm Hg at the conclusion of the procedure. Courtesy of John Lasala, M.D., Ph.D., Cardiac Catheterization Laboratory, Barnes Hospital-Washington University School of Medicine, St. Louis, Missouri.

Surgical Treatment

Mitral Stenosis

Mitral stenosis was among the first valvular cardiac lesions to be treated surgically. Surgical treatment was made feasible by the ingenious recognition that the mitral valve could be approached in the closed, beating heart without extracorporeal circulation—the so-called closed mitral commissurotomy (Figure 25.3). This procedure was pioneered simultaneously by Harken and by Bailey in the 1940s[16,17] and later refined by Glenn[18] and others. A variety of specific techniques and surgical implements (including a sewing thimble borrowed from Dr. Glenn's wife) were described to facilitate closed commissurotomy. The principle was to break open the commissural fusion, to relieve the stensosis, without disturbing the subvalvular apparatus and inducing unwanted regurgitation. Dr. Glenn reported 100 consecutive patients operated by closed commissurotomy without a single mortality—a remarkable accomplishment for that or any era. Relief of stenosis was effective and durable with this technique. We still see patients of Dr. Glenn's, who were operated two to three decades ago, enjoying continued good relief of their stenosis.

Closed commissurotomy has been largely supplanted by open mitral valve surgery. The generation of surgeons trained and experienced in closed commissurotomy has largely reached retirement age. Concomitantly, techniques for open cardiac surgery have advanced to the point that use of the heart–lung machine is very well tolerated and quite routine. Currently, commissurotomy is almost always performed by the open technique. The open technique allows for direct visualization of the fused leaflets and precisely applied surgical commissurotomy (Figure 25.4). The open technique also allows

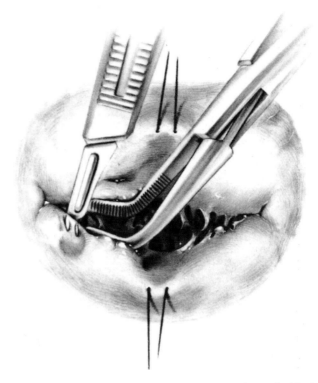

FIGURE 25.4. Open mitral commisurotomy, performed with the heart–lung machine. Reprinted with permission from Harlan et al.[20]

surgical relief of the subvalvular fusion (of thickened chordae) that so frequently accompanies rheumatic leaflet fusion.

When the leaflets are too severely damaged to permit commissurotomy, as is the case in severe leaflet calcification, the valve must be replaced by a prosthesis, either biologic or mechanical. The diseased valve is excised, sutures are placed around the annulus, and the prosthetic valve is lowered into the annulus and seated in position (Figure 25.5). This procedure is well standardized. The most frequent problem for the surgeon is extensive calcification of the mitral annulus, especially posteriorly. This can present a vexing and, at times, life-threatening problem. The general options, outlined by Mills,[21] in the scenario of extreme calcification of the posterior annulus include (1) decalcifying the annulus, with the attendant danger to the circumflex coronary artery and coronary sinus; (2) attaching the posterior portion of the prosthetic valve onto the left atrial wall, rather than the annulus proper; (3) leaving part of the posterior leaflet intact and attaching the valve sewing ring to the free edge of the posterior leaflet; and (4) surgically drilling the calcified leaflet/annulus to permit placement of individual sutures. Thanks to the pioneering accomplishments of Carpentier[22] (see later) many surgeons are currently comfortable with decalcifying the annulus without fear of disrupting adjacent structures or impairing atrial–

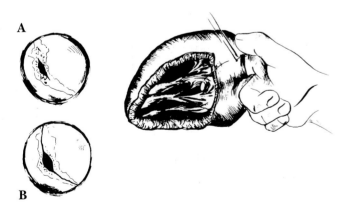

FIGURE 25.3. Closed mitral commisurotomy. The finger is inserted without cardiopulmonary bypass through the left atrial appendage into the mitral valve, which is fractured to convert from the preoperative stenotic state (**A**) to the postoperative relieved state (**B**). Reprinted with permission from Ionescu and Cohn.[19]

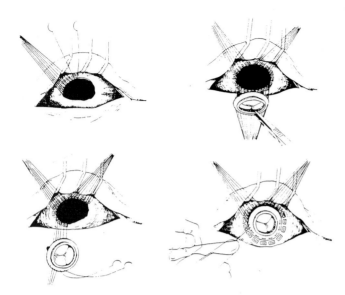

FIGURE 25.5. Mitral valve replacement. The diseased valve is excised, sutures are placed around the annulus, the valve is lowered into place, and the sutures tied to secure the new valve. Reprinted with permission from Ionescu and Cohn.[19]

ventricular continuity. Vander Salm[23] has reported ultrasonic decalcification of the calcified annulus, which may be less likely to cause disruption of the atrial–ventricular continuity.

Indications for surgery in mitral stenosis consist largely of the presence of stenosis and associated symptoms of mild or greater severity. Surgery is recommended for patients with class II or higher symptoms. Untreated mitral stenosis not only progressively impairs quality of life but also leads to pulmonary hypertension, right ventricular failure, and death. Mitral stenosis does, however, unlike other valvular lesions, protect the left ventricle, which sees only a small volume load and no increased pressure load. A valve area of less than 1.5 cm^2 is usually considered severe enough for surgical intervention. An area less than 1.0 cm^2 is considered critical mitral stenosis unequivocally requiring surgical intervention.

Mitral Regurgitation

The appropriate indications for surgical treatment of mitral regurgitation have been the subject of debate. It is known that in many patients, unchecked severe mitral regurgitation leads to inexorable left ventricular dilatation and dysfunction based on the inherent increased volume load. Some of the debate has been predicated on uncertainty regarding the natural history of asymptomatic or minimally symptomatic mitral regurgitation. It is generally accepted that the presence of severe mitral regurgitation and severe symptoms (class III or IV) warrants surgery. Until recently, for patients with no or mild symptoms (class I or II), the recommendation was to

avoid surgery unless evidence indicated progressive enlargement of the left ventricle or a progressive fall in ejection fraction. Very recent evidence[24,25] indicates that even with mild symptoms, severe mitral regurgitation is a serious cardiac illness, with a 6.3% yearly mortality and a progression to death or surgery in fully 90% of patients over 10 years (Figure 25.6). Accordingly, current recommendations are for earlier intervention, usually at the time when the ejection fraction approaches the lower limits of normal (50%–55%).[26,27] Cardiologists are becoming more comfortable with earlier mitral valve surgery because risks of surgery have fallen with modern techniques, and many patients can undergo repair rather than replacement. The recent advent of chordal-sparing valve replacement (see later) further encourages earlier surgical intervention.

For decades, the standard treatment for mitral regurgitation was mitral valve replacement. Most surgeons considered the wispy mitral valve leaflets too ephemeral to permit direct corrective procedures. Although a few surgeons[28,29] persisted in exploring reparative techniques, it was not until the germinal contributions of Carpentier that mitral valve repair became a widespread clinical reality. Carpentier's methodical and imaginative development of techniques for repair of the mitral apparatus in regurgitant lesions, culminating in the address to the American Association for Thoracic Surgery in 1983 entitled "Cardiac Valve Surgery—the 'French correction,'"[30] is certainly one of the most significant contributions in the history of cardiac surgery. The precise communication of these findings and techniques to the community of cardiac surgeons via direct, televised operative sessions constitutes one of the greatest achievements in the history of medical communication.

Carpentier's reparative techniques are based on his precise delineation of the pathology of the mitral apparatus in regurgitant lesions. Carpentier classified the etiology of regurgitation into three categories (Figure 25.7): (1) normal leaflet motion, (2) restricted leaflet

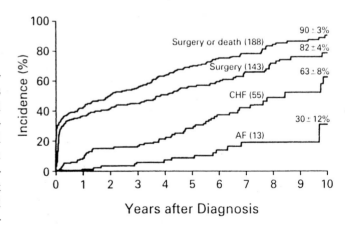

FIGURE 25.6. Outlook after detection of mitral insufficiency. Reprinted with permission from Ling et al.[24]

FIGURE 25.7. The classification of regurgitant lesions into those with normal, restricted, and excessive leaflet motion. Reprinted with permission from Carpentier.[30]

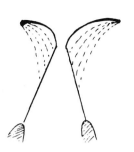
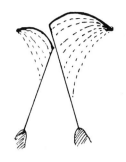
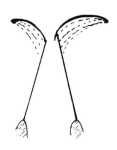

Type I
Normal Leaflet Motion

Type II
Leaflet Prolapse

Type III
Restricted Leaflet Motion

motion, and (3) excessive leaflet motion. When leaflet motion is normal, regurgitation results from dilatation of the annulus, usually as a consequence of left ventricular dysfunction and dilatation. Because of the dilatation, the leaflets can no longer coapt centrally, leading to regurgitation. This can be corrected by restoration of the size and shape of the annulus by placement of a prosthetic ring (Figure 25.8). Restricted leaflet motion is usually seen as part of the pattern of rheumatic disease and can often be corrected by relief of subvalvular chordal fusion. Excess leaflet motion is usually caused by primary degenerative disease of the mitral leaflets and chordae.

Carpentier further subclassifies the pathology in excessive leaflet motion according to the sites affected. The classification includes a letter (A for the anterior leaflet and B for the posterior) and a number (1 to 3 for the first, second, or third scallop, numbered from the surgeon's left to right). The recognition of the pathophysiology of mitral insufficiency progressed in lockstep with

the advancement of echocardiographic techniques, especially the advent of transesophageal echocardiography. The echocardiogram can be used to predict a specific pathophysiology, such as P2 prolapse. P2 prolapse, from elongated or ruptured chordae, is the commonest and best-known specific lesion. Confirmation of echocardiographic findings is made after the valve is surgically exposed, by comparison of leaflet motion with a reference point, usually the P1 scallop, which does not prolapse in clinical disease. Multiple pathophysiologic abnormalities frequently coexist.

The cornerstone of Carpentier repair is the quadrangular resection of the prolapsed posterior leaflet (Figure 25.9). After resection of the prolapsed portion of the posterior leaflet, the annulus is reapproximated with heavy sutures to support the delicate leaflet edges, which are then reapproximated with fine sutures. A prosthetic ring reinforces the repair, taking the hemodynamic load off the leaflets themselves and even off the annulus. Competence is assessed by gentle instillation of saline solution. Not only watertight retention of the saline in the ventricle, but also leaflet coaptation in a smooth "smile" parallel to the posterior annulus, are indicative of a successful repair (Figure 25.10). The repair is reassessed by echocardiogram after the left atrium is closed and the patient weaned from cardiopulmonary bypass. If the operative criteria indicated are met, the echocardiogram will confirm the successful repair.

Central to Carpentier's method is the principle that the anterior annulus, because it is part of the central fibrous infrastructure of the heart, does not dilate. As a corollary, the anterior leaflet cannot be resected in case of excessive leaflet motion, because the annulus could not possibly be imbricated at the site of leaflet resection. A different set of techniques, including chordal shortening and chordal transfer from the posterior leaflet, has been developed for correction of excessive motion of the anterior leaflet.

Carpentier's techniques have evolved and continue to evolve. Others[31-35] have validated the principles of mitral valve repair and extended or elaborated on the tech-

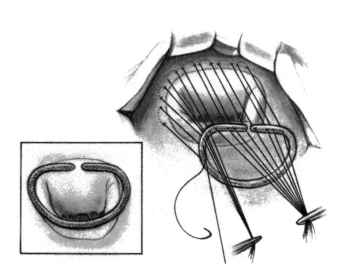

FIGURE 25.8. Placement of Carpentier's annuloplasty ring to correct annular dilatation. Reprinted with permission from Carpentier.[30]

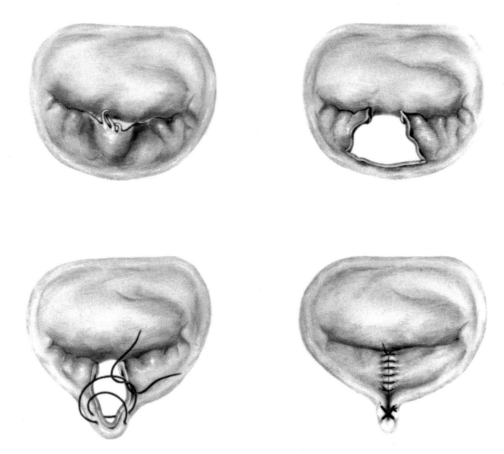

FIGURE 25.9. Quadrangular resection of the posterior leaflet for repair of mitral regurgitation. Reprinted with permission from Carpentier.[30]

niques. Multiple newer annuloplasty rings[36-38] have been developed with specific properties in mind. In particular, there is a belief, based on careful echocardiographic analysis, that flexibility of the prosthetic ring, more closely mimicking nature's original architecture, may be of considerable importance. Dr. Carpentier's own long-term data confirms the excellent effectiveness of his techniques[35] (Figure 25.11). Long-term survival, freedom from thromboembolism, and freedom from anticoagulant-related hemorrhage are superb.

Repair is superior to replacement in several important ways. Evidence, both experimental and clinical, has been accumulating that indicates that repair is hemodynamically superior by virtue of its preservation of the chordal-papillary muscle apparatus. Elegant studies by Dr. Miller and colleagues at Stanford University have shown the importance of the chordal-papillary apparatus in the laboratory.[39,40] Studies by Phillips[41] and others have shown better preservation of left ventricular systolic function with sparing of the papillary apparatus. Studies have been published that demonstrate an advantage in long-term survival in patients who have repair rather than replacement.[42-44] Another advantage of repair over placement of a mechanical valve is that long-term anti-

coagulation is not required; most surgeons do, however, administer an anticoagulant for several months after repair to allow the prosthetic ring to endothelialize. Biologic valves, like repaired valves, do not in and of themselves require long-term anticoagulation.

Not all regurgitant lesions can or should be repaired. Valve replacement is the procedure of choice if repair is complex or unlikely to remain secure. As with mitral stenosis, either a biologic or mechanical prosthesis may be selected.

Dr. Carpentier has recently shown[45] that repair techniques are indeed effective in the mitral valve disease of Marfan's syndrome. Prior concerns had centered on the possibility of early disruption of the repair due to intrinsic structural weakness of the Marfan's mitral leaflet connective tissue. Dr. Carpentier demonstrated excellent short-term and long-term results without recurrence of mitral insufficiency.

Techniques have now been developed that allow some of the benefits of repair when replacement is necessary. Specifically, multiple techniques have been described[46-48] that permit retention of the chordal apparatus, in its entirety, despite placement of a biological or mechanical valve. Formerly, concerns about potential interference

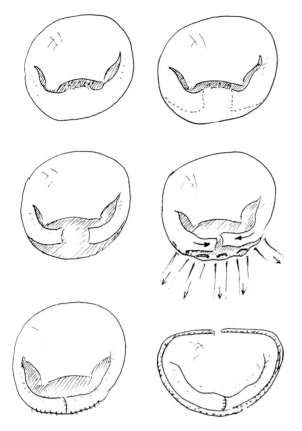

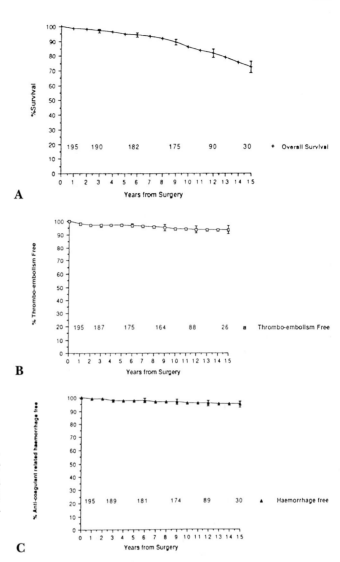

FIGURE 25.10. Assessement of adequacy of mitral valve repair. Above, saline is injected to test visually for residual prolapse or leak. Below, the line of leaflet coaptation should resemble a smooth "smile" (left). An asymmetric smile, like that of facial palsy, results in improper leaflet coaptation and residual regurgitation. Reprinted with permission from Carpentier.[30]

FIGURE 25.11. Long-term results after mitral valve repair with Carpentier techniques. **A, B,** and **C** demonstrate, respectively, long-term survival, freedom from thromboembolism, and freedom from hemorrhage after valve repair. Reprinted with permission from Deloche et al.[35]

with prosthetic valve function prevented surgeons from saving the chordal attachments. It is now well demonstrated that the chordal apparatus can be preserved in its entirety without impingement on the prosthetic valve.

A difficult problem facing the surgeon has to do with the moderately severe mitral insufficiency observed in the patient presenting primarily for coronary revascularization. Frequently, these patients have depressed left ventricular function, with mitral insufficiency resulting from ventricular dilatation. If the insufficiency is grade I to II, most surgeons perform only coronary revascularization, recognizing that revascularization alone, by improving wall motion and function of the mitral papillary apparatus, is likely to improve the mitral insufficiency.[49] If the regurgitation is grade IV, especially if there is evidence of congestive heart failure, pulmonary edema, or acute hemodynamic compromise, most surgeons correct the mitral valvular abnormality by repair or replacement. In moderately severe mitral regurgitation (grade III), controversy exists. Many surgeons perform coronary

revascularization alone, whereas others[50] advocate concomitant valve repair.

Results of Mitral Valve Surgery: Effectiveness, Complications, and Outcome

Mitral valve replacement carries a mortality risk of 4% to 12%.[33,51] Replacement for regurgitation carries a higher risk than replacement for stenosis. Advanced age, emergency operation, advanced heart failure status, prior myocardial infarction, and hepatic dysfunction raise the risk of mitral valve surgery. Mitral repair surgery carries

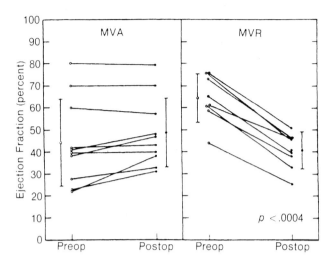

FIGURE 25.12. Influence of mitral valve surgicalon ejection fraction in patients with mitral regurgitation. Left, repair; right, replacement. Data from Goldman et al.[43]

a lower mortality than surgery for replacement, with risk in the range of 0% to 4%.[32]

The incidence of paravalvular leak after mitral valve replacement approaches zero when surgery is carried out at centers with experienced staff. After mitral valve repair, about 1 in 20 patients requires early reoperation for residual mitral insufficiency of clinical significance. Thrombembolic events occur at a rate of 2% to 4% per year after mitral valve replacement but are exceedingly rare after valve repair.[35]

The available data indicates that ejection fraction does fall after replacement of the mitral valve, reflecting loss of the important supporting effect of the mitral papillary-chordal apparatus[41,52] (Figure 25.12A.) This fall in ejection fraction is not seen after valve repair (Figure 25.12B).[42,43] Preliminary data regarding the chordal-sparing replacement techniques discussed earlier indi-

cate that ventricular function is preserved by this type of replacement, perhaps to the same extent as with valve repair. These developments add another tool to the surgeon's armamentarium for preserving ventricular function in valve surgery: valve replacement with complete chordal preservation.

An important complication of mitral valve repair is left ventricular outflow tract obstruction (Figure 25.13). Outflow tract obstruction can produce severe hemodynamic decompensation with life-threatening consequences; when less severe, the phenomenon can produce clinical symptoms late after operation, necessitating reoperation. This phenomenon, which occurs in about 2% of repair procedures, is thought to be the consequence of anterior displacement of the line of coaptation of the two leaflets. The underlying abnormality is excess tissue in the posterior leaflet, which forces the line of coaptation toward the left ventricular outflow tract, whereby the anterior leaflet tissue produces mechanical obstruction during ventricular systole. Preoperative echocardiographic examination can detect those patients with large, redundant posterior leaflets who are likely to be prone to this serious complication. Dr. Carpentier has developed a "sliding plasty" technique in which part of the remaining posterior leaflet (after resection of the prolapsed portion) is removed to decrease the height of the posterior leaflet. This maneuver prevents undue anterior displacement of the line of closure and, thus, discourages systolic anterior motion and outflow tract obstruction.

Acute myocardial infarction occurs in about 5% of patients undergoing mitral valve surgery.[53] The infarct is often inferior and is thought to reflect air embolism to the right coronary artery. Cosgrove and colleagues found this phenomenon to be more common after repair than replacement and incriminated the insufflation of fluid into the left ventricular cavity to check valve competence as a possible cause.

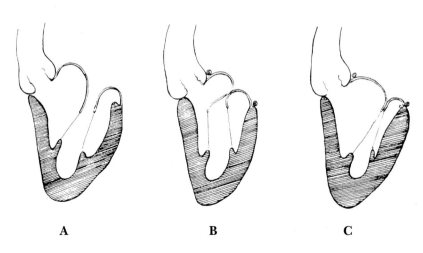

A   B   C

FIGURE 25.13. Schematic representation of the mechanism of left ventricular outflow tract obstruction after mitral valve repair. **A,** Preoperatively, excess tissue of anterior and posterior leaflet is seen, together with a dilated mitral annulus. **B,** After repair and ring placement (shown in cross section), the line of closure is displaced toward the left ventricular outflow tract, whereby the anterior leaflet may produce obstruction. **C,** Surgical reduction of the height of the posterior leaflet at the time of mitral valve repair restores the closure line to an appropriate distance from the left ventricular outflow tract, preventing systolic anterior motion and left ventricular outflow tract obstruction. Modified with permission from Carpentier et al.[37]

One of the most dreaded complications of mitral valve surgery is the disruption of the anatomic left atrial–left ventricular connection that can occur from debridement of the posterior annulus, from excess tension on the annulus, or from trauma from the high-profile struts of a biologic prosthetic valve. This often-lethal complication is seen most commonly after debridement of the calcified mitral valve annulus. Options and techniques for management of the calcified mitral annulus have already been discussed.

Another feared complication of mitral valve surgery is occlusion of the circumflex coronary artery where it runs posteriorly in the atrioventricular groove behind the posterior mitral valve annulus. The proximity of the circumflex artery should be kept in mind while placing all posterior sutures during both valve repair and replacement.

On occasion, the placement of sutures in the mitral annulus in its anterior, cephalad portion can inadvertently ensnare a leaflet of the adjacent aortic valve, resulting in iatrogenic aortic insufficiency. This is an unusual complication that may be seen more frequently in the face of severe mitral annular scarring after multiple valve replacements.

Long-term outcome after mitral valve surgery depends to a large extent on the antecedent level of ventricular function (Figure 25.14). Patients with a normal preoperative ejection fraction have excellent postoperative survival, whereas those with a moderately to severely depressed ejection fraction do much more poorly.

Mitral Valve Surgery in the "Bad" Ventricle

A common, difficult problem faced by the cardiologist and the surgeon has to do with the patient who manifests severe mitral insufficiency in the face of advanced left ventricular dysfunction. It is well known that left ventricular dysfunction and dilatation can lead to mitral insufficiency by impairment of the function of the mitral papillary apparatus. In particular, the transition from the normal ellipsoid shape of the left ventricle to a spherical shape has been shown to adversely affect mitral valve competence.[55] Conversely, severe chronic mitral insufficiency can lead to left ventricular failure because of unsustainable volume overload of the left ventricle. In cases presenting with advanced left ventricular failure and severe mitral insufficiency, it is difficult to know which is the "chicken" and which the "egg." Nonetheless, most authorities agree that continued severe mitral insufficiency in the face of advanced left ventricular dysfunction leads to further worsening of left ventricular function and a downward spiral ending in death. A very recent publication[24] pinpoints the lethal effects of mitral insufficiency over the long-term. It has not been clear, however, whether mitral valve repair or replacement is safe or of benefit in the patient with advanced left ventricular dysfunction.[52]

A recent report[56] on a relatively large group of patients with severe mitral insufficiency and advanced left ventricular dysfunction (mean ejection fraction 29%) finds that (1) surgery is relatively safe (4% risk), (2) ejection fraction does *not* decrease in these patients (despite theoretical concerns that elimination of the low-pressure "blow-off" into the left atrium would overwhelm the failing left ventricle), (3) symptomatic state is markedly improved (with 90% of patients restored to class I or II status), and (4) fair long-term survival (50% at 5 years) is attained following surgery. Survival in this range was felt to be favorable in comparison with that expected with medical management alone. In that study, patients with the lowest ejection fractions (those below 25%) had higher operative mortality and poorer long-term survival, especially in the presence of concomitant severe ischemic disease; cardiac transplantation was recommended for that subset of patients.

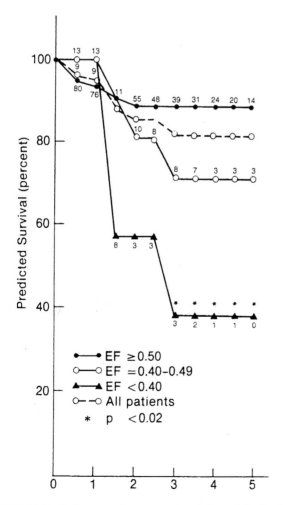

FIGURE 25.14. Influence of preoperative left ventricular function on late survival after mitral valve replacement. Reprinted with permission from Elefteriades et al.[54]

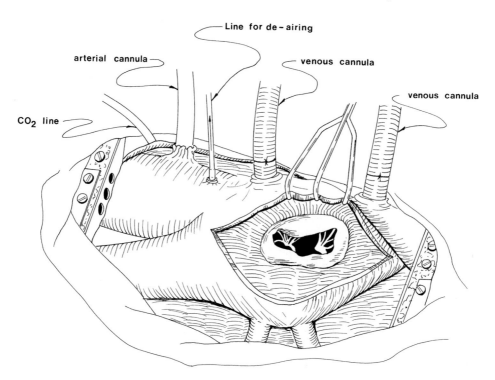

FIGURE 25.15. Approach to re-do mitral valve replacement through a "keyhole" left anterior thoracotomy approach. Reprinted with permission from Braxton et al.[59]

Alternate Approaches for Mitral Valve Surgery

Mitral valve surgery has traditionally been performed through a median sternotomy and an approach through the left atrium posterior to the interatrial groove on the right side of the heart. Recently, alternate approaches—often harking back to earlier historic techniques—have been advocated for particular situations or because of specific advantages. Guiradon[57] has validated an approach through the right atrium with subsequent incision of the interatrial septum. This approach provides excellent exposure with minimal retraction and obviates the occasional difficulties encountered with closure of a direct left atriotomy. Kron[58] and Braxton from our group[59] have reported on performance of mitral valve replacement through a right thoracotomy (Figure 25.15). This approach was found especially useful for mitral reoperations; it avoided bleeding complications and preserved hemodynamics better than the traditional approach of re-do sternotomy. The recent interest in minimally invasive approaches to open heart surgery has produced a number of reports on access through a smaller right thoracotomy.[60,61] Carpentier has taken this one step further, employing a microincision supplemented by video techniques for visualization.[62]

The advances described have transformed mitral valve surgery from the feared high-risk undertaking of two decades ago to a safe, effective procedure that can be performed with a variety of techniques through a number of different approaches.

References

1. Tompkins DG, Boxerbaum B, Liebman J. Long-term prognosis of rheumatic fever patients receiving regular intramuscular benzathine penicillin. *Circulation.* 1972;45: 543–551.
2. Committee on the Prevention of Rheumatic Fever and Bacterial Endocarditis of the American Heart assocation. Prevention of rheumatic fever. *Circulation.* 1988;78: 1082–1086.
3. Dajani AS, Bisano AL, Chung KJ. Prevention of bacterial endocarditis. *JAMA.* 1990;264:2919–2922.
4. Lin M, Chiang HT, Lim SL et al. Vasodilator therapy in chronic asymptomatic aortic regurgitation: enalapril versus hydralazine. *J Am Coll Cardiol.* 1994;24:1046–1053.
5. Scognamiglio R, Rahimtoola SH, Fasoli G. Nifedipine in asymptomatic patients with severe aortic regurgitation and normal left ventricular function. *N Engl J Med.* 1994;331: 689–694.
6. Harshaw CW, Grossman W, Munro AB, Mc Laurin LP. Reduced systemic vascular resistance as therapy for severe mitral regurgitation of valvular origin. *Ann Intern Med.* 1975; 83(3):312–316.
7. Braunwald E, Baunwald NS, Ross J, et al. Effects of mitral valve replacement on the pulmonary vascular dynamics of patients with pulmonary hypertension. *N Engl J Med.* 1965; 273:509–514.
8. Tuzcu EM, Block PC, Palacios IF. Comparison of early versus late experience with percutaneous mitral balloon valvuloplasty. *J Am Coll Cardiol.* 1991;17:1121–1124.

9. Vahanian A, Michel PL, Cormier B, et al. Results of percutaneous mitral commissurotomy in 200 patients. *Am J Cardiol.* 1989;63:847–852.

10. Setaro JF, Clemen MW, Remetz MS. The right ventricle in disorders causing pulmonary venous hypertension. *Cardiol Clin.* 1992;10:165–183.

11. Block PC, Palacios IF. Pulmonary vascular dynamics after percutaneous mitral valvotomy. *J Thorac Cardiovasc Surg.* 1988;96:39–43.

12. Fawzy ME, Choi WB, Mimish L, et al. Immediate and long-term effect of mitral balloon valvotomy on left ventricular volume and systolic function in severe mitral stenosis. *Am Heart J.* 1996;132:356–360.

13. Abascal VM, Wilkins GT, O'Shea JP, et al. Prediction of successful outcome in 130 patients undergoing percutaneous balloon mitral valvotomy. *Circulation.* 1990;82:448–456.

14. Berman AD, McKay RG, Grossman W. Ballon valvuloplasty. In: Baim DS, Grossman W, eds. *Cardiac Catheterization, Angiography, and Intervention.* 5th ed. Baltimore, Md: Williams & Wilkins; 1996:659.

15. Reyes VP, Raju BS, Wynne J, et al. Percutaneous balloon valvuloplasty compared with open surgical commissurotomy for mitral stenosis. *N Engl J Med.* 1994;331:961–967.

16. Bailey CP. The surgical treatment of mitral stenosis. *Chest.* 1949;15:377–392.

17. Harken DE. Surgery of the mitral valve. In: Brest AN, Harken DE, eds. *Cardiovascular Clinics of North America: Cardiac Surgery, 1..* Philadelphia, Pa: FA Davis; 1976: 215–220.

18. Glenn WW, Goodyear AV, Stansel HC Jr, et al. Mitral valvulotomy, II: Operative results after closed valvulotomy: a report of 500 cases. *Am J Surg.* 1969;117:493–501.

19. Ionescu M, Cohn LH. *Mitral Valve Disease: Diagnosis and Treatment.* London: Butterworths; 1985:140.

20. Harlan BJ, Starr A, Harwin FM. *Manual of Cardiac Surgery.* Vol 1. New York: Springer-Verlag; 1980:142.

21. Mills NL, McIntosh IL, Mills LJ. Techniques for management of the calcified mitral annulus. *J Card Surg.* 1986;1:347–355.

22. Carpentier AF, Pellerin M, Fuzellier J-F, Relland JYM. Extensive calcification of the mitral valve annulus. Pathology and surgical management. *J Thorac Cardiovasc Surg.* 1995;111:718–729.

23. Vander Salm TJ. Mitral annular calcification: a new technique for valve replacement. *Ann Thorac Surg.* 1989;48:437–439.

24. Ling LH, Enriques-Sarano M, Seward JB, et al. Clinical outcome of mitral regurgitation due to flail leaflet. *New Engl J Med.* 1996;335:1147–1423.

25. Ross J Jr. The timing of surgery for severe mitral regurgitation. *New Engl J Med.* 1996;335:1156–1458.

26. Enriquez-Sarano M, Tajik AJ, Schaff HV, et al. Echocardiographic prediction of left ventricular function after correction of mitral regurgitation: results and clinical implications. *J Am Coll Cardiol.* 1994;24:1536–1543.

27. Stewart WJ. Choosing the "golden moment" for mitral valve repair. *J Am Coll Cardiol.* 1994;24:1544–1546.

28. Kay JH, Zubiate P, Mendez AM, et al. Mitral valve repair for patients with pure mitral insufficiency. *JAMA.* 1976;236:1584–1586.

29. Duran CG, Pomar JL, Revuelta JM, et al. Conservative operation for mitral insufficiency: critical analysis supported by postoperative hemodynamic studies in 72 patients. *J Thorac Cardiovasc Surg.* 1980;79:326–332.

30. Carpentier A. Cardiac valve surgery—the "French correction." *J Thorac Cardiovasc Surg.* 1983;86:323–337.

31. Cohn LH. Mitral valve surgery: replacement vs. reconstruction. *Hosp Pract.* 1991;26:49–58.

32. Cosgrove DM, Chavez AM, Lytle BW, et al. Results of mitral valve reconstruction. *Circulation.* 1986;74(suppl 1): 82–87.

33. Chavez AM, Cosgrove DM III, Lytle BW, et al. Applicability of mitral valvuloplasty techniques in a North American population. *Am J Cardiol.* 1988;62:253–256.

34. Duran CM. Present status of reconstruction surgery for aortic valve disease. *J Card Surg.* 1993;8:443–452.

35. Deloche A, Jebara VA, Relland JYM, et al. Valve repair with Carpentier techniques: the second decade. *J Thorac Cardiovasc Surg.* 1990;99:990–1002.

36. Cosgrove DM III, Arcidi JM, Rodriguez L, et al. Initial experience with the Cosgrove-Edwards annuloplasty system. *Ann Thorac Surg.* 1995;60:499–503.

37. Carpentier AF, Lessana A, Relland JYM, et al. The "Physio-Ring": an advanced concept in mitral valve annuloplasty. *Ann Thorac Surg.* 1995;60:1177–1186.

38. Gorton M, Piehler JM, Killen DA, et al. Mitral valve repair using a flexible and adjustable annuloplasty ring. *Ann Thorac Surg.* 1993;55:860–863.

39. Sarris GE, Cahill PD, Hansen DE, et al. Restoration of left ventricular systolic performance after reattachment of the mitral chordae tendineae. The importance of valvular-ventricular interaction. *J Thorac Cardiovasc Surg.* 1988;95:969–979.

40. Hansen DE, Sarris GE, Niczyporuk MA, et al. Physiologic role of the mitral aparatus in left ventricular regional mechanics, contraction synergy, and global systolic performance. *J Thorac Cardiovasc Surg.* 1989;97:521–533.

41. Phillips HR, Levine FH, Carter JE, et al. Mitral valve replacement for isolated mitral regurgitation: analysis of clinical course and late postoperative left ventricular ejection fraction. *Am J Cardiol.* 1981;48:647–654.

42. David TE, Uden DE, Strauss HD. The importance of the mitral apparatus in left ventricular function after correction of mitral regurgitation. *Circulation.* 1985;68(suppl II):II76–II82.

43. Goldman ME, Mora F, Guarino T, et al. Mitral valvuloplasty is superior valve replacement for preservation of left ventricular function: an intraoperative two-dimensional echocardiographic study. *J Am Coll Cardiol.* 1987;10:568–575.

44. Galloway AC, Colvin SB, Baumann FG, et al. A comparison of mitral valve reconstruction with mitral valve replacement: intermediate-term results. *Ann Thorac Surg.* 1989;47:655–662.

45. Fuzellier JF, Chauvaud S, Fornes P, et al. Surgical and pathological characteristics of mitral valve in patients with Marfan syndrome operated on for mitral regurgitation. *Circulation.* 1996;94(suppl):I534.

46. Vander Salm TJ, Pape LA, Mauser JF. Mitral valve replacement with complete retention of native leaflets. *Ann Thorac Surg.* 1995;59:52–55.

47. Rose EA, Oz MC. Preservation of anterior leaflet chordae tendineae during mitral valve replacement. *Ann Thorac Surg.* 1994;57:768–769.

48. Rousou J. Mitral valve replacement with chordal preservation. *Video J Cardiothorac Surg.* 1996;10(4).

49. Elefteriades JA, Morales DL, Gradel C, et al. Results of coronary artery bypass grafting by a single surgeon in patients with left ventricular ejection fractions < or =30%. *Am J Cardiol.* 1997;79:1573–1578.

50. Hendren WG, Nemec JJ, Lytle BW, et al. Mitral valve repair for ischemic mitral insufficiency. *Ann Thorac Surg.* 1991;52:1246–1251.

51. Scott WC, Miller DC, Haverich A, et al. Operative risk of mitral valve replacement: discriminant analysis of 1329 procedures. *Circulation.* 1985;72:II108–119.

52. Bonow RO, Nikas D, Elefteriades JA. Valve replacement for regurgitant lesions of the aortic or mitral valve in advanced left ventricular dysfunction. In: Elefteriades JA, Lee FA, Letsou GV, eds. *Advanced Treatment Options for the Failing Left Ventricle: Cardiology Clinics.* Philadelphia, Pa: WB Saunders; 1995:73–83.

53. Obarski TP, Loop FD, Cosgrove DM, et al. Frequency of acute myocardial infarction in vavle repairs versus valve replacement for pure mitral regurgitation. *Am J Cardiol.* 1990;65:887–890.

54. Elefteriades JA, Lee IA, Letsou GV. *Cardiology Clinics.* Philadelphia, Pa: WB Saunders; 1995:80.

55. Nass O, Rosman H, Al-Khaled N, et al. Relation of left ventricular chamber shape in patients with low (≤40%) ejection fraction to severity of functional mitral regurgitation. *Am J Cardiol.* 1995;76:402–404.

56. Elefteriades JA, Jones MF, Fleigner K, et al. Mitral valve procedures in advanced left ventricular dysfunction. *Circulation.* 1996;94(suppl):I533.

57. Guiradon GM, Ofiesh JG, Kaushik R. Extended vertical transatrial septal approach to the mitral valve. *Ann Thorac Surg.* 1991;52:1058–1062.

58. Tribble CG, Killinger WA Jr, Harman PK, et al. Anterolateral thoracotomy as an alternative to repeat median sternotomy for replacement of the mitral valve. *Ann Thorac Surg.* 1987;43:380–382.

59. Braxton JM, Higgins RS, Schwann TA, et al. Reoperative mitral valve surgery via right thoracotomy: decreased blood loss and improved hemodynamics. *J Heart Valve Dis.* 1996;5:169–173.

60. Galloway AC, Ribakove GH, Schwartz DS, et al. Limited thoracotomy mitral valve surgery [abstract]. *Circulation.* 1999. In press.

61. Pompili MF, Yakub A, Siegel LC, et al. Port-access mitral valve replacement: initial clinical experience. *Circulation.* 1996;94(suppl):3122.

62. Loulmet D, Carpentier A, Le Bret E. Less invasive techniques for mitral valve surgery. *J Thorac Cardiovasc Surg.* 1998;115(4):772–779.

26

Prosthetic and Homograft Heart Valves

Ozuru O. Ukoha and John A. Elefteriades

Tuffier performed an aortic valvulotomy in 1912, and Cutler, a mitral commissurotomy in 1923, but it wasn't until 1953, when cardiopulmonary bypass was developed, that surgeons, by direct visualization of valvular pathology, began in earnest to explore the range of possibilities in the treatment of these abnormalities. Prosthetic valves were placed initially in the descending aorta, but in 1960 Harken et al. achieved much better outcomes by placing them proximally into the aortic annulus.[1] During the same year, Starr replaced the mitral valve with a mechanical ball-and-cage valve.[2] Since then, prosthetic valve surgery has enjoyed ever-increasing success. Following mitral valve replacement, pulmonary hypertension is relieved[3–6] and following aortic valve replacement, the compensatory mechanisms of hypertrophy and/or ventricular dilatation regress[7,8] and impaired ventricular performance improves.[8,9] Thousands of patients undergo valve replacement annually worldwide.

In order to replace the native valve, the ideal prosthetic valve must have excellent hemodynamic characteristics that provide unimpeded forward flow with minimal transvalvular gradient upon opening. The ideal prosthesis must produce a competent valve with minimal regurgitation upon closing. The valve must be non-thrombogenic, resistant to infection, nondestructive to blood elements, structurally sound and durable, easy to implant and explant, and readily available at reasonable cost.[10] Despite many years of technologic advancement and improved valve performance, with consequent decline in patient morbidity, the ideal prosthetic valve is yet to be manufactured. The success of prosthetic valve surgery has favorably changed the natural history of patients with valvular heart disease, but mechanical prosthetic valve–related problems have also emerged. These include thromboembolism, thrombosis, anticoagulant-related hemorrhage, insufficient durability, hemolysis, and prosthetic valve endocarditis. To overcome these problems, not only are valves constantly undergoing modifications in structural design, but several types of valves are now available to choose from: mechanical, bioprosthetic, homograft, and autograft.

The use of bioprosthetic valves grew rapidly when they were introduced in the 1970s because of the aforementioned problems with mechanical valves. A decade later, when limited durability emerged as a significant problem with bioprostheses, interest in mechanical valves was rekindled, especially with the availability of the second-generation series that offered better hemodynamic performance and lower thromboembolic rates. Surgeons loved the durability of the mechanical valves, and although there was a definite decline in the rate of morbidity with these devices, the associated complications could not be completely eradicated. Hence, the persistent search for the perfect replacement valve continued and included resurrection of the homograft and the autograft, which had been around as long as the mechanical valves but were abandoned because of the increased mortality rate associated with them. The use of the homograft in the aortic position is more technically demanding than prosthetic valve replacement. Because the homograft is not a totally viable tissue, definite concerns persisted regarding its long-term durability, although it showed an excellent hemodynamic profile. Autograft valve replacement was even more difficult to popularize within the surgical community. Earlier on, when subcoronary implantation was the usual method and an unacceptably high mortality rate was associated with this procedure, surgeons had reasons to wonder about the prudence of replacing two valves instead of one. But with the aortic root replacement method in use since 1976, better results have been realized along with a lower mortality rate. The autograft is once more enjoying a resurgence.

Tables 26.1 through 26.3 show, in the following order, valves approved for use in the United States in 1996 by

TABLE 26.1. Valves approved for use in the United States by the US Food and Drug Administration in 1996.

Mechanical	Bioprosthetic	Other
Caged-ball valve	Porcine valve (stented)	Homograft
Starr–Edwards	Carpentier–Edwards	
(2160, 6120)	Hancock	
Bileaflet valve		Pulmonary
St Jude Medical		autograft
Carbomedics	Bovine pericardial valve	
	Carpentier–Edwards	
Single tilting-disk valve		
Medtronic–Hall		
Omniscience		

TABLE 26.2. Valves used outside the United States in 1996 but not approved by the US Food and Drug Administration.

Bioprosthetic valves
Stented valves (porcine)
    Carpentier–Edwards supra-annular
        Hancock II
Stentless valves (porcine/bovine pericardial)
    Toronto SPV
    Bravo 300

TABLE 26.3. Mechanical valves not approved by the US Food and Drug Administration.

Alvarez	Harken–Surgitool
Barnard–Goosen	Hufnagel
Beall–MV	Hufnagel–Brunswick
Beall–Surgitool	Hufnagel trileaflet
Björk–Shiley	Kay–Shiley
Braunwald–Morrow	Kay–Suzuki
Cooley–Bloodwell–Cutter	Lillehei–Kaster
Cooley–Bloodwell–Liotta–Cromie	Magovern–Cromie
Cooley–Cutter	Nakib toroidal
Cross–Jones	Pemco–Cartwright
DeBakey–Surgitool	Smeloff–Cutter
Duromedics	Smeloff–Cutter–Davy–Kaufman
Gott–Daggett	Starr–Edwards ball (other than 1260, 2160)
Hammersmith	Starr–Edwards disk
Harken ball and cage	Wada–Cutter

Some of these valves have been implanted in patients in the United States; others are not approved because the companies have chosen not to invest in the expense and time required to gain approval.

In the bioprosthetic group is the Ionescu–Shiley pericardial valve implanted in more than 80,000 patients in the United States but now discontinued.

Reproduced with permission from Akins.[11]

the Food and Drug Administration (FDA); valves used commonly outside the United States but not approved by the FDA; and valves not approved for use by the FDA.

Mechanical Valves

As a group (Figure 26.1 and Table 26.4), the mechanical valve is the most frequently used heart valve prosthesis worldwide, enjoying a 65% to 35% market-share advantage over the bioprosthetic prostheses.[12] This has occurred as a result of comparatively greater durability, ease of implantation, proven hemodynamic reliability, and overall effectiveness. The single most important deterrent to use, is the continued need for lifetime anticoagulation. Warfarin administration is begun as soon as the patient can take oral medications. Heparin therapy may be instituted by the first postoperative day at a subtherapeutic dose until the international normalized ratio (INR) comes into appropriate range. If by the fifth postoperative day the INR is still not within range, the heparin can be administered at therapeutic

dosages. Design modifications over the 35 years since introduction have limited the occurrence of structural failure, thrombosis, hemolysis, and other valve-related complications.

The most commonly used valve is the bileaflet St Jude Medical: over 600,000 have been implanted worldwide in its 19 years of availability. The basic component of the valve mechanism is unchanged since its introduction. The pyrolytic carbon discs pivot inside a pyrolytic carbon housing to which a Dacron sewing ring is attached. The two leaflets of the valve open to 85° from the horizontal axis.[11] In smaller sizes of 21 mm or less, modification of the sewing ring to decrease transvalvular gradient led to the introduction of the Hemodynamic Plus (HP) series. Further design modifications of the sewing ring (St Jude Medical Masters series) allow rotation of the device as in the Carbomedics and the Medtronic–Hall valves. This feature makes these second-generation valves very useful in circumstances in which leaflet excursion is impeded either by native heart structures or by valvular debris, islands of calcium in the periphery of the annulus, suture tails, or subvalvular pledgets.

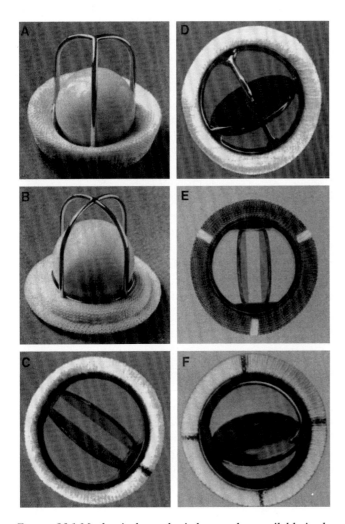

FIGURE 26.1 Mechanical prosthetic heart valves available in the United States in 1995. **A,** Starr–Edwards model 1260; **B,** Starr–Edwards model 6120; **C,** Carpentier–Edwards; **D,** Medtronic–Hall; **E,** Carbomedics; **F,** Omniscience.

and, on full excursion, open to 78° to the plane of the ring. The pivots of the leaflets are designed to provide continuous washing.[13]

The Medtronic–Hall valve is a single tilting disc valve. Its circular disc is coated with pyrolytic carbon, which pivots over a central strut inside a housing, machined from one solid piece of titanium to which is attached a sewing ring.[12] The aortic valve disc is designed to have an open disc angle of 75°, and the mitral disc, an open angle of 70°. The translation of the Medtronic–Hall disc downsteam in systole aids in washing the valve housing of microthrombi. In addition, the machining of the support struts and the central post from one piece of titanium avoids possible weakness caused by welding.[14]

The second-generation design of the original Lillehei–Kaster valve, is the Omniscience valve. It has a single pyrolytic carbon disc inside a titanium housing, to which is attached a seamless Teflon sewing ring. The disc is designed to open at an angle of 80°.[11]

The Starr–Edwards valve is a ball-and-cage prosthesis with a barium-impregnated silastic ball riding inside a stellite cage, to which is attached a seamless cloth sewing ring. The ball is removable from the aortic prosthesis, but not from the mitral prosthesis.

Methods of insertion have become standardized. They include the most commonly employed mattress sutures with or without teflon pledgets, figure-of-eight sutures, simple sutures, and running sutures.[10] In order to limit the confusion that may result from sorting sutures lying unorganized on the operative field, alternating color sutures are usually employed. The currently available cylindrical valve sizers provide an exact duplicate of the size of the valve at the valve–tissue junction: stretching the annulus or forcing the sizer may therefore place the surgeon and the patient at risk for a poor fit. The general recommendation for the valves is to use the valve size that slides easily through the native annulus because oversizing is unnecessary and can make implantation very difficult. Sutures should be passed through the sewing ring some distance back from the edge of the outflow housing so that when the knots are tied in the suture, they will lie away from the housing to avoid disc impingement.[14] Some surgeons cut the tied implantation sutures with a miniature thermal cautery, thereby fusing the suture tails and preventing leaflet or disc impingement. Extreme caution must be observed not to scratch

The other bileaflet valve is the Carbomedics valve. Its graphite substrate contains 20% tungsten, and the stiffening ring is made of titanium, making both of these components advantageously radiopaque.[13] The stiffening ring prevents deformation of the annulus of the prosthesis by the patient valve annulus. In suspected cases of valve dehiscence, the ability to visualize the valve and its leaflets under fluoroscopy is beneficial. The leaflets sit at a 25° angle to the plane of the valve ring

TABLE 26.4. Mechanical cardiac valvular prosthesis approved by the US Food and Drug Administration in 1995.

Valve	Year approved	Design	Number inserted	List price ($)
Starr–Edwards (1260, 6120)	1965	Caged ball	150,000	4300
Medtronic–Hall	1977	Single tilting disk	170,000	4000
St Jude Medical	1977	Bileaflet	600,000	4010
Omniscience	1978	Single tilting disk	45,000	3800
Carbomedics	1993	Bileaflet	110,000	4250

Reproduced with permission from Akins.[12]

the valve or disc of pyrolyte carbon prostheses because this can serve as a nidus for later fatigue fractures.

Functional Characteristics of the Mechanical Valves

Table 26.5 contains a subjective assessment of the functional characteristics of the mechanical valves as reported by Akins.[12]

The Starr–Edwards valves have the highest profile because of their ball-and-cage design. The Carbomedics valve has the lowest profile, followed closely by the St Jude Medical valve. The two single-disc valves—Omniscience and Medtronic–Hall—have a low profile in the closed position but in the open position, their profile exceeds that of the bileaflet valves.

Freedom from occluder impingement is poorest for the Medtronic–Hall valve because its occluder seats horizontally at the equator of the housing and therefore can be immobilized by retained valve remnants or sutures tails that have been left too long.

The gradient relief characteristics of the Starr–Edwards valves are almost unacceptable, especially in smaller sizes. This is followed by the Omniscience, the Carbomedics, and equally the St Jude Medical and the Medtronic–Hall valves.

Complete opening of a mechanical valve is either a function of the completeness of rotation or translation of the occluder from the closed to the open position, or the length of time that the occluder stays open during that portion of the cardiac cycle when it is intended to be open. In the aortic position, the bileaflet valves open uniformly and remain open during systole, but in the mitral position, an important percentage of these valves demonstrate biphasic partial closure of both leaflets during diastole ("diastolic fluttering") in patients with atrial fibrillation.[16,17] Complete opening of the Medtronic–Hall valve is virtually always achieved, whereas the disc of the Omniscience valve has been reported to not rotate to the open position completely.[18,19] Ball rebound off the distal cage can affect the secondary orifice of the ball-and-cage design. Also, the inertia of the ball may keep the valve from completely opening or closing at high heart rates. However, complete opening of this valve design is the norm.

That part of valvular regurgitation that occurs before the occluder becomes seated in the housing is known as the dynamic regurgitant fraction. It is lowest in the single-disc valves, followed by the bileaflet designs. The inertia of a Starr–Edwards ball delays its closure.[12] Static leak rate is that part of valvular regurgitation that occurs once the occluder is seated. The single-disc valves have a moderate built-in leak rate to flush the disc and housing. The bileaflet valves have a somewhat higher static leak rate because of the increased length of the lines of closure between the discs and the housing, in conjunction with the tolerance needed to fulfill the engineered requirements for washing the valve components. Static leak rate is nonexistent for the Starr–Edwards valves.

Long-Term Complications

The composite linearized rate of complication, which is the total number of all events from all applicable studies, divided by the total patient-years of the follow-up (percent per patient-year), from the work of Akins[12] is cited repeatedly in this section. Standardized definitions have been proposed for the reporting of valve-related complications to compare the performance of valve prostheses implanted in patients at different centers.[15]

Thromboembolism

A prosthetic-related thromboembolic event is defined as any new, permanent, or transient, focal or global neurologic deficit or peripheral embolus in the absence of another clear-cut source. A thrombus can form on the polished metal components of the mechanical valves, the sewing rings, areas of pannus ingrowth, or areas of tissue valve degeneration and calcification. Lifelong anticoagulation is required.[10] Aspirin is not recommended as a concomitant form of therapy in patients taking warfarin because of its unpredictable elevation in bleeding time

TABLE 26.5. Mechanical valve functional characteristics.*

Characteristics	Starr–Edwards	Medtronic–Hall	St Jude Medical	Omniscience	Carbomedics
Structural integrity	4+	5+	3+	5+	5+
Profile	1+	3+	4+	3+	5+
Rotatability[†]	0	5+	0	5+	5+
Interference with occluder	4+	2+	4+	3+	3+
Transvalve gradient	1+	5+	5+	4+	4+
Complete opening	4+	5+	4+	3+	4+
Dynamic regurgitate fraction	3+	5+	4+	5+	4+
Static leak rate	5+	4+	3+	4+	3+

*A grade of 5+ is the best and 0 the worst.
[†]St Jude Medical Masters series, recently introduced, rotates.
Reproduced with permission from Akins.[12]

TABLE 26.6. Aortic valve replacement: thromboembolism.

Valve and year	Composite linearized rate (range)	Follow-up (patient years)	Percentage free after 5 yr	Percentage free after 10 yr
Starr–Edwards				
1991	2.1 (1.4–3.3)	19,324	89–95	76–91
1995	2.1 (1.4–3.3)	19,324	89–95	76–91
Medtronic–Hall				
1991	1.8 (0.8–4.7)	6411	82–96	—
1995	1.4 (0.7–4.7)	9433	82–96	87
St Jude Medical				
1991	1.6 (0.7–2.8)	6351	88–98	—
1995	2.0 (0.9–2.8)	17,242	88–98	67–90
Omniscience				
1991	3.0 (1.9–5.1)	766	84–93	—
1995	2.7 (0–5.1)	863	84–93	—
Carbomedics				
1995	1.9 (1.9)	1533	94	—

Reproduced with permission from Akins.[12]

and therefore increased risk of the precipitation of bleeding episodes. However, the risk of thromboembolism may be reduced by concomitant dipyridamole therapy.[20] Among the various prosthetic valves, there may be subtle differences in the degree of anticoagulation required to avoid thromboembolism.

The use of the INR as a measurement for anticoagulation may provide uniform standard monitoring of the dosage of warfarin among hospitals and across countries. Lower dose INR target levels, which have minimized anticoagulant-related hemorrhage and thromboembolism, have been advocated.[21,22] In general, thromboembolism is more common for valves in the mitral position than for those in the aortic position, and thromboembolism is more common with mechanical valves, even with anticoagulation, than with tissue valves without anticoagulation. The risk of thromboembolism increases threefold if anticoagulation is stopped. The composite linearized rate for the incidence of thromboembolism in aortic and mitral valve replacement is shown in Tables 26.6 and 26.7, respectively. In the aortic position, the highest rate of thromboembolism is reported for the Omniscience valve, whereas the lowest rate is seen with the Medtronic–Hall valve. Just slightly higher incidence is reported for the other three valves—the St Jude Medical, Starr–Edwards, and Carbomedics. In the mitral position, the lowest rate of thromboembolism is reported for the Medtronic–Hall valve, followed by the St Jude Medical.

TABLE 26.7. Mitral valve replacement: thromboembolism.

Valve and year	Composite linearized rate (range)	Follow-up (patient years)	Percentage free after 5 yr	Percentage free after 10 yr
Starr–Edwards				
1991	3.6 (1.5–5.7)	18,155	62–81	55–91
1995	3.6 (1.5–5.7)	18,155	62–81	55–91
Medtronic–Hall				
1991	1.8 (0.5–4.2)	6637	82–89	—
1995	1.8 (0.5–4.2)	8183	84–91	91
St Jude Medical				
1991	2.4 (0.4–4.0)	5237	89–99	—
1995	2.5 (0.4–4.4)	17,696	89–99	77–90
Omniscience				
1991	5.1 (1.7–12.8)	942	90–97	—
1995	4.4 (1.7–12.8)	1202	90–97	—
Carbomedics				
1995	3.3 (3.3)	1101	91	—

Reproduced with permission from Akins.[12]

TABLE 26.8. Aortic valve replacement: thrombosis.

Valve and year	Composite linearized rate (range)	Follow-up (patient years)	Percentage free after 5 yr	Percentage free after 10 yr
Starr–Edwards				
1991	0.2 (0.1–0.2)	15,072	95	76–91
1995	0.2 (0.1–0.2)	15,070	95	76–91
Medtronic–Hall				
1991	0.2 (0–1.1)	6248	94–100	—
1995	0.2 (0–1.1)	8263	94–100	100
St Jude Medical				
1991	0.2 (0–0.7)	4737	99	—
1995	0.2 (0–0.3)	13,710	99	—
Omniscience				
1991	0.5 (0–0.8)	611	96–100	—
1995	0.4 (0–0.8)	708	96–100	—
Carbomedics				
1995	0 (0)	1553	100	—

Reproduced with permission from Akins.[12]

The rates for the Carbomedics and the Starr–Edwards valves are increased further, whereas the highest rates are seen with the Omniscience valve.

Valve Thrombosis

Thrombosis of a mechanical valve is quite rare. Occasionally, a disastrous outcome of acute congestive heart failure, pulmonary edema, and cardiogenic shock may result. The most commonly employed diagnostic modality, because of its ease of application, is echocardiography, but cardiac catheterization can also be used to evaluate disc mobility and define transvalvular gradient. Fluoroscopy, advocated by some, may detect impairment of disc excursion in valves that are radiopaque. Auscultation usually reveals loss of valve clicks. In acute valve thrombosis, thrombolytic therapy may be lifesaving, but the risks of this modality include systemic embolization, persistent thrombosis after thrombolytic therapy is withdrawn, and persistent valve dysfunction from tissue ingrowth or organized thrombus.[10] More often than not, emergency surgery for valve rereplacement is required to treat this problem, and it carries a high mortality rate of up to 50%. The risk of mechanical valve thrombosis is highest in the tricuspid position (where many authors feel mechanical valves should be avoided if possible), followed by the mitral position, and then the aortic position. The composite linearized rate for aortic and mitral valve prosthetic thrombosis is shown in Tables 26.8 and 26.9, respectively. The risk of valve thrombosis is increased 5- to 10-fold if anticoagulation is stopped.[23]

TABLE 26.9. Mitral valve replacement: thrombosis.

Valve and year	Composite linearized rate (range)	Follow-up (patient years)	Percentage free after 5 yr	Percentage free after 10 yr
Starr–Edwards				
1991	0.4 (0–0.5)	9726	—	96
1995	0.4 (0–0.5)	9726	—	96
Medtronic–Hall				
1991	0.3 (0–1.1)	4762	96	—
1995	0.3 (0–1.1)	5915	96–100	—
St Jude Medical				
1991	0.5 (0–0.8)	3231	96	—
1995	0.2 (0.1–0.9)	14,437	96	—
Omniscience				
1991	2.9 (0.4–9.4)	942	95–100	—
1995	2.3 (0.4–9.4)	1202	95–100	—
Carbomedics				
1995	0.8 (0.8)	1101	97	—

Reproduced with permission from Akins.[12]

TABLE 26.10. Aortic valve replacement: anticoagulation complications.

Valve and year	Composite linearized rate (range)	Follow-up (patient years)	Percentage free after 5 yr	Percentage free after 10 yr
Starr–Edwards				
1991	1.9 (0.8–3.1)	19,324	87–95	74–93
1995	1.9 (0.8–3.1)	19,324	87–95	74–93
Medtronic–Hall				
1991	0.8 (0.7–2.6)	5490	91	—
1995	0.9 (0.7–1.7)	6027	91–94	80
St Jude Medical				
1991	2.5 (0.2–7.9)	5107	89	—
1995	2.2 (0–7.9)	14,845	82–92	73–95
Omniscience				
1991	2.3 (2.3)	42	97	—
1995	0.7 (0–2.3)	139	97	—
Carbomedics				
1995	2.3 (2.3)	1553	92	—

Reproduced with permission from Akins.[12]

In the aortic position, the Carbomedics valve has no reported cases of thrombosis. Very low rates are reported for the St Jude Medical, Starr–Edwards, and Medtronic–Hall valves. The incidence of thrombosis with the Omniscience valve is increased. In the mitral position, the rate of valve thrombosis is very low for the St Jude Medical, Medtronic–Hall, and Starr–Edwards valves. The rate is somewhat elevated for the Carbomedics and is highest for the Omniscience valve.

Anticoagulant-Related Hemorrhage

When the patient is physically examined and his or her history is taken, the search for potential contraindications to anticoagulation must be very thorough, because any pertinent findings usually influence valve selection.

The use of anticoagulation to decrease the risk of thromboembolism may result in minor or major, even life-threatening bleeding complications that could lead to cerebrovascular accident, internal bleeding, reoperation, hospitalization, blood transfusions, and even death. The risk of bleeding is highest in the elderly population, approximating 9% per year in patients more than 70 years of age: the annual risk of minor bleeding is 4.8%, major bleeding 1% to 2%, and fatal outcome 0.5%.[24] The composite linearized rate for anticoagulant-related hemorrhage with prosthetic valves in aortic and mitral valve positions is shown in Tables 26.10 and 26.11, respectively. In the aortic position, the incidence of anticoagulant-related hemorrhage is lowest for the Omniscience valve, followed by the Medtronic–Hall, and then the St Jude

TABLE 26.11. Mitral valve replacement: anticoagulation complications.

Valve and year	Composite linearized rate (range)	Follow-up (patient years)	Percentage free after 5 yr	Percentage free after 10 yr
Starr–Edwards				
1991	1.7 (1.0–3.7)	16,026	82–93	67–90
1995	1.7 (1.0–3.7)	16,026	82–93	67–90
Medtronic–Hall				
1991	1.1 (0.5–4.8)	3286	—	—
1995	1.2 (0.5–4.8)	3732	91	86
St Jude Medical				
1991	1.8 (0.3–2.9)	4466	91–97	—
1995	1.7 (0.2–6.4)	16,679	90–97	81–98
Omniscience				
1991	2.7 (2.7)	222	94	—
1995	3.5 (2.7–4.2)	482	94	—
Carbomedics				
1995	2.2 (2.2)	1101	95	—

Reproduced with permission from Akins.[12]

TABLE 26.12. Aortic valve replacement: prosthetic valve endocarditis.

Valve and year	Composite linearized rate (range)	Follow-up (patient years)	Percentage free after 5 yr	Percentage free after 10 yr
Starr–Edwards				
1991	0.7 (0.4–1.1)	18,761	95	92–97
1995	0.7 (0.4–1.1)	18,761	95	92–97
Medtronic–Hall				
1991	0.4 (0–1.2)	5490	100	—
1995	0.5 (0.3–1.2)	6323	96–100	96
St Jude Medical				
1991	0.5 (0.1–2.1)	4110	99	—
1995	0.4 (0.1–1.7)	12,084	99	94–99
Omniscience				
1991	1.6 (0–1.9)	255	94–96	—
1995	1.4 (0–1.9)	352	94–96	—
Carbomedics				
1995	0.4 (0.4)	1553	98	—

Reproduced with permission from Akins.[12]

Medical, Starr–Edwards, and Carbomedics valves. In the mitral position, the rate is lowest for the Medtronic–Hall valve and a bit higher for the Starr–Edwards and the St Jude Medical valves. The rate is increased further for the Carbomedics and is highest for the Omniscience valve.

Prosthetic Valve Endocarditis

The incidence of prosthetic valve endocarditis (PVE) is 1% to 2% per year.[25] PVE is considered "early" if it manifests within the first 2 months after surgery. The infectious organism is usually *Staphylococcus aureus,* which carries a poor prognosis, with a mortality rate approaching 50% even when treated with antibiotics and surgery. Prosthetic valve endocarditis that develops after the first

2 months is "late PVE." The organisms are usually similar to those encountered with native valve endocarditis. Antibiotics alone may be used to treat it. The mortality rate for this state is still considerable at 25%. Infections involving mechanical valves tend to produce periannular abscesses and nearly always require surgical intervention. The composite linearized rate for PVE in aortic and mitral positions is presented in Tables 26.12 and 26.13. In the aortic position the reported rates for all the valves is very low, with the Omniscience valve showing a slightly higher rate. In the mitral position, the rate is low for the St Jude Medical, Starr–Edwards, and Medtronic–Hall valves. It is minimally higher for the Carbomedics and remains substantially elevated for the Omniscience valve.

TABLE 26.13. Mitral valve replacement: prosthetic valve endocarditis.

Valve and year	Composite linearized rate (range)	Follow-up (patient years)	Percentage free after 5 yr	Percentage free after 10 yr
Starr–Edwards				
1991	0.4 (0.3–0.8)	16,026	95–97	92–98
1995	0.4 (0.3–0.8)	16,026	95–97	92–98
Medtronic–Hall				
1991	0.4 (0–1.7)	3286	100	—
1995	0.5 (0–1.7)	3939	95–100	88
St Jude Medical				
1991	0.4 (0.1–2.2)	3559	98	—
1995	0.5 (0–2.2)	14,903	98	98–99
Omniscience				
1991	2.4 (0–5.4)	507	98	—
1995	1.8 (0–5.4)	767	98	—
Carbomedics				
1995	0.7 (0.7)	1101	96	—

Reproduced with permission from Akins.[12]

TABLE 26.14. Aortic valve replacement: nonstructural dysfunction.

Valve and year	Composite linearized rate (range)	Follow-up (patient years)	Percentage free after 5 yr	Percentage free after 10 yr
Starr–Edwards				
1991	0.2 (0.1–1.4)	7681	—	—
1995	0.2 (0.1–1.4)	7681	—	—
Medtronic–Hall				
1991	0.5 (0–0.9)	1761	100	—
1995	0.5 (0.1–1.4)	3276	95–100	99
St Jude Medical				
1991	0.5 (0–3.4)	2281	—	—
1995	0.4 (0–3.4)	10,234	—	97
Omniscience				
1991	2.4 (0.9–6.7)	746	98	—
1995	2.1 (0–6.7)	843	98	—
Carbomedics				
1995	0.8 (0.8)	1553	95	—

Reproduced with permission from Akins.[12]

Hemolysis

Hemolysis is the result of periprosthetic leak or a stenotic or regurgitant valve, therefore reoperation is usually required. Perivalvular leak can sometimes be repaired with a few additional sutures, but valve rereplacement is usually required. Hemolysis can be detected by elevated lactic dehydrogenase levels, decreased serum haptoglobin, hemoglobinuria, or a transfusion requirement.[10] With current valve prostheses, even in the presence of significant gradients, cellular destruction from normal transvalvular forward flow or regurgitation is unusual.

Nonstructural Dysfunction

Nonstructural dysfunction comprises largely paravalvular leak and, to a lesser extent, hemolysis. The composite linearized rate for nonstructural dysfunction for the aortic and mitral positions is shown in Tables 26.14 and 26.15, respectively.

In the aortic position, the rate of nonstructural dysfunction is lowest for the Starr–Edwards valve, followed by the Medtronic–Hall and the St Jude Medical valves. The rate is a little higher for the Carbomedics valve and is further elevated for the Omniscience valve. In the mitral position, the lowest rate is recorded for the Starr–

TABLE 26.15. Mitral valve replacement: nonstructural dysfunction.

Valve and year	Composite linearized rate (range)	Follow-up (patient years)	Percentage free after 5 yr	Percentage free after 10 yr
Starr–Edwards				
1991	0.3 (0.1–0.8)	9051	—	—
1995	0.3 (0.1–0.8)	9051	—	—
Medtronic–Hall				
1991	0.4 (0.3–0.6)	2171	100	—
1995	0.7 (0–2.1)	2824	93–100	83
St Jude Medical				
1991	1.0 (0.7–2.2)	1344	—	—
1995	0.6 (0–2.2)	12,341	—	98
Omniscience				
1991	1.0 (0.4–1.9)	673	99	—
1995	0.8 (0–1.9)	933	99	—
Carbomedics				
1995	1.4 (1.4)	1101	95	—

Reproduced with permission from Akins.[12]

TABLE 26.16. Aortic valve replacement: reoperation.

Valve and year	Composite linearized rate (range)	Follow-up (patient years)	Percentage free after 5 yr	Percentage free after 10 yr
Starr–Edwards				
1991	0.7 (0.4–3.7)	19,324	95	90–98
1995	0.7 (0.4–3.7)	19,324	95	90–98
Medtronic–Hall				
1991	1.8 (0.4–2.1)	1021	100	—
1995	1.5 (0.6–3.0)	2536	90–100	97
St Jude Medical				
1991	0.3 (0–0.9)	2914	98	—
1995	0.4 (0–1.4)	10,417	98–99	92–99
Omniscience				
1991	2.4 (2.4)	42	—	—
1995	0.7 (0–2.4)	139	—	—
Carbomedics				
1995	0.6 (0.6)	1553	97	—

Reproduced with permission from Akins.[12]

Edwards valve, followed by the St Jude Medical valve, Medtronic–Hall, and Omniscience valves. The rate for the Carbomedics valve is somewhat higher.

Reoperation

Determinants of surgical death after reoperation include higher New York Heart Association class, poor hemodynamic status, poor nutritional status, older age, emergency operation, prosthetic valve infection, right heart failure, number of previous heart operations, and the need for concomitant surgical procedures such as combined mitral and aortic valve replacement, left ventricular aneurysmectomy, and ascending aortic surgery. The composite linearized rate for reoperation for the aortic

and mitral positions is presented in Tables 26.16 and 26.17.

The rates of reoperation for aortic prosthesis is lowest for the St Jude Medical valve. It is minimally elevated for the Carbomedics, Starr–Edwards, and Omniscience valves. It is highest for the Medtronic–Hall valve. In the mitral position, reoperation is lowest for the St Jude Medical valve, a little higher for Starr–Edwards valve, and slightly higher for the Medtronic–Hall and the Carbomedics valves. It is considerably higher for the Omniscience valve.

The St Jude Medical valve and, to a lesser extent, the Medtronic–Hall valve are the popular mechanical valve prostheses in the United States because of their low rates

TABLE 26.17. Mitral valve replacement: reoperation.

Valve and year	Composite linearized rate (range)	Follow-up (patient years)	Percentage free after 5 yr	Percentage free after 10 yr
Starr–Edwards				
1991	1.0 (0.6–1.7)	13,410	93–94	84–95
1995	1.0 (0.6–1.7)	13,410	93–94	84–95
Medtronic–Hall				
1991	1.5 (1.3–1.7)	1614	94	—
1995	1.6 (1.3–1.9)	2267	92–94	88
St Jude Medical				
1991	0.9 (0.6–3.0)	2871	97–99	—
1995	0.6 (0.2–3.0)	14,132	92–99	94–98
Omniscience				
1991	5.4 (5.4)	222	—	—
1995	2.5 (0–5.4)	482	—	—
Carbomedics				
1995	1.4 (1.4)	1101	93	—

Reproduced with permission from Akins.[12]

of valve-related complications and their documented excellent and comparable hemodynamic performance. The Carbomedics valve ranks behind these two on the basis of somewhat higher transvalvular gradient and increased incidence of thromboembolism despite adequate anticoagulation, especially in the mitral position. Various reports do not favor the hemodynamic performance or the freedom from complications of the Omniscience valve. The Starr–Edwards valves are not competitive with current disc prostheses because of poorer gradient relief and an increased incidence of valve-related complications, despite impressive durability.

Bioprosthetic Valves

The bioprosthetic valves include the stented porcine valves, pericardial valves (Figure 26.2), and stentless porcine valves.

Stented Porcine Valves

The first generation Hancock (standard) porcine bioprosthetic valve was introduced in 1970; a year later, the Carpentier–Edwards (standard) porcine bioprosthetic valve was introduced in an effort to overcome the need for lifelong anticoagulation and the related complications seen with mechanical valves. These valves are the aortic valves of pigs. They are both treated with glutaraldehyde, but the Hancock valve incorporates a polypropylene stent with a thin Stellite ring added to the annulus for rigidity, whereas the Carpentier–Edwards

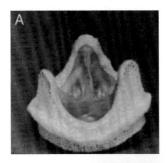 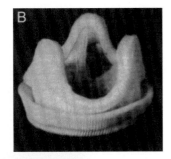

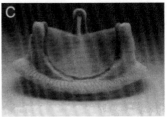

FIGURE 26.2. Bioprosthetic heart valves available in the United States in 1995. **A,** Carpentier–Edwards porcine (standard); **B,** Hancock porcine (standard); **C,** Carpentier–Edwards pericardial.

valve uses a flexible Elgiloy wire frame that is intended to reduce the stresses on the leaflets.[26]

Durability has remained the Achilles heal of porcine bioprosthetic valves, and the advantage offered by these valves in eliminating prolonged anticoagulation was offset by inferior hemodynamic performance (especially in smaller sizes of 21 mm or less). In 1977, the Hancock modified orifice (MO) aortic prosthesis (model 250) was introduced in the United States: the septal muscular shelf at the base of the right leaflet, which reduced the effective orifice area (EOA) in the standard aortic prosthesis (model 242), had been eliminated. The right leaflet was replaced with a noncoronary leaflet from a second porcine valve.[26] Despite the larger effective orifice area and the lower peak valve gradients, the difference in hemodynamic performance of the Hancock MO series is not statistically significant,[27] nor was there an improvement in durability.[28,29] In the early 1980s, the second-generation porcine bioprosthetic supra-annular valves (compared with intra-annular placement of the standard valves) became available—the Carpentier–Edwards Supra-annular and the Hancock II. These valves were intended to reduce the incidence of structural valve deterioration, so both are fixed with glutaraldehyde first at low pressure, then the Hancock II is fixed at physiologic pressure in an attempt to maintain normal collagen crimp waveforms. To retard calcification, the Carpentier–Edwards valve is treated with the surfactant polysorbate-80, whereas the Hancock II is treated with sodium dodecyl sulfate.[26] Although widely used in Canada and Europe, these second-generation valves are not available in the United States. Currently available data fail to show any distinct advantage in their performance compared with the first-generation valves.[30,31]

With respect to the competitive first-generation valves, no statistically significant differences were observed when the following indices were examined: freedom from structural deterioration,[32] overall patient survival, and incidence of valve-related death and reoperation.[33]

Higher surgical risk may be incurred in older patients, during emergency operation, with concomitant coronary artery disease,[34,35] or with mitral instead of aortic disease. The overall performance of these valves is significantly better in the aortic position.[36,37] The incidence of structural valve failure is extremely low during the first 5 years of follow-up but then begins to increase 5 to 6 years after implantation[38,39]: rates of freedom from structural deterioration are 76% to 91% at 10 years and 37% to 58% at 14 to 15 years.[37–42] The younger the age at operation, the higher the incidence of structural deterioration. Differences in calcium metabolism and hemodynamics have been proposed to explain the increased rate of valvular fibrocalcific degeneration observed in patients of younger age, during pregnancy, and with renal failure.[41–44] However, Magilligan et al.[38] speculate that the primary event may not be calcification but the mechanical stresses that compromise the structural integrity of the valve. Valve performance heretofore has been assessed using actuarial analysis but, according to Grunkemeier et al., this does not provide truly accurate data because the risk described for nonfatal events (e.g., valve failure) is the risk a patient would experience if he or she were immortal; moreover, this statistical modality was originally devised to describe freedom from death, not freedom from nonfatal complications.[45] A more accurate estimate of *actual* failure is the percentage of patients whose valve will actually fail before they die. Because older patients have a lower risk of tissue failure and a higher risk of death than younger patients, the difference between the actual and actuarial estimates increases with the patient's age.

Compared with the mechanical valves, bioprosthetic valves are not as susceptible to thromboembolism; however, in the early postoperative period their sewing ring may be a nidus for thrombus formation. Most centers treat patients with warfarin for anticoaulation for 3 months, followed by aspirin therapy if the patient is in sinus rhythm.[46] Anticoagulation is recommended indefinitely following mitral valve replacement if the patient is in atrial fibrillation or has a history of thromboembolism, or if a large left atrium is present.

Infections involving bioprosthetic valves are infrequent; the incidence is similar to that seen with mechanical valves (1% to 2% per patient-year).[47] The infection may be limited to the valve leaflets and can occasionally be sterilized with antibiotic therapy. Poorly treated or advanced tissue valve PVE often involves the sewing ring and periannular tissues. Based on multivariate analysis, older age is a significant risk factor for PVE.[36]

Stentless Porcine Bioprosthetic Valves

Even though some improvements in valve material and valve design have optimized the hemodynamic characteristics of heart valve prostheses in recent years,[48] the presence of a stent always results in a reduction of the effective orifice area, which becomes more hemodynamically significant in the small aortic root. After promising experimental results using stentless porcine valves in sheep,[49] David et al. started a controlled clinical trial[50] several years after the first pioneering experiences.[51,52]

Two forms of the stentless valve are available for implantation: the porcine aortic valve and the bovine pericardial aortic valve. Neither is available in the United States. (This is changing as this chapter goes to press.) Both are treated with glutaraldehyde.

The renewed interest in the use of stentless bioprostheses comes as a result of their proven superior hemodynamic performance[53] and perceived usefulness in the small aortic annulus, where they offer a lower gradient when compared with either biological stented valves or mechanical valves.[53,54]

Implantation of the stentless aortic valves requires more skill. Misjudgement in the commissure positioning and alignment in the aortic root, or the wrong choice of the valve size will result in an incompetent prosthesis. Hemodynamic performances also may depend on the type of valve and the tissue employed. The improved durability said to be achieved by using the aortic wall as a valve stent awaits long-term follow-up.

Pericardial Valves

Pericardial valves are man-made from the pericardial tissue of a cow. The major advantage of porcine valves is their low incidence of thromboembolism even without anticoagulation,[55,56] but their limited durability, structural deterioration of 20% at 10 years,[57] and poor hemodynamic performance in small sizes,[58-61] have combined to restrict their use. In 1971, Ionescu et al[62] introduced the first pericardial valves as an alternative to the glutaraldehyde-treated porcine valves. Despite excellent hemodynamic performance,[63] they were doomed by early structural failure.[64,65]

The most commonly used pericardial valve, the Carpentier–Edwards model, was introduced in 1971. The significant design modification is the two pieces of pericardium of adjacent cusps that pass between the two arms of the stent, rather than over the stent.[66] The stent is flexible, and the shape of the pericardial cusps is the product of finite element analysis. The cusps are matched for thickness and treated with surfactant to retard calcification.[67] Both in vitro and in vivo studies along with echocardiographic data have shown this valve to have excellent hemodynamics. It opens at a lower flow rate and to a greater extent than the porcine valves at all flow rates. In addition, it has a lower mean gradient and larger orifice area than either the standard Carpentier–Edwards valve or the supra-annular Carpentier–Edwards valve.[67-69]

The downfall of all previous biologic valves has been structural deterioration. With a 10-year actuarial freedom from structural deterioration of 91%[70] and intermediate-term follow-up figures approaching 100%,[66,67,71] valve durability for the current pericardial valve is better than that of porcine valves.[36,72] The implication for the surgeon is that this valve now provides an excellent alternative for young patients who do not desire anticoagulation and for patients over the age of 65.

Homografts

It wasn't until 1962 that Sir Donald Ross and G. Barrat Boyes independently and simultaneously replaced the aortic valve with a homograft—an aortic valve taken from a deceased human being. To achieve sterility and for convenience of storage, chemical processing was the initial method. Since then, other methods have evolved including antibiotic processing, fresh implantation (Homovital), and finally, cryopreservation. Cryopreservation made aortic homografts readily available for use by many surgeons. All methods of preservation are less than perfect and result in some deterioration of the tissues.

The homograft tissue is pliable and versatile and conforms to irregular surfaces. There are four different surgical techniques that may be utilized to implant an aortic homograft: (1) the 120° rotation freehand technique, (2) the intact noncoronary sinus freehand technique, (3) aortic root enlargement with or without use of the anterior leaflet of the mitral valve, and (4) aortic root replacement techniques that may comprise an inclusion technique ("miniroot") or a free-standing root replacement.[73]

Most of the experience is in younger patients (<55 years of age). Perioperative deaths are quite rare; so is thromboembolism. Actuarial survival is 94% at 7.5 years, and clinical follow-up extended to the same time interval shows 87% of the patients to be in NYHA functional class 1. In patients with endocarditis, a cure can usually be expected after operation with a homograft. At 7.5 years, actuarial freedom from reoperation for any reason is 89%, and for structural failure it is 93%. Critics of the homograft point out that late follow-up is limited and that the homograft is "just another dead valve" like the pericardial and the porcine valves, doomed to fail as the nonliving collagen breaks eventually under the strain of performance.

The anterior leaflet of the donor mitral valve is usually left attached to the aortic homograft at harvesting. This may be very valuable in some clinical situations, such as the presence of subvalvular left ventricular outflow tract obstruction. Here, the anterior leaflet of the mitral valve of the aortic homograft may be used to widen the outflow tract in association with the aortic valve replacement. Posterior enlargement of the left ventricular outflow tract into the anterior leaflet of the mitral valve augmented by mitral tissue from the homograft will provide relief of obstruction caused by fibromuscular membranes that significantly involve the anterior leaflet of the mitral valve, which cannot be adequately resected.[73] The extra mitral leaflet tissue of the homograft can also be used to repair structural defects related to endocarditis.

Pulmonary Autograft

At the time when degenerative changes in homografts were first becoming evident, Sir Donald Ross in 1967 replaced the aortic valve with the patient's autogenous pulmonary valve, and the missing pulmonary valve with a homograft, thus ushering in the procedure bearing his name: the Ross procedure.[74] Until 1976, the pulmonary valve was implanted in the aortic root in the subcoronary position. By the 10-year mark, the reoperation rate was 22%. This high failure rate was reduced to only 5% in the past 20 years because the technique was modified to include insertion of the entire pulmonary trunk. The operation was based on the premise that the pulmonary valve is anatomically identical to the aortic valve and, being autogenous, is completely viable. The concept worked, providing superior and unmatched hemodynamic performance, but the extended length and complexity of the operation led to higher early mortality and a 10-year mortality rate of 9%. Today, after many years of mastering the operation, the surgical mortality rate is less than 1%[75] at expert centers. Aortic valve replacement with a pulmonary autograft is an ideal operation for patients with life expectancy of more than 20 years. When patients are in the age range of 55 to 75 years, it may be preferable to use a mechanical prosthesis because these patients may have less reserve and more associated medical conditions, unless there is a contraindication to anticoagulation, in which case an aortic homograft may be desirable.

Contraindications to the use of pulmonary autograft include comorbid medical problems such as coronary artery disease; obesity; long-term pulmonary, hepatic, or renal disease; corticosteroid therapy, Marfan's syndrome, and other connective tissue disorders such as systemic lupus erythematosus or rheumatoid arthritis. A great deal of caution is required in patients who need aortic valve replacement for rheumatic disease, especially if the patient is young and the active phase of the disease is recent. Primary abnormalities of the pulmonary valve such as leaflet thickening, prolapse, and regurgitation preclude its use. The use of a competent bicuspid pulmonary valve remains controversial. Pulmonary autograft valves injured during excision from the right ventricular outflow tract should not be repaired; a double homograft, with one each in the aortic and pulmonary valve positions constitutes a reasonable alternative.

In some patients with asymmetric septal hypertrophy or complete subvalvular left ventricular outflow tract obstruction also requiring aortic valve replacement, an excellent treatment option is resection and incision of the septum anteriorly, supplemented by augmentation of the septum using a pulmonary autograft to which a generous portion of the right ventricular outflow tract is left attached.

The tensile strength of the pulmonary valve leaflets equals or exceeds that of the aortic valve leaflet tissues.[76] Calcification, tears, or thinning of explanted pulmonary valves have not been found.[75] The pulmonary trunk is autogenous and viable and therefore has growth potential, as already documented in children,[77] with enlargement of the pulmonary autograft proportional to the somatic growth. The pulmonary homograft may not last a lifetime because it is cryopreserved or chemically treated in all cases. The expectation is that late degeneration will be at a slower rate and with more delayed consequences as a result of thinner walls and lower calcium and elastin content than seen in the degeneration of homograft aortic valves in the aortic position.[75] So far, intermediate-term follow-up data is quite encouraging. Reoperation is one source of concern. At the 20-year mark, Ross et al. report an actuarial freedom from reoperation of 85%.[75] Reasons for reoperation include implant technique (which favors aortic root replacement), bacterial endocarditis (rare), aortic annular dilation (which argues for the use of annular support), and pulmonary homograft stenosis. The pulmonary autograft has the potential to function well for perhaps the lifetime of the patient, depending on whether the operative technique achieves a perfect implant, free of any distortion of the valve.

Surgeons individually vary in their viewpoint regarding the Ross procedure, especially because aortic valve replacement with a mechanical prosthesis is such a straightforward procedure with excellent long-term results. Some feel that it converts a rather simple operation into a more complex one; whereas others think it is still investigational because the number of patients reaching late follow-up is relatively small and the degree to which Ross procedure can be generalized is limited.

portant consideration only when a small-sized valve is implanted. All prosthetic valves will manifest some resting gradient because the valve's sewing ring reduces its *EOA* to one that is smaller than the native orifice. This discrepancy has been termed *valve prosthesis–patient mismatch.*[22] The normal valve area is 2.5 to 3.5 cm^2 (aorta), and 4.0 to 6.0 cm^2 (mitral); a substantial gradient will usually not be present unless the *EOA* is less than 1 cm^2 because of the curvilinear relationship between the mean systolic gradient and the aortic valve area (Figure 26.3).

Mitral valve sizes of 25 to 27 mm give an *EOA* of 1.5 to 2.0 cm^2, which is equivalent to mild to moderate mitral stenosis. Porcine valves demonstrate suboptimal leaflet opening, with high pressure drops and narrow jet-type flows. For these reasons, their hemodynamic performance is inferior to that of mechanical valves. In general, all the currently available mechanical tilting disc valves demonstrate comparable hemodynamic function in equivalent sizes, except that the HP series has demonstrated some definite advantage in smaller sizes.

The diameter of the pulmonary annulus exceeds that of the natural aortic annulus by about 2 mm. The Ross procedure achieves a slight upsizing of the left ventricular outflow tract, which translates into excellent hemodynamic performance superior to any other method of aortic valve replacement, except perhaps aortic root replacement with a homograft.[79]

Hemodynamics

The hemodynamic performance of prosthetic valves is an exceedingly important aspect of their overall function; hemodynamic amelioration is the primary goal in the effort to replace the native valve. Performance is determined by the transvalvular gradient, and the transvalvular energy loss that occurs during systole, during valve closure and after valve closure from leakage. Assessment of in vitro hemodynamic performance using pulse duplicators provides comparative data for different valves in various sizes and at various cardiac outputs. Also, a performance index *(PI),* defined as the ratio of the effective orifice area *(EOA)* to the sewing ring area *(SWA)* has been proposed to compare various prosthetic valves. This ratio becomes more clinically relevant at smaller valve sizes (< 25 mm mitral and < 21 mm aortic). This concept was employed in the design of the Hemodynamic Plus (HP) series of the St Jude Medical and the Omniscience valves. The tilting disc valves have the highest *PI* (0.65–0.70), followed by the pericardial valves (0.65), then the supra-annular valves (0.54), and finally the porcine valves (0.35–0.40).[10] The hemodynamic performance of a prosthetic valve becomes an im-

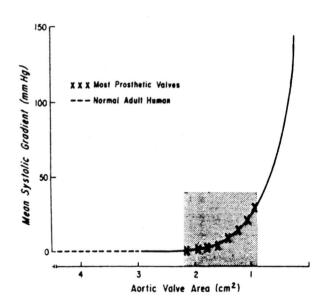

FIGURE 26.3. Relationship between the mean systolic gradient and the aortic valuve area. Note that the gradient begins to increase once the *EOA* is less than 50% of the normal valve area and rises steeply when the *EOA* is less than 1 cm^2. Reproduced with permission of the American Heart Association, Inc. from Rahimtoola.[78]

Durability

Of the five mechanical prostheses in use in the United States, there are very rare reported cases of structural failure; isolated cases of structural deterioration of the ball-and-cage valve have been reported. The lifespan of a mechanical valve is usually limited by the development of structural deterioration, but occasionally, thromboembolism, PVE, or anticoagulant-related bleeding that requires reoperation will limit the lifespan of a prosthesis. The Bjork-Shiley convexoconcave 60° model available from 1967 to 1987 was implanted in more than 80,000 patients. Patients who have this valve should be followed closely because the incidence of strut fracture is 0.295% per year for 29- to 33-mm valves manufactured between February 1, 1981, and June 30, 1982; it is 0.087% per year for similar-sized valves manufactured thereafter. Elective replacement is not advised because the risk of reoperation far exceeds the risk of strut fracture.[80] The Beall MV, a disc-in-cage prosthesis implanted in more than 17,000 patients between 1969 and 1975 has a teflon disc, teflon-covered metal struts, and a cloth seating area. The wear of these areas has led to significant hemolysis and eventual disc embolization in many patients.

Tissue valves may require reoperation for PVE or thromboembolism. Their lifelong durability is compromised predominantly by the development of structural deterioration caused by collagen degeneration and calcification of the leaflets. This appears to be related primarily to mechanical stress on the leaflets and may account for the slightly greater rate of deterioration of mitral prostheses, which are routinely subjected to greater ventricular pressure during leaflet closure than prostheses in the aortic position.[36] In patients more than 35 years of age, the incidence of structural failure necessitating reoperation approximates 1% to 2% per year for the first 7 years. Thereafter, an accelerating pattern of degeneration develops, with about 25% of patients requiring reoperation at 10 years, and 65% at 15 years. In young patients, the rate of valve failure is worse, approximating 50% at 10 years for those under 35 years of age,[81] 75% at 10 years for patients under 30 years of age,[82] and as high as 80% at 6 years for those under 20 years of age.[83] Failure rates are low in patients more than 65 years of age.[84]

Preservation techniques for homografts have evolved from chemical treatment and irradiation, through antibiotic sterilization and refrigeration at 4°C, to cryopreservation. About 90% of cryopreserved valves are free of degeneration at 10 years, possibly because the process preserves viable donor fibroblasts.[85] Reoperation-free survival of 90% at 10 years and nearly 50% at 19 years has been reported for the Ross procedure.[86]

Selection

Whereas it is oftentimes clear which type of valve is best suited for a particular patient, not infrequently, patients fall into the "gray zone" in which there is more than one choice. Factors to consider in making the selection may be patient related, valve related, or anatomic. A comprehensive list of these factors is provided in Table 26.18.

Patient-related factors are extremely important in influencing long-term survival and, hence, valve selection. Valve-related factors, on the other hand, tend to determine patient morbidity; the incidence of most complications and the mortality associated with their development is greater in older patients.[87-89]

Tissue valves have a lower rate of valve-related complications during the first 5 years, but after 7 years, the intrinsic rate of structural valve failure begins to manifest. In mechanical valves, the risk is constant with time. Two basic considerations are crucial in valve selection: (1) the ability to anticoagulate safely and (2) the anticipated life span of the patient. The selection criteria favoring each type of valve prosthesis are indicated in Tables 26.19 through 26.22.

TABLE 26.18. Factors to consider in selecting prosthetic valves.

Patient related	Valve related	Anatomical
Personal preference	Anticipated Prosthetic valve	Morphological configuration and size of the aortic root
Age	Hemodynamic performance	
Gender	Risk of thromboembolism	
Life expectancy	Risk of infection	
Occupation	Durability	
Lifestyle	Cost	
Bleeding history		
Coexisting medical illness		
Socioeconomic status		
Etiology of valve disease		
Desire to bear children		

TABLE 26.19. Selection criteria favoring mechanical cardiac valvular prosthesis.

No anticoagulation contraindications
Anticipated life expectancy of more than 10 yr
No plans for childbearing
Aortic valve replacement in the small aortic root (tilting disk); third choice to autograft/homograft in young patient
Mitral valve replacement in the small, hypercontractile, or hypertrophic left ventricle (to avoid left ventricular rupture—seen more with Carpentier–Edwards valve)

TABLE 26.20. Selection criteria favoring bioprosthetic cardiac valvular prosthesis.

Women of childbearing age (third choice in aortic position to autograft/homograft; first choice in mitral position)
Contraindication to anticoagulation
Unreliable, noncompliant patient
Lack of access to medical care facility
Anticipated life expectancy of less than 10 yr
Age more than 70 yr
Age more than 60 yr with comorbid illness
Endocarditis (stentless valve third choice to homograft/autograft)

TABLE 26.21. Selection criteria favoring homograft aortic valves.

Small aortic root (second choice to autograft in young patients)
Women of childbearing age (second choice to autograft)
Endocarditis (first choice)

TABLE 26.22. Selection criteria favoring pulmonary autograft.

Children, young adults who require tissue valve in aortic position
Life expectancy of more than 20 yr
Endocarditis (second choice to homograft)

Many surgeons now believe that the Ross procedure is the operation of choice when aortic valve replacement is required in young patients. When not feasible it is important to remember that in the small aortic root, the valve with the highest *PI* should be selected so as to minimize the degree of valve prosthesis–patient mismatch. It is generally accepted that tilting disc valves have the best hydraulic function in the 19- to 21-mm sizes, followed by the pericardial valves and then the porcine. Enlargement of the aortic annulus to avoid the placement of prosthetic valves with an *EOA* of less than 1 cm² should be performed when necessary.

The majority of prosthetic valves currently cost between $3,500.00 and $4,500.00. The overall cost of a homograft is approximately one and one-half times that of a prosthetic valve.

Conclusion

For the mechanical valves, each prosthetic design has some strong mechanical advantage but also some very

important limitations. The overall clinical performance of each valve type is reflected in the estimates of freedom from valve-related mortality, which is the likelihood of a patient dying of any valve-related complication including sudden death or nonsudden death from cardiac failure, or unexplained early or late deaths. Long-term performance of the porcine bioprosthesis is satisfactory in older patients for whom the incidence of structural failure is offset by limited survival time.

The ultimate goal of perfection in the search for more durable and less thrombogenic tissue and/or mechanical valves will undoubtedly remain elusive for years to come. In the meantime, safer anticoagulation and greater awareness of specific factors associated with valve-related complications, and more accurate anticipation of specific surgical outcome will assist in the most prudent valve selection for a given patient.

References

1. Harken DE, Soroff HS, Taylor WJ, et al. Partial and complete prosthesis in aortic insufficiency. *J Thorac Cardiovasc Surg.* 1960;44:744–762.
2. Starr A, Edwards ML. Mitral replacement: a clinical experience with the ball valve prosthesis. *Ann Surg.* 1961;154: 726–740.
3. Ellis FH, Kirklin JW, Parker RK, et al. Mitral commissurotomy: an overall appraisal of clinical and hemodynamic results. *Arch Intern Med.* 1954;94:774–784.
4. Selzer A, Malmborg RO. Some factors influencing changes in pulmonary vascular resistance in mitral valvular disease. *Am J Med.* 1962;32:532–544.
5. Braunwald E, Braunwald NS, Ross J Jr, Morrow AG. Effects of mitral valve replacement on the pulmonary vascular dynamics of patients with pulmonary hypertension. *N Engl J Med.* 1965;273:509–514.
6. Dalen JE, Matloff JM, Evans GL, et al. Early reduction of pulmonary vascular resistance after mitral valve replacement. *N Engl J Med.* 1967;277:387–394.
7. Kennedy JW, Doces J, Stewart DK. Left ventricular function before and following aortic valve replacement. *Circulation.* 1977;56:944–950.
8. Pantley G, Morton MJ, Rahimtoola SH: Effects of successful, uncomplicated valve replacement on ventricular hypertrophy, volume, and performance in aortic stenosis and aortic incompetence. *J Thorac Cardiovac Surg.* 1978;75: 383–391.
9. Smith N, McAnulty J, Rahimtoola SH. Severe aortic stenosis with impaired left ventricular function and clinical heart failure: results of valve replacement. *Circulation.* 1978;58:255–264.
10. Bojar RM. Valvular heart disease, including hypertrophic cardiomyopathy. In: Bojar RM. *Adult Cardiac Surgery.* Cambridge, Mass: Blackwell Scientific Publications; 1992: 154–240.
11. Akins CW. Mechanical cardiac valvular prosthesis. *Ann Thorac Surg.* 1991;52:161–172.
12. Akins CW. Results with mechanical cardiac valvular prosthesis. *Ann Thorac Surg.* 1995;60:1836–1844.

13. Copeland JG. The Carbomedics prosthetic heart valve: a second generation bileaflet prosthesis. *Sem Thorac Cardiovasc Surg.* 1996;8:237–241.

14. Akins CW. Medtronic–Hall prosthetic aortic valve. *Sem Thorac Cardiovasc Surg.* 1996;8: 242–248.

15. Edmunds LH Jr, Clark RE, Cohn LH, Miller DC, Weisel RD. Guidelines for reporting morbidity and mortality after cardiac valvular operations. *Ann Thorac Surg.* 1988;46: 257–259.

16. Feldman HJ, Gray RJ, Chaux A, et al. Noninvasive in-vivo and in-vitro study of the St Jude Medical mitral valve prosthesis. *Am J Cardiol.* 1982;49:1101–1109.

17. Panidis IP, Ren JF, Kotler MN, et al. Clinical and echocardiographic evaluation of the St Jude cardiac valve prosthesis following 126 patients. *J Am Coll Cardiol.* 1984;4: 454–462.

18. Kazui T, Komatsu S, Inoue N. Clinical evaluation of the Omniscience aortic disc valve prosthesis. *Scand J Thorac Cardiovac Surg.* 1987;21:173–174.

19. Carrier M, Martineau JP, Bonan R, Polletier LC. Clinical and hemodynamic assessment of the Omniscience prosthetic heart valve. *J Thorac Cardiovasc Surg.* 1987;93: 300–307.

20. Chesebro JH, Fuster V, Elveback LR, et al. Trial of combined warfarin plus dipyridamole or aspirin therapy in prosthetic heart valve replacement: danger of aspirin combined with dipyridamole. *Am J Cardiol.* 1983;51: 1537–1541.

21. Butchart EG, Lewis PA, Bethel JA, Breckenridge JM. Adjusting anticoagulation to prosthesis: thrombogenicity and patient risk factors. Recommendations for the Medtronic–Hall valve. *Circulation.* 1991;84(suppl III): III61–III69.

22. Stein PD, Alpert JS, Copeland J, et al. Antithrombotic therapy in patients with mechanical and biologic prosthetic heart valves. *Chest.* 1992;102:445S–455S.

23. Eckman MH, Beshansky JR, Durand-Zaleski I, et al. Anticoagulation for noncardiac procedures in patients with prosthetic heart valves. Does low risk mean high cost? *JAMA.* 1990;263:1513–1521.

24. Rahimtoola SH. Valvular heart disease: a perspective. *J Am Coll Cardiol.* 1983;1:199–215.

25. Cowgill LD, Addonizio VP, Hopeman AR, Harken AH. A practical approach to prosthetic valve endocarditis. *Ann Thorac Surg.* 1987;43:450–457.

26. Fann JI, Miller DC. Porcine valves: Hancock and Carpentier–Edwards aortic prostheses. *Sem Thorac Cardiovasc Surg.* 1996;8:259–268.

27. Rossiter SJ, Miller DC, Stinson EB, et al. Hemodynamic and clinical comparison of the Hancock Modified Orifice and standard orifice bioprosthesis in the aortic position. *J Thorac Cardiovasc Surg.* 1980;80:54–60.

28. Cohn LH, Couper GS, Aranki SF, et al. The long-term follow-up of the Hancock Modified Orifice porcine bioprosthetic valve. *J Cardiac Surg.* 1991;6:557–561.

29. Cohn LH, DiSesa VJ, Collins JJ Jr. The Hancock Modified Orifice porcine bioprosthetic valve; 1976–1988. *Ann Thorac Surg.* 1989;48:S81–S82.

30. Fernandez J, Chen C, Gu J, et al. Comparison of low pressure versus standard pressure fixation Carpentier–Edwards bioprosthesis. *Ann Thorac Surg.* 1995;60:S205–S210.

31. David TE, Armstrong S, Sun E. The Hancock II bioprosthesis at 10 years. *Ann Thorac Surg.* 1995;60:S229–S234.

32. Sarris GE, Robbins RC, Miller DC, et al. Randomized prospective assessment of bioprosthetic valve durability: Hancock versus Carpentier–Edwards valves. *Circulation.* 1993;88(pt 2):55–64.

33. Bolooki H, Kaiser GA, Mallon SM, Palatianos GM: Comparison of long-term results of Carpentier–Edwards and Hancock bioprosthetic valves. *Ann Thorac Surg.* 1986;42: 494–499.

34. Jones EL, Weintraub WS, Craver JM, et al. Interaction of age and coronary disease after valve replacement: implications for valve selection. *Ann Thorac Surg.* 1994;58: 378–385.

35. Lytle BW, Cosgrove DM, Taylor PC, et al: Primary isolated aortic valve replacement: early and late results. *J Thorac Cardiovasc Surg.* 1989;97:675–694.

36. Burdon TA, Miller DC, Oyer PE, et al. Durability of porcine valves at fifteen years in a representative North American population. *J Thorac Cardiovasc Surg.* 1992;103: 238–252.

37. Akins CW, Carroll D, Buckley MJ, et al. Late results with Carpentier–Edwards porcine bioprosthesis. *Circulation.* 1990;82(suppl 4):65–74.

38. Milligan DJ Jr, Lewis JW, Stein P, Alam M: The porcine bioprosthetic heart valve: experience at 15 years. *Ann Thorac Surg.* 1989;48:324–330.

39. Cohn LH, Collins JJ Jr, DiSesa V, et al. Fifteen-year experience with 1678 Hancock porcine bioprosthetic heart valve replacements. *Ann Surg.* 1989;210:435–443.

40. Jones EL, Weintraub WS, Craver JM, et al. Ten-year experience with the porcine bioprosthetic valves: Interrelationship of valve survival and patient survival in 1050 valve replacements. *Ann Thorac Surg.* 1990;49:370–384.

41. Milano AD, Bortolotti U, Mazzucco A, et al. Performance of the Hancock porcine bioprosthesis following aortic valve replacement: considerations based on a 15 year experience. *Ann Thorac Surg.* 1988;46:216–222.

42. Jamieson WRE, Munro AI, Miyagishima RT, et al. Carpentier–Edwards standard porcine bioprosthesis: clinical performance to seventeen years. *Ann Thorac Surg.* 1995;60: 999–1007.

43. Glower DD, White WD, Hatton AC, et al. Determinants of reoperation after 960 valve replacements with Carpentier–Edwards prostheses. *J Thorac Cardiovasc Surg.* 1994; 107:381–393.

44. Pelletier LC, Carrier M, Leclerc Y, et al. Influence of age on late results of valve replacement with porcine bioprostheses. *J Thorac Cardiovasc Surg.* 1992;33:526–533.

45. Grunkemeier GL, Jamieson WRE, Miller DC, Starr A: Actuarial versus actual risks of porcine structural valve deterioration. *J Thorac Cardiovasc Surg.* 1994;108:709–718.

46. Bernal JM, Rabasa JM, Lopez R, et al. Durability of the Carpentier–Edwards porcine bioprosthesis: role of age and valve position. *Ann Thorac Surg.* 1995;60:S248–S252.

47. Papello DF, Bessone LN, Hiro SP, et al. Bioprosthetic valve longevity in the elderly: an 18-year longitudinal study. *Ann Thorac Surg.* 1995;60:S270–S275.

48. Carpentier A, Dubost C, Lane E. Continuing improvement in valvular prostheses. *J Thorac Cardiovasc Surg.* 1982;83: 27–42.

49. David TE, Ropchan GC, Butany JW. Aortic valve replacement with stentless porcine bioprostheses. *J Cardiac Surg.* 1988;3:501–505.

50. David TE, Pollick C, Bos J. Aortic valve replacement with stentless porcine aortic bioprostheses. *J Thorac Cardiovasc Surg.* 1990;99:113–118.

51. Binet JP, Duran CG, Carpentier A, Langlois J. Heterologous aortic valve transplantation *Lancet.* 1965;2:1275.

52. O'Brein MF, Clarebrough JK. Heterograft aortic valve transplantation for human valve disease. *Med J Aust.* 1966; 2:228–230.

53. Jin XY, Gibson DG, Yacoub MH, Pepper JR: Perioperative assessment of aortic homograft, Toronto stentless valve and stented valve in the aortic position. *Ann Thorac Surg.* 1995;60:S395–S401.

54. Casabona R, DePaulis R, Zattera GF, et al. Stentless porcine and pericardial valve in aortic position. *Ann Thorac Surg.* 1992;54:681–685.

55. Cohn LH, Koster JK, Mee RBB, Collins JJ Jr. Long-term follow-up of the Hancock bioprosthetic heart valve: a 6-year review. *Circulation.* 1979;60(suppl):187–192.

56. Davila JC, Magilligan DJ Jr, Lewis JW Jr. Is the Hancock porcine valve the best cardiac valve substitute today? *Ann Thorac Surg.* 1978;26:303–316.

57. Craver JM, King SB III, Douglas JS, et al. Late hemodynamic evaluation of Hancock modified orifice aortic bioprosthesis. *Circulation.* 1979;60(suppl):193–197.

58. Hannah H III, Reis RL. Current status of porcine heterograft prosthesis: a 5-year appraisal. *Circulation.* 1976; 54 (suppl):27–31.

59. Johnson A, Thompson S, Vieweg WVR, et al. Evaluation of the in-vivo function of the Hancock porcine xenograft valve. *J Thorac Cardiovasc Surg.* 1978;76:599–605.

60. Morris DC, King SB III, Douglas JJ Jr, et al. Hemodynamic results of aortic valvular replacement with the porcine xenograft valve. *Circulation.* 1977;56:841–844.

61. Jones EL, Craver JM, Morris DC, et al. Hemodynamic and clinical evaluation of the Hancock xenograft bioprosthesis for aortic valve replacement (with emphasis on management of the small aortic root). *J Thorac Cardiovasc Surg.* 1978;76:300–308.

62. Ionescu MI, Tandon AP, Mary DAS, Abid A. Heart valve replacement with the Ionescu- Shiley pericardial xenograft. *J Thorac Cardiovasc Surg.* 1977;73:31–42.

63. Becker RM, Strom J, Fishman W, et al. Hemodynamic performance of the Ionescu-Shiley valve prosthesis. *J Thorac Cardiovasc Surg.* 1980;80:613–620.

64. Willey VM, Keon WJ. Patterns of failure in Ionescu-Shiley bovine pericardial bioprosthetic valves. *J Thorac Cardiovasc Surg.* 1987;93:925–933.

65. Gonzalez-Levin L, Chi S, Blair C, et al. Five-year experience with the Ionescu-Shiley bovine pericardial valve in the aortic position. *Ann Thorac Surg.* 1983;36:270–280.

66. Frater RWM, Salomon NW, Rainer WG, et al. The Carpentier–Edwards pericardial aortic valve: intermediate results. *Ann Thorac Surg.* 1987;94:200–207.

67. Cosgrove DM. Carpentier pericardial valve. *Sem Thorac Cardiovasc Surg.* 1996;8:269–275.

68. Pelletier LC, Leclerc Y, Bonan R, et al. Aortic valve replacement with the Carpentier– Edwards pericardial bio-

prosthesis: clinical and hemodynamic results. *J Cardiac Surg.* 1988;3:405–412.

69. Gabbay S, Frater RWM. In-vitro comparison of the newer heart valve bioprosthesis in the mitral and aortic positions. In: Cohn LH, Galluccci V, eds. *Cardiac Prostheses. Proceedings of the Second International Symposium.* Stoneham, Mass: York Medical Books; 1982:456–468.

70. Cosgrove DM, Lytle BW, Taylor PC. The Carpentier–Edwards pericardial aortic valve: 10-year results. *J Thorac Cardiovasc Surg.* 1995;110:651–662.

71. Perier P, Mihacleanu S, Fabiani JN, et al. Long-term evaluation of the Carpentier–Edwards pericardial valve in the aortic position. *J Card Surg.* 1991;6(suppl):589–594.

72. Burdon TA, Miller DC, Oyer PE, et al. Durability of porcine valves at 15 years in a representative North American population. *J Thorac Cardiovasc Surg.* 1992;103: 238–252.

73. Doty DB. Aortic valve replacement with homograft and autograft. *Sem Thorac Cardiovasc Surg.* 1996;8:249–258.

74. Ross DN. Replacement of aortic and mitral valves with pulmonary autograft. *Lancet.* 1967;2:956–958.

75. Ross D, Jackson M, Davies J. Pulmonary autograft aortic valve replacement: long-term results. *J Card Surg.* 1991;6: 529–533.

76. Gorczynski A, Trenkner M, Anisimowicz L, et al. Biomechanics of the pulmonary autograft valve in the aortic position. *Thorax.* 1982;37:535–539.

77. Elkins RC, Knott-Craig CJ, Ward KE, et al. Pulmonary autograft in children: realized growth potential. *Ann Thorac Surg.* 1994;57:1387–1394.

78. Rahimtoola SH. The problem of valve prosthesis–patient mismatch. *Circulation.* 1978;58:20–24.

79. Kouchoukos NT, Davila-Roman VG, Spray TL, et al. Replacement of the aortic root with a pulmonary autograft in children and young adults with aortic valve disease. *N Engl J Med.* 1994;330:1–6.

80. Hiratzka LF, Kouchoukos NT, Grunkemeier GL, et al. Outlet strut fracture of the Bjork–Shiley 60° convexo-concave valve: current information and recommendation for patient care. *J Am Coll Cardiol.* 1988;11:1130–1137.

81. Magilligan DJ Jr, Lewis JW Jr, Tilley B, Peterson E. The porcine bioprosthetic valve. Twelve years later. *J Thorac Cardiovasc Surg.* 1985;89:499–507.

82. Jamieson WRE, Rosado LJ, Munro, et al. Carpentier–Edwards standard porcine bioprosthesis: primary tissue failure (structural valve deterioration) by age groups. *Ann Thorac Surg.* 1988;46:155–162.

83. Antunes MJ, Santos LP. Performance of glutaraldehyde-preserved porcine bioprosthesis as a mitral valve substitute in a young population group. *Ann Thorac Surg.* 1984;37: 387–392.

84. Jamieson WRE, Burr LH, Munro AI, et al. Cardiac valve performance in the elderly: clinical performance of biologic prostheses. *Ann Thorac Surg.* 1989;48:173–185.

85. O'Brien MF, Stafford EG, Gardner MAH, et al. A comparison of aortic valve replacement with viable cryopreserved and fresh allograft valves, with a note on chromosomal studies. *J Thorac Cardiovasc Surg.* 1987;94:812–823.

86. Matsuki O, Okita Y, Almeida RS, et al. Two decades' experience with aortic valve replacement with pulmonary autograft. *J Thorac Cardiovasc Surg.* 1988;95:705–711.

87. Mitchell RS, Miller DC, Stinson EB, et al. Significant patient-related determinants of prosthetic valve performance. *J Thorac Cardiovasc Surg*. 1986;91:807–817.

88. Hammermeister KE, Henderson WG, Burchfield CM , et al. Comparison of outcome after valve replacement with a bioprosthesis versus a mechanical prosthesis: initial 5-year results of a randomized trial. *J Am Coll Cardiol*. 1987;10: 719–732.

89. Hammond GL, Geha AS, Kopf GS, Hahim SW. Biologic versus mechanical valves. Analysis of 1116 valves inserted in 1012 adult patients with a 4818 patient-year and a 5327 valve-year follow-up. *J Thorac Cardiovasc Surg*. 1987;93: 182–198.

27

Techniques for Interventional Catheterization Guided by Transesophageal Echocardiography

Faruk Erzengin and Kemalettin Büyüköztürk

Transesophageal echocardiography (TEE) was first used clinically by anesthesiologists for intraoperative monitoring of cardiac functions. Later, intraoperative TEE has been accepted by cardiologists, cardiac surgeons, and anesthesiologists as a basic tool to evaluate the immediate hemodynamic results of a surgical procedure.[1,2]

Transseptal catheterization technique was first developed in 1960.[3] Further investigations of this technique showed that procedural mortality and complications were relatively rare.[4] The transseptal puncture has traditionally been performed with fluoroscopic guidance, but this method is not always easy and safe because of the technical difficulties in recognizing the correct three-dimensional structure of the interatrial septum. Although transthoracic echocardiography (TTE) may be helpful as a guide to localize the interatrial septum, it has limited value because of well-known technical difficulties. During percutaneous mitral balloon valvuloplasty (PMBV), it is possible to visualize the interatrial septum and foramen ovale by using advanced (multiplane and pediatric) TEE probes. The correct localization of these structures guides the operator through the interatrial septum to the left atrium. Also, the TEE technique helps the operator with evaluation of the mitral valve, mitral apparatus, and mitral orifice size and helps selection of the appropriate balloon size. During the procedure, it is possible to follow the results step-by-step after each balloon inflation and, in this way, avoid causing significant mitral regurgitation. Currently, TEE and fluoroscopic guidance are used routinely in combination in PMBV applications as well as in other interventional catheterization techniques such as balloon atrial septostomy, atrial septal defect, patent ductus arteriosus closure, and percutaneous cardiopulmonary support with left atrial cannulation for severe left ventricular failure.[5]

PMBV with TEE in the Catheterization Laboratory

PMBV is a still-developing technique and is an alternative to surgical closed valvotomy in the treatment of pure mitral stenosis. In 1982, Inoue et al. first applied PMBV using a special balloon catheter and recommended echocardiographic monitoring.[6,7] In the currently used technique, the left atrium is catheterized through the interatrial septum. The interatrial septum has to be punctured in the area of fossa ovale by a modified Brockenbrough needle to form a passage for the balloon catheter to enter the left atrium. This stage of the procedure requires correct orientation of the interatrial septum by the operator, otherwise it may not be safe and can lead to catheter-related complications. X-ray guidance alone is not sufficient for clear visualization of the interatrial septum and localization of the level of the foramen ovale. Today, both fluoroscopy and TEE guidance are recommended for a safe and successful procedure in interventional cardiology.

The aims of performing conventional echocardiography or TEE before and/or during PMBV are as follows:

1. To recognize the presence of thrombi or spontaneous contrast in the left atrium
2. To evaluate the morphologic characteristics of the mitral valve and the subvalvular apparatus
3. To determine the severity of mitral stenosis by planimetry and continuous wave Doppler imaging using the pressure half-time method
4. To assess the degree of mitral regurgitation
5. To search for an interatrial shunt by color flow Doppler imaging
6. To correctly calculate the stenotic mitral valve score (refer to Chapter 28)

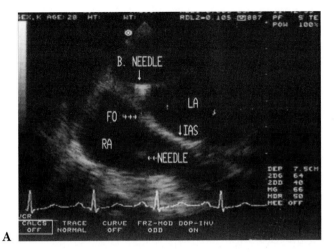

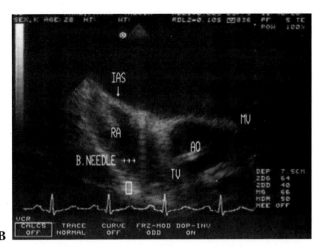

FIGURE 27.1. TEE images showing puncture of the interatrial septum. **A,** Brockenborough needle on the interatrial septum showing tent formation; **B,** Brockenborough needle visualized in both left and right atrium after passing through the intra- trial septum. In **A,** IAS indicates interatrial septum; RA, right atrium. In **B,** needle indicates Brockenborough needle; TV, tri- cuspid valve; AO, aortic root; MV, mitral valve; FO, foramen ovale.

The patients must be in a fasting state for at least 6 hours before the procedure. Before swallowing the probe, the patient's throat is locally anesthesized with li- docaine aerosol. Immediately after hemodynamic angio- graphic study for PMBV, the TEE probe is swallowed by the patient while in the left lateral decubitus position. Af- ter introduction of a Brockenbrough needle, the tent formation of the interatrial septum must be clearly seen by means of the TEE probe so that transseptal puncture may be accomplished (Figure 27.1). Left atrial pressure and oxygen saturation must be recorded immediately af- ter this procedure. Saline is injected into the catheter to create contrast echoes in the left atrium to confirm the positioning of the catheter through the interatrial sep- tum. After this procedure, to avoid aspiration or irrita- tion of the esophagus, we prefer to remove the probe from the patient until the mitral commissurotomy bal- loon is inflated. Before inflation of the balloon in the mi- tral orifice, reintroduction of the TEE probe is recom- mended.

The second important part of the PMBV procedure is the dilatation of the stenotic mitral valve with the appro- priate size balloon to avoid mitral regurgitation due to the rupture of mitral annulus or chordae tendineae, or other complications (Figure 27.2).[8] It is very easy to use TEE or TTE for measuring mitral valve area to detect a possible mitral regurgitation after each balloon dilata- tion procedure. It is also possible to use TEE images ob- tained after PMBV to detect and evaluate the degree of the shunt produced by atrial septal cannulation. By us- ing more advanced probes (biplane or multiplane) it is possible to obtain more detailed images and therefore better and quicker evaluation of the mitral valve before, during, and after the procedure. All these advantages of

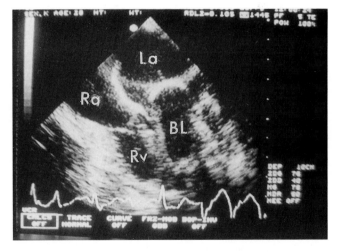

FIGURE 27.2. TEE image during inflation of Inoue balloon in the orifice of the mitral valve.

TEE guidance provide better and safer PMBV results with improved residual mitral valve anatomy and intra- operative mortality and morbidity. Experience has shown that mortality and morbidity are clearly reduced in procedures guided by TEE.[9,10]

Closure of Atrial Septal Defect with TEE Guidance in the Catheterization Laboratory

A technique for closure of atrial septal defect with TEE guidance in the catheterization laboratory has been developed and applied by Hellenbrand et al. whose first results were published in 1990.[11] In this procedure, a guidewire is passed through the atrial septal defect to the left atrium, and a special catheter with a closed clamshell umbrella at the tip is introduced on this guide wire. Then the umbrella is opened and the catheter withdrawn until the umbrella is installed on the atrial septal defect. This method is especially successful in small ostium secundum–type defects. However, residual leaks through the closed defect may be detected following the procedure in some patients. These leaks may be hemodynamically significant, require a repetition of the procedure, and cause troublesome hemolytic anemia and embolization.

TEE performance before closure of the atrial septal defect provides a better evaluation of the size, location, shape, and number defects, and assists with the calculation of the degree of shunt required (pulmonary blood flow/systemic blood flow [Q_p/Q_s]). This information is especially important for selecting the appropriate size umbrella. It is possible to clearly visualize the atrial septum and to see and control the final position of the umbrella by using TEE during the procedure. Following closure of the defect, TEE is the most sensitive method for the detection of even very small residual leaks around the edges of the umbrella. As a result, TEE guidance provides more information and a confortable, safe setting both for the patient and the operator.

Closure of Patent Ductus Arterious with TEE Guidance in the Catheter Laboratory

A similar technique to the one used for atrial septal defect closure is being used for closure of patent ductus arteriosus with a Rashkind device.[12] It is well known that TTE is not as sensitive as TEE, especially in detecting the residual leaks after closure of the defect. Therefore, TEE guidance enables the operator to manipulate the device to optimize results, check the presence and degree of residual leaks to avoid postprocedural hemolytic anemia, and minimize hemodynamically significant residual shunt.

Balloon Atrial Septostomy

Balloon atrial septostomy is the most commonly applied procedure for patients with critical cyanotic congenital heart disease. This intervention has been traditionally performed with fluoroscopic monitoring in the catheter laboratory. Currently it is possible to apply this tech-

nique with TTE or TEE guidance at bedside in the critical care unit. Echocardiography is useful to confirm the position of the balloon in the left atrium and for determination of the appropriate balloon size. It is also possible to evaluate the size of the defect and the flow through the enlarged atrial septal defect by means of echocardiography. TEE guidance may be helpful in preventing serious complications related to balloon atrial septostomy. Although TTE is usually sufficient to guide the operator, TEE provides some additional advantages such as permitting continuous monitoring of cardiac function in these critically ill patients and keeping the operative field sterile. However, if the patient is not intubated, it is not appropriate to apply a TEE probe because of the aspiration risk. As a result, TEE guidance is preferred in the intubated patient, and TTE monitoring should be applied to avoid aspiration if the patient is not intubated.

Future Aspects of TEE Use During Interventional Cardiology

The latest advances in TEE include three-dimensional reconstruction and panoramic echocardiography.[9] However, there are some problems with the real timing of the three-dimensional images. Technical studies are continuing to solve this problem. As the techniques develop, these two systems can be used successfully to guide interventional catheterization methods.

Acknowledgment
We would like to thank Dr. Nevnihal Eren for her kind assistance.

References

1. Matsumoto M, Oka Y, Strom J. Application of transesophageal echocardiography to continuous intraoperative monitoring of left ventricular performance. *Am J Cardiol.* 1980;46:95–105.
2. Schiller N, Quinones M, Cahalan M, et al. Who are candidates for intraoperative TEE? When do you need a cardiologist in the OR? Who should read intraoperative studies? Symposium on Transesophageal Echocardiography 1991. Frenchmen's Reef Beach Resort St. Thomas, U.S. Virgin Islands April 11–13.
3. Brockenbrough EC, Braunwald E. A new technique for left ventricular angiography and transseptal left heart catheterization. *Am J Cardiol.* 1960;6:1062.
4. Conti CR, Grossman W. Percutaneous approach and transseptal catheterization. In: Grossman W, ed. *Cardiac Catheterization and Angiography.* Philadelphia, Pa: Lea & Febiger; 1974:59–75.

5. Foster, E, Schiller BN. The role of transesophageal echocardiography in critical care: UCSF experience. *J Am Soc Echocardiogr.* 1992;5:368–374.

6. Inoue K, Nakamura T, Kitamura F. Nonoperative mitral commissurotomy by a new balloon catheter [abstract]. *Jpn Circ J.* 1982;46:877.

7. Inoue K, Owaki T, Nakamura T. Clinical application of transvenous mitral commissurotomy by a new balloon catheter. *J Thorac Surg.* 1984;87:394–402.

8. Manga B, Singh S, Brandis S. Left ventricular perforation during percutaneous mitral balloon valvuloplasty. *Cathet Cardiovasc Diagn.* 1992;25:317–319.

9. Kyo S, Omoto R, Mototyama T, et al. Transesophageal echocardiography during catheter interventions. In: Maurer G, ed. *Transesophageal Echocardiography.* New York: McGraw-Hill; 1994:215–233.

10. Jaarsma W, Visser CA, Suttorp MJ, et al.: Transesophageal echocardiography during percutaneous balloon mitral valvuloplasty. *J Am Soc Echocardiogr.* 1990;3:384–391.

11. Hellenbrand WE, Fahey JT, Mc Gowan FX. Transesophageal echocardiography guidance of transcatheter closure of atrial septal defect. *Am J Cardiol.* 1990;66:207–213.

12. Rashkind WJ, Mullins CE, Hellenbrand WE, et al. Nonsurgical closure of patent ductus arteriosus: clinical application of the Rashkind PDA Occluder system. *Circulation.* 1987;75:583–592.

28

Percutaneous Mitral Balloon Valvuloplasty

Mehmet Meriç, Nevres Koylan, and Kemalettin Büyüköztürk

Since it was first introduced in 1982 by Inoue et al.,[1] percutaneous balloon mitral valvuloplasty (PMBV) has become established as an important nonsurgical alternative for the management of patients with mitral stenosis.[2] Another technique using a single-balloon[3] or double-balloon[4] through transseptal left atrial catheterization quickly followed. Variations of this technique using transarterial balloon introduction[5] and retrograde left atrial catheterization[6] have also been reported. Today, the most commonly used technique is the antegrade approach with a single and double balloon, or a specially designed Inoue balloon. The mechanism of this procedure is similar to that of surgical commissurotomy for the splitting of the fused commissures.

Technique

Retrograde Approach

In this technique (Figure 28.1), the guidewire is introduced from the femoral vein through the inferior vena cava, right atrium, left atrium, and left ventricle, and out the aorta using a transseptal technique performed by means of the puncture of the interatrial septum. The wire is drawn out from the femoral artery with a wire loop or a retriever catheter. The balloon catheter is introduced percutaneously through the femoral artery and aorta to the mitral valve.[5-7] Today, the use of this technique is limited.

Antegrade Approach Single- and Double-Balloon Techniques

In these techniques, the mitral valve is dilated by one or two polyethylene balloons. Access to left atrium is by the transseptal route from the right atrium. A single bifoil or trefoil balloon on a single guidewire, or two balloons (two monofoil balloons or a monofoil and a trefoil balloon) (Schneider Europe; Mansfield Scientific Inc, Boston, Mass) on separate guidewires may be used. When using two balloons, both left and right femoral veins must be punctured.

The left atrium is catheterized through the interatrial septum by standard transseptal puncture.[8] The atrial septum is punctured in the area of the fossa ovalis from the right femoral vein using a modified Brockenbrough needle and an 8-Fr Mullin's sheath and dilator (USCI, Billerica, Mass). During puncture of the atrial septum, the guidance of a pigtail catheter at the level of the aortic valve may be helpful. Echocardiographic guidance may also be useful for this purpose. When the needle enters the left atrium, the localization is confirmed by oximetry, pressure measurement, and contrast injection. The needle and dilator are then removed, leaving the Mullin's sheath in the left atrium.

Following left atrial catheterization, 100 U/kg of heparin is administered intravenously. A 7-Fr balloon wedge catheter is advanced through the sheath into the left atrium and then into the left ventricle. Simultaneous recording of left atrial and left ventricular pressures are performed to calculate the mitral valve area. A flow-directed balloon wedge catheter is inserted from femoral vein to left atrium and left ventricle, and is deflected through the aortic valve into the ascending and descending aorta. One or two (according to the number of balloons that will be used) 0.038-inch guidewires can be advanced through each lumen so that J-tips of the guidewires lie in the descending aorta at the level of the diaphragm. The double-lumen catheter is then removed, leaving guidewires.[8]

A 5-mm dilating balloon catheter can be advanced over one of the guidewires to the interatrial septum, the balloon is inflated to further dilate the atrial septum in the puncture area, and then the balloon is removed. The dilating balloon catheter(s) are then advanced over the transfer guidewires and cautiously positioned across the mitral valve. The transfer guidewires in the left ventricle

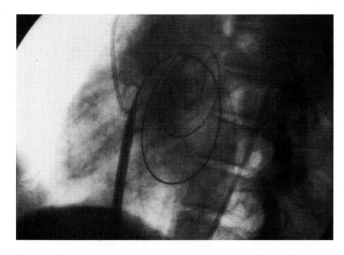

FIGURE 28.1. Cineangiographic view showing guidewire located in left atrium and a 5-mm balloon being inserted over the guidewire to dilate interatrial septum.

should be large enough to allow the dilating balloon catheters to pass smoothly across the mitral valve. Two balloons are inflated together with a hand-held syringe, then quickly deflated and withdrawn into the left atrium. Inflation–deflation must be quick to avoid prolonged hypotension. During inflation, the indentation of the stenotic mitral valve on the balloons appears and quickly disappears (Figure 28.2).

Following dilatation, any dilating balloon catheters are removed, and a double lumen floating balloon wedge catheter is advanced to the left atrium to measure the gradient across the mitral valve. Mitral valve gradient and cardiac output measurements are again performed to calculate postprocedural mitral valve area. To evaluate the presence of mitral regurgitation, left ventriculography is performed in either left lateral or right anterior oblique projection. Finally, pressure measurements and oximetric studies of the left and right heart are per-

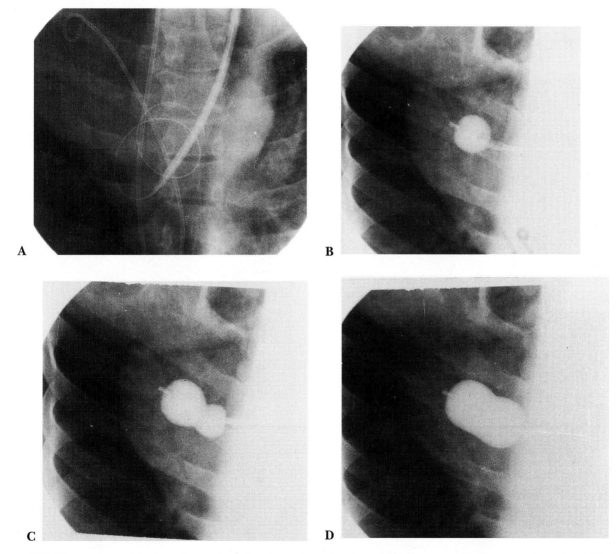

FIGURE 28.2. Cineangiographic view of an antegrade approach balloon at the mitral valve level. The indentations of the stenotic mitral valve on the balloon appear and quickly disappear. The labels **A, B, C,** and **D** show the sequence of operation.

formed to determine the pressure changes and left-to-right shunting through the atrial septum. Arterial and venous sheaths are pulled immediately following the procedure.[8]

Inoue Technique

The Inoue technique is an antegrade approach technique developed by Kanji Inoue and colleagues in 1982,[2] and a special balloon, named after Inoue, is used. The Inoue balloon (Toray Inc, New York) is made of latex and nylon and has many unique properties. It has a segmental hourglasslike inflation profile. The distal portion of the balloon is inflated first, then the proximal portion. The balloon is easily inserted from the femoral vein and is easily advanced through the mitral valve by means of its low profile; progressively larger inflation is possible by virtue of the balloon's high compliance. High compliance also makes shorter inflation–deflation times possible. The balloon tip is steerable, making manipulation easier. Left atrial pressure can be measured after the inflation–deflation by means of the central lumen, and finally, no guidewire is necessary in the left ventricle, thus reducing arrhythmia risk. These characteristics make the procedure simpler and faster.[9]

In this technique, the left atrium is catheterized by the standard transseptal approach and the interatrial septum is dilated as already described. The Inoue balloon is introduced transseptally into the left atrium from the femoral vein and, with the aid of an internal steering stylet, is advanced across the mitral valve to left ventricle. With initial inflation, only the proximal portion of the balloon enlarges. The balloon is then pulled back against the valve, away from the left ventricular apex. With further inflation, the proximal and middle sections are inflated, respectively, thus fixing the balloon in position and dilating the valve (Figure 28.3).

Mitral valve opening and the presence of mitral regurgitation are evaluated with the aid of pressure measurements (Figure 28.4), two-dimensional echocardiography and Doppler echocardiography (Figure 28.5). If necessary, further inflation can be performed before the device is removed.[10] Recently, transesophageal echocardiography has also been used to evaluate the performance of PMBV.[11] Moreover, a study performed by Kültürsay et al.[12] reports that PMBV can be safely performed with transesophageal echocardiography and without using fluoroscopy.

Results of the studies comparing conventional single- and double-balloon antegrade approach techniques and

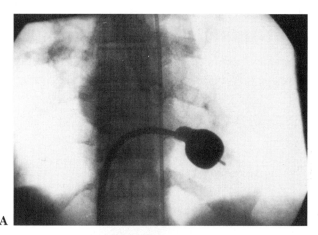

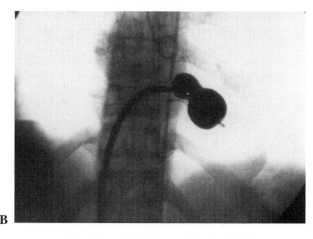

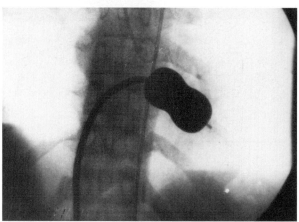

FIGURE 28.3. Cineangiographic view of the three phases of the inflation of an Inoue balloon at the level of the mitral valve during PMBV. **A,** Inoue balloon passed through the mitral valve and left ventricular portion, inflated to position the balloon on the mitral valve. **B,** Both left atrial and left ventricular portions of the Inoue balloon are inflated and the indentation of the stenotic mitral valve can be seen on the balloon. **C,** The indentation on the fully inflated Inoue balloon disappears, indicating commissural tear of the stenotic mitral valve.

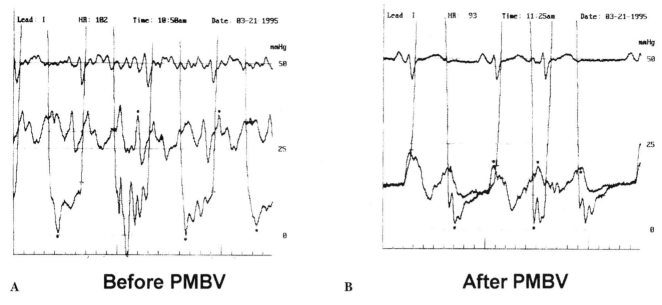

FIGURE 28.4. Pressure gradient across the mitral valve before and after PMBV in a patient with rheumatic mitral stenosis.

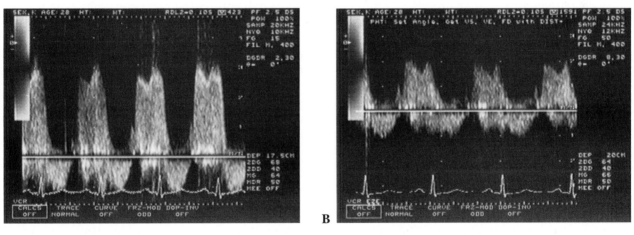

FIGURE 28.5. Transthoracic pulsed-wave Doppler echocardiographic flow of the stenotic mitral valve before (**A**) and just after (**B**) PMBV.

the Inoue technique show that both techniques are similarly effective, but the Inoue technique is easier and safer.[13–15] A study describing the use of the Inoue balloon catheter via retrograde nontransseptal route has been published, but the reliability of this technique needs further investigation.[16]

Patient Selection

All patents with symptomatic mitral stenosis are potential candidates for PMBV. Clinical parameters predictive of a successful PMBV include normal sinus rhythm and young age, but with increasing experience, successful results are also reported with older patients.[17,18]

The echocardiographic examination of the mitral valve and subvalvular apparatus were reported to be the most important predictors of procedural outcome. An echocardiographic score, which is being used to screen potential candidates, has been developed based on mitral valve leaflet mobility, thickness, calcification, and subvalvular fibrosis[19] (Table 28.1). These parameters were graded from 1 to 4, and a total score ranging from 4 to 16 was obtained by summing these parameter scores. The severity of the disease increases with the total score. If the total score is 8 or less, the procedural outcome is generally good; such patients are good candidates for PMBV. In patients whose total scores range from 9 to 12, the results of PMBV are variable. If the total echocardiographic score is 12 or more, PMBV should be

TABLE 28.1. Echocardiographic grading of morphological mitral valve characteristics.

Characteristic	Grade I	Grade II	Grade III	Grade IV
Leaflet mobility	Highly mobile valve with restriction only at the leaflet tips	Reduced mobility at midportion and base of leaflets	Mainly basal diastolic forward movement of the valve leaflets	No or minimal diastolic forward movement of the valve leaflets
Valvular thickening	Near normal leaflets (4–5 mm)	Midleaflet thickening, marked thickening at the margins	Thickening through the entire leaflets (5–8 mm)	Marked thickening through all leaflet tissue (≥8–10 mm)
Subvalvular thickening	Minimal thickening of the chordal structures just below the valve	Thickening of the chordae extending up to one third of chordal length	Chordal thickening extending up to two thirds of the chordae	Extensive thickening and shortening of all chordae extending down to the papillary muscle
Valvular calcification	Single area of increased echocardiographic brightness	Scattered areas of brightness confined to leaflet margins	Brightness extending to the middle of the leaflets	Extensive brightness through most of the leaflet tissue

Adopted from Wilkins et al.[19]

performed only in patients for whom open heart surgery is contraindicated.[20,21]

Evidence of left atrial thrombus assessed by echocardiographic examination (transthoracic and/or transesophageal), or a recent embolic event is accepted to be a major contraindication for PMBV. However, in some studies with limited numbers of patients, PMBV performed with the Inoue balloon was feasible and safe in patients with left atrial thrombus.[22,23] However, because of limited experience, this option should be used only for patients for whom surgery is contraindicated and treatment is urgent. It has to be kept in mind that if the thrombus is free-floating or located in the left atrial cavity, PMBV is certainly contraindicated. In the presence of thrombus in the left atrial appendage, a recent embolic event, or in patients with atrial fibrillation, anticoagulant therapy must be given for at least two months. The disappearance of the thrombus must then be demonstrated with repeat new transesophageal echocardiography.[23,24] The procedure is also contraindicated in patients with left ventricular thrombus within an area of old myocardial infarction.

In case of severe mitral calcification, severe subvalvular thickening, or the presence of mitral regurgitation of grade II or higher, the chance of success is low and the complication rate is higher, thus limiting the use of this technique only to patients who carry a high risk for surgical intervention.[20,21,25] On the other hand, the presence of mild mitral[26] or aortic regurgitation[27] is not regarded as a contraindication for PMBV.

Percutaneous mitral balloon valvuloplasty may be an alternative for patients in whom surgery is regarded to have high risk because of suprasystemic pulmonary hypertension.[28,29] Limited experience also suggest that PMBV can be applied safely during pregnancy.[30,31] On the other hand, PMBV is the only chance for patients for whom surgery is prohibited because of a number of clinical conditions including renal, hepatic, and respiratory insufficiency.[32]

Immediate Results

The technical success rate of PMBV is generally high. According to unpublished data from our institution, the primary success rate was found to be 90% for 60 patients who had the procedure performed by the double-balloon technique, and 96.4% for 56 patients who had the Inoue technique. Published results are similar.[25,32–34]

TABLE 28.2. Immediate results of percutaneous mitral balloon valvuloplasty.

	Number of patients	MV gradient (mm Hg)		MV area (cm²)	
		Before PMBV	After PMBV	Before PMBV	After PMBV
Meriç M et al. 1993 (single balloon antegrade)	60	18.0 ± 4.2	2.45 ± 1.47	1.13 ± 0.18	2.29 ± 0.37
Meriç M et al. 1993 (Inoue)	56	15.8 ± 5.0	1.8 ± 0.9	1.13 ± 0.36	1.98 ± 0.32
Hung et al.[32] (Inoue)	204	13.0 ± 5.1	5.7 ± 2.6	1.0 ± 0.3	2.0 ± 0.7
NHLBI registry[33]	517	14.0 ± 6.0	6.0 ± 3.0	1.0 ± 0.3	2.0 ± 0.8
Inoue[34]	527	11.9 ± 0.27	5.5 ± 0.14	1.13 ± 0.02	1.97 ± 0.04
Rihal et al.[38]	50	15.7 ± 7.1	7.5 ± 3.9	1.06 ± 0.32	2.01 ± 0.7
Stefanidis et al.[7] (retrograde approach)	86	16 ± 6	5 ± 2	0.92 ± 0.22	2.14 ± 0.54
Dai et al.[39] (Inoue)	200	25.49 ± 10.22	6.71 ± 4.87	1.08 ± 0.28	2.20 ± 0.47
Chinese multicenter study[40] (Inoue)	4832	18.3 ± 5.1	5.4 ± 3.1	1.1 ± 0.3	2.1 ± 0.2

PMBV, percutaneous mitral balloon valvuloplasty; MV, mitral valve.

Immediate hemodynamic and clinical improvement are obtained after PMBV (Figure 28.4). According to National Heart, Lung, and Blood Institute Registry results,[33] the pressure gradient across the mitral valve decreased from 14 to 6 mm Hg, and mitral valve area increased from 1.0 to 2.0 cm². Similar results were obtained by Hung et al.[32] using the Inoue technique. Our results using both techniques and results from various institutions are also comparable (Table 28.2). Plasma catecholamines rapidly decrease both at rest[35] and during exercise[36] after PMBV, whereas exercise capacity, ventilation, and skeletal muscle oxygenation increase.[37]

Echocardiographic grading seems to be the most important factor for determining the immediate outcome. The patients with low echocardiographic scores present with better results, whereas patients with high echocardiographic scores have poorer results.[20,25,41]

Complications

The complications of PMBV can be classified in two main categories: those related to transseptal catheterization and those related to balloon dilatation of the valve. The primary complication rates at various institutions, including death rates, are given in Table 28.3. PMBV appears to be an effective and safe intervention, especially when compared with complications from both closed chest[42] and open heart[43] surgical procedures (e.g., comparing infection, operative morbidity and mortality, problems of general anesthesia, postoperative pericarditis, and late consequences of valve replacement). It is generally accepted that operator experience and patient selection criteria are the two most important determinants of the complications following PMBV.[38,44]

Mortality

Death occurring during the procedure is generally related to acute right heart failure secondary to an acute increase in pulmonary artery pressure in patients with severe pulmonary hypertension, unrecognized pericardial tamponade due to transmural transseptal catheterization, or ventricular perforation due to guidewires or balloon catheters. Procedural mortality of PMBV is about 1% (0%–3%). Both mortality and complication rates decrease as experience increases.[32,33,44,45]

Cardiac Tamponade

Cardiac tamponade, or hemopericardium, which generally occurs in less than 1% (0.5%–7%) of patients, is the main complication of transseptal catheterization.[32,33,45] It may be the result of a tear of the atrial wall with either the Brockenborough needle or the septal dilator. It is generally self-limited and can be treated by pericardial aspiration in the catheterization laboratory. Surgical intervention is rarely required. The operator should be aware of symptoms and signs of cardiac tamponade during transseptal puncture, and pericardial aspiration must be performed under fluoroscopic control. In rare instances, cardiac tamponade is due to ventricular perforation caused by the guidewires or the balloon itself, especially in patients with poor general condition; this complication is generally fatal.[32,48]

Systemic Embolism

Systemic embolism (including stroke) and severe mitral regurgitation are the two most frequent complications of PMBV. The incidence of systemic embolism is about 1% to 2% and is generally related to the displacement of left atrial thrombus during transseptal puncture or manipulation of the guidewires or balloon within the left atrium, or debris from the mitral valve. Care should be taken to avoid manipulating guidewires in the left atrial appendage, which is the commonest site of thrombus formation. Transesophageal echocardiography performed before the procedure is the most useful tool to exclude the presence of left atrial thrombus, especially in patients with atrial fibrillation. Left atrial spontaneous echocardiographic contrast is also accepted as an important marker of increased thromboembolic risk, but it may resolve after PMBV.[49] In addition, patients with atrial fibrillation must have full anticoagulation therapy for at least two months before the procedure. The administration of heparin during the procedure is also very important, especially for the prevention of embolism during transseptal catheterization.[50,51]

TABLE 28.3. Complication rates of percutaneous mitral balloon valvuloplasty.

	Number of patients	Mortality (%)	Cardiac tamponade (%)	Embolism (%)	Severe MR (%)
Meriç M et al. 1993 (unpublished data)					
Double balloon antegrade	60	0	6.7	0	0
Inoue	56	0	0	0	0
Tuzcu et al.[44]	311	1.7	—	—	8.7
Vahanian et al.[45]	600	0.5	0.8	3.3	3.8
NHLBI registry[46]	738	3	4	3	3
Nobuyoshi et al.[47]	106	0	2	0	5

MR, mitral regurgitation.

Mitral Regurgitation

Mitral regurgitation after PMBV is not rare (the frequency is 3% to 11%), and some mitral regurgitation or a slight increase in mitral regurgitation may occur during the procedure.[52] Small tears in the leaflet, rigidity of a leaflet leading to incomplete closure, localized rupture of the chordae, or shortened chordae prohibiting the complete closure of the leaflets may be the causes for mitral regurgitation. Prolapse of the anterior leaflet may also be responsible for mild mitral regurgitation in patients with pliable valves.[53] However, severe mitral regurgitation is rare and is frequently related to noncommissural tearing of the leaflets.[46,54] Other causes of severe mitral regurgitation include excessive commissural tearing and rupture of the papillary muscle.[55] The main preprocedural determinant of severe mitral regurgitation is unfavorable anatomy, especially severely calcified leaflets or extensive subvalvular disease, again pointing out the importance of echocardiographic grading before the procedure.[56] Although a case report of spontaneous resolution of PMBV-related severe mitral regurgitation[57] offers encouragement to patients and physicians who find themselves confronting acute mitral regurgitation, the frequency of this type of spontaneous resolution is unclear, and severe mitral regurgitation generally leads to deterioration of left ventricular performance.[58] Although there are data to suggest that more modest improvement in procedure-related mitral regurgitation occurs frequently,[59] valve replacement is generally required within 1 year in most patients with severe mitral regurgitation. However, conservative surgical repair combining the suture of the tear and commissurotomy may be adequate in cases where valve deformity is not too severe.[60]

Atrial Septal Defect

Patency of the transseptal puncture site is observed in most cases, but its frequency varies greatly with the technique used to detect it. The best method for the detection of left-to-right shunts after PMBV is color Doppler echocardiography by the transesophageal approach[61]; oximetry seems to be the least sensitive method.[47] Despite the presence of a left-to-right shunt, ratio of pulmonary blood flow (Q_p) to systemic blood flow (Q_s) rarely exceeds 1.5 and is very seldom over 2. In our unpublished series of patients evaluated by oximetry in the catheterization laboratory, the incidence of left-to-right shunt was found to be 13%, and Q_p/Q_s was below 1.5 for all of them. During the 3-year follow-up, Doppler echocardiography showed that the left-to-right shunt disappeared in half of the patients. In the series published by Casale et al.,[62] the incidence of atrial septal defect after PMBV was 19%. Advanded age, high NYHA class,

high echocardiographic score, the presence of valve calcification, and low cardiac output were determined as the predictors of atrial septal defect in the same patients. Right-to-left shunts are very rare and occur only in patients with right heart failure and pulmonary hypertension.[63] Hemodynamically significant shunting after PMBV is mainly related to technical factors rather than clinical and hemodynamic parameters.[64] Excessive dilatation of the valve,[65] forceful pullback of the balloon during balloon dilatation,[66] and inadequate deflation of the balloon during pullback from the left atrium[67] seem to be the principal causes. The incidence of left-to-right shunting is lower when the Inoue technique is used.[68,69]

Other Complications

Complete heart block may be seen during septal puncture or dilatation of the valve, but it is generally transient, and the need for permanent pacemaker implantation is very rare.[70] Cardiac catheterization complications such as inguinal hematomas may also be seen, but they are rarely seen with antegrade approach techniques.

Midterm and Long-term Follow-up After PMBV

Most patients have marked clinical improvement following PMBV. The NYHA class of these patients changes to I or II, and improvement persists for a long time. Generally, lower echocardiographic scores and good immediate results provide good follow-up results,[18,20,32,45] but low preoperative echocardiographic scores seem to be more important than good operative outcome.[18,20,71] If the increase in mitral valve area is not satisfactory after PMBV, valve replacement is generally performed because of the unfavorable valve anatomy that caused the failure of first intervention.

Long-term results after successful PMBV are generally good. In the study of Block et al.,[72] a small decrease was observed in mitral valve area 2 years after PMBV. Similarly, in our series of 32 patients followed for 3 years, mean mitral valve area decreased from 2.44 ± 0.40 cm^2 to 1.83 ± 0.83 cm^2 ($P < .01$). The 4-year clinical follow-up results of Palacios et al.[73] showed that 4-year survival after PMBV was over 90%, and mitral valve replacement was performed in only 13% of the patients. In our series, mitral valve replacement was performed in only 12.5% of the patients during the following 3 years. According to the long-term results recorded in the National Heart, Lung, and Blood Institute Balloon Valvuloplasty Registry,[74] intervention-free and event-free survival was 80% at 1 year, 71% at 2 years, 67% at 3 years, and 60% at 4 years.

Restenosis after PMBV may be defined as a loss of 50% or more of the increase obtained, with a valve area of 1.5

cm² or less.[20] The incidence of restenosis is between 10% and 20%. Age, mitral valve area after PMBV, and echocardiographic valve anatomy are the main predictors of restenosis.[20,45,75] In our series, the restenosis rate was 12.5% over a period of 3 years, and restenosis was three times more frequent in patients whose echocardiographic scores were over 8. Similar results were obtained by Palacios et al.[73] The restenosis rate was 5.2% over a follow-up period of 32.2 ± 14.2 months in the more recent Chinese multicenter study[40] that investigated a very large number of patients. Limited experience on repeat PMBV after restenosis indicates good results.[76] However, it is necessary to remember that preprocedure echocardiographic grading must indicate appropriate conditions for intervention.

The degree of postprocedure mitral regurgitation generally remains stable or decreases slightly during follow-up[75,77] in patients who develop mild-to-moderate mitral regurgitation after PMBV. In our patients who had mild-to-moderate mitral regurgitation after PMBV, regurgitation showed a slight increase in 25%, remained stable in 50%, and decreased in 25%. On the other hand, patients with severe mitral regurgitation after PMBV usually needed surgical treatment in the ensuing months.

PMBV Versus Mitral Valve Surgery

The good initial and long-term results of PMBV make the need for surgical intervention for mitral stenosis questionable in patients whose condition is suitable for PMBV. Results of the studies comparing the short-term and long-term outcome of PMBV and mitral valve surgery imply that mitral valve surgery should be considered only for those patients with unfavorable mitral valve anatomy. Patel et al[78] prospectively investigated the immediate clinical and hemodynamic results and found that the increase in mitral valve area and exercise capacity was better in the group that received PMBV than in the group that received closed mitral commissurotomy. Complication rates were similar in both groups. A study by Cohen et al[79] prospectively compared the 36-month survival of patients who underwent PMBV, open surgical commissurotomy, or mitral valve replacement and found that 36-month survival rates are similar in the three groups, but the need for subsequent mitral valve procedures was higher in the PMBV group. A randomized trial comparing PMBV and open surgical mitral commissurotomy in patients with mitral stenosis showed comparable initial results and low rates of restenosis. The authors point out that PMBV should be considered for all patients with favorable mitral valve anatomy because of its better hemodynamic results at 3 years, lower cost, and elimination of the need for thoracotomy.[59]

PMBV and Particular Clinical Conditions

PMBV in the Elderly and the High-Risk Patient

Current data suggest that PMBV may be a useful method for treating the elderly and patients with high surgical risk. This method excludes the risks of surgery and its risk is acceptable, but the results are less favorable than they are for younger patients. Although the limited anatomic improvement may be adequate for symptomatic improvement, the probability of restenosis is high, and long-term benefit is limited because of associated disease. On the other hand, valve anatomy in the elderly may not be suitable for PMBV because of the high incidence of valvular calcification in these patients. Conversely, long-term prognosis seems to be better following successful surgery. Decisions must be made on an individual basis, and results and risks of both surgery and PMBV have to be taken into account.[21,30,31]

PMBV for Restenosis Following Surgical Commissurotomy

Because of the increased life expectancy after surgical commissurotomy, there is increase interest in mitral restenosis. Reoperation is not preferred in these patients because of the incidence of adhesions, but valve replacement may be necessary. Published data point out that PMBV may be the method of choice in this setting.[80,81] This intervention significantly increases valve area and improves symptoms, as it does in patients with primary mitral stenosis, and midterm results also seem to be good. However, all the limitations of the procedure that we discussed in the sections on "Patient Selection" and "Complications" are still valid. In addition, the procedure may be more difficult to perform in these patients because of increased thickness of the interatrial septum caused by previous surgery, or the funnel-shaped structure of the mitral valve that is frequent in these patients. On the other hand, it has been reported that the risk of pericardial tamponade is low in these patients because of pericardial adhesions.[80–82]

References

1. Inoue K, Nakamura T, Kitamura F. Nonoperative mitral commissurotomy by a new balloon catheter [abstract]. *Jpn Circ J.* 1982;46:877.
2. Inoue K, Owaki T, Nakamura T, et al. Clinical application of transvenous mitral commissurotomy by a new balloon catheter. *J Thorac Cardiovasc Surg.* 1984;87:394–402.
3. Lock JE, Khalilulah M, Shrivastava S, et al. Percutaneous catheter commissurotomy in rheumatic mitral stenosis. *N Engl J Med.*1985;313:1515–1518.

4. Al Zaibag MA, Kasab SA, Ribeiro PA, et al. Percutaneous double-balloon mitral valvulotomy for rheumatic mitral-valve stenosis. *Lancet*. 1986;1:757–761.

5. Babic UU, Pejcic P, Djurisic Z, et al. Percutaneous transarterial balloon valvotomy for mitral valve stenosis. *Am J Cardiol*. 1986;57:1101–1104.

6. Orme EC, Wray RB, Mason JW. Balloon mitral valvuloplasty via retrograde left atrial catheterization. *Am Heart J*. 1989;117:680–683.

7. Stefanidis C, Stratos C, Pitsavos C, et al. Retrograde non-transseptal balloon mitral valvuloplasty: immediate results and long-term follow-up. *Circulation*. 1992;85:1760–1767.

8. Palacios IF, Lock JE, Keane JF, et al. Percutaneous transvenous balloon valvotomy in a patient with severe calcific mitral stenosis. *J Am Coll Cardiol*. 1986;7:1416–1419.

9. Bassand JP, Schiele F, Bernard Y, et al. The double balloon and Inoue techniques in percutaneous mitral valvuloplasty. *J Am Coll Cardiol*. 1991;18:982–989.

10. Dietz WA, Waters JB, Ramaswamy K, et al. Use of balloon inflations in combination with serial evaluation by color flow Doppler minimizes mitral regurgitation as a complication of percutaneous mitral valvuloplasty [abstract]. *J Am Coll Cardiol*. 1991;17 (suppl. A):82A.

11. Kronzon I, Tunick PA, Schwinger ME, et al. Transesophageal echocardiography during percutaneous mitral valvuloplasty. *J Am Soc Echocardiogr*. 1989;2:380–385.

12. Kültürsay H, Türkoglu C, Payzin S, et al. Mitral balloon valvuloplasty with transesophageal echocardiography without using fluoroscopy [abstract]. *Eur Heart J*. 1992;13:227.

13. Chen CR, Huang ZD, Lo ZX, et al. Comparison of single rubber–nylon balloon and double polyethylene balloon valvuloplasty in 94 patients with rheumatic mitral stenosis. *Am Heart J*. 1990;119:102–111.

14. Bassand JP, Schiele F, Bernard Y, et al. The double balloon and Inoue techniques in percutaneous mitral valvuloplasty: comparative results in a series of 232 cases. *J Am Coll Cardiol*. 1991;18:982–989.

15. Shim WH, Jang YS, Yoon JH, et al. Comparison of outcome among double, bifoil and Inoue balloon techniques for percutaneous mitral valvuloplasty in mitral stenosis. *Yongsei Med J*. 1992;33:48–53.

16. Stefanadis C, Stratos C, Kallikazaros I, et al. Retrograde nontransseptal balloon mitral valvuloplasty using the Inoue balloon catheter [abstract]. 67th Scientific Sessions of the American Heart Association, November 14–17, 1994, Dallas, Tx, USA. Abstract 338.

17. Michel PL, Vahanian A, Maroni JP, et al. Percutaneous mitral comissurotomy in patients over 70 years of age [abstract]. *Eur Heart J*. 1990;11:223.

18. Tuzcu EM, Block PC, Griffin PB, et al. Immediate and long-term outcome of percutaneous mitral valvotomy in patients 65 years and older. *Circulation*. 1992;85:963–971.

19. Wilkins GT, Weyman AE, Abascal VM, et al. Percutaneous mitral valvotomy: an analysis of echocardiographic variables related to outcome and the mechanism of dilatation. *Br Heart J*. 1988;60:299–308.

20. Palacios IF, Block PC, Wilkins GT, et al. Follow-up of patients undergoing mitral balloon valvotomy: analysis of factors determining restenosis. *Circulation*. 1989;79:573–579.

21. Scortichini D, Bonan R, Mickel M, et al. Balloon mitral commissurotomy in surgical high risk patients: results from the NHLBI balloon valvuloplasty registry [abstract]. *Circulation*. 1991;84(suppl II):II203.

22. Hung JS, Lin FC, Chiang CW. Successful percutaneous transvenous catheter balloon mitral commissurotomy after warfarin therapy and resolution of left atrial thrombus. *Am J Cardiol*. 1989;64:126–128.

23. Chen WJ, Chen MF, Liau CS, et al. Safety of percutaneous transvenous balloon mitral commissurotomy in patients with mitral stenosis and thrombus in left atrial appendage. *Am J Cardiol*. 1992;70:117–119,.

24. Vahanian A, Michel PL, Ghanem G, et al. Percutaneous mitral balloon valvotomy in patients with a history of embolism [abstract]. *Circulation*. 1991;84(suppl II):II205.

25. Tuzcu EM, Block PC, Griffin B, et al. Percutaneous mitral balloon valvotomy in patients with calcific mitral stenosis—immediate and long-term outcome. *J Am Coll Cardiol*. 1994;23:1604–1609.

26. Alfonso F, Macaya C, Hernandez R, et al. Early and late results of percutaneous mitral valvuloplasty for mitral stenosis associated with mild mitral regurgitation. *Am J Cardiol*. 1993;71:1304–1310.

27. Chen CR, Cheng TO, Chen JY, et al. Percutaneous balloon mitral valvuloplasty for mitral stenosis with and without associated aortic regurgitation. *Am Heart J*. 1993;125:128–137.

28. Wisenbaugh T, Essop R, Middlemost S. Is severe pulmonary hypertension a risk factor for poor outcome with balloon mitral valvotomy? [abstract]. *J Am Coll Cardiol*. 1992;19(suppl A):363A.

29. Bahl VK, Chandra S, Talwar KK, et al. Balloon mitral valvotomy in patients with systemic and suprasystemic pulmonary artery pressures. *Cathet Cardiovasc Diagn*. 1995;36:211–215.

30. Esteves CA, Ramos AI, Braga SN, et al. Effectiveness of percutaneous balloon mitral valvotomy during pregnancy. *Am J Cardiol*. 1991;68:930–934.

31. Gangbar EW, Watson KR, Howard RS, et al. Mitral balloon valvuloplasty in pregnancy: advantages of a unique balloon. *Cathet Cardiovasc Diagn*. 1992;25:313–316.

32. Hung JS, Chern MS, Wu JJ, et al. Short- and long-term results of catheter balloon percutaneous transvenous mitral comissurotomy. *Am J Cardiol*. 1991;67:854–862.

33. The National Heart, Lung, and Blood Institute Balloon Valvuloplasty Registry Participants Multicenter Experience with Balloon Mitral Comissurotomy. NHLBI balloon valvuloplasty registry report on immediate and 30-day follow-up results. *Circulation*. 1992;85:448–461.

34. Inoue K, Noboyushi M, Chen C, Hung JS: Advantage of Inoue balloon (self-positioning balloon) in percutaneous transvenous mitral comissurotomy [abstract]. *Circulation*. 1988;78(suppl II):II490.

35. Tsuchihashi K, Sawai N, Takizawa H, et al. Plasma noradrenaline as an indicator of functional state in hearts with mitral stenosis—the influence of acutely reduced left atrial pressure by balloon mitral commissurotomy. *Heart Vessels*. 1993;8:85–90.

36. Ikeda J, Furuyama M, Sakuma T, et al. Effects of percutaneous transluminal mitral valvuloplasty on plasma cate-

cholamine levels during exercise. *Am Heart J.* 1993;126: 130–135.

37. Marzo KP, Herrmann HC, Mancini DM. Effect of balloon mitral valvuloplasty on exercise capacity, ventilation and skeletal muscle oxygenation. *J Am Coll Cardiol.* 1993;21: 856–865.

38. Rihal CS, Nishimura RA, Holmes DR Jr. Percutaneous balloon mitral valvuloplasty—the learning curve. *Am Heart J.* 1991;122:1750–1756.

39. Dai R, Jiang S, Huang L, et al. Percutaneous transseptal balloon valvuloplasty for dilating mitral valve stenosis (report of 200 cases). *Chin Med Sci J.* 1993;8:191–196.

40. Chen CR, Cheng TO. Percutaneous balloon mitral valvuloplasty using Inoue technic: a multicenter study of 4832 patients in China [abstract]. 67th Scientific Sessions of the American Heart Association, November 14–17, 1994, Dallas, Tx, USA. Abstract 342.

41. Lin SL, Chang MS, Lee GW, et al. Usefulness of echocardiography in the prediction of early results of catheter balloon mitral valvuloplasty. *Am Heart J.* 1990;31:161–174.

42. Turi ZG, Reyes VP, Soma Raju B, et al. Percutaneous balloon versus surgical closed commissurotomy for mitral stenosis. *Circulation.* 1991;83:1179–1185.

43. Reyes VP, Soma Raju B, Turi ZG, et al. Percutaneous balloon vs. open surgical commissurotomy for mitral stenosis: a randomized trial [abstract]. *Circulation.* 1990;82(suppl III):III545.

44. Tuzcu EM, Block PC, Palacios IF. Comparison of early versus late experience with percutaneous mitral balloon valvuloplasty. *J Am Coll Cardiol.* 1991;17:1121–1124.

45. Vahanian A, Michel PL, Cormier B, et al. Immediate and midterm results of percutaneous mitral commisurotomy. *Eur Heart J.* 1991;12(suppl B):84–89.

46. The National Heart, Lung, and Blood Institute Balloon Valvuloplasty Registry. Complications and mortality of percutaneous balloon mitral commissurotomy. *Circulation.* 1992;85:2014–2024.

47. Nobuyoshi M, Hamasaki N, Kimura T, et al. Indications, complications, and short-term clinical outcome of percutaneous transvenous mitral commissurotomy. *Circulation.* 1989;80:782–792.

48. Berland J, Gerber L, Gamra H, et al. Percutaneous balloon valvuloplasty for mitral stenosis complicated by fatal pericardial tamponade in a patient with extreme pulmonary hypertension. *Cathet Cardiovasc Diagn.* 1989;17:109–111.

49. Leung DY, Black IW, Cranney GB, et al. Resolution of left atrial spontaneous echocardiographic contrast after percutaneous mitral valvuloplasty—implications for thromboembolic risk. *Am Heart J.* 1995;129:65–70.

50. Drobinski G, Montalescot G, Evans J, et al. Systemic embolism as a complication of percutaneous mitral valvuloplasty. *Cathet Cardiovasc Diagn.* 1992;25:327–330.

51. Milner MR, Goldstein SA, Lindsay J, et al. Transesophageal echocardiographic guidance for percutaneous balloon mitral valvuloplasty [abstract]. *Circulation.* 1990; 82(suppl III):III81.

52. Harrison JK, Wilson JS, Hearne SE, Bashore TM. Complications related to percutaneous transvenous mitral commissurotomy. *Cathet Cardiovasc Diagn.* 1994;2(suppl.): 52–60.

53. Essop MR, Wisenbaugh T, Skoularigis J, et al. Mitral regurgitation following mitral balloon valvotomy: differing mechanisms for severe versus mild-to-moderate lesions. *Circulation.* 1991;84:1669–1679.

54. Serra A, Bonan R, Vanderperren O, et al. Anatomical and pathological study of mitral valve rupture following percutaneous mitral commissurotomy [abstract]. *Circulation.* 1990;82(suppl III):III546.

55. Vahanian A, Michel PL, Michel X, et al. Features of severe mitral regurgitation following percutaneous mitral commissurotomy [abstract]. *J Am Coll Cardiol.* 1989;13(suppl A):55A.

56. Vahanian A, Michel PL, Cormier B, et al. Surgery for complications following percutaneous mitral commissurotomy [abstract]. *Circulation.* 1990;82(suppl III):III546.

57. Kannan P, Jeyamalar R. Severe mitral incompetence following balloon mitral valvuloplasty: complete resolution during follow-up. *Cathet Cardiovasc Diagn.* 1995;34: 220–221.

58. Wisenbaugh T, Berk M, Essop R, et al. Effect of abrupt mitral regurgitation after balloon mitral valvuloplasty on myocardial load and performance. *J Am Coll Cardiol.* 1991; 17:872–879.

59. Reyes VP, Raju BS, Wyenne J, et al. Percutaneous balloon valvuloplasty compared with open surgical commissurotomy for mitral stenosis. *N Engl J Med.* 1994;331:961–967.

60. Acar C, Deloche A, Tibi PR, et al. Operative findings after percutaneous mitral dilatation. *Ann Thorac Surg.* 1990; 49: 959–963.

61. Vilacosta I, Iturralde E, San Roman IA, et al. Transesophageal echocardiography monitoring of percutaneous mitral balloon valvotomy. *Am J Cardiol.* 1992;70: 1040–1044.

62. Casale P, Block PC, O'Shea JP, et al. Atrial septal defect after percutaneous mitral balloon valvuloplasty: immediate results and follow-up. *J Am Coll Cardiol.* 1990;15: 1300–1304.

63. Goldberg N, Roman CF, Docha S, et al. Right to left interatrial shunting following balloon mitral valvuloplasty. *Cathet Cardiovasc Diagn.* 1989;16:133–135.

64. Watson KR, Crisholm RJ, Azoiri JR, et al. Elevated left atrial pressure does not cause left-to-right shunting after balloon valvuloplasty. *Cathet Cardiovasc Diagn.* 1991;24: 173–175.

65. Cequier A, Bonan R, Dyrda I, et al. Atrial shunting after percutaneous mitral valvuloplasty. *Circulation.* 1990;81: 1190–1197.

66. Chen CH, Lin SL, Hsu TL, et al. Iatrogenic Lutenbacher's syndrome after percutaneous transluminal mitral valvotomy. *Am Heart J.* 1990;119:209–211.

67. Fields CD, Slovenkai GA, Isner JM. Atrial septal defect resulting from mitral balloon valvuloplasty: relation of defect morphology to transseptal catheter delivery. *Am Heart J.* 1990;119:568–576.

68. Thomas MR, Monaghan MJ, Metcalfe JM, et al. Residual atrial septal defects following balloon mitral valvuloplasty using different techniques. A transthoracic and transesophageal echocardiographic study demonstrating an advantage of the Inoue balloon. *Eur Heart J.* 1992;13: 496–502.

69. Nigri A, Alessandri N, Martuscelli E, et al. Clinical significance of small left-to-right shunts after percutaneous mitral valvuloplasty. *Am Heart J.* 1993;125:783–786.

70. Carlson MD, Palacios IF, Thomas JD, et al. Cardiac conduction abnormalities during percutaneous balloon mitral or aortic valvotomy. *Circulation.* 1989;79:1197–1203.

71. Palacios IF, Tuzcu ME, Weyman AE, et al. Clinical follow-up of patients undergoing percutaneous mitral balloon valvotomy. *Circulation.* 1995;91:671–676.

72. Block PC, Palacios IF, Block EH, et al. Late (two-year) follow-up after percutaneous mitral valvuloplasty. *N Engl J Med.* 1991;327:1329–1335.

73. Palacios IF, Tuzcu EM, Newell JB, et al.Four year clinical follow-up of patients undergoing percutaneous mitral balloon valvotomy [abstract]. *Circulation.* 1990;82(suppl III): III545.

74. Dean LS, Mickel M, Bonan R, et al. Long-term follow-up of patients undergoing percutaneous balloon mitral commissurotomy—a report from the NHLBI Balloon Valvuloplasty Registry [abstract]. 67th Scientific Sessions of the American Heart Association, November 14–17, 1994, Dallas, Tx, USA. Abstract 342.

75. Desideri A. Vanderperren O, Serra A, et al. Long term (9 to 33 months) echocardiographic follow-up of after successful percutaneous mitral commissurotomy. *Am J Cardiol.* 1992;69:1602–1606.

76. Gupta S, Vora A, Lokhandwalla Y, et al. Percutaneous balloon mitral valvotomy in mitral restenosis. *Eur Heart J.* 1996;17:1560–1564.

77. Pan JP, Lin SL, Go JU, et al. Frequency and severity of mitral regurgitation one year after balloon mitral valvuloplasty. *Am J Cardiol.* 1991;67:264–268.

78. Patel JJ, Shama D, Mitha AS, et al. Balloon valvuloplasty versus closed commissurotomy for pliable mitral stenosis—a prospective hemodynamic study. *J Am Coll Cardiol.* 1991;18:1318–1322.

79. Cohen JM, Glower DD, Harrison JK, et al. Comparison of balloon valvuloplasty with operative treatment for mitral stenosis. *Ann Thorac Surg.* 1993;56:1254–1262.

80. Rediker DE, Block PC, Abascal PM, et al. Mitral balloon valvuloplasty for mitral restenosis after surgical commissurotomy. *J Am Coll Cardiol.* 1988;11:252–256.

81. Medina A, Delezo JS, Hernandez E, et al. Balloon valvuloplasty for mitral restenosis after previous surgery. A comparative study. *Am Heart J.* 1990;120:568–571.

82. Davidson CJ, Bashore TM, Mickel M, et al. Balloon mitral commissurotomy after previous surgical commissurotomy. *Circulation.* 1992;86:91–99.

Atherosclerosis: Understanding the Relationship Between Coronary Artery Disease and Stenosis Flow Reserve

Richard M. Fleming

The first study to look at the flow of fluids through tubular structures was published by Jean Leonard Marie Poiseuille in 1840.[1] He described what became the basic model of blood flow:

$$(1) \quad Q = \frac{\pi \, (P_i - P_o) \, d^4}{128 \, \eta \, l}$$

where Q is flow, π is the constant 3.14, $P_i - P_o$ is the difference of the input pressure and output pressure, d is the diameter of the tube, η is the viscosity of fluid, and l is the length of the tube.

There was no further investigation until the 1920s when researchers[2-11] began looking at blood flow in various animal species and different vascular beds. These studies demonstrated that blood flow in a specific vascular bed (e.g., that of the coronary arteries) is different from blood flow in other vascular beds(e.g., those of the brain, legs, and kidneys) and that information from one could not easily be extrapolated to another. Likewise, these studies revealed that blood flow in a specific vascular bed of one species (e.g., that of the coronary artery of a dog) is different from blood flow in the same vascular bed of another species (e.g., that of the coronary artery of a human). Despite these limitations, research continued with available animal models and aided in defining human blood flow.

Until recently[12,13] assumptions about the coronary artery blood flow of humans was almost entirely based upon animal models[14-16] and not on information obtained directly from human coronary blood flow. After the development of quantitative coronary arteriography (QCA)[12,17] it became possible to accurately determine the various parameters of atherosclerotic disease in humans.[12,17,18]

Whereas Poiseuille's original work was concerned with the flow of fluids through rigid tubes, the concept of stenosis flow reserve (SFR) was developed to describe the ability of an artery to increase blood flow upon demand. Typically a human coronary artery can carry 65 to 100 mL of blood/min per 100 g of myocardium. A normal artery without evidence of atherosclerosis can increase the amount of blood flowing through it by a factor of five to meet the increased demands for oxygen by the heart, which occurs as a result of increased exertion. This increase in available blood supply is known as *flow reserve*, or, in a stenotic (atherosclerosed) artery *stenosis flow reserve*, which is defined as

$$(2) \quad \text{SFR} = 5(Q_{\text{stenosed}}) / Q_{\text{unstenosed}},$$

where Q is flow.

Because the heart extracts essentially all of the oxygen flowing through the coronary arteries at any given time, the ability of the heart to receive additional oxygen is dependent upon its flow reserve. As we see later in the chapter, this is determined primarily by the percent diameter stenosis (%DS) of an atherosclerotic lesion and is much less dependent upon the other variables. Before proceeding further we must first look at the multiple independent variables that contribute to coronary artery disease (CAD) as we now know it to exist as measured by QCA methods.

Coronary Artery Disease

Initial interpretation of stenosis severity defined as percent DS is typically based upon visual estimates of CAD after the injection of contrast agents into the coronary arteries. This procedure, known as coronary arteriography or coronary angiography, primarily utilizes visual estimates of stenosis severity and is flawed by multiple problems that result in the misinterpretation of stenosis severity.[18,19] The development of QCA, as shown in Figure 29.1, has made it possible to more accurately describe and define CAD, including %DS, percent area stenosis (%AS), absolute diameter measurement (mm), absolute length (mm) of the lesion, angle of entry (α) to and from a narrowing (Ω), and the density (percent of maximum) of contrast within the stenotic lesion.

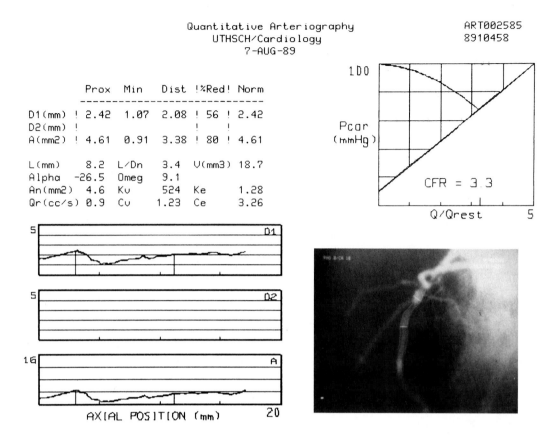

FIGURE 29.1. Example of automated quantitative coronary arteriogram. An example of a stenotic first diagonal coronary artery is outlined. The table shows that this artery has a 56% DS and an 80% AS. The artery also has an entry angle (Alpha) of −26.5 degrees and an exit (Omega) angle of +9.1 degrees. A indicates the cross-luminal area; An, the normal cross-sectional area; CFR, stenosis flow reserve from QCA measurements; Ce and Kv, coefficients of viscosity losses; D1 and D2, orthogonal diameters; Dist, distal; L, length; L/Dn, length/diameter; Min, minimal; Norm, normal; Pcor, coronary perfusion reduction; Prox, proximal; Q/Qrest, coronary flow reserve; Qr, rest flow; and V, intraluminal volume. Reprinted with permission from Fleming et al.[12]

Although all of these independent variables have some importance in the overall definition of atherosclerotic CAD, they do not all play a major role in determining SFR. The range for each of these variables was first reported in 1994[12] after studying 1040 arteries by QCA. Table 29.1 shows some of the information obtained during that study. Stenosis flow reserve ranges from 5 to 0 as stenosis severity increases. As we see later, %DS is the primary determinant of stenosis severity and, subsequently, SFR. Typically %DS is thought to range from 0 to 100 percent. However, when the true %DS is measured by computer, it actually ranges from 0 to 89. According to the accuracy of computer measurements (QCA), once a stenosis exceeds 89% DS, the vessel closes, suggesting that turbulent, thrombotic, vasospastic, neurohumoral, and/or other factors precipitate complete closure of the coronary artery. What is visually reported as 90% to 99% DS truly represents %AS, as has recently been demonstrated.[19] This misinterpretation of %DS occurs because the visual interpretation of %DS actually represents the density of the contrast flowing through the artery as seen during coronary arteriography. When QCA results of density (4% to 99%) information are compared with the %AS (0% to 99%) results obtained by QCA measurement, the two sets of results agree. When the results of %DS visually reported by angiographers are compared with the %AS reported by QCA,[18] the results revealed that angiographers are visually reading density and reporting it as %DS.

The development of significant atherosclerosis also appears to be somewhat related to specific arteries. Although not fully understood, the 1040 arteries analyzed[12,13] by QCA revealed only one patient whose left circumflex artery was significantly (≥ 50% DS) diseased in the absence of significant disease in either the left anterior descending and/or right coronary artery. This may represent differences in branching patterns (number or angle) or other properties not yet defined.

Also as shown in Table 29.1, the absolute length of stenotic lesions ranges from 1.8 mm to 4.84 cm. Presum-

TABLE 29.1. Descriptive statistics of 1040 coronary artery stenoses.*

Variable	Mean	Minimal value	Maximal value
Stenosis flow reserve	3.45	0.30	5.00
Percent diameter stenosis	48.06	0.00	89.00
Percent area stenosis	69.10	0.00	99.00
Length (mm)	15.24	1.80	48.40
Absolute diameter (mm)	1.54	0.40	6.36
Entry angle (degrees)	−12.08	2.00	−39.00
Exit angle (degrees)	12.14	0.00	35.00
Density (percentage of maximum)	0.72	0.04	0.99

*Excluding 39 arteries, which were totally occluded.

ably, as with the limitations seen with %DS, once the length of a stenosis exceeds these values, complete occlusion occurs. Similarly, angles of entry (α) and exit (Ω) are limited, most likely because of turbulent factors (shear force, etc.) that result in thrombotic occlusion from platelet activation. Because of differences in the physical properties of fluids flowing through narrowings of 90 degrees as opposed to narrowings of 39 degrees, extrapolations from animal models or human models using occlusive devices producing 90 degrees angles of entry and exit cannot be depended upon to provide accurate interpretation of fluid flow in atherosclerotic coronary arteries or SFR.

In human coronary arteries, entry angles into a stenosis range from +2 to −39 degrees. This means that nonaneurysmic stenotic lesions may have an entry angle between slightly dilated (+2 degrees) and −39 degrees at entry. (The minus sign indicates the angle of entry into the stenosis.) Likewise, the angle leaving a stenosis can range up to but not exceed 35 degrees. The visual estimate[12,13,18–20] of stenosis severity is unreliable. Now that we have examined the different independent variables involved in describing atherosclerosis, it is time to look at the impact each has on determining SFR.

Stenosis Flow Reserve

Prior to 1994 the models developed to describe SFR required the use of expensive instrumentation,[14,15,17,19,20] additional personnel, and complicated mathematical models that are not easily adaptable to most if not all clinical settings. Given the work of Poiseuille[1] more than 150 years ago, it should be easier to understand the properties of blood flow through a stenotic lesion because

$$(2)\ \text{SFR} = 5(Q_{\text{stenosed}})/Q_{\text{unstenosed}}$$

or

$$(3)\ \text{SFR} = \frac{\text{maximum flow}}{\text{resting flow}}$$

If all the variables already mentioned in Table 29.1 are considered in light of Poiseuille's equation (Equation 1), it becomes obvious that even though there are many independent variables that determine the appearance of atherosclerotic CAD, the effect of most of these independent variables on flow reserve is only minimal. Regardless of whether blood flow is being considered during maximal or resting conditions, the mathematical constant π remains a mathematical constant (3.14159265 . . .). Likewise, the viscosity (η) of the blood does not change between maximal and resting flow, because the viscosity is determined primarily by properties of the blood itself and not what it is flowing through. Given no changes in the patients hemodynamic status (blood pressure, heart rate, blood volume, etc.), there should be no appreciable changes in pressure ($P_i - P_o$) of input and output through the coronary vascular bed. Similarly the overall length (*l*) should not appreciably change, leaving the primary effect to be determined by some factor reflecting the diameter of the narrowing itself compared with the normal diameter. For Poiseuille, differences in the diameter (d^4) of the tube had the most dramatic effect. If the original theories of Poiseuille are correct, then differences between maximal and resting blood flow (flow reserve) in a stenotic artery should be determined primarily by some determinant of diameter change (%DS or absolute diameter) from the normal to the stenotic artery.

With the use of QCA, the effect of each independent variable (Table 29.1) was investigated and the results published for the first time in 1994.[12,13] The results are summarized in Table 29.2 where the effect of each independent variable and the interactive effect on SFR are described. Clearly the variable with the greatest impact on SFR is %DS ($p \le 0.001$), which we now know to be extremely important. None of the remaining variables, including %AS, absolute diameter of stenosis (which does not take into account the expected diameter as %DS does), or absolute length demonstrated any statistically significant relationship with SFR. Not present in the table are the relationships between entry and exit angles and SFR, because their effect was even less.

TABLE 29.2. Results of general linear model of analysis of variance for stenosis flow reserve.

Source	P (statistical significance)
%DS	0.001***
%AS	NS
Length	NS
Abs	NS
%DS × %AS	0.001***
%DS × Length	0.019***
%DS × Abs	0.001***
%AS × Length	0.031***
%AS × Abs	NS
Length × Abs	NS
%DS × %AS × Length	NS
%DS × %AS × Abs	0.001***
%DS × Length × Abs	NS
%AS × Length × Abs	NS
%DS × %AS × Length × Abs	NS

%DS, percent diameter stenosis; %AS, percent area stenosis; Length, absolute length; Abs, absolute diameter; ***, statistical significance; NS, not statistically significant.

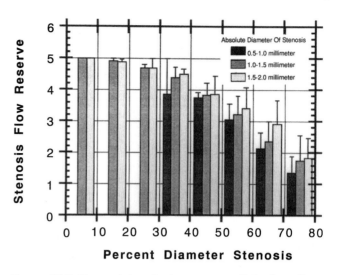

FIGURE 29.2. Determining the importance of absolute diameter. When the absolute diameters (mm) of stenotic arteries are subdivided into 0.5-mm increments ranging from 0.5 to 2.0 mm, there is no significant difference in SFR for any given %DS. Therefore, subdividing absolute diameter did not affect SFR calculations.

Theoretically one could ask whether there would be any difference in the predictability of SFR if certain ranges of absolute diameter or absolute length are used. As demonstrated in Figures 29.2 and 29.3, respectively, the answer is no. Figure 29.2 shows the relationship between SFR and %DS for lesions with absolute diameters ranging from 0.5 to 2.0 mm, using increments of 0.5 mm. Differences in SFR were not statistically different for these subgroups, demonstrating that regardless of the absolute diameter considered there was no change in the predictability of SFR. The same result is seen in Figure 29.3, where atherosclerotic lesions are subgrouped by 5-mm increments ranging in length from 5 to 25 mm. These ranges were selected because the vast majority of lesions fit these criteria.

The interactions of each variable were then compared to determine the relationship between each combination of variables and SFR. In all but one instance, the interactions included the independent variable %DS and were no more predictive of SFR than %DS itself. In the one combination of independent variables where %DS was not involved (%AS by length, p ≤ 0.031), the result was less significant than %DS alone or any other combination of variables. In fact, the more variables factored in, the less predictive the results, as shown in Table 29.2.

Given the significance of %DS on predicting SFR, the relationship was studied first graphically then mathematically. The relationship between %DS and SFR is graphically depicted in Figure 29.4, where a curvilinear relationship is shown. This curvilinear relationship was discovered to be a quadratic function of %DS. Attempts to mathematically manipulate both %DS and SFR resulted in no additional improvement in mathematical modeling. This model revealed that SFR is a quadratic

function of %DS, just as flow through rigid tubes is a quadratic function of diameter. The complete quadratic equation is published here for the first time, as seen in Equation 4.

(4) $SFR = 5.134 - (3.4151 \times \%DS) + (19.083 \times \%DS^2) - (53.312 \times \%DS^3) + (33.495 \times \%DS^4)$

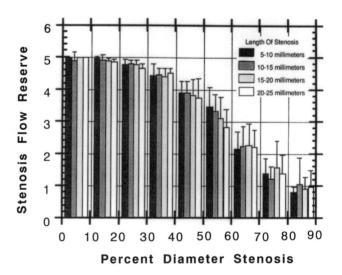

FIGURE 29.3. Determining the importance of absolute length. When the absolute lengths (mm) of stenotic arteries are further subdivided into 5-mm increments ranging from 5 to 25 mm, there is no significant difference in SFR for any given %DS. Therefore, subdividing absolute length did not affect SFR calculations.

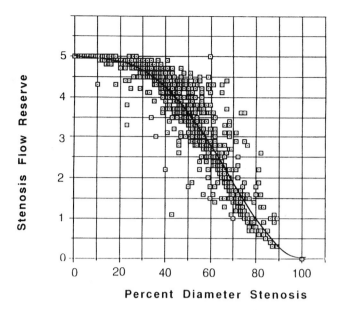

FIGURE 29.4. Comparison of %DS with SFR. When the SFR of 1040 lesions was plotted against %DS, the results revealed a quadratic relationship. No apparent decrease in SFR was observed until a 15% to 20% reduction in diameter was reported. SFR then progressively decreased until %DS reached 80%, after which SFR was less than 1.

As with all mathematical models, it should be possible to test this relationship against any currently accepted model or standard. This was done and reported for the first time in 1994.[13] Using 100 different atherosclerotic

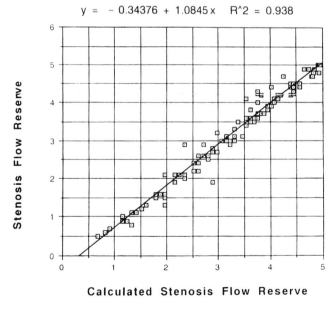

$$y = -0.34376 + 1.0845x \quad R^2 = 0.938$$

FIGURE 29.5. Comparison of measured and calculated SFR. When the results of QCA-determined SFR are plotted against the results obtained from Equation 4 there is excellent agreement ($r = 0.97$, $R^2 = 0.94$) between the two methods. Reprinted with permission from Fleming and Harrington.[13]

plaques, QCA measurement provided not only the independent variables, but the SFR, using the previously reported models. When %DS alone was used to determine SFR based upon the Fleming model (Equation 4), the results were almost identical to that determined by QCA, as shown in Figure 29.5, confirming the quadratic relationship between SFR and %DS. The ability to understand the physiologic parameters of coronary artery blood flow (SFR) as they relate to anatomic parameters (%DS) is now possible. This should shed light on the relationship between SFR and %DS in the clinical management of patients and help us understand how the results of nuclear studies (physiologic information) relate to results seen on coronary (anatomic information) arteriograms, assuming objective and not subjective measurements.

Understanding the Relationship Between Angina, Coronary Artery Stenosis, and SFR

The onset of angina begins with the development of atherosclerosis. Whereas half of the people with CAD unfortunately discover the severity of their problem by sudden death, the other half present with symptoms that typically occur over a period of time, becoming worse as the disease progresses. The reasons for this are obvious after looking at Figure 29.4. The development of exertional angina occurs when the demand for more blood flow during exertional (physical, psychological, and pharmacological) periods cannot adequately be met by the coronary arteries. Physiologically this occurs when the flow reserve decreases to the point that adequate blood flow through a stenosis (SFR) cannot be sufficiently increased to meet the increased demand.

Initially the development of atherosclerotic plaque formation narrows the artery with little if any effect upon SFR, although, as Figure 29.4 demonstrates, some people experience reductions in SFR with as little as 10% to 20% DS. For the majority however, the drop in SFR begins when narrowing of the artery reaches 30% to 40% DS. This explains why what is sometimes perceived as no disease[18,19,21] on visual interpretation of coronary angiograms may in fact be consistent with exertional angina and flow abnormalities as demonstrated with nuclear imaging of the heart (see Chapter 31 on nuclear cardiology). With recent advances in nuclear cardiac imaging, it has become obvious that physiologic changes, as detected by single photon emission computed tomography or positron emission tomography imaging, first reflect changes seen in the small- and medium-sized coronary arteries and not the larger epicardial arteries that are visualized at the time of coronary angiography.[22]

This entire phenomenon has been given the term *syndrome X*.

Once narrowing exceeds 40% DS, there is an almost linear decrease in flow reserve until the narrowing reaches 70% to 80% DS. This period of progressive disease with relatively rapid decline in SFR explains why the progression of symptoms can occur so rapidly, why the reversal of disease (see Chapter 30 on cholesterol) can yield such dramatic reductions in symptoms, and why aggressive treatment of lipid abnormalities is so important in the treatment of patients with CAD. As the disease progresses, reductions in SFR result in less and less exercise tolerance until an SFR of 1 is reached. At this point, the patient is unable to increase coronary blood flow above resting levels, and rest angina ensues. This typically occurs with 75% to 85% DS. As we learned earlier in this chapter, once %DS exceeds 89 as objectively measured (QCA, not visual estimates), the stenotic artery appears to totally close, probably for the reasons discussed earlier.

Conclusion

Although the initial determination of fluid flow through tubular structures was described in 1840 by Poiseuille, it required more than 150 years of further investigation to begin to understand the relationship between angina, SFR, and the severity of atherosclerosis. Models to describe blood flow in the coronary arteries must come from experiments performed in coronary arteries, not other vascular beds. Likewise, complete understanding can be achieved only from work with human coronaries because the differences between species prevents precise extrapolation of conclusions about human coronary arteries. Similarly, because the properties of fluid flow through narrowings are significantly influenced by entry and exit angles, studies should not exceed the parameters normally seen in humans.

The discovery of the quadratic relationship (Equation 4) described in this chapter provides the first working model that relates %DS and SFR in a manner that is practical for clinical investigation and patient care. The relationship between SFR and %DS explains discrepancies reported on nuclear imaging and coronary arteriography. It also explains the physiologic reasons for the development of exertional and rest angina in the majority of cases. The ability to obtain one piece of information (e.g., %DS) calculate the other parameter (e.g., SFR) via the quadratic equation may alleviate the need for additional tests . Alternatively, invasive testing (coronary arteriography) may not be necessary with improved standardization of nuclear cardiac imaging,[22] except when revascularization procedures are planned and, perhaps, not even then as our techniques and understand evolve.

In the interim, this mathematical model not only explains the relationship between the anatomy and physiology of CAD, but it is practical in the clinical setting because it does not require additional equipment, personnel, or financial resources.

References

1. Poiseuille JLM. Recherches experimentales sur le mouvement des liquides dans les tubes de tres petits diametres. *Comptes Rendus Academy of Science (Paris)*. 1840;2:961–1041.
2. Gregg DE, Green HD, Wiggers CL. Phasic variations in peripheral coronary resistance and their determinants. *Am J Physiol*. 1935;112:362–373.
3. Mann FC, Herrick JF, Essex HE, et al. The effect on the blood flow of decreasing the lumen of a blood vessel. *Am J Physiol*. 1938;4:249–252.
4. Gregg DE, Green HD. Phasic blood flow in coronary arteries obtained by a new differential manometer method. *Am J Physiol*. 1939;41:597–598.
5. Shipley RE, Gregg DE, Schroeder EF. An experimental study of flow patterns in various peripheral arteries. *Am J Physiol*. 1942;138:718–730.
6. Pritchard WH, Gregg DE, Shipley RE, et al. A study of flow and pattern responses in peripheral arteries to the injection of vasomotor drugs. *Am J Physiol*. 1942;138:731–740.
7. Shipley RE, Gregg DE. The effect of external constriction of a blood vessel on blood flow. *Am J Physiol*. 1944;141:289–296.
8. May AG, DeWeese JA, Rob CG. Hemodynamic effects of arterial stenosis. *Surgery*. 1963;53:513–524.
9. May AG, DeBerg LV, DeWeese JA, et al. Critical arterial stenosis. *Surgery*. 1963;54:250–259.
10. Fiddian RV, Byar D, Edwards EA. Factors affecting flow through a stenosed vessel. *Arch Surg*. 1964;88:83–90.
11. Berguer R, Hwang NHC. Critical arterial stenosis: a theoretical and experimental solution. *Ann Surg*. 1974;180:39–50.
12. Fleming RM, Harrington GM, Gibbs H, et al. Quantitative coronary arteriography and its assessment of atherosclerosis, I: examining the independent variables. *Angiology*. 1994;45:829–833.
13. Fleming RM, Harrington GM: Quantitative coronary arteriography and its assessment of atherosclerosis, II: calculating stenosis flow reserve from percent diameter stenosis. *Angiology*. 1994;45:835–840.
14. Gould KL, Lipscomb K, Hamilton GW. Physiologic basis for assessing critical coronary stenosis. *Am J Cardiol*. 1974;33:87–93.
15. Gould, Kirkeeide RL, Buchi M. Coronary flow reserve as a physiologic measure of stenosis severity. *J Am Coll Cardiol*. 1990;15:459–474.
16. Kirkeeide RL. Coronary obstructions, morphology and physiologic significance. In: Reiber JHC, Serruys PW, eds. *Quantitative Coronary Arteriography*. Dordrecht, The Netherlands: Kluwer Academic Publishers; 1991:229–244.
17. Brown BG. Response of normal and diseased epicardial coronary arteries to vasoactive drugs: quantitative arteriographic studies. *Am J Cardiol*. 1985;56:23E–29E.

18. Fleming RM, Kirkeeide RL, Smalling RW, et al. Patterns in visual interpretation of coronary arteriograms as detected by quantitative coronary arteriography. *J Am Coll Cardiol.* 1991;18:945–951.

19. Fleming RM, Fleming DM, Gaede R. Training physicians and health care providers to accurately read coronary arteriograms. A training program. *Angiology.* 1996;47:349–359.

20. Fleming RM, Kirkeeide RL, Taegtmeyer H, et al. Comparison of technetium-99m teboroxime tomography with automated quantitative coronary arteriography and thallium-201 tomographic imaging. *J Am Coll Cardiol.* 1991;17:1297–1302.

21. Fleming RM. Improving our interpretation of true percent diameter stenosis and stenosis flow reserve from visually reported percent diameter stenosis obtained at the time of cardiac catheterization. *Int J Angiol.* Submitted.

22. Fleming RM. The importance of physiologic information from cardiac PET in assessing coronary artery disease in people with "normal" coronary angiograms. *Int J Angiol.* Submitted.

30

Cholesterol, Triglycerides, and the Treatment of Hyperlipidemias

Richard M. Fleming

Prior to the discovery of antibiotics in the mid twentieth century, the number one cause of death involved infectious diseases. After the discovery of penicillin by Sir Alexander Fleming and the development of newer antibiotics, coronary artery disease (CAD) became the number one cause of death among North Americans and Europeans alike. In the United States, CAD kills more people than all other diseases combined. In 1998, CAD killed more people *worldwide* than any other illness or cause of death.

The initial relationship between dietary cholesterol and CAD can be traced back to the early 1900s, if not before. Approximately 30 years ago, research into atherosclerotic plaques began first with rhesus and cynomolgus monkeys[1-10] and showed that cholesterol plaqueing occurred when animals were placed on diets high in cholesterol. These studies also showed that the disease could be reversed if the animals where later placed on diets low in cholesterol.

Beginning in the late 1970s, epidemiologic data began to accumulate[11-14] that showed a positive correlation between dietary intake of cholesterol and the subsequent development of atherosclerosis. During the same period of time,[15-29] studies were conducted to determine the impact of various medications designed to reduce cholesterol (antihyperlipemics and hypolipemics), with little if any attention being paid to the effect of dietary modification. Some of these studies are listed in Table 30.1, representing more than 70,000 people.

Attempts to document changes in atherosclerotic plaques by coronary arteriography (cardiac catheterization) began during the 1970s. Some of these studies[30-38] demonstrated improvement (regression), whereas others did not. Multiple reasons exist for the discrepancy in these results, including but not limited to (1) inadequate changes in dietary restriction of cholesterol, triglycerides (fat), and total calorie intake; (2) inadequate methods for determining changes in cholesterol plaques; and (3) problems with various medications used for the treatment of hyperlipidemia and hypertension.

Most of the studies to date[39-58] have not differentiated between the effect obtained with dietary modification and that obtained with hypolipemic medications. Distinction between the effects obtained with dietary restriction, hypolipemic medications, and the combination of both waited until the early 1990s[59-69] and has included studies on both older (> 65 years of age) and younger (< 65 years of age) individuals. In this chapter we review the screening of hyperlipidemia and the importance of both dietary and medical management.

Routine Screening of Hyperlipidemia

Beginning in the late 1980s the American Heart Association proposed routine screening of cholesterol levels in an attempt to identify individuals at increased risk for CAD and begin treatment to reduce elevated lipid levels. Multiple algorithms exist, including the one shown in Figure 30.1. The initial screening of cholesterol levels does not require that the patient fast, however, fasting is necessary if the cholesterol is to be fractionated to determine the levels of low-density lipoprotein (LDL-C) cholesterol, high-density lipoprotein (HDL-C) cholesterol, triglycerides, and total cholesterol (TC). Although opinions vary, a TC level exceeding 240 mg/dL is considered to place a person at increased risk for CAD. However, if we look at populations of people[11-14] who live relatively long life spans and are healthy and active, we discover that their TC levels are below 150 mg/dL, with relatively low HDL-C levels. It now appears that TC levels ≥ 150 mg/dL, LDL-C levels ≥ 100 mg/dL (and probably ≥ 80 mg/dL), or triglyceride levels ≥ 150 mg/dL increase a person's risk for heart disease and stroke. An in-depth review of cholesterol is beyond the scope of this chapter and can be found elsewhere.[70,71]

Individuals with TC levels between 200 and 239 mg/dL are particularly at increased risk for CAD if they have two or more additional risk factors for atherosclero-

TABLE 30.1. Examples of studies looking at morbidity and mortality.

Reference	Number of patients	Age range	Sex
Dewar et al.[15]	497	<65 yr	Both
Alstead et al.[16]	717	40–69 yr	Both
Coronary Drug Project Research Group[17]	8341	30–64 yr	Male
Puska et al.[18]	1683	25–59 yr	Both
Kornitzer et al.[19]	19,390	40–59 yr	Male
Shekelle et al.[20]	1900	40–55 yr	Male
Kjelsberg[21]	12,866	35–57 yr	Male
Lipids Research Clinics Program[22]	3806	35–59 yr	Male
Goldbourt et al.[23]	10,059	>40 yr	Male
Miettinen et al.[24]	1825	50–65 yr	Male
Brunner et al.[25]	2992	35–64 yr	Both
Frick et al.[26]	4081	40–55 yr	Male
Carlson and Rosenhamer[27]	555	<70 yr	Both
Assmann et al.[28]	2754	40–65 yr	Male
Alderman et al.[29]	101	36–73 yr	Both

sis, as listed in Table 30.2. In fact, for each 1% increase in serum cholesterol, there is a 2% increased risk for CAD. Although most algorithms advise that dietary changes should be initiated first and then hypolipemic medications, there is little if any useful information in the medical literature regarding the appropriate dietary changes necessary to reduce elevated cholesterol levels. In many cases both the patient and doctor are confused about what constitutes an appropriate diet. Many individuals are inclined to be too liberal in their saturated fat, calorie, and cholesterol intake. This can be like trying to put out a fire (cholesterol) with gasoline. If you see a fire and you add a pint of gasoline (less cholesterol in the diet), as opposed to a gallon of gasoline (regular diet),

you are not going to put out the fire. In fact you will just have added more fuel.

Two books recently published for the lay public[70,71] are excellent references for patients, physicians, and other health care providers as they seek to understand and lower cholesterol levels. Table 30.3 lists the recommended dietary guidelines according to the American Heart Association, however, as we discuss later, patients who modify their diets by eliminating cholesterol and reducing calories and saturated fat are able to achieve dramatic reductions in their TC levels, with few exceptions. The Fleming guidelines[68–71] are also shown in Table 30.3, with the major difference being that the total caloric need for an individual is calculated first, and then the amount of protein, fat, and carbohydrate needed is determined, making the dietary guidelines useful for people with high cholesterol and triglyceride levels, high blood pressure, and excess weight, as well as people with diabetes mellitus. As noted in Chapter 29 on atherosclerosis, the successful reduction of percent diameter stenosis by regression of cholesterol plaques can produce a significant improvement in exercise tolerance and other symptoms.

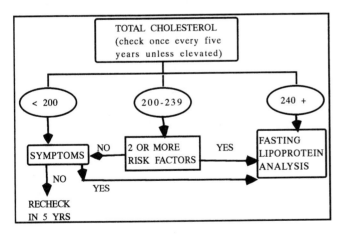

FIGURE 30.1. *Old algorithm* for cholesterol screening. Patients with no prior history of heart disease or who have never had their cholesterol checked should undergo testing at least every 5 years. Further determinations concerning the need for fasting lipoprotein profiles should be based on the total cholesterol level, presence of other risk factors, and the presence or absence of symptoms.

TABLE 30.2. Independent risk factors for coronary artery disease.

Prior heart attack
Angina pectoris
Men or postmenopausal women
Family history
Smoking
Hypertension
Diabetes mellitus
Severe obesity

TABLE 30.3. Comparison of the current US diet, the American Heart Association (AHA) guidelines, and the Fleming guidelines.

Nutrient	Current US diet	Step 1 AHA diet	Step 2 AHA diet	Fleming guidelines
Cholesterol	500 mg	<300 mg	<200 mg	<200 mg
Total fat	~42%	<30%	<30%	15%
Saturated fat	~17%	<10%	<7%	<5%
Carbohydrates	—	50%–60%	50%–60%	70%
Protein	—	15%–20%	15%–20%	15%

Dietary Changes

When making changes in an individual's dietary habits, several factors must be kept in mind. First, if the serum cholesterol level is elevated, the person is at increased risk for heart disease. Failure to understand that prior eating habits have led to elevated lipids is the first problem you and the patient must overcome. As mentioned in Chapter 29 on atherosclerosis, the progression of atherosclerosis from 40% to 80% diameter stenosis results in significant reductions in the flow reserve of the heart. Cholesterol is not the patient's friend, and like anything else that threatens the patient's life, it should be avoided like the plague. Good reference sources for fat, calorie, and cholesterol contents of foods, along with recipes, are now available[70,71] for patients and doctors alike. For an individual who is less likely to adhere to changes in their diet, the physician should (with the assistance of a registered dietitian and/or nutritionist) strive to have the patient change his or her diet to either the step I or step II American Heart Association diet. The general guidelines for this diet are listed in Table 30.3. However, remember that this diet merely pours a pint of gasoline on the fire instead of a gallon of gasoline. Obviously there is less fuel for the fire, but the fire is not likely to go out. Later we review what happens when patients adhere to either the AHA step II or Fleming guidelines.

Second, the overall fat intake must be reduced to control cholesterol level and body weight. Triglycerides, which are part of the overall lipid component, are made from fats. When dietary fat is increased there is an increase in triglyceride levels and, subsequently, an increase in cholesterol, regardless of whether any cholesterol is consumed in the diet. Particularly alarming is the amount of saturated (animal and processed foods) fat eaten by most people. One of the major problems with most dietary regimens, once the patient adheres to eliminating cholesterol in the diet, is a failure to watch the amount of fat and calories in the diet. As noted in Figure 30.2, adequate reductions in cholesterol levels require control of cholesterol, fats, and calories.

Third, the number of calories the patient eats in a day should not exceed his or her caloric needs.[70,71] When this amount is exceeded, the excess calories will be stored as glycogen, cholesterol, and triglycerides for future needs. Of course, if one does not draw on these stored calories, they will continue to accumulate. Adipose tissue is one area where excess calories are stored. Another area is the coronary arteries, where this stored energy can be rapidly broken down and supplied to the heart during emergencies. This makes perfect sense when preparing for fight-or-flight situations, but most individuals do not tap into these stores. So the stored energy continues to accumulate, eventually leading to problems with atherosclerosis.

Finally, the time of day the patient eats is also important.[68–70] If one eats the required number of calories per day and no more, one might assume there will be no problem. However, this is not so. Eating just before going to bed, or eating a major meal within a few hours of going to bed, will not give the body enough time to use those calories before going to sleep. As the metabolism slows for sleep, the body perceives the additional calories as excessive and store them as glycogen, cholesterol, and triglycerides. Although some of these calories may be catabolized by the body the following day, it is unlikely that all of these calories will be used, and the slow but steady accumulation of cholesterol and triglycerides continues, leading to increased risk of atherosclerotic heart disease and other potential health problems.

Hypolipemic Medications

Over the last 30 years a variety of medications have been developed and utilized in an attempt to reduce serum

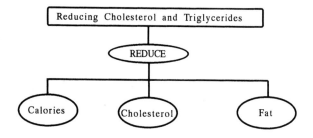

FIGURE 30.2. Control of hyperlipidemia means reducing calories and cholesterol, and saturated fat intake. Adequate reduction of serum lipids (cholesterol and triglycerides) is dependent on the modification of dietary calorie, cholesterol, and saturated fat intake.

TABLE 30.4. Commonly available hypolipemic medications.

Group of medications	Medication	Dosage per day
Bile acid sequestrants	Colestid	5–30 g
	Questran	4–24 g
		(1–6 scoops)
Fibric acid derivatives	Atromid-S	2 g
	Lopid	600–1200 mg
	Tricor	67–201 mg
3-hydroxy-3-methylglutaryl–	Lescol	20–40 mg
coenzyme A	Mevacor	20–80 mg
reductase inhibitors	Pravachol	10–40 mg
	Zocor	5–40 mg
	Lipitor	5–40 mg
	Baycol	0.2–0.3 mg
Nicotinic acid	Nicobid	250–1000 mg
	Nicolar	1–6 g
Other	Lorelco	500–1000 mg

cholesterol and triglyceride levels. A list of many of the currently available medications for the treatment of elevated cholesterol and triglyceride levels is shown in Table 30.4.

Bile Acid Sequestrants

The bile acid sequestrants, which consist primarily of colestipol hydrochloride and cholestyramine, have been available for approximately 20 years. As shown in Figure 30.3, these drugs, which are bile acid resins, work in the intestines and absorb bile salts, including cholesterol. Several forms of these medicines have been available, including mixes and bar forms. Because they are active only while passing through the intestines, they must be taken two or three times each day and have been associated with gastrointestinal bloating. Additionally, medications (e.g., digoxin) that are taken within a couple hours of these drugs may be bound by the bile acid sequestrant and not absorbed as they should be.

As shown in Figure 30.3, once ingested (step 1), these resin drugs bind with available bile salts that are also in the intestine (step 2), resulting in less LDL-C in the liver. The liver is then able to receive more LDL-C from the blood (step 3). As a result of increased uptake of LDL-C by the liver from the blood, the liver may actually increase its production of very low density lipoprotein cholesterol (VLDL-C), causing as much as a 20% percent increase in TC.

Other potential problems include gastrointestinal problems such as gallstones, constipation, and hemorrhoid exacerbation, in addition to dizziness, headaches, myalgias, weakness, and other symptoms. In addition, patients with phenylketonuria should not use colestipol hydrochloride because it contains phenylalanine.

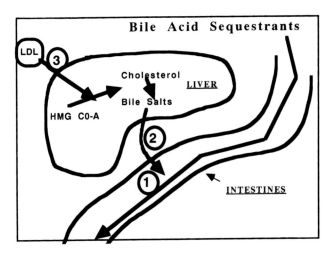

FIGURE 30.3. How bile acid sequestrants work: Once ingested, bile acid sequestrants bind bile salts (including cholesterol). This causes further production of bile salts by the liver and release of these bile salts from the gallbladder into the gastrointestinal tract. Once this occurs, LDL-C can be removed from the bloodstream by the liver, which may then increase its production of cholesterol. HMG Co-A, 3-hydroxy-3-methylglutaryl-coenzyme A.

Fibric Acid Derivatives

There are three principal fibric acid medications available for prescription by most physicians: clofibrate, gemfibrozil, and fenofibrate. These medications are used for the treatment of elevated triglyceride levels, although there have been intermittent reports that some beneficial reduction in LDL-C may also occur. As shown in Figure 30.4, these medications work by increasing the activity of the enzyme lipoprotein lipase, which converts VLDL-C to intermediate lipoprotein cholesterol, which is then converted to LDL-C.

Clofibrate and gemfibrozil, like the bile acid sequestrants, must be taken more than once a day to have an ef-

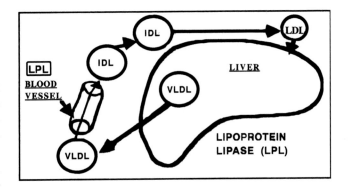

FIGURE 30.4. How fibric acid derivatives work: fibric acid derivatives increase the activity of lipoprotein lipase, which increases the catabolism of VLDL cholesterol to intermediate lipoprotein (IDL) cholesterol, and finally to LDL cholesterol.

fect. Typically they are taken twice a day before meals. Fenofibrate is taken once daily. The most common problems reported with these medications include hepatobiliary (e.g., cholelithiasis) problems and myalgias. Frequent checking of liver function tests and creatine kinase levels is recommended to detect problems with muscle and liver irritation. This is particularly important because of the increased rate of deaths from cancers and pancreatitis among patients taking clofibrate. Fibric acid medications can be particularly problematic if taken with 3-hydroxy-3-methylglutaryl-coenzyme A (HMG Co-A) reductase inhibitors. Other problems include elevation of blood sugar and blurry vision, particularly in diabetic individuals. Patients taking coumadin should be monitored closely because the combination of fibric acid medications and coumadin has been associated with an increased tendency to bleed.

HMG Co-A Reductase Inhibitors (Statins)

The HMG Co-A reductase inhibitors have been shown not only to improve LDL-C levels but also to improve total triglyceride and HDL-C levels. The drugs in this newest class of hypolipemic medicines include fluvastatin, lovastatin, pravastatin sodium, simvastatin, atorvastatin, and cerivastatin. Each works by slowing down but not stopping the production of cholesterol in the liver by inhibiting the enzyme HMG Co-A. This enzyme is the rate limiting step in the production of cholesterol by the liver. Figure 30.5 shows the site of action of these drugs in the liver. Many of these medications are taken with the evening meal or at bedtime. By taking these medications at this time of day, they have their maximum impact on cholesterol synthesis while the patient is sleeping. Because the majority of cholesterol synthesized by the liver is made during sleep, taking the medications

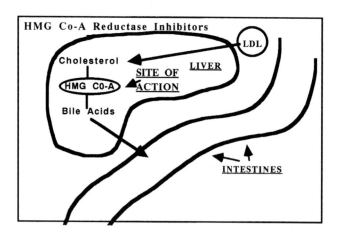

FIGURE 30.5. How HMG Co-A reductase inhibitors work: HMG Co-A reductase inhibitors work by reducing the rate at which cholesterol is synthesized in the liver by slowing the rate-limiting enzyme HMG Co-A.

earlier in the day has less effect on cholesterol production, although some physicians prescribe these medicines twice a day.

As mentioned earlier, the combined use of these medications with fibric acid derivatives has been associated with increased myalgias and liver abnormalities. The combination has, however, demonstrated greater reductions in cholesterol than either group of medicines alone. Caution should be used when these medicines are taken with other drugs that are metabolized in the liver, such as erythromycin (macrolide antibiotics), niacin, cyclosporine, and FK-506 (tacrolimus), to name a few. Frequent monitoring of liver function tests and creatine kinase levels is recommended.

Nicotinic Acid

Neither of the two medications (niacin and timed-release niacin) in this class of drugs contains nicotine. Instead they both contain niacin, whose primary effect is to increase HDL-C levels up to 25%. Little if any effect on the other lipid components is seen. The most frequent side effect is skin flushing, which is caused by the release of prostaglandins and can be blocked by taking an aspirin one-half hour before the niacin. Because of the associated stomach irritation, niacin should be taken with food, although caution needs to be exercised in diabetic patients because of niacin's tendency to increase blood glucose. Patients with gout should be cautioned about an increased tendency to precipitate gouty episodes. Although most of the problems associated with these medicines are minor, fatal dysrhythmias have been reported, and caution should be exercised in any patient with cardiac dysrhythmias, as well as in patients with liver disease or inflammatory bowel disease. Patients should be carefully monitored while taking these drugs.

Other Hypolipemics

Probucol has been shown to decrease LDL-C levels via its antioxidation effect. However, it also decreases HDL-C levels. Because of this effect and its potential for fatal dysrhythmias, it is seldom used. Any patient who is considered for this drug should have a resting electrocardiogram to determine if there is QT prolongation. Probucol should not be given to people taking tricyclic antidepressants because of potential problems with QT prolongation and rhythm abnormalities. Patients with low potassium and magnesium levels also should not be placed on this drug. In general, patients who have bradycardia or conduction problems, are taking digoxin, or have recently had a myocardial infarction should find alternative treatment. Other problems include syncope and lightheadedness.

Other medications that have been associated with reductions in TC levels but are not primarily designed to treat hyperlipidemia include the angiotensin-converting enzyme inhibitors. Some but not all of these drugs reduce TC levels by a pathway not yet elucidated.

Comparing Dietary Change and Hypolipemic Drugs in the Management of Hyperlipidemia

Beginning in 1992 our group began investigating both dietary and drug effects in the treatment of hyperlipidemia.[59–70] Throughout the 18-month study and since, 70 individuals were enrolled into one of four treatment groups designed to determine the effect of diet, diet and drug, drug only, and no treatment. The first group received routine suggestions to reduce their dietary intake of fats and cholesterol, and to control the total number of calories they were eating to maintain an ideal body weight. Reading material was available but no additional counseling or medications were provided. Over the following 18 months, these patients increased their TC levels by 15%, which represented a 30% increased risk for CAD.

During this same time interval, the second group of subjects received dietary counseling with specific instructions to assist in reducing or eliminating foods with cholesterol and saturated fats. Additionally, patients were counseled regarding their caloric intake. By the completion of the study all patients had attained a step II (see Table 30.3) diet or better despite their original belief that they could not make the necessary changes in their diet. As a result the average TC level dropped by 13% during the first 6 months, and 30% by the end of the study. This represents a 26% and 60% reduction in the risk of heart disease at 6 and 18 months, respectively.

The third group of individuals received 6 months of dietary counseling identical to that received by the second group. However, after the first 6 months of the study, these patients stopped receiving dietary counseling and subsequently returned to their prior eating habits. Additionally, this group also received hypolipemic medications at the beginning of the study, with increased dosages as determined by the primary care physician. During the first 6 months these people not only showed an average reduction in their TC levels of 27%, representing a 54% reduced risk for heart disease, but many were able to discontinue antianginal medications. This undoubtedly represents an improvement in flow reserve as explained in Chapter 29 on atherosclerosis. Unfortunately, after the dietary counseling was discontinued, the overall TC levels increased from the 6-month level. The TC levels demonstrated an overall reduction of 12% by the end of the study as compared with the beginning of the study. This 12% reduction is

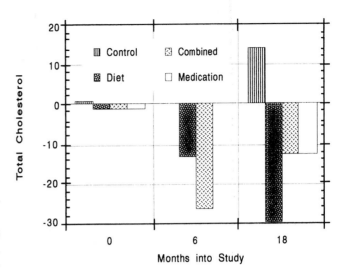

FIGURE 30.6. The effect of changed diet, hypolipemic medications, and the combination of diet and medication. Reductions in TC levels can be achieved either by dietary changes, hypolipemic medications, or a combined approach. When dietary modification to either a step 2 American Heart Association diet or Fleming guidelines occured, cholesterol levels were decreased by 30%. Hypolipemic medications resulted in a 12% reduction, whereas the combined approach yielded even greater reductions (in as little as 3 to 6 months) than either approach used alone.

typical of what is seen and reported in the literature when patients receive medications but do not change their diet. The results during the first 6 months of the study suggest, however, that even greater strides could have been made if dietary counseling and improved dietary habits had been maintained.

The final group consisted only of people receiving medications to treat hyperlipidemia. There was no dietary counseling. By the completion of the study, the average reduction in TC levels was 12%. This is identical to the results obtained by group 3 after dietary counseling had ceased and patients had returned to their prior dietary habits. The results of this study are graphically shown in Figure 30.6.

Conclusion

Atherosclerotic CAD is the number one killer of people worldwide. More people die each year in the United States from heart disease and strokes than would have died in 20 Vietnam Wars. This means that each day more than 8000 people (one every 10 s) will die from heart disease in the United States (more than half will be women), with one third to one half having no prior symptoms or warning signs. Additionally, one American has a stroke every minute, and every 4 min a person dies from a stroke-related problem. The current recommendations are to reduce total serum cholesterol levels to less than 150 mg/dL, or LDL-C levels to less than 100 mg/dL. Likewise, triglyceride levels should be reduced to 150 mg/dL or less. Studies over the past 30 years have shown that hyperlipidemia can and should be treated and that CAD can be reversed, at least to some extent, depending on the severity of the disease, when it is detected, and the motivation of the patient and doctor. Until recently, little information has been available to assist with the dietary changes necessary to significantly reduce elevated cholesterol and triglyceride levels. We now know that diet or diet and drug therapy can dramatically reduce elevated lipids and reduce the risk of CAD and stroke. This information[70,71] is now available for the general public and the clinician to assist them in better understanding the diagnosis and treatment of hyperlipidemia.

Although cholesterol and calcium (atherosclerosis) are two factors involved in CAD, the Fleming theory[71–73] (as explained in Chapter 64) proposes that other factors may be important in individual cases. The first of these is the inflammatory process that is initiated with damage to coronary endothelium. This can occur as a result of cholesterol deposition, ulceration of plaques, interventional procedures, and oxidative stress. A second is bacterial involvement, including *Streptococcus pneumoniae*, *Chlamydia pneumoniae*, and *Helicobactor pylori*. Once these bacteria infiltrate a coronary plaque they may precipitate further damage and ulceration in addition to increasing the inflammatory process. Once the initial screening for hyperlipidemia is completed it is important that repeat evaluations continue to monitor the patient's progress and, when appropriate, markers of inflammation and bacterial involvement, including fibrinogen, lipoprotein (a), C-reactive protein, interleukins, and homocysteine.

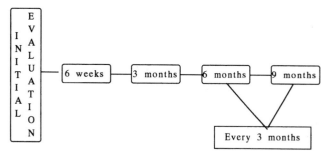

FIGURE 30.7. Recommended follow-up evaluations for patients with hyperlipidemia. Once patients undergo dietary and/or hypolipemic drug management for hyperlipidemia, close monitoring of results with dietary and drug modifications is necessary to optimize results. Patients should have fasting lipoprotein analysis (LDL-C, HDL-C, TC, and total triglycerides) performed at each visit, along with appropriate liver function tests, monitoring of creatine kinase (if taking hypolipemic medications), and other tests as outlined in Chapter 64.

Adjustments in dietary habits and medications can be made during these visits, along with monitoring of the effects of the medications on the liver and muscles. The recommended schedule for office visits and blood work is shown in Figure 30.7.

References

1. Tucker CF, Catsulis C, Strong JP, Eggen DA. Regression of early cholesterol-induced lesions in rhesus monkeys. *Am J Pathol.* 1971;65:493–514.
2. Eggen DA, Strong JP, Newman WP, et al. Regression of diet-induced fatty streaks in rhesus monkeys. *Lab Invest.* 1974;31:294–301.
3. Kokatnur MG, Malcom GT, Eggen DA, Strong JP. Depletion of aortic free and ester cholesterol by dietary means in rhesus monkeys with fatty streaks. *Atherosclerosis.* 1975; 21:195–203.
4. Strong JP. Reversibility of fatty streaks in rhesus monkeys. *Primates Med.* 1976;9:300–320.
5. Armstrong ML, Megan MB. Arterial fibrous proteins in cynomolgus monkeys after atherogenic and regression diets. *Circ Res.* 1975;36:256–261.
6. Malinow MR, McLaughlin P, Papworth L, et al. A model for therapeutic intervention on established coronary atherosclerosis in a nonhuman primate. *Adv Exp Med Biol.* 1976;67:3–31.
7. Vesselinovitch D, Wissler RW, Hughes R, et al. Reversal of advanced atherosclerosis in rhesus monkeys, I: light-microscopic studies. *Atherosclerosis.* 1976;23:155–176.
8. Weber G, Fabbrini P, Resi L, et al. Regression of arteriosclerotic lesions in rhesus monkey aortas after regression diet. Scanning and transmission electron microscope observations of the endothelium. *Atherosclerosis.* 1977;26: 535–547.
9. Chakravarti RN, Kumar BS, Nair CR, et al. Reversibility of cholesterol adrenaline-induced atherosclerosis in rhesus monkeys. Evaluation of safflower oil and low-fat low-calorie diet. *Atherosclerosis.* 1977;28:405–416.
10. Hollander W. Studies on the progression and regression of coronary and peripheral atherosclerosis in the cynomolgus monkey, I: effects of dipyridamole and aspirin. *Exp Mol Pathol.* 1979;30:55–73.
11. Connor WE, Cerqueira MT, Connor RW, et al. The plasma lipids, lipoproteins, and diet of the Tarahumara Indians of Mexico. *Am J Clin Nutr.* 1978;31:1131–1142.
12. McGill HC. The relationship of dietary cholesterol to serum cholesterol concentration and to atherosclerosis in man. *Am J Clin Nutr.* 1979;32:2664–2702.
13. Glueck CJ. Dietary fat and atherosclerosis. *Am J Clin Nutr.* 1979;32:2703–2711.
14. Simons LA. Interrelations of lipids and lipoproteins with coronary artery disease mortality in 19 countries. *Am J Cardiol.* 1986;57:5G–10G.
15. Dewar HA, Arthur JB, Ashby WR, et al. Trial of clofibrate in the treatment of ischaemic heart disease. Five-year study by a group of physicians of the Newcastle upon Tyne region. *Br Med J.* 1971;4:767–775.
16. Alstead S, Aitchison JD, Barr JB, et al. Ischaemic heart disease: a secondary prevention trial using clofibrate. Report

by a research committee of the Scottish Society of Physicians. *Br Med J.* 1971;4:775–784.

17. Coronary Drug Project Research Group. Clofibrate and niacin in coronary heart disease. The Coronary Drug Project Research Group. *JAMA.* 1975;231:360–381.

18. Puska P, Virtamo J, Tuomilehto J, et al. Cardiovascular risk factor changes in a three-year follow-up of a cohort in connection with a community programme (the North Karelia Project). *Acta Med Scand.* 1978;204:381–388.

19. Kornitzer M, Backer GD, Dramaix M, et al. The Belgian Heart Disease Prevention Project. Modification of the coronary risk profile in an industrial population. *Circulation.* 1980;61:18–25.

20. Shekelle B, Shryock AM, Paul O, et al. Diet, serum cholesterol, and death from coronary heart disease. The Western Electric study. *N Engl J Med.* 1981;304:65–70.

21. Kjelsberg MO. Multiple risk factor intervention trial. Risk factor changes and mortality results. *JAMA.* 1982;248:1465–1477.

22. Lipids Research Clinics Program. The lipid research clinics coronary primary prevention trial results, I: reduction in incidence of coronary heart disease; II: the relationship of reduction in incidence of coronary heart disease to cholesterol lowering. *JAMA.* 1984;251:351–374.

23. Goldbourt U, Holtzman E, Neufeld HN. Total and high density lipoprotein cholesterol in the serum and risk of mortality: evidence of a threshold effect. *Br Med J.* 1985;290:1239–1243.

24. Miettinen TA, Huttunen JK, Naukkarinen V, et al. Multifactorial primary prevention of cardiovascular diseases in middle-aged men. Risk factor changes, incidence, and mortality. *JAMA.* 1985;254:2097–2102.

25. Brunner D, Weisbort J, Meshulam N, et al. Relation of serum total cholesterol and high-density lipoprotein cholesterol percentage to the incidence of definite coronary events: twenty-year follow-up of the Donolo Tel Aviv Prospective Coronary Artery Disease study. *Am J Cardiol.* 1987;59:1271–1276.

26. Frick JH, Elo O, Haapa K. Helsinki heart study: primary prevention trial with gemfibrozil in middle-aged men with dyslipidemia. Safety of treatment, changes in risk factors, and incidence of coronary heart disease. *N Engl J Med.* 1987;317:1237–1245.

27. Carlson LA, Rosenhamer G. Reduction of mortality in the Stockholm Ischaemic Heart Disease Secondary Prevention study by combined treatment with clofibrate and nicotinic acid. *Acta Med Scand.* 1988;223:405–418.

28. Assmann G, Schulte H, Munster DR. The Prospective Cardiovascular Monster (PROCAM) study: prevalence of hyperlipidemia in persons with hypertension and/or diabetes mellitus and the relationship to coronary heart disease. *Am Heart J.* 1988;116:1713–1724.

29. Alderman JD, Pasternak RC, Sacks FM, et al. Effect of a modified, well-tolerated niacin regimen on serum total cholesterol, high density lipoprotein cholesterol and the cholesterol to high density lipoprotein ratio. *Am J Cardiol.* 1989;64:725–729.

30. Cohn K, Sakai FJ, Langston MF. Effect of clofibrate on progression of coronary disease: a prospective angiographic study in man. *Am Heart J.* 1975;89:591–598.

31. Kuo PT, Hayase K, Kostis JB, et al. Use of combined diet and colestipol in long-term (7–7 and 1/2 years) treatment of patients with type II hyperlipoproteinemia. *Circulation.* 1979;59:199–211.

32. Nash DT, Gensini G, Esente P. Effect of lipid-lowering therapy on the progression of coronary atherosclerosis assessed by scheduled repetitive coronary arteriography. *Int J Cardiol.* 1982;2:43–55.

33. Levy RI, Brensike JF, Epstein SE, et al. The influence of changes in lipid values induced by cholestyramine and diet on progression of coronary artery disease: results of the NHLBI Type II Coronary Intervention study. *Circulation.* 1984;69:325–337.

34. Nikkila EA, Viikinkoski P, Valle M, et al. Prevention of progression of coronary atherosclerosis by treatment of hyperlipidemia: a seven year prospective angiographic study. *Br Med J.* 1984;289:220–223.

35. Arntzenius AC, Kromhout D, Barth JD, et al. Diet, lipoproteins, and the progression of coronary atherosclerosis. The Leiden Intervention Trial. *N Engl J Med.* 1985;312:805–811.

36. Blankenhorn DH, Nessim SA, Johnson RL, et al. Beneficial effects of combined colestipol-niacin therapy on coronary atherosclerosis and coronary venous bypass grafts. *JAMA.* 1987;257:3233–3240.

37. Blankenhorn DH, Johnson RL, Nessim SA, et al. The Cholesterol Lowering Atherosclerosis Study (CLAS): design, methods, and baseline results. *Control Clin Trials.* 1987;8:354–387.

38. Gould KL, Buchi M, Kirkeeide RL, et al. Reversal of coronary artery stenosis with cholesterol lowering in man followed by arteriography and positron emission tomography [abstract]. *J Nucl Med.* 1989;30:845.

39. Brown BG, Lin JT, Schaefer SM, et al. Niacin or lovastatin, combined with colestipol, regress coronary atherosclerosis and prevent clinical events in men with elevated apolipoprotein B [abstract]. *Circulation.* 1989;80(suppl II):II266.

40. Ornish DM, Brown SE, Scherwitz LW, et al. Can lifestyle changes reverse coronary heart disease? *Lancet.* 1990;336:129–133.

41. Gould KL, Buchi M, Kirkeeide RL, et al. Reversal of coronary artery stenosis with cholesterol lowering in man followed by arteriography and positron emission tomography [abstract]. *J Nucl Med.* 1989;30:845.

42. Brown BG, Bolson EL, Dodge HT. Arteriographic assessment of coronary atherosclerosis. Review of current methods, their limitations, and clinical applications. *Arteriosclerosis.* 1982;2:2–15.

43. Buchwald H, Moore RB, Varco RL. Surgical treatment of hyperlipidemia. *Circulation.* 1974;49(suppl 1):1–22.

44. Rafflenbeul W, Smith LR, Rogers WJ, et al. Quantitative coronary arteriography. Coronary anatomy of patients with unstable angina pectoris reexamined 1 year after optimal medical therapy. *Am J Cardiol.* 1979;43:699–707.

45. Roth D, Kostuk WJ. Noninvasive and invasive demonstration of spontaneous regression of coronary artery disease. *Circulation.* 1980;62:888–896.

46. Gohlke H, Sturzenhofecker P, Gornandt L, et al. Progression and regression der koronaren Herzerkrankung im

chronischen Infarkstadium bei Patienten unter 40 Jahren [Progression and regression of coronary heart disease in chronic infarction stage in patients under 40]. *Schweiz Med Wochenschr.* 1980;110: 1663–1665.

47. Buchwald H, Moore RB, Rucker RD, et al. Clinical angiographic regression of atherosclerosis after partial ileal bypass. *Atherosclerosis.* 1983;16:117–128.

48. Brensike JF, Levy RI, Kelsey SF, et al. Effects of therapy with cholestyramine on progression of coronary arteriosclerosis: results of the NHLBI Type II Coronary Intervention Study. *Circulation.* 1984;69:313–324.

49. Lardinois CK, Neuman SL. The effects of antihypertensive agents on serum lipids and lipoproteins. *Arch Intern Med.* 1988;148:1280–1288.

50. Bredie SJ, de Bruin TW, Demacker PN, et al. Comparison of gemfibrozil versus simvastatin in familial combined hyperlipidemia and effects on apolipoprotein-B-containing lipoproteins, low-density lipoprotein subfraction profile, and low-density lipoprotein oxidizability. *Am J Cardiol.* 1995;75:348–353.

51. Byington RP, Furberg CD, Crouse JR III, et al. Pravastatin, lipids, and atherosclerosis in the carotid arteries (PLAC-II). *Am J Cardiol.* 1995;75:455–459.

52. Pollare T, Lithell H, Berne C. A comparison of the effects of hydrochlorothiazide and captopril on glucose and lipid metabolism in patients with hypertension. *N Engl J Med.* 1989;321:868–873.

53. Kuo PT. Inducing regression of atherosclerosis. *Choices in Cardiology.* 1989;3:308–309.

54. Parmley WW, Blumlein S, Sievers R. Modification of experimental atherosclerosis by calcium-channel blockers. *Am J Cardiol.* 1985;55:165B–171B.

55. Parmley WW. Calcium channel blockers and atherogenesis. *Am J Med.* 1987;82(suppl 3B):3–8.

56. Atkinson JB, Swift LL. Nifedipine suppresses atherogenesis in cholesterol-fed heterozygous WHL rabbits [abstract]. *Circulation.* 1989;80(suppl II):II382.

57. Loaldi A, Polese A, Montorsi P, et al. Comparison of nifedipine, propranolol and isosorbide dinitrate on angiographic progression and regression of coronary arterial narrowings in angina pectoris. *Am J Cardiol.* 1989;64: 433–439.

58. Gottlieb SO, Brinker JA, Mellits ED, et al. Effect of nifedipine on the development of coronary bypass graft stenoses in high-risk patients: a randomized double-blind, placebo-controlled trial [abstract]. *Circulation.* 1989;80(suppl II): II228.

59. Fleming RM, Rater D, Ketchum K. Reducing cholesterol and triglycerides in the elderly patient by diet alone. Paper presented at: Council on Arteriosclerosis for the 66th Scientific Sessions of the AHA; November 8–11, 1993; Atlanta, Ga.

60. Fleming RM, Rater D. Dietary changes without medication can equally reduce cholesterol in both the young and older patient. Paper presented at: Council on Arteriosclerosis for the 66th Scientific Sessions of the AHA; November 8–11, 1993; Atlanta, Ga.

61. Fleming RM, Rater D, Ketchum K. Studying the effect of medications on cholesterol and triglycerides in subjects not receiving dietary counseling. Paper presented at: Council on Arteriosclerosis for the 66th Scientific Sessions of the AHA; November 8–11, 1993; Atlanta, Ga.

62. Fleming RM, Ketchum K. Dietary reinforcement is an integral component of cholesterol reduction. Paper presented at: Council on Arteriosclerosis for the 66th Scientific Sessions of the AHA; November 8–11, 1993; Atlanta, Ga.

63. Fleming RM, Fleming DM, Gaede R. Hyperlipidemic elderly patients: comparing diet and drug therapy. Paper presented at: Council on Arteriosclerosis for the 67th Scientific Sessions of the AHA; November 14–17, 1994; Dallas, Tex.

64. Fleming RM, Fleming DM, Gaede R. Treatment of hyperlipidemic patients: diet versus drug therapy. Paper presented at: Council on Arteriosclerosis for the 67th Scientific Sessions of the AHA; November 14–17, 1994; Dallas, Tex.

65. Fleming RM, Ketchum K, Fleming DM, Gaede R. Controlling hypercholesterolemia by diet and drug therapy in the elderly. Paper presented at: 1st Annual Scientific Session on Cardiovascular Disease in the Elderly; March 18, 1995; New Orleans, La.

66. Fleming RM: Reducing cholesterol and triglyceride levels in both the young and elderly patient, by dietary changes: with and without hyperlipidemic medications. Paper presented at: 17th World Congress of the International Union of Angiology; April 3–7, 1995; Westminister, London.

67. Fleming RM, Ketchum K, Fleming DM, Gaede R. Investigating differences in cholesterol and triglyceride levels as influenced by diet and hyperlipidemic medications. Paper presented at: 42nd Annual World Assembly of the American College of Angiology; October 18, 1995; Maui, Hawaii.

68. Fleming RM, Ketchum K, Fleming DM and Gaede R.: Treating hyperlipidemia in the elderly. *Angiology.* 1995;46: 1075–1083.

69. Fleming RM, Ketchum K, Fleming DM, et al. Assessing the independent effect of dietary counseling and hypolipidemic medications on serum lipids. *Angiology.* 1996;47: 831–840.

70. Fleming RM. How to Bypass Your Bypass: What Your Doctor Doesn't Tell You About Cholesterol and Your Diet. Bethel, Conn: Rutledge Books; 1997.

71. Fleming RM. *The Diet Myth and Keeping Your Heart Forever Young. What you need to know and why!* Austin, Tex: Windsor House Publishing Group; 1998. In press.

72. Fleming RM. The Fleming theory: a link between atherosclerosis, inflammation and bacterial infection and their role in the overall pathogenesis of coronary artery disease. *Int J Angiol.* Submitted.

73. Fleming RM. The natural progression of atherosclerosis in an untreated patient with hyperlipidemia. *Int J Angiol.* Submitted.

31

Nuclear Cardiology: Its Role in the Detection and Management of Coronary Artery Disease

Richard M. Fleming

Nuclear imaging of the heart began with the discovery of x-rays emitted from uranium salts by Henry Becquerel in 1896. Radioactive materials were first used in 1926 when Herman Blumgart injected radon gas into arm veins and recorded the time necessary for the radioactivity to appear in the blood of the opposite arm.[1] This was known as the *circulation time*, which was prolonged in patients with heart disease. The first use of radioisotope scanning occurred in 1958 to detect pericardial effusion with a rectilinear scanning method.[2] The first attempt to detect myocardial infarction met with limited success because of too much tracer uptake in the stomach.[3] With the advent of the anger circuit,[4] the way was cleared for improved detection of cardiac abnormalities, particularly when coupled with technetium 99m imaging agents.

In the early 1970s[5] potassium 43 chloride was used to image the myocardium, and the search for more appropriate potassium analogs lead to the discovery of thallium 201 and rubidium 82. Despite popular misconceptions about thallium 201, this radionuclide follows regional blood flow as demonstrated in dogs.[6] Since then several additional isotopes[7-17] have been developed for use with planar and single photon emission computed tomography (SPECT) imaging of the heart. Additional investigation concerning the reversibility[7-10,18-32] of coronary atherosclerosis, using both SPECT and positron emission tomography (PET) imaging, has been possible in recent years with improvements in available isotopes and imaging techniques. This chapter focuses on the methods used to determine changes in coronary blood flow and the assessment of normal, ischemic, and infarcted myocardium using planar, SPECT, and PET imaging.

terpreting test results. The different types of tests available as well as their interpretation are discussed here. Before ordering a nuclear study, the physician must make three decisions. *First*, one must decide what type of camera (planar, SPECT, or PET) will best answer the question. *Second*, one must determine which form of stress will best bring out differences in blood flow between resting and physiologically stressed conditions. Of course, this is not a consideration when ordering a resting ventriculogram (RVG), which has other names including multiple gated analysis (MUGA). (*Gated* means that images are matched with electrocardiogram activity to differentiate systole from diastole.) The MUGA can be either a resting or stressed (usually bicycle) study used to determine the ejection fraction of either the right (first-pass) side of the heart or the left ventricle. These studies can also be used to determine if there are shunts (atrioseptal defect, ventriculoseptal defect, patent ductus arteriosus, etc.), regurgitant valves (mitral, etc.), or regional wall motion abnormalities (Figure 31.1) such as would be seen with atherosclerotic heart disease. *Finally*, a decision must be made about the type of radionuclide to be used. Radionuclides are the radioactive compounds injected into the patient and subsequently detected by the camera. These radioactive materials are not called *radionucleotides* (radioactively labeled nucleic acids), but *radionuclides*.

For the purpose of this chapter we do not further address RVG/MUGA studies. Instead we focus our attention on planar, SPECT, and PET imaging of the heart, allowing us to develop a better understanding of these tests.

The Components of Nuclear Cardiac Imaging

There are several components to nuclear imaging of the heart that can lead to confusion when ordering and in-

Types of Cameras

There are currently three major types of cameras available for cardiac imaging. These include planar, SPECT, and PET cameras. Each uses photomultiplier tubes

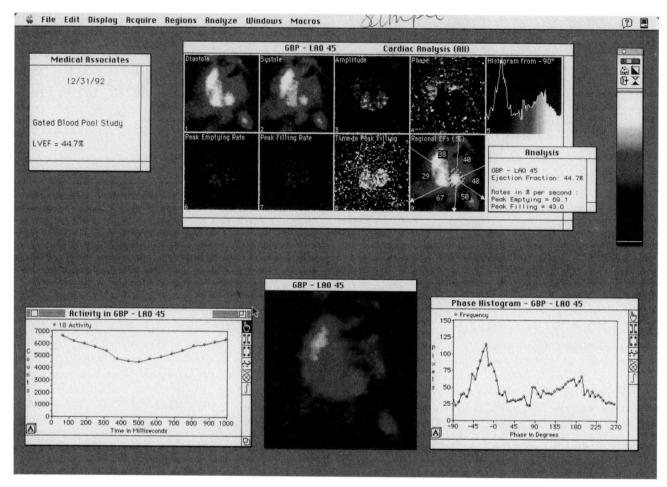

FIGURE 31.1. Gated blood pool imaging. Regional wall motion abnormalities, first-pass (right ventricle ejection fraction) and multiple-gated analysis of the left ventricle was assessed using 1 mCi of "cold" pyrophosphate and 26 mCi of technitium 99m. Initial imaging of the right ventricle demonstrated a right ventricle ejection fraction of 22% (not shown here). Imaging of the left ventricle is statically displayed here showing the diastolic and systolic activity and histogram curves that are used to assess left ventricle ejection fraction, which was 44.7%. The images represented here were obtained from the left anterior oblique position and are divided into specific regions (regional ejection fractions) as shown in the last square of the top two rows of images. These regional ejection fractions demonstrate mildly depressed ejection fractions anteriorly, consistent with left anterior artery disease.

(PMTs) designed to absorb different levels of energy (photons) and convert them into electrical signals interpreted by the computer as radioactivity. Planar and SPECT cameras also utilize crystals and collimators designed to reduce extraneous information and improve their accuracy. The radioactivity being detected by the cameras presumably comes from the patient who has been injected with an appropriate radioactive compound. However, neither planar nor SPECT imaging has a mechanism to totally exclude other sources of radiation from being interpreted by the computer as coming from the patient. The primary difference between planar and SPECT imaging is that in SPECT imaging, the camera moves around the patient, whereas the camera operator must position the camera for planar imaging.

Figure 31.2 shows how radioactivity from outside the patient could be recognized by the camera as coming from the patient and how radioactivity coming from the patient may not be detected but may be absorbed or sufficiently diminished by the time it reaches the collimators. The energy released by radioisotopes that can be

TABLE 31.1. Planar and single photon emission computed tomography isotopes.

Isotope	Radionuclide	Physical half-life (h)	Imaging energy
Thallium 201	Ti 201	73	67–82 KeV
Teboroxime	Tc 99m	6	140 KeV
Sestamibi	Tc 99m	6	140 KeV

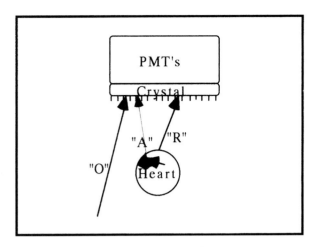

FIGURE 31.2. Planar and SPECT imaging. Radioactivity (R) passes through the collimator and is then detected by the scintillation crystal, after which it is converted to electrical information by photomultiplier tubes (PMTs). The computer records these events as coming from the patient following the injection of radioactive isotopes. Other sources of radioactivity may be interpreted as coming from the patient (O) when in fact they are not. Similarly, activity coming from the patient (A) may not be detected because of energy loss en route to the SPECT camera.

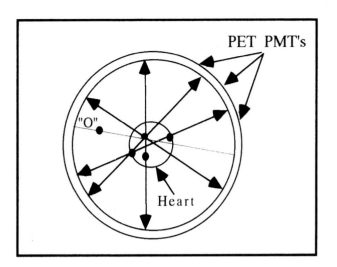

FIGURE 31.3. PET imaging. Patients are placed within circular rings of PMTs that detect positron–electron annihilation events (filled circles) and record these events as coming only from the patient. Those events originating outside the region of the heart (O) are excluded. Attenuation is corrected for by gallium scanning earlier in the study. See text for full details.

Types of Physiologic Stress

best detected by planar and SPECT systems ranges from 60 to 180 keV. This means that technetium compounds (Table 31.1), which have a photon energy of 140 keV are ideal for SPECT imaging.

Unlike planar and SPECT systems, the PET camera is designed to detect two different photons released simultaneously when a positron (antimatter electron) from a PET isotope (Table 31.2) injected into the patient collides with an electron from the patient. When this happens, the mass of the positron and the mass of the electron are converted into two photons of energy ($E = mc^2$), each having 511 keV and traveling in essentially opposite directions (Figure 31.3). These photons are almost simultaneously detected by two opposing PMTs. Because photons travel at the speed of light, the time necessary for both photons to reach PMTs on opposite sides of the patient can be calculated by knowing how far the heart is from the PMTs. Using this information (time-of-flight) virtually eliminates errors in determining the source of radioactivity, which increases the sensitivity and specificity of PET imaging as compared with either SPECT or planar methods.

Many clinicians still consider there to be only one method for inducing changes in coronary artery blood flow; such changes are frequently referred to as *stressing the heart*. In reality there are two major approaches available. The first is to increase the heart rate and blood pressure by walking on a treadmill or bicycling, thereby increasing the heart's demand for blood, as described in Chapter 29 on atherosclerosis. Using well-established protocols, the intensity of the exercise is gradually increased until one of several things happen. These events include but are not limited to reaching at least 85% of the patient's maximal predicted heart rate (determined by age [Table 31.3]); developing a hypertensive response to exercise (e.g., diastolic blood pressure greater than 100 to 110 mm Hg); cerebrovascular accident; developing a potentially fatal dysrhythmia; developing angina; ischemia or infarction as demonstrated on the electrocardiogram, regardless of symptoms; exertional dyspnea; hypotensive response to exercise (indicative of left ventricular dysfunction); leg fatigue; or physical exhaustion. In all but the first of these scenarios (reaching 85% of the maximal predicted heart rate), the patient does not attain the necessary hemodynamic response required to produce sufficient changes in coronary blood flow to detect differences between the stressed and resting states.

Alternatively, pharmacologic approaches have been developed[7–10] to cause sufficient changes in blood pressure and heart rate to elicit a meaningful stress response in patients, while minimizing potential problems and side effects. A comparison of the expected hemody-

TABLE 31.2. Position emission tomography isotopes.

Isotope	Source	Physical half-life (h)	Imaging energy
18-Fluoro-2-deoxyglucose	Cyclotron	110 min	511 keV
Ammonia 13	Cyclotron	10 min	511 keV
Rubidium 82	Generator	75 s	511 keV

TABLE 31.3. Maximum predicted heart rate by age.

Age	20	25	30	35	40	45	50	55	60	65	70	75	80	85
Heart rate	197	195	193	191	189	187	184	182	180	178	176	174	172	170

TABLE 31.4. Hemodynamic results of different stressors.*

	Percent change in heart rate	Percent change in systolic pressure	Percent change in diastolic pressure
Dipyridamole	45.5 ± 22.2	−8.3 ± 11.3	−9.6 ± 8.0
Dobutamine	77.0 ± 28.8	19.4 ± 31.4	−8.9 ± 14.3
Treadmill	89.5 ± 35.1	31.3 ± 18.5	4.22 ± 11.3

*Values are displayed as mean plus or minus standard deviation.

namic results as well as the possible side effects for both dobutamine and high-dose dipyridamole (HDD) are listed in Tables 31.4 and 31.5, respectively. The protocols for using these agents are shown in Figures 31.4 and 31.5, which also include the approach used with exercise (treadmill) testing, in addition to minor differences in timing needed for each of the available isotopes used with planar, SPECT, and PET imaging. Patients should not receive dipyridamole if there is any evidence of pulmonary disease or allergies to the drug. Full details of these approaches are discussed elsewhere.[7]

Because differences in blood flow between resting and stressed states should be maximized, the clinician must carefully choose the approach to be used, otherwise the study will provide little or no useful information. The cost and risks to the patient in these circumstances cannot be totally justified if meaningful results are not obtained. The results of exercise (treadmill) testing and SPECT imaging are usually reported together. Discrepancies between the treadmill tests and nuclear imaging results are well known[9,10] and should be considered in light of the limitations of each method.

PET imaging protocols have an added component that is used to improve the accuracy of the information obtained as compared with SPECT and planar imaging. This is seen in protocol A of Figure 31.5, which shows the various PET protocols used for assessing coronary artery blood flow and myocardial viability. This additional component (attenuation correction) determines the effect of tissue energy loss (attenuation) and corrects

for diminished photon energy reaching the PMTs as a result of the effect of individual patient body mass and air surrounding the patient. Planar and SPECT imaging may have artifacts from both diaphragmatic (inferior wall of heart) and breast (anterior wall) attenuation, resulting in false positive results.

To determine the PET attenuation correction, a Plexiglas ring is placed around the patient; 3 mCi of gallium 68 is administered, and counts are collected until 200 million counts are recorded. This information is used by the computer to determine how much energy attenuation is occurring, thereby improving the accuracy of the detection of attenuated photons from different regions of the heart (as detected by each PMT surrounding the patient). The full procedure for PET imaging is shown in Figure 31.5.

Radionuclides (Tracers)

There are numerous radionuclides currently available, and their use depends on the clinical question being asked and the type of camera system being employed. The radionuclides are used in conjunction with a specific stress protocol (Figures 31.4 and 31.5) to obtain resting and stress images. Interestingly, when PET is employed, the rest image is obtained first, giving useful information regarding any prior myocardial infarction, whereas planar and SPECT protocols almost always begin with the stress component, which has the potential to precipitate problems in the absence of baseline information. At our institute, we perform all nuclear cardiac studies using the rest/stress approach.

The availability of 18-fluoro-2-deoxyglucose (FDG) has made it possible to determine myocardial viability when given to patients who are not fasting. When a fasting state exits, the results are uninterpretable because the heart obtains its energy from the metabolism of fatty acids while suppressing the metabolism of glucose. For FDG to be useful, the patient must be in a nonfasting state so that glucose will be taken up by myocardial cells and used for cellular metabolism. This is why patients (who must be

TABLE 31.5. Percentage of patients reporting side effects with pharmacological stress.

	Dipyridamole	Dobutamine
Chest pressure	41.3	20.0
ST-segment depression	25.3	20.0
Headache	9.3	0.0
Nonspecific ST changes	6.7	0.0
Nausea	6.7	0.0
Dyspnea	5.3	0.0
Increased ventricular ectopy	4.0	40.0
Flush	2.7	0.0

FIGURE 31.4. Stress protocols used for planar and SPECT imaging. Protocols A and B utilize high-dose dipyridamole (HDD) for the radionuclides thallium, Tc 99m hexakis-2-methoxy-2-isobutyl isonitrile (sestamibi), and Tc 99m chloromethyl-boron(1-)-tris[1,2-cyclohexane-dionedioxime(1)] (teboroxime). Protocols C and D are used for exercise treadmill testing and intravenous dobutamine, respectively.

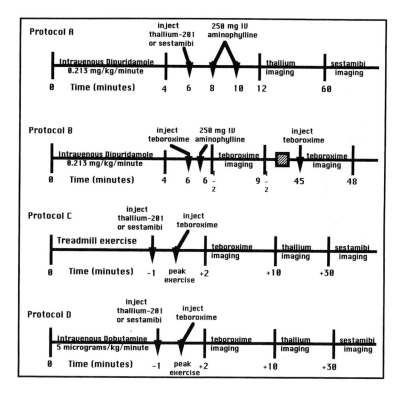

fasting for protocols B and C) are given 50 grams of glucose at the beginning of protocol D. Since FDG can be taken up by both viable and ischemic myocardium, blood flow must also be determined with ammonia-13 to determine if the region has normal or ischemic blood flow. After a myocardial infarction, a region of the heart occluded from the blood supply shifts to the anaerobic metabolism of glucose, leading to intense uptake of glucose in that region. Additional FDG activity in this region may be related to phagocytosis of myocardial cellular debris by white blood cells. It is probably for these reasons that patients who have recently undergone a myocardial in-

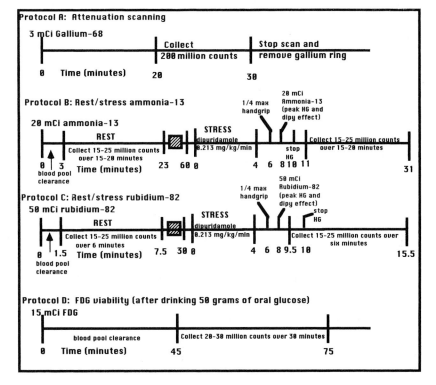

FIGURE 31.5. PET imaging protocols for determining attenuation correction, coronary blood flow, and myocardial viability. Protocol A illustrates the procedure for attenuation correction, which must be done before protocol B, C, or D. Protocols B and C display the procedure used for assessing coronary artery blood flow using ammonia 13 and rubidium 82. The hand grip needed to increase sympathetic nervous system activity is determined by having the patient demonstrate maximum grip strength prior to the study. The patient is then asked to exhibit a grip strength (measured) of one-quarter maximum during the stress component of the study to augment the dipyridamole effect. Protocol D demonstrates the procedure for assessing myocardial viability using 18-fluoro-2-deoxyglucose (FDG). See text for full details.

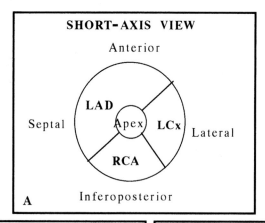

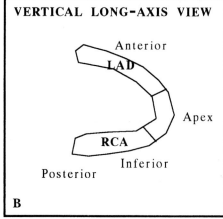

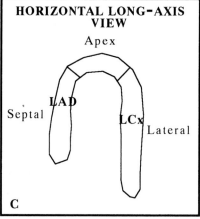

FIGURE 31.6. Relative regions of myocardial blood flow in relationship to reconstructed images from nuclear imaging. **A** represents a reconstructed short-axis view of the heart showing the anterior, septal, apical, inferoposterior, and lateral walls. This same presentation is used for bull's-eye displayed images. **B** represents a reconstructed vertical long-axis view along with the locations of the anterior, apical, inferior, and posterior regions. Likewise, **C** shows the septal, apical, and lateral walls of the heart as represented on the horizontal long-axis view. The correlating arterial distributions are shown as RCA (right coronary), LAD (left anterior descending), and LCx (left circumflex) arteries. The apex is frequently supplied by the LAD, but this may vary depending on the coronary anatomy of the patient.

farction may demonstrate a false positive uptake of FDG when the tissue is in fact necrotic.

Diabetic individuals may also give unpredictable FDG uptake patterns, whether they have taken their usual dose of insulin or not, suggesting that they have nonviable tissue because of failure to take up glucose (FDG) even though the myocardium has normal perfusion and function.

Review of images using planar, SPECT, and PET approaches is accomplished via computer reconstructions that are displayed as short-axis, vertical long-axis, and horizontal long-axis views. Diagrams of these three different views are shown in Figure 31.6, along with the most common arterial distribution found in each specific region. Regions of the myocardium are then compared for the amount of tracer activity present, which is defined as normal, reduced, or absent. These ratings are subjective and vary depending[8] on reader interpretation and experience. Once the rest and stress images are interpreted individually, they are compared to determine if the different regions of myocardium are normal, ischemic, or infarcted, as shown in Table 31.6. Based on the experience and training of the individual and the type of camera (planar, SPECT, or PET) used, the sensi-

TABLE 31.6. Interpretation of nuclear cardiac imaging.

Planar and single photon emission computed tomography image interpretation

Resting image	Stress image	Interpretation	
Normal	Normal	Normal	
Normal	Decreased or absent	Ischemia	
Decreased or absent	Decreased or absent	Infarcted	

Positron emission tomography image interpretation

Resting image	Stress image	FDG* result	Interpretation
Normal	Normal	Normal	Normal and viable
Normal	Decreased or absent	Normal	Ischemic but viable
Normal	Decreased or absent	Decreased or absent	Ischemic and necrotic
Decreased or absent	Decreased or absent	Decreased or absent	No flow and necrotic

FDG, 18-fluoro-2-deoxyglucose.

TABLE 31.7. Sensitivity and specificity of nuclear imaging techniques.

	Percent sensitivity	Percent specificity
Planar	60–70	50–60
Single photon emission computed tomography	70–90	60–80
Positron emission tomography	92–96	92–100

tivity and specificity of the results can vary widely, as shown in Table 31.7. Recently, it has been shown that PET is not only more cost-effective in the detection of coronary artery disease,[33] but results in greater extension of quality-adjusted life years as a result of treatment based on the test results. However, with the use of HDD protocols and attenuation correction of SPECT imaging, SPECT results are approaching that of PET.

Interpretation of test results must be considered as a physiologic parameter of atherosclerosis, as described in Chapter 29. Reductions in stenosis flow reserve as detectable by nuclear imaging may not be well appreciated on coronary arteriography[34–36] because of coronary angiography's inherent limitations in the detection of anatomic changes. When PET was compared with coronary arteriography,[33] individuals with less than 70% pretest probability of coronary artery disease demonstrated a lower cost per effect with PET than with coronary arteriography and both SPECT and PET can detect "early" CAD that angiograms can miss.

Examples of Nuclear Cardiac Perfusion Studies

A comparison of resting coronary artery blood flow is made with maximally obtainable (stress) blood flow, regardless of camera type, form of radionuclide, or type of stress used to induce changes in coronary blood flow. The reconstructed images are compared (Table 31.6) and results reported for each region of the myocardium. The regions are designed to yield useful information regarding the blood flow in each coronary artery (Figure 31.6).

Figure 31.7 shows the results of a patient who underwent stress imaging with dipyridamole using a technetium 99m compound. The images shown represent short-axis (coronal) images that have been reconstructed by the computer. Rows 1 (top) and 3 (second from the bottom) display the relative tracer activity during dipyridamole-induced stress. Rows 2 (second from the top) and 4 (bottom) show the same regions of myocardium during the resting component of the study. Each image (slice) shows the anterior (A), lateral (L), inferoposterior (P), and septal (S) walls. To the right of the images is a gray scale ranging from highest flow (greatest isotope activity, top) to the least amount of activity (bottom). The central part of most of the images is blue-green, which represents the

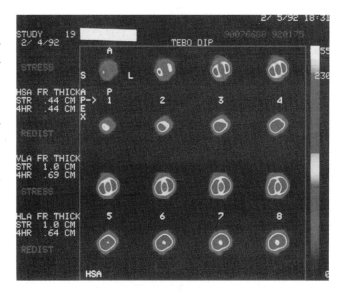

FIGURE 31.7. Example of SPECT imaging. Reconstructed short-axis images are seen in rows 1 through 4. Rows 1 and 3 reveal stress images, whereas rows 2 and 4 show rest images of the same regions. Images are compared using the qualitative scale to the right of the images, ranging from the highest blood flow (top) to the least (bottom). This study demonstrates ischemia in the anterior and inferior regions of the heart, consistent with coronary artery disease. See text for full details.

left ventricular chamber where there are no coronary arteries.

Image slices 1 through 8 represent matched stress and rest images beginning at the apex of the heart and proceeding upward to the base of the heart. Stress images in rows 1 and 3 demonstrate less tracer activity in the anterior (A) and inferoposterior (P) distributions of the heart. This same patient had a 64% narrowing of the proximal left anterior descending artery (A), a 72% narrowing of the right coronary artery (P), and a 26% narrowing of the left circumflex artery (L), as measured by quantitative coronary arteriography as described in Chapter 29 on atherosclerosis. The resting images reveal normal blood flow. These findings of normal blood flow at rest and decreased blood flow under stress represent ischemia in the right coronary and left anterior descending coronary arteries.

Figure 31.8 shows the results of a patient who underwent dipyridamole PET imaging using ammonia 13 and FDG to determine myocardial blood flow and viability, respectively. Assessment of myocardial blood flow was performed using the protocols shown in Figure 31.5, with reconstructed images displayed using bull's-eye equivalent images as explained in Figure 31.6. Images are compared using the qualitative scale at the bottom of the reconstructed images: the right represents the highest blood flow and the left the least. The stress image is displayed on the left of Figure 31.8; the corresponding rest image is displayed in the center. Intensity

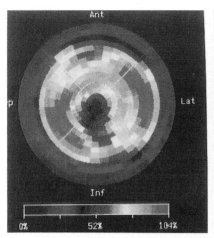
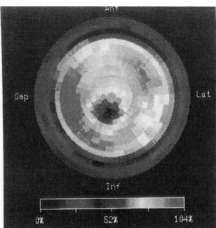
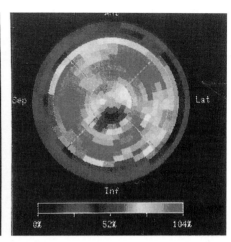

FIGURE 31.8. Example of PET perfusion imaging using ammonia 13. Images are presented using a bull's-eye equivalent approach, with the apex at the center of each image, the anterior wall at 12 o'clock, the lateral wall at 3 o'clock, the inferior wall at 6 o'clock, and the septum at 9 o'clock. The tracer activity is depicted using the qualitative scale at the bottom, where the greatest activity is represented on the right and the least on the left. The first image (left) shows the result after injection of 20 mCi of ammonia 13 following high-dose dipyridamole and handgrip-induced stress. The center image represents the corresponding resting image after 20 mCi are injected at rest. The stress image shows decreased tracer activity in the anterior, apical, and inferior walls of the heart when compared with the resting image. See text for full details. Assessment of myocardial viability using FDG (right) was performed at rest after the ingestion of 50 grams of oral glucose and 15 mCi of FDG. Image acquisition began 45 min after injection with FDG, providing adequate time for blood pool clearance of FDG. Normal tracer activity is detected in all but the apical distribution of the myocardium, indicating that the apex is necrotic and the remainder of the myocardium is viable. See text for full details.

Image Number _____

Reader Number 0 1 2 3 4 5 6

Please circle the reader ID# and record the image # above.

Please circle the appropriate myocardial perfusion image (MPI) result for each region.

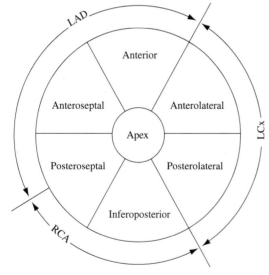

	Myocardial perfusion rating*					
Anterior	0	1	2	3	4	5
Anteroseptal	0	1	2	3	4	5
Posteroseptal	0	1	2	3	4	5
Inferoposterior	0	1	2	3	4	5
Posterolateral	0	1	2	3	4	5
Anterolateral	0	1	2	3	4	5
Apex	0	1	2	3	4	5

* 5 = normal, 4 = probaby normal, 3 = mild defect,
2 = moderate defect, 1 = severe defect, 0 = no perfusion

LAD = Left Anterior Descending Artery
LCx = Left Circumflex Artery
RCA = Right Coronary Artery

REST

the Center for Clinical Cardiology & Research

FIGURE 31.9. Protocols used at the Fleming Heart & Health Institute for qualitative reporting of myocardial perfusion imaging or myocardial viability. Each image (rest, stress, and viability) is evaluated to determine tracer activity in each of seven regions of the myocardium. These regions correlate to each of the three major (LAD, LCx, and RCA) epicardial arteries. Tracer activity is reported on a continuum from no perfusion (0) to normal perfusion (5).

of tracer activity (representing coronary blood flow) is decreased in the inferoposterior and apical regions during the stress component of the study, but improves during the rest imaging. This is consistent with ischemia in this region of the myocardium but does not define whether the heart is viable or infarcted.

The far-right image in Figure 31.8 represents myocardial viability assessment using FDG in the same patient. All images occurred at rest using the same approach to reconstruct images as previously discussed. The inferoposterior regions demonstrate normal FDG uptake, indicating ischemic but viable (Table 31.6) myocardium. In contrast, the apical region does not metabolize FDG and represents ischemic or infarcted myocardium.

Conclusion

The role of nuclear cardiology is continuing to expand as needs for improved, noninvasive assessment of coronary artery disease increase. The ability to qualitatively (Figure 31.9) determine myocardial perfusion imaging and myocardial viability with PET and SPECT[37-41] provides physiologic information that coronary arteriography cannot provide. Recent improvements in available isotopes, better and safer approaches to physiologically stress the heart, and improvements in both SPECT and PET imaging have increased the utility and diagnostic accuracy of these tests. The ability to detect subtle changes in stenosis flow reserve before changes in percent diameter stenosis can be detected on coronary arteriography (see Chapter 29) has resulted in many physicians recognizing an increased need and role for nuclear cardiac imaging using either SPECT or PET technologies. Additionally, myocardial perfusion imaging (MPI) also allows the physician to determine if angioplasty or bypass surgery will benefit myocardium which is supplied by a stenosis artery.

References

1. Blumgart HL, Weiss S. Studies on the velocity of blood flow, III: the velocity of blood flow and its relation to other aspects of the circulation in patients with rheumatic and syphilitic heart disease. *J Clinic Invest.* 1927;4:149–171.
2. Rejali AM, MacIntyre WJ, Friedell HL. A radioisotopic method of visualization of blood pools. *Am J Roentgenol.* 1958;79:129–137.
3. Dreyfuss F, Ben-Porath M, Menczel J. Radioiodine uptake in the infarcted heart. *Am J Cardiol.* 1960;6:237–245.
4. Anger HO. Scintillation camera. *Rev Sci Instrum.* 1958; 29:27.
5. Hurley PJ, Cooper M, Reba RC, et al. Potassium-43: a new radiopharmaceutical for imaging the heart. *J Nucl Med.* 1971;12:516–519.
6. Forman R, Kirk ES: Thallium-201 accumulation during reperfusion of ischemic myocardium: dependence on re-gional blood flow rather than viability. *Am J Cardiol.* 1984; 54:659–663.
7. Fleming RM, Rose CH, Feldmann KM: Comparing a high-dose dipyridamole SPECT imaging protocol with dobutamine and exercise stress testing protocols. *Angiology.* 1995; 46:547–556.
8. Fleming RM, Kirkeeide RL, Taegtmeyer H, et al. Comparison of technetium-99m teboroxime tomography with automated quantitative coronary arteriography and thallium-201 tomographic imaging. *J Am Coll Cardiol.* 1991;17: 1297–1302.
9. Fleming RM, Gibbs HR, Swafford J. Using quantitative coronary arteriography to redefine SPECT sensitivity and specificity. *Am J Physiol Imaging.* 1992;7:59–65.
10. Fleming RM. Detecting coronary artery disease using SPECT imaging: a comparison of thallium-201 and teboroxime. *Am J Physiol Imaging.* 1992;7:20–23.
11. Seldin DW, Johnson LL, Blood DK, et al. Myocardial perfusion imaging with technetium-99m SQ 30217: comparison with thallium-201 and coronary anatomy. *J Nucl Med.* 1989;30:312–319.
12. Hendel RC, McSherry B, Karimeddini M, et al. Diagnostic value of a new myocardial perfusion agent, teboroxime (SQ 30,217), utilizing a rapid planar imaging protocol: preliminary results. *J Am Coll Cardiol.* 1990;16:855–861.
13. Iskandrian AS, Heo J, Nguyen T, et al. Myocardial imaging with Tc-99m teboroxime: technique and initial results. *Am Heart J.* 1991;121:889–894.
14. Iskandrian AS, Heo J, Kong B, et al. Use of technetium-99m isonitrile (RP-30A) in assessing left ventricular perfusion and function at rest and during exercise in coronary artery disease, and comparison with coronary arteriography and exercise thallium-201 SPECT imaging. *Am J Cardiol.* 1989;64:270–275.
15. Sinusas AJ, Beller GA, Smith WH, et al. Quantitative planar imaging with technetium-99m methoxyisobutyl isonitrile: comparison of uptake patterns with thallium-201. *J Nucl Med.* 1989;30:1456–1463.
16. Gibbons RJ, Verani MS, Behrenbeck T, et al. Feasibility of tomographic technetium-99m-hexakis-2-methoxy-2-methylpropyl-isonitrile imaging for the assessment of myocardial area at risk and the effect of acute treatment in myocardial infarction. *Circulation.* 1989;80:1277–1286.
17. Trobaugh GB, Wackers FJTh, Sokole EB, et al. Thallium-201 myocardial imaging: an interinstitutional study of observer variability. *J Nucl Med.* 1978;19:359–363.
18. Ornish D, Brown SE, Scherwitz L, et al: Can lifestyle changes reverse coronary heart disease? *Lancet.* 1990;336: 129–133.
19. Fleming RM, Ketchum K, Fleming DM, et al. Treating hyperlipidemia in the elderly. *Angiology.* 1995;46:1075–1083.
20. Fleming RM., Ketchum K, Fleming DM, et al. Assessing the independent effect of dietary and hypolipemic medications on serum lipids. *Angiology.* 1996;47:831–840.
21. Fleming RM. *How to Bypass Your Bypass: What Your Doctor Doesn't Tell You About Cholesterol and Your Diet.* Bethel, Conn: Rutledge Books; 1997.
22. Fleming RM, Rater D, Ketchum K. Reducing cholesterol and triglycerides in the elderly patient by diet alone. Paper presented at: Council on Arteriosclerosis for the 66th Scientific Sessions of the AHA; November 8–11, 1993; Atlanta, Ga.

23. Fleming RM, Rater D. Dietary changes without medication can equally reduce cholesterol in both the young and older patient. Paper presented at: Council on Arteriosclerosis for the 66th Scientific Sessions of the AHA; November 8–11, 1993; Atlanta, Ga.

24. Fleming RM, Rater D, Ketchum K. Studying the effect of medications on cholesterol and triglycerides in subjects not receiving dietary counseling. Paper presented at: Council on Arteriosclerosis for the 66th Scientific Sessions of the AHA; November 8–11, 1993; Atlanta, Ga.

25. Fleming RM, Ketchum K. Dietary reinforcement is an integral component of cholesterol reduction. Paper presented at: Council on Arteriosclerosis for the 66th Scientific Sessions of the AHA; November 8–11, 1993; Atlanta, Ga.

26. Fleming RM, Fleming DM, Gaede R. Hyperlipidemic elderly patients: comparing diet and drug therapy. Paper presented at: Council on Arteriosclerosis for the 67th Scientific Sessions of the AHA; November 14–17, 1994; Dallas, Tex.

27. Fleming RM, Fleming DM, Gaede R. Treatment of hyperlipidemic patients: diet versus rug therapy. Paper presented at: Council on Arteriosclerosis for the 67th Scientific Sessions of the AHA; November 14–17, 1994; Dallas, Tex.

28. Fleming RM. Comparing the results of SPECT imaging using high-dose dipyridamole, dobutamine and treadmill stress. Paper presented at: Council on Arteriosclerosis for the 67th Scientific Sessions of the AHA; November 14–17, 1994; Dallas, Tex.

29. Fleming RM. Arteriosclerosis as defined by quantitative coronary arteriography. Paper presented at: Council on Arteriosclerosis for the 67th Scientific Sessions of the AHA; November 14–17, 1994; Dallas, Tex.

30. Fleming RM, Ketchum K, Fleming D, et al. Controlling hypercholesterolemia by diet and drug therapy in the elderly. First Annual Scientific Session on Cardiovascular Disease in the Elderly; March 18, 1995; New Orleans, La.

31. Fleming RM. Reducing cholesterol and triglyceride levels in both the young and elderly patient, by dietary changes: with and without hyperlipidemic medications. 17th World Congress of the International Union of Angiology; April 3–7, 1995; Westminister, London.

32. Fleming RM, Ketchum K, Fleming DM, et al. Investigating differences in cholesterol and triglyceride levels as influenced by diet and hyperlipidemic medications. 42nd Annual World Assembly of the American College of Angiology; October 15–20, 1995; Maui, Hawaii.

33. Patterson RE, Eisner RL, Horowitz SF. Comparison of cost-effectiveness and utility of exercise ECG, single photon emission computed tomography, positron emission tomography, and coronary arteriography for diagnosis of coronary artery disease. *Circulation.* 1995;91:54–65.

34. Fleming RM, Kirkeeide RL, Smalling RW, et al. Patterns in visual interpretation of coronary arteriograms as detected by quantitative coronary arteriography. *J Am Coll Cardiol.* 1991;18:945–951.

35. Fleming RM, Fleming DM, Gaede R. Training physicians and health care providers to accurately read coronary arteriograms: a training program. *Angiology.* 1996;47:349–359.

36. Fleming RM, Harrington GM. Quantitative coronary arteriography and its assessment of atherosclerosis, II: calculating stenosis flow reserve from percent diameter stenosis. *Angiology.* 1994;45:835–840.

37. Reske SN, Knapp FF, Winkler C. Experimental basis of metabolic imaging of the myocardium with radioiodinated aromatic free fatty acids. *Am J Physiol Imaging.* 1986; 1:214–229.

38. Fleming RM, Feldmann KM, Fleming DM. Comparing a high dose dipyridamole SPECT imaging protocol with dobutamine and exercise stress testing protocols, II: using high-dose dipyridamole to determine lung-to-heart ratio. *Int J Angiol.* 1988;7:325–328.

39. Fleming RM, Feldmann KM, Fleming DM. Comparing a high-dose dipyridamole SPECT imaging protocol with dobutamine and exercise stress testing protocols, III: using dobutamine to determine lung-to-heart ratios, left ventricular dysfunction, and a potential viability marker. *Int J Angiol.* 1999;8:22–26.

40. Fleming RM. The clinical importance of risk factor modification: looking at both myocardial viability (MV) and myocardial perfusion imaging (MPI). *Int J Angiol.* Submitted.

41. Fleming RM. The importance of physiologic information from cardiac PET in assessing coronary artery disease in people with "normal" coronary angiograms. *Int J Angiol.* Submitted.

32

Defining and Treating Heart Failure

Richard M. Fleming

In many aspects the term *congestive heart failure* is a misnomer that continues to be used in the vernacular and the medical literature. Congestive heart failure, which is due to the inability of the heart to maintain adequate cardiac output, should be viewed as either left sided (left ventricle, LV) or right sided (right ventricle, RV), and systolic and/or diastolic in character. Despite suggestions that differences between systolic and diastolic failure can be made clinically, few physicians (if any) can correctly distinguish between the two 100% of the time. Successful distinction between systolic and diastolic dysfunction requires the use of noninvasive tests such as echocardiography (transthoracic or transesophageal) and radionuclide ventriculograms as discussed in Chapter 31, and invasive testing such as ventriculography performed during cardiac catheterization. The importance of coronary artery disease as a cause of death is well established, but many clinicians underestimate the significance of death in patients with class IV congestive heart failure (Table 32.1) for which the average survival time (5 years) is less than that for a patient who has recently developed acquired immunodeficiency syndrome (7 years).

In this chapter we discuss many of the various forms of heart failure, define right-sided and left-sided causes as well as systolic and diastolic failure, and review available treatment options.

TABLE 32.1. New York Heart Association classification of heart failure.

Class	Symptom
I	No symptom
II	Comfortable at rest; may have exertional symptoms
III	Fairly comfortable at rest; symptomatic with activity
IV	Symmptomatic at rest; symptoms worse with exertion

What Is Heart Failure?

Heart failure is the inability of the heart to adequately supply blood flow (cardiac output) to itself and the rest of the body. The workload placed on the heart is determined by a number of factors that can be grouped into three different categories: preload, contractility, and afterload. Each factor applies to both the right side and left side of the heart, as shown in Figures 32.1 and 32.2, respectively. Decisions concerning drug treatment and the use of mechanical assist devices such as an intra-aortic balloon pump (IABP) are based on these factors (Figure 32.3) and the patient's response to treatment. We now look at each of these independent variables.

Preload

Preload is the return of venous blood to the heart, which is then pumped out of the heart through the arteries of the body. On the right side of the heart, blood is returned via the superior and inferior vena cava, with smaller amounts returning from the lungs (azygos and bronchial veins) and heart (coronary sinus). Venous return to the left side of the heart arrives via the pulmonary vein. If the right side of the heart is unable to accept or receive this blood, or if it is unable to pump the blood into the lungs, volume overload (Figure 32.1) will occur. This is accompanied by distention of neck veins and leg edema. The patient will report leg swelling and possibly weight gain. Clinically there will be evidence of lower extremity and/or sacral edema, depending on whether the patient has been bedridden. Other evidence of RV volume overload includes elevated right atrial pressures (>8–10 mm Hg) and an increased lift over the left lower sternal border that can best be appreciated by the heel of the examiners hand. Sternal lifts re-

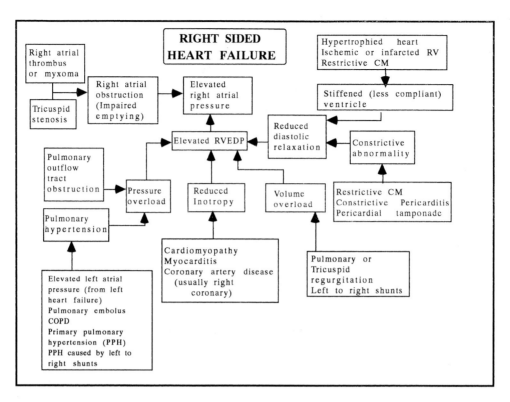

FIGURE 32.1. Right-sided heart failure. Problems that result in right-sided heart failure cause elevations in right atrial pressure either as a result of right atrial obstruction or problems with volume overload, pressure overload, inotropic or chronotropic problems, and/or diastolic dysfunction.

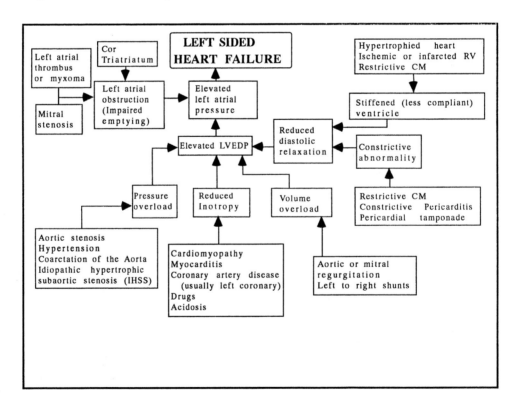

FIGURE 32.2. Left-sided heart failure. Elevations in left atrial pressure or obstruction to left atrial emptying can result in increased left atrial pressure, precipitating left-sided heart failure. Obstructions to left atrial emptying include masses, congenital abnormalities, or stenotic valves. Additional problems arise from preload, inotropic, chronotropic, and afterload disorders.

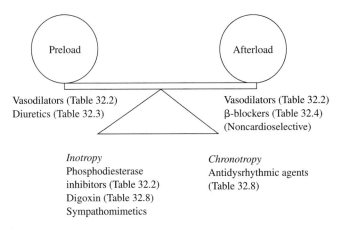

Vasodilators (Table 32.2)
Diuretics (Table 32.3)

Vasodilators (Table 32.2)
β-blockers (Table 32.4)
(Noncardioselective)

Inotropy
Phosphodiesterase
inhibitors (Table 32.2)
Digoxin (Table 32.8)
Sympathomimetics

Chronotropy
Antidysrhythmic agents
(Table 32.8)

FIGURE 32.3. Determinants of myocardial workload. Workload on the heart increases with increased preload and afterload. Reduced inotropy or increased rhythm problems (chronotropy) may exacerbate myocardial dysfunction.

sulting from volume overload are brisk in character, whereas lifts resulting from pressure overload have a slow, sustained lift. Third heart sounds (S_3) are associated with volume overload (increased preload) states, although they may occasionally be heard in healthy individuals ($<35–40$ years of age) or during the last trimester of pregnancy. When an S_3 occurs from right ventricular overload, it is heard over the left lower sternal border where the RV is normally positioned. Enlargement of the RV can also be seen as an enlarged cardiac silhouette (5 o'clock position) on posteroanterior chest radiographs. Lateral views demonstrate a concomitant loss of retrosternal airspace.

An example of acute RV overload is seen in patients who have an acute anteroseptal myocardial infarction (anteroseptal MI) with rupture of the interventricular septum, known as a ventricular septal defect (VSD). This acute anteroseptal MI with associated VSD accounts for approximately 2% of all MI–related deaths. Unless systemic vascular resistance (SVR) is reduced, the blood pressure, which is greater in the LV than in the RV, will cause a shunting of blood from the LV to the RV into the pulmonary artery, finally returning it to the left side of the heart where the entire process can repeat itself.

This increased blood flow from the LV through the VSD into the RV and finally into the pulmonary artery will be represented by increased RV and pulmonary capillary occlusion/wedge pressures (PCOP/PCWP), and by increased vascular markings on the chest radiograph. Initial findings of pulmonary edema begin with cephalization (increased vascular markings in the apices of the lungs) and perivascular cuffing (fluid accumulation immediately around the pulmonary vessels) once the PCOP exceeds 15 to 18 mm Hg. This is the necessary pressure needed to overcome the osmotic pressure that serves to maintain serum within blood vessels of the body.

The holosystolic murmur associated with a VSD can sometimes be confused with an acute rupture of the mitral valve apparatus (acute mitral regurgitation), but can be differentiated clinically by the "thrill" felt over the RV when the examiner places the palm of his/her hand on the patient's chest, and/or by echocardiogram. An S_4 will be heard over the less compliant (stiffened) left ventricle as a result of the MI, whereas an S_3 will be heard over the fluid-overloaded RV. As fluid continues to accumulate in the lungs, perihilar prominence, perivascular cuffing, cephalization, Kerley's B-lines, and pleural effusions will be seen on the chest radiograph. Effusions are more common in the right costophrenic angle when unilateral but are frequently seen bilaterally. Such an effusion is transudative in character.

Management of an acute anteroseptal MI with VSD requires simultaneous mechanical and medical treatment. This requires the placement of an IABP to improve the LV cardiac output by decreasing aortic resistance to forward blood flow, thereby decreasing the shunting of blood from the LV to the RV. Dopamine is needed concomitantly to reduce SVR. Caution must be exercised when dosing the dopamine because treatment is aimed at reducing the SVR (blood pressure), thereby enhancing blood flow from the LV to the aorta, minimizing the shunting of blood through the VSD to the RV as described above. Low-dose dopamine (1–5 mg/kg per minute) activates the dopaminergic and $β_2$-receptors, producing vasodilation of the renal and mesenteric arteries, with lesser dilatation of the coronary and cerebral arteries. This effectively lowers SVR, improves the movement of blood from the LV to the aorta, and reduces the shunting of blood through the VSD. When the amount of dopamine is increased (5–10 mg/kg per minute), the $β_1$-receptors are activated, which increases the contractility of the heart (Figure 32.3) but does not improve the SVR. When even higher doses of dopamine are used, the α-receptors are activated, which produces vasoconstriction and increases the SVR and shunting of blood from the LV through the VSD into the RV, which in turn causes further deterioration of the patient.

A team approach including a cardiologist or angiologist, cardiovascular surgeon, and others must decide on the best time for surgical repair of the VSD. The best outcome is usually obtained if surgery can be delayed until sufficient healing has occurred for a surgical patch to be secured into place. However, deterioration of the patient may require emergent surgery at less than optimal times even though this has been associated with a greater than 50% mortality.

Medical and surgical treatment of almost everything in medicine must focus on both the cause and the associated symptoms. Many cases of fluid overload (increased preload) can be treated using medications that reduce the preload of the heart by vasodilatation or diuresis.

These medications include but are not limited to those shown in Tables 32.2 and 32.3, which list many of the available angiotensin-converting enzyme inhibitors, nitrates, phosphodiesterase inhibitors, antihypertensive agents, and diuretics currently available. Many of these medications may need to be given intravenously if there is evidence of gastrointestinal edema (frequently seen with peripheral edema), because edema of the gastrointestinal wall is associated with decreased absorption of oral medicines. Caution must be exercised when using diuretics, particularly when patients are also receiving β-adrenergic blocking agents (Table 32.4) or digitalis glycosides. If too much fluid is removed from a patient (e.g., in the treatment of peripheral edema) by diuretic agents, the patient could experience electrolyte abnormalities and/or hypovolemic shock. Digitalis toxicity can easily occur when hypokalemia, hypomagnesemia, hypercalcemia, and hypercapnia exist and is particularly a problem when patients are receiving diuretic therapy or anything else that may adversely affect electrolyte levels. In the end you cannot treat electrocardiogram results, Swan–Ganz catheter readings, blood test results, or anything else and forget about the patient without having potential adverse effects on the patient.

Other causes of elevated right atrial pressure include impaired atrial emptying, which may be caused by stenotic valves, intra-atrial masses, or chamber abnormalities, as shown in Figures 32.1 and 32.2. These are most easily detected with an echocardiogram, although computed tomography, magnetic resonance imaging, and auscultory changes may be present. Figures 32.1 and 32.2 also list various causes of pressure overload, reduced inotropy, and diastolic dysfunction, some of which we discuss later.

Myocardial Contractility

Myocardial contractility, the pumping action of the heart, is dependent on two independent factors: inotropy and chronotropy. Inotropy is the "force" of contraction and is sometimes expressed as the pressure produced by the ventricle (usually the LV) in a given amount of time (dP/dT). This is frequently equated to the ejection fraction of a ventricle (RV or LV), which can be detected by echocardiography, radionuclide ventricu-

TABLE 32.2. Vasodilators used to treat preload and afterload.

Medication	Preload*	Afterload*	Usual daily dose	Peak effect	Duration of effect
Angiotensin-converting enzyme inhibitors					
Captropril	3	4	12.5–25 mg	1–2 h	4–8 h
Enalapril	3	4	5–40 mg	4–8 h	18–30 h
Lisinopril	3	4	5–40 mg	4–6 h	18–30 h
Quinapril	3	4	5–40 mg	2–3 h	24 h
Fosinopril	3	4	20–40 mg	3 h	12 h
Moexipril	3	4	10–80 mg	1–2 h	12–14 h
Nitrates					
Sublingual nitroglycerin	4	1	0.4 mg	1–3 min	30–60 min
Oral, sustained release	4	1	2.5–9 mg	60 min	8–12 h
Paste	4	1	1–2 in	15 min	4 h
Transdermal	4	1	2.5–15 mg/24 h	30 min	24 h
Intravenous	4	1	25–500 µg/min	Minutes	Minutes
Phosphodiesterase inhibitors					
Milrinone	4	2	12.5 µg/kg loading dose; 0.2–0.7 µg/kg/min	5–15 min	6–12 h
Amrinone	4	2	5–10 µg/kg/min	5 min	6 h
Direct-acting vasodilators					
Hydralazine	0	3	10–100 mg every 6 h	1–4 h	12–24 h
Minoxidil	0	3	10–40 mg	1–3 h	24–48 h
Nitroprusside	3	3	5–150 µg/min	Minutes	1–3 min
Prostacyclin	3	3	5–15 ng/kg/min	Research	Research
Adrenergic blockers					
Phenoxybenzamine	2	2	10–20 mg every 8 h	1–2 min	24 h
Phentolamine	2	2	50 mg every 6 h	1–2 min	20 min
Prazosin	3	2	1–5 mg every 6 h	3 h	6–8 h
Terazosin	2	3	1–5 mg	2–3 h	12–24 h
Calcium channel blockers					
Nifedipine, sustained release	2	4	30–90 mg	1–3 h	8–12 h
Diltiazem, sustained release	1	1	60–120 mg	1–3 h	8–12 h
Verapamil, sustained release	0	2	40–120 mg	1–3 h	8–12 h

*Preload and afterload graded from 0 (no effect) to 4 (greatest effect).

TABLE 32.3. Diuretics used to treat preload.

Medication	Site of action	Usual daily dose	Peak effect	Duration of effect
Thiazides				
Chlorothiazide	Distal tubule	250–500 mg	4 h	6–12 h
Hydrochlorothiazide	Distal tubule	25–100 mg	4 h	>12 h
Chlorthalidone	Distal tubule	25–100 mg	6 h	24 h
Metolazone	Distal and proximal tubule	2.5–20 mg	2 h	12–24 h
Trichlormethiazide	Distal tubule	4–8 mg	6 h	24 h
Loop diuretics				
Furosemide	Ascending limb, loop of Henle	20–80 mg	1–2 h	6 h
Ethacrynic acid	Ascending limb, loop of Henle	25–100 mg	2 h	6–8 h
Bumetanide	Ascending limb, loop of Henle	0.5–2 mg	1–2 h	4–6 h
Potassium-sparing agents				
Spironolactone	Distal tubule	50–200 mg	2–3 d	2–3 d
Triamterene	Distal tubule	100–200 mg	6–8 h	12–16 h
Amiloride	Distal tubule	5–10 mg	6–10 h	24 h

TABLE 32.4. β-Adrenergic blocking agents used to treat heart rate and afterload.

Medication	Cardioselective (β_1)	Usual daily dose	Peak effect	Duration of effect
Acebutolol	Yes	200–1200 mg	3–8 h	≤24 h
Atenolol	Yes	25–200 mg	2–4 h	24–48 h
Labetalol*	No	400–800 mg	2–4 h	8–12 h
Metoprolol	Yes (up to 100 mg)	50–300 mg	2–4 h	24–48 h
Nadolol	No	20–120 mg	2–4 h	24–48 h
Pindolol	No	20–60 mg	1–2 h	<24 h
Propranolol	No	40–480 mg	2–4 h	24–48 h
Timolol	No	20–60 mg	2 h	20–24 h

*Also has alpha (vasoconstrictive) effect.

lograms, or cardiac catheterization (of the LV). Chronotropy is the rate and rhythm of the heart as influenced by the sympathetic and parasympathetic nervous system, thyroid function, atrial and/or ventricular irritability (ischemia or MI), medications, and so forth.

The overall strength (inotropy) of myocardial muscle fibers can be weakened by any of a number of factors.

These include the dilated cardiomyopathies (DCMs), which are shown in Table 32.5, along with hypertrophic cardiomyopathy (HCM), restrictive cardiomyopathy (RCM), and obliterative cardiomyopathy (OCM). An example of iatrogenically induced DCM includes patients who have received more than 450 mg/m^2 of one of the two anthracycline agents: doxorubicin and daunorubicin.

TABLE 32.5. Cardiomyopathies (CM).

	Dilated CM	Hypertrophic CM	Restrictive CM	Obliterative CM*
Morphology[†]	Biventricular dilatation	Hypertrophy of involved regions	Thickened noncompliant heart	Space-occupying lesions
Chamber size	Increased	Normal or decreased	Normal or increased	Frequently decreased
LVEDP	Increased	Normal or increased	Increased	Usually increased
SV	Decreased	Normal or increased	Normal or decreased	Normal or decreased
EF	Decreased	Increased	Normal or decreased	Normal or decreased
CO	Decreased	Normal	Normal or decreased	Normal or decreased
Diastolic compliance	Normal or decreased	Decreased	Decreased	Decreased
Causes	Adriamycin	Aortic stenosis	Amyloidosis	
	Alcohol	Idiopathic hypertrophic subaortic stenosis	Friedreich's ataxia	Hypereosinophilic syndromes
	Amyloidosis		Glycogen storage diseases	
	Diabetes mellitus	Mitral stenosis		
	Hypophosphatemia		Infiltrative disease	
	Rheumatic fever		Löffler's endocarditis	
	Viral infection/myocarditis			

*Restrictive–obliterative cardiomyopathies (considered by many to be an extension of restrictive CM).
[†]LVEDP, left ventricular end-diastolic pressure; SV, stroke volume; EF, ejection fraction; CO, cardiac output.

Other causes of DCM include diabetes (diabetic patients have four to five times the prevalence of DCM compared with nondiabetic individuals) and other endocrine disorders such as Cushing's disease, thyrotoxicosis, acromegaly, myxedema, pheochromocytoma, and uremia. Various chemicals (lead, cobalt, alcohol, steroids, and chemotherapy agents) and infectious agents (viruses and *Trypanosoma cruzi*, which causes Chagas' disease), as well as hypophosphatemia can also cause DCM. DCM disorders also include postpartum cardiomyopathy and acquired immune deficiency syndrome cardiomyopathy. Although specific treatments for postpartum cardiomyopathy and acquired immune deficiency syndrome cardiomyopathy produce unimpressive results, patients should still receive symptomatic treatment.

Acute MI is an example of an injury to the heart that affects both inotropic and chronotropic function. During an MI, part of the heart muscle goes without adequate blood flow for a sufficient amount of time (1–4 hours) to result in permanent damage to the heart. Early intervention (within 1–4 hours) with thrombolytic agents may reduce the amount of damage done and improve early survival, although it is questionable whether long-term survival is increased unless lifestyle changes and control of risk factors (see Chapters 30 and 64) are successfully implemented.[1,2] Successful thrombolysis results in rapid washout of creatine kinase–myocardial band and dysrhythmias, and resolution of electrocardiographic abnormalities (Table 32.6). Changes in coronary blood flow can be documented in the cardiac catheterization laboratory (Table 32.7) or by myocardial perfusion imaging (see Chapter 31).

Coronary artery bypass graft surgery and/or the use of an IABP may be indicated, depending on the patient's presentation and clinical course. The use of other ventricular assist devices (hemopump, etc.) and intravenous medications such as glucose–insulin–potassium have not demonstrated any additional benefit despite initial hopes. In fact, the use of glucose–insulin–potassium has been associated with significant hypokalemia, dysrhythmias, and death in the clinical setting. Patients who have

recently had an MI should not be prophylactically treated with lidocaine unless they demonstrate ventricular ectopy. Patients who have been given lidocaine but do not have ventricular premature beats have demonstrated increased mortality.

Additional approaches to treating DCMs include removal of offending agents; anticoagulation if a thrombus is present or is expected; and treatment of associated dysrhythmias (Table 32.8), including digitalis if either atrial fibrillation is present of if the left ventricular ejection fraction is less than 30%. In the absence of atrial fibrillation or systolic dysfunction (reduced left ventricular ejection fraction) there is no evidence to support the use of digitalis glycosides at this time, and potential problems can occur in patients with hypercapnia or those with electrolyte abnormalities, as noted above. Likewise, digitalis should not be used in patients with amyloidosis because of potential toxicity problems. Additional treatments for DCMs include preload and afterload reduction when appropriate.

In addition to inotropic problems, chronotropic issues must also be addressed. A list of many of the current antidysrhythmic agents used today is included in Table 32.8. Some patients are extremely dependent upon the "atrial kick" that occurs at the end of diastole and provides the final one-third of ventricular filling from the atria immediately preceding systole. These patients may benefit from implantation of atrial-ventricular sequential pacemakers. Other patients with dysrhythmias refractory to medical therapy may benefit from implantation of an automatic implantable cardiofibrillator device, which can both sense and defibrillate lethal dysrhythmias.

Afterload

Afterload is the resistance against which the heart must work to eject blood from the ventricles into the arteries of the body. As shown in Figures 32.1 and 32.2, resistance can be provided by stenotic valves, obstructions, hypertension, and shunts. Afterload can best be understood by considering the law of La Place (Figure 32.4), where *T* is the tension (work) placed on the heart, *P* is the ventricular pressure, *r* is the radius of the ventricular cavity, and *h* is the height (thickness) of the ventricular wall. Hypertrophy of the ventricular wall can be either a primary problem or secondary to volume overload and so forth, as shown in Table 32.9.

In addition to increasing the workload on the heart, myocardial thickening impairs blood flow through the coronary arteries. Because coronary arteries receive most of their blood flow during diastole, any increase in wall tension of the heart will increase the resistance to blood flow, subsequently decreasing coronary blood flow and its delivery of oxygen to the heart, further limiting the amount of work the heart is able to do.

TABLE 32.6. Sequence of electrocardiographic changes occurring during transmural (Q-wave) myocardial infarction.

Hyperacute (peaked) T waves
ST-segment elevation
Q-wave development
T-wave inversion
Resolution of ST segments

TABLE 32.7. Thrombolysis in myocardial infarction flow.

0	No flow
1	Minimal flow distal to stenosis
2	Complete but sluggish flow distal to stenosis
3	Normal flow

TABLE 32.8. Antiarrhythmic agents.*

Medication	Onset of action	Duration of action	Half-life ($t_{1/2}$)	Indication
Class IA agents (sodium channel blockers)				
Moricizine	2 h	10–24 h	1.5–3.5 h	Life-threatening VT, VPB
Quinidine	0.5 h	6–8 h	6–7 h	APBs, VPBs, SVT, VT
Procainamide	0.5 h	>3 h	2.5–4.5 h	APBs, VPBs, SVT, VT
Disopyramide	0.5 h	6–7 h	4–10 h	APBs, VPBs, SVT, VT
Class IB agents (shorten repolarization)				
Lidocaine (intravenous)	1–5 min	0.25 h	1–2 h	VPBs, VT
Phenytoin	0.5–1 h	24 h	22–36 h	VPBs, VT, Digitalis toxicity
Tocainide	0.5–2 h	6–12 h	11–15 h	VPBs, VT
Mexiletine	30–120 min	6–12 h	10–12 h	VPBs, VT
Class IC agents (depress repolarization)				
Flecainide†	1–6 h	12–24 h	12–27 h	Life-threatening VT
Encainide†	0.5–1.5 h	Variable	1–2 h	Life-threatening VT
Propafenone‡	3.5 h	12–24 h	2–10 h	Life-threatening VT, SVT, AF
Class II agents (β-blockers, slow atrioventricular conduction)				
Propranolol	0.5 h	3–5 h	2–3 h	SVT
Esmolol (intravenous)	<5 min	Very short	0.15 h	SVT
Acebutolol	2–3 h	24–30 h	3–4 h	VPBs
Class III agents (prolong action potential)				
Bretylium (intravenous)	1–5 min	6–8 h	5–10 h	VF, VT
Amiodarone	Days to weeks	Weeks to months	26–107 d	Refractory VT, SVT
Sotalol	2–4 h	12 h	12 h	VT
Class IV agents (slow calcium channel blockers)				
Verapamil	0.5 h	6 h	3–7 h	SVT
Other agents				
Digoxin	0.5–2 h	>24 h	30–40 h	AF
Adenosine (intravenous)	34 s	1–2 min	<10 s	SVT

*Dosage depends on clinical scenario.
†May precipitate heart failure.
‡Propafenone is also a weak calcium channel blocker.
AF, atrial fibrillation; APB, atrial premature beats; SVT, supraventricular tachycardia; VF, ventricular fibrillation; VPB, ventricular premature beats; VT, ventricular tachycardia.

TABLE 32.9. Primary and secondary causes of cardiac hypertrophy.

Primary causes	
Right sided	Left sided
Left heart failure	Aortic stenosis
Primary pulmonary disease	Coarctation of the aorta
Pulmonary stenosis	Hypertension

Secondary causes
Volume overload
Athletic heart
Aortic regurgitation
Mitral regurgitation
Reactive hypertrophy
Ischemic cardiomyopathy
Myocardial infarction

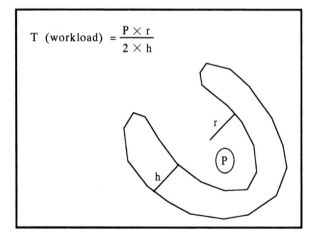

$$T \text{ (workload)} = \frac{P \times r}{2 \times h}$$

FIGURE 32.4. La Place's law. The workload (tension) on the heart is increased when LV pressure increases or the LV dilates. The heart attempts to compensate by hypertrophy of the ventricle (increased wall thickness, *h*). Both increased preload *(r)* and afterload *(P)* can increase the workload on the heart, resulting in myocardial hypertrophy. See text for full details.

HCMs include abnormalities that may or may not cause obstruction of the aortic outflow tract (Figures 32.1 and 32.2). Clinical thickening of a ventricular chamber resulting from hypertension is usually associated with an increased intensity in valve closure for either the aortic or pulmonic valve. This increased intensity is caused by differences in pressure on either side of the valve. Stenotic valves, which may cause HCM, have less mobility and are therefore associated with less intense valve closure.

Stenotic valves on the left side of the heart are relatively easy to distinguish because mitral stenosis presents as a diastolic rumble best auscultated at the apex with the bell of the stethoscope while the patient lies in the left lateral decubitus position. Mitral stenosis is frequently associated with dypsnea, angina, hemoptysis, hoarseness, and cough. On auscultation there is an opening snap when the stenotic mitral valve opens. The more severe the stenosis, the shorter the S2–opening snap interval.

In contrast to mitral stenosis, aortic stenosis is a systolic murmur heard best at the right upper sternal border and typically radiates to both carotid arteries. Aortic sclerosis sounds similar but does not tend to radiate to the carotid arteries. Distinction between the two is best made by echocardiography. Aortic stenosis is associated with syncope, angina, and dyspnea. The onset of dyspnea suggests left ventricular dysfunction and is indicative of patient mortality within 6 to 18 months unless successfully relieved. As aortic stenosis worsens, there is further delay in the opening of the aortic valve, with delayed peaking of the systolic ejection murmur occurring later and later in the murmur. This produces a delayed carotid upstroke known as *parvus et tardus* and a decrease in the intensity of aortic valve (A2) closure.

For the patient with HCM a distinction must be made between aortic stenosis and idiopathic hypertrophic subaortic stenosis, which produces outflow tract obstruction. Idiopathic hypertrophic subaortic stenosis is also known as asymmetric septal hypertrophy and hypertrophic obstructive cardiomyopathy. The distinction between aortic stenosis and idiopathic hypertrophic subaortic stenosis frequently requires the use of echocardiography, but differences in the hemodynamics of these murmurs can be detected clinically by performing maneuvers that change LV blood volume, as shown in Table 32.10. Treatment of mitral stenosis, aortic stenosis, and idiopathic hypertrophic subaortic stenosis may be accomplished medically or surgically, depending on the severity of the disease.[3,4]

In addition to the three previous determinants of cardiac workload (preload, contractility, and afterload), failure of the heart to adequately relax can also lead to right-sided and left-sided failure, as shown in Figures 32.1 and 32.2, respectively. Examples include stiffened and constrictive abnormalities such as RCM. The classic feature of RCM disorders is impedance of diastolic filling of the ventricle(s) with subsequent abnormal diastolic function. As shown in Table 32.5, there are a variety of diseases that can lead to RCM, including but not limited to amyloidosis, pseudoxanthoma elasticum, radiation damage (from treatment of lymphomas or other tumors), endomyocardial fibrosis (also known as Löffler's endocarditis), tumors (primary or secondary), glycogen storage diseases, and hemochromatosis.

An important distinction in the evaluation of RCM is to differentiate between "constrictive pericarditis," which may respond to pericardial stripping, and "restrictive cardiomyopathy." Evaluation of left and right ventricular chamber pressures will reveal the classical diastolic dip and plateau morphology known as the *square root sign*. Diastolic dysfunction is evidenced by an elevation in the diastolic pressures. Although it may be necessary to perform an endomyocardial biopsy to distinguish between these two disorders and their cause, some important clues can be provided by comparing the left and right ventricular chamber pressures. If diastolic pressures are equal for both ventricular chambers then the patient typically has a constrictive pericarditis, whereas patients with RCM will usually have greater end-diastolic pressures in the LV.

It is also important to differentiate between constrictive pericarditis and cardiac tamponade. Differentiation between the two is important because cardiac tamponade requires removal of the pericardial effusion to prevent hemodynamic collapse. This occurs when right atrial and RV filling are impaired because of the greater pressure generated by the LV, resulting in a bulging of the interventricular septum into the RV cavity, which impedes RV filling. Reduced RV filling results in less blood reaching the LV, which subsequently results in decreased cardiac output and hemodynamic collapse. Removal of the pericardial fluid can be done by either pericardiocentesis or a surgical window. True differentiation between constrictive pericarditis and cardiac tamponade may require echocardiography, but they should normally be distinguishable clinically, as shown in Table 32.11.

TABLE 32.10. Differentiation aortic stenosis (AS) from idiopathic hypertrophic subaortic stenosis (IHSS).

| | | *Murmur intensity* | | | |
	Carotid upstroke	After ventricular premature beat	Isoprel of hand grip	Valsalva's maneuver	Amyl nitrate
AS	Parvus et tardus (slow and delayed)	Increased	Normal or decreased	Decreased	Increased
IHSS	Bisferiens (spike and dome)	Decreased	Increased	Increased	Increased

TABLE 32.11. Differentiating between cardiac tamponade and constrictive pericarditis.

Clinical findings	Cardiac tamponade	Constrictive pericarditis
Elevated jugular venous pulse	Yes	Yes
Kussmaul's sign	No	Yes
Pulsus paradoxus	Yes	No
Clear lungs	Yes	Yes
Heart sounds	Normal to decreased	Pericardial knock
Ascites	No	Yes
Edema	No	Yes
Chest x-ray—cardiomegaly	Often	No (may see pericardial calcification)
Swan-Ganz catheter	Prominent X-descent	Prominent Y-descent
Electrocardiogram (electrical alternans)	Yes	No
Echocardiogram (pericardial fluid)	Yes	No

The fourth and final group of cardiomyopathies (Table 32.5) includes the OCMs and comprises any process that produces a mass effect within any chamber of the heart. This includes tumors, asymmetric septal hypertrophy, Löffler's endocarditis at the apex of the heart, and so forth. Treatment is directed at eliminating the obstruction (obliteration) to blood flow and providing symptomatic relief.

Clinically a thickened, less compliant ventricle will have a fourth heart sound (S_4). This is caused by blood entering a stiffened ventricle that has increased ventricular end-diastolic pressure (LVEDP or RVEDP) that the incoming blood must move against. Pressure overload in the ventricles (S_4) can result in hypertrophy of the ventricle, whereas volume-overloaded ventricles (S_3) first experience dilatation, although the presence of one state can eventually lead to the other. Treatment must be focused on both the primary cause and the resulting symptoms.

There are a wide variety of medications available for the treatment of systemic hypertension (defined in millimeters of mercury or as SVR), but there has been limited success in the treatment of pulmonary hypertension (defined in millimeters of mercury or as pulmonary vascular resistance). Medications useful for the treatment of SVR include those listed in Tables 32.2, 32.3, and 32.4. The use of β-adrenergic blocking agents (Table 32.4) may also be of use in the treatment of certain atrial dysrhythmias (Table 32.8). Caution should be exercised when using these drugs when there is evidence of systolic dysfunction either clinically, echocardiographically, by nuclear imaging, or by cardiac catheterization.

Systolic Versus Diastolic Failure

Classically, ventricular function has been looked at in many ways including volume–pressure curves. Although initially somewhat difficult to understand, step-by-step analysis makes them quite easy to follow and understand. Figure 32.5 shows the volume–pressure loop for a normal LV. Blood volume inside the LV is represented on the x-axis, whereas LV pressure is displayed on the y-axis. Systole begins with mitral valve closure (MVC), preventing additional blood from entering the left ventricle. At this time the ventricle begins contraction, but blood is not ejected from the ventricle until the aortic valve opens (AVO). This period of contraction is known as isovolumetric contraction (IVC) because there is no change in blood volume within the LV. During the IVC the pressure in the ventricle rises until it exceeds the aortic pressure. Once this happens the aortic valve opens (AVO) and left ventricular ejection of blood begins. With the ejection of blood into the aorta the LV blood volume drops from 100 mL to 35–40 mL. Left ventricular ejection continues until the pressure in the aorta exceeds that in the ventricle and the aortic valve closes (AVC), ending systole.

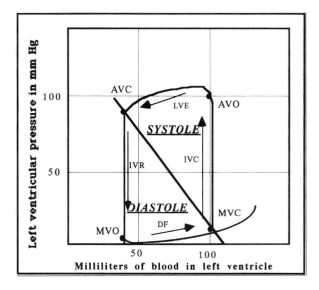

FIGURE 32.5. Volume–pressure relationships of a normal left ventricle. Systole begins with MVC and concludes with AVC, at which time diastole begins. Diastole ends with MVC, where LVEDP and left ventricular end-diastolic volume (LVEDV) are seen. See text for full details.

With the end of systole, ventricular contraction has been completed and ventricular relaxation (diastole) begins. During this time, known as isovolumetric relaxation (IVR), blood does not enter the ventricle although the pressure decreases due to relaxation of the ventricle. Diastolic filling of the LV begins when the left atrial pressure exceeds the left ventricular pressure, resulting in mitral valve opening (MVO) because of the pressure of the left atrial blood. The volume of blood in the LV increases from 35 to 40 mL to approximately 100 mL. The last part of ventricular diastolic filling occurs with atrial contraction, and diastole is completed with MVC, and systole begins again.

When systolic failure occurs, there is an increase in both left ventricular end-diastolic volume (LVEDV) and LVEDP, as represented by the example in Figure 32.6. In this example, increased LVEDV is evidenced by comparing the volume present at MVC, which is greater for the systolic failure loop (A_1MVC) than the normal volume–pressure loop (A_2MVC), 125 and 100 mL, respectively. Because

$$(1)\ \% \text{LVEF} = [(\text{LVESV} - \text{LVEDV})/\text{LVEDV}] \times 100$$

where LVEF is the left ventricular ejection fraction, LVESV is the left ventricular end-systolic volume, and LVEDV is the left ventricular end-diastolic volume, we can now calculate the LVEF for each of the two ventricles in question.

$$\text{Normal ventricle: LVEF} = (\text{LVESV} - \text{LVEDV})/$$
$$\text{LVEDV} = (100 - 35)/100 = 65\%$$

$$\text{Systolic failure ventricle: LVEF} =$$
$$(\text{LVESV} - \text{LVEDV})/\text{LVEDV} = (125 - 80)/125 = 36\%$$

As expected, the ventricle with an increased LVEDV represents a ventricle with reduced systolic function (LVEF). It is also obvious from the volume–pressure loop that to increase the LVEF we must reduce the SVR and/or increase the contractility of the ventricle.

An increase in LVEDP (A_1MVC) is also seen when pressure at end-diastole (MVC) is compared with the normal (A_2MVC) end-diastolic pressure. In this example LVEDP is 20 mm Hg for the systolic failure ventricle, as opposed to 10 mm Hg for the normally functioning ventricle. With an LVEDP of 20 mm Hg (which should represent PCOP), the patient will be dyspneic and have pulmonary edema, which requires preload reduction.

In contrast to systolic failure, diastolic dysfunction is caused by a failure of the ventricle to adequately relax. As a result, LVEDP is elevated as shown in Figure 32.7. Because the ventricle is stiffened, the pressure within the left ventricle increases rapidly during diastolic filling, resulting in early closure of the mitral valve (MVC) once pressure in the LV exceeds that in the left atria. This reduces the LVEDV without decreasing the LVEF.

$$\text{Diastolic failure ventricle: LVEF} =$$
$$(\text{LVESV} - \text{LVEDV})/\text{LVEDV} = (80 - 35)/35 = 56\%$$

Although LVEF is normal, the actual stroke volume (SV = LVESV − LVEDV) is reduced, with an SV of 45 mL for the LV with diastolic failure and 65 mL for the

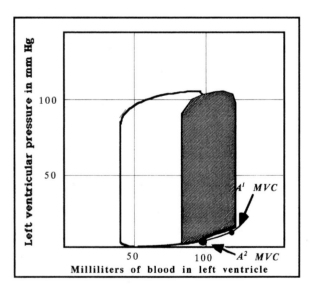

FIGURE 32.6. Systolic failure as represented by the volume–pressure loop. The normally functioning LV is represented by the open loop, and the ventricle with impaired systolic function is represented by the hashed loop. Both the LVEDV and LVEDP are elevated with systolic failure. See text for full details.

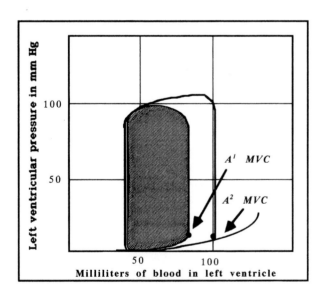

FIGURE 32.7. Diastolic failure as represented by the volume–pressure relationships. The hashed loop represents a ventricle with diastolic failure with an elevated LVEDP and reduced LVEDV as compared with the normally functioning LV, represented by the open loop.

normal ventricle. Therefore, treatment of diastolic dysfunction must focus on improving ventricular relaxation and not on increasing contractility, as many people mistakenly attempt with digitalis or inotropic agents. LVEF should be determined in each case to decide if inotropic support is needed. Similar volume–pressure loops can be drawn for RV function, although the pressures are lower for the right side of the heart.

Right-Sided Versus Left-Sided Heart Failure

By examining and understanding these volume–pressure relationships it is easy to see that treatment of systolic failure should focus on reducing both the LVEDV and LVEDP, whereas treatment of diastolic function should focus on decreasing the LVEDP without further compromising LVEDV, which could make matters worse. Successful treatment requires recognition of the underlying cause, assessment of systolic and diastolic function, and a determination as to whether the problem is right sided, left sided, or biventricular. A classic example of how important this becomes is in the treatment of an acute MI. Treatment typically includes oxygen, morphine sulfate for pain control and diuretic effect, heparin and thrombolytic agents, pressor support (dopamine, dobutamine, isoproterenol, etc.) if needed, alternative medications where available,[5,6] interventional techniques (angioplasty, stents, atherectomy, etc.), and mechanical support (IABP) and/or bypass surgery. If the left ventricle is involved, then diastolic dysfunction along with decreased inotropy and chronotropy frequently occur. In this setting, pulmonary edema (increased PCOP) may easily happen, worsening the overall scenario. Diuretics may be required but must be given cautiously so as not to deplete the intravascular volume, which could worsen the LVEDV and systolic function.

Patients who have an inferior wall MI should routinely have right precordial leads placed so they may be tested for evidence of RV infarction. This can occur in 20% to 30% of the cases of inferior wall MI. Inferior wall MIs have also been associated with the Bezold-Jarisch reflex, which consists of bradycardia, vasodilatation, and hypotension due to involvement of the parasympathetic (phrenic) nerve running along the inferior aspect of the heart/diaphragm. Patients presenting with these symptoms should not receive β-adrenergic blocking agents because of an already slowed heart rate. In patients with a RV MI, the right atrial and RV end-diastolic pressure (RVEDP) may be elevated but the PCOP will usually be low or normal. This is because the RV is a passive conduit (volume pump under low pressure) to the lungs, in contrast to the LV, which is a pressure pump. Part of the overall treatment of RV MI includes cautiously giving intravenous fluid to increase the PCOP and secure LV fill-ing to maintain adequate LV cardiac output. The distinction between right-sided and left-sided infarction of the heart becomes extremely important, as evidenced by this example.

Cardiac Transplantation

Unfortunately heart failure, from whatever cause, may ultimately be untreatable despite changes in dietary habits, adjustment in medications, pacemakers, artificial valves, mechanical assist devices, and/or emergency surgery. As mentioned at the beginning of this chapter, patients with New York Heart Association class IV failure can have shorter lifespans than patients in the early stages of acquired immunodeficiency syndrome.

Once the available treatments have been exhausted, the one remaining hope for many patients remains cardiac transplantation.[7] The overall 1-year survival rate for transplant recipients remains at 70%. Many factors are involved in determining whether a person is an appropriate transplant candidate and whether an organ is available. Combination heart–lung transplants are frequently reserved for patients with congenital heart disease, pulmonary hypertension, or Eisenmenger's syndrome. Despite considerable work in the field of artificial hearts, latissimus dorsi muscle flap surgeries, and other valiant efforts, the vast majority of patients die while awaiting a heart transplant, with one third of these dying suddenly.

Conclusion

An adequate approach to the treatment of heart failure requires that one understand the mechanism behind the problem. To do this it is important to distinguish between right ventricular, left ventricular, and biventricular failure, as well as systolic and diastolic dysfunction. Physical examination skills, history-taking skills, and the use of appropriate diagnostic tests to elucidate the underlying pathology while looking for treatable and perhaps reversible causes are all required. Focusing on appropriate interventions for preload, contractility (inotropy and chronotropy), and afterload dysfunction can improve the overall management of the patient's condition. Careful monitoring of a patient's response to treatment is extremely important because it allows the physician to maximize patient benefit and minimize problems. It is important to remember that it is the patient you are treating and not pressure measurements obtained from a Swan–Ganz catheter or a laboratory report. Successful treatment of heart failure requires a team approach that includes a cardiologist or angiologist, a cardiovascular surgeon, and others.

References

1. Fleming RM. *How to Bypass Your Bypass: What Your Doctor Doesn't Tell You About Cholesterol and Your Diet.* Bethel, Conn: Rutledge Books; 1997.

2. Fleming RM. *The Diet Myth.* Austin, Tex: Windsor House Publishing Group; 1998.

3. Ross J Jr. Left ventricular function and the timing of surgical treatment in valvular heart disease. *Ann Intern Med.* 1981; 94:498–504.

4. Passick CS, Ackerman DM, Pluth JR, et al. Temporal changes in the causes of aortic stenosis: a surgical pathologic study of 646 cases. *Mayo Clin Proc.* 1987;62:119–123.

5. Goldstein RA, Fleming RM. Clinical Aspects of Phosphodiesterase Inhibitors. Heart Failure, Basic Science and Clinical Management. New York, NY: Marcel Dekker; 1993.

6. Pollesello P, Kaivola J, Tilgmann C, et al. Binding of a new Ca^{2+}-sensitizer levosimendan, to recombinant human cardiac troponin C. Paper presented at: International College of Angiology Meetings; July 1995; Helsinki, Finland.

7. Rickenbacher PR, Haywood G, Fowler MB. Selecting candidates for cardiac transplantation: how to assess exclusion criteria and predict who will benefit. *Journal of Critical Illness.* 1995;10:199–206.

33

Role of Fibrinogen as a Vascular Risk Factor in Atherogenesis and Thrombogenesis

P. Pola, P. Tondi, M. Serricchio, and R. Pola

Human fibrinogen is a symmetrical dimeric glycoprotein (molecular weight 340,000 d) synthesized in the liver. Each dimer consists of three different polypeptide chains—alpha, beta, and gamma—held together by interdimeric (alpha–alpha, gamma–gamma) and intradimeric (beta–gamma, gamma–alpha) disulfide bridges (—S—S—). Thrombin cleaves fibrinopeptides A and B to transform fibrinogen into fibrin monomers. The fibrin monomers are then polymerized to form fibrin.[1–3] Normal plasma levels range from 2.0 to 4.0 g/L.

Fibrinogen, through interaction with endothelial cells, and fibrin can alter the organization and permeability of endothelial cells, stimulate the proliferation of smooth muscle cells, and favor lipid adhesion to the vessel wall, which starts the atherogenic process.

Fibrinogen before and fibrin after constitute the basic matrix for the blood clotting process. In particular, hyperfibrinogenemia, which increases clotting activity and aggregation of erythrocytes, leukocytes, and platelets, can be an important factor in the thrombotic event.

Epidemiology of Fibrinogen

The presence of high levels of fibrinogen in atherosclerosis was suggested many years ago. Because it is not known whether hyperfibrinogenemia is a cause, a consequence, or simply an incidental factor in cardiovascular disease, in the last 30 years many large epidemiological studies have been carried out in order to define the role of fibrinogen as an independent vascular risk factor in the development of atherosclerosis.

Prospective Studies

The first prospective study on the role of fibrinogen in the development of atherosclerosis was the Northwick Park Heart Study,[4,5] which began in 1976 in the United Kingdom and was carried out for 10 years on 1510 men aged 40 to 64 years. In these subjects the incidence of cardiovascular events was recorded in relation to coagulation factors and other known cardiovascular risk factors. In particular, fibrinogenemia, cholesterolemia, and plasma concentrations of factors VII and VIII were taken into consideration over a 4- and 10-year follow-up period. After 4 years 27 deaths from cardiovascular illness occurred, and after 10 years 68 deaths occurred. In both follow-up evaluations it was observed that cardiovascular events were strictly associated with a simultaneous increase of plasma concentration of fibrinogen and of factor VIII and that this association was much higher than the already known association with cholesterol, particularly in subjects under age 60.

Studies carried out in Wales at Speedwell in 1979 and at Caerphilly in 1982[6,7] with an average follow-up period of 5.1 and 3.2 years, respectively, to evaluate the incidence in the sample population of ischemic cardiopathy and the possible association of serum lipoproteins in male subjects between 45 and 64 years of age also took into consideration other blood characteristics, such as fibrinogenemia, plasma viscosity, and leukocyte count. In the period considered 251 major coronary events occurred. Various analyses demonstrated that fibrinogenemia represented an independent risk factor in the onset of ischemic cardiopathy and had a predictive role equal to that of other important known risk factors, such as cholesterolemia, diastolic blood pressure, and body mass index.

In the Gothenburg Study,[8] which began in 1963, clotting factors, blood pressure, total cholesterol, and smoking habits were taken into account in a sample of 792 male patients born in 1913. After 13.5 years 92 cases of myocardial infarction and 37 cases of stroke occurred. Univariate analysis demonstrated that the degree of smoking, systolic pressure, and cholesterol and fibrinogen levels evaluated at the beginning of the study were related to the onset of myocardial infarction, whereas stroke was related to the levels of systolic pressure and fibrinogenemia. In multivariate analysis, however, only the association between fibrinogenemia and stroke was significant.

419

Another important study was carried out at Framingham beginning in 1948.[9,10] Fibrinogen as a risk factor was taken into account after 1968,[11] and its levels were measured in 1315 subjects without cardiovascular disease. In the following 12 years cardiovascular disease appeared in 165 men and 147 women. Through univariate analysis this pathology (except stroke for women) was shown to be positively related, for both sexes, to levels of fibrinogenemia at the beginning of the study. Also in this study the importance of fibrinogenemia as an independent variable proved to be equal to that of known and accepted main risk factors. Multivariate analysis demonstrated a correlation between fibrinogenemia and cardiovascular disease, including stroke, in both sexes, but the correlation was more evident in men. These data have been confirmed by two other studies, the Prospective Cardiovascular Muenster Study,[12,13] which began in 1982 and involved 2187 male patients aged 40 to 65 years, and the Goettingen Risk Incidence and Prevalence Study,[14] which began in 1987 and involved 5239 men aged 40 to 60 years. In all trials univariate and multivariate analyses demonstrated that fibrinogenemia was strictly related to cardiovascular events and represented a constantly present risk factor.

Cross-Sectional Studies

Many cross-sectional studies described variations in fibrinogen levels in relation to factors such as race, age, sex, lifestyle, and pathology.

Race

Low levels of plasma fibrinogen have been found in Asians; intermediate levels in Anglo-Saxons, Czechs ,and North American whites; and high levels in Finns, Scots, African Americans, and some American Indian tribes.[15,20] The presence of high fibrinogen levels in populations with low cardiovascular risk, such as certain rural African populations, is explained by the fact that endemic disease and poor life conditions do not permit the development of atherosclerosis.[17]

Age

We have demonstrated,[21] and others have confirmed, that fibrinogenemia increases with age at a constant rate estimated to be about 0.1 to 0.2 g/L per decade in adults of both sexes.[15,18,19,22–24]

Sex

Fibrinogen levels are significantly higher in fertile women compared with men,[15,18,19,22–24] whereas, after menopause, the levels coincide in the two sexes.[18,22]

Lifestyle

The most significant lifestyle variable associated with hyperfibrinogenemia is cigarette smoking, especially in men.[15,18–20,22–31] Those who smoke have an average fibrinogen level increase of 10% compared with those who do not smoke. Fibrinogenemia seems to be definitely and linearly related to the average consumption of cigarettes. When smoking ceases, fibrinogen levels progressively fall and return to normal levels within 5 years.[15] Even second-hand smoke seems to increase the risk of fibrinogenemia. The mechanism through which smoking leads to an increase in fibrinogen levels is still not clear; however, it is not likely to be caused by the greater incidence of respiratory infection or by the reduction of plasma volume typical in individuals who smoke.

Obese subjects of both sexes have higher fibrinogen levels with respect to control subjects.[15,18,19,22,24–26] However, longitudinal studies[30,32] could not demonstrate a reduction of fibrinogenemia associated with a decrease in body weight. The mechanism is unclear.

The use of oral contraceptives increases plasma fibrinogen levels.[15,19,24,25] A negative correlation with fibrinogenemia has been observed in the case of degree of physical activity,[18,19,27,33,34] of moderate consumption of alcohol,[15,16,18,19,23,25,26,30] and of a diet rich in polyunsaturated fatty acids.[16,22,35] Lower levels of plasma fibrinogen have also been observed in individuals of high social class and those who are highly educated.[15,22,27,36,37]

Pathology

Various pathological conditions, such as diabetes mellitus[15,17–19] and hypertension,[19,22] are associated with high levels of fibrinogenemia, although it has not yet been demonstrated whether these levels are secondary to the disease or to the intervention of other risk factors. A slight positive correlation to fibrinogenemia has also been observed with plasma levels of lipoprotein(a), triglycerides, low-density lipoprotein and total cholesterol,[18,19,22,27] homocysteine,[38] insulin,[18] and microalbuminuria.[15] A negative association has been shown with high-density lipoprotein cholesterol.[18,19,27]

Because fibrinogen is an acute phase reactant, its plasma concentration increases markedly in all acute stresses (e.g., myocardial infarction, stroke, infection, trauma, and invasive procedures). Consequently, in the early studies on acute myocardial infarction and stroke, hyperfibrinogenemia was supposed to be an epiphenomenon and not a casual factor.[39] More recently, however, it has been shown that subjects with unstable angina or with transient ischemic attacks present high fibrinogen levels before acute cardiovascular events. Therefore a strongly predictive role has been attributed to fibrinogen levels in coronary, cerebral, and systemic ischemic pathology.[40]

Fibrinogen and Atherogenesis

Hyperfibrinogenemia can cause disorganization and functional alteration of vascular endothelial cells. It exerts this action by promoting the deposit of atherogenic substances and stimulating the proliferation of smooth muscle cells, thus participating in the early phase of the atherogenic process. Fibrinogen can act on the vascular wall in two ways: (1) endothelial deposition of fibrin that induces edema of the intimal surface[41-44] and (2) alteration of endothelial permeability by means of fibrinopeptides cleaved by thrombin. These peptides, which cause disorganization of endothelial cells, would impair the barrier function and promote accumulation on the intimal surface of low-density lipoprotein and fibrinogen components (E fragment, which seems to be the most active, and X fragment). Fibrinogen is trapped within the subendothelial connective tissue in the early phases of the lesion; later the thrombin not inactivated by antithrombin III present on the intimal surface transforms fibrinogen into fibrin.[45]

Fibrin and intramural microthrombi have been observed in the apparently normal intimal surface.[46-50] It is not yet known whether intimal fibrin derives from the endothelial deposits or is formed within the endothelial surface. However, that fibrin promotes enlargement of primitive endothelial lesions and represents a fundamental factor in atherogenesis is well known. In fact, fibrin acts as a mitogen by three different mechanisms: (1) bridge formation, with migration and consequent proliferation of smooth muscle cells; (2) binding with thrombin, which amplifies the mechanisms recruiting other fibrin[51,52]; and (3) release of fibrin degradation products by fibrinolysis.[53,54] Furthermore, fibrin is atherogenic in that it favors accumulation of low-density lipoproteins and lipoprotein(a) on the intimal surface and binds these substances with a very high affinity to displace plasminogen.[41,54] Fibrin also provides direct or indirect stimulation for synthesis and release of growth factors (from leukocytes and platelets) that determine smooth muscle cell proliferation and migration.[55] Activation of leukocytes and platelets by fibrinogen activity, which plays a key role in atherogenesis, is described in the section on fibrinogen's thrombogenic action.

All activities of fibrinogen are enhanced when its plasma concentration is high. Hyperfibrinogenemia is caused by interlinked genetic and behavioral factors. The genotype modulates individual responses to environmental conditions. An interaction has been shown, for example, between genotype and smoking in the determination of fibrinogen plasma concentration.[56] In this sense, the genotype effect is particularly evident in individuals who smoke and in practice is absent in those who do not smoke. Some studies show that plasma fib-rinogen variations can be explained with BclI polymorphism of the B fibrinogen gene.[57-59]

Fibrinogen and Thrombogenesis

In both physiological and pathological conditions, fibrin derives from fibrinogen through the action of thrombin. The proteolytic cleavage of fibrinogen produces the formation of fibrinopeptides A and B and fibrin monomers. The latter then polymerize by stable linkage noncovalent but to form soluble and removable fibrin. At this point, circulating thrombin also activates factor XIII, which acts as a transamidase and forms stabilizing bonds between fibrin monomers to ultimately produce insoluble and stable fibrin.[60] The fibrinogen level modulates the degree of activation of these mechanisms and consequently the amount of fibrin produced.

A direct relation exists between fibrinogenemia and fibrin formation, so that in hyperfibrinogenemia there is more fibrin formation than normal. When fibrin formation exceeds the capacity of its removal by local or general fibrinolytic systems, the excess fibrin is deposited on vessels to generate a possible atherogenetic lesion or to favor thrombogenesis.[61]

The interaction between fibrinogen and blood cells in thrombogenesis and its effect on blood and plasma viscosity are very important. Interaction with platelets is another way through which fibrinogen participates in thrombus formation. Binding to specific membrane receptors (complex GP IIb–IIIa) induces the formation of bridges, which contribute to platelet activation by increasing sensibility to aggregation agents, promoting adhesion to subendothelium, and releasing stimulating platelet-derived growth factor.[62]

Experimental studies have confirmed these mechanisms and have shown that the effect of fibrinogen on platelet aggregation has an inverse relationship with adenosine diphosphate concentration. Because of a competitive mechanism, a high adenosine diphosphate concentration corresponds to a lower aggregating activity of fibrinogen.[63]

Fibrinogen thrombogenic activity also develops through white blood cell activation. Fibrinogen is thought to induce release of adhesive molecules and cytokines after binding to leukocyte surface receptors.[64] These molecules induce adhesion of leukocytes to the endothelium, activate T lymphocytes, modulate fibroblast displacement, and stimulate cytokines and tumor necrosis factor release from endothelial cells and leukocytes.[65-67]

Many cytokines are released from leukocytes; among them interleukin 1 plays a key role in thrombogenic activity.[68] In fact, along with other activities, this cytokine is capable of shifting in a thrombogenic way the clotting–

fibrinolytic balance. It thus promotes microvessel occlusion by (1) reduction of local fibrinolytic activity after endothelial inhibition of tissue-type plasminogen activator and increased release of plasminogen activator inhibitor 1 and (2) increase of blood clotting after inhibition of thrombomodulin, with consequent functional decrease of protein C concentration and exposure of factor VII and tissue factor as well as an increase of the intrinsic activation of blood clotting and activation of factor X. The functions of tumor necrosis factor on the blood clotting and fibrinolytic system are similar to those of interleukin 1.[69]

Another important action of fibrinogen is its interaction with red blood cells, which develops through three mechanisms:

1. *Reduction of membrane deformability.* It has been demonstrated that hyperfibrinogenemia induces an alteration in erythrocyte function similar to that caused by aging of red blood cells, because of the reduction of Na^+,K^+–adenosine triphosphatase activity.
2. *Enhancement of red blood cell adhesion to endothelium.* In experimental studies employing cultured human vascular endothelial cells under standardized conditions,[70] purified human fibrinogen enhanced adhesion of washed red cells to vascular endothelium in a concentration-dependent fashion in normal subjects, in diabetics,[71] and in patients with sickle cell anemia,[72] whereas the adhesion of erythrocytes to glass tubes was not significantly increased.[70] Fibrinogen, which seems to be the plasma protein mainly responsible for amplification of erythrocyte adhesion, is more effective than fibronectin, albumin, or γ-globulins. The binding of fibrinogen to endothelium suggests a reaction with a surface component of endothelial cells or a substance secreted by endothelial cells. Further studies are required to clarify this reactivity. Clotting alterations recorded in vivo during vascular occlusive episodes could potentiate erythrocyte–endothelial cell interactions, and the formation of fibrin degradation products capable of enhancing vascular permeability by modifing endothelial cell junctions may further increase red cell adhesion.[73]
3. *Red blood cell aggregation.* Many experimental and clinical studies have shown that fibrinogen also modifies red blood cell aggregability, which enhances intercellular bindings and thus causes abnormalities in hemodynamics.[74–76]

Fibrinogen, because of its shape and size, is thought to be the plasma protein mainly responsible for plasma viscosity.[77]

These concentration-dependent actions of fibrinogen on plasma viscosity, deformability, adhesivity, and aggregability of erythrocytes, reactivity and aggregability of platelets, and reactivity and adhesivity of leukocytes may explain the fact that high fibrinogen levels increase blood viscosity and resistance to blood flow and may have important deleterious consequences for tissue perfusion and tissue oxygenation.[74]

It has been observed that the activity of fibrinogen on blood viscosity is expressed in both the microcirculation (especially by interaction with leukocytes and platelets) and the macrocirculation (by interaction with erythrocytes). To confirm this hypothesis, clinical studies have demonstrated relief of symptoms in vasculopathic patients after reduction of plasma fibrinogen level and subsequent reduction of hyperviscosity and red blood cell aggregation.[78,79]

Fibrinogen and Venous Stasis

A new mechanism capable of increasing the plasma concentration of fibrinogen is represented by venous stasis. Our recent studies have shown that stasis, regardless of how it is provoked (by standing, immobilization, experimental induction, etc.), in healthy subjects and in patients whith venous insufficiency of the lower limbs, produces an increase in fibrinogenemia noticeable not only locally (i.e., in areas where the stasis is present) but also at a distance.[80] These observations demonstrate that hyperfibrinogenemia provoked by stasis represents not only a local thrombogenic risk factor but also a general risk factor for both atherogenesis and thrombogenesis. Our studies have also demonstrated that an increase in fibrinogen level is associated with an increase of tissue-type plasminogen activator and a reduction of plasminogen activator inhibitor 1, which counteract the action of hyperfibrinogenemia. However, the action of fibrinogen remains uncontested because the variations of local fibrinolytic activity are reduced over time.[81]

Variations in fibrinogenemia can also result from orthostatic stasis of a few hours. Because stasis takes place daily in every subject, hyperfibrinogenemia is becoming the most frequent and important vascular risk factor.

Reduction of Fibrinogenemia: Modification of Lifestyle and Therapeutic Intervention

Based on what has been described so far, it is evident that lowering high levels of plasma fibrinogen is an important step in reducing vascular risk. Hyperfibrinogenemia can be reduced by administration of drugs and change of lifestyle.

Drugs

Many drugs reduce the plasma level of fibrinogen, as demonstrated during the treatment of other diseases. These drugs include the following:

1. *Fibrates.* Fibrates lower fibrinogen levels more markedly than any other drug class. In patients with hyperfibrinogenemia the decline may be even more pronounced. Clofibrate[82,84] and bezafibrate[82–84] cause a 17% to 43% decrease in fibrinogen levels. Fenofibrate and ciprofibrate[84,85] are less effective, producing a 20% and 18% reduction, respectively, of fibrinogen levels. Two possible mechanisms have been proposed as an explanation for the fibrate-induced fibrinogen effect: interaction with apolipoprotein A and direct inhibition of hepatic fibrinogen synthesis.[84]
2. *β-Adrenergic receptor blockers.* Propranolol[86] and celiprolol[87] have been reported to lower fibrinogen concentration.
3. *Platelet inhibitors.* Ticlopidine has been shown to induce a 11% to 20% reduction in fibrinogen levels.[88,89] Dipyridamole and aspirin have also been found to lower fibrinogen concentration,[84] but confirmation of these findings is awaited.
4. *Defibrotide.* This oral profibrinolytic and antithrombotic drug has been reported to markedly reduce fibrinogenemia.[90]
5. *Vasodilatators.* Vasodilators are less effective than the other classes in reducing fibrinogenemia. Pentoxifylline,[75,91–94] naftidrofuryl,[95] suloctidil,[96] troxerutin,[97] xanthinol niacinate,[98] prazosin,[99] niceritrol,[100] vinburnine,[101] and calcium dobesilate[102] are widely used, but their effect on fibrinogen levels needs to be confirmed in controlled trials.
6. *Anabolic steroids.* Stanozolol lowers fibrinogen levels in both healthy volunteers and vasculopathic patients.[103]
7. *Other drugs.* Allium sativum (garlic),[104] sulfinpyrazone,[105] tamoxifen,[106] and nisoldipine[107] have all been reported to lower fibrinogen levels.

Lifestyle

Changes in lifestyle that could lead to a reduction of fibrinogenemia include the following:

1. Cessation of smoking: fibrinogenemia is normalized after 5 years[15,20,22]
2. Normalization of body mass index[15,22,23]
3. Moderate and regular physical activity: a program of regular physical exercise can lower fibrinogenemia by approximatively 0.4 g/L, with a consequent reduction of vascular risk estimated at approximatively 60%[18]
4. Withdrawal of oral contraceptives[15,19,23,24]

5. Regular and moderate consumption of alcohol[15,16,18,19,21,22,24,26,30]
6. Control of stress: stress factors increase fibrinogen values, but no evidence suggests that relaxation programs can normalize them.

To our knowledge there are two possible ways of lowering fibrinogenemia: changes in lifestyle and use of drugs, of which fibrates are the most effective. Much research is still being conducted to better define the physiological mechanisms through which fibrinogenemia is controlled and to identify specific agents capable of reducing plasma fibrinogen concentration. However, further research is necessary to determine whether the reduction of fibrinogenemia reduces the incidence of cardiovascular events and to establish the exact role of fibrinogen as a risk factor.

References

1. Doolittle RF. Fibrinogen and fibrin. *Sci Am.* 1981;245: 92–101.
2. Henschen A. Fibrinogen-Blutgerinnungsfaktor I. Biochemische Aspekte. *Haemostaseologie.* 1981;1:30–40.
3. Hermans J, McDonagh J. Fibrin: structure and interactions. *Semin Thromb Hemost.* 1982;8:11–24.
4. Meade TW, Chakrabarti R, Haines AP, et al. Haemostatic function and cardiovascular death: early results of a prospective study. *Lancet.* 1980;1:1050–1053.
5. Meade TW, Brozovic M, Chakrabarti R, et al. Haemostatic function and ischaemic heart disease: principal results of the Northwick Park Heart Study. *Lancet.* 1986;2:533–537.
6. Baker IA, Eastham R, Elwood PC, et al. Haemostatic factors associated with ischaemic heart disease in men aged 45 to 64 years. *Br Heart J.* 1982;47:490–494.
7. Yarnell JWG, Baker IA, Sweetnam PM, et al. Fibrinogen, viscosity, and white blood cell count are major risk factors for ischaemic heart disease: the Caerphilly and Speedwell Collaborative Heart Disease Studies. *Circulation.* 1991;83: 836–844.
8. Wilhelmsen L, Svardsudd K, Korsan-Bengtsen K, et al. Fibrinogen as a risk factor for stroke and myocardial infarction. *N Engl J Med.* 1984;311:501–505.
9. Gordon T, Moore FE, Shurtleff D, et al. Some methodologic problems in the long-term study of cardiovascular diseases: observations from the Framingham Study. *Journal of Chronic Diseases.* 1959;10:186–206.
10. Shurtleff D. Some Characteristics Related to the Incidence of Cardiovascular Diseases and Death: Framingham Study. 18-years Follow-up. Section 30. Washington, DC: Government Printing Office; 1974. DHEW publication NIH 74-599.
11. Kannel W, Wolf PA, Castelli WP, et al. Fibrinogen and risk of cardiovascular disease. *JAMA.* 1987;258:1183–1186.
12. Ballestein L, Schulte H, Assmann G, et al. Coagulation factors and the progress of coronary heart disease. *Lancet.* 1987;1:461.

13. Heinrich J, Schulte H, Ballestein L, et al. Predictive value of haemostatic variables in the PROCAM Study. *Thromb Haemost.* 1991;65:815.

14. Cremer P, Nagel D, Boettcher B, Seidel D. Fibrinogen: ein koronarer Risickofactor. *Diagnose and Labor.* 1992;42: 28–35.

15. Folsom AR: Epidemiology of fibrinogen. *Eur Heart J.* 1995; 16(suppl A):21–24.

16. Iso H, Folsom AR, Sato S, et al. Plasma fibrinogen and its correlates in Japanese and US population samples. *Arterioscler Thromb.* 1993;13:783–790.

17. Meade TW, Stirling Y, Thompson SG, et al. An international and interregional comparison of haemostatic variables in the study of ischaemic heart disease: report of a working group. *Int J Epidemiol.* 1986;15:331–336.

18. Folsom AR, Wu KK, Davis CE, et al. Population correlates of plasma fibrinogen and factor VII: putative cardiovascular risk factors. *Atherosclerosis.* 1991;91:191–205.

19. Folsom AR, Qamhieh HT, Flack JM, et al., for the investigators of the Coronary Artery Risk Development in Young Adults (CARDIA) Study. Plasma fibrinogen: levels and correlates in young adults. *Am J Epidemiol.* 1993;138: 1023–1036.

20. Folsom AR, Johnson KM, Lando EA, et al. Plasma fibrinogen and other cardiovascular risk factors in urban American Indian smokers. *Ethnicity Dis.* 1993;3:344–350.

21. Pola P, Savi L. Fibrinogenemia, determined immunonephelometrically, as a possible parameter in the evaluation of peripheral arteriosclerotic arteriopathy. *Atherosclerosis.* 1978;29:205–216.

22. Lee AJ, Smith WCS, Lowe GDO, et al. Plasma fibrinogen and coronary risk factors: the Scottish Heart Health Study. *J Clin Epidemiol.* 1990;43:913–919.

23. Krobot K, Hense HW, Cremer P, et al. Determinants of plasma fibrinogen: relation to body weight, waist-to-hip ratio, smoking, alcohol, age, and sex: results from the Second MONICA Augsburg Survey 1989–90. *Arterioscler Thromb.* 1992;12:780–788.

24. Ballaisen L, Bailey J, Epping PH, et al. Epidemiological study on factor VII, factor VIII, and fibrinogen in an industrial population: baseline data on the relation to age, gender, body-weight, smoking, alcohol, pill-using, and menopause. *Thromb Haemost.* 1985;54:475–479.

25. Meade TW, Chakrabarti R, Haines AP, et al. Characteristics affecting fibrinolytic activity and plasma fibrinogen concentrations. *BMJ.* 1979;1:153–156.

26. Yarnell JWG, Fehily AM, Milbank J, et al. Determinants of plasma lipoproteins and coagulation factors in men from Caerphilly, South Wales. *J Epidemiol Community Health.* 1983;37:137–140.

27. Moller L, Kristensen TS. Plasma fibrinogen and ischaemic heart disease risk factors. *Arterioscler Thromb.* 1991;11: 344–350.

28. Yarnell JWG, Sweetnam PM, Rogers S, et al. Some long term effects of smoking on the haemostatic system: a report from the Caerphilly and Speedwell Collaborative Surveys. *J Clin Pathol.* 1987;40:909–913.

29. Kannel WB, D'Agostino RB, Belanger AJ. Fibrinogen, cigarette smoking, and risk of cardiovascular diasease: insights from the Framingham Study. *Am Heart J.* 1987;113: 1006–1010.

30. Meade TW, Imeson J, Stirling Y. Effects of changes in smoking and other characteristics on clotting factors and the risk of ischaemic heart disease. *Lancet.* 1987;2: 986–988.

31. Feher MD, Rampling MW, Brown J, et al. Acute changes in atherogenic and thrombogenic factors with cessation of smoking. *J R Soc Med.* 1990;83:146–148.

32. Folsom AR, Qamhieh HT, Wing RR, et al. Impact of weight loss on plasminogen activator inhibitor (PAI-1), factor VII, and other haemostatic factors in moderately overweight adults. *Aterioscler Thromb.* 1993;13:162–169.

33. Connelly JB, Cooper JA, Meade TW. Strenuous exercise, plasma fibrinogen, and factor VII activity. *Br Heart J.* 1992; 67:351–354.

34. Lakka TA, Salonen JT. Moderate to high intensity conditioning leisure time physical activity and high cardiorespiratory fitness are associated with reduced plasma fibrinogen in eastern Finnish men. *J Clin Epidemiol.* 1993;46: 1119–1127.

35. Hostmark AT, Bjerkedal T, Kierulf P, et al. Fish oil and plasma fibrinogen. *BMJ.* 1988;297:180–181.

36. Rosengren A, Wilhelmsen L, Welin L, et al. Social influences and cardiovascular risk factors as determinants of plasma fibrinogen concentration in a general population sample of middle-aged men. *BMJ.* 1990;300:634–648.

37. Markowe HLJ, Marmot MG, Shipley MJ, et al. Fibrinogen: a possible link between social class and coronary heart disease. *BMJ.* 1985;291:1312–1314.

38. Von Eckardstein A, Malinow MR, Upson B, et al. Effects of age, lipoproteins, and haemostatic parameters on the role of homocyst(e)inemia as a cardiovascular risk factor in men. *Arterioscler Thromb.* 1994;14:460–464.

39. Ernst E. Fibrinogen as a cardiovascular risk factor: interrelationship with infections and inflammation. *Eur Heart J.* 1993;14(suppl K):82–87.

40. Ernst E, Matrai A, Marshall M. Blood rheology in patients with transient ischaemic attacks. *Stroke.* 1988;19:634–636.

41. Smith EB, Thompson WD. Fibrin as a factor in atherogenesis. *Thromb Res.* 1994;73:1–19.

42. Smith EB, Crosbie L. Fibrinogen and fibrin in atherogenesis. In: Ernst E, Koenig W, Lowe GDO, Meade TW, eds. *Fibrinogen: A "New" Cardiovascular Risk Factor.* Vienna: Blackwell-MZV; 1992:4–10.

43. Smith EB. Fibrin deposition and fibrin degradation products in atherosclerotic plaques. *Thromb Res.* 1994;75: 329–335.

44. Stirk CM, Kochhar A, Smith EB, et al. Presence of growth-stimulating fibrin degradation products containing fragment E in human atherosclerotic plaques. *Atherosclerosis.* 1993;103:159–169.

45. Kaplan KL, Bini A, Feroglio J, et al. Fibrin and vessel wall. In: Lui CY, Chien S, eds. *Fibrinogen, Thrombosis, Coagulation and Fibrinolysis.* New York: Plenum Press; 1990:313–318.

46. Duguid JB. Thrombosis as a factor in the pathogenesis of coronary atherosclerosis. *J Pathol Bacteriol.* 1946;58: 207–222.

47. Duguid JB. Thrombosis as a factor in the pathogenesis of aortic atherosclerosis. *J Pathol Bacteriol.* 1948;60:57–61.

48. Haust MD. The morphogenesis and fate of potential and early atherosclerotic lesions in man. *Hum Pathol.* 1971;1: 1–29.

49. Movat HZ, Haust MD, More RH. The morphologic elements in the early lesions of arteriosclerosis. *Am J Pathol.* 1959;35:93–97.

50. Jorgensen L, Packham MA, Rowsell HC, et al. Deposition of formed elements of blood on the intima and signs of intima injury in the aorta of rabbit, pig, and man. *Lab Invest.* 1972;27:341–350.

51. Chen LB, Buchanan JM. Mitogenic activity of blood components, I: thrombin and prothrombin. *Proc Natl Acad Sci U S A.* 1975;72:131–135.

52. Bar-Shavit R, Benezra M, Eldor A, et al. Thrombin immobilised to extracellular matrix is a potent mitogen for vascular smooth muscle cells: nonenzymatic mode of action. *Cell Regulation.* 1990;1:453–463.

53. Smith EB, Ashall C. Fibrinolysis and plasminogen concentration in aortic intima in relation to death following myocardial infarction. *Atherosclerosis.* 1985;55:171–185.

54. Smith EB, Crosbie L. Does lipoprotein(a) (Lp(a)) compete with plasminogen in human atherosclerotic lesions and thrombi? *Atherosclerosis.* 1991;89:127–136.

55. Godspodarowicz D. Growth factors and their action in vivo and in vitro. *J Pathol.* 1983;141:201–233.

56. Green F, Hamsten A, Blomback M, et al. The role of beta-fibrinogen genotype in determining plasma fibrinogen levels in young survivors of myocardial infarction and healthy controls from Sweden. *Thromb Haemost.* 1993;70:915–920.

57. Thomas A, Kelleher C, Green F, et al. Variation in the promoter region of the beta-fibrinogen gene is associated with plasma fibrinogen levels in smokers and non-smokers. *Thromb Haemost.* 1991;65:487–490.

58. Thomas A, Lamlum H, Humphries S, et al. Linkage disequilibrium across the fibrinogen locus as shown by five genetic polymorphism, G/A^{-455} (HaeIII), C/T^{-148} (HindIII/AluI), T/G^{-1689} (AvaII), BClI (beta-fibrinogen), and TaqI (alfa-fibrinogen), and their detection by PCR. *Hum Mutat.* 1994;3:79–81.

59. Heinrich J, Funke H, Rust S, et al. Impact of polymorphism in the alpha- and beta-fibrinogen gene on plasma fibrinogen concentrations of coronary heart disease patients. *Thromb Res.* 1995;77:203–215.

60. Henschen A, McDonagh J. Fibrinogen, fibrin, and factor XIII. In: Zwaal RDF, Hemker HC, eds. *Blood Coagulation.* Amsterdam: Elsevier; 1986:171–239.

61. Smith EB. Fibrinogen, fibrin, and the arterial wall. *Eur Heart J.* 1995;16(suppl A):11–15.

62. Hawiger J. Mechanisms involved in platelet vessel wall interaction. *Thromb Haemost.* 1995;74:369–372.

63. Meade TW, Vickers MV, Thompson SG, et al. The effects of physiological levels of fibrinogen on platelet aggregation. *Thromb Res.* 1985;38:527–534.

64. Langler EG, van Hinsbergh VWM. Endothelial cytokines. *Am J Physiol.* 1991;260:e1052–e1053.

65. Adams D, Show S. Leukocyte-endothelial interaction and regulation of leukocyte migration. *Lancet.* 1994;343:831–836.

66. von Adrian UH, Chambers JD, McEvoy L, et al. Two step model of leukocyte-endothelial cell interaction in inflammation: distinct roles for Lecam-1 and the leukocyte β_2 integrins in vivo. *Proc Natl Acad Sci U S A.* 1991;88:7538–7542.

67. Andersen DC: Adhesion molecule in clinical disease. In: Anderson DC, ed. *Cell Adhesion Molecules.* San Francisco: Anderson DC. Edition; 1996:13–14.

68. Dinariello CA, Wolf SM. The role of interleukin-1 in disease. *N Engl J Med.* 1993;328:106–113.

69. Liblau RS, Fugger MT. Tumor necrosis factor and disease progression in multiple sclerosis. *N Engl J Med.* 1992;326:272–273.

70. Wautier JL, Pintigny D, Wautier MP, et al. Fibrinogen, a modulator of erythrocyte adhesion to vascular endothelium. *J Lab Clin Med.* 1983;101:911–920.

71. Wautier JL, Paton RC, Wautier MP, et al. Increased adhesion of erythrocytes to endothelial cells in diabetes mellitus and its relation to vascular complications. *N Engl J Med.* 1981;305:237–262.

72. Hebbel RP, Yamada O, MoldoW C, et al. Abnormal adherence of sickle erythrocytes to cultured vascular endothelium: possible mechanism for microvascular occlusion in sickle cell disease. *J Clin Invest.* 1980;65:154–160.

73. Busch CH, Gerdin B. Effect of low molecular weight fibrin degradation products to endothelial cells in culture. *Thromb Res.* 1981;22:33–39.

74. Kaibara M. Rheology of blood coagulation. *Biorheology.* 1996;33:101–117.

75. Pribush A, Meyerstein D, Meyerstein N. Study of red blood cell aggregation by admittance measurements. *Biorheology.* 1996;33:139–151.

76. Vicaut E. Opposite effects of red blood cell aggregation on resistence to blood flow. *J Cardiovasc Surg.* 1995;36:361–368.

77. Pola P, Flore R, Tondi P. Blood and plasma viscosity in experimentally induced hyper- and hypofibrinogenaemia. *Int J Tissue React.* 1986;8:333–336.

78. Triebe G, Muennich U, Liebold F. Haemodilution or pentoxifylline in the treatment of peripheral vascular diseases. *Dtsch Med Wochenschr.* 1992;117:523–530.

79. Walzl B, Walzl M, Valentitsch H, et al. Increased cerebral perfusion following reduction of fibrinogen and lipid fractions. *Haemostasis.* 1995;25:137–143.

80. Pola P, Tondi P, De Martini D, et al. Influence of stasis in fibrinogen values. *Int J Angiol.* 1994;3:180–182.

81. Pola P, Tondi P, De Martini D, et al. Is the stasis induced by orthostasism a vascular risk factor for arteries as well as for veins? *Int J Angiol.* 1996;5:144–148.

82. Cook NS, Tapparelli C, Dryer M, et al. Effect of bezafibrate and other drugs on plasma fibrinogen levels in rats. *Thromb Haemost.* 1991;65:202–205.

83. Almèr LO, Kjellstrom T. The fibrinolytic system and coagulation during bezafibrate treatment of hypertriglyceridaemia. *Atherosclerosis.* 1996;61:81–85.

84. Ernst E, Resh KL. Therapeutic interventions to lower plasma fibrinogen concentration. *Eur Heart J.* 1995;16 (suppl A):47–53.

85. Simpson JA, Lorimer AR, Walker ID, et al. Effect of ciprofibrate on platelet aggregation and fibrinolysis in patients with hypercholesterolaemia. *Thromb Haemost.* 1985;54:442–444.

86. Mehotra TN, Mital HS, Singh VS, et al. Platelet adhesiveness plasma fibrinogen and fibrinolytic activity in angina pectoris before and after propanolol treatment. *J Assoc Physicians India.* 1983;31:641–643.

87. Herrmann JM, Mayer EO. A long term study of the effects of celiprolol on blood pressure and lipid associated risk factors. *Am Heart J.* 1988;116:1416–1421.

88. Aukland A, Hurlow RA, George AJ, et al. Platelet inhibition with ticlopidine in atherosclerotic intermittent claudication. *J Clin Pathol.* 1982;35:740–743.

89. Conrad J, Lecrubier C, Scarabin P, et al. Effects of long term administration of ticlopidine on platelet function and haemostatic variables. *Thromb Res.* 1980;20:143–148.

90. Pola P, Tondi P, De Martini D, et al. Variazioni della fibrinogenemia, del tPA e del PAI-1 dopo somministrazione parenterale di defibrotide (Engl Abs). *Giornale Italiano di Angiologia.* 1994;14:14–18.

91. Ward A, Clissold SP. Pentoxifylline. *Drugs.* 1987;34:50–57.

92. Ott E, Lechner H. Haemorheologic conditions in patients with pentoxifylline. *Research in Clinic and Laboratory.* 1981; 11(suppl 1): 253–256.

93. Ernst E, Matrai A, Weihmayr T, et al. Behandlung der arteriellen Verschlusskrankheit. *Munchener Medizinische Wochenschrift.* 1985;127:917–919.

94. Bachet P, Lancrenon S, Chassoux G. Fibrinogen and pentoxifylline. *Thromb Res.* 1989;55:161–163.

95. Kiesewetter H, Jung F, Schwab J, et al. Periphere arterielle Verschlusskrankheit. *Munchener Medizinische Wochenschrift.* 1987;129:21–24.

96. Roba J, Roncucci R, Lambelin G. Pharmacological properties of suloctidil. *Acta Clin Belg.* 1977;32:3–7.

97. LeDevehat C, Lemoine A. Haemorheological changes induced by troxerutin in patients affected by venous insufficiency of lower legs [abstract]. *Clin Hemorheol.* 1985;5:740.

98. Davis E, Rozov H. The effect of xantinol nicotinate on small blood vessels. *Bibliotheca Anatomica.* 1973;11: 334–339.

99. Letcher RL, Chien S, Laragh JH. Changes in blood viscosity accompanying the response to prazosin in patients with essential hypertension. *J Cardiovasc Pharmacol.* 1977;9 (suppl 6):S8–S20.

100. Hamazaki T, Hasunuma K, Kobayashi S, et al. The effects on lipids, blood viscosity, and platelet aggregation of combined use of niceritrol and a low dose of acetyl salicylic acid. *Atherosclerosis.* 1985;55:107–113.

101. LeDevehat C, Vimeux M. Pharmacological study of the action of vinburnine versus placebo. *Int Angiol.* 1989;8: 57–61.

102. Benarroch JS, Brodsky M, Rubinstein A, et al. Treatment of blood hyperviscosity with calcium dobesilate in patients with diabetic retinopathy. *Ophthalmic Res.* 1985;17: 131–138.

103. Preston FE, Burakowski BK, Portes MR, et al. The fibrinolytic response to stanazolol in normal subjects. *Thromb Res.* 1981;22:543–551.

104. Harenberg J, Giese C, Zimmermann R. Effect of dried garlic on blood coagulation, fibrinolysis, platelet aggregation, and serum cholesterol levels in patients with hyperlipoproteinaemia. *Atherosclerosis.* 1988;74:247–249.

105. Johnston RV, Lowe GDO, Drummond MM, et al. A study of the effect of sulphinpirazone ("Anturan") on blood viscosity. *Curr Med Res Opin.* 1979;6:271–273.

106. Love RR, Surawicz TS, Williams EC. Antithrombin III level, fibrinogen level, and platelet count changes with adjuvant tamoxifen therapy. *Arch Intern Med.* 1992;152: 317–320.

107. Salmasi AM, Salmasi S, MacDonald G, et al. Improvement of silent myocardial ischaemia and reduction of plasma fibrinogen during nisoldipine therapy in occult coronary arterial disease. *Int J Cardiol.* 1991;31:71–80.

34

Oxygen Free Radicals and Peripheral Vascular Disease

Kailash Prasad

Oxygen free radicals (OFRs) are becoming a popular topic of research. They have been implicated in the pathophysiology of various disease processes including ischemia–reperfusion injury, heart failure, hypercholesterolemic atherosclerosis, diabetes mellitus, hemorrhagic and endotoxic shock, burn, Parkinson's disease, Alzheimer's disease, cataract, and peripheral vascular disease. In this chapter I give a brief description of the definition of OFRs; their formation, sources, and effects; and antioxidants and the role of OFRs in peripheral vascular disease.

Definition

An atom contains a nucleus, around which electrons usually move in pairs. A free radical is an atom or molecule that contains one or more unpaired electrons. The unpaired electron alters the chemical reactivity of an atom or molecule, making it reactive. An *oxygen free radical* is defined as any compound derived from molecular oxygen that has acquired fewer than four electrons. The superoxide anion (O_2^-) and hydroxyl radicals $(\cdot OH)$ are OFRs, but hydrogen peroxide is not. Hence, sometimes the term *reactive oxygen metabolites* is used for all of these. However, free radicals and other reactive species are not confined to derivatives of O_2.

Formation of Oxygen-Derived Free Radicals

Oxygen-derived free radicals include the superoxide anion (O_2^-), and hydroxyl $(\cdot OH)$, peroxyl $(ROO\cdot)$, alkoxyl $(RO\cdot)$, and hydroperoxyl $(HOO\cdot)$ radicals. Oxygen metabolites that contain an even number of electrons, such as H_2O_2 and hypochlorous acid (HOCl), are not OFRs.

The Superoxide Anion

Univalent reduction of molecular oxygen generates O_2^-, which is very unstable. It can act as both oxidant and reductant. It oxidizes ascorbate, sulfhydryl-containing compounds, sulfate, and catecholamines. It reduces ferric iron and quinones. It inactivates a variety of enzymes (e.g., tRNase, RNase, glyceraldehyde-3-phosphate dehydrogenase, and aconitase[46]). O_2^- is not highly toxic, and most of the damaging effects are due to highly toxic $\cdot OH$. Oxygen is metabolized as shown in Figure 34.1.

Hydrogen Peroxide

H_2O_2 is formed by dismutation of O_2^-, a process accelerated by superoxide dismutase (SOD). It is a relatively stable oxidant and very lipophilic and hence crosses cell membrane rapidly. It can inactivate some enzymes by oxidizing their reactive sulfhydryl groups. Catalase and glutathione peroxidase (GSH-P_X) convert it to $H_2O + O_2$.

The Hydroxyl Radical

O_2^- and H_2O_2 in the presence of metal (iron or copper) generate $\cdot OH$ via the Haber–Weiss or Fenton reaction. It is a highly reactive species. Other modes of formation of $\cdot OH$ are described in the section on sources of OFRs.

Singlet Oxygen

In addition to its reduction to free radicals, the activity of molecular oxygen can be increased in another way. Reactivity is increased during the course of certain reactions involving molecular oxygen that invert the spin of

427

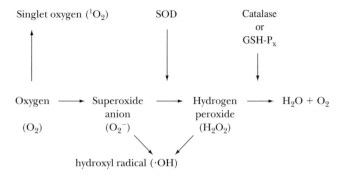

FIGURE 34.1. Generation of OFRs. SOD, superoxide dismutase; GSH-P$_X$, glutathione peroxidase.

one of the electrons of the two outer orbitals. This process produces singlet oxygen, which is highly reactive.[64] There are two types of singlet oxygen, the very short-lived sigma and the long-lived delta singlet oxygen. Singlet oxygen ($^1O_2$) is formed by the action of light on molecular oxygen in the presence of a photosensitizer. Singlet oxygen is also generated during an iron-catalyzed Haber–Weiss reaction, spontaneous dismutation of O_2^-, and oxidation of halides by hydrogen peroxides. Delta singlet oxygen is not a free radical, but it is capable of rapidly oxidizing many molecules including membrane polyunsaturated fatty acids.[95] Sigma singlet oxygen is very highly reactive when compared with delta singlet oxygen. Many compounds such as beta carotene, 1,4-diazabicyclooctane, and azide are effective quenchers of $^1O_2$. Singlet oxygen has a longer lifetime as D_2O than H_2O. Amino acids react rapidly with $^1O_2$. Histidine, tryptophan, and methionine quench $^1O_2$ effectively.

Peroxyl Radicals

Hydroxyl radicals react with certain carbohydrates, proteins, nucleotide bases, and lipids to produce peroxyl radicals (ROO·) that are slightly less reactive than ·OH and have a half-life of seconds instead of nanoseconds. Peroxyl radicals damage biomolecules.

Hypochlorous Acid and Halogenated Amines

Hypochlorous acid and halogenated amines are free radicals but not oxygen-derived free radicals. They are very potent oxidants. Potentially cytotoxic species of oxygen include O_2^-, H_2O_2, ·OH, ROO·, and $^1O_2$.

Sources of OFRs

There are various sources of OFRs in the body.

Mitochondria

Under normal physiological conditions, 95% of the oxy-

gen inhaled is utilized by a tetravalent pathway yielding no free radicals; however, about 5% of oxygen is metabolized by a univalent pathway, which results in highly reactive OFRs.[24] In the univalent pathway, oxygen gains one electron (e$^-$) at a time and is reduced to O_2^-. The ubiquinone–cytochrome b region of the electron transport chain is a major site of O_2^- production.[95] H_2O_2 is produced by spontaneous dismutation of O_2^-, the rate of this dismutation being considerably increased by SOD. H_2O_2 is metabolized to water by catalase and GSH-P$_X$. The whole reaction is summarized in the following:

$$O_2 + e^- \rightarrow O_2^- \rightarrow$$

$$O_2^- + O_2^- + 2H^+ \xrightarrow{\text{SOD}} H_2O_2 + O_2$$

$$2GSH + H_2O_2 \xrightarrow{\text{GSH-P}_X} GSSG + 2H_2O$$

$$2H_2O_2 \xrightarrow{\text{catalase}} 2H_2O + O_2,$$

where SOD is superoxide dismutase; GSH, reduced glutathione; GSSG, oxidized glutathione and GSH-P$_X$, glutathione peroxidase. Hydroxyl radicals (·OH) are formed in various ways, as described in the following.

Fenton Reaction

In the Fenton reaction, H_2O_2, in the presence of ferrous or cupric ions, is converted to ·OH as follows:

$$Fe^{2+} + H_2O_2 \rightarrow Fe^{3+} + \cdot OH + OH^-.$$

Haber–Weiss Reaction

The formation of ·OH is based on the interaction between H_2O_2 and O_2^- in the presence of transition metals.[3]

$$Fe^{3+} + O_2^- \rightarrow Fe^{2+} + O_2$$

$$Fe^{2+} + H_2O_2 \rightarrow Fe^{3+} + \cdot OH + OH^-.$$

O_2^- and Nitric Oxide

The superoxide anion reacts with nitric oxide (NO·) to generate peroxynitrite (ONOO$^-$), which at physiological pH gives rise to peroxynitrous acid (ONOOH). It is very unstable and rapidly decomposes to ·OH:[4]

$$O_2^- + NO\cdot \rightarrow ONOO^-$$

$$ONOO^- + H^+ \rightarrow ONOOH \rightarrow \cdot OH + NO_2\cdot.$$

Hypochlorous Acid

Hypochlorous acid (HOCl) also gives rise to ·OH, as shown in the following:

$$O_2^- + HOCl \rightarrow \cdot OH + O_2 + Cl^-.$$

Polymorphonuclear Leukocytes

The NADPH oxidase system is a membrane-associated enzyme complex that lies dormant in unstimulated polymorphonuclear leukocytes (PMNLs). Activated PMNLs rapidly activate NADPH oxidase, a flavoprotein complex that acts as an electron transport chain. PMNLs are stimulated by activated complement component C5 (C5a), N-formyl-Met-Leu-Phe, immune complexes, and leukotriene B4. These ligands interact with specific receptors in PMNLs. NADPH oxidase catalyzes the reduction of O_2 to O_2^- by way of NADPH derived from the pentose phosphate pathway:

$$2O_2 + NADPH \xrightarrow[\text{oxidase}]{\text{NADPH}} 2O_2^- + NADP^+ + H^+.$$

O_2^- undergoes dismutation to produce H_2O_2, which is metabolized to either H_2O or ·OH through the Haber–Weiss or Fenton reaction.[1,104] PMNLs and, to a lesser extent, monocytes also contain myeloperoxidase (MPO) in their azurophilic granules; it is released into the phagocytic vacuole or into extracellular fluid following stimulation of PMNLs.[45] In the presence of H_2O_2, myeloperoxidase catalyzes the oxidation of the halides chloride (Cl^-), bromide (Br^-), and iodide (I^-), as well as thiocyanate to their corresponding hypohalous acids.[46] Because Cl^- is most abundant (present at levels a thousand times that of other halides) in biological systems, HOCl is the most common hypohalous acid formed by PMNLs. HOCl can chlorinate amines, amino acids, thioethers, and aromatic and other unsaturated carbon groups. HOCl can also chlorinate endogenous and exogenous amino acids to N-chloramines,[104] which are long-lived and very potent oxidizing species. HOCl is the most powerful oxidant and is generated in large quantities by PMNLs.

Oxidation of Cl^- by the enzyme-substrate complex (MPO + H_2O_2) proceeds as follows:

$$H_2O_2 + Cl^- + H^+ \rightarrow HOCl + H_2O.$$

HOCl and hypochlorite (OCl^-) are powerful oxidizing and chlorinating agents and are approximately 100 times more reactive than O_2^- and H_2O_2.

Eosinophil peroxidase preferentially catalyzes the formation of hypobromous acid (HOBr).[104] HOBr is as potent as HOCl at oxidation, halogenation, and cytotoxic activities.[105] Human saliva, tears, and milk contain high concentrations of peroxidase, thiocyanate, and H_2O_2. Hypothiocyanous acid formed from H_2O_2 and thiocyanate is a potent oxidant and known to control bacterial growth in exocrine secretions.

Enzymatic Sources

Xanthine Oxidase

In healthy tissue, xanthine oxidase exists as the nicotinamide adenine dinucleotide (NAD+)–reducing enzyme called *xanthine dehydrogenase*. NAD+ accepts electrons without producing any superoxide anions. Xanthine dehydrogenase is converted to xanthine oxidase by various mechanisms. During ischemia, it is converted to xanthine oxidase by calcium-dependent proteases and sulfhydryl group oxidation.[19] During ischemia, adenosine triphosphate (ATP) is catabolized to adenine nucleotides (adenosine diphosphate, adenosine monophosphate, and inosine). Adenine nucleotides are further metabolized to hypoxanthine and xanthine.[13] Biochemical changes during ischemia are the basis of production of OFRs, as shown later.[59] Generation of oxygen radicals from an adenine nucleotide and xanthine oxidase is shown in Figure 34.2.

Xanthine + xanthine oxidase gives $O_2^- + H_2O_2 +$ uric acid. Whereas xanthine dehydrogenase reduces NAD+ and cannot transfer electrons to molecular oxygen, xanthine oxidase transfers electrons from hypoxanthine to oxygen to form a superoxide anion radical. At neutral pH, 80% of O_2 metabolized is converted to H_2O_2 via divalent reduction of O_2, whereas 20% is converted

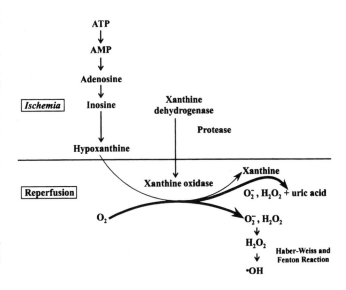

FIGURE 34.2. Schematic diagram for the formation of oxygen radicals with interaction of an adenine nucleotide and xanthine oxidase. ATP indicates adenosine triphopshate, AMP, adenosine monophosphate.

to O_2^- via univalent reduction.[23] During ischemia without reperfusion, OFRs can be produced, but in limited amounts. Some oxygen has been found within the lipid bilayer of cell membranes in quantities sufficient to allow the production of OFRs. Evidence of these early free radicals came from the study by Rao et al.[84]

Aldehyde Oxidase

Aldehyde oxidase, which has properties similar to those of xanthine oxidase, produces O_2^-. Dehydroorotate dehydrogenase, flavoprotein dehydrogenase, and tryptophan dioxygenase also produce O_2^-.

Auto-oxidation of Small Molecules

Molecules capable of undergoing auto-oxidation include catecholamines, hydroquinones, thiols, and flavins. When undergoing auto-oxidation they generate O_2^-. Catecholamine undergoes oxidation to form quinone radicals, which react with oxygen to form O_2^-.[60]

Oxidative deamination of dopamine by monoamine oxidase leads to formation of $H_2O_2^-$:

$$\text{Dopamine} + O_2 + H_2O \rightarrow$$
$$\text{3,4-dihydroxyphenylacetaldehyde} + NH_3 + H_2O_2.$$

Oxidative deamination of 5-hydroxytryptamine also gives rise to H_2O_2:

$$\text{5-hydroxytryptamine} + H_2O + O_2 \rightarrow$$
$$\text{5-hydroxyindoleacetic acid} + H_2O_2 + NH_3.$$

Arachidonic Acid Metabolism

Arachidonic acid is metabolized to prostaglandins via the cyclooxygenase pathway. In this process of metabolism a carbon-centered free radical is formed by cyclooxygenase-mediated abstraction of one of the methylene hydrogens of arachidonic acid.[22] An oxygen-centered free radical ($\cdot OH$) is probably formed during breakdown of hydroperoxide to prostaglandin G_2.[18] During conversion of prostaglandin G_2 to prostaglandin H_2 a number of free radicals including O_2^- are generated.[51] During conversion of prostaglandin H_2 to thromboxane, OFRs are generated.[91]

During synthesis of leukotrienes from arachidonic acid via the lipoxygenase pathway, $\cdot OH$ is also generated.[62]

The Endoplasmic Reticulum and Nuclear Membrane

Endoplasmic reticulum and nuclear membranes contain cytochrome P-450 and cytochrome b_5, both of which can oxidize xenobiotics and fatty acids and reduce dioxygen.[22] O_2^- is directly formed by a one-electron transfer reaction by microsomal and nuclear membrane cytochromes. H_2O_2 is formed by dissociation of peroxycytochrome complexes. Auto-oxidation of flavoproteins containing cytochrome P-450 and cytochrome b_5 is also a source of O_2^- and H_2O_2. Microsomal $\cdot OH$ may be derived from an iron-catalyzed Haber–Weiss reaction.

Peroxisomes

Oxidases present in peroxisomes, which are specialized cells or organelles, generate H_2O_2 via divalent reduction of molecular oxygen.[22] H_2O_2 generated is metabolized by peroxisomal catalases. H_2O_2 is free to diffuse out of peroxisomes and into the cytoplasm where it may be converted into $\cdot OH$.

Antioxidants

Antioxidants are substances that, when present at a low concentration compared with the concentration of an oxidizable substrate, significantly delay or inhibit oxidation of that substrate. The body is equipped with a variety of antioxidants to protect against excessive radical generation and the consequences thereof. Intracellular antioxidants scavenge aberrant free radicals locally. Extracellular antioxidants break the chain of radical reaction propagation and remove metal ions and heme proteins by sequestering them and making them incapable of generating free radicals. There are two classes of antioxidants: enzymatic and nonenzymatic.

Enzymatic Antioxidants

SOD, catalase, GSH-P_X, and other peroxidases are enzymatic antioxidants.

Superoxide Dismutase

There are two types of SOD: copper–zinc SOD is present in cytosol, and Mn-SOD is present in mitochondria. Both Cu,Zn-SOD and Mn-SOD are also found in extracellular fluid.[58] Both enhance dismutation of O_2^- to H_2O_2 and O_2. Synthesis of SOD may be increased in cells in response to hyperoxidant states.[25]

Catalase

Catalase enzymatically converts $2H_2O_2$ to $2H_2O + O_2$. It is present in all tissues, but intestine contains very little activity. It becomes more important when H_2O_2 is present in high concentration. O_2^- inhibits catalase and GSH-P_X; H_2O_2 inactivates SOD. There is a mutually supportive interaction among the enzymes that provide defense against OFRs.[56]

GSH-P$_X$

GSH-P$_X$ is a selenium-containing enzyme and converts H_2O_2 to water and oxidized glutathione (GSSG) using reduced glutathione (GSH) as a hydrogen donor:

$$2\ GSH + H_2O_2 \xrightarrow{\text{GSH-P}_X} GSSG + 2H_2O.$$

Glutathione reductase (GSH-Rd) regenerates GSH from GSSG by using NADPH:

$$GSSG + NADPH + H \xrightarrow{\text{GSH-Rd}} 2\ GSH + NADP^+.$$

At low concentration, most of the H_2O_2 is removed by GSH-P$_X$. This also catalyzes reduction of lipid peroxides and hence prevents the propagation reaction of lipid peroxidation.[95] The ratio of GSH to GSSG determines the capacity to counter oxidative stress. Supplementation of selenium in the diet increases the activity of GSH-P$_X$.

Nonenzymatic Antioxidants

The nonenzymatic antioxidants include those that are water soluble (ascorbic acid, uric acid, glucose, pyruvate, bilirubin, and sulfhydryl groups), lipid soluble (alpha tocopherol, beta carotene, ubiquinol 10), and plasma protein–bound (transferrin, albumin, ceruloplasmin, haptoglobin, and hemopexin molecules).

Free radical scavengers are substances that donate an electron to a free radical thus inactivating the radical species.

Ascorbic Acid (Vitamin C)

During its antioxidant action, ascorbic acid undergoes a two-electron oxidation to dehydroascorbate, with intermediate formation of an ascorbyl radical. Dehydroascorbate is relatively unstable and can be reduced back to ascorbate or hydrolyzed to diketogulonic acid. Ascorbic acid reacts with O_2^- and H_2O_2 and scavenges O_2^-, hydroperoxyl, ·OH, and singlet oxygen.[29] Auto-oxidation of ascorbic acid in the presence of Fe^{3+} and Cu^{2+} results in production of H_2O_2. Agents that retard auto-oxidation of ascorbic acid (e.g., EDTA, citrate, oxalate, histidine, urate, and flavonoids) inhibit production of H_2O_2. Ascorbic acid also scavenges HOCl and acts as an alternate substrate for MPO.[29] Ascorbate peroxidase converts ascorbate to dehydroascorbate (DHA) using H_2O_2. Ascorbate is continuously regenerated from DHA by DHA-reductase, with GSH as the electron donor. In do-

ing so, GSH is oxidized to glutathione disulfide (GSSG) that is reconverted to GSH by GSSG-reductase. Ascorbic acid helps in the regeneration of vitamin E from its oxidized form. Ascorbic acid is both a prooxidant and antioxidant.[107] At low concentrations it is prooxidant but at higher concentrations it is antioxidant.[55]

Alpha Tocopherol (Vitamin E)

Alpha tocopherol is the major lipid-soluble, chain-breaking antioxidant in plasma and cell membranes.[10] It breaks the propagating lipid peroxidation chains by reducing peroxyl radicals to hydroperoxides. It scavenges O_2^-, singlet oxygen, and triplet carboxyl compounds. The alpha tocopherol radical can become alpha tocopherol by reaction with ascorbic acid. Besides being a powerful antioxidant, vitamin E enhances the body's immune responses, inhibits conversion of nitrite to nitrosamine (a carcinogenic agent in the stomach), and inhibits platelet adhesion and aggregation.

Beta Carotene

In humans, beta carotene, alpha carotene, and cryptoxanthine are converted to vitamin A. The carotenoids lutein and lycopene are not converted to vitamin A. Beta carotene quenches singlet oxygen and triplet sensitizers and scavenges free radicals. Lycopene is the most efficient quencher of singlet oxygen.

Ubiquinol 10

Ubiquinol 10 is a chain-breaking antioxidant and free radical scavenger.[29]

Glucose and Pyruvate

Glucose scavenges ·OH, whereas pyruvate scavenges H_2O_2.[29]

Uric Acid, Sulfhydryl Groups, and Bilirubin

Uric acid and sulfhydryl groups scavenge free radicals and hypochlorous acid. Urate also chelates active iron. Bilirubin scavenges free radicals (peroxyl radicals and singlet oxygen).[29,97]

Haptoglobin and Hemopexin

Haptoglobin binds the free hemoglobin released from erythrocytes. Therefore it prevents iron from being available for free radical generation and prevents heme from propagating lipid peroxidation. Hemopexin binds free heme and therefore prevents propagation of lipid peroxidation.[29]

Transferrin and Albumin

Transferrin binds iron and thus prevents radical reactions. Albumin binds copper.[29]

Ceruloplasmin

Ceruloplasmin oxidizes ferrous iron to ferric iron, which then is removed by transferrin.[29]

Other Antioxidants

There are numerous antioxidants of dietary origin that are very effective. Of importance are some components of garlic and flaxseed. Fresh garlic extract and extract-of-garlic tablets provide a potent scavenger of ·OH.[77,78] However, the active principle of garlic (allicin) does not scavenge ·OH.[76]

Flaxseed has recently been used as a dietary supplement for the prevention of cancer and hypercholesterolemic atherosclerosis.[69,81] Secoisolariciresinol diglucoside, a lignan in the meal of flaxseed, is a scavenger of ·OH and O_2^-.[70]

OFRs and Cellular Damage

Free radicals vary in their reactivity, acting as both oxidizing and reducing agents. When free radicals react with nonradical compounds, other free radicals can be formed, thus inducing chain reactions. The initial free radicals produce only local effects, but the secondary radicals can have biologic effects distant from the initial site of formation.

The superoxide anion is not a particularly reactive species but is potentially toxic. It is capable of initiating and propagating free radical chain reactions and damaging cell components by direct and indirect actions. It oxidizes a variety of biomolecules such as ascorbate, sulfhydryl group–containing compounds, sulfite, and catecholamines and can reduce ferric iron and certain quinones. It inactivates the NADH dehydrogenase complex of the mitochondrial electron transport chain.[30] The pronated form of O_2^-, under acid conditions, can oxidize amino acids, fatty acids, and alpha tocopherol. O_2^- generated by xanthine and xanthine oxidase releases lysosomal enzymes from cardiac lysosomes; this release is independent of pH.[38,40] O_2^- reacts with nitric oxide to produce peroxynitrite, which decomposes to produce ·OH. High levels of H_2O_2 can inactivate glycolytic enzymes.[30] Other actions of H_2O_2 are detailed in the previous section.

·OH is a very unstable but extremely powerful oxidant and can interact with almost all biological substrates.[95] It is involved in addition reactions, hydrogen extraction, and electron transfers. It reacts with substrates at or close to the site of its generation because of its very short half-life (nanoseconds). However, it may produce substances that are stable and toxic, and they can diffuse to a considerable distance to damage cells. Toxic effects of ·OH include lipid peroxidation of polyunsaturated fatty acids (PUFAs) in organelles and plasma membranes; oxidation and inactivation of biological enzymes; polysaccharide depolymerization; mutation; and inhibition of protein, nucleotide, and fatty acid synthesis.[95]

Protein

Proteins that contain amino acids with unsaturated bonds or sulfur groups are easily attacked by OFRs and undergo free radical–mediated modification.[95] Amino acids at risk include phenylalanine, tyrosine, tryptophan, histidine, cysteine, and methionine. Enzymes such as glyceraldehyde-3-phosphate dehydrogenase that depend on these amino acids are inhibited by OFRs. Glyceraldehyde-3-phosphate dehydrogenase is essential for glycolysis, and its inhibition results in decreased production of ATP.

Nucleic Acid

Mutation and cell death from ionizing radiation are due primarily to free radical reactions with DNA.[22] ·OH alone has been implicated in causing more than 80% of radiation-induced cell deaths. Cytotoxicity of OFRs is a direct consequence of chromosomal aberrations mediated by scission of DNA strands and chemical modification of the nucleic acid bases.[8] Damage to nucleic acid leads to inhibition of nucleotide and protein synthesis that are essential for production of ATP and various enzymes.[95]

Membrane Lipids

Biomemebranes and subcellular organelles contain PUFAs in their membrane phospholipids, which are extremely susceptible to free radical attack.[22,27] PUFAs react with OFRs and undergo peroxidation. Lipid peroxidation can be initiated by ·OH, the hydroperoxyl radical, and perhaps singlet oxygen, but not by less reactive O_2^- and H_2O_2.[95] Lipid peroxidation is commonly represented as consisting of chain initiation, propagation, and termination steps:

Initiation: $LH + R· → L· + RH$
                $L· + O_2 → LOO·$
Propagation: $LOO· + LH → LOOH + L·$
Termination: $LOO· + LOO· → LOOL + O_2$
                $LOO· + L· → LOOL,$

where LH is PUFAs R· is free radicals L· is carbon-centered radicals LOO· is peroxy radicals LOOH is lipid hydroperoxides LOOL is nonradical products.

The chain reaction in lipid peroxidation and the termination by an antioxidant are shown in Figure 34.3. OFRs attack the double bonds of PUFAs in phospho-

FIGURE 34.3. Diagram showing the free radical chain reaction in lipid peroxidation, and natural termination or termination with an antioxidant (alpha tocopherol). PUFA indicates polyunsaturated fatty acids; R·, free radicals; L·, carbon-centered radicals; LOOH, hydroperoxide; LOO·, peroxy radicals; LOOL, nonradical products; α-TO-H, alpha tocopherol; α-TO·, alpha tocopherol radicals.

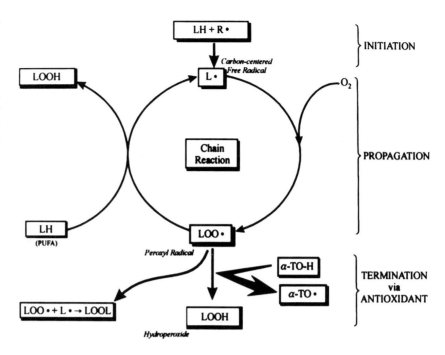

lipids and cause lipid peroxidation. The initiating radicals extract hydrogen from the lipid (LH) and form a lipid radical (L·). This is followed by a bond rearrangement that results in formation of conjugated dienes, which then react with molecular oxygen to form peroxy radicals (LOO·). The peroxy radicals in turn attack new lipids (LH) to form more lipid radicals (L·) and lipid hydroperoxide (LOOH). This propagation reaction can be repeated many times. Thus, an initiation of lipid peroxidation will persist as long as oxygen supplies and unoxidized fatty acid chains are available. Propagation is terminated when two peroxy radicals (LOO·) collide to form a nonradical product. The presence in membranes of chain-breaking antioxidants such as alpha tocopherol interrupt the propagation phase by scavenging peroxy radicals. Oxidized alpha tocopherol can be reduced to alpha tocopherol in the presence of vitamin C.

Lipid hydroperoxides are fairly stable molecules under physiological conditions, but their decomposition is catalyzed by transition metal ions or heme–protein complexes to form alkoxyl and peroxy radicals, which in turn initiate and propagate other chain reactions. The breakdown products of lipid peroxidation, alkanals (malondialdehyde [MDA]), alkenals (4-hydroxynonenal), and alkanes (pentane and ethane), are toxic. They diffuse and cause damage away from the site of production. Lipid peroxides stimulate prostaglandin synthesis by activating cyclooxygenase, control cell proliferation, affect cell growth, and modulate activity of phospholipases. Epoxy fatty acids affect hormone secretion. 4-Hydroxynonenal affects phospholipase C and adenyl cyclase activity, reduces cell growth, promotes cell differentiation, inhibits platelet

aggregation, blocks macrophage action, and is a substrate for GSH-P$_X$.[87]

MDA can initiate cross-linking reactions in structural proteins, enzymes, RNA, DNA, and phospholipids, leading to plasma membrane and intracellular damage. It can alter membrane properties, ion transport, and enzyme activity.[22] It modifies low-density lipoproteins and their route of degradation. It is mutagenic, genotoxic, and carcinogenic.

The potential consequences of peroxidation of membrane lipids include cell damage, loss of PUFAs, decreased lipid fluidity, altered membrane permeability, effects on membrane-associated enzymes, altered ion transport, release of materials from subcellular compartments, and generation of cytotoxic lipid hydroperoxides.

Vascular Responses to OFRs

Oxygen free radicals have varying effects on the vascular system. Those of O_2^-, H_2O_2, and ·OH are discussed here in brief. OFRs generated exogenously by xanthine plus xanthine oxidase, and activated PMNLs increase systemic and pulmonary vascular resistance.[73,74]

Superoxide Anions

Superoxide anions generated by xanthine and xanthine oxidase increase tone in isolated bovine pulmonary artery[14] and rabbit aorta.[6] However, oxygen radicals so generated produced relaxation in dog coronary artery.[89] Kontos et al[48] reported a sustained dilation of cat pial arterioles. A biphasic effect of OFRs, contraction followed by relaxation, has been observed in mouse pial vessels.[88]

Hydrogen Peroxide

H_2O_2 produces contraction[31,85,86] and relaxation,[9,14,99] but low concentrations produce only contraction, whereas higher concentrations produce biphasic effects: relaxation followed by contraction.[5] H_2O_2-induced contraction is completely abolished by catalase and is endothelium independent.[5,6] Relaxation is endothelium dependent and is mediated by endothelium-derived relaxing factor.[6]

Hydroxyl Radicals

Exogenously generated ·OH produces a concentration-dependent relaxation of rabbit aorta.[7] This is prevented by ·OH scavengers, is endothelium dependent, and is partly mediated by an endothelium-derived relaxing factor, vasodilatory arachidonic acid metabolites, and ATP-sensitive K^+ channels.[7] It is of interest that acetylcholine-induced vascular relaxation is mediated by ·OH derived from interaction of nitric oxide (NO·) and O_2^-.[71]

When using exogenous agents to generate particular OFRs, one has to keep in mind that other OFRs are also generated and that the effects could be an algebraic sum of the effects of those OFRs. It is apparent that relaxation is due to ·OH, whereas contraction is due to O_2^- and H_2O_2.

Endothelial Dysfunction and Vascular Responses to Vasodilator and Constrictor Agents

As described previously, OFRs are toxic to endothelial cells which may become dysfunctional or may even be damaged. Acetylcholine produces contraction in blood vessels that contain dysfunctional endothelium or when the endothelium is completely removed.[7,26] The effects of norepinephrine and other vasoconstrictor agents are enhanced in the presence of dysfunctional endothelium because vasodilator substances from endothelium will be absent or reduced and there is unopposed action of vasoconstrictors. This has implications for coronary artery and peripheral vascular diseases. In presence of dysfunctional endothelium, circulating vasoconstrictors have enhanced effects, and the organs supplied by it will suffer ischemic insult. In coronary and peripheral vascular atherosclerosis, when endothelium is damaged, vasoconstrictors have enhanced activity. Vasodilators such as acetylcholine also have vasoconstrictor effects in blood vessels with dysfunctional endothelium. This may be due to damage to the endothelium with inability to produce endothelium-derived relaxing factor.

Peripheral Vascular Disease and OFRs

OFRs have been implicated in various peripheral vascular diseases. Here the description is restricted to only a few important disease conditions.

Hypercholesterolemic Atherosclerosis

OFRs have been implicated in hypercholesterolemic atherosclerosis.[69,72,75,79–81,86] Antioxidants, vitamin E,[72] probucol,[75] purpurogallin,[79] garlic,[80] flaxseed,[69] and CDC-flaxseed[81] have been reported to retard development of hypercholesterolemic atherosclerosis. The atherosclerosis decreases the antioxidant reserve and increases the concentration of OFRs. Antioxidant-induced retardation of the hypercholesterolemic atherosclerosis is associated with decrease in the concentration of OFRs and with normalization of antioxidant reserve. Hypercholesterolemic atherosclerosis and OFRs is discussed further in the section on atherosclerosis and its mechanism.

Hypertension

High blood pressure is often associated with other pathology related to oxidative stress such as atherosclerosis, diabetes mellitus, alcohol consumption, and smoking. Imbalance between oxidants and antioxidants may lead to hypertension. The superoxide anion—a vasoconstrictor—may play a significant role in essential hypertension.[63] The blood pressure of spontaneously hypertensive rats was decreased by SOD. Furthermore, because O_2^- inactivates the endothelium-dependent relaxing factor, NO, it may be responsible for impairment of endothelium-dependent relaxation in patients with essential hypertension.[66] Acute hypertension induced by vasopressor agents is associated with generation of O_2^- at the sites of blood vessels.[103] OFRs have been implicated in morphological and functional damage following acute hypertension.[49,103] Inhibitors of OFRs prevent both vascular damage and functional alterations in cerebral circulation.[103] Pontremoli et al[68] reported a high rate of OFR production by PMNLs on stimulation in patients with essential hypertension. There is an increase in the OFR-producing activity of PMNLs, and a decrease in antioxidant enzymes (SOD and GSH-P_X) in patients with essential hypertension.[90] Sharma et al[93] reported abundant antioxidant activity (SOD, catalase, and GSH-P_X) in the arterial wall of rabbits with early hypertension. An acute antihypertensive effect of three antioxidants (vitamin C, glutathione, and thiopronine) has been reported in subjects with hypertension.[12] OFRs are capable of releasing Ca^{2+} from intracellular stores such as the sarcoplasmic reticulum and mitochondria[65] and are known to depress the Na^+–K^+ pump,[57] with resultant increase in intracellular Ca^{2+} and, hence, increased vascular tone.

Diabetes Mellitus and Hypertension

Association of diabetes mellitus and hypertension suggests a role for OFRs in hypertension. Increased plasma and tissue glucose in diabetes mellitus is the primary source of increased OFRs. Various mechanisms that contribute to increased concentration of OFRs include glucose oxidation, glycated proteins or auto-oxidative glycosylation, and alteration in sorbitol pathway activity.[2,33] There is an increase in lipid peroxidation products in the blood of patients and experimental animals with diabetes.[34,36,92] Oxidative injury may also be increased in diabetes because of weakened defenses due to reduced endogenous antioxidants (vitamin E and GSH).[28] Oxidation of plasma lipoproteins and cellular membranes is associated with vascular disease in diabetes.[92,98] Antioxidants such as vitamin E, SOD, catalase, glutathione, and ascorbic acid are all decreased in diabetic tissue and blood.[41,109] Activity of the antioxidant enzymes has been reported to increase in experiemental diabetes.[36,37] This could be due to induction of antioxidant enzymes as a result of oxidative stress and also related to the duration of diabetes. Endothelium-dependent relaxation is impaired in diabetic aorta.[67] Hypertension in diabetic patients may be due to dysfunctional endothelium, which may enhance the effect of circulating vasopressor agents and also convert the vasodilatory effects of acetylcholine to vasopressor.

Cigarette Smoking and Hypertension

The evidence incriminating cigarette smoking in coronary artery and occlusive peripheral vascular disease is now substantial. Cigarette smoke contains reactive peroxy radicals[15] and can activate PMNLs by directly activating the alternate pathway of the complement component C5.[43] Nicotine enhances PMNL responsiveness to C5a.[101] Kalra et al.[39] have shown an increase in the OFR-producing activity of PMNLs, which is associated with an increase in lipid peroxidation product (MDA) in cigarette smokers. Thus, cigarette smoking would produce dysfunctional endothelium and, hence, may lead to hypertension through mechanisms already alluded to.

Alcohol and Hypertension

There are various possible sources of OFRs from alcohol consumption:

1. *Metabolism of acetyldehyde (a metabolic product of ethanol) by xanthine oxidase.* This is supported by the increase in blood uric acid concentration in primary alcoholics.[82]
2. *Microsomal ethanol-oxidizing system.* The microsomal ethanol-oxidizing system has been shown to be a source of OFRs.[11,47,108]

3. *PMNLs.* The plasma membrane of hepatocytes altered by acetyldehyde has been shown to stimulate PMNLs to produce superoxide anions.[106]

Lipid peroxidation products (MDA,[102] conjugated dienes,[20] ethane, and pentane) in breath[21,61] have been shown to increase after alcohol consumption. Chronic alcohol consumption increases the rate of reaction between radicals and alpha tocopherol, resulting in an increased concentration alpha tocopherol quinone.[42] Animals given ethanol and a diet poor in vitamin E released larger amounts of pentane and had high plasma concentrations of MDA.[54] Chronic alcoholism in humans leads to lower hepatic and circulating concentrations of glutathione.[35,52]

Defective endothelium-dependent vascular relaxation has been found in an animal model of hypertension and in hypertensive patients. An imbalance due to reduced production of nitric oxide or increased production of free radicals (mainly O_2^-) may facilitate development of an arterial spasm.

Intermittent Claudication and Other Peripheral Vascular Diseases

An increase in the plasma concentration of malondialdehyde has been reported in patients with intermittent claudication.[53] For these patients, exercise results in generation of OFRs and endothelial damage.[32]

There is a decrease in the O_2^- production by PMNLs and SOD activity in the blood of patients with venous stasis. This may cause capillary plugging and possibly damage the microcirculatory vessel wall in the venous disease.[16]

There is an increase in generation of OFRs and cytokines during conventional aortoaortic aneurysm repair, but no such changes with endovascular aneurysmal repair.[100] There is a depletion of antioxidants during aortic aneurysm repair.[44] This may have significant consequences because OFRs and cytokines have been implicated in the development of systemic organ failure following aortic surgery.

OFRs have been implicated in the development of lower limb edema after femoropopliteal bypass grafting. Edema was associated with an increase in blood concentration of MDA. Allopurinol (an inhibitor of xanthine oxidase) reduced the lower limb swelling and decreased the MDA concentration.[94]

Aortic cross-clamping may lead to spinal cord injury.[17] Qayumi et al.[83] have shown that OFRs play a role in the pathophysiology of spinal cord injury induced by aortic cross-clamping in animal models. They have also shown that antioxidants (allopurinol and SOD) retard the degree of spinal cord injury following aortic cross-clamping.

There is an increase in the generation of OFRs or a reduction in the antioxidant activity, as evidenced by an increase in plasma MDA levels in patients undergoing iliac or femoral artery reconstruction and amputation of limb at the thigh.[53]

The data to date suggest that OFR levels are elevated in peripheral vascular disease and during peripheral vascular surgery. The use of antioxidants may be beneficial in these disease processes to prevent or treat the disease or to retard the associated complications and those of surgical manipulation.

Acknowledgment
The excellent secretarial assistance of Ms. Gloria Schneider is gratefully acknowledged.

References

1. Babior BM. The respiratory burst of phagocytes. *J Clin Invest.* 1984;73:599–601.

2. Baynes JW. Perspectives in diabetes, role of oxidative stress in development of complications of diabetes. *Diabetes.* 1991;40:405–412.

3. Beauchamp C, Fridovich I. A mechanism for the production of the hydroxyl radical by xanthine oxidase. *J Biol Chem.* 1970;245:4641–4646.

4. Beckman JS, Beckman TW, Chen J, et al. Apparent hydroxyl radical production by peroxynitrite: implication for endothelial injury from nitric oxide and superoxide. *Proc Natl Acad Sci U S A.* 1990;87:1620–1624.

5. Bharadwaj LA, Prasad K. Mediation of H_2O_2-induced vascular relaxation by endothelium-derived relaxing factor. *Mol Cell Biochem.* 1995;149/150:267–270.

6. Bharadwaj LA, Prasad K. The role of oxygen-derived free radicals in the modulation of vascular smooth muscle tone [abstract]. *Proceedings of the 36th Annual World Congress of the International College of Angiology.* 1995;7:13.

7. Bharadwaj LA, Prasad K. Mechanism of hydroxyl radical-induced modulation of vascular tone. *Free Radic Biol Med.* 1997;22:381–390.

8. Brawn K, Fridovich I. DNA strand scission by enzymatically generated oxygen radicals. *Arch Biochem Biophys.* 1981;206:414–419.

9. Burke TM, Wollin MS. Hydrogen peroxide elicits pulmonary arterial relaxation and guanylate cyclase activation. *Am J Physiol.* 1987;21:H721–H732.

10. Burton GW, Ingold KU. Vitamin E as in vitro and in vivo antioxidant. *Ann N Y Acad Sci.* 1989;570:7–22.

11. Cederbaum AI, Dicker E, Rubin E, et al. The effect of dimethyl sulfoxide and other hydroxyl-radicals scavengers on the oxidation of ethanol by rat liver microsomes. *Biochem Biophys Res Commun.* 1977;78:1254–1262.

12. Ceriello A, Giugliano D, Quantraro A, et al. Antioxidants show an antihypertensive effect in diabetic and hypertensive subjects. *Clin Sci.* 1991;81:739–742.

13. Chamber DE, Parks DA, Patterson G, et al. Xanthine oxidase a source of free radical damage in myocardial ischemia. *J Mol Cell Cardiol.* 1985;17:145–152.

14. Cherry PD, Omar HA, Farrell KA, et al. Superoxide anion inhibits cyclic guanosine monophosphate associated bovine pulmonary arterial relaxation. *Am J Physiol.* 1990;259:H1056–H1062.

15. Church DF, Pryor WA. Free radical chemistry of cigarette smoke and its toxicological implications. *Environ Health Perspect.* 1985;64:111–126.

16. Ciuffetti G, Mannarino E, Paltriccia R, et al. Leukocyte activity in chronic venous insufficiency. *Int Angiol.* 1994;13:312–316.

17. Costello TG, Fisher A. Neurological complications following aortic surgery. Case reports and review of literature. *Anaesthesia.* 1983;38:230–236.

18. Egan RW, Paxton J, Kuehl FA. Mechanism for irreversible self deactivation of prostaglandin synthesis. *J Biol Chem.* 1976;251:7329–7335.

19. Engerson TD, McKelvey TG, Rhyne DB, et al. Conversion of xanthine dehydrogenase to oxidase in ischemic rat tissue. *J Clin Invest.* 1987;79:1564–1570.

20. Fink R, Marjot DH, Cawood P, et al. Increased free-radical activity in alcoholics. *Lancet.* 1985;2:291–294.

21. Frank H, Hintze T, Bimboes D, et al. Monitoring lipid peroxidation by breath analysis: endogenous hydrocarbons and their metabolic elimination. *Toxicol Appl Pharmacol.* 1980;56:337–344.

22. Freeman BA, Crapo JD. Biology of disease: free radical and tissue injury. *Lab Invest.* 1982;47:412–426.

23. Fridovich I. Quantitative aspects of production of superoxide anion radical by milk xanthine oxidase. *J Biol Chem.* 1970;245:4053–4057.

24. Fridovich I. The biology of oxygen radicals. *Science.* 1978;201:875–879.

25. Fridovich I. Superoxide radical: an endogenous toxicant. *Annu Rev Pharmacol Toxicol.* 1983;23:241–244.

26. Furchgott RF, Zawadski JV. The obligatory role of endothelial cells in relaxation of arterial smooth muscle by acetylcholine. *Nature.* 1980;288:373–376.

27. Girotti AW. Mechanism of lipid peroxidation. *Free Radic Biol Med.* 1985;1:87–95.

28. Giugliano D, Ceriello A, Paolisso G. Diabetes mellitus, hypertension, and cardiovascular disease: which role for oxidative stress? *Metabolism.* 1995;44:363–368.

29. Halliwell B, Gutteridge JMC. Antioxidants of human extracellular fluids. *Arch Biochem Biophys.* 1990;280:1–8.

30. Halliwell B, Gutteridge JMC, Cross CE. Free radicals, antioxidants and human disease: where are you now? *J Lab Clin Med.* 1992;598–620.

31. Heinle H. Vasoconstriction of carotid artery by hydrogen peroxides. *Arch Int Physiol Biochem.* 1984;92:1–5.

32. Hickman P, Harrison DK, Hill A, et al. Exercise in patients with intermittent claudication results in the generation of oxygen-derived free radicals and endothelial damage. *Adv Exp Med Biol.* 1994;361:565–570.

33. Hunt JV, Smith CCT, Wolff SP. Auto-oxidative glycosylation and possible involvement of peroxides and free radicals in LDL modification by glucose. *Diabetes.* 1990;39:1420–1424.

34. Jain SK, Levine SN, Duett J, et al. Elevated lipid peroxidation levels in red blood cells of streptozotocin treated rats. *Metabolism.* 1990;39:971–975.

35. Jewell SA, Di Monte D, Gentile A, et al. Decreased hepatic glutathione in chronic alcoholic patients. *J Hepatol.* 1986;3:1–6.

36. Kakkar R, Kalra J, Mantha SV, et al. Lipid peroxidation and activity of antioxidant enzymes in diabetic rats. *Mol Cell Biochem.* 1995;151:113–119.

37. Kakkar R, Mantha SV, Kalra J, et al. Time course study of oxidative stress in aorta, heart and blood in diabetic rats. *Clin Sci.* 1996;91:441–448.

38. Kalra J, Chaudhary AK, Prasad K. Role of oxygen free radicals and pH on the release of cardiac lysomal enzymes. *J Mol Cell Cardiol.* 1989;21:1125–1136.

39. Kalra J, Chaudhary AK, Prasad K. Increased production of oxygen free radicals in cigarette smokers. *Int J Exp Pathol.* 1991;72:1–7.

40. Kalra J, Lautner D, Massey L, et al. Oxygen free radical-induced release of lysosomal enzymes in vitro. *Mol Cell Biochem.* 1988;84:233–338.

41. Karpen CW, Pritchard KA Jr, Arnold JH, et al. Restoration of the prostacyclin/thromboxane A_2 balance in the diabetic rat: influence of vitamin E. *Diabetes.* 1982;31:947–951.

42. Kawase T, Kato S, Lieber CS. Lipid peroxidation and antioxidant defense systems in rat liver after chronic ethanol feeding. *Hepatol.* 1989;10:815–821.

43. Kew RR, Ghebrehiwet B, Janoff A. Cigarette smoking can activate the alternative pathway of complement in vitro modifying the third component of complement. *J Clin Invest.* 1985;75:1000–1007.

44. Khaira HS, Maxwell SR, Thomason H, Thorpe GH, Green MA, Shearman CP. Antioxidant depletion during aortic aneurysm repair. *Br J Surg.* 1996;83;401–403.

45. Klebanoff SJ. Oxygen metabolism and the toxic properties of phagocytes. *Ann Intern Med.* 1980;93:480–489.

46. Klebanoff SJ. Phagocytic cells: products of oxygen metabolism. In: Gallin JI, Goldstein IM, Snyderman R, eds. *Inflammation: Basic Principles and Clinical Correlates.* New York, NY: Raven Press; 1988:391–444.

47. Klein SM, Cohen G, Lieber CS, et al. Increased microsomal oxidation of hydroxyl radical scavenging agents and ethanol after chronic consumption of ethanol. *Arch Biochem Biophys.* 1983;223:425–432.

48. Kontos HA, Wei EP, Christman CW, et al. Free radicals in cerebral vascular responses. *Physiologist.* 1983;26:165–172.

49. Kontos HA, Wei EP, Dietrich WD, et al. Mechanism of cerebral arteriolar abnormalities after acute hypertension. *Am J Physiol.* 1981;240:H511–H527.

50. Kontos HA, Wei EP, Povlishock JT. Inhibition by arachidonate of cerebral arteriolar dilation from acetylcholine. *Am J Physiol.* 1989;256:H665–H671.

51. Kontos HA, Wei EP, Povlishock JT, et al. Cerebral arteriolar damage by arachidonic acid and prostaglandin G_2. *Science.* 1980;209:1242–1245.

52. Lauterburg BH, Velez ME. Glutathione deficiency in alcoholics: risk factor for paracetamol hepatotoxicity. *Gut.* 1988;29:1153–1157.

53. Ledwozyw A, Michalak J, Stepien A, et al. The relationship between plasma triglycerides, cholesterol, total lipids and lipid peroxidation products during human atherosclerosis. *Clin Chem Acta.* 1986;155:275–284.

54. Litov RE, Irving DH, Downey JE, et al. Lipid peroxidation: a mechanism involved in acute ethanol toxicity as demonstrated by in vivo pentane production in rat. *Lipids.* 1978;13:305–307.

55. Mak IT, Weglicki WB. Characterization of iron-mediated peroxidative injury in isolated hepatic lysosomes. *J Clin Invest.* 1985;75:58–63.

56. Mantha SV, Prasad M, Kalra J, et al. Antioxidant enzymes in hypercholesterolemia and effects of vitamin E in rabbits. *Atherosclerosis.* 1993;101:135–144.

57. Maridonneau I, Braquet P, Garay RP. Na^+ and K^+ transport damage induced by oxygen free radicals in human red cell membranes. *J Biol Chem.* 1983;258:3107–3113.

58. Marklund S. Distribution of Cu-Zn-superoxide dismutase and Mn-superoxide dismutase in human tissues and extracellular fluid. *Acta Physiol Scand.* 1980;492:19–23.

59. McCord JM, Roy RS. The pathophysiology of superoxide: notes on inflammation and ischemia. *Can J Physiol Pharmacol.* 1982;60:1346–1352.

60. Mishra HP, Fridovich I. The role of superoxide anion in the autoxidation of epinephrine and a simple assay of superoxide dismutase. *J Biol Chem.* 1972;247:3170–3175.

61. Muller A, Sies H. Alcohol, aldehyde and lipid peroxidation: current notions. *Alcohol-Alcohol.* 1987;suppl I:67–74.

62. Murota S, Morita I, Suda N. The control of vascular endothelial cell injury. *Ann N Y Acad Sci.* 1990;598:182–187.

63. Nakazano K, Watanabe N, Matsumo K, et al. Does superoxide underlie the pathogenesis of hypertension? *Proc Natl Acad Sci U S A.* 1991;88:10045–10048.

64. Ogryzlo EA. The nature of singlet oxygen. In: Ranby B, Rabek JF, eds. *Singlet Oxygen: Reactions With Organic Compounds and Polymers.* New York, NY: John Wiley & Sons; 1978:4–11.

65. Orrenius S, McConkey DJ, Nicotera P. Mechanism of oxidant-induced cell damage. In: Cerruti PA, Fridovich I, McCord JM, eds. *Oxyradicals in Molecular Biology and Pathology.* New York, NY: Alan R. Liss; 1988:327–339.

66. Panza JA, Quyyumi AA, Brush JE Jr, et al. Abnormal endothelium-dependent vascular relaxation in patients with essential hypertension. *N Engl J Med.* 1990;323:22–27.

67. Piper GM, Gross G. Oxygen derived free radicals abolish endothelium-dependent relaxation in diabetic rat aorta. *Am J Physiol.* 1988;255:H825–H833.

68. Pontremoli S, Salamino F, Sparatore B, et al. Enhanced activation of respiratory burst oxidase in neutrophils from hypertensive patients. *Biochem Biophys Res Commun.* 1989;758:966–972.

69. Prasad K. Dietary flaxseed in the prevention of hypercholesterolemic atherosclerosis. *Atherosclerosis.* 1997;132:69–76.

70. Prasad K. Hydroxyl radical scavenging property of secoisolariciresinol diglucoside (SDG) isolated from flaxseed. *Mol Cell Biochem.* 1997;168:117–123.

71. Prasad K, Bharadwaj LA. Hydroxyl radical—a mediator of acetylcholine-induced vascular relaxation. *J Mol Cell Cardiol.* 1996;28:2033–2041.

72. Prasad K, Kalra J. Oxygen free radicals and hypercholesterolemic atherosclerosis: effect of vitamin E. *Am Heart J.* 1993;125:958–973.

73. Prasad K, Kalra J, Chan WP, Chaudhary AK. Effect of oxygen free radicals on cardiovascular function at organ and cellular level. *Am Heart J.* 1989;117:1196–1202.

74. Prasad K, Kalra J, Chaudhary AK, Debnath D. Effect of polymorphonuclear leukocyte-derived oxygen free radicals and hypochlorous acid on cardiac function and some biochemical parameters. *Am Heart J.* 1990;119:538–550.

75. Prasad K, Kalra J, Lee P. Oxygen free radicals as a mechanism of hypercholesterolemic atherosclerosis: effects of probucol. *International Journal of Angiology.* 1994;3:100–112.

76. Prasad K, Kungle J, Raney B, Mantha SV, Kalra J, Laxdal VA. Evaluation of antioxidant activity of allicin in garlic. *Proceedings of the International Symposium on Free Radicals in Medicine and Biology,* Chaudhary Offset Pvt. Ltd., Udaipur, India, 22–24 September, 1997. pp. 29–30.

77. Prasad K, Laxdal VA, Yu M, et al. Antioxidant activity of allicin, an active principle in garlic. *Mol Cell Biochem.* 1995; 148:183–189.

78. Prasad K, Laxdal VA, Yu M, et al. Evaluation of hydroxyl radical scavenging property of garlic. *Mol Cell Biochem.* 1996;154:55–63.

79. Prasad K, Mantha SV, Kalra J, et al. Purpurogallin in the retardation of hypercholesterolemic atherosclerosis. *International Journal of Angiology.* 1996;6:157–166.

80. Prasad K, Mantha SV, Kalra J, et al.. Prevention of hypercholesterolemic atherosclerosis by garlic an antioxidant. *Journal of Cardiovascular Pharmacology and Therapeutics.* 1997;2:239–242.

81. Prasad K, Mantha SV, Muir AD, et al. Reduction of hypercholesterolemic atherosclerosis by CDC-flaxseed with very low alpha-linolenic acid. *Atherosclerosis.* 1998;136:367–375.

82. Puig JG, Fox IH. Ethanol-induced activation of adenine nucleotide turnover. Evidence for a role of acetate. *J Clin Invest.* 1984;74:936–941.

83. Qayumi AK, Janusz MT, Jamiesen WR, et al. Pharmacologic interventions for prevention of spinal cord injury caused by aortic cross clamping. *J Thorac Cardiovasc Surg.* 1992;104:256–261.

84. Rao PS, Cohen MV, Mueller HS. Production of free radicals and lipid peroxides in early experimental myocardial ischemia. *J Mol Cell Cardiol.* 1983;15:713–716.

85. Rhoades RA, Packer CS, Meiss RA. Pulmonary vascular smooth muscle contractility effect of free radicals. *Chest.* 1988;93:945–955.

86. Rhoades RA, Packer CS, Roepke DA, et al. Reactive oxygen species alter contractile properties of pulmonary arterial smooth muscle. *Can J Physiol Pharmacol.* 1990;68:1581–1589.

87. Rice-Evans C, Baurdon R. Free radical–lipid interactions and their pathological consequences. *Prog Lipid Res.* 1993;32:71–110.

88. Rosenblum WI. Effects of free radical generation on mouse pial arterioles: probable role of hydroxyl radicals. *Am J Physiol.* 1983;14:H139–H142.

89. Rubanyi GM. Vascular effects of oxygen-derived free radicals. *Free Radic Biol Med.* 1988;4:107–120.

90. Sagar S, Kallo IJ, Kaul N, et al. Oxygen free radicals in essential hypertension. *Mol Cell Biochem.* 1992;111:103–108.

91. Salvador M, Bonting S, Mullane K, et al. Imidazole, a selective inhibitor of thromboxane synthetase. *Prostaglandins.* 1977;13:611–618.

92. Sato Y, Hotta H, Sakatomota N. Lipid peroxide level in plasma of diabetic patients. *Biochem Med.* 1981;25:373–378.

93. Sharma RC, Crawford DW, Kramsch DM, et al. Immunolocalization of native antioxidant scavenger enzymes in the early hypertensive and atherosclerotic arteries. Role of oxygen free radicals. *Arterioscler Thromb.* 1992;12:403–415.

94. Soong CV, Young IS, Lightbody JH, et al. Reduction of free radical generation minimises lower limb swelling following femoropopliteal bypass surgery. *European Journal of Vascular Surgery.* 1994;8:435–440.

95. Southorn PA, Powis G. Free radicals in medicine, I: Chemical nature and biological reactions. *Mayo Clin Proc.* 1988; 63:381–389.

96. Steinberg D. Antioxidants and atherosclerosis. A current assessment. *Circulation.* 1991;84:1420–1425.

97. Stocker R, Ames B. Potential role of conjugated bilirubin and copper in the metabolism of lipid peroxides in bile. *Proc Natl Acad Sci U S A.* 1987;84:8130–8134.

98. Stringer MD, Gorg PG, Freeman A, et al. Lipid peroxides and atherosclerosis. *Br Med J.* 1989;298:281–284.

99. Thomas G, Ranwell P. Induction of vascular relaxation by hydrogen peroxides. *Biochem Biophys Res Commun.* 1986;139:102–108.

100. Thompson MM, Nasim A, Sayers RD, et al. Oxygen free radical and cytokines generation during endovascular and conventional aneurysm repair. *Eur J Vasc Endovasc Surg.* 1996;12:70–75.

101. Totti N, McCusker KT, Campbell E, et al. Nicotine is chemotactic for neutrophils and enhances neutrophil responsiveness to chemotactic peptides. *Science.* 1984;223:169–171.

102. Vendemiale G, Altomare E, Grattagliano I, et al. Increased plasma levels of glutathione and malondialdehyde after acute ethanol ingestion in humans. *J Hepatol.* 1989;9:359–365.

103. Wei EP, Kontos HA, Christman CW, et al. Superoxide generation and reversal of acetylcholine-induced cerebral arteriolar dilation after acute hypertension. *Circ Res.* 1985;57:781–787.

104. Weiss SJ. Tissue destruction by neutrophils. *N Engl J Med.* 1989;320:365–376.

105. Weiss SJ, Test ST, Eckmann CM, et al. Brominating oxidants generated by human eosinophils. *Science.* 1986;234:200–203.

106. Williams AJK, Barry RE. Superoxide anion production and degranulation of rat neutrophils in response to acetaldehyde-altered liver cell membranes. *Clin Sci.* 1986;71:313–318.

107. Wills ED. Effects of iron overload on lipid peroxide formation and oxidative demethylation by the liver endoplasmic reticulum. *Biochem Pharmacol.* 1972;21:239–247.

108. Winston GW, Cederbaum AI. A correlation between hydroxyl radical generation and ethanol oxidation by liver, lung and kidney microsomes. *Biochem Pharmacol.* 1982;31:2031–2037.

109. Wohaeib SA, Godin DV. Alteration in free radical tissue defense mechanisms in streptozotocin-induced diabetes in rat. Effect of insulin treatment. *Diabetes.* 1987;36:1014–1018.

35

Regulation of Vascular Tone and Capillary Perfusion

Silvia Bertuglia, Antonio Colantuoni, and Marcos Intaglietta

The regulation of tissue perfusion takes place in the microcirculation, where the delivery of blood is controlled at the level of arterioles. These vessels contract and relax over a wide range of luminal dimensions; this property, termed *tone*, constitutes the primary mechanism for the control of blood flow in the peripheral circulation. This active diameter variability is due to smooth muscle present in the arteriolar wall that responds to differentiated stimuli, namely (1) a pressure-dependent response termed *myogenic* property, (2) a neural mechanism due to the activity of the autonomic nervous system, (3) a hormonal mechanism due to circulating hormones, (4) a local metabolic regulation, (5) endothelial products, and (6) flow-mediated diameter variability.

Summation of all or some of these arterial tone modulators sets a microvascular perfusion pressure that maintains fluid balance and results in a level of capillary perfusion that meets tissue metabolic demand. That homeostatic mechanisms are wholly dependent on a single mechanical event, namely varying smooth muscle cell tension and therefore arteriolar diameter, suggests that the level of tone prevailing at any given physiological or pathophysiological condition is a complex function of many variables. To the extent that tissue perfusion is a variable controlled by arteriolar tone, and also a signal that influences tone, it is apparent that tissue perfusion and arteriolar tone must ultimately be analyzed as a whole.

Capillary perfusion has been considered the passive consequence of events occurring in the arterioles. This view was largely supported by the assumption that capillaries do not have anatomical components endowed with contractility and therefore would be unable to control their diameter. Recent studies showed that endothelial cells possess contractile fibers and regulate their volume in response to physicochemical stimuli.[16] Furthermore, growing evidence suggests that they respond to changes in blood pressure so that capillary diameter

decreases during hypotension to the extent that red blood cell transit is inhibited.[74]

Arteriolar tone modulation and the consequent regulation of capillary perfusion is the normal physiological mechanism that ensures fulfillment of the metabolic need in the different organs. This process results from a condition of balance between different mechanisms that act on the arteriolar wall; the balance is disrupted in pathophysiological conditions and, unless reestablished, leads to the demise of the tissue. Therefore, it becomes critically important to consider the different aspects of blood flow regulation in the tissue when dealing with diseased conditions; therapeutic interventions can thus lead to a positive outcome instead of reenforcing potentially negative feedback mechanisms whose presence is intrinsic to the existence of such a multitude of phenomena aimed at controlling tissue perfusion.

Myogenic Mechanism

Although many mechanisms exist to ensure that blood flow matches the tissue demand for oxygen, there is also a form of regulation that maintains constant blood flow in the presence of varying arterial blood pressure, a process termed *autoregulation*. This process, present in virtually all tissues, and in organs such as brain, kidney, and myocardium and skeletal muscle at rest, is able to maintain constant blood flow over a range of perfusion pressures ranging from 50 to 150 mm Hg. Mechanisms proposed to drive autoregulation have been explained in terms of metabolic and myogenic factors. According to the metabolic theory, fluctuations in blood flow due to varying arterial pressure cause the change of concentration of vasoactive materials present in the tissue, which affects vascular tone. The difficulty with this explanation is that in some tissues autoregulation is so strong and rapid that flow changes are virtually nonexistent, even with substantial pressure variations. This mechanism thus requires a very high sensitivity of the vasculature to vasoactive metabolites, an effect that has not been observed.[35] Furthermore, such a metabolic mechanism requires that information be transmitted to vessels upstream from the point of release of the metabolites.

A control mechanism based on sensing blood pressure rather than flow-dependent effects could provide a more direct input for autoregulation. Such a mechanism is present, to varying degrees, in virtually all blood vessels, because they show a contractile response in reaction to increased vascular pressure and vice versa. This phenomenon was first described in 1852 by Jones,[63] who reported that bat wing venular contractile activity increased with increasing pressure. In 1902 Bayliss[6] introduced the myogenic concept as a drive for the autoregulation process on the basis of experiments carried out with isolated arteries; he drew a parallel with the contractile response to stretch found in other muscles. That reduction of ambient pressure around the limbs leads to sustained vasoconstriction, a situation that does not involve flow or metabolic changes, is conclusive proof of the existence of pressure-sensitive control of vessel caliber.[62]

For an autoregulatory mechanism to be operational, it must be activated under both decreased and increased pressure conditions, which implicitly requires that blood vessels be able to contract and relax. Consequently, we may assume that in the normal basal condition, blood vessels are at an intermediate state of contraction, implying that the vessel wall is under a basal state of tension or tone. Folkow[39] demonstrated that complete denervation of blood vessels did not abolish vascular tone, which suggests that basal tone is in part a consequence of intravascular pressure.

It is difficult to conceive of a system in which all functions are regulated so precisely that metabolism, flow, and pressure are optimally related over time. When we observe microcirculation in a tissue whose macroscopic blood flow is constant, the pattern of blood flow is continuously variable. Such a variability is more readily explained in terms of a myogenic process in which vasoconstriction of feed vessels causes vasodilatation in the daughter vessel because local blood pressure is reduced in the latter. Conversely, in a metabolic scheme of regulation, signals that lead to vessel constriction should cause a compensatory increase in diameter (or flow) in neighboring vessels. The metabolite related to conditions that lead to a local decrease in flow must thus cause an opposite effect when reaching a different vessel. Such a process would also require the release of a vasoconstricting flow-dependent metabolite whose existence is still under debate.

Steady Versus Oscillatory Myogenic Control

Both in vivo and in vitro studies show that resting basal tone is primarily of myogenic origin and results from stretch of the vessel wall.[81] This property is characteristic of resistance vessels[50,81,89] and is not evident in arteries, veins, or capillaries. Myogenic tone is steady in the larger vessels, becomes time dependent, and causes oscillatory and random patterns of diameter variation in the smallest arterioles, giving rise to the phenomenon of vasomotion (i.e., the rhythmic contraction and relaxation of arterioles). Oscillatory tone is also found in the experimental studies of larger vessels such as the hamster aorta and rat portal vein, but this activity has not been reported in the intact animal.[89,112]

In most tissues oscillatory tone is characteristic of arterioles. Larger vessels with a diameter on the order of 50 to 100 μm exhibit luminal contraction and relaxation at a frequency of two to three cycles per minute and amplitude oscillation of 10% to 20% of mean diameter. The activity becomes progressively faster and of a greater relative amplitude as vessel diameter decreases, and in the terminal arterioles frequency is 10 to 25 cycles per minute and amplitude can be 100% of mean diameter; these factors lead to the periodic opening and closing of the vessels.[28]

Periodic contraction and relaxation of the vessel wall originates from the intrinsic ability of smooth muscle cells to become periodically depolarized. This electrical event appears to propagate and through the phenomenon of frequency entrapment[105] synchronizes the activity of groups of cells located predominantly at arteriolar bifurcations. These cells act as pacemakers for periodic vessel wall motion[30,80] and cause waves of contraction and relaxation to move along the microvessels. The pacemaker mechanism has been shown to be omnipresent, although it may not always engage the contractile system of smooth muscle, because lowered local arterial pressure and decreased vessel tone, due to the myogenic response, translate into the appearance of periods of impeded contraction in skeletal muscle terminal arterioles.[79]

Myogenic Tone and Reactivity

The condition of sustained constriction present in blood vessels that allows them to dilate following a decrease in intraluminal pressure is termed *basal tone*. However, this steady-state condition is not the necessary consequence or identical to the mechanism underlying the response of vascular smooth muscle to a stretch input, which is termed *myogenic reactivity*. This difference becomes evident in studying isolated vessels that react to the sudden increase in distension with the development of force over some time; this phenomenon underlies basal or intrinsic tone and is stable for hours.

Myogenic tone is the direct consequence of calcium influx, as shown by the fact that a calcium-free environment or calcium channel blockers lead to the disappearance of tone. Conversely, myogenic reactivity is modulated by special stretch-dependent calcium channels present in the smooth muscle cell membrane.[11] Basal tone does not appear to be endothelium dependent because it is present in denuded vessels.[67] This independence, however, cannot be asserted for myogenic reactivity, because the endothelium is sensitive to the difference between steady and pulsatile pressure, as evidenced by its production of prostacyclin,[41] and consequently exhibits some degree of pressure sensitivity. The experimental evidence, however, is inconclusive and appears to depend in part on the technique used to remove or inactivate the endothelium.[91]

Neural Mechanism

The central nervous system controls the diameter of larger arterioles and the tone of smooth muscle cells through sympathetic vasoconstrictor fibers that maintain systemic blood pressure by modulating vascular resistance. Sympathetic fibers invest the aorta, large and small arteries, and, to a variable degree, the network of arteriolar vessels.[112] In some tissues, such as skeletal muscle, skin, stomach, intestine, liver, salivary glands, and kidney, most of the arterial network is well innervated. There is no direct innervation of the capillary network. Sympathetic fibers are usually superimposed on the smooth muscle cells: catecholamines are released from varicosities in the nerve fiber and into the vicinity of smooth muscle cells.

Norepinephrine and epinephrine produce their effects by activating α- and β-adrenoceptors on target tissue. These receptors can be further subdivided into α_{1A}, α_{1B}, α_{1C}, α_{2A}, α_{2B}, and α_{2C} and β_1, β_2, and β_3 based on their affinities for selective agonists and antagonists.[68] The action of neurotransmitters begins with their interaction with specific receptors located in plasma membranes. Such interaction initiates a complex series of membrane processes that leads to the generation of intracellular signals or to changes in ionic conductance. Two signal transduction systems have received considerable attention in recent years: adenylate cyclase and phosphoinositide calcium signaling.[13,58]

In most blood vessels innervated by sympathetic neurons, norepinephrine activates postjunctional α-adreno- ceptors. Arterioles generally respond to the sympathetic transmitter norepinephrine with vasoconstriction, and innervation appears to be extended down to the terminal arterioles in some microvascular network. In general, the level of sympathetic discharge sets the state of vascular smooth muscle contraction (basal tone) and hence vascular resistance,[90] which is also modulated by circulating and local vasoactive influences (e.g., endothelial-derived relaxant factor [EDRF], endothelin, and vasoactive substances released from parenchymal cells) and myogenic tone.[15,89]

Most vascular smooth muscle contains both α_1- and α_2-adrenoceptor subtypes, with the exception of the cerebral circulation, in which α_2-adrenoceptors predominate over α_1-adrenoceptors.[68] Intracellular calcium availability is fundamental to smooth muscle contraction, and α-adrenoceptors are linked to membrane channels that regulate this availability. Voltage-dependent Ca^{2+} channels, the L-type Ca^{2+} channels, are involved in excitation contraction coupling in vascular smooth muscle.[76,87] However, these channels, which are particularly sensitive to calcium channel blockers,[21] are opened by various constrictor substances such as angiotensin II and norepinephrine. Therefore depolarization is not obligatory for calcium influx, and contraction can occur independently of voltage change. The latter occurrence has been termed *pharmacomechanical coupling* to distinguish it from *electromechanical coupling*, which describes contractions associated with membrane depolarization. Despite the explosion of knowledge, we are probably at the beginning in the quest to understand the properties and modulation of smooth muscle calcium channels.

The α_1-adrenoceptor mechanism is through G protein regulation of phosphatidylinositol 4,5-bisphosphate (PIP_2) hydrolysis. The initial hormone-binding mechanism that generates the second messenger adenosine $3',5'$-cyclic adenosine monophosphate (cAMP) is modulated, in stimulatory and inhibitory fashions, by the proteins G_s and G_i. α_1-Adrenoceptors increase intracellular calcium concentration. The mechanism of signal transduction of α_2-adrenoceptors differs from that of α_1-adrenoceptors. α_2-Adrenoceptors are modulated by guanine nucleotides coupled to adenylate cyclase.[17,20,98] Activation of the receptor results in inhibition of adenylate cyclase and a fall in cAMP levels.

All three β-adrenoceptor subtypes appear to be linked to adenylate cyclase activation through a stimulatory G protein. The stimulation of β-adrenergic receptors and cAMP and the increase in amplitude of L-type Ca^{2+} channel activity in vascular smooth muscle is still controversial.[87] β-Adrenoceptors invariably determine relaxation of vascular smooth muscle and have been found in arterioles and venules of many microvascular networks. β_1-Adrenoceptors predominate in coronary smooth muscle, and β_2-adrenoceptors are more common in systemic vessels.[112]

Cholinergic sympathetic vasodilator fibers that supply resistance vessels of skeletal muscle and the coronary system are present in rats, primates, and humans.[111] However, whether acetylcholine released from postganglionic sympathetic terminals in small arteries that supply skeletal muscle acts by activating postjunctional muscarinic receptors or prejunctional receptors located on noradrenergic terminals is still debated. From a functional point of view, it appears that cholinergic nerves are usually inactive and increase blood flow during exercise. They become functional after stimulation of hypothalamic areas that produce defense reactions or in anticipation of muscular exercise.

Parasympathetic nerves are known to supply arterioles of different organs including brain, erectile tissue of the genitalia, and various glands in the gastrointestinal tract. The vasodilative effects of these fibers do not appear to participate in significant homeostatic reflexes.

Hormonal Mechanism

Circulating hormones may induce vasodilation, vasoconstriction, or sometimes both, depending on their concentration. These systemic hormones are released into the circulation by homeostatic reflexes. They are represented by catecholamines, the renin–angiotensin system, vasopressin, and atrial natriuretic peptide.

Catecholamines such as norepinephrine and epinephrine are released from the adrenal medulla, and norepinephrine is released predominantly by postganglionic adrenergic neurons. The level of circulating epinephrine is increased during stress, exercise, hyperthermia, and hypoglycemia. In organs with arterioles that contain β_2-adrenoceptors, the effect of epinephrine is predominantly vasodilation.[25]

The renin–angiotensin system has become established as an endocrine system that plays an important role in the physiological regulation of cardiovascular, renal, endocrine, and other functions. Recent studies have suggested the existence of a vascular wall renin–angiotensin system independent of the renal baroreceptor system.[99] Vascular renin may originate from uptake of circulating renin, uptake and subsequent activation of inactive renin by endothelial cells, or local synthesis in endothelial or vascular smooth muscle cells. Renin is contained within the secretory granules of juxtaglomerular cells, located near the glomerular end of the renal afferent arteriole. Angiotensin II is a potent vasoconstrictor, formed in the plasma when the proteolytic enzyme renin (which is released from the kidney) acts on angiotensinogen in the plasma to release angiotensin I. In the pulmonary circulation, angiotensin I is cleaved by angiotensin-converting enzyme to generate angiotensin II. Endothelial cells, which have been shown to synthesize and express angiotensin-converting enzyme, are thus important participants in the regulation of vasomotor tone. Angiotensin II constricts arterioles to cause an increase in total peripheral resistance and arterial blood pressure. In the vessel wall the binding of angiotensin II is highly specific, reversible, saturable, and of high affinity. Angiotensin II determines the coupling of the receptor with an inhibitory guanine nucleotide–regulatory protein, similar to that described for α_2-adrenoceptors, that inhibits adenylate cyclase. In vascular smooth muscle cells, inositol 1,4,5-triphosphate is thought to initiate cellular responses to angiotensin II and thus induce vasoconstriction.

The actions of angiotensin II on the brain, sympathetic ganglia, adrenal medulla, and sympathetic nerve endings to enhance sympathetic activity may contribute to the pressor response to the peptide. Renin release and sympathetic discharge are both increased in hypotensive and hypovolemic states; the former results in part from increases in renal sympathetic nerve activity and circulating catecholamine levels. In contrast to its direct vasoconstrictor effect, angiotensin II can induce vasodilation of renal and cerebral arteries, an effect apparently mediated by prostacyclins.

The neurohormone vasopressin, or antidiuretic hormone, is released from the posterior lobe of the neurohypophysis of the pituitary gland.[1] Release of vasopressin is stimulated by a change in plasma osmolarity, which is detected by osmosensitive neurons in the hypothalamus and baroreceptor mechanisms.[53] V_1 receptors present on vascular smooth muscle have been differentiated from renal tubule V_2 receptors.[1] Inositol–lipid turnover and calcium mobilization contribute to V_1-mediated contraction. The occasional vasodilative response may be mediated by a V_2 receptor coupled with adenylate cyclase. Vasodilation may result from the effects of vasodilative prostaglandins from V_1-induced arachidonate release.[33]

Atrial natriuretic peptide is a cardiac hormone secreted primarily by atrial myocytes in response to local wall stretch. Atrial natriuretic peptide elicits a decrease in blood pressure that is mediated in part by direct relaxation of vascular smooth muscle, an increase in salt and water excretion, and an inhibition of the release or action of several hormones, such as aldosterone, angiotensin II, endothelin, renin, and vasopressin.[101] The action of atrial natriuretic peptide on vasculature, kidneys, adrenals, and other organs reduces both acutely and chronically increased systemic blood pressure and intravascular volume. Specific receptors that bind atrial natriuretic peptide are found in many tissues, and there is evidence that its cellular action involves increased formation of cyclic guanosine monophosphate because of activation of a particulate guanylate cyclase.[73] Agents that increase cyclic guanosine monophosphate level decrease intracellular calcium concentration by accelerating cellular calcium efflux in smooth muscle cells.

Many hormones and neuropeptides are frequently coreleased along with the classical neurotransmitters or other neuropeptides.[23] Vasoactive intestinal peptide is thought to be a cotransmitter with acetylcholine in postganglionic parasympathetic neurons of many tissues. It is a potent vasodilator, and like β-adrenergic receptors vasoactive intestinal peptide receptors are coupled with a membrane-bound adenylate cyclase. In some vessels relaxation induced by vasoactive intestinal peptide may be endothelium dependent. Substance P, widely distributed in the sensory nerve endings of small arterioles, has a strong vasodilative effect that appears to be endothelium dependent.

Calcitonin gene–related peptide tends to coexist with substance P in primary sensory afferents. Depending on the vascular bed, calcitonin gene–related peptide exerts its relaxing effects either directly on the vascular smooth muscle or through an endothelium-dependent mechanism.[106]

Neuropeptide Y is localized throughout the central and peripheral nervous systems and has been reported to coexist with norepinephrine in sympathetic nerves. In many vessels neuropeptide Y is a potent vasoconstrictor and may enhance the effect of norepinephrine at the terminal nerve endings.[92]

Local Metabolic Regulation

In addition to neural and humoral mechanisms that regulate the function of the cardiovascular system, mechanisms intrinsic to the various tissues operate independently of neurohumoral influences.[34,60,62] Common examples of local control processes are reactive hyperemia and functional hyperemia.[35] Reactive hyperemia describes the elevated blood flow that follows a period of circulatory arrest. Dilation during hyperemia is preferentially located at small arterioles in which complete relaxation is observed after 20 seconds of occlusion. A graded but less pronounced dilatation that occurs in large arterioles, resistance vessels, and veins reaches a maximum about 120 seconds after the vessel is no longer occluded. The recovery phase is characterized by an active myogenic constrictor component on the arterial side, whose promptness also serves to protect capillaries from excessive pressure load due to the sudden increase in arterial pressure.

Cells have a continuing need for oxygen and also produce metabolic wastes, some of which are vasoactive.[108] It has been accepted that in most vascular networks decreased tissue oxygen tension leads to increased blood flow. Therefore oxygen directly or indirectly contributes to local regulation of blood flow. Inadequate energy production by vascular smooth muscle does not appear to be a factor, and no oxygen sensor for vascular smooth muscle has been identified. Jackson and Duling found that arteriolar responses to oxygen did not depend on tissue-derived metabolites.[59] It was recently found that rat cremaster arterioles constrict in response to increases in oxygen tension by reducing the synthesis of endothelium-derived dilator prostaglandins.[82]

In conditions in which an imbalance exists between O_2 supply and demand, some adjustments may cause vasodilation and thus lower resistance to blood flow. A number of candidates that can be produced locally within surrounding tissues have been proposed. The list includes hydrogen, potassium, and phosphate ions, carbon dioxide, adenine nucleotide (adenosine triphosphate [ATP], adenosine diphosphate, AMP), and lactate. Development of lactic acidosis is essential in performance of heavy work. Hydrogen ions, locally produced with lactate during inadequate O_2 flow to tissues, raise capillary Po_2 and facilitate O_2 diffusion to mitochondria. Increased CO_2 levels have been shown to cause vasodilation in many tissues. However, arteriolar sensitivity to lactic acid is not evident, and this mechanism may be related to a decrease of tissue Po_2. Increased potassium ion and interstitial fluid osmolarity (i.e., more osmotically active particles) transiently cause vasodilation under physiological conditions associated with increased tissue activity.

Adenosine, considered to be a mediator of vasodilation, is formed by hydrolysis of AMP through the action of 5′-nucleotidase.[97] The effects of adenosine are mediated predominantly by extracellular membrane purinergic-type receptors classified as P_1 and P_2 and generally found in the myocardium and coronary vasculature. Adenosine binds to P_1 receptors and activates cAMP to cause relaxation, and adenosine diphosphate and ATP bind to P_2 receptors that are coupled with phosphoinositide hydrolysis. Stimulation of P_2 receptors on endothelial cells results in an increase in intracellular Ca^{2+} concentration and a release of EDRF/prostacyclin (PGI_2), and P_2 receptors on vascular smooth muscle mediate contraction.[88] Adrenergic nerve stimulation causes release of purine compounds in different vascular networks that inhibit adrenergic neurotransmission at the prejunctional level. The inhibitory effect of ATP on noradrenergic transmission is caused by rapid breakdown of ATP to adenosine. The most detailed evidence for adenosine as mediator of blood flow was obtained in the coronary system, particularly during hypoxia, reactive hyperemia, and increased heart activity.[36] Inhibition of adenosine-induced vasodilation in arterioles <200 μm was obtained by blocking large-conductance Ca^{2+}-activated K^+ channels.[18] Adenosine has also been proposed as a mediator of skeletal muscle microcirculation during exercise and in control of cerebral flow.[7,83]

Many hormones are locally active, and their effects are not involved in systemic regulation of blood pressure. Kallikreins are a group of serine proteases found in glandular cells, neutrophils, and biological fluids.[12] Kallikreins release the vasoactive peptides kinins from endogenous substrates called kininogens by enzymatic action. Tissue kallikreins release kallidin (Lys-bradykinin), which is converted to bradykinin. The release of kinins increases local blood flow or may reduce peripheral resistance and lower the blood pressure under particular pathophysiological conditions. Evidence suggests that the kidneys are a source of kinins. Vascular smooth muscle is an additional source of kinins, which raises the possibility that it plays an active role in local blood flow regulation. The arteriolar dilation by bradykinin is mediated by the release of prostaglandins and/or EDRF. The cyclooxygenase inhibitor indomethacin inhibits the vasodilative effect of bradykinin on the coronary circulation of isolated perfused rabbit heart. Endothelium removal from the dog coronary artery affects the kinin relaxation response.

Histaminergic receptors have been identified on vascular smooth muscle; the predominant effect of histamine in vivo is vasodilation.[70] However, depending on the vessel type, species, and concentration, histamine can determine constriction or relaxation by virtue of its direct effect on smooth muscle. Contraction is mediated by H_1 receptors and relaxation by H_2 receptors, the nature of the response being determined by the dominance of H_1 versus H_2 receptor activation. Histamine is an important mediator of vasodilation accompanying inflammatory reactions, presumably because of its combined action on smooth muscle, adrenergic nerves, and endothelial cells.

5-Hydroxytryptamine (5-HT), or serotonin, is both a central neurotransmitter and a vasoactive agent in many microvascular networks.[114] High concentrations of 5-HT receptors are found in chromaffin cells in the gastrointestinal tract and in circulating platelets. Recently $5-HT_1$ (differentiated in five subtypes), $5-HT_2$, $5-HT_3$, and $5-HT_4$ receptors have been distinguished. $5-HT_2$ receptors predominate on smooth muscle cells of arteries, smaller arteries, and veins and induce vasoconstriction. Endothelial cells also present 5-HT receptors that mediate vasodilation. The vascular effects of 5-HT are different according to vessel type, sympathetic nervous activity, and metabolic conditions. In the microcirculation the constriction of venules predominates over the effects on arterioles.[112]

Endothelium-Dependent Mechanism

Since Furchgott and Zawadzki's demonstration of the phenomenon of endothelium-dependent vascular smooth muscle relaxation in 1980, much information has been gained on the pharmacological and biochemical factors that control release and production of EDRF.[44,45] Several recent reviews have highlighted the importance of endothelium in arterioles (10–100 µm), where 50% to 80 of vascular resistance resides. The microvascular endothelium produces many vasoactive substances that help to maintain proper tissue perfusion.[65,107] It secretes relaxing factors such as nitric oxide (NO) and PGI_2 and constrictor factors such as endothelin.[84,85] Dilation by NO is blocked or attenuated by several substances including methylene blue, hemoglobin, oxygen free radicals, and inhibitors of NO synthesis.[91] Endothelial cells are important regulators of all aspects of vascular homeostasis, a process based on the basal release of NO and PGI_2 and the secretion of high molecular weight proteins, such as von Willebrand's factor, tissue plasminogen activator, and cell surface proteins (e.g., thrombomodulin and specific leukocyte adhesion molecules).[47,52,65] The synthesis or secretion of these agents is induced or repressed by a variety of external stimuli that act on surface receptors.[19] In particular, PGI_2 is a prostanoid derived from the action of cyclooxygenase on arachidonic acid. It is released from endothelium and causes relaxation of smooth muscle cells by increasing intracellular cAMP content. Bradykinin, substance P, and adenine nucleotide stimulate formation of PGI_2, an antithrombotic agent that suppresses platelet aggregation.

The transduction mechanisms of receptor-induced EDRF/NO release and/or production are thought to initially involve a guanine nucleotide transducing protein (G protein). NO easily crosses the smooth muscle cell membrane and binds to the heme moiety of soluble guanylate cyclase, thereby enhancing the formation of cyclic guanosine monophosphate.[49,73] Cyclic guanosine monophosphate reduces intracellular Ca^{2+} concentrations, which leads to dephosphorylation of the myosin light chain and relaxation. Deficient NO release is an important contributing factor of vasospasm. In addition to endothelial cells, NO formation has been demonstrated in macrophages, neutrophils, and cells from adrenal glands, the central nervous system, and vascular smooth muscle.[52] NO plays a role in the maintenance of blood pressure and autonomic nonadrenergic noncholinergic neurotransmission.[85] Furthermore, shear forces exerted by the circulating blood induce the endothelium- and flow-dependent vasodilation, an important adaptive response of the vasculature during metabolic hyperemia.[5]

Endothelial-derived hyperpolarizing factor is a yet unidentified EDRF that causes hyperpolarization of vascular smooth muscle.[113] It was described in guinea pig mesenteric arteries, isolated arteries, vein preparations, and coronary arteries.[113] Inhibitors of L-arginine–NO production do not reduce endothelial-derived hyperpolarizing factor activity despite effectively inhibiting EDRF/NO activity. However, depending on the species, endothelium-dependent hyperpolarizations are mediated by the activation of either K_{Ca} or K_{ATP} channels on vascular smooth muscle. Therefore, several endothelial-derived hyperpolarizing factors may exist.[26]

Endothelins, a family of regulatory peptides, were found in at least four distinct isoforms (ET-1, ET-2, ET-3, and a vasoactive intestinal contractor).[22] Endothelin is synthesized by endothelial cells and by a variety of other cells in diverse tissues such as those of the central and peripheral nervous systems, kidney, lung, heart, gut, adrenal gland, and eye. The sustained contraction induced by endothelins in smooth muscle cells appears to be the result of activation of the phosphoinositide–protein kinase C signaling pathway and opening of voltage-dependent L-type channels.

Some endothelial-derived contracting factors appear to depend on the activity of cyclooxygenase. One likely candidate liberated during fatty acid metabolism is the superoxide anion, because arachidonic acid is generated whenever cell membranes are perturbed. These observations imply that under a number of physiologic and pathologic conditions that cause deformation of the cell membrane, endothelial cells may become a source of vasoconstrictor signals.

Cyclooxygenase-independent endothelial-derived contracting factors are present in cerebral, coronary, and pulmonary blood vessels, where acute anoxia increases contraction determined by norepinephrine and serotonin. This contraction is markedly reduced or abolished if endothelial cells are removed. This endothelial-derived contracting factor is different from that released by arachidonic acid, stretch, or acetylcholine, because endothelium-dependent hypoxic contraction is not prevented by inhibitors of cyclooxygenase.

A variety of pharmacological agents directly influence the EDRF/NO system. This includes the semiessential amino acid L-arginine, which acts as a substrate for NO, which in turn protects against damage in ischemia and reperfusion injury.[116,118] Superoxide dismutase, which scavenges superoxide radicals and thus prevents destruction of NO, protects the tissue in splanchnic ischemic shock and in myocardial ischemic reperfusion. Also, NO donors that replace NO are protective in ischemia and shock.[69]

Therefore, the endothelium may modulate vasoconstrictor responses of vascular smooth muscle cells acting as a physical barrier between smooth muscle cells and circulating hormones or causing release of EDRF/NO. Norepinephrine, angiotensin II, and serotonin cause endothelium-dependent relaxation in femoral and pulmonary arteries and veins.

How endothelial cells perceive and transduce mechanical forces is not known, but cytoskeletal elements may play a central role. It is unclear whether the same shear stress receptors transduce rapid endothelial cell signals, such as production of NO, and slower signals, such as changes in cell morphology and proliferation. Between these acute and chronic responses are many interacting components. F-actin microfilaments, through their network of connections to focal adhesion sites, intercellular adhesion proteins, and membrane proteins of the integrin family, are positioned to confer tension to the cell and act as mechanotransducers at diverse sites within the cell.[32] Two transcription factor families are present in the cytoplasm of mast cells and endothelium: Rel-related nuclear factor kappa B (NF_kB) and nuclear factor activator protein 1. Both are stimulated by shear stress; NF_KBp50–p65 complex binds to a recently described shear stress response element identified as a consensus sequence found in several flow-responsive genes.

Fluid shear stress causes directional remodeling of focal adhesion sites that may be associated with protein tyrosine kinase activity.[2] Therefore, endothelium-dependent vasodilation is mediated, at least in part, by a signaling pathway that involves a tyrosine kinase.[86] The endothelium appears functionally impaired in patients with hypertension, atherosclerosis, and a number of cardiovascular diseases that may cause microvascular spasms and abnormal neurohumorally mediated responses.

Flow-Mediated Diameter Variability

Endothelial cells sense changes in blood flow. Hemodynamic forces elicit a range of endothelial responses that regulate tone and vascular structure. Early responses to shear stress include rapid changes in ionic conductance, inositol phosphate generation, guanosine monophosphate concentration, activation of guanosine triphosphate–binding protein, and in some circumstances elevation of intracellular free calcium concentration. The release of neurotransmitters such as acetylcholine, substance P, and ATP within a few seconds of flow causes the release of substantial amounts of the potent vasoactive agents PGI_2 and NO[107](Figure 35.1).

Both EDRFs and prostaglandin metabolites of arachidonic acid have been suggested as mediators of flow-dependent dilator response.[65] Much recent work has focused on the signal transduction mechanisms in the endothelial cells that regulate specific cellular responses to shear stress.[32] Flow-induced dilation ensures continuous regulation of hydraulic resistance, which causes a rapid and immediate response during functional and other types of hyperemia. As a consequence, decreases in pressure in arteries are stable over a wide range of flow rates and optimal organ blood flow distribution is ensured.

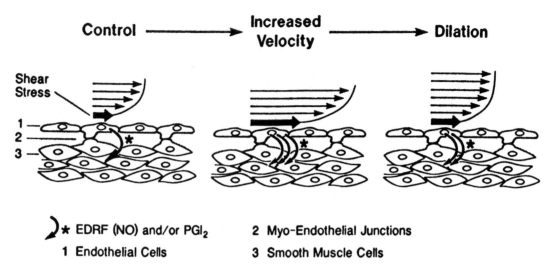

FIGURE 35.1. Schematic diagram of current concept of flow-induced dilatation showing changes that occur during a period of increased blood flow velocity. Under control conditions (left), there is a continuous release of endothelial-derived relaxant factor (EDRF) and/or prostacyclin (PGI$_2$). When blood velocity increases (middle), rise in shear stress of the blood stream acting on the endothelial layer of the blood vessel causes greater release of EDRF and/or PGI$_2$ and possibly vasodilator signals through the myoendothelial junctions, leading to vessel dilation (right) and partial return of shear stress toward control state. NO, nitric oxide. (Reprinted with permission from Smiesko and Johnson.[107])

Coordination of Vasomotor Responses

Because many tissues can vary their metabolism by as much as 10-fold, the resistance vessels must be able to alter their caliber to accommodate a comparable change in flow. Given that the resting nutritional demand is minimal when compared with the maximum metabolic activity, it follows that at rest a substantial level of myogenic vascular tone generates a large flow reserve. This flow reserve is mobilized through inhibition of basal tone by vasodilators, which are now mostly identified with materials released from the endothelium. In this context, Folkow[40] has compared transmural pressure with a positive feedback mechanism in which increased pressure causes vasoconstriction, which further increases pressure. Locally produced vasodilators and lowered Po$_2$ and pH may constitute negative feedback, because decreased blood flow would increase the concentration of chemical factors. Because the ultimate target of autoregulation is the regulation of flow, it is logical to assume that this process entails a flow-sensitive component that modulates or interacts with the pressure-dependent signals.

Evidence for the interaction between pressure and flow signals is found in experiments that explore autoregulation by changes in venous pressure.[3,48,62,64] These studies show that myogenic response is overridden in part by flow-related factors. Because the mechanical effect of flow is shear stress, and the cells affected by this stimulus are endothelial, it would appear that these cells should participate in the myogenic–flow interaction that sets tone. This interaction is expressed as a summation, and substantial evidence supports the concept that flow and pressure effects are sensed by independent cellular mechanisms.[11]

When the microcirculation is analyzed in terms of its branching components, it becomes apparent that there cannot be a unique myogenic response because vasoconstriction, at any given location, will increase pressure upstream. It will thus induce what could be interpreted to be a counterflow-propagated vasoconstriction while lowering pressure downstream and promoting vasodilation. These phenomena can be readily observed in microvascular preparations in which systemic perturbations are induced in awake animals, such as the acute lowering of central blood pressure consequent to hemorrhagic shock.[29] Within the microvascular network there is only one group of vessels that responds in a manner consistent with the myogenic hypothesis, whereas preceding or following vessels in the branching hierarchy present contrary behavior. It is thus apparent that although the myogenic response should have a predictable outcome, it is superposed by vasoconstrictor and/or vasodilator effects spreading from the active site, which are nonmechanical signals.[104]

Experimental evidence suggests that the myogenic response is modulated by changes in sympathetic activity,[61] and therefore the nervous system plays an enhancement role that leads to superregulation of flow. The myogenic control regulates flow, because it is well established that arteries and small arterioles have important flow-dependent diameter regulation. The only circumstance in which well-defined evidence exists for exclusive pressure (myogenic) regulation is in conditions of constant flow, a situation that can be achieved only in experimental studies. The interaction between endothelium and smooth muscle cells during sympathetic activation leads to the summation of effects due to myogenic, neurogenic, and endothelium-derived factors; these effects become the basis for the oscillatory pattern of diameter variation normally seen in arterioles. Therefore, the key component in controlling the time-dependent redistribution of capillary perfusion is related to oscillatory mechanisms generated in the microvascular network.

Oscillatory tone may be a feature necessary for the economic management and regulation of blood flow. Tone per se determines three major homeostatic mechanisms (i.e., peripheral vascular resistance, blood flow distribution, and fluid balance) by causing a single mechanical event—the constriction and relaxation of the vessels whose vascular walls are endowed with smooth muscle.[57] The accomplishment of such a complex process by constricting and relaxing blood vessels is a remarkable occurrence that may not yield the desired homeostatic outcome in all circumstances without additional hemodynamic features. One of these features appears to be the time-dependent pattern of activity of individual vessels whose spatially and temporarily averaged effects yield the required conditions. The time scale over which these adjustments take place must be short and commensurate with the metabolic need of the cells, which may not be deprived of oxygenated blood over periods exceeding their capacity to survive anoxia.

Arterioles show vasomotion that has been described in different microvascular beds, such as skeletal muscle, skin, retina, and mesentery, and in the renal microcirculation. Arterioles show periodic self-sustained oscillation and random diameter fluctuations without any evident periodicity.[8,10,80] The physiological significance of vasomotion is not yet completely understood. Vasomotion may reduce fluid filtration from the intravascular compartment because arteriolar closure reduces distal pressure and promotes fluid uptake through an osmotic effect. The final effect is to reduce the filtration rate relative to that under steady conditions. Vasomotion has also been suggested to promote uniformity in oxygen delivery to tissues by extending its range of spatial diffusion. Terminal arteriolar vasomotion produces a continuous interdependent adjustment of capillary blood hematocrit and velocity whereby red blood cells flow through capillaries at higher than average velocity.[54,56]

Vasomotion causes periodic flow variations termed *flowmotion* (Figure 35.2) that have been observed at different frequencies in adjacent regions of the same tissue.[31,79] The different frequencies indicate that oscillations are not controlled by a central pacemaker. Evidence from experimental animal preparations shows that vasomotion is a local phenomenon, similar to myogenic autoregulation, because different vessels in a network have independent frequencies and phase. Although vasomotion is not centrally driven, central mediation cannot be precluded, because some stimuli produce synchronized vasomotion over large portions of the skin.[102] Reactive hyperemia following the occlusion of a major arterial vessel causes a related flowmotion effect in the human skin.[117] Hemorrhagic shock and hypoxia result in a similar effect in rabbit skeletal muscle and dog visceral circulation when investigated by microcirculatory methods.[115,119]

Vasomotion does not appear to depend on systemic factors, because it is readily observed in isolated vessel in vitro.[100] Vasomotion appears to originate from pacemaker regions within the arterioles, mainly at the bifurcations, and is then propagated to the other downstream arterioles.[30] A high density of voltage-activated calcium channels arranged in a sphincterlike pattern in the smooth muscle cells at the origin of the daughter vessels has been observed. Some investigators suggest that activation of Ca^{2+} channels in the membrane of vascular smooth muscle through stretch (myogenic mechanism) or agonist stimulation results in an increased Ca^{2+} influx. The elevation in Ca^{2+} level can cause the change in the contractile machinery that drives vasomotion. Such systems of branching points of resistance arteries could provide more refined control of the capillary feeding pressure. Studies also show that vasomotion is blocked by calcium entry blockers, suggesting an important role for channel-mediated Ca^{2+} entry.[27]

EDRF/NO is an important factor in the modulation of vasomotion (Figure 35.3), even if the presence of arteriolar vasomotion does not appear to be directly related to its production in conscious animals.[10] However, EDRF/NO plays a role in balancing vasoconstrictor stimuli that arise primarily from the sympathetic drive because it can induce large changes in the vasomotion pattern. Flow-dependent dilation, by modulating the resistance of each vessel, exerts a significant influence on the spatial distribution of blood flow within an intact vascular network and thus plays an important role in the overall coordination of blood flow. Consequently the interaction between the endothelium and smooth muscle cells is the integrative mechanism of vasomotion.

Capillary Perfusion

Blood flow regulation, capillary perfusion, and oxygen delivery to the tissues are intertwined. Blood flow to many organs is closely regulated to ensure that the parenchymal cells receive an adequate supply of oxygen under a wide variety of circumstances, and the same

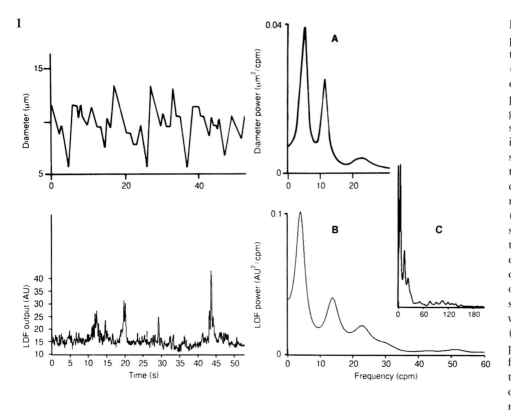

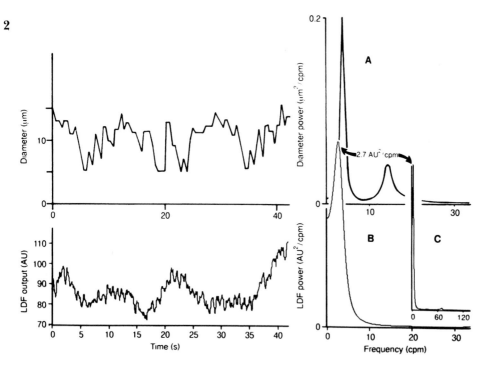

FIGURE 35.2. **1,** In the upper part a typical vasomotion pattern of an order 2 arteriole (according to Strahler classification) and corresponding power spectrum with autoregressive modeling (A) are shown. In the lower part there is a laser Doppler fluxmetry signal derived from a daughter order 1 arteriole and corresponding autoregressive modeling power spectrum (enlarged scale B and normal scale C) under control conditions in hamster skeletal muscle. **2,** In the upper part a typical vasomotion pattern of an order 3 arteriole and corresponding power spectrum with autoregressive modeling (A) are shown. In the lower part there is a laser Doppler fluxmetry signal derived from the same order 3 arteriole and corresponding autoregressive modeling power spectrum (enlarged scale B and normal scale C) under control conditions in hamster skeletal muscle. The fundamental frequencies (i.e., the frequencies with the highest amplitude) were coincident in both examples. Note that all of the graphs are scaled to the maximum value. (Reprinted with permission from Colantuoni et al.[31])

mechanisms also prevent an overabundance of oxygen delivery. Concepts of oxygen distribution to tissue have been dominated for many years by the Krogh model, which considers the capillary to be the site of oxygen transfer from blood to the surrounding tissue cylinder.[66] The oxygenation of the tissue as a whole has been extrapolated from the characteristics of these unitary com-ponents. This analysis leads to the concept of a "lethal corner," the tissue site most distant from the capillary that autoregulation of blood supply is designed to prevent from becoming anoxic.

Capillaries were first perceived as the connection between the arteriolar and venous system. Their role as suppliers of oxygen to the tissue was a direct conse-

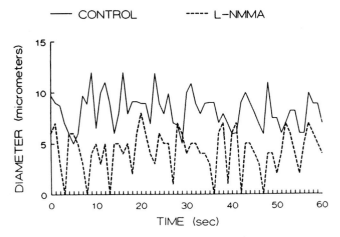

FIGURE 35.3. A typical vasomotion pattern of an order 1 arteriole (according to Strahler classification) in skeletal muscle microcirculation in control conditions (solid line) and 3 minutes after intravenous injection of the NO synthesis inhibitor NG-monomethyl-L-arginine (L-NMMA) (0.3 mg/100 g body weight) in unanesthetized hamster (dashed line). (Reprinted with permission from Bertuglia et al.[10])

quence of observations in the lung, where these conduits were found to be the structures responsible for delivering atmospheric oxygen to blood. Because capillaries were soon also found to be present in tissue, it was automatically assumed that their function in tissue would be a mirror image, or reversal, of that in the lung, namely that of unloading blood oxygen to tissue. This conclusion may be only partially applicable in normal conditions and not viable in extreme circumstances. The lung is the only organ whose tissue is composed mostly of capillaries, which may not be capillaries in the sense of tubes as they appear in tissues but actually surfaces held together by tethers. Thus, lung and tissue capillaries may also have different functions, particularly regarding transmission of oxygen to and from the tissue. Duling and Berne showed that a significant amount of oxygen is delivered from the arterioles,[35] and some evidence suggests that venules serve as sinks for capillary oxygen.[93]

The parameter that characterizes the role of capillaries as a system for the exchange of materials between blood and tissue is functional capillary density (FCD), defined as the number of capillaries capable of red blood cell transit.[9] Although the natural variability in FCD has been established, no systematic attempts have been undertaken to determine mechanisms underlying the fluctuations in the number of capillaries with blood flow. Failure to identify an anatomical "precapillary sphincter" and the notion that capillaries are relatively rigid structures have led to the assignation of control of capillary flow to arterioles, which are presumed to regulate the entrance of red blood cells into the capillary network. The muscle perfusion during exercise "recruits"

capillaries (i.e., increases FCD), but there is no specific information on the state and condition of these conduits when the demand was not present.

From a clinical viewpoint, it is well established that FCD is a critical parameter in the diagnosis of ischemic necrosis and gangrene and an index of chronic arterial and venous insufficiency.[37,38] FCD and capillary red blood cell velocity are also correlated to the degree of ischemia reperfusion injury in different tissues.[72,77,94] This relationship arises because ischemia and tissue reoxygenation during reperfusion initiate oxygen-dependent biochemical reactions that cause endothelial cell damage and lead to capillary blood flow stoppage and the reduction in FCD and tissue perfusion. This process, called *capillary no-reflow*, leads to irreversible tissue damage.[9,78,118]

Mechanisms that alter FCD either have a structural origin related to capillary diameter changes or are due to hydrodynamic effects and flow conditions that prevent red blood cells from entering capillary branches. Thus the reduction in capillary lumen size is determined by a combination of mechanical and cellular factors, with intravascular pressure determining diameter because of the elastic properties of the capillary tissue system. This finding is supported by studies in muscle[71] in which FCD decreases with lower perfusion pressure. Pressure–flow studies in isolated organs show that flow hindrance increases as perfusion pressure decreases, a behavior attributed to shear dependence of blood viscosity and diameter changes in the distensible segments of the vasculature. Edema of the precapillary tissue and cellular volume regulation of the endothelium are additional factors. Some evidence suggests that endothelial cells possess contractility and that this phenomenon has spontaneous dynamics. Consequently, FCD results from passive and active processes present at the level of individual capillaries.

Capillary Distensibility and Decompression

Capillary distensibility was studied experimentally by Baez et al.,[4] who increased pressure in the rat mesoappendix to 200 mm Hg without detecting diameter changes; they thus concluded that these vessels are rigid. Characterization of the capillary tissue environment by experimental and mathematical modeling in the mesentery supported this finding and led to the conclusion that capillary mechanical properties are due to the medium in which they are embedded.[43] These studies were superseded by analysis of red blood cell motion in occluded capillaries due to pulsatile pressure[24] and led to the conclusion that capillaries are distensible within the physiological range of blood pressure manifested in the microcirculation.[54,55,110]

These changes, although small, become significant when the fact that blood viscosity increases sharply in capillary diameters of <5 μm is considered.[103] This phenomenon determines that for human blood the limiting deformation that cells may undergo corresponds to that necessary to pass through 2.8-μm diameter conduits.[51,103] Data on capillary diameter heterogeneity are scarce and limited to small segments; in skeletal and cardiac muscle approximately 10 of the capillaries measured in histological sections have a diameter less than 3 μm.[95] Consequently, this population of capillaries is affected by small changes in capillary pressure. This group, however, does not portray the potential significance of decreasing perfusion pressure, because it is sufficient that only narrow portions in each capillary undergo elastic recoil, or decompression, for the whole capillary to become inoperative. Thus, lowering capillary pressure can significantly decrease FCD solely on the basis of mechanical considerations, a phenomenon supported by experimental evidence.[24]

Endothelial Component of Capillary Luminal Changes

Capillary diameter is also a function of effects in the cellular lining and endothelial volume. Changes in endothelial configuration and particularly volume are present in ischemia and hemorrhagic shock,[46,74] which cause the influx of sodium and water. Endothelial volume changes can be accommodated only by luminal invasion and therefore have an important effect on FCD.

Endothelium has an actin-myosin–based contractile system[47] that responds to mediators that also activate smooth muscle cell contraction.[16] Given an active contractile machinery within the endothelium, we may assume that tone is also a factor in these cells and therefore the capillaries may exhibit this property to a varying degree in normal conditions.[15,16]

The importance of cellular events that regulate the volume and shape of the endothelium is apparent when analyzing hemorrhagic shock, ischemia, and reperfusion injury, which lower FCD. Electron microscopy studies and direct in vivo observations of single capillaries during control and in reduced- or no-flow conditions show that the capillary lumen is reduced whereas the interstitium is unaltered. This phenomenon is attributed to the alteration in cell volume regulation. In ischemia the process is sporadic, with swollen cells interspersed among normal cells.[46] In shock there is a more uniform thickening of the endothelium.[96] This latter response is also present when endothelial cell cultures are subjected to osmotic transients.[75]

Capillary Hemodynamics and FCD

FCD changes are also temporary in nature and encompass naturally occurring flow cessation due to vasomo-

tion. Furthermore, a capillary does not necessarily need to be occluded to be nonfunctional (i.e., void of red blood cells) because this situation can result from factors that prevent red blood cells from entering a capillary. Bifurcating tubes with flow divide the incoming stream into daughter conduits in an inverse proportion to their hydraulic resistance. This process also partitions flow of the parent vessel according to the dividing streamline, which directs the majority of the fluid of the parent vessel into the branch with greater flow. This causes the concentration of blood cells to be greater in the faster-moving stream of the lower-resistance branch. In extreme conditions a very high resistance capillary side branch will receive only the plasma layer void of cellular elements; a nonfunctional capillary is the result.

This hydrodynamic phenomenon is the reason for the decrease of hematocrit in the microcirculation and shows why small variations in capillary diameter due to lowered intravascular pressure produce significant changes in FCD. For instance, a bifurcation with branches of different diameter and length shows a significant increase in hydraulic resistance in the branch with the smaller diameter if the elastic recoil of the endothelium is uniform.[54]

Capillaries respond passively to pressure, distending and allowing for red blood cell flow when capillary pressure is high and vice versa. Substantial evidence suggests that capillaries actively and continuously regulate their flow in a fashion that may be termed *capillary flowmotion;* this regulation corresponds to the presence of contractile fibers within the endothelium.[15,16] Capillaries have been excluded from the process of autoregulation because of the presumed lack of active components. However, they have been implicated in the local regulation of blood flow in response to increased oxygen availability.[14,42] Passive and active control of capillary conductivity suggests the existence of capillary flow functions in addition to the function of supplying oxygen to the tissue.[109]

Tissue perfusion is ultimately determined by the production of metabolites in the capillary network and the parenchymal cells, a factor dependent on functional capillary density. These metabolites regulate arteriolar responsiveness through the interaction of flow- and pressure-dependent mechanisms that modulate vessel tone in concert with neurogenic controls. Consequently, capillary dynamics, integrated with all of the mechanisms that affect arteriolar reactivity, is an important component in the control of tissue perfusion.

References

1. Altura BM, Altura BT. Actions of vasopressin, oxytocin, and synthetic analogs on vascular smooth muscle. *Fed Proc.* 1984;43:80–86.
2. Ayajiki K, Kindermann M, Kecker M, et al. Intracellular pH and tyrosine phosphorylation but not calcium deter-

mine shear-stress induced nitric oxide production in native endothelial cells. *Circ Res.* 1996;78:750–758.

3. Baez S, Laidlaw Z, Orkin LR. Localization and measurement of microcirculatory response to venous pressure elevation in the rat. *Blood Vessels.* 1974;11:260–276.

4. Baez S, Lamport H, Baez A. Pressure effects in microscopic blood vessels. In: Copley AL, Stainsby G, eds. *Flow Properties of Blood and Other Biological Systems.* Oxford, England: Pergamon Press; 1960:122–136.

5. Bassenge E, Heusch G. Endothelial and neurohumoral control of coronary blood flow in health and disease. *Rev Physiol Biochem Pharmacol.* 1990;116:79–163.

6. Bayliss WM. On the local reaction of the arterial wall to changes in internal pressure. *J Physiol Lond.* 1902;28: 220–321.

7. Berne RM, Winn HR, Rubio R. Metabolic regulation of cerebral blood flow. In: Vanhoutte PM, Leusen I, eds. *Vasodilation.* New York, NY: Raven Press; 1981:231–241.

8. Bertuglia S, Colantuoni A, Coppini G, et al. Hypoxia- or hyperoxia-induced changes in arteriolar vasomotion in skeletal muscle microcirculation. *Am J Physiol.* 1991;260: H362–H372.

9. Bertuglia S, Colantuoni A, Intaglietta M. Effect of leukocyte adhesion and microvascular permeability on capillary perfusion during ischemia-reperfusion injury in hamster cheek pouch. *Int J Microcirc Clin Exp.* 1993;13:13–27.

10. Bertuglia S, Colantuoni A, Intaglietta M. Effects of L-NMMA and indomethacin on arteriolar vasomotion in skeletal muscle microcirculation of conscious and anesthetized hamsters. *Microvasc Res.* 1994;48:68–85.

11. Bevan JA. Selective action of diltiazem on cerebral vascular smooth muscle in the rabbit: antagonism of extrinsic but not intrinsic maintained tone. *Am J Cardiol.* 1982;49: 52–59.

12. Bhoola KD, Figueroa CD, Worthy K. Bioregulation of kinins: kallikreins, kininogens, and kininases. *Pharmacol Rev.* 1992;44:1–80.

13. Bolton TB. Mechanism of action of transmitters and other substances on smooth muscle. *Physiol Rev.* 1979;59: 606–718.

14. Bosman J, Slaaf DW, Tangelder GJ, et al. Oxygen tension influences the flow cessation phenomenon and capillary diameter in skeletal muscle capillaries of anesthetized rabbits [abstract]. *Int J Microcirc Clin Exp.* 1992;11(suppl 1):42.

15. Boswell CA, Joris I, Majno G. The concept of cellular tone: reflection on the endothelium, fibroblasts, and smooth muscle cells. *Perspect Biol Med.* 1992;36:79–86.

16. Boswell CA, Majno G, Joris I, et al. Acute endothelial cell contraction in vitro: a comparison with fibroblasts and smooth muscle cells. *Microvasc Res.* 1992;43:178–191.

17. Brown AM, Birnbaumer L. Direct G protein gating of ion channels. *Am J Physiol.* 1988;254:H401–H410.

18. Cabell F, Weiss DS, Price JM. Inhibition of adenosine-induced coronary vasodilatation by block of large conductance Ca^{2+}-activated K^+ channels. *Am J Physiol.* 1994; 267:H1455–1460.

19. Carter TD, Hallam TJ, Pearson JD. Protein kinase C activation alters the sensitivity of agonist stimulated endothelial cell prostacyclin production to intracellular ionised calcium. *Biochem J.* 1989;262:431–437.

20. Casey PJ, Gilman AG. G protein involvement in receptor effector coupling. *J Biol Chem.* 1988;263:2577–2580.

21. Cauvin C. Theoretical bases for vascular selectivity of Ca^{2+} antagonists. *J Cardiovasc Pharmacol.* 1984;6:S630–S638.

22. Christie PT, Simonson MS, Dunn MJ. Endothelin: receptors and transmembrane signals. *News in Physiological Sciences.* 1992;7:207–212.

23. Christophe J, Waelbroek M, Chatelain P, et al. Heart receptors for VIP, PHI, and secretin are able to activate adenylate cyclase and mediate inotropic and chronotropic effects: species variations and physiopathology. *Peptides.* 1984;5:341–353.

24. Clough G, Fraser PA, Smaje LH. Compliance measurements in single capillaries of the cat mesentery. *J Physiol.* 1974;240:1–2.

25. Clutter WE, Bier DM, Shah SD, et al. Epinephrine plasma metabolic clearance rates and physiologic thresholds for metabolic and hemodynamic actions in male. *J Clin Invest.* 1980;66:94–101.

26. Cohen RA, Vanhoutte PM. Endothelium-dependent hyperpolarization beyond nitric oxide and cyclic GMP. *Circulation.* 1995;92:3337–3349.

27. Colantuoni A, Bertuglia S, Intaglietta M. The effects of α- or β-adrenergic receptor agonists and antagonists and calcium entry blockers on the spontaneous vasomotion. *Microvasc Res.* 1984;28:143–158.

28. Colantuoni A, Bertuglia S, Intaglietta M. Quantitation of rhythmic diameter changes in arterial microcirculation. *Am J Physiol.* 1984;246:H508–H517.

29. Colantuoni A, Bertuglia S, Intaglietta M. Microvessel diameter changes during hemorrhagic shock in unanesthetized hamsters. *Microvasc Res.* 1985;30:133–142.

30. Colantuoni A, Bertuglia S, Intaglietta M. Variations of rhythmic diameter changes at the arterial microvascular bifurcations. *Pflügers Arch.* 1985;403:289–295.

31. Colantuoni A, Bertuglia S, Intaglietta M. Microvascular vasomotion: origin of laser Doppler fluxmotion. *Int J Microcirc Clin Exp.* 1994;14:151–188.

32. Davies PF, Barbie KA, Valen MV, et al. Spatial relationship in early signaling events of flow-mediated endothelial mechanotransduction. *Annu Rev Physiol.* 1997;59:527–549.

33. Doyle VM, Ruegg UT. Vasopressin induced production of inositol triphosphate and calcium influx in smooth muscle cell line. *Biochem Biophys Res Commun.* 1985;131:469–476.

34. Duling BR. Control of striated muscle blood flow. In: Crystal RG, West JB, eds. *The Lung: Scientific Foundations.* New York, NY: Raven Press; 1980:1497–1505.

35. Duling BR, Berne RM. Longitudinal gradients in periarteriolar oxygen tension a possible mechanism for the participation of oxygen in local regulation of blood flow. *Circ Res.* 1970;27:669–678.

36. Ely SW, Berne RM. Protective effects of adenosine in myocardial ischemia. *Circulation.* 1992;85:893–904.

37. Fagrell B. Vital microscopy: a clinical method for studying changes of skin microcirculation in patients suffering from vascular disorders of the leg. *Angiology.* 1972;23: 284–298.

38. Fagrell B. The skin microcirculation and the pathogenesis of ischemic necrosis and gangrene. *Scand J Clin Lab Invest.* 1977;37:473–476.

39. Folkow B. A study of the factors regulating the tone of denervated blood vessels perfused at various pressure. *Acta Physiol Scand.* 1952;27:99–117.

40. Folkow B. Description of the myogenic hypothesis. *Circ Res.* 1964;15(suppl 1):279–287.

41. Frangos JA, Eskin SG, McIntire LV, et al. Flow effect on prostacyclin production in cultured human endothelial cells. *Science.* 1985;227:1477–1479.

42. Friesenecker B, Tsai AG, Intaglietta M. Capillary perfusion during ischemia reperfusion in subcutaneous connective tissue and skin muscle. *Am J Physiol.* 1994;267: H2204–H2212.

43. Fung YC, Zweifach BW, Intaglietta M. Elastic environment of the capillary bed. *Circ Res.* 1966;19:441–461.

44. Furchgott RF. Studies on the relaxation of rabbit aorta by sodium nitrite: the basis for the proposal that acid-activable inhibitory factor from bovine retractor penis is inorganic nitrite and the endothelium-derived relaxing factor is nitric oxide. In: Vanhoutte PM, ed. *Vasodilation: Vascular Smooth Muscle, Peptides, Autonomic Nerves, and Endothelium.* New York, NY: Raven Press; 1988:101–114.

45. Furchgott RF, Zawadzki JV. The obligatory role of endothelial cells in the relaxation of arterial smooth muscle by acetylcholine. *Nature.* 1980;288:373–376.

46. Gidlof A, Lewis DH, Hammersen F. The effect of total ischemia on the ultrastructure of human skeletal muscle capillaries: a morphometric analysis. *Int J Microcirc Clin Exp.* 1987;7:62–67.

47. Gotlieb AI, Wong MKK. Current concepts on the role of endothelial cytoskeleton in endothelial integrity, repair, and dysfunction. In: Ryan US, ed. *Endothelial Cells.* Boca Raton, Fla: CRC Press; 1988:81–101.

48. Greenfield ADM, Patterson GC. Reactions of the blood vessels of the human forearm to increases in transmural pressure. *J Physiol Lond.* 1954;125:508–524.

49. Griffith TM, Edwards DH, Lewis MJ, et al. Evidence that cyclic guanosine monophosphate (cGMP) mediated endothelium-dependent relaxation. *Eur J Pharmacol.* 1985; 112:195–202.

50. Harper S, Bohelen H, Rubin M. Arterial and microvascular contribution to cerebral cortical autoregulation in rats. *Am J Physiol.* 1984;246:H17–H24.

51. Henquell L, La Celle PL, Honig GR. Capillary diameter in rat heart in situ: relation to erythrocyte deformability, O_2 transport, and transmural O_2 gradients. *Microvasc Res.* 1976;12:259–274.

52. Hibbs JB Jr. Synthesis of nitric oxide from L-arginine: a recently discovered pathway induced by cytokines with antitumour and antimicrobial activity. *Res Immunol.* 1991;142: 565–569.

53. Hirsch A, Majzoub T, Ren CJ, et al. Contribution of vasopressin to blood pressure regulation during hypovolemic hypotension in humans. *J Appl Physiol.* 1993;75:1984–1988.

54. Intaglietta M. Measurement of fluid exchange between single capillaries and tissue *in vivo.* In: Kaley G, Altura B, eds. *Microcirculation.* Vol 3. Baltimore, Md: University Park Press; 1980:393–406.

55. Intaglietta M. Vasomotor activity, time dependent fluid exchange, and tissue pressure. *Microvasc Res.* 1981;21: 153–164.

56. Intaglietta M, Breit GA. Chaos and microcirculatory control. In: Messmer K, ed. *Capillary Functions and White Cell Interaction.* Prog Appl Microcirc 18. Basel, Switzerland: S. Karger; 1991:22–32.

57. Intaglietta M, Richardson DR, Tompkins WR. Blood pressure, flow, and elastic properties of microvessels of cat omentum. *Am J Physiol.* 1971;221:922–928.

58. Ishikawa T, Hume JR, Keef KD. Regulation of Ca^{2+} Channels by cAMP and cGMP in vascular smooth muscle. *Circ Res.* 1993;73:1128–1137.

59. Jackson WF, Duling BR. The oxygen sensitivity of hamster cheek pouch arterioles: in vitro and in vivo studies. *Circ Res.* 1983;53:515–525.

60. Johnson PC. The myogenic response. In: Bohr DF, Somlyo AP, Sparks HV Jr, eds. *Handbook of Physiology. The Cardiovascular System: Vascular Smooth Muscle.* Bethesda, Md: American Physiological Society; 1980:409–442.

61. Johnson PC. The myogenic response: *in vivo* studies. In: Bevan JA, Halpern W, Mulvany MJ, eds. *The Resistance Vasculature.* Totawa, NJ: Humana Press; 1988:159–168.

62. Johnson PC, Intaglietta M. Contribution of pressure and flow sensitivity to autoregulation in mesenteric arterioles. *Am J Physiol.* 1976;231:1686–1698.

63. Jones TW. The discovery that veins of the bat's wing (which are furnished with valves) are endowed with rhythmical contractility and the onward flow of blood is accelerated with each contraction. *Phil Trans.* 1852;1:131–136.

64. Kiel JW, Riedel GL, Shepherd AP. Local control of canine gastric mucosal blood flow. *Gastroenterology.* 1987;93: 1041–1053.

65. Koller A, Kaley G. Prostaglandins mediate arteriolar dilatation to increased blood flow velocity in skeletal muscle microcirculation. *Circ Res.* 1990;67:529–534.

66. Krogh A. *The Anatomy and Physiology of Capillaries.* New York, NY: Hafner; 1959.

67. Kuo L, Davis MJ, Chilian WM. Endothelium-dependent, flow induced dilation of isolated coronary arterioles. *Am J Physiol.* 1990;259:H1063–H1070.

68. Langer SZ, Schoemaker H. α-Adrenoceptor subtypes in blood vessels: physiology and pharmacology. *Clin Exp Hypertens.* 1989;11:21–30.

69. Lefer AM, Lefer DJ. Pharmacology of endothelium in ischemia reperfusion and circulatory shock. *Annu Rev Pharmacol Toxicol.* 1991;33:71–90.

70. Leusen I, Van de Voorde J. Endothelium-dependent responses to histamine. In: Vanhoutte PM, ed. *Vasodilatation: Vascular Smooth Muscle, Peptides, Autonomic Nerves, and Endothelium.* New York, NY: Raven Press; 1988:469–474.

71. Lindbom L, Arfors KE. Mechanism and site of control for variation in the number of perfused capillaries in skeletal muscle. *Int J Microcirc Clin Exp.* 1985;4:121–127.

72. Maekiti J. Microvasculature of rat striated muscle after temporary ischemia. *Acta Neuropathol.* 1977;37:247–253.

73. Martin W, White DG, Henderson AH. Endothelium-derived relaxing factor and atriopeptin II elevates cyclic GMP levels in pig aortic endothelial cells. *Br J Pharmacol.* 1988;93:229–239.

74. Mazzoni MC, Borgstrom P, Intaglietta M, et al. Lumenal narrowing and endothelial cell swelling in skeletal muscle capillaries during hemorrhagic shock. *Circ Shock.* 1989;29: 27–39.

75. Mazzoni MC, Lundgren E, Arfors KE, et al. Volume changes of an endothelial cell monolayer on exposure to anisotonic media. *J Cell Physiol.* 1989;140:272–280.

76. McDonald TF, Pelzer S, Trautwein W, et al. Regulation and modulation of calcium channels in cardiac muscle, skeletal muscle, and smooth muscle. *Phys Rev.* 1994;74: 365–463.

77. Menger MD, Sacks FU, Barker JH, et al. Quantitative analysis of microcirculatory disorders after prolonged ischemia in skeletal muscle: therapeutic effects of prophylactic isovolemic hemodilution. *Res Exp Med.* 1988;188: 151–165.

78. Menger MD, Steiner D, Messmer K. Microvascular ischemia-reperfusion injury in striated muscle: significance of no reflow. *Am J Physiol.* 1992;263:H1892–H1900.

79. Meyer JU, Borgstrom M, Lindbom L, et al. Vasomotion patterns in skeletal muscle arterioles during changes in arterial pressure. *Microvasc Res.* 1988;35:193–203.

80. Meyer JU, Lindbom L, Intaglietta M. Coordinated diameter oscillations at arteriolar bifurcations in skeletal muscle. *Am J Physiol.* 1987;253:H568–H573.

81. Mellander S, Johansson B. Control of resistance, exchange, and capacitance functions in the peripheral circulation. *Pharmacol Rev.* 1968;20:117–196.

82. Messina EJ, Sun D, Koller A, et al. Increases in oxygen tension evoke arteriolar constriction by inhibiting endothelial prostaglandin synthesis. *Microvasc Res.* 1994;48:151–160.

83. Mohrman DE. Adenosine handling in interstitia of cremaster muscle studied by bioassay. *Am J Physiol.* 1988;254: H369–H376.

84. Moncada S, Palmer RMJ, Higgs EA. Biosynthesis of nitric oxide from L-arginine. *Biochem Pharmacol.* 1989;3: 1867–1869.

85. Moncada S, Palmer RMJ, Higgs EH. Nitric oxide: physiology, pathophysiology, and pharmacology. *Pharmacol Rev.* 1990;43:109–142.

86. Muller JM, Davis MJ, Chilian WM. Coronary arteriolar flow-induced vasodilation signals through tyrosine kinase. *Am J Physiol.* 1996;270:H1878–1884.

87. Nelson MT, Patlak JB, Worley JF, et al. Calcium channels, potassium channels, and voltage dependence of arterial smooth muscle tone. *Am J Physiol.* 1990;259:C13–C18.

88. O'Connor SE, Wood BE, Leff P. Characterization of P_{2x}-receptors in rabbit isolated ear artery. *Br J Pharmacol.* 1990;101:640–644.

89. Osol G. Myogenic properties of blood vessels *in vivo.* In: Bevan JA, Halpern W, Mulvany MJ, eds. *The Resistance Vasculature.* Totawa, NJ: Humana Press; 1988;143–157.

90. Owen M, Walmsley J, Mason M, et al. Adrenergic control in three segments of diminishing diameter in rabbit ear. *Am J Physiol.* 1983;245:H508–H517.

91. Palmer RMJ, Ferrige AG, Moncada S. Nitric oxide release accounts for the biological activity of endothelium derived relaxing factor. *Nature.* 1987;327:524–526.

92. Pernow J, Lundberg JM. Release and vasoconstrictor effects of neuropeptide Y in relation to non-adrenergic sympathetic control of renal blood flow in the pig. *Acta Physiol Scand.* 1989;136:507–517.

93. Popel AS. Theory of oxygen transport to tissue. *Crit Rev Biomed Eng.* 1989;17:257–321.

94. Potter RJ, Dietrich HH, Tyml K, et al. Ischemia reperfusion induced microvascular dysfunction in skeletal muscle: application of intravital microscopy. *Int J Microcirc Clin Exp.* 1993;13:173–186.

95. Potter RF, Groom AC. Capillary diameter and geometry in cardiac and skeletal muscle studied by means of corrosion casts. *Microvasc Res.* 1983;25:68–84.

96. Quinones-Baldrich WJ, Chervu A, Hernandez JJ, et al. Skeletal muscle function after ischemia: "no-reflow" versus reperfusion injury. *J Surg Res.* 1991;51:5–12.

97. Rankumar V, Pierson G, Stiles GL. Adenosine receptors: clinical implications and biochemical mechanisms. *Prog Drug Res.* 1988;32:196–245.

98. Rapoport MD, Murad F. Agonist induced endothelium-dependent relaxation in rat thoracic aorta may be mediated through cGMP. *Circ Res.* 1983;52:352–357.

99. Reid IA. Interactions between ANG II, sympathetic nervous system, and baroreceptor reflexes in regulation of blood pressure. *Am J Physiol.* 1992;262:E763–E778.

100. Rusch NJ, Hermsmeyer K. Vasopressin induced rhythmic activity in rat basilar artery. *Ann Biomed Eng.* 1985;13: 295–302.

101. Ruskoaho H. Atrial natriuretic peptide: synthesis, release, and metabolism. *Pharmacol Rev.* 1992;44:479–602.

102. Salerud GE, Tenland T, Nilsson GE, et al. Rhythmical variations in human skin microcirculation. *Int J Microcirc Clin Exp.* 1983;2:91–102.

103. Secomb TW, Fleischman GJ, Papenfuss HD, et al. Effects of reduced perfusion and hematocrit on flow distribution in capillary networks. In: Messmer K, Hemmezsen F, eds. *Microcirculation and Inflammation: Vessel Wall-Inflammatory Cells-Mediator Interactions.* Prog Appl Microcirc 12. Basel, Switzerland: S. Kruger; 1987;205–211.

104. Segal SS, Duling BR. Propagation of vasodilation in resistance vessels of the hamster: development and review of a working hypothesis. *Circ Res.* 1987;61:20–25.

105. Siegel G, Ebeling BJ, Hofer HW. Foundation of vascular rhythm. *Ber Bunsenges Phys Chem.* 1980;84:403–406.

106. Skoftisch G, Jacobowitz D. Calcitonin gene related peptide coexists with substance P in capsaicin sensitive neurons and sensory ganglia of the rat. *Peptides.* 1985;6: 747–754.

107. Smiesko NPS, Johnson PC. The arterial lumen is controlled by flow related shear stress. *NIPS.* 1993;8:34–38.

108. Sparks HV. Effect of local metabolic factors on vascular smooth muscle. In: Bohr DF, Somlyo AP, Sparks HV Jr, eds. *Handbook of Physiology. The Cardiovascular System: Vascular Smooth Muscle.* Bethesda, Md: American Physiological Society; 1980:475–513.

109. Suval WD, Hobson RW, Boric MP, et al. Assessment of ischemia reperfusion injury in skeletal muscle by macromolecular clearance. *J Surg Res.* 1987;42:550–559.

110. Swayne GTC, Smaje LH, Bergel DH. Distensibility of single capillaries and venules in the rat and frog mesentery. *Int J Microcirc Clin Exp.* 1989;8:25–42.

111. Üvnas B. (1988) Cholinergic vasodilator nerves. *Fed Proc.* 1966;25:1618–1622.

112. Vanhoutte PM. Heterogeneity in vascular smooth muscle. In: Kaley G, Altura BM, eds. *Microcirculation.* Vol 2. Baltimore, Md: University Park Press; 1978:181–309.

113. Vanhoutte PM. *Endothelium-Derived Hyperpolarizing Factor.* Richmond, Calif: Berlex Biosciences; 1997.

114. Vanhoutte PM, Luscher TF. Serotonin and the blood vessel wall. *J Hypertens.* 1986;4:29–36.

115. Weiner RM, Borgstrom P, Intaglietta M. Induction of vasomotion by hemorrhagic hypotension in rabbit tenuissimus muscle. In: Intaglietta M, ed. *Vasomotion and Flowmotion in the Microcirculation.* Basel, Switzerland: Karger; 1989:93–99.

116. Weyrich A, Ma XI, Lefer AM. The role of L-arginine in ameliorating reperfusion injury following myocardial is-

chemia in the cat. *Circulation.* 1992;86:2665–2674.

117. Wilkin JK. Periodic cutaneous blood flow during post occlusive reactive hyperemia. *Am J Physiol.* 1986;250: H756–H768.

118. Wright JG, Fox D, Kerr JC, et al. Rate of reperfusion blood flow modulates reperfusion injury in skeletal muscle. *J Surg Res.* 1988;44:754–763.

119. Zweifach BW, Lee RE, Hyman C, et al. Omental microcirculation in morphinized dogs subjected to graded haemorrhage. *Ann Surg.* 1944;120:250–273.

Section 2
Occlusive Disease

36

Atherosclerosis

Graziana Lupattelli and Elmo Mannarino

Definition and Sites of Atherosclerosis

Atherosclerosis, a chronic disease of the large- and medium-caliber arteries, is currently considered inflammatory. This process, which begins in the intima, includes (1) focal lipid accumulation; (2) cell proliferation; and (3) production and deposition of connectival matrix, which leads to the formation of the fibrous–fatty lesion that evolves into an atheroma. In advanced atheromatous lesions, not only the intima but also the adjacent media and adventitia are involved.

In the evolution of atherosclerosis four stages can be identified: (1) the initial stage (with intracellular lipids and the accumulation of a few foam cells), (2) the fatty streaks stage (with even more foam cells stratified in layers), (3) the intermediate stage (with extracellular lipid accumulation), and (4) the atheroma stage (atheromas have a lipid core).

In the last 20 years the atherogenic cascade has been identified as not merely a degenerative process but a multifactorial inflammatory disorder that is initially triggered by endothelial injury and that actively involves cell migration and proliferation and the production of substances such as growth factors, cytokines, nitric oxide, oxidized lipids, and so forth, all of which modulate cell functions.[65]

Atherogenesis, in the form of initial lesions, known as fatty streaks, begins very early in life, but related symptoms (e.g., coronary heart diseases, cerebrovascular diseases, and peripheral arterial occlusive disease) do not appear until the vessel lumen is partially or totally obstructed by plaque, which occurs after several decades.

Although the atherosclerotic process is ubiquitous, lesion-prone sites, such as arterial branches and bifurcations in the aorta and carotid, coronary, and peripheral arteries, have been identified. Brachial arteries are very rarely affected. Hemodynamic stresses that reflect the geometry of the arterial system account for the topographic distribution of atherosclerotic plaques.[69]

In the coronary arteries initial lesions, such as fatty streaks, are present even in infancy; after the age of 15 they can be found in both the left and right coronary arteries. Advanced lesions tend to occur first on the left anterior descending coronary artery.[71–73]

Initial lesions are also visible in the aortas of children[78] and tend to increase in number in the descending aorta until the age of approximately 20 years.[21] Advanced lesions are mainly localized in the abdominal tract of the aorta, between the orifice of the inferior mesenteric artery and the bifurcation of the common iliac arteries.[73]

In the peripheral arteries atherosclerotic lesions occur in the aortoiliac, femoral, and more distal segments, such as femoropopliteal and tibioperoneal segments.[18] The carotid bifurcations and internal carotid, middle cerebral, anterior cerebral, posterior cerebral, and vertebrobasilar arteries are affected in cerebrovascular disease. Tables 36.1 through 36.4 show the major clinical pictures associated with atherosclerosis.

TABLE 36.1. Coronary heart disease.

Affected vessels
Coronary vessels

Clinical pictures
Silent ischemia
Angina pectoris
    Stable
    Unstable
Myocardial infarction
Arrhythmias
Heart failure
Sudden death

TABLE 36.2. Cerebrovascular disease.

Affected vessels
Carotid territory
Vertebrobasilar territory

Clinical pictures
Transient ischemic attack
Progressing stroke
Completed stroke

TABLE 36.3. Peripheral arterial occlusive disease.

Affected vessels
Aorta
Iliac–femoral arteries
Popliteal–distal arteries

Clinical pictures
Aneurysm (rupture, thrombosis, embolization)
Leriche's syndrome
Intermittent claudication
Critical limb ischemia
Gangrene

TABLE 36.4. Renal and visceral occlusive disease.

Affected vessels
Superior mesenteric artery
Inferior mesenteric artery
Celiac artery
Renal arteries

Clinical pictures
Acute gastrointestinal ischemia
Chronic gastrointestinal ischemia
Ischemic colitis
Hypertension

Epidemiology

Cardiovascular disease is the main cause of death in the developed countries (United States, Canada, Northern European countries, New Zealand, and Australia), and atherosclerosis is the most frequent underlying disease process. When assessing the epidemiology of atherosclerosis, morbidity and mortality rates for each single correlated disease—ischemic heart disease (IHD), cerebrovascular disease, and peripheral arterial occlusive disease (PAOD)—should be approached from the perspective that atherosclerosis is a systemic disease that affects the entire arterial system. The patient with PAOD generally dies of coronary heart disease rather than gangrene.

The prevalence of IHD in 1985 in the United States was 61 per 1000 for adults and rose to 138 per 1000 in persons over 65 years of age. IHD is still the main cause of death in the United States and is responsible of nearly 520,000 deaths annually, which is more than the total number of deaths caused by cancer. This prevalence is despite the fact that the IHD mortality rate has dropped in the past two decades due to changes in lifestyle (e.g., reducing animal fat intake and cigarette smoking) and

that more effective treatment for hypertension and hypercholesterolemia, which is the major risk factor for IHD, is available.[12,55,82]

Cerebrovascular disease is the third main cause of death in the United States after IHD and cancer; prevalence in the general population is around 4 to 6 per 1000. The incidence is closely related to age and doubles in each successive decade for people over age 55; in the population aged 65 the prevalence is 45 per 1000. In the United States it accounts for 150,000 deaths per year. The mortality rate is still particularly high in Asia and Eastern Europe, but in developed countries antihypertensive therapy has reduced the mortality rate by 50% since 1972. This reduction has been most marked in Japan.[55,79,82]

Data on prevalence and incidence of PAOD are conflicting and depend largely on age, sex, country, and the diagnostic criteria used, either Rose's questionnaire (the standardized Rose's questionnaire defines claudication as exercise calf pain not present at rest that is relieved only by rest within 10 minutes) or the ankle/arm pressure index (which, when below 0.8, is diagnostic of PAOD). Prevalence ranges from 0.4% to 14% if the diagnosis is made with Rose's questionnaire and from 4.2% to 35% using the ankle/arm pressure index.[4]

Some reports show a prevalence of PAOD of 12% to 15% in the population over age 50, whereas in the Basel study incidence of PAOD ranged from 0.6% in younger subjects (age 35–44) to 7.5% in older subjects (age 60–64).[14,77,84]

Risk Factors

Atherosclerosis is not linked only to aging but can be initiated and potentiated by a group of risk factors. It can therefore be controlled and attenuated by identification and optimal treatment of these factors. Cigarette smoking, hypertension, diabetes, and hypercholesterolemia are considered the major risk factors; the largest body of evidence implicates hypercholesterolemia in the development of coronary atherosclerosis.

TABLE 36.5. Atherosclerosis risk factors.

- Cigarette smoking
- Hypertension
- Diabetes mellitus
- Hypercholesterolemia
- Family history of vascular disease
- Male sex
- Abdominal obesity
- Elevated lipoprotein(a) levels
- Hyperuricemia
- Physical inactivity
- Personal lifestyle
- Menopause
- Oral contraceptive use

The subject's family history and genotype deserve particular mention, because many genes responsible for lipoprotein disorders and apolipoprotein polymorphism, which can therefore influence the development of atherosclerotic disease, have been identified. Male sex, abdominal obesity, elevated levels of lipoprotein(a) (Lp[a]), hyperuricemia, physical inactivity, and personal lifestyle are also strongly associated factors (Table 36.5).

Cigarette Smoking

Cigarette smoking is closely linked to atherosclerosis of coronary, carotid, and peripheral arteries and the abdominal aorta.[26,33,58] Smoking is associated with a twofold to fourfold increased risk of IHD; 70% of all PAOD patients smoke, and both active and passive smoking seem to be related to carotid artery atherosclerosis.[37,45]

The cardiovascular risk increases with the number of cigarettes, the depth of inhalation, and the number of years accumulated in patients of all ages.[35] Stopping smoking greatly reduces cardiac morbidity and mortality in both younger and older populations.[35]

Cigarette smoke contains thousands of components, but carbon monoxide and nicotine have been implicated most in vascular disease. Carbon monoxide probably acts as an initiating factor by injuring the endothelium, and nicotine induces platelet activation and adhesion to the vessel wall, thus contributing to lesion progression. Both compounds modify the oxygen supply–demand ratio: nicotine increases oxygen demand by increasing heart rate and blood pressure, and carbon monoxide reduces oxygen availability to body tissues.[45,64]

Levels of high-density lipoproteins (HDLs), which are known to exert a protective role, are constantly lower in those who smoke than in those who do not.[52] The hypoxemia induced by carboxyhemoglobin causes secondary polyglobulinemia, which increases blood viscosity.

Hypertension

Patients with hypertension are at increased risk of cerebrovascular disease and of IHD. Hypertension is by far the most important risk factor for stroke, and its treatment is linked to greatly reduced incidence of cerebrovascular disease. A statistically significant reduction in IHD is less evident, probably because the importance of hypertension as a risk factor for myocardial infarction depends on the presence of other risk factors such as hypercholesterolemia.[38,39,49]

Hypertension itself produces structural abnormalities in the vessel wall that lead to atherosclerosis. Increased pressure stress is responsible for endothelial lesions and also induces hypertrophia of the media smooth muscle cells, which causes their migration from the media to the intima, with a corresponding loss of contractile power. The phenotype of the smooth muscle cells changes from contractile to synthetic, and the cells are transformed into synthesizers of interstitial matrix (e.g., collagen, elastin, and mucopolysaccharides). Moreover, several growth factors such as those derived from platelets, the endothelium, and smooth muscle cells are involved in smooth muscle cell proliferation. Finally, when hypertension is present, lipoprotein infiltration into the vessel wall accelerates and thus contributes to plaque development.[6,20]

Diabetes

Before insulin was available, most diabetic patients died of diabetic coma. Since the advent of insulin therapy, atherosclerosis has become the main cause of death in patients with diabetes mellitus, because vascular diseases, in particular IHD and PAOD, are frequent complications of diabetes. The diabetic patient with PAOD tends to present a prevalently distal atherosclerotic plaque localization in the femoral, popliteal, or tibioperoneal arteries.[18,51,68]

It is not clear whether reduced tolerance of carbohydrates is an independent risk factor for vascular disease in diabetic patients or whether it is secondary to increased lipoprotein plasma concentrations or to concomitant pathologies such as hypertension. High glycemic levels cause apolipoprotein glucosylation, particularly of apolipoprotein B in the low-density lipoproteins (LDLs) and very-low-density lipoproteins (VLDLs). These altered lipoproteins are not catabolized through the LDL receptor but principally through the nonreceptor means of macrophages, which leads to plaque formation.[75]

The lack of insulin in insulin-dependent diabetes mellitus and insulin resistance in non–insulin-dependent diabetes mellitus greatly modify lipid metabolism. Lack of insulin diminishes lipoprotein lipase activity and causes hyperchylomicronemia. Lipolysis is increased, which leads to higher hepatic levels of fatty acids and consequently to elevated triglyceride synthesis. Insulin resistance stimulates adipose tissue lipase and increases hepatic VLDL synthesis because of the excess of free fatty acids in the liver. Increased VLDL production is associated with reduced catabolism (mediated by reduced lipoprotein lipase) and consequently with high triglyceride levels and low HDL formation.[36,60]

Insulin resistance is frequently associated with the atherogenic lipoprotein phenotype. This phenotype is characterized by increased levels of VLDLs, reduced levels of HDLs, and higher density and smaller LDLs (average diameter of 24.8 nm) than average LDL particles. Atherogenic lipoprotein phenotype is associated with a higher risk of myocardial infarction. This small LDL pattern is also called pattern B. In pattern A, which is more frequently encountered in the general population, LDLs are larger and less dense (26.6 nm). The gene responsible for the atherogenic lipoprotein phenotype has recently been identified on chromosome 19 and has linkages with the insulin receptor gene and the LDL receptor gene.[3,22,56,61]

In diabetic patients Lp(a) and plasminogen activator inhibitor 1 levels are frequently elevated and predispose individuals to thromboembolic complications. Similar in structure to LDL and plasminogen, Lp(a) is composed of a lipid core and two protein subunits: apolipoprotein B and apolipoprotein(a), which are linked by a disulfuride bridge.[23] Lp(a) is atherogenic, probably because of its structural similarities with apolipoprotein B (which is found in the atheromatous plaque) and thrombogenic because it competitively inhibits plasminogen–fibrin binding and fibrinolysis.[53] Several epidemiological studies have shown that Lp(a) plays a predictive role in IHD and that Lp(a) levels are higher in patients with ischemic stroke and vascular dementia.[15,81] Elevated Lp(a) levels are also found in patients with insulin-dependent diabetes mellitus but not in those with non–insulin-dependent diabetes mellitus.[13]

Plasminogen activator inhibitor 1 inhibits plasminogen tissue activator, which initiates fibrinolysis. Elevated plasminogen activator inhibitor 1 concentrations may be associated with insulin resistance[28] and are frequently found in patients with hypertriglyceridemia; high concentrations thus create conditions favorable to the development of thromboembolic disease.[30,31,83]

The clinical condition that illustrates the association of many risk factors for atherosclerosis in concomitance with non–insulin-dependent diabetes mellitus is known as syndrome X. Worth noting is insulin resistance clustering with high triglyceride levels, low HDL cholesterol concentrations, hypertension, and abdominal obesity.[60]

Hypercholesterolemia

Cholesterol has long been identified as a risk factor in the onset and progression of atherosclerosis. In the nineteenth century Von Rokitansky believed atherosclerosis was due to lipid deposits on the endothelium and in the intima. Later Anitchkov was the first to observe lipid accumulation in the intimal matrix of arteries in hypercholesterolemic rabbits. In the past decades studies on animal models and genetic, epidemiological, and interventional investigations have clearly demonstrated a cause–effect relationship between high cholesterol levels and atherosclerosis. High plasma LDL cholesterol levels cause endothelial lesions, increase LDL infiltration into the subendothelial space, and thus lead to the formation and accumulation of monocyte/macrophage foam cells that form a fatty streak and stimulate smooth muscle cell proliferation and migration.

Experimental Studies

Many animal species including nonhuman primates develop atherosclerosis if fed high-cholesterol diets. As in humans, hypercholesterolemic animals develop intimal lesions (fatty streaks) that evolve into fibrous–lipid plaques that eventually ulcerate. In several animal species dietary or pharmacological intervention to lower cholesterol levels can cause lesions to regress.[85]

Atherosclerosis regression has been studied extensively in the Macaca rhesus monkey, because its capacity for developing lesions is very similar to that of humans, as are the clinical complications such as myocardial infarction, stroke, and xantomas. Coronary lesion regression in this species was first observed in the 1970s, and recent reports have shown that regression is mainly due to reductions in cholesterol esters and only in a very small part to a fall in collagen and elastin vessel wall contents. Many anatomical changes in plaques have been observed in animals during regression: the lipid content drops, the damaged endothelium is repaired, fibrous elements are remodeled and condensed, and cell proliferation is reduced.[85] In the Macaca rhesus monkey plaques are reported to regress independently of both the hypolipemic therapy administered and the stage of the lesion.

Genetic Studies

Evidence that severe hypercholesterolemia alone causes atherosclerosis of the coronary arteries even in the young comes from patients affected by familial hypercholesterolemia in whom a mutation exists on chromosome 19 of the gene encoding the apolipoprotein B-100/E receptor. In homozygote subjects there is no receptor activity, and LDL cholesterol cannot be catabolized by the receptor pathway. From birth these subjects present high cholesterol levels and even as preschool children suffer from angina and myocardial infarction. If untreated, most die before the age of 30.[27] Although in the heterozygote form of familial hypercholesterolemia 50% receptor activity is normal and LDL cholesterol levels are lower than in the homozygote form, IHD is present much more often in these patients than in the general population.[27] The Watanabe rabbit, which provides an animal model of familial hypercholesterolemia, develops systemic atherosclerosis even if fed a low-cholesterol diet.[27]

Transgenic mice have a human gene that codifies a certain apolipoprotein or the corresponding mutant allele inserted into their genome to provide further evidence of the effects of variations in quantitative and/or phenotypical apolipoprotein abnormalities in the development of atherosclerosis. Examples of transgenic mice include animals with an apolipoprotein E deficiency and high apolipoprotein(a) or apolipoprotein A-II levels.

Apolipoprotein E–deficient mice develop widespread atherosclerotic lesions localized in the aorta and proximal coronary, carotid, mesenteric, renal, and femoral arteries. Apolipoprotein A-II and apolipoprotein(a) transgenic mice have an increased susceptibility to atherosclerosis; in apolipoprotein(a) mice this atherosclerosis is usually localized in the aortic sinus.[8,29]

Epidemiological Studies

International epidemiological studies have shown that high cholesterol levels are strongly linked with and are predictive of IHD.[1,40,41,50] The Multiple Risk Factor Intervention Trial[70] observed a population of 350,000 for more than 6 years. When divided on the basis of cholesterol levels the mortality rate for IHD was observed to rise constantly with each quintile, reaching its maximum with the passage from the fourth to the fifth quintile. The correlation between cholesterol levels and IHD is constant and progressive, with no plateau or risk threshold. In other words, the lower the cholesterol levels, the lower the risk of IHD.

Interventional Studies

Since the 1970s diets and hypolipemic agents have been tested in an attempt to reduce morbidity and mortality rates for IHD. Depending on whether patients are affected by IHD at enrollment, interventional studies are classified as primary or secondary. Meta-analysis of approximately 20 primary prevention trials has concluded that reducing total cholesterol and LDL cholesterol levels is associated with approximately a 9% reduction in the risk of fatal myocardial infarction and a 19% drop in the risk of nonfatal infarction.[1,24,44] The results of secondary prevention trials indicate that aggressive hypolipemic therapy reduces cardiovascular disease morbidity and mortality and the overall mortality rate, and angiographic studies have demonstrated that coronary lesions progress more slowly and regression occurs in 25% of patients.[9,24,44,66]

All of this experimental, genetic, epidemiological, and interventional evidence refers to the role of total and LDL cholesterol in the genesis and development of coronary atherosclerosis. However, in the lipid hypothesis of atherogenesis, factors other than total and LDL cholesterol levels must be taken into consideration.[32] These factors include low HDL cholesterol, high triglyceride (although the correlation between triglyceridemia and IHD is weaker if HDL is included), non-HDL cholesterol (i.e., the cholesterol contained in all apolipoprotein B–containing lipoproteins), oxidized LDL, Lp(a), and LDL pattern B levels. Although only a few studies have correlated Lp(a) and pattern B with cardiovascular risk, all preliminary results have shown that patients with elevated Lp(a) levels (>20–30 mg/dL) and subjects with pattern B are at increased risk for IHD.[3,15]

Pathogenesis

Endothelial injury and lipid infiltration are the most important steps in early plaque formation. Stimuli such as increased shear stress, viruses, toxins, antibodies, and so forth can act as initiating factors. These factors cause endothelial injury, which thus induces platelet adhesion, degranulation, and production of growth factors such as platelet-derived growth factor (PDGF), which stimulate smooth muscle cell growth. The most recent hypotheses on endothelial injury concur that injured endothelial cells, even if not exfoliated, express more adhesion molecules and secrete cytokines that are chemotactic for leukocytes and smooth muscle cells, the migration and proliferation of which is a key event in plaque development.[64,65,73]

In the majority of cases LDLs are the initiating factors, particularly when oxidized. They accumulate in the intima, predominantly in areas exposed to high mechanical stress, especially when blood pressure is high. Oxidized lipoproteins then induce a series of reactions, the most important of which is the formation of macrophage foam cells[34,86] (see later section "Role of Lipoproteins").

Until the 1990s there was no consensus on classification of the stages of atherosclerotic lesions. In 1958 the World Health Organization proposed the terms *fatty streak, atheroma, fibrous plaque,* and *complicated plaque.* In 1968 the International Atherosclerosis Project adopted only the terms *fatty streak, fibrous plaque,* and *complicated plaque.* In 1994 a special committee of the American Heart Association defined preatheroma lesions as initial, or type I; fatty streaks, or type II; and lesions between fatty streaks and atheroma, or type III.[73]

Type I: Initial Lesions

Initial lesions, which are not visible to the naked eye, are usually found in autopsies on infants. Composed of lipid deposits in the intima, they are associated with cell reactions that form isolated groups of macrophages containing lipid droplets (macrophage foam cells). Accumulation of macrophages or macrophage-derived foam cells is also the earliest atherosclerotic lesion in laboratory animals fed a hypercholesterolemic diet.

Type II: Fatty Streaks

Type II lesions include fatty streaks, or sudanophilic lesions, which can be seen by the naked eye. They are made up of macrophage-derived foam cells that are no longer isolated as in type I lesions but stratified in adjacent laminae of intimal-derived smooth muscle cells containing lipid droplets, of macrophages without lipid droplets, and of T lymphocytes with monoclonal antibodies. In type II lesions cholesterol esters, cholesterol, and phospholipids are found inside the cells.

The lack of precise correlation between sites of fatty streaks and atheromas is provided by autopsy reports that show that subjects with large fatty streaks did not present advanced lesions and vice versa. This finding has led to the hypothesis that an intermediate lesion (type III) links the two stages. Type II lesions have been reclassified on the basis of whether they will evolve toward type III lesions: type IIa lesions are called progression prone or advanced lesion prone, and type IIb lesions are called progression resistant or advanced lesion resistant. Type IIa lesions have different features than type IIb lesions: more smooth muscle cells are involved, accumulation of lipoproteins and macrophages is greater, foam cells and extracellular lipids are localized deeper in the intima, and macrophages that are not filled with lipids are found mainly close to the endothelium surface. Type IIb lesions do not progress, progress very slowly, or progress only in subjects with extremely high lipoprotein levels.

Type III: Intermediate Lesions

Type III lesions are transitional or preatheroma lesions found mainly in the progression-prone regions of arteries, where the atheromas will eventually be found. Characteristic of type III lesions are extracellular lipids that are mainly localized between layers of macrophages and foam cells. More free cholesterol, fatty acids, sphingomyelin, lysolecithin, and triglycerides are present than in the fatty streak, but the type III lesion is made up of the same types of cells.

Advanced Lesions

The advanced plaque, or atheroma, has a lipid core, a disrupted and thickened intima, and arterial deformation and may be complicated by ulceration, thrombosis, calcification, and intraplaque hemorrhage. Derived from the fusion of extracellular lipid drops, the lipid core is found within the intimal elastic muscle lamina, which is consequently thickened. Fewer intimal smooth muscle cells are present in the advanced plaque, and the foam cells are distributed along its edge. The term *fibroatheromatous plaque* refers to a type of lesion with a fibrous or collagenous cap (i.e., a proteoglycan lamina with numerous smooth muscle cells in a large collagen–capillary matrix). *Fibrous plaques* are advanced lesions with few lipids but many cells and collagens.[71]

Role of Endothelium

The endothelium plays a central role in the development of atherosclerosis because it modifies its functions in response to injury by changing from a quiescent state to an activated state. This initial insult does not necessarily lead to endothelial stripping (initial lesions occur where the endothelium is intact[65]) but does change endothelial cell functioning. The endothelium reacts to the injury by suppressing its physiological functions, including the synthesis of the anticoagulants thrombomodulin and heparin, of fibrinolytic tissue-type plasminogen activator, and of substances that regulate vascular tone (nitric oxide and prostacyclin). Factors that injure or activate the endothelium include viruses, changes in shear stress, oxygen free radicals, oxidized lipoproteins, and homocysteine.[19]

Oxidized lipoproteins play a major role in endothelial injury, because they induce endothelial release of adhesion molecules such as vascular cell adhesion molecule 1, which stimulates endothelial leukocyte adhesion and leukocyte migration into the subendothelial space.[5,43] Oxidized lipoproteins also modulate vascular tone because they inhibit the effects of endothelial-derived relaxant factor or nitric oxide[46] and induce release of endothelin 1, a potent vasoconstrictor.[7]

The activated endothelium initiates a series of mechanisms that trigger and promote atherosclerosis. These mechanisms include reducing the synthesis of anticoagulating substances such as heparin and tissue-type plasminogen activator, modifying the release of vasoactive molecules by reducing nitric oxide and prostacyclin production, increasing permeability to macromolecules, augmenting monocyte adhesion by releasing chemotactic factors such as vascular cell adhesion molecule 1 and colony-stimulating factor M, and producing cell growth factors such as the release of PDGF.[73] Its release is modified by factors such as increased osmolarity, which occurs in the course of diabetes mellitus, and by increased shear stress.[54,63–65] As lesions evolve from type I to type III the endothelium also undergoes a series of morphological changes: loss of blood flow orientation, a rounded shape, and increased proliferation.[73]

Role of Lipoproteins

Lipoprotein accumulation in the vessel intima is a key event in atherogenesis. Once they have penetrated the intima, lipoproteins are either trapped in the matrix or catabolized by macrophages and smooth muscle cells, a process that leads to the formation of foam cells.

Lipoprotein flux through the vessel wall depends on LDL, VLDL, and intermediate-density lipoprotein plasma concentrations (plasma levels and flux are positively correlated[57]) and on vessel permeability. Although the latter has great interindividual variability, it is increased in several conditions including atherosclerosis.[76] Lipoprotein size is another important factor. The vessel wall is practically impermeable to chylomicrons and larger VLDL molecules, but HDLs, LDLs (especially the smaller molecules), intermediate-density lipoproteins, and Lp(a) pass more easily. Lipoproteins penetrate the endothelial wall through intercellular spaces or by means of endocytosic vesicles.

In the past decade attention has been focused on oxidized lipoproteins, which are of primary importance in the development of atherosclerosis.[34,59] Even when LDL plasma levels are normal, the presence of circulating oxidized LDLs has been hypothesized to increase the risk of atherosclerosis because of their increased uptake by macrophages.[34,86] Although LDL oxidation and interaction with different cells involved in atherosclerosis have been studied to date only in vitro, their existence in vivo has been confirmed by the presence of antioxidized LDL antibodies,[67] and antioxidant therapy has been considered to induce atheromatous plaque regression.[74]

LDL oxidation is catalyzed by endothelial cells, smooth muscle cells, and monocytes through three mechanisms: release of oxygen reactive agents such as superoxide anions, lipoperoxide intracellular generation, and oxidizing enzymes acting directly on LDLs when they come into contact with plaque cells.[59] The oxidized LDLs have great atherogenic potential. They have a direct toxicity on the endothelium and increase monocyte migration into the subendothelial space. They potentiate the release of adhesion molecules such as vascular cell adhesion molecule 1. Through the scavenger pathway macrophages take up oxidized LDLs more avidly, which leads to the formation of foam cells.[34,86] Increased susceptibility of LDLs to oxidization has been observed in subjects with pattern B, who are considered more prone to atherosclerosis.[42,80]

Role of Cells

The endothelial cells, monocytes/macrophages, smooth muscle cells, and T lymphocytes are most involved in atherosclerotic plaque development. Macrophages are present in the plaque in all stages of its development. Derived from circulating monocytes, they penetrate the intima at both the microvascular and macrovascular levels. Their recruitment and adhesion are regulated by adhesion molecules; in the intima macrophages are transformed into foam cells as they accumulate cholesterol esters that take up oxidized lipoproteins through specific membrane receptors known as scavenger receptors. The macrophage role in the immune response to atherosclerosis is extremely important because these cells present the antigen to the T lymphocyte and thus trigger the immune cascade. T lymphocytes and macrophages

that express the class II histocompatibility antigen have been observed within plaques.[47] Monocytes and macrophages release growth factors (e.g., PDGF, which stimulates the proliferation and migration of smooth muscle cells, the basic fibroblast growth factor, a mitogen that triggers smooth muscle cell replication, the macrophage colony-stimulating factor, and interleukin 1).[48]

Smooth muscle cells are present at all stages of plaque development but predominate in the fibrous plaques.[64] Their proliferation begins within the tunica media and is followed by migration to the intima, where proliferation continues.[62]

Smooth muscle cells exist as two phenotypes, the contractile and the synthetic, differentiated according to the quantity of myosine filaments and of rough endoplasmic reticula inside the cells. These phenotypes represent different states of cell activity and susceptibility to mitogens.[11] The contractile state responds to physiological vasoconstrictive and vasodilating stimuli. The synthetic state is a cellular phenotype that expresses specific growth factor receptors to basic fibroblast growth factor, PDGF, and angiotensin II. It synthesizes interstitial matrix including elastic fibers, proteoglycans,[65] and from 25 to 48 times more collagen than the contractile phenotype.[2]

Increased production of extracellular matrix is observed as lesions progress from type I to type III.[73] Stimuli that trigger smooth muscle cell proliferation and transform the cells from contractile to synthetic phenotypes include oxidized LDLs, which stimulates PDGF release, and macrophages, which release several growth factors. T lymphocytes are also found within atherosclerotic plaques; monoclonal T lymphocytes in stage II lesions have been reported, but whether they are monoclonal is open to discussion. Maximum concentrations of T lymphocytes are found in plaques in transplanted coronary arteries, which could be the expression of an immunological mechanism that has not yet been fully defined.

Role of Growth Factors

In the genesis and development of lesions, growth factors and cytokines are the source of complex interactions with all the other types of cells. They stimulate chemotaxis and stimulate or even inhibit cell proliferation.[65,73]

Many growth factors have been discovered. Those that stimulate chemotaxis and those that act as mitogens for monocytes are colony-stimulating factors produced by the endothelium; transforming growth factor β, which is produced by macrophages, lymphocytes, and smooth muscle cells; monocyte chemotactic protein, which is produced by the monocytes; and oxidized LDLs.

Smooth muscle cell proliferation is stimulated by PDGF, whose main sources are platelets, endothelial cells, macrophages, and the smooth muscle cells themselves; by the β-fibroblast growth factor, produced by the smooth muscle cells; by the insulinlike growth factor 1 and the heparin-binding epidermal growth factor, both of which are released by smooth muscle cells; by leukocyte-derived cytokines such as interleukin 1 and the tumor necrosis factor; and by oxidized LDLs.

Acting through a network of interactions with target cells, the release of one growth factor stimulates the production of a second or third growth factor, which amplifies the response. Atherosclerosis is thus not merely a degenerative but also a proliferative process.

Complicated Plaques

The most common complications of advanced plaques are a fissured or ulcerated surface with an overlying thrombus. Nonthrombotic mechanical occlusion of vessels secondary to internal hemorrhage or to protrusion of intraplaque contents are more rare. Calcified deposits and intraplaque hemorrhage are further complications that render plaques unstable and more at risk of fissuring and ulcerating. Endothelial injury, monocyte activation, platelet adhesion and aggregation, and release of procoagulating factors all contribute to thrombus formation on the denudated endothelium surface.

In advanced plaques the endothelium is almost always practically denudated even if the plaque is not fissured. Deposits of platelets and fibrinogen that are responsible for further lesion growth through smooth muscle cell stimulation are always present,[10] which leads to thrombus formation on the denudated surface. Apart from simple endothelial denudation, the plaque may develop fissures, or splits, or ulcerate.

Plaques most at risk of rupture are known to have a high lipid content, a large lipid core if eccentric, and a high macrophage density (i.e., they are highly inflammatory lesions).[16,17] These plaques are more likely to rupture if exposed to high shear rate in a stenotic area or in parts of the vessel with brusque changes in pressure.[25]

When blood penetrates the lipid core and comes into contact with thrombogenic material, a thrombus, which may be either mural, involving part of the vessel wall, or occlusive, involving the vessel itself to an extent that it is completely occluded, is suddenly formed.[16] When small atherosclerotic plaques develop fissures and mural thrombi followed by fibrosis, the process contributes to the development of the plaque and to the narrowing of the vessel lumen and leads to clinical signs of the onset of ischemia. The occlusive thrombus on the other hand often provokes signs of acute ischemia.

Plaque complications are responsible for acute and/or chronic ischemia, with arterial thrombosis being the trig-

TABLE 36.6. Predictive factors for thrombosis.

- Fibrinogen
- Hematocrit
- Leukocyte count
- Blood viscosity
- Plasminogen activator inhibitor 1
- Lipoprotein(a)
- Lupus anticoagulant
- Proteinuria
- Left ventricular hypertrophy
- Homocystinemia
- Factor VII
- Protein S

gering agent in most cases of myocardial and cerebral infarction and in PAOD. Besides the condition of the plaque itself, other abnormalities in blood factors and organs contribute to the development of the thrombus. Table 36.6 lists predictive factors for thrombus formation. The success in combating atherothrombotic disease lies first in risk factor treatment from the early stages and second in antithrombotic therapy when signs of plaques are clinically present or when they have been visualized by ultrasonography or angiography.

Acknowledgments
Translation by Dr. G. A. Boyd.

References

1. American Heart Association. The cholesterol facts: a summary of the evidence relating to dietary fats, blood cholesterol, and coronary artery disease. A joint statement by the AHA and the NHLBI. *Circulation.* 1990;81:1721–1733.
2. Ang AH, Tachas G, Campbell JH, et al. Collagen synthesis by cultured rabbit aortic SMCs: alteration with phenotype. *Biochem J.* 1990;265:461–469.
3. Austin MA, King MC, Vranizan KM, et al. Atherogenic lipoprotein phenotype: a proposed genetic marker for coronary heart disease risk. *Circulation.* 1990;82:495–506.
4. Balkau B, Vray M, Eschwege E. Epidemiology of peripheral arterial disease. *J Cardiovasc Pharmacol.* 1994;23(suppl 3P):S8–S16.
5. Berliner JA, Territo MC, Sevanian A, et al. Minimally modified low density lipoprotein stimulates monocyte endothelial interaction. *J Clin Invest.* 1990;85:1260–1266.
6. Bondjers G, Glukhova M, Hasson GK, et al. Hypertension and atherosclerosis: cause and effect, or two effects with one unknown cause? *Circulation.* 1991;84(suppl 6):2–16.
7. Boulanger CM, Tanner FC, Bea ML, et al. Oxidized low density lipoproteins induce messenger RNA expression and release of endothelin from human and porcine endothelium. *Circ Res.* 1992;70:1191–1197.
8. Breslow JL. Transgenic mouse models of lipoprotein metabolism and atherosclerosis. *Proc Natl Acad Sci U S A.* 1993;90:8314–8318.
9. Brown RG, Zhao XQ, Sacco DE, et al. Lipid lowering and plaque regression: new insights into prevention of plaque

disruption and clinical events in coronary disease. *Circulation.* 1993;87:1781–1791.

10. Burrig K. The endothelium of advanced arteriosclerotic plaques in humans. *Arterioscler Thromb.* 1991;11:1678–1689.

11. Chamley-Campbell JH, Campbell GR, Ross R. Phenotype-dependent response of cultured aortic smooth muscle toserum miogens. *J Cell Biol.* 1981;89:379–383.

12. Consensus Conference. Lowering blood cholesterol to prevent heart disease. *JAMA.* 1985;253:2080–2086.

13. Couper JJ, Bates DJ, Cocciolone R, et al. Association of lipoprotein (a) with puberty in IDDM. *Diabetes Care.* 1993; 16:869–873.

14. Criqui MH, Fronek A, Barret-Connor E, et al. The prevalence of peripheral arterial disease in a defined population. *Circulation.* 1985;71:510–515.

15. Dahlen G, Guyton JR, Attar M, et al. Association of levels of lipoprotein Lp(a), plasma lipids, and other lipoproteins with coronary heart disease documented by angiography. *Circulation.* 1986;74:758–762.

16. Davies MJ. Pathology of arterial thrombosis. *Br Med Bull.* 1994;4:789–802.

17. Davies MJ, Thomas AC. Plaque fissuring: the cause of acute myocardial infarction, sudden ischemic death, and crescendo angina. *Br Heart J.* 1985;53:363–373.

18. De Palma RG. Patterns of peripheral atherosclerosis: implication for treatment. In: Shepherd JC, Morgan PD, Packard M, eds. *Atherosclerosis: Developments, Complications, and Treatment.* Amsterdam: Excerpta Medica; 1987: 161–174.

19. DiCorleto PE, Soyombo AA. The role of endothelium in atherogenesis. *Curr Opin Lipidol.* 1993;4:364–372.

20. Dzau VZ. Atherosclerosis and hypertension: mechanisms and interrelationship. *J Cardiovasc Pharmacol.* 1990;15 (suppl 5):59–64.

21. Eggen DA, Solberg LA. Variation of atherosclerosis with age. *Lab Invest.* 1968;18:571–579.

22. Feingold KR, Grunfeld C, Pang M, et al. LDL subclass phenotypes and triglyceride metabolism in non insulin dependent diabetes. *Arterioscler Thromb.* 1992;12:1496–1502.

23. Fless GM, Rolich CA, Scanu AM. Heterogeneity of human plasma lipoprotein (a). *J Biol Chem.* 1984;258:11470–11474.

24. Frohlich JJ. Blood cholesterol is causally related to atherosclerosis. *Card Res.* 1994;28:574–578.

25. Fuster V, Stein B, Ambrose JA, et al. Atherosclerotic plaque rupture and thrombosis. *Circulation.* 1990;82(suppl 2): 47–59.

26. Giral P, Phitois-Merli I, Filitti V, et al. Risk factors and early extracoronary atherosclerotic plaques detected by three sites ultrasound imaging in hypercholesterolemic men. *Arch Intern Med.* 1991;151:950–956.

27. Goldstein JL, Brown MS. Familial hypercholesterolemia. In: Scriver CR, Beaudet AL, Sly WS, Valle D, eds. *The Metabolic Basis of Inherited Disease.* New York, NY: McGraw-Hill; 1989:1215–1250.

28. Grant PJ, Kruithof EKO, Felley CD, et al. Short-term infusion of insulin, triacylglycerol, and glucose do not cause acute increases in plasminogen activator inhibitor-1 concentration in man. *Clin Sci.* 1990;79:513–516.

29. Guyton JR. The arterial wall and the atherosclerotic lesion. *Curr Opin Lipidol.* 1994;5:376–381.

30. Hamsten A, De Faire U, Waldius G, et al. Plasminogen activator inhibitor in plasma: risk factor for recurrent myocardial infarction. *Lancet.* 1987;2:3–9.

31. Hamsten A, Wiman B, De Faire U, et al. Increased plasma levels of rapid inhibitor of tissue plasminogen activator in young survivors of myocardial infarction. *N Engl J Med.* 1985;313:1557–1563.

32. Havel RJ, Rapaport E. Management of primary hyperlipidemia. *Drug Ther.* 1995;332:1491–1498.

33. Heiss G, Sharrett AR, Barnes R, et al. Carotid atherosclerosis measured by B mode ultrasound in populations: associations with cardiovascular risk factors in the ARIC study. *Am J Epidemiol.* 1991;3:250–256.

34. Henriksen T, Mahoney EM, Steinberg D. Enhanced macrophage degradation of low density lipoprotein previously incubated with cultured endothelial cells: recognition by the receptor for acetylated low density lipoproteins. *Proc Natl Acad Sci U S A.* 1981;78:6499–6503.

35. Hermanson B, Gilbert S, Omenn MD, et al. Beneficial six year outcome of smoking cessation in older men and women with coronary artery disease. *N Engl J Med.* 1988; 319:1365–1369.

36. Howard BV. Lipoprotein metabolism in diabetes mellitus. *J Lipid Res.* 1987;28:613–628.

37. Howard G, Burke GL, Szklo M, et al. Active and passive smoking are associated with increased carotid wall thickness: the Atherosclerosis Risk in Communities Study. *Arch Intern Med.* 1994;154:1277–1282.

38. Hypertension Detection and Follow Up Group. The effect of treatment on mortality in "mild" hypertension. *N Engl J Med.* 1982;307:976–980.

39. Hypertension Detection and Follow-up Program Cooperative Group. Five-year findings of the hypertension detection and follow-up program. *JAMA.* 1979;242: 2562–2567.

40. Kannel WB, Castelli WP, Gordon T. Serum cholesterol, lipoproteins, and risk of coronary heart disease: the Framingham Study. *Ann Intern Med.* 1971;74:1–9.

41. Keys A. Coronary heart disease in seven countries. *Circulation.* 1970;41(suppl):211–218.

42. Krauss RM. Heterogeneity of plasma low density lipoproteins and atherosclerosis risk. *Curr Opin Lipidol.* 1994;5: 339–349.

43. Kume N, Cybulski MI, Gimbrone MA Jr. Lysophosphatydylcoline, a component of atherogenic lipoproteins, induces mononuclear leucocyte adhesion molecules in cultured human and rabbit arterial endothelial cells. *J Clin Invest.* 1992;90:1138–1144.

44. La Rosa JC, Cleeman JI. Cholesterol lowering as a treatment for established coronary heart disease. *Circulation.* 1992;85:1229–1235.

45. Lakier JB. Smoking and cardiovascular disease. *Am J Med.* 1992;93(suppl IA):8–12.

46. Lefer AM, Ma X. Decreased basal nitric oxide release in hypercholesterolemia increases neutrophil adherence to rabbit coronary artery endothelium. *Arterioscler Thromb.* 1993;13:771–776.

47. Libby P. Inflammatory and immune mechanisms in atherogenesis. *J Immunol.* 1990;144:2343–2350.

48. Libby P, Clinton SK. The role of macrophages in atherogenesis. *Curr Opin Lipidol.* 1993;4:355–363.

49. Lithell H. Pathogenesis and prevalence of atherosclerosis in hypertensive patients. *Am J Hypertens.* 1994;7:2–6.

50. Marmot MG, Syme SL, Kagan A, et al. Epidemiologic studies of coronary heart disease and stroke in Japanese men living in Japan, Hawaii, and California: prevalence of coronary and hypertensive heart disease and associated risk factors. *Am J Epidemiol.* 1975;102:514–519.

51. Maser RE, Wolfson SK, Ellis D, et al. Cardiovascular disease and arterial calcification in insulin dependent diabetes mellitus: interrelations and risk factor profiles. *Arterioscler Thromb.* 1991;11:958–996.

52. McGill HC Jr. Potential mechanism for the augmentation of atherosclerosis and atherosclerotic disease by cigarette smoking. *Prev Med.* 1979;8:390–393.

53. Miles LA, Plow EF. Lp(a): an interloper in the fibrinolytic system. *Thromb Haemost.* 1990;63:331–334.

54. Mizutani M, Okuda Y, Yamaoka T, et al. High glucose and hyperosmolarity increase platelet derived growth factor mRNA levels in cultured human vascular endothelial cells. *Biochem Biophys Res Commun.* 1992;187:664–669.

55. National Center for Health Statistics. Advance Report of Final Mortality Statistics, 1986. Hyattsville, Md: Public Health Service; 1988. DHHS publication PHS 88-1220.

56. Nishina PM, Johnson JP, Naggert JK, et al. Linkage of atherogenic lipoprotein phenotype to the low density lipoprotein receptor locus on the short arm of chromosome 19. *Proc Natl Acad Sci U S A.* 1992;89:708–712.

57. Nordestgaard BG, Tybjaerg-Hansen A, Lewis B. Influx in vivo of low density lipoproteins into aortic intimas of genetically hyperlipidemic rabbits: role of plasma concentration, extent of aortic lesion, and lipoprotein particle size as determinants. *Arterioscler Thromb.* 1992;12:6–18.

58. P-Day Research Group. Relationship of atherosclerosis in young men to serum lipoprotein cholesterol concentration and smoking. *JAMA.* 1990;264:3018–3024.

59. Parthasarathy S, Steinberg D. Cell-induced oxidation of LDL. *Curr Opin Lipidol.* 1992;3:313–317.

60. Reaven GM. Banting lecture: role of insulin resistance in human disease. *Diabetes.* 1988;37:1595–1607.

61. Reaven GM, Chen YDI, Jeppesen J, et al. Insulin resistance and hyperinsulinemia in individuals with small, dense, low density lipoprotein particles. *J Clin Invest.* 1993;92:141–146.

62. Reidy AM, Bowyer DE. Control of arterial smooth muscle cell proliferation. *Curr Opin Lipidol.* 1993;4:349–354.

63. Resnick N, Collins T, Atkinson W, et al. Platelet derived growth factor B chain promoter contains a *cis*-acting fluid shear-stress-responsive element. *Proc Natl Acad Sci U S A.* 1993;90:4591–4595.

64. Ross R. The pathogenesis of atherosclerosis: an update. *N Engl J Med.* 1986;314:488–499.

65. Ross R. The pathogenesis of atherosclerosis: a perspective for the 1990s. *Nature.* 1993;362:801–809.

66. Rossow JE, Lewis B, Rifkind BM. The value of lowering cholesterol after myocardial infarction. *N Engl J Med.* 1990;323:1113–1119.

67. Salonen JT, Yla-Herttuala S, Yamamoto R, et al. Autoantibody against oxidized LDL and progression of carotid atherosclerosis. *Lancet.* 1992;339:883–887.

68. Schettler FG, Wollenweber J. Clinical aspect. In: Schettler FG and Boyd A, eds. *Atherosclerosis.* Amsterdam: Elsevier; 1969:633–672.

69. Schwartz CJ, Kelley JL, Nerem RM, et al. Pathophysiology of the atherogenic process. *Am J Cardiol.* 1989;64: 23G–30G.

70. Stamler J, Wentworth MPH, Neaton JD. Is the relationship between serum cholesterol and risk of premature death from coronary heart disease continuous and graded? Findings in 356222 primary screens of Multiple Risk Factor Intervention Trial (MRFIT). *JAMA.* 1986;256: 2823–2830.

71. Stary HC. Evolution and progression of atherosclerosis: implication for treatment. In: Shepherd JC, Morgan PD, Packard M, eds. *Atherosclerosis: Developments, Complications, and Treatment.* Amsterdam: Excerpta Medica; 1989: 161–174.

72. Stary HC. Evolution and progression of atherosclerotic lesions in coronary arteries of children and young adults. *Arteriosclerosis.* 1989;9(suppl 1):19–32.

73. Stary HC, Chadler AB, Glagov S, et al. A definition of initial, fatty streak, and intermediate lesions of atherosclerosis: a report from the Committee on Vascular Lesions of the Council on Arteriosclerosis, American Heart Association. *Circulation.* 1994;89:2462–2478.

74. Steinberg D, Workshop Participants. Antioxidants in the prevention of human atherosclerosis: summary of the proceedings of a National Heart, Lung, and Blood Institute Workshop: September 5–6, Bethesda, Maryland. *Circulation.* 1992;85:2337–2344.

75. Steinbrecher UP, Witztum JL, Kesaniemi YA, et al. Comparison of glucosylated LDL with methylated or cyclohexanedione-treated LDL in the measurement of receptor-independent LDL catabolism. *J Clin Invest.* 1983;7: 960–964.

76. Stender S, Hjelms E. In-vivo influx of free and esterified plasma cholesterol into human aortic tissue without atherosclerotic lesions. *J Clin Invest.* 1984;74:1871–1881.

77. Strandness DE, Didisheim P, Clowes AW, et al., eds. *Vascular Diseases: Current Research and Clinical Application.* Orlando, Fla: Grune & Stratton; 1987.

78. Strong JP, McGill HC Jr. The pediatric aspects of atherosclerosis. *J Atheroscl Res.* 1969;32:251–265.

79. Thom TJ. Stroke mortality trends: an international perspective. *Ann Epidemiol.* 1993;5:509–518.

80. Tribble DL, Holl LG, Wood PG, et al. Variations in oxidative susceptibility among six low density lipoprotein subfractions of differing density and particle size. *Atherosclerosis.* 1992;93:189–199.

81. Urakami K, Mura T, Takahashi K. Lp(a) lipoprotein in cerebrovascular disease and dementia. *Jpn J Psychiatry Neurol.* 1987;41:743–746.

82. US Department of Health and Human Services. *Current Estimates from the National Health Interview Survey, United States, 1985.* Hyattsville, Md: National Center for Health Statistics; 1986.

83. Vague JI, Vague PH, Alessi MC, et al. Relationship between plasma insulin, triglyceride, body mass index, and plas-

minogen activator inhibitor. *Diabete Metab.* 1987;13:
331–336.

84. Widmar LK, Greensher A, Kannel WB. Occlusion of peripheral arteries: a study of 6400 working subjects. *Circulation.* 1964;30:836–842.

85. Wissler RW, Vesselinovitch D. Can atherosclerotic plaques regress? Anatomic and biochemical evidence from non human animal models. *Am J Cardiol.* 1990;65:33F–40F.

86. Witztum JL, Steinberg D. Role of oxidized low density lipoprotein in atherogenesis. *J Clin Invest.* 1991;88:21785–21792.

37

Inflammatory Vascular Disease

Gaetano Vaudo and Elmo Mannarino

Vascular inflammation, in the form of vasculitis, has long been recognized as one cause of arterial thrombosis, but a precise overall estimate of vasculitis is difficult to obtain.[60] Some rare forms such as Wegener's granulomatosis and classical nodular polyarteritis present an incidence of 0.2 to 1.8 per 100,000 annually.[77] Partial estimates of the incidence of vasculitis in the course of other pathologies are available. In the United Kingdom, for example, the annual incidence of vasculitis associated with rheumatoid arthritis (RA) is 12.5 per million (15.8 per million in men and 9.4 per million in women).[86]

Clinical signs and symptoms of vascular involvement appear only when the lungs, kidneys, heart, brain, or skin are extensively affected. Vasculitis is classified according to the caliber of the vessel involved (see Table 37.1) and may be primary (e.g., giant cell arteritis, Takayasu's arteritis, classical nodular polyarteritis, Kawasaki's syndrome, Wegener's granulomatosis, Churg–Strauss syndrome, Schönlein–Henoch purpura, and mixed essential cryoglobulinemia) or secondary to systemic lupus erythematosus (SLE), RA, mixed connective tissue disease, polymyositis/dermatomyositis, scleroderma, Sjögren's syndrome, or Behçet's syndrome.

Pathophysiology

In the vessel wall vasculitis provokes lesions that may become necrotic, lumen thickening, and occlusion due to overlying thrombi. Aneurysms may form, and hemorrhage may occur. Because connective tissue and vessel wall tissue both originate in mesenchymal cells, their ultrastructure is similar. One feature of chronic systemic vascular inflammation is an abnormal functioning of the immune system.[85] Evidence in support of immune-mediated pathogenesis includes the presence of immunoglobulins (Ig) in the vessel wall, circulating immunocomplexes, and associated hypocomplementemia.[84] Cell-mediated immunity may also be activated.[22]

Ig deposits in the vessel wall can be detected through immunofluorescence and immunoperoxidases. These tests are positive only when large quantities of Ig, antigens, and specifically related antibodies are present. Ig, complement factors, and deposits that contain both the IgG and IgM rheumatoid factor[56] have been found in the small-artery walls of patients with RA-associated vasculitis[17]; patients with RA who develop vasculitis are those with the highest levels of circulating IgG and IgM.[58]

TABLE 37.1. Vasculitis: clinical and anatomical criteria.

Vessel	Primary	Secondary
Large-caliber vessels	Giant cell arteritis	Rheumatoid arthritis–associated aortitis
	Takayasu's arteritis	Infections (syphilis)
Medium-caliber vessels	Classic nodular polyarteritis	Infections (hepatitis B)
	Kawasaki's disease	
Medium-to-small–caliber vessels	Wegener's granulomatosis	Systemic lupus erythematosus, rheumatoid arthritis, and
	Churg–Strauss syndrome	systemic sclerosis
	Microscopic polyangitis	Drugs
		Infections (HIV)
Small-caliber vessels (leukocytoclastic)	Schönlein–Henoch purpura	Drugs (sulphonamides, penicillin, diuretics, etc.)
	Mixed essential cryoglobulinemia	Infections

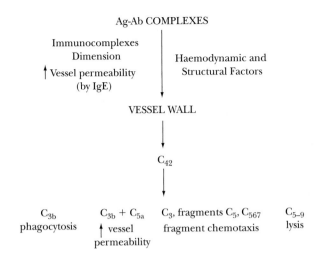

Ag-Ab COMPLEXES

Immunocomplexes
Dimension

↑ Vessel permeability
(by IgE)

Haemodynamic and
Structural Factors

VESSEL WALL

C_{42}

| C_{3b} phagocytosis | $C_{3b} + C_{5a}$ ↑ vessel permeability | C_3, fragments C_5, C_{567} fragment chemotaxis | C_{5-9} lysis |

FIGURE 37.1. Mechanism of immunocomplex-mediated damage in vasculitis.

Deposits of Ig and complement factors C3, C1q, and C5–C9 are present in small cutaneous vessels affected by vasculitis in patients with SLE,[9,28,76] but the values do not correlate with the severity of inflammation.[78] In necrotizing vasculitis associated with SLE, bioptic samples from different organs and tissues have contained deposits of IgM, IgG, and C3 in the arterioles, capillaries, and venules,[10] which indicates that vasculitis is systemic. In Wegener's granulomatosis, IgM, C3, and fibrin deposits have been observed in the venules[36] and small arterioles.[71] Figure 37.1 illustrates the chain of events and factors that mediate inflammatory damage to the vessel wall as hypothesized by the immunocomplex theory.

Hypocomplementemia is frequently encountered in patients with SLE, RA, and other connective tissue diseases and is a direct consequence of Ig deposits on the vessel walls and high levels of circulating immunocomplexes.[92] Figure 37.2 illustrates the chain of events and factors that mediate vasculitis-induced injury to the vessel wall as hypothesized by the cell-mediated theory. Takayasu's arteritis is an example of vascular inflamma-

tion in which clinical findings and laboratory tests tend to suggest an autoimmune process[11,28] mediated by both anti–vessel wall antibodies[82] and a cellular component, although the cause is unknown.[69] Other possible pathophysiological mechanisms include a genetic defect because of the high frequency of particular types of histocompatibility antigens (HLA-Bw52 and HLA-DR2).[54,66] Sexual hormones,[82] infections,[33] and increased endothelin 1 levels[91] have also been implicated.

Thrombosis associated with vasculitis may be caused by the antiphospholipid syndrome, which can be diagnosed by the anticardiolipin antibody test. Antiphospholipid antibodies bind with the phospholipid anions in the prothrombin complex and are clinically associated with recurrent arterial and venous thrombosis. When the antiphospholipid syndrome is not associated with any other disease, it is considered primary; the secondary form is usually concomitant with connective tissue disease or neoplasias.[48]

Thrombosis is found in 23% to 54% of patients with SLE, and three classes of antibodies have been identified: (1) reagins, which produce a false-positive syphilis test result; (2) IgG or IgM lupus anticoagulant; and (3) anticardiolipin antibodies. All of these antibodies bind with negatively charged phospholipid coagulants and interfere with the ability of protein S to bind to the endothelial cells. They also interact with platelets, endothelial cells, thrombomodulin, or its associated phospholipids. Impairments in platelet–endothelial cell interactions lead to the release of platelet-derived growth factor (which stimulates fibroblasts and collagen proliferation) and an abnormally high release of interleukin 1 (which also stimulates fibroblast proliferation). This ensuing mechanical injury to the vessel wall is the trigger for thrombus formation.[47]

Histology

Three connected stages in the development of inflammatory vascular lesions have been observed microscopically. Stage I, the acute stage, is characterized by fibri-

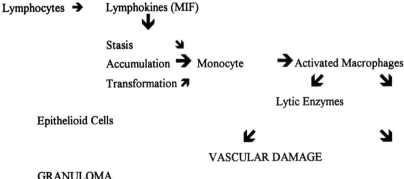

FIGURE 37.2. Mechanism of cell-mediated damage in vasculitis.

Lymphocytes ➔ Lymphokines (MIF)

Stasis
Accumulation ➔ Monocyte ➔ Activated Macrophages
Transformation ↗

Lytic Enzymes

Epithelioid Cells

VASCULAR DAMAGE

GRANULOMA

noid necrosis. Constituents are acellular, homogeneous eosinophil matter, histologically similar to fibrin, which accumulates in the intima on the entire wall thickness and may lead to aneurysms. Neutrophils are the most frequently involved cells and have been found along with a varying percentage of mononuclear leukocytes, lymphocytes, histiocytes, and epithelioid cells in the perinuclear spaces. In infiltrated areas leukocytes undergo leukocytoclasis (i.e., nuclear fragments are formed within the leukocytes).[16]

In stage II lesions are healing, and areas of proliferation rather than of necrosis can be seen. Fibrosis tends to engulf the vasa vasorum and the adventitial nerves. Neocapillaries proliferate in the media. Macrophages and plasma cells may be observed. Fibroblasts, often arranged in concentric circles in the tunica intima, cause internal thickening and narrowing of the vessel lumen. When they proliferate into the adventitia, vascular irregularity and nodular formation result; when proliferation is in the intima, overlying thrombi are formed.

In stage III vascular damage is stabilized. Stabilized fibrosis involves the entire adventitia and the other two thirds of the media. The vasa vasorum are totally obliterated; fibrous tissue takes the place of the outer elastic lamina. Irregular and thickened, the intima determines varying degrees of vessel lumen stenosis. Fibrous tissue mixed with a few lymphocytes, plasma cells, and occasionally calcium deposits are responsible for ischemic areas or parenchymal infarction.[43,74]

Granulomata can be observed in some patients with vasculitis (e.g., Wegener's granulomatosis and Takayasu's arteritis).[24] Identified histologically as panarteritis, the entire thickness of the artery wall is inflamed, even though only segments may be involved. Panarteritis is found in the aorta, its main branches, and the pulmonary artery. Early lesions appear in the tunica media, spread to the adventitia and the intima, and result in an abnormal artery wall repair process. In the final stages lesions cause stenosis and/or occlusion alternating with aneurysms along the affected tract. In any segment the demarcation between affected and healthy areas is clearly evident.

Severe granuloma-type inflammation between the tunica media and the adventitia leads to the destruction of the outer elastic lamina, but the inner third of the media and the inner elastic lamina are unaffected. A marked inflammatory cellular infiltration mainly of mononucleates and giant cells and the fragmentation of the internal elastic lamina are common features.[21] Another histopathological aspect of Wegener's granulomatosis is extravessel necrotizing granulomata, up to 5 to 6 cm in diameter, which are made up of fibrinoid or granular necrosis without leukocyte invasion. In their final stages they are surrounded by a stockade of histiocytes and mononuclear giant cells.[2]

Clinical Features

Primary

Clinical features in all primary forms of vasculitis may overlap, but there is no single sign or symptom that can be considered an unequivocal marker of vascular inflammation. Clinical signs of giant cell arteritis are linked to its localization in the temporal arteries, the most frequently affected site. Two thirds of patients with monolateral temporal involvement complain of a pulsing headache; monolateral temporal involvement is also associated with sudden blindness in 20% of patients and signs and symptoms of rheumatic polymyalgia (e.g., rigidity and muscular pain in the shoulders, neck, pelvic area, hips, and thighs) in 50%.[64] Giant cell arteritis may also involve large- and medium-caliber arteries[14]; typical signs include intermittent claudication of the limbs and masticatory muscles but rarely of the tongue and deglutitory muscles.

Named after the Japanese ophthalmologist who first drew attention to its associated ocular abnormalities, Takayasu's arteritis is an inflammation of the aorta, its principal branches, and the pulmonary artery. Because the brachiocephalic vessels are often occluded, the disease is also known as pulseless disease or the aortic arch syndrome. Although most cases have been observed in the Far East, Takayasu's arteritis has been detected worldwide.[87] Although 70% to 80% of patients develop the disease in their 20s or 30s, cases have also been described in childhood and middle age.[13,70] The incidence is eight to nine times higher in women than in men.[77] The preocclusive stage is associated with aspecific signs and symptoms such as fever, night sweats, malaise, weight loss, arthralgia, nausea, and vomiting.[52] The erythrocyte sedimentation rate is elevated, and anemia and serum protein abnormalities are associated with splenomegaly, cutaneous lesions, Raynaud's phenomenon, and occasionally serum positivity for SLE or RA.[59]

As long as 10 years later, the preocclusive stage is followed by the occlusive stage, which is characterized by signs of ischemia.[35] Symptoms may rapidly worsen because of acute poussés. Cardiovascular signs include the absence of pulses, dyspnea during exercise, hypertension (caused by the loss of arterial elasticity), renal hypoperfusion, and carotid sinus insensibility. Peripheral vessel involvement is manifested in intermittent claudication of the upper and lower limbs and subclavian steal. Heart disease such as angina pectoris and myocardial infarction may be due to coronary occlusion, even though the coronary origin is predominantly affected, or to aortic insufficiency due to aortic valve deformation or inflammation-induced aortic root dilation. Although pericarditis has only occasionally been described, signs of healed pericarditis are common autopsy findings.

Syncope, originally attributed to carotid sinus hypersensitivity, may be a sign of cerebral ischemia caused by obstruction of the brachiocephalic arteries. Syncope may also be caused by hypotension when associated with even a slight degree of stenosis. Headache, dizziness, and hemiparesis may also be present, but the central nervous system is rarely directly involved.

Spiral anastomoses around the optic pupils (which first attracted Takayasu's attention) cause prolonged ischemia of the retina. Signs of ocular ischemia are scotoma, loss of vision, and transient blindness; cataracts, corneal opacity, and atrophy of the iris are common in advanced stages.

Prognosis is poor; survival in the advanced stage ranges from a few months to 3 to 5 years. Cerebrovascular, cardiac, or renal failure[40] is usually the cause of death. Prognosis depends on complications such as hypertensive retinopathy, hypertension, aortic insufficiency, and aneurysms. Life expectancy is better for patients with no complications or only one, because they respond better to therapy.[38]

In classic nodular polyarteritis, purpura, ulcers, and gangrene are signs of cutaneous vasculitis. The mesenteric, renal, hepatic, splenic, and pulmonary arteries are frequently and more seriously affected. The early signs—fever, asthenia, weight loss, and headache—tend to be aspecific, but renal failure (70%), hypertension (54%), abdominal pain (44%), heart failure (33%), gastric ulcer, and peripheral neuropathy later develop.[25,43]

In Kawasaki's syndrome oral ulcers and fistulae, palmar and plantar erythema, exanthema of the trunk, edema, and periungual desquamation are signs of cutaneous vasculitis. Associated signs are fever, conjunctivitis, and widespread (particularly cervical) lymph node disease. Although vasculitis affects the coronary arteries in all patients with Kawasaki's syndrome it is not always symptomatic and is the cause of death in only 1% to 2% of affected individuals.[44]

In Wegener's granulomatosis, in which the upper airways are affected, epistaxis, scabby lesions, and deafness may occur. The lungs are affected in 50% of patients, with symptoms ranging from cough and sputum with blood to dyspnea.[45] Cutaneous signs of vasculitis include purpura rash, ulcers, nodules, and blisters. Renal involvement is a sign of poor prognosis. Cardiac, pituitary, and gastroenteric involvement is possible.[30,62,73]

In the Churg–Strauss syndrome (allergic angiitis) a history of atopy and/or allergic asthma long precedes the onset of vasculitis in small-caliber arteries and veins. Aspecific signs include fever, weight loss, respiratory distress, and pulmonary infiltrate that may be transitory (Löffler's syndrome) or persistent. Infiltrate may be found in the heart, nervous system, gastrointestinal tract, and skin.[11,68] Microscopic granulomata (necrotic cores with eosinophil infiltration, surrounded by epithelioid and giant cells) may join to form large lesions known as extravascular granulomata.[5]

Schönlein–Henoch purpura is systemic hypersensitive vasculitis that affects small vessels.[55] With an onset in childhood after even minor infections, cutaneous signs include urticaria and/or rash on the buttocks and limbs. In 70% of patients arthralgia and gastrointestinal disorders (e.g., nausea, vomiting, fecal bleeding, and abdominal colic) may be present. In 50% of the adult patients who develop Schönlein–Henoch purpura, renal involvement (e.g., hematuria, glomerular nephritis, and renal failure) is predominant.[79]

In mixed cryoglobulinemia, vasculitis is systemic and involves mainly small blood vessels, where amorphous cryoprecipitate can be detected. In 50% of patients with proliferative membrane glomerular nephritis, it is believed to be of viral origin (e.g., Epstein-Barr, hepatitis B, or cytomegalovirus). Cutaneous purpura, caused by exposure to cold, stress, and prolonged standing, is often associated with arthralgia and asthenia. Signs of lung involvement, which is rare, include bloody sputum and dyspnea.[18]

Secondary to Connective Tissue Disease

The clinical aspects of vasculitis in the course of connective tissue disease are closely linked to the type and site of affected vessels, with damage being very different in the connective tissue of skin and in the internal organs.[7]

In SLE, the typical "butterfly" rash on the face, limbs, and trunk that worsens on exposure to sunlight is a clear sign of vasculitis. Erythema, pain in the fingertips and palms, nailbed bleeding, and perinailbed infarction often develop. When associated with cryoglobulinemia, a network of irregular blue–red patches (livedo reticularis) may be seen on the legs but rarely on the arms. Cryoglobulinemia worsens on contact with cold water and may evolve into ulcers or be associated with vascular thrombosis (Sneddon's syndrome), antiphospholipid antibodies, and thrombocytopenic purpura.[23,27,39] Painful superficial lesions, often infected by *Candida albicans*, frequently appear in the genital and oral mucosa; ulcers in the soft palate or nasal mucosa tend to be deeper and complicated by epistaxis and/or septum perforation. Vasculitis may also involve the heart (angina pectoris), lungs (pulmonary hypertension and sputum containing blood), gastrointestinal tract (infarction and bowel perforation), and nervous system (psychosis, dementia, epilepsy, ischemic and hemorrhagic stroke, and meningitis).[35,63]

In RA small brownish spots that lead to ulceration in the nailbed, perinailbed area, fingertips, and perimalleolar area are evidence of vasculitis.[50] Occlusive endoarteritis of the digital arteries has also been observed and is probably the final stage of the necrotizing arteritis found in the most virulent forms of RA.[17] When internal organs are involved, vasculitis predominantly affects the nervous system (cerebral infarction, polyneuropathy), the heart (infarction), the respiratory system (pulmonary hypertension), and the gastrointestinal tract (multiple infarctions).[3,72]

In mixed connective tissue disease Raynaud's phenomenon is the most frequently observed symptom of vascular involvement. The lupuslike rash typical of vasculitis rarely occurs. The kidneys are affected in 20% of patients, but renal failure is rarely observed.

In dermatomyositis, whether primary or secondary to vasculitis and/or connective tissue disease, cutaneous lesions are present in 90% of patients. Onset usually occurs at a young age, even in childhood, and is manifested by a widespread or localized erythema, pustules, eczema-type dermatitis, and occasionally exfoliate dermatitis. A heliotrope purple rash appears on the eyelids, nose, knees, knuckles, and nailbed. Lesions may be associated with persistent itchiness but rarely ulcerate. Electrocardiographic abnormalities may occur, but no other internal organ besides the heart is affected.[42] Alveolar hemorrhage can occur.[67]

In scleroderma, cutaneous involvement is manifested by arteriolar intimal thickening, and in 95% of patients Raynaud's phenomenon is the first symptom. Necrotic or ulcerating areas on the fingertips are frequent, but the entire finger is rarely affected. Vasculitis, which affects mainly the lungs, causes pulmonary hypertension that usually progresses slowly. Cases of isolated pulmonary hypertension associated with cutaneous scleroderma have been reported as occurring 15 to 30 years after the original diagnosis. In these cases dyspnea soon worsens and patients often die within 2 years. The kidneys are affected in 20% of patients with malignant hyperreninemic hypertension, which leads to acute renal failure.[46] When the gastrointestinal tract is affected, esophageal dysphagia may be associated with widespread telangiectasia and hemorrhage.

Primary Sjögren's syndrome is seen in only 25% of patients with a cutaneous sign of vasculitis: a nodular purpura on the legs. In some patients, systemic necrotizing vasculitis is associated with fever, a cutaneous rash, and intestinal infarction. Vasculitis is usually episodic and rarely becomes chronic. Systemic vasculitis usually affects the kidney (nephrovascular hypertension), the central nervous system (sensory polyneuropathy or multiple mononeuritis), and the heart (electrocardiographic abnormalities).[49]

In Behçet's syndrome, cutaneous, oral, and genital ulcers (2–10 mm in diameter) are evidence of vasculitis and occur in 87% to 100% of patients. Although extremely painful, the ulcers heal spontaneously within 2 weeks.[37] In 56% of patients the eyes may be affected by iritis, uveitis, retinal thrombosis, and optic nerve neuritis, which may lead to blindness. Large- and medium-caliber arteries (e.g., aorta and femoral and pulmonary arteries) may be affected, and venous involvement (migrating superficial thrombophlebitis or deep vein thrombosis) is found 40.5% of patients.[4] In the lungs pain, cough, and bleeding when coughing are signs of vasculitis; pulmonary vasculitis is the main cause of death in patients with Behçet's syndrome.[80] Signs of cerebral vasculitis are neurological, motor, or sensory deficits that are usually focal and consequent to infarction and endocranial hypertension. Depression has been observed in some patients with Behçet's syndrome.[32]

Diagnostic Tests

Laboratory tests show a high erythrocyte sedimentation rate that tends to normalize in the chronic or quiescent stages, an increase in α_2-globulins, and in some cases antiarterial wall antibodies.

Chest x-rays may show heart enlargement, usually of the left ventricle. When large-caliber vessels are involved, the aorta is longer, calcified, and pushed upward by supra-aortic vessel sclerosis and retraction. Examination of the fundus oculi, field of vision, and fluoroangiography reveal abnormalities in the eyes. Stenosis in peripheral vessels may be detected by means of Doppler velocimetry and Doppler echocardiography. When large-caliber vessels are affected, carotid stenosis or occlusion and hypertrophy of the vertebral arteries are common. Stenotic lesions are also frequently found in the pulmonary and renal arteries.[70] Angiography, preferably total body angiography or digital subtraction angiography,[89] is mandatory because it reveals single or multiple segments of narrowed arteries that are often associated with aneurysm. Occasionally widespread narrowing of the entire descending and abdominal aortic tracts or coarctation in the supradiaphragm or iuxtarenal segments may be observed.

In giant cell arteritis high alkaline phosphatase, aspartate transaminase, and glutamic–pyruvic transaminase values, indicative of liver involvement, are sometimes found. A biopsy of the temporal artery after the most suitable segment has been identified through ultrasound scans or angiography will show the giant cells.[74]

In the active phase of Takayasu's arteritis the erythrocyte sedimentation rate is increased and a moderate anemia is frequent; serum γ-globulin levels are increased. Widening or irregularity of the aorta on chest x-rays and electrocardiographic signs of hypertension are common findings. Arteriograms show restricted or extended narrowed vascular segments in the aorta and its branches. Involved arteries may not be biopsied because of the risk of creating vascular insufficiency, but any part of the le-

TABLE 37.2. Antibodies in connective tissue diseases.

Connective tissue disease	Specific antibodies
Systemic lupus erythematosus	Anti-dsDNA
	Anti-Sm
	Antihistones
	Anti-RNP
Rheumatoid arthritis	Anti-Ig (RF)
Mixed connective tissue disease	Antinucleolar RNP (ENA)
Scleroderma	Anti–Scl-70
Polymyositis	Anti–Jo-1
Sjögren's syndrome	SS-A/Ro
	SS-B/La

sion excised at the time of surgical bypass should be examined for histological confirmation of the disease.

In classic nodular polyarteritis systemic vasculitis is frequently associated with a high eosinophil count and a low complement titer, cryoglobulins, rheumatoid factor, and occasionally disseminated intravascular coagulation. Diagnosis is confirmed by the presence of necrotizing vasculitis in the affected organ, which is usually the kidney, on biopsy.[43]

In Kawasaki's syndrome an increased number of immature blood cells and high aspartate transaminase and glutamic–pyruvic transaminase levels are common. Anti–endothelial cell antibodies are often found during the acute phase. All of the following diagnostic criteria must be met to confirm that a patient has Kawasaki's syndrome: conjunctivitis, inflammation of upper airway mucosa, rash on the trunk, palmar and plantar erythema, and widespread lymph node disease.[44]

In Wegener's granulomatosis high serum titers of antibodies to cytoplasm neutrophil antigens are present in 75% of patients. Two different immunofluorescence patterns are found: the widespread cytoplasma pattern, stimulated by antigens such as serinic proteinases, is more specific than the perinuclear cytoplasm pattern. Antinuclear antibodies and cryoglobulins are usually absent. Biopsy of tissue from accessible affected sites confirms the diagnosis.[8,74]

In Churg–Strauss syndrome an extremely high eosinophil count that ranges from 5000 to 20,000 per mm^3, particularly in acute stages, is usual.[5] In Schönlein–Henoch purpura increases in serum Ig, particularly IgA, are associated with proteinuria and hematuria. Biopsy on skin or kidney tissue showing IgA deposits in vessel walls confirms the diagnosis.[6] In a mixed cryoglobulinemia biopsy of cutaneous lesions is essential to confirm diagnosis, which is suggested by the presence of cryoglobulins in the blood.[74]

Because the clinical signs and symptoms of vasculitis secondary to different diseases may overlap, a definitive diagnosis must be based on laboratory tests. Identifying the various autoantibodies differentiates the pathologies (Table 37.2), but vasculitis is confirmed only by biopsy findings.

In vasculitis secondary to connective tissue disease the antinuclear antibodies are specific autoantibodies for SLE. Antinuclear antibodies act as opsonins for the nuclear antigens and cause LE phenomenon. Immunofluorescence patterns are classified as homogeneous, speckled, nucleolar, and rim. All patterns may be seen in serum from patients with SLE, but the rim pattern, produced by antibodies to double-stranded DNA, is the most specific for SLE. Table 37.3 shows the antinuclear antibodies divided into subgroups according to their specificity for diseases.

Longer prothrombin times, paradoxically associated with an increased incidence of arterial and venous thrombosis, are often found in patients with antiphospholipid syndrome. Circulating antibodies to coagulating factors VIII, IX, XI, and XII may be observed. A low complement activation level due to both reduced synthesis and increased complement request is typical of SLE.

Serum levels of total hemolytic complement activity of C3 and C4 are reduced and indicate active disease. Circulating Ig, particularly IgG and IgM, may be increased; gammopathy has occasionally been observed. Cryoglobulins are present in patients with Raynaud's phenomenon and are usually associated with moderate non-

TABLE 37.3. Antigens linked to connective tissue diseases.

Antigen	Percentage	Clinical significance
DNA		
Double stranded	60	Highly specific; active disease
Single stranded	60	Nonspecific
Histones	70	Drug-induced SLE (90%)
Ribonucleoproteins		
Sm	30	Found only in SLE
U1-RNP	40	Frequent in overlapping syndromes
Ro (SS-A)	30	SLE associated with Sjögren's syndrome; subacute cutaneous SLE
La (SS-B)	15	SLE associated with Sjögren's syndrome
Ribosomal P	5	SLE-induced psychosis

SLE, systemic lupus erythematosus.

hemolytic anemia, a positive Coombs' test, leukopenia, neutrophil–endothelial adhesion, and modest thrombocytopenia.[17,74]

Nailbed capillaroscopy reveals functional and structural abnormalities in the microcirculation. Capillary flow may be fast or corpusculated and granular, and in severe cases stasis may be present.[19] Capillaries may reach 1 mm in length and be dilated or corkscrew in form. Lesions may cause microhemorrhages. The venular plexus is often visible near damaged capillaries.[29]

Although rheumatoid factor (IgM) is present in 70% of patients with RA, it is not specific. At least 25% of patients who test positive for RA have increased antinuclear antibodies, which usually present a homogeneous immunofluorescence pattern. Tests are false-positive in 5% to 10% of patients with syphilis. Although usually rare in RA, complement levels are constantly low in systemic forms of the disease.[65,74] In RA capillary abnormalities are classified as (1) short capillaries and loops, in shoal-of-fish (banc des poissons) formation; (2) long capillary loops in stockade formation, with a clearly visible venous plexus; and (3) anarchic capillary formation.[20]

In mixed connective tissue disease speckled pattern antinuclear antibodies are usually strongly positive. Specifically the differentiating factor is the high antiribonucleoprotein component of the extractable nuclear antigen antibody levels. More than 50% of patients test positive for circulating rheumatoid factor, and the level is often very high. Polyclonal hypergammaglobulinemia is frequent, and low complement titers, leukocyte count, and anemia are observed in 30% of patients.[74]

No specific antibodies exist for the diagnosis of dermatomyositis; when associated with polymyositis, anti-Jo-1 nonisotonic antiprotein antibodies (of the antinuclear antibody group) are found in 30% to 50% of patients.[90] In dermatomyositis enlarged capillaries are observed in glomerular formation and cause cutaneous microtelangiectasia.[51]

Although 95% of patients with scleroderma test positive for antinuclear antibodies, serum antibody findings are nonspecific. Diagnosis is confirmed in 85% of patients by the presence of seven identified antibodies that are specific for the organ involved; for example, the anti-centromero antibody is found in 60% of patients with cutaneous involvement and the antithymus (with a nucleolar pattern) is found in 10% of patients. Anti-ribonucleic acid polymerase III and antitopoisomerase I antibodies are found in 80% of patients with systemic scleroderma. The anti–U_3 ribonucleoprotein and anti–U_1 ribonucleoprotein are frequently found in overlapping forms of connective tissue disease. Two specific antibodies are rarely found in the same patient, which suggests that genetic factors may be involved.[74]

Only in scleroderma are enormous capillaries with rigid, irregular-shaped walls found at a density of 3 to 4 capillaries per millimeter versus the normal 10 capillaries per millimeter. Ramifications, anastomoses, and microhemorrhages are common.[83]

In Sjögren's syndrome the anti–SS-A antibodies are sensitive but not highly specific markers and are indicative of serious systemic involvement. The anti–SS-B antibodies are more specific but are present in only 50% of patients. Polyclonal hypergammaglobulinemia and high levels of circulating immunocomplexes, rheumatoid factor, and antinuclear antibodies may also be found.

Sjögren's syndrome can be diagnosed on the basis of the following criteria: (1) signs and symptoms of ocular dryness (Schirmer's test, pink Bengal test, and fluorescein), (2) dryness in the oral cavity (little saliva and abnormal salivary gland biopsy results), and (3) evidence of autoimmune diseases (rheumatoid factor >1:320; antinuclear antibody >1:320; positive for anti–SS-A and anti–SS-B antibodies). In secondary forms, signs and symptoms of Sjögren's syndrome associated with clinical features that lead to a diagnosis of SLE, RA, polymyositis, or scleroderma are sufficient for diagnosis.

In all forms of primary vasculitis, markers of inflammation (see Table 37.4) present constantly abnormal levels. Each form has its own specific clinical pattern that, together with biopsy results, confirms the differential diagnosis.

In Behçet's syndrome histocompatibility antigens, particularly HLA-B5, are frequently found. Fundamental to diagnosis of the syndrome is evidence of vasculitis obtained by biopsy of internal organs or of samples of skin and/or mucosa affected by the disease.[74]

TABLE 37.4. Diagnosing vasculitis.

Inflammation
Urine analysis (proteinuria, hematuria, cylinders)
Renal function (creatinine clearance, 24-h proteinuria profile)
Blood tests (total, WBC, eosinophil count)
Aspecific markers (ESR, PCR, FR)

Immunological tests
Autoantibodies (ANA, nDNA, ENA, Scl-70, ANCA)
Complement and circulating immunocomplexes
Cryoglobulins

Differential diagnosis
Blood cultures
Viral infection (serum) HBV, CMV
Echocardiogram

Specific tests
Chest and nasal sinus x-rays
Biopsy of involved tissue (kidney)
Angiography

WBC, white blood count; ESR, erythrocyte sedimentation rate; PCR, polymerase chain reaction; RF, rheumatoid factor; ANA, antinuclear antibody; nDNA, nuclear deoxyribonucleic acid; ENA, extractable nuclear antigens; Scl-70, antibody against nuclear enzyme DNA topoisomerase I; ANCA, anti–neutrophil-cytoplasm-antibodies; HBV, hepatitis B virus; CMV, cytomegalovirus.

Treatment

Therapy for vasculitis aims at long-term disease remission and identification of the earliest signs of relapse.[2,53] Medication should be kept to the minimum effective dosage to limit the serious toxic side effects of those drugs.[12]

Assessing the effects of therapy in most forms of primary vasculitis is difficult because of the chronic course of the disease. Cardiovascular complications such as cardiac insufficiency and hypertension (which is usually symptomatic) should be treated using the standard approach. Steroids, particularly oral prednisone (30–50 mg/d), are administered in the acute stage, with the dosage gradually being reduced to maintenance levels of 10 to 20 mg/d.[70] Besides normalizing the erythrocyte sedimentation rate, steroids sometimes control the course of the disease by slowing or even inhibiting its progression.[34] Antiaggregation and anticoagulant agents may also be prescribed because, independently of the stage of the disease, they prevent thrombus formation, which is often an additional complication.[81]

Surgery to remove chronic vascular obstruction is the last resort and is used only in extremely advanced stages of Takayasu's arteritis.[61] Aortic aneurysms and stenotic lesions of the epiaortic, renal, and abdominal vessels can generally be treated with surgery, but the presence of chronic inflammation increases the frequency of postoperative complications such as ruptures or pseudo-aneurysms on the sites of parietal sutures, which increase perioperative mortality rates. The bypass is the most successful approach because it is less influenced by lesion inflammation; thrombectomy and percutaneous angioplasty often yield only partial results and are successful only in the short term because of vessel wall inflammation.[41,70,75]

Therapy for vasculitis secondary to connective tissue disease depends on the type and caliber of affected vessels. Because prognosis is good for nonnecrotizing lesions in small vessels, they can be treated conservatively, and patients usually respond well to steroid administration (oral prednisone, 20–60 mg/d) for a short period (e.g., less than 3 months). Vasculitis in medium- and large-caliber vessels also responds well to steroid therapy (oral prednisone, 40–60 mg/d) for at least 1 year. As results of laboratory tests improve, the dosage can later be reduced over a 6-month period to ≤10 mg/d.[2,26]

The advent of cyclophosphamide, at an oral or intravenous dosage of 3 mg/kg daily, has dramatically improved prognosis, particularly in systemic, necrotizing vasculitis. Cyclical oral administration is better than continuous therapy because the potentially toxic side effects (e.g., episodes of hemorrhagic cystitis, the development of bladder neoplasias, and infertility), which are often dose dependent, are attenuated.[26]

Therapy should be continued for up to 6 months after remission of vasculitis. Oral azatioprine (2–3 mg/kg daily) is a valid alternative to cyclophosphamide and can be substituted for it in patients who experience serious side effects. Weekly cycles of oral methotrexate (5–30 mg/wk) may be substituted for azathioprine in patients in remission.[57,88] Because a high percentage (about 50%) of relapses occur even in patients on cyclophosphamide therapy, repeated cycles may be required for 5 to 10 years after diagnosis.[1]

Plasmapheresis is indicated when systemic advanced vasculitis is associated with predominantly marked involvement of the lungs and kidney.[31] Side effects are the risk of pulmonary hemorrhage and rapid renal failure.

Intravenous administration of Ig (400 mg/kg daily for 4 days) is of real benefit only in vasculitis associated with Kawasaki's syndrome.[44] Its efficacy in other forms of vasculitis remains to be determined.

Acknowledgment
Translation by Dr. G. A. Boyd.

References

1. Abe C. Application of immunosuppressants for therapy of patients with vasculitis. *Nippon Rinsho.* 1994;52:2177–2181.
2. Abe T. Steroid and non-steroidal anti-inflammatory drug therapy of vasculitis. *Nippon Rinsho.* 1994;52:2173–2176.
3. Achkar AA, Stanson AW, Johnson CM, et al. Rheumatoid vasculitis manifesting as intra-abdominal hemorrhage. *Mayo Clin Proc.* 1995;70:565–569.
4. Alpsoy E, Yilmaz E, Basaran E. Interferon therapy for Behçet disease. *J Am Acad Dermatol.* 1994;31:617–619.
5. Amitani R, Kuze F. Churg-Strauss syndrome. *Rheumatol Int.* 1994;52:2072–2076.
6. Araque A, Sanchez R, Alamo C, et al. Evolution in immunoglobulin A nephropathy into Henoch-Schönlein purpura in an adult patient. *Am J Kidney Dis.* 1995;25:340–342.
7. Barber HS. Myalgic syndrome with constitutional effects: polymyalgia rheumatica. *Ann Rheum Dis.* 1957;16:230–237.
8. Barksdale SK, Hallahan CW, Kerr GS, et al. Cutaneous pathology in Wegener's granulomatosis: a clinicopathologic study of 75 biopsies in 46 patients. *Am J Surg Pathol.* 1995;19:161–172.
9. Biesecker G, Lavin L, Siskind M. Cutaneous localization of the membrane attack complex in discoid and systemic lupus erythematosis. *N Engl J Med.* 1982;306:264–267.
10. Brentjens J, Ossi E, Albini B. Disseminated immune deposits in lupus erythematosus. *Arthritis Rheum.* 1977;20:962–964.
11. Burke AP, Sobin LH, Virmani R. Localized vasculitis of the gastrointestinal tract. *Am J Surg Pathol.* 1995;19:338–349.
12. Calabrese LH, Hoffman GS, Guillevin L. Therapy of resistant systemic necrotizing vasculitis: polyarteritis, Churg-Strauss syndrome, Wegener's granulomatosis, and hyper-

sensitivity vasculitis group disorders. *Rheum Dis Clin North Am.* 1995;21:41–57.

13. Chen CC, Kerr GS, Carter CS, et al. Lack of sensitivity of indium-111 mixed leukocyte scans for active disease in Takayasu's arteritis. *J Rheumatol.* 1995;22:478–481.

14. Citron P, Halpern M, McCarron M. Necrotizing angiitis associated with drug abuse. *N Engl J Med.* 1970;283: 1003–1006.

15. Ciuffetti G, Pasqualini L, Fuscaldo G, et al. Neutrophil-derived adhesion molecules in human digital ischemia and reperfusion. *Vasa.* 1995;24:155–158.

16. Cochrane CG, Weigle WO, Dixon FJ. The role of polymorphonuclear leukocytes in the initiation and cessation of the Arthus vasculitis. *J Exp Med.* 1959;100:481–494.

17. Conn DL, McDuffie FC, Dyck PJ. Immunopathologic study of sural nerves in rheumatoid arthritis. *Arthritis Rheum.* 1972;15:135–139.

18. Dammacco F, Sansonno D, Han JH, et al. Natural interferon-alpha versus its combination with 6-methyl-prednisolone in the therapy of type II mixed cryoglobulinemia: a long-term, randomized, controlled study. *Blood.* 1994;84: 3336–3343.

19. Davis E, Landau J, Ivry M. Vasomotion in health and disease. *Bibl Anat.* 1964;6:195–200.

20. Dequeker J, Rosberg G. Digital capillaritis in rheumatoid arthritis. *Acta Rheum Scand.* 1967;13:299–307.

21. Epstein WL. Granulomatosis hypersensitivity. *Prog Allergy.* 1967;11:36–88.

22. Fauci AF, Wolff SM. Wegener's granulomatosis and related diseases. In: Dowling HF, ed. *Disease-a-Month.* Vol 23, No 7. Chicago, Ill: Chicago Year Book Medical Publishers; 1977: 1–9.

23. Fetoni V, Berti E, Cecca E, et al. Sneddon's syndrome: clinical and immunohistochemical findings. *Clin Neurol Neurosurg.* 1994;96:310–313.

24. Fienberg R. The protracted superficial phenomenon in pathergic (Wegener's) granulomatosis. *Hum Pathol.* 1981; 12:458–461.

25. Fortin PR, Larson MG, Watters AK, et al. Prognostic factors in systemic necrotizing vasculitis of the polyarteritis nodosa group: a review of 45 cases. *J Rheumatol.* 1995;22: 78–84.

26. Genereau T, Lortholary O, Leclerq P, et al. Treatment of systemic vasculitis with cyclophosphamide and steroids: daily oral low-dose cyclophosphamide administration after failure of a pulse intravenous high-dose regimen in four patients. *Br J Rheumatol.* 1994;33:959–962.

27. Geschwind DH, FitzPatrick M, Mischel PS, et al. Sneddon's syndrome is a thrombotic vasculopathy: neuropathologic and neuroradiologic evidence. *Neurology.* 1995;45:557–560.

28. Gianetti A, Serri F, Bernasconi C. Immunofluorescent studies of the skin in mixed cryoglobulinemia and Schönlein-Henoch purpura. *Acta Derm Venereol.* 1976;56: 211–214.

29. Gilje O. Capillary microscopy in the differential diagnosis of skin disease. *Acta Derm Venereol.* 1953;33:303–317.

30. Goodfield NE, Bhandari S, Plant WD, et al. Cardiac involvement in Wegener's granulomatosis. *Br Heart J.* 1995; 73:110–115.

31. Hashimoto H. Vascular involvements in systemic lupus erythematosus. *Nippon Rinsho.* 1994;52:2109–2113.

32. Hashimoto T, Haraoka H. Vasculo-Behçet's disease. *Nippon Rinsho.* 1994;52:2138–2142.

33. Hernandez-Pando R, Reyes P, Espitia C, et al. Raised agalactosyl IgG and antimycobacterial humoral immunity in Takayasu's arteritis. *J Rheumatol.* 1994;21:1870–1876.

34. Hoffman GS. Treatment of resistant Takayasu's arteritis. *Rheum Dis Clin North Am.* 1995;21:73–80.

35. Hotchi M. Intractable vasculitis: general consideration, concept, and classification: pathological aspects. *Nippon Rinsho.* 1994;52:1963–1969.

36. Hu CH, O'Loughlin S, Winkelmann RK. Cutaneous manifestations of Wegener's granulomatosis. *Arch Dermatol.* 1977;113:175–178.

37. Inoue C, Itoh R, Kawa Y, et al. Pathogenesis of mucocutaneous lesions in Behçet disease. *J Dermatol.* 1994;21: 474–480.

38. Ishikawa K, Maetani S. Long-term outcome for 120 Japanese patients with Takayasu's disease: clinical and statistical analyses of related prognostic factors. *Circulation.* 1994;90: 1855–1860.

39. Jain R, Chartash E, Susin M, et al. Systemic lupus erythematosus complicated by thrombotic microangiopathy. *Semin Arthritis Rheum.* 1994;24:173–182.

40. Jennette JC, Falk RJ. The pathology of vasculitis involving the kidney. *Am J Kidney Dis.* 1994;24:130–141.

41. Joseph S, Mandalam KR, Rao VR, et al. Percutaneous transluminal angioplasty of the subclavian artery in nonspecific aortoarteritis: results of long-term follow-up. *J Vasc Interv Radiol.* 1994;5:573–580.

42. Kadoya A, Akahoshi T, Sekiyama N, et al. Cutaneous vasculitis in a patient with dermatomyositis without muscle involvement. *Intern Med.* 1994;33:809–812.

43. Kasukawa R, Sakuma F, Oshima Y. Polyarteritis nodosa. *Nippon Rinsho.* 1994;52:2066–2071.

44. Kato H, Nishiyori A, Sugimura T, et al. Kawasaki vasculitis. *Nippon Rinsho.* 1994;52:2095–2102.

45. Katzenstein AL, Locke WK. Solitary lung lesions in Wegener's granulomatosis: pathologic findings and clinical significance in 25 cases. *Am J Surg Pathol.* 1995;19: 545–552.

46. Kobayashi M, Saito M, Minoshima S, et al. A case of progressive systemic sclerosis with crescentic glomerulonephritis associated with myeloperoxidase-antineutrophil cytoplasmatic antibody (MPO-Anca) and anti-glomerular basement membrane antibody. *Nippon Jinzo Gakkai Shi.* 1995;37:207–211.

47. Lie JT. Vasculopathy in the antiphospholipid syndrome: thrombosis or vasculitis, or both? *J Rheumatol.* 1989;16: 713–715.

48. Lie JT. Vasculitis in the antiphospholipid syndrome: culprit or consort? *J Rheumatol.* 1994;21:397–399.

49. Lindgren S, Hansen B, Sjoholm AG, et al. Complement activation in patients with primary Sjögren's syndrome: an indicator of systemic disease. *Autoimmunity.* 1993;16: 297–300.

50. McRorie ER, Jobanputra P, Ruckley CV, et al. Leg ulceration in rheumatoid arthritis. *Br J Rheumatol.* 1994;33: 1078–1084.

51. Merlen JF. Phénomène de Raynaud et sclérodermie. *Baillerie Clin Rheum.* 1980;29:333–337.

52. Meyers KE, Thomson PD, Beale PG, et al. Gallium scintig-

raphy in the diagnosis and total lymphoid irradiation of Takayasu's arteritis. *S Afr Med J.* 1994;84:685–688.

53. Niimi H, Nakajima Y, Nosaka S, et al. CT and MRI findings of refractory vasculitis. *Nippon Rinsho.* 1994;52:2047–2053.

54. Nishimura Y. HLA-linked susceptibility to intractable vasculitis syndrome. *Nippon Rinsho.* 1994;52:2000–2005.

55. Nota ME, Gokemeijer JD, van der Laan JG. Clinical usefulness of abdominal CT-scanning in Henoch-Schönlein vasculitis. *Neth J Med.* 1995;46:142–145.

56. Nowoslawsky A. Immunopathological features of rheumatoid arthritis. In: Muller W, Harverth HG, Fehrk W, eds. *Rheumatoid Arthritis.* New York, NY: Academic Press; 1971: 325–361.

57. Ohno T, Matsuda I, Furukawa H, et al. Recovery from rheumatoid cerebral vasculitis by low-dose methotrexate. *Intern Med.* 1994;33:615–620.

58. Onyewotu II, Johnson PM, Johnson GD. Enhanced uptake by guinea-pig macrophages of radio-iodinated human aggregated immunoglobulin G in the presence of sera from rheumatoid patients with cutaneous vasculitis. *Clin Exp Immunol.* 1975;19:267–271.

59. Pariser KM. Takayasu's arteritis. *Curr Opin Cardiol.* 1994;9: 575–580.

60. Park JH, Chung JW, Im JG, et al. Takayasu arteritis: evaluation of mural changes in the aorta and pulmonary artery with CT angiography. *Radiology.* 1995;196:89–93.

61. Robbs JV, Abdool-Carrim AT, Kadwa AM. Arterial reconstruction for non-specific arteritis (Takayasu's disease): medium to long term results. *Eur J Vasc Surg.* 1994;8: 401–407.

62. Roberts GA, Eren E, Sinclair H, et al. Two cases of Wegener's granulomatosis involving the pituitary. *Clin Endocrinol.* 1995;42:323–328.

63. Robson MG, Walport MJ, Davies KA. Systemic lupus erythematosus and acute demyelinating polyneuropathy. *Br J Rheumatol.* 1994;33:1074–1077.

64. Salvarani C, Gabriel SE, Gertz MA, et al. Primary systemic amyloidosis presenting as giant cell arteritis and polymyalgia rheumatica. *Arthritis Rheum.* 1994;37:1621–1626.

65. Sany J. Clinical and biological polymorphism of rheumatoid arthritis. *Clin Exp Rheumatol.* 1994;12(suppl 11P): S59–S61.

66. Sato R, Sato Y, Ishikawa H, et al. Takayasu's disease associated with ulcerative colitis. *Intern Med.* 1994;33:759–763.

67. Schwarz MI, Sutarik JM, Nick JA, et al. Pulmonary capillaritis and diffuse alveolar hemorrhage: a primary manifestation of polymyositis. *Am J Respir Crit Care Med.* 1995; 151:2037–2040.

68. Sehgal M, Swanson JW, De Remee RA, et al. Neurologic manifestations of Churg-Strauss syndrome. *Mayo Clin Proc.* 1995;70:337–341.

69. Seko Y, Yazaki Y. Cytotoxic factor in vascular injury. *Nippon Rinsho.* 1994;52:2018–2023.

70. Sharma BK, Siveski-Iliskovic N, Singal PK. Takayasu arteritis may be underdiagnosed in North America. *Can J Cardiol.* 1995;11:311–316.

71. Shasby DM, Schwarz MI, Forstot JZ. Pulmonary immune complex deposition in Wegener's granulomatosis. *Chest.* 1982;81:338–341.

72. Singleton JD, West SG, Reddy VV, et al. Cerebral vasculitis complicating rheumatoid arthritis. *South Med J.* 1995;88: 470–474.

73. Spiera RF, Filippa DA, Bains MS, et al. Esophageal involvement in Wegener's granulomatosis. *Arthritis Rheum.* 1994; 37:1404–1407.

74. Sugiura H, Hosoda Y. Histopathological and immunohistochemical diagnosis of intractable vasculitis syndromes. *Nippon Rinsho.* 1994;52:2034–2040.

75. Tada Y. Surgical treatment of intractable vasculitic syndromes with special reference to Buerger disease, Takayasu arteritis, and so-called inflammatory abdominal aortic aneurysm. *Nippon Rinsho.* 1994;52:2192–2202.

76. Tan EM, Kunkel HG. An immunofluorescent study of the skin lesions in systemic lupus erythematosus. *Arthritis Rheum.* 1966;1:37–41.

77. Tanabe T. Intractable vasculitis syndromes: incidence and epidemiology. *Nippon Rinsho.* 1994;52:1987–1991.

78. Theofilopoulos AN. Evaluation and clinical significance of circulating immune complexes. *Prog Clin Immunol.* 1980;4:63–66.

79. Tomino Y. Hypersensitivity angiitis, Henoch-Schönlein purpura. *Nippon Rinsho.* 1994;52:2077–2081.

80. Tunaci A, Berkmen YM, Gokmen E. Thoracic involvement in Behçet disease: pathologic, clinical, and imaging features. *American Journal of Roentgenology.* 1995;164:51–56.

81. Vanoli M, Miani S, Amft N, et al. Takayasu's arteritis in Italian patients. *Clin Exp Rheumatol.* 1995;13:45–50.

82. Van Vollenhoven RF. Adhesion molecules, sex steroids, and the pathogenesis of vasculitis syndromes. *Curr Opin Rheumatol.* 1995;7:4–10.

83. Vayssairat M, Fiessinger JN, Housset E. Place de la capillaroscopie dans les acrosyndromes. *Ann Med Interne (Paris).* 1980;131:41–42.

84. Voskuyul AE, Martin S, Melchers L, et al. Levels of circulating intercellular adhesion molecule-1 and -3 but not circulating endothelial leucocyte adhesion molecule are increased in patients with rheumatoid vasculitis. *Br J Rheumatol.* 1995;34:311–315.

85. Waksman BH. Delayed (cellular) hypersensitivity. In: Samter M, ed. *Immunological Diseases.* Vol 1. Boston, Mass: Little, Brown; 1971:220–231.

86. Watts RA, Carruthers DM, Symmons DP, et al. The incidence of rheumatoid vasculitis in the Norwich Health Authority. *Br J Rheumatol.* 1994;33:832–833.

87. Weyand CM, Goronzy JJ. Molecular approaches toward pathologic mechanisms in giant cell arteritis and Takayasu's arteritis. *Curr Opin Rheumatol.* 1995;7:30–36.

88. Wilson K, Abeles M. A 2 year, open ended trial of methotrexate in systemic lupus erythematosus. *J Rheumatol.* 1994; 21:1674–1677.

89. Yamada I, Himeno Y, Suzuki S. Angiography in vasculitis. *Nippon Rinsho.* 1994;52:2041–2046.

90. Yamamoto T, Ohkubo H, Katayama I, et al. Dermatomyositis with multiple skin ulcers showing vasculitis and membrano-cystic lesion. *J Dermatol.* 1994;21:687–689.

91. Yamane K. Endothelin and collagen vascular disease: a review with special reference to Raynaud's phenomenon and systemic sclerosis. *Intern Med.* 1994;33:579–582.

92. Yoshinoya S. Immune complex and vasculitis. *Nippon Rinsho.* 1994;52:1992–1999.

38

Hyperviscosity Syndromes

Giovanni Ciufetti and Rita Lombardini

Rheology is the study of how matter is deformed or flows when force is applied. Hemorheology is the study of the flow properties of one fluid—blood—circulating in a closed system that is subjected to a tangential force originating in a pulsing pump—the heart. Clinical hemorheology is the study of blood flow during physiological changes in normal circulation and the syndromes or diseases that develop under pathological conditions.

In this section we briefly describe the physics of blood flow, fluid resistance to flow (blood viscosity), and the elastic behavior of blood in terms of deformation, adhesion, aggregation, and activation of individual blood cells (blood deformability). Hyperviscosity syndromes are described, and the techniques for measuring parameters of blood rheology for routine use in a clinical hemorheology laboratory are included.

The Physics of Blood Flow

Blood flows along an energy gradient and passes from high energy levels in the aorta through the arteries and microcirculation to low energy levels in the veins and venules. Pressure, gravity, and potential and kinetic energy all contribute to the total fluid energy during flow, and the difference in the energy levels at any two points determines the direction and rate of flow. Blood flow also depends on the vessel diameter and its changes during constriction and dilation, on vessel bifurcations and junctions, on the pressure difference between the arterial and venous ends of blood vessels, and on blood fluidity.

Blood flow rate is governed by the Hagen–Poisseuille equation:

$$\text{volume flow rate} = \frac{\text{pressure gradient} \times \text{vessel radius}^4}{8 \times \text{vessel length} \times \text{fluid viscosity}}$$

which, for a simple liquid in a straight tube, shows that an inverse linear relationship exists between flow rate

and viscosity. Viscosity, the reciprocal of fluidity, is the frictional flow resistance between layers that must be overcome by a driving force to cause shearing and hence flow.

In large blood vessels, blood moves in a streamlined fashion known as *laminar flow,* and velocity is parabolic in shape. Adjacent layers move parallel to each other, and the difference in velocity (velocity gradient) between any two layers quantifies shearing, or the *shear rate,* which is expressed as units of inverse seconds (s^{-1}). The force required to produce the flow velocity and hence the internal shearing of the liquid is termed *shear stress,* expressed as units of milliPascals (mPa). Yield stress is the minimum shear stress necessary to produce a minimum shear rate or flow.

The ratio of shear stress to shear rate defines the *coefficient of viscosity.*

$$\text{Viscosity (mPa} \cdot \text{s}^{-1}) = \frac{\textit{shear stress (mPa)}}{\text{shear rate (s}^{-1})}$$

Because the viscosity of whole blood is not constant, but increases markedly at low shear rates (Figure 38.1), blood is defined as a non-Newtonian fluid. Its non-Newtonian behavior is principally due to red cell aggregation at low shear rates and red cell deformation at high shear rates (Figure 38.2).

Laminar blood flow becomes turbulent when, by moving radially or reversing direction, part of the blood stream flows in a different manner from the main stream, thus causing eddies or vortices that may damage vessel walls. Turbulent flow dissipates energy not only in the form of noise and heat but also in overcoming the resistance of laminar flow. The ratio of inertial to viscous forces is expressed by

$$\text{Reynolds' number (R}_e) = \frac{\textit{flow velocity} \times \textit{tube diameter} \times \textit{fluid density}}{\text{fluid viscosity}}$$

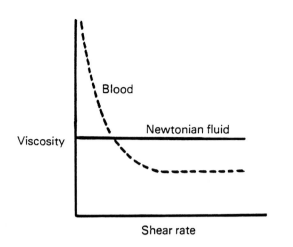

FIGURE 38.1. Relationship between shear rate and viscosity in a Newtonian fluid and blood.

and when it exceeds approximately 700, flow changes from laminar to turbulent. This probably never occurs in normal circulation but almost certainly does under pathological conditions, particularly when blood viscosity is low, because Reynolds' number is inversely related to viscosity.

Laminar blood flow loses its streamline properties in the microcirculation because of axial migration. In axial flow, red blood cells migrate from the vessel wall to its axis; platelets and plasma are diffused toward the wall; and, when vessels are less than 300 μm in diameter, blood becomes less viscous. In capillaries smaller than 10 μm in diameter, blood viscosity equals plasma viscosity. The Fahraeus–Lindqvist phenomenon[65] links reduced vascular bore with a reduction in the number of blood cells entering the capillary (screening effect)[34] and with an increase in red blood cell deformability. When capillary bore is 5 μm or less, a transition from the Fahraeus–Lindqvist phenomenon to the inversion phe-

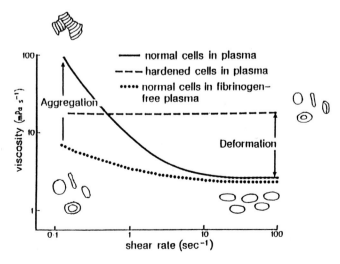

FIGURE 38.2. Mechanism of shear rate dependence of blood viscosity. (Adapted from Chien.[20])

nomenon occurs, and blood viscosity decreases suddenly with the capillary radius.

Blood Viscosity and Deformability

Blood is a suspension of erythrocytes, leukocytes, and platelets in plasma, which is a water-based solution of proteins and inorganic constituents. Serum is the fluid that remains after blood is allowed to clot and the solid material is removed. Although serum is a solution of ions and inorganic and organic molecules in water, its viscosity depends on its protein fractions, changing with their molecular size and the departure of their shape from the spherical (as indicated by the length-to-diameter ratio).[23] Close to serum in composition, plasma includes some of the clotting factors and fibrinogen, which makes a 22% contribution to plasma's viscosity. α_2-Macroglobulins and immunoglobulins also influence plasma viscosity because of their nonspherical shape and large size.[23] Because whole blood is a suspension of cells in plasma, its viscosity is a function of plasma viscosity.[102,142] When levels of plasma proteins—particularly fibrinogen—are increased, the corresponding rise in plasma viscosity influences whole blood viscosity. Besides fibrinogen, hematocrit (or packed cell volume) is a major determinant of blood viscosity, which also varies with shear rate, red cell aggregation in slow flow, and red cell deformation in rapid flow.

At any shear rate, a linear increase in hematocrit within the 20% to 60% range leads to logarithmic increases in blood viscosity. Normal high-shear blood viscosity (3.5–7.5 mPa s^{-1} at 37°C) largely reflects the normal range of hematocrit (37%–51%). Increases in hematocrit within the normal range greatly increase red cell aggregation and hence low-shear blood viscosity and yield stress.[20] At abnormally high hematocrit levels, the close proximity of red cells, resulting from a decrease in free fluid volume, reduces the effects of aggregation.[20] At low hematocrit levels, aggregation is limited because of the small number of red cells available.[20]

At high shear rates (above 100 s^{-1}), normal whole blood behaves as a Newtonian fluid because all the erythrocyte forces are dispersed by shear forces. At intermediate shear rates (16–100 s^{-1}), the Newtonian to non-Newtonian behavior exhibited by whole blood occurs over the entire range.[106] At low shear rates (below 16 s^{-1}), red cells tend to aggregate (i.e., to stack end to end), forming structures known as rouleaux, which decrease the fluidity of whole blood and increase the erythrocyte sedimentation rate[63] and blood viscosity.[64] The effect of shear rate on red cell aggregation is shown in Figure 38.1. Aggregation depends on plasma protein changes, especially elevated fibrinogen concentrations and a high ratio of globulin to albumin.[20] An increased packed cell volume within the normal to slightly elevated range also markedly increases aggregation.

The rouleaux and networks that are formed when zero or low shear conditions exist, are broken up as the shear rate rises, which lowers cell volume and hence blood viscosity.[20] In normal blood, the aggregates are completely broken down at a shear rate of 50 s[-1] (shear stress 0.2 mPa).[14,65,126] As shear rate rises, the red cells deform, changing from a biconcave disk to an ellipsoid shape in axial orientation, which results in a further drop in blood viscosity to an asymptomatic maximum value at a shear rate of 100 to 200 s[-1].

The ability of the red cell to deform in response to external stresses[90] is one aspect of blood deformability (defined as the capacity of blood to flow through nutritive capillaries [mean diameter 5 mm] when the resting diameter of blood cells is 7.5 mm) that depends essentially on the viscoelastic properties of erythrocytes, leukocytes, and platelets.

Erythrocytes

At rest, the erythrocyte is a biconcave disk with an average diameter of 7.2 to 8.3 μm, a surface area of 128 to 160 μm^2, and a volume of 76 to 96 μm^3. To traverse microcirculation vessels, the erythrocyte flattens and lengthens into a parachute—or, in smaller vessels, torpedo-type—shape, and the increasing shear rates produce axial orientation of red cells with ellipsoid deformation.[20,21]

There are three main intrinsic determinants of erythrocyte deformability. (1) Cell shape is regulated by the surface/volume ratio. When the ratio is high, the erythrocyte forms the more deformable biconcave disk; when it is low, erythrocytes are rounded in shape and consequently less deformable. (2) Cell membrane flexibility depends on structural changes in protein (spectrin) and lipid (cholesterol/phospholipid ratio) contents. (3) Internal viscosity is determined by cell hemoglobin concentration and by any intracellular inclusions.[21] High hemoglobin levels alter volume hemostasis mechanisms and increase cytoplasma viscosity, which impairs erythrocyte deformability.[21]

Factors that are extrinsic to the erythrocyte and that influence deformability are increases in the velocity gradient in the extracellular fluid and, consequently, in the shear rate at the cell fluid junction; cell concentrations affected by plasma protein levels; and vessel diameter, which influences viscosity on the basis of the Fahraeus–Lindqvist phenomenon.[21]

Leukocytes

Although of similar diameter to the erythrocyte (6.2–7.5 μm), the leukocyte has twice the volume (because it is

spherical), whereas its elasticity is decreased 4-fold and its cellular viscosity is more than 1000-fold greater because of the nucleus, the granular cytoplasm, and the active contractile elements that lie beneath the membrane with its ruffled surface.[24] Precapillary arterial–venous shunts usually prevent leukocytes from traversing the nutritive capillaries, but when they do, deformation starts rapidly. Although deformation is partial in the first stage, it is followed by a slower final adaptation of the cell to the form of a cylinder capped with hemispherical ends to the capillary lumen.[6] Within the lumen, leukocytes proceed more slowly than erythrocytes, which tend to stack up behind, forming what is often called *train flow*.[6] Endothelial cell nuclei bulging into the capillary lumen may delay or stop leukocyte transit, causing capillary plugging, which must not be confused with adhesion of the leukocytes to the capillary walls.[6] Adhesion is mediated by activated leukocytes expressing adhesion molecules such as LFA-1, Mac-1, and p150,95, which interact with corresponding endothelial ligands.[3] When the number of leukocytes is increased, they are potential blockers of nutritive flow in low-flow states if they become stiffer or if the driving pressure is decreased.[95]

Platelets

Although platelets are small (2–4 μm), occupy less than 0.5% of blood volume, and have negligible effects on blood viscosity, platelet adhesion to the subendothelium and subsequent aggregation alter flow in vivo. Adhesion and aggregation are each influenced by chemical mediators in the blood and vessel wall and by rheological factors. Increases in flow rate (specifically with shear rate at vessel wall, up to shear rates of 700 s[-1]),[138] in packed cell volume,[138] in erythrocyte concentration, and in mean erythrocyte volume,[1] together with a loss of erythrocyte deformability,[2] contribute to platelet aggregation and adhesion to the subendothelium, which follows platelet activation. This is triggered by chemical stimuli such as thrombin, collagen, adenosine diphosphate, serotonin, and thromboxane A_2 and by shear forces. A procoagulant activity of platelets (platelet factor 3, attributed to membrane phospholipids) is also sensitive to shear stress on platelets[143]; this may explain why blood clotting time shortens with increasing shear rate.[43,60]

Clinical Hemorheology

Several diseases impair the rheological properties of blood. In acute rheumatic disorders such as gout, rheumatic fever, transient synovitis, and polymyalgia rheumatica, the abnormal plasma viscosity and erythrocyte sedimentation rate are largely due to increased fibrinogen levels; serum viscosity is rarely increased.[25] By contrast, rheumatoid arthritis is associated with increased serum viscosity, correlating with gamma globulin concentration and the rheumatoid factor.[128] Increased plasma viscosity, erythrocyte sedimentation rate, and whole blood viscosity have been observed in patients with systemic lupus erythematosus,[74,132] temporal arteritis,[25,57] ankylosing spondylitis,[61] and scleroderma with Raynaud's syndrome.[7] Patients with these conditions also show a decreased blood filterability,[7,83] which may reflect the effect of plasma or serum factor on red cell behavior[83] and may also contribute to cardiac microangiopathy. In primary Raynaud's phenomenon, a drop in temperature is associated with abnormal response of blood viscosity,[72] and leukocyte–endothelial adhesive interactions correlate with a significant degree of neutropenia.[31]

Rheological changes in blood contribute to the development of thrombotic occlusive disease. In the macrocirculation where blood flow streamlines separate from the mainstream (e.g., arterial bifurcations, such as the carotid sinus), low velocity flow reverses and recirculates and the low shear vortices increase erythrocyte aggregation and hematocrit and fibrinogen concentrations. Blood viscosity levels are raised; flow stagnation and endothelial interactions with activated platelets and leukocytes are facilitated, as is the selective deposition of fibrinogen. Thus, arterial disease is promoted; in fact, early intimal thickening and atherosclerotic plaques are often localized at arterial bifurcations.

In the microcirculation, contraction of plasma volume and loss of plasma proteins raise viscosity and lower blood filterability through the capillaries, leading to thrombosis formation. In the presence of venous or arterial disease,[92] surgery,[51,107,108,139] trauma,[10,88] burns,[4,5,37,129,144] hypotension, and shock[17,19,61,70,130] may impair microvascular perfusion and perpetuate a positive feedback cycle of decreased flow and increased blood flow resistance. The ensuing high blood viscosity probably increases shear stresses on cells and proteins flowing through the stenosis with a local viscosity increase in the low shear, poststenotic area, promoting activated cell–coagulant protein interactions.[55] By contrast, large-scale increases in proteins, cell mass, and the internal viscosity of blood cells—particularly the erythrocytes, which occur in the course of pure hyperviscosity syndrome—also reduce blood flow, causing stasis and thrombus formation.[48]

Hyperviscosity States and Atherosclerosis

Risk Factors

All the major cardiovascular risk factors are associated with elevated blood and/or plasma viscosity levels,[93] which may be the common denominator promoting atherogenesis and ischemia.[92]

1. *Age.* The slight age-related rise in blood viscosity is probably due to the increase of plasma fibrinogen with aging,[13] but it may result from older subjects having occult chronic disease, which is usually associated with high fibrinogen concentrations.[13]

2. *Sex.* Blood viscosity and hematocrit are lower in women than in men; this sex difference, like the risk of ischemic heart disease, disappears after menopause.[103] Abnormalities in blood rheology have been observed in women taking oral contraceptives.

3. *Cigarette smoking.* Smokers have reversible increases in blood viscosity compared with nonsmokers because of high hematocrit and plasma viscosity.[101,103] The latter is largely due to increases in fibrinogen and other acute-phase reactant proteins such as α_{-2} macroglobulin.[101]

4. *Obesity.* Although overweight is associated with elevated blood viscosity, hematocrit, plasma viscosity, and fibrinogen levels,[101,103] the causes are unknown.

5. *Sedentary lifestyle.* Little or no physical activity may be associated with increased blood viscosity.[18]

6. *Blood groups.* Differences in blood rheology factors in A, B, and O blood groups may be relevant to the epidemiological findings of excess arterial disease in blood group A compared with blood group O.[44]

7. *Hyperlipemia.* Patients with type II or type IV hyperlipoproteinemia have higher blood viscosity, hematocrit, plasma viscosity, serum viscosity, and red cell aggregation levels than control subjectss.[12,87,143] The increased plasma viscosity and red cell aggregation reflect direct effects of abnormal lipoproteins[87,131] as well as hyperfibrinogenemia, which may be a chronic-phase reaction to cholesterol-induced endothelial damage.[92] In population studies, blood viscosity, hematocrit, plasma viscosity, serum viscosity, and fibrinogen correlated with both plasma cholesterol and plasma triglyceride levels.[100] Elevated red cell membrane cholesterol and a high cholesterol/phospholipid ratio increase membrane rigidity and decrease red cell deformability[36]; however, whole blood filtration is normal in patients with hyperlipoproteinemia.[92]

8. *Diabetes.* Compared with nondiabetics, diabetics have higher levels of plasma and serum viscosity, red cell aggregation, low-shear blood viscosity, and high-shear blood viscosity at standard hematocrit. Hematocrit varies more because of increased plasma fluid transfer to the interstitial compartment through leakier capillaries.[85] It also varies because the osmotic and diuretic effects of blood glucose fluctuations[69] are higher in younger diabetics[95] and in patients with ketoacidotic or hyperosmolar dehydration[9] and lower in longer-duration diabetics with renal impairment. These rheological abnormalities are greater in patients with macrovascular or microvascular complications, because of their higher fibrinogen levels.[105,128] Blood

viscosity, plasma viscosity, and blood filterability are predictive of deterioration in retinopathy over a 3-year follow-up period,[9] and improved glycemic control is associated with a reduction in blood viscosity[9] and improved blood filterability. The causes of impaired blood filterability are controversial and may include plasma protein effects, leukocytosis,[136] and decreased white[59] and red cell deformability[59,128]; blood filterability impairment is reversed by insulin administration both in vitro and ex vivo.[136]

9. *Hypertension.* Chronic arterial hypertension is due to increased total peripheral resistance, with vascular and viscous components both contributing. Blood pressure correlates significantly and independently with both plasma and whole blood viscosity,[81,82,100] with the blood viscosity/blood pressure association being largely due to plasma viscosity. Blood viscosity may play a pathogenic role because (1) the viscous and vascular components of total peripheral resistance are multiplicative,[23] (2) left ventricular hypertrophy in hypertensive patients shows a closer correlation with blood viscosity than with blood pressure,[39] and (3) blood viscosity may promote the ischemic diseases that account for most of the morbidity and mortality in hypertension.[68] The effects of antihypertensive drugs on blood rheology require further study. At present, it appears that vasodilators improve rheology, β-adrenergic blockers have no effect, and diuretics may have adverse effects.[68]

Acute Ischemic Syndromes

In the acute (stroke or myocardial infarction) and chronic (cerebrovascular disorders, coronary heart disease, or critical limb ischemia) clinical pictures associated with atherosclerosis, compensation for rheological abnormalities is absent.[135] Not only is the hematocrit level inappropriately high, but blood flow rate and shear rate are reduced distal to arterial stenosis, allowing red cell aggregation, white cell plugging of capillaries, and venular obstruction by adherent white cells to promote or perpetuate ischemia.

Rheological factors are more important in acute rather than in chronic ischemia, and intervention must be prompt and adequate to prevent irreversible tissue necrosis. In acute ischemia, flow conditions rapidly deteriorate. Flow rates and shear rates falling toward zero are associated with impaired vasodilation. Plasma volume contracts, and acute-phase increases in fibrinogen, other globulins, and leukocytes impair the flow properties of blood[93] and lead to leukocyte plugging of the nutritive capillaries, trapping, activation, and the release of leukocyte-derived free radicals. Further impairment, plugging, and so forth ensue with the progressive exacerbation of ischemia.[114]

The low shear rates that occur during ischemia as a consequence of the low perfusion pressure are associated with a reduction in the washout of endogenous endothelial proinflammatory agents such as prostaglandins, cytokines, proteolytic enzymes, and so on.[123] Activated leukocytes express adhesion molecules such as LFA-1, Mac-1, and p150,95. An accumulation of the secretory products could well facilitate interactions of leukocyte surface receptors with corresponding endothelial ligands. Furthermore, again as a result of the low perfusion pressure in the ischemic area, contact time between the adhesive molecules is longer, the adhesion process is facilitated, and increased leukocyte adherence has been observed in venules.[86,123] Neutrophil involvement in functional alterations and/or damage to remote organs is part of an acute systemic inflammatory response[27] and may, for example, contribute to the high mortality rate from cardiovascular events that is associated with peripheral arterial occlusive disease.[113]

Ischemic Stroke

Increased blood viscosity in acute stroke is associated with rises in hematocrit, fibrinogen, plasma viscosity, and red cell aggregation levels.[56,96] Blood filterability is decreased,[89] partly reflecting decreased deformability of both granulocytes and mononuclear cells.[26] Cerebral blood flow correlates inversely with fibrinogen and hematocrit, levels of which also correlate with infarct size. When the hematocrit measurement is greater than 0.50, mortality rates are doubled in younger patients.[115] Mortality risk is also related to values of blood viscosity, fibrinogen, globulin/albumin ratio, erythrocyte sedimentation rate, mean red cell volume, and white cell count.[96,99,115]

Therapy

Hemodilution[71] and defibrination with ancrod[76] are suitable in some cases of acute stroke. Antiaggregation agents such as ticlopidine[118] and acetylsalicylic acid[48] may safely be prescribed but are often of little clinical benefit. Because the extension of ischemic damage and clinical outcome are correlated with the leukocyte count,[30] research has recently focused on the role of the white blood cells. Drugs acting as oxygen free radical scavengers, specific monoclonal antibodies against granulocyte adhesion receptors, and agents that protect the endothelium may prove to be the therapeutical strategy of the future.

Myocardial Infarction

Blood viscosity is increased in acute myocardial infarction as a result of hemoconcentration from pulmonary edema formation and high plasma concentrations of fibrinogen and other globulins that increase plasma viscosity and erythrocyte aggregation.[80] The decrease in blood filterability probably reflects these plasma protein changes and leukocytosis, because specific measurement of red cell and white cell filterability in buffer is normal.[92] In a comparative study, patients with unstable angina had elevations of fibrinogen, plasma viscosity, and white cell count levels that were intermediate between patients with myocardial infarction and control subjects. Blood viscosity, fibrinogen, and white cell count correlate with infarct size[92] and, together with blood filterability,[92] are all predictive of poor prognosis.

Therapy

Animal studies of hemodilution[94] and lowering the white cell count[94] have shown infarct size and complications[94] are reduced, but in patients with acute infarction, controlled studies of hemodilution have provided conflicting results.[49] Streptokinase reduces not only total mortality risk but also pulmonary and systemic arterial pressures,[62] possibly by decreasing blood viscosity[137] and hence pulmonary, systemic, and coronary total peripheral resistance,[22] as well as lysing coronary thrombosis. Reperfusion injury nonetheless appears to be the major complication. Again, experimental studies are investigating whether drugs preventing leukocyte adhesion are feasible.

In patients with chronic coronary, peripheral, or cerebral arterial disease,[54,103,119] high hematocrit levels appear to be due to contracted plasma volume rather than increased red cell mass,[33] and they may reflect the high prevalence of smokers[92] in these patients. Increased fibrinogen and plasma viscosity levels are due to high levels of catecholamines and free fatty acids.[135]

The influence of rheology on blood flow is much greater when circulation is compromised.[1] In ischemic organs, decreased perfusion pressure may be insufficient to overcome the flow resistance of even normal blood while compensatory vasodilation reaches a maximum. Under these conditions, even relatively small increases in packed cell volume and fibrinogen levels may have marked effects on erythrocyte aggregation and blood viscosity, and they may reduce residual perfusion even more. Microcirculatory plugging by erythrocyte aggregates and rigid leukocytes contributes to ischemia and impairments in whole blood filterability, probably because of the effects of erythrocytes on lactic acidosis and because of the release of products from activated platelets or white cells.[66] Activation of leukocytes increases their adhesiveness and decreases their deformability.[58]

When patients with risk factors for atherosclerosis or acute or chronic vessel disease are affected concomitantly by infection,[111,112] tumors,[41] alcoholism (Guegen), liver disease,[8,25,35,36,67,120] kidney disease,[40,78,95,104,121,140]

or thyroid disease,[45] a complete hemorheological profile should be monitored because all these conditions impair blood rheology.

Chronic Ischemic Syndromes

Cerebrovascular Disorders

Reduced erythrocyte deformability and increased blood viscosity have been observed in 70% of patients with chronic cerebrovascular disorders and are correlated with impairments in cognitive and psychobehavioral functions.[127]

Coronary Artery Disease

Patients with angina pectoris have higher hematocrit measurements, fibrinogen levels, and blood and plasma viscosity than healthy controls.[135] Cycle ergometer exercise is associated with abnormalities in the rheological properties of leukocytes[27,29] in patients with stable angina pectoris who also have increased platelet aggregation.[101] The prognostic significance of these abnormalities is not known. In unstable angina, transient lymphocyte activation may be responsible for the instability,[116] and monocyte activation has been linked to the role of extraplatelet thromboxane A_2 in this pathology.[117]

Intermittent Claudication

Chronic ischemia of the lower limbs is associated with abnormally high blood viscosity in about 25% of patients.[52] The mechanism is not always clear, but, in the majority of patients, it is due to hyperfibrinogenemia and a relatively high hematocrit level. The onset of prohibitive calf pain is associated with abnormalities in leukocyte deformability, activation, and expression of adhesion molecules.[28]

Retinal Vascular Disorders

The susceptibility of the retinal circulation to arterial and venous occlusion, diabetic microangiopathy, and increased intraocular pressure exemplifies how relatively small increases in hematocrit, plasma viscosity, and rigid cell measurements reduce capillary perfusion, thus promoting visual disturbances. Retinal arterial occlusion and/or venous diabetic retinopathy and glaucoma have all been associated with rheological abnormalities, which are most marked in ischemic/proliferative retinopathy.[97]

Deafness

The inner ear has a specialized circulation that may be susceptible to rheological disturbances. Tinnitus and deafness have been reported in all overt hyperviscosity syndromes and respond to viscosity reduction. In patients with idiopathic hearing loss, hearing impairment correlates with relative high-shear blood viscosity.[15] Sudden deafness is also associated with impairments in erythrocyte deformability.[32]

Therapy

Because these states are linked with abnormalities in several biohumoral and cellular factors—none of which, apart from fibrinogen concentrations, may present excessively high levels—no standard therapeutical approach can be recommended. Defibrinating agents appear to be a good option, at least in theory, when chronic arterial disease is associated with elevated fibrinogen concentrations.[98]

The two main defibrinating agents, ancrod (Arvin) and batroxobin (Defibrase), are proteolytic enzymes purified from snake venom. Conventional contraindications to anticoagulant therapy should be observed because the main side effect is bleeding; other adverse reactions are rare.

Defibrination reduces blood and plasma viscosity and probably also decreases erythrocyte aggregation.[91] Moderate transient falls in the platelet count and decreased levels of platelet factors 3 and 4 have been observed during the initial infusion.[98] Systemic fibrinolytic activity is usually not increased, but plasma plasminogen levels fall by about 50%; activated plasminogen, secondary to intravascular fibrin formation, contributes to the breakdown of fibrin, which is also mediated by the reticuloendothelial system.[98] Unfortunately, after 4 to 6 weeks of therapy, ancrod and batroxobin are inactivated by the formation of antibodies, which clearly limits the duration of treatment.

Long-term therapy is possible with agents that act on several parameters and can safely be administered with no adverse reactions or counterindications (apart from individual lack of tolerance) in chronic or acute arterial disease. Pentoxifylline,[141] buflomedil,[53] and ticlopidine[118] all improve blood rheology by reducing blood viscosity and improving filterability, through their concomitant action on several factors. However, the clinical benefits are often disappointing. In recent reports, prostaglandins have emerged as a promising new approach.

Pure Hyperviscosity Syndrome

Pure hyperviscosity syndrome is associated with large-scale changes in blood composition and specific clinical evidence involving different organs and systems. It occurs in the course of other pathologies, which, by augmenting whole blood viscosity, act as the pathogen.[47] Increases in proteins, cell mass, and the internal viscosity of blood cells, particularly the erythrocytes, significantly alter internal attrition; ex vivo potential resistance to deformation is enhanced, and whole blood viscosity levels

are markedly higher than normal. Levels higher than 6 cP cause symptoms in 60% of patients, and levels higher than 7 cP cause symptoms in 80% of patients.[47] Although there is no correlation between clinical effects and blood viscosity levels, the measurement of the blood or serum viscosity is of considerable predictive value because in each patient there is remarkable reproducibility in the type and degree of symptoms for a given viscosity. For many patients the viscosity level may be accurately predicted from the accompanying clinical picture.

Clinical Features

Nasal bleeding and oozing from gums are the most common symptoms but postsurgical or gastrointestinal bleeding may occur. Flame-shaped retinal hemorrhages and papilledema may be seen, and the patient may complain of blurring or loss of vision. Neurological symptoms include dizziness, headache, vertigo, nystagmus, hearing loss, ataxia, paraesthesias, diplopia, and drowsiness.[84] When untreated, the pure hyperviscosity syndrome can cause stroke, myocardial infarction, and critical limb ischemia.

The three forms of pure hyperviscosity syndrome are serum, polycythemic, and sclerocytemic.

Serum Hyperviscosity Syndrome

Blood rheology is irreversibly altered by an increase in circulating immunoglobulins caused by dysproteinemia (the continuous release of M, G, and A immunoglobulins, with an electrophoretic affinity but no antibody activity). Dysproteinemia occurs in the course of diseases such as Waldenström's macroglobulinemia and benign monoclonal gammopathy by cryoglobulinemia (cryoglobulins are proteins that precipitate when cooled and dissolve when heated), which occurs in the presence of multiple myeloma or solid tumors[41,47] and in the presence of 4% to 10% of all proliferative disorders.[47] Modifications in density, charge, size, and shape of the protein molecules that are released in excess lead to the formation of a fluid structure made up of cell protein (i.e., cell bridges and rouleaux). Thrombus plugging of small blood vessels ensues as a consequence of the abnormal blood rheology and protein cell interactions.[47]

Patients are usually asymptomatic when serum viscosity levels are 3 cP or lower (normal range: 1.8 cP or lower). Levels higher than 4 cP cause symptoms in 60% of patients;levels higher than 5 cP affect 75% of patients.[85] When untreated, serum hyperviscosity aggravates congestive heart disease, and somnolence may deteriorate into coma or general convulsions.[85]

Polycythemic Syndrome

Polycythemic syndrome includes all cases of blood hyperviscosity that are caused by an increased circulating cell mass. Usually caused by a rise in the number of erythrocytes, polycythemic syndrome may be the consequence of an elevated leukocyte count but never an increase in platelet numbers.[47] Primary erythrocytosis may be caused by polycythemia vera rubra (i.e., abnormal erythroid progenitor cell proliferation resulting from disturbances in erythropoiesis) or by familiar erythrocytosis arising from an intrinsic cellular defect. Secondary erythrocytosis includes hypoxic erythrocytosis (i.e., hypobaric hypoxia), chronic pulmonary disease, chronic carbon monoxide intoxication, cyanotic congenital heart disease, and high-oxygen-affinity hemoglobins. Physiological compensation for impaired tissue oxygenation is the primary cause of the syndrome. Erythrocytosis associated with renal disease or tumors is caused by inappropriate erythropoietin secretion. Relative or spurious erythrocytosis is due to a normal red cell mass with an abnormally high packed cell volume, secondary to, for example, acute dehydration caused by diarrhea, diaphoresis, diuretics, deprivation of water, chronic stress, or Gaisböck's syndrome.[47]

When untreated, polycythemic hyperviscosity causes deep venous thrombosis in the lower limbs; pulmonary embolism; or cerebrovascular, coronary, and peripheral vascular occlusions. Thrombosis may develop at unusual anatomic sites such as the splenic, hepatic, portal, and mesenteric vessels. Neurological abnormalities in almost 60% to 80% of patients include transient ischemic attacks, cerebral infarction, cerebral hemorrhage, fluctuating dementia, confusional states, and choreic syndromes.[75]

When, in case of acute and/or chronic myeloid or lymphoid leukemia, the total leukocyte count rises above 200×10^9 per liter, blood hyperviscosity may ensue.[87] This is a relatively rare complication, occuring in 1% of patients.[77] Neurological symptoms are not uncommon in patients with leukemia but are usually related to leukemic infiltration or hemorrhage within the central nervous system.[77] Patients complain of profound lethargy, unsteady gait, visual disturbances, deafness, headaches, and coma. Significant hearing loss appears to be more prominent in patients with cellular rather than abnormal paraprotein hyperviscosity. Fundal investigation reveals congested and tortuous retinal vessels with or without associated retinal hemorrhages.[11] Urgent leukopheresis and chemotherapy are required. High-dose hydroxyurea is safe and effective at doses up to 4 g/d.[11]

Sclerocytemic Syndrome

Sclerocytemic syndrome includes all forms of erythrocyte-induced hyperviscosity not due to increased packed-cell volume. Because of irreversible, usually genetic, abnormalities, red blood cell deformability is reduced and causes impairments in blood rheology,[47] leading to ves-

sel occlusion, which is associated with pain, organ dysfunction, and organ failure. Almost every organ system in the body can be affected by vascular occlusion. Growth failure, increased susceptibility to infection, and psychosocial problems are common. The pattern of illness is also characterized by aplastic crises and splenic sequestration crises. Cardiac and renal symptoms and cerebral hemorrhage are often noted in adults, and vaso-occlusive–related strokes are seen in children. Loss of erythrocyte deformability is due to changes in cell shape or geometry (which determines the ratio of cell surface to cell volume), changes in cytoplasmic viscosity (which is regulated by intracellular hemoglobin concentrations), and membrane deformability. Hemolytic anemias frequently cause sclerocytemic hyperviscosity by means of a mechanism of red blood cell injury.[47] Sclerocytosis is a common inherited hemolytic disorder of erythrocyte membrane and shape; hemoglobinopathies such as sickling disorders cause abnormalities in hemoglobin structure,[125] whereas thalassemia is a hereditary abnormality in hemoglobin synthesis.[47]

Therapy

The aim of any therapy is to lower plasma or whole blood viscosity levels. This is usually achieved by hemodilution in polycythemic syndrome, plasmapheresis or plasma exchange in serum hyperviscosity syndrome, and drugs modifying erythrocyte deformability in sclerocytemic syndrome.

Hemodilution can be defined as the absolute or relative reduction in the cellular component of the circulating mass of blood.[110] Because it stimulates any increase in plasma volume, it is the simplest and most effective technique for lowering blood viscosity as long as it does not compromise the blood's oxygen-carrying capacity.[109] Maintenance of a hematocrit level at 30% to 35% should restore the fluidity of blood and guarantee satisfactory oxygenation.[127] Counterindications include coronary heart disease, cardiac or respiratory insufficiency, renal or liver failure, and coagulation disorders. Hemodilution is termed hypovolemic, normovolemic, or hypervolemic according to whether blood volume is not replaced, replaced in equal measure, or replaced in excess.

Hypovolemic hemodilution is recommended in the polycythemic syndrome and in secondary hyperviscosity states only to prevent cerebral arterial disease. Therapy schedule: phlebotomy (250–300 cc) is repeated daily until an optimal hematocrit level (30%–35%) is achieved. If hematocrit levels subsequently rise, phlebotomy is repeated as required.

Normovolemic (isovolemic) hemodilution is indicated for secondary hyperviscosity states during and after surgery and in the advanced stage of peripheral arterial occlusive disease. Therapy schedule: first day, 300 mL of blood are drawn and a plasma substitute infused after allergy testing. Usually 300 mL dextran 40, 5% dextran-albumin, 5% gelatin, and 5% saline solutions are viable alternatives. The procedure is repeated every 3 to 4 days until the hematocrit level falls to approximately 30%. When the hematocrit level rises above 35%, a new cycle is begun. Therapy may last for 8 to12 weeks and may be administered on an outpatient basis or in a day hospital.

Hypervolemic hemodilution is recommended for patients with peripheral occlusive arterial disease in its intermediate stages. After allergy testing, 300 to 500 mL dextran 40 or one of the alternatives cited earlier is infused over 30 minutes daily for 21 days. The aim is to increase blood volume, cardiac output, and hence circulation in the affected limb, with a concomitant reduction in peripheral resistance. Although hematocrit levels generally fall, the benefit of improved peripheral circulation is achieved independently of an optimal hematocrit level.

Plasmapheresis, or removal of plasma, is recommended for treatment not only of serum hyperviscosity syndrome but also of autoimmune diseases (e.g., pemphigus, myasthenia gravis, Goodpasture's syndrome, Guillain-Barré syndrome, cold agglutinin disease, cryoglobulinemia, and immune thrombocytopenic purpura), metabolic disorders (familial hypercholesterolemia), and poisoning.[16] Counterindications are the same as for hemodilution. For removal of less than 500 mL, no plasma replacement is required, but large-volume plasmapheresis is not possible without replacement of whole or fractioned plasma or plasma substitutes (*plasma exchange),* with the frequency of exchange depending on total body burden, rate of synthesis, and plasma concentration of the solute.[79] The replacement solution should maintain intravascular volume, restore important plasma proteins and trace minerals, and maintain the electrolyte balance. In moderately well-nourished subjects, homeostatic mechanisms obviate the need for precise plasma replacement. Otherwise, solutions should be prepared to meet individual requirements, but routine calcium, potassium, and immunoglobulin supplements are unnecessary.[79] Side effects, reported in about 10% of procedures, are mainly due to the replacement solution and include chills, nausea, vomiting, syncope, hypocalcemia, and hypotension. Frequent plasma exchange reduces immunoglobulin levels and some plasma proteins (complement system) and depletes coagulation factors, leading to mild thrombocytopenia.[133] Vasovagal reactions, the clotting of fistulae and catheters, and urticaria may also be observed. Major complications such as air embolism or hemolysis are rare, but because of the high risk of adverse side effects, plasma exchange should always be carried out under close medical supervision.

The effects of plasma exchange on blood rheology are complex, depending mainly on the extent of fibrinogen depletion and the removal of abnormal plasma components. If the fluid balance is not maintained, changes in hematocrit may occur; a reduced blood viscosity may lower blood pressure.[50]

In sclerocytemic syndrome, recommended therapy is based on drugs acting on erythrocyte deformability, which depends on the quality of the lipid membrane, intracellular calcium levels, and adenosine triphosphate.[52] Agents that improve red cell flexibility by directly influencing membrane composition are atidin-phosphocholine and sulfo-adenosine-methionine.[52] An indirect effect on the erythrocyte membrane is achieved by lecithin acting on the plasma lipid concentrations, which determine cholesterol and phosphatidylcholine membrane content.[52] Under pathological conditions, the erythrocyte membrane may increase its permeability to calcium (Ca^{2+}), and the intracell calcium content increases. This can be counteracted by administering calcium antagonists such as cinnarizine and flunarizine[38] and β-blockers (e.g., alprenolol[44]) or vasodilators such as isoxsuprine,[46] which are reported to reduce whole blood viscosity and improve erythrocyte deformability.[52] Pentoxifylline increases erythrocyte adenosine triphosphate content by enhancing glycolysis, which is caused by increased membrane permeability to glucose and/or by the conversion of xanthine derivates to purine derivates that the erythrocyte cannot synthesize de novo.[52]

Differential Diagnosis

A pure hyperviscosity state may be suspected if, besides the symptoms already described, the circulatory impairment seems out of proportion to the vessel or cardiac disease. A normal peripheral arterial pulse does not necessarily guarantee good blood flow; it merely indicates the absence of a major mechanical block between the heart and the point at which the pulse is felt. In pure hyperviscosity syndrome, the peripheral pulse is normal even though blood flow is decreased. In small-vessel disease distal to the pulse, the pulsation may even be exaggerated. A frequent clinical problem is how to exclude a hyperviscosity component from the circulatory impairment. The best safeguard is the clinician's constant awareness of the possibility of an underlying hyperviscosity situation, followed by a request for the appropriate screening tests. Serum viscosity measurement is rarely required for diagnosis.

Routine blood tests—the erythrocyte sedimentation rate, hematocrit levels, total bilirubin and bilirubin fractions, and total protein concentrations—support a putative diagnosis of pure hyperviscosity syndrome, which is confirmed by high plasma and whole blood viscosity levels. See Table 38.1 for differential diagnosis of pure hyperviscosity syndromes.

In secondary hyperviscosity states, a complete hemorheological profile is necessary. Chronic arterial and venous disease may or may not be associated with instru-

TABLE 38.1. Differential diagnosis of hyperviscosity states and pure hyperviscosity syndrome.

	Pure hyperviscosity syndromes			Secondary hyperviscosity states
	Serum	Polycytemic	Sclerocytemic	
Total proteins	+++			= / +
Packed-cell volume		+++		+
Erythrocyte sedimentation rate	+++			= / +
Fibrinogen				+
Plasma and serum viscosity	+++			+
Whole blood viscosity		+++	+++	+

+, increased; ++, greatly increased; +++, extremely increased; =, unchanged.

mentally overt signs of hyperviscosity but with slight to moderate rheological abnormalities in several parameters. They should be treated because, in the presence of chronic vascular disease, impairments in the flow properties of blood may act as precipitating factors for acute ischemic events or thrombus formation.

In acute ischemic events, a complete hemorheological profile is also necessary. All patients should be treated with specific agents to control leukocyte activation, free radical release, and adhesive interactions because abnormal leukocyte functioning has been implicated in the extension of the ischemic area.[58] Any other rheological impairment should also be corrected.

In nonatherogenic, nonthrombotic states, secondary hyperviscosity and the hemorheological stress syndrome[124] become important and should be monitored in patients with risk factors for atherosclerosis and acute or chronic arterial or venous disease when they are affected concomitantly by clinical conditions such as infection, surgery, trauma, burns, kidney disease, and rheumatic disorders.

Acknowledgment
Translation by Dr. G. A. Boyd.

References

1. Aarts PA MM, Bolhis PA, Sakariassen KS, Heether RM, Sixma JJ. Red blood cell size is important for adherence of blood platelets to artery subendothelium. *Blood.* 1983; 62:214–217.
2. Aarts PA MM, Heether RM, Sixma JJ. Red blood cell deformability influences platelets–vessel wall interaction in flowing blood. *Blood.* 1984;64:1228–1233.
3. Arnaout MA. Structure and function of the leukocyte adhesion molecules CD11/CD18. *Blood.* 1990;75:1037–1050.
4. Baar S. Water movement in red cells from burned patients: its relationship to sodium retention and red cell filterability. *Acta Clinical Chemistry.* 1979;94:181–190.
5. Baar S. The influence of catecholamines and prostaglandins on calcium efflux and filterability of thermally damaged erythrocytes: an in vivo study. *British Journal of Experimental Pathology.* 1982;63:644–654.
6. Bagge U, Branemark PL. White blood cell rheology: an intravital study in man. *Advances in Microcirculation.* 1977; 7:1–17.
7. Bareford D, Coppock JS, Stone PCW, Bacon PA, Stuart J. Abnormal blood rheology in Raynaud's phenomenon. *Clinical Hemorheology.* 1986;6:53–60.
8. Bareford D, Stone PCW, Caldwell NM, Stuart J. Erythrocyte morphology as a determinant of abnormal erythrocyte deformability in liver disease. *Clinical Hemorheology.* 1985;5:473–481.
9. Barnes AJ. Blood viscosity in diabetes mellitus. In: Lowe GDO, Barbenel JC, Forbes CD, eds. *Clinical Aspects of Blood Viscosity and Cell Deformability.* Berlin: Springer-Verlag; 1981:151–162.
10. Bergentz SE, Gelin L, Rudenstam G, Zederfeld B. The viscosity of whole blood in trauma. *Acta Chirugica Scandinavica.* 1965;126:289–293.
11. Bloch KJ, Maki DG. Hyperviscosity syndromes associated with immunoglobulin abnormalities. *Semin Hematol.* 1973; 10:113–121.
12. Bottiger LE, Carlson LA, Ekelund LG, Olsson AC. Raised ESR is asymptomatic hyperlipoproteinaemia. *BMJ.* 1973;2: 681–683.
13. Bottiger LE, Svedberger CA. Normal erythrocyte sedimentation rate and age. *BMJ.* 1967;2:85–87.
14. Brooks DE, Goodwin JW, Seaman GVT. Interactions among erythrocytes under shear. *J Appl Physiol.* 1970;28: 172–174.
15. Browning GG, Gatehouse S, Lowe GDO. Blood viscosity as a factor in sensorineural hearing impairment. *Lancet.* 1986;1:121–123.
16. Buskard NA. Plasma exchange and plasmapheresis. *Can Med Assoc J.* 1978;119:681–683.
17. Cade DC, O'Donovan JE, Panelli D, Galbally BP. Volume replacement in shock. *Medicine.* (3rd series) 1980;28: 1463–1467.
18. Charm SE, McComis W, Tejada C, Kurland G. Effect of a fatty meal on whole blood and plasma viscosity. *J Appl Physiol.* 1963;18:1217–1220.
19. Chien S. Blood rheology and its relation to flow resistance and transcapillary exchange, with special reference to shock. *Advances in Microcirculation.* 1969;2:89–103.
20. Chien S. Present state of blood rheology. In: Messmer K, Schmid-Schoenbein H, eds. *Hemodilution: Theoretical Basis and Clinical Application.* Basel: Karger; 1972:1–40.
21. Chien S. Principles and techniques for assessing erythrocyte deformability. *Blood Cells.* 1978;3:71–74.

22. Chien S. Hemorheology in disease: pathophysiological significance and therapeutic implications. *Clinical Hemorheology.* 1981;1:419–442.

23. Chien S, Dormandy JA, Ernst E, Matrai A. *Clinical Hemorheology.* Dordrecht: Martinus Nijhoff; 1987.

24. Chien S, Schmid-Schoenbein H, Sung KLP, Schmalzer EA, Skalak R. Viscoelastic properties of leucocytes. In: Meiselman HJ, Lichtmann KA, LaCelle PL, eds. *White Cell Mechanics: Basic Science and Clinical Aspects.* New York, NY: Alan R. Liss; 1984:19–51.

25. Chien S, Usami S, Taylor HM, Lundberg J, Gregersen MI. Effects of haematocrit and plasma proteins on human blood rheology at low shear rates. *J Appl Physiol.* 1966;21: 81–85.

26. Ciuffetti G, Balendra R, Lennie SE, Anderson J, Lowe GDO. White blood cell rheology in acute stroke. *BMJ.* 1989;298:930–931.

27. Ciuffetti G, Corea L, Mannarino E, Mercuri M, Lombardini R, Santambrogio L. Leucocytes and free radicals in stable angina pectoris. *Jpn Heart J.* 1992;33:145–157.

28. Ciuffetti G, Lombardini R, Paltriccia R, Santambrogio L, Mannarino E. Human leucocyte-endothelial interactions in peripheral arterial occlusive disease. *Eur J Clin Invest.* 1994;24:65–68.

29. Ciuffetti G, Mercuri M, Lombardini R, et al. Stable angina pectoris and controlled ischaemia: what causes the abnormalities in whole blood filterability? *Am Heart J.* 1990; 119:54–56.

30. Ciuffetti G, Mercuri M, Lombardini R, Paltriccia R, Ott C. Human leucocyte rheology after acute infection. *Haematologica.* 1990;75:94.

31. Ciuffetti G, Pasqualini L, Fuscaldo G, Piccioni N, Paltriccia R, Mannarino E. Neutrophil-derived adhesion molecules in human digital ischaemia and reperfusion. *Vasa.* 1995;24:155–158.

32. Ciuffetti G, Scardazza A, Serafini G, Lombardini R, Mannarino E, Simoncelli C. Whole blood filterability in sudden deafness. *Laryngoscope.* 1991;101:65–67.

33. Cohn LH, Klovekorn P, Moore FD, Collins JJ Jr. Intrinsic plasma volume deficits in patients with coronary artery disease: effects of myocardial revascularization. *Arch Surg.* 1974;108:57–60.

34. Cokelet GR. Macroscopic rheology and tube flow of human blood. In: Grayson BJ, Ziugg KJ, eds. *Microcirculation.* New York, NY: Plenum Publishing Co; 1976:9–31.

35. Cooper RA. Hemolytic syndromes and red cell membrane abnormalities in liver disease. *Seminari Hematologica.* 1980; 17:103–112.

36. Cooper RA, Leslie MH, Fischkoff S, Shinitzky M, Shattil SJ. Factors influencing the lipid composition and fluidity of red cell membranes in vitro: production of red cells possessing more than two cholesterols per phospholipid. *Biochemistry.* 1978;17:327–331.

37. Davies JWL. *Physiological Response to Burning Injury.* London: Academic Press Inc; 1982.

38. De Cree J, De Cock W, Geukens H, De Clerck F, Beerens M, Verhaegen H. The rheological effects of cinnarizine and flunarizine in normal and pathological conditions. *Angiology.* 1979;30:505–525.

39. Devereaux RB, Drayer JJM, Chien S, et al. Whole blood viscosity as a determinant of cardiac hypertrophy in systemic hypertension. *Am J Cardiol.* 1984;54:592–595.

40. Dintenfass L. *Rheology of Blood in Diagnostic and Preventive Medicine.* London: Butterworth; 1976:49–58.

41. Dintenfass L. Some aspects of haemorheology of metastasis in malignant melanoma. *Haemotologia.* 1977;11:301–304.

42. Dintenfass L. Haemorheology of cancer metastases: an example of malignant melanoma. *Clinical Hemorheology.* 1982; 2:259–271.

43. Dintenfass L, Forbes CD, McDougall IR. Blood viscosity in hyperthyroid and hypothyroid patients. *Haemostasis.* 1974;3:348–352.

44. Dintenfass L, Lake B. Beta-blockers and blood viscosity. *Lancet.* 1976;1:1026.

45. Dintenfass L, Ibels LS. Blood viscosity factors and occlusive arterial disease in renal transplant recipients. *Nephron.* 1975;15:456–465.

46. Di Perri T, Forconi S, Agnusdei D, Guerrini M, Laghi Pasini F. The effect of intravenous isoxsuprine on blood viscosity in patients with occlusive arterial disease. *Br J Clin Pharmacol.* 1978;5:255–260.

47. Di Perri T, Forconi S, Di Lollo F, Porza G. La sindrome da iperviscosità ematica: fisiologia, patologia e clinica. In: *Atti 84 Congresso Società Italiana Medicina Interna.* Rome: Edizione Luigi Porri; 1983:193–294.

48. Di Perri T, Vittoria A, Guerrini M, et al. Action of ASA on hemorheological changes of ischemic patients. In: Segre FA, Ohnmeiss WL, eds. *ASA International Symposium on Present State of Acetylsalicylic Acid in Research and Therapeutic Application.* Florence, Italy: OIC Medical Press; 1982: 81–84.

49. Ditzel J. Hemodilution in myocardial infarction. In: Messmer K, Schmid-Schoenbein H, eds. *Hemodilution: Theoretical Basis and Clinical Application.* Basel: Karger; 1972: 264–270.

50. Dodds AJ. Plasma exchange? In: Lowe GDO, Barbenel JC, Forbes CD, eds. *Clinical Aspects of Blood Viscosity and Cell Deformability.* Berlin: Springer-Verlag; 1981:227–234.

51. Dodds AJ, Matthews PN, Bailey MJ, Flute PT, Dormandy JA. Changes in red cell deformability following surgery. *Thromb Res.* 1980;18:561–566.

52. Dormandy JA. Drug modification of erythrocyte deformability. In: Lowe GDO, Barbenel JC, Forbes CD, eds. *Clinical Aspects of Blood Viscosity and Cell Deformability.* Berlin: Springer-Verlag; 1981:251–256.

53. Dormandy JA, Ernst E. Effects of buflomedil on erythrocyte deformability. *Angiology.* 1981;32:714–717.

54. Dormandy JA, Hoare E, Colley J, Arrowsmith DE, Dormandy TL. Clinical haemodynamic, rheological, and biochemical findings in 126 patients with intermittent claudication. *BMJ* 1973;4:576–581.

55. Douglas JT, Lowe GDO, Hillis WS, Rao R, Hogg KJ, Gemmill JD. Blood and plasma hyperviscosity in acute myocardial infarction compared to unstable angina: rapid reversal by thrombolysis. *Thromb Haemost.* 1989;62:590–592.

56. Eisenberg S. Blood viscosity and fibrinogen concentration following cerebral infarction. *Circulation.* 1966;33–34 (suppl 2):10–14.

57. Ellis ME, Ralston S. The ESR in the diagnosis and management of the polymyalgia rheumatica/giant cell arteritis syndrome. *Ann Rheum Dis.* 1983;42:168–172.

58. Ernst E, Hammerschmidt DE, Bagge U, Matrai A, Dormandy JA. Leucocytes and the risk of ischemic diseases. *JAMA.* 1987;257:2318–2324.

59. Ernst E, Matrai A. Altered red and white blood cell rheology in type II diabetes. *Diabetes.* 1986;35:1412–1415.

60. Ernst E, Matrai A, Dormandy JA. Shear dependence of blood coagulation. *Clinical Hemorheology.* 1984;4:395–399.

61. Ernst E, Roloff C, Magyarosy I, Matrai A. Hemorheological abnormalities in ankylosing spondylitis. *Clinical Hemorheology.* 1985;5:109–114.

62. European Collaborative Study Group. Streptokinase in acute myocardial infarction. *N Engl J Med.* 1979;301:797–802.

63. Fahraeus R. The suspension stability of blood. *Physiol Rev.* 1929;9:241–274.

64. Fahraeus R. Influence of the rouleaux formation of the erythrocytes on the rheology of the blood. *Acta Medica Scandinavica.* 1958;161:151–159.

65. Fahraeus R, Lindqvist T. The viscosity of the blood in narrow capillary tubes. *Am J Physiol.* 1931;96:562–568.

66. Forconi S, Pieragalli D, Guerrini M, Di Perri T. Hemorheology and peripheral arterial diseases. *Clinical Hemorheology.* 1987;7:145–158.

67. Garnier M, Hanss M, Paraf A. Erythrocytes filterability reduction and membrane lipids in cirrhosis. *Clinical Hemorheology.* 1983;3:45–52.

68. Goldsmith HL, Karino T. Microrheology and clinical medicine: unravelling some problems related to thrombosis. *Clinical Hemorheology.* 1982;2:143–156.

69. Gordon W. The effect of ingested glucose and intravenous injections of glucose on the viscosity of whole blood in man. *Clin Sci (Colch).* 1969;36:25–39.

70. Goslinga H. *Blood Viscosity and Shock.* Berlin: Springer-Verlag; 1984.

71. Gottstein U. Normovolemic and hypervolemic hemodilution in cerebrovascular ischemia. *Biblioteca Haematologica.* 1981;47:127–138.

72. Goyle KB, Dormandy JA. Abnormal blood viscosity in Raynaud's phenomenon. *Lancet.* 1976;1:1317–1318.

73. Guegen M, Delamaire D, Durand F, Deugnier Y, Bourel M, Genetet B. Haemorheological abnormalities in chronic alcoholism. *Clinical Hemorheology.* 1984;4:327–340.

74. Hazelton RA, Lowe GDO, Forbes CD, Sturrock RD. Increased blood and plasma viscosity in systemic lupus erythematosus (SLE) [letter]. *J Rheumatol.* 1985;12:616.

75. Hoffman R, Boswell HS. Polycythemia vera. In: Hoffman R, Benz EJ Jr, Shattil SJ, Furie B, Cohen HJ, eds. *Hematology Basic Principles and Practice.* New York, NY: Churchill Livingstone; 1991:834–854.

76. Hossmann V, Heiss WD, Bewermeyer H, Wiedemann G. Controlled trial of ancrod in ischemic stroke. *Arch Neurol.* 1983;40:803–808.

77. Hughes TP, Goldman JM. Chronic myeloid leukemia. In: Hoffman R, Benz EJ Jr, Shattil SJ, Furie B, Cohen HJ, eds. *Hematology Basic Principles and Practice.* New York, NY: Churchill Livingstone; 1991:854–869.

78. Inauen W, Staubli M, Descoeudres C, Galeazzi RL, Straub PW. Erythrocyte deformability in dialyzed and non-dialyzed uremic patients. *Eur J Clin Invest.* 1982;12:173–176.

79. Isbister JB, Biggs JL. Reactions to rapid infusion of stable plasma protein solution during large volume plasma exchange. *Anaesth Intensive Care.* 1976;4:105–107.

80. Jan KM, Chien S, Bigger JT Jr. Observations on blood viscosity changes after acute myocardial infarction. *Circulation.* 1975;51:1079–1084.

81. Koenig W, Sund M, Ernst E, Keil U, Rosenthal J, Hombach V. Association between plasma viscosity and blood pressure. Results from the MONICA-Project Augsburg. *Am J Hypertens.* 1991;4:529–536.

82. Koenig W, Sund M, Ernst E, Matrai A, Keil U, Rosenthal J. Is increased plasma viscosity a risk factor for high blood pressure? *Angiology.* 1989;40:153–163.

83. Kovacs IB, Sowemimo-Coker SO, Kirby JDT, Turner P. Altered behaviour of erythrocytes in scleroderma. *Clin Sci (Colch).* 1983;65:515–519.

84. Kyle RA. Plasma cell proliferative disorders. In: Hoffman R, Benz EJ Jr, Shattil SJ, Furie B and Cohen J, eds. *Haematology Basic Principles and Practice.* New York, NY: Churchill Livingstone; 1991:1021–1038.

85. Langer L, Bergentz SE, Bjure J, Faberberg SE. The effect of exercise on haematocrit, plasma volume, and viscosity in diabetes mellitus. *Diabetologia.* 1971;7:29–33.

86. Lawrence MB, Smith CW, Eskin SG, McIntire LV. Effect of venous shear stress on CD18–mediated neutrophil adhesion to cultured endothelium. *Blood.* 1990;75:227–237.

87. Leonhardt H, Arntz HR, Klemens U. Studies of plasma viscosity in primary hyperlipoproteinaemia. *Atherosclerosis.* 1977;28:29–40.

88. Long DM, Rosen AL, Malone LVW, Meier MA. Blood rheology in trauma patients. *Surg Clin North Am.* 1972;52:19–30.

89. Lorient-Roudaut MF, Manuau JP, Bricaud H, Boisseau MR. Filterability and cerebrovascular thrombosis. *Scand J Clin Lab Invest.* 1981;41(suppl 156):203–208.

90. Lowe GDO. Report on Working Group Meeting: red cell deformability—methods and terminology. *Clinical Hemorheology.* 1981;1:513–515.

91. Lowe GDO. Defibrination, blood flow, and blood rheology. *Clin Hemorheol.* 1984;4:15–28.

92. Lowe GDO. Blood rheology in arterial disease. *Clin Sci (Colch).* 1986;71:116–137.

93. Lowe GDO. Blood rheology and hyperviscosity syndromes. *Baillière's Clin Haematol.* 1987;1:798–867.

94. Lowe GDO. Blood rheology in vitro and in vivo. *Baillière's Clin Haematol.* 1987;1:597–636.

95. Lowe GDO. Blood rheology in general medicine and surgery. *Baillière's Clin Haematol.* 1987;9:827–861.

96. Lowe GDO, Anderson J, Barbanel JC, Forbes CD. Prognostic importance of blood rheology in acute stroke. In: Hartmann HL, Kuschinsky TK, eds. *Cerebral Ischemia and Hemorheology.* Berlin: Springer-Verlag; 1987:496–501.

97. Lowe GDO, Forbes CD, Foulds WS. Haemorheology and retinal disorders. *Clinical Hemorheology.* 1987;7:181–188.

98. Lowe GDO, Forbes CD, Prentice CRM. Defibrinating agents. In: Lowe GDO, Barbenel JC, Forbes CD, eds. *Clini-*

cal Aspects of Blood Viscosity and Cell Deformability. Berlin: Springer-Verlag; 1981.

99. Lowe GDO, Jaap AJ, Forbes CD. Relationship of atrial fibrillation and high haematocrit to mortality in acute stroke. *Lancet.* 1983;1:784–786.

100. Lowe GDO, Smith WCS, Tunstall-Pedoe H, et al. Cardiovascular risk and haemorheology: results from the Scottish Heart Health Study and the MONICA-Project, Glasgow. *Clinical Hemorheology.* 1988;8:517–524.

101. Lowe GDO, Wood DA, Douglas JT, et al. Relationships of plasma viscosity, coagulation, and fibrinolysis to coronary risk factors and angina. *Thromb Haemost.* 1991;65: 339–343.

102. Matrai A, Whittington RB, Ernst E. A simple method of estimating whole blood viscosity at standardized hematocrit. *Clinical Hemorheology.* 1987;7:261–265.

103. Mayer GE. Blood viscosity in healthy subjects and patients with coronary heart disease. *Can Med Assoc J.* 1964;91: 951–954.

104. McGinley E, Lowe GDO, Boulton-Jones M, Forbes CD, Prentice CRM. Blood viscosity and haemostasis in the nephrotic syndrome. *Thromb Haemost.* 1983;49:155–157.

105. McMillan DE. Two roles for plasma fibrinogen in the production of diabetic microangiopathy. *Diabetes.* 1975;24 (suppl 2):438–440.

106. Merrill EW, Pellietier GA. Viscosity of human blood: transition from Newtonian to non-Newtonian. *J Appl Physiol.* 1967;23:178–181.

107. Messmer KFW. Acceptable hematocrit levels in surgical patients. *World J Surg.* 1987;11:41–46.

108. Messmer KFW. The use of plasma substitutes with special attention to their side effects. *World J Surg.* 1987;11:69–74.

109. Messmer KFW, Schmid-Schoenbein H. Hemodilution, theoretical basis, and clinical application. Basel: Karger; 1972.

110. Messmer KFW, Schmid-Schoenbein H. International hemodilution. In: Dintenfass L, Copley AL, eds. *Proceedings Second International Symposium Biblioteca Hematologica.* Basel: Karger; 1975.

111. Miller AK, Whittington RB. Plasma viscosity in pulmonary tuberculosis. *Lancet.* 1942;2:510–511.

112. Miller LH, Usami S, Chien S. Alteration in the rheologic properties of *Plasmodium knowlesi*-infected red cells: a possible mechanism for capillary obstruction. *J Clin Invest.* 1971;50:1451–1460.

113. Nash GB, Shearman CP. Neutrophils and peripheral arterial disease. *Crit Ischaemia.* 1992;2:15–21.

114. Nash GB, Thomas PRS, Dormandy JA. Abnormal flow properties of white blood cells in patients with severe ischaemia of the leg. *BMJ.* 1988;296:1699–1701.

115. National Institute of Neurological and Communicative Disorders and Stroke. The National Survey of Stroke. *Stroke.* 1981;12(suppl):23–24.

116. Neri Serneri GG, Abbate R, Gori AM, Gensini GF. A transient, intermittent lymphocyte activation is responsible for the instability of angina. *Circulation.* 1992;85:1200–1220.

117. Neri Serneri GG, Gensini GF, Poggesi L, et al. The role of extraplatelet thromboxane A$_2$ in unstable angina investigated with a dual thromboxane A$_2$ inhibitor: importance of activated monocytes. *Coron Artery Dis.* 1994;5:137–145.

118. Newmann V, Cove DH, Shapiro LM, et al. Effect of ticlopidine on platelet function and blood rheology in diabetes mellitus. *Clinical Hemorheology.* 1983;3:13–16.

119. Nicolaides AN, Bowers R, Horbourne T, Kidner PH, Bestermann EM. Blood viscosity, red cell flexibility, haematocrit, and plasma fibrinogen in patients with angina. *Lancet.* 1977;2:943–945.

120. Owen JS, Bruckdorfer KR, Day RC, McIntyre N. Decreased erythrocyte membrane fluidity and altered lipid composition in human liver disease. *J Lipid Res.* 1982;23: 124–132.

121. Ozanne P, Francis RB, Meiselman HJ. Red blood cell aggregation in nephrotic syndrome. *Kidney Int.* 1983;23: 519–525.

122. Parnetti L, Ciuffetti G, Senin U. Chronic cerebrovascular disorders: hemorheological and psychobehavioural aspects. *Gerontology.* 1986;32:228–230.

123. Perry MA, Granger DN. Role of CD11/CD18 in shear rate dependent leukocyte-endothelial interactions in cat mesenteric venules. *J Clin Invest.* 1991;87:1798–1804.

124. Reizenstein P. The haematological stress syndrome. *Br J Haematol.* 1979;43:329–334.

125. Richardson SGN, Matthews KB, Stuart J, Geddes AM, Wilcox RM. Serial changes in coagulation and viscosity during sickle cell crisis. *Br J Haematol.* 1979;41:95–103.

126. Schmid-Schoenbein H, Gaehtgens P, Hirsch H. On the shear rate dependence of red cell aggregation in vitro. *J Clin Invest.* 1968;47:1447–1500.

127. Schmid-Schoenbein H, Rieger H. Isovolaemic Haemodilution. In: Lowe GDO, Barbenel JC, Forbes CD, eds. *Clinical Aspects of Blood Viscosity and Cell Deformability.* Berlin: Springer-Verlag; 1981:211–226.

128. Schmid-Schoenbein H, Teitel P. In vitro assessment of "covertly abnormal" blood rheology; critical appraisal of presently available microrheological methodology. A review focussing on diabetic retinopathy as a possible consequence of rheological occlusion. *Clinical Hemorheology.* 1987;7:203–238.

129. Schoen RG, Wells CH, Kolman SN. Viscometric and microcirculatory observations following flame injury. *J Trauma.* 1971;11:619–626.

130. Scholz PM, Karis JH, Gump FE, Kinney JM, Chien S. Correlation of blood rheology with vascular resistance in critically ill patients. *J Appl Physiol.* 1975;39:1008–1011.

131. Seplowitz AH, Chien S, Smith FR. Effects of lipoproteins on plasma viscosity. *Atherosclerosis.* 1981;38:89–95.

132. Shearn MA, Epstein WV, Engleman EP. Serum viscosity in rheumatic diseases and macroglobulinaemia. *Arch Intern Med.* 1963;112:98–100.

133. Solomon A, Fahey IL. Plasmapheresis therapy in macroglobulinemia. *Ann Intern Med.* 1963;58:799–804.

134. Stoltz JF, Gaillard S, Rousselle D, Voisin P, Drouin P. Rheological study of blood during primary hyperlipoproteinaemia. *Clinical Hemorheology.* 1981;1:227–234.

135. Stuart J. The acute phase reaction and haematological stress syndrome in vascular disease. *Int J Microcirc Clin Exp.* 1984;3:115–129.

136. Stuart J, Juhan-Vague I. Erythrocyte rheology in diabetes mellitus. *Clinical Hemorheology.* 1987;7:239–245.

137. Theiss W, Volger E, Wirtzfeld A, Kiesel I, Bloemer H. Coagulation studies and rheological measurements during streptokinase therapy of myocardial infarction. *Klinische Wochenschrift.* 1980;58:607–609.

138. Turitto VT, Baumgartner HR. Platelet adhesion. In: Harker GF, Zimmermann BD, eds. *Measurements of Platelet Function.* Edinburgh: Churchill Livingstone; 1983:46–63.

139. Twigley AJ, Hillmann KM. The end of the crystalloid era? A new approach to perioperative fluid administration. *Anaesthesia.* 1985;40:860–871.

140. Udden MM, O'Rear EA, Kegel H, McIntire LV, Lynch EC. Decreased deformability of erythrocytes and increased intracellular calcium in patients with chronic renal failure. *Clinical Hemorheology.* 1984;4:473–481.

141. Ward A, Clissold SP. Pentoxifylline: a review of its pharmacodynamic and pharmacokinetic properties, and its therapeutic efficacy. *Drugs.* 1987;34:50–97.

142. Whittington RB, Harkness J. Whole blood viscosity, as determined by plasma viscosity, hematocrit, and shear. *Biorheology.* 1982;19:175–184.

143. Wurzinger LJ, Opitz R, Blasberg P, Eschweiler H, Schmid-Schoenbein H. The role of hydrodynamic factors in platelet activation and thrombotic events: the effects of shear stress of short duration. In: Schettler AC, Nerem FJ, Schmid-Schoenbein H, Morl R, Diehm C, eds. *Fluid Dynamics as a Localizing Factor in Atherosclerosis.* Berlin: Springer-Verlag; 1983:91–102.

144. Zingg W, Suler JC, Morgan CD. Relationship between viscosity and hematocrit in blood of normal persons and burn patients. *Can J Physiol Pharmacol.* 1970;48:202–210.

39

Hemorheology

Giovanni Ciufetti and Rita Lombardini

Details of patient preparation, blood sampling and handling before measurement, and measurement techniques have been published by the International Committee for Standardization in Haematology.[8]

Viscosity

Blood Sample Collection

Samples for any hemorheological test are obtained in the same way.[8] Venous blood is used routinely, avoiding stasis, usually after an overnight fast. Because excess trauma to the blood during withdrawal must be avoided, a wide-bore needle and minimum suction on the syringe should be used. To prepare a whole blood specimen the sample is placed in an anticoagulant container and gently mixed. The most commonly used anticoagulant is ethylenediaminetetraacetic acid (EDTA). For a plasma specimen the whole blood sample anticoagulated with EDTA is centrifuged at 3000 rpm for 10 minutes. The supernatant (plasma) is removed. To prepare a serum specimen the whole blood sample is left at room temperature for approximately 30 minutes and then centrifuged at 3000 rpm for 10 minutes and the supernatant (serum) is removed.

Storage

If the sample is kept at room temperature, all measurements should be carried out within 4 to 8 hours, because the metabolic changes that occur in blood outside the circulation influence whole blood viscosity, which begins to change unpredictably a few hours after withdrawal. However, blood can be stored at 4°C for up to 12 hours.

Viscosity Instruments

Two types of viscosimeters—capillary and rotational—are currently in use. Capillary viscosimeters measure the rate of flow through a narrow glass tube of specified dimensions. As the sample travels under gravity along a tube at changing pressure leads it is exposed to a whole range of shear rates, and it is impossible to define a single shear rate at which measurements are made. Since whole blood is non-Newtonian and its viscosity varies with the shear rate, capillary viscosimeters are not suitable for measuring whole blood viscosity.

Capillary viscosimeters (e.g., the Coulter Harkness viscosimeter [Coulter Electronics, Dunstable, UK]) with standard capillary dimensions, constant driving pressure, and accurate temperature control (60.5°C) are recommended by the International Committee for Standardization in Haematology.[7] The Harkness viscosimeter is accurate (0.03 mPa s^{-1}) and reproducible (coefficient of variation <1%), uses a small sample volume (0.5 mL), and takes less than 1 minute per sample, with no need to clean and dry the capillary between samples. It can even be used to measure whole blood viscosity at high shear rates. Other instruments (e.g., the Kapillarsclauch Plasmaviskometer and the Luckham viscosimeter [Luckham Ltd, Burgess Hill, UK]) are acceptable provided they give results comparable to the standard method.

Rotational viscosimeters are also more expensive, more tedious, and less accurate than capillary viscosimeters in routine use. They can have cone and plate sensor systems and/or coaxial cylinder sensor systems. In all rotational viscosimeters the sample is sheared between two surfaces that move in relation to each other. One surface is usually static, and the other can be rotated at different speeds equivalent to single shear rates. The Wells–Brookefield viscosimeter, the first commercial rotational viscosimeter, has a cone and plate sensor system that ensures the whole sample is exposed to the same shear rate. The velocity difference between the two surfaces will increase toward the periphery but so will the distance between them, thereby ensuring that the velocity gradient remains constant. The main disadvantage of this viscosimeter is that the cone and plate sensor system has small cone angles and is reliable only at medium to high shear sensors, an unsuitable range for research purposes.

The Contraves viscosimeter, with its coaxial cylinder sensor system, is more sensitive than the Wells–Brookefield model because one component of the sample chamber is used to apply the shear rate and the stress is measured by the other. Because this viscosimeter measures very low shear rates (even 0.01 s^{-1}) it is suitable for determining whole blood viscosity. The Haake Rotovisco viscosimeter is basically the same as the Contraves model. Precise and reliable, it is easy to use and requires smaller samples. Because it measures very low shear rates (0.01 s^{-1}) it appears to be the ideal instrument for sensitive routine measurements in clinical use and research.

A rolling-ball viscosimeter has recently been marketed for plasma and serum viscosity measurement (Haake Messtechnik, Karlsruhe, Germany). The sample viscosity is linearly related to the time taken by a gold-plated ball to roll a defined distance through the sample, which is aspirated into a syringe. Only a small volume (60 μL) is required, but further evaluation is awaited. In the Weissenberg rheogoniometer either cone and plate or coaxial cylindrical configurations are available for use with blood. It is the most accurate of the commercially available viscosimeters, but it is correspondingly delicate and requires more technical skill to use reliably. It has the added disadvantage of requiring larger sample volumes than most other viscosimeters. For these reasons it is not used much in medical research and is not suitable for routine tests. The Deer rheometer is fundamentally different from those previously described. It applies a constant torque to a cylinder suspended in the sample and measures the resultant rate of rotation of the cylinder. Yield stress and the viscoelastic properties of blood can be measured more directly. Very few published results using this viscosimeter are available.

Measurements of viscosity are usually carried out at the physiological temperature of 37°C. Temperature should fluctuate only by ±1°C because viscosity increases as the temperature falls. Measurements at lower temperatures may be necessary when investigating Raynaud's syndrome or cryoglobulinemia. Because the normal ranges of whole blood, plasma, and serum viscosities vary with the viscosimeter, the range of hematocrit of the sample, and the shear rate at which measurements are carried out, each laboratory should establish its own reference range.

Serum and Plasma Viscosity

Plasma viscosity and serum viscosity are usually measured in capillary or tube viscosimeters, in which the liquid is sheared by flow past the tube wall. Although shear stress and shear rate vary across the tube diameter, these varia-

tions are unimportant because plasma and serum are Newtonian fluids.

Plasma and serum viscosity can also be measured in rotational viscosimeters. A guard ring is essential to prevent surface film formation at the air–liquid interface, which causes artifactually high readings. Using the Haake Rotovisco, our normal ranges for plasma and serum viscosity, at 37°C and a shear rate of 300 s^{-1}, are 1.38 ± 0.03 cP and 1.27 ± 0.04 cP, respectively.

Whole Blood Viscosity

An important consideration in measurements of whole blood viscosity is that aggregation of erythrocytes at low shear rates causes the separation of plasma from cell aggregates and facilitates erythrocyte sedimentation. Therefore, the blood sample must be well mixed immediately before the viscosity measurement, and the high shear measurement should be taken before the low shear measurement.

Whole blood viscosity should be measured at the patient's own (native) hematocrit because hematocrit is an important determinant. To assess the contributions of factors other than hematocrit, the test viscosity can be compared with a laboratory reference curve for hematocrits between 0.20 and 0.70.[8] Alternatively, blood viscosity can be corrected to a standard hematocrit of 0.45 using a convenient and validated formula.[4,10] Results with the rotational viscosimeter appear higher than results with capillary viscosimeters.

Because whole blood viscosity is potentially sensitive to erythrocyte deformability and erythrocyte aggregation, these two indices can be quickly calculated in routine tests using the following formula:

$$\text{RBC deformability} = \frac{\text{whole blood viscosity at high shear and normal PCV}}{\text{plasma viscosity}}$$

$$\text{RBC aggregation} = \frac{\text{whole blood viscosity at low shear and normal PCV}}{\text{plasma viscosity}}$$

where RBC refers to red blood cells and PCV refers to packed-cell volume.

Hematocrit

The hematocrit level corresponds to the packed-cell volume and can be measured by the Wintrobe macromethod (blood samples anticoagulated with EDTA in 2.5- to 3-mm bore test tubes are centrifuged at 2000 rpm for 30 minutes); the micromethod (blood samples anticoagulated with EDTA in 1-mm bore test tubes are centrifuged at 12,000 rpm for 5 minutes; this method is used for routine blood tests because the sample is collected directly from the capillary); or an electronic system, using automatic instruments. Results from an electronic system are usually 2% to 3% lower than those from the other methods because there is no plasma entrapment in the packed-cell volume. All results are expressed as the percentage of erythrocytes in total blood volume. Normal values for men are 45% ± 7% and for women 42% ± 5%.

Erythrocyte Sedimentation Rate

In a column of anticoagulated blood, red cell aggregation increases the rate of settling of the red cell column within the plasma.[5] Two techniques are commonly used. In the Westergren method,[6] four parts of blood are anticoagulated and diluted with one part of sodium citrate. Blood is aspirated into a specially calibrated pipette placed in the vertical position, and the results are read in millimeters after 1 hour at the interface between the plasma surface and the upper meniscus of the sedimented erythrocyte column. The Wintrobe method uses anticoagulation and minimal hemodilution with EDTA. The procedure is identical to the original Westergren method, but shorter pipettes are used. Katz proposed reading the erythrocyte sedimentation rate after 1 and 2 hours and expressing the results as Katz's Index (IK) according to the following formula:

$$IK = \text{reading at first hour} + \frac{\text{reading at second hour}}{2}$$

Normal erythrocyte sedimentation rate values change with age. In the newborn the erythrocyte sedimentation rate is rarely higher than 2 mm/h, probably because of the high erythrocyte count; in adolescents and adults it ranges from 1 to 10 mm/h in men and from 1 to 15 mm/h in women. Erythrocyte sedimentation rate values are usually higher in the elderly, ranging from 0 to 38 mm/h in men and from 0 to 53 mm/h in women.

Fibrinogen

Several methods that measure fibrinogen plasma concentration by means of the conversion times of fibrinogen to fibrin are available. Fibrin is measured by gravimetry, nephelometry, chemical analysis, or precipitation with ammonium sulfate. Radial immunodiffusion on Partigen plates, which exploits the precipitation of specific antiserum in vitro on contact with their antigens, is the most commonly used method. The normal range is 2.0 to 4.5 g/L.[14]

Albumin/Globulin Ratio

Until recently albumin and globulin levels and the albumin/globulin ratio were determined using the Howe method. A saline solution was added to the serum sample and the globulin precipitation observed. Today serum protein levels are determined by means of electrophoresis on paper or cellulose acetate.[14]

Deformability

Whole Blood

Suspend whole blood at 10% hematocrit in a 2% phosphate buffered saline (PBS).

Erythrocytes

The whole blood sample is anticoagulated with EDTA. After centrifugation at 3000 rpm for 10 minutes the plasma, buffy coat, and upper 10% of packed erythrocytes are aspirated and discarded. Erythrocytes from the middle part of the erythrocyte column are suspended in PBS at a 10% hematocrit. Leukocyte contamination is checked in a Neubauer counting chamber using a light microscope.

Unfractionated Leukocytes

The whole blood sample is anticoagulated with EDTA and centrifuged at 1500 rpm for 10 minutes. After removing the plasma and the buffy coat, the uppermost red cells are aspirated and resuspended in 2 mL of plasma. After 15 minutes the erythrocyte sedimentation occurs and leukocyte-rich plasma is aspirated and diluted with PBS. It is centrifuged twice and the final pellet suspended in 2 mL of PBS for filtration.[11]

Polymorphonuclear and Mononuclear Leukocyte Subpopulations

Fractionation of leukocyte subpopulations is carried out by layering these samples onto a two-step density gradient made up of Ficoll–Hypaque preparations. After centrifugation at 1400 rpm at 20°C for 40 minutes, the leukocyte subpopulations appear as two distinct bands, the upper layer being mononuclear leukocytes and the lower layer polymorphonuclear leukocytes. Each fraction is harvested, and after adding PBS the cells are washed twice by centrifugation at 1000 rpm for 10 minutes. Cells are then made up to the desired concentrations in PBS, with the addition of 0.5% bovine serum albumin (BSA), and used immediately for filtration studies.[9]

Monocytes and Lymphocytes

Monocytes and lymphocytes are prepared by suspending the mononuclear fraction in PBS and placing it in a plastic Petri dish for 40 minutes. The lymphocytes are removed with a pipette, and the monocytes that adhere to the plastic surface are removed with trypsin. The cells are then suspended in PBS or BSA for filtration measurements.

Filtration Instruments

Filtrometers either measure filtration pressure of the different blood cells through membrane pores at constant flow rates or measure flow when different pressures, whether constant or changing, are applied. In both systems flow resistance increases with filtration time because rigid cells clog the pores. Nuclepore filters, usually with 5-μm diameter channel pores at least 10 μm in length, are used in all filtration instruments. Because there is batch-to-batch variation in the geometry and distribution of filter pores, all filters used in a clinical or experimental study should be taken from the same batch and the batch number stated.

There are two types of filtrometers currently in use for assessing blood cell rheology. St. George's blood filtrometer[3] operates on the principle of creating a constant low differential pressure that will cause any cell suspension present in the system to pass through a filter. The rate of filtration is determined after introducing the suspension into a capillary tube and following the meniscus along the bore of the capillary tube through four pairs of fiber-optic light sources and detectors. Because this filtrometer is capable of measuring the filterability of whole blood, erythrocyte, or leukocyte suspensions, it is eminently suitable for routine clinical use. It is relatively inexpensive, easy to use, accurate, and sensitive. The Vickers apparatus[9] consists of a syringe pump connected to a "pop-top" filter holder that contains the Nuclepore filter and to a pressure transducer linked to a pressure indicator/amplifier. Pressure changes are traced as continuous pressure–time curves. Filtration of PBS or BSA buffer used to suspend the cells produces a constant pressure reading. Subsequent filtration of the cell suspension in buffer through the same filter gives a time-dependent increase in pressure due to progressive occupation of pores by slowly passing cells.

Expression of Results

Filtration results for cell suspensions should be expressed as a ratio of the flow resistance of the cell suspension to that of the suspending medium, with the ratio being expressed as a function of time of filtration. Because each laboratory needs to develop its own procedures and reproducibility standards, at least five successive filtrations of cell suspensions of the same normal blood sample must be studied to estimate the coefficient of variation.

Erythrocyte, Leukocyte, and Platelet Counts

Cells can be counted directly under the light microscopy after the blood sample has been diluted in a neutroisotonic solution. Cells will be deposited in the counting chamber. The more advanced method is to use an electronic counter, such as the Coulter counter, which gives more accurate results more quickly.[14]

Leukocyte Activation

Morphological Assessment

A small proportion of unfractioned leukocytes (obtained as described earlier) in suspension is fixed in 1% glutaraldehyde and observed under light microscopy. The percentage of cells with pseudopodia or cytoplasmic irregularities is calculated and classified as active.[12]

Functional Assessment

Functional assessment includes quantifying polymorphonuclear leukocyte production of oxygen free radicals and observing the phenotypical expression of adhesion receptors on activated leukocytes. The production of superoxide anions from polymorphonuclear leukocytes, after in vitro stimulation by phorbol-12-myristate-13-acetate,[13] is assessed as the superoxide dismutase inhibitable reduction of ferricytochrome C^2 as read on the spectrophotometer. Superoxide release is expressed in nanomoles $O_2^2/4 \times 10^6$ leukocytes/15 min.

The phenotypical expression of adhesion receptors (LFA-1 [CD11a/CD18], Mac-1 [CD11b/CD18], and p150,95 [CD11c/CD18]) is observed by indirect immunofluorescence using monoclonal antibodies for these cell receptors. Visualization of the receptor–antibody complex is achieved by adding a fluorescein isothiocyanate–goat antimouse immunoglobulin G. Fluorescent intensity is read on a fluorescence-activated cell sorter flow cytometer. The results are expressed as changes in relative fluorescence intensity.[1,3]

Acknowledgment

Translation by Dr. G. A. Boyd; technical notes by R. Lombardini MSc (Biol).

References

1. Anderson DC, Schmalstieg FC, Finegold MJ, et al. The severe and moderate phenotypes of heritable MAC-1, LFA-1,

p150,95 deficiency: their quantitative definition and relation to leukocyte dysfunction and clinical features. *J Infect Dis.* 1995;152:225–234.

2. Capsoni F, Venegani E, Minonzio F, Ongazi AM, Maresca V, Zanussi C. Inhibition of neutrophil oxidative metabolism by nimesulide. *Agents Action.* 1987;21:1–2.

3. Dormandy JA, Flute P, Matrai A, Bogar L, Mikita J. The new St. George's blood filtrometer. *Clinical Hemorheology.* 1985;5:975–983.

4. Ernst E, Matrai A. Software package CH-001-S84: hematocrit correction for blood viscosity. *Clinical Hemorheology.* 1985;5:1–8.

5. Fahraeus R. The suspension stability of blood. *Physiol Rev.* 1929;9:241–274.

6. International Committee for Standardization in Haematology. Recommended measurement of erythrocyte sedimentation rate of human blood. *Am J Clin Pathol.* 1977; 68:505–507.

7. International Committee for Standardization in Haematology. Recommendation for a selected method for the measurement of plasma viscosity. *J Clin Pathol.* 1984;37: 1147–1152.

8. International Committee for Standardization in Haematology, Expert Panel on Blood Rheology. Guidelines for measurements of blood viscosity and erythrocyte deformability. *Clinical Hemorheology.* 1986;6:439–453.

9. Lennie SE, Lowe GDO, Barbanel JC, Forbes CD, Fould WS. Filterability of white blood cell subpopulations, separated by an improved method. *Clinical Hemorheology.* 1987; 7:811–816.

10. Matrai A, Whittington RB, Ernst E. A simple method of estimating whole blood viscosity at standardized hematocrit. *Clinical Hemorheology..* 1987;7:261–265.

11. Mikita J, Nash GB, Dormandy JA. A simple method of preparing white blood cells for filterability testing. *Clinical Hemorheology.* 1986;6:635–639.

12. Nash GB, Thomas PRS, Dormandy JA. Abnormal flow properties of white blood cells in patients with severe ischaemia of the leg. *BMJ.* 1988;296:1699–1701.

13. Newburger PE, Chovanick ME, Cohen HJ. Activity and activation of the granulocyte superoxide generating system. *Blood.* 1980;55:85–92.

14. Pasquinelli F. *Diagnostica e Tecniche di Laboratorio.* Rosini, Italy: Firenze; 1979.

40

Lipid Pattern

Graziana Lupattelli

Because lipids play a major role in the development and progression of the atherosclerotic plaque, lipid, apolipoprotein, and lipoprotein analysis is a fundamental step in the study of any patient affected by, or at risk of, atherosclerotic disease. Lipid analysis is necessary to assess the patient's vascular risk and to diagnose primary hyperlipidemias (e.g., polygenic hypercholesterolemia, familial hypercholesterolemia, familial combined hyperlipidemia, familial hypertriglyceridemia, and hyperchylomicronemia). When used with screening examinations, it identifies secondary forms of hyperlipidemias (e.g., hypercholesterolemia due to nephrotic syndrome, hypothyroidism, connective tissue diseases, myeloma, and Cushing's syndrome and hypertriglyceridemia due to diabetes, alcoholism, and liver diseases).

Any investigation into the lipid pattern starts with measuring lipid levels—total cholesterol, triglycerides, high-density lipoprotein (HDL) cholesterol, and low-density lipoprotein (LDL) cholesterol—before carrying out more specialized tests, which include lipoprotein electrophoresis, lipoprotein separation by means of ultracentrifuge, apolipoprotein isoelectrofocusing, evaluation of LDL receptor activity, and analysis of the apolipoprotein genes and enzymes involved in lipid metabolism.

Who should undergo lipid examination? Patients with atherosclerotic disease of the heart and/or of the peripheral arteries, patients with other risk factors (e.g., smoking, hypertension, or diabetes), and healthy patients with a family history of hyperlipemia or vascular disease. The National Cholesterol Education Program recommends total and HDL cholesterol measurements in all adults 20 years or older at least every 5 years. If a hyperlipemic state is shown, regular tests are required to verify the efficacy of hypolipemic therapy.[1,17]

Before undergoing baseline lipid analysis patients should maintain their usual lifestyle and diet and suspend all drugs that could influence lipid metabolism for 3 weeks before the tests. Hypolipemic drugs should not be withdrawn if checkup tests are prescribed to monitor drug efficacy. The results of lipid tests have no diagnostic validity during pregnancy, inflammation that has not been fully resolved, and within 6 months of acute vascular diseases, because all of these conditions can modify lipid concentrations.

Analysis should be scheduled in the morning after a 12- to 14-hour overnight fast. The fasting condition is extremely important, especially for triglyceride determination, because levels have a high intraindividual variability and are significantly modified by eating time: blood samples drawn after a 12- to 14-hour fast and during the early hours of the morning guarantee the most homogeneous result.[20]

Blood samples should be drawn after the patient has been seated for 5 minutes because orthostatism increases total cholesterol level by approximately 10%. The tourniquet should be removed as soon as blood starts to flow into the test tube because venous stasis modifies triglyceride concentrations.[11,20]

Lipid parameters can be measured in either serum or plasma. Samples can be stored at 4°C for no more than 4 days. Samples should be stored at −70°C if they must be held for longer periods.

Total Cholesterol

Total cholesterol levels vary widely within the individual, so the test should be performed on at least two different occasions at a 2-month interval. As for all determinations on the lipid pattern, pretest procedures should be carefully standardized. Many methods are currently available, but the enzymatic colorimetric technique based on commercial tests is used in 95% of laboratories. Values >240 mg/dL are considered indicative of hypercholesterolemia in adults, but the limits above which dietary and pharmacological therapy are required are 200 mg/dL in adults and 180 mg/dL in children.[1,17]

Triglycerides

Triglycerides present the highest intraindividual variability of all the lipids, but a 12- to 14-hour fast guarantees the most homogeneous results. In the hours immediately before drawing the blood sample, patients should refrain from smoking, exercising, and drinking alcohol, because all three factors significantly modify triglyceride concentrations.[7,20] Triglycerides are measured by enzymatic methods. The first step is a complete triglyceride hydrolysis using different lipases either with or without adding protease or esterase. Using the enzymatic method, their normal value is <200 mg/dL.[11] No consensus has yet been reached on hypertriglyceridemia as a risk factor for ischemic heart disease. Although high plasma concentrations are predictive of premature heart disease, the correlation weakens when other risk factors, such as HDL cholesterol levels, are considered.[9]

HDL Cholesterol

High HDL cholesterol levels are known to be a protective factor for ischemic heart disease, because HDLs are involved in the centripetal transport of cholesterol from the peripheral tissues to the liver.[6] HDL cholesterol is measured by dextran–sulfate precipitation of lipoproteins that contain apolipoprotein B (very-low-density lipoprotein [VLDL] and LDL) and by determining cholesterol level in the supernatant.[3] HDL cholesterol values are lower in those who smoke, the obese, and the sedentary. Protective values are 35 mg/dL for adults.[17]

HDL particles are polymorphic: of particular interest are HDL_2 and HDL_3. Liver and gut synthesize mainly HDL_3 particles, which are later transformed into HDL_2, a fraction that is larger and less dense than HDL_3. Although some studies have shown that low levels of HDL_2 are better predictors of myocardial infarction than low concentrations of HDL_3, the results of other reports are conflicting.[15] HDL_2 and HDL_3 can be determined by using ultracentrifuge separation followed by the enzymatic colorimetric method.[18]

LDL Cholesterol

LDL cholesterol plays a key role in the onset and development of atherosclerotic plaque. LDL cholesterol levels are measured directly by determining the quantity of cholesterol bound to LDL, as calculated by Friedewald's formula:

$$\text{LDL cholesterol} = \text{total cholesterol} - (\text{triglycerides}/5 + \text{HDL cholesterol}).$$

Friedewald's formula cannot be used in patients with hypertriglyceridemia because of chylomicrons and remnants of VLDL in the serum. In these cases LDL cholesterol should be measured by ultracentrifuge.[10] Recommended values are <130 mg/dL in healthy adults and <100 mg/dL in patients with ischemic heart disease.[1]

Lipoprotein(a)

Lipoprotein(a) has recently been recognized as an independent risk factor for atherosclerotic disease and should be measured to assess the cardiovascular risk, particularly when there is a strong family or personal history of vascular disease. The most common methods for measuring lipoprotein(a) are enzyme-linked immunosorbent assay, radio-immuno assay, radial immunodiffusion, and nephelometry, which are all based on apolipoprotein(a) binding with monoclonal or polyclonal antibodies. Despite recent improvements, specificity and sensitivity problems remain with all of these techniques, particularly with regard to immunoreactivity of antibodies to the different isoforms of apolipoprotein(a). Values considered indicative of vascular risk are those >20 to 30 mg/dL. Dietary and pharmacological treatments are almost completely ineffective in reducing plasma lipoprotein(a) levels.[2,14]

Apolipoproteins A-I and B

Apolipoprotein A-I, a protein structure made up of a single chain of 245 amino acids and with a molecular weight of 28,300 d, is the HDL structural protein and its vehicle. Apolipoprotein B-100—with a molecular weight of 512,000 d—is the VLDL and LDL structural and vehicle protein and plays an important role in LDL catabolization. Apolipoprotein A-I and apolipoprotein B concentrations correspond to plasma HDL and LDL concentrations. However, using these values as predictive of ischemic heart disease is not recommended because all epidemiological data on ischemic heart disease are based on lipid measurements. The most common methods for measuring apolipoprotein A-I and apolipoprotein B are nephelometry, radial immunodiffusion, and radio-immuno assay using commercial kits.[16] The apolipoprotein B level should be <100 mg/dL, and the apolipoprotein A-I level should be >130 mg/dL.

Lipoprotein Electrophoresis

Lipoprotein separation by electrophoresis occurs after seeding samples on agarose gel or cellulose acetate. With their different electrical charges and particle diameters, all lipoproteins have different electrophoretic mobility patterns that correspond to the density of the lipoprotein classes.

The lipoproteins separate into four principal classes in order of increasing mobility: chylomicrons, which, when present, remain at the origin; β-lipoproteins (corresponding to LDLs) with a mobility pattern similar to plasma globulins; pre-β-lipoproteins (corresponding to VLDLs); and α-lipoproteins (corresponding to HDLs). Electrophoresis can be used to identify some hyperlipemic phenotypes. It differentiates phenotype III (characterized by hypercholesterolemia, hypertriglyceridemia, and a broad band with β-mobility) from phenotype IIB (characterized by hypercholesterolemia and hypertriglyceridemia but with two distinct bands, β and pre-β). It also detects chylomicrons, which are indicative of phenotypes I and V.[13]

Ultracentrifuge

Ultracentrifugation separates lipoproteins by their density.[10] A saline solution with a known density (NaCl, density 1006 g/mL) is added to the plasma sample and centrifuged at 100,000 rpm for 18 hours. VLDLs are harvested from the supernatant. The infranatant still contains lipoproteins with a density of more than 1006 g/mL (i.e., HDL and LDL). To separate LDL from the HDL another saline solution with a density of 1063 g/mL is added. After 24 hours of centrifugation the LDL can be collected in the supernatant and the HDL in the infranatant.

Lipids and apolipoproteins are measured in each fraction, and different apolipoprotein isoforms and mutant apolipoproteins can be identified. Ultracentrifugation is used mainly for research purposes but is also essential for diagnosing different forms of hyperlipidemia (e.g., familial combined hyperlipidemia, which exhibits high apolipoprotein B levels in VLDL, or broad b-band disease in which the cholesterol/triglyceride ratio is 0.3 in the VLDL).

Isoelectrofocusing

Isoelectrofocusing is used to identify apolipoprotein isoforms or mutant apolipoproteins. It can be carried out on whole serum samples or on lipoprotein fractions after ultracentrifugation and delipidation.[19]

Isoelectrofocusing is particularly useful for studying apolipoprotein E isoforms. There are three known phenotypes: E2, E3, and E4, each of which is encoded by a specific allele. Any patient may be heterozygote or homozygote for each one of these alleles. The most common patterns in the general population are E3/E3 and E3/E4. The least frequently encountered pattern is E2/E2, which is responsible for type III hyperlipidemia.

Isoelectrofocusing has also been used to identify structural variations in apolipoprotein A-I, generally associated with lower HDL cholesterol levels (apolipoprotein A-I Milano), and in apolipoprotein C-II, which causes hypertriglyceridemia and hyperchylomicronemia.[4]

Apolipoprotein B-100/E Receptor Activity

Apolipoprotein B-100/E receptor activity is studied when heterozygote or homozygote familial hypercholesterolemia is suspected.[5] Receptor activity is assessed on fibroblasts from a patient's skin or on blood lymphocytes through uptake of LDL radiolabeled with [125]I. Receptor activity is absent in the homozygote form of familial hypercholesterolemia and is present at about 50% in the heterozygote form.[58]

Genetic Studies

Molecular biology techniques identify the molecular basis of several abnormalities in the genes that encode apolipoproteins, enzymes, and receptors. Mutations in genes that encode apolipoprotein B-100, apolipoprotein A-I, the apolipoprotein B-100 receptor, and several enzymes that regulate lipoprotein metabolism have been identified. Progress in this field has increased the possibility of a correct diagnosis of the different types of hyperlipidemia, particularly of the rarer forms.[12,21]

Acknowledgments
Translation by Dr. G. A. Boyd.

References

1. Adult treatment Panel II, National Cholesterol Education Program. Second report of the expert panel on detection, evaluation, and treatment of high blood cholesterol in adults. *Circulation.* 1994;89:1333–1445.
2. Albers JJ, Marcovina SM. Lp(a) quantification: comparison of methods and strategies for standardization. *Curr Opin Lipidol.* 1994;5:417–421.
3. Bachorik PS, Albers JJ. Precipitation methods for quantification of lipoproteins. In: Albers FG, Segrest RH, eds. *Methods in Enzymology.* London: Academic Press; 1986:129: 78–100.
4. Breslow JL. Human apolipoprotein molecular biology and genetic variation. *Annu Rev Biochem.* 1985;54:699–727.
5. Brown MS, Goldstein JL. A receptor mediated pathway for cholesterol homeostasis. *Science.* 1986;232:34–40.

6. Castelli WP, Garrison RJ, Wilson PWF, Abbott RD, Kalousdian S, Kannel WB. Incidence of coronary heart disease and lipoprotein cholesterol levels. *JAMA*. 1986;256: 2835–2838.

7. Cooper GR, Mayers GL, Smith SJ, Sampson EJ. Standardization of lipid, lipoprotein, and apolipoprotein measurements. *Clin Chem*. 1988;34:B95–B105.

8. Cuthbert JA, East CA, Bilheimer DW, Lipsky PE. Detection of familial hypercholesterolemia by assaying functional low density lipoprotein receptors on lymphocytes. *N Engl J Med*. 1986;314:879–883.

9. Havel RJ. Role of triglyceride rich lipoproteins in progression of atherosclerosis. *Circulation*. 1990;81:694–696.

10. Havel RJ, Eder HA, Bragdon JH. The distribution and chemical composition of ultracentrifugally separated lipoproteins in human serum. *J Clin Invest*. 1955;34: 1345–1353.

11. International Task Force for Prevention of Coronary Heart Disease. Prevention of coronary heart disease: scientific background and new clinical guidelines. *Nutrition Metabolism and Cardiovascular Diseases*. 1992;2:113–156.

12. Lalouel JM. Linkage approach to dyslipidemia. *Curr Opin Lipidol*. 1991;2:86–89.

13. Noble RP. Electrophoretic separation of plasma lipoprotein in agarose gel. *J Lipid Res*. 1968;9:693–700.

14. Scanu AM. Update on lipoprotein (a). *Curr Opin Lipidol*. 1991;2:253–258.

15. Silverman DI, Ginsburg GS, Pasternak RC. High density lipoprotein subfractions. *Am J Med*. 1993;94:636–645.

16. Smith SJ, Cooper GR, Henderson LO, Hannor WH, and the Apolipoprotein Standardization Group. An international collaborative study on standardization of apolipoprotein AI and B, I: evaluation of lyophilized candidate reference and calibration material. *Clin Chem*. 1987;33: 2240–2249.

17. National Cholesterol Education Program Expert Panel on Detection, Evaluation, and Treatment of High Blood Cholesterol in Adults. Report. *Arch Intern Med*. 1988;148: 36–69.

18. Von Eckardstein A, Huang Y, Assmann G. Physiological role and clinical relevance of high density lipoprotein subclasses. *Curr Opin Lipidol*. 1994;5:404–416.

19. Warnick GR, Mayfield C, Albers JJ, Hazzard WR. Gel isoelectrofocusing method for specific diagnosis of familial hyperlipoproteinemia type III. *Clin Chem*. 1979;25:279–284.

20. Waseniaus A, Stugaard M, Otterstad JE. Diurnal and monthly intraindividual variability of the concentration of lipids, lipoproteins, and apoproteins. *Scand J Clin Lab Invest*. 1990;50:87–93.

21. Zannis VI, Kardassis D, Cardot P, Hadzopoulou-Cladaras M, Zanni EE, Cladaras C. Molecular biology of the human apolipoprotein genes: gene regulation and structure/function relationship. *Curr Opin Lipidol*. 1992;3:96–113.

41

Blood Coagulation

Salvatore Innocente

Blood Coagulation

Blood coagulation is envisaged as a series of stepwise reactions whereby an inactive proenzyme is converted to the active enzymatic form, which, in turn, converts another proenzyme to its active form; the cycle continues until fibrinogen is converted to fibrin and the fibrin is cross-linked.

In the absence of tissue factor blood is capable of generating its own procoagulant activity. This is designated the *intrinsic* system of coagulation, in contrast to the *extrinsic* system, which is the pathway used when tissue extracts are added to whole blood.

Primary hemostasis is assessed by means of the bleeding time and the platelet count. The so-called coagulation factors may be evaluated by means of partial thromboplastin times, prothrombin times, thrombin times, fibrinogen concentration, and fibrinogen degradation products (FDP). The activity of coagulation inhibitors can be assessed by means of protein C, protein S, and antithrombin III (AT III).

Patient Preparation

Any blood samples for coagulation tests should be taken after an overnight fast and, except for samples for capillary tests, should be drawn from a forearm vein.

Bleeding Time

The bleeding time is the time that elapses between infliction of a standard wound and arrest of bleeding. Bleeding stops because platelets, which have adhered to exposed basement membrane and tissue collagen at the site of injury, undergo aggregation that results in the formation of the hemostatic plug. The bleeding time test is therefore a measure of the number and function of circulating platelets, although red cells also play a role in the arrest of bleeding. The bleeding time is thus influenced by the actual hemostatic level of the patient.

Materials

The following materials are needed to assess bleeding time:

1. A sphygmomanometer
2. Three stopwatches
3. Disposable sterile lancets (no. 433)
4. Disposable sterile surgical blades (no. 11)
5. Filter paper disks
6. A device consisting of a polystyrene template with a slit (11 mm long), a lancet holder, and a gauge that allows the lancet to protrude exactly 1 mm through the slit of the template
7. Sterile disposable bleeding time devices

The Ivy Method

The sphygmomanometer cuff is applied around the upper arm and inflated to 40 mm Hg. After disinfecting the forearm skin three 2-mm– to 5-mm–deep punctures are made about 5 cm distal to the antecubital fossa, taking care to avoid superficial veins. As soon as the first drop of blood issues from the puncture site a stopwatch is started and the blood is removed by filter paper at 30-second intervals. Care is taken to avoid touching the edge of the wound. As soon as the blood stops staining the filter paper the stopwatch is stopped; the bleeding time is represented by the mean value of three observations. Normal value is <4 minutes.

Comments

The bleeding time is prolonged in hereditary and acquired platelet function defects, in thrombocytopenia of various origins, in hereditary and acquired von Willebrand's disease, and in patients with low hematocrit lev-

501

els. A prolonged bleeding time may also occur in patients with connective tissue disorders, congenital factor V or VII deficiency, or afibrinogenemia.

Platelet Count

Blood is mixed with a compound that lyses the red cells and leaves the platelets intact.

Materials

The following materials are needed to assess platelet count:

1. Ammonium oxalate (1 g) dissolved in distilled water (100 mL) and filtered
2. A Neubauer counting chamber
3. White cell pipettes
4. A humid chamber
5. A leveling table

Method

Ammonium oxalate is drawn to the 0.5-mL mark in a white cell pipette. Well-mixed Na_2 ethylenediaminetetraacetic acid–anticoaculated blood is then drawn up until the pipette is filled to the 0.1-mL mark, enough diluent is then added so that the pipette is filled to the 11-mL mark (1:20 dilution). The pipette is vigorously shaken for 3 minutes. The first few drops are discarded, and the counting chamber is filled. The counting chamber is left to settle for 20 minutes in a humid chamber (Petri dish that contains moist filter paper). Platelets are counted in 80 small squares by phase contrast or ordinary light microscopy. At least 100 platelets should be counted. If the platelet count is low, two sets of squares are counted or blood is diluted at 1:10 instead of 1:20. The platelet count is calculated by multiplying the number of platelets counted by 100 (i.e., volume times dilution), which gives the number of platelets per microliter. The normal range is 150,000 to 350,000 platelets.

Comments

In general, abnormal results are obtained in conjunction with a prolonged bleeding time.

Prothrombin Time Test

Collection of Blood

Collect venous blood, using a polystyrene syringe fitted with a 20- or 21-gauge needle, into a suitable capped plastic vessel that contains a freshly prepared solution of 3% to 13% trisodium citrate ($Na_3C_6H_5O_7 2H_2O$) (one volume of anticoagulant to nine volumes of blood). Mix several times by gentle inversion.

Separation of Plasma

Centrifuge blood as soon as possible after collection to obtain platelet-poor plasma (1500–2000 g for 15 minutes). Using a silicone Pasteur pipette, transfer plasma to a second dry container. Store at 4°C in crushed ice. Plasma samples should be tested as soon as possible and not more than 2 hours after collection.

Performance of Test

1. Reagents: calcium chloride 0 to 0.25 M; prepare from an M/1 solution
2. Glassware: use chemically clean, unscratched glass tubes; finely calibrated 0.1-mL pipettes (E-MIL type) should be used.
3. Method: into a water bath at 37°C place the following to warm:
   a. Sufficient glass tubes for testing samples
   b. An aliquot of calcium chloride (0–0.25 M)
4. Into a glass tube add the following:
   a. 0.1 mL thromboplastin
   b. 0.1 mL plasma
   c. 0.1 mL calcium chloride solution
5. Warm together for 1 to 2 minutes

Start stopwatch. Tilt the test tube evenly and gently until a clot is formed. The speed and angle of tilting should be standardized to minimize the cooling effect caused by withdrawal from the 37°C water bath. Tilting three times every 5 seconds, at an angle of 90 degrees, is recommended. Excessive cooling may result in prolongation of the prothrombin time. Tests should be performed twice. If the discrepancy between duplicate tests is more than 5% of the mean clotting time, the tests should be repeated. Results may be expressed in seconds, with normal times ranging from 28 to 33 seconds, or as a percentage of prothrombin activity, with the normal range being 70% to 100%.

Comments

Prolonged prothrombin times are indicative of either hypoprothrombinemia, caused by low vitamin K levels due to insufficient liver synthesis or excessively high dosages of oral anticoagulant agents, or pseudohypoprothrombinemia, caused by defects in factors V and VII as found, for example, in Owren's disease.

Thrombin Time

The thrombin time test measures the clotting time of citrated plasma in the presence of thrombin. It explores the last phase of the clotting cascade (fibrin formation) except for factor XIII activity.

Test Sample

The test sample consists of fresh or fresh frozen plasma from a normal subject.

Reagents

Veronal or Tris buffer (pH 7.35, ionic strength 0.15) thrombin (generally bovine) is the usual reagent. Thrombin is kept in a freeze-dried form or frozen as a solution in buffer at a high concentration (at least 100 NIH units/mL). It is diluted at the time of testing to a concentration of 5 to 10 NIH units, which should control plasma clotting in 18 to 20 seconds. During the test, the thrombin solution is kept on ice to prevent progressive inactivation.

Procedure

Into a standard glass tube prewarmed for 1 minute in a water bath at 37°C, use a pipette to remove 0.2 mL of a patient's plasma or control plasma (duplicate tubes for each sample). After 1 minute, add 0.1 mL thrombin solution; mix by shaking the tube and record the clotting time. Clotting may be detected by regularly tilting or dipping a glass loop into the sample. The latter method may be preferable because in this test (unlike others such as that for prothrombin time) the end point can by marked by formation of wispy strands of fibrin rather than a full clot.

Technical Notes

Satisfactory results can be obtained on samples that have been stored for several months at −20°C. Clotting times of less than 15 seconds should be avoided. If necessary, the thrombin solution can be further diluted.

Comments

Normal values for thrombin times are in the range of 18 to 25 seconds. Longer thrombin times may be due to low fibrinogen concentration (<80 mg/100 mL in plasma), defective fibrinogen function (congenital or acquired dysfibrinogenemias) (Table 41.1), the presence of an abnormal antithrombin activity, heparin therapy, or the

TABLE 41.1. Congenital dysfibrinogenemias associated with thrombosis.

Name	Year
Fibrinogen Baltimore	1964
Fibrinogen Oslo I	1967
Fibrinogen Paris II	1968
Fibrinogen Wiesbaden	1971
Fibrinogen Chapel Hill I	1975
Fibrinogen New York	1975
Fibrinogen Charlottesville	1977
Fibrinogen Marburg	1977
Fibrinogen Naples	1977
Fibrinogen Copenhagen	1979
Fibrinogen Dusard	1984
Fibrinogen Bergamo II	1986
Fibrinogen Nijmegen	1988

presence of an inhibitor of fibrin monomer polymerization (such as paraproteins of fibrinogen or fibrin degradation products). Severe hyperbilirubinemia, hypoalbuminemia, and hemolysis may prolong the thrombin time aspecifically.

FDP Assays

Principles

Because most of the common methods for measuring FDP are based on characteristics (immunological or other) common to the parent fibrinogen molecule, fibrinogen must be removed from the sample before starting the test. The sample to be tested is collected with aprotinin (100 KIE units/mL final concentration) and incubated for 4 hours with a solution that contains 0.0125 M $CaCl_2$, 1.0 NIH unit/mL thrombin, and 0.05 M ε-aminocaproic acid. If heparin is suspected in the sample, 0.1 mL reptilase-R or thrombin coagulase can be added to each milliliter of the clotting mixture. The tube that contains the clot is centrifuged at 3000 g for 15 minutes and the supernatant is used for FDP assay. This supernatant may be stored at −20°C for several days before testing. Note that when measuring circulating FDP, it is preferable to clot citrated platelet-poor plasma rather than whole blood to prevent artifactual in vitro fibrinolysis. Normal plasma, defibrinated in these conditions, has FDP levels <2 μg/mL.

The general principle of tests for routine evaluation of FDP is that red cells or latex particles coated with an antigen can be visibly agglutinated when the corresponding antibody is added. This agglutination is inhibited if antiserum is preincubated with a sample that contains the antigen (agglutination-inhibited techniques). Alternatively, latex particles can be coated with antibody and agglutinated when adding the antigen (direct agglutination techniques). The test that best meets both rapidity and specificity requirements is the latex particle agglutination inhibition technique, which comprises two steps:

1. Serial dilutions of the sample are incubated with anti-fibrinogen antiserum.
2. The presence of the free antibody is detected by the addition of latex particles coated with fibrinogen.

Reagents

All of the necessary reagents and accessories are available in commercial kits, which contain the following:

1. Albumin–glycine buffered saline, pH 8.2, that contains 0.1 M glycine and 2% bovine albumin for dilution of the test samples
2. Antihuman fibrinogen antiserum already diluted to the concentration that provides optimal agglutination of latex particles
3. Latex particles coated with human fibrinogen
4. Lyophilized fibrinogen for use as a standard

For the standard, in view of the possible lack of stability of purified fibrinogen preparations, it is preferable to use a normal plasma pool of known fibrinogen concentration prepared in the laboratory. This pool can be stored at $-20°C$ in small aliquots thawed at the time of use.

Procedure

The following procedure is used in measuring FDP:

1. Prepare double dilutions of standard and test samples in albumin–glycine buffer.
2. Place one drop of each on a convenient glass surface such as a microscope slide against a black background.
3. Add one drop of antifibrinogen serum to each dilution sample on the glass slide and mix with a wooden stick (to form a spot not larger than 1 cm in diameter); leave for 2 minutes.
4. Add one drop of latex to each sample, mix again, and rock gently for 2 minutes.
5. Record the highest dilution at which agglutination is prevented in standard and test samples.

FDP result (μg/mL fibrinogen equivalents):

$$\frac{\text{test sample dilution}}{\text{standard sample dilution}} \times \text{fibrinogen in standard sample}$$

Comments

The presence of FDP is indicative of disseminated intravascular coagulation or reduced liver clearance.

Fibrinogen Assay

Principle

The fibrinogen assay method is based on the kinetics of fibrinogen-to-fibrin conversion. In the presence of an exceedingly large amount of thrombin, the clotting time is inversely proportional to the amount of fibrinogen present in the system, provided the fibrinogen level is low. In these conditions the time required for the proteolytic step of fibrinogen-to-fibrin conversion is extremely short and can be considered as reduced to a constant minimal value. Because the rate of polymerization depends on the concentration of fibrin monomers in the system, the more fibrinogen in the sample, the shorter the time needed to form the first fibrin strand. The clotting time in this system therefore depends mainly on the fibrin polymerization time. The optimal conditions for the kinetics of the reaction are obtained with a very high concentration of enzyme (thrombin) and a very low concentration of substrate (fibrinogen).

Test Sample

The test sample should consist of venous or capillary whole blood or fresh or fresh citrated platelet-poor plasma. When plasma must be used, blood is collected with 100 KIE units/mL of aprotinin to prevent in vitro proteolysis during preparation of the sample.

Reagents: Thrombin

The concentration of thrombin has been experimentally fixed at 400 NIH units/mL in Tris-HCL buffer (pH 7.4, ionic strength 0.15). Thrombin from various manufacturers can be used. Thrombin solutions of 400 NIH units/mL can be stored in small aliquots at $-20°C$ in plastic tubes for at least 3 months. Once thawed, the solutions must be used immediately and kept on ice during the experiment. Diluent for blood or plasma may be the special reagent FPT-Dil citrate buffered solution that contains aprotinin (FPT-Dil, Christiaens, Brussels, Belgium). This diluent can be stored at 4°C.

Procedure

The procedure for calculating fibrinogen concentration is as follows:

1. Prewarm 0.2 mL of the test sample (generally diluted 1:10 for blood and 1:20 for plasma) in a water bath at 37°C for 1 minute.
2. Add 0.2 mL of thrombin and shake rapidly.
3. Monitor the clotting time using a glass hook to detect formation of the first fibrin strand as an end point; because of the low fibrinogen concentration in the di-

luted pooled plasma sample, the whole sample clots slowly.
4. From the clotting time, calculate the concentration of fibrinogen

Antithrombin III

Principle

AT III is a glycoprotein purified by electrophoresis and more recently by affinity chromatography on heparin sepharose. The half-life has been found to be 2.83 days in humans. AT III essentially reacts with thrombin.[1]

Immunological Tests

Immunological tests determine the AT III antigen concentrations and are based on the development of specific polyclonal (rarely monoclonal) heterologous antibodies for human AT III. With an appropriate dilution of plasma, immunophelometry in liquids and radial immunodiffusion, electroimmunodiffusion, or immunoenzymatic techniques (enzyme-linked immunosorbent assay [ELISA]) in solids form an antibody–antigen complex, the quantity of which is directly proportional to the quantity of AT III in the plasma specimen. Radial immunodiffusion is the simplest but least sensitive method. Electroimmunodiffusion is more complex and requires more equipment and more experienced laboratory staff but is more sensitive. ELISA provides improved sensitivity.[2,5]

Bidimensional immunoelectrophoresis estimates AT III qualitatively. AT III is separated from plasma by electrophoresis on agarose gel (first dimension) and identified using a specific heterologous antibody (second dimension). AT III migration velocity is assessed and gross structural abnormalities identified. When heparin is dissolved in the first-dimension agar, two forms of AT III with either high or low affinity for heparin can be distinguished. In normal subjects 90% of plasma AT III possesses heparin affinity.[2,5]

Limitations

Although immunological methods for determining AT III are very simple, they cannot be used alone for laboratory investigation because the antigen concentration may be normal even in cases of congenital or acquired AT III deficiency. A typical example is when AT III is synthesized at a normal rate but a certain quota is functionally inactive because of a genetic mutation in perhaps only one amino acid. This does not affect AT III antigen concentrations, which are all within the normal range, but does reduce the protein's functional activity.

Functional Tests

Functional tests, which assess only the quantity of biologically active AT III in plasma, provide a good estimate of the antithrombin potential of the patient. They are all based on the principle of AT III inhibiting the biological activity of one of the target serum proteases (i.e., thrombin or activated factor X). The diluted plasma sample reacts with one of the two enzymes, and the excess residue is quantified by means of a specific chromogenic substrate. Assays performed in the presence of heparin thus provide data on the heparin cofactor activity; in the absence of heparin they estimate progressive AT III activity.[1,5]

Technical Notes

The AT III inhibitory activity is faster than normal condition when heparin is present (in normal conditions one result is the equivalent of the other). All commercial kits measure the heparin cofactor activity using thrombin as the target enzyme; they are suitable for screening patients with a congenital or acquired AT III deficit. In order to estimate the AT III inhibitory activity, we use the bovine thrombin and incubation times between plasma and thrombin (30–60 seconds); in these conditions the interference of heparin cofactor II, which also inhibits thrombin, is reduced. Using activated factor X as the target enzyme avoids HCII interference completely.

AT III inhibitory activity is usually expressed as a percentage. The pool of normal values obtained in plasma from 20 normal subjects provides a calibration curve and gives an average of 100% activity. Each pool can be calibrated against the international reference standard of the National Institute for Biological Standards, London, UK. Unlike the other anticoagulants, the normal values of AT III have been well defined and range from 80% to 120%.

Protein C

Principle

Protein C may be activated with thrombin, thrombin thrombomodulin, or a protein extracted from snake venom. When thrombin or thrombin thrombomodulin is used for protein C activation, the protein C sample must be extracted from the plasma specimen.[6]

Immunological Tests

Protein C antigen concentrations can also be measured by immunological methods (e.g., electroimmunodiffusion, ELISA, and bidimensional immunoelectrophoresis).[5,7]

TABLE 41.2. Syndromes of thrombosis associated with anticardiolipin antibodies.

Type I syndrome
Deep vein thrombosis with or without pulmonary embolism

Type II syndrome
Coronary artery thrombosis
Peripheral artery thrombosis
Aortic thrombosis

Type III syndrome
Retinal artery thrombosis
Retinal vein thrombosis
Cerebrovascular thrombosis
Transient cerebral ischemic attacks

Type IV syndrome
Mixtures of types I, II, and III
Type IV syndrome is rare

Limitations

In cases of congenital dysfunctional deficits and acquired protein C deficits, immunological methods yield discrepant results that are often at variance with the results of functional tests. For example, in patients administered oral anticoagulant therapy, electroimmunodiffusion usually measures higher concentrations of protein C than ELISA. Both ELISA and electroimmunodiffusion measure higher levels than functional texts because of a deficit in protein C carboxylation induced by the oral anticoagulants. Discrepancies in immunological tests occur in patients with disseminated intravascular coagulation because of the differing capacity of the heterologous antibodies to recognize complexes that include activated protein C and its natural inhibitors, which are generated in plasma after coagulation activation (Table 41.2). Functional methods are therefore preferable.

Functional Methods

Many different types of functional methods with varying degrees of difficulty exist, but they can be divided into anticoagulant and amyloid methods. The anticoagulant techniques measure the capacity of activated protein C to inhibit its natural substrates (factors VIIIa and Va) by prolonging coagulation times of normal plasma through the addition of activated protein C. In the amyloid methods the amyloid activity of activated protein C is measured with specific chromogenic substrates.

The main advantage of the protac techniques is that the protein is activated directly in the plasma. All of these techniques are suitable for screening patients with congenital protein C deficits, even though diagnosis may be difficult because of the overlap in the values of patients and normal control subjects. This overlap usually occurs independently of the method and is due to the wide biological variability of protein C in the normal population. A congenital heterozygote deficiency (values around 50%) is difficult to distinguish from a nor-

mal value at the lower tail end of the distribution curve. Studies on the genealogical tree are needed in these patients.[5,7]

Technical Notes

Many commercial kits are available; those based on an anticoagulant method are preferable because they better reflect in vivo activity. Each laboratory therefore needs to establish its own standard for protein C values for each level in the therapeutic range.

Protein C values are usually expressed as a percentage of the normal level, with the calibration curve based on a pool of normal subjects. Because of the extreme biological variability of protein C, the pool needs to be as representative as possible of the general population and its value of 100% must be in direct proportion to the number of subjects included. Each laboratory can calibrate its pool against the International Reference Standard of the Natural Institute for Biological Standards, London, UK.

Protein S

Principle

Determining protein S plasma concentrations is complicated by the fact that 60% binds to C4b-BP, a complement regulating protein. Because only the free 40% has the cofactor properties of activated protein C, any laboratory method should determine the functional activity of only the free quota. All functional methods exploit protein S's capacity to lengthen the coagulation times of plasma with a protein S deficiency when activated protein C is added.[3,4]

Immunological Tests

Immunological methods quantify the protein S antigen by using polyethylene glycol to precipitate the protein S–C4b-BP complex. The quantity of free protein S in the supernatant is determined. This method does not assess the protein S functional activity and is not very specific because not all bound protein S may be precipitated and/or varying quantities of free protein S may also be precipitated. Results are also influenced by the quantity of C4b-BP in the plasma, because high levels of C4b-BP indicate less free protein S circulation. If the ELISA method is used this problem can be overcome by prolonging the incubation time to more than 6 hours.[3,4]

Functional Tests

Techniques that use monoclonal antibodies to separate free and bound protein S are complicated. Although all of these methods satisfy specificity and sensitivity criteria, they are subject to variables such as the quality of the plasma with protein S deficiency, the quantity of activated protein C used, and the basic procoagulant potential of the plasma under analysis, which make it difficult to correctly interpret the results. A recent study that compared four of these methods on plasma from patients with a congenital or acquired protein S deficiency showed that results were satisfactory in patients with a quantitative congenital deficiency but discrepant in the few cases of a congenital dysfunctional deficit. Diagnosis was not confirmed in any of the latter patients.[3,4]

Technical Notes

The results are usually expressed as a percentage of the normal concentration in a pool of normal plasma. Protein S concentrations vary greatly, and the normal pool cannot be calibrated because no international standard has yet been established.

Lupus Anticoagulants

Multiple lupus anticoagulant assays are commonly used. The first consists of a prothrombin time in which the thromboplastin is diluted to give a "normal time" of 60 seconds; when a time of 65 seconds or longer is noted, a lupus anticoagulant is considered to be present. This test may miss immunoglobulin M lupus anticoagulants. A superior test is a modified dilute Russel viper venom time in which the venom is diluted to give a "normal" time of 23 to 27 seconds and the phospholipid is then diluted down to a minimal level that will continue to support this range; a prolongation of the dilute Russel viper venom time will not be corrected with a mixture of patient and normal plasma, and this test detects both immunoglobulin G and immunoglobulin M lupus anticoagulant. If the dilute Russel viper venom time is prolonged, a lupus anticoagulant is confirmed by neutralizing (shortening) prolonged tests with a phospholipid void of platelet material, such as cephalin.[8,9] The failure of plasma infusion to correct an isolated factor II defi-

ciency in lupus patients suggests that an anti–factor II antibody may be present.[8]

Comment

Biologic false-positive tests for syphilis are seen in up to 40% of patients with systemic lupus and between 50% and 90% of patients with systemic lupus plus the lupus anticoagulant. Almost 40% of patients with biologic false-positive tests for syphilis have a lupus anticoagulant that should be searched for.[8]

Acknowledgment
Translation by Dr. G. A. Boyd.

References

1. Abildgaard U. Purification of two progressive antithrombins of human plasma. *Scand J Clin Lab Invest.* 1967;19:190–196.
2. Chan V, Chan TK, Wong Z. The determination of antithrombin III by radioimmunoassay and its clinical application. *Br J Haematol.* 1979;41:563–572.
3. Comp PC. Laboratory evaluation of protein S status. *Semin Thromb Hemost.* 1990;16:177–191.
4. Comp PC, Doray D, Patton D. An abnormal plasma distribution of protein S occurs in functional protein S deficiency. *Blood.* 1986;67:504–515.
5. Comp PC, Nixon R, Esmon CT. Determination of functional levels of protein C, an antithrombotic protein, using thrombin/thrombomodulin complex. *Blood.* 1984;63:15–28.
6. Esmon CT. Protein C: biochemistry, physiology, and clinical implications. *Blood.* 1983;62:1155–1167.
7. Griffin JH, Bezaud A, Evatt B. Functional and immunologic studies of protein C in thromboembolic disease. *Blood.* 1983;62:301a–310a.
8. Mannucci PM, Caciani MT, Mari D. The varied sensitivity of partial thromboplastin and prothrombin time reagent in the demonstration of lupus-like anticoagulants. *Scand J Haematol.* 1979;22:423–433.
9. Sammaritano LR, Gharavi AE, Lockshin MD. Antiphospholipid antibody syndrome: immunologic and clinical aspects. *Semin Arthritis Rheum.* 1990;20:81–97.

42

Critical Limb Ischemia

Leonella Pasqualini and Elmo Mannarino

Definition

Critical limb ischemia (CLI) is defined as a condition that endangers all or part of the limb if no radical improvement in blood flow can be achieved by means of surgery, interventional radiology, or medical treatment[163] (Figure 42.1).

Although acute critical ischemia is easily identified clinically, diagnosing chronic critical ischemia can be difficult. The term *chronic critical limb ischemia* was first introduced at the International Vascular Symposium in 1982 when the following instrumental and clinical criteria defining it were established[11]:

- Rest pain, with ankle systolic pressure (ASP) below 40 mm Hg
- Tissue necrosis (ulcer or gangrene) of the foot or toes with ASP below 60 mm Hg

Although this definition is recommended by the Ad Hoc Committee on Reporting Standards, the Society for Vascular Surgery, and the International Society for Cardiovascular Surgery,[138] its major limitation is the lack of specific reference to diabetic patients, who make up a large percentage of patients with CLI and who have a different clinical picture and fate.

In 1989, on the basis of two largely surgical studies,[3,11] the First Consensus Document on Critical Limb Ischaemia adopted criteria that are valid for both diabetic and nondiabetic patients[57]:

- Persistent rest pain that requires regular analgesia for more than 2 weeks and/or ulcerations or gangrene of the foot
- ASP below 50 mm Hg and/or the absence of palpable pulses; published in 1991, the Second Consensus Document suggested identifying CLI according to one of the following criteria[58]:

  1. Persistent rest pain requiring analgesia for more than 2 weeks with ASP equal to or below 50 mm Hg and/or toe systolic pressure (TSP) equal to or below 30 mm Hg
  2. Ulceration or gangrene of the foot or toes with the ASP equal to or below 50 mm Hg or the TSP equal to or below 30 mm Hg

Rest pain must conform to the classical description of this symptom.[42] An ASP value of 50 mm Hg was chosen as the cutoff because this level includes most patients with rest pain and trophic lesions who do not improve spontaneously without therapy.[182] TSP measurement is recommended particularly for diabetic patients because ankle pressure readings may be misleadingly high due to the calcified arteries that are often associated with diabetes or less commonly with other pathologies such as Mönckeberg's arteriosclerosis. The TSP reading of 30 mm Hg was accepted because most diabetic patients with this value have a very poor prognosis.[3,24,25] Fontaine's classification, which is based on easily determined clinical criteria and has been largely adopted in Europe, was subdivided into two subgroups in stage III:

- Stage IIIa: patients with rest pain and ASP above 50 mm Hg or TSP above 30 mm Hg
- Stage IIIb: patients with rest pain and ASP below 50 mm Hg or TSP below 30 mm Hg

A patient can be diagnosed as affected by CLI if classified at Fontaine's stage IIIb or IV. Stage IIIa is excluded because the limb is not in any immediate danger.

In the United States and Great Britain the term *critical limb ischemia* is gradually being substituted for the corresponding stages of Fontaine's classification for two fundamental reasons: to judge prognosis more precisely and to compare the results of therapy obtained in different centers using different types of treatment.

In recent years the term *subcritical limb ischemia* has also been introduced to identify patients with established ischemic rest pain, ulcers, or gangrene, with proven arterial disease, who have systolic pressure above the limits

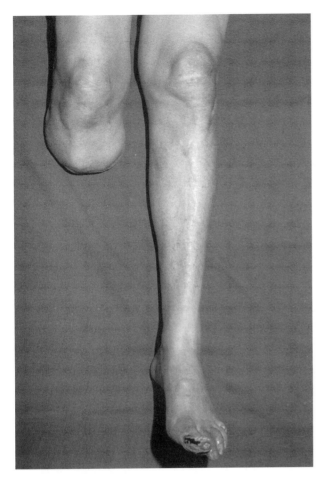

FIGURE 42.1. Critical ischemia of the left foot in a diabetic 75-year-old woman, with previous below-knee amputation of the right leg because of gangrene.

currently set for CLI. These patients are at less risk of losing limbs than patients with CLI.

Epidemiology

Incidence and Prevalence

There is little direct information on the incidence or prevalence of CLI using the preceding definition. Inferences can be drawn to CLI from the incidence and prevalence of asymptomatic peripheral arterial occlusive disease (PAOD) and intermittent claudication and their patterns of deterioration. Additional data derived from amputation rates can be used to estimate the incidence of CLI.

The accepted prevalence of PAOD in the general population is approximately 1% to 1.5%. A review of data showed that about 1.5% of woman under age 50 and 5% of men over age 50 are affected by symptomatic PAOD,[49] with a 0.3% to 7.7% range in prevalence.[63] The Framing-

ham Study assessed the incidence of symptomatic PAOD as 0.5% in men between 55 and 65 years of age,[92] and the Basel Study estimated it as 0.6% in younger subjects ranging in age from 33 to 44 and as 7.5% in subjects between 60 and 64 years of age.[177]

Differences in estimates of incidence and prevalence are mainly due to features such as age, sex, job, and the like (which varied in the populations under study), to diverse methods of investigation, and to different diagnostic criteria. A British study of patients over the age of 60 that used only the absence of palpable toe pulse as a diagnostic criterion showed a prevalence of 22.7% in men and 9.8% in women.[105] A similarly high prevalence (31.6% in men, 19.5% in women) also emerged in a US study that used the same diagnostic criterion.[140] Noninvasive instrumental methods make diagnosis of PAOD more reliable. A Danish study on a population of 666 subjects over age 60 showed a prevalence of 16% in men and 15% in women when an ankle/arm pressure index below 0.9 was used as the criterion for diagnosis.[149] In the Edinburgh Artery Study 4.5% of the population aged 54 to 75 were, on the basis of the World Health Organization Rose Questionnaire,[134] affected by intermittent claudication. Noninvasive techniques, such as a reduced ankle/brachial pressure index and reactive hyperemia test, provided evidence of PAOD in a further 8% of the population.[64] These studies show that the true prevalence of PAOD in the general population is often underestimated. According to Criqui and coworkers the prevalence of PAOD is at least five times greater than the estimated figure and reaches 27.7% when instrumental techniques capable of revealing large- and small-vessel disease are employed.[36]

A progressive worsening of the clinical picture with the onset of rest pain and gangrene occurs in 15% to 25% of patients with intermittent claudication;[48,77,87] a 3% to 10% amputation rate was found within 15 years of the diagnosis.[161,167] Considerable discrepancies can be noted in the results of different studies. Two large epidemiological studies on the general population calculated progression at 2.5% and showed that 1.5% of patients with intermittent claudication require amputation.[127,176] Recently PAOD was estimated to progress in 41% of 195 patients with intermittent claudication 8 years after diagnosis.[135] Therefore, assuming that in about 20% of patients with intermittent claudication the disease progresses to CLI, approximately 1% of men over age 50 are affected by CLI.

The prevalence of CLI can also be assessed from the number of amputations, assuming that most limbs are amputated because of ischemia and that about 25% of patients with CLI require amputations. In the United States the incidence of amputations in nondiabetic patients is 200 per million of habitants but rises to 3900 per million in patients with diabetes.[118] In the United King-

TABLE 42.1. Incidence of major amputation.

Estimated incidence (per yr)	Sources
150/million	Referrals to limb fitting centers in the UK[42]
280/million	Danish hospital survey—nondiabetic patients[39]
3000/million	Danish hospital survey—diabetic patients[39]
200/million	Nondiabetic US patients[117]
3900/million	Diabetic US patients[117]
112–172/million	North Italian hospital survey[26]

dom the incidence of amputations, extrapolated from the patients attending limb fitting centers, is 150 per million per year.[42,43] The Danish Hospital Survey calculated an annual incidence of 280 amputations per million in nondiabetic patients and 3000 per million in diabetics.[39] From these figures the annual incidence of CLI in the United States and Europe can be estimated as ranging between 500 and 1000 per million.[58] In Northern Italy a recent epidemiological study assessed the incidence of CLI as 459 to 652 per million and amputations as 112 to 172 per million, which are much lower figures than seen elsewhere[26] (Table 42.1).

Prognosis

Although the prognosis for patients with ischemic rest pain and gangrene depends to some extent on the specialized units they attend and the type of therapy, within 1 year of diagnosis of CLI more than 90% of patients undergo percutaneous transluminal angioplasty (PTA), revascularization surgery, or major amputation.[180] The UK Joint Vascular Group reported that 61% of 409 patients with CLI underwent surgical revascularization procedures or PTA, 17% underwent primary amputation, and 22% underwent sympathectomy or conservative therapy.[180] One year after diagnosis 26% had undergone major amputations, 8% had died, and only 56% were still alive and had both legs.[180] A Zurich investigation on 124 patients with CLI who had undergone PTA and, if unsuccessful, revascularization procedures showed that within 6 months of hospitalization 20% of patients had undergone amputation and 18% had died.[146]

Results of a study carried out between 1979 and 1989 in Maryland showed that the amputation rate remained constant at around 30 per 100,000, despite the dramatic increase in PTA and the twofold increase in bypass surgery.[166] Similar figures were reported in the Danish county of Aalborg from 1961 to 1971.[28] A larger elderly population may partially explain these reports, even if the age-standardized rate of amputations also increased fourfold. The use of insulin therapy and consequently the increased survival rate of diabetic patients is another factor, but when diabetic patients are excluded, a threefold increase in the age-standardized incidence of amputations still remains. The high incidence of amputations might also be a trend toward a conservative approach to

CLI that has determined an increase in PTA and revascularization procedures and consequently a drop in the number of primary amputations but not in the overall amputation rate.[128] Progress in the development of noninvasive techniques means that today PAOD is diagnosed at an earlier stage at which revascularization procedures can be carried out before more radical surgery. In the United States the total number of procedures for PAOD rose from 1 to 2 per patient in 1974 to 18 per patient in 1989.[170]

The high cardiovascular mortality rate, which is directly linked to concomitant coronary and cerebrovascular disease, also contributes to the extremely poor prognosis of patients with CLI.[49,159] The prevalence of ischemic heart disease in patients with PAOD is two to four times higher than in subjects without PAOD.[64] In the Edinburgh Artery Study 54% of patients with asymptomatic PAOD and 71% of those with symptoms also suffered from associated ischemic heart disease.[64,137] Angiography has visualized severe ischemic heart disease in 27% to 29% of patients with intermittent claudication or CLI.[77] Ischemic heart disease is responsible for 40% to 57% of deaths in patients with PAOD and for 63% of deaths in patients with intermittent claudication. A further 7% to 17% of deaths can be attributed to stroke.[49] Patients with CLI are also at greater risk of arterial thromboembolism and, when bedridden, of venous thromboembolism.

The prognosis for patients with CLI also depends on the mortality rate associated with revascularization surgery and amputations. The early postoperative mortality rate after reconstructive surgery is 4.5%, which rises to 18% within 1 year.[180] The mortality rate immediately after below-knee amputation is approximately 5% to 10% and increases to 15% to 20% for above-knee amputation. Particularly alarming is the long-term mortality rate in these patients, which ranges from 25% to 30% 2 years after surgery to 50% to 75% after 5 years.[50]

Pathophysiology

Although atherosclerosis is the primary cause of CLI, microcirculatory abnormalities that follow large-vessel occlusion, hemorheological alterations, and hemostatic alterations play an important role. The onset of rest pain and trophic lesions, which are typical of CLI, are hypothesized to be due to cutaneous nutritive microcirculation deterioration.

Hemodynamic Alterations

Macrocirculation

CLI is caused by stenosis or obstruction of one or more of the main arteries, which increases proximal limb vascular resistance and reduces flow and distal perfusion pressure to a level insufficient to satisfy the nutritive needs of the limb at rest. The onset of CLI often results from multiple arterial occlusions and lesions in critical collateral branches or in terminal arteries and implies that the mechanism compensates for chronic ischemia (i.e., the development of collateral circulation and arteriolar vasodilation have failed).[33,159]

Atherosclerosis, or, more rarely, inflammatory arteritis (e.g., thromboangiitis obliterans), an embolism, or distal diabetic angiopathy are the causes of arterial damage in CLI (Figure 42.2). An acute complication of atherosclerosis, such as plaque rupture or thrombosis, is often responsible of the onset of CLI. The success of thrombolysis and evidence of fresh thrombi, which are often found during revascularization surgery, seem to confirm this hypothesis. High levels of plasma cross-linked fibrin degradation products in patients with CLI are further evidence that thrombosis may be the precipitating factor in the genesis of critical ischemia.[102]

Arterial vasospasm can also increase vascular resistance in the proximal arteries. Angiography has visualized vasospasm in the coronary arteries and in cerebrovascular arteries during subarachnoid hemorrhage. In peripheral arteries of the leg vasospasm has been observed during diagnostic and therapeutic catheterization. Apart from these examples of mechanical or chemical insult, there is little direct evidence that vasospasm alone precipitates critical ischemia.

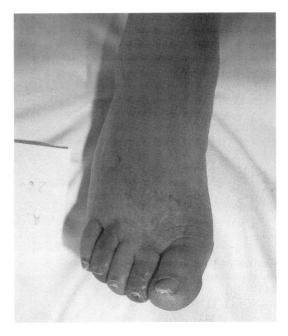

FIGURE 42.2. Critical ischemia of the right foot caused by thromboangiitis obliterans in a 38-year-old woman who smokes.

As the source of embolisms that occlude limb circulation, the heart may be involved in the genesis of hemodynamic alterations in CLI. More frequently, a decrease in cardiac output due to arrhythmias or abnormal myocardial contractility reduces peripheral perfusion pressure to a critical level.[101] Antihypertensive therapy may induce a similar effect. Increased venous hydrostatic pressure and edema in the lower limbs, both associated with heart failure, contribute to reduce nutritive capillary flow.[91,101]

The reduced perfusion pressure typical of critical ischemia and a consequence of insufficient arterial blood flow may, in some cases, be caused by venous obstruction. Deep vein thrombosis may obstruct venous return, determine the onset of edema, and even reduce capillary perfusion, which ultimately lead to cutaneous trophic damage (venous gangrene or phlegmasia cerulea dolens). Urgent thrombolysis or thrombectomy is essential for treating this type of critical ischemia. Widespread thrombosis of cutaneous venules may cause CLI in the course of purpura fulminans, coumarin-induced skin necrosis, and protein C deficiency (see Chapter 41, "Blood Coagulation").[101]

Microcirculation

Although segmental systolic blood pressure readings are essential for defining the level and severity of PAOD[73] and for identifying CLI, values of ankle and toe systolic pressure widely overlap in patients with and without CLI.[59,80,182] Some patients with zero toe blood pressure do not develop critical ischemia, whereas others with relatively high blood pressure levels do develop critical ischemia.[117] These observations suggest that microcirculatory blood flow may be important in the pathogenesis of CLI, and the development of new diagnostic techniques has focused attention on microcirculatory abnormalities.

The microcirculation includes arterioles, capillaries, and venules and functionally may be divided into thermoregulatory and nutritional vessels. Deterioration of skin nutritive blood flow is probably the principal cause of the onset of trophic lesions because, although the microcirculation can compensate for extreme hypoperfusion, critical ischemia is rapidly triggered once nutritive blood flow is compromised. One of the main compensatory mechanisms aimed at maintaining adequate nutritive flow, despite occlusion of the proximal arteries, is arteriolar vasodilation, which is induced by local hypotension and ischemic tissue release of vasoactive metabolites.[14,15]

In critical ischemia arterioles are maximally dilated and unresponsive to normal vasoconstrictive and vasodilative stimuli (vasomotor paralysis).[111,116] Paradoxically, probably because of vasodilation in tissue around the ischemic area, some patients with CLI present an increased total blood flow in the ischemic foot.[116] Approximately 90% of distal blood flow in the limbs is thermoregulatory flow that passes through the arteriovenous anastomoses and bypasses the nutritive vessels. Therefore, despite an increase in total blood flow, impaired perfusion of the nutritive vessels may result from a maldistribution of microvascular blood.

In patients with CLI a marked dysfunction in microcirculatory vasomotility has been reported. In healthy tissue the nutritive capillaries are rhythmically perfused by means of regular precapillary arteriole contraction and release; laser Doppler fluxmetry shows low-frequency waves (3–12 per minute). Under conditions of critical ischemia, low-frequency waves are reduced and high-frequency waves (21 ± 4 per minute) appear.[30,31] Furthermore, in distal areas of ischemic limbs capillaroscopy has visualized several morphological abnormalities of nutritive capillaries such as a reduction in capillary density, poorly defined capillaries, hemorrhage, and interstitial edema.[59,113]

Studies that used both fluorescent capillaroscopy and transcutaneous oxygen pressure measurements (TcPO$_2$) have shown that CLI may be associated with an anatomically normal capillary density but with a functionally reduced capillary density (i.e., patent capillaries with impaired perfusion). In abnormally perfused capillaries fluorescence appears significantly later and is associated with increased transcapillary diffusion and a significant reduction in TcPO$_2$ values (0–8 mm Hg) in the corresponding cutaneous areas.[65]

Of the many explanations for these morphological and functional abnormalities that have been proposed, endothelial disturbance is one possible initiating factor for microvascular damage. In normal conditions the endothelium plays a key role in maintaining vascular patency by removing active mediators of thombosis (e.g., adenosine diphosphate, adenosine triphosphate, and thrombin) from the circulation and by releasing prostacyclin and endothelial-derived relaxant factor, which prevent vasoconstriction and platelet aggregation.[101] Under ischemic conditions, the imbalance in release of endothelial-derived relaxant factor and endothelial-derived constricting factor causes vasospasm and platelet aggregation, and increased von Willebrand's factor levels promote platelet–endothelial adhesion. Hypoxic endothelial damage is also associated with increased capillary permeability, edema, and collapse of patent capillaries.[101] Increased erythrocyte aggregation and stiffness, increased platelet aggregation, and increased leukocyte stiffness and adhesivity have also been observed in patients with CLI and may lead to microthrombosis.[30,104,120,131] All of these abnormalities may result in a vicious circle of interactions between vessel wall and blood cells, which leads to severe malfunctioning and/or occlusion of the microvascular bed (Figure 42.3).

Hematological and Biochemical Factors

Several hematological and biochemical factors are abnormal in patients with critical or noncritical limb ischemia.[48] Blood viscosity, which is determined by hematocrit, plasma viscosity, and blood cell deformability, is a major factor that determines blood flow, particularly in the microcirculation (see Chapter 38, "Hyperviscosity Syndromes"). In PAOD, blood viscosity is increased because of high hematocrit and fibrinogen levels, which in most patients may be due to cigarette smoking. In CLI, because of tissue necrosis and occasionally infection, fibrinogen levels, plasma viscosity, and erythrocyte aggregation are even higher.[101] These patients also experience a pronounced fall in perfusion pressure, overall blood flow rate, and shear stress. Therefore the passage of erythrocytes and leukocytes through the nutritive capillaries is more difficult. Acidosis, hyperosmolarity, and calcium accumulation in the ischemic area may reduce erythrocyte and leukocyte deformability even further and consequently increase whole blood viscosity.[101] Blood filterability is impaired in patients with PAOD, and the reduction is greater in patients with CLI than in those with intermittent claudication.[131] The contribu-

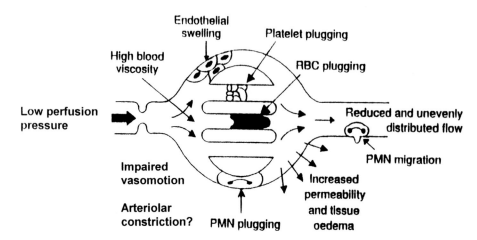

FIGURE 42.3. Hypothesized mechanisms of microvascular injury in critical limb ischemia. RBC, red blood cell; PMN, polimorphonuclear.

tion of hemorheological factors to CLI is confirmed by the adverse prognostic significance of blood viscosity and fibrinogen levels in intermittent claudication and CLI,[48] the adverse prognostic significance of hemoglobin levels in healing of amputation,[4] and the beneficial effect of hemodilution in some patients with CLI.[132]

Critical and noncritical limb ischemia are associated with a significantly increased leukocyte count[3,120] and impaired leukocyte filterability and activation. That similar findings have been shown in patients with acute cerebral infarction or chest infarction suggests white blood cell activation may be a nonspecific response to tissue injury.[29] Activated leukocytes occlude the capillary because of their greater stiffness and adhesivity, and by releasing platelet activating factor, leukotrienes, superoxide anions, and proteolytic enzymes they also injure the endothelium. Furthermore, they exert a chemotactic action on other leukocytes and facilitate vasospasm. As yet, no prospective studies on leukocytes or their activation products in PAOD have been undertaken, although the white blood cell count was found to be adversely predictive of reocclusion of distal bypass.[101]

Several alterations in platelet behavior have been described in patients with PAOD, but their prognostic significance and relation to CLI is unknown. In vivo and in vitro studies on blood samples of patients with PAOD indicated increased levels of platelet products such as β-thromboglobulin, serotonin, and thromboxane A_2; shortened platelet survival time; decreased platelet count; and increased platelet adhesiveness and aggregability.[62,103,104,183] These abnormalities may reflect either activation at atherosclerotic plaques or local activation in the microcirculation and may be due to high shear stresses at arterial stenosis, increased hematocrit levels, or increased plasma fibrinogen levels. By releasing platelet-derived growth factor, activated platelets facilitate the progression of the atherosclerotic lesions and worsen tissue ischemia by forming microaggregates, releasing vasoconstrictive substances (serotonin, thromboxane A_2), inhibiting fibrinolysis, activating leukocytes, and so forth.[35,155] Evidence confirming these observations can be drawn from thrombocythemia, in which the number of circulating platelets is increased and associated with increased platelet aggregation in vitro. In these patients microcirculatory ischemia and tissue necrosis may develop even in the absence of occlusive disease in large vessels.[103] Angiographic studies provide evidence that acetylsalicylic acid and dipyridamole, which induce platelet inhibition, delay the progression of peripheral atherosclerosis.[78]

Patients with PAOD often present many biochemical abnormalities. Imbalances in lipid and glycemic metabolism as risk factors for atherosclerosis have been discussed elsewhere (see Chapter 36, "Atherosclerosis"); in this chapter we examine some pathogenic mechanisms in diabetic patients with CLI.

Diabetes greatly modifies fibrinolytic activity, plasminogen and tissue plasminogen activator inhibitor concentrations, prostacyclin synthesis and fibrinogen levels,[32] red blood cell and platelet aggregation, and endothelial and white blood cell functions.[32] These abnormalities facilitate not only atherosclerotic macroangiopathy but also the development of microcirculatory abnormalities typical of CLI.

Hyperglycemia in itself determines the onset of diabetic microangiopathy and neuropathy. The real importance of small-vessel disease in determining microvascular disease in diabetic patients is still open to discussion. Some evidence shows a thickening of the capillary wall but without luminal reduction.[100] Functional abnormalities of the capillary that result from autonomic neuropathy more than anatomical obstruction seem to contribute to diabetic ulcer formation.

Peripheral neuropathy has a high prevalence in diabetic patients[75] and involves sensory, motor, and autonomic nerve fibers. As a consequence of sensory impairment diabetic patients may not be able to notice small thermal trauma, pressure from shoes, and other trauma. More important local consequences of autonomic abnormalities may result in vasomotor instability with increased arteriovenous shunting that may lead to capillary ischemia.[53]

Assessment

The primary cause of CLI is stenosis or occlusion of the main leg arteries, but the final cause for the symptoms is a marked reduction or abolition of the local nutritional circulation. Patients with CLI are often affected by widespread atherosclerosis, and their prognosis is poor within the first 2 years of diagnosis because of associated cardiovascular disease. Therefore a complete clinical, instrumental, and laboratory evaluation of the entire vascular system is necessary.

Clinical History and Examination

A detailed case history should include information on the onset, duration, and evolution not only of symptoms linked to PAOD (e.g., intermittent claudication and rest pain) but also of those linked to coronary or cerebral atherosclerosis. Any family history of cardiovascular disease or deaths and all risk factors (e.g., smoking, diabetes, hypertension, and hyperlipemia) should be recorded along with all current drug therapy or previous amputation or vascular surgery.

The clinical examination should start with notation of changes in skin color (pallor, cyanosis, or redness), temperature (hotter or colder than normal), and trophism (loss of hair, ulcers, or gangrene). Most errors in interpretation are made in the diagnostic and prognostic evaluation of tissue defects in the extremities. A distinction must be made between cutaneous trophic damage associated with PAOD and that caused by PAOD. Patients with arterial occlusive disease and claudication may have tissue defects as a result of trauma (e.g., excessively tight footwear, corn removal, nail extraction, or other minor injuries) that is not indicative of CLI but rather of complicated stage II PAOD.

An elevation test should be performed by raising the leg to a 45-degree angle from the horizontal plane and asking the patient to perform dorsal and plantar flexions of the foot for 1 minute. The test is indicative of ischemia if the foot becomes pale, because discoloration shows that distal perfusion pressure is too low to counteract the effects of increased gravitational pressure on blood flow. In the ischemic limb, the sitting position with the limb dependent is associated with a passive distension of the vascular bed, intensive reddening, and an increased temperature.

Femoral, popliteal, posterior tibial, and pedal pulses should be taken and the abdomen palpated and auscultated to detect abdominal aorta aneurysm and stenosis of the renal arteries. Radial, ulnar, omeral, subclavian, and carotid pulses should also be taken. In diabetic patients the clinical examination should include a complete neurological checkup with particular attention to sensitivity to heat, pain, and vibrations and to osteotendon reflexes.

Laboratory Investigation

Macrocirculation

Several noninvasive techniques, including segmentary systolic blood pressure readings by means of Doppler velocimetry, are currently available for studying the micro-

circulation. Ankle systolic blood pressure equal to or below 50 mm Hg and associated with rest pain and/or gangrene supports a diagnosis of CLI.[58] Besides being essential for a diagnosis of CLI, pressure readings are also a reliable prognostic index because an ASP below 50 mm Hg appears to be a reliable indicator of poor wound healing,[133] and an ankle/brachial pressure index below 0.30 is associated with an increased mortality rate.[37,84]

In about 10% of diabetic patients, however, calcification of the arterial wall may give falsely high pressure readings. Segmental pressure readings and a pressure gradient above 20 mm Hg in two contiguous levels in the limb provides information on the site of the lesion and distinguishes between iliac, femoral, and popliteal distal lesions. Analysis of Doppler velocimetry waveform and duplex scanning provide more details.

Duplex scanning combines information obtained from spectral analysis of the Doppler signal with ultrasound imaging and provides excellent visualization of the abdominal aorta and the iliac, femoral, and popliteal arteries. Its resolution is poor for distal vessels. At the proximal level duplex devices offer increased sensitivity, specificity, and versatility in detecting, localizing, and characterizing the extent of vascular lesions.

Details such as the presence of stenosis or occlusion, the length of the lesion, and the presence of calcium, hemorrhage, or ulceration of the plaque may determine the feasibility of interventional versus surgical therapy even before angiography[6] (Figure 42.4). Ultrasound scanning of the abdominal aorta is also mandatory because approximately 10% of patients with PAOD also present with abdominal aortic aneurysm.[22]

Plethysmography, whether air, water, impedance, or strain gauge, measures segmental systolic–diastolic variations in the volume of the limb. This technique quantifies total segmental blood flow and, by means of hyperemic tests, assesses the compensatory activity of collateral

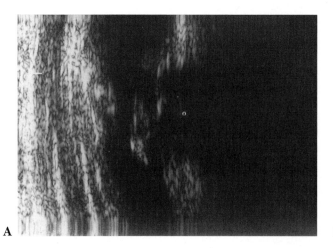

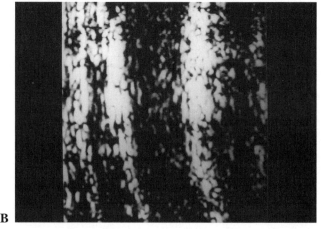

A   **B**

FIGURE 42.4. B-mode echotomography shows a short, calcified stenosis of the superficial femoral artery (A) and recent occlusion of the popliteal artery (B) in a 60-year-old male smoker with recent onset of ischemic rest pain.

circulation.[158] Photoplethysmography is essential for studying toe blood flow in patients with CLI. For diabetic patients in whom systolic ankle pressure readings may be unreliable, systolic toe pressure <30 mm Hg and the absence of arterial toe pulse after vasodilation are considered diagnostic criteria.[58]

Angiography is mandatory in all patients with CLI to establish whether revascularization procedures through surgery or interventional radiology are feasible. CLI usually results from multiple arterial stenoses and occlusions, and angiography helps to localize and quantify these lesions. A map of the entire peripheral arterial bed is essential for assessing distal runoff and formulating a prognosis after revascularization.[60]

Arterial digital subtraction angiography is an extremely precise technique for defining distal runoff, particularly in patients with extensive proximal occlusion and reduced cardiac output. Because it maps arterial circulation in the foot and the distal part of the limb, it not only provides decisive information for selecting the most suitable revascularization procedure but also identifies the best site for the anastomosis[136] (Figure 42.5).

Intraoperative angiography can be used to obtain more details of the vascular bed and its potential capacity to receive and distribute adequate blood flow to an ischemic foot. This method is useful when deciding between limb salvage and primary amputation and may help the surgeon determine which vessel to use for reconstruction and to test graft patency.[74,154]

Peripheral magnetic resonance angiography (MRA) has been successfully employed to assess deep vein thrombosis of the leg, peripheral arterial occlusive disease, arteriovenous malformations, and vascular abnormalities in the hands and feet.[99] In patients with CLI, MRA provides the surgeon with excellent anatomical images on the location and length of occlusion and the degree of collateralization, which are essential for planning surgical or angioplastic procedures.

Studies comparing MRA and other conventional imaging methods have been performed. The detection of sig-

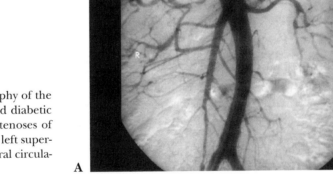

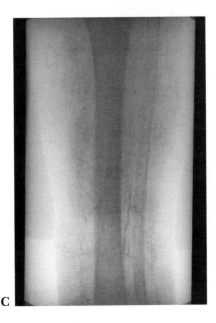

FIGURE 42.5. Arterial digital subtraction angiography of the abdominal aorta and its branches in a 72-year-old diabetic women with foot gangrene. Note the multiple stenoses of the renal arteries, obstruction at the origin of the left superficial femoral artery, and poor below-knee collateral circulation.

A

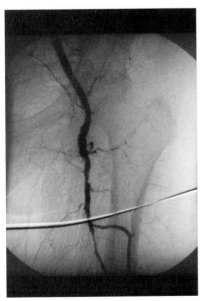

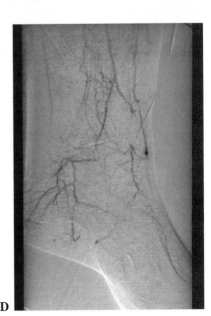

B

C

D

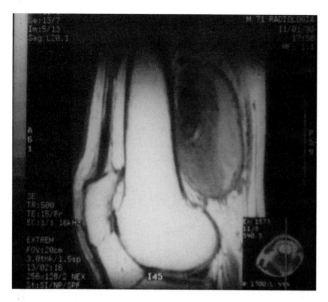

FIGURE 42.6. Magnetic resonance image of a large aneurysm in the right popliteal artery in an 80-year-old man with progressive ischemic rest pain of the omolateral foot.

nificant (>50%) stenosis by MRA and ultrasound agreed with angiography 71% and 93% of the time, respectively.[119] The image quality of MRA is superior to ultrasound, and in the popliteal and tibial vessels in particular MRA is more effective in assessing stenosis[51] (Figure 42.6). Although arteriography remains a popular vascular imaging method, MRA is preferable in patients in whom contrast administration is contraindicated.

Angioscopy also provides the vascular surgeon with important data. Direct images of the lesion that show the real dimension of stenosis and whether calcification and/or overlying thrombi are present make the choice of recanalization procedures more precise. Even though angioscopy provides more detailed information than angiography when studying an anastomosis or endoarterectomy, it is not necessary for routine vascular bypasses and remains very much a research technique.[125,142]

Microcirculation

Assessing local microcirculation of the ischemic limb by means of vital capillaroscopy, $TcPO_2$ measurement, and laser Doppler flowmetry is recommended for a more precise description and follow-up of patients with CLI and is also useful for designing and reporting on clinical trials. Vital capillaroscopy directly and noninvasively evaluates blood filling and morphology of the nutritional skin capillaries. A three-stage classification of capillaroscopic patterns in the ischemic foot is usually adopted[59,61,113] (Figure 42.7):

Stage A: clearly defined blood-filled papillary capillaries
Stage B: interstitial edema, poorly defined capillaries, and capillary hemorrhage
Stage C: no or few perfused capillaries

If normal capillary structure and blood filling are seen the patient's risk of developing skin necrosis in the next 3 months is less than 10% independent of the macrocirculatory status. The presence of only a few or no blood-filled capillaries has an 87% sensitivity and a 95% specificity for the development of cutaneous necrosis, and the predictive value of TSP is increased.[61]

Fluorescein angiography, videomicroscopy, and videodensitometry can be used to follow the appearance intravenously of injected sodium fluorescein in capillary areas, its transcapillary diffusion, and its interstitial distribution. Abnormalities observed in ischemic areas of skin include delayed inflow (fluorescein appearance time longer than 55 seconds) and increased capillary permeability.

$TcPO_2$ measurement reflects hyperemic skin blood supply in the ischemic limb and is clinically relevant in patients with more severe PAOD. CLI may be assumed if the supine and dependent foot $TcPO_2$ values are less than 10 mm Hg and 45 mm Hg, respectively, and do not increase with inhalation of oxygen.[108,133]

The $TcPO_2$ value may also predict ischemic ulcer healing and help determine amputation level.[66,93] Oxymetric values above 40 mm Hg are normally associated with

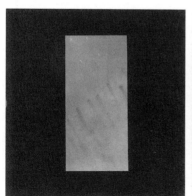
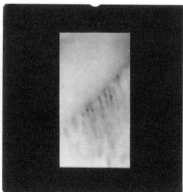
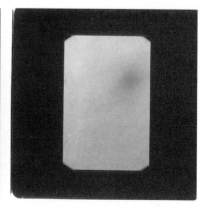

FIGURE 42.7. Nailbed capillaroscopic patterns in ischemic limbs.

early stump healing.[21] TcPO$_2$ levels can also be used to monitor the efficacy of revascularization procedures and/or pharmacological therapy[109,126] (Figure 42.8). The disadvantage of TcPO$_2$ measurement is the great variability that has been observed in repeated tests on the same patient.[124]

Laser Doppler flowmetry measures skin perfusion at a depth penetration of approximately 1 mm, and both nutritive and thermoregulatory flow are assessed. In patients with CLI this technique has revealed several alterations in vasomotion including a reduction in low-frequency motion waves (3–12 per minute), the appearance of high-frequency motion waves (21 ± 4 per minute), and disturbed postural vasoconstriction.[81,152,174] These ischemic-related vasomotion patterns are indicative of microvascular flow maldistribution (see earlier section titled "Pathophysiology") and disappear after successful revascularization.[82,167]

Cardiovascular System

The elevated cardiovascular mortality rate and the high incidence of atherosclerotic disease of coronary and carotid arteries associated with CLI indicate that these vascular areas should also be investigated. Instrumental assessment of coronary circulation should include an electrocardiogram at rest to exclude severe coronary ischemia and arrhythmia, a chest x-ray, and when possible an electrocardiogram exercise test. These results not only assess the risk for surgery but also show whether intervention in the coronary circulation is required before peripheral revascularization procedures. Radionuclide scintigraphy and/or Doppler echocardiography provide further data on the patient's suitability for surgery. A heart ejection fraction below 30% may be contraindicative for aorta reconstruction but not necessarily for femoropopliteal or distal bypass, which can be per-

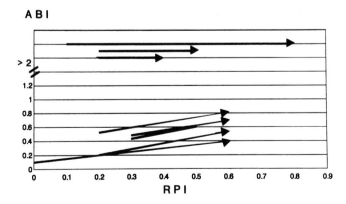

FIGURE 42.8. Improvements in ankle/brachial pressure index (ABI) and regional perfusion index (RPI) (i.e., foot TcPO$_2$/chest TcPO$_2$) after successful percutaneous transluminal angioplasty in eight limbs with rest pain. PAOD, peripheral arterial occlusive disease. Data from Mannarino et al.[109]

formed under regional or local anesthesia.[136] Duplex scanning and, when required, carotid angiography should be performed on all patients with CLI, even if they are asymptomatic for cerebrovascular disease.

Blood Tests

Besides routine blood tests, parameters that should be tested in patients with CLI include lipid levels, particularly triglycerides (high levels of which are one of the major risk factors for PAOD); total cholesterol, and high-density lipoprotein cholesterol (see Chapter 40, "Lipid Pattern"). A 24-hour glycemic profile, glycosylated hemoglobin A$_1$, glycosuria, and ketonuria are also needed in diabetic patients. CLI patients' blood tests should also routinely include a complete profile of hematocrit; hemoglobin; red blood cell, white blood cell, and platelet counts; the erythrocyte sedimentation rate, plasma viscosity; and fibrinogen levels (see "Laboratory Assessment: Hemorheology"). Some coagulation tests, such as the partial thromboplastin time and the prothrombin time, should also be performed, and certain patients may require measurement of protein C and protein S levels or antiphospholipid antibodies (see "Laboratory Assessment: Coagulation").

Treatment

General Management

Concomitant Disease

Cardiovascular Disease

Cardiac insufficiency or severe arrhythmias should be promptly treated in patients with CLI because reduced cardiac output and edema impair perfusion in the ischemic limb. These diseases may also render the subjects unable to undergo surgery, general anesthesia, or even arteriography. The coexisting coronary insufficiency and symptomatic carotid stenosis should be investigated to assess the need for coronary bypass or carotid endoarterectomy before peripheral arterial surgery. Several drugs, such as β-blockers, that are useful in coronary heart disease may be contraindicated in CLI and vice versa (e.g., isovolemic hemodilution may have an unfavorable effect in patients with severe ischemic heart disease).

Hypertension

Hypertension must be carefully managed because although high blood pressure levels increase the incidence of stroke, their reduction may trigger or worsen CLI. The Second Consensus Document on Critical Limb Ischaemia recommends that antihypertensive drugs be prescribed in the acute early stage of CLI only when orthostatic systolic pressure is above 180 mm Hg and the diastolic pressure is more than 100 mm Hg. When the blood pressure levels are below these values, the antihypertensive drugs might be suspended because a rise of 10 to 20 mm Hg in systolic pressure increases poststenosis perfusion pressure and may improve symptoms of ischemia. After the early critical period of leg ischemia, antihypertensive therapy should aim at maintaining a blood pressure of no higher than 165/95 mm Hg. β-Blockers should be avoided and preference given to vasodilating agents such as calcium antagonists, angiotensin-converting enzyme inhibitors, α-blockers, and so forth.

Hyperlipidemias

Hypertriglyceridemia, associated with an increase in very-low-density lipoprotein cholesterol and a decrease in high-density lipoprotein cholesterol, is frequently encountered in patients with PAOD.[151] Controlling lipid metabolism is beneficial for symptomatic peripheral atherosclerosis[52] and also improves peripheral bypass patency and limb salvage after angioplasty.[114] High lipoprotein(a) levels have recently been reported to correlate with early graft occlusion.[179]

Diabetes

Although no prospective studies have confirmed that good glycemic control increases the chances of limb salvage, the general consensus holds that all diabetic patients with CLI should be treated with insulin. Fasting glucose levels should range from 80 to 120 mg/dL; postprandial values should be below 200 mg/dL, with no glycosuria and a normal glycosylated hemoglobin A_1. Insulin therapy controls glycemia and improves lipid metabolism by reducing very-low-density and low-density lipoprotein cholesterol plasma concentrations and increasing high-density lipoprotein cholesterol concentrations.[97,98]

Ischemic Limb

Walking should be restricted in patients with rest pain and/or foot ulcers because it causes trauma in ischemic tissue. Because ulcerating necrotic lesions are prevalently localized on the first, second, and fifth toes where footwear often compresses, patients should wear soft, loose shoes, preferably with foam rubber insoles so that pressure is evenly distributed while walking.[60]

To increase cutaneous perfusion in the distal areas, the ischemic limb should be kept dependent. Patients should be advised to contract calf muscles periodically to facilitate venous return and to prevent edema, which must be counteracted, if necessary, even by administering diuretics.

Bacterial infections are one of the greatest dangers for ischemic limbs because they increase the size of lesions and can hinder healing. Ischemic areas surrounding lesions should be kept dry. Damp bandages, which damage the skin and help microorganisms proliferate, should be avoided. Mechanical cleaning of the ulcerated area and removal of dead necrotic material is also essential. Because infections spread rapidly in ischemic tissue, systemic antibiotic therapy should be initiated at the first sign of infection; however, indiscriminate routine administration of systemic antibiotics should be avoided to prevent bacterial resistance. When ulcers are profound and fistulas are present, swabs should be taken of the infected areas to establish specific antibiotic therapy. Local administration of antibiotics is of little use because the infected tissue cannot be reached by this route. Even intravenous or intra-arterial antibiotic therapy may be problematic if arterial circulation of the infected limb is poor. Retrograde venous administration has been used experimentally in patients with diabetic gangrene[147] because infection in these patients occurs more frequently and local and systemic complications are more severe. Infection may be complicated by abscesses or osteomyelitis and may trigger toxemia, ketoacidosis, or hyperosmolar nonketotic coma.

Percutaneous Reopening Procedures

PTA

PTA alone or in association with local thrombolysis has become accepted therapy for PAOD. Because it is performed under local anesthesia, the overall risk is less than that of surgery,[8] and PTA may be the only revascularization procedure possible in patients for whom surgery is contraindicated. Although 65% to 85% of PTAs are performed on patients with intermittent claudication, its most important clinical application is limb salvage in patients with CLI. About 22% of limbs affected by CLI are suitable candidates for PTA, and a clinical improvement is seen in 11% of those thus treated[34] (Figure 42.9).

Indications

PTA is primarily indicated for monolateral or bilateral iliac stenosis, single or multiple stenoses in the femoral and popliteal arteries, and occlusions of 10 cm or less in the femoropopliteal tract.[185] PTA may also be performed on longer occlusions or more distal popliteal lesions when reconstructive surgery is not recommended or has little chance of success.[173] PTA may be associated with reconstructive surgery to dilate iliac stenoses before femoropopliteal bypass, to improve distal runoff, or to dilate stenoses at the anastomosis.

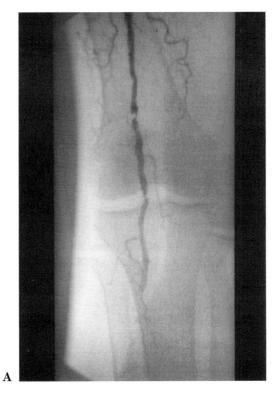 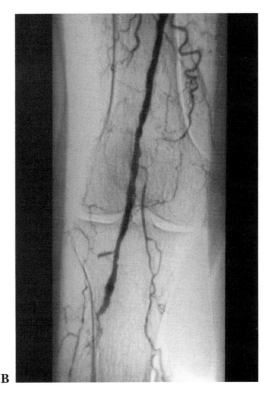

A   B

FIGURE 42.9. Arterial digital subtraction angiography before (A) and after (B) percutaneous transluminal angioplasty of the right popliteal artery. Even with nonoptimal recanalization rest pain disappeared and the toe ulcer gradually healed.

Contraindications

Serious coagulation disorders, thrombocytopenia, and thrombosed aneurysm are absolute contraindications to PTA. Relative contraindications, because of technical difficulties or high risk of complications, are obesity, long iliac occlusion, eccentric plaque, extensive vessel wall calcification, and extensive tibial disease with multiple occlusions.

Complications

The most frequent complications of PTA are hemorrhage, thromboembolism, and early thrombotic occlusion.[184] These complications are significantly more frequent in patients with CLI than in those with intermittent claudication, although the rates vary greatly. Zeitler reported that 1% to 2% of patients with intermittent claudication require surgery for complications following PTA compared with the 2% to 3% of patients with stages III to IV PAOD.[186] Complications are more frequent after femoropopliteal PTA (2.7%) and when PTA is used to treat long occlusions (6.7%).[184,185] Review data show that general complications range from 3% to 15%, complications that require surgery range from 1% to 5%, and the mortality rate may be as high as 7%.[96]

Results

Few long-term studies have been undertaken on the effects of PTA in patients with gangrene or rest pain, and no study has included patients with CLI as defined by the Second Consensus Document. Furthermore, criteria of success and/or patency after PTA vary greatly. Schmidtke et al. reported a PTA success rate of 71% in patients with rest pain and 40% in those with gangrene with subsequent stabilization at stage II. In a follow-up period ranging from 6 to 30 months 25.3% of segments remained patent.[145] Most authors report poorer results in CLI than in stage II PAOD. Limb salvage in patients with stage III and stage IV PAOD is reported as 48% after 1 year and 33% after 5 years, compared with 74% and 52%, respectively, in patients with intermittent claudication.[90]

The results of limb salvage by means of PTA overlap with those of reconstructive surgery in many types of lesions including stenoses in the femoropopliteal axis and short occlusions (<12 cm) in the femoral and popliteal arteries. Surgery provides better results in the case of long occlusions of the femoropopliteal tract and crural occlusion.[178,184,185]

Results of recent studies on PTA carried out in arteries such as the tibioperoneal trunks and anterior tibial, posterior tibial, and peroneal arteries seem encouraging, with an immediate postoperative success rate of 83% that drops to 82% after 1 year.[173]

Variables that determine the limb salvage ratio after PTA include lesion type (stenosis or occlusion), the number of affected segments that were treated, and the type of distal runoff. Diabetes, high fibrinogen concentrations, and low high-density lipoprotein cholesterol levels are predictive factors for poor limb salvage ratio after PTA.[115] Thromboembolic prophylaxis with antiplatelet agents should be administered for 1 to 3 days before PTA. Administration of acetylsalicylic acid (500–1000 mg/d) is widely recommended for at least 6 months after recanalization procedures, particularly if performed in the femoropopliteal tract. Lower dosages (100 mg/d) have not been shown to be efficacious. Anticoagulant therapy may be required in some patients, but it is in any case mandatory in the immediate postoperative period to prevent acute thrombotic complications.[96]

PTA and Thrombolytic Therapy

Local thrombolysis, whether alone or associated with PTA, is preferable to systemic thrombolysis in patients with CLI. Urokinase is more efficacious than streptokinase; the effects of new thrombolytic agents such as tissue-type plasminogen activator are still under study. Recommended dosages range from 30,000 UI to 50,000 UI for streptokinase and from 100,000 UI to 200,000 UI for urokinase; the higher dosages may be accompanied by systemic effects. It is not clear whether repeated single doses or continuous infusion of the fibrinolytic agent is more effective.

Indications

Thrombolysis is primarily indicated in cases of acute occlusion due to thrombosis or embolism. In PAOD, unlike coronary occlusion, thrombi can be lysed up to 12 months after their formation. When thrombolysis is performed before PTA, it may transform a long occlusion into a short stenosis that is susceptible to dilation. Thrombolysis is also indicated in graft occlusion.

Contraindications and Complications

Contraindications are the same as those for PTA but are extended to include stroke within the previous 2 months, gastrointestinal bleeding, and pregnancy. Compared with PTA the complications in terms of local bleeding and microembolisms have the highest incidence, ranging from 1%–1.5% to 5.3% and 7% to 10%, respectively.[96]

Results

Reports on the percentage of patency after thrombolysis vary greatly because of the extreme heterogeneity of patients and procedures. Review data show success rates of 70% for femoropopliteal occlusion and 50% to 55% for surgical graft occlusions. Results are generally better in patients with intermittent claudication than in those with advanced ischemia.[153] Five years after thrombolysis, Hess reported patency in 94% of patients at stage IIA, in 70% at stage IIB, in 62% at stage III, and in 50% at stage IV.[79]

PTA and Laser Recanalization

One recent advance in angioplasty techniques is laser-assisted angioplasty in which the laser beam vaporizes the plaque. Results are encouraging in long and short occlusions, particularly when calcified,[76,143,175] but randomized studies are necessary to establish the efficacy and safety of laser-assisted PTA in patients with CLI. When PTA is thermally induced by laser, results are disappointing and the incidence of perforation is high (33%).[181]

Surgical Revascularization

Before the development of PTA and suitable drug therapy, surgery was the only way to treat CLI. Revascularization procedures such as bypass surgery or, less commonly, endoarterectomy are still often the first choice of therapy for patients with CLI and long, multiple, or distal occlusions that cannot be treated otherwise.

For bypass surgery as for PTA, results should be assessed not only in terms of graft patency percentages but also, and above all, in terms of limb salvage, because a limb remains vital for several months after graft occlusion. The success of surgical revascularization depends mainly on the lesion site and the bypass length. Synthetic grafts provide excellent results when inserted above the inguinal ligament. In below-knee bypasses the patency percentage is significantly better when an autologous vein is used.[139,164]

Aortobifemoral Bypass

Lesions in the aorta or iliac vessels alone rarely cause critical ischemia but are frequently part of a multisegmental process. An aorta–bifemoral bypass may save the limb without additional revascularization procedures for distal lesions.[10]

The synthetic material used in aorta–bifemoral bypasses gives excellent results for patients with CLI. After 1 year patency is 90%, after 5 years it ranges from 74% to 90%, and after 10 years it ranges from 59% to 69%.[16] The mortality rate is approximately 5%.[139]

In patients for whom major abdominal surgery is contraindicated alternative surgical approaches may be used. The retroperitoneal approach is less traumatic than standard transperitoneal surgery and may provide equally satisfactory results. Extra-anatomic bypasses such as femorofemoral crossover or axillofemoral bypass are also possible.[89]

Femoropopliteal Bypass

Femoropopliteal bypass is used rarely in patients with critical ischemia and an isolated occlusion of the femoral artery longer than 10 cm that cannot be treated with PTA. When distal anastomoses are above the knee, synthetics such as Dacron or polytetrafluoroethylene can be successfully grafted.[10] For a bypass with distal anastomosis below the knee the first choice of graft material is an autologous vein (e.g., the saphena in situ or reversed or the cephalic vein). One year after femoropopliteal bypass with distal anastomosis above the knee, patency is approximately 75% for autologous vein grafting and 65% when synthetic materials are used.[85]

In below-knee bypasses the percentages fall to 70% and 60%, respectively. In a retrospective study on 600 patients with CLI who underwent 695 femoropopliteal bypasses, Merzelle reported that graft patency and limb salvage after 5 years were 50% and 70%, respectively.[114]

Femorocrural and Pedal Bypasses

Femorocrural bypasses are frequently performed on patients with CLI even though results are greatly inferior to those obtained with femoropopliteal bypasses. After 1 year, the patency of femorotibial bypasses is around 70% when autologous vein is used. The patency drops to 40% when synthetic materials are used. Results when anastomoses are distal to the ankle or in the foot are encouraging, with an overall limb salvage rate of 84% at 3 years[164] (Table 42.2).

Graft Occlusion

Graft occlusion may occur in the early postoperative period (within 30 days) or later. Early occlusions are usually due to erroneous grafting techniques, the wrong surgical choice, poor runoff, low blood flow through the graft, or thrombus formation on the graft surface. Most early occlusions can be avoided with an accurate preoperative assessment of distal runoff and by intraoperative angiographic check of graft patency.

Late graft occlusion may be due to thrombosis, fibrointimal hyperplasia in the distal anastomosis, or further evolution of the atherosclerotic processes. Besides the type of material used and the graft site, factors that negatively influence graft patency include age, poor clinical condition, smoking, diabetes, and high lipoprotein(a) and fibrinogen concentrations.[17,114,179]

Amputation

Although destructive and invalidating major amputation of the leg is often necessary in patients with CLI, especially if they are diabetic. Besides causing permanent invalidity and often loss of self-sufficiency, amputation is associated with a high perioperative mortality rate (see earlier section titled "Epidemiology"). Amputees also have a very poor prognosis for survival, and about 40% die within 2 years of major amputation.[50]

Indications

Primary amputation should be performed only if revascularization procedures are unfeasible because of a lack of distal vessels or very poor distal runoff. Primary amputation is also indicated in cases of necrotic lesions in a functionally impaired limb or in the presence of necrosis-induced toxemia.[74] When considering amputation, every case should be evaluated individually, bearing in mind the increased risk associated with distal femoral reconstruction failure and that below-knee amputation might be better than a series of bypass or recanalization procedures with little chance of success and increased morbidity and mortality risks.

Preoperative Evaluation

A simple method for detecting patent vessels and distal runoff preoperatively is by Doppler ultrasound.[7] Angiography should always be performed before major amputation to determine the presence or absence of patent dis-

TABLE 42.2. Patency after surgical reconstruction for critical limb ischemia.

Bypass	After 1 yr[150]	After 5 yr[16]	After 10 yr[16]
Aortoiliac–femoral	90%	74%–90%	59%–69%
Above-knee femoropopliteal			
With vein	75%		
With synthetic graft	65%		
Below knee femoropopliteal			
With vein	70%		
With synthetic graft	60%		
Femorocrural			
With vein	70%		
With synthetic graft	40%		

tal vessels. In the presence of extensive proximal occlusions preoperative angiography even with digital enhancement of the images can fail to demonstrate poorly perfused but patent distal arteries. Direct surgical exploration of the vessels at the ankle supplemented by intraoperative angiography is the most certain way of assessing the situation accurately but has obvious disadvantages.[144] $TcPO_2$ determinations are essential for a preoperative assessment of primary healing after below-knee amputation because the prognosis of primary stump healing when $TcPO_2$ values are below 40 mm Hg is very poor.[21]

Below-Knee Versus Above-Knee Amputation

Below-knee amputations have several advantages over above-knee procedures. Average intraoperative mortality rates are approximately 7% versus 20%; rehabilitation is satisfactory in 54% of below-knee amputations versus 20% of above-knee amputations. Disadvantages include a lower percentage of stump healing and a more frequent need of further surgery (only 70% of cases heal primarily, 15% require a second intervention, and the other 15% later require above-knee amputation).[50]

After major amputation some patients, particularly the elderly, may tend not to use the artificial limb. This situation can be avoided by early and appropriate rehabilitation and follow-up. Early mobilization and rehabilitation are essential, particularly after below-knee amputations, to prevent muscle contraction and joint stiffness that could annul the benefits of preserving the knee joint. Because there is a high risk of pulmonary embolism after amputation, patients should receive routine prophylaxis with subcutaneous heparin.[12]

Other Procedures

Iliac Endoarterectomy

Patients with CLI and monolateral iliac occlusive disease are suitable candidates for endoarterectomy. However, PTA is currently preferred for this type of lesion, and endoarterectomy has gradually been phased out because of technical difficulties and the risk of early recurring thombosis.

Sympathectomy

Surgical or chemical (phenol or pure alcohol) sympathectomy is occasionally proposed for patients with rest pain or gangrene, even though no controlled clinical studies are available to justify the use of this technique. Sympathectomy may offer advantages for patients with occlusion of the foot arteries or small foot ischemic ulcerations without hemodynamic critical ischemia (i.e.,

ankle systolic pressure >50 mm Hg and/or systolic toe pressure >30 mm Hg).[169]

Satisfactory results have also been obtained in patients with CLI associated with thromboangiitis obliterans.[10] Although sympathectomy alone rarely increases the chances of limb salvage by raising the temperature in the ischemic foot, it may attenuate symptoms.[70] The benefit of lumbar sympathectomy associated with surgical revascularization procedures to increase distal runoff has never been confirmed.[169]

Epidural Spinal Electrostimulation

Epidural spinal electrostimulation may relieve rest pain, but the data available are insufficient for unreserved recommendation of this technique for patients with CLI. Recent reports have, however, suggested that epidural spinal electrostimulation may be a valid alternative when revascularization procedures are technically impossible.[71,86] Analyzing the results of these studies shows that the overall percentage of limb salvage after 1 and 2 years is 80% and 56%, respectively. In responsive patients capillaroscopy has shown a significant improvement in capillary density and erythrocyte flow rate.[86]

Pharmacotherapy

Pharmacological treatment of CLI should be considered when catheter procedures and reconstructive surgery are not technically possible, are contraindicated, have failed, or carry an unacceptable risk–benefit ratio. Drugs that act on platelet activation and aggregation (e.g., antiplatelet drugs and prostanoids) or on coagulative factors (e.g., heparin, oral anticoagulant agents, and thrombolytic agents) are normally prescribed for patients with CLI, either in association with or as an alternative to surgical revascularization, even though no study has justified the use of primary drug therapy.

Antiplatelet Agents

Acetylsalicylic acid and ticlopidine seem to delay the progress of atherosclerotic lesions in the peripheral arteries. A significant delay in progression of femoroiliac lesions has been reported in patients treated with acetylsalicylic acid (1 g/d) compared with a placebo-treated group.[77,147] Unlike Schoop, Hess reports better results when acetylsalicylic acid was administered with dipyridamole (1 g/d and 225 mg/d): the active treatment was even more beneficial in hypertensive patients and smokers, in whom PAOD progresses rapidly if left untreated.[78,148]

Ticlopidine, which inhibits fibrinogen binding to the glycoprotein IIb/IIIa and modifies platelet adenosine diphosphate receptors, has been reported to slow the progress of atherosclerotic lesions in patients with intermittent claudication as visualized by angiography.[156] Because none of these trials had any specific clinical end point for CLI, no definitive conclusions about the efficacy of these drugs can be drawn.

The use of antiplatelet agents in patients with CLI is recommended because the drugs reduce the incidence of myocardial infarction and stroke and consequently cardiovascular mortality. Support for a beneficial impact of antiplatelet agents comes from a meta-analysis of 28 trials that involved a total of 3864 patients, many of whom had undergone reconstructive surgery.[1] Graft patency was also improved.[2] Most data refer to acetylsalicylic acid, but ticlopidine has recently been shown to reduce fatal and nonfatal cardiovascular events.[171]

Unfractionated and Low Molecular Weight Heparin

No data from clinical trials using heparin to treat patients with CLI are available. In our experience, 6-month therapy with low molecular weight heparin (15,000 units anti-Xa subcutaneously) compared with placebo significantly improved walking capacity in patients with intermittent claudication.[110] Fraciparin (CY 216), a low molecular weight heparin fraction, when tested in an open trial, was reported to alleviate rest pain and promote healing of ulcers that were previously resistant to therapy.[68] Recently low molecular weight heparin has been indicated as better than aspirin and dipyridamole in maintaining femoropopliteal graft patency in CLI patients undergoing salvage surgery.[54]

Oral Anticoagulants

Long-term therapy with oral anticoagulant agents is theoretically the best approach to prevent thrombosis in PAOD patients. However, although the results of the few clinical trials seem to indicate a positive trend, no definitive evidence has emerged (see Buonameaux [20] for review). Oral anticoagulants seem to improve survival rate in patients with CLI who have undergone femoro-popliteal bypass.[95]

Vasoactive Drugs

Although oral administration of vasodilators increases muscle blood flow and capillary flow in normal limbs, clinical results in patients with PAOD are disappointing.[172] In double-blind trials, pentoxifylline, buflomedil, and naftidrofuryl, vasodilators that also improve blood rheology or cell oxygenation, have been tested in patients with intermittent claudication and those with CLI. Improvements in walking capacity and oxygen delivery have been observed.[106,112,129] Although Ketanserin has recently been reported to lengthen walking distance and increase calf blood flow in patients with intermittent claudication,[40] these data have not been confirmed in other trials.[19,130]

Prostanoids

Powerful antiplatelet and vasodilating agents that inhibit leukocyte adhesion to integral or damaged endothelium and leukocyte–platelet interactions, prostanoids also possess profibrinolytic properties.[40] By stimulating cholesterol ester hydrolysis metabolism and inhibiting smooth muscle cell proliferation, prostanoids exert an antiatherosclerotic effect.[41]

Prostaglandin PGE₁

In 1973 Carlson and Erikson first reported the beneficial effects of intra-arterial infusion of PGE_1 (10 mg/kg per hour) for 1 to 3 days in four patients who required amputation.[23] Since then large controlled trials have administered prostanoids (PGE_1, prostacyclin [PGI_2], or the stable prostacyclin analog iloprost) to patients with severe arterial disease, rest pain, and ulcers.

Table 42.3 reports the results of several controlled trials.[13,45,55,88,140,141,162,165] The one with the highest number of patients ($N = 120$)[150] failed to demonstrate a consistent efficacy of either intra-arterial or intravenous PGE_1 in reducing pain or in ulcer healing. Short-term PGE_1 intra-arterial or intravenous infusion, either intermittent or continuous, was considered insufficient to achieve a long-lasting clinical benefit. Moreover, the question of whether PGE_1, when given intravenously, escapes pulmonary metabolism and reaches the peripheral tissues remains to be answered.

Prostacyclin

PGI_2, a natural prostaglandin produced by vascular cells that possesses greater antiplatelet and vasodilative properties than PGE_1, was first tested in five patients with ischemic ulcers. Results were encouraging: rest pain disappeared during the second day of infusion and ulcers healed in three patients within 2 months and markedly improved in the other two.[160] Data obtained from controlled trials showed a therapeutic benefit of PGI_2 in some but not all cases.[9,38,83,94,121,122] Intermittent or continuous infusion for 72 hours was generally associated with poor clinical results, whereas positive results were obtained when the drug was continuously administered for more than 72 hours (Table 42.4). There was apparently no advantage of intra-arterial or intravenous infusion, even though these two administration routes were not directly compared in any trial.

Iloprost

Iloprost infusion dramatically benefited diabetic patients for whom limb amputation had been planned.[27]

TABLE 42.3. PGE$_1$ in critical limb ischemia.

Author	Number of patients	Dosage and schedule	End points	Results	Statistical significance
Sakaguchi[140]	65	0.05 or 0.15 ng/kg per min (IA) 24 d	Ulcer size Pain	Reduced by higher dose	$P = .039$
Eklund[55]	24	20 µg × 7 h/d (IV) 3 d	Ulcer size Pain	Negative Negative	
Schuler[149]	120	20 ng/kg per min (IV) 72 h	Ulcer size Pain	Negative Negative	
Telles[162]	30	10 ng/kg per min (IV) 72 h	Ulcer size, pain Amputation	Negative Negative	
Jogestrand[87]	16	2 ng/kg per min (IV) 72 h	Ulcer size Calf blood flow	Negative Negative	
Böhme[13]	34	10–20 µg/h per d (IA) 23 d	Ulcer size, pain Stage regression Amputation Death	Negative Positive Negative Reduced	NS NS
Trübestein[165]	51	20 µg/h per d (IA) 21 d	Pain, ulcer size Clinical stage Amputation Analgesic cons.	NA	
Diehm[45]	23	60 µg/4 h per d (IV) 21 d	Pain Analgesic cons. Clinical stage	Reduced Reduced Positive	NS NS NS

IA, intra-arterial; IV, intravenous; NA, data not available due to lack of objective evaluation; NS, not significant.

Dormandy[46,47] reviewed data from five randomized prospective placebo-controlled European studies of iloprost in a total of 728 patients with stage III or IV PAOD in whom revascularization was impracticable or had failed (Table 42.5). Overall, 51.5% of patients treated with iloprost responded: pain was relieved or signs of ulcers healing were observed.[5,18,44,72,123,168] In three studies a 6-month follow-up showed that iloprost had significantly reduced the need for amputation.[69] Studies are in progress to determine whether long-term oral administration of prostaglandin analogs is tolerable, safe, relieves pain, aids ulcer healing, and reduces the amputation and mortality rates of these patients.

Normovolemic Hemodilution

Normovolemic hemodilution, by reducing hematocrit to 35% to 40% and consequently achieving a lower blood viscosity level, improves local perfusion.[56] Although benefits have been reported in patients with intermittent claudication,[56,107] there is little evidence that hemodilution improves the clinical picture in those with CLI. In a group of patients with ischemic ulcers who were not suitable candidates for surgical revascularization and who were mostly diabetic, Stolz reported that above-knee amputations fell from 56% to 41% after dextran therapy.[157]

TABLE 42.4. PGI$_2$ in critical limb ischemia.

Author	Number of patients	Dosage (ng/kg per min) and schedule	End points	Results	Statistical significance
Belch[9]	28	2-5-10 (IV) 96 h	Pain Analgesic cons. Ankle pressure	Early benefit Long-term reduction Negative	
Hossmann[82]	12	5 (IV) 7 d	Ulcer size Pain	Reduced Negative	$P < .05$
Nizankowski[121]	30	2.5–5 (IA) 72 h	Ulcer size Pain	Reduced Negative	$P < .02$
Cronenwett[38]	26	6 (IV) 72 h	Ulcer size Pain	Negative Negative	
Karnik[93]	20	5 (IV) 10 h × 5 d	Ulcer size Pain	Negative Negative	
Negus[120]	29	8 (IA) 72 h	Ulcer size Pain	Negative Negative	

TABLE 42.5. Iloprost in critical limb ischemia.

Author	Number of patients	Dosage and schedule	End points	Results (%)
Diehm[44] Brock[18]	210	≤2 ng/kg per min (IV) 28 d	Pain, ulcer size Amputation (6 mo)	IL 58 vs PL 20 NA
Norgren[122]	103	≤2 ng/kg per min (IV) 14 d	Pain, ulcer size Amputation (6 mo)	IL 40 vs PL 24 IL 33 vs PL 45
UK Severe Limb Ischaemia Study[168]	151	≤2 ng/kg per min (IV) 28 d	Pain, ulcer size Amputation (6 mo)	IL 45 vs PL 29 IL 19 vs PL 38
Guilmot[71]	128	≤2 ng/kg per min (IV) 21 d	Pain, ulcer size Amputation (6 mo)	IL 55 vs PL 36 IL 12 vs PL 19
Balzer[4]	136	≤2 ng/kg per min (IV) 14 d	Pain, ulcer size Amputation (6 mo)	IL 55 vs PL 42 NA

IL, iloprost; PL, placebo; NA, data not available.

Hyperbaric Oxygen

Hyperbaric oxygen therapy for patients with CLI is recommended on the grounds that inhaling oxygen at 3 atm increases oxygen plasma levels and improves oxygen delivery to interstitial fluid. No definitive evidence of clinical benefit has been published. In over 2000 patients treated in more than 7000 sessions, Fredenucci reported relief of rest pain and ulcer healing in one third of patients after 4 to 6 weeks of treatment, but the contributions of local therapy and heparin infusion to these results remains to be clarified.[67] The main drawback to hyperbaric oxygen therapy is the cumbersome, expensive equipment required.

Pain Relief

Pain relief is an important step in managing patients with advanced PAOD. Usually patients with CLI keep the limb dependent to relieve pain, but nonsteroidal anti-inflammatory drugs and morphine derivatives may be required. In some cases a nerve block or epidural anesthesia may be considered.

Acknowledgment
Translation by Dr. G. A. Boyd.

References

1. Antiplatelet Trialist's Collaboration. Collaborative overview of randomised trials of antiplatelet therapy: prevention of death, myocardial infarction, and stroke by prolonged antiplatelet therapy in various categories of patients. *BMJ.* 1994;308:81–106.

2. Antiplatelet Trialist's Collaboration. Collaborative overview of randomised trials of antiplatelet therapy, II: maintenance of vascular graft or arterial patency by antiplatelet therapy. *BMJ.* 1994;308:159–168.

3. Apelqvist J, Castenfors J, Larsson J, Stenstron A, Agardh CD. Prognostic value of systolic ankle and toe blood pressure levels in outcome of diabetic foot ulcer. *Diabetes Care.* 1989;12:115–120.

4. Bailey MJ, Yates CJP, Johnston CLW. Preoperative haemoglobin as predictor of outcome of diabetic amputation. *Lancet.* 1979;2:168–170.

5. Balzer K, Bechara G, Bisler H, Clevert HD, Diehm C. Reduction of ischaemic rest pain in advanced peripheral arterial occlusive disease: a double blind placebo controlled trial with iloprost. *Int Angiol.* 1991;10:229–232.

6. Barnes RW. Noninvasive diagnostic assessment of peripheral vascular disease. *Circulation.* 1991;83(suppl 1):20–27.

7. Beard JD, Scott DJ, Evans JM, Skidmore R, Horrocks M. Pulse generated run off: a new method of determining calf vessel patency. *Br J Surg.* 1988;74:361–363.

8. Becker GJ, Katzen BT, Dake MD. Noncoronary angioplasty. *Radiology.* 1989;170:921–940.

9. Belch JJF, McKay A, McArdle BM, et al. Epoprostenol (prostacyclin) and severe arterial disease: a double-blind trial. *Lancet.* 1983;1:315–317.

10. Bell PRF. Surgical reconstruction for critical limb ischaemia. In: Dormandy JA, Stock G, eds. *Critical Leg Ischaemia: Its Pathophysiology and Management.* Berlin: Springer-Verlag; 1990:73–84.

11. Bell PRF, Charlesworth D, DePalma RG. The definition of critical ischaemia of a limb: Working Party of International Vascular Symposium. *Br J Surg.* 1982;69(suppl):S2.

12. Berqvist D. Postoperative Thromboembolism: Frequency, Etiology, Prophylaxis. Berlin: Springer-Verlag; 1983.

13. Böhme H, Brülisauer M, Härtel U, Bollinger A. Kontrollierte Studie zur Wirksamkeit von i.a. Prostaglandin E₁ Infusionen bei peripherer arterieller Verschlußkrankheit im stadium III und IV. *Vasa.* 1987;20(suppl):206–208.

14. Bollinger A, Barras JP, Mahler F. Measurement of foot artery blood pressure by micromanometry in normal sub-

jects and in patients with arterial occlusive disease. *Circulation*. 1976;53:506–512.

15. Bollinger A, Fagrell B. Clinical Capillaroscopy: A Guide to Its Use in Clinical Research and Practice. Toronto: Hogrefe & Huber; 1990.

16. Branchereau A, Colonna MA, Magnan PE. Resultants des pontages artériels après dix ans. In: Chigot JP, et al., eds. *Chirurgie Spécialités*. Paris: Expansion Scientifique; 1990: 62–65.

17. Brewster DC, La Salle AJ, Robinson JG. Factors affecting patency of femoro-popliteal bypass graft. *Surgery Gynecology and Obstetrics*. 1983;157:473.

18. Brock FE, Abri O, Baitsch G, et al. Iloprost in der Behandlung inschämischer Gewebsläsionen bei Diabetikern. Ergebnisse einer placebokontrollierten Multizentrenstudie mit einem stabilen Prostazyklinderivat. *Schweiz Med Wochenschr*. 1990;20:1477–1482.

19. Buonameaux H, Holditch T, Hellemans H, Berent A, Verhaeghe R. Placebo-controlled, double-blind, two-centre trial of Ketanserin in intermittent claudication. *Lancet*. 1985;2:1268–1271.

20. Buonameaux H, Verhaeghe R, Verstraete M. Thromboembolism and antithrombotic therapy in peripheral arterial disease. *J Am Coll Cardiol*. 1986;8:98B–103B.

21. Burgess ME, Matsen FA, Wyss CR, Simmons CW. Segmental transcutaneous measurement of Po_2 in patients requiring below-the-knee amputation for peripheral vascular insufficiency. *J Bone Joint Surg*. 1982;64A:378–382.

22. Carbellon S, Moncrief C, Pierre C, Cavanaugh DG. Incidence of abdominal aortic aneurysms in patients with atheromatous arterial disease. *Am J Surg*. 1983;146: 575–576.

23. Carlson LA, Eriksson I. Femoral-artery infusion of prostaglandin E_1 in severe peripheral vascular disease. *Lancet*. 1973;1:155–156.

24. Carter SA. The relationship of distal systolic pressures to healing of skin lesions in limbs with arterial occlusive disease, with special reference to diabetes mellitus. *Scand J Clin Lab Invest*. 1973;31(suppl):239–243.

25. Carter SA, Lezack JD. Digital systolic pressures in the lower limb in arterial disease. *Circulation*. 1971;43:905–914.

26. Catalano M. Epidemiology of critical limb ischaemia: North Italian data. *European Journal of Medicine*. 1983;2: 11–14.

27. Chiesa R, Vicari A, Mari G, Galimberti M, Di Carlo V, Pozza G. Use of stable prostacyclin analogue ZK36374 to treat lower limb ischaemia. *Lancet*. 1985;2:95–96.

28. Christensen S. Lower extremity amputations in the county of Aalborg 1961–1971. *Acta Orthop Scand*. 1976;47: 329–334.

29. Ciuffetti G, Balendra R, Lennie SE, Anderson J, Lowe GDO. Impaired filterability of white cells in acute cerebral infarction. *BMJ*. 1989;289:930–931.

30. Ciuffetti G, Mannarino E, Pasqualini L, Mercuri M, Lennie SE, Lowe GDO. The haemorheological role of cellular factors in peripheral vascular disease. *Vasa*. 1988;17: 168–170.

31. Ciuffetti G, Mercuri M, Mannarino E, Robinson MK, Lennie SE, Lowe GDO. Peripheral vascular disease: rheo-

logic variables during controlled ischaemia. *Circulation*. 1989;80:348.

32. Colwell JA, Lopes-Virell MF. A review of the development of large vessel disease in diabetes mellitus. *Am J Med*. 1988;85(suppl):113–118.

33. Conrad MC. Abnormalities of the digital vasculature as related to ulceration and gangrene. *Circulation*. 1968;38: 568–581.

34. Cooper JC, Welsh CL. The role of percutaneous transluminal angioplasty in the treatment of critical ischaemia. *European Journal of Vascular Surgery*. 1991;5:261–264.

35. Crawford N, Scrutton MC. Biochemistry of the blood platelet. In: Bloom AL, Thomas DP, eds. *Haemostasis and Thrombosis*. Edinburgh: Churchill Livingston; 1987:47–77.

36. Criqui MH, Coughlin SS, Fronek A. Noninvasively diagnosed peripheral arterial disease as a predictor of mortality: result from a prospective study. *Circulation*. 1985;72: 768–773.

37. Criqui MH, Fronek A, Klauber MR, Barret-Connor E, Gabriel S. The sensitivity, specificity, and predictive value of traditional clinical evaluation of peripheral arterial disease: results from non invasive testing in a defined population. *Circulation*. 1985;71:516–522.

38. Cronenwett JL, Zelenock GB, Whitehouse WM, Lindenauer SM, Graham LM, Stanley JC. Prostacyclin treatment of ischaemia ulcers and rest pain in unreconstructible peripheral arterial occlusive disease. *Surgery*. 1986;100: 369–375.

39. Danish Amputation Register. Herlev Hospital, Copenhagen; 1989.

40. De Cree J, Leempoels J, Geukens H, Verhaegen H. Placebo-controlled double-blind trial of ketanserin in the treatment of intermittent claudication. *Lancet*. 1984;1: 606–609.

41. De Gaetano G, Bartelè V, Carletti C. Mechanism of action and clinical use of prostanoids. In: Dormandy JA, Stock G, eds. *Critical Leg Ischaemia: Its Pathophysiology and Management*. Berlin: Springer-Verlag; 1990:117–137.

42. de Wolfe VG. Chronic occlusive arterial disease of the lower extremities in clinical vascular disease. *Cardiovascular Clinic*. 1983;13:15–35.

43. DHSS Statistics and Research Division. Amputation statistics for England, Wales, and Northern Ireland. London: Department of Health and Social Security; 1976–1986.

44. Diehm C, Abri O, Baitsch G, Bechara G, Beck K. Iloprost, ein stabiles Prostazyklinderivat, bei arterieller Verschlusskrankheit im stadium IV. Eine placebo-kontrollierte Multizentrenstudie. *Dtsch Med Wochenschr*. 1989;114: 783–788.

45. Diehm C, Stammler F, Hübsch-Müller C, Eckstein HH, Simini B. Clinical effects of intravenously administered prostaglandin E_1 in patients with rest pain due to peripheral obliterative arterial disease (POAD): a preliminary report on a placebo-controlled double-blind study. *Vasa*. 1987;(suppl 17):52–56.

46. Dormandy J. Use of the prostacyclin analogue iloprost in the treatment of patients with critical limb ischaemia. *Therapie*. 1991;46:319–322.

47. Dormandy JA. Clinical Experience with iloprost in the

treatment of critical leg ischaemia. Cardiovascular significance of endothelium-derived vasoactive factors. 1991: 335–347.

48. Dormandy JA, Hoare E, Colley J, Arrowsmith DE, Dormandy TL. Clinical, haemodynamic, rheological, and biochemical findings in 126 patients with intermittent claudication. *BMJ*. 1973;4:576–581.

49. Dormandy J, Mahir M, Ascady G, et al. Fate of the patient with chronic leg ischaemia. *J Cardiovasc Surg*. 1989;30: 50–57.

50. Dormandy JA, Thomas PRS. What is the natural history of critically ischaemic patients with and without his leg? In: Greenhalgh RM, Jameson CW, Nicolaides AN, eds. *Limb Salvage and Amputation for Vascular Disease*. Philadelphia, Pa: WB Saunders; 1988:11–26.

51. Dousset V, Wehrli RS, Louie A. Popliteal artery hemodynamics: MR imaging US correlation. *Radiology*. 1991;179: 437–441.

52. Duffield RGM, Miller NE, Brunt JNH. Treatment of hyperlipidaemia retards progression of symptomatic femoral atherosclerosis: a randomised controlled trial. *Lancet*. 1983;2:639–642.

53. Edmonds ME. The neuropathic foot in diabetes. Part I: Blood flow. *Diabet Med*. 1986;3:111–115.

54. Edmondson RA, Cohen AT, Das SK, Wagner MB, Kakkar VV. Low-molecular-weight heparin versus aspirin and dipyridamole after femoro-popliteal bypass grafting in patient with critical leg ischaemia. *Lancet*. 1994;384:914–918.

55. Eklund AE, Eriksson G, Olsson AG. A controlled study showing significant short term effect of prostaglandin E₁ in healing of ischaemic ulcers of the lower limb in man. *Prostaglandins Leukotr Essent Fatty Acids*. 1982;8:265–271.

56. Ernst E, Kollar L, Matrai A. Placebo-controlled, double-blind study of hemodilution in peripheral arterial disease. *Lancet*. 1987;1:1449–1451.

57. European Working Group on Critical Limb Ischemia. European consensus on critical limb ischemia. *Lancet*. 1989; 1:737–738.

58. European Working Group on Critical Limb Ischemia. Second European consensus document on chronic critical leg ischaemia. *Circulation*. 1991;84(suppl 4):1–22.

59. Fagrell B. Vital capillary miscroscopy: a clinical method for studying changes of the nutritional skin capillaries in legs with arteriosclerosis obliterans. *Scand J Clin Lab Invest*. 1973;133 (suppl):1–50.

60. Fagrell B. Investigation and general management: commentary. In: Dormandy JA, Stock G, eds. *Critical Leg Ischaemia: Its Pathophysiology and Management*. Berlin: Springer-Verlag; 1990:41–48.

61. Fagrell B, Lundberg G. A simplified evaluation of vital capillary microscopy for predicting skin viability in patients with severe arterial insufficiency. *Clin Physiol*. 1984; 4:403.

62. FitzGerald GA, Smith B, Pedersen AK, Brash AR. Increased prostacyclin biosynthesis in patients with severe atherosclerosis and platelet activation. *N Engl J Med*. 1984; 310:1065–1068.

63. Fowkes FGR. Epidemiology of atherosclerotic arterial disease in the lower limb. *Eur J Vasc Endovasc Surg*. 1988;2: 282–291.

64. Fowkes FGR, Howsley E, Cawood EHH. Edinburgh Artery Study: prevalence of asymptomatic and symptomatic peripheral arterial disease in the general population. *Int J Epidemiol*. 1991;20:384–392.

65. Franzeck UK, Liebethal R, Diehm C. Mikrovaskulare Flußverteilung und transcutaner4Sauerstoffpartialdruck der HautKapillaren von Patienten mit peripherer arterieller Verschlußkrankheit im Stadium III und IV. *Vasa*. 1987;20(suppl):309–310.

66. Franzeck UK, Talke P, Bernstein EF. Transcutaneous Po₂ measurements in health and peripheral arterial occlusive disease. *Surgery*. 1982;91:156–163.

67. Fredenucci P. Oxygénothérapie hyperbare et artériophaties. *J Mal Vasc*. 1985;10:166–172.

68. Gauthier O. Efficacy and safety of CY 216 in the treatment of specific leg ulcers. In: Breddin K, Fareed J, Samama M, eds. *Fraxiparine. Analytical and Structural Data, Pharmacology, Clinical Trials*. Stuttgart: Schattauer; 1987:21.

69. Grant SM, Goa KL. Iloprost: a review of its pharmacodynamic and pharmacokinetic properties, and therapeutic potential in peripheral vascular disease, myocardial ischaemia, and extracorporeal circulation procedures. *Drugs*. 1992;43:889–924.

70. Greenstein D, Brown TF, Kester RC. Assessment of chemical lumbar sympathectomy in critical limb ischaemia using thermal imaging. *Int J Clin Monit Comput*. 1994;11:31–34.

71. Guarnera G, Furgiuele S, Camilli S. Spinal cord electric stimulation vs femoro-distal bypass in critical ischaemia of the legs. Preliminary results in a randomized prospective study. *Minerva Cardioangiol*. 1994;42(5):223–227.

72. Guilmot J-L, Diot E. Treatment of lower limb ischaemia due to atherosclerosis in diabetic and nondiabetic patients with iloprost, a stable analogue of prostacyclin: results of a French multicentre trial. *Drug Invest*. 1991;3:351–359.

73. Gundersen J. Segmental measurements of systolic blood pressure in the extremities including the thumb and the great toe. *Acta Chirurgia Scandinavica*. 1972;426(suppl): 1–90.

74. Harris PL, Moody P. Amputations. In: Dormandy JA, Stock G, eds. *Critical Leg Ischaemia: Its Pathophysiology and Management*. Berlin: Springer-Verlag; 1990:87–95.

75. Hatary Y. Diabetic peripheral neuropathy. *Ann Intern Med*. 1987;107:546–559.

76. Heintzen MP, Neubaur T, Klepzig M. Laser angioplasty of iliac and femeropopliteal obstructive lesions. In: Höfling B, Pölnitz A, eds. *Interventional Cardiology and Angiology*. Darmstadt: Springer-Verlag; 1989:153–161.

77. Hertzer NR. The natural history of peripheral vascular disease: implications for its management. *Circulation*. 1991; 83(suppl):12–19.

78. Hess H, Mietaschk A, Deichsel G. Drug-induced inhibition of platelet function delays progression in peripheral occlusive arterial disease: a prospective double-blind arteriographically controlled trial. *Lancet*. 1985;1:415–419.

79. Hess H, Mietasschk W, Brück H. Peripheral arterial occlusions: a 6-year experience with local low-dose thrombolitic therapy. *Radiology*. 1987;163:753–758.

80. Hirai M, Kawai S. Clinical significance of segmental blood pressure in arterial occlusive disease of lower extremity. *Vasa*. 1978;7:383–388.

81. Hoffman U, Bollinger A. Laser-Doppler. In: Kriesman A, ed. *Aktuelle Diagnostik und Therapie in der Angiologie.* Stuttgart: Thieme; 1988:56–60.

82. Hoffman U, Saesseli B, Geiger M, Schneider E, Bollinger A. Vasomotion in patients with severe ischaemia before and after percutaneous transluminal angioplasty (PTA). *Int J Microcirc Clin Exp.* August 1988(special issue): 89.

83. Hossman V, Auel H, Rücker W, Schrör K. Prolonged infusion of prostacyclin in patients with advanced stages of peripheral vascular disease: a placebo-controlled crossover study. *Klin Wochenschr.* 1984;62:1108–1114.

84. Howell MA, Colgan MP, Seeger RW, Ramsey DE. Relationship of severity of lower limb peripheral vascular disease to mortality and morbidity: a six-year follow-up study. *J Vasc Surg.* 1988;9:691–697.

85. Hunink MG, Donaldson MC, Meyerovitz MF, et al. Risks and benefits of femoropopliteal percutaneous balloon angioplasty. *J Vasc Surg.* 1993;7:183–192.

86. Jacobs MJHM, Slaaf DW, Reneman RS. Dorsal column stimulation in critical limb ischaemia. *Vascular Medicine Review.* 1990;1:215–220.

87. Jelnes R, Gardstang O, Jensen HK, Baekgaard N, Tonnesen KH, Schroeder T. Fate in intermittent claudication: outcome and risk factors. *BMJ.* 1986;293:1137–1140.

88. Jogestrand T, Olsson AG. The effect of intravenous prostaglandin E_1 on ischaemic pain and on leg blood-flow in subjects with peripheral artery disease: a double-blind controlled study. *Clin Physiol.* 1985;5:495–502.

89. Johnson JN, McLoughlin GA, Wake PN. Comparison of extraperitoneal and transperitoneal methods of aortoiliac reconstruction: twenty years experience. *J Cardiovasc Surg.* 1986;27:561–565.

90. Johnston KW, Raew M, Hogg-Johnston SA, et al. Five-year result of a prospective study of percutaneous transluminal angioplasty. *Ann Surg.* 1987;206:403.

91. Jünger M, Frey-Schnewlin G, Bolliger A. Microvascular flow distribution and trans-capillary diffusion at the forefoot in patients with peripheral ischaemia. *Int J Microcirc Clin Exp.* 1989;8:3–24.

92. Kannel WB, Skinner JJ, Schwartz MJ, Shurtleff D. Intermittent claudication: incidence in the Framingham Study. *Circulation.* 1970;41:857–883.

93. Karanfilian RG, Lynch TG, Zirul VT. The value of laser Doppler velocimetry and transcutaneous oxygen tension determination in predicting healing of ischaemic forefoot ulcerations and amputations in diabetic and nondiabetic patients. *J Vasc Surg.* 1986;4:511.

94. Karnik R, Valentin A, Slany J. Prostacyclin versus naftidrofuryl. *Herz/Kreislauf.* 1987;1:23–26.

95. Kretschmer G, Wenzl E, Schemper M, et al. Influence of postoperative anticoagulant treatment on patient survival after femoropopliteal vein bypass surgery. *Lancet.* 1988;1: 797–799.

96. Krings W, Peters PE. Percutaneous reopening procedures. In: Dormandy JA, Stock G, eds. *Critical Leg Ischaemia: Its Pathophysiology and Management.* Berlin: Springer-Verlag; 1990:53–68.

97. Krolewski AS, Warren JH. Epidemiology of diabetes mellitus. In: Marble A, Krall LP, Bradley RS, Christlieb AR,

Souldner JS, eds. *Joslin's Diabetes Mellitus.* 12th ed. Philadelphia, Pa: Lea & Febiger; 1989:12–42.

98. Krone W, Müller-Wieland D. Special problems of the diabetic patient. In: Dormandy JA, Stock G, eds. *Critical Leg Ischaemia: Its Pathophysiology and Management.* Berlin: Springer-Verlag; 1990:145–157.

99. Loehr S, Link KM, Martin EM, Baker MB, Lesko NM, Loehr WJ. Peripheral magnetic resonance angiography. *Critical Ischaemia.* 1993;3:7–18.

100. LoGerfo FW, Coffman JD. Vascular and microvascular disease of the foot in diabetes. *N Engl J Med.* 1984;311: 1615–1619.

101. Lowe GDO. Pathophysiology of critical limb ischaemia. In: Dormandy JA, Stock G, eds. *Critical Leg Ischaemia: Its Pathophysiology and Management.* Berlin: Springer-Verlag; 1990:17–38.

102. Lowe GDO, Dugla JT, Zahrani H, et al. Plasma D-dimer antigen in chronic peripheral arterial disease and in population study. *Fibrinolysis.* 1988;2(suppl):1–37.

103. Lowe GDO, Prentice CRM. Haemostatic and haemorheological factors in peripheral vascular disease. In: Pollok JG, ed. *Topical Review in Vascular Surgery.* Vol 1. London: Wright, Bristol; 1982:25–48.

104. Lowe GDO, Reavey MM, Johnston RV, Forbes CD, Prentice CRM. Increased platelet aggregates in vascular and non-vascular illness: correlation with plasma fibrinogen and effect of ancrod. *Thromb Res.* 1979;14:377–386.

105. Ludbrook J, Clark AM, McKenzie JK. Significance of absent ankle pulse. *BMJ.* 1962;1:1724–1728.

106. Maas H, Amberger HG, Böhme H. Naftidrofuryl bei arterieller Verschlußkrankheit. Kontrollierte multizentrische Dopplerblinstudie mit oraler Applikation. *Dtsch Med Wochenschr.* 1984;109:745–750.

107. Mannarino E, Ciuffetti G, Maragoni G, Pasqualini L, Selvi A. Clinical and hemorheological implications of normovolemic hemodilution in peripheral vascular disease: results of a pilot study. *Progress in Angiology.* Torino, Italy: Minerva Medica; 1985:545–547.

108. Mannarino E, Maragoni G, Pasqualini L, Sanchini R, Rossi P, Orlandi U. Transcutaneous oxygen tension behavior in the different stages of peripheral vascular disease and its correlation with ankle/arm pressure ratio and calf blood flow. *Angiology.* 1987;38:463.

109. Mannarino E, Pasqualini L, Innocente S, Vaudo G, Scricciolo V, Ciuffetti G. Modifications in transcutaneous oxygen pressure in ischaemic limbs after successful PTA. *Int Angiol.* 1994;3:113.

110. Mannarino E, Pasqualini L, Innocente S, et al. Efficacy of low-molecular-weight heparin in the management of intermittent claudication. *Angiology.* 1991;42:1–7.

111. Mannarino E, Pasqualini L, Maragoni G. Vasospasm: its role in peripheral vascular disease patients. In: Crepaldi G, ed. *Atherosclerosis.* Vol VIII. Elsevier; 1989:547–551.

112. Mannarino E, Paqualini L, Maragoni G, Orlandi U. Effect of buflomedil chlorhydrate on local oxygen delivery in peripheral vascular disease. *Angiology.* 1989;40:559–562.

113. Mannarino E, Pasqualini L, Scricciolo V, Fedele F, Innocente S. Nailfold capillaroscopy in the assessment of peripheral arterial occlusive disease. *Arch Gerontol Geriatr.* 1991;2(suppl):389.

114. Marzelle J, Fichelle JM, Alimi G, et al. Femoro-distal revascularization for critical chronic atheromatous ischemia. 695 cases. *Presse Med.* 1992;21:253–257.

115. Matsi PJ, Manninen HI, Laakso M, Jaakkola P. Impact of risk factors on limb salvage after angiopalsty in chronic critical lower limb ischaemia: a prospective trial. *Angiology.* 1994;45:797–804.

116. McEwan AJ, Ledingham IM. Blood flow characteristics and tissue nutrition in apparently ischaemic feet. *BMJ.* 1971;3:220–224.

117. Morris-Jones W, Preston E, Greaves M, Duleep K. Gangrene of the toes with palpable peripheral pulses. *Ann Surg.* 1981;193:402–466.

118. Most RS, Sinnock P. The epidemiology of lower extremity amputations in diabetic individuals. *Diabetes Care.* 1983; 6:87–91.

119. Mulligan SA, Matsuda T, Langer P, et al. Peripheral arterial occlusive disease: prospective comparison of MR angiography and color duplex US with conventional angiography. *Radiology.* 1991;178:695–700.

120. Nash GB, Thomas PRS, Dormandy JA. Abnormal flow properties of white cells in patients with severe ischaemia of the leg. *BMJ.* 1988;296:1699–1701.

121. Negus D, Irving JD, Friedgood A. Intra-arterial prostacyclin compared to praxilene in the management of severe lower limb ischaemia: a double-blind trial. *J Cardiovasc Surg.* 1987;28:196–199.

122. Nizankowsky R, Krolikowsky W, Beiltowicz J, Szczeklik A. Prostacyclin for ischemic ulcers in peripheral arterial disease: a random-assignment, placebo-controlled study. *Thromb Res.* 1985;37:21–28.

123. Norgen L, Alwmark A, Angqvist KA, et al. A stable prostacyclin analogue (iloprost) in the treatment of ischaemic ulcers of the lower limb: a Scandinavian-Polish placebo controlled, randomised multicenter study. *Eur J Vasc Surg.* 1990;4:463–467.

124. Oishi CS, Fronek A, Golbranson FI. The role of noninvasive vascular studies in determining levels of amputation. *J Bone Joint Surg.* 1988;70:1520–1530.

125. Olcott C. Clinical applications of video angioscopy. *J Vasc Surg.* 1987;5:664–666.

126. Pasqualini L, Vaudo G, Piccioni N, Ciuffetti G, Clerici G, Mannarino E. Effects of oral defibrotide on transcutaneous oxygen pressure and leukocyte rheology in stage II peripheral arterial occlusive disease. *Advances in Therapy.* 1994;11:85.

127. Peabody CN, Kannel WB, McNamara PM. Intermittent claudication: surgical significance. *Arch Surg.* 1974;109: 693–697.

128. Pell JP, Fowkes FGR. Epidemiology of critical limb ischaemia. *Critical Ischaemia.* 1992;2:23–29.

129. Porter JM, Cutler BS, Lee BY. Pentoxifylline efficacy in the treatment of intermittent claudication: multicenter controlled double-blind trial with objective assessment of chronic occlusive arterial disease patients. *Am Heart J.* 1982;104:66–72.

130. Prevention of Atherosclerotic Complications with Ketanserin Trial Group. Prevention of atherosclerotic complications: controlled trial of ketanserin. *BMJ.* 1989;298: 424–430.

131. Reid HL, Dormandy JA, Barnes AJ. Impaired red cell deformability in peripheral vascular disease. *Lancet.* 1976;1: 666–668.

132. Rieger H, Kohler M, Schoop W. Hemodilution (HD) in patients with ischemic skin ulcers. *Klin Wochenschr.* 1979; 57:1153–1161.

133. Rieger H, Scheffler D. Diagnosis of advanced stages of PAOD. *Critical Ischaemia.* 1990;1:15–21.

134. Rose GA. The diagnosis of ischaemic heart pain and intermittent claudication in field surveys. *Bull Who.* 1962; 27:645–658.

135. Rosenbloom MS, Flanigan DP, Schuler JJ. Risk factors affecting the natural history of intermittent claudication. *Arch Surg.* 1988;123:867–870.

136. Ruckley CV. Investigation and general management: commentary. In: Dormandy JA, Stock G, eds. *Critical Leg Ischaemia: Its Pathophysiology and Management.* Berlin: Springer-Verlag; 1990:49–51.

137. Ruckley CV. Symptomatic and asymptomatic disease. In: Fowkes FGR, ed. *Epidemiology of Peripheral Vascular Disease.* London: Springer-Verlag; 1991:326–331.

138. Rutherford RB, Flanigan DP, Gupta SK, and the Ad Hoc Committee on Reporting Standards SVS/ISCVS. Suggested standards for reports dealing with lower extremity ischaemia. *J Vasc Surg.* 1986;4:80–94.

139. Rutherford RB, Jones DN, Bergentz SE. Factors affecting the patency of infrainguinal bypass. *J Vasc Surg.* 1988;8: 236–246.

140. Sackett KL, Winkelstein W. The epidemiology of aortic and peripheral atherosclerosis: a selective review. *Journal of Chronic Diseases.* 1965;18:775–793.

141. Sakaguchi S, Kusaba A, Mishima Y, et al. A multi-clinical double blind study with PGE₁ (α-cyclodextrin clathrate) in patients with ischemic ulcers of the extremities. *Vasa.* 1978;7:263–267.

142. Salenius JP. Experience of peripheral angioscopy in Scandinavia. *Int Angiol.* 1995;4:65–68.

143. Sanborn TA. Technical success, clinical success, and patency in laser angioplasty. *Radiology.* 1989;170: 576–577.

144. Scarpato R, Gembarowicz R, Forber R. Intraoperative pre-reconstruction arteriography. *Arch Surg.* 1981;116: 1953–1955.

145. Schmidtke I, Roth F-J, Schoop W, Cappius G. Perkutane transluminale Katheterbehandlung bei Kranken mit arteriellen Duchblutungsstörungen im Stadium III unf IV. In: Müller-Wiefel H, ed. *Mikrozirkulation und Blutrheologie: Therapie der arteriellen Verschlußkrankheit.* Baden-Baden: Verlag Gerhard Witzstrock; 1980:411.

146. Schneider E, Grüntzig A, Bolliger A. Die perkutane tranluminale Angioplastie (PTA) in den Stadien III und IV der peripheren arteriellen Verschlüsskrankheut. *Vasa.* 1982;11:336–339.

147. Schoop W. A new path for antibiotic therapy of ischaemic lesions? *Critical Ischaemia.* 1992;2:3–4.

148. Schoop W, Levy H, Schoop B, Gaentzsch A. Experimentelle und klinische Studien zu der sekundären Prävention der peripheren Arteriosklerose. In: Bollinger A, Rhyner K, eds. *Thrombozytenfunktionshemmer.* Stuttgart: Thieme; 1983:49–58.

149. Schroll M, Munck O. Estimation of peripheral arteriosclerotic disease by ankle blood pressure measurements in a population study of 60 year old men and women. *Journal of Chronic Diseases*. 1981;34:261–269.

150. Schuler JJ, Flanigan DP, Holcroft JW, Ursprung JJ, Mohrland JS, Pyke J. Efficacy of prostaglandin E$_1$ in the treatment of lower extremity ischemic ulcers secondary to peripheral vascular occlusive disease. *J Vasc Surg*. 1984;1: 160–170.

151. Seeger JM, Silverman SH, Flynn TC, et al. Lipid risk factors in patients requiring arterial reconstruction. *J Vasc Surg*. 1989;10:418–424.

152. Seifert H, Jager K, Bollinger A. Analysis of flow motion by the laser Doppler technique in patients with peripheral arterial occlusive disease. *Int J Microcirc Clin Exp*. 1988;7: 223.

153. Serradimigni A, Villain PH. Traitements anticoagulants et fibrinolytiques. In: Rouffy J, Natali J, eds. *Artériopathies Athéromateuses des Membres Inférieurs*. Paris: Masson; 1989: 314–330.

154. Simms MH. Is pedal arch patency a prerequisite for successful reconstruction? In: Greenhalgh RM, Jamieson CW, Nicolaides AN, eds. *Limb Salvage and Amputation for Vascular Disease*. London: WB Saunders; 1988:49–62.

155. Smith JB. Prostaglandins in platelet aggregation and haemostasis. In: Bloom AL, Thomas DP, eds. *Haemostasis and Thrombosis*. Edinburgh: Churchill Livingston; 1987: 78–89.

156. Stiegler H, Hess H, Mietaschk A, Tramppisch HJ, Ingrisch H. Einfluβ von Ticlopin auf die periphere ablitierende Arteriopathie. *Dtsch Med Wochenschr*. 1984;109:1240–1243.

157. Stoltz J, Bartel M. Einfluβ einer adjuvanten Infusionstherapie von niedermolekularen Dextranen (Infukoll M40) und deproteinisiertem Haemoderivat (Activegin) bei chronisch arteriellen Durchblutungsstörungen im Stadium IV nach Fontaine. *Zentralbl Chir*. 1988;113: 1044–1055.

158. Strandness DE, Bell JW. Peripheral vascular disease: diagnosis and objective evaluation using mercury strain gauge. *Ann Surg*. 1965;4(suppl):161.

159. Strandness DE Jr, Sumner DS, eds. *Haemodynamics for Surgeons*. New York: Grune and Stratton; 1975:278–281.

160. Szczeklik A, Skawinski S, Gluszko P, Nizankowski R, Szczeklik J, Gryglewski RJ. Successful therapy of advanced arteriosclerosis obliterans with prostacyclin. *Lancet*. 1979; 1:1111–1114.

161. Taylor GW, Calo AR. Atherosclerosis of arteries of lower limbs. *BMJ*. 1962;1:507–510.

162. Telles GS, Campbell WB, Wood RFM, Collin J, Baird RN, Morris PJ. Prostaglandin E$_1$ in severe lower limb ischaemia: a double-blind controlled trial. *Br J Surg*. 1984; 71:506–508.

163. Thompson MM, Sayers RD, Varty K, Reid A, London JM, Bell PRF. Chronic critical leg ischaemia must be redefined. *Eur J Vasc Endovasc Surg*. 1993;7:420–426.

164. Tordoir JH, van der Plas JP, Jacobs MJ, Kitslaar PJ. Factors determining the outcome of crural and pedal revascularisation for critical limb ischaemia. *Eur J Vasc Surg*. 1993;7: 82–86.

165. Trübestein G, Diehm C, Gruss JD, Horsch S. Prostaglandin E$_1$ in chronic arterial disease: a multicenter study. *Vasa*. 1987;17(suppl):39–43.

166. Tunis SR, Bass EB, Steinberg EP. The use of angioplasty, bypass surgery, and amputation in the management of peripheral vascular disease. *N Engl J Med*. 1991;325: 556–562.

167. Ubbink DTH, Kitslaar PJEHM, Tordoir JHM, Tangelder GJ, Reneman RS, Jacobs MJHM. The relevance of posturally induced microvascular contriction after revascularisation in patients with chronic leg ischaemia *Eur J Vasc Endovasc Surg*. 1992;6:525–532.

168. UK Severe Limb Ishaemia Study Group. Treatment of limb-threatening ischaemia with intravenous iloprost: a randomised double-blind placebo-controlled study. *Eur J Vasc Endovasc Surg*. 1991;5:511–516.

169. Vayssairat M, Gouny P, Baudot N, Gaitz JP, Nussaume O. Distal arteritis of the legs: lumbar sympathectomy. *J Mal Vasc*. 1994;19(suppl):174–177.

170. Veith FJ, Bupta SK, Wengerter KR. Changing arteriosclerotic disease patterns and management strategies in lower-limb threatening ischaemia. *Ann Surg*. 1990;212: 402–414.

171. Verhaeghe R. Antiplatelet drugs in critical limb ischaemia. *Critical Ischaemia*. 1992;2:26–29.

172. Verstraete M. Current therapy for intermittent claudication. *Drugs*. 1982;24:240–247.

173. Wack C, Wolfle KD, Loeprecht H, Tietze W, Bohndorf K. Percutaneous balloon dilatation of isolated lesions of the calf arteries in critical ischemia of the leg. *Vasa*. 1994;23: 30–34.

174. Walden R, Bass A, Balaciano M, Moldan M, Zulty L, Adar R. Laser Doppler flowmetry in lower extremity ischaemia: application and interpretation. *Ann Vasc Surg*. 1992;6: 511–516.

175. Weber HP, Neufeld KH, Ringelmann W, et al. Laser recanalization of peripheral arteries. *Int Angiol*. 1995;4: 74–82.

176. Widmer LK, Biland L, DaSilva A. Risk profile and occlusive periphery artery disease (OPAD). In: *Proceedings of the 13th International Congress of Angiology*. Athens, Greece; 1985:28.

177. Widmer LK, Greensher A, Kannel WB. Occlusion of peripheral arteries: a study of 6400 working subjects. *Circulation*. 1964;30:836–842.

178. Wilson SE, Wolf GL, Cross A. Percutaneous transluminal angioplasty versus operation for peripheral atherosclerosis: report of a randomised trial in a selected group of patients. *J Vasc Surg*. 1989;9:1–9.

179. Wiseman S, Kenchington G, Dain R, et al. Influence of smoking and plasma factors on patency of femoropopliteal vein graft. *BMJ*. 1989;299:643–646.

180. Wolfe JHN. Defining the outcome of critical ischaemia: a one year prospective study. *Br J Surg*. 1986;73:321.

181. Wright JG, Belkin M, Greenfield AJ. Laser angioplasty for limb salvage: observations on early results. *J Vasc Surg*. 1989;10:29–38.

182. Yao ST. Haemodynamic studies in peripheral arterial disease. *Br J Surg*. 1970;57:761–766.

183. Zahavi J, Zahavi M. Enhanced platelet release reaction, shortened platelet survival time, and increased platelet aggregation and plasma thromboxane B_2 in chronic obstructive arterial disease. *Thromb Haemost.* 1985;53: 105–109.

184. Zeitler E. Primary and late results of percutaneous trans- luminal angioplasty (PTA) in iliac and femoro-popliteal obliterations. *Int Angiol.* 1984;4:81–85.

185. Zeitler E. Transluminal catheter dilatation: indications, technical aspects, results. *Int Angiol.* 1986;5:137–150.

186. Zeitler E, Richter EI, Roth F-J. Results of percutaneous transluminal angioplasty. *Radiology.* 1982;146:57–60.

43

Embolic Arterial Occlusion

Sibu P. Saha

Embolic arterial occlusion is a common vascular surgical problem whose incidence[1,5] appears to be increasing. This apparent increase in incidence has been attributed to better diagnosis and a larger number of elderly patients with cardiovascular diseases. There are many sources and causes of emboli in the arterial system:

1. *Arterial embolism of cardiac origin.* Approximately 80% of all emboli originate in the heart. Rheumatic heart disease used to be a frequent cause of arterial embolism of cardiac origin. Currently, atrial fibrillation, myocardial infarction, ventricular aneurysm, and cardiomyopathy are the main causes of cardiac emboli. Other cardiac causes include valvular heart disease, prosthetic cardiac valve, subacute bacterial endocarditis,[21] and myxomas of the heart.
2. *Arterial embolism of arterial origin.* The well-known arterial source of emboli is aneurysm, mostly abdominal and popliteal[1] aneurysms; however, embolization from other sites of arterial aneurysms has been reported. An increasing number of embolic problems secondary to severe ulcerative atheromatous lesions of the descending thoracic and abdominal aorta have also been reported. Microembolism secondary to cholesterol or atherothrombotic particles is called atheroembolism.[8,10,23] The term *blue toe syndrome* is used to describe atheroembolism in the foot. The patient presents with painful toes with areas of mottled blue discoloration in the presence of palpable pedal pulses.
3. *Arterial embolism of venous origin (paradoxical embolism).*[7,11] The term *paradoxical embolism* is used to describe arterial occlusion by an embolus that originates from the deep venous system or the right heart and passes through a septal defect into systemic circulation. The patient may present with a stroke or ischemic limbs.
4. *Unusual embolism.* Embolic arterial occlusion may result from foreign particles such as a bullet[18,19] or dislodged prosthetic device. Stroke due to air embolism is a rare but well-known complication in open heart surgery.

The effect of arterial occlusion depends on the site of occlusion, the organ involved, the degree of obstruction, and the adequacy of the collateral circulation. Approximately 20% to 30% of the emboli involve the carotid or visceral arteries, and approximately 70% involve arteries of the extremities. The most frequent sites of embolism are the femoral artery, the aortoiliac segment, and the popliteal artery, respectively. Approximately 15% of emboli are reported to involve the brachial artery. Duration of ischemia has a tremendous impact on overall patient outcome. The skin and subcutaneous tissue seem to tolerate ischemia longer than the muscles and nerves. Ischemia of extremities over 4 to 6 hours (golden period) is very poorly tolerated. Early interventions improve limb salvage and patient survival rates. Prompt administration of heparin prevents propagation of clots to collaterals and in many cases allows expansion of the golden period.

Acute arterial occlusion causes local and systemic complications. Among the local complications, muscle necrosis remains the most serious problem. Awareness of reperfusion injury[14,22] that follows revascularization is important. The suspected offender is toxic oxygen free radicals. Endothelial swelling and sludging of microcirculation with blood cells and particles also contribute to progressive muscle necrosis after reperfusion. Toxic metabolites released from a reperfused ischemic limb may cause metabolic acidosis, hyperkalemia, and renal failure, which is often described as myonephropathic metabolic syndrome. This syndrome remains the primary cause of high mortality rates in elderly patients with peripheral embolism. In some cases, severe arterial ischemia results in venous thrombosis, perhaps due to sluggish flow or damaged intima of the veins in an ischemic area. Venous thrombosis may aggravate limb ischemia or cause pulmonary embolism.

Diagnosis

The five classic signs and symptoms of acute arterial embolus in a limb are pain, pulselessness, pallor, paresthesia, and paralysis. Patients should undergo a comprehensive evaluation with special focus on cardiac evaluation and examination of the limb with a Doppler echocardiogram. Rutherford et al.[17] have recommended categorization of acute limb ischemia into three groups: viable, threatened viability, and reversible ischemic changes. This type of assessment is very helpful in initiating appropriate treatment in a timely manner. Differential diagnosis[4] of emboli arterial occlusion includes arterial thrombosis, acute aortic dissection, and low output syndrome. Patients with thrombosis are often older, and the onset of symptoms is usually gradual. They often give a history of claudication, and the area of ischemia is poorly demarcated. Angiogram usually reveals diffuse atheromatous disease with well-developed collaterals. Patients with emboli are usually young, and the onset is sudden; angiogram shows a sharp area of demarcation (Figure 43.1) and a sharp cutoff in an otherwise fairly normal vessel with very few collaterals. Patients with

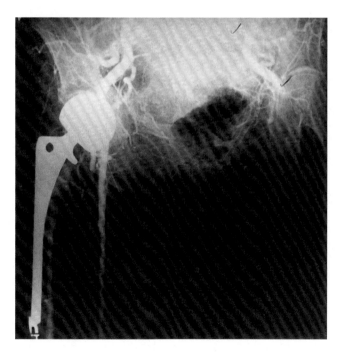

FIGURE 43.1. Angiogram that shows multiple emboli (left femoral, left internal iliac, and right profunda femoris arteries).

acute aortic dissection often give a history of hypertension and sudden severe back pain that radiates downward. Computed tomography and magnetic resonance imaging are extremely helpful in establishing a diagnosis of acute aortic dissection.

Treatment

Surgical treatment[24] for embolic arterial occlusion has been popular since the introduction of the balloon-tip Fogarty[6] catheter in 1963. Use of this instrument has brought a remarkable improvement in limb salvage and patient survival. However, a recent report has indicated that mortality and morbidity rates have not declined in the last 10 to 15 years. This may be due to a patient population of advancing age with multiple organ dysfunction. As soon as the diagnosis of acute arterial ischemia is made, patients should be given heparin and a complete evaluation should be carried out promptly. The laboratory tests should include a complete blood count, chemistry-24, chest x-ray, arterial blood gases, coagulation profile, blood type, and cross-matching. An echocardiogram[2] may give a clue to the origin of this embolus. Noninvasive Doppler examination is essential to categorize the limb ischemia as described by Rutherford.[17] We recommend placement of a Swan–Ganz catheter and arterial line in all critically ill patients and also in patients with a history of cardiac disease. This approach provides necessary hemodynamic information for perioperative management.

Transfemoral embolectomy[9] is performed under local anesthesia for iliac and femoral embolism. Both femoral arteries are exposed in patients with saddle emboli.[3] Completion angiography is undertaken when blood flow is fully restored. Popliteal embolism is approached through an infrapopliteal incision through which the clots from all trifurcation vessels can be retrieved successfully. In rare cases, distal tibial embolectomy[25] is performed. Surgical embolectomy is cost-effective and more successful than thrombolytic therapy.[12,15] In rare cases, intraoperative thrombolytic therapy[13] may be beneficial when all of the emboli cannot be retrieved by balloon catheter. The brachial artery cutdown technique[16] is often used for upper extremity embolism; proper perioperative care is very important to patient survival. Patients are administered low doses of heparin[20] for the first 2 to 3 days or until fully coumadinized. Thrombolytic therapy (Figure 43.2) is advocated in a limited number of patients in whom operative risk would be prohibitive. Patients with irreversible ischemia should undergo prompt primary amputation to avoid the metabolic consequences of massive tissue necrosis. In spite of all the advances, limb loss remains in the range of 10% to 15%, and the mortality rate is about 10% to 20%.

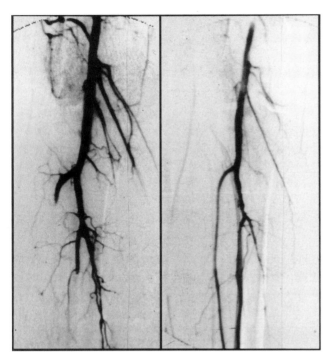

Pre   **Post**

FIGURE 43.2. Angiogram showing successful thrombolytic therapy for embolic occlusion of trifurcation vessels.

Acknowledgment

I greatly appreciate the assistance of Ms. Connie Powell in the preparation of this chapter.

References

1. Abbott WM, Maloney RD, McCabe CC, Lee CE, Wirthlin LS. Arterial embolisms: a 44 year perspective. *Am J Surg.* 1982;143:460–464.

2. Aschenberg W, Schulter M, Kremer P, Schroder E, Siglow V, Bleifield W. Transesophageal two-dimensional echocardiography for the detection of left atrial appendage thrombus. *J Am Coll Cardiol.* 1956;7:163–166.

3. Busuttil RW, Keehn G, Milliken J, et al. Aortic saddle embolus. *Ann Surg.* 1983;197:698–706.

4. Dale WA. Differential management of acute peripheral arterial ischemia. *J Vasc Surg.* 1984;1:269–278.

5. Elliot JP, Hagerman JH, Szilagyi E, Ramakrishman V, Bravo JJ, Smith RF. Arterial embolization: problems of source, multiplicity, recurrence, and delayed treatment. *Surgery.* 1980;88:833–845.

6. Fogarty TJ, Krause RJ, Hafner CD. A method for extraction of arterial emboli and thrombi. *Surgery, Gynecology and Obstetrics.* 1963;116:241–244.

7. Gazzangia AB, Dalen JE. Paradoxical embolism: its pathophysiology and clinical recognition. *Ann Surg.* 1970;171: 137–142.

8. Kaufman JL, Stark K, Brolin RE. Disseminated atheroembolism from extensive degenerative atherosclerosis of the aorta. *Surgery.* 1987;102:63–70.

9. Kendrick J, Thompson BW, Read RC, Campbell GS, Walls RC, Casali RE. Arterial embolectomy in the leg. *Am J Surg.* 1981;142:739–743.

10. Kwaan JH, Molen RV, Stemmer EA, Connolly JE. Peripheral embolism resulting from unsuspected atheromatous aortic plaque. *Surgery.* 1975;78:583–588.

11. Laughlin RA, Mandel SA. Paradoxical embolization: case report and review of the literature. *Arch Surg.* 1977;112: 648–650.

12. Nilsson L, Albrechtsson U, Jonung T, et al. Surgical treatment vs. thrombolysis in acute arterial occlusion: a randomized controlled study. *European Journal of Vascular Surgery.* 1992;6:189–193.

13. Parent FN, Bernhard VM, Pabst TS, McIntyre KE, Hunter GC, Malone JM. Fibrinolytic treatment of residual thrombus after catheter embolectomy for severe lower limb ischemia. *J Vasc Surg.* 1989;9:153–160.

14. Perry MO, Fantini G. Ischemia, profile of an enemy: reperfusion injury of skeletal muscle. *J Vasc Surg.* 1987;6: 231–234.

15. Porter JM, Taylor LM. Current status of thrombolytic therapy. *J Vasc Surg.* 1985;2:239–249.

16. Ricotta JJ, Scudder PA, McAndrew JA, Deweese JA, May AJ. Management of acute ischemia of the upper extremity. *Am J Surg.* 1983;145:661–666.

17. Rutherford RB, Flanigan DP, Gupta SK, et al. Suggested standards for reports dealing with lower extremity ischemia. *J Vasc Surg.* 1986;64:80–94.

18. Shannon JJ, Nghia MV, Stanton PE, Dimler M. Peripheral and arterial missile embolization: a case report and 22-year literature review. *J Vasc Surg.* 1987;5:773–778.

19. Symbas PN, Harlaftis N. Bullet emboli in the pulmonary and systemic arteries. *Ann Surg.* 1977;185:318–320.

20. Tawes RL, Beare JP, Scribner RG, Sydorak GR, Brown WH, Harris EJ. Value of postoperative heparin therapy in peripheral arterial thromboembolism. *Am J Surg.* 1983;146: 213–215.

21. Vo NM, Russell JC, Becker DR. Mycotic emboli of the peripheral vessels: analysis of forty-four cases. *Surgery.* 1981; 90:541–545.

22. Walker PM, Lindsay TF, Labbe R, Mickle DA, Romaschin AD. Salvage of skeletal muscle with free radical scavengers. *J Vasc Surg.* 1987;5:68–72.

23. Williams GM, Harrington D, Burdick J, White RI. Mural thrombus of the aorta: an important, frequently neglected cause of large peripheral emboli. *Ann Surg.* 1981;194: 737–744.

24. Yeager RA, Moneta GL, Taylor LM, Hamre DW, McConnell DB, Porter JM. Surgical management of severe acute lower extremity ischemia. *J Vasc Surg.* 1992;15: 385–393.

25. Youckey JR, Clagett GP, Cabellon S, Eddleman WL, Salander JM, Rich NM. Thromboembolectomy of arteries explored at the ankle. *Ann Surg.* 1984;199:367–371.

44

Thromboangiitis Obliterans

Hisao Masaki and Tatsuki Katsumura

Thromboangiitis obliterans (TAO) is a typical chronic arterial obstruction similar to arteriosclerosis obliterans that forms thrombi in the appendicular peripheral arteries and veins. Its causes remain unknown.

The disease was named *endarteritis* in 1878 by von Winiwarter,[1] who found hyperplastic wall and angiostenosis of arteries in the amputated limb of a 57-year-old male patient with chronic arterial obstruction of the lower extremities. Buerger,[2] who found acute angiitis with thrombogenesis in the arteries of 11 amputated limbs in 1908 and acute phase lesions of veins in 1909, defined TAO as a unit of disease that resulted in angiostenosis due to thrombus formation following changes in the vascular wall.[3] Although TAO had been studied mainly histopathologically, its relation to arteriosclerosis was then discussed. In 1960 Wessler et al.[4] investigated the age at onset of these diseases, appearance of the clinical symptoms of arteriosclerosis, and lack of cases with characteristic acute lesions in TAO; they consequently suggested that the existence of the disease was questionable. However, later studies confirmed the existence of juvenile peripheral artery obstruction with proliferative and inflammatory changes different from arteriosclerosis or thrombosis. Therefore, most of the angiologists in Asia and Europe and many of those in the United States categorize TAO as an independent unit of disease.

Pathophysiology

In Japan, TAO occurs more frequently in men than in women (8:1), and the age at onset ranges from the third to fifth decades. The disease accounts for only a small percentage of chronic arterial obstructions in the United States and Europe. Although in Japan the incidence of TAO previously was higher than that of arteriosclerosis obliterans, recent data show either no marked changes or a tendency toward fewer cases of TAO with the rapid increase in arteriosclerosis obliterans.[5]

The pathogenesis of TAO remains unknown, although bacterial infection, changes in blood components, allergy, autoimmunity, and abnormal hormone levels have been discussed as possible causes of the disease. Because TAO occurs more frequently in smokers and laborers, the pathological findings of angiitis peculiar to this disease may result from vascular disorder caused by repeated dull trauma to the extremities; damage of vascular endothelium, an increase in blood coagulability, and hypofibrinolysis, which lead to thrombus formation in those who smoke; and involvement of an autoimmune mechanism. Smoking is noted as a causative or deteriorative factor. Both passive and active smoking make therapeutic effects insignificant.[6]

Buerger classified TAO into the following three stages according to the histopathological features:

Stage I: acute cell filtration spreading to the whole tunicae of vessels, effusion, appearance of giant cells, and thrombus formation

Stage II: disappearance of acute inflammation and organization of thrombus

Stage III: hyperplasia of the tunica intima and connective tissues in and around the arterial wall

Hyperplasia of the intima, inflammatory cell filtration in the media and adventitia, and repeated contraction probably develop during onset. A thrombus is then formed in the primary stage, followed by organization of the thrombus, recanalization, destruction of the interior elastic tunica, and increased inflammatory cell filtration; as a result, penetrating thromboangiitis occurs. Arterial lesions are commonly found in the muscular arteries of the legs, but some arterial obstructions are also found in the upper limbs, particularly in the forearms. Approximately 40% of patients with TAO have three to four affected limbs (Table 44.1).

TABLE 44.1. Summary of the diagnostic criteria for thromboangiitis obliterans.

1. Arterial obstruction is found in a lower limb or several limbs including a lower limb.
2. Thromboangiitis obliterans occurs frequently in men, with an age at onset of less then 40 years.
3. Many of the patients are smokers at the time of onset or have a history of smoking.
4. Multiple segmented obstructions are observed in the peripheral main arteries of the lower limb (not larger than popliteal artery) by arteriography.
5. Patients with migrating phlebitis (or a history of it) are frequently observed.
6. No findings of arteriosclerotic changes or diabetes are generally observed.

Clinical Features and Their Bases

The system created by Fontaine,[7] a vascular surgeon in France, is used for the pathological classification of chronic arterial obstruction. The degree of ischemia becomes more severe from grade I to grade IV.

Grade I: Slight Ischemia in Skin

When the blood supply decreases, skin becomes pale and cold. Persistent arterial obstruction causes vascular relaxation at sites peripheral to the obstruction, and congestion with venous obstruction and finally cyanosis develop. Because of the capillarectasia caused by arterial obstruction, slowed blood flow, and congestion, acromelic skin often turns reddish-violet.

Grade II: Intermittent Claudication

Because arterial obstruction prevents the increase in muscular blood flow needed during exercise, metabolites caused by anaerobic metabolism accumulate. Muscle pain then occurs but disappears after exercise is stopped. This symptom is frequently observed in the legs because peripheral arterial obstruction commonly develops in patients with TAO.

Grade III: Rest Pain

In grade III chronic arterial obstruction, patients have severe pain in their fingers and toes while sleeping.

Grade IV: Ulcer and Gangrene

Ulcer and gangrene are induced by acromelic nutritional disorders due to ischemia, trauma, and infection (Figure 44.1). In TAO, small ulcers tend to develop in fingers and toes during a relatively early stage.

Migrating Phlebitis

In migrating phlebitis inflammatory lesions are observed in both extremital veins and extremital arteries. This thrombophlebitis develops mainly in the superficial veins of lower limbs: indurations develop along the veins

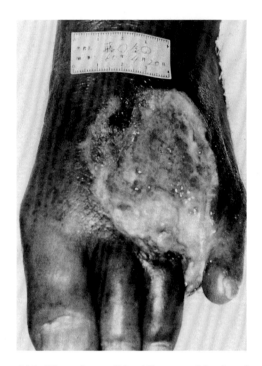

FIGURE 44.1. Thromboangiitis obliterans with ulcer formation on the dorsalis portion of the left foot.

and inflammation is found on the skin above them, accompanied by pain. Because these lesions disappear in 2 to 3 weeks (except for dermal pigmentation) but recur at different sites, the disease is referred to as *migrating phlebitis*. Migrating phlebitis is observed in about half of all patients with TAO and occurs either before or during development of the arterial lesions. The period during which the disease is observed is considered an active state of the angiitis; therefore, the progression of TAO must be carefully noted before it is treated.

Diagnostic Tests

Results of Physical Tests

Palpation of a Peripheral Artery

Palpation of a peripheral artery for the existence of a pulse is the most basic and simplest test to determine obstructed sites.

Lower Limb Elevating and Descending Tests

In lower limb elevating and descending tests, patients who are in a dorsal position perform bending and stretching exercises of their toes for 30 to 60 seconds; both lower limbs are elevated before the color tone of the soles is compared. Normal limbs show normal color, and affected limbs turn pale. This test is fairly clear and reliable. After the elevation test, patients sit on the edge of a bed and let their limbs hang down. Whereas normal limbs turn reddish in about 10 seconds, color may not return to the affected limbs for some time. Finally, affected limbs flush when they are kept down. Because this tendency is promoted by decreased venous reflux, the latter finding is not so clear and reliable as the former.

Blood Flowmetry

Ultrasonic Doppler Flowmetry

Ultrasonic Doppler flowmetry uses the Doppler effect for blood flowmetry. Because the instrument is inexpensive and easy to operate, it is the most frequently used technique in medical institutions that treat vascular disease.

A probe connected with the instrument is percutaneously applied to a vessel at an angle of 45 to 60 degrees to the direction of the blood flow and measures at the position where the strongest sounds are audible. Normal sounds reveal regular beats in accordance with pulses, whereas in obstruction more central than where the measurement was taken, beats disappear and a murmur is audible. An experienced researcher can thus determine whether lesions are present by the difference in tone quality alone. The method is usually used for measuring blood pressure and analyzing both flow rate and waveform but can be utilized more easily for measuring blood pressure.[8]

Pressure Measurement

As shown in Figure 44.2, a blood pressure cuff is wrapped around the ankle, and through a Doppler probe a plateau wave is observed. Because blood pressure is measured in the dorsal artery of the foot, it is called ankle blood pressure; its ratio to systolic pressure is called the ankle pressure index. Normal values range between 1.0 and 1.2, values less than 1.0 (particularly less than 0.9) may be due to arterial stenosis or obstruction, and values less than 0.3 suggest a severe decrease in blood flow. In addition, the blood pressure cuff may be wrapped around the thigh or calf to estimate lesion site and measure blood pressure at those sites.

Analysis of Flow Velocity Waveform

As shown in Figure 44.3, type 0 shows normal flow; type I presents moderate stenosis; type II shows severe stenosis;

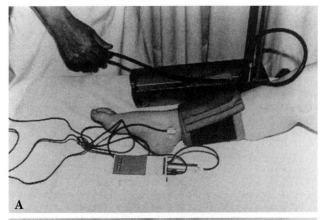

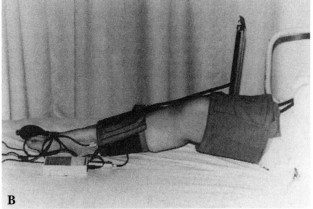

FIGURE 44.2. Measurement of ankle blood pressure and thigh blood pressure using Doppler flowmetry. **A,** Ankle blood pressure. **B,** Ankle and thigh blood pressure.

and type III demonstrates the obstruction existing more centrally than the measurement site. Ultrasound Doppler flowmetry is useful for qualitative analysis.

Other diagnostic methods include the pulsed-wave Doppler system to diagnose whether lesions are present and, in combination with ultrasound and tomography, to determine the extent of the lesions by examining the changes in blood flow rates.

Volume Pulse Wave

Cardiac conduction causes a wave in inner arteries. The wave is a volume pulse wave, which is mainly measured at the tips of fingers or toes. Photoplethysmography (Figure 44.4) is used most frequently to determine volume pulse wave, although other forms of plethysmography are available. For example, a certain light is applied to the tip of the finger, and then the changes in blood content in the site are determined according to the changes in the amount of transmitted or reflected light.

A normal pulse wave, as seen in Figure 44.5, has a sharply elevated wave, whereas lesions located more centrally than the site measured produce a wave of lower height and ultimately a plateau wave. However, because

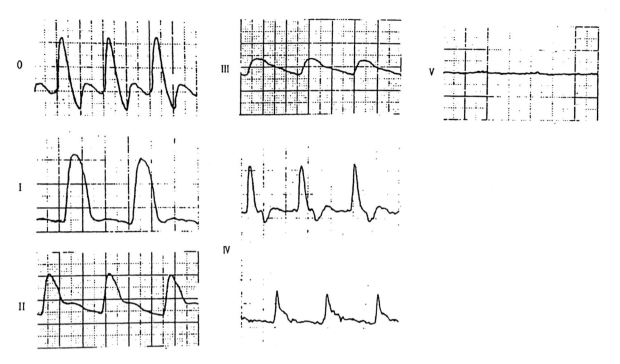

FIGURE 44.3. Doppler flow velocity waveform.

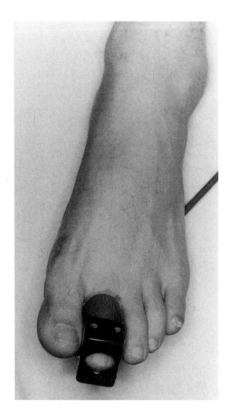

FIGURE 44.4. Photoplethysmography.

the pulse wave is affected by factors such as cardiac output, diagnosis should be made after the waves obtained from the toes of normal and affected limbs are compared. Therefore, a strain gauge, which detects the changes in flow volume, may have some advantages for reactive hyperemia studies.

Thermography

Thermography represents the changes in dermal temperature as an image according to a principle of infrared radiation. Inhibited blood flow decreases dermal blood flow, which is accompanied by a decline in dermal temperature; the image thus turns green or blue. However, when dermal temperature rises, or blood flow increases, the image turns red. Thermography is affected by factors such as temperature, environment, and mental state, and consequently dermal blood flow can change. Therefore the analysis should be performed in a controlled environment such as a thermoregulated room; otherwise, its diagnostic value is limited. It is suitable for investigating a drug's efficacy in a patient as well.

Arteriography

Arteriography is essential not only for definitive diagnosis of TAO but also for selection of a surgical technique suitable for its treatment, including arterial reconstruction (Figures 44.6 and 44.7). TAO has characteristic

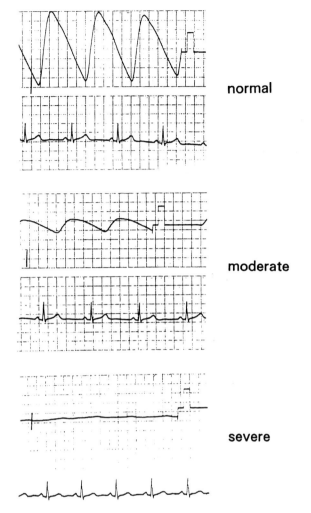

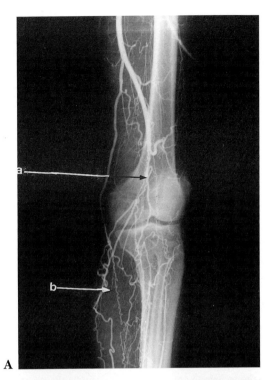

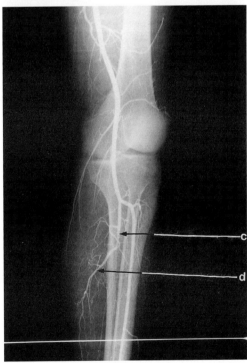

FIGURE 44.5. Moderate occlusive lesions or severe stenosis lesions located in a more centrally located site than the site at which measurements were taken. Severe occlusive lesions located in the proximal site.

findings on arteriography that include abrupt, tapering, and corkscrew images (Table 44.2).

Therapy

Without strict instructions lifestyle changes, treatment may be ineffectual even if drug therapy or reconstruction of blood vessels is undertaken. Discussions about lifestyle should include the following instructions:

1. Do not smoke and avoid secondhand smoke (in the home, office, vehicle, and so on).
2. Keep the whole body, especially the affected limbs, warm.
3. Clean the affected limbs and protect them from trauma.
4. Walk regularly for exercise.

FIGURE 44.6. Femoral arteriogram. **1,** Left femoral arteriogram demonstrates occlusion of the left popliteal artery. **A,** Abrupt appearance. **B,** Corkscrew appearance. **2,** Left femoral arteriogram demonstrates occlusion of the left posterior tibial artery. **C,** Tapering appearance. **D,** Tree root appearance.

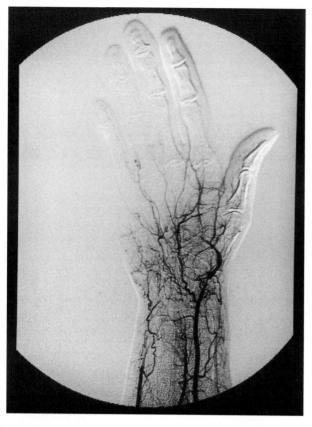

FIGURE 44.7. Arteriogram of right upper limbs demonstrates occlusion of the ulnar and digital arteries.

Guidelines for Treatment

The previously mentioned Fontaine's classification based on the extent of inhibition of blood flow is convenient to select the most appropriate therapy for chronic arterial obstruction.

Fontaine's Grade I

Drugs are administered orally for about 3 months; if symptoms do not improve or instead deteriorate, drugs should be administered intravenously for 2 to 3 weeks. When no improvement is observed, surgical treatment should be considered; however, drug therapy is usually effective for the symptoms in this grade.

Fontaine's Grade II

Medication is administered orally for patients with slight symptoms (intermittent claudication >300 meters). When the symptoms remain stable or worsen, angiography is warranted. Blood vessels should be reconstructed if possible, and medication is administered intravenously if reconstruction is impossible because of peripheral vascular lesions.

For severe cases (intermittent claudication <200 meters), surgery is considered the best treatment. After angiography is performed, vessels are reconstructed when the operation is thought to be possible; if impossible, drugs should be administered orally or intravenously.

TABLE 44.2. Differential diagnosis for thromboangiitis obliterans and arteriosclerosis obliterans.

	Thromboangiitis obliterans	Arteriosclerosis obliterans
Age at onset	Usually less than 40	Usually more than 40
Sex	Mostly male	Male > Female
Race	Asians, Jews	No difference
Smoking	Deteriorating factor (strongly related)	Deteriorating factor
Wounds	Joint flexion sites	Not related
Cold changes	Yes	Yes
Major symptoms	Ulcer and necrosis	Intermittent claudication
Migrating phlebitis	About 20%–40%	No
Sites of lesions	Medium- and small-caliber arteries (popliteal, tibial, radial, and ulnar arteries)	Large- and medium-caliber arteries (aorta to popliteal artery and subclavian artery to brachial artery)
	Lower limbs > upper limbs	Mainly lower limbs
	Occasionally more than three limbs	Usually one to two limbs
	Usually segmented, peripheral	Continued. discontinued
	Wide range	Central
Diabetes	Not related	20%–40%
Hyperlipidemia	Not related	Yes
Hypertension	Rare	Yes
Vascular lesions in other organs	Rare	Yes
Arteriography	Abrupt	Moth eaten
	Tapering	Stenosis
	Corkscrew	Calcification

Fontaine's Grades III and IV

For patients with grades III and IV chronic arterial obstruction, surgical treatment is necessary. After angiography, blood circulation is rerouted if possible; if impossible because of severe peripheral lesions, a sympathectomy is performed or drugs are administered orally or intravenously.

Medical Treatment

Drugs

Prostaglandin E₁–CD

Prostaglandin E_1–CD (PGE_1) is the injection most commonly used and has both vasodilative and platelet aggregation inhibitory effects. Although it is effectively administered intravenously, for severe cases it is administered by continuous arterial injection. Side effects may include phlebitis.

Lipo-PGE₁

Most PGE_1 is quickly inactivated in the pulmonary circulation. Lipo-PGE_1 contains PGE_1 in fat particles in lipid emulsion to prevent inactivation. Its main advantages are that it is long acting and can be administered with one intravenous injection.[9]

Argatroban

Argatroban is an anticoagulant that selectively inhibits thrombin and also has a platelet aggregation inhibitory effect.

Batroxobin

Batroxobin is a snake venom formulation that decreases blood viscosity by decreasing fibrinogen level and as a result improves microcirculation.

Sodium Veraprost

Sodium veraprost, a prostacyclin derivative, has strong vasodilative and platelet aggregation inhibitory effects. It is the drug used most commonly in this situation.

Ticlopidine

Ticlopidine is a cyclic adenosine monophosphate phosphodiesterase inhibitor that has both vasodilative and platelet aggregation inhibitory effects.

Cilostazol

Cilostazol is thought to inhibit the function of fibrinogen receptors on the activated human platelets without changing cyclic adenosine monophosphate levels in them. The drug thus has a strong platelet aggregation inhibitory effect.

Selection of Drugs

Because a variety of drugs are available, how and which drugs are selected remain controversial issues. Because the symptoms of inhibited blood circulation due to chronic arterial obstruction are caused by the reduction of blood flow, increasing blood flow is most important for improvement of the symptoms; therefore, a drug with a vasodilative effect should be selected. However, like PGE_1, the drugs with vasodilative effects occasionally result in the steal phenomenon, which is found especially in patients with Fontaine's grade III or IV chronic arterial obstruction. In our investigations, the steal phenomenon was observed in severe cases with bilateral lesions. The causes still remain unknown, although some have tried to elucidate them by using angiography. To discover the steal phenomenon as quickly as possible, changes in the blood flow in toes and dermal temperature measured by thermography are determined after PGE_1 is administered; we then select a suitable drug. When PGE_1 treatment increases blood flow, a drug in the prostaglandin group is selected; if blood flow decreases, a drug without vasodilative effect is chosen. Molecular markers in the aggregation and fibrinogenolysis systems should be determined by a simultaneous blood examination to select an appropriate drug. If such a measuring instrument is not available, PGE_1 should be given first. If side effects of PGE_1 including pain occur or no improvement is observed after PGE_1 is administered for 2 weeks, a different drug should be tried.

Surgical Treatment

Bypass

Femoropopliteal bypass or femorotibial bypass is performed in patients with TAO. Because bypass is intended mainly for areas below the knees due to the specificity of the disease, autologous vein is generally used for grafting. If autologous vein is not available because it has a caliber of less than 4 mm or migrating phlebitis is present, the use of an artificial vessel made of Goretex or Dacron may be necessary. For reconstruction using autologous vein, reverse and in situ methods are available. In the latter, the venous valve must be split with a valvulotome. When a very long bypass is needed, the in situ method is performed because a difference in caliber between the graft and artery occurs in the reverse method. Because the in situ method is used only if the operated limb has an intact great saphenous vein, which may be unlikely due to migrating phlebitis, it must be determined whether the vein is suitable for grafting.[10] In the reverse method, a venous graft can be obtained from either the operated limb, the other lower limb, or the upper limbs; veins from the upper limbs occasionally must be formed into one graft with venous–venous anastomosis. If a venous graft cannot be obtained, a composite of the graft and an artificial vessel is used.

Sympathectomy

Sympathectomy is used in patients who are unable to undergo blood vessel reconstruction and have rest pain or ulcer to increase cutaneous blood flow. Because it increases cutaneous but not muscular blood flow, sympathectomy is not effective in patients with intermittent claudication.

In lumbar sympathectomy, the second to fourth sympathetic ganglions are resected. Dysspermia, which is especially common in bilateral sympathectomy of the first sympathetic ganglion, may occur postoperatively. Thoracic sympathectomy is used in removing the second and third thoracic sympathetic ganglions as well as the lower one third of the satellite ganglion. Recently it has been performed with a thoracoscope.

Amputation

Amputation is indicated in patients whose limbs are necrotic or who have intractable ulcers that do not improve by any treatment. These patients usually require minor rather than major amputation.

Others

Thromboendarterectomy is frequently performed in patients with arteriosclerosis obliterans but not in patients with TAO, because few lesions are localized in TAO and after thromboendarterectomy the lesions often remain, increasing reobstruction rates. At present, endovascular surgery, such as percutaneous transluminal angioplasty or laser angioplasty, which was recently used in patients with arteriosclerosis obliterans, is rarely indicated in patients with TAO because of the presence of diffuse lesions.

References

1. Winiwarter F. Uber eine eigenthumliche Form von Endarteritis und Endphlebitis mit Gangran des Fusses. *Archiv Für Klinische Chirurgie*. 1878;23:202–226.
2. Buerger L. Thrombo-angiitis obliterans: a study leading to presenile spontaneous gangrene. *Am J Med Sci*. 1908;136: 567–580.
3. Buerger L. The association of migrating thrombophlebitis with thromboangiitis obliterans. *International Clinics*. 1909; 19:84–105.
4. Wessler S, Ming SC, Gurewich V, Freiman DG. A critical evaluation of thromboangiitis obliterans: the case against Buerger's disease. *N Engl J Med*. 1960;262:1149–1162.
5. Katsumura T, Masaki H. Buerger disease [in Japanese]. *Sogorinsho*. 1992;41:888–892.
6. Shionoya S. Buerger's disease. In: Shionoya S, ed. *Pathology, Diagnosis, and Treatment*. Nagoya, Japan: University of Nagoya Press; 1990:38.
7. Fontaine R, Kim M, Kieny R. Die Chirurgische Behandlung der peripheren Durchblutungsstorungen. *Helvetica Chirurgica Acta*. 1954;21:499–533.
8. Kathumura T, Masaki H. Therapy of peripheral arterial occlusive disease in foot [in Japanese]. *Orthopaedics*. 1990;31: 79–88.
9. Masaki H, Katsumura T, Fujiwara T, Miyake T. Clinical evaluation of the effect of lipoPGE$_1$ on peripheral circulation in patients with chronic arterial occlusive disease. *J Jpn Coll Angiol*. 1994;34:419–424.
10. Katsumura T, Masaki H. Surgical treatment of chronic arterial occlusive disease [in Japanese]. *Geka*. 1985;27: 176–181.

Section 3
Visceral Arterial Occlusion

45

Visceral Arterial Obstructive Disease

Raymond A. Dieter, George Kuzycz, Ray A. Dieter, III, and Robert Dieter

The gastrointestinal tract makes up a large portion of the intracavitary abdominal organs. The arterial and venous supply of the lower esophagus, stomach, duodenum, small bowel, and colon seldom cause major ischemic problems. However, major ischemic problems are cause for significant concern when they occur on an acute basis. The chronic vascular obstructive process is much less dramatic and may go unnoticed until profound effects (e.g., weight loss and abdominal pain) take place. The liver, pancreas, and spleen may also have occlusive vascular disease on both arterial and venous bases. We concentrate in this chapter on the gastrointestinal tract and to a lesser degree on the liver and pancreas.

The etiology of these problems may be classified in a number of ways. The acute process, as seen with an embolus, is very dramatic. The chronic process may be more subtle and more difficult to diagnose. Table 45.1 lists a number of the etiological causes for intestinal arterial obstructive problems.

The symptomatology depends on the artery involved and the structure thus affected. Therefore, the celiac artery occlusive phenomenon is usually a chronic progressive problem and creates upper abdominal pain and postprandial difficulties due to gastric involvement. Bending, stretching, sagging, or occlusion of the superior mesenteric artery may create another set of complaints. Inferior mesenteric artery occlusion on a chronic basis due to aneurysmal formation and thrombosis may progress without any symptomatology at all. However, in the acute situation (such as a ligature) patients may develop ischemic colitis including gangrene with secondary slough that requires colostomy and colectomy.

Because of the uncommon nature of visceral vascular occlusive processes no individual treats a large series of these patients. Standardized operative techniques have not been well publicized, and reconstructive surgery has been rather uncommon for these syndromes. The surgical correction depends to a great extent on whether the diagnosis is made preoperatively, intraoperatively, or postoperatively. Further, a vascular surgeon may not always be available to perform the corrective procedure. The surgical procedures performed for visceral obstructive symptoms include both resectional and reconstructive surgery.

Anatomy of the Abdominal Visceral Arteries

The aorta provides the major vascular supply of the intra-abdominal organs. The visceral branches of the abdominal aorta that supply these organs include the celiac trunk, the superior mesenteric artery, the inferior mesenteric artery, and the middle suprarenal, renal, testicular, and ovarian branches. The first three vessels and their branches (the celiac trunk and the superior and inferior mesenteric arteries) are unpaired vessels, whereas the middle suprarenal, renal, testicular, and ovarian arteries are paired vessels. The terminal branches of the aorta, the iliac vessels, provide the vascular supply to the organs of the pelvis and the lower extremities and are also paired.

The celiac axis (trunk) arises from the aorta just below the aortic hiatus of the diaphragm (Figure 45.1). This arcuate ligament, or muscular anatomy, helps define the level of the celiac artery. It is a short, thick vessel and usually measures approximately 8 mm (7–15 mm) in diameter. It arises just below the entrance of the aorta into the abdomen and is flanked by the celiac ganglia and the crus of the diaphragm. After a length of only 1 to 2 cm, the celiac artery usually divides into three branches: the hepatic, the left gastric, and the splenic arteries. Congenital anomalies, such as the left gastric artery arising from the aorta or from the hepatic or splenic arteries, may occur. The hepatic artery may also arise from

TABLE 45.1. Visceral arterial obstructive etiologies.

Arteriosclerosis obliterans
Most common
Celiac artery
Superior mesenteric artery
Inferior mesenteric artery

Embolus: usually superior mesenteric artery

Thrombosis
Aortic
Small-vessel aneurysms

Vascular dissection
With aortic
Spontaneous (superior mesenteric artery)

Iatrogenic
Celiac artery (usually with no symptoms) concomitant to tumor
    surgery
Superior mesenteric artery, especially after pancreatic surgery with
    small bowel gangrene
Inferior mesenteric, at the time of aneurysm surgery
Midcolic: colon slough
Splenic: infarct of spleen
Hepatic: liver necrosis
Vessel dissection: during stent placement angioplasty or tumor
    catheter insertion

Anatomic
Median arcuate (celiac axis compression) syndrome
Neurofibromatosis
Radiation
Congenital hypoplasia/coarctation

Nonocclusive ischemia
Cardiac
Steal

Other
Systemic lupus
Rheumatoid arthritis
Allergic vasculitis
Possibly fibromuscular hypertrophy

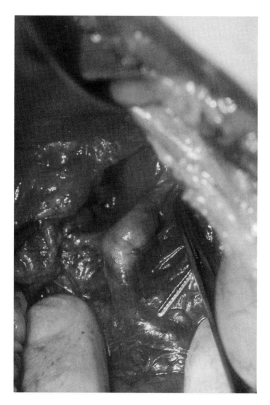

FIGURE 45.1. Celiac axis with poststenotic dilatation.

the aorta, and the splenic artery may rarely arise from the aorta or the superior mesenteric artery. Rarely are the celiac trunk and the superior mesenteric arteries combined. The first branch of the celiac axis is usually the left gastric artery (a vessel 5 mm in diameter), the smallest branch of the celiac trunk. It supplies the cardioesophageal, ventral, and dorsal branches of the left gastric artery. On occasion, an aberrant left hepatic artery may arise from the left gastric artery; this possibility should be considered when ligating the left gastric artery or infusing intrahepatic chemotherapy.

The next celiac branch, the hepatic artery, usually measures about 7 mm in diameter (Figure 45.2). This artery courses along the head of the pancreas to the portal triad and then parallels the common bile duct and the portal vein into the hilum of the liver, giving off the right and left hepatic arteries from the common hepatic artery. Behind the duodenum, it gives rise to the gastroduodenal artery as it enters the portal triad. As it travels

anterior to the portal vein, before its division into its three terminal branches (the right, left, and middle hepatic arteries), it is called the proper hepatic artery. Aberrant hepatic arteries are seen in 40% of patients. The right gastroepiploic artery takes origin from the gastroduodenal artery, which takes origin from the common hepatic artery. The right gastric artery originates from the proper hepatic artery or the distal common hepatic artery. At times, the gastroduodenal artery may arise from a hepatic artery that is the sole blood supply to one of the lobes of the liver. The gastroduodenal artery gives off the supraduodenal and retroduodenal branches, the right gastroepiploic artery, and the superior pancreaticoduodenal arteries. The right hepatic artery branches from the proper hepatic artery after the gastroduodenal branch near the porta hepatis. About one quarter of patients have aberrant right hepatic arteries with aberrant origins, including an origin from the superior mesenteric artery, aorta, celiac trunk, gastroduodenal artery, and left hepatic vessels. The right hepatic artery supplies the cystic artery (Figure 45.3). The left hepatic artery, which usually supplies the posterior liver, the caudate lobe, and the left lobe, is aberrant in 25% of patients. Most aberrant left hepatic arteries originate from the left gastric artery.

The splenic artery is the largest branch of the celiac trunk. Just after its origin, it curves slightly to the right up to the pancreas and then follows a tortuous course to

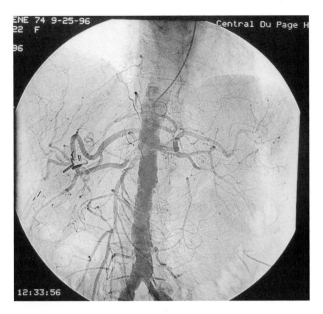

FIGURE 45.2. Angiogram demonstrating celiac, renal, and mesenteric vessels.

the left along the pancreas. The second part of the splenic artery lies in the groove of the upper part of the dorsal surface of the body of the pancreas. The splenic artery gives off branches to the pancreas and then crosses the anterior surface of the pancreas to the hilum of the spleen. The fourth portion of the splenic vessel is that portion between the pancreas and the hilum of the spleen that divides into five or more branches. The branches of the splenic artery include the pancreatic, left gastroepiploic, short gastric, and splenic branches.

The superior mesenteric artery takes origin from the anterior surface of the aorta approximately 1 to 1.5 cm below the celiac trunk in most patients. The superior mesenteric artery is a large vessel that supplies the entire

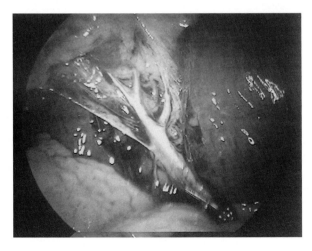

FIGURE 45.3. Cystic artery branch of right hepatic artery as visualized through laparoscope.

small intestine (except the superior, or proximal, portion of the duodenum), the cecum, the ascending colon, and approximately one half of the transverse colon. It takes origin at approximately the level of the first lumbar vertebra and is crossed at its origin by the splenic vein and the neck of the pancreas. It passes downward under the body of the pancreas over the uncinate process of the pancreas and over the transverse portion of the duodenum, through the mesentery, to supply the entire small bowel. It lies anterior to the inferior vena cava, right ureter, and iliopsoas muscles and may form large connecting arches with its own ileocolic branch. Running parallel with it is the superior mesenteric vein and a superior mesenteric neuroplexus. We have also seen the superior mesenteric artery come off of the aorta, below the level of the renal vessels, which complicates the repair of abdominal aortic aneurysms. The superior mesenteric artery branches into the inferior pancreaticoduodenal, jejunoileal, ileocolic, right colic, and middle colic vessels, which serve their respective visceral organs. Access to the superior mesenteric artery and celiac axis may be obtained through the lesser sac. Access to the superior mesenteric artery alone usually is simplified by following the mesenteric artery under the pancreas up to the aorta. Access to the celiac axis alone may be obtained through the superior approach above the lesser curvature and dissecting downward to the celiac axis in that area. A large collateral circulation may occur between the midcolic arterial branch from the superior mesenteric artery and the left colic branch of the inferior mesenteric artery (artery of Drummond).

The inferior mesenteric artery usually takes origin from the anterior lateral aspect of the aorta approximately halfway from the renal arteries to the bifurcation of the aorta into the iliac system. This is at the level of the midportion of the third lumbar vertebra and the lower border of the transverse duodenum and is about 3 to 4 cm above the iliac bifurcation. It is smaller than the superior mesenteric artery, crosses the left iliac artery medial to the left ureter, and branches into the left colic artery, sigmoid vessels, and superior rectal vessels. As mentioned, the ascending branch of the left colic artery may unite or form the marginal artery (of Drummond) to collateralize with the midcolic branch of the superior mesenteric artery. An arterial anastomotic system develops through these branches to the colon. However, a critical area of vascular anastomosis also occurs between the field supplied by the sigmoid vessels and the superior rectal vessels.[1,2]

Etiology

The etiology of visceral arterial obstructive disease may be divided into acute and chronic situations. Usually the acute patient has an associated malady (e.g., atrial fibrillation or myocardial infarction) that leads to the current symptoms. Such a patient is a candidate for the development of endocardial thrombi, which may then embolize to the extremities, brain, kidneys, or bowel (particularly the superior mesenteric artery) and require urgent diagnosis and treatment. The patient with hypertension or medial necrosis may develop aortic dissection and vascular stenosis or occlusion with resultant ischemia. Similarly, iatrogenic dissection of the celiac artery, as well as spontaneous dissection, may occur in selected patients.[3,4]

The patient with thrombosis of the aorta, particularly one that extends above the diaphragm, presents with an acute catastrophic problem including abdominal symptoms. This situation is seldom rectified even if a thrombectomy is performed. We have been unable to save patients in this situation. The embolic patient presents with acute abdominal pain and may elicit the exact time and activity level when pain began. Dissection and resection of large gastrointestinal tumors (e.g., esophagogastrectomy), in our experience, has not led to concomitant ischemic symptoms from ligation and division of the celiac axis. With congenital abnormalities ever present, the possibility of such symptoms certainly must be a consideration. We have consulted with patients who had pancreatic surgery, including Whipple's operation, and major para-aortic surgery with acute occlusion of the superior mesenteric artery. The inability to reconstruct this damaged or transected artery almost invariably leads to infarction of the small bowel and usually the demise of the patient. Other iatrogenic causes such as ligation of the inferior mesenteric artery at the time of abdominal or thoracoabdominal aneurysm surgery are possible. This has led to colectomy and colostomy formation in a number of patients.

Ligation of the midcolic artery at the time of pancreatic surgery, with secondary infarction and slough of the colon, may also occur. In our experience splenic artery ligation has not been a source of infarction of the spleen but has been reported after splenorenal bypass.[5] We have seen patients with untreatable hepatic artery ligation develop liver necrosis. Also, acute traumatic thrombosis of the mesenteric vessel in severe abdominal trauma with vessel wall damage has occurred. Lastly, acute thrombosis of small visceral artery aneurysms has caused symptomatology that requires operative intervention.

Chronic Etiologies

By far the most common etiology for visceral arterial obstruction and visceral ischemia revolves around arteriosclerosis obliterans and its progressive etiology (Figure 45.4). Despite the high frequency of atherosclerosis, symptomatic intestinal ischemia, or angina, is very un-

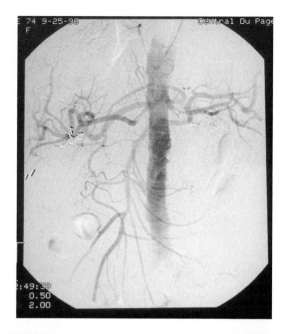

A

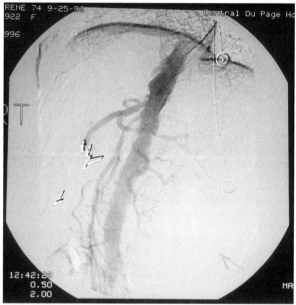

B

FIGURE 45.4. Anterioposterior and lateral views demonstrate bilateral renal and superior mesenteric artery stenosis.

common. Usually, this requires the involvement of two vessels rather than just one. Occasionally the patient is asymptomatic, and yet at autopsy all three vessels are occluded and collateral circulation had been feeding the involved viscera. These patients have usually had coexisting atherosclerotic symptomatology involving other locations, including the heart, brain, kidneys, and legs. Many of these individuals have coexisting aortic lesions or lesions of the branches of the aorta. Thus, multiple visceral arterial branches may be involved in a majority of the patients. Superior and inferior mesenteric artery occlusion alone rarely leads to symptomatology, whereas the occasional celiac artery lesion may lead to symptomatology. Chronic malabsorption rarely develops from this condition. When atherosclerotic plaques lead to chronic dissection, the renal arteries, both mesenteric arteries, and the celiac axis may be in jeopardy. Usually, inferior mesenteric artery occlusion is totally asymptomatic and may be found frequently during surgery on the aorta (for either aneurysm or occlusive disease) without pulsation, flow, or lumen.

Chronic compression of the celiac axis may lead to upper abdominal symptoms. This concern was much more common in the past than it has been more recently. The median arcuate ligament has been implicated in this etiology. We have rarely seen this problem. However, one striking example was a 47-year-old woman who benefited greatly from surgical correction of the problem. External compression by the median arcuate ligament has even been suggested to involve the superior mesenteric artery with compression. These patients are usually young, slender, and have pain as the major symptom, with weight loss being a less common symptom.

Other etiologies for the chronically afflicted patient include a chronic dissection of the aorta and congenital hypoplasia of the aorta and the visceral vessels (particularly in association with abdominal coarctation). Radiation fibrosis and neurofibromatosis have also been implicated in the etiology of this syndrome. Other reported causes of these intestinal ischemic syndromes include associated diseases such as systemic lupus erythematosus (especially difficult to treat in our experience) and rheumatoid arthritis. Fibromuscular hypertrophy has also been implicated, but little evidence of its involvement is available. Allergic vasculitis may also be a rare cause.[6]

TABLE 45.2. Arterial occlusive disease symptomatology.

Celiac artery
Celiac artery syndrome
Acute upper gastrointestinal symptomatology

Superior mesenteric artery
Acute
    Acute ischemic symptoms or gangrene of the small bowel
      Superior mesenteric artery syndrome
Chronic weight loss and postprandial pain

Colic vessel
Midcolic artery: acute occlusion leads to gangrene of the colon
Inferior mesenteric
    Acute abdominal distention and colonic gangrene
      Chronic and usually without symptoms

ated with a cardiac source and may also be associated with emboli in other areas such as the extremities, brain, or kidneys, thus causing additional symptoms. Distention, sepsis, and deterioration are all common. Abdominal tenderness develops. There is not time for collaterals to develop. Flat plate x-ray films of the abdomen demonstrate a gasless abdomen until much later in the course. At surgery, the diagnosis may not be found in the early acute situation.

Chronic visceral ischemia is usually caused by atherosclerosis, and affected patients may have other concomitant atherosclerotic syndromes, especially of the aorta and its branches. In the chronic situation, abdominal bloating, distention, and diarrhea may all develop. The patient may have unexplained weight loss. Abdominal discomfort may develop, especially after eating, and extensive evaluation may fail to demonstrate the cause of the problem. Many patients have no symptoms at all until

Symptomatology

The symptom complex of visceral arterial obstruction and visceral ischemia (Table 45.2) again depend on the structure involved and the type of obstruction present, particularly whether it is an acute or chronic situation and whether there is total or partial obstruction. Acute occlusion of the visceral vessels is a highly lethal situation that requires urgent evaluation and consideration of emergency surgery. The diagnosis of an acutely occluded visceral artery (thrombotic or embolic) is very serious (Figures 45.5 and 45.6). Patients with acute embolic phenomenon experience marked pain. Due to its sudden onset patients often can remember the exact minute the incident happened. They complain of severe periumbilical abdominal pain, which may be associated with emptying of the gastrointestinal tract. Physical examination may demonstrate active bowel sounds and minimal tenderness until later in the course of the attack. The acute embolic phenomenon is usually associ-

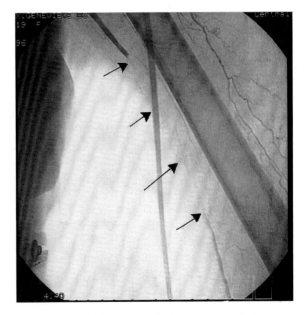

FIGURE 45.5. Brachial artery occlusion due to embolus.

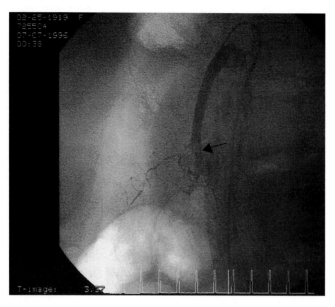

FIGURE 45.6. Embolic superior mesenteric artery occlusion in same patient as Figure 45.5 with catheter in place.

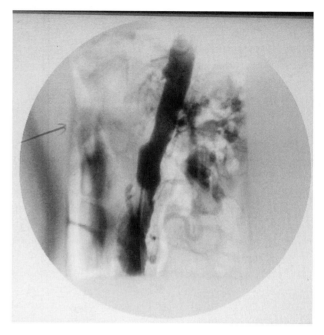

FIGURE 45.7. Occluded visceral vessels in a patient with typical symptoms.

the process becomes extensive, at which time treatment options are limited. Many patients who are asymptomatic have only a single lesion and do not experience symptoms until they develop a second stenosis or obstruction. In the chronic situation, one, two, or three mesenteric vessels may be occluded without symptomatology. In our experience, the symptom complex has been more common in women than in men, but because of the larger vessel size in men, they are easier to treat. Usually individuals are in the fifth or sixth decade of life or older.

As they become symptomatic, typical postprandial abdominal pain usually develops; some physicians believe that a steal syndrome from the intestines to the stomach may occur. Postprandial abdominal pain is the most common symptom. If the pain is chronic, it usually develops 30 to 45 minutes after a meal and lasts for 1 to 3 hours. The symptoms, which become recurrent, may first occur with large meals but then may develop even after small meals. Bloating, weight loss, and diarrhea ensue, and the patient becomes very frustrated when the workup fails to delineate the problem. Pain may be colicky, cramping, or dull. Weight loss becomes evident, and patients may lose 20 to 30 pounds, probably primarily on the basis of decreased intake due to "food fear" rather than malabsorption (Figure 45.7). Nausea, vomiting, diarrhea, and constipation may all be present as a result of motility disturbances.

Patients with chronic celiac axis compression syndrome may have associated emotional, psychiatric, or alcohol abuse problems. The bruit may vary with respiration. Many chronic patients have associated conditions (e.g., smoking and hypertension) that may exacerbate

their problems. Coronary artery disease is a frequent concomitant finding. Less often the pain localizes in the lower abdomen rather than the epigastrium. A physical examination that demonstrates weight loss and abdominal bruit, in conjunction with the patient history, is significant. Most patients who develop chronic intestinal ischemia have occlusion of at least two of the three main vessels. Autopsy reports demonstrate a higher incidence of the occlusive process than seen in clinical practice because of collateralization.[7,8] Thus, affected patients see many physicians until, with escalation of the symptomatology, infarction eventually occurs. Infarction then creates the acute symptomatology seen in toxic patients.

Diagnosis

Correctly diagnosing patients with visceral arterial obstructive disease may be very difficult, particularly early in the ischemic bowel syndrome when atypical nondirectional symptomatology may be more an annoyance than true discomfort. Also, the patient may not be able to relate a precise history regarding the problem. However, as the symptomatology complex progresses, the history becomes more significant and may thus delineate the problem. A careful, precise history should reveal the direction of the diagnostic and therapeutic program (Table 45.3). Physical examination may or may not reveal any abnormalities. The most common finding may be a bruit heard over the abdomen. However, many affected patients have soft abdomens, show weight loss, and have

TABLE 45.3. Diagnostic approach for visceral obstructive lesions.

History

Physical examination

Laboratory (limited value)
Complete blood count
Multichannel chemistry analysis
Amylase

Radiological
Noninvasive
    Upper gastrointestinal/small bowel series
    Barium enema
    Magnetic resonance imaging
    Ultrasound
Invasive
    Angiography
      • Aortic flush
      • Selective
      • Anteroposterior and lateral views
      • Catheter or translumbar technique
      • Rapid changing film sequence
    Intraoperative Doppler
    Blood flow studies

Endoscopy
Upper gastroduodenoscopy
Colonoscopy

Surgical Exploration

no bruit. In the acute situation a bloody mucoid discharge may be present.

Initially, many patients may undergo an upper gastrointestinal and small bowel series that occasionally may delineate compression of the first part of the small bowel (duodenum) by the superior mesenteric artery. However, this finding is rarely significant and usually only positional. Barium enemas are commonly performed and, in our experience, usually provide normal results. Occasionally, the thumbprinting changes of ischemia characteristic of visceral arterial occlusion of the colon are seen. Upper and lower gastrointestinal endoscopy is also frequently performed in the chronic situation. Again, only on rare occasions are ischemic bowel patterns (discoloration or bleeding) noted—particularly in the colon. Otherwise, endoscopic examinations have had little value. Hematologic studies may demonstrate an elevated white cell count—especially in the acute phase. Anemia or hemoconcentration (acute) may be present. Multichannel chemistry studies may reveal a depletion of proteins (both total and albumen) and show the depleted condition of the patient with diminished cholesterol and blood urea nitrogen levels.

Radiologic Techniques

Duplex ultrasonography has been used by some to evaluate the flow and characteristics of the mesenteric vessels.

If severe disease is present in two of the three major mesenteric vessels, then additional concerns and angiography must be considered. Thus, as an initial diagnostic step, duplex ultrasonography of the celiac axis and of the superior mesenteric artery may be considered. The celiac artery duplex features are similar to those of the internal carotid artery, with a high resting flow component during diastole that persists after ingestion of a test meal. The velocity pattern of the superior mesenteric artery resembles more closely those of a peripheral artery, with a flow reversal component during diastole that suggests high peripheral resistance. After ingestion of a test meal, the shape of the waveform normally changes with the increased superior mesenteric flow and loss of the reversed flow component. With the development of stenosis in the superior mesenteric artery and celiac axis, the peak systolic frequency shifts and spectral broadening develops throughout the cycle. These results suggest that the study should be performed in the resting or fasting state.[6]

The "gold" standard for the diagnosis of visceral ischemia or vascular obstructive phenomenon is angiography (Figure 45.8). We generally prefer a transfemoral catheter arteriogram to delineate the evolving vascular anatomy. Many times a supine study is adequate. However, lateral films (especially with the patient lying on his or her side) are frequently necessary, particularly for the superior mesenteric and celiac arteries. Then one may obtain both anteroposterior and lateral film series. Most such obstructive phenomena occur at the visceral artery origin or slightly beyond. Thus, selective angiography usually is not necessary and may not demonstrate the obstructing process if the catheter tip passes beyond the obstruction. Translumbar aortography and visceral angiography have been performed in a patient with total occlusive disease of the distal aorta and iliac system. This is not the method of choice, but lateral films have been demonstrative using this technique. On occasion, we have also performed mesenteric angiography studies through the brachial artery approach. Whether newer modalities such as magnetic resonance angiography will prove of value has yet to be determined.

Intraoperative Doppler studies may also eventually further define the lesion. Flow studies to determine the area of ischemia and the potential new source of blood flow for that area will hopefully be available in the future. Rapid sequence film or video studies during angiography are important in these patients, as are the volume of contrast material used (use caution in renal failure or the allergic patient), the x-ray technician, and defining the correct injection–exposure delay time for the angiogram. We prefer not to puncture previous grafts (especially synthetic grafts in the groin) for passage of the angiographic catheter because of the risks of infection and thrombosis.

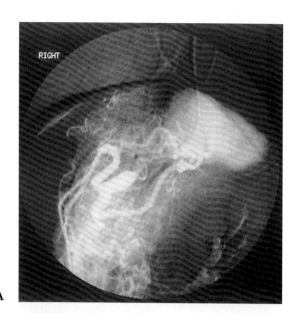

A

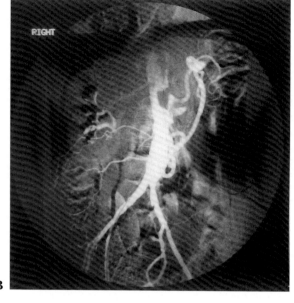

B

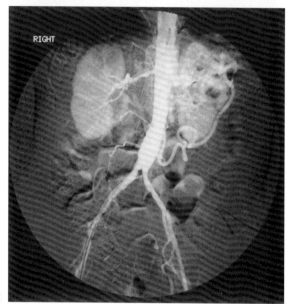

C

FIGURE 45.8. Views demonstrating collateral from inferior mesenteric circulation in patient with occluded celiac and superior mesenteric artery.

Therapeutic Considerations

Acute Occlusion

The patient with an acute process requires surgical consideration early in the course or drastic consequences may develop. The acutely occluded patient, on average, has high mortality and complication rates. A nonoperative palliative hospital course is rarely helpful for these patients. Once a diagnosis is established, patients almost always proceed to surgery (Table 45.4). Many undergo an open exploration that finds gangrene of the entire bowel and no chance for salvage (Figure 45.9). These patients' wounds are closed, and the outcome is universally fatal. Others may be potentially salvageable with early aggressive management. Each artery requires careful evaluation, as well as review of the angiogram (Figure 45.10). On the acute basis, we have performed embolectomy (Figure 45.11) after appropriate dissection of the mesenteric artery, usually from beneath the pancreas but at times through the lesser sac. Recognizing that these are not strong vessels, one must be careful with the amount of tension and traction placed on them. Once the embolectomy has been completed, the bowel is allowed to stabilize. Patients may be brought back at a later time to evaluate whether there are viable areas in the bowel that may be salvaged and other areas that must be resected. We have used this "second-look" concept on a number of occasions for patients with acute occlusive processes.

TABLE 45.4. Surgical procedures.

Reconstructive
Graft: synthetic or autologous
    Bypass
    Patch
    Interposed segment
    Y grafts
    Multiple
Endarterectomy: trapdoor
Angioplasty: operative
Anastomosis
    End to end
    End to side
    To branch vessel
Transplantation of origin

Resectional
Small or large bowel resection
Enterostomy

Adhesions or bands
Lysis
Resection

Open angioplasty/vascular dilation
Through aorta
Through side
Through primary vessel

If acute occlusive thrombosis is found, the problem becomes much more difficult, because insertion of a graft, whether synthetic or autologous, is a more prolonged process. In our experience, grafting has not been a particularly successful operation for the acutely thrombosed or occluded artery, except when we are readily available for surgery and the occlusion has been noticed at the time of the initial surgery. At this point, we have been able to reimplant the inferior mesenteric artery or an anomalous superior mesenteric origin in ruptured aortic aneurysm patients. In several patients with iatrogenic complications, we have proceeded to perform colostomies or descending colectomies. For inferior mesenteric occlusion and midcolic artery occlusion, we have

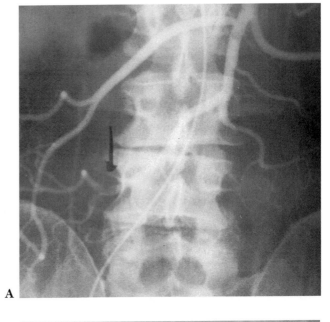

A

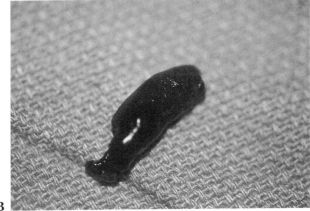

B

FIGURE 45.10. **A,** Superior mesenteric artery embolus on selective angiography. **B,** Embolus from same artery.

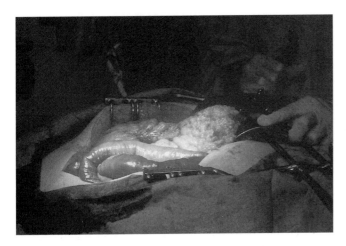

FIGURE 45.9. Gangrene bowel due to acute ischemia.

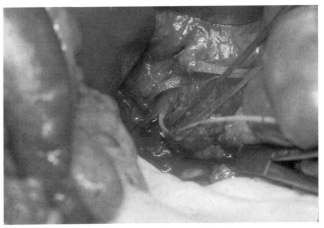

FIGURE 45.11. Fogarty thrombectomy of the superior mesenteric artery.

performed colostomies and colectomies. Pancreatic surgical patients with vascular complications have universally been very difficult to treat and to obtain viable bowel. When the etiology is an acutely thrombosed aneurysm, attempts at correction of the aneurysm and thrombectomy or resection have been carried out. Again, these approaches have not been met with uniform success.

A number of newer approaches have been utilized for the acutely occluded or dissected visceral vessel (Table 45.5). We have used enzymatic therapy for emboli in the superior mesenteric artery in the acutely ill patient after myocardial revascularization and carotid endarterectomy. However, this approach has not been universally successful, and determining whether it is a viable therapeutic consideration in the long run requires additional investigation. In iatrogenic dissections of the celiac and hepatic arteries, spontaneous healing may occur.[3] Stent placement following an aortic dissection in both the celiac and superior mesenteric arteries to restore vascular perfusion has been reported to have successful results.[4] With time, we would expect that endovascular techniques may lead to further utilization of this approach. The technique of percutaneous transluminal angioplasty (PTA) has been used even for patients with hepatic artery stenosis after transplantation.[9] In the absence of peritoneal signs, nonsurgical treatment may include the infusion of streptokinase or urokinase intraarterially and a vasodilator. Repeat arteriography is necessary in these patients, and laparotomy should be initiated if worrisome peritoneal signs develop. Percutaneous transfemoral catheter extraction has been attempted in individuals with emboli with some success.

A number of surgical procedures have been developed for visceral arterial occlusive problems (Table 45.4). Acutely, aortic bypass procedures to the celiac, hepatic, or mesenteric arteries have not had a high success rate. Revascularization of the celiac artery alone may preserve the patient's bowel in some cases. Revascularization, with bypass graft or transplantation, should be performed after distal thrombectomy. The infection rate appears to be less when the graft comes from above the celiac axis.

TABLE 45.5. Nonoperative therapy.

Expectant observation

Anticoagulants
Heparin, acute
Coumadin, chronic

Enzymatic

Angiographic
Angioplasty
Stent
Future endarterectomy
Embolectomy

However, in the face of bowel necrosis, gangrene, or perforation, an autogenous saphenous vein bypass rather than a synthetic or prosthetic material is usually recommended. We prefer to avoid the thoracoretroperitoneal approach in these patients due to their serious condition. If obvious infarcted bowel is present at the time of completion of the revascularization procedure and observation, the infarcted bowel with multiple ostomies or anastomoses may be resected before closure. Otherwise, a second-look procedure is utilized. The foul serosanguinous (morbid) odor and exudate found in most acute patients at the time of exploration foreshadows what is to come. With a high postoperative problem list, poor survival is the rule.

Chronic Treatment and Surgery

To date, treatment of patients with chronic visceral arterial occlusions remains a challenge. The first successful revascularization procedure was reported by Shaw and Maynard in the *New England Journal of Medicine* in 1958; they performed a thromboendarterectomy.[10] Until that time, the treatment of these patients was largely unsuccessful. Since the 1958 report, interest has been piqued and new techniques have been used to treat chronic visceral arterial occlusions. The majority of patients with only one vessel chronic stenosis or occlusion do not require surgical intervention. An occasional celiac compression patient may require surgical intervention. A patient's symptoms dictate the course of treatment. The technical options therefore have been expanded and more widely used. However, they still carry a significant risk to the patient, particularly in the early postoperative period. If patients are able to tolerate the surgery, from the pulmonary and cardiac aspect, and avoid the complications often seen in these high-risk individuals, long-term survival may be possible.

Antibiotics are frequently used in these individuals beginning preoperatively (when possible) and continuing for 2 to 3 days postoperatively. Cardiologic and pulmonary consultation and intraoperative monitoring (including electrocardiogram, arterial lines, and Swan–Ganz catheters) are provided as necessary. Adequate exposure and surgical instrumentation are important. Cross-clamping at the diaphragm (supraceliac artery) may lead to an increased ischemic risk for marginal patients, especially from the myocardial aspect. At any rate, intraoperative evaluation of the reconstruction may be very valuable in patients to ensure all vessels are open. Therefore, wide palpation of the mesenteric vessels, angiography, and duplex ultrasonography may all be helpful. Digital subtraction angiography or aortography is sometimes used to evaluate these vessels before discharge.

More recently, with use of the catheter technique as a therapeutic modality, angioplasty (PTA) has been utilized safely and effectively for the treatment of visceral ischemia. This technique has been used for the three major vessels—the celiac, superior mesenteric, and inferior mesenteric vessels—by Hallisey et al.[11] They found no instances of acute vessel reocclusion, rupture, or distal embolization and no major or minor complications secondary to the transaxillary route. Their mortality and morbidity rates were low. However, their summary of a number of articles in the literature demonstrated a mortality rate after PTA of 0% to 10% with a recurrence of 0% to 63% by a number of authors from 1980 to 1994. The use of this modality for transplantation hepatic artery stenosis demonstrates the versatility of this concept.[9] Others such as Crotch-Harvey et al. have reported the utilization of PTA for inferior mesenteric artery chronic mesenteric ischemia.[12]

When the angioplasty, enzymatic, and stent insertion approaches are not acceptable, surgery may be considered. We have primarily used a transabdominal midline approach with these patients because the exposure is excellent. The ability to dissect the celiac, superior mesenteric, and inferior mesenteric arteries is enhanced, and the anesthesia personnel feel very comfortable with the supine position. Following the long midline incision, the vessel to be approached is delineated. The celiac trunk is usually approached through the lesser curvature gastrohepatic tissue or through the lesser sac by retracting the stomach upward. The superior mesenteric artery may be exposed either through the lesser sac or by retracting the colon upward and following the superior mesenteric artery out of the mesentery down to the aorta. The superior mesenteric artery and the celiac arteries originate very close to each other and thus may be confused (Figure 45.12). The inferior mesenteric artery may be exposed by approaching the aorta approximately 3 to 4 cm above its bifurcation and dissecting the inferior mesenteric artery free.

The triangular ligament may be divided to allow retraction of the liver to the right if approaching the celiac axis. The diaphragmatic curve and the arcuate ligament may be divided to provide exposure of the lower thoracic and upper abdominal aorta. Nerve fibers and paravesicular tissue may be divided as appropriate, and the superior mesenteric artery may also be located at this point. Some institutions have used the retroperitoneal thoracoabdominal approach for delineation of the thoracoabdominal aorta and its major visceral and renal branches. The patient is positioned with the left chest elevated. Following appropriate skin preparation, an incision is made in the eighth intercostal area and is carried down through the abdominal muscles to open the retroperitoneum. A portion of the diaphragm may be divided and the kidney retracted. The celiac ganglion fibers are divided and the pancreas retracted upward. The celiac axis, superior mesenteric artery, and inferior mesenteric artery may all be exposed and approached. Concomitant renal artery procedures may be performed through the thoracoabdominal-retroperitoneal approach as well. This approach requires a patient of adequate health. We have not used a laparoscopic approach for the splenic artery or splenic artery aneurysms, but these and other techniques may become available in the future.[13]

Surgical Techniques

A number of surgical techniques are available to the surgeon and the patient. The variety of options were reviewed in 1992 by Calderon et al.,[8] who defined approximately 20 different techniques for their patients. Thromboendarterectomy of the visceral arteries, particularly their orifices, requires an extensive incision that uses the thoracoabdominal approach through the retroperitoneum. This is a very extensive approach, but one may endarterectomize the origins of multiple vessels with one trapdoor type of procedure. An endarterectomy of the renal arteries may be performed simultaneously. This may be accompanied by additional patch grafts or bypass procedures for the endarterectomized vessels. However, the patients must be of adequate physical health to undergo such a procedure.

More commonly, aortovisceral bypass grafting is performed to accommodate or eliminate the patient's problem. Antegrade flow through the obstructed vessel or vessels is the desired result. Autogenous vein, synthetic grafts, such as Dacron or Goretex, and interposed arterial conduits may be used. A reverse saphenous vein grafting procedure in the aortoceliac or aortomesenteric (superior or inferior) position or an aorto–left gastric or aortohepatic bypass may be performed. Polytetrafluo-

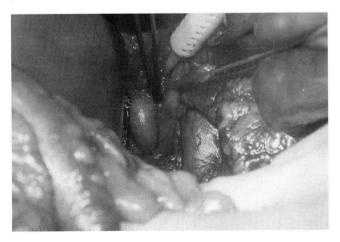

FIGURE 45.12. Superior mesenteric artery next to the celiac artery; these vessels may be confused with each other.

roethylene grafts have been utilized for aortic or iliac bypass to the superior mesenteric, celiac, or hepatic artery. These grafts may be end-to-side or interposed techniques. Y grafts may be used for bypass to renal arteries and mesenteric vessels. Autogenous grafts with retrograde orientation have been abandoned to a great extent because of high failure rates both early and late. When possible, the grafts should be placed in a disease-free aorta, so that an antegrade alignment of the vessel to be approached is created. Some individuals have utilized an elliptical aortotomy to create the approximate anastomosis. In general, we have not used this approach. Many of these grafting procedures require access through a synthetic aortic graft. For example, an aortic aneurysm is repaired and then a bypass graft may be taken from the aneurysm to the obstructed mesenteric vessel. Again, these may be end-to-side or end-to-end anastomoses, depending on the situation and the grafting material available. Many patients require a double bypass rather than a single bypass technique. If these patients develop unusual abdominal pain or deteriorate, a second look must be considered to rule out graft thrombosis and to resect the appropriate bowel that may be involved.

The usual postoperative considerations must be given to these high-risk individuals, including renal failure and cardiac concerns. The infrarenal aorta, where accessible, has been utilized successfully by a number of institutions with the development of a retrograde bypass. However, at the supraceliac level, the antegrade bypass technique is more common. The latter requires additional dissection for a difficult exposure. Some have felt that occlusion of a saphenous vein or Goretex retrograde graft was due to the complexity of the disease rather than the graft material or the retrograde flow. The use of polytetrafluoroethylene, however, may minimize the possible kinking of the graft caused by intestinal movements. Autogenous vein has been recommended for these grafts in the face of intra-abdominal infection. These patients do not usually require preoperative nutritional support.[8] The suprarenal aorta generally has less disease present and theoretically may be a better access point to the aorta; the infrarenal aorta may require additional surgery in the future and may also enhance the chance of buckling of the graft. Thus, some individuals, such as Ward and Cormier,[7] recommend the use of the supraceliac aorta for an antegrade grafting technique using any of the three graft materials (saphenous vein, Dacron, or polytetrafluoroethylene). Ward and Cormier generally prefer prosthetics for mesenteric artery bypass because of their durability. Retraction of the esophagus and division of crural fibers may be required in these patients.

Celiac revascularization may be accomplished through decompression of the celiac trunk by freeing up the muscle and arcuate ligament, by decompression and dilatation of the lumen, or by decompression and celiac artery reconstruction. When decompressing the celiac trunk, the celiac ganglion fibers should also be resected. Dilatation of the lumen of the artery may be performed by passing a retrograde catheter or dilator through the splenic artery. The celiac axis may then be revascularized through an aortic graft by either an end-to-side or end-to-end anastomosis to the celiac stump. Further revascularization, which may be carried out to the hepatic or splenic artery, accomplishes the same goal without dissecting the celiac origin; a wide distal anastomosis is thus ensured. The superior mesenteric artery may be revascularized after administering heparin to the patient by endarterectomy, by transplantation of its origin, or by bypass grafting with an appropriate substitute. We have used the superior mesenteric artery as a source of flow to the celiac axis in a single patient by transecting the celiac artery at its origin and anastomosing it to the origin of the superior mesenteric artery when there was a poststenotic dilatation in the celiac vessel (Figure 45.13). Both antegrade and retrograde grafts have been used for the superior mesenteric artery. Endarterectomy is not commonly performed for the celiac or mesenteric vessels. To avoid creating a flap or a dissection, which would be difficult to control, we have used this technique only rarely. Reimplantation of the superior mesenteric artery may be carried out after division distal to the plaque. The stump of the superior mesenteric artery is oversewn, and then the distal artery is sutured caudal to the left renal vein. This is a limited value procedure, however, because of the amount of aortic disease that may be present, as well as the anatomical branches of the superior mesenteric artery.

The inferior mesenteric artery presents a special consideration. We have seen many patients with abdominal

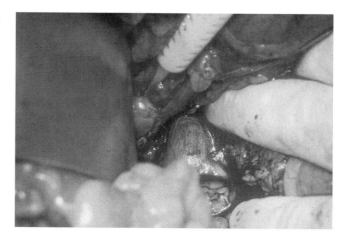

FIGURE 45.13. Transected atherosclerotic occluded celiac artery anastomosed to the thrombectomized superior mesenteric artery end to side.

aortic aneurysms in whom the sigmoid colon appeared devascularized and morbid white in color when we have cross-clamped the inferior mesenteric artery. In these patients we have utilized a swatch of aneurysm tissue with the origin of the inferior mesenteric artery to re-anastomose the inferior mesenteric artery to the synthetic graft. On occasion, however, even when the colon appeared healthy and when there was an occluded mesenteric artery from thrombus or plaque, we have seen ischemia of the colon. In these patients, if recognized at the time of surgery, a bypass graft utilizing a saphenous vein or an endarterectomy has been carried out with reanastomosis to the synthetic graft. Usually, however, the inferior mesenteric artery is occluded and no additional surgery is required for this vessel.

Postoperatively, the patients are taken to the recovery room, where they are stabilized, their blood count is checked, and their respiratory condition is monitored. Most patients are then moved to the intensive care unit, where they are carefully monitored and maintained without oral nutrition with a Nasogastric sump tube until the gastrointestinal tract develops function, the abdomen is soft, and the patients are ambulatory.

Visceral Ischemia of Other Causes

It would be remiss for us not to mention a few nonvisceral artery obstructive causes of ischemic symptoms and gangrene of the intestines. A number of differential diagnoses should be considered when gangrenous changes of the large and small bowel occur. Patients with venous thrombosis, protein C or protein S deficiency, or infarction of the intestines as a result of mesenteric venous occlusive disease may be seen occasionally (Figure 45.14). Fortunately this is an uncommon process because successful treatment of these individuals is difficult.[14,15]

Nonobstructive ischemic changes may also occur as a result of hypoperfusion. We have reported on a series of patients at two meetings that focused on the steal syndrome and the iatrogenic steal syndrome.[16,17,18] Two of these patients had LeRoche's syndrome. The first patient had an aortobifemoral bypass graft and postoperatively developed spinal cord ischemia and descending colon ischemia as a result of hypoperfusion of the spinal and colonic vessels. The second patient had a large superior mesenteric artery with what appeared to be collateral circulation eventually supplying the lower extremity. When the obstruction was removed through an aorto-bifemoral Dacron bypass graft, the patient developed gangrene of the small bowel as a result of hypoperfusion of the superior mesenteric artery, felt to be based on a steal syndrome or diminished perfusion with the distal obstruction removed. Both patients unfortunately died postoperatively. Other differential diagnoses of these gangrenous patients would include adhesive changes and spontaneous twisting of the viscera.

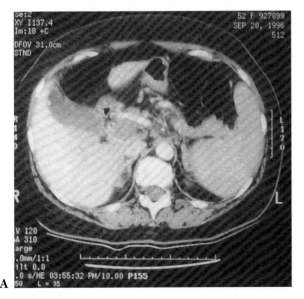
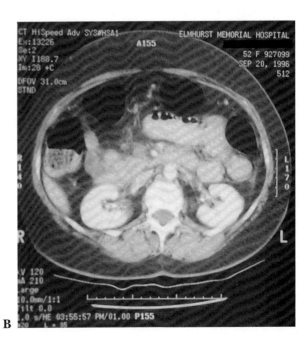

FIGURE 45.14. Partial mesenteric, splenic, and portal vein thrombosis viewed on computed tomography scan in a patient with protein C deficiency.

References

1. Clemente CD. *Gray's Anatomy.* 30th American Ed. Philadelphia, Pa: Lea & Febiger; 1985:732–746.

2. Netter FH. *Atlas of Human Anatomy.* Summit, NJ: Ciba-Geigy Corp; 1989 (plates 323–333).

3. Yoon DY, Park JH, Chung JW, Han JK, Han MC. Iatrogenic dissection of the celiac artery and its branches during transcatheter arterial embolization for hepatocellular carcinoma outcome in 40 patients. *Cardiovasc Intervent Radiol.* 1995;18:16–19.

4. Connell DA, Thomson KR, Gibson RN, Wall, AJ. Stent placement in coeliac and superior mesenteric arteries to restore vascular perfusion following aortic dissection. *Aust Radiol.* 1995;39:68–70.

5. Valentine RJ, Rossi MB, Myers SI, Clagett GP. Splenic infarction after splenorenal arterial bypass. *J Vasc Surg.* 1993; 17:602–606.

6. Ernst CB. Renal artery reconstruction. In: Haimovici H, et al., eds. *Vascular Surgery: Principles and Techniques.* Norwalk, Conn: Appleton & Lange; 1989:763–780.

7. Ward AS, Cormier JM. Surgery of the visceral arteries. In: *Operative Techniques in Arterial Surgery.* Chicago, Ill: Precept Press Inc; 1986:305–328.

8. Calderon M, Reul GJ, Gregoric ID, et al. Long term results of the surgical management of symptomatic chronic intestinal ischemia. *J Cardiovasc Surg.* 1992;33:723–728.

9. Mondragen RS, Karani JB, Heaton ND, et al. The use of percutaneous transluminal angioplasty in hepatic artery stenosis after transplantation. *Transplantation.* 1994;57: 228–231.

10. Shaw RS, Maynard EP III. Acute and chronic thrombosis of the mesenteric arteries associated with malabsorption: a report of two cases successfully treated by thromboendarterectomy. *N Engl J Med.* 1958;258:874–878.

11. Hallisey MJ, Deschaine J, Illescas FF, et al. Angioplasty for the treatment of visceral ischemia. *J Vasc Intervent Radiol.* 1995;6:785–791.

12. Crotch-Harvey MA, Gould DA, Green AT. Case report: percutaneous transluminal angioplasty of the inferior mesenteric artery in the treatment of chronic mesenteric ischemia. *Clin Radiol.* 1993;46:408–409.

13. Saw EC, Kie W, Ramachandra S. Laparoscopic resection of a splenic artery aneurysm. *J Laparoendosc Surg.* 1993;3: 167–171.

14. Klein HM, Lensing R, Kloserhalfen B, Tons C, Gunther RW. Diagnostic imaging of mesenteric infarction. *Radiology.* 1995;197:79–82.

15. Rhee RY, Gloviezki P, Mendenca CT, et al. Mesenteric venous thrombosis: still a lethal disease in the 1990s [review]. *J Vasc Surg.* 1994;20:688–697.

16. Dieter RA Jr. Steal syndrome. Paper presented at: Annual Meeting of International College of Surgeons; September 23–25, 1983; Cleveland, Ohio.

17. Dieter RA Jr, Kucycz G. The iatrogenic steal syndrome. Paper presented at: Annual Meeting of the International College of Surgeons; February 14–15, 1988; New Orleans, La.

18. Dieter RA Jr, Kucycz G. The steal syndrome. Iatrogenic causes. *Int. Surg.* 1998; 83:355–357.

46

Acute Mesenteric Ischemia

Chittoor B. Sai Sudhakar, Jeffrey S. Pollock, and Bauer E. Sumpio

Ischemic intestinal disorders account for 0.1% of patient referrals to hospitals and 1% of patients with acute abdominal pain.[15,58,77,79] Acute mesenteric ischemia has a mortality rate of 55% to 90%[9–11,47,48,52,86] and is a source of significant morbidity. The high mortality rates are attributed primarily to the inability to make an early diagnosis due to diffuse symptoms and lack of definitive diagnostic methods. Mesenteric ischemia has been termed the "enigma among abdominal diseases."[56]

Clinical Features of Acute Mesenteric Ischemia

The four pathologically distinct causes of acute mesenteric ischemia are occlusion of the superior mesenteric artery (SMA) secondary to thrombosis or embolism, mesenteric vein thrombosis (MVT), and a distinct entity termed *nonocclusive mesenteric ischemia* (NOMI). Acute mesenteric ischemia occurs in three phases: (1) an initial phase of severe abdominal pain with paucity of clinical signs; (2) an intermediate phase with few characteristic symptoms; and (3) a terminal phase with necrosis of bowel, sepsis, and death within 12 to 48 hours.[56]

Mesenteric arterial thrombosis accounts for 8% to 20% of cases of acute mesenteric ischemia. It is insidious in onset and characterized by a history of chronic postprandial abdominal discomfort preceding the acute abdominal pain[3] and loss of weight secondary to a decreased appetite. The patients may have histories of myocardial infarction, congestive heart failure, chronic mesenteric ischemia, or other evidence of atherosclerotic heart disease. The mean age at onset is 66.8 years (range 52–86 years). Guaiac-positive stools are observed in 66% and peritoneal signs are present in 75% of patients at the time of presentation.[96] The nonspecificity of clinical findings on initial abdominal examination contributes to a delay in diagnosis and the institution of appropriate therapeutic measures.

Mesenteric ischemia may be caused by an embolus in 20% to 40% of patients presenting with acute mesenteric ischemia. The embolus is usually from the heart and rarely from the proximal aorta. Diagnostic angiographic procedures can rarely cause acute mesenteric ischemia by releasing a shower of emboli into the mesenteric circulation.[96,115] Occasionally there is a history of previous embolic episodes in the region of the cerebral or extremity circulation.[100] Atrial fibrillation is present in a significant number of patients.[96] Patients present with sudden onset of acute abdominal pain associated with nausea, vomiting, diarrhea, or bloody stools. Peritoneal signs are present in less than 45% of patients.[96] Late stages are complicated by acidosis, hypovolemia, hemoconcentration,[100] and definitive peritoneal signs. Presence of peritoneal signs is an indication for surgical exploration, and studies have yielded conflicting conclusions about its usefulness as a predictor of survival.[16]

Acute mesenteric venous thrombosis accounts for <5% of cases of acute mesenteric ischemia, with a male to female ratio of 1.5:1 to 1:1.[33] The disease is common in the sixth and seventh decades of life. It is classified as primary or secondary based on the absence or presence of a predisposing factor, respectively. The incidence of primary MVT is decreasing as a result of better understanding of the coagulation pathways and increasing diagnostic capabilities for the more recently described coagulopathies.[22,72] About 80% of patients have associated illnesses such as hypercoagulable states (antithrombin III deficiency, protein S or C deficiency, use of oral contraceptives, polycythemia vera, and thrombocytosis), portal hypertension, inflammation (pancreatitis or peritonitis), or a postoperative state or trauma. Sclerotherapy for esophageal varices or selective transhepatic portal angiography occasionally causes MVT in addition to splenic or portal vein thrombosis.[6] Clinical features are nonspecific. Most patients have a history of intermittent, colicky progressively increasing abdominal discomfort lasting weeks or months. Hematemesis or hematochezia is present in 15% of patients. Frank gastrointestinal bleeding may occur secondary to variceal hemorrhage. Presence of nausea, vomiting, and occult blood in stools is variable. Abdominal distension with tenderness, ascites, hypoactive bowel sounds, and pyrexia form part of the clinical picture. Guarding, rigidity, rebound tenderness, hypotension, and shock occur in the later stages of the disease.[1]

Low flow syndrome, spastic mesenteric insufficiency, and functional mesenteric infarction are synonyms that indicate the pathophysiology of NOMI. NOMI accounts for 15% to 50% of all cases of acute mesenteric ischemia.[53,84,111] Better monitoring of patients in cardiogenic shock and decreasing the periods of hypotension associated with acute cardiac events has led to a decrease in the incidence of NOMI. The use of calcium channel blockers and nitrates in patients with myocardial ischemia also protects the mesenteric vasculature from vasospasm. The low flow state that causes NOMI could be secondary to heart failure, hypotension (shock or sepsis), and hypovolemia (dehydration, bleeding, or diuretic therapy). Initially, autoregulation of intestinal blood flow maintains intestinal viability. A prolonged decrease in the cardiac index eventually leads to vasoconstriction due to failure of the autoregulatory mechanisms. The vasoconstriction persists even after correction of the low flow state. Following reperfusion, further bowel injury is mediated by oxygen free radicals. A number of drugs have been implicated in the pathogenesis of NOMI. A history of digoxin therapy is present in 57% to 90% of patients.[21] Digoxin is a potent mesenteric vasoconstrictor. Other drugs associated with NOMI include furosemide, ergotamine, vasopressors, cocaine, and β-blockers.[49] Diuretic usage results in stimulation of antidiuretic hormone and renin secretion, both of which cause splanchnic vasoconstriction.

Patients may present with any one of the features of abdominal pain, nausea, vomiting, diarrhea, or melena stools. Abdominal tenderness (96%), hypoactive bowel sounds (69%), dehydration (69%), hypotension (13%), sepsis, and shock are present in the advanced stages of the disease.[69]

Diagnostic Studies

Laboratory Investigations

In evaluating patients with acute abdominal pain, laboratory tests including blood count, serum electrolyte levels, liver function tests, and pancreatic enzyme levels are usually obtained. A careful analysis of these initial tests in combination with a thorough history and physical examination may help direct the surgeon's attention to the differential diagnosis of mesenteric ischemia. Unfortu-

nately these tests lack the accuracy to diagnose mesenteric ischemia.

Leukocytosis is present in 85% to 90% of patients with mesenteric ischemia.[17,57] However, it is not of diagnostic significance in differentiating ischemic bowel from other causes of acute abdominal pain.[35] Significant metabolic acidosis and associated base deficit complicate mesenteric ischemia.[23,55] Lactic acid and inorganic phosphate released from the ischemic bowel are the source of the base deficit. Lactic acid is produced during periods of anaerobic metabolism and accumulates due to excess production of lactate from ischemic tissues or decreased clearance. High serum lactate levels (>5 mmol/L) are present in mesenteric infarction. Although its sensitivity as a marker for mesenteric ischemia is 100%, its specificity is only 42%. The bowel wall contains high levels of inorganic phosphate (1.8215 mg/g bowel) in comparison to other tissues (0.03955 mg/g lung).[55] In a study of 18 patients by Feretis et al., 17 patients had elevated serum phosphate levels (6.12 + 0.75 mg/dL) between 4 and 12 hours after the onset of symptoms, and the degree of elevation correlated with duration of symptoms (up to 12 hours after onset of symptoms) and the length of infarcted bowel. As little as 12 cm of necrotic bowel raised phosphate levels in the peripheral circulation.[35] Serum transaminases, alkaline phosphatase, lactic dehydrogenase, and creatinine kinase levels are elevated in a variety of clinical conditions and are nonspecific markers for mesenteric ischemia.[45,46,55,61,67,82]

N-acetylhexosaminidase is a lysosomal acid hydrolase found in a number of tissues, including the intestine.[93,106] It exists in two isozymic forms, HEX A and HEX B.[59] HEX B activity has been reported to be elevated in patients with mesenteric infarction.[88] Diamine oxidase (DAO, histaminase) is a histamine catabolizing enzyme[64,65] present in the intestinal mucosa in large amounts, especially in the surface mucosal cells.[8,75,102] DAO is released into the intestinal lymph and peripheral circulation during acute intestinal ischemia in experimental animals.[65,66] In clinical studies serum DAO activity was elevated in a patient with acute necrosis of the intestinal mucosa.[19] Because DAO is transported to the blood mainly via the lymphatic vessels, elevated serum DAO levels could also be utilized in the diagnosis of mesenteric infarction secondary to mesenteric venous thrombosis.

Intestinal fatty acid–binding protein is a 15-kd protein located at the tips of small intestinal mucosal villi and constitutes 2% of the total mucosal protein.[80] It is normally not detected in peripheral circulation. Kanda et al. retrospectively analyzed serum samples from two patients with mesenteric ischemia. Serum intestinal fatty acid–binding protein levels were elevated even at the time of admission and were undetectable after bowel resection.[59] Malondialdehyde (a stable product of lipid peroxidation generated by the action of oxygen derived free radicals on the polyunsaturated fatty acids in cellular membranes)[83] and D(−)-lactate (a stereoisomer of the mammalian L[+]-lactate)[78] have been investigated to elucidate their role in the diagnosis of acute mesenteric ischemia.

Imaging Studies

Serum markers alone lack the accuracy to diagnose mesenteric infarction. A number of radiologic methods have been utilized to aid in the diagnosis of mesenteric ischemia. Early in the course of mesenteric ischemia, the plain radiographs are essentially normal[57] and help to exclude other causes of abdominal pain. Nonspecific findings include air fluid levels, dilated loops, gasless abdomen, free intraperitoneal fluid, gas in the intestinal wall and portal vessels, and ileus.[17] Thumbprinting of the bowel is a late finding in mesenteric ischemia and occurs due to edematous mucosal folds. Small bowel series may demonstrate thickening of the bowel wall due to congestion and edema that cause narrowing of the lumen, separation of small bowel loops by thickened mesentery, and thumbprinting. In addition, there may be dilated bowel with thickened folds, scalloped bowel contour, ulceration, stenosis, and mucosal effacement. However, gastrointestinal contrast studies are not performed to evaluate acute mesenteric ischemia.

Ultrasound scan of the abdomen may demonstrate dilated fluid-filled loops,[57] thickening of the small bowel wall, free abdominal fluid, and intramural gas, all of which are nonspecific for acute mesenteric ischemia.[63] Duplex color sonography may help in evaluating flow in mesenteric vessels. A lack of flow in the superior mesenteric–portal vein system is indicative of mesenteric vein thrombosis. In addition, duplex scan may reveal an intraluminal thrombus and wormlike vascular channels in the area of the portal vein, which suggests cavernomatous transformation from prior portal vein thrombosis. Enlargement of splanchnic veins, lack of compressibility, and absence of respiratory variation in vein size are other findings observed in MVT. The presence of normal mesenteric arteries on Doppler ultrasonography or mesenteric angiography decreases the clinical suspicion of mesenteric ischemia as the cause of abdominal pain but not vice versa because significant disease of the SMA and celiac axis is present in 18% of people over the age of 65 years without evidence of mesenteric ischemia.[94,108]

The role of computed tomography (CT) in the diagnosis of mesenteric infarction is controversial.[2,74,110,112] In at least one study, there was no statistical difference between the ability of the CT scan of the abdomen and arteriography to diagnose mesenteric infarction (82% versus 87.5%).[63] CT scans may help to rule out other important causes of acute abdominal pain in the elderly.[27,40] In mesenteric ischemia CT may demonstrate bowel wall thickening, dilation of the ischemic segments, mesenteric edema, intramural gas, and free intraperitoneal fluid. Administration of intravenous contrast results in mural enhancement only in normal bowel segments and not in ischemic bowel segments[62] and nonenhancement of the SMA lumen. An occluding embolus is hypoattenuating. Focal zones of low attenuation in infarcted bowel after intravenous contrast could be secondary to focal ischemic edema or the inability of contrast to reach the ischemic zones.[28,63]

CT scan has a sensitivity of 100% in detecting any of the abnormalities associated with acute MVT (thrombus in either the splenic or portal vein in 35% of cases each, bowel wall thickening, pneumatosis,[103] and streaky mesentery in 70%). Other findings suggestive of MVT include ascites, persistent bowel wall enhancement, sharply defined vein wall with a rim of increased density (due to the flow of contrast around a thrombus or in the vasa vasorum in the vessel wall) associated with a central area of low attenuation,[41] and dilated collateral vessels in the mesentery. In addition, contrast enhancement of mucosa (target phenomenon) may be present. Hepatic portal venous gas may be seen in patients with mesenteric ischemia, but other conditions associated with portal venous gas include trauma, liver abscess, and intraabdominal sepsis. Improved techniques, including spiral CT scans, have led to an increase in the sensitivity of CT to diagnose acute mesenteric ischemia from 33% to 82%.[2,63,85]

Angiography establishes the diagnosis of mesenteric ischemia. It has a sensitivity of 90%,[63] determines the site and nature of the occlusion, and differentiates between occlusive and nonocclusive ischemia. It can also facilitate the treatment of some patients with localized delivery of vasodilators[15,18] or fibrinolytic agents (streptokinase and urokinase). Lateral aortography must be done before selective catheterization of SMA.

There are several classic arteriographic findings in patients with acute mesenteric ischemia. Thrombosis of the mesenteric artery (Figures 46.1 and 46.2) occurs within the first 3 cm of the origin of the blood vessel, and there are associated features of atherosclerosis. Collateral blood flow (meandering artery) may be present between the visceral arteries. Emboli (Figure 46.3) appear as rounded filling defects with high-grade obstruction to distal flow. More than 50% of the emboli are distal to the origin of the middle colic artery. The radiologic features that favor emboli are the absence of gross atherosclerotic changes in the vascular tree, multiple lesions in the SMA branches, and the presence of extramesenteric emboli (which occurs in 50% of patients with SMA embolism).

Segmental ischemia secondary to NOMI (Figures 46.4, 46.5, and 46.6) is diagnosed based on the features of nar-

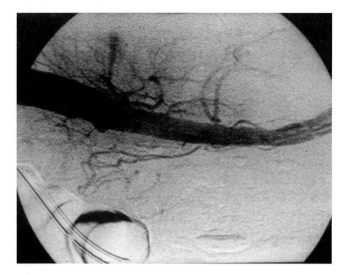

FIGURE 46.1. Acute mesenteric arterial thrombosis. Lateral aortography shows occlusion of the celiac and superior mesenteric arteries and a severe stenosis at the origin of the inferior mesenteric artery.

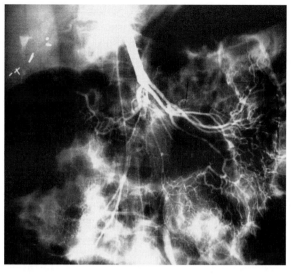

FIGURE 46.3. Embolus (filling defect) in the mid and distal superior mesenteric artery distal to the origin of the second jejunal branch.

rowing of origins of multiple branches of SMA, string of sausage sign, spasm of mesenteric arcades, and impaired filling of intramural vessels, frequently in a patchy fashion. Involvement of the entire vascular bed is demonstrated as a pruned appearance of the entire mesenteric vasculature. These features should exist in the absence of systemic hypotension, acute congestive heart failure, or systemic vasoconstrictor drug therapy.

In MVT (Figures 46.7, 46.8, 46.9, and 46.10), angiographic findings include the demonstration of a partially or completely occluding thrombus, slow or absent filling of the mesenteric vein, arterial spasm, prolongation of the arterial phase, failure of arterial arcades to empty, reflux of contrast into the artery, prolonged blush in the involved bowel segment, and failure to visualize the superior mesenteric vein or portal vein. In addition, collateral mesenteric veins may be present.

The criticism leveled against angiography is that although it delineates the blood vessels in the mesentery with accuracy, it provides very little further information about the pathology in the bowel wall. Moreover, NOMI is undetected in a significant number of patients.[29,50] In

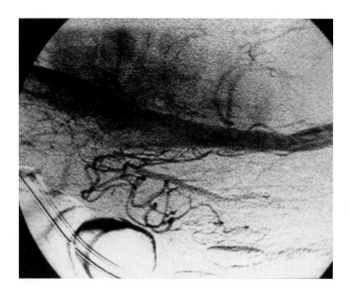

FIGURE 46.2. Acute mesenteric arterial thrombosis. Acute thrombosis of the superior mesenteric artery. Collateral flow from the inferior mesenteric artery reconstitutes the superior mesenteric artery.

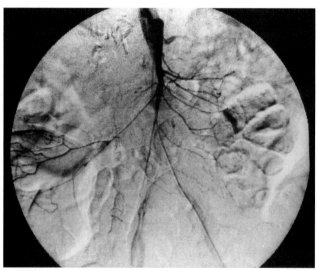

FIGURE 46.4. Nonocclusive mesenteric ischemia. Diffusely narrowed superior mesenteric artery with lesser involvement of the right colic artery.

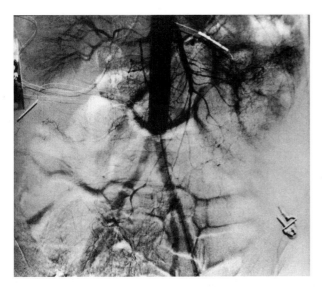

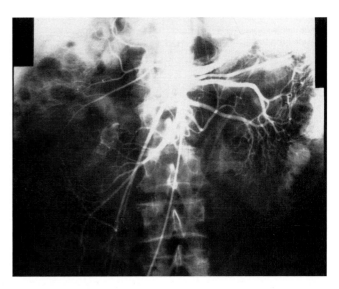

FIGURE 46.5. Nonocclusive mesenteric ischemia in a 72-year-old man 9 days after aortic valve replacement. Angiography demonstrates diffusely narrowed superior mesenteric artery, slow transit of the contrast, and gaps in the perfusion of the ileum and right colon. A papaverine infusion was started.

FIGURE 46.7. Acute mesenteric vein thrombosis. Arterial phase of the superior mesenteric angiogram shows decreased perfusion to the distal small bowel.

magnetic resonance imaging features suggestive of bowel ischemia are thickening of the bowel wall, a twofold to threefold increase in signal intensity from bowel on T_2-weighted images, and slightly increased signal intensity within the bowel wall on T_1-weighted images.[60] Bowel ischemia causes intracellular and intercellular fluid accumulation[24] and an increase in tissue water.[38] The increased signal intensity seen on T_2-weighted pulse sequences is due to increased water content within the bowel wall, which represents bowel wall edema and may be a nonspecific marker because inflammatory bowel disease, hypoproteinemia, and massive fluid resuscitation also cause bowel wall edema. Increased signal intensity on T_1-weighted images is due to hemorrhage within the bowel wall secondary to ischemia. Parenteral administration of a paramagnetic contrast agent gadolinium diethyltriamine pentaacetic acid increases the signal intensity in T_1-weighted images in normal bowel in comparison to the ischemic areas.[62]

Ischemia alters intracellular metabolism and the concentration of intracellular phosphorylated compounds.

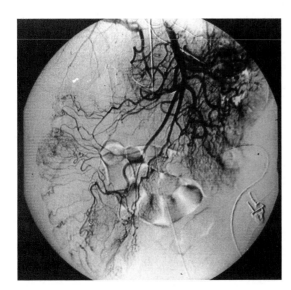

FIGURE 46.6. Repeat angiography in patient in Figure 46.5 3 hours after papaverine infusion. There is marked improvement in the caliber and flow through the mesenteric artery, although there are still some areas of poor perfusion in the ileum and ascending colon.

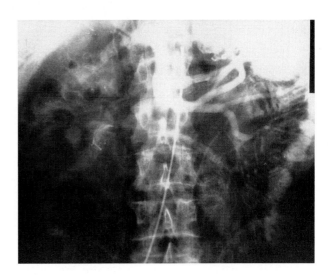

FIGURE 46.8. Acute mesenteric vein thrombosis. Venous phase shows no venous return from the distal small bowel.

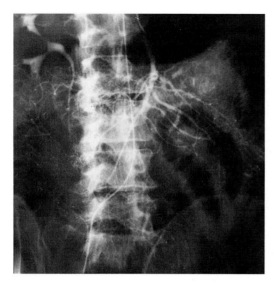

FIGURE 46.9. Acute mesenteric vein thrombosis. Arterial phase of superior mesenteric angiogram demonstrates narrowed arteries that taper distally.

Phosphonuclear magnetic resonance spectroscopy is a noninvasive method of monitoring intracellular metabolism. The intracellular phosphorylated compounds are visualized as characteristic spectroscopic peaks, and ischemic bowel segments are differentiated from normal bowel based on differences in the peaks of phosphorylated compounds.[13,107]

Orally administered contrast agents are not absorbed, and their appearance in serum and urine reflects disruption of the intestinal mucosal barrier. In occasional patients, following gastrointestinal contrast studies, there is an opacification of the renal system; in such instances, disruption of the mucosal barrier with entry into the systemic circulation should be suspected.[4,105]

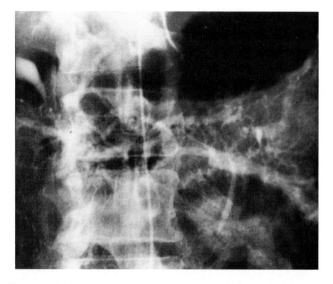

FIGURE 46.10. Acute mesenteric vein thrombosis. Venous phase shows a near occlusive filling defect in the first large jejunal vein that extends into the superior mesenteric vein.

In summary, plain abdominal x-ray films are not sufficiently sensitive. Ultrasound scan and CT are readily available tools in most institutions and have an important role in investigating acute abdominal pain. Angiography is the mainstay in the diagnosis of mesenteric ischemia. Both magnetic resonance imaging and magnetic resonance spectroscopy have yielded encouraging results but are not readily available.

Other Investigations

The value of peritoneal fluid analysis in mesenteric ischemia is debatable; consequently, it is rarely used in critically ill patients with dilated bowel because of its attendant risks of perforation and hemorrhage while obtaining a sample.[95,97] Tonometry is a minimally invasive procedure used for indirect measurement of intramural pH in the gastrointestinal tract. The tonometer (Tonomitor, Tonometrics, Bethesda, MD) consists of a semipermeable silastic balloon attached to a polyester elastomer catheter placed in the intestinal lumen. Saline solution (2.5 mL) is instilled into the balloon, and after a period of equilibration (ranging from 10 to 20 minutes) with intraluminal CO_2, the saline is withdrawn. The initial 1.0 mL of saline representing the catheter dead space is discarded, and CO_2 content in the remaining 1.5 mL is determined. Tonometry is based on the principle that the intraluminal P_{CO_2} equilibrates with intramural P_{CO_2} and HCO_3^- in the intestinal wall equilibrates with arterial HCO_3^-. Depending on the duration of the equilibration period a correction factor is required to adjust the measured P_{CO_2} of the tonometric saline because equilibration across the semipermeable membrane of the balloon is only 70% even at 20 minutes.[37] The corrected partial pressure of CO_2 in the tonometric fluid sample and the HCO_3^- of the arterial blood are utilized in the Henderson–Hasselbach equation to determine the intramucosal pH.[76]

Sigmoid and gastric tonometric measurement of intramucosal pH reveals a drop during the clamp application at the time of infrarenal abdominal aortic aneurysm repair and reflected ischemia of the bowel.[34] Low colonic intramural pH and the duration of intramural acidosis accurately predict the development of ischemic colitis after aortic surgery.[36,99]

However, tonometry suffers from certain limitations. A prolonged equilibration period (up to 60 minutes) is necessary for the saline in the tonometer balloon to equilibrate with the intramucosal pH. Moreover, an additional factor is the overestimation of intramural HCO_3^- based on arterial HCO_3^-. In low flow states, HCO_3^- delivery to ischemic tissues is limited and the available HCO_3^- is utilized to buffer protons generated by ischemic tissues.[5]

In intensive care units, laparoscopy is 96% accurate, with a procedure-related morbidity rate of only 8%[20]

when used to evaluate patients with acute abdominal pain. Laparoscopy can be successfully used to objectively review the clinical course of a patient on intra-arterial fibrinolytic therapy[89] and in the diagnosis of MVT.[101] For postoperative evaluation of patients after initial surgery for mesenteric ischemia, a second-look laparoscopy with provision to convert to a full laparotomy may be helpful.[43,107] At completion of the initial laparotomy, a midline peritoneal drain is placed.[70] During the second procedure the drain is exchanged for a Veress needle to create pneumoperitoneum and the bowel is examined laparoscopically. The criticism against laparoscopy in evaluating mesenteric ischemia is that laparoscopy visualizes only the serosal surface of the bowel[32] and early events in the pathology of mesenteric ischemia occur in bowel mucosa. Moreover, introduction of pneumoperitoneum increases intra-abdominal pressure and may theoretically worsen mesenteric ischemia when pressure of pneumoperitoneum exceeds the already low perfusion pressures in critically perfused segments of the bowel.

Early changes in mesenteric ischemia affect mucosa, and endoscopy is well suited for the evaluation of the gastrointestinal tract for evidence of ischemia. However, the lengths of esophagogastroduodenoscopes and colonoscopes do not permit evaluation of the small bowel.

The frequency of slow waves in the small bowel decreases and irregular fibrillary activity is present during the ischemic period; findings return to normal after reperfusion.[42] A superconducting quantum interference device magnetometer is capable of detecting magnetic fields that are only one billionth the strength of Earth's magnetic field. It contains four niobium pickup coils arranged at the corners of a 4.4-mm square and is housed within the vacuum space of a liquid helium–filled Dewar. This arrangement maintains the coils below the critical temperature of 9 K at which niobium wires become superconducting.[44] A superconducting quantum interference device magnetometer can measure the basic electric rhythm of the small bowel and the changes in the slow waves that appear during ischemia. By using a large number of channels spontaneous activity of the entire gastrointestinal tract can be observed.[26] Although the superconducting quantum interference device magnetometer has been used in animal experiments in the detection of mesenteric ischemia,[42,91] further investigations and refinements in technology need to be clarified to find a clinical application.

Management

The treatment of acute mesenteric ischemia is based on the principles of resuscitation, revascularization, resection, and reoperation. The goals of therapy are optimization of hemodynamic parameters, restoration of pulsatile blood flow to the bowel, resection of nonviable intestine, and salvage of ischemic but viable bowel. Revascularization should precede resection so that borderline ischemic but viable bowel can be salvaged and intestinal resection can be limited to the frankly necrotic bowel; the problems associated with short bowel syndrome can thus be avoided.

Resuscitation

Acute mesenteric ischemia is complicated in the later stages by hypotension, sepsis, shock, respiratory insufficiency, oliguria, and renal failure. Hemodynamic resuscitation with invasive monitoring is instituted to optimize the cardiac indices. Correction of hypovolemia, hypotension, and anemia enhances the blood flow in the mesenteric vasculature. Broad-spectrum antibiotic coverage is started empirically. Additional therapeutic measures include the discontinuation of agents known to cause mesenteric vasoconstriction and the treatment of cardiogenic shock with afterload-reducing agents and vasodilators.

Restoration of Blood Flow

Early restoration of intestinal blood flow is of critical importance in limiting intestinal resection and plays a major role in decreasing the mortality and morbidity associated with acute mesenteric ischemia. Minimally invasive procedures attempted before the onset of peritoneal signs include the infusion of papaverine or fibrinolytic agents or percutaneous transluminal angioplasty, depending on the etiology of acute mesenteric ischemia. The presence of peritoneal signs is an absolute indication for laparotomy and revascularization by techniques such as embolectomy, thromboendarterectomy, or bypass surgery.

Embolectomy carried out within the first few hours after the onset of symptoms results in the return of mesenteric circulation and either limits the area of infarction or in some cases prevents infarction and necrosis and resection of any portion of the small bowel. Embolectomy is performed by laparotomy and exposure of the SMA at the junction of mesenteries of the small bowel and the transverse colon along the inferior border of the pancreas.[114] For a proximal embolectomy, a 3- or 4-F balloon catheter is introduced over a guide wire via a longitudinal or transverse arteriotomy and the embolus is removed. Pulsatile inflow from the aorta is established, and a distal embolectomy is carried out with a 2-F catheter. Following thromboembolectomy, a residual clot may remain in the peripheral arcades. Although not widely practiced, an intra-arterial catheter may be placed intraoperatively for postoperative infusion of fibrinolytic agents. Because the amount of fibrinolytic agents administered by this route is small, systemic enhancement of the fibrinolytic system does not occur, bleeding is uncommon, and angiography can be periodically performed through the catheter to monitor the mesenteric circulation. Following the reestablishment of mesenteric circulation, bowel viability is reassessed and intestinal continuity is restored after resection of gangrenous bowel segments. Occasionally, the ends of the small bowel are brought to the surface as stomas with reestablishment of continuity at a second surgery.

Cases have been reported of successful fibrinolysis of SMA thromboembolism with local delivery of fibrinolytic agents such as recombinant tissue plasminogen activator (two boluses of 20 mg each at 12 hourly intervals followed by heparinization), streptokinase, and urokinase in the absence of clinical evidence of mesenteric infarction.[39,73,87] Recent cerebrovascular accident within the previous 2 months and active hemorrhage are absolute contraindications to the use of thrombolytic therapy. Other prerequisites to thrombolytic therapy include the complete absence of peritoneal signs and the 24-hour availability of angiographic facilities. The duration of the abdominal pain is also important if a conservative line of management is adopted. If duration of pain is more than 6 hours infarction is presumed to have occurred. Following therapy, the patient should have complete resolution of symptoms and persistent normal abdominal examination.

Revascularization procedures performed in the management of SMA thrombus include reimplantation, endarterectomy, and mesenteric bypass. Reimplantation of the SMA is performed by transecting the SMA distal to the occlusion and anastomosing the stump directly to the aorta. The short length of the SMA and atherosclerosis in the abdominal aorta pose technical difficulties in performing an effective procedure to reestablish circulation to the small bowel. Endarterectomy of the SMA thrombus may be done by either the transarterial or transaortic route using a trapdoor aortic incision. The transarterial route is difficult and usually unsuccessful because the most proximal extent of the SMA occlusion is difficult to remove safely. Moreover, this procedure also entails the removal of the thickened aortic intima adjacent to the visceral artery orifice by blind extraction. Transaortic endarterectomy could be performed by either an abdominal approach or the thoracoretroperitoneal approach; in an emergency, the abdominal approach is preferred. The ventral origin of the SMA from the aorta may make this procedure difficult, and the need to cross-clamp the aorta above the celiac vessels increases the risk of ischemic renal injury. In addition to the technical difficulties during endarterectomy, embolization to the distal vascular beds is a risk.[104]

In comparison to the previously described methods, mesenteric bypass is a preferred method in view of its simplicity and effectiveness in revascularization. The conduits selected for this procedure include autografts (arterial or venous) and prosthetic grafts (polytetrafluorourethane or Dacron). The endarterectomized external iliac artery has been used in the past, with the donor site arterial defect being replaced with a Dacron graft. Autologous reversed saphenous vein grafts may be utilized in the presence of abdominal sepsis. Although a saphenous vein conduit is preferred by some surgeons, others have successfully performed bypass procedures using prosthetic grafts even in the presence of peritoneal contamination. The advantages of the prosthetic grafts include ready availability and decreased risk of deformity and kinking in comparison to vein grafts. In addition, the short, rigid grafts exposed to high flow rates from the aorta have excellent patency rates and are easy to work with at the anastomotic sites. Retroperitoneal positioning of these grafts allows for more stability and less chance of kinking than a free-floating intraperitoneal location and also excludes them from potentially contaminated surroundings.

The distal anastomosis is performed to the side of the SMA distal to the occlusion. The proximal anastomotic site to the aorta is selected to permit either antegrade or retrograde flow. The proximal anastomosis to the supraceliac portion of the distal thoracic aorta is done by splitting and retracting the posterior fibers of the diaphragm. At this site there is minimal atherosclerotic involvement of the thoracic aorta and such an anastomosis favors antegrade flow. Retrograde flow is achieved by constructing an anastomosis in the infrarenal aorta, thereby avoiding suprarenal cross-clamping of the aorta, which is necessary if the anastomosis is performed in the thoracic aorta. Though easy to perform, the disadvantages include progression of atherosclerotic disease in the infrarenal aorta and kinking of the graft with movement of the mesentery. In cases of excessive aortic calcification, the common iliac artery can be used as the proximal takeoff point. Following revascularization procedures, the viability of the bowel is reassessed. With return of mesenteric circulation, there is often a dramatic improvement in the appearance of the bowel. Frankly necrotic bowel segments are resected. The decision to perform a second-look procedure is made at the initial surgery to avoid resecting large amounts of small bowel of borderline viability and to eliminate the risk of leaving necrotic bowel behind. In some cases further abdominal explorations are warranted.

Percutaneous transluminal angioplasty has occasionally been used to successfully treat acute mesenteric ischemia secondary to thrombotic occlusion of the SMA by passing a guide wire across the occlusion and dilation with a 6-mm balloon catheter followed by close clinical observation and repetition of the angiography.[14] Although percutaneous transluminal angioplasty may have a role in early ischemia without peritoneal signs and in intestinal angina,[81,92,109] a laparotomy is mandatory if there is clinical evidence of mesenteric infarction. A significant complication of percutaneous transluminal angioplasty is the potential for thrombus dislodgment and embolization of the distal mesenteric vasculature.

In patients with mild abdominal symptoms secondary to NOMI, correction of the low flow state is sufficient to reverse the ischemic events, angiography is not necessary, and the patient can be managed conservatively by careful clinical observation and monitoring. Severe abdominal pain with peritoneal findings is an indication for laparotomy without preliminary angiographic studies. Angiography is unreliable in the presence of shock because mesenteric vasoconstriction will be present even in the absence of mesenteric ischemia. In patients whose clinical picture is of an intermediate nature, angiography is followed by placement of the catheter tip in the SMA for papaverine infusion. Papaverine is a phosphodiesterase inhibitor that increases the concentration of cyclic adenosine monophosphate and produces vasodilation. It is infused directly into the SMA at a rate of 30 to 60 mg/h for at least 24 hours, and additional 24-hour periods of infusion are continued based on the clinical and radiologic response.[69,100] SMA infusion of papaverine does not cause hypotension because it is effectively cleared by the liver during the first passage. However, catheter dislodgment may result in papaverine entry into the systemic circulation, which may cause hypotension. Hence, when a patient undergoing papaverine infusion develops hypotension, catheter dislodgment must be ruled out angiographically.

With papaverine therapy radiologic and clinical resolution occurs in 1 to 5 days in early cases of NOMI.[58] If the clinical condition deteriorates and peritoneal signs develop, laparotomy with resection of the necrotic bowel is the appropriate course of action and is followed by continuation of papaverine in the postoperative stage. In some cases, infusion can be continued during surgery to salvage the borderline ischemic segments. Heparin is incompatible with papaverine, and thus the drugs are not used concomitantly. Other pharmacological agents that have been investigated to relieve vasospasm include intra-arterial prostaglandin E_1, tolazolin, glucagon, phenoxybenzamine, and levadosine and intravenous urokinase.[7] Initial resection is limited to definitely gangrenous segments because vasodilator therapy and correction of low flow state improve the perfusion of the bowel of questionable viability and a second-look surgery can be performed to verify the blood supply of the bowel.

Resuscitation, resection, postoperative anticoagulative therapy, and correction of any predisposing factors form the cornerstones in the management of MVT. Blood volume is expanded with effective resuscitation. In the absence of peritoneal signs, a combination of intravenous heparin and streptokinase is occasionally successful. Surgery is indicated when peritoneal signs are present. Intraoperative findings suggestive of MVT are cyanotic discoloration of the affected segments of the intestine, segmental intestinal infarction with sparing of the colon, palpable pulsations in the SMA or mesentery, extrusion of a thrombus from the veins in the divided edges of the mesentery, and poor demarcation between viable and nonviable tissues. Venous thrombosis usually extends beyond the margins of macroscopically involved intestinal segments. The state of the collateral circulation is a critical factor in determining the extent of bowel involvement. If it is poorly developed, then after superior mesenteric vein thrombosis there is vascular engorgement of the bowel that results in a dark-reddish appearance without any clear demarcation between viable and nonviable bowel, extravasation of blood into the bowel wall and adjacent mesentery, and finally infarction of the small bowel.[33]

At surgery, access is gained to the lumen of the superior mesenteric vein by a linear venotomy and clots are milked from the veins. Fogarty balloon catheters are utilized for the larger veins. Occasionally, portomesenteric venous thrombectomy has been successfully performed in patients with acute intestinal ischemia secondary to MVT. All infarcted bowel is resected with wide margins. Anticoagulation therapy is mandatory and should be started either preoperatively or intraoperatively when the diagnosis is made during the course of surgery.[90] It effectively reduces the incidence of recurrence, which occurs in a third of the patients, and improves survival rates. Therapy is started with heparin and continued with coumadin. Long-term anticoagulation therapy is indicated in patients with primary MVT and the coagulation disorders. Anticoagulation therapy is imperative even in the presence of cirrhosis, portal hypertension, or varices[30,71]. As with other forms of mesenteric ischemia, a second-look procedure often prevents massive bowel resection during the initial surgery. Lytic therapy with recombinant tissue-type plasminogen activator has been reported to be useful in anecdotal cases.[113] The mortality risk from MVT is around 30%, and anticoagulation therapy improves survival rates.[68,90]

Intraoperative Evaluation of Bowel Ischemia

In SMA thrombosis the entire small bowel is ischemic, but the stomach and duodenum and distal portions of the colon are spared. In contrast, ischemia due to embolus manifests itself by sparing of the proximal jejunum because the embolus is lodged beyond the first few branches of the SMA and distal to the origin of the middle colic artery. The physical appearance of ischemic intestine includes loss of normal sheen, dull gray discoloration, lack of peristalsis, absence of pulses in proximal

SMA or in the mesenteric vascular arcades, and absence of pulse on Doppler examination. The presence of foul-smelling fluid in the peritoneal cavity is not an indicator of necrotic bowel because it is present in early bowel ischemia without necrosis. The standard clinical criteria that indicate healthy, viable bowel are normal intestinal color, palpable mesenteric pulsations, visible peristalsis, and bleeding from the cut edge of the intestine. Clinical and experimental studies have demonstrated that clinical assessment is inaccurate. Necrosis and perforation of the bowel could still occur even after arterial pulsation and color return to the bowel after prolonged ischemia. Various methods to determine the viability of the bowel (e.g., use of Doppler probes, fluorescein perfusion, surface oximetry, infrared photoplethysmography, and laser Doppler velocimetry) have been investigated.

In a prospective controlled trial to compare the various methods of determining small bowel viability, Bulkley et al.[25] concluded that the fluorescein method and standard clinical judgment were better than Doppler assessments in sensitivity, specificity, predictive value, and accuracy, with the fluorescein method superseding clinical judgment. In the fluorescein perfusion method, fluorescein (10–15 mg/kg) is injected intravenously, the operating room is darkened, and a handheld Wood's lamp emitting ultraviolet light is used to differentiate viable bowel from nonviable segments. Patchy fluorescence and nonfluorescence indicate nonviability, and homogeneous or reticular distribution suggests viable bowel. The disadvantages of this method are the potential for anaphylaxis, difficulty in interpretation of the different patterns, and the inability to use the dye at second-look surgery due to its excretion characteristics. Surgeons overwhelmingly use the standard clinical criteria and err on the side of caution by resecting viable bowel rather than leaving behind bowel of questionable viability.

Second-Look Procedure

The decision to reoperate is made during the initial procedure.[114] Some centers advocate this procedure regardless of the findings on initial surgery or the condition of the patient as a way of limiting the extent of bowel resection at initial surgery. Other institutions have specific indications (e.g., lack of clear demarcation zone at the initial operation, extensive small bowel ischemia without evidence of necrosis, and nonresection of bowel of questionable viability at initial surgery) for second-look surgery.[68]

Summary

Acute mesenteric ischemia is the cause of considerable morbidity and mortality.[90] The inability to make an early diagnosis[31,51,54,98] prevents rapid institution of the corrective measures necessary to reverse the ischemic process.

Angiography remains the gold standard in the diagnosis of mesenteric ischemia. Adopting an aggressive approach of early angiography and selective papaverine infusion, Boley et al. were able to significantly decrease the mortality rate from 70% to 80% down to 46%[16,58] in patients with acute mesenteric ischemia. About 30% of patients investigated by Boley et al. did not have acute mesenteric ischemia and had a negative study. Although angiography detects the state of flow in the mesentery, it does not provide information about changes within the bowel wall. In this regard contrast-enhanced CT and magnetic resonance imaging scans appear to be useful in detecting mesenteric ischemia. The problem in obtaining magnetic resonance imaging scans on a 24-hour basis in an emergency situation limits the value of this test. A combination of contrast-enhanced CT scan and early angiography may further decrease the risk of morbidity in patients with mesenteric ischemia. Moreover, CT scans are helpful to rule out other important causes of acute abdominal pain and are important components in the diagnostic armamentarium of the physician.

In the absence of peritoneal signs, adequate resuscitation with careful follow-up may help to avoid an unnecessary laparotomy in an already ill individual. In the presence of peritoneal signs the principles of revascularization and resection should be strictly adhered to. With a high index of suspicion, better diagnosis, and early intervention, the mortality and morbidity rates of acute mesenteric ischemia can be further reduced.

References

1. Abdu RA, Zakhour BJ, Dallis DJ. Mesenteric venous thrombosis: 1911 to 1984. *Surgery.* 1987;101:383–388.
2. Alpern MB, Glazer GM, Francis IR. Ischemic or infarcted bowel: CT findings. *Radiology.* 1988;166:149–152.
3. Altman KA. Superior mesenteric artery occlusion: a review and case report. *Am J Gastroenterol.* 1971;152:1971–1974.
4. Andersen R, Stordahl A, Hoyseth H, et al. Increased intestinal permeability for the isoosmolar contrast medium iodixanol during small bowel ischemia in rats. *Scand J Gastroenterol.* 1995;30:1082–1088.
5. Antonsson JB, Boyle CC III, Kruithoff KL, et al. Validation of tonometric measurement of gut intramural pH during endotoxemia and mesenteric occlusion in pigs. *Am J Physiol.* 1990;259(suppl):G519–G523.
6. Ashida H, Kotoura Y, Nishioka A, et al. Portal and mesenteric venous thrombosis as a complication of endoscopic sclerotherapy. *Am J Gastroenterol.* 1988;84:306–310.
7. Athanasoulis CA, Wittenberg J, Bernstein R, Williams LF. Vasodilatory drugs in the management of nonocclusive bowel ischemia. *Gastroenterology.* 1975;68:146–150.
8. Baylin SB, Beaven MA, Buja LM, Keiser HR. Histaminase activity: a biochemical marker for medullary carcinoma of the thyroid. *Am J Med.* 1972;53:723–733.

9. Bergan JJ, Dean RH, Conn J, Yao JST. Revascularization in treatment of mesenteric infarction. *Ann Surg.* 1975;182: 430–438.

10. Bergan JJ, Dry L, Conn J, Trippel OH. Intestinal ischemic syndrome. *Ann Surg.* 1969;169:120–126.

11. Bergan JJ, Yao JST. Acute intestinal ischemia. In: Rutherford RB, ed. *Vascular Surgery.* Philadelphia, Pa: WB Saunders; 1977:825–842.

12. Beyer D, Horsch S, Bohr M, Schmitz T. Roentgenographic findings of experimental bowel ischemia in dogs following occlusion of the superior mesenteric artery. *Fortschritte auf dem Gebiete der Rontgenstrahlen und der Nuklearmedizin.* 1980;132:377–385.

13. Blum H, Chance B, Buzby GP. In vivo noninvasive observation of acute mesenteric ischemia in rats. *Surgery, Gynecology and Obstetrics.* 1987;164:409–414.

14. Bocchini T, Hoffman J, Zuckerman D. Mesenteric ischemia due to an occluded superior mesenteric artery treated by percutaneous transluminal angioplasty. *J Clin Gastroenterol.* 1995;20:86–88.

15. Boley SJ, Brandt LJ, Veith FJ. Ischemic disorders of the intestine. *Curr Probl Surg.* 1978;15:1–98

16. Boley SJ, Sprayregan S, Siegelman SS, Veith FJ. Initial results from an aggressive roentgenological and surgical approach to acute mesenteric ischemia. *Surgery.* 1977;82: 848–855.

17. Bottger T, Jonas J, Weber W, Junginger T. Sensitivity of preoperative diagnosis in mesenteric vascular occlusion [in German]. *Bildgebung.* 1991;58:192–198.

18. Bottger T, Schafer W, Weber W, Junginger T. Value of preoperative diagnostics in acute mesenteric vascular occlusion: a prospective study. *Langenbecks Arch Chir.* 1990;375: 278–282.

19. Bounous G, Echave V, Vobecky SJ, Navert H, Wollin A. Acute necrosis of the intestinal mucosa with high serum levels of diamine oxidase. *Dig Dis Sci.* 1984;29:872–874.

20. Brandt CP, Priebe PP, Eckhauser ML. Diagnostic laparoscopy in the intensive care patient: avoiding the nontherapeutic laparotomy. *Surg Endosc.* 1993;73:168–172.

21. Britt LG, Cheek RC. Non-occlusive mesenteric vascular disease: clinical and experimental observations. *Ann Surg.* 1969;169:704–711.

22. Broekmans AW, Van Rooyen W, Westerveld BD, Briet E, Bertina RM. Mesenteric venous thrombosis as presenting manifestation of hereditary protein S deficiency. *Gastroenterology.* 1987;92:240.

23. Brooks DH, Carey LC. Base deficit in superior mesenteric artery occlusion. *Ann Surg.* 1973;177:352–356.

24. Brown RA, Chiu CJ, Scott HJ, Gurd FN. Ultrastructural changes in the canine ileal mucosal cell after mesenteric arterial occlusion. *Arch Surg.* 1970;101:290–297.

25. Bulkley GB, Zuidema GD, Hamilton SR, O'Mara C, Klacsmann PG, Horn SD. Intraoperative determination of small intestinal viability following ischemic injury. *Ann Surg.* 1981;193:628–637.

26. Cabot R, Kohatsu S. The effects of ischemia on the electrical contractile activities of the canine small intestines. *Am J Surg.* 1976;136:242–246.

27. Catalono O. Computed tomography in the diagnostic approach to acute mesenteric ischemia. *Radiol Med (Torino).* 1995;89:440–446.

28. Clark RA. Computed tomography of bowel infarction. *J Comput Assist Tomogr.* 1987;11:757–762.

29. Clark RA, Gallant TE. Acute mesenteric ischemia: angiographic spectrum. *AJR Am J Roentgenol.* 1984;142:555–562.

30. Clavien PA, Durig M, Harder F. Venous mesenteric infarction: a particular entity. *Br J Surg.* 1988;75:252–255.

31. Deehan DJ, Heys SD, Brittenden J, Eremin O. Mesenteric ischaemia: prognostic factors and influence of delay upon outcome. *J R Coll Surg Edinb.* 1995;40:112–115.

32. Duh QY. Laparoscopic procedures for small bowel disease [review]. *Baillieres Clin Gastroenterol.* 1993;7:833–850.

33. Ellis DJ, Brandt LJ. (1994) Mesenteric venous thrombosis. *Gastroenterologist.* 1994;2:293–298.

34. Englund R, Lalak N, Jacques T, Hanel KC. Sigmoid and gastric tonometry during infrarenal aortic aneurysm repair. *Austr N Z J Surg.* 1996;66:88–90.

35. Feretis CB, Koborozos BA, Vyssoulis GP, Manouras AJ, Apostolidis NS, Golematis BC. Serum phosphate level in acute bowel ischemia: an aid to early diagnosis. *Am Surg.* 1985;51:242–244.

36. Fiddian-Green RG, Amelin PM, Herrmann JB, et al. Prediction of the development of sigmoid ischemia on the day of aortic operations: indirect measurements of intramural pH in the colon. *Arch Surg.* 1986;121: 654–660.

37. Fiddian-Green RG, McCough E, Pittenger G, Rothman E. Predictive value of intramural pH and other risk factors for massive bleeding from stress ulceration. *Gastroenterology.* 1983;85:613–620.

38. Fine J. The intestinal circulation in shock. *Gastroenterology.* 1967;52:454–458.

39. Flickinger EG, Johnsrude IS, Ogburn NL, Weaver MD, Pories WJ. Local streptokinase infusion for superior mesenteric artery thrombo-embolism. *AJR Am J Roentgenol.* 1983;140:771–772.

40. Fock CM, Kullnig P, Ranner G, Beaufort-Spontin F, Schmidt F. Mesenteric arterial embolism: the value of emergency CT in diagnostic procedure. *Eur J Radiol.* 1994; 18:12–14.

41. Franquet T, Bescos JM, Reparaz B. Noninvasive methods in the diagnosis of isolated superior mesenteric vein thrombosis: US and CT. *Gastrointestinal Radiology.* 1989;14: 321–325.

42. Garrard CL, Halter S, Richards WO. Correlation between pathology and electrical activity during acute intestinal ischemia. *Surg Forum.* 1994;45:368–371.

43. Glattli A, Seiler C, Metzger A, Stirnemann P, Baer HU. Second look laparoscopy after mesenteric infarct. *Langenbecks Arch Chir.* 1994;379:66–69.

44. Golzarian J, Wikswo JP Jr, Friedman RN, Richards WO. First biomagnetic measurements of intesinal basic electric rhythms (BER) *in vivo* using a high-resolution magnetometer. *Gastroenterology.* 1992;103(suppl):A1385.

45. Graeber GM, Wolf RE, Harmon JW. Serum creatinine kinase and alkaline phosphatase in experimental small bowel infarction. *J Surg Res.* 1984;37:25–32.

46. Graeber GM, Wukich DK, Cafferty PJ, et al. Changes in peripheral serum creatine phosphokinase and lactic dehydrogenase in acute experimental colonic infarction. *Ann Surg.* 1981;194:708–715.

47. Gusberg R, Gump F. Combined surgical and nutritional management of patients with acute mesenteric vascular occlusion. *Ann Surg.* 1974;179:358–361.

48. Haglund U, Lundgren O. Nonocclusive acute intestinal vascular failure. *Br J Surg.* 1979;66:155–158.

49. Harris MT, Lewis BS. Systemic diseases affecting the mesenteric circulation. *Surg Clin North Am.* 1992;72:245–261.

50. Herr FW, Silen W, French SW. Intestinal gangrene without apparent vascular occlusion. *Am J Surg.* 1965;110:231–238.

51. Heys SD, Brittenden J, Crofts TJ. Acute mesenteric ischemia: the continuing difficulty in early diagnosis. *Postgrad Med J.* 1993;69:48–51.

52. Hibbard JS, Swenson PC, Levin AG. Roentgenology of experimental mesenteric vascular occlusion. *Arch Surg.* 1933;26:20–26.

53. Hirner A, Haring R, Hofmeister M. Akute mesenterialgefabverschlusse. *Chirurg.* 1987;58:577–584.

54. Howard TJ, Plaskon LA, Wiebke EA, Wilcox MG, Madura JA. Non occlusive mesenteric ischemia remains a diagnostic dilemma. *Am J Surg.* 1996;171:405–408.

55. Jamieson WG, Lozon A, Durand D, Wall W. Changes in serum phosphate levels associated with intestinal infarction and necrosis. *Surgery, Gynecology and Obstetrics.* 1975;140:19–21.

56. Jamieson WG, Marchuk S, Rowson J, Durand D. The early diagnosis of massive acute intestinal ischemia. *Br J Surg Suppl.* 1977;69:552–553.

57. Jonas J, Bottger T. Diagnosis and prognosis of mesenterial infarct [in German]. *Med Klin.* 1994;89:68–72.

58. Kaleya RN, Sammartano RJ, Boley SJ. Aggressive approach to mesenteric ischemia. *Surg Clin North Am.* 1992;72:157–181.

59. Kanda T, Fujii H, Fujita M, Sakai Y, Ono T, Hatakeyama K. Intestinal fatty acid binding protein is available for diagnosis of intestinal ischemia: immunochemical analysis of two patients with ischemic intestinal diseases. *Gut.* 1995;36:788–791.

60. Kaufman AJ, Tarr RW, Holburn GE, McCurdy M, Partain CL, James AE Jr. Magnetic resonance imaging of ischemic bowel in rabbit model. *Invest Radiol.* 1988;23:93–97.

61. Kazmierczak SC, Lott JA, Caldwell JH. Acute intestinal infarction or obstruction: search for better laboratory tests in an animal model. *Clin Chem.* 1988;34:281–288.

62. Klein HM, Klosterhalfen B, Kinzel S, et al. CT and MRI of experimentally induced mesenteric ischemia in a porcine model. *J Comput Assist Tomogr.* 1996;20:254–261.

63. Klein H, Lensing R, Klosterhalfen B, Tons C, Gunther RW. Diagnostic imaging of mesenteric infarction. *Radiology.* 1995;197:79–82.

64. Kusche J, Richter H, Schmidt J, Hesterbert R, Friedrich A, Lorenz W. Diamine oxidase in rabbit small intestine: separation from a soluble monoamine oxidase. Properties and pathophysiological significance in intestinal ischemia. *Agents and Action.* 1975;5:431–439.

65. Kusche J, Stahlknecht CD, Lorenz W, Reichert G, Dietz W. Comparison of concentrations in the histamine-diamine oxidase system during acute intestinal ischemia in pigs, dogs, and rabbits: evidence for a uniform pathophysiological mechanism. *Agents and Action.* 1979;9:49–52.

66. Kusche J, Stahlknecht CD, Lorenz W, Reichert G, Richter H. Diamine oxidase activity and histamine release in dogs following acute mesenteric artery occlusion. *Agents and Action.* 1977;7:81–84.

67. Lange H, Jackel R. Usefulness of plasma lactate concentration in the diagnosis of acute abdominal disease. *Eur J Surg.* 1994;160:381–384.

68. Levy PJ, Krauz MM, Manny J. The role of second-look procedure in improving survival time for patients with mesenteric venous thrombosis. *Surgery, Gynecology and Obstetrics.* 1990;170:287–291.

69. Lock G, Scholmerich J. Non-occlusive mesenteric ischemia [review]. *Hepatogastroenterology.* 1995;42:234–239.

70. MacSweeney STR, Postlethwaite JC. 'Second-look' laparoscopy in the management of acute mesenteric ischaemia. *Br J Surg.* 1994;81:90.

71. Mathews J, White RR. Primary mesenteric venous occlusive disease. *Am J Surg.* 1971;122:579–583.

72. Maung R, Kelly JK, Schneider MP, Poon MC. Mesenteric venous thrombosis due to antithrombin III deficiency. *Arch Pathol Lab Med.* 1988;112:37–39.

73. McBride KD, Gaines PA. Thrombolysis of a partially occluding superior mesenteric artery thromboembolus by infusion of streptokinase. *Cardiovasc Intervent Radiol.* 1994;17:164–166.

74. Mishima Y, Horie Y. Experimental studies of ischemic enterocolitis. *World J Surg.* 1980;4:601–608.

75. Mizuguchi H, Imamura I, Takemura M, Fukui H. Purification and characterization of diamine oxidase (histaminidase) from rat small intestine. *J Biochem.* 1994;116:631–635.

76. Montgomery A, Hartmann M, Jonsson K, Haglund U. Intramucosal pH measurement with tonometers for detecting gastrointestinal ischemia in porcine hemorrhagic shock. *Circulatory Shock.* 1989;29:319–327.

77. Moore WM, Hollier LH. Mesenteric artery occlusive disease. *Cardiol Clin.* 1991;9:535–541.

78. Murray MJ, Gonze MD, Nowak LR, Cobb CF. Serum D(−)-lactate levels as an aid to diagnosing acute intestinal ischemia. *Am J Surg.* 1994;167:575–578.

79. Nozaki E, Kohno A, Narimatsu A, Shigeta A, Nakagawa T, Suzuki T. Superior mesenteric artery occlusion: an unenhanced CT finding. *J Comput Assist Tomogr.* 1991;15:866–867.

80. Ockner RK, Manning JA. Fatty acid binding protein in small intestine: identification, isolation, and evidence for its role in cellular fatty acid transport. *J Clin Invest.* 1974;54:326–338.

81. Odurny A, Sniderman KW, Colapinto RF. Intestinal angina: percutaneous transluminal angioplasty of the celiac and superior mesenteric arteries. *Radiology.* 1988;167:59–62.

82. Okoye MI, Verrill HL, Mueller WF. Marked concomitant elevations in serum creatinine kinase and lactic dehydrogenase in a patient with bowel necrosis. *Am Surg.* 1983;49:612–615.

83. Otamiri TA, Tagesson C, Sjodahl R. Increased plasma malondialdehyde in patients with small intestinal strangulation obstruction. *Acta Chir Scand.* 1988;154:283–285.

84. Ottinger LW, Austen WG. A study of 136 patients with mesenteric infarction. *Surgery, Gynecology and Obstetrics.* 1967;124:251–261

85. Perez C, Llauger J, Puig J, Palmer J. Computed tomographic findings in bowel ischemia. *Gastrointestinal Radiology.* 1989;14:241–245.

86. Pierce GE, Brockenbrough ED. The spectrum of mesenteric infarction. *Am J Surg.* 1970;119:233–238.

87. Pillari G, Doscher W, Fierstein J, Ross W, Loh G, Berkowitz BJ. Low dose streptokinase in the treatment of celiac and superior mesenteric artery occlusion. *Arch Surg.* 1983;118:1340–1342.

88. Polson H, Mowat C, Himal HS. Experimental and clinical studies of mesenteric infarction. *Surgery, Gynecology and Obstetrics.* 1981;153:360–362.

89. Regan F, Karlstad RR, Magnuson TH. Minimally invasive management of acute superior mesenteric artery occlusion: combined urokinase and laparoscopic therapy. *Am J Gastroenterol.* 1996;91:1019–1021.

90. Rhee RY, Gloviczki P, Mendonca CT, et al. Mesenteric venous thrombosis: still a lethal disease in the 1990s. *J Vasc Surg.* 1994;20:688–697.

91. Richards WO, Garrard CL, Allos AH, Bradshaw LA, Staton DJ, Wikswo JP Jr. Noninvasive diagnosis of mesenteric ischemia using a SQUID magnetometer. *Ann Surg.* 1995;221:696–705.

92. Roberts L, Wertman DA, Mills SR, Moore AV, Heaston DK. Transluminal angioplasty of the superior mesenteric artery: an alternative to surgical revascularization. *AJR Am J Roentgenol.* 1983:141:1039–1042.

93. Robinson D, Stirling JL. N-Acetyl glucosaminidases in human spleen. *Biochem J.* 1968;107:321–327.

94. Roobottom CA, Dubbins PA. Significant disease of the celiac and superior mesenteric arteries in asymptomatic patients: predictive value of Doppler sonography. *AJR Am J Roentgenol.* 1993;161:985–988.

95. Rush BF, Host WR, Fewel J, Hsieh J. Intestinal ischemia and some organic substances in serum and abdominal fluid. *Arch Surg.* 1972;105:151–157.

96. Sachs SM, Morton JH, Schwartz SI. Acute mesenteric ischemia. *Surgery.* 1982;92:646–653

97. Sawer BA, Jameison WG, Durand D. The significance of elevated peritoneal fluid phosphate level in intestinal infarction. *Surgery, Gynecology and Obstetrics.* 1978;146:43–45.

98. Scheppach W, Langenfeld H, Schultz G, Wittenberg G, Hahn D, Kochsiek K. Non obstructive mesenteric ischemia: a diagnostic problem in internal medicine. *Z Gastroenterol.* 1995;33:214–218.

99. Schiedler MG, Cutler BS, Fiddian-Green RG. Sigmoid intramural pH for prediction of ischemic colitis during aortic surgery: a comparison with risk factors and inferior mesenteric artery stump pressure. *Arch Surg.* 1987;122:881–886.

100. Schneider TA, Longo WE, Ure T, Vernava AM III. Mesenteric ischemia: acute arterial syndromes. *Dis Colon Rectum.* 1994;37:1163–1174.

101. Serreyn RF, Schoofs PR, Baetens PR, Vandekerckhore D. Laparoscopic diagnosis of mesenteric venous thrombosis. *Endoscopy.* 1986;18:249–250.

102. Shakir KMM, Margolis S, Baylin SB. Localization of histaminase (diamine oxidase) in rat small intestinal mucosa: site of release by heparin. *Biochem Pharmacol.* 1977;26:2343–2347.

103. Sommer A, Jaschke W, Georgi M. CT diagnosis of acute mesenteric vein thrombosis with intestinal infarction. *Aktuelle Radiol.* 1994;4:344–347.

104. Stoney RJ, Ehrenfeld WK, Wylie EJ. Revascularization methods in chronic visceral ischemia caused by atherosclerosis. *Arch Surg.* 1977;186:468–476.

105. Stordahl A. Urinary excretion of iohexol after intestinal administration in rats with bowel ischemia: the effects of mesenteric arterial and/or venous occlusion. *Acta Radiol.* 1989;30:87092–87097.

106. Swallow DM, Stokes DC, Corney G, Harris H. Differences between the N-acteyl hexosaminidase isoenzymes in serum and tissues. *Ann Hum Genet.* 1976;37:287–302.

107. Temes T, Kauten RJ, Schwartz MZ. Nuclear magnetic resonance as a noninvasive method of diagnosing intestinal ischemia: technique and preliminary results. *J Pediatr Surg.* 1991;26:775–779.

108. Volteas N, Labropoulos N, Leon M, Kalodiki E, Chan P, Nicolaides AN. Detection of superior mesenteric and celiac artery stenosis with colour flow duplex imaging. *European Journal of Vascular Surg.* 1993;7:616–620.

109. Warnock NG, Gaines PA, Beard JD, Cumberland DC. Treatment of intestinal angina by percutaneous transluminal angioplasty of superior mesenteric artery occlusion. *Clin Radiol.* 1992;45:18–19.

110. Wilkerson DK, Mezrich R, Drake C, Sebok D, Satina MA. Magnetic resonance imaging of acute occlusive intestinal ischemia. *J Vasc Surg.* 1990;11:567–571.

111. Williams LF Jr, Wittenberg J, Grimes ET, Byrne JJ. Ischemic diseases of the bowel. *Dis Colon Rectum.* 1970; 13:275–282.

112. Wolf E, Sprayregen S, Bakal CW. Radiology in intestinal ischemia: plain film, contrast, and other imaging studies. *Surg Clin North Am.* 1992;72:107–124.

113. Yankes RJ, Uglietta JP, Grant J. Percutaneous transhepatic recanalization and thrombolysis of the superior mesenteric vein. *AJR Am J Roentgenol.* 1988;151:289–290.

114. Zuidema GD. Surgical management of superior mesenteric arterial emboli. *Arch Surg.* 1961;82:267–270.

115. Zuidema GD, Reed D, Turcotte JG, Fry WJ. Superior mesenteric artery embolectomy. *Ann Surg.* 1964;159:548–553.

Section 4
Arterial Aneurysms

47

Aneurysms

Jose Alemany, Hartmut Görtz, and Klaus Schaarschmidt

Introduction and Historical Aspects

Successful surgical treatment of arterial aneurysms by extirpation or exclusion with subsequent graft interposition was not reported before the early twentieth century. Even in the pre-Christian era aneurysmal vascular dilatation was observed; Galen described expansive pulsation as the principal symptom of aneurysms.

About 1300 Antyllus proposed proximal ligation of the artery with subsequent incision and excavation of the aneurysm. In 1567 Vesalius reported on the first abdominal aortic aneurysm, and in 1893 Rudolf Matas was the first to successfully perform a proximal ligature of an abdominal aorta with an infrarenal aneurysm. Although numerous conservative and surgical treatments were attempted earlier, the beginning of modern aneurysm surgery lies in the early twentieth century.

Goyanes[1] is credited with the first successful resection and graft interposition for an aneurysm of the popliteal artery in 1906. One year later Lexer performed the same operation in a patient suffering from an axillary artery aneurysm. But it was not until 1951 that Charles Dubost[2] completed the first successful resection of an infrarenal abdominal aortic aneurysm with reconstruction of the continuity by interposition of a free graft of the homologous thoracic aorta. The breakthrough in surgical treatment of infrarenal abdominal aortic aneurysms came with the introduction and universal availability of alloplastic grafts of high quality and unlimited quantity.

Gradually the morbidity and mortality rates of aneurysm surgery decreased to well below 2% due to the refinements in surgical technique as well as the advances of anesthesia and intensive care medicine[3] (the first intensive care unit was introduced in Baltimore in 1958,[4] artificial respiration and blood gas checks in the mid 1960s,[5] parenteral nutrition in 1968 by Dudrick et al.,

positive end-expiratory pressure ventilation in 1970,[6] pulmonary artery catheters by Swan and Ganz in 1975,[7] and pulse oximetry in the late 1980s[8,9]). Further developments in the operative treatment of aneurysms were initiated by the first clinical reports on the successful transarterial implantation of stented intraluminal grafts into abdominal aortic aneurysms.

Pathology and Pathophysiology

An aneurysm is a permanent localized dilatation of an arterial lumen. This dilatation is limited to a well-defined segment of an artery, which distinguishes the aneurysm from both ectasia and elongation. If the whole arterial segment is dilated evenly, the aneurysm is called a fusiform aneurysm, whereas a dilatation confined to only part of the arterial circumference is termed a saccular aneurysm.

A *true aneurysm* is formed by all layers of the arterial wall. Conversely, the term *false aneurysm* denotes a periarterial hematoma connected to the lumen of an opened vessel and separated by no more than a membrane of organized fibrin. Most of these false aneurysms are of infectious or traumatic origin.

The *dissecting aneurysm* is not an aneurysm proper but arises from a split tunica media subsequent to an intimal tear. A dissecting aneurysm may result in an adventitial tear with profuse hemorrhage, spontaneous thrombosis, reentry through a second intimal tear, or obstruction of aortic branches with subsequent peripheral ischemia. A further complication is aortic valve insufficiency caused by dissection of the ascending aorta.

An aneurysm arises from a persistent disproportion between blood pressure and vessel wall resilience. A healthy artery sustains no damage from normotone pulsatile blood pressure. However, increased vessel wall compliance combined with chronic hypertension favors the development of an aneurysm. The factors reported to cause aneurysms most frequently include the following:

1. Arteriosclerosis
2. Activation of proteolytic enzymes
3. Genetic predisposition
4. Hemodynamic influences

According to classical theory, the elastomuscular lamellae of the aortic tunica media are nourished by diffusion from the aortic lumen, because there are few vasa vasorum in this aortic segment. In arteriosclerosis, intimal plaque formation increases the diffusion distance and thus progressively compromises nutrition of the tunica media. However, the influence of arteriosclerosis on aneurysm formation is not entirely clear. Arteriosclerotic changes might be the consequence of deteriorated media nutrition rather than its cause.[10,11]

Increased activity of proteolytic enzymes may also cause aneurysm formation. This theory is supported by the finding of increased elastase and collagenase activities in the walls of rapidly growing and ruptured abdominal aortic aneurysms. So far it is unclear whether this rise represents a cause or the enzyme activities are stimulated by other factors.[12]

More than 15% of all patients who suffer from an aneurysm have been reported to have a positive family history for the condition.[13] Genetic studies suspect mutations on the gene for type III collagen. Several gene mutations have already been described for the Ehlers-Danlos and Marfan's syndromes (fibrillin genes on chromosomes 3, 5, and 15). However, genetic changes are highly unlikely to be a major or sole cause of aneurysm formation in more than a few patients.

Blood flow quantity and velocity have a strong bearing on the arterial diameter because high shear stress increases the arterial lumen size. According to Laplace's law arterial wall tension and thus the risk of rupture increase with the second power of the arterial diameter. As a result, the development of an aneurysm must be assumed to be a multifactorial process in the vast majority of patients so that none of the mentioned factors can be identified as the sole cause.

Inflammatory Aneurysms

Inflammatory aneurysms of the aorta represent a special form of aneurysms recognizable by their marked fibrotic thickening of the aortic wall and adhesion to the surrounding tissues and organs. Frequently the aortic wall is found to be infiltrated by lymphocytes and plasma cells. The etiology and pathogenesis of these inflammatory aneurysms are yet unknown but have been attributed by some authors to an autoimmune reaction and by others to a severe inflammatory reaction secondary to arteriosclerosis.[14]

Localization

The most frequent site of aneurysms is the infrarenal aorta, followed by the popliteal and common femoral arteries. In up to 25% of all patients who suffer from aortic aneurysms there are concurrent aneurysms of the popliteal artery and in 15% concurrent aneurysms of the common femoral artery.

The higher incidence of aneurysm in the abdominal aorta compared with the thoracic aorta is attributed to the marked paucity of elastomuscular lamellae in the tunica media of the abdominal aorta and its decreased perfusion and fewer vasa vasorum.[11] The following aneurysms can be distinguished by site:

Central aneurysms
    Thoracic aneurysms
    Thoracoabdominal aneurysms
    Abdominal aneurysms
    Visceral aneurysms
Peripheral aneurysms
    Aneurysms of the brachiocephalic arteries
    Aneurysms of the upper extremity
    Aneurysms of the lower extremity

Abdominal Aneurysms

About 95% of all abdominal aneurysms originate below the renal arteries. In 4% to 5% the aneurysm is located in the juxtarenal or suprarenal portion of the abdominal aorta. The preferred site of abdominal aneurysms in the infrarenal aorta is explained by the anatomical and hemodynamic properties of this vascular region. These aneurysms develop as a rule in the direction of lowest resistance (i.e., to the left-sided retroperitoneal tissue) (Figure 47.1). The inferior vena cava and the mesenteric root form an obstacle to right-sided aortic expansion. In more than half of these aneurysms there is a coexisting dilative, rarely obliterative arteriopathy of the central pelvic arteries. Concurrent peripheral aneurysms, particularly of the popliteal and common femoral artery, are common. Saccular peripheral aneurysms are rarer but more prone to rupture than fusiform peripheral aneurysms. Different authors report the overall incidence of infrarenal abdominal aortic aneurysms to be between 0.3% and 2.8%. A mean annual increase in diameter between 0.2 and 0.4 cm has been observed but is influenced by several factors including wall calcification, parietal thrombus formation, peripheral fibrosis, and the degree of hypertension.[15,16]

The mean age of our patients who underwent surgery for abdominal aortic aneurysms from 1985 through 1995 was 64 years, with a male to female ratio of 10:1. Coronary vascular disease and hypertension were the leading concurrent diseases. More than 75% of abdominal aortic aneurysms are asymptomatic and diagnosed by chance on routine ultrasonograms, laparotomies, or post-

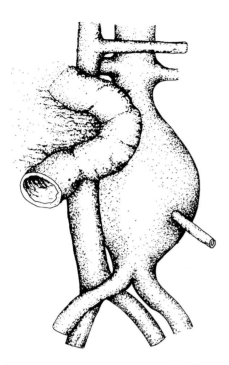

FIGURE 47.1. Abdominal aortic aneurysm development.

mortem examinations.[17] Only the largest aneurysms become symptomatic when they compress adjacent organs, obstruct important arterial branches, penetrate into vertebral bodies, or perforate (Figure 47.2).

Clinically, patients with abdominal aortic aneurysms present with diffuse abdominal pain sometimes accompanied by sensations of repletion (full or bloated feeling), back pain, and pulsatile swellings. This pain is of particular intensity and rarely combined with spinal nerve paresis if the aneurysm has eroded the vertebral column or compresses the spinal roots leaving the spinal canal at this level.

Aneurysms that extend into the iliac bifurcation rarely lead to compression of the ureters and subsequent hydronephrosis.[18] If visceral, renal, or pelvic arteries have been occluded, signs of mesenterial, renal, or peripheral ischemia may predominate. The most frequent clinical mistakes are erroneous diagnoses of ileus or appendicitis.

Clinical Features and Their Bases

Symptoms

Small aneurysms (<4 cm) may remain hidden until death. In 10% of patients abdominal aortic aneurysmal emboli that originate from aneurysmal thrombi engender acute lower extremity ischemia. Rupture is the most severe complication of abdominal aortic aneurysms; surgeons usually encounter it in the retroperitoneal space, because rupture into the free abdominal cavity leads to almost immediate death. Perforations into adjacent organs are rare but may occur in the ascending duodenum, the inferior vena cava, or the internal iliac veins in aortoiliac aneurysms (Figure 47.3). Patients who suffer from a central arteriovenous fistula subsequent to such an event frequently develop cardiopulmonary decompensation and may be admitted to the hospital for suspected myocardial infarction. It is well known that survival between 24 hours and 9 days can be attained in a patient with a ruptured abdominal aortic aneurysm by conservative measures. It has been shown, however, that the prospects for successful surgical management deteriorate rapidly when more than 8 hours pass after rupture.

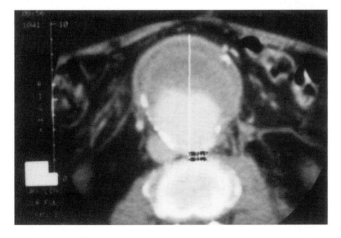

FIGURE 47.2. Computed tomography scan: aneurysm penetration into the vertebral body.

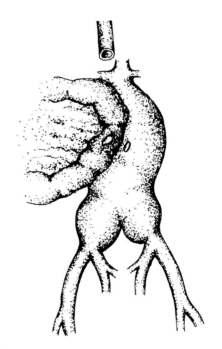

FIGURE 47.3. Perforation in the duodenum.

Diagnostic Measures

Unfortunately the diagnosis of an abdominal aortic aneurysm is rarely made clinically, because only large aneurysms are palpable (Figure 47.4). Conversely, in very slim patients the physiological pulsations of the normal aorta may be misinterpreted.

The aim of diagnostic measures is not only to establish the diagnosis of an abdominal aortic aneurysm but also to gain sufficient information on local operability, extent, and possible invasions into adjacent organs. Plain abdominal or renal x-ray films are of very limited use. Usually they are ordered for other reasons, and the incidental detection of a calcareous sickle that projects onto the spine draws attention to the abdominal aortic aneurysm (Figure 47.5).

The following imaging procedures have attained special diagnostic value in abdominal aortic aneurysms:

Abdominal ultrasound examination
Nuclear magnetic resonance imaging
Computed tomography
Digitally subtracted arteriography

Abdominal ultrasonic examination is the simplest method to verify the clinical suspicion of an abdominal aortic aneurysm. The advantages are general availability, low cost, and the ease of repeated examinations for the patient. The sensitivity of abdominal ultrasound examination approximates 98% for modern color duplex scans. The sole application of ultrasonography is not adequate, because it yields only very limited information on the relation of the aneurysm to visceral and iliac arteries. Moreover, intraluminal fresh thrombi are not depicted accurately, particularly if they form only a narrow fringe or if the aorta has undergone marked atheromatous changes. However, ultrasonography has established its role in follow-up examinations with both conservatively and surgically managed abdominal aortic aneurysms.[19,20]

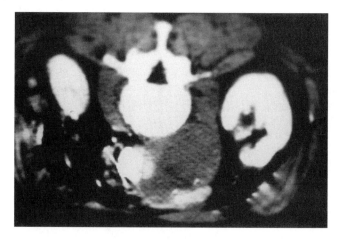

FIGURE 47.5. Computed tomography scan: abdominal aortic aneurysm sublined by calcium.

Computed tomography (preferably spiral computed tomography) is indispensable for determining local operability. It provides accurate information on the exact extent and topographical relation to the renal arteries, suprarenal aorta, and adjacent organs such as the duodenum, vena cava, or ureters and is required for reliable recognition of penetrations. The extent of wall calcifications is visible, which helps in determining preoperatively the optimal site of anastomosis. Finally, in addition to accurate delineation of peripheral fringes, the computed tomography scan accurately differentiates between inflammatory and symptomatic aneurysms.

Magnetic resonance imaging allows the most accurate depiction of aneurysms in all three planes. Drawbacks are the inability to delineate calcifications, the high cost, the lengthy examination, and the fact that it is not suitable for all patients. Thus magnetic resonance imaging is indicated in special cases if both ultrasonography and computed tomography fail to supply sufficient preoperative information on aneurysmal morphology and if the information is critical for operative planning.[21]

Angiography is required for every patient who undergoes surgery because it is the only investigation that depicts exactly parietal and visceral aortic branches. In particular, angiography can detect anatomical anomalies and obliterating disease of the renal, superior and inferior mesenteric, and iliac arteries. This information is invaluable, because complications such as renal insufficiency, ischemic colitis, and gluteal ischemia can thus be avoided.[22]

Apart from these specific investigations the general operability, in particular cardiopulmonary and renal functions, should be evaluated carefully. A duplex ultrasonography of the supra-aortic branches is recommended.

If the patient suffers from severe coronary disease or symptomatic carotid stenosis, an aortocoronary bypass operation or carotid desobliteration must be given prior-

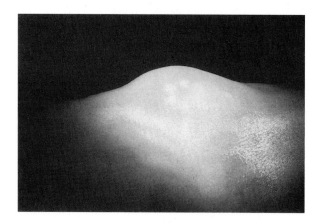

FIGURE 47.4. Large aneurysms are palpable.

ity to elective repair of an abdominal aortic aneurysm.[23] If the abdominal aortic aneurysm is symptomatic as well, prioritizing is difficult and requires considerable personal experience because simultaneous reconstructions raise the total mortality rate disproportionately. Acute abdominal inflammations such as appendicitis, cholecystitis, and diverticulitis should not be treated surgically in the same session but rather should be dealt with before elective reconstruction for an abdominal aortic aneurysm. Incidental appendectomies or cholecystectomies without acute inflammation bear no increased risk in our experience and can be performed in the same session with adequate perioperative antibiotic prophylaxis. If colorectal tumors are detected during elective surgery for an abdominal aortic aneurysm, a second session is strongly recommended, because a simultaneous operation increases the likelihood of infection of the alloplastic graft.[24,25]

Medical Treatment and Risk of Rupture

The advances in diagnosis and surgical therapy have considerably improved the prognosis of abdominal aortic aneurysm, partly because aneurysms are now diagnosed very early by screening examination and partly because the mortality rate from rupture does not increase before the aneurysms have reached a certain size. The mortality rate for an emergency operation for a ruptured abdominal aortic aneurysm has changed little during recent decades and is still in the range of 50% as opposed to 1% to 2% for an elective operation. As a result, there are conflicting opinions on the ideal timing of elective reconstruction. Whether the diagnosis of an abdominal aortic aneurysm requires immediate surgery or whether the patient can be managed conservatively at first depends on the following[26]:

Life expectancy
Operative risk
Risk of spontaneous rupture

The aim is to perform the operation when the risk of rupture exceeds the operative risk and life expectancy is higher than the likelihood to succumb to a ruptured aneurysm. Although life expectancy and operative risk are gauged by scores (for example, American Society of Anaesthesiologists literature[27]) that depend on age and associated morbidity, the risk of spontaneous rupture is the critical parameter in determining when surgery is warranted.

Investigations on the growth of aneurysms have shown an annual increase of 0.2 cm/y for small but more than 3 cm/y for large aneurysms exceeding a diameter of 4 cm. The speed of aneurysmal growth is influenced by the arterial wall structure (e.g., calcifications, thrombi, and perianeurysmal fibrosis) and wall tension. According to Laplace's law ($r = P \cdot r_i / h$, where r = wall tension, P = intraluminal pressure, r_i = inner radius, and h = wall thickness) the pulsatile aortal wall tension increases exponentially with the increase in radius. A dilatation of the aorta with only 3-fold increase of the original aortal diameter results in 12-fold increase in wall tension at the same blood pressure.

Risk of spontaneous aneurysmal rupture is reported to lie between 6% and 20% per year at a diameter exceeding 5 cm. But even aneurysms of diameters less than 5 cm have a risk of spontaneous rupture that amounts to 18% within 5 years.[28-30] Saccular aneurysms and aneurysms with a history of excessive growth during recent months are particularly prone to spontaneous rupture.

Although whether an operation is necessary in a certain patient depends on the mentioned parameters, the following guidelines may also be helpful:

1. Patients with normal operative risk, normal life expectancy, and aneurysms larger than 4 cm in diameter should be treated surgically.
2. Patients with significantly increased operative risk or markedly reduced life expectancy and aneurysms larger than 4 cm in diameter should only be treated surgically if signs indicate imminent rupture of the aneurysms.
3. Patients with aneurysms smaller than 4 cm in diameter can be managed conservatively at first.

Conservative management includes observing the aneurysm through imaging procedures and instructing the patient on necessary lifestyle changes (i.e., no carrying of heavy loads) and about the symptoms of imminent or actual rupture of the aneurysm. Concurrent hypertension should be treated immediately. An indispensable prerequisite to conservative management is adequate availability of emergency vascular surgery facilities.

Surgical Treatment

The operative treatment of choice is extirpation or exclusion of the aneurysm (Figure 47.6). The implantation of an endovascular stent is currently being developed as an alternative method; initial results have been encouraging, but this surgical therapy has not yet passed the experimental stage. Therefore, it is used only in patients in whom aneurysmal rupture is imminent but for whom surgery is not an option. The development of exact differential indications for endovascular stents must be left to the results of the large studies currently under way. Even if the new technique offers significant benefit to individual patients, open surgical extirpation or exclu-

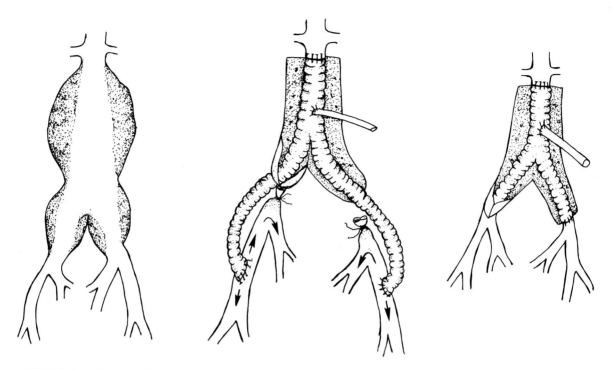

FIGURE 47.6. Extirpation or exclusion of the abdominal aortic aneurysm and subsequent graft implantation.

sion will remain the gold standard by which new procedures must be judged. Reliable long-term results are
available only for open surgery at present.[31,32]

Nonruptured Abdominal Aortic Aneurysm

Sufficient experience in operative indications, optimal
perioperative care, and above all an experienced surgical team determine success or failure in the treatment of
abdominal aortic aneurysms.

Access

We prefer the transperitoneal access by a median laparotomy from the xiphoid process to the pubic symphysis.
Some surgeons prefer a transverse laparotomy, but this
approach is likely to raise problems if the operation has
to be extended into the pelvic region. Retroperitoneal
access may be chosen if many intraperitoneal adhesions
are anticipated.

Dissection

After opening the retroperitoneum laterally to the ascending duodenum, the left renal vein is dissected. If the
distance between the aortic aneurysm and the left renal
vein is less than 2 cm the vein should be mobilized by
severing the suprarenal, testicular, or ovarian veins between ligatures, which as a rule yields sufficient area for
a reliable aortic clamp below or above the origin of the
renal arteries.

To avoid possible injury to nerve fibers that supply the
genitourinary system the retroperitoneum should not be
opened near the aortic bifurcation. If the aneurysm
reaches the iliac vessels the retroperitoneum directly
overlying them is split longitudinally (i.e., caudally) to
the cecal pole on the right and caudally to the sigmoid
colon on the left[33] (Figure 47.7).

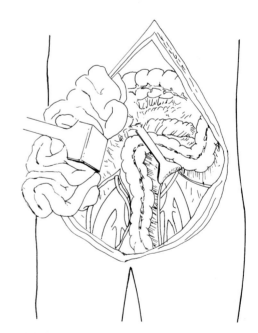

FIGURE 47.7. Dissection of the external iliac and hypogastric
artery.

Resection or Exclusion

Small or intermediate aneurysms less than 5 cm in diameter without any significant adhesions to the retroperitoneum or the venae cavaeare partially or totally resected after direct ligature and severing of the lumbar arteries to minimize blood loss. Moreover, the rear wall of the aorta can be mobilized completely and the posterior row of the anastomosis can be performed entirely under visual control. This technique has little effect on operating time.

Inflammatory or large aneurysms with a diameter of more than 5 cm, particularly if they display massive adhesions to the retroperitoneum, are corrected by the inlay technique. After incision of the anterior aneurysmal wall the thrombi, including the altered intima, are removed and the lumbar vessels are oversewn.

Vascular Reconstruction

An entirely infrarenal abdominal aortic aneurysm without any extension into the pelvic vessels is reconstructed by implanting a tube prothesis (Figure 47.8). If the aorta displays severe atheromatous plaques at the bifurcation that compromise the distal anastomosis with a tube prothesis, a bifurcated graft with distal anastomoses in the upper third of the common iliac artery is preferable. The inferior mesenteric artery is reimplanted if it has shown a satisfactory orthograde flow and a sufficient caliber (i.e., >2 mm). If a concurrent aneurysm or a severe stenosis of the common iliac artery is found, the artery is reconstructed by a bifurcated graft with distal end-to-side anastomoses between the middle and distal thirds of the external iliac artery. The common iliac artery is ligated proximal to its bifurcation and oversewn. Thus the inter-

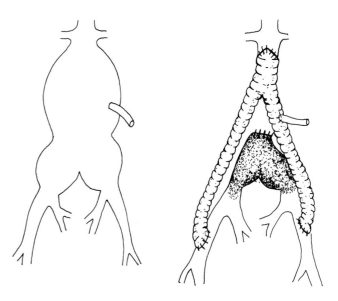

FIGURE 47.9. Surgical treatment of an abdominal aortoiliac aneurysm.

nal iliac artery receives retrograde perfusion (Figure 47.9). The complication of aneurysmal common iliac artery stump dilatation has not occurred in more than 400 reconstructions performed with this technique.[34]

If in addition to the aortoiliac aneurysm an aneurysmal dilatation of the internal iliac artery is detected, this aneurysm should be excised and reconstructed as well (Figure 47.10). In this situation the bifurcated graft limbs are anastomosed to the external iliac arteries.

After extirpation of the internal iliac artery aneurysm, which as a rule does not extend beyond the first bifurcation of the internal iliac artery, a smaller Dacron tube graft is interposed between one of the bifurcated graft limbs and the internal iliac artery. After severing the internal iliac artery at its origin the internal iliac artery aneurysm can be easily dissected and excised up to the bi-

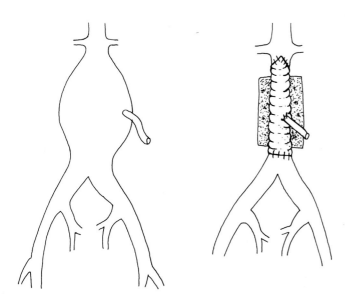

FIGURE 47.8. Surgical treatment of an infrarenal abdominal aortic aneurysm.

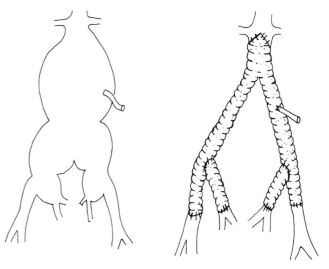

FIGURE 47.10. Surgical treatment of an abdominal aortoiliac aneurysm including an aneurysm of the hypogastric artery.

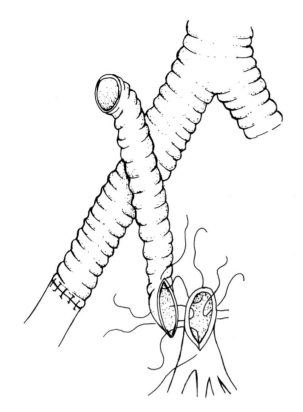

FIGURE 47.11. Reconstruction of the hypogastric artery.

furcation. The 8- or 9-mm Dacron tube graft is anastomosed end to end to the distal internal iliac artery using a four-point technique; then the internal iliac artery revascularization is completed by proximal end-to-side anastomosis to the bifurcated graft limb (Figure 47.11).[34] A patient's donation of blood before reconstruction by elective operation and intraoperative autotransfusion by cell saver minimize the risk due to foreign blood transfusions and thus further reduce the total morbidity of the elective operation.

Results

The described technique has proven its efficiency in more than 530 abdominal aortic aneurysm reconstructions in recent years (1987–1994). Thus the complications of gluteal gangrenous changes, ischemic colitis, or the lumbar portion of the spinal cord in cases of retained internal iliac artery perfusion have never recurred with this technique. Postoperative mortality rates were reduced significantly by 2.5% to a current rate of 1.2%.[34–37]

Ruptured Infrarenal Abdominal Aortic Aneurysm

Aneurysmal rupture is the most severe complication of abdominal aortic aneurysms; they rupture into the retroperitoneal space in more than 80% of patients, rarely into the free abdominal cavity, and only occasionally into the gastrointestinal tract or the inferior vena cava.[38] The rupture of an aneurysm always necessitates immediate operation. The prognosis, however, depends on the interval between rupture and operation, the patient's general condition, and the experience of the operating team. The most important initial step of the operation is control of hemorrhage. After opening the abdominal cavity and the retroperitoneum, the abdominal aorta can be clamped immediately distal to the origin of the renal arteries. If the neck of the aneurysm cannot be delineated reliably within the retroperitoneal hematoma, infradiaphragmatic clamping of the abdominal aorta is preferable in the beginning to secure temporary control of hemorrhage. For dissection of the aorta, the minor omentum is severed and the diaphragmatic crura spread.

After clamping the iliac arteries, the renal veins and arteries can be identified quickly so that the aorta can be clamped proximally to the renal arteries and the clamp on the abdominal aorta can be removed. Infradiaphragmatic clamping time usually does not exceed 15 minutes. Because operating time has a strong bearing on the patient's prognosis, a tube prothesis is implanted if possible. The rest of the operative course is identical to the elective operation.[39]

In case of an aortoduodenal fistula, the fistula is excised and oversewn after meticulous dissection of the bowel. If an aortojejunal fistula is found, a segmental resection of the affected jejunum with subsequent end-to-end jejunojejunostomy may be the easiest procedure. The second step is anatomical aortic reconstruction; extra-anatomical reconstruction does not seem to be warranted in this situation, because we have not observed a single graft infection in any of our patients.

In the rare event of an aortosigmoidal fistula, anatomical reconstruction of the right pelvic vascular system is combined with exclusion of the aneurysm. Subsequently the graft is covered by omentum and retroperitoneal tissue and the sigmoid colon is oversewn. After closing the laparotomy the left pelvic vascular system is reconstructed by means of an extra-anatomical cross-over bypass.

A new method of managing arterial reconstructions in an infected area is the use of homologous grafts in an anatomical position. Recent studies have shown encouraging results.[40] In spite of the advances in operative technique, anesthesia, and postoperative intensive care, the mortality rate of an emergency operation in a ruptured abdominal aortic aneurysm still lies in the range of 30% to 60% due to the frequent development of multiorgan failure. Timely elective reconstruction in patients suffering from infrarenal abdominal aortic aneurysms is thus important.

References

1. Goyanes DJ. Substitucion plastica de las arterias por las venas o arterioplatia venosa aplicada como nuevo metodo al tratamiento de los aneurismas. *Siglo Medico.* 1906;53:346.
2. Dubost C, Allary M, Oeconomas N. Resection of an aneurysm of the abdominal aorta: re-establishment of the continuity by a preserved human arterial graft, with results after five months. *Arch Surg.* 1952;64:405.
3. Larwin P. Die Entwicklung der Intensivmedizin, eine kritische Übersicht. *Anästhesist.* 1985;34:329.
4. Safa P, Dekornfeld TJ, Pearson JW, Redding JF. Intensive care unit. *Anaesthesia.* 1961;16:275.
5. Holmdahl MH. The respiratory care unit. *Anaesthesiology.* 1962;23:559.
6. Hicking KG. Ventilatory management of ARDS: can it affect the outcome? *Intens Care Med.* 1990;16:226.
7. Swan HJC, Ganz W, Forrester J, Markus M, Diamond G, Chonette D. Catheterisation of the heart in man with the use of flow-directed balloon-tipped catheter. *New Engl J Med.* 1970;283:447–451.
8. Payne JP, Severinghaus JW. *Pulse-oxymetry.* Berlin: Springer-Verlag; 1986.
9. Tremper KK, Barker SJ. Pulse-oxymetry. *Anaestesiology.* 1989;70:98–108.
10. Reed D, Reed C, Stemmermann G, Hayasi T. Are aortic aneurysms caused by atherosclerosis? *Circulation.* 1992; 85:205.
11. Heistad DD, Marcus ML, Carsen GE, et al. Role of vasa vasorum in nourishment of the aortic wall. *Am J Physiol.* 1981;240(suppl):H781.
12. Cohen JR, Mandell C, Margois I, et al. Altered aortic protease and antiprotease activity in patients with ruptured aortic aneurysms. *Surgery, Gynecology and Obstetrics.* 1987; 164:355.
13. Kuivaniemi H, Tromp G, Prockop DG. Genetic causes of aortic aneurysms: unlearning at least part of what the textbooks say. *J Clin Invest.* 1991;88:1441.
14. Boontje AH, van den Dugen JJ, Blanksma C. Inflammatory abdominal aortic aneurysms. *J Cardiovasc Surg.* 1990;31: 661.
15. Bernstein EF, Dilley RB, Goldberger LE, et al. Growth rates of small abdominal aortic aneurysms. *Surgery.* 1980; 80:765.
16. Deling A, Ohlsen H, Swedenborg J. Growth rate of abdominal aortic aneurysms as measured by computed tomography. *Br J Surg.* 1985;72:230.
17. Szilagyi DE, Eliott JP, Smith RF. Clinical fate of the patient with asymptomatic abdominal aortic aneurysm and unfit for surgical treatment. *Arch Surg.* 1972;104:600.
18. Safran R, Sklenicka R, Kay H. Iliac aneurysms: a common cause of ureteral obstruction. *J Urol.* 1975;113:605.
19. Gomez MN, Hakkal HG, Sellinger D. Ultrasonography and CT scanning: a comparative study of abdominal aortic aneurysms. *Computed Tomography.* 1978;2:99.
20. Lederle FA, Walker JM, Reinke DB. Selective screening for abdominal aortic aneurysms with physical examination and ultrasound. *Arch Int Med.* 1988;148:1753–1756.
21. Rieber A, Wrazidlo W, Brambs HJ, Allenberg JR. Stellenwert der Kernspintomographie in der Diagnostic der infrarenalen Bauchaortenaneurysmen. *Digitale Bilddiagnose.* 1990;10:101.
22. Bunt TJ, Cropper L. Routine angiography for abdominal aortic aneurysms: the case for informed operative selection. *J Cardiovasc Surg.* 1986;27:725.
23. Hertzer NR, Beven EG, Young JR, et al. Coronary artery disease in peripheral vascular patients. *Ann Surg.* 1988; 223:1983.
24. Nora JD, Pairolero PC, Nivatvongs S, et al. Concomitant abdominal aortic aneurysms and colorectal carcinoma: priority of resection. *J Vasc Surg.* 1989;9:630–635.
25. Alemany J, Görtz H, Wozniak G. Simultane abdominelle Eingriffe bei Aortoiliakalen Rekonstruktionen. In: Bürger K, ed. *Grenzfälle der Gefäßchirurgischen Praxis.* Darmstadt: Steinkopff Verlag; 1993:161–163.
26. Lijeqvist L, Ekeström S, Nordhus O. Abdominal aortic aneurysms, II: long term follow up of operated and unoperated patients. *Acta Chir Scand.* 1979;145:529.
27. American Society of Anaesthesiologists. New Classification of Physical Status. *Anaesthesiology.* 1963;24:111.
28. Imig H, Horsch S, Pichlmair H. Überlebenssrate mit einem Bauchaortenaneurysma nach Resektion und Spontanverlauf. *Langenbecks Arch Chir.* 1980;325:545–548.
29. Bernstein EF, Chang EL. Abdominal aortic aneurysm in high risk patients: outcome of selective management based in size and expansion rate. *Ann Surg.* 1984;200: 255–263.
30. Darling RC. Ruptured arteriosclerotic abdominal aortic aneurysms: a pathological and clinical study. *Am J Surg.* 1970;119:397–401.
31. DeBakey ME, Cooley DA. Surgical treatment of aneurysm of abdominal aorta and restoration of continuity with homograft. *Surgery, Gynecology and Obstetrics.* 1953;97:257.
32. DeBakey ME, Crawford ES, Cooley DA, et al. Aneurysms of the abdominal aorta: analysis of results of graft replacement therapy one to eleven years after operation. *Ann Surg.* 1964;160:622.
33. Alemany J, Teubner K, Montag H, Tannous R. Indikation zur operative Revaskularisation der A. iliaca interna. *Angio Archiv.* 1988;11:56.
34. Alemany J, Marsal T, Reim T. Importance of the revascularization of the hypogastric artery in reconstruction of infrarenal aortic aneurysms. *Vasc Surg.* 1991;25:587–594.
35. Alemany J, Montag H. Die Bedeutung der Revaskularisation der A. iliaca interna bei der Rekonstruktion des aorto-iliakalen Aneurysmas. *Helvetica Chirurgica Acta.* 1992; 58:595–599.
36. Biedermann H. Diagnose und Therapie vaskulär bedingter Erektionsstörunen. *Angio.* 1984;11:215–225.
37. Gloviczki P, Cross SA, Stanson AW, et al. Ischemic injury to the spinal cord or lumbosacral plexus after aorto-iliac reconstruction. *Am J Surg.* 1991;162:131–136.
38. Johansson G, Schwedenborg J. Ruptured abdominal aortic aneurysms: a study of incidence and mortality. *Br J Surg.* 1986;73:101.
39. Crawford ES. Ruptured abdominal aortic aneurysms: an editorial *J Vasc Surg.* 1991;13:348.
40. Hickey NC, Douwnung R, Hamer JD, Asston F, Stanley G. Abdominal aortic aneurysms complicated by iliocaval or duodenal fistulae. *J Cardiovasc Surg.* 1991;32:181.

48

Peripheral Arterial Aneurysms

Jose Alemany, Hartmut Görtz, and Klaus Schaarschmidt

More than 90% of all peripheral arterial aneurysms affect the popliteal and common femoral arteries and much more rarely the subclavian and brachial arteries. In a large proportion of these patients there are coexisting aneurysms of other locations as well, particularly in the infrarenal abdominal aorta.[1]

Aneurysm of the Popliteal Artery

Constituting nearly 70% of all peripheral aneurysms, the popliteal artery is the most frequent site of peripheral arterial aneurysms. Most authors assume arteriosclerosis to be the main cause of aneurysm formation.[2] More rarely anomalies such as the entrapment syndrome, local trauma, or infections can provoke aneurysms. Rupture of popliteal aneurysms is unusual, but recurrent peripheral emboli are frequent and compression of adjacent structures such as the popliteal vein, peroneal nerve, or tibial nerve may be observed occasionally.[3]

The clue to diagnosis is clinical examination by the physician. He or she may find a pulsating swelling on palpation of the knee that can be confused with a Baker's cyst. The diagnosis can be substantiated by duplex ultrasonography. Angiography and a computed tomography scan should be obtained for assessment of local operability, influx, and runoff.

Two principal sites of aneurysms in the popliteal artery are distinguished:

1. The proximal and middle third of the popliteal artery (Figure 48.1)
2. The distal third of the popliteal artery (Figure 48.2)

Aneurysms in the proximal and middle third of the popliteal artery are observed most frequently; they are rarely seen in the distal portion of the popliteal artery.

Aneurysms in the distal third of the popliteal artery are rarer and frequently accompanied by aneurysmal di-latations of the tibiofibular truncus. These aneurysms are considerably more prone to thromboses of the popliteal trifurcation and to recurrent peripheral emboli.[4]

All symptomatic peripheral aneurysms are an indication for surgery,[4–6] particularly if thrombosis or embolization have led to critical peripheral ischemia. However, asymptomatic peripheral aneurysms that cause dilatation of the popliteal artery to more than 3 cm should be corrected surgically, especially if they lie in the proximal or middle third of the popliteal artery where reconstruction is technically easy. The operative risk is low, and early and late results are very satisfactory.

Aneurysms in the distal third of the popliteal artery should be treated conservatively if no parietal thrombosis has supervened. In patients who suffer from general aneurysms expectant management is warranted, and regular ultrasonographical follow-up examinations are indispensable; in all other cases, however, surgical repair should be the goal.[7] Surgical therapy of aneurysms of the proximal and middle third of the popliteal artery consists of extirpation or exclusion of the aneurysm and restoration of perfusion by interposing a vascular graft or bypass (Figure 48.3).

Alloplastic material is considered only in isolated aneurysms of the proximal popliteal artery. Extensive aneurysms in the proximal and middle third of the popliteal artery warrant vascular reconstruction with autologous vascular transplants. After resection or exclusion of the aneurysm we prefer vascular reconstruction with a distal end-to-side anastomosis immediately proximal to the popliteal bifurcation, where anastomosis seems technically easier (Figure 48.4).

Revascularization of the distal third of the popliteal artery is more challenging, however. The anterior tibial artery and the tibiofibular truncus usually experience aneurysmal dilatation close to their origin and moreover may contain parietal thrombi. In these cases a distal femorocrural reconstruction is inevitable. If ischemia is

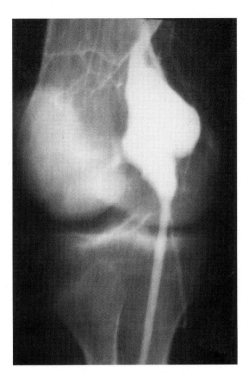

FIGURE 48.1. Aneurysm of the proximal third of the popliteal artery.

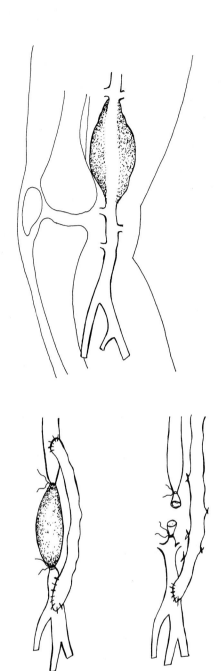

FIGURE 48.3. Surgical treatment of aneurysms of the proximal and middle third of the popliteal artery.

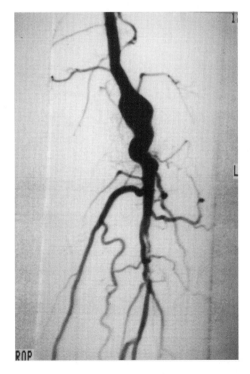

FIGURE 48.2. Aneurysm of the distal third of the popliteal artery.

present, both the anterior tibial artery and the tibiofibular truncus should be revascularized if possible, because in this situation extensive aseptic necroses of the nonreconstructed segment have been observed. If marked adhesions are present or the surgeon has insufficient operative experience the aneurysm should be excluded rather than extirpated.

Division of the medial popliteal tendon apparatus is warranted only rarely. If acute ischemia has developed some authors recommend treating the acute emergency by local thrombolysis and deferring operative recon-

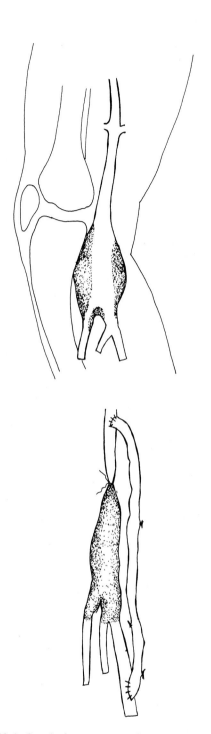

an ischemic stage subsequent to recurrent peripheral emboli produces significantly worse results.

Aneurysm of the Femoral Artery

The femoral artery is the second most frequent site of peripheral arterial aneurysms. However, isolated aneurysms of the superficial or deep femoral artery are rare. Only 25% of all femoral artery aneurysms are symptomatic.[12,13] The following sites of femoral artery aneurysms are distinguished (Figure 48.5):

1. Isolated aneurysms of the common femoral artery
2. Aneurysms of the common femoral artery with aneurysmal dilatations of the superficial or deep femoral arteries at their origin

The principal sign of femoral artery aneurysms is a pulsating swelling of the inguinal region. The differential diagnosis of an inguinal hernia can usually be excluded by clinical examination. The inguinal mass may lead to compression of adjacent structures such as the femoral vein and femoral nerve with subsequent thrombosis or neurological defects.

The diagnosis is verified by conventional or duplex ultrasonography, which excludes parietal thrombi of the aneurysm. Local operability should be judged by means of an angiography and a computed tomography scan. All

FIGURE 48.4. Surgical treatment of aneurysms of the distal third of the popliteal artery.

struction. Early and late results of operative reconstructions in nonischemic limbs are excellent, and perioperative morbidity and mortality rates have been very low.[8-11] After the implantation of an autologous vascular graft the 5-year patency rate for revascularization of the proximal and middle thirds of the popliteal artery is greater than 90%, and in the distal third of the popliteal artery the patency rate is 60%. Obviously, revascularization in

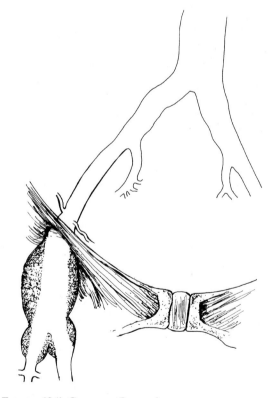

FIGURE 48.5. Common femoral artery aneurysms.

aneurysms of a diameter of more than 2.5 cm or with evidence of parietal thrombi require surgical repair. If expectant management is preferred, however, regular ultrasonographical follow-up examinations are essential.[14] If abdominal aortic or iliac artery aneurysms are found, reconstruction of the more proximal aneurysms has unequivocal priority. The popliteal artery aneurysm may be repaired in either the same or a second session.

Operative therapy of common femoral artery aneurysms is easy to perform by extirpation and interposition of usually alloplastic material. The inguinal ligament can be mobilized to facilitate comfortable clamping of the distal external iliac artery. In large or perforated inguinal aneurysms a retroperitoneal dissection of the external iliac artery may be necessary (Figure 48.6). If the aneurysm extends beyond the femoral bifurcation the perfusion of both the superficial and the deep femoral artery should be preserved, if possible. In this case we prefer an end-to-end anastomosis with the deep femoral artery and reimplantation of the superficial femoral artery into the graft or the deep femoral artery. According to the recommendations for critical extremity perfusion due to popliteal artery aneurysms, initial local thrombolysis has been advocated by several authors. Correspondingly, surgical treatment requires a second procedure.

The results of surgical treatment for femoral artery aneurysms are very satisfactory, and the reconstruction is an excellent option. The 5-year patency rate is greater than 90%, and morbidity and mortality rates are very low.

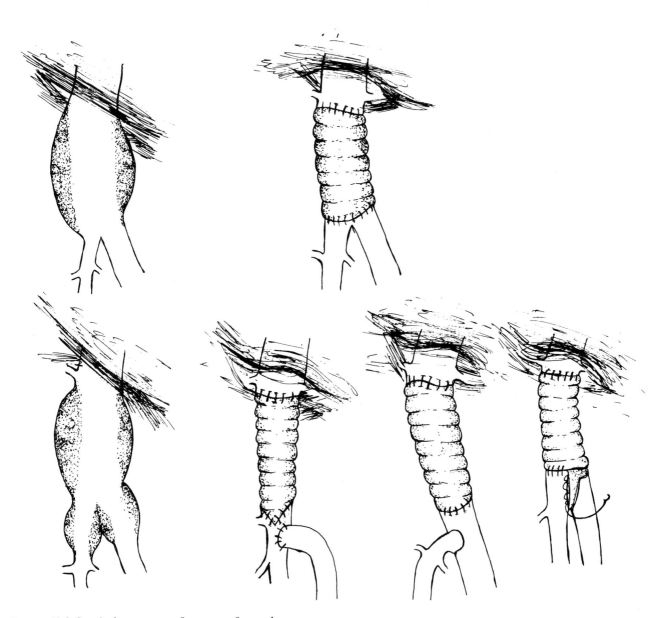

FIGURE 48.6. Surgical treatment of common femoral artery aneurysms.

References

1. Evans WE, Hayes JP. Popliteal and femoral aneurysms. In: Rutherford RB, ed. *Vascular Surgery*. Philadelphia, Pa: WB Saunders; 1989:951–957.

2. Farina C, Cavallaro A, Sultz RD, et al. Popliteal aneurysms. *Surgery, Gynecology and Obstetrics*. 1991;169:7.

3. Gillespie DL, Cantelmo NL. Traumatic popliteal artery pseudoaneurysms: case report and review of the literature. *J Trauma*. 1991:31:412.

4. Alemany J. Problemas de diagnostico y tratamiento de los aneurismas de la arteria poplitea. *Angiologia*. 1972;24:9.

5. Cutler BS, Darling RC. Surgical management of arteriosclerotic femoral aneurysms. *Surgery*. 1973;74:764.

6. Gaylis H. Popliteal arterial aneurysms: a review and analysis of 55 cases. *S Afr Med J*. 1974;48:75.

7. Bowyer RC, Cawthorn SJ, Walker WJ, Giddings AE. Conservative management of the asymptomatic popliteal aneurysm. *Br J Surg*. 1990;77:1132–1135.

8. Wychulis AR. Popliteal aneurysms. *Surgery*. 1970;68:942.

9. Hand LJ, Collin J. Infra-inguinal aneurysms: outcome for patient and limb. *Br J Surg*. 1991;78:32.

10. Halliday AW, Taylor PR, Wolfe JH, Mansfield AO. The management of popliteal aneurysms: the importance of early surgical repair. *Ann R Coll Surg Engl*. 1991;73:253.

11. Shortell CK, DeWeese JA, Ouriel K, Green RM. Popliteal arterial aneurysms: a 25-year surgical experience. *J Vasc Surg*. 1991;14:771.

12. Cutler BS, Darling RC: Surgical management of arteriosclerotic femoral aneurysms. *Surgery*. 1973;74:764.

13. Graham LR, Rubin JR. Arteriosclerotic femoral artery aneurysm. In: Ernst Calvin B and Stanley James C, eds. *Current Therapy in Vascular Surgery*. Philadelphia, Pa: BC Decker; 1991:347.

14. Adiseshiah M, Babey DA. Aneurysms of the femoral artery. *Br J Surg*. 1972;59:614.

49

Visceral Aneurysms: Splenic, Hepatic, Mesenteric, and Renal

Ricardo Gesto Castromil and Jose Porto Rodriguez

Aneurysm of the visceral arteries is an uncommon disease entity of multiple etiologies that affects the large branches of the abdominal aorta: the splanchnic and renal arteries. Until the 1960s, practically all of the cases described were ruptured aneurysms or autopsy findings. The availability of computed tomography (CT) and magnetic resonance imaging (MRI) and, above all, the widespread use of angiography have led to a significant increase in the diagnosis of these lesions. The more than 3000 cases reported in the literature to date have given us further insight on the incidence, natural history, and treatment of these aneurysms. Aneurysms of the visceral arteries account for approximately 5% of all aneurysms treated in vascular surgery units.[24] The incidence of splanchnic artery aneurysm is twice that of renal artery aneurysm. The marked differences in etiology, clinical features, natural history, and complications warrant a separate description of each type of lesion.

Aneurysms of the Splanchnic Arteries

Aneurysms of the splanchnic arteries involve the celiac, superior mesenteric, and inferior mesenteric arteries and their branches. They are usually asymptomatic[54] and present as a surgical emergency in slightly more than 20% of patients.[45] In decreasing order of frequency, they affect the splenic (60%); hepatic (20%); superior mesenteric (5.5%); celiac (4%); gastric and gastroepiploic (4%); jejunal, ileal, and colic (3%); pancreatic and pancreatoduodenal (2%); and gastroduodenal (1.5%) arteries.[17,48] Aneurysms of the inferior mesenteric artery are extremely rare; only 13 cases were described before 1988.[26]

Aneurysms of the Splenic Artery

Aneurysms of the splenic artery are the most common visceral aneurysms and account for 60% of all splanchnic aneurysms. Their incidence in autopsy studies has been reported to range from 0.098% to 10.4%,[6,37] which reflects the different criteria used in the definition of aneurysm, differences in the population studied, and how specifically aneurysm is searched for in each particular study. In a series of 3500 unselected abdominal arteriograms, aneurysm of the splenic artery was found in 0.78%,[46] which is considered to be a good estimate of its incidence in the general population. The age of presentation of these aneurysms has a peak incidence around age 60, and only 20% of patients are diagnosed before age 50.[54] There is a higher prevalence in women, with a female to male ratio of 4:1, a ratio that is even higher (10:1) for patients under 50 years.[54] Splenic artery aneurysms (SAAs) are usually single and saccular; less than 20% are multiple and located in the bifurcation of the distal third of the splenic artery.[54] On average, SAAs are 1.3 to 2 cm in size. An incidence of 12% of associated aneurysms has been reported at other sites.[54]

Pathophysiology

Unlike with aortic aneurysms, atherosclerosis is not considered to be a factor that triggers SAA. Although changes compatible with calcified atherosclerosis are frequently found within the walls of these aneurysms, the remaining artery is usually free of atherosclerosis.[51] Why the splenic artery is predisposed to aneurysmal dilatations has not yet been elucidated; this predisposition has been ascribed to fragmentation of the elastic fibers, loss of arterial smooth muscle, and rupture of the elastic layer of the media. Three clinical conditions have been clearly associated with increased risk for SAA:

1. Fibromuscular dysplasia
2. Numerous pregnancies (multiparity)
3. Portal hypertension with splenomegaly

The incidence of SAA is six times higher in patients with fibromuscular dysplasia than in the general population[46]; one out of eight female patients with SAA has fibromuscular disease at other sites.[10] Because of the known involvement of the arterial wall in fibrodysplasia, a cause–effect relationship can be assumed.

The second important factor associated with these aneurysms is the number of pregnancies.[17] About 40% of the women with SAA in the University of Michigan series[46] and 25% in the Mayo Clinic series[54] had six or more pregnancies, and the incidence of SAA in the multipara is six times that of the general population. This increased incidence may be ascribed to the increased splanchnic blood flow, reduced peripheral resistance, and hormonal changes that occur during pregnancy.[51] Splenic blood flow in cirrhotic patients is twice normal,[53] and this increased flow, which is common in portal hypertension with splenomegaly[22,46] or portal-systemic shunts,[53] has been classically associated with SAAs. Of 181 patients with SAAs, 30% showed evidence of portal hypertension with splenomegaly,[22] and 7% to 10% of patients with portal hypertension are known to have SAAs.[41,46] Patients undergoing liver transplantation belong to this subset of patients with an increased incidence of SAAs.[2,7] Because the first two factors described are practically exclusive to women, it is not surprising to find a higher prevalence of SAAs in the female population.

The relationship of pancreatitis with peripancreatic aneurysms has been well established[29,46] and affects 10% of patients with pancreatic pseudocysts. One of the arteries frequently involved in these patients is the splenic artery. Iatrogenic or noniatrogenic trauma and fungal embolisms, particularly in drug addicts, are rare causes of SAAs. Connective disorders, especially panarteritis nodosa, cause multiple intrasplenic microaneurysms.

Clinical Features

Most of the SAAs remain asymptomatic until they rupture or are incidentally discovered. Only 20%[46,54] present with nonspecific epigastric and/or left hypochondrial pain that usually becomes more severe and radiates to the left scapular region with sudden enlargement of the aneurysm. Rupture of the aneurysm is the most common and severe complication of SAAs. Bleeding usually occurs in the retrogastric area and posteriorly goes through Winslow's hiatus to the free peritoneal cavity. In 25% of cases the hemorrhage is initially contained within the lesser sac, giving rise to a double-rupture phenomenon that may permit diagnosis and surgical treatment before progressing to massive intraperitoneal hemorrhage.

The symptoms of ruptured SAAs in pregnant women may mimic other obstetric emergencies such as uterine rupture, abruptio placentae, or embolism of amniotic fluid. Rupture presents during the third trimester of pregnancy in most patients and during labor in approximately 20%.[32,38] In very few patients, almost always those with an underlying inflammatory condition, SAAs may rupture into adjacent structures, including the gastrointestinal tract, pancreatic pseudocysts, pancreatic duct, or splenic vein.[28,31,42]

The incidence of ruptured noninflammatory splenic aneurysms in the nonpregnant population is approximately 2%[46] and does not appear to be affected by parietal calcifications, age, or hypertension.[46,54] Pregnancy probably increases the risk of rupture. In fact, 95% of the SAAs in pregnancy are diagnosed under these circumstances.[32,38,46] However, this figure does not reflect the true risk of rupture of SAAs, because its incidence in pregnancy is unknown due to a lack of cross-sectional studies. The other factors associated with a higher incidence of rupture of SAAs are pancreatitis with pancreatic pseudocyst and liver transplantation.[2,8] A relationship between cocaine use and SAA rupture has recently been suggested.[39]

Diagnosis

The clinical features (absent or nonspecific) and physical examination usually do not provide information that permits the diagnosis of SAA before rupture. Early diagnosis is usually an incidental finding during abdominal radiologic evaluation. The plain abdominal film shows a typical ring-shaped calcification of left hypochondrium in 70% of patients.[54] SAAs may be a secondary finding in ultrasonography, CT, MRI, or duplex scan, although the majority are usually diagnosed during abdominal angiographic evaluation for other pathologies.[46] Nonetheless, arteriography is the method of choice for confirming the diagnosis, determining the aneurysm type, and planning surgery. CT and recently MRI have proved useful in determining whether pancreatic disease is a coexisting condition and in the follow-up of these aneurysms if surgery is not indicated.

Treatment

Patients with noninflammatory aneurysm of the splenic artery are at a 3% to 10% risk of aneurysmal rupture.[46,54] The surgical mortality rate of noninflammatory ruptured SAAs in the nonpregnant population is approximately 25%. Rupture of an aneurysm in pregnancy carries a mortality rate of 75% for the mother and 95% for the fetus.[5,11,54] In fact, before 1993, only 12 cases in which both mother and fetus survived after aneurysmal rupture were reported.[11]

On the other hand, mortality resulting from prophylactic surgery of noninflammatory SAA is practically nonexistent.[46,48,54] It is widely accepted that surgery is indicated in all cases of symptomatic SAAs and those diagnosed during pregnancy or in women of childbearing age. Although classically a third indication for surgery is a SAA more than 1.5 to 2.5 cm in diameter,[49] performing surgery from the outset, regardless of the size of the aneurysm, achieves the best results and is probably safest in patients at low surgical risk.

The surgical technique varies according to the location of the SAA. Those in the proximal or medial third of the artery are generally submitted to resection and ligation of the proximal and distal arterial segments, without arterial reconstruction or splenectomy, because splenic blood supply is assured by gastric and pancreatic collateral blood flow. In case of compromise of the distal third or the splenic hilius, the approach has generally been resection of the aneurysm and splenectomy. Because of the current interest in preserving the spleen there is a tendency in these cases to do a simple ligation, endoaneurysmorrhaphia, or simple arterial repair or grafting. Patients at high surgical risk have been treated with success by intra-arterial embolization or ligation of the proximal and distal segments of the artery by laparoscopy.[40,43]

SAA secondary to pancreatitis is a special problem. The mortality rate for these aneurysms was more than 30% in a historical series.[44] In these patients, in whom even accessing the artery for simple ligation is extremely difficult, percutaneous embolization appears to be indicated.[34]

Aneurysm of the Hepatic Artery

Hepatic artery aneurysms (HAAs) are second in frequency of all splanchnic aneurysms, accounting for 20%.[17,48] Excluding those that arise from trauma, the maximum incidence of these aneurysms is found after age 60. HAA is more prevalent in men, with a 2:1 male to female ratio. Aneurysm of the hepatic artery is usually single, except those associated with connective disorders. It is fusiform if less than 2 cm in diameter and saccular otherwise. About 80% are located in the extrahepatic artery; intrahepatic lesions are generally found in cases of trauma. In 63% of patients, the extrahepatic lesions involve the common or proper hepatic artery, the right hepatic in 28%, the left hepatic in 5%, and both in 4%.[48] The predisposition of the right hepatic artery to aneurysm has not been explained. In a recent study,

75% of 12 patients with HAA had aneurysms at other sites,[18] which indicates the need for a routine search.

Pathophysiology

Slightly more than 30% of HAAs are associated with atherosclerosis. Whether there is a cause–effect relationship or merely secondary changes has not yet been elucidated.[51] In 24% of patients there was evidence of degenerative disease of the media similar to that found in SAAs. Unlike SAAs, however, it is not known which factors, if any, can favor the development of aneurysms of this nature. Open or blunt trauma has been increasingly incriminated in the etiology of these aneurysms and accounts for 22% of cases. Trauma generally causes false aneurysms and is the first cause of intrahepatic aneurysms. Open cholecystectomy has been classically associated with sporadic cases of iatrogenic lesions in the proper and right hepatic arteries. HAAs have recently been associated with liver transplantation and endoscopic cholecystectomy.[23,33] The availability of sophisticated diagnostic and therapeutic techniques via the transparietohepatic route has led to an increasing number of false intrahepatic aneurysms secondary to these techniques.[35]

Mycotic aneurysms currently account for 10% of all HAAs and are generally associated with intravenous drug users. Rare causes of HAA are panarteritis nodosa and other nonatherosclerotic artery diseases. Cases secondary to adjacent inflammatory disease (cholecystitis and pancreatitis) have been reported very rarely.

Clinical Features

Many HAAs remain asymptomatic. Some patients present with vague discomfort in the region of the right hypochondrium or epigastrium that is usually ascribed to gallbladder pathology, although unrelated to intake. The sudden enlargement of these aneurysms is generally accompanied by intense epigastric pain that may or may not radiate to the back and mimics gallbladder colic or pancreatitis. Large HAAs can impinge on the adjacent structures, usually the biliary tree, and cause jaundice. Extrahepatic portal hypertension secondary to compression of the portal vein has been described.

The incidence of rupture has varied over time[9,48] and is currently estimated to be approximately 20%[45,51]; the mortality rate has remained stable at approximately 35%.[9,45] Rupture into the bile ducts or free peritoneal cavity presents with the same frequency. The former, usually secondary to intrahepatic aneurysms, causes hemobilia and is accompanied by pain and jaundice in 30% of patients.[15] Rupture into the abdominal cavity presents with severe hypovolemic shock. On rare occasions, the aneurysm communicates with the adjoining structures, including the gastrointestinal tract, pancreatic duct, and portal vein. Cases of thrombosis of HAAs have been reported rarely.[1]

Diagnosis

As in SAAs the clinical features or findings at physical examination do not provide information that permits diagnosis of HAAs. Early diagnosis is usually incidental during radiologic abdominal evaluation. Angiography continues to be the diagnostic method of choice and is irreplaceable for planning the surgical strategy for these aneurysms because it provides information on anatomical variations of the hepatic vasculature, which are seen in 40% of patients (Figure 49.1). Projections of the superior mesenteric artery should be done because of the large number of asymptomatic ostial lesions in patients over age 60.[36]

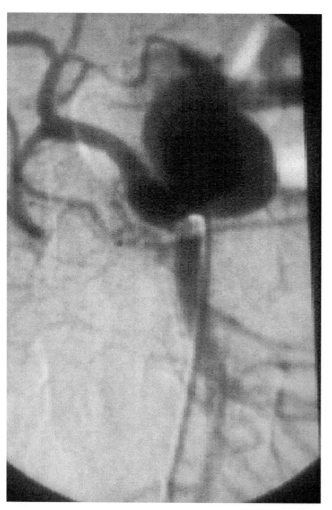

FIGURE 49.1. Aneurysm at the origin of the common hepatic artery.

Treatment

The high incidence of rupture, because it is unpredictable and associated with high mortality rates, makes surgical treatment of HAA advisable once it has been diagnosed and whenever the patient is at an acceptable level of surgical risk.[51] The surgical technique depends on the location of the aneurysm. Hence, for aneurysms of the common hepatic artery, double ligation and complete, partial, or no resection are sufficient. In these patients revascularization is generally not required because of the excellent collateral blood supply of the liver from the gastroduodenal and right gastric arteries. In case of liver disease or insufficient collateral blood supply, the artery must be revascularized. Most groups prefer the use of inguinal saphenous vein grafts, with origin in the proximal hepatic artery, celiac artery, or supraceliac or infrarenal aorta. In selected patients with saccular aneurysms, repair may suffice with or without the use of a patch. HAAs that affect the proper hepatic artery or its branches warrant revascularization techniques, although occasionally portal blood flow is sufficient to keep the liver viable. The elective surgery mortality rate is less than 10%.[18] Intrahepatic aneurysms and some extrahepatic aneurysms in patients at high risk warrant embolization procedures, either percutaneous or transparietohepatic, depending on the situation.[3,35]

Aneurysms of the Superior Mesenteric Artery

Aneurysms of the superior mesenteric artery account for approximately 5.5% of all splanchnic aneurysms reported in the literature.[17,48] The age at onset of these aneurysms varies according to the etiology and is under 50 years for the fungal aneurysms and over 60 years for those arising from other causes.[21,51] Superior mesenteric artery aneurysms (SMAAs) are single lesions, fusiform or saccular, and usually involve the first 5 cm of the artery. There is no predisposition according to sex in the incidence of SMAAs.

Pathophysiology

Approximately 60% of SMAAs are mycotic,[5] and, unlike in other visceral arteries, their frequency has remained unchanged in recent decades. Microbiological features of these aneurysms have changed, however. Currently, nonhemolytic *Streptococcus* and *Staphylococcus* (generally associated with intravenous drug users) are the most common pathogens.[21] Atherosclerosis is present in 20% of patients. As in other splanchnic arteries, it is uncertain whether the foregoing is incidental. Although uncommon, degenerative disease of the tunica media affects the superior mesenteric artery in a special manner and causes aneurysms and spontaneous dissection.[14] Trauma is a very rare cause of aneurysms at this site.

Clinical Features

Unlike other splanchnic aneurysms, many SMAAs are symptomatic. The clinical features of this aneurysm depend on its etiology. Hence, in those associated with atherosclerosis, most patients have a clinical picture compatible with chronic mesenteric ischemia before the aneurysm's diagnosis or rupture. Mycotic SMAAs are usually accompanied by epigastric abdominal pain that increases with enlargement of the aneurysm. In patients with bacterial endocarditis, the appearance of abdominal pain warrants assessment to identify this condition.

Mycotic aneurysms enlarge and rupture in almost all cases. The natural history of atherosclerotic aneurysms of the superior mesenteric artery is unknown, although it is assumed that slow enlargement following thrombosis or rupture must be their logical course.

Diagnosis

Mycotic SMAAs are palpated as pulsatile and movable masses in almost 50% of patients.[51] Based on the clinical history and findings of noninvasive imaging techniques or as an incidental finding, the diagnosis can often be suspected based on the plain film and confirmed by ultrasound, duplex scan, CT, or MRI (Figures 49.2 and 49.3). The definitive diagnosis is by arteriography, which also shows the exact location and the presence and quality of collateral blood supply (inferior pancreatoduodenal and midcolic arteries), basic points for determining surgical technique (Figure 49.4).

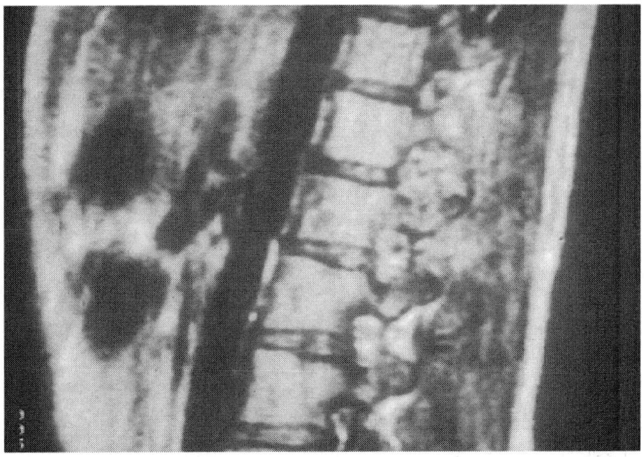

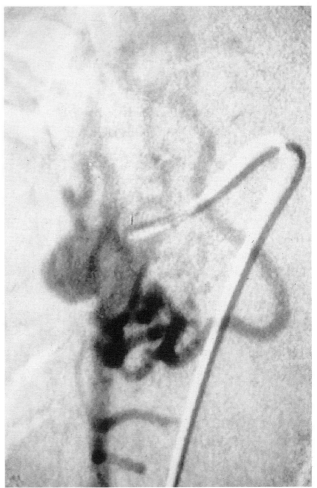

FIGURE 49.3. MRI of an SMA aneurysm.

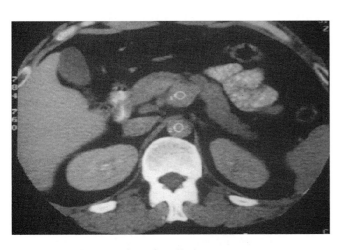

FIGURE 49.2. CT scan view of an SMA aneurysm.

FIGURE 49.4. Arteriography. Lateral view of an SMA aneurysm.

Treatment

SMAAs usually result in thrombosis or rupture, and elective surgery is therefore advisable in all patients at a reasonable surgical risk.[51] The surgical technique is based on the etiology, morphology, location, and presence or absence of collateral blood supply. Although the majority of these aneurysms can be approached by the inframesenteric route, those that lie very proximal to the ostium of the SMA must be approached by a combination technique that includes visceral rotation or the retroperitoneal approach.

Mycotic aneurysms with sufficient blood supply warrant proximal and distal ligation with complete resection, if technically possible, of the aneurysmal sac and long antibiotic coverage. In case of ischemic compromise, revascularization of the distal artery can be achieved by interpositioning saphenous vein grafts with aortic or extra-anatomic origin. Saccular aneurysms in many cases benefit from resection and direct closure or closure with a venous patch graft. Large atherosclerotic SMAAs in a patent arteries are amenable to endoaneurysmal repair with proximal and distal control; this approach diminishes the risk of injury to adjoining structures. Finally, the thrombosed aneurysms should be managed following the same criteria for revascularization as in chronic mesenteric ischemia, adding resection in case of symptoms of compression. The mortality rate associated with these techniques in elective surgery is less than 15%.[51] There are no clear indications for treatment by percutaneous embolization, and although it may be useful in the management of certain saccular aneurysms in patients at high risk, it is not without complications.[3]

Aneurysms of the Celiac Artery

Aneurysms of the celiac artery account for 4% of all splanchnic aneurysms. The mean age of patients with celiac artery aneurysms (CAAs) is 52 years at the time of diagnosis.[25] The distribution according to sex was 2:1 (male to female ratio) from 1950 to 1970[48]; this ratio has not been confirmed in more recent studies.[25] CAAs are visceral aneurysms most frequently associated with aneurysms at other sites: 18% are associated with abdominal aorta aneurysms and 38% with splanchnic aneurysms[25]; hence these lesions should be routinely sought.

Pathophysiology

More than 25% of CAAs are associated with atherosclerosis and, less frequently, with degenerative disease of the media. Congenital weakness of the artery wall at bifurcations accounts for 17% of cases. Trauma and poststenotic dilatation of the celiac artery (atherosclerotic or not) are uncommon. Fungal aneurysms are very rare at this site.[25]

Clinical Features

Most CAAs are asymptomatic. About 60% of symptomatic patients present with nonspecific epigastric pain that becomes more intense with sudden enlargement of the aneurysm, mimicking pancreatitis (pain radiating to the back, nausea, and vomiting).[25] The incidence of rupture of the aneurysm has been less than 15% in recent decades. It usually occurs in the free abdominal cavity and carries an estimated mortality rate of 40%.[25,49]

Diagnosis

Although clinical features do not usually provide useful information in the diagnosis of CAAs, physical examination discloses a pulsatile epigastric mass in 30% of patients. Only 20% have calcifications and may be incidentally discovered by abdominal plain films. However, a vast majority of CAAs (65%) are secondarily diagnosed on abdominal angiographic evaluation.[25]

Treatment

Like most splanchnic aneurysms, CAAs warrant prophylactic management for all patients with a reasonable surgical risk and life expectancy.[25,49,51] Most CAAs can be resected through a wide longitudinal laparotomy with or without resection of the xyphoid process or by a Chevron-type transverse laparotomy, although some patients may require a retroperitoneal or thoracoabdominal approach for proximal control.

Ligation with or without resection of the aneurysm has been used in 35% of the reported cases,[25] although the current approach is revascularization. Bypass with the origin from the aorta or proximal celiac artery to the distal celiac or hepatic artery depends on the situation. In selected patients, resection with direct anastomosis may be indicated. Some saccular aneurysms warrant resection and artery repair with or without a patch. The mortality rate of elective surgery ranges from 5% to 15%.[25,49]

Aneurysms of the Gastric and Gastroepiploic Arteries

About 4% of splanchnic aneurysms affect the perigastric arteries; the gastric artery is affected 10 times more frequently than the gastroepiploic arteries.[52] Perigastric artery aneurysms are generally single lesions. Most patients are diagnosed after age 60, and the male to female ratio is 3:1.[51]

Pathophysiology

Aneurysms of the gastric and gastroepiploic arteries, initially considered congenital or atherosclerotic in origin,[48] are mostly secondary to medial degeneration or periarterial inflammation.[51] Arterial dissection and congenital anomalies are rare causes of these aneurysms.

Clinical Features and Diagnosis

Less than 10% of gastric and gastroepiploic artery aneurysms are asymptomatic when diagnosed. About 90% present clinically as massive hemorrhage, which, unlike other splanchnic aneurysms, occurs in the gastrointestinal tract in 70% of patients.[48,51] Approximately 30% present as intraperitoneal hemorrhage. The mortality rate from rupture of these aneurysms is approximately 70%.[48] Due to the form of presentation, most of these aneurysms are diagnosed at surgery or, less frequently, during arteriographic evaluation for gastrointestinal hemorrhage.

Treatment

Perigastric aneurysms are not amenable to revascularization procedures. The extramural types are treated by ligation with or without resection. Intramural aneurysms and those communicating with the gastrointestinal tract additionally require partial gastric resections.

Aneurysms of the Jejunal, Ileal, and Colic Arteries

Aneurysms of the jejunal, ileal, and colic arteries account for 3% of all splanchnic aneurysms and commonly affect patients in the seventh decade of life. They affect men and women equally.[51] Apart from those that are secondary to vasculitis, they are frequently single lesions and less than 1 cm in diameter.[45]

Pathophysiology

Aneurysms of the jejunal, ileal, and colic arteries are secondary to congenital or acquired disorders of the media. Multiple aneurysms are generally secondary to vasculitis and, less frequently, to infectious arteritis.

Clinical Features and Diagnosis

About 70% of aneurysms of the jejunal, ileal, and colic arteries are silent and are incidentally discovered during angiographic evaluation.[45] The remaining 30% remain asymptomatic until they rupture. Rupture of the aneu-

rysm leads to intraluminal bleeding more frequently than mesenteric hematoma or hemiperitoneum and carries a mortality rate of 20%.[45,48]

Treatment

As with other splanchnic aneurysms, due to the risk of rupture and the high mortality rate, prophylactic surgical management is advised.[51] The major difficulty entailed in surgical management of this condition is the location of the aneurysm. However, identification can be facilitated by the intramural hematoma and preoperative or even perioperative arteriography.[45] Aneurysms of the intestinal arteries require ligation with or without aneurysmectomy. This procedure must be combined with intestinal resection for aneurysms located in the artery wall, intraluminal bleeding, intramural hematoma, and/or ischemia following artery ligation.[45]

Aneurysms of the Gastroduodenal, Pancreatic, and Pancreatoduodenal Arteries

Gastroduodenal and pancreatoduodenal artery aneurysms account for 1.5% and 2% of all splanchnic aneurysms, respectively. These lesions are diagnosed more frequently in patients over age 60. The distribution according to sex varies according to the etiology. Aneurysms related to pancreatitis have a male to female ratio of 4:1. There is no sex prevalence for the noninflammatory type.[19]

Pathophysiology

About 60% of gastroduodenal and 30% of pancreatoduodenal artery aneurysms are secondary to acute or chronic pancreatitis.[19] Degenerative disease of the media, atherosclerosis, and conditions that cause increased blood flow to these arteries when functioning as collateral supply channels are less common causes of these aneurysms.

Clinical Features and Diagnosis

Many aneurysms of the gastroduodenal, pancreatic, and pancreatoduodenal arteries cause epigastric pain that cannot be distinguished from that of pancreatic disease. Rupture of the aneurysm is the most severe and most common complication. It occurs in 70% of aneurysms associated with pancreatitis and causes gastrointestinal hemorrhage in 90% of patients. Approximately 50% of the noninflammatory aneurysms are diagnosed during rupture; of these intraluminal or intraperitoneal bleeding occurs in 50% of patients. The rupture-related mortality rate is 50% for inflammatory and 20% for noninflammatory aneurysms. Gastrointestinal hemorrhage in a patient with chronic pancreatitis or pancreatic pseudocyst may indicate the presence of these aneurysms. Gastrointestinal tract endoscopy is useful in excluding other causes of bleeding. CT and MRI scans can be diagnostic of aneurysm and are fundamental for the evaluation of this condition and to identify or exclude pancreatic disease as the problem. Angiography is necessary for diagnosis and planning the therapeutic strategy.

Treatment

Some type of therapy is indicated for all viable patients. Intra-arterial embolization has been reported to achieve a success rate of 79% without mortality,[34] and surgery has been reported to have a mortality rate of more than 20%.[19,43] Therefore, the percutaneous techniques are perhaps the procedures of choice for bleeding and prophylactic management of these aneurysms. Surgery should be reserved in case these procedures fail and to treat the underlying pancreatic disease.

Aneurysms of the Renal Artery

True macroaneurysms of the renal artery are the second most common visceral artery aneurysms and are surpassed only by SAAs. Their incidence in the general population is estimated to be 1 per 1000, as shown by two large nonselected angiographic series: 0.3% of 10,000 patients[27] and 0.09% of 8500 patients[47] had renal artery aneurysms (RAAs). RAAs are seen most commonly in the fifth decade of life.[30,47] If aneurysms associated with fibrodysplasia are excluded, there is no prevalence according to sex or side.[30,47] The average size of these aneurysms is 1.3 to 1.5 cm.[50] RAAs are saccular in most cases, and, unlike the fusiform types, they affect the lobar and segmental divisions of the renal artery in 75% of patients. Only 10% are intrarenal aneurysms.

Pathophysiology

True macroaneurysms of the renal artery, particularly the saccular types, are usually secondary to degenerative disease of the tunica media of the artery; they may or may not be associated with fibrodysplasia or atherosclerosis.[47,50] The fusiform types are usually associated with stenotic disease of the renal artery and may or may not be atherosclerotic.

Clinical Features

Most RAAs are silent and are incidentally discovered during abdominal arteriographic evaluation, frequently for arterial hypertension. They occasionally cause flank pain and may mimic renal colic. The pain and hematuria that usually accompany this condition cannot be easily explained in relation to the aneurysm[50] but are considered to be signs of impending rupture.

Hypertension is present in 50% of patients with saccular and 80% with fusiform aneurysms. Whether this association has a cause–effect relationship or is incidental is debated. The relationship has been explained by the following three conditions: (1) distal atheroembolism from the aneurysm, (2) compression of arterial branches produced by the aneurysm, and (3) associated intrinsic renal artery stenosis. The first two conditions are rare and account for less than 5% of cases in large series.[47] Demonstrating the cause–effect relationship between aneurysm and hypertension requires performing functional tests (renin test and scintiscan with captopril). Unfortunately, most of the large surgical series were reported before these tests became widely used.

Rupture is the most severe complication of RAAs and accounts for less than 3% of the cases.[27,45,50] Pregnancy appears to increase the risk of rupture, and the maternal and fetal mortality rates are 55% and 85%, respectively.[13] Hypertension, partial or no calcification, and diameter greater than 1.5 cm do not increase the risk of rupture in a statistically significant way.[50] Mortality due to rupture in the nonpregnant population is 10%, although it carries a higher incidence of kidney loss.

Diagnosis

As with other visceral aneurysms, ultrasonography, duplex scan, CT, and MRI can be diagnostic under certain circumstances and are useful for noninvasive follow-up of these aneurysms if surgery is not indicated. Arteriography is necessary to confirm the diagnosis and for planning the surgical strategy (Figure 49.5).

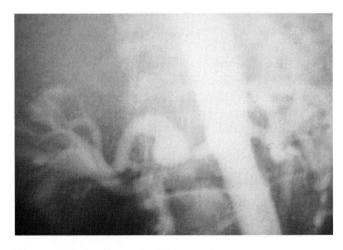

FIGURE 49.5. Arteriography. Right renal artery aneurysm.

Treatment

The clear indications for surgery in RAAs include rupture; sudden enlargement with clinical symptoms that indicate imminent rupture; vasculorenal hypertension demonstrated by functional studies secondary to associated stenosis, compression, or atheroembolism; women of childbearing age; and aneurysms that have enlarged during regular follow-up.

The size criteria are a subject of discussion, although clearly asymptomatic RAAs less than 2 cm in diameter do not warrant operation and can be regularly followed by noninvasive imaging techniques and close control of arterial pressure. Treatment of larger-sized aneurysms depends on the patient, location, technical difficulties, and surgical risk.

Surgical technique depends on the location of the aneurysm. Aneurysms that affect the main segment of the renal artery require resection or exclusion combined with reconstructive techniques. In this location, saphenous vein grafts from the aorta are the most widely used. When vein is unavailable for grafting or the distal artery diameter does not match, synthetic grafts may be used with excellent results. Hepatic or splenic artery bypass is useful in patients at high risk or those with hostile aortas. Some patients can benefit from reimplantation procedures or angioplasty. These two techniques are usually the procedures of choice for RAAs located at the first bifurcation of the renal artery.[12] More complex or distal lesions warrant ex vivo surgery.[4,16] Intra-arterial embolization achieves the best results for intraparenchymal aneurysms.

Conclusions

Aneurysms of visceral arteries are rare. Unlike the more common aortoiliac aneurysms, atherosclerosis is not considered a common etiological factor. Degenerative disease of the media, periarterial inflammation, and mycotic embolism are common causes of these aneurysms, which as a group are more prevalent in women. Except for the mycotic or traumatic types, the peak incidence of visceral aneurysms is in the sixth decade of life. Located deeply, supplying or surrounded by vital organs, insidious, and generally small in size, these aneurysms cause no symptoms and are rarely palpable. Rupture is not common as a presenting feature. Aneurysms are frequently discovered incidentally due to the widespread use of arteriography, which continues to be important for confirming and assessing aneurysms. They may be difficult to identify intraoperatively, difficult to manage, and generally skill demanding when revascularization becomes necessary. The new percutaneous therapeutic modalities may be useful in isolated cases and indispensable in aneurysms for which surgery, including prophy-

lactic surgery, carries high morbidity and mortality rates. Endoprostheses have not yet been reported in the management of these aneurysms, but they are likely to have a place in the therapeutic armamentarium in the future.

References

1. Alexander DJ, Madan M. Hepatic artery aneurysm: an unusual presentation. *Br J Clin Pract.* 1993;47:269–270.
2. Ayalon A, Wiesner RH, Perkins JD. Splenic artery aneurysms in liver transplant patients. *Transplantation.* 1988; 45:386–389.
3. Baker KS, Tisnado J, Cho SR, Beachley MC. Splanchnic artery aneurysms and pseudoaneurysms: transcatheter embolization. *Radiology.* 1987;163:135–139.
4. Barral X, Faure JP, Gourmier JP. Lesions anneurismales des branches de l'artere renale: chirurgie ex situ. *J Med Vasc.* 1994;19(suppl A):118–123.
5. Barrett JM, Caldwell BH. Association of portal hypertension and ruptured splenic artery aneurysm in pregnancy. *Obstet Gynecol.* 1981;57:255–257.
6. Bedford PD, Lodge B. Aneurysms of the splenic artery. *Gut.* 1960;1:321–326.
7. Brems JJ, Hiatt JR, Klein AS, Colonna JO, Busuttil RW. Splenic artery aneurysm rupture following orthotopic liver transplantation. *Transplantation.* 1988;45:1136–1137.
8. Bronsther O, Merhav H, van Thiel D, Starzl TE. Splenic artery aneurysms occurring in liver transplant recipients. *Transplantation.* 1991;52:723–724.
9. Busuttil RW, Brin BJ. The diagnosis and management of visceral artery aneurysms. *Surgery.* 1980;88:619–630.
10. den Butter G, van Bockel JH, Aarts JC. Arterial fibrodysplasia: rapid progression complicated by rupture of a visceral aneurysm into the gastrointestinal tract. *J Vasc Surg.* 1988;7:449–453.
11. Caillouette JC, Merchant EB. Ruptured splenic aneurysm in pregnancy: twelfth reported case with maternal and fetal survival. *Am J Obstet Gynecol.* 1993;168:1810–1813.
12. Cairols MA, Gimenez A, Gost AL, Miralles M. Aneurismas de las ramas de la arteria renal secundarios a fibrodisplasia intimal. *Arch Esp Urol.* 1993;46:453–457.
13. Cohen JR, Shamash FS. Ruptured renal artery aneurysms during pregnancy. *J Vasc Surg.* 1987;6:51–59.
14. Cormier F, Ferry J, Artru B, Wechsler B, Cormier JM. Dissecting aneurysms of the main trunk of the superior mesenteric artery. *J Vasc Surg.* 1992;15:424–430.
15. Countryman D, Norwood S, Register D, Torma M, Andrassy R. Hepatic artery aneurysm: report of an unusual case and review of the literature. *Am Surg.* 1983;49:51–54.
16. Dean RH, Meacham PW, Weaver FA. Ex vivo renal artery reconstructions: indications and techniques. *J Vasc Surg.* 1986;4:546–552.
17. Deterling RA. Aneurysms of the visceral arteries. *J Cardiovasc Surg.* 1971;12:309–314.
18. Dougherty MJ, Gloviczki P, Cherry KJ Jr, Bower TC, Hallet JW, Pairolero PC. Hepatic artery aneurysms: evaluation and current management. *Int Angiol.* 1993;12:178–184.
19. Eckhauser FE, Stanley JC, Zelenock GB, Borlaza GS, Freier DT, Lindenauer SM. Gastroduodenal and pancreaticoduodenal artery aneurysms: a complication of pancreatitis

causing spontaneous gastrointestinal hemorrhage. *Surgery.* 1980;88:335–355.

20. Eidus LB, Rasuli P, Manion D, Heringer R. Caliber-persistent artery of the stomach (Dieulafoy's vascular malformation). *Gastroenterology.* 1990;99:1507–1510.

21. Friedman SG, Pogo GJ, Moccio CG. Mycotic aneurysm of the superior mesenteric artery. *J Vasc Surg.* 1987;6:87–90.

22. Fukunaga Y, Usui N, Hirohashi K, et al. Clinical courses and treatment of splenic artery aneurysms: report of 3 cases and review of literatures in Japan. *Osaka City Med J.* 1990;36:161–173.

23. Genyck YS, Keller FS, Halpern NB. Hepatic artery pseudoaneurysm and hemobilia following laser laparoscopic cholecystectomy: a case report. *Surg Endosc.* 1994;8: 201–204.

24. Gesto R, Porto J. Aneurismas de las arterias viscerales. In: Barguño J, ed. *Tratamiento de las Lesiones Vasculares Asintomáticas.* Barcelona: Sobregrau-Auge; 1995:63–72.

25. Graham LM, Stanley JC, Whitehouse WM Jr, et al. Celiac artery aneurysms: historic (1745–1949) versus contemporary (1950–1984) differences in etiology and clinical importance. *J Vasc Surg.* 1985;2:757–764.

26. Greene DR, Gorey TF, Tanner WA, Lane BE, Collins PG. The diagnosis and management of splenic artery aneurysms. *J R Soc Med.* 1988;81:387–388.

27. Hageman JH, Smith RF, Szilagy DE, Elliot JP. Aneurysms of the renal artery: problems of prognosis and surgical management. *Surgery.* 1978;84:563–572.

28. Harper PC, Gamelli RL, Kaye MD. Recurrent hemorrhage into the pancreatic duct from a splenic aneurysm. *Gastroenterology.* 1984;87:417–420.

29. Hofer BO, Ryan JA Jr, Freeny PC. Surgical significance of vascular changes in chronic pancreatitis. *Surgery, Gynecology and Obstetrics.* 1987;164:499–505.

30. Hubert JP Jr, Pairolero PC, Kazmier FJ. Solitary renal artery aneurysm. *Surgery.* 1980;88:557–565.

31. Lambert CJ Jr, Williamson JW. Splenic artery aneurysm: a rare cause of upper gastrointestinal bleeding. *Am Surg.* 1990;56:543–545.

32. Mac Farlane JR, Thorbjarnason B. Rupture of splenic artery aneurysm during pregnancy. *Am J Obstet Gynecol.* 1966;95:1025–1037.

33. Madariaga J, Tzakis A, Zajko AB, et al. Hepatic artery pseudoaneurysm ligation after orthotopic liver transplantation: a report of 7 cases. *Transplantation.* 1992;54: 824–828.

34. Mandel SR, Jaques PF, Mauro MA, Sanofsky S. Nonoperative management of peripancreatic arterial aneurysm: a 10-year experience. *Ann Surg.* 1987;205:126–128.

35. Merhav H, Zajzo AB, Dodd GD, Pinna A. Percutaneous transhepatic embolization of an intrahepatic pseudoaneurysm following liver biopsy in a liver transplant patient. *Transpl Int.* 1993;6:239–241.

36. Moneta GL, Lee RW, Yeager RA, Taylor LM, Porter JM. Mesenteric duplex scanning: a blinded prospective study. *J Vasc Surg.* 1993;17:79–86.

37. Moore SW, Guida PM, Schumacher HW. Splenic artery aneurysm. *Bull Soc Int Chir.* 1970;29:210–219.

38. O'Grady JP, Day EJ, Toole AL, Paust JC. Splenic artery aneurysm ruptured in pregnancy: a review and case report. *Obstet Gynecol.* 1977;50:627–630.

39. Park H. Rupture of splenic artery aneurysm. *Am J Forensic Med Pathol.* 1992;13:230–232.

40. Probst P, Castaneda-Zuniga WR, Gomes AS, Yoheniro EG, Delaney JP, Amplatz K. Nonsurgical treatment of splenic artery aneurysms. *Radiology.* 1978;128:619–623.

41. Puttini M, Aseni P, Brambilla G, Belli L. Splenic artery aneurysms in portal hypertension. *J Cardiovasc Surg.* 1982; 23:490–493.

42. Revhaug A, Flatmark A, Enge I. Splenic artery aneurysm with bleeding oesophageal varices. *Acta Chir Scand.* 1978; 144:403–404.

43. Saw EC, Ku W, Ramachandra S. Laparoscopic resection of a splenic artery aneurysm. *J Laparoendosc Surg.* 1993;3: 167–171.

44. Spittel JA, Fairbairn JF, Kincaid OW, Remine VH. Aneurysm of the splenic artery. *JAMA.* 1961;175:452–459.

45. Stanley JC. Abdominal visceral aneurysm. In: Haimovici H, ed. *Vascular Emergencies.* New York, NY: Appleton-Century-Crofts; 1981:387–397.

46. Stanley JC, Fry WJ. Pathogenesis and surgical significance of splenic artery aneurysms. *Surgery.* 1974;76:898–909.

47. Stanley JC, Rhodes EL, Gewertz BL, Chang CY, Walter JF, Fry WJ. Renal artery aneurysms: significance of macroaneurysms exclusive of dissections and fibrodysplastic mural dilatations. *Arch Surg.* 1975;110:1327–1333.

48. Stanley JC, Thompson NW, Fry WJ. Splanchnic artery aneurysms. *Arch Surg.* 1970;101:689–697.

49. Stanley JC, Wakefield TW, Graham LM, Whitehouse WM Jr, Zelenock GB, Lindenauer SM. Clinical importance and management of splanchnic artery aneurysms. *J Vasc Surg.* 1986;3:836–840.

50. Stanley JC, Whitehouse WM Jr. Renal artery macroaneurysms. In: Bergan JJ, Yao JST, eds. *Aneurysms: Diagnosis and Treatment.* New York, NY: Grune & Stratton; 1982: 417–431.

51. Stanley JC, Zelenock GB. Splanchnic artery aneurysms. In: Rutherford RB, ed. *Vascular Surgery.* Philadelphia, Pa: WB Saunders; 1995:1124–1139.

52. Thomford NR, Yurko JE, Smith EJ. Aneurysm of gastric arteries as a cause of intraperitoneal hemorrhage: review of literature. *Ann Surg.* 1968;168:294–297.

53. Tam TN, Lai KH, Tsai YT, et al. Huge splenic aneurysm after portocaval shunt. *J Clin Gastroenterol.* 1988;10:565–568.

54. Trastek VF, Pairolero PC, Joyce JW, Hollier LH, Bernatz PE. Splenic artery aneurysms. *Surgery.* 1982;91:694–699.

55. Witte JT, Hasson JE, Harms BA, Corrigan TE, Love RB. Fatal gastric artery dissection and rupture occurring as a paraesophageal mass: a case report and literature review. *Surgery.* 1990;107:590–594.

50

Aneurysms of the Brachiocephalic Arteries as a Source of Brain Embolization

John D. Corson, Roderick T. A. Chalmers, Jamal J. Hoballah, Chittur R. Mohan, William J. Sharp, and Timothy F. Kresowik

The presence of atherosclerotic plaque at the carotid bifurcation is recognized as a frequent cause of transient ischemic attacks (TIAs) and strokes that involve the anterior cerebral circulation. More rarely, these symptoms may be due to atherosclerotic plaque in the common carotid arteries or the innominate artery. Usually the plaque is at the origin of these vessels. Similarly, in the posterior cerebral circulation, atherosclerotic disease of the vertebral arteries may be a source of TIAs and strokes. The symptoms of cerebral ischemia from extracranial arterial disease are thought to be related mainly to embolization rather than hypoperfusion unless the involved extracranial artery is thrombosed. Although atherosclerotic embolic disease of the aforementioned extracranial arteries is the major etiology of TIAs and strokes, cerebral embolization from a cardiac source accounts for a large number of such events. Another potential but rare source of cerebral embolization is from intraluminal thrombus present in an aneurysm of the brachiocephalic arteries. This latter problem forms the basis of this review.

Innominate Artery Aneurysms

Innominate artery aneurysms are rare. In recent reports from two large institutions a total of only nine innominate artery aneurysms that required surgery were identified.[1,2] The etiologies of these nine aneurysms were atherosclerosis (seven), blunt chest trauma (one), and infection (one). Other possible etiologies of innominate artery aneurysms include hereditary factors, iatrogenic trauma, and aortic dissection.[3–8] Luetic aneurysms are now a rarity. Seven of the nine innominate artery aneurysms in the Massachusetts General Hospital and Mayo Clinic series were associated with the presence of an arterial aneurysm at other sites—four in the abdominal aorta, three in the thoracic aorta, and one each in the femoral, popliteal, and subclavian arteries.[1,2]

Usually innominate artery aneurysms present in older patients, and there is a male predominance.[1] A large aneurysm may present as an expansile mass at the suprasternal notch or above the right costoclavicular joint. Symptoms are due to either cerebral embolization causing TIAs and stroke or compression of the surrounding structures.[9,10] Innominate vein compression presents as cyanosis of the head and neck. Tracheal compression may lead to dyspnea or stridor. Compression of the recurrent laryngeal nerve may cause hoarseness, and involvement of the sympathetic chain may give rise to Horner's syndrome. Occasionally brachial plexus compression causes upper extremity pain and/or paresis. A false aneurysm may present as a pulsatile mass or enlarging hematoma in association with a bruit and thrill and diminished distal pulses. Alternatively, an innominate artery aneurysm can be asymptomatic and present incidentally as a superior mediastinal or paratracheal mass on a chest x-ray.

Both magnetic resonance imaging and computed tomography can be useful studies to demonstrate the extent of the aneurysmal process and especially involvement of the aortic arch. Additionally, compression of the trachea or erosion into the posterior aspect of the sternum are important features to look for in these studies. Preoperative arteriography demonstrates the arterial anatomy and any associated disease of the other arch vessels. In a stable patient, following trauma to these vessels, an arteriogram is a very useful study because it defines the exact site of injury and helps guide the operative approach.

The surgical approach to innominate arterial aneurysms is straightforward.[1,2,10] Invasive cardiovascular monitoring is required to maintain a stable blood pressure. A radial artery line is preferentially placed on the left side. A median sternotomy provides excellent exposure and may be extended into the right neck if necessary. In rare cases, with a large aneurysm eroding into the sternum, a patient may require emergency femorofemoral bypass if a median sternotomy cannot be safely performed. Division of the innominate vein is not usually necessary, but if it needs to be divided to facilitate the procedure it should be repaired after completion of the arterial reconstruction. A femoral venous line is useful to provide adequate intravenous access if the innominate vein is divided. Distal arterial clamping is performed first to minimize embolic complications. Shunting does not appear to be necessary in most patients who undergo replacement of an innominate artery aneurysm due to the excellent collateral circulation. However, the use of electroencephalographic monitoring may be helpful in the event of simultaneous interruption of the left and right common carotid artery blood flow due to either the proximity of the origin of the left common carotid to the innominate artery or the takeoff of the left common carotid artery from a common innominate trunk. In addition, it may also be useful to detect inadequate perfusion of the brain if blood pressure is decreased.

After opening the aneurysm and removing the laminated thrombus a 10- or 12-mm-diameter prosthetic tube graft is anastomosed proximally to the disease-free origin of the innominate artery. If this is aneurysmal or the aortic arch is involved, the graft can be taken either directly from a normal portion of the ascending aorta or from an aortic prosthetic patch or graft that replaces the diseased aorta. To facilitate placing a side-biting clamp on the ascending aorta, the systemic blood pressure may need to be temporarily reduced by administration of nitroprusside or nitroglycerin. Great care should be taken with the proximal aortic anastomosis, and a nondiseased or minimally diseased portion of the aortic arch should preferentially be clamped to minimize disastrous complications from embolization or an aortic dissection.[10] After this portion of the operation is completed and a hemostatic suture line is obtained, the distal end of the graft is anastomosed to the distal innominate artery. If this segment is diseased, it is anastomosed end to end to the divided right common carotid artery and a side arm is anastomosed from the tube graft to the right subclavian artery. Alternatively, some authors recommend the use of a small bifurcated prosthetic graft.[2,11,12] Ruel et al. stress the need to place the origin of a bifurcated graft on the proximal right side of the ascending aorta to prevent kinking or compression.[11] Controversy exists over whether a tube or bifurcation graft is the better approach. It is not easy to reach any definitive conclusion because, even in the largest reported series, patient numbers are small. Certainly large bifurcated grafts should be avoided because they may be compressed.

A false aneurysm may be repaired by a variety of techniques (e.g., simple sutures, patch closure, aortic transection and end-to-end arterial anastomosis, or resection and graft interposition) depending on the situation.[3,7,8,10]

In infected cases, successful autogenous reconstructions using either saphenous vein grafts or arterial allograft have been reported.[9,10,13] Pasic et al. recently reported the successful use of a prosthetic bypass in situ for the treatment of a mycotic innominate artery aneurysm with the implantation of antibiotic-releasing carriers around the graft.[14]

Cardiopulmonary bypass may need to be utilized when the arch of the aorta and great vessels are involved in an associated aneurysmal process that requires replacement. Deep hypothermia and total circulatory arrest is another option that can be utilized. Mild hypothermia (35°C) may also be useful in selected cases.

In 1978 Schumacher and Wright reviewed the literature on 47 cases of nontraumatic innominate artery aneurysms, 18 of which were reported from 1946 to 1978, and found an overall mortality rate of 41.7%.[9] Bower et al. more recently reported no operative deaths in their six cases.[1] However, one patient with preoperative vertebrobasilar TIAs sustained a brain stem infarction on the 10th postoperative day and two patients had significant pulmonary complications. Several reports describe successful repairs of traumatic innominate artery aneurysms and define some of the complexities of dealing with these problems.[6-8]

Extracranial Carotid Artery Aneurysms

Fusiform, saccular, false, and mycotic arterial aneurysms may be found in the extracranial carotid circulation. Extracranial carotid aneurysms comprise 0.4% to 4% of all peripheral artery aneurysms.[15] The external carotid artery is rarely involved in the aneurysmal process.[16] In a review of 5000 carotid arteriograms by Houser and Baker, only eight extracranial carotid artery aneurysms were found.[17] In a series of 1500 carotid procedures performed over an 8-year period at the Cleveland Clinic, Painter et al. found only six patients who underwent surgical treatment of an extracranial carotid artery aneurysm.[18] Busuttil et al. reported a series of 19 extracranial carotid artery aneurysms: 59% were localized to the carotid bifurcation and 26% to the high cervical internal carotid artery, and 16% had diffuse ectatic changes of the common and internal carotid arteries.[19] These aneurysms are usually secondary to atherosclerosis, infection, fibromuscular dysplasia, congenital arterial weakness, or spontaneous carotid dissection.[1,18-26] False aneurysms are also seen after carotid artery surgery or trauma.[19,27] The etiologies of 145 extracranial carotid artery aneurysms reported in five series are shown in Table 50.1. Busuttil et al. noted that 26% of their patients had other aneurysms elsewhere.[19]

TABLE 50.1 Etiology of extracranial cartoid aneurysms.

	ASCVD	FMD	Spontaneous dissection	Prior CEA	Trauma	Mycotic	Unknown
McCollum et al.[27]	16 (44%)	—	—	19 (51%)	2 (5%)	—	—
Rhodes et al.[23]	16 (70%)	—	—	3 (13%)	4 (17%)	—	—
Busuttil et al.[19]	5 (26%)	—	—	5 (26%)	6 (34%)	1 (5%)	2 (11%)
Bower et al.[1]	3 (12%)	3 (12%)	6 (24%)	2 (8%)	8 (32%)	2 (8%)	1 (4%)
Welling et al.[24]	21 (51%)	—	26 (39%)	3 (7%)	—	1 (2%)	—

Proximal aneurysms are usually atherosclerotic or a complication of carotid endarterectomy, whereas distal aneurysms are most likely due to trauma, dissection, or infection and are seen in younger patients more frequently. Proximal fusiform extracranial atherosclerotic carotid artery aneurysms usually involve the bifurcation and may be bilateral in up to 21% of cases.[19,22,23] They are found most frequently in late middle age, and affected individuals usually have hypertension.[18,22,23] There is also a relative male preponderance.[22] In Bower and coworkers' recent report concerning extracranial carotid artery aneurysms there was a 1.8:1 male/female ratio,[1] and in Painter and coworkers' series the ratio was 2:1.[18] Cerebrovascular symptoms, secondary to distal embolization or thrombosis, can occur in up to 50% of patients with untreated extracranial carotid artery aneurysms. Winslow reviewed 106 cases of extracranial carotid artery aneurysms detected before 1925 and found that 71% of the untreated patients died of related causes.[28] Zwolak et al. noted a 50% stroke rate in a group of six patients with atherosclerotic carotid aneurysms that were followed for a mean interval of 6.3 years after diagnosis.[22] In the Cleveland Clinic series preoperative cerebrovascular symptoms referable to the treated carotid aneurysm had occurred in 43% of the patients.[18] Moreau et al. noted preoperative evidence of cerebral ischemia in 74% of their patients.[29]

A patient with an atherosclerotic extracranial carotid artery aneurysm usually has a palpable, expansile, well-circumscribed neck mass.[30] More distal aneurysms do not usually present as a neck mass but rather as an endobuccal mass.[29] Symptoms are due to cerebral embolization, thrombosis, or expansion, with high lesions causing compression of cranial nerves IX, X, and XI and less commonly rupture and hemorrhage. Local pain is occasionally present over a carotid artery aneurysm.[23] Rupture is an unusual complication of an extracranial atherosclerotic carotid aneurysm. A false or infected aneurysm is more prone to rupture. There are occasional reports of rupture into the oropharynx, ear canal, and the soft tissues of the neck; these occurrences are associated with significant morbidity and mortality rates.[31-33] The airway may be compromised and endotracheal intubation may be difficult due to significant edema and anatomical distortion. Hence the establish-ment of a satisfactory airway is a major priority in managing such patients.

A color duplex scan is very useful in determining the location and size of these aneurysms as well as the extent of the intraluminal thrombus (Figure 50.1). A preoperative arch and four-vessel arteriogram including intracranial views is valuable in planning appropriate surgical therapy (Figure 50.2).

A false aneurysm may develop following a carotid endarterectomy or trauma.[18,19,23,27,34] The latter are usually high aneurysms, and the mechanism is thought to be acute hyperextension and rotation of the neck that lead to compression of the internal carotid artery at the level of the first and second cervical vertebrae or alternatively compression of the internal carotid artery against the transverse process of the atlas from forces applied to the angle of the mandible.[19,23] A false aneurysm may also develop after a bypass that involves an anastomosis to the carotid artery. The incidence of carotid aneurysmal degeneration after endarterectomy is less than 1%[35]; the majority have a false aneurysm. Recurrent carotid artery stenosis may also be associated with aneurysmal degeneration of the arterial wall, and affected patients are thought to be at an increased risk for cerebrovascular

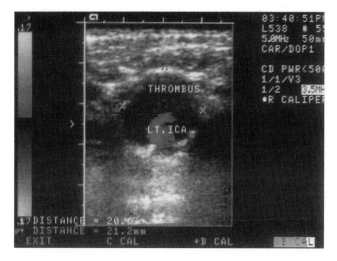

FIGURE 50.1. The extent of thrombus in this extracranial internal carotid artery aneurysm is clearly defined by a color duplex scan.

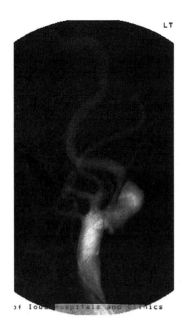

FIGURE 50.2. This large saccular aneurysm of the proximal internal carotid artery was replaced by an interposition vein bypass graft.

symptoms. In a series of 21 false aneurysms following carotid endarterectomy reported by McCollum et al., 16 were in patients with a Dacron carotid patch.[27] Prosthetic patch angioplasty closure of a carotid endarterectomy increases the risk of a false aneurysm fourfold compared with simple closure.[18] The incidence of a false aneurysm after the use of a vein patch is quite low. A false aneurysm following carotid endarterectomy without use of a patch is unusual but does occur occasionally.

A carotid artery aneurysm may be a late result of spontaneous carotid artery dissection.[36] A carotid dissection occurs in individuals between 25 and 45 years of age, and two thirds of the patients are men.[26,36,37] Characteristically the patient with an acute dissection presents with pain over the carotid artery and evidence of a neurological or visual deficit.[36] Horner's syndrome can be found in up to 50% of patients. Duplex studies may show an echogenic intraluminal flap or hypoechoic thrombus with Doppler velocities that show narrowing of the internal carotid artery.[38] Proximal to the dissection there is evidence of a resistive, damped, or biphasic blood flow by Doppler. The presence of such findings alone may be diagnostic of a high dissection. Arteriography usually demonstrates an irregular long stenosis of the internal carotid artery or a tapered occlusion or "string" sign.[24,36,38,39] The arteriogram may also show occlusion of an intracerebral branch artery due to distal embolization or fibromuscular dysplasia.[40]

Once the diagnosis is suspected, a computed tomographic or magnetic resonance imaging study of the brain should be performed to exclude the presence of a hemorrhagic infarct. The majority of patients with spontaneous carotid dissection do well with conservative therapy that consists of intravenous administration of

heparin initially followed by oral administration of coumadin for a total of at least 6 weeks of anticoagulation therapy.[36,37,41,42] Longer periods of anticoagulation therapy may be required depending on the symptomatology and the status of the carotid artery as seen by duplex or arteriographic follow-up studies. Welling et al. reported resolution with recanalization in 11 of 16 patients treated in this manner.[24]

If symptoms persist or the neurological deficit progresses despite anticoagulation therapy, the occasional patient may benefit from surgery.[36] Those with hypoperfusion-related symptoms require some type of revascularization. Patients with embolic symptoms may be cured by carotid ligation or endovascular occlusion, especially if the dissection extends very high and limits access for a safe bypass and if there is adequate collateral circulation. Occasionally an associated extracranial-to-intracranial bypass may be required.[43] A small number of patients may require early surgery if they cannot tolerate anticoagulation therapy.

The treatment of an extracranial carotid artery aneurysm depends on its accessibility, size, and symptomatology; the status of the collateral circulation; and the etiology of the aneurysm. Since Sir Astley Cooper first successfully treated an internal carotid artery aneurysm by ligation in 1808, a variety of surgical procedures have been utilized for the treatment of extracranial carotid artery aneurysms.[44] Resection with reestablishment of arterial continuity by end-to-end anastomosis was first performed in 1952 and remains the preferred treatment option.[6,23,45] Great care must be taken intraoperatively to minimize embolization by not manipulating the aneurysm during dissection and clamping the distal internal carotid artery as soon as feasible. On occasion, after internal carotid artery aneurysm resection, arterial continuity may be restored by anastomosing the external carotid artery to the distal internal carotid artery. An arterioplasty after resection of the aneurysm may also be used to restore flow to both the internal and external carotid arteries. Aneurysmorrhaphy can be used to treat a saccular aneurysm. The defect is then closed primarily or by a patch graft.

High extracranial carotid artery aneurysms pose a significant technical challenge due to the difficulty of exposure and distal control. Balloon occlusion shunts are extremely useful to obtain distal control and provide cerebral protection. Hans et al. divided the cervical internal carotid artery into three zones.[46] Zone I extends from the carotid bifurcation to the superior margin of the third cervical vertebra, zone II extends from the superior margin of the third cervical vertebra to the inferior margin of the first cervical vertebra, and zone III extends from the inferior margin of the first cervical vertebra to the base of the skull. These zones are not the same as those used to categorize the level of cervical trauma. Zone III aneurysms pose the most difficulty. Previously many such "inaccessible" extracranial carotid artery aneurysms were observed without surgical intervention if they were small and asymptomatic. Large or symptomatic and inaccessible aneurysms were treated by proximal ligation or graded carotid occlusion with a Selverstone clamp.[47] Such patients had a significant incidence of stroke in spite of concomitant anticoagulation therapy.[18,31,47,48] Hence consideration in selected cases should be given to an extracranial-to-intracranial artery bypass.

Surgical access to high lesions may be improved by the use of nasotracheal intubation and mandibular subluxation or rarely dislocation. Surgical exposure of the distal internal carotid artery at the skull base may be required in some patients for interposition vein grafting.[49–51] Exposure is enhanced by removal of portions of the styloid process and division of the stylohyoid and digastric muscles.[49] Additionally mastoidectomy, modified mandibular osteotomies, and resection of the temporomandibular joint articulation are other methods used to enhance exposure of the distal internal carotid artery.[51] Fisch et al.[52] described the use of the technique of subtotal petrosectomy with permanent anterior displacement of the facial nerve and middle ear obliteration for safe exposure of the temporal course of the internal carotid artery. Due to the morbidity of this procedure, it is seldom used.

Selected patients may be managed by endovascular techniques with placement of small intraluminal detachable balloons for permanent arterial occlusion.[53] This method of occlusion may be better than surgical ligation because the balloon can be placed just proximal to the ophthalmic artery and thus avoids the potential embolic source of a long cul de sac invariably present after proximal surgical ligation. Larson et al. reported satisfactory results on long-term follow-up of 58 patients treated with this technique.[54] The majority of the aneurysms they treated were intracranial. Preoperative temporary balloon occlusion of the internal carotid artery combined with cerebral blood flow monitoring and induced hypotension were used to determine tolerance for occlusion in this series.

Mycotic extracranial carotid aneurysms are usually due to *Staphylococcus aureus, Streptococcus pyogenes,* or rarely *Salmonella enteritidis.*[22] Other organisms reported in carotid aneurysms include *Escherichia coli, Proteus mirabilis, Klebsiella* species, *Corynebacterium* species, and *Yersinia enterocolitica.* Infected aneurysms should be treated by a primary autogenous reconstructive procedure under appropriate intravenous antibiotic coverage with radical debridement of infected tissues and coverage of the reconstruction with vascularized muscle. Because infection is often associated with a false carotid artery aneurysm, an autogenous reconstruction is also the treatment of choice for such lesions.[27] Excising the diseased portion of the artery and placing an interposition vein graft are the preferred treatment.

The limited data available suggest that the risk of serious complications from extracranial carotid artery aneurysms can be reduced by timely or early surgical intervention. The morbidity and mortality rates following treatment of extracranial carotid artery aneurysms are quite high compared with those found in current reports of carotid endarterectomies for both symptomatic and asymptomatic carotid artery atherosclerosis.[55–57] The results are not strictly comparable, however, due to a lack of synchronicity, but they do raise some questions about the risk of management of these lesions. Painter et al. reported a 7.6% incidence of transient neurological deficits, a 7.6% incidence of permanent stroke, and an operative mortality rate of 4.5% in a group of 66 patients who underwent surgical treatment of extracranial carotid artery aneurysms as reported in the literature from 1975 to 1985.[18] Zwolak et al. noted transient perioperative neurological deficits in 17% and a permanent deficit in 5%.[23]

Although these figures seem high, they should be considered in light of the significant morbidity and mortality risks from the natural history of untreated extracranial carotid artery aneurysms. The morbidity risk due to cranial nerve palsies can be expected to be higher than that following carotid artery endarterectomy, especially when treating large extracranial carotid aneurysms that distort the normal anatomy. This morbidity risk can be limited by leaving the back wall of the aneurysm intact. Because these injuries occur frequently, all patients with extracranial carotid artery aneurysms should have a careful evaluation of cranial nerve function both preoperatively and postoperatively.

Subclavian Artery Aneurysms

Subclavian artery aneurysms can be classified as either extrathoracic or intrathoracic.[58] The most common etiology, particularly for intrathoracic subclavian artery aneurysms, is atherosclerosis, which accounts for 34% of the aneurysms in the series reported by Bower et al., 72% of cases reported by Coselli and Crawford, and 50% of the patients in the series reported by McCollum et al.[1,58,59] However, for extrathoracic subclavian artery aneurysms, thoracic outlet syndrome and trauma are other important etiological factors.[60,61] Other etiologies encountered less frequently include infection, medial degeneration, arteritis, and congenital arterial wall weakness in conditions such as Ehlers-Danlos and Marfan's syndromes.[4,5,62,63]

Although subclavian artery aneurysms may be bilateral, there is a predilection for occurrence on the right side for nonatherosclerotic subclavian artery aneurysms.[60] The cause of this right-sided predominance is unclear. Extrathoracic subclavian artery aneurysms due to thoracic outlet compression are seen more frequently where there is an occupational etiology (e.g., in dock laborers and coal heavers, who are predominantly right-handed). Additionally, false aneurysms are more common on the right side, and many are related to iatrogenic injury.[60] Hence the higher right-sided incidence of nonatherosclerotic subclavian artery aneurysms may also reflect the physician's preference for central venous access as well as an occupational predilection.

The mean age in Bower and coworkers' series of subclavian artery aneurysms was 51.7 years.[1] An atherosclerotic subclavian artery aneurysm may be associated with the presence of an aneurysm elsewhere.[1,58,59] The usual male predominance of aneurysmal disease is not seen in the subclavian artery unless the aneurysm is associated with an aberrant right subclavian artery.[64] The majority of subclavian artery aneurysms are symptomatic.[60] A characteristic clinical feature of a subclavian artery aneurysm is local pain due to expansion and compression of neighboring structures. Horner's syndrome or phrenic nerve palsy may occur due to local compression.[58] An aneurysm of the subclavian artery occasionally gives rise to symptoms in the ipsilateral upper limb due to arterial embolism or thrombosis. Rarely, cerebrovascular symptoms have been identified in patients with proximal subclavian artery aneurysms, presumably due to vertebral artery embolization.[61] Retrograde embolization up the right common carotid artery is another possibility. Ruptured subclavian artery aneurysms may be encountered occasionally.[1,64] Dealing with rupture of an aberrant subclavian artery aneurysm may be quite taxing due to its location.

Usually an extrathoracic subclavian artery aneurysm can be detected clinically as a palpable, pulsatile mass in the supraclavicular fossa, whereas an intrathoracic subclavian artery aneurysm is apparent only on a chest x-ray as a mass in the superior mediastinum.[58] If the site of the aneurysm is amenable for study by B-mode ultrasound, the size of the aneurysm and the presence of the mural thrombus can be documented. A cervical rib is seen occasionally on plain films of the chest and neck and may be associated with the presence of an extrathoracic subclavian artery aneurysm.[61] Either computed tomography or magnetic resonance imaging can be used to evaluate a chest lesion that raises suspicion of an intrathoracic subclavian artery aneurysm. However, a conventional arteriogram (or magnetic resonance angiogram) is necessary to define coexisting arterial disease or anatomical variants.[65] A complete arteriographic runoff study of the extremity including the hand also detects evidence of prior distal extremity embolization.

The surgical treatment of most subclavian artery aneurysms can be undertaken with minimal morbidity and with good long-term results.[1,58] Hence, the definitive treatment for the majority of subclavian artery aneurysms is operative unless the patient is considered to be at high risk. The surgical approach to a subclavian artery aneurysm depends on its location. A right-sided intrathoracic aneurysm is approached via a median ster-

notomy, which ensures adequate proximal arterial control.[58] This incision can always be extended to the supraclavicular area if necessary. A left-sided intrathoracic aneurysm is best approached through a left anterolateral thoracotomy for safe proximal control and exposure. Early clamping of the vertebral artery and gentle handling of the lesion should limit any intraoperative embolization. The vertebral artery can be either ligated or revascularized as necessary by either reimplantation or bypass. An extrathoracic aneurysm on either side can usually be reached satisfactorily via a supraclavicular approach.[59,60] Involvement of the proximal axillary artery may require an associated infraclavicular incision and occasionally resection of the medial portion of the clavicle. The clavicular defect can be repaired following the vascular procedure with anticipation of a good long-term functional result. If repair of the clavicle is not planned, the periosteum of the resected portion of the clavicle should be removed completely to prevent bony regrowth and the possibility of later extrinsic vascular compression.[60]

An atherosclerotic subclavian artery aneurysm is preferentially treated by resection and replacement with a prosthetic graft.[59] A saccular aneurysm may be amenable to aneurysmorrhaphy whereby the defect is closed directly or with a patch.[60] A mycotic aneurysm may require exclusion and arterial ligation.[58,59] If no revascularization is done, 25% of patients may have arm claudication.[60] In a patient with a subclavian artery aneurysm secondary to thoracic outlet compression, the current therapeutic recommendation is thoracic outlet decompression and graft replacement of the aneurysmal artery.[60] However, an artery with only a small degree of poststenotic aneurysmal dilatation, no intraluminal thrombus, and a smooth lumen does not require replacement after decompression of the thoracic outlet. Intraoperative B-mode ultrasound evaluation may be helpful in assessing the need to replace a portion of the subclavian artery with a bypass graft.

The outcome of surgery for subclavian artery aneurysms is good. Coselli and Crawford reported an operative mortality rate of 6% for a series of 16 patients with 18 operated intrathoracic subclavian artery aneurysms.[58] The results are excellent given that these patients frequently had been treated for associated complex aneurysmal disease. Bower et al. reported a 12.2% mortality rate.[1] Two patients with ruptured aneurysms died, and three other patients died from complications associated with other concomitant major cardiovascular procedures. Survival rates were 87% after 5 years and 62% after 10 years, which are less than those for age-matched controls. Consequently, in all but high-risk patients with small stable aneurysms, operative repair should be undertaken. A patient with ultrasound evidence of mural thrombus within a subclavian artery aneurysm should be treated preferentially by surgical replacement of the aneurysmal artery due to the risk of embolism, even if the aneurysm is small and asymptomatic.

Vertebral Artery Aneurysms

Extracranial vertebral artery aneurysms are encountered very infrequently and are mainly related to trauma or dissection.[66-68] Occasionally they are associated with neurofibromatosis.[69] As with any aneurysm that contains a laminated thrombus, embolic cerebrovascular events may occur either as presenting symptoms or as a complication of the treatment. Direct surgical repair is associated with high morbidity and mortality risks, and hence vertebral artery ligation is frequently utilized if there is adequate collateral blood flow.[68,70,71] An extracranial-to-intracranial bypass is sometimes required.[72] Endovascular techniques are satisfactory methods of treatment in selected cases.[73] Duplex directed manual compression is another option that has been used to treat vertebral false aneurysms.[74]

Conclusions

Surgery of the aortic arch and great vessels comprises less than 7% of the procedures performed on the cerebral vasculature. Aneurysms of the brachiocephalic and carotid arteries are relatively unusual lesions. Because there is a high incidence of stroke or TIAs and also a chance of rupture, brachiocephalic artery aneurysms pose a major threat to life if left untreated. Due to their location, they present insidiously and give rise to challenging surgical problems. The results of surgical intervention are justifiable given the natural history of these lesions. Because they may be associated with the presence of aneurysmal disease elsewhere, continued follow-up is advised to detect further significant aneurysmal disease.

References

1. Bower TC, Pairolero PC, Hallet JW, Toomey BJ, Gloviczki P, Cherry KJ. Brachiocephalic aneurysm: the case for early recognition and repair. *Ann Vasc Surg.* 1991;5:125–132.
2. Brewster DC, Moncure AC, Darling RC, Ambrosino JJ, Abbott WM. Innominate artery lesions: problems encountered and lessons learned. *J Vasc Surg.* 1985;2:99–112.
4. Valverde A, Tricot JF, de Crepy B, Bakdach H, Djabbari K. Innominate artery involvement in type IV Ehlers-Danlos syndrome. *Ann Vasc Surg.* 1991;1:41–45.
5. Austin MG, Schafer RF. Marfan's syndrome with unusual blood vessel manifestations: primary medionecrosis dissec-

tion of right innominate, right carotid, and left carotid arteries. *Arch Pathol.* 1957;64:205–209.
6. Follis F, Miller KB, Paone RF, Wernly JA. Iatrogenic pseudoaneurysm of the innominate artery. *Texas Heart Inst J.* 1992;19:294–296.
7. Kraus TW, Paetz B, Richter GM, Allenberg JR. The isolated posttraumatic aneurysm of the brachiocephalic artery after blunt thoracic contusion. *Ann Vasc Surg.* 1993;7:275–281.
8. Edwards JD, Sapienza P, Lefkowitz DM, et al. Post-traumatic innominate artery aneurysm with occlusion of the common carotid artery at its origin by an intimal flap. *Ann Vasc Surg.* 1993;7:368–373.
9. Schumacher PD, Wright CB. Management of arteriosclerotic aneurysm of the innominate artery. *Surgery.* 1979;5:489–494.
10. Grecula JC, Clark TW, Horattas MC, Oddi MA, Evans MJ. Innominate artery aneurysms. *Surg Rounds.* 1994;17:95–102.
11. Reul GJ, Jacobs MJ, Gregoric ID, et al. Innominate artery occlusive disease: surgical approach and long term results. *J Vasc Surg.* 1991;14:405–412.
12. Vogt DP, Hertzer NR, O'Hara PJ, Beven EG. Brachiocephalic arterial reconstruction. *Ann Surg.* 1982;196:541–552.
13. Schuch D, Wolff L. Repair of mycotic aneurysm of the innominate artery with homograft tissue. *Ann Thorac Surg.* 1992;52:863–864.
14. Pasic M, Vonsegesser L, Turina M. Implantation of antibiotic-releasing carriers and in situ reconstruction for treatment of mycotic aneurysm. *Arch Surg.* 1992;127:745–746.
15. Moosa HH, Higgins R, Shapiro SP, Harrison AM. Isolated extracranial internal carotid artery aneurysm in a 22 year old patient. *Contemporary Surgery.* 1992;40:40–44.
16. Schecter DC. Cervical carotid aneurysms. *New York State Journal of Medicine Part I.* 1979;7:892–901.
17. Houser OW, Baker HL. Fibromuscular dysplasia and other uncommon diseases of the cervical carotid artery: angiographic aspects. *Am J Roentgenol.* 1968;104:201–212.
18. Painter TA, Hertzer NR, Beven EG, O'Hara PJ. Extracranial carotid aneurysms: report of six cases and review of the literature. *J Vasc Surg.* 1985;2:312–318.
19. Busuttil RW, Davidson RK, Foley KT, Livesay JT, Barker WF. Selective management of extracranial carotid arterial aneurysms. *Am J Surg.* 1980;140:85–91.
20. Margolis MT, Stein RL, Newton TH. Extracranial aneurysms of the internal carotid artery. *Neuroradiology.* 1972;4:78–89.
21. Grossi RJ, Onofrey D, Tvetenstrand C, Blumenthal J. Mycotic carotid aneurysm. *J Vasc Surg.* 1987;6:81–83.
22. Zwolak RM, Whitehouse WM, Knake JE, et al. Atherosclerotic extracranial carotid artery aneurysms. *J Vasc Surg.* 1984;1:415–422.
23. Rhodes EL, Stanley JC, Hoffman GL, Cronenwett JL, Fry WJ. Aneurysms of extracranial carotid arteries. *Arch Surg.* 1976;111:339–343.
24. Welling RE, Taha A, Goel T, et al. Extracranial carotid artery aneurysms. *Surgery.* 1983;93:319–323.
25. Chamberlain EN. Bacterial aneurysm. *Br Heart J.* 1943;5:121–125.

26. Nass R, Hays A, Chutorian A. Intracranial dissecting aneurysms in childhood. *Stroke.* 1982;11:204–207.

27. McCollum CH, Wheeler WG, Noon GP, DeBakey ME. Aneurysms of the extracranial carotid artery: twenty-one years experience. *Am J Surg.* 1979;137:196–200.

28. Winslow N. Extracranial aneurysms of the internal carotid artery. *Arch Surg.* 1926;13:689–729.

29. Moreau P, Albat B, Thevenet A. Surgical treatment of extracranial internal carotid aneurysm. *Ann Vasc Surg.* 1994; 8:409–416.

31. Rittenhouse EA, Radke HM, Sumner DS. Carotid artery aneurysm: review of the literature and report of a case with rupture into the oropharynx. *Arch Surg.* 1972;105: 786–789.

32. Harrison DFN. Two cases of bleeding from the ear from carotid aneurysm. *Guys Hosp Rep.* 1954;103:207–212.

33. Morki B, Piepgras DG, Sundt TM, Pearson BW. Extracranial internal carotid artery aneurysm. *Mayo Clin Proc.* 1982;57:310–321.

34. Shipley AM, Winslow N, Walker WW. Aneurysm in the cervical portion of the internal carotid artery. *Ann Surg.* 1937; 105:673–699.

35. Bergamini TM, Seabrook GR, Bandyk DF, Towne JB. Symptomatic recurrent carotid stenosis and aneurysmal degeneration after endarterectomy. *Surgery.* 1993;113: 580–586.

36. Lutz B, Horsch S, DeVleeschauer P. Surgical management of isolated dissection of the internal carotid artery: a review of the literature. In: Chang JB, ed. *Modern Vascular Surgery.* Vol 4. New York, NY: PMA Publishing Corp; 1989: 115–123.

37. Linskey ME, Sekhar LN, Hirsch W Jr, et al. Aneurysms of the intracavernous carotid artery: clinical presentation, radiographic features, and pathogenesis. *Neurosurgery.* 1990; 26:71–79.

38. Gardner DJ, Gosink BB, Kallman CE. Internal carotid artery dissection: duplex ultrasound imaging. *J Ultrasound Med.* 1992;10:607–614.

39. Mokri B, Sundt TM, Houser W, et al. Spontaneous dissection of the internal carotid artery. *Ann Neurol.* 1986;19: 126–138.

40. Carrascal L, Mashiah A, Charlesworth D. Aneurysms of the extracranial carotid arteries. *Br J Surg.* 1978;65: 590–592.

40. Hart RG, Easton JD. Dissection of cervical and cerebral arteries. *Neurol Clin.* 1983;1:155–182.

43. Ausman JI, Pearch JE, DeLos Reyes RA, Schanz G. Treatment of a high extracranial carotid artery aneurysm with CCA-MCA bypass and carotid ligation. *J Neurosurg.* 1983; 58:421–424.

44. Cooper A. Account of the first successful operation performed on the common carotid artery for aneurysm in the year of 1808 with postmortem examination in the year 1821. *Guys Hosp Rep.* 1836;1:53.

45. Dimtza A. Aneurysms of the carotid arteries: report of two cases. *Angiology.* 1956;7:218–227.

46. Hans SS, Shah S, Hans B. Carotid endarterectomy for high plaques. *Am J Surg.* 1989;157:431–434.

47. McCann RC. Basic data related to peripheral artery aneurysms. *Ann Vasc Surg.* 1990;4:411–414.

48. Ohara I. Surgery of the cervical carotid artery. Neurological sequelae following unilateral occlusion of the carotid artery. *J Cardiovasc Surg.* 1970;11:175–182.

49. Otero-Coto E, Orozco M, Collado ML. Giant aneurysm of the high internal carotid artery: surgical treatment. *Surgery.* 1992;11:348–351.

50. Fisch UP, Oldring DJ, Senning A. Surgical therapy of internal carotid artery lesions of the skull base and temporal bone. *Otolaryngol Head Neck Surg.* 1980;88:548–554.

51. Nelson SR, Schow SR, Stein SM, Read LA, Talkington CM. Enhanced surgical exposure for the high extracranial internal carotid artery. *Ann Vasc Surg.* 1992;6:467–477.

52. Fisch UP, Oldring DJ, Senning A. Surgical therapy of internal carotid artery lesions of the skull base and temporal bone. *Otolaryngol Head Neck Surg.* 1980;88:548–554.

53. Higashida RT, Hieshima GB, Halbach, et al. Intravascular detachable balloon embolization of intracranial aneurysms. *Acta Radiol.* 1986;369:594.

54. Larson JJ, Tew JM Jr, Tomsick TA, Van Loveren HR. Treatment of aneurysms of the internal carotid artery by intravascular balloon occlusion: long-term follow-up of 58 patients. *Neurosurgery.* 1995;36:26–30.

55. Hobson RW II, Weiss DG, Fields WS, and VA Cooperative Study Group 167. Efficacy of carotid endarterectomy for asymptomatic carotid stenosis. *N Engl J Med.* 1993;328: 221–227.

56. North American Symptomatic Carotid Endarterectomy Trial Collaborators. Beneficial effect of carotid endarterectomy in symptomatic patients with high-grade carotid stenosis. *N Engl J Med.* 1991;325:445–507.

57. Executive Committee for the Asymptomatic Carotid Atherosclerosis Study. Endarterectomy for asymptomatic carotid artery stenosis. *JAMA.* 1995;273:1421–1428.

58. Coselli JS, Crawford ES. Surgical treatment of aneurysms of the intrathoracic segment of the subclavian artery. *Chest.* 1987;91:705–708.

58. Follis F, Miller KB, Paone RF, Wernly JA. Iatrogenic pseudoaneurysm of the innominate artery. *Texas Heart Inst J.* 1992;19:294–296.

59. McCollum CH, DaGama AD, Noon GP, DeBakey ME. Aneurysm of the subclavian artery. *J Cardiovasc Surg.* 1979; 20:159–164.

60. Pairolero PC, Walls JT, Payne WS, Hollier LH, Fairbairn JF. Subclavian-axillary artery aneurysms. *Surgery.* 1981;90: 757–763.

61. Davis JM, Golinger D. Cervical rib, subclavian artery aneurysm, axillary and cerebral emboli. *Proceedings of the Royal Society of Medicine.* 1966;59:1002–1003.

62. Bjork VO. Aneurysm and occlusion of the right subclavian artery. *Acta Chirurgica Scandinavica.* 1965;356(suppl): 103–108.

63. Persand V. Subclavian artery aneurysm and idiopathic cystic medionecrosis. *Br Heart J.* 1968;30:436–440.

64. Hobson RW, Sarkaria J, O'Donnell JA, Neville WE. Atherosclerotic aneurysms of the subclavian artery. *Surgery.* 1978; 85:368–371.

65. Deutsch L. Anatomy and angiographic diagnosis of extracranial and intracranial vascular disease. In: Rutherford RB, ed. *Vascular Surgery.* Vol 2. Philadelphia, PA: WB Saunders; 1989:1314–1334.

66. Sorek PA, Silbergleit R. Multiple asymptomatic cervical cephalic aneurysms. *Am J Neuroradiol.* 1994;14:31–33.

67. Egnor MR, Page LK, David C. Vertebral artery aneurysm: a unique hazard of head banging by heavy metal rockers. Case report. *Pediatr Neurosurg.* 1991–1992;17:135–138.

68. Andoh T, Shirakami S, Nishimura Y, et al. Clinical analysis of a series of vertebral aneurysm cases. *Neurosurgery.* 1992; 31:987–993.

69. Okbata N, Ikota T, Tashiro T, Okamote K. A case of multiple extracranial vertebral artery aneurysms associated with neurofibromitosis. *Neurologic Surgery.* 1994;22:637–641.

70. Hanakita J, Suna H, Nishihara K, Lihara K, Sakaida H. Giant pseudoaneurysm of the extracranial vertebral artery successfully treated using intraoperative balloon catheters. *Neurosurgery.* 1991;28:738–742.

71. Pritz MB. Evaluation and treatment of aneurysm of the vertebral artery: different strategies for different lesions. *Neurosurgery.* 1991;29:247–256.

72. Nagasawa S, Ohta T, Kajimoto Y, Tanaka H, Kawanishi M, Tada Y. Giant thrombosed vertebral artery aneurysm treated by extracranial-intracranial bypass and aneurysmectomy: case report. *Neurol Med Chir (Tokyo).* 1994;34: 311–314.

73. Halbach VV, Higashida RT, Dowd CR, et al. Endovascular treatment of vertebral artery dissections and pseudoaneurysms. *J Neurosurg.* 1993;79:183–191.

74. Feinberg RC, Sorrell K, Wheeler JR, et al. Successful management of traumatic false aneurysm of the extracranial vertebral artery by duplex directed manual occlusion: a case report. *J Vasc Surg.* 1993;18:889–894.

Section 5
Abdominal Aortic Aneurysm

Indications, Management, and Long-term Outcome of Abdominal Aortic Aneurysms

John B. Chang and Theodore A. Stein

Without intervention, abdominal aortic aneurysms (AAAs) continue to grow and eventually rupture. When rupture occurs, nearly one half of patients die before reaching the operating room, and of those who have an aneurysmal repair, the 1-month survival rate is only 53%.[1] In the United States, approximately 15,000 deaths per year are caused by AAAs.[2] Ruptured and symptomatic aneurysms must be treated as soon as possible, and even asymptomatic aneurysms larger than 5 cm in diameter should be attended to, because 25% to 41% of these aneurysms will rupture within 5 years.[2–7] Surgical reconstruction has been an effective treatment for AAAs but has a mortality risk of approximately 5%.[8,9] In some patients, endovascular stented grafts have been used to exclude the infrarenal AAAs, but the long-term benefit is still unclear. Although smaller aneurysms (less than 4 cm in diameter) can rupture,[10,11] it is less clear when to reconstruct these aneurysms. Some vascular surgeons advocate watchful waiting until the aneurysm reaches a critical size or the rate of expansion increases.[12–15]

Although rupture is the ultimate outcome of an expanding aorta, it is not entirely clear why some AAAs suddenly rupture. Rupture of the aneurysm has been associated with rapid expansion of the aorta.[16,17] Limet and colleagues have determined that when the expansion rates exceeded a critical value, rupture of the aneurysm was likely to occur, and that patients with rapidly expanding AAAs should be considered as being at high risk.[16] Thus, urgent repair is necessary for ruptured and symptomatic aneurysms, and early surgical repair of the aneurysm should be considered in patients who have accelerated aorta growth.

Pathophysiology

The etiology of abdominal aortic aneurysms is related to hereditary and biochemical factors. Aneurysms can be classified as fusiform, saccular or dissecting and are related to the weakening of the vessel's wall as a result of the loss of collagen and elastin. Dobrin and colleagues have shown that expansion rates are related to the decrease in elastin content, but that rupture is related to the decrease in collagen content.[18] When the rate of collagen degradation exceeds the rate of collagen synthesis, the tensile strength of the aortic wall declines, and the wall is predisposed to rupture.[19] Expansion increases with the increase in the size of the aorta.[5–7] Rapid expansion can occur with any size of aneurysm, is not related to the size of the AAA, and is associated with rupture.[16,20] Increased collagenolytic protease activities are probably involved in the rapid expansion of the aneurysm, and a critical decrease in collagen content results in the rupture of the aneurysm.

Diagnosis

AAAs can be detected by several different methods. Historically, diagnosis has been made by physical examination. However, the diameter of the aorta should be measured above, at, and below the aneurysm. We have used B-mode ultrasonography (AutoSector, Technicare Ultrasound, Englewood, Colo. from 1982 to 1990, and the Acuson 128XP, Mountain View, Calif. from 1990 to 1994) with transducers of 3.5 MHz. Our accuracy for repetitive measurements of the aorta is ±0.3 cm and is similar to that reported by others.[2] Images are obtained suprarenally and infrarenally, just above the aortic bifurcation, and the anteroposterior diameter is determined. The aorta is considered aneurysmally dilated when the diameter is larger than 3.5 cm in young females and 4.5 cm in older males.[21,22] Usually the vessel is calcified and the anterior and posterior walls can be seen by abdominal x-rays taken from the lateral view. Computed tomography and magnetic resonance imaging could also be used for the initial diagnosis, but these techniques are relatively expensive. Computed tomography, however, has been found useful in determining the potential for rupture and should be considered for patients with pain.[23–25]

Risk Factors

High-risk patients can be identified and should have increased surveillance of their aneurysm to help determine when to reconstruct the aorta. The risk factors for rapid expansion are advanced age, the initial size of the aorta, severe cardiac disease, cigarette smoking, hypertension, a previous stroke, chronic obstructive pulmonary disease, and high pulse pressures .[7,20,25] Diabetes mellitus, angina alone, and alcohol ingestion are not related to the growth of the aorta. Aging has been found to be an important risk factor for rapid expansion in our study of 514 patients.[20] The incidence of rapid expansion increases with age, going from 7.8% in patients under 60 years of age to 21.4% in patients above 80 years of age. Cigarette smoking increases aortic wall elastase activity[26] and results in elastin degradation in the media. The elastin breakdown products further injure the wall, and collagen degradation ensues.[27] Although some patients have these risk factors without experiencing rapid expansion and rupture of their aneurysm, it would be prudent to follow these patients closely to determine the appropriate time for elective repair.

Surveillance

We do routine ultrasonographic surveillance at 6- to 12-month intervals for larger AAAs (>4 cm in diameter) and at 12-month intervals for smaller dilations. Measurements are done more frequently for faster-growing aortas. We determine growth of the aorta from the slope of the best-fit line, which is determined from sequential measurements of the diameter, when the rate of growth is steady. However, when the rate of growth increases suddenly, the expansion rate of the aorta is calculated by dividing the growth of the aorta by the time interval between the last two consecutive size measurements.

Screening and surveillance of the growth of the aorta has been suggested by others to reduce the mortality rate associated with ruptured AAAs.[2,13,14,28–31] Most AAAs are small and asymptomatic, and the growth of the aorta in patients with these aneurysms should be followed by periodic ultrasound examination.[32,33] The need for an elective reconstruction of large or symptomatic AAAs is clear, but smaller aneurysms should be watched for rapid or sudden expansion in the diameter of the aorta. The frequency for appropriate surveillance of small aneurysm is unknown because rupture occurs in only a few.[2,5] Thus, the cost-benefit for surveillance of these aneurysms may not be economical for all patients.

Our surveillance of 514 patients has determined a mean expansion rate of 0.70 ± 0.11 cm/year for all patients.[20] The expansion rates were <1.0 cm/year in 452 (88%) patients and the mean expansion rate was 0.11 ± 0.01 cm/year. The expansion rates were ≤0.5 cm/year in 339 patients (66%), and between 0.5 and 1.0 cm/year in 113 patients (22%). In 63 (12%) patients who had a rapid expansion (≥1.0 cm/year) of their aorta, the mean expansion rate was 3.08 ± 0.51 cm/year. Others have reported mean expansion rates from 0.26 to 0.74 cm/year.[2,7,16,25,28,31] The expansion rate is determined, in part, the initial size of the aorta. Small aneurysms grow more slowly than large aneurysms.[2,17,28] Aorta diameters that are less than 4 cm expand at a rate of 0.08 ± 0.12 cm/year, and those that are greater than 4 cm expand at a rate of 0.33 ± 0.12 cm/year.[13] Thus, the size of the aneurysm is a good indicator of further expansion and is probably the most important factor for determining the time for elective surgery.

Our younger patients, who are less than 70 years of age, have had mean expansion rates of 0.49 cm/year. Our older patients have had a mean expansion rate of 1.02 cm/year. Patients with advanced age have faster-growing aortas, and should be followed at shorter intervals. Younger patients have smaller aortas and can be followed at longer intervals. Our surveillance of small aneurysms in some patients has reached 14 years, and expansion rates remain low. When the initial size is <3.0 cm in diameter, the age of the patient has no effect on the growth rate, but when it is between 3.0 and 4.0 cm, older patients are more likely to have rapid growth.[20] When the initial size is >4.0 cm in diameter, patients of any age can have rapid growth. Rapid expansion has occurred in 25% of our patients with aneurysms that measure between 4 and 5 cm in diameter and in 46% of patients with aneurysms that measure more than 5 cm in diameter. High-risk patients who are over 70 years of age with aneurysms greater than 3.0 cm in diameter and all patients with aneurysms greater than 4.0 cm in diameter should be followed at 6-month intervals to improve survival.

In a study that compared elective surgery to watchful waiting, the investigators suggested that surgery should be done on aneurysms greater than 4.7 cm in diameter to improve survival.[12] However, other investigators have reported that 13% of aneurysms <4.0 cm in diameter rupture, and that 44% of aneurysms between 4 and 6 cm rupture.[10] It is clear that some smaller aneurysms can expand rapidly, and these patients should have elective surgery before impending rupture to reduce perioperative mortality. Our criteria for scheduling patients for elective repair of their AAAs include a sudden rapid expansion (>0.25 cm in 3 months or 1 cm/year) of the aneurysm, reaching or exceeding a critical size, or symptoms. The critical size varies from 4.0 to 7.0 cm in diameter and depends on the patient's age, gender, health,

TABLE 51.1. Calculation of the critical size (cm)* of the aneurysmal abdominal aorta for surgical intervention.

Criteria for the numerical value given to the factors in the equation:
Age factor: 0 for <50 y, 0.25 for 50–70 y, and 0.5 for >70 y
Gender factor: 0 for women and 0.5 for men
Health factor: 0 for low-risk patients, 1 for moderate-risk patients, and 2 for high-risk patients or patients with serious life-threatening illnesses, such as cancer
Growth factor: 0 for expansion rates (ER) between 0.5 and 1.0 and 0.5 for ER <0.5; when the ER is >1, surgical intervention needs to be considered to prevent possible rupture

Examples
A young, healthy woman with an ER from 0.5 to 1 would have a critical size of 4 cm, or critical size = 4 + 0 + 0 + 0 + 0 = 4 cm
An older, healthy man with an ER from 0.5 to 1 would have a critical size of 5 cm, or critical size = 4 + 0.5 + 0.5 + 0 + 0 = 5 cm
An older man with metastatic cancer and an ER from 0.5 to 1 would have a critical size of 7 cm, or critical size = 4 + 0.5 + 0.5 + 2 + 0 = 7 cm

*Critical size = 4 + age factor + gender factor + health factor + growth factor.

and aneurysm expansion rate.[6] We use an equation to help estimate the critical size for surgical intervention. This equation is shown in Table 51.1. The critical size is then determined from the clinical status of the patient and the equation. Our estimate of critical size with the equation is 4.0 cm in diameter in healthy young (<50 years of age) females and 5.0 cm in diameter in healthy older (>70 years of age) males. Critical size would be higher for patients who have another severe coexisting disease that could increase the operative morbidity/mortality risk or who have a terminal illness would be followed longer before scheduling surgical repair. When there is a rapid expansion of the aneurysm or the patient becomes symptomatic, operative repair should be done expeditiously. Elective repair of rapidly growing aneurysms in our 63 patients has been accomplished without severe complications.

Surgical Intervention

To maintain low mortality and morbidity rates, the surgical team must be attentive to anesthesia, the patient's condition, the operative technique, and the postoperative care. Blood pressure must be maintained and fluid needs to be replaced during cross-clamping. Some patients are at a higher mortality risk because of advanced age (≥85 years), pulmonary or renal complications, or significant cardiac disease.[34] The aneurysm can be reached either by a celiotomy or by a retroperitoneal approach. Although the transperitoneal incision is commonly used, a left retroperitoneal approach may be advantageous in some patients.[35,36]

Polyester grafts are being widely used for reconstruction of the abdominal aorta. Many vascular surgeons

have used an albumin-impregnated prosthetic graft to prevent the leakage of blood through the material's pores and possibly reduce the need for high-volume blood transfusions. However, albumin-impregnated grafts have not been found to decrease perioperative blood loss and have no effect of the patency rate or infection.[37] A gelatin coating on a graft may be better at preventing blood loss than a collagen coating, but further studies are necessary to determine its true value.[38] The application of linear stapling devices to the exclusion of AAAs has been found to be safe and without aneurysm expansion or rupture, and 97% of the excluded aneurysms thrombose by 5 years after treatment.[39]

Exclusion of infrarenal AAAs with endovascular stented grafts has become feasible. Several types of malleable metallic or plastic stents are available; some have hooks to securely fix the stent, and others are self-expanding.[40] However, it is still unclear how to achieve long-term success.[41,42] A durable graft depends on the stability of the stent without proximal and distal dilation. The absence of a distal aneurysmal neck or involvement of the iliac arteries may preclude the placement of an aortoaortic stent.[43] In a series of 50 patients, 80% of the procedures were considered successful at a mean time of 17 months postsurgery, with complete exclusion of the aneurysm and restoration of normal blood flow.[44] The remaining 20% of procedures were failures because of death, improper placement of the stent, or leakage of blood into the aneurysmal sac. A self-expanding, modular, bifurcated stent has been shown to be clinically effective in reducing aortic diameters within 6 months.[45] One complication of endovascular grafts is that many patients can have perigraft leakage; computed tomography has shown that 42% of the grafts leaked and one half of these had leakage that persisted for more than 1 year.[46] In time the appropriate selection of patients, the ideal graft type, and the long-term success of endovascular stented grafts will be known.

Survival

After diagnosing an AAA, the 15-year survival has been estimated to be only 15%.[9] Death from myocardial infarction or congestive heart failure occurred in 19.3% and from stroke in 5.4%.[9] Coronary artery disease has been found in 69% of patients, and their 5-year survival is 84%.[47] Survival after AAA repair has been reported to be 67% at 5 years and is lower than the survival of a normal population control group.[46] The 5-year survival rate is 48% in octogenarians, and 80% in younger patients.[48] The higher mortality and morbidity rates are related to concomitant cardiovascular disease. Coexisting carotid artery disease or lower extremity arterial occlusive disease has been associated with a poorer survival.[47] Our 5-, 10-, and 15-year survival rates after AAA repair are 77%,

54%, and 36%, respectively.[20] For our patients, survival after AAA repair is better than the survival with unoperated, small AAAs. Coronary artery disease remains the primary cause of death in our patients. Performing a timely aortic repair achieves good survival rates for these patients. The long-term survival rate after placement of endovascular stented grafts in the aneurysmal aorta is unknown at this time.

References

1. Koskas F, Kieffer E. Surgery for ruptured abdominal aortic aneurysm: early and late results of a prospective study by the AURC in 1989. *Ann Vasc Surg.* 1997;11:90–99.
2. Ernst CB. Abdominal aortic aneurysm. *N Engl J Med.* 1993;328:1167–1172.
3. Abernathy CM Jr, Baumgartner R, Butler HG, et al. The management of ruptured abdominal aneurysms in rural Colorado. *JAMA.* 1986;256:597–600.
4. Johansson G, Nydahl S, Olofsson P, Swedenborg J. Survival of patients with abdominal aortic aneurysms: comparison between operative and non-operative management. *Eur J Vasc Surg.* 1991;4:497–502.
5. Glimaker H, Holmberg L, Elvin A, et al. Natural history of patients with abdominal aneurysm. *Eur J Vasc Surg.* 1991;5:125–130.
6. Hollier LH, Taylor LM, Ochsner J. Recommended indications for operative treatment of abdominal aortic aneurysms: report of a subcommittee of the Joint Council of the Society for Vascular Surgery and the North American Chapter of the International Society for Cardiovascular Surgery. *J Vasc Surg.* 1992;15:1046–1056.
7. Cronenwett JL, Sargent SK, Wall MH, et al. Variables that affect the expansion rate and outcome of small abdominal aortic aneurysms. *J Vasc Surg.* 1990;11:260–269.
8. Trotter MC, Ilabaca PA. Ruptured abdominal aortic aneurysms: a retrospective look at a ten-year interval. *Vasc Surg.* 1993;27:183–186.
9. Perko MJ, Olsen PS, Schroeder TV, Sorensen S, Lorentzen JE. Abdominal aortic aneurysm: age as a risk factor influencing postoperative survival. *Vasc Surg.* 1993;27:176–182.
10. Gloviczki P, Pairolero PC, Mucha P Jr, et al. Ruptured abdominal aortic aneurysms: repair should not be denied. *J Vasc Surg* 1992;15:851–859.
11. Darling RC, Messina CR, Brewster DC, Ottinger LW. Autopsy study of unoperated abdominal aortic aneurysms: the cases for early resection. *Circulation.* 1977;56(suppl 2):161–164.
12. Katz DA, Littenberg B, Cronenwett JL. Management of small abdominal aortic aneurysms. Early surgery vs watchful waiting. *JAMA.* 1992;268:2678–2686.
13. Bengtsson H, Nilsson P, Bergqvist D. Natural history of abdominal aneurysm detected by screening. *Br J Surg.* 1993;80:718–720.
14. Collin J, Heather B, Walton J. Growth rates of subclinical abdominal aortic aneurysms—implications for review and rescreening programmes. *Eur J Vasc Surg.* 1991;5:141–144.
15. Crawford ES, Hess KR. Abdominal aortic aneurysm. *N Engl J Med.* 1989;321:1040–1042.
16. Limet R, Sakalihassan N, Albert A. Determination of the expansion rate and incidence of rupture of abdominal aortic aneurysms. *J Vasc Surg.* 1991;14:540–548.
17. Delin A, Ohlsen H, Swedenborg J. Growth rate of abdominal aortic aneurysms as measured by computed tomography. *Br J Surg.* 1985;72:530–532.
18. Dorbin PB, Baker WH, Gley WC. Elastolytic and collagenolytic studies of arteries. *Arch Surg.* 1984;119:405–409.
19. Satta J, Juvonen T, Haukipuro K, Juvonen M, Kairaluoma MI. Increased turnover of collagen in abdominal aortic aneurysms, demonstrated by measuring the concentration of the aminoterminal propeptide of type III procollagen in peripheral and aortic blood samples. *J Vasc Surg.* 1995;22:155–160.
20. Chang JB, Stein TA, Liu JP, Dunn ME. Risk factors associated with rapid growth of small abdominal aortic aneurysms. *Surgery.* 1997;121:117–122.
21. Johnston KW, Rutherford RB, Tilson MD, Shah DM, Hollier L, Stanley JC. Suggested standards for reporting on arterial aneurysms. *J Vasc Surg.* 1991;13:452–458.
22. Siegel CL, Cohan RH. CT of abdominal aortic aneurysms. *AJR.* 1994;163:17–29.
23. Pillari G, Chang JB, Zito J, et al. Computed tomography of abdominal aortic aneurysm. *Arch Surg.* 1988;123:727–732.
24. Mehard WB, Heiken JP, Sicard GA. High-attenuating crescent in abdominal aortic aneurysm wall at CT: a sign of acute or impending rupture. *Radiology.* 1994;192:359–362.
25. Wolf YG, Thomas WS, Brennan FJ, Goff WG, Sise MJ, Bernstein EF. Computed tomography scanning findings associated with rapid expansion of abdominal aortic aneurysms. *J Vasc Surg.* 1994;20:529–538.
26. Cohen JR, Sarfati I, Wise L. The effect of cigarette smoking on rabbit elastase activity. *J Vasc Surg.* 1989;9:580–582.
27. Nevitt MPH, Ballard DJ, Hallett JW Jr. Prognosis of abdominal aneurysms: a population-based study. *N Engl J Med.* 1989;321:1009–1014.
28. Bergqvist B, Bengtsson H. Should screening for abdominal aortic aneurysm be advocated? *Acta Chirurgica Scandinavica.* 1990;555(suppl):89–97.
29. Holmes DR, Shixiong L, Parks WC, Thompson RW. Medial neovascularization in abdominal aortic aneurysms: A histopathologic marker of aneurysmal degeneration with pathophysiologic implications. *J Vasc Surg.* 1995;21:761–772.
30. Russel JGB. Is screening for abdominal aortic aneurysm worthwhile? *Clin Radiol.* 1990;41:182–184.
31. O'Kelly TL, Heather BP. General practice based population screening for abdominal aneurysm: a pilot study. *Br J Surg.* 1989;76:479–480.
32. Bernstein EF, Dilley RB, Goldberger LE, Gosink BB, Leopold GR. Growth rates of small abdominal aneurysms. *Surgery.* 1976;80:765–773.
33. Guirguis EM, Barber CC. The natural history of abdominal aortic aneurysms. *Am J Surg.* 1991;162:481–483.
34. Pairolero PC. Repair of abdominal aortic aneurysms in high-risk patients. *Surg Clin N Am.* 1989;69:755–763.
35. Komori K, Okazaki J, Kawasaki K, et al. Comparison of retroperitoneal and transperitoneal approach for reconstruction of abdominal aortic aneurysm in patients with

previous laparotomy. *International Journal of Angiology*. 1997;6:230–233.

36. Shah DM, Paty PSK, Chang BB, Kaufman JL, Leather RP. The retroperitoneal approach for abdominal aorta replacement. *Comtemp Surg*. 1990;37:9–15.

37. Chakfe N, Beaufigeau M, Nicolini P, et al. Albumin-impregnated prosthetic graft for infrarenal aortic replacement: effects on the incidence and volume of perioperative blood transfusion. *Ann Vasc Surg*. 1997;11:588–595.

38. Ukpabi P, Marois Y, King M, et al. The Gelweave polyester arterial prosthesis. *Canadian Journal of Surgery*. 1995;38: 322–331.

39. Blumenberg RM, Skudder Jr PA, Gelfand ML, Bowers CA, Barton EA. Retroperitoneal nonresective staple exclusion of abdominal aortic aneurysms: clinical outcome and fate of the excluded abdominal aortic aneurysms. *J Vasc Surg*. 1995;21:623–634.

40. Veith FJ, Abbott WM, Yao JST, et al. Guidelines for development and use of transluminal placed endovascular prosthetic grafts in the arterial system. *J Vasc Surg*. 1995;21: 670–685.

41. Diethrich EB. What do we need to know to achieve durable endoluminal abdominal aortic aneurysm repair? *Tex Heart Inst J*. 1997;24:179–184.

42. Matsumura JS, Pearce WH, McCarthy WJ, Yao JS. Reduction in aortic aneurys size: early results after endovascular graft placement. *J Vasc Surg*. 1997;25:113–123.

43. White RA, Donayre CE, Walot I, Kopchok GE, deVirgilio C, Mehringer CM. Aortic aneurysm morphology for planning endovascular procedures. *Tex Heart Inst J*. 1997;24: 160–166.

44. Parodi JC. Endovascular repair of abdominal aortic aneurysms and other arterial lesions. *J Vasc Surg*. 1995;21: 549–557.

45. White RA, Donayre CE, Walot I, et al. Modular bifurcation endprosthesis for treatment of abdominal aortic aneurysms. *Ann Surg*. 1997;226:381–391.

46. Koskas F, Kieffer E. Long-term survival after elective repair of infrarenal abdominal aortic aneurysm: results of a prospective multicentric study. *Ann Vasc Surg*. 1997;11: 473–481.

47. Starr JE, Hertzer NR, Mascha EJ, et al. Influence of gender on cardiac risk and survival in patients with infrarenal aortic aneurysms. *J Vasc Surg*. 1996;23:870–880.

48. O'Hara PJ, Hertzer NR, Krajewski LP, Tan M, Xiong X, Beven EG. Ten-year experience with abdominal aortic aneurysm repair in octogenarians: early results and late outcome. *J Vasc Surg*. 1995;21:830–838.

52

Inflammatory Abdominal Aortic Aneurysms

Igor Huk, Joseph Nanobashvili, Georg Kretschmer, and Peter Polterauer

Inflammatory aneurysms of the abdominal aorta (inflammatory AAAs) are a distinct clinicopathological entity, different from typical atherosclerotic abdominal aneurysms (atherosclerotic AAAs).[1] Marked lamellar and perianeurysmal fibrosis, a thick aneurysm wall, and adhesions to the surrounding organs are characteristic pathological features of inflammatory AAAs.[2,3]

The term *inflammatory aneurysm* was introduced by Walker et al[1] in 1972. They reported that 10% of their 187 aneurysmectomies had excessive thickening of the aneurysm wall and perianeurysmal adhesions.

Incidence and Natural History

Inflammatory AAAs account for 1.9% to 19.0% of all abdominal aortic aneurysms[4,5] and occur predominantly in males.

The probability of rupture of an inflammatory AAA in the natural course was reported to range from 15% to 25%, which is apparently not less than the probability of rupture of atherosclerotic AAAs.[6,7]

Macroscopic and Histological Aspects

The macroscopic characteristics of inflammatory AAAs are a porcelaneous appearance, excessive thickening of the aortic wall (thickness greater than 0.5 cm), and perianeurysmal adhesions. Inflammatory AAAs are characteristically covered on their anterior and lateral sides with thick, white fibrous tissue.

Histological examination shows signs of atherosclerosis of the media and marked fibrotic thickening of the adventitia, with the presence of lymphocyte aggregates—a sign of chronic inflammation.[8]

Histopathological studies usually reveal two components: an inflammatory infiltrate and a diffuse fibrosis.

The lympho-, mono-, and plasmacellular infiltrate and the interstitial deposits of collagen define the histological picture of inflammatory AAA.

Fibrosis around nerves or ganglia at the outer margin of mural fibrosis, and the thickness of the combined fibrotic media and adventitia allow satisfactorily high discrimination between atherosclerotic AAAs and inflammatory AAAs.[9]

Because prominent atherosclerotic lesions are consistently observed, inflammatory AAAs may be inferred to be a variant of atherosclerotic AAAs, characterized by a particular prominence of inflammation and fibrosis.[10]

Etiopathogenesis

In spite of the increasing number of observations reported in recent years, the etiopathogenesis of inflammatory AAAs has not been defined. The lesion can present in an acute, subacute, or chronic manner.[11]

It is suggested that an immune reaction against some antigen components in the aneurysm wall may lead to the pronounced inflammatory response that is characteristic of inflammatory AAAs.[12] Chronic periaortitis was shown to be accompanied by autoallergy to the breakdown products of apolipoprotein B that resulted from the oxidation of low-density lipoprotein within human atherosclerotic plaques.[13] Increased numbers of activated T cells were found in peripheral blood, the aortic aneurysm wall, and the perianeurysmal tissue. After aneurysm repair, peripheral blood analysis demonstrated normalization of the T-cell subsets. These data suggest that inflammatory abdominal aortic aneurysm is associated with an immune response in peripheral blood and aneurysm tissue, and the immune response regresses after aneurysm repair.[14]

Factors other than immune-mediated mechanisms may play an important role in the development of inflammatory AAAs:

616

1. Mechanical mechanisms such as chronic contained rupture of the aneurysm with following reactive lymphatic hyperplasia.[15]
2. Atheroemboli in the aortic vasa vasorum. It is suggested that ischemic injury to the media, caused by lesions such as these and by other features of atherosclerosis, may be an initiating factor in some cases of idiopathic chronic periaortitis.[16]
3. Stasis and fibrosis, then the rupture of the lymphatic components into the aneurysmal wall have been described for inflammatory AAAs. This lymphatic etiology might explain the inflammatory character of these aneurysms.[17] The frequent occurrence of dilation of both periaortic lymphatic vessels and lymph node sinuses, even in "incipient" aneurysms, support the hypothesis that it may be the lymphatic stasis that determines periaortic fibrosis.[10]
4. Periaortal fibrosis, as a manifestation of retroperitoneal fibrosis (Ormond's disease), can result in an inflammatory aneurysm with chronic dissection.[18]

Clinical Picture and Diagnosis

The inflammatory AAA is often symptomatic. The most important differential diagnosis concerns the covered perforation and the dissecting aortic aneurysm, as well as Ormond's disease, periaortal lymphomas, and other retroperitoneal tumors.

The following clinical signs are characteristic of inflammatory AAAs[19]:

- Significantly frequent abdominal pain in patients with inflammatory AAAs compared with patients with atherosclerotic AAAs
- Weight loss and anorexia
- Increased erythrocyte sedimentation rate (≈ 40 mm/h)
- Lumbago and low-grade fever, probably due to deterioration of the inflammatory AAA
- Obstructive uropathy (see later)

Until the advent of modern radiologic imaging modalities, inflammatory AAA was usually discovered only at the time of surgery. Computed tomography (CT) and magnetic resonance imaging (MRI) provide adequate information to diagnose inflammatory AAAs before surgery and thus allow for better surgical planning.[20]

A correct diagnosis was made in 73% of the patients that were examined preoperatively by CT.[21] Aortic rupture, aortic dissection, and retroperitoneal lymphoma may produce similar appearances on CT, nevertheless CT remains the method of choice for the diagnosis of inflammatory AAA because of its high sensitivity.[21]

MRI is superior to CT with respect to many diagnostic requirements. MRI diagnosis was found to correspond to the surgical and pathological diagnosis in all cases. There were no false positives among those patients with simple aneurysms, and no false negatives.[3] MRI showed sclerosis in regions that appeared normal with CT. Occlusion of large vessels and collateral circulation were better depicted with MRI.[22]

Ultrasonographic findings are nonspecific, but ultrasound is the screening method of choice. If ultrasonographic findings show a sonolucent zone anterior or anterolateral to an atherosclerotic aneurysm, CT should be used to delineate the perivascular abnormalities.[23]

Involvement of Adjacent Organs in Inflammatory AAA

Periaortic adhesions and congestion of neighboring structures are characteristic features of inflammatory AAAs. The organs most frequently involved in adhesions are the duodenum (in 79% of cases), the inferior caval vein, the left renal vein (32%), the ureter, and the transverse mesocolon.[24,25]

One may expect ureteral congestion (unilateral or bilateral) in 20% to 41.2% of cases.[26,27] Patients with inflammatory AAAs reveal a significant difference with respect to hydronephrosis, compared with patients with atherosclerotic AAAs.

Inflammatory AAA can masquerade as an occlusion of the inferior caval vein or may present as bilateral hydroceles.

Conservative Treatment

Some reports indicate that steroid therapy of inflammatory AAAs can be successful in resolving the inflammatory process and alleviating symptoms.[28,29] However, surgery is considered the method of choice once the diagnosis is made, as opposed to waiting for steroid therapy to reduce the extent of inflammation, because of the well-known risk of rupture and the controversial efficacy of medical therapy.[4]

Steroid therapy and ureterolysis may occasionally be indicated when the situation is considered inoperable or when the patient declines surgery.[30,31]

Surgical Treatment

Conventional Surgery

Aortic replacement with a tube graft or bifurcation Y graft is advocated as the treatment of choice for the prevention of rupture of the inflammatory AAA.[26,32]

Surgery of inflammatory AAAs is rendered difficult due to periaortic fibrosis, which may spread into the retroperitoneum.[33] Surgical treatment requires a specific technique that includes clamping of the supracoeliac aorta[34] and minimal dissection with maximum care not to dissect the adjacent viscera.[15,35] Attempts to isolate the aneurysm can lead to operative injuries of these structures, thus increasing the rates of complications and mortality.[36]

A standard, midline transperitoneal approach is the method of choice for aneurysm resection and grafting. However, the retroperitoneal approach may have advantages over the transabdominal approach for the following reasons: (1) the posterolateral aspect of the aorta is characteristically not significantly involved by the inflammatory process, whereas the anterior aspect is; (2) the duodenum does not need to be dissected away from the aorta and, in fact, is not seen; (3) the left renal vein moves up off the neck of the aneurysm with forward mobilization of the kidney, facilitating proximal control.[37]

Preoperative nephrostomy, ureteral catheter placement, or ureteral stenting, as well as intraoperative ureterolysis, are advocated for resolution of hydronephrosis.[7,26] Hydronephrosis was found to subside spontaneously after resection of the aneurysm[6,38] because aortic replacement was shown to reverse the perianeurysmal inflammatory process.[27,32]

Chylos ascites caused by injuries to the intestinal lymphatics or to their recipients, the left lateroaortic lymph nodes or the cisterna chyli, were reported after the surgery. If ascites persists after 4 to 6 weeks of conservative treatment, a peritoneojugular derivation or a direct lymphoanastomosis may be contemplated.[17]

In contrast to atherosclerotic AAAs, surgical repair of inflammatory AAAs is associated with higher rates of mortality and morbidity that are a result of higher operational risk. Thus, the perioperative mortality rate in elective cases was reported to range from 6% to 37%.[25,39,40]

Endovascular Grafting

Transluminal placement of an endovascular graft offers an alternative approach to the treatment of the potentially high-risk group of patients with typical atherosclerotic AAAs because it decreases the morbidity and mortality associated with extensive retroperitoneal dissection and prolonged aortic cross-clamping.[41] The acceptance of endovascular placement of stented grafts in cases of atherosclerotic AAA is increasing worldwide with the accumulation of the clinical experience. Reports on long-term results have been obtained from only a few centers so far. In our preliminary experience with more than 40 patients treated for atherosclerotic AAA using the endoluminal graft placement technique, we encountered no perioperative or immediate postoperative mortality. We found the technique to be a feasible alternative to stan-

dard surgical procedures in the treatment of selected patients with an aneurysm of this type.

Patients with atherosclerotic AAAs and high operative risk represent the main population suitable for endovascular aortic grafting.[42,43] An inflammatory AAA, even without severe comorbidity, represents a high technical risk per se.

While planning endovascular implantation of stented grafts in patients with inflammatory AAA, specific potential problems should be considered before intervention.

First, retrograde blood flow from small arteries originating from the aneurysm lumen and/or paraprosthetic leaks may create elevated pressure between the aneurysm wall and the inserted graft, threatening a delayed rupture.[41] Such small arteries and leaks are expected to be thrombosed spontaneously, but a careful evaluation is mandatory.

Another important question that has not yet been clarified is whether a periaortic inflammation process is a possible response to endoaortic insertion of a stented graft. Conventional surgery with aneurysm resection and graft replacement was noted to reverse the inflammatory process.[27,44]

We now present a case of inflammatory AAA successfully treated by endovascular implantation of a stented graft. A patient with inflammatory AAA and a high risk for aortic surgical replacement by the conventional technique was offered a transfemoral, endovascular, stented bifurcated Y graft repair of the inflammatory AAA.

Report of a Case

A 69-year-old man was hospitalized because of gastrointestinal complaints (obstipation), constant back pain, weight loss (the patient has lost 15 kg in the previous 3 months) and edema of both legs. An aortocoronary bypass had been performed 2 years previous because of coronary artery disease. Sufficient cardiac function was found at the time of admission. The patient showed an increased erythrocyte sedimentation rate (from 65 to 120 mm/h). Elevated blood plasma creatinine levels (2.1 mg/100 mL) indicated impaired renal function. This was considered to be a result of left ureteral obstruction, which was confirmed by intravenous pyelography. Deep vein thrombosis was excluded by sonography. Abdominal sonography showed an AAA 6 cm in diameter. A CT scan was performed and demonstrated a large infrarenal AAA with enormous thickening of the aneurysmal wall and a large mass of periaortic tissue ventral and lateral to the aorta outside the calcified aortic wall (Figure 52.1). The duodenum, the left ureter, and the inferior vena cava were involved in perianeurysmal adhesions, which explained the edema of both legs. The CT image was considered to be typical for inflammatory AAA. Aortography documented a 2.3-cm region of normal-sized aorta

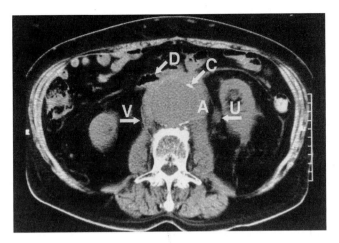

FIGURE 52.1. Contrast-enhanced CT scan demonstrates an excessively thickened aortic wall (A) and a thick mass of periaortic tissue ventral and lateral to the aorta outside the calcified (C) aortic wall. The duodenum (D), the inferior vena cava (V), and the left ureter (U) are involved in perianeurysmal adhesions.

between the left renal artery and the distal abdominal aortic aneurysm.

The possible treatment measures and potential complications were assessed preoperatively, and an endovascular repair of the aneurysm was proposed to the patient. It was stressed that this new technique constituted a minimally invasive alternative to conventional surgery.

The first intervention was the treatment of hydronephrosis. Percutaneous nephrostomy was performed on March 15, 1995. Blood plasma creatinine levels returned to normal within two days after the intervention. The nephrostomy catheter was then removed and substituted by a ureteral splint.

The procedure of endovascular aortic repair was carried out in the operating theater under general anesthesia on March 17, 1995. We used a bifurcated Y graft (Cragg Endo Pro System 1, Min Tec Inc, Freeport, Grand Bahamas) containing a nitinol stent covered with polyester fabric (the diameter of the central part was 20 mm and that of the limbs was 10 mm). The central part of the graft with the fixed left limb was inserted in a retrograde fashion through a left femoral open arteriotomy. Then, the right graft limb was brought and attached to the inserted graft through a percutaneous right transfemoral puncture. The graft was fixed to the wall of aorta and iliac arteries using a balloon catheter. Intraluminal manipulations were performed under digital fluoroscopic control by a Siremobil 2000 imager (Siemens, Germany). Completion arteriography showed the correct position of the graft and complete exclusion of the aneurysm (Figure 52.2). There were no perioperative or postoperative complications.

The follow-up sonographies of the abdomen showed gradual regression of the thickness of the aortic wall.

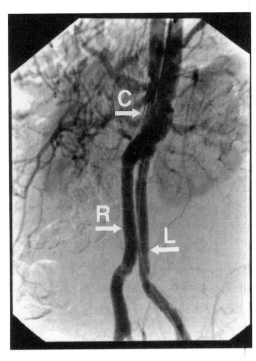

FIGURE 52.2. Completion arteriogram after endovascular insertion of a bifurcated Y graft. C indicates the central part of the graft; and R and L, right and left limbs of the graft, respectively. The arteriogram demonstrates the graft in correct position and the complete exclusion of the aneurysm.

The control CT scan performed 6 months after graft implantation showed a functioning graft and no signs of blood leakage outside the graft. Regression of inflammatory infiltration around the aorta and release of compression of the inferior vena cava were also easily detectable on the CT image (Figure 52.3). On the

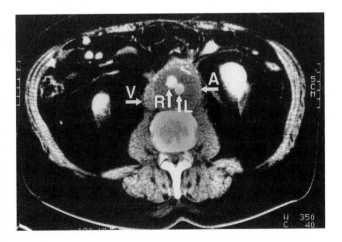

FIGURE 52.3. This follow-up contrast-enhanced CT scan of the patient 6 months after stented graft insertion shows regression of the fibrosis around the aorta (A) and a functioning graft (R and L, right and left limbs of the graft, respectively) without signs of blood leakage. The inferior vena cava (V) is no longer encased and compressed by periaortic adhesions.

intravenous pyelogram, hydronephrosis was shown to have nearly disappeared. The ureteral splint catheter was removed on June 7, 1995. No further signs of ureteral obstruction or obstructive nephropathy were observed thereafter. The patient's erythrocyte sedimentation rate levels returned to almost normal (19 to 32 mm/h). He recovered his usual weight and noted a decrease of edema in his legs.

Advances in vascular imaging, exact preoperative diagnosis, and clinical feasibility of endovascular techniques now offer an excellent alternative to conventional surgical repair in patients with inflammatory AAAs. However, meticulous planning and a high-grade interdisciplinary cooperative approach are mandatory to achieve good results from endovascular surgery of this type.

References

1. Walker DI, Bloor K, Williams G, Gillie I. Inflammatory aneurysms of the abdominal aorta. *Br J Surg.* 1972;59: 609–614.
2. Rieber A, Kauffman GW, Allenberg JR, Mattfeldt T. Die radiologische Diagnostik des inflammatorischen Aneurysmas. *Radiologie.* 1989;29:620–624.
3. Tennant WG, Hartnell GG, Baird RN, Horrocks M. Inflammatory aortic aneurysms: characteristic appearance on magnetic resonance imaging. *Eur J Vasc Surg.* 1992;6: 399–402.
4. Arpesani A, Giorgetti PL, Giordanengo F, Miani S, Rampoldi V, Franch L. Considerazioni cliniche su 38 casi di aneurisma inflammatorio dell'aorta addominale su un totale di 2.014 AAA operati. *Minerva Cardioangiol.* 1991;39: 135–140.
5. Tennant WG, Hartnell GG, Baird RN, Horrocks M. Radiologic investigation of abdominal aortic aneurysm disease: comparison of three modalities in staging and the detection of inflammatory change. *J Vasc Surg.* 1993;17: 703–709.
6. Ruckert R, Inderbitzi R, Picco Ch, Schwarz H. Inflammatorisches Bauchaortenaneurysma und Ureterobstruktion. *Helvetica Chirurgica Acta.* 1989;56:629–632.
7. Lindblad B, Almgren B, Bergqvist D, et al. Abdominal aortic aneurysm with perianeurysmal fibrosis: experience from 11 Swedish vascular centers. *J Vasc Surg.* 1991;13: 231–239.
8. Fiorani P, Bondanini S, Faraglia V, et al. Clinical and therapeutical evaluation of inflammatory aneurysms of the abdominal aorta. *Int Angiol.* 1986;5:49–53.
9. McMahon JN, Davies JD, Scott DJ, et al. The microscopic features of inflammatory abdominal aortic aneurysm: discriminant analysis. *Histopathology.* 1990;16:557–564.
10. Bernucci P, D'Amati G, De-Santis F, et al. Aneurismi inflammatori dell'aorta addomonale: studio anatomo-clinico su 16 casi e ipotesi patogenetiche. *G Ital Cardiol.* 1992; 22:1381–1388.
11. Giordanengo F, Trimarchi S, Franch L, et al. Gli aneurismi inflammatori dell'aorta sottorenale. Aspetti istopatho-logici, diagnostici e terapeutici. *Minerva Cardioangiol.* 1994; 42:351–357.
12. Stella A, Gargiulo M, Pasquinelli G, et al. The cellular component in the parietal infiltrate of inflammatory abdominal aortic aneurysms (IAAA). *Eur J Vasc Surg.* 1991; 5:65–70.
13. Parums DV, Brown DL, Mitchinson MJ. Serum antibodies to oxidized low-density lipoprotein and ceroid in chronic periaortitis. *Arch Pathol Lab Med.* 1990;114:383–387.
14. Lieberman J, Scheib JS, Googe PB, et al. Inflammatory abdominal aortic aneurysm and the associated T-cell reaction: a case study. *J Vasc Surg.* 1992;15:569–572.
15. Sterpetti AV, Hunter WJ, Feldhaus RJ, et al. Inflammatory aneurysms of the abdominal aorta: incidence, pathologic and etiologic considerations. *J Vasc Surg.* 1989; 9:643–649.
16. West AB, Ryan PC, O'Briain DS, Keane FB. Inflammatory aortic aneurysm: report of a case suggesting athero-ischaemic aetiology. *J Cardiovasc Surg (Torino).* 1988;29: 213–215.
17. Combe J, Buniet JM, Douge C, et al. Chylothorax et chyloperitoine apres chirurgie d'un anevrysme aortique inflammatoire. Un cas avec revue de la litterature. *J Mal Vasc.* 1992;17:151–156.
18. Kacl GM, Bino M, Salomon F, et al. Thorakale periaortale Fibrose und Morbus Ormond. *Aktuelle Radiologie.* 1995;5: 169–172.
19. Stella A, Gargiulo M, Faggioli GL, et al. Inflammatory abdominal aortic aneurysms: does an early stage exist? *J Cardiovasc Surg (Torino).* 1991;32:732–736.
20. Duckett G, Laperriere J, Fontaine S, Bruneau L, Choquet A, Gregoire A. Anevrisme inflammatoire de l'aorte. Utilite de la tomodensitometrie et de l'echographie dans le diagnostic d'un cas et revue de la litterature. *J Radiol.* 1986;67: 911–915.
21. Koch JA, Grützner G, Jungblut RM, et al. Computertomographische Diagnostik des inflammatorischen Bauchaortenaneurysmas. *Fortschritte auf dem Gebiete der Röntgenstrahlen und der neuen bildgebenden Verfahren.* 1994;161:31–37.
22. Bachmann G, Bauer T, Rau WS. MRT und CT in Diagnose und Verlaufskontrolle der idiopathischen (retoperitonealen) Fibrosen. *Radiologie.* 1995;35:200–207.
23. Liu CI, Cho SR, Brewer WH, et al. Inflammatory aneurysm of the abdominal aorta: diagnosis by computerized tomography and ultrasonography. *South Med J.* 1987;80: 1352–1354.
24. Kaschner AG, Sandmann W, Kniemeyer HW, Borchard F. Das inflammatorische Bauchaortenaneurysma. *Langenbecks Arch Chir.* 1985;366:327–329.
25. Moosa HH, Peitzman AB, Steed DL, Julian TB, Jarrett F, Webster MW. Inflammatory aneurysms of the abdominal aorta. *Arch Surg.* 1989;124:673–675.
26. Boontje AH, van den Dungen JJ, Blanksma C. Inflammatory abdominal aortic aneurysms. *J Cardiovasc Surg (Torino).* 1990;31:611–616.
27. Leseche G, Schaetz A, Arrive L, Nussaume O, Andreassian B. Diagnosis and management of 17 consecutive patients with inflammatory abdominal aortic aneurysm. *Am J Surg.* 1992;164:39–44.

28. Yasuda K, Sakuma M, Goh K, et al. Surgical treatment of "inflammatory" aneurysms of the abdominal aorta. *Nippon Geka Gakkai Zasshi.* 1987;88:1503–1508.

29. Tjon A, Meeuw L, Bollinger A. Aneurysma der Bauchaorta. Diagnostik und Therapieindikationen. *Schweiz Med Wochenschr.* 1991;121:683–692.

30. Cheatle T, Hickman P, Grimley RP. Inflammatory abdominal aortic aneurysms. *J R Soc Med.* 1987;80:757–758.

31. Bainbridge ET, Woodward DA. Inflammatory aneurysms of the abdominal aorta with associated ureteric obstruction or medial deviation. *J Cardiovasc Surg (Torino).* 1982;23:365–370.

32. Sethia B, Darke SG. Abdominal aortic aneurysm with retroperitoneal fibrosis and ureteric entrapment. *Br J Surg.* 1983;70:434–436.

33. Curci JJ. Modes of presentation and management of inflammatory aneurysms of the abdominal aorta. *J Am Coll Surg* 1994;178:573–580.

34. Nypaver TJ, Shepard AD, Reddy DJ, Elliott JP Jr, Ernst CB. Supraceliac aortic cross-clamping: determinants of outcome in elective abdominal aortic reconstruction. *J Vasc Surg.* 1993;17:868–875.

35. Goldstone J, Malone JM, Moore WS. Inflammatory aneurysms of the abdominal aorta. *Surgery.* 1978;83:425–430.

36. Fiorani P, Faraglia V, Speziale F, et al. Extraperitoneal approach for repair of inflammatory abdominal aortic aneurysm. *J Vasc Surg.* 1991;13:692–697.

37. Metcalf RK, Rutherford RB. Inflammatory abdominal aortic aneurysm: an indication for the retroperitoneal approach. *Surgery.* 1991;109:555–557.

38. Valesky A, Liepe B, Gmelin E, Sellin D, Schildberg FW. Neuere Aspekte zur Diagnostik und Therapie des inflammatorischen Bauchaortenaneurysmas. *Chirurg.* 1984;55:464–468.

39. Tovar Martin E, Acea Nebril B. Aneurismas inflamatorios de aorta abdominal. *Angiologia.* 1993;45:107–111.

40. Pennell RC, Hollier LH, Lie JT, et al. Inflammatory abdominal aortic aneurysms: a thirty-year review. *J Vasc Surg.* 1985;2:859–869.

41. Parodi JC, Marin ML, Veith FJ. Transfemoral, endovascular stented graft repair of an abdominal aortic aneurysm. *Arch Surg.* 1995;130:549–552.

42. Volodos NL, Karpovich IP, Troyan VI, et al. Clinical experience of the use of self-fixing synthetic prostheses for remote endoprosthetics of the thoracic and the abdominal aorta and iliac arteries through the femoral artery and as intraoperative endoprosthesis for aorta reconstruction. *Vasa.* 1991; 33(suppl):93–95.

43. Parodi JC, Palmaz JC, Barone HD. Transfemoral intraluminal graft implantation for abdominal aortic aneurysms. *Ann Vasc Surg.* 1991;5:491–499.

44. Siebenmann R, Schneider K, von Segesser L, Turina M. Das inflammatorische Bauchaortenaneurysma. *Schweiz Med Wochenschr.* 1988;118:881–888.

53

Aortic Aneurysm Repair: Endovascular Grafts

Dieter Raithel

Rapid development of endovascular techniques and instrumentation have led to the development of treating abdominal and thoracic aneurysms by transluminal graft techniques. In 1991 Parodi, from Argentina, described the first six cases of human endoaortic graft insertion.[1] One graft was inserted for aortic dissection, the other five patients had abdominal aortic aneurysms. In 1991 Volodos reported on other initial clinical use of a graft–stent combination in a small number of patients with aortic aneurysms.[2] Many other balloon-expanded systems are currently under development, several of which integrate the structural properties of the stent into components of the graft.

In 1993 Chuter[3] described his initial laboratory experience with a new endovascular delivery system for straight bifurcated grafts, and in 1994 described his first clinical endovascular placement of a bifurcated graft for abdominal aortic aneurysm.[4]

In 1993 the first implantation of Endovascular Technologies' (EVT) endoluminal prostheses occurred at the UCLA Medical Center.[5] They used the Lazarus/S concept of a self-expanding attachment device with fixation pins that are driven into the wall of the abdominal aorta.[6]

In June 1993 White et al used the Sydney endovascular graft (White–Yu endograft) for the first time in a patient with a symptomatic abdominal aortic aneurysm.[7]

Semba and Dake reported on endoluminal stent grafting in patients with thoracic aortic aneurysms.[8] They used two different devices and found that self-expandable stents were better suited for the thoracic aorta. Their stents were custom-built for each patient based on dimensions obtained from spiral computer tomographic (CT) data.

In 1995 Miale reported on a multicenter trial with a balloon-expanded system (the Nitinol stent).[9] We have had experience with this and other devices since June 1994.[10,11]

Anatomical Criteria

For a proximal anchoring site, the aorta must have a nondilated segment with a length of at least 50 mm below the most caudated renal artery. For distal anchoring of a tube graft, the distal aorta proximal of the aortic bifurcation must also have a nondilated segment. If there is no distal cuff, a bifurcated endograft must be implanted. For adequate graft anchoring, a nondilated common iliac artery segment 10 mm in length on both sides is required.

Extremely elongated or stenotic iliac arteries are a contraindication for endovascular treatment because the rigid endovascular graft cannot be inserted through these extremely diseased vessels. Therefore the minimum diameter of the iliac artery must be 7 mm, with a maximum diameter of 12 mm.

The maximum diameter of the proximal aorta is 24 to 26 mm.

Patient Selection

Careful selection of patients by angiography of the aorta using a spiral CT scan and by additional conventional angiography is necessary.

Operative Technique

Due to the fact that this is a new procedure and there is a possibility of causing iliac aortic trauma as a result of introducing the device, the procedure should be carried out in an operating theater that allows emergency conversion. Endograft implantation can be performed under general or spinal anaesthesia; in special cases local anaesthesia may be adequate. We prefer general anaesthesia. The endograft implantation is monitored by x-ray imaging; adequate images can be obtained with a mobile C-arm.

For implantation of tube grafts, only one common femoral artery is exposed through a short longitudinal incision distal from the inguinal ligament; for bifurcated grafts, both common femoral arteries must be exposed. After exposure of one or both femoral arteries, the most caudated renal artery and the aortic bifurcation are marked on the x-ray monitor. After removal of the angiography catheter, the endovascular device with a prosthesis can be introduced. During graft deployment the mean arterial blood pressure should be lowered to about 70 mmHg. After deployment of the endovascular graft, the exact position of the renal arteries and the aortic bifurcation must be verified by contrast-medium injection.

Implantation Techniques for Different Devices

All of the different devices consist of a graft–stent combination.

The Parodi device is a transluminal graft–stent combination that consists of a modified Palmaz balloon expandable stent sutured onto the particle-overlapping end of a tubular, knitted Dacron graft.[1] This is done in such a way that stent expansion presses the graft against the aortic wall, creating a water-tight seal.

In the Chuter–Gianturco system, graft attachment relies on self-expanding Gianturco-Z stents. The straight graft has two stents on the inside, one at each end. The stent–graft prosthesis is mounted on a carrier system of coaxial catheters. Attachment to this carrier system depends on the presence of the innermost catheter. When this is removed, the prosthesis is released from the carrier. The bifurcated graft has an already-attached left limb that can be pulled into position by a catheter or su-

ture, which is accessible at the femoral level after the graft has been inserted.

Chuter Straight Grafts

Straight graft insertion can be performed entirely through one femoral artery.

The angiographic catheter is replaced over a guide wire for the delivery system. Correct graft position is maintained by manipulation of the central carrier as the introducer sheath is withdrawn.[3,4] The stents expand spontaneously as soon as they leave the confinement of the introducer sheath. Then the graft is released from the carrier by removal of the inner catheter, permitting removal of the delivery system.

Chuter Bifurcated Grafts

After systemic heparinization, both common femoral arteries are incised transversally. After inserting a cross-femoral catheter through the left iliac artery into a waiting stone retrieval basket, the catheter is pulled down the right iliac artery to the right groin (Figure 53.1). A double-lumen dilator is inserted over the cross-femoral catheter. Then a guide wire is passed through the double-lumen dilator into the proximal aorta.

After the cross-femoral catheter and the guide wire are separated on removal of the double-lumen catheter, the delivery system is inserted over the guide wire (Figure 53.2). Then an angiogram is performed with the delivery system in place. Next, the graft can be extruded by withdrawing the sheath to its fullest extent, after which the left limb of the graft is pulled into the left iliac artery.

Removal of the delivery system initiates the release of the right limb stent, and removing the left limb catheter releases the left limb stent from its sheath. The aortic stent carries eight barbs, and they penetrate the aortic

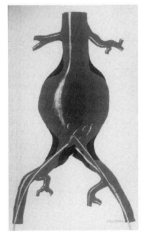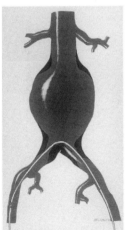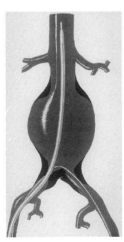

FIGURE 53.1. Operative technique for implaniting a Chuter device.

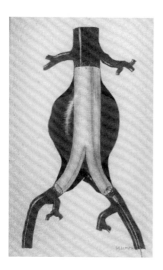

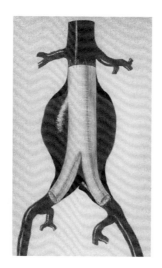

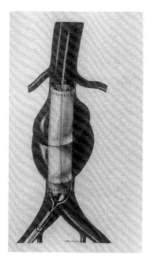

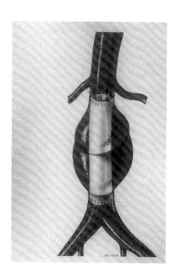

FIGURE 53.2. Operative technique for implanting a Chuter device (step 2).

FIGURE 53.4. Operative technique for implanting an EVT device (step 2).

wall and act as anchors only if the open stent starts moving downstream. A completion angiogram is performed after withdrawal of the entire system to document the presence or absence of proximal or distal graft leaks.

EVT Device

The procedure used for the EVT device is similar to the procedure already described.

After the self-expanding system is deployed proximally, an implantation balloon is advanced to the proper location. This is identified by a marker in the balloon system that will allow the balloon to be centered in the area of the attachment system. Then the balloon is inflated to 2 atm. With the proximal balloon inflated, the sheath is withdrawn, thus exposing the distal attachment system. After the distal attachment system is deployed, it is also secured with the balloon (Figures 53.3 and 53.4).

The EVT device has a superior and inferior attachment system, and the graft has radiopaque markers. The self-expanding frame of the attachment system is intended to spring out of the diameter of the vessel to actively hold the graft against the vessel wall and circumferentially seal the space between the vascular graft and the vessel wall. The angled hooks hold the self-expanding frame tightly against the vessel wall (Figure 53.5).

MinTec/Vanguard Device

The MinTec/Vanguard device is a modular system with a nitinol stent. This nitinol stent has a shape memory and super elasticity (Cragg stent)[9] and is covered with a thin, woven polyester fabric.

The three-stage delivery system enables individual deployment of each section of the device. The delivery sys-

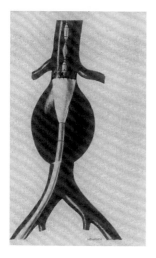

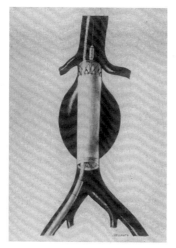

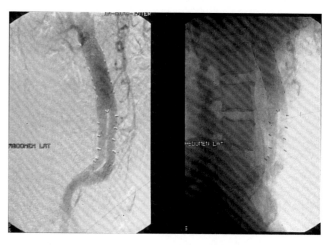

FIGURE 53.3. Operative technique for implanting an EVT device (step 1).

FIGURE 53.5. Postoperative angiogram showing the EVT bifurcated device.

tem is an 18 F device. After deployment of the endoluminal graft, a balloon is used to ensure proper fixation of the device against the aortic wall. Tube and bifurcated endografts are available.

Since the autumn 1996 the MinTec graft has been improved by the Boston Scientific Company and is now called the Vanguard stent.

Perioperative Quality Control

During surgery, the entire implantation procedure is monitored with an image intensifier. On the following day an ultrasound examination of the abdomen is performed. Furthermore, CT scans and an angiographic control are necessary to document any evidence of leaks, thromboses, or changes in the aneurysm (Figures 53.6 and 53.7).

Discussion

Endovascular graft training is necessary for the physicians caring for patients with abdominal aortic aneurysms. Endovascular grafts must be placed only by surgeons skilled in the management of patients with abdominal aortic aneurysms, and we feel strongly that an operating room environment is preferable for endovascular aneurysm grafting. This is critically important if, on occasion, urgent conversion to transabdominal aortic aneurysm repair becomes necessary. Complications of the endovascular grafting procedure are likely to require

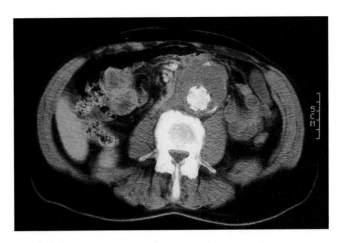

FIGURE 53.7. Postoperative CT scan shows complete exclusion of the aneurysm by the MinTec/Vanguard device.

prompt surgical intervention, and the surgeon can make the decision, if the procedure fails, to convert the operation to conventional graft repair. Furthermore the vascular surgeon is person who can treat further perioperative complications.

We hold the view that in the long run, about 15% of aortic aneurysms can be treated endovascularly with a straight graft, and another 15% to 20% can be treated with a bifurcated graft.

Complications in transfemoral endovascular aneurysm treatment include inadequate access to the iliac artery or poor positioning of the attachment system. Therefore, good preoperative and perioperative imaging techniques are necessary to minimize these complications. Furthermore, during application there is a possibility of damaging the iliac vessels or the aorta. If this occurs, a laparotomy should be performed immediately.

Poor positioning of the endografts results in an endoleak. Endoleaks can be documented at the proximal neck and at the distal cuff in tube grafts and at the iliac limb attachment system. Accurate patient selection is important for avoiding or reducing such leaks.

We can also see extra graft flow after graft implantation. This extra graft flow can be documented by postoperative examinations with duplex or CT scan, and sometimes by a postoperative angiogram. The extra flow occurs due to a persisting collateral circulation through the inferior mesenteric artery and the lumbar arteries, but often disappears spontaneously.

Follow-up Imaging

Follow-up imaging includes serial CT scan, duplex ultrasonography, plain abdominal radiography, and angiography to check for perigraft leakage, graft stenosis, stent migration, and aneurysm enlargement.

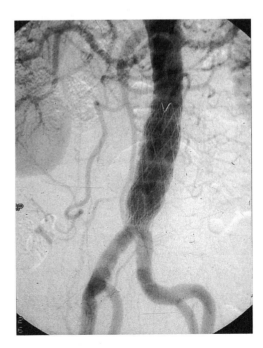

FIGURE 53.6. Postoperative angiogram (Vanguard device).

The first postoperative study is done before discharging the patient and includes duplex ultrasonography and CT scan; this is repeated at 3- and 6-month intervals. Color-coded duplex ultrasound scanning is used to screen for endoleaks and graft stenosis. Any abnormal findings in duplex scanning should be assessed by CT scan and/or angiography.

In our series of more than 130 endovascular grafts for abdominal aortic aneurysm repair, at follow-up we have seen patients who still have an endoleak, and they show a shrinking of the aneurysm sack. On the other hand, we have patients with no endoleak and a growth of the aneurysm sack. An increase in the aneurysm diameter or volume is always an indication for reoperation because growth of the aneurysm probably means that there is a risk of aneurysm rupture.

Conclusion

Endovascular aneurysm repair techniques are evolving rapidly, and we think this enables a wider range of patients to be treated with better results. Although the results of endovascular grafting are promising, we need to see much longer follow-up periods before drawing any conclusion about the durability of this technique of aneurysm repair. We need careful follow-up combined large studies in which the selection criteria and the apparatus have been standardized to provide a statistical basis for comparing this technique to conventional surgery. Due to our experience we believe that endovascular grafting of aneurysms should be limited to a few departments of vascular surgery. The members of these departments should have adequate experience to avoid potential complications or, at least, to reduce the complication rate.

References

1. Parodi JC, Palmaz JC, Barone HD. Transfemoral intraluminal graft implantation for abdominal aortic aneurysm. *Ann Vasc Surg.* 1991;5:491–499.

2. Volodos NL, Karpovich IP, Troyan VI, et al. Clinical experience of the use of a self-fixing prosthesis for remote endoprosthetics of the thoracic and the abdominal aorty and iliac arteries through the femoral artery and as intraoperative endoprosthesis for aorta reconstruction. *Vasa.* 1991;33(suppl):93–95.

3. Chuter TAM, Green RM, Ouriel K, Fiore WM, DeWeese JA. Transfemoral endovascular aortic graft placement. *J Vasc Surg.* 1993;18:185–197.

4. Scott RAP, Chuter TAM. Clinical endovascular placement of bifurcated graft in abdominal aortic aneurysm without laparotomy. *Lancet.* 1994;343:413.

5. Quinones-Baldrich WJ. The EVT endoluminal prosthesis: clinical experience and results. In: Chuter TAM, Donayre CE, White RA, eds. *Endoluminal Vascular Prostheses.* Boston, Mass: Little, Brown & Company; 1995:93–105.

6. Lazarus HM. The EVT prosthesis: development concepts and design. In: Chuter TAM, Donayre CE, White RA, eds. *Endoluminal Vascular Prostheses.* Boston, Mass: Little, Brown & Company; 1995:81–91.

7. White GH, May J, Yu W. Stented and nonstented endoluminal grafts for aneurysmal disease: the Australian experience. In: Chuter TAM, Donayre CE, White RA, eds. *Endoluminal Vascular Prostheses.* Boston, Mass: Little, Brown & Company; 1995:107–152.

8. Semba CP, Dake MD. Endoluminal stent-grafting in the thoracic aorta. In: Chuter TAM, Donayre CE, White RA, eds. *Endoluminal Vascular Prostheses.* Boston, Mass: Little, Brown & Company; 1995:153–171.

9. Mialhe C, Amicabile C. Endovascular treatment of aneurysms of the subrenal aorta using the Stentor endoprosthesis. *J Mal Vasc.* 1995;20:290–295.

10. Raithel D, Heilberger P, Ritter W, Zeitler E. Wertigkeit differenzierter Systeme in der endovaskulären Therapie von Aortenaneurysmen. Paper presented at: Meeting of the 113th Kongress der Deutschen Gesellschaft für Chirurgie; April 9–13, 1996; Berlin, Germany.

11. Raithel D. Indication for endovascular stent grafting of aortic aneurysms or arterio-venous fistula—selection of patients according to different devices. Paper presented at: Meeting of the 38th Annual World Congress of the International College of Angiology; June 16–22, 1996; Cologne, Germany.

Section 6
Aortic Arch and Major Arteries

54

Subclavian Steal Syndrome

Raymond A. Dieter Jr, Robert O. Maganini, and Robert Dieter

The normal blood flow to the brain occurs through both the carotid and vertebral systems, flowing distally from their more proximal origins from the aorta, the innominate or the subclavian vessels. When there is a reversal in this flow pattern such that blood flows away from the brain rather than toward the brain, the potential for the development of symptoms exists. When the flow reversal affects an organ to the degree that symptoms (for example headache, dizziness, or anginal chest pain) develop, the patient may be defined as having the subclavian steal syndrome.

History

The first angiographic demonstration of vertebral flow reversal was reported in 1960 by Contorni.[1] Subsequent to this, additional reports and consideration were given when this reversed flow was correlated with the symptomatology. Other authors began to develop the concept and recognize the potential for such a syndrome. We reported on the treatment of anomalous right subclavian artery origin and described the potential for the reversed flow and subclavian steal syndrome.[2] Various definitions and terminology for the diagnosis have been presented. The terms *reversed cerebral flow,* the *vertebral steal syndrome,* and the *subclavian steal syndrome* were all discussed. Fischer originally presented the term *subclavian steal syndrome* in an editorial.[3] With increased awareness, the recognition of the reversal of flow in the vertebral system, the subclavian obstruction, and the subclavian steal syndrome have been further reviewed, discussed, and reported.

Definition

The definition and the significance of subclavian steal and the subclavian steal syndrome have been repeatedly discussed. Subclavian steal implies and is the result of the reversal of flow in branches of the arteries normally supplied by the subclavian artery. Having this reversal of flow does not necessarily imply or mean that there are symptoms or other problems in the patient. In fact, on a number of occasions we have found such a reversal in patients without the patient having any complaints or symptoms of the steal syndrome except for the physical finding of a diminished pulse and demonstration of the reversed flow on vascular studies.

Patients with symptomatology referable to the cerebral system, extremity, or heart, when associated with the subclavian steal, are defined as having the subclavian steal syndrome. In other words, when a patient has reversal of flow in the vascular system, with arterial blood flowing away from the brain or from the heart to perfuse the extremity, and the patient develops symptoms from this (such as chest pain, angina, dizziness, headaches, or syncope with use of the extremity), the patient is then described as having the subclavian steal syndrome. Such patients more frequently require interventional therapy as compared with patients with asymptomatic subclavian steal findings.

Anatomy and Physiology

The anatomic location of the obstructing process that creates or leads to the development of the subclavian steal syndrome is most commonly the left subclavian artery (Table 54.1). When the subclavian artery becomes severely stenotic or occluded, the structures distal to the lesion retain their requirement for blood and oxygen. Therefore the blood must be supplied through collateral circulation. These routes may include the carotid artery and its branches, the vertebral artery through the circle of Willis and its branches, and the distal subclavian vessels through the chest wall, as well as other collaterals (Table 54.2). Thus, when the organ affected is the brain,

TABLE 54.1. Etiology of subclavian steal.

Arteriosclerosis obliterans
Most common
Takayasu's disease
Atheromatous plaques

Traumatic occlusion of subclavian artery

Iatrogenic
Ligation of anomalous origin, subclavian artery
Blalock–Taussig operation with division of distal subclavian artery

TABLE 54.2. Collateral circulatory channels.

Internal carotid to vertebral communication via circle of Willis
External carotid, vertebral, thyrocervical trunk, and costocervical
    trunk communications
Transcervical anastomosis between the inferior thyroid arteries
Indirect vertebral-to-vertebral spinal branch anastomosis
Internal thoracic or aorto–internal thoracic artery communications
    through intercostal vessels

TABLE 54.3. Symptoms of subclavian steal syndromes.

Auditory

Vertebral basilar insufficiency
Dizziness
Syncope/vertigo
Headache
Weakness
Nausea and vomiting
Ataxia
Drop attacks

Occular
Blurred vision
Diplopia

Cardiac
Chest pain
Anginal symptoms

Shoulder and arm pain
Claudication
Paresthesia
Rest pain
Gangrene

Other
Exercise induced (is uncommon)
Hemiparesis/hemisensory dysfunction suggest carotid disease

the blood may flow up the right innominate, the right carotid, or the right vertebral artery to the brain and then to the circle of Willis. At this point, the blood flows away from the brain, down the left vertebral artery to the distal subclavian artery, especially on the left, and out into the axillary and brachial vessels. When the patient is at rest or not overutilizing the extremity, usually no symptoms develop. However, when the blood volume requirements of the extremity reach such a degree that the body is taking more blood away from the circle of Willis, the base of the brain, and the cerebellum, than the brain can afford to give up, the patient may develop symptomatology that results from a net deficit of cerebral blood flow and ischemia.

Some studies have suggested, however, that proximal subclavian artery obstruction and reversal of the vertebral blood flow actually cause no difference in the amount of cerebral blood flow.[4] Others believe that auditory symptoms and vertebral basilar symptoms (including dizziness, syncope, and headaches) may all develop as a result of this anatomic variant (Table 54.3) In our experience the disabling neurologic symptoms that have been reported by others have not been noted in most of our patients. In fact, most of our patients have been totally asymptomatic, and the finding of a subclavian steal has only been an incidental occurrence. This is the case even with patients who had a Blalock–Taussig operation for treatment of tetralogy of Fallot. However, the development of headaches does occur in some of these individuals as they reach maturity.[2]

The question does arise whether a subclavian steal concomitant with other cerebral-circulation–limiting arterial lesions may predispose the patient to significant neurologic symptoms. We consider this to be the case with a number of our patients. At times, we have even wondered if the correction of the other cerebral vascular lesions may enhance the subclavian steal and potentiate

the possibility for a subclavian steal syndrome. Whether a patient develops symptoms as a result of the subclavian steal would seem to depend on multiple considerations including the collateral circulation, the presence of other cerebral arterial lesions, the circle of Willis and its anatomy, and the size of the vertebral arteries—especially the contralateral vertebral artery. A large amount of information regarding the medical and surgical treatment and complications of this syndrome was reported from the joint study of extracranial arterial occlusion.[5]

With the development of better diagnostic techniques, angiography, and coronary surgery, a large number of innovative bypass procedures have been utilized for the treatment of coronary artery occlusive disease. As a result of this, internal mammary artery and saphenous vein bypass graft procedures have been utilized. When patients who have undergone these procedures develop subclavian artery disease with occlusion, their symptomatology may revert back to that of the presurgical prebypass condition of chest pain and angina. On restudy, these patients may be demonstrated to have subclavian artery occlusion. A steal phenomenon from the coronary artery into the jump graft, and retrograde flow to the distal subclavian artery and the extremity may occur. Interventional therapy thus is warranted in these iatrogenically developed steal syndromes.

Diagnosis

Most patients, in our experience, have been suspected to have a subclavian steal syndrome on the basis of history and physical exam. If the patient is having symptoms compatible with the subclavian steal syndrome, whether from an atherosclerotic lesion or a reversed flow resulting from another etiology such as coronary steal, one may suspect it from the medical history. Then, on examination of the patient, with emphasis on bilateral upper extremity examination of the pulse and the blood pressure, the suspicion of a subclavian stenosis or occlusion arises. With further details of the patient's history, one may have a very high suspicion of an occluded vessel and subclavian steal. When the patient's symptoms suggest that additional evaluation is warranted, we perform noninvasive and/or invasive evaluation of the patient. Doppler study of the carotid vessels may be performed. Simultaneously, vertebral artery evaluation may be carried out with particular reference to the direction of blood flow.

Depending on the patient's symptoms and the noninvasive evaluation, including any nuclear studies, a patient may then proceed to magnetic resonance angiography or digital subtraction angiography (Table 54.4). Both have proven helpful in patients for whom noninvasive evaluation is indicated or who decline interventional review. Most patients with atherosclerosis demonstrate both the occlusive process in the subclavian artery and additional atherosclerotic changes in the carotid system, in the internal, external, or common carotid vessels. Occasionally an aneurysm or other degenerative vascular process may be noted in the innominate system on the right. If the patient is younger and has had previous anomalous subclavian origin surgery, particularly subclavian ligation but without subclavian grafting, we then proceed to angiography, especially if the patient's symptoms are severe. The patient who has had previous internal mammary artery bypass procedures or subclavian saphenous vein procedures and have a diminished pulse on the left side certainly should be considered for angiography including the coronary system (Table 54.5).

TABLE 54.4. Diagnosis of subclavian steal.

History: suspicion

Physical examination
Absence or diminished radial pulse
Unequal arm blood pressures
Subclavian bruit

Noninvasive studies
Cervical duplex scanning: reversal of flow
Digital subtraction angiography (DSA) or digital vascular imaging (DVI)
Magnetic resonance imaging
Nuclear medicine studies
Transcranial Doppler (ultrasound) studies

Invasive
Arch angiography
Carotid–subclavian selective studies

TABLE 54.5. Types of subclavian steal.

Vertebral vertebral
Carotid basilar
External carotid to vertebral
Carotid subclavian (right side only with proximal brachiocephalic occlusion)
Coronary–subclavian artery via mammary artery or jump graft

Anatomic consideration would also suggest that the patients who have had the Blalock–Taussig procedure should be considered for evaluation and angiography when they develop complaints, such as headaches, consistent with those found in the subclavian steal syndrome.

Therapy

In most patients, the subclavian steal syndrome is an incidental finding and is not symptomatic. Therefore, only a few patients require surgical intervention. When a patient is aware of the physical findings and the potential steal syndrome, he or she may alter work or other activities in accordance. The treatment of these patients is usually confined to serial follow-up and avoidance of interventional therapy unless the symptoms become significant. The risks of surgery, including the high incidence of stroke and mortality, have been published extensively. When the patient becomes symptomatic, the patient should be reevaluated to determine the best type of surgical procedure to reverse the flow of blood, keeping in mind both general and regional considerations. Table 54.6 presents the flow abnormalities one is able to see with angiography.

If the patient is at high risk for complications from surgery, a procedure under local anesthesia may be more beneficial, for example, an axillary procedure or an interventional endovascular approach through the groin. Subclavian artery angioplasty and stent placement may be the optimal choice for some patients, especially for stenosis. As the symptoms and severity of the patient's condition increase, more extensive intervention may be required, or a potentially longer-lasting procedure may be considered (Table 54.7). In the younger individuals who otherwise are in good health, we have considered a thoracotomy utilizing either a midsternotomy or lateral chest approach. Depending on the pathology present, (whether it is an atherosclerotic lesion or an anomalous congenital lesion), we have utilized end-

TABLE 54.6. Flow abnormalities of vertebral artery.

Stage I reduced forward (antegrade)
Stage II reversal of flow during exercise
Stage III permanent reversed (retrograde)

TABLE 54.7. Surgical approaches for correction of the subclavian steal syndrome.

Extrathoracic
Graft interposition (synthetic or vein)
    Carotid subclavian
    Carotid axillary
    Carotid vertebral
    Subclavian subclavian
    Femoral axillary
    Axilloaxillary bypass graft
Direct anastomosis
    Subclavian carotid
    Vertebral carotid
Endarterectomy (transcervical, vertebral, subclavian or brachiocephalic
    vessels)
Combinations of preceding

Intrathoracic
Endarterectomy with patch graft
Aortosubclavian or aorta–innominate bypass
Correction of aortic arch abnormalities
Ligation of vertebral artery or branches thereof
Aorta subclavian bypass

Percutaneous
Transluminal angioplasty
Stent placement
Directional atherectomy

arterectomy, patch grafting, or aortosubclavian bypass. Many authors, including ourselves, have an interest in this topic. The subclavian arteries may be difficult to suture and to perform grafting techniques upon due to their friability and the tendency of these vessels to tear. We have had very good results with the left thoracotomy approach, in selected individuals, with graft coverage by the pleura at the termination of the procedure after utilizing a partial occluding clamp on the aorta. The aortosubclavian bypass has also been utilized in a group of patients with subclavian steal and Takayasu's disease when more than one vessel was affected. When performing the Blalock–Taussig procedure, consideration for simultaneous ligation of the vertebral artery or the branches of the subclavian artery has been given to avoid the subclavian steal syndrome. The long-term consequences of the subclavian steal syndrome in these patients is yet to be completely delineated.

A large percentage of the older patients requiring surgical intervention also have internal carotid artery disease with ulceration and stenosis. Most patients who have transient ischemic attacks or strokes as a result of vascular disease have them consequent to their carotid artery disease and not their subclavian steal. Therefore, when considering options for these individuals, one should consider either a carotid endarterectomy or patch graft, with correction of the carotid lesion and then secondary correction of the subclavian steal. Usually, correcting the carotid lesion will eliminate the patient's symptoms.

Stroke is usually not a result of the subclavian steal. Therefore, if the only vascular lesion is a subclavian artery occlusion, one should consider a surgical procedure that minimizes the risk of stroke as a result of the surgery. A number of authors have suggested the performance of a carotid subclavian bypass graft using the supraclavicular approach, with a single transverse incision made in the lower neck. The phrenic nerve is preserved and the scalenus anticus muscle is resected. With careful dissection, an end-to-end carotid to graft and graft-to–subclavian artery bypass can be performed. Others have performed direct anastomosis between the subclavian and the carotid artery. Reports have suggested that direct anastomosis or the synthetic Dacron/ polytetraflouroethylene approach have a longer life span than a saphenous vein interposition. This, in effect, creates a new left brachioinnominate vessel. The common carotid appears to have the ability to carry adequate blood supply to both the brain and the arm in these individuals. The chance for development of a carotid steal in these situations seems to be minimal. The mortality and complication rates of these extrathoracic procedures do not appear to be any less than those of intrathoracic procedures, when patients are properly selected.

Other individuals prefer not to operate on the common carotid artery in an effort to minimize the chance of an iatrogenic stroke and choose a subclavian-to-subclavian bypass graft using the supraclavicular approach. This is a somewhat more tedious procedure on rather friable vessels. Because of the difficulty of suturing these vessels in the supraclavicular approach, the possibility of kinking of the grafts, and the limited exposure provided, Thompson et al, have suggested utilization of an interposition vein cuff between the subclavian artery and the synthetic prosthesis, as has been used in femoral distal grafts.[6]

Because of its difficulties, we have preferred not to perform the subclavian-subclavian bypass. When performing access from one upper extremity to the other, we have preferred the axilloaxillary approach rather than a femoral axillary graft. The axilloaxillary bypass procedure has had a low operative mortality in our experience and has been an easier operation to perform in elderly patients. This approach is particularly valuable for the patient with the brachiocephalic occlusion on the right, or the tracheobrachiocephalic fistula, as well as those with extensive scarring in the neck. One must be certain that the donor vessel is widely patent and not stenotic. As reported by Sumner, this procedure may be performed relatively easily with good access under local anesthesia and is not usually affected by arm motion.[7] The complications suggested by previous reports, including vascular obstruction due to the patient's sleeping in a prone position and a bulge across the sternum, have not been of high incidence.

As mentioned, we fortunately have not had to open the sternum in these patients for coronary surgery. If such a procedure should need to be performed, the donor anastomosis may be transferred to the ascending aorta. It is important to note that when performing arteriography for delineation of this syndrome, arch aortography with a single view demonstrates the obstructing subclavian lesion. However, serial studies with the rapid film-changing technique are valuable in delineating carotid artery disease and the potential for opposite-side obstructions or aneurysmal lesions and demonstrating the reversal of flow in the vertebral vessels. Both axillo-axillary incisions and the subclavian-subclavian bypass require two incisions but do minimize the chance of stroke or embolic innominate phenomenon. Mannick comments on the excellent results of corrective operative procedures for the hemodynamic abnormalities of the subclavian steal, with the relief of the associated cerebral symptoms in 75% to 80% of patients.[8]

With the development of percutaneous angiography and percutaneous endovascular or endoluminal surgery, angioplastic techniques have been developed for the subclavian vessels. The approach may be performed transfemorally under local anesthesia in elderly patients, with amazing results. Initial reports have suggested that the long-term patency of transluminal angioplasty is less optimal than that of surgical procedures. With additional experience and the addition of stents, hopefully, the immediate complication rate, particularly that of bleeding and the long-term patency rate, will improve, and we will see the restenosis rate diminished significantly. Restenosis in some instances may again be handled by angioplasty utilizing the transluminal balloon technique. Delaney et al. discussed the need for future prospective randomized data for evaluation of this procedure.[9] Combining noninterventional techniques, such as the xenon-computed tomography technique described by Webster, with the lesser invasive procedures, we hope it will be possible to diagnose, define the indications, and treat affected individuals with fewer complications.[10]

Coronary Subclavian Steal Syndrome

With the increased awareness of coronary artery disease and the ability to demonstrate the coronary lesion, we have seen a proliferation of coronary flow–enhancing procedures. These have included endarterectomy, the saphenous vein bypass procedure, the internal mammary bypass, balloon angioplasty, and the placement of intra-arterial stents. Recurrence of coronary symptomatology, especially angina, may be noted when the left internal mammary artery was utilized for coronary artery bypass and subclavian occlusion developed. A number of articles have been published describing the development of the coronary subclavian steal syndrome in patients who had concomitant subclavian artery stenosis or developed subclavian artery stenosis or occlusion subsequent to the surgical bypass procedure.[11-14]

Subsequent to the angiographic demonstration of the lesion and the reversed flow, a number of these patients have had surgical correction. Feld, Beltz, Crowe, and Georges have utilized percutaneous transluminal angioplasty for the correction of the subclavian stenosis and to treat the coronary subclavian steal syndrome.[14-17] Other approaches have also been utilized. Rossum found an occluded carotid subclavian conduit in a patient along with additional coronary disease.[18] Breall et al[19] performed a directional atherectomy using the percutaneous transfemoral approach for treatment of the coronary subclavian steal syndrome. Raschkow performed an axillo-axillary gortex graft for treatment of the subclavian coronary steal.[20]

With new and innovative surgical techniques also come surgical problems as the disease process advances. The subclavian coronary steal syndrome delineates the need to be alert for future concerns and innovative techniques concerning the development and treatment of subclavian steal syndrome. As we stated in our presentation at the annual meeting of the International College of Surgeons in 1988, a number of vascular steal syndromes, including iatrogenic, are now being seen and should be considered in symptomatic patients following surgery.[21-23]

References

1. Contorni L. Il circolo collaterale vertebraovertebrale nella obliterazione dell'arterio subclavia all sua origine. *Minerva Chir.* 1960;15:268–271.
2. Piffare R, Dieter RA Jr, Neidballa RLG. Definitive surgical treatment of the aberrant retroesophageal right subclavian artery in the adult. *Thorac Cardiovasc Surg.* 1971;61:154–159.
3. Fisher CM. Editorial comment: a new vascular syndrome—the subclavian steal. *N Engl J Med.* 1961;265:912–913.
4. Eklof B, Schwartz SI. Effects of subclavian steal and compromised cephalic blood flow on cerebral circulation. *Surgery.* 1970;68:431–441.
5. Fields WS, Lemak NA. Joint study of extracranial arterial occlusion. *JAMA.* 1972;222:1139–1143.
6. Thompson MM, Beard JD, Bell PRF. Subclavian to subclavian bypass facilitated by the use of an interposed vein cuff. *Br J Surg.* 1991;78:630–631.
7. Sumner DS. Axillo axillary bypass graft. In: Nyhus LM, Baker RJ. *Mastery of Surgery.* Boston, Mass: Little, Brown & Company; 1992:1648–1654.
8. Mannick JA. Subclavian steal syndrome. In: Sabiston DC Jr. *Textbook of Surgery. The Biological Basis of Modern Surgical Practice.* Philadelphia, Pa: WB Saunders; 1991:1584–1588.

9. Delaney CP, Couse NF, Mehigan D, et al. Investigation and management of subclavian steal syndrome. *Br J Surg.* 1994; 81:1093–1095.

10. Webster MW, Downs L, Yonas H, et al. The effect of arm exercise on regional cerebral blood flow in the subclavian steal syndrome. *Am J Surg.* 1994;168:91–93.

11. Breall JA, Kim D, Baim DS, et al. Coronary subclavian steal. An unusual cause of angina pectoris after successful internal mammary-coronary artery bypass grafting. *Cathet Cardiovasc Diagn.* 1991;24:274–276.

12. Latific-Jasnic D, Zorman D, Cijan A, et al. Unusual subclavian steal phenomenon. *Tex Heart Inst J.* 1994;21:236–237.

13. Samoil D, Schwartz JL. Coronary subclavian steal syndrome. *Am Heart J.* 1993;126:1463–1466.

14. Feld H, Nathan P, Raninga D, et al. Symptomatic angina secondary to coronary subclavian steal syndrome treated successfully by percutaneous transluminal angioplasty of the subclavian artery. *Cathet Cardiovasc Diagn.* 1992;26: 12–14.

15. Belz M, Marshall JJ, Cowley MJ, et al. Subclavian balloon angioplasty in the management of the coronary-subclavian steal syndrome. *Cathet Cardiovasc Diagn.* 1992;25:161–163.

16. Crowe KE, Iannone LA. Percutaneous transluminal angioplasty for subclavian artery stenosis and patients with subclavian steal syndrome and coronary subclavian steal syndrome. *Am Heart J.* 1993;126:229–233.

17. Georges NP, Ferretti JA. Percutaneous transluminal angioplasty of subclavian artery occlusion for treatment of subclavian steal. *AJR.* 1993;161:399–400.

18. Rossum AC, Weinstein E, Holland M. Angiographic evaluation of a carotid subclavian bypass graft in a patient with subclavian artery stenosis and left internal mammary artery bypass graft. *Cathet Cardiovasc Diagn.* 1994;32: 178–181.

19. Breall JA, Grossman W, Stillman IE, et al. Atherectomy of the subclavian artery for patients with symptomatic coronary subclavian steal syndrome. *J Am Coll Cardiol.* 1993; 21:1564–1567.

20. Rashkow AM. Angina pectoris caused by subclavian coronary steal. *Cathet Cardiovasc Diagn.* 1993;30:230–232.

21. Dieter RA Jr, Hamouda F, McCray R, et al. Surgically induced iatrogenic steal syndrome. Paper presented at: International College of Surgeons Annual Meeting; February 15; 1988; New Orleans, La.

22. Dieter RA Jr, Kuzycz G. The steal syndrome iatrogenic causes. 1998;83:355–377. *International Surgery.*

23. Harty RS, Heuser RR. Embolization of IMA side branch for post-CABG ischemia. *Ann Thorac Surg.* 1997;63: 1765–1766.

55

Thoracic Outlet Syndrome

Raymond A. Dieter, Jr, Timothy O'Brien, and Raymond A. Dieter, III

The thoracic outlet syndrome (TOS) presents a concern for both the patient and the physician diagnostician and therapist. Patients with TOS are seen by multiple physicians in multiple specialties in an attempt to delineate their problems. The physician, in many ways, is attempting to diagnose a syndrome or problem that in most patients has no definitive laboratory diagnostic test to define the diagnosis and potential therapy. Some physicians even question whether the syndrome exists. Yet, other physicians feel very strongly about its presence and the need for therapy. Part of the dilemma that physicians face is the symptomatology correlation with the physical findings of absent or diminished radial artery pulsation found in many individuals.

We have attempted to divide our patients into two groups. First, we select those in whom we feel there is a positive physical finding upon performance of specific vascular compression maneuvers while checking for radial artery pulsation. In these individuals, the hypermilitary position or the Adson maneuver may eliminate or block the transmission of a pulse to the radial artery. But, these same individuals may have no symptoms at all or they may have marked symptoms. We then attempt to diagnose the cause of the symptoms and appropriately categorize the patient: are the symptoms due to a thoracic outlet problem or, possibly, due to another problem such as a neoplastic or metastatic process to the cervical spine? Thus, we have subdivided our original group into two subgroups that we call *thoracic outlet obstruction, asymptomatic* and *thoracic outlet obstruction with the thoracic outlet syndrome*. This may be a rather artificial division, but it has helped to clarify the patient's situation in our minds. The thoracic outlet syndrome is a diagnosis of exclusion in many instances, thus making the understanding and consideration of the individual patient's condition more difficult. A third, much larger group consists of those patients in whom we feel there is no indication that their symptoms relate to TOS.

Historical Aspects

The thoracic outlet syndrome and its treatment options have slowly progressed over the years. The initial description of a cervical rib was apparently made by Galen and Vesalius.[1] Early in the nineteenth century the symptoms ascribed to the cervical ribs were treated medically. It was not until 1861 that Coote resected the offending cervical rib to eliminate the patient's symptoms.[2] As time progressed, additional awareness of the components and various aspects of the syndrome became more apparent. Subclavian artery occlusion or poststenotic dilation consequent to the cervical rib, and the soft tissue etiologies for the syndrome, including ligamentous and scalenus muscle involvement, began to become apparent. The value of division of the scalenus anticus was then championed. During the late 1930s and early 1940s, this syndrome was treated primarily by sectioning of the muscle.[3] As time progressed, the bony components of this syndrome became more and more apparent. In addition to resection of the cervical rib, resection of the clavicle and the first rib were advocated to a greater extent. Various approaches (anterior, posterior, and axillary) were utilized for this surgery. As one of us (RD Jr.) was finishing his training program, Roos popularized the transaxillary resection with a small axillary incision below the hairline.[4] Other approaches were also being popularized, including the anterior subclavicular, the supraclavicular, and the posterior thoracoplastic approaches. As time progressed, each of these approaches has been popularized, evaluated, and followed a utilization curve.

Potential complications and technical difficulty tended to delineate which technique was most acceptable.

Anatomical Considerations

The anatomy of the relevant area has been variously described and reviewed by a large number of individuals from various perspectives including pure anatomical descriptions, functional review, and surgical anatomical considerations.[5] Each aspect has its merits and concerns. Even the definition of the term *thoracic outlet* should be reviewed because it actually represents a conglomeration of a number of etiologic factors that are brought together under the one term *thoracic outlet syndrome*. However, the etiology of the problems may originate from a fractured clavicle, a congenital variant of the first, or cervical, rib, or from structures lateral to the first rib (Table 55.1.) Thus, we present general description and a concern for the technical aspects.

The subclavian arteries and veins leave the thoracic inlet to traverse the cervicoaxillary canal and enter the upper extremity. The vein passes through the space between the subclavius and anterior scalene muscle, whereas the artery and the lower trunk of the brachial plexus pass between the anterior and the middle scalene muscles. Each step of the way, as the vascular structures leave the chest to unite with the neurologic structures, one is confronted with another concern for possible creation of the symptoms affecting the patient. Proximally, the scalene triangle is divided from the costoclavicular space, and distally or laterally one encounters the axillary space. The neurovascular compression occurs most commonly in the costoclavicular space, which is outlined by the clavicle, the first rib, and the costoclavicular ligament. Posteriorly, one finds the scalenus medius and the long thoracic nerve. The scalene tubercle and the scalenus anticus divide this space into the anterior space in which we note the subclavian vein and, posteriorly, the subclavian artery and the brachial plexus (in the scalene

triangle). As various portions of this area become diseased or pathologic, they may create problems by compressing the brachial plexus, the subclavian artery, or the subclavian vein. Patients, therefore, are seen with a multitude of symptoms that result from various activities performed during their usual daily routines. For example, computer operators working in certain positions may have a great deal of difficulty because they hold their arms and shoulders in a certain position and angle. Others may have symptoms caused by heavy breasts with sagging shoulders. Depending on the structure affected, the patient develops neurologic-, arterial-, or venous-related symptoms. In our experience, most of the symptoms relate to neurologic rather than vascular (arterial or venous) compression.

Signs and Symptoms

Most of the patients that we see are referred because of pain or paresthesias in their upper extremities (Table 55.2). A large percentage of these patients are noted to have developed their symptoms because of certain work-related efforts. Ironing clothes, long-distance truck driving while holding the steering wheel, washing and drying dishes, working overhead on an automobile, washing windows, or painting walls may create the necessary anatomic condition to initiate the patient's visit to a

TABLE 55.1. Causes of thoracic outlet obstruction syndrome.

Bony
Cervical rib
First rib (fracture, rudimentary, exostosis)
Enlarged C7 transverse process
Dislocation of head of humerus
Clavicle (fracture, exostosis, bifid)
Cervical spondylosis
Crushing injury to upper thorax

Soft tissue
Fibrous bands
Scalene muscles
Omohyoid muscle
Sudden muscular shoulder girdle efforts
Large, pendulous breasts

TABLE 55.2. Signs and symptoms.

Neurological
Peripheral
    Pain
    Numbness
    Paresthesia
Sympathetic
    Raynaud's disease
    Color
Central: transient blindness

Muscular
Weakness
Atrophy
Dropping items

Vascular
Venous
    Edema
    Venous distentions
    Thrombosis (Paget–Schroetter syndrome)
Arterial
    Coldness
    Absent pulse
    Ulceration
    Claudication
    Pain

Other
Chest pain
Cervical tenderness

physician and the subsequent referral to us. Generally, these symptoms are relieved in a few hours or days after the patient decreases or eliminates the activity to which he or she ascribes the etiology. Switching from ironing to using drip-dry clothes, and not washing windows may help. The dishwasher, the typist, and the long-distance automobile or truck driver have all learned methods to improve their situation and relieve pains and other symptoms. The modification of any repetitive action, whether it be work related, sleeping in an unusual position, or entertainment such as bowling, may improve the paresthesias, numbness, and pain.

However, approximately 10% of these patients will be seen with weakness in the upper extremity, particularly in the interosseous muscles of the fingers. Muscular atrophy and weakness in lifting have been noted. Some patients develop such weakness that they are unable to carry their child, a sack of groceries, or a pack sack, or lift a bucket. These individuals, particularly when they have demonstrably diminished function of the nerves and muscles, require greater consideration and quicker intervention than those who are able to modify their activity levels. For most patients, the discomfort has developed over a long period of time and a specific date, time, or incident that initiated the problem cannot be pinpointed. The exception to this is the individual who has been in an accident or some other acute stress situation, including exercise, that clearly initiated the problem and brought them to the physician. It may be very difficult to differentiate among C7 to C8, the median nerve, and herniated cervical disc compression as the source of many of these symptoms (Table 55.3). It may become particularly difficult in those individuals who have a cervical rib, as this rib may compress components of the lower cervical and T1 nerves.

Other symptoms of TOS include development of chest pain and shoulder discomfort on the side of the abnormality. On occasion the chest pain may be more prominent than the extremity discomfort, and therefore evaluation may be directed away from the neck, thoracic outlet, and upper extremity, and more toward the chest and the heart. In fact, over the years, cardiac catheterization and even cardiac surgical procedures have been performed in individuals to treat the chest pain, without relief. On further evaluation, some of these individuals have been found to have the TOS. Symptoms involving the shoulder, arm, and hand may be correlated with a headache or cervical pain on the affected side.[6-8] In a large percentage of patients, the ipsilateral supraclavicular or lower cervical area is tender to the touch.

Occasionally patients complain of symptoms that emanate from vascular compression or compromise.[9] These individuals may have an acutely thrombosed vein (thrombosis of effort), with a markedly swollen arm, a reddened or a cord-like structure near the axilla, and pain in the extremity. Others may develop acute arterial

TABLE 55.3. Thoracic outlet syndrome: differential diagnosis.

Arterial
Embolic
Raynaud's disease
Occlusive vascular disease
Aneurysms
Atherosclerosis
Reflex, vasomotor

Venous
Thrombosis of effort
Superior vena caval obstruction
Malignant compressive syndrome

Cervical spine and spinal cord
Spinal cord tumor
Ruptured intervertebral disk
Severe arthritis
Neurologic disorders (such as Lou Gehrig's disease)

Compressive syndromes
Carpal tunnel or median nerve syndrome
Entrapment of an ulnar nerve at the elbow
Radial nerve
Traumatic syndromes (hyperextension, whiplash)
Brachial plexus effects of Pancoast's tumor
Traumatic brachial plexus injuries
Shoulder tear or instability
Orthosis appliances

Atypical or other
Coronary artery disease
Lung—pancoast tumors
Chest wall injury or boney abnormality
Esophageal pain

ischemic symptoms with a white, painful extremity or even a functionless extremity. Fortunately, these symptoms are uncommon. More usual is the individual who complains of a cold hand that is weak and fatigues readily. In these individuals, the pain has a different distribution than one ordinarily sees with a neurologic compression. In these individuals, absence of a pulse or the discoloration of the extremity, including the shoulder, arm, or hand, should lead one to consider thoracic outlet vascular compression.

Diagnostic Criteria

The patient's history and physical findings are certainly the most important aspects of the diagnosis of TOS and the differentiation of this syndrome from other potential causes. Again, we believe that, for many patients, this is a matter of exclusion rather than a matter of being able to perform a specific test that leads to a specific diagnosis. In fact, for many patients complaining of neurologic symptoms, it has been very difficult for us to determine whether the symptoms arose from the spinal cord, the spinal neuroexits (foramena), the brachial plexus, or the extremity and its specific nerve. Therefore, the history and physical examination may need to be performed from a number of aspects including primary care, the neurosurgical, the orthopedic, the vascular, and the thoracic surgical. The practitioners of each specialty examine the patient with a different concept and consideration.

From the physical aspect, neurologic examination by a qualified neurologist or neurosurgeon may be most important in delineating the underlying causative agent. However, the surgeon performing corrective treatment on the thoracic outlet should also perform a neurologic examination of the patient. We routinely test for function and strength of the upper and lower extremities, for reflexes, for light touch and deep pain sensation, for pinprick determination, and for gait and other neurologic problems. The most commonly performed studies for TOS are the vascular compressive maneuvers (Table 55.4).[10,11] The studies that we most frequently perform include the following:

1. We examine the patient while he or she is in the position in which he or she most frequently notes the problem, including the radial pulse, to see if there is a compression, a diminution, or an obliteration of the pulse. At the same time, we will examine the neck for any mass, tenderness, or cervical rib abnormalities, and for change in color of the extremity or lack of sensation of the extremity.

2. The Adson maneuver, as described in 1951, in which the scalenus anticus and medius are tightened, decreases the interscalene space and compresses the subclavian artery and the brachial plexus.[12,13] With the neck extended, the patient turns his or her head toward the opposite side while taking a deep breath; in this position, one is able to evaluate the radial pulse. Quite commonly, it is absent on both the symptomatic and the nonsymptomatic sides. This suggests a bilateral compression obstruction and unilateral compression syndrome.

3. In the hypermilitary position (the costoclavicular test), the shoulders are thrown backward and downward. The patient may or may not take a deep breath at the same time. With the narrowing of the costoclavicular space, we may again evaluate the pulse for the

effect of compression on the neurovascular bundle and the potential for producing symptoms.

4. The hyperabduction test is performed when the arm is at 180 degrees. With the arm in this position the structures around the pectoralis minor tendon, coracoid process, and head of the humerus may be compressed. We may also have the patient turn his or her head to the side in an attempt to exaggerate these positions.

5. The arm is routinely pulled downward when the patient is in a neutral position; the radial artery is examined for any effect on the pulse.

6. Quite frequently, patients notice symptoms while their arms are in certain positions, particularly when their arms are overhead. Therefore, we also have the patient place his or her arms overhead and check the pulse. If the radial pulse diminishes and these are the positions in which symptoms develop, we believe we have a positive result from a highly correlative test.

Laboratory studies may be performed to further evaluate the patient and help avoid operating on an individual who may have a different problem that will not benefit from first rib resection or scalenotomy. Therefore, electromyography and nerve conduction studies may be performed. These studies, most often, are normal in individuals with minimal or lesser symptomatology. The individual who has weakness or atrophy almost always has significantly abnormal electromyography and nerve conduction results. The average ulnar nerve conduction velocity may be measured across the thoracic outlet, the elbow, the forearm, and the wrist (Table 55.5). Patients with TOS may have reduction in ulnar nerve velocity. Many times one may also find an abnormality suggestive of a carpal tunnel syndrome or ulnar nerve compression. These individuals should have those problems corrected prior to thoracic outlet surgery because the risk of surgery for those conditions is less than for thoracic outlet surgery. On occasion, the patient requires more than one type of surgical procedure to relieve symptoms. Abnormal electromyography results, particularly with fasciculations, are found only on occasion, but when they are found they are rather significant. Once again, one should remember that most diagnoses are based primarily on the patient's history and physical examination and may or may not be confirmed with laboratory studies. Sometimes, somatosensory evoked potentials are used to evaluate these patients. We use them only on occasion.

TABLE 55.4. Diagnostic criteria.

History and physical
Examine in position creating problem
Outlet or compression maneuvers
    Adson (scalene)
    Anticus (costoclavicular)
    Hyperabduction
    Overhead
Laboratory
    Antinuclear antibody
    Electromyography
    Nerve conduction
    Somatosensory evoked potential

TABLE 55.5. Normal ulnar nerve conduction studies.

	Mean (m/s)	Normal limit (m/s)
Erb's point to axilla	68	58
Axilla to elbow	63	53
Elbow	51	43
Elbow to wrist	61	51

TABLE 55.6. X-ray procedures.

Chest x-ray
Cervical/thoracic spine
Clavicle
Previous x-rays
Cervical myelography
Computerized tomography (C-T)
Magnetic resonance imaging (MRI)
Angiograms: in various positions
    Arch
    Retrograde subclavian
    Venogram
    Cardiac or coronary catheterization
    Intravenous digital subtraction angiograms
Stress test
    Thallium
    Exercise
Duplex scanning

X-ray Studies

A large percentage of patients have multiple x-ray procedures performed (Table 55.6). The symptoms and the physical findings may lead one to perform cervical and upper thoracic spine x-rays to look for bony abnormalities. One may also x-ray the clavicles and the chest, particularly in patients who have had previous trauma to the upper chest or lower neck. These x-rays may be particularly important when bony abnormalities are noted; these may be of a congenital nature. Obtaining previous x-rays may assist in allaying concerns of a possible neoplasm when the patient has felt a hard mass in the neck and developed symptoms. The patient may assume that it is a malignancy when in reality it is an abnormal first or cervical rib with a large synostosis.

Recently we have used Magnetic resonance imaging in a number of our patients to delineate their anatomy and their problem, as well as to see if there is a specific mass or deformity that may be creating the problem. Computed tomography scans of the neck and spine as well as cervical myelography are common studies performed in an attempt to determine whether the patient's symptoms arise from the spinal cord, a ruptured disc, or an extra spinal thoracic outlet process.

Angiographic Studies

In the 1960s and 1970s, a large percentage of patients with a thoracic outlet problem were evaluated by both physical examination and diagnostic angiography. Both venography of the subclavian and the axillary veins and arteriography were performed. The arteriograms were performed with archograms in the antegrade fashion, or retrograde studies on the extremity to evaluate the subclavian and innominate vessels. One can inject the dye, with the arm in different positions, to evaluate the func-

tion and the possible obstruction of these vessels. Certainly the presence of a bruit would be suggestive of possible vascular involvement. Angiographic studies are usually not necessary for the majority of patients. As mentioned earlier, coronary angiography and cardiac catheterization studies, Thallium stress tests, and exercise stress tests have been performed on occasion in the evaluation of these patients.

Other diagnostic studies, including experimental microcirculation or quantitative vascular studies involving the extremity are usually not necessary.

Differential Diagnosis

The differential diagnosis is very long, very difficult, and varies with the type of symptoms the patient has. Patients may be seen because of pain, paresthesias, or vascular or cardiac symptoms. Thus, the evaluation and differential diagnosis is extended and includes the spinal cord, cervical spine, brachial plexus, peripheral nerve complex, and thoracic and cardiac problems, as shown in Table 55.3.[14,15]

Treatment

The initial goal for care of the patient with upper extremity symptoms concerns obtaining an adequate diagnosis. Once the diagnosis has been established, the treatment can be determined. If the patient and the physician realize that many patients with TOS have symptoms that wax and wane, the symptoms will be easier to treat. In some patients, the symptoms may continue to worsen without ever returning to a normal level or plateau. In our practice, we take a conservative approach to treatment, utilizing appropriate laboratory and radiologic evaluation and an understanding review of the patient's situation. Many times, when one takes the necessary appropriate time—up to an hour of discussion—particularly at either the first or second visit, pointing out possible ways to reduce or eliminate the discomfort or the situation without an interventional approach, the patient may experience relief and at the same time avoid the risk of a surgical procedure.

If a diagnosis of mild TOS or a radiculopathy (or neuropathy) has been made without this being ascribed to the thoracic outlet obstruction, the patient should be followed with a conservative nonoperative approach that uses analgesics (preferably nonnarcotic), muscle relaxants, physiotherapy, and change of lifestyle and job activities (Table 55.7). Lifestyle and job changes might mean raising or lowering the level of a typewriter or computer, washing a few dishes and then drying a few, changing to drip-dry clothing, changing jobs, changing from long-distance driving to "short hops," hiring someone to wash

TABLE 55.7. Nonoperative therapy of the patient with thoracic outlet syndrome.

Physiotherapy
Posture improvement
Heat
Exercise to strengthen and stretch

Medication
Analgesics (nonnarcotic)
Muscle relaxants
Anticoagulants
Thrombolytics

Change in lifestyle
Workplace
Home chores

Psychiatric
Patience/understanding
Therapy (where warranted)

walls and ceilings, altering sleep positions and so forth. Utilizing this conservative approach, most patients will not require surgical intervention. We see a moderate number of new patients with the potential diagnosis of TOS and yet we seldom operate on these patients because of our patience and understanding of the individual's circumstances. The patient who has escalating symptoms without improvement under conservative treatment, especially if the symptoms have been ongoing for more than a year, will be considered for surgical intervention. Patients who have suffered whiplash or other types of trauma, have had symptoms for only a few weeks, and in whom no previous symptoms occurred are less likely candidates for surgery. Massage, heat and cold therapy, and various exercises have all been used with some degree of benefit. No single approach has been uniformly successful for these patients.[16,17]

Surgical Intervention

For patients who have neurologic or vascular symptoms without vascular thrombosis or aneurysm formation, a number of surgical techniques are available.[5,17,18] When warranted, resection and correction of the underlying

TABLE 55.8. Surgical approaches.

Rib resection (first or cervical)
Transaxillary
Anterior
  Supraclavicular
  Infraclavicular
Posterior (thoracoplasty approach)
Thoracoscopic

Clavicle resection

Soft tissue transsection or resection
Scalene
Pectoralis minor tendon
Breast reduction

anatomic pathology, using the approaches listed in Table 55.8, have been undertaken.

Transaxillary Rib Resection

This is the most common procedure that we perform, especially in young, thin females. The patient is placed on his or her back with the symptomatic side elevated approximately 15 to 20 degrees on a sand bag. The patient's effected extremity is then held up by an individual, such that the arm is flexed at the elbow and there is light to moderate traction or tension. The assistant, if short, should stand on a low platform for their ease and comfort in holding up the extremity. The patient's extremity, axilla, anterior chest, supraclavicular area, and area posterior to the axilla are then surgically prepped using a paint-on material (Duraprep). A loose stockinette is placed over the hand and arm, up to near the axilla. The assistant holding the arm should, every 5 or 10 minutes, relax the arm so that there is not undue pressure on the neurovascular bundles. A physician provides retraction in the axilla. The surgeon makes an incision approximately three to four inches in length in the axilla beneath the hairline. This is carried down to the lateral thoracic fascia. Dissection is carried upward along the chest wall to the area of the first rib, using care to avoid the intercostal brachiocutaneous nerve exiting from the second interspace.

We approach the first rib with blunt dissection, using the tip of the finger and a blunt "gray mixter" rather then a sharp, right-angle mixter. We then approach the first rib from below and encircle it extraperiosteally, pushing the parietal pleura off the rib. We then go around the top of the rib and locate and encircle the scalenus anticus muscle. The scalenus anticus is then divided. The first rib is cleaned anteriorly to its costoclavicular junction and transected at that point. Any sharp edge is removed with a rongeur. The first rib is then dissected posteriorly with blunt dissection—usually the finger. At this point, with the gray mixter, the scalenus medias muscle is encircled posteriorly and divided under direct vision, being sure to avoid any nerve fibers and to preserve the long thoracic nerve. The first rib is then transected far posteriorly near the transverse process and removed. If there is a cervical rib present, this also is cleared with blunt dissection. At times it is necessary to use the periosteal elevator. We then check for bleeding. Throughout the procedure we lift the arm for periods of only 5 to 10 minutes to avoid any tension on the nerves. Utilizing this technique, one can usually complete the entire procedure in 45 to 60 minutes. If a hole or rent has been made in the pleura, a chest tube is placed and brought out of the lower margin of the incision, then placed under water until the wound is closed. The tube is then removed in most instances. The wound is closed with running 2-O Chromic sutures and running subcuticular 4-O undyed Vicryl. Steri-strips are applied. A postoperative chest x-ray and blood count (CBC) are done. The patient will usually go home on the second or third day.

Supraclavicular Approach

There are a number of physicians, including ourselves, who have used the supraclavicular approach in the past for either first rib resection or scalenotomy. Some individuals believe that the scalene muscle should first be transected through a small supraclavicular incision and that no rib resection should be performed unless there is gross abnormality or if the scalenotomy does not provide the symptomatic relief the patient desires. We have found this approach to be difficult for adequate resection of the first rib and, in addition, have found mobilization of the neurovascular structures to be more complicated.

Infraclavicular Approach

With the patient supine and adequately prepped, an approach to the first rib may be made beneath the clavicle with a transverse incision. The incision may be somewhat disturbing to patients concerned about the cosmetic appearance of the scar. With this approach, anatomic considerations become more difficult, particularly when one performs it on a very infrequent basis. This procedure has been championed by some surgeons.

Posterior Thoracoplasty Approach

The posterior thoracoplasty incision has been used on occasion by ourselves in individuals who had previous transaxillary first rib surgery. The patient is positioned on the side opposite to the side where the surgery takes place and may be somewhat rotated toward the anterior. Access to the first rib may be obtained readily with a high incision. Again, it is an incision that is somewhat less cosmetically acceptable and, in our opinion, results in a more major surgical procedure than the transaxillary approach.

Vascular Surgery

For those patients with acute vascular thrombosis, particularly arterial occlusion with ischemia, loss of function, or ulceration of the digits, we, as others, have used a number of surgical procedures.[19] If possible, we prefer the resection of the first rib, followed by revascularization (thrombectomy, embolectomy, thromboendarterectomy, and/or bypass). With this technique, our patients have been fortunate to avoid the loss of any digit, extremity, or function. Venous thrombosis or occlusion has

TABLE 55.9. Other surgical approaches.

Arterial
Thrombectomy
Embolectomy
End-to-end anastomosis
Bypass graft (vein or synthetic)
Concomitant bony resection

Neural
Dorsal sympathectomy
Video assisted or open
Neurolysis

Venous: thrombectomy (uncommon)

Soft tissue

been a more difficult problem to treat. On a short-term basis we have utilized anticoagulant therapy, rest, and avoidance of the causative exercise or activity. Most of these patients, on follow-up, have resolved the thrombus, opened up the subclavian vein, or developed collateral circulation so that no further intervention is necessary. Thrombolytics have been given to some of these individuals, and subclavian or cephalic vein thrombectomy in association with first rib resection has also been considered. However, only a minority of patients are likely to need such therapy.

Other Surgical Approaches

We have performed resection of the clavicle in those individuals who have had previous trauma to the clavicle and marked deformity (Table 55.9).We believe that we are able to expose the clavicle and the bony abnormality more readily in this fashion than with a deep approach.

Resection of the coracoid process and the proximal humerus have been carried out by some surgeons. We have not performed either of these procedures. More recently, video-assisted thoracic surgery resection of the first rib has been accomplished for TOS and dorsal sympathectomy.[20,21] Neurolysis of the brachial plexus has also been utilized.[22,23]

Complications

The definition of a complication and concerns for the patient vary somewhat with the individual performing the therapy or surgery. One of the more difficult considerations for this syndrome is whether the patient will find symptomatic relief.[24] This is particularly true for individuals who do not have any gross abnormalities discernible from x-ray, EMG, and nerve conduction tests, or physical examination. We caution these people prior to surgery as to their potential for improvement. Many of these patients are asked to see a psychiatrist prior to surgery. In addition, we caution the patient that there will be more discomfort for a few weeks after surgery than there was preoperatively. Presumably this occurs because of potential stretching and pulling on the neurovascular bundle, as well as the postoperative surgical incision discomfort. Therefore, we are slow to judge whether the operation has been beneficial until 6 to 8 weeks or longer after surgery.

Neurologic complications are discussed with each patient, including the potential for injury to the nerve transversing the axilla and potential for permanent or transient numbness of the axilla and the inner arm depending, on whether the nerve is stretched, severed, or severely traumatized (Table 55.10). Further, we discuss the potential for postoperative brachial plexus injuries and loss of function of the extremity as a result of the surgery, particularly if there are extensive adhesions and bands around the neurovascular bundle. In order to avoid these consequences, the arm is retracted or held by an assistant rather than being hung on a standard. We then relax the arm frequently to avoid prolonged tension. We are aware of the rare person who has lost partial or complete function of the extremity after this surgery. Fortunately, we ourselves have not had patients with these difficulties.

Vascular injury and bleeding must be a concern for each surgeon performing this type of surgery. The vein may occasionally be entrenched in an adhesive fibrous tissue, which makes it difficult to dissect free. We have had to suture the subclavian vein on one occasion. Arterial injuries are a possibility. Again we have been fortunate, even with the patients requiring reconstruction, to not have any iatrogenic or arterial complications. One person who required postoperative heparinization bled into the right chest after a right transaxillary approach when the pleura was opened. This patient had a chest tube inserted for removal of the intrapleural blood and received a blood transfusion.

The most common complication that we have seen with the transaxillary approach has been the occurrence of pneumothorax when the pleura develops a rent or opening. This is almost always a benign condition and rarely requires postoperative chest tube drainage. Resolution is usually obtained by an intraoperative tube that is removed at the end of surgery while positive pressure is applied by the anesthesiologist on the endotracheal tube. Wound infection has been uncommon. An occasional suture granuloma resolves on removal of the absorbable subcuticular suture knot.

Results

The treatment and diagnosis of TOS have varied. A large portion of our patients do not receive any surgical intervention and are treated with a conservative nonoperative approach that uses the measures discussed in this chapter. Most patients are able to maintain or improve their condition with the noninvasive approach. Many of them eventually become symptom free following changes in posture and activity (Table 55.11). The occasional person who has required surgical intervention, by and large, has had a good result. However, approximately 20% may return with persistent, recurrent, or new symptoms. In this group, consideration of potential recurrent TOS or a misdiagnosis must be entertained. We routinely perform postoperative chest x-rays to be sure that the correct rib and appropriate amount of the rib was resected. We have seen patients in consultation who had the second rib resected rather than the first rib. These individuals almost always require a second procedure to resect the remaining first rib or cervical rib.

It is of interest that the patients with recurrent or persistent TOS may have had no radial artery pulse palpable prior to the first surgery, and after surgery they may have a good pulsation during all compression maneuvers. Yet, despite the return of a good pulse, their symptoms have not decreased. These individuals warrant additional evaluation to exclude another diagnoses. Most patients are very pleased with the surgical procedure and are much improved compared with their preoperative condition. Accurate clinical and laboratory evalua-

TABLE 55.10. Complications.

Neural
Brachial plexus
Long thoracic nerve
Intercostal brachiocutaneous
Traction

Arterial
Rupture
Thrombosis

Venous: tear

Symptomatology
No improvement
Worsening
Recurrent

Pneumothorax

Bleeding

Wound: suture granuloma

Bony
Removal of wrong rib
Inadequate removal of rib
Regrowth of rib

TABLE 55.11. Results.

75–80%	Good
10–15%	Fair
10%	No improvement
3–5%	Reoperation

tion, with a tendency toward conservatism, will relieve the physician of a large of number patients who do not benefit from surgery. On occasion, a psychiatric referral prior to surgical treatment is appropriate. Our goal is to avoid a negative result and work toward a higher success rate.

Dr. Esteban Noda of Puerto Rico has written and spoken extensively on the cerebellar thoracic outlet syndrome (CTOS). He describes neck and brain transitory vascular compression causing neurological lesions.[25] He has postulated a relationship between TOS and central neurologic symptoms including Parkinson's disease and ipsilateral paralysis. We have no experience in the diagnosis and treatment of CTOS. Dr. Noda presents his experience with positron emission tomography scans and single photon emission computed tomography, as well as his surgical experience with bilateral scalenotomy.

References

1. Borchardt M. Symptomatologie und therapie der halsrippen. *Berliner Klinische Wochenschrift.* 1901;38:1265.

2. Coote H. Pressure on the axillary vessels and nerve by an exostosis from a cervical rib: interference with circulation of the arm; removal of the rib, exostosis: recovery. *Medical Times Gazette.* 1861;2:108.

3. Naffziger HC, Grant WT. Neuritis of the brachial plexus mechanical in origin: the scalenus syndrome. *Surgery, Gynecology and Obstetrics.* 1938;67:722–730.

4. Roos DB. Transaxillary approach for first rib resection to relieve thoracic outlet syndrome. *Ann Surg.* 1966;163:354–358.

5. Urschel HC Jr, Razzuk MA, Baue AE. Thoracic outlet syndrome. In: Baue AE, Geha AS, Hammond GL, Laks H, Naunheim KS, eds. *Glenn's Thoracic and Cardiovascular Surgery.* Norwalk, Conn: Appleton and Lange; 1991:495–505.

6. Dawson DM. Entrapment neuropathies of the upper extremities. *N Engl J Med.* 1993;329:2013–2018.

7. Urschel JD, Hameed SM, Grewal RP. Neurogenic thoracic outlet syndromes. *Postgrad Med J.* 1994;70:785–789.

8. Levin LS, Dellon AL. Pathology of the shoulder as it relates to the differential diagnosis of thoracic outlet compression. *J Reconst Microsurg.* 1992;8:313–317.

9. Sill JJ, Rael JR, Orrison WW. Rotational vertebro-basilar insufficiency as a component of thoracic outlet syndrome resulting in transient blindness. *J Neurosurg.* 1994;81:617–619.

10. Novak CB, Mackinnon ES, Patterson GA. Evaluation of patients with thoracic outlet syndrome. *J Hand Surg.* 1993;18A:292–299.

11. Harding A, Silver D. Thoracic outlet syndrome. In: Sabiston DC Jr, ed. *Textbook of Surgery.* Philadelphia, Pa: WB Saunders; 1991:1757–1761.

12. Adson AW. Cervical ribs: symptoms, differential diagnosis for section of the scalenus anticus muscle. *Journal of the International College of Surgeons.* 1951;16:546–559.

13. Urschel HC Jr, Razzuk HA. Thoracic outlet syndrome. In: Sabiston DC Jr, Spencer FC, eds. *Surgery of the Chest.* Philadelphia, Pa: WB Saunders; 1990:536–553.

14. Hama H, Matsusue Y, Ite H, et al. Thoracic outlet syndrome associated with an anomalous coracoclavicular joint. *J Bone Joint Surg.* 1993;75-A:1368–1369.

15. Deck KL, Vasquez BR. The vannini rizzoli orthosis. A unique case of thoracic outlet syndrome. *Arch Phys Med Rehabil.* 1993;74:441–444.

16. Kenny RA, Traynor GB, Withington D, et al. Thoracic outlet syndrome: A useful exercise treatment option. *Am J Surg.* 1993;165:228–284.

17. Leffert RD. Thoracic outlet syndrome. *Hand Clinics.* 1992;8:285–297.

18. Carty NJ, Carpenter R, Webster JHH. Continuing experience with transaxillary excision of the first rib for thoracic outlet syndrome. *Br J Surg.* 1992;79:761–762.

19. Sander RJ, Haug C. Review of arterial thoracic outlet syndrome with a report of five new instances. *Surgery, Gynecology and Obstetrics.* 1991;173:415–425.

20. Green R. Thoracoscopic first rib resection [video]. First Annual Symposium of Vascular and Endovascular Techniques. June 2, 1995, Grand Hyatt Hotel, New York.

21. Urschel HC Jr. Dorsal sympathectomy and management of thoracic surgery. *Ann Thorac Surg.* 1993;56:717–720.

22. Wood VE, Ellison DW. Results of upper plexus thoracic outlet syndrome operation. *Ann Thorac Surg.* 1994;58:458–461.

23. Dellon AL. The results of supraclavicular brachial plexus neurolysis (without first rib resection) in management of post-traumatic "thoracic outlet syndrome." *J Reconstr Microsurg.* 1993;9:11–17.

24. Cherington M, Cherington C. Thoracic outlet syndrome: reimbursement patterns and patient profiles. *Neurology.* 1992;42:943–945.

25. Noda E, Nunez-Arguelles J, Silva F, et al. Neck and brain transitory vascular compression causing neurological lesions. Results of surgical treatment on 900 patients. *Clin Pharmacol Ther.* 1993;3:789–803.

56

Surgery and the Vertebral Arteries

Egidijus M. Barkauskas and Povilas A. Pauliukas

Introduction

The diagnostic procedures, indications for surgery, and operative techniques for carotid artery occlusive diseases are well established. The role of the vertebral arteries (VAs) in supplying blood to the brain, and the value of surgical repair of stenotic lesions of the VAs are still underestimated by neurologists and most vascular surgeons.

For a long time, reconstructive surgery of the VAs was performed only occasionally by a few vascular surgeons. In the 1980s and 1990s, experience with VA surgery developed in several vascular surgery centers. In recent years most vascular surgery centers have begun to operate on VAs. Neurologists and angiologists have also begun to appreciate the relationship between stenotic lesions of the VAs and symptoms of ischemia in vertebrobasilar territory, as well as the effectiveness of surgical correction of the VAs in these cases. With improved surgical techniques, VA surgery is no longer considered too difficult and dangerous. Nevertheless, there is still a lot of controversy concerning surgical treatment of vertebrobasilar insufficiency (VBI). In cases of multiple carotid artery and VA lesions, understanding the role of the circle of Willis in the redistribution of the blood supply to the brain and appreciation of this structure's abnormalities are the keys to deciding which artery to operate.

The anomalies of the VAs emerge as a distinct pathology in patients with VBI. In these patients the circle of Willis is typically disconnected posteriorly (both posterior communicating arteries are absent), so it can't compensate for insufficient blood flow from the carotid arteries in the vertebrobasilar region.

This information in this chapter is based on our 25-year experience in VA surgery; to May 1995 1142 VA operations were performed on 1112 patients with VBI.

History

Cate and Scott were pioneers in VA surgery. In 1953 they performed the first direct operation on a VA: a transsubclavian endarterectomy.[13] In 1958 Crawford and De Bakey were the first to publish their experience in VA surgery.[17] The results of anatomic studies on cadavers made by Hutchinson and Yates in 1956 provided great impetus for the development of VA surgery.[32] They found that approximately 70% of patients who had died due to vertebrobasilar stroke, had atherosclerotic stenotic or occlusive lesions in their VAs, most of which were at their origins at the subclavian arteries. Clinical and angiographic studies showed that such lesions cause a decreased blood flow in the vertebrobasilar territory of the brain and, therefore, the neurological symptoms of VBI described by Denny-Brown in 1953.[19] Contorni in 1960[16] described the subclavian steal syndrome as including symptoms of VBI, associated with a reversed flow in the VA supplying the blood to the arm in cases where the proximal part of the subclavian artery is occluded. He proposed a surgical repair in these cases to restore normal blood flow in the subclavian artery, which in turn reverses to normal the flow of blood in the VA. Powers et al[50] described the lateral and posterior branching of the VA from the subclavian artery and successfully corrected this pathology by excision of the scalenus anterior muscle, ligation and transection of the thyrocervical trunk, and desympatization of the VA. Hardin and Poser[26] were the first to describe the extravasal compression of the first portion of the VA by the fascial bands. They proved the hemodynamic significance of this pathology by angiography: the first portion of the VA was stenosed or even occluded while rotating the head to the opposite side. At operation they found the fibrous bands crossing and compressing the first portion of the VA. Their surgical procedure included scalenotomy, transection of fibrous bands crossing the VA, transection of the thyrocervical trunk, and fixation of the subclavian artery using the thyrocervical stump to the scalenus anterior stump on the first rib. They used the same procedure for the straightening of the kinked VAs. They stated that straightening the VA in this way was a safer procedure than direct reconstructive shortening of the VA. After these operations, angiography revealed normal lumen of the VA in all head positions. Hurvitz[31] described the extraluminal compressions of the VAs in cases of VBI and successfully cured these patients by surgical decompression and desympatization of the VAs. He found that the sympathetic trunk or its branches were often the causes of VA compression. The hemodynamic importance of VA kinks were appreciated and surgically managed by Imparato,[33] Imparato and Lin,[35] Wesolowski et al,[62] and Barkauskas.[3] The anatomic studies by Daseler and Anson[18] showed that anomalies of the VAs are encountered often. Husni et al[29,30] described the entrapment of the VA between the scalenus anterior and longus colli muscles just below its entrance into the transverse process of the sixth cervical vertebra. He proposed a surgical procedure to excise the scalenus anterior muscle and the lateral edge of longus colli muscle and then interposition adipose tissue between these muscles to prevent scarring. Postoperative angiography showed normal VAs on the operated side, whereas preoperative angiography had shown stenosis or even occlusion with the neck extended and head rotated to the opposite side. They stressed the importance of functional angiography in such cases. The clinical importance and surgical treatment of VA anomalies have been studied by us intensively since 1977.[4,46–48] Atherosclerotic lesions of the VAs at their origins have been managed in different ways: vertebral artery endarterectomy with an autovenous patch,[33–35,58] autovenous shunt from the subclavian artery to the side of vertebral artery,[6] reimplantation of the VA into the subclavian artery,[3,5,45] and transposition of the VA into the common carotid artery.[7–9,11,14,20,21,39] In cases of thrombosed V1 and V2 segments of the VA or when the VA has multiple stenotic lesions of the V2 segment due to atherosclerosis or cervical osteochondrosis, revascularization of the distal VA between C1–C2 transverse processes has been increasingly used by vascular surgeons.[6–9,25,34,39] Neurosurgeons have also performed direct endarterectomies on the V4 segment of the VA and created extraintracranial anastomoses to the arteries of the vertebrobasilar region.[28,36,44,55,57]

The surgical treatment of VBI is still lagging behind surgical treatment of the carotid artery. Much controversy exists among vascular surgeons concerning the indications, tactics, and even techniques for surgical treatment of VBI.

Normal Anatomy of the Vertebrobasilar System and Anomalies of the VAs

Normally the left and the right VA are the first branches of subclavian arteries. The left VA originates from the aortic arch in 2.5% of the population (anatomic studies by E. Daseler and B. Anson[18]). The right VA originates from the aortic arch in only 0.1% of angiographically studied patients.[47,48] Normally both VAs enter the canalis transversarius at the C6 transverse process. The VA enters the canalis transversarius at the C5 transverse process in 6.6% of the population.[18] The incidence of this anomaly is the same for both left and right VAs. The VA enters the canalis transversarius at the C4 level in 0.5% of the population.[18]

For practical purposes the VA is divided into four portions. The V1 portion commences at the orifice of the vertebral artery and continues to its into the canalis transversarius at the C6 transverse process. The V2 portion constitutes the segment of the VA that is in the canalis transversarius from the C6 transverse process to the C2 transverse process. The V3 portion constitutes the section from the C2 transverse process to the atlanto-occipital membrane. The V4 portion is the intracranial part of the VA. The V4 portions of the VAs obliquely cross the ventral surface of the medulla oblongata and join to form a basilar artery that is ventral to the pons cerebri. The basilar artery branches into two posterior cerebral arteries, which are connected with intracranial internal carotid arteries by posterior communicating arteries. The right and left anterior cerebral arteries are connected by the anterior communicating artery.

Normally, the main intracranial arteries (anterior, middle, and posterior cerebral arteries) are connected together by the circle of Willis. The blood flow can be shifted from one carotid artery to another through the anterior communicating artery and from carotid arteries to the vertebrobasilar territory through the posterior communicating arteries or, vice versa, from the vertebrobasilar territory to the carotid (anterior) circulation. The impressive ability of the circle of Willis to distribute the blood flow is illustrated in Figure 56.1. Both internal carotid arteries are occluded in this patient; the reconstructed dominant left VA supplies blood to all six main cerebral arteries. However, only 50% of the population have a normal circle of Willis.[1,51] The most common abnormality of the circle of Willis is absence of one or both posterior communicating arteries.[1] In these cases the posterior cerebral artery sometimes originates from the internal carotid artery (so-called posterior trifurcation of internal carotid artery). The so-called anterior trifurcation of the internal carotid artery (both anterior cere-

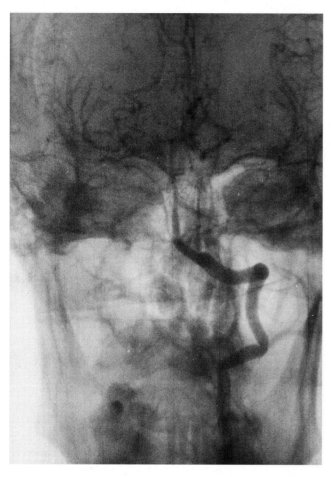

FIGURE 56.1. Six main cerebral arteries supplied from the reconstructed left VA.

bral arteries are branches of the same internal carotid artery, and the contralateral carotid artery has only one branch—the middle cerebral artery) is encountered in 0.5% of angiographically studied patients.[47,48] The anterior communicating artery is absent in these cases. There can be "quadrifurcation" of the internal carotid artery when both anterior, ipsilateral middle, and posterior cerebral arteries originate from the same internal carotid artery.

The VA usually has no branches in its first portion. However, we have encountered one small VA branch that supplied blood to the deep neck muscles in approximately 1% of operated cases. In its second portion, the VA has segmental rami spinales that supply blood to the medulla spinalis and its cervical roots. The third portion of the VA usually has several muscular and collateral branches connecting it with the cervical ascendens and occipital arteries. In cases of proximal occlusion of the VA they can supply a significant blood flow to the distal vertebral artery. The first branches of V4 portion of the VA are the posterior and anterior spinal branches, which supply blood to the medulla spinalis. The posterior cere-

bellar artery is an important branch of the VA. Occlusion of this branch usually causes significant cerebellar infarct and sometimes lateral medullary infarct, the clinical manifestations of which were described by Wallenberg.[61] The large branches of the basilar artery are the anterior inferior and superior cerebellar arteries. An important branch is arteria labyrinthi. At its distal end, the basilar artery divides into two main branches: the posterior cerebral arteries. Normally they are connected by posterior communicating arteries with the intracranial part of internal carotid arteries. The small penetrating branches of the basilar artery supply blood to the pons cerebri. Small, deep (lacunar) infarcts in the brain stem are caused by the disruption of these small arteries or, less commonly, by occlusion of these arteries in hypertensive and diabetic patients. The hypoplasia (diameter < 2 mm) of one vertebral artery is encountered in 10% of angiographically studied patients).[47] Anatomic studies by Stopford[56] revealed an incidence of 14.7% of one hypoplastic VA. The hypoplasia of the right VA is more common (ratio 2:1) in comparison with the left VA.[47] Hypoplasia of both vertebral arteries is encountered in 0.3% of angiographically studied patients.[47] Aplasia of one vertebral artery is encountered in 0.3% of angiographically studied patients.[47] Out of more than 2000 angiographically studied patients we had one patient with aplasia of both VAs[47]; he had a compensating anomaly: a basilar artery was a continuation of the left hypertrophied occipital artery.[47]

Surgically Important Anomalies of the VAs

Only in patients with a totally posteriorly disconnected circle of Willis are these anomalies of clinical and surgical importance. Otherwise, insufficient blood flow is compensated through the posterior communicating arteries from the carotid arteries. In addition, the contralateral VA in most cases is hypoplastic or anomalous. The spasm of extrinsically compressed VAs is a very important pathogenetic mechanism in developing VBI or even vertebrobasilar stroke.

Lateral Branching of the VA

The VA originates more lateral than normally from the subclavian artery, sometimes even lateral to the thyrocervical trunk. This anomaly is encountered in 3% of the population (anatomic studies by Daseler and Anson[18]) and in 4.2% of patients with VBI evaluated by angiography.[48] In these cases the VA is under the scalenus anterior muscle and can be compressed by the scalenus anterior muscle if the muscle is also compressing the subclavian artery. The augmented linear flow in the proximal VA is revealed by duplex Doppler scanning in these cases.[22] Over one third of these patients have a systolic bruit over the proximal part of the VA; approximately half have upper thoracic outlet symptoms.

Posterior Branching of the VA From the Subclavian Artery

The VA branches from the dorsal aspect of the subclavian artery and kinks just distal to its orifice. The right VA is affected more often that the left, with a ratio of 3:2. The hemodynamic significance of this pathology can be estimated by duplex Doppler scanning and angiographic studies. The posterior branching of the VA from the subclavian artery is easily visualized by duplex Doppler sonography, and its hemodynamic significance is estimated by measuring the blood flow velocity at the kink. Increased flow velocity at the kink (systolic >150 cm/s) and poststenotic turbulent blood flow with dampening of the systolic part of the curve in the V2 segment of the VA are the criteria for hemodynamic significance of posterior branching of the VA from the subclavian artery. The contrast material is injected into the subclavian artery and anterioposterior and oblique views of the proximal part of the VA are visualized on angiograms. The posterior branching is best seen on oblique views. The hypertrophied cervical ascendens artery serving as a collateral is usually seen in these cases.[47,48]

High Entrance of the VA Into the Canalis Transversarius

Longus colli and anterior scalene muscles join together, and their lower fibers intercross and insert onto the C6 transverse process. Normally, the VA enters the canalis transversarius through the C6 transverse process just below the joining of the muscle tendons just mentioned. When the VA enters the canalis transversarius at a point that is higher than the C6 vertebra, it is compressed dorsally between the C6 transverse process and ventrally between the longus colli tendon. The symptoms of VBI manifest when the VA becomes spasmophilic: its reaction to the compression is a vasospasm, which can last minutes, hours, or even days. Entrapment of the VA between the longus colli and scalenus anterior muscles is encountered even in patients with normal entrance of the VA into the canalis transversarius.[29,30,41,47,48] In these cases the tendons of the longus colli and scalenus anterior muscles join lower (below the C6 transverse process) and tightly compress the VA during the retractions of these muscles. Again, spasm of the VA is a dominant pathogenetic mechanism. This type of VA entrapment was recognized and proved angiographically by Husni,[29,30] Kojima et al,[30] and Pauliukas et al.[46–48] Figure 56.2 illustrates a tightly stenosed left VA between the longus colli and scalenus anterior muscles, and the vasoconstricted extracanal part (V1 segment) of the VA. Figure 56.3 illustrates the compression of the VA between the longus colli and scalenus anterior muscles in cases with normal and high

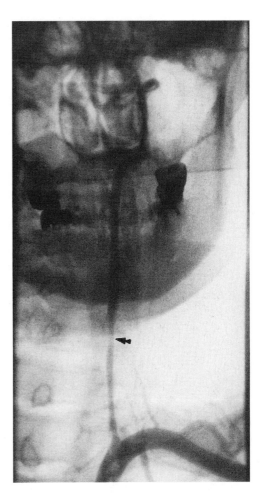

FIGURE 56.2. Compression of the left VA between the longus colli and scalenus anterior muscles (arrow). Note the vasoconstricted extracanal part (V1 segment) and normal V2 segment of the VA.

entrance of the VA into the canalis transversarius, and the typical surgical procedure used for these cases.

Extrinsic Compression of the First Portion of the VA

The most common cause of extrinsic compression of the first portion of the VA is the sympathetic trunk or its lateral branches. The angiographic appearance of this pathology is illustrated in Figure 56.4. Fibrous or fascial bands may also be the cause of extrinsic compression of the VA. During the operation in these cases the VAs are found to be very spasmophilic.

Extrinsic Compression of the VA Between the C1 and C2 Transverse Processes

The short ventral branch of the C2 nerve can be a cause of extrinsic compression).[48,59] Division of the ventral branch of the second cervical nerve in these cases was curative for patients.

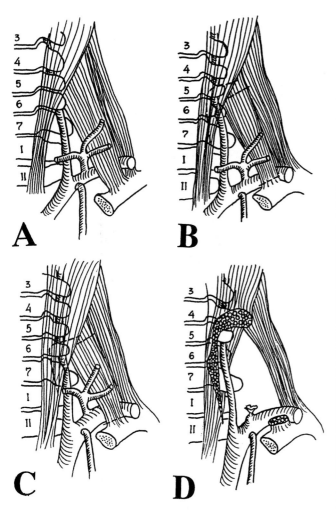

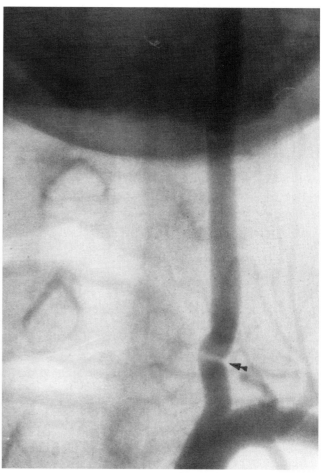

FIGURE 56.4. Extrinsic compression of the first portion of the left VA (arrow) by the sympathetic nerve.

FIGURE 56.3. **A,** Normal anatomical relations between the VA and longus colli and anterior scalenus muscles. **B,** The compression of the VA between the longus colli and the transverse process of the C6 vertebra in a case where the VA enters into the transverse process of the C5 vertebra. **C,** Compression of the VA in a case of abnormal placement of the longus colli muscle and normal entry of the VA into the transverse process of the C6 vertebra. **D,** Typical surgical procedure performed on the patients described in **B** and **C:** total excision of the anterior scalenus muscle and excision of the lateral edge of the longus colli muscle.

Etiology and Pathophysiology

The most common cause of stenotic and occlusive lesions of the VAs is atherosclerosis, and the most common site of involvement is the orifice of the VA. The typical atherosclerotic plaque begins in the subclavian artery several millimeters proximal to the VA and it thickens at the orifice of the VA. The plaque usually ends 3–5 mm distal to the VA orifice. On rare occasions the plaque extends distally, close to the entrance of the VA into the bony canal; sometimes even the V2 segment of the VA is diseased. The V3 segment is usually spared. The intracranial part of the VA or basilar artery is seldom involved. Atherosclerotic stenosis of the basilar artery affects all three of its segments with equal frequency. The proximal stenoses or occlusions of the VAs are more benign than intracranial ones due to the preserved collateral blood supply to the brain through the contralateral VA or through the cervical ascendens and occipital arteries. The pathophysiologic mechanism of VBI in these cases is hypoperfusion of the vertebrobasilar region. The tight

Origin of the VA From the Aortic Arch

When the VA originates from the aortic arch, there are no direct hemodynamic consequences. However, in 86% of cases, these anomalous VAs exert extrinsic compression by means of the sympathetic fibers or longus colli muscle. During operation, high entrance of the VA into the bony canal is often seen and is most likely the ultimate cause of the compression. The angiographic appearance of high entrance of the VA into the canalis transversarius is illustrated in Figure 56.5.

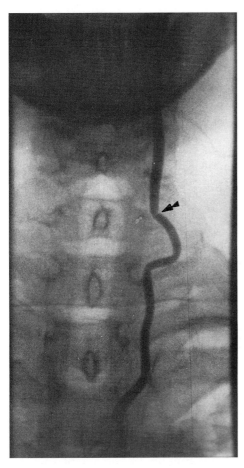

FIGURE 56.5. The left VA originates from the aortic arch and enters the bony canal into the transverse process of the C5 vertebra (arrow).

stenosis or occlusion of the innominate artery and both subclavian arteries causes the so called subclavian steal phenomenon: the arm is supplied by the retrograde blood flow in the ipsilateral VA. The direction of blood flow is normal, and flow is augmented in the opposite VA and is retrograde on diseased side. When the opposite VA is occluded or hypoplastic, reversed blood flow is seen in the basilar artery: the blood to the arm on the diseased side in these cases is supplied from the carotid arteries through the posterior communicating arteries of the circle of Willis. The subclavian steal can be asymptomatic, provided the contralateral VA is normal and the circle of Willis is normal also.[27,39,42] However, when posterior communicating arteries are absent, symptoms manifest as headache, dizziness, chronic VBI, vertebrobasilar transient ischemic attacks (TIAs), or even stroke, pain, or claudication of the ischemic arm. The cause of VBI in these cases is hypoperfusion. Nevertheless, these symptoms rarely result in permanent neurologic damage. Symptoms of VBI and subclavian steal can be present despite ipsilateral VA occlusion. The blood flow in these cases is reversed in the collateral neck arteries sup-

plying the blood to the arm.[49] When the subclavian steal phenomenon is asymptomatic, it does not require surgical correction.[27,42] If the symptoms of VBI or arm ischemia are present, caroticosubclavian bypass is the procedure of choice.[39,54]

Recently, due to magnetic resonance imaging and more widely used digital subtraction four-vessel angiography of brain arteries, the embolic mechanism of vertebrobasilar ischemic stroke is better understood. The source of emboli may be the heart (atrial fibrillation, valvular diseases, myocardial infarction, etc.) and atherosclerotic atheromatous disease of aortic arch, innominate artery, subclavian arteries, and atheromatous plaques in the origins of the VAs. The incidence of embolism arising from the VAs is not known. Berguer[9] and Caplan and Shifrin[12] feel that the embolic mechanism is quite common in vertebrobasilar ischemia. Our experience suggests that the hypoperfusion mechanism prevails in vertebrobasilar ischemia even in patients with atherosclerosis.

In osteochondrosis the V2 segment of the VA can be compressed by osteophytes or by a ruptured intervertebral disc.[53] Herniation of the VA from the bony canal can be the cause of VBI. While turning the head, the VA can be stenosed or even occluded in these cases. Due to compression, intimal damage with or without embolization to the brain vessels or VA thrombosis can occur. Kinks and coils of the V1 portion of the VAs cause hypoperfusion in vertebrobasilar region. Anomalies, extrinsic compressions, and spasm of the VAs are also causes of vertebrobasilar hypoperfusion. Trauma, intimal dissection, fibromuscular dysplasia, arteriovenous malformations, and aneurysms are uncommon lesions of the VAs. Takayasu's arteritis involving subclavian and vertebral arteries is quite common in some Asian countries, and surgical repair of aortic arch branches and, less commonly, VAs is required in some cases.

Clinical Manifestations

Clinical manifestations in vertebrobasilar disease depend on the pathogenetic mechanism of ischemia: embolic/thrombotic or hypoperfusion. The symptoms can arise from the entire vertebrobasilar territory in state of hypoperfusion. The nuclei that are most sensitive to ischemia in the hindbrain are the vestibular and oculomotor nuclei.[41] Hence, the first and most common symptoms in vertebrobasilar hypoperfusion are related to these nuclei: dizziness, vertigo, nausea, vomiting, and diplopia. Ataxia, a common symptom, is related to hypoperfusion of the cerebellum. Hypoperfusion in the area of the posterior cerebral arteries (occipital lobes) manifests as visual disturbances. Common symptoms are headache (mostly occipital) and hearing disturbances

TABLE 56.1. Incidence of symptoms in 1099 patients, who underwent surgery for vertebrobasilar disease.

Symptoms	Number of patients	Percentage
Dizziness	1002	91.2
Visual disturbances	923	84.0
Headache (mostly occipital)	793	72.2
Ataxia	780	71.0
Vertigo episodes	563	51.2
Nausea (vomiting)	553	50.3
Hearing disturbances	538	49.0
Sensory disturbances	512	46.6
Memory deterioration	471	42.9
Episodic or continuous arterial hypertension	406	36.9
Syncopal episodes	203	18.5
Motor disturbances	195	17.7
Dysarthria	180	16.4
Drop attacks	94	8.6

(tinnitus and hypoacusis). Sensor and motor disturbances are less common in vertebrobasilar hypoperfusion. The symptoms resulting from vertebrobasilar hypoperfusion fluctuate and manifest as vertebrobasilar TIAs, chronic VBI, and less commonly, as vertebrobasilar stroke. In most cases, TIAs precede the vertebrobasilar stroke. In two thirds of patients with basilar artery stenosis, TIAs occur before brain stem stroke.[12] In chronic VBI of hypoperfusion origin, memory deterioration progresses, and compensating arterial hypertension of cerebroischemic origin is present in most patients. Despite the high incidence of disease, serious brain stem or posterior circulation strokes are rarely caused by occlusive disease which is limited to the extracranial portion of the VA. Occlusive disease of the intracranial portion of the VA is much more serious than extracranial disease. When the only VA is occluded (the contralateral VA is hypoplastic or occluded), the resulting syndrome is indistinguishable from occlusion of the basilar artery. The mortality in basilar artery thrombosis ranges between 50% and 80%.[12] However, the clinical syndromes related to specific infarcted areas of the brain due to thrombotic or embolic occlusions of intracranial arteries of the vertebrobasilar system are not the subject of this chapter. From the surgical point of view it is important to determine the source of the embolism. When it is an atheromatous plaque in the subclavian or vertebral arteries, it should be surgically repaired. The incidence of symptoms encountered in 1099 patients with vertebrobasilar disease operated by us is given in Table 56.1.

Diagnostic Evaluation

The diagnosis of VBI is a clinical challenge because most of its manifestations are subjective and difficult to quantify. In the early years of VA surgery the clinical evaluation of the patient and the sole objective instrumental evaluation—aortic arch angiography—were used to select patients for VA repair. Recently, ultrasonic noninvasive diagnostic techniques have become widely used for the evaluation of blood flow in the VAs.

Continuous Wave Doppler Studies of Blood Flow in the VAs

Continuous wave Doppler ultrasonography was widely used in our clinic before the era of duplex scanners. We still use it as a primary tool for the selection of patients for duplex and angiographic studies. The blood flow in the V2 portion of the VAs between the transverse processes is assessed. Then the V1 segments of the VAs are evaluated. When the symptoms of VBI are present and continuous wave Doppler studies detect occlusive or stenotic lesions of the VAs, duplex scanning is performed.

Duplex Scanning

Duplex scanning is the most widely used noninvasive diagnostic technique for evaluating patients with VBI. In most cases it is possible to assess the blood flow in the VAs in the bony canal (V2 segment) and to estimate the diameter of the VAs.[60] Hence, aplasia, hypoplasia, or occlusion of the VAs can be diagnosed. The characteristics of the blood flow in the V2 segment of a VA enable diagnosis of proximal (poststenotic blood flow) or distal (prestenotic blood flow) stenotic lesions of the VAs. Evaluation of the extracanal (V1) part of the VAs by duplex scanner using B-mode visualization and blood flow measurements enables the examiner to diagnose the atherosclerotic stenoses, kinks, and even hemodynamically significant anomalies of the VAs. We have been using duplex scanning since 1991 have evaluated more than 10,000 patients with this method. In our clinic, the accuracy of duplex scanning in the evaluation of VA pathology is over 80%. Accuracy depends on the experience of the examiner. The normal values of linear blood flow in the orifice of the VA, according to our data, are as follows: systolic, 83 ± 14 cm/s; and diastolic, 18 ± 3 cm/s. The normal linear blood flow values in the extracanal (V1) and osseous (V2) portions of the VAs are as follows: systolic, 65 ± 11 cm/s; and diastolic, 21 ± 4 cm/s. Hemodynamically important lesions of the proximal part of the VAs were considered when the systolic blood flow velocity was more than 150 cm/s.

Transcranial Doppler Imaging

The data from transcranial Doppler (TCD) studies combined with data from duplex scanning enable one to diagnose stenotic lesions from the orifice of the VAs up to the posterior cerebral arteries. Stenotic lesions of the V4 segment of the VAs, of the basilar artery, and of the posterior cerebral arteries can also be revealed with this combination. The presence of the posterior communicating arteries of the circle of Willis and the direction of blood flow in these arteries can be detected also. Monitoring of the flow in the middle cerebral artery is widely used by vascular surgeons in carotid artery surgery while clamping the internal carotid artery. TCD is very useful in monitoring blood flow in the ipsilateral posterior cerebral artery while clamping the only VA (when the contralateral VA is occluded, hypoplastic, or aplastic).

Color Doppler Imaging

Color Doppler imaging is the most advanced ultrasonic technique used for the evaluation of vessel blood flow. The blood flow toward the probe is coded in red, and the flow away from the probe is blue. The flow velocity is coded by color intensity. The apparatus has B-mode ultrasonic visualization of the vessels, pulsed Doppler linear flow estimation, and real-time spectral analysis of the Doppler signal. The flow abnormalities (flow changes and turbulence) are recognized easily with color Doppler imaging.

Electroencephalography

Electroencephalography reflects the functional status of the brain. The computer-assisted analysis of spectral and pathological changes in brain electric potentials enables one to localize the infarction area or even the hypoperfusion area. It is not a diagnostic technique with regard to changes in brain blood flow but is the most valuable means for diagnosis of generalized or localized epileptic activity of the brain. Electroencephalography can also indicate possible brain tumors.

Computed Tomography and Magnetic Resonance Imaging

Computed tomography (CT) scans and magnetic resonance imaging (MRI) are both very valuable in differentiating brain infarction from hemorrhagic stroke, brain tumors, and other brain diseases. MRI is a more advanced and sensitive method of imaging than CT and enables the detection of very small, clinically silent areas of brain infarction. It is very important to know an infarction's location, size, and relation to the diseased VA when considering surgical repair of the VA. When vertebrobasilar TIAs are caused by low flow (hypoperfusion) episodes, there may be no infarcted areas seen on CT or MRI scans. However, severe and long-lasting hypoperfusion can cause large areas of ischemic brain damage.

Angiography

Biplane selective four-vessel digital subtraction angiography is the "gold standard" for diagnosing lesions of the arteries supplying blood to the brain. Angiographic evaluation should visualize the subclavian arteries, the VAs from their orifices to their joining with the basilar artery, the basilar artery, and all intracranial branches of the VAs and basilar arteries. The left VA may be absent on the left subclavian angiogram, because in 3% of population it originates from the aortic arch. To obtain good visualization of the entire left VA and the branches of the VA and basilar artery, selective angiography of the left VA should be performed. Next, angiography of the aortic arch should be done to visualize the orifice of the left VA. The aortic arch angiogram is also useful when stenotic lesions of the innominate artery and/or both common carotid and subclavian arteries are suspected or have been diagnosed by duplex scanning. The proximal part of the VA is the most common site of atherosclerotic stenotic lesions in the vertebrobasilar system. Figure 56.6 illustrates typical atherosclerotic stenosis of the left VA. The kinks and coils of the VAs may be congenital or ac-

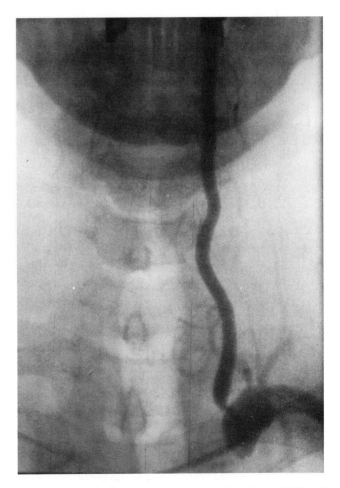

FIGURE 56.6. Typical atherosclerotic stenosis of the left VA orifice.

quired due to aging and loss of elasticity in hypertensive patients and are located in the V1 segment. Figure 56.7 illustrates a kinked first portion of the left VA. On rare occasions the V3 segment may be kinked. Sometimes the VA is kinked at the distal end of an atherosclerotic plaque. Atherosclerotic lesions of the V2 segment are uncommon. Osteophytes usually compress the VA in the bony canal. This pathology can be diagnosed by duplex scanning and verified by angiography. Sometimes, functional angiography of the VAs while the head is turned to each side is required to estimate the degree of compression or stenosis of the VA at the V2 segment.

TCD and angiographic studies were performed in our clinic for 100 patients with VBI. We formed the following conclusions from the data: (1) If the carotid and vertebral arteries are normal and pressures in the carotid and vertebrobasilar systems are equal, then the posterior communicating arteries are not functioning and not visualized on angiograms. Compression of the common carotid artery is required to detect the flow in the posterior communicating artery by TCD and by selective angiogram of the ipsilateral VA. (2) When the symptoms of VBI are present and hypoperfusion of the vertebrobasi-

lar territory exists, the pressure in the vertebrobasilar ystem is lower than that in the carotid territories. As a result, the posterior communicating arteries are redistributing the blood flow from the carotid arteries to the vertebrobasilar territory and can be visualized on conventional selective carotid angiograms. Figure 56.8 illustrates a functioning posterior communicating artery in a patient with an occluded left VA. The posterior trifurcation of the internal carotid artery (when the posterior cerebral artery is a branch of the internal carotid artery) should be recognizable on the angiogram. In this case the posterior cerebral artery has a straight course (Figure 56.9). It should be kept in mind that in these cases the infarction area in the occipital lobe and clinical manifestations related to it will be due to emboli arising through the internal carotid artery, or due to stenotic lesions of the latter, causing hypoperfusion in the territory of the posterior cerebral artery.

Here, we present the algorithm that we use when selecting patients for VA surgery (Figure 56.10).

Our comments concerning this algorithm include the following: (1) The patient must have the symptoms of

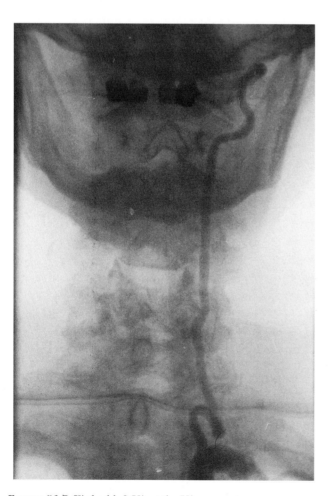

FIGURE 56.7. Kinked left VA at the V1 segment.

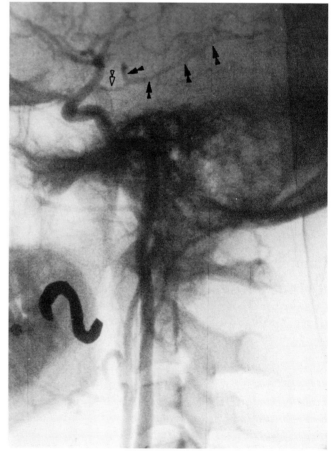

FIGURE 56.8 Posterior communicating artery (open arrow) supplying blood to the posterior cerebral artery (arrows) in a patient with an occluded left VA.

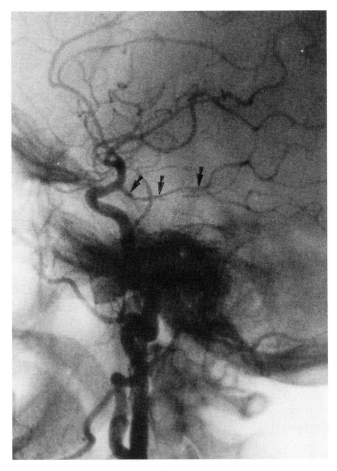

FIGURE 56.9. Posterior trifurcation of the left internal carotid artery. Arrows point to the posterior cerebral artery.

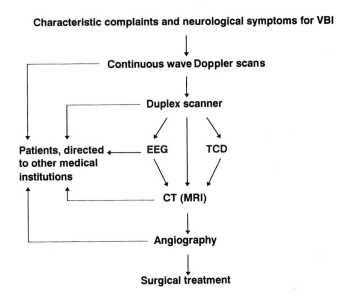

FIGURE 56.10. Algorithm for selecting patients for VA surgery.

VBI. (2) If normal blood flow in the V1 and V2 segments of both VAs is revealed by continuous wave Doppler scans, the patient is excluded from further evaluation. (3) When pathology of the VA is suspected as a result of continuous wave Doppler scans, the patient is evaluated with duplex scanning. (4) If the duplex scans reveal that both VAs are normal, the patient is excluded from further evaluation. Sometimes TCD or EEG studies are required to determine if the patient should be excluded from further evaluation. (5) CT or MRI studies are done in most patients to exclude brain tumors, hemorrhagic strokes, and other pathology of the brain and to estimate the infarction size and location. (6) If the patient has not been excluded at this point, he or she is a possible candidate for VA surgery; biplane digital subtraction selective angiographic studies of all four main brain arteries are performed. The indications and angiographic criteria for VA surgery are discussed next.

Indications for Surgical Treatment

Reconstruction of the VAs is a relatively new area of vascular surgery. Until the 1980s, few vascular surgeons performed surgery on the VAs. The indications for VA surgery were not obvious for neurologists and vascular surgeons. Even now few vascular surgeons routinely operate on VAs.

In patients with symptoms of VBI and vertebrobasilar strokes, 30% have an embolic disease.[8] These patients have recurrent ischemic events that usually involve different areas of the vertebrobasilar territory, and the malignant course of the disease is characterized by massive neurologic deficits and high morbidity and mortality. To determine the embolic mechanism, one must see the offending source (atheroma, thrombus, dissection) and the end organ damage (brain infarctions in the vertebrobasilar territory). The most common source of emboli is the heart (atrial fibrillation, rheumatic valve diseases, myocardial infarction). Atheromatous lesions of the innominate, subclavian, and vertebral arteries must be repaired if they are the source of embolization. Recently it has been appreciated that stenotic plaques of the VA origins can be atheromatous and embolize to the brain vessels.[12] Small infarctions in the vertebrobasilar territory cannot be detected with CT scans. Visualization of such small infarcts is possible only with MRI. Surgery is indicated if the source of the emboli is detected and the embolic infarction areas related to this source in the vertebrobasilar territory are revealed by MRI. In embolic disease, indications for surgery are irrelevant with respect to the status of the opposite VA and the anatomical variations of the circle of Willis. Surgery for asymptomatic patients can be advised when there is an aneurysm, which is likely to lead to embolization or thrombosis in the vertebrobasilar system. Traumatic lesions of the VAs as well as aneurysms and traumatic arteriovenous fistulae are definite indications for surgical repair. The indications for surgical repair of atherosclerotic stenosing lesions of the VAs in cases of hypoperfusion are still controversial. Berguer[9] proposes following indications: a 75% diameter stenosis of both VAs if they are both complete and of equivalent size. If one VA is hypoplastic, a 75% diameter stenosis of the dominant VA is required. These anatomic requirements apply also to the kinks and extrinsic compressions of the VA during head rotation/extension that cause symptoms during angiography. The same strict definition of indications for VA surgery are proposed by Imparato,[34] Imparato and Lin,[35] Deriu et al,[20] and Giangola et al.[24] Our definition of indications for VA surgery differs from these. We believe that the key to deciding on surgical repair lies in the posterior communicating arteries of the circle of Willis. Only half of the population have a normal circle of Willis.[1,51] In these patients stenosis or even occlusion of one VA will be asymptomatic. They will survive even with extracranial occlusion of both VAs. The opposite will hold for patients with absent posterior communicating arteries. Even one tightly stenosed VA can be the cause of VBI, despite a normal contralateral VA. The same point of view is supported by Benedetti-Valentini et al,[5] Nagashima et al,[41] Comerota et al,[15] and many others. Even one kinked VA can be the cause of VBI.[3,43,47,48] Extrinsic compression of the VA can be the cause of VBI if the contralateral VA is abnormal and one or both posterior communicating arteries are absent.[22,26,31,41,47,48,50] In cases of extrinsic compression of the VAs, spasming of the VA plays a major role (Figure 56.2); this can be revealed by duplex scans during the TIA related to the spasm. On duplex scan images, the artery will show a normal lumen except at the site of extrinsic compression in an asymptomatic period. Extrinsic compression of the VA will be seen during dynamic angiography, and in some cases, vasospasm of the compressed VA is also seen on angiograms (Figure 56.2). For patients with normal carotid arteries, we define the indications for VA surgery as follows : (1) Patients must have symptoms of VBI. (2) All other pathological conditions of the brain that can result in similar symptoms must be ruled out. (3) Duplex scanning and TCD studies must reveal stenotic or occlusive lesions in the V1 to V3 region of the VA, with impaired poststenotic blood flow distal to the stenotic lesion. (4) Angiography must reveal more than 75% stenosis or a kink of the VA. (5) If symptoms of VBI are present despite a normal contralateral VA, the diseased VA should be repaired. (6) Critical stenosis of the dominant VA even in asymptomatic patients should be repaired if the mortality plus morbidity of VA reconstructions is lower than 1% in the vascular surgery center.

In patients with multiple lesions of the carotid and vertebral arteries, the decision concerning which artery to repair depends on the presenting symptoms (hemispheric or vertebrobasilar) and the presence or absence of the posterior communicating arteries of the circle of Willis. If the patient has vertebrobasilar symptoms and both posterior communicating arteries are absent on angiogram, the VA must be repaired. When posterior communicating arteries are functioning, repair of a tightly stenosed internal carotid artery clears the vertebrobasilar symptoms. Hence, in patients with normal circle of Willis, hemodynamically significant stenoses of the internal carotid arteries should be repaired first. On the other hand, when internal carotid arteries are occluded or stenosed intracranially, repair of the tightly stenosed vertebral artery clears hemispheric symptoms (Figure 56.1). The same data are presented by Archie.[2]

Extensive experience, knowledge of brain hemodynamics, appreciation of the role of the circle of Willis, and long-term follow up data enable the physician to make the right decision for each patient. Those who are just beginning VA surgery should adhere strictly to the indications defined by Berguer.[9]

Surgical Management

The most common site of VA stenosis is the V1 segment. Atherosclerosis typically affects its orifice. Kinks and extrinsic compression of the VA by the sympathetic nerve or fascial bands are also found in this portion. Over 90% of VA reconstructions are performed on the V1 segment.

Our Technique of Surgical Repair of the V1 Segment of the VA

The patient is placed in a supine position with the neck slightly hyperextended; this is accomplished by placing a folded sheet under the shoulder on the side of operation with the head gently rotated to the opposite side. The rotation and hyperextension of the neck is accomplished after intubation. General anesthesia is preferred. A horizontal supraclavicular incision 10 cm long (1 to 2 cm above the medial half of the clavicle and laterally along the skin crease) is made. This incision is adequate for freeing the VA up to the fifth cervical vertebra. In cases of high entry of the VA into the C4 or C3 transverse processes, a vertical incision of reverse T configuration is made as high as needed. The platysma is transsected. The supraclavicular nerves in the lateral corner of the wound are preserved. The heads of the sternocleidomastoid muscle are divided. The omohyoid muscle is freed and pulled upward or divided. The prescalene fat pad is divided along the scalenus anterior muscle, and its medial and lateral flaps are retracted by traction sutures. The arteria suprascapularis is ligated and divided. The phrenic nerve is isolated, encircled with a tape, and mobilized from its origin at the C5 cervical nerve root well below the point where it crosses the subclavian artery. The medial and lateral edges of the anterior scalene muscle are dissected from the muscle's insertion to the transverse process of the C6 vertebra to the point below the subclavian artery. This maneuver makes scalenectomy easier. Then, a right-angle hemostat is gently passed behind the scalenus anterior muscle at the level of the subclavian artery. The muscle is divided with a scalpel as the right-angle hemostat pulls the muscle away from the subclavian artery. The anterior scalene muscle is excised to the level of the transverse process of C6 vertebra. All the branches of the thyrocervical trunk are ligated and divided. The internal mammary artery can be preserved. The next step is mobilization of the vertebral vein. The vein is encircled with a tape and all its tributaries are ligated as far as its entry into the bony canal. This maneuver facilitates the ligation of the vertebral vein tributaries and enables mobilization of the VA up to its entrance into the bony canal. After ligation of all the tributaries, the vertebral vein is ligated at both ends and excised. Ligation of the vertebral vein itself, before its tributaries, creates difficulty in mobilizing the VA because the vein branches encircle the VA. The VA is encircled with a tape and mobilized from its origin to the entrance into the bony canal. The white tendon of the lateral edge of the longus colli muscle is seen crossing the transverse process of the C6 vertebra. If the VA enters the bony canal at a higher point, it is always compressed by the longus colli tendon against the transverse

process of C6 vertebra. Our technique (Figure 56.3) requires the total excision of the anterior scalene muscle and the lateral edge of longus colli muscle to the level C6 transverse process, completely exposing the entrance of the VA into the bony canal for all repairs of VA anomalies and kinks. With atherosclerotic lesions the exposure of the VA entrance is not obligatory. In operations for VA kinks and certain types of anomalies, the redundant VA is clamped below the C6 transverse process, the subclavian artery is cross-clamped proximal and distal to the VA, and the VA is divided at its orifice, shortened, and reimplanted back into the enlarged orifice, using the parachute technique for the posterior part of the anastomosis. Atherosclerotic lesions of the proximal part of the VA are managed by transposing the VA to the site of the thyrocervical trunk, or if this site is diseased and atherosclerotic plaque is surrounding its orifice, the VA is transposed to the subclavian artery where it is free from atherosclerosis. Typically, the thyrocervical trunk is divided obliquely, leaving its posterior wall longer than the anterior. An elliptical hole 5 to 7 mm in diameter, in accordance with the VA diameter, is made in the anterior wall of the subclavian artery. The parachute technique is used for the posterior portion of the anastomosis. Both ends of the suture are joined and tied on the anterior line of the anastomosis. Over 90% of atherosclerotic lesions of the VA orifice can be repaired by this technique. If the VA has no extra length, our approach allow the mobilization of the subclavian artery, and the VA can be transposed easily. Figure 56.11 illustrates our preferred

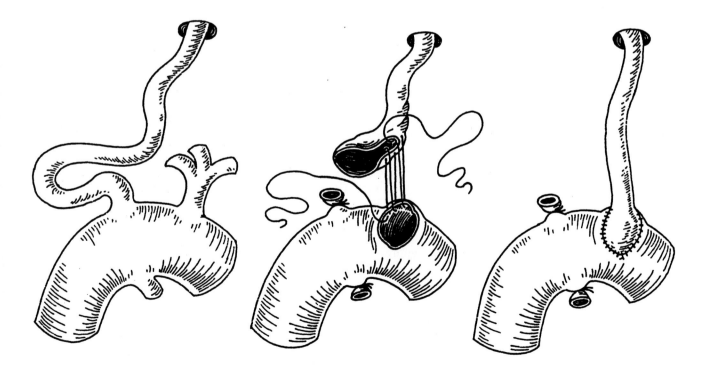

FIGURE 56.11. Technique for transposing the VA to the site of thyrocervical trunk.

technique of VA transposition to the site of the thyrocervical trunk. When the VA is not long enough for reimplantation, we prefer angioplasty of the VA with a saphenous vein patch. The VA is transposed to the common carotid artery only when the subclavian artery is stenosed or the arterial wall has an atherosclerotic plaque involving all of the subclavian artery. Our surgical approach to the proximal part of the VA is suitable for all reconstructive techniques used in the reconstruction of the first portion of the VA. When the VA repair is completed, the brachial plexus and VA are covered by the prescalene fat pad, and the sternocleidomastoid muscle is reattached. Skin sutures are subcuticular. Reimplantation of the VA into the subclavian artery is preferred for the following reasons: (1) It avoids the clamping of two arteries (vertebral and common carotid) that supply blood to the brain; clamping is dangerous with multiple atherosclerotic lesions of the brachiocephalic arteries. (2) Unlike with various bypass operations, only one anastomosis is required, and it is easy to accomplish. (3) After reconstruction the blood flow is physiological. (4) When the arteries are redundant, the common carotid artery is very mobile, and it is very difficult to appropriately adjust the length of the VA when transposing it to the common carotid artery. In hypertensive patients, whose arteries tend to elongate, a common follow-up finding is a kink in the transposed VA. Reimplantation of the VA into the subclavian artery is preferred by Ogawa et al[45] and Benedetti-Valentini et al.[5]

When the contralateral VA is occluded, TCD monitoring of the flow in the posterior cerebral artery on the side of the operation is obligatory. When the posterior cerebral artery is a branch of the internal carotid artery (so-called posterior internal carotid trifurcation is present) on the side of the VA reconstruction, the blood flow in the opposite posterior cerebral artery should be monitored if it is a branch of the basilar artery. In our clinic since 1993, when both posterior cerebral arteries are branches of the internal carotid arteries, we have monitored the blood flow in the basilar artery. We used TCD to monitor the blood flow in posterior brain circulation in 36 patients while clamping the only vertebral artery or when the contralateral artery was hypoplastic. We have not yet estimated the critical level of blood flow in the posterior cerebral artery or basilar artery, but the following conclusions can be drawn: (1) The patients tolerate VA clamping for the time (10 to 20 minutes) required to perform VA reconstruction even if the contralateral artery is hypoplastic but joins the contralateral vertebral artery and its diameter is more than 2 mm. (2) If one or both posterior communicating arteries are present and seen on angiograms, patients tolerate clamping of the only VA. When the only VA is diseased, the posterior communicating arteries must be seen on conventional internal carotid angiograms as a result of the differences

in blood pressures in the carotid and vertebrobasilar systems, provided the internal carotid artery has no hemodynamically significant stenosis. We have monitored seven cases in which both posterior communicating arteries were absent and the contralateral VA occluded. In four the blood flow in the posterior cerebral artery dropped to zero (undetectable by TCD) while clamping the only VA. In one case the hole in the subclavian artery was prepared distal to the VA, then the VA was clamped and transposed to the prepared hole. The VA was clamped for 7 minutes. Bradycardia (30 beats/min) and arterial hypotension (70 mm Hg systolic) developed. Restoration of blood flow through the VA returned the heart rate and blood pressure to normal values. In the second patient the reconstruction of the only VA was abandoned. In the third case the kinked VA was straightened by resection of the distal portion of the subclavian artery. In the fourth case the kinked VA was straightened by pulling the subclavian artery down and fixing it with the thyrocervical stump to the stump of the scalenus anterior muscle. We need more experience with TCD monitoring to estimate the safe level of blood flow in the posterior cerebral arteries. However, when the blood flow drops to an undetectable level, the Senters[52] technique of using an internal shunt for reconstruction of the VA at any level (V1 through V3) should be used. Since 1993, when monitoring of posterior brain circulation while clamping the only VA was introduced in our clinic, we have had only one perioperative vertebrobasilar stroke in over 300 VA operations. Berguer[9] and Kieffer[39] do not use TCD monitoring of posterior brain circulation while operating the only VA and never use internal shunting in these cases. They even clamp the VA and ipsilateral internal carotid artery at the same time while performing transposition of the distal VA into the side of the internal carotid artery. Kieffer[39] reported 3.8% perioperative strokes (half of them lethal). Berguer and Kieffer prefer direct transposition of the VA into the site of the common carotid artery in proximal (V1) VA reconstructions. This type of repair is used by Kieffer[39] in over 80% and by Berguer[7] in over 90% of proximal VA reconstructions. This technique can be used successfully in atherosclerotic lesions of the VAs and is described by Berguer in detail.[9] Here we briefly describe Berguer's technique.

A low neck incision that obliquely crosses the insertion of both sternocleidomastoid heads is carried out. The approach to the VA is between the two sternocleidomastoid heads; these are separated. The jugular vein and vagus nerve are identified and retracted laterally. The common carotid artery stays medial. The thoracic duct is identified (on the left side), ligated, and divided between ligatures. The vertebral vein is identified and ligated. The VA is found beneath it. During dissection of the VA care is taken to protect the sympathetic fibers that run medial to the VA and across it. Distally the artery is dissected up to the transverse process of sixth cervical vertebra, and proximally to its origin on the subclavian artery. The adjacent common carotid artery is mobilized. Heparin (5 units) is administered intravenously. The VA is occluded at the C6 transverse process by means of vascular clamp. Proximally the VA is ligated at its origin, divided above the ligature, pulled out from the loop formed by the sympathetic fibers, and brought to the site selected for carotid anastomosis. The common carotid artery is cross-clamped, and an arteriotomy is performed on its posterior wall with a 5-mm aortic punch. The VA is anastomosed to the carotid artery with continuous 6-0 polypropylene suture, which is parachuted at the beginning of the anastomosis.

Alternatives to vertebral–carotid transposition include reimplantation of the VA to a different subclavian site, and a subclavian-to-vertebral artery autogenous vein bypass. Berguer[7] uses these two techniques when the common carotid artery is not a suitable donor vessel because of its disease or occlusion, or when the contralateral internal carotid artery is occluded. These two alternative techniques require the exposure of the second (retroscalene) segment of the subclavian artery. To accomplish this, the incision already described is drawn more laterally. The prescalene fat pad is dissected and reflected to the outer border of the wound. The transverse scapular artery and vein are divided. The phrenic nerve is identified and preserved. The scalenus anterior muscle is divided, exposing the second segment of the subclavian artery, which is then encircled with a tape and cleared for anastomosis. The VA is dissected from its origin up to the C6 transverse process, ligated at its origin, divided, brought laterally, and implanted into the subclavian artery. If the operation is a subclavian–vertebral bypass, the VA is dissected near the C6 transverse process, and an adequate length of VA for anastomosis is prepared. The origin of the VA does not need to be dissected. After the vein graft is prepared, anastomosis to the side of the subclavian artery is performed, and then the vein graft is anastomosed to the side of the VA. The VA proximal to the anastomosis is occluded with a hemoclip.

Imparato[34] uses a neck skin incision along the lower third of the anterior edge of the sternocleidomastoid muscle, extended to the level of the head of the clavicle, where it is then curved laterally and parallel to the clavicle for approximately 10 cm. He divides the sternal head of the sternocleidomastoid muscle. The prescalene fat pad is divided. The phrenic nerve is identified and preserved, the scalenus anterior muscle is divided, and all branches of the thyrocervical trunk are ligated and divided. The subclavian artery is cross-clamped as is the VA at the C6 transverse process. An ellipse of the anterior wall of the subclavian artery surrounding the origin of the VA is excised, and the arteriotomy is continued

along the anterior wall of the VA to its normal lumen. If there is a redundancy of the VA, plication is used to correct it, suturing the normal intima of the VA to the intima of the subclavian artery; the VA is shortened as much as required, and its redundancy is exteriorized.[35] The "dog ears" created by this plication technique of the VA are closed. The newly created vertebral ostium is made funnel shaped by suturing patch of saphenous vein over it. Imparato and Lin[35] very rarely use VA transposition to the common carotid artery or a saphenous vein bypass from the subclavian artery to the side of the V1 or V2 segment of the VA. Deriu et al[20] also prefer the VA transposition to the common carotid artery, whereas we and others[5,45] prefer VA reimplantation into the subclavian artery. There are several other techniques for reconstruction of the V1 portion of the VA.

VA Resection With End-to-End Anastomosis When the VA is Kinked

VA resection with end-to-end anastomosis requires meticulous technique and is more demanding than VA transposition techniques; therefore, it is not recommended.

Straightening of the Kinked VA by Resection of the Distal Subclavian Artery

Resection of the distal subclavian artery to straighten a kinked VA was proposed by Wesolowski.[62] We now use this technique for straightening a kinked VA when the subclavian artery is elongated and situated high in the neck close to the entrance of the VA into the bony canal. Sometimes, additional shortening and transposition of the VA to the more proximal part of the subclavian artery is required.

Vertebral Artery Replacement by an Autologous Vein

We have used autologous vein replacement for VA reconstruction in only 12 cases when other VA reconstruction techniques failed (cases with stenosis, intimal flap at the site of anastomosis, dissection of intima, etc.) or in cases when only the distal portion of the V1 segment of the VA was free of disease.

Surgical Techniques for Correction of VA Anomalies

The modified Powers technique is used for lateral branching of the VA from the subclavian artery.[50] Scalenectomy, ligation of the thyrocervical trunk, and fixation of the subclavian artery by the thyrocervical stump to the stump of the scalenus anterior muscle on the first rib clears vertebrobasilar and thoracic outlet symptoms. Excision of the scalenus anterior muscle up to the C6 transverse process, as well as excision of the lateral edge of the longus colli muscle, exposing the entrance of the VA into the bony canal, are required in all operations for VA anomalies to ensure that the high entrance of the VA into the bony canal is not left uncorrected because tandem anomalies of the VAs are often encountered.

Posterior branching of the VA from the subclavian artery is repaired by transposing the VA from the dorsal to the upper aspect of the subclavian artery, using the technique illustrated in Figure 56.11. When moderate posterior branching of the VA is present, ligation of the thyrocervical trunk and other muscular branches of the subclavian artery and rotation and fixation to the stump of scalenus anterior muscle on the first rib by the thyrocervical stump corrects the position and hemodynamics of the VA.

The excision of the scalenus anterior muscle and the lateral edge of the longus colli muscle, exposing the entrance of the VA into the bony canal, is required for the correction of the VA entrapment between these muscles when there is normal entrance of the VA. When the VA enters the bony canal higher than normally, at C5, C4, or even C3, it must be freed up to its entrance by excising all the muscle tissue (the intercrossing longus colli, longus capitis, and scalene muscles) in front of it, creating a free pathway for the VA.

When the cause of VBI is an extrinsic compression of the first segment of the VA, as seen on angiogram, the VA is freed from its origin up to the C6 transverse process, dividing all the structures in front of it. Usually fibrous and fascial bands or the small branch of the sympathetic trunk are found to be compressing the VA. They can be divided without sequelae. When all the sympathetic trunk or its thick branch is crossing the VA, or the latter is embedded in the sympathetic ganglion, the artery is divided at its origin and freed from all attachments between the sympathetic nerves and the adventitia of the artery, without damaging either. The artery is pulled out, placed in front of the sympathetic nerves, and reimplanted back into the subclavian artery. The VA is very spasmophilic at operation in these cases. Hence, desympatization of the entire length of the extracanal VA is performed, and moistening with 2% papaverine solution completes the procedure.

VA Transposition From the Aortic Arch to the Subclavian Artery

The surgical approach to the subclavian artery is the same as described by us for all operations on the V1 segment of the VA. The VA is identified close to the C6

transverse process and dissected distally to its entrance into the bony canal. According to data published by Pauliukas et al,[47,48] in 74% of operations, the VA originating from the aortic arch entered the bony canal higher than normally, into the C5, C4, or even C3 transverse process. Hence, the VA must be freed up to its entrance into the bony canal by the technique just described. Then the VA is freed proximally to the point where its length is sufficient to transpose it to the subclavian artery. The VA is implanted into the subclavian artery by the same technique used in all cases of VA reimplantation into the subclavian artery (Figure 56.11). Sometimes, identification of the VA is difficult because it takes a more medial course than usual. Intraoperative Doppler scanning is very helpful in locating the VA in these cases.

Simultaneous Reconstructions of the Vertebral and Subclavian Arteries

When the proximal part of the subclavian artery is occluded or tightly stenosed and the VA is stenosed at its orifice, the latter should be reconstructed first, by transposing it to the subclavian artery or common carotid artery, by autovenous bypass from the subclavian artery to the VA, by autovenous replacement of the VA, or by other techniques. Then, the caroticosubclavian bypass, using a vascular prosthesis, is constructed. When it is possible to transpose the subclavian artery into the side of the common carotid artery, the VA can be repaired afterward. The reconstruction of the VA simultaneously with the subclavian artery in combined lesions is of the utmost importance, because later it is very difficult or impossible to repair the first segment of the VA due to the scarring and the vascular prosthesis lying in front of the VA.

Percutaneous transluminal angioplasty (PTA) of the carotid, subclavian, and vertebral arteries is used in several vascular surgery centers as an alternative to surgical management. Kachel[37] strongly advocates the use of PTA for these arteries. Strict adherence to the indications for PTA is necessary to keep the complication rate (due to embolization to the brain from the atherosclerotic plaques) as low as that in surgical patients. The role of PTA in the revascularization of the vertebrobasilar region and the carotid territories is not yet established.

Surgical Access and Reconstruction of the VA at Its Distal (V3) Segment

When the VA is occluded, stenosed, or compressed in the intraosseous (V2) segment, the easiest way to reestablish normal blood flow to the VA between the C1 and C2 transverse processes, when there is sufficient distance between them, is to perform the anastomosis to the side of the VA or an end-to-end anastomosis. Surgical exposure of the VA between the C1 and C2 transverse processes is described in detail by Elkin and Harris,[23] and has been adapted and refined for revascularization of the V3 segment of the VA by Berguer[7,9] and Kieffer et al.[39] Kieffer and his associates have the most extensive experience with surgery of distal VA; they have performed over 300 operations on the V3 segment.[39]

The skin incision is along the anterior edge of the sternocleidomastoid muscle from the mastoid process to the middle of the neck. The dissection proceeds between the anterior edge of the sternocleidomastoid muscle and the internal jugular vein. The accessory spinal nerve is identified, encircled with a tape, and mobilized. The digastric muscle is divided at its tendon and reattached during wound closure. The accessory nerve is dissected up to the point where it crosses the transverse process of atlas. This prominent bony landmark is easily identified by finger palpation. The fibrofatty tissue that covers the levator scapulae muscle is removed. The anterior and posterior edges of this muscle are identified. The anterior ramus of the C2 nerve, emerging from the anterior edge of levator scapulae muscle, is identified and used as a guide to divide the levator scapulae muscle. The latter is cut immediately below its insertion on the C1 transverse process and is excised distally, exposing the anterior ramus of the C2 nerve, which is gently dissected from the VA lying immediately beneath it. The nerve is cut, and the VA is seen between the C1 and C2 transverse processes. The vertebral venous plexus surrounds the VA. These small veins are coagulated with bipolar cautery. The VA is encircled with a tape and freed from the C2 to the C1 transverse process. Now the VA is ready for anastomosis. The most common revascularization procedure at this VA level is a saphenous vein bypass from the side of the common carotid artery to the side or distal end of the VA. The anastomosis to the VA is made first. If it is end-to-side anastomosis, then both ends of the VA are backbled, flow is resumed through the VA, and the vein is clamped close to the anastomosis. The vein is passed under the jugular vein to the common carotid artery well bellow the bifurcation, where it is seldom affected by atherosclerosis. An end-to-side anastomosis between the vein graft and the lateral aspect of the common carotid artery is constructed. After the backbleeding from both ends of the common carotid artery and the VA, the anastomosis is completed and the blood flow is resumed into the distal carotid artery and then into the VA. When the contralateral internal carotid artery is occluded, clamping of the common or internal carotid arteries must be avoided. In these cases and when the ipsilateral common carotid artery is occluded, the proximal end of the vein graft is anastomosed to the side of the subclavian artery, provided it is not diseased.

The subclavian artery is exposed through the supraclavicular horizontal incision, as already described for the reconstruction of the V1 segment of the VA. The vein graft is passed under the sternocleidomastoid muscle to the subclavian artery. We and Imparato[34] prefer to perform the distal anastomosis of the vein graft to the side of the VA between the C1 and C2 transverse processes. There is no need to unroof the C2 transverse process, as described by Imparato,[34] to perform the end-to-side anastomosis. The flow in the vein graft is lower in this configuration of anastomosis than in the end-to-end type, but it is still several times higher than in femoropopliteal bypass, and its patency is determined by the quality of the anastomosis rather than the flow velocity. If there is no suitable vein, the most common procedure is transposition of the external carotid artery to the distal VA. For this operation the VA is dissected as already described. The common carotid artery and its bifurcation are exposed. The superior thyroid artery is ligated. The external carotid artery is dissected, ligating all its branches up to the internal maxillary artery. The digastric muscle is divided. The external carotid artery is divided at the point where it has adequate length to make an anastomosis to the distal VA between the C1 and C2 transverse processes. The external carotid artery is passed under the jugular vein. Anastomosis can be end-to-side or end-to-end between the external carotid and the VA. End-to-end anastomosis is easier to perform. In this procedure the common carotid artery and its bifurcation must be dissected to allow rotation of the external carotid artery from the medial to the lateral aspect of the wound.

The transposition of the distal VA to the internal carotid artery requires the same exposure as described for the distal VA. This operation requires simultaneous clamping of the ipsilateral internal carotid and vertebral arteries. Hence, it cannot be done in patients who have an occluded contralateral internal carotid artery. Even if it is patent, the risk of brain ischemia is too great, and TCD monitoring of the flow in the ipsilateral middle cerebral artery and posterior cerebral artery should be used. Berguer[7,9] and Kieffer[39] widely use this technique. For this type of reconstruction, the internal carotid artery is dissected at the level of the C1 vertebra, immediately above the superior cervical sympathetic ganglion, and displaced posteriorly to reach the VA. The VA is clamped below the C1 transverse process, ligated above the C2 transverse process, and divided just above the ligature. Then it is brought forward and anastomosed to the side of the internal carotid artery.

Access to the Suboccipital VA

Access to the suboccipital VA is required for arteriovenous aneurysm that involve the VA above the C1 transverse process, for acute traumatic lesions of the VA at the

V3 segment, for intimal dissections of the C1 to C2 segment that do not respond to anticoagulation, for extrinsic compression of the VA between the atlas and the occipital bone, and when anastomosis to the VA between the C1 and C2 vertebra fails and repair cannot be accomplished at this level.

The patient is placed in the park-bench position. The skin incision is parallel to the lower border of the occipital bone. It begins from the midline of the neck and is extended laterally to the mastoid process, then is curved down along the anterior edge of the sternocleidomastoid muscle. The sternocleidomastoid muscle is divided close to the mastoid process. The C1 transverse process is identified as an important landmark early in the dissection. The splenius capitis and longissimus capitis muscles are divided. Then, over a right-angle hemostat, the obliqus capitis superior muscle is carefully divided. The VA is identified immediately below the obliqus capitis superior muscle on the posterior arch of the atlas and is encircled with a tape. The multiple veins, forming a venous plexus around the VA, are coagulated with bipolar cautery. Sometimes, for better exposure, the rectus capitis posterior major muscle is incised or divided. If the posterior arch of the atlas is very close to the occipital bone, the posterior lamina of the atlas arch must be removed. To do this, the lamina is isolated from the VA using a periosteum elevator, and laminectomy is performed with an appropriate rongeur. If the VA is to be reconstructed, the saphenous vein bypass from the side of the common carotid artery to the side or end of the suboccipital VA is constructed. Berguer[9] advocates vein bypass to the side of the VA from the side of the internal carotid artery.

Repair of VA Injuries and Arteriovenous Aneurysms

The most common injuries to the extracranial part of the VAs encountered by vascular surgeons are gunshot and, less commonly, stab wounds. The cupula of the pleura can be damaged in penetrating wounds of the lower neck and injuries to the proximal part of the VA and/or subclavian artery. Exsanguinating bleeding into the pleural cavity is present in these cases. A straightforward operation must be undertaken And control of the subclavian and vertebral arteries obtained. The VA is transposed to the common carotid artery, if possible.

When the VA injury is close to the entrance into the bony canal, a vein interposition graft is used or the VA is ligated, and a bypass from the common carotid to the distal VA between the C1 and C2 transverse processes is performed. If the subclavian artery is injured, it is repaired. A lateral thoracotomy in the fourth intercostal space is performed, the blood flow from the pleural cavity is eliminated, the lung is inspected and, if injured, repaired. The pleural cavity is drained and the wound closed. When the proximal part of the left subclavian artery is injured, an emergency anterolateral thoracotomy for control of the left subclavian artery is performed. Injuries to the V2 segment of the VA are rare and usually manifest later as arteriovenous fistulae, which are managed intra-arterially by a detachable balloon. Bleeding of injuries to the V3 segment of the VA can usually be controlled by means of extrinsic compression. Angiography can be performed to localize the site of injury. Bleeding can be controlled by detachable balloon or inflated balloon. Surgical repair afterward is straightforward and accomplishes ligation of the proximal VA to obtain control distal to the injured part of the VA and create a bypass to the distal VA from the common carotid artery. Usually, isolated VA lesions are not exsanguinating and manifest as traumatic arteriovenous fistulae or aneurysms. Most of them can be successfully managed percutaneously with an intra-arterial detachable balloon. Surgical repair is required when the blood flow in the injured VA must be restored (the only VA is injured) or when intra-arterial management is impossible due to tortuosity of the injured VA.

Personal Experience

From 1970 to May 1995, 1142 operations on VAs were performed in 1112 patients. The patients comprised three groups distinguished according to VA pathology (Table 56.2). Patients with kinked or coiled VAs constituted the largest group. This is due to the more benign natural history of this pathology. Almost all patients in this group had a long history of vertebrobasilar TIAs. Hence, these patients had a good chance of being directed by neurologists to our institution for evaluation and surgical management. The number of patients in the group with atherosclerosis has been increasing because of the increasingly wider use of duplex scanning by neurologists. Overall, 26.8% of patients underwent oper-

TABLE 56.2. Patient distribution according to sex and the type of vertebral artery pathology.

Sex	Atherosclerosis	Kinks and coils	Anomalies	Total
Male	168	121	116	405 (36.4%)
Female	138	387	182	707 (63.6%)
Total	306 (27.5%)	508 (45.7%)	298 (26.8%)	1112 (100%)

TABLE 56.3. Age (in years) distribution of 1112 patients who underwent surgery for vertebrobasilar disease.

Age group (yr)	Men		Women		Total	
	Number	Percentage	Number	Percentage	Number	Percentage
1–9	2	0.5	1	0.1	3	0.3
10–19	24	5.9	26	3.7	50	4.5
20–29	31	7.7	55	7.8	86	7.7
30–39	68	16.8	102	14.4	170	15.3
40–49	85	21	164	23.2	249	22.4
50–59	111	27.4	183	25.9	294	26.4
60–69	67	16.5	150	21.2	217	19.5
Over 70	17	4.2	26	3.7	43	3.9
Total	405	100	707	100	1112	100

ation because of VA anomalies. We have been intensively working in this field since 1977, evaluating the majority of children, teenagers, and young adults in Lithuania with vertebrobasilar symptoms. We have accumulated extensive experience in diagnostic evaluation and surgical management of these young patients. Only a small percentage of them require surgery, and only when medical treatment fails and vertebrobasilar symptoms are expressed and interfere with work and life activities. The age distribution of patients undergoing surgery for VA pathology is given in Table 56.3. All children and teenagers and most of the patients younger than 30 years were treated by surgery because of VA anomalies. Kinks and coils as the indication for surgery prevailed in the fifth and sixth decades of life. Most patients with atherosclerosis were in the sixth and seventh decades of life.

Neurological indications for VA repair are presented in Table 56.4. For 13 (4.2%) of the patients in the group with atherosclerosis, the goal of the surgery was to improve anterior circulation through the posterior communicating arteries because both internal carotid arteries were occluded or inoperable.

The surgical techniques we used in VA repair are presented in Table 56.5. Transsubclavian VA endarterectomy was used in the first operations we performed but is no longer used. VA resection with end-to-end anastomosis also was used during the first year for reconstruction of the kinked VAs but is no longer used. Fifteen re-

constructions of the distal VA were vein bypasses from the common carotid artery to the distal VA. In one case the external carotid artery was anastomosed end to end to the distal VA. In cases with occluded ipsilateral common and internal carotid arteries, a vein bypass from the subclavian artery to the distal VA was performed.

Arteriovenous aneurysms and malformations are rarely encountered in the extracranial part of the VAs. We encountered only four patients with this type of VA pathology. In one case, due to a stab injury to the neck, a large arteriovenous aneurysm developed between the V3 portion of the left VA and the internal jugular vein. It was successfully managed percutaneously with an intra-arterial detachable balloon. In the second case an arteriovenous fistula between the V1 portion of the VA and the vertebral vein caused by a stab injury to the neck was surgically repaired, preserving the blood flow in the VA. In the third case, the arteriovenous malformations (multiple fistulae) involving the first portion of the VA were successfully excised, preserving the blood flow in the VA. Direct surgical repair was undertaken in case of an arteriovenous aneurysm on the posterior arch of the atlas due to a gunshot injury to the suboccipital VA; the intra-arterial procedure was impossible due to tortuosity of the injured VA (Figure 56.12). The VA was ligated between the C1 and C2 transverse processes. Then all large, tortuous veins were ligated and the lesser ones coagulated with bipolar cautery. The distal end of the VA at

TABLE 56.4. Indications for surgery in 1112 patients according to vertebral artery pathology.

Indications	Atherosclerosis		Kinks and coils		Anomalies	
	Number	Percentage	Number	Percentage	Number	Percentage
VB TIAs	66	21.6	157	30.9	30	10.1
Chronic VBI and TIAs	105	34.3	162	31.9	177	59.4
VB stroke (per history)	112	36.6	187	36.8	90	30.2
Acute VB stroke	10	3.3	2	0.4	1	0.3
Hemispheric stroke	9	2.9	—	—	—	—
Hemispheric TIAs	4	1.3	—	—	—	—
Total	306	100	508	100	298	100

VB, vertebrobasilar; TIAs, transient ischemic attacks; VBI, vertebrobasilar insufficiency.

TABLE 56.5. Types of surgical repair of vertebral arteries (1142 operations).

Surgical technique	Number of operations	Thrombosis of reconstructed VA	Died
Transsubclavian VA endarterectomy	12	1	1
VA endarterectomy with vein patch angioplasty	49	1	2
VA transposition to the SA	164	1	1
VA transposition to the site of thyrocervical trunk	672	2	3
Vertebral artery replacement by autologous vein	12	1	1
VA transposition to the common carotid artery	10	0	1
VA transposition from the aortic arch to the SA	36	0	0
Straightening of the VA by resection of the distal SA	32	0	0
VA resection with end-to-end anastomosis	16	1	1
Scalenectomy and SA fixation (S. Powers procedure)	104	0	1
Reconstruction of the distal VA (V3 segment)	17	2	0
Simultaneous VA and SA reconstructions	14	0	0
Arteriovenous VA aneurysms	4	0	0
Total	1142	9 (0.8%)	11 (1%)

VA, vertebral artery; SA, subclavian artery.

the atlanto-occipital membrane was tortuous and aneurysmatic. Hence, revascularization of the VA could not be performed. The distal end of the VA was ligated

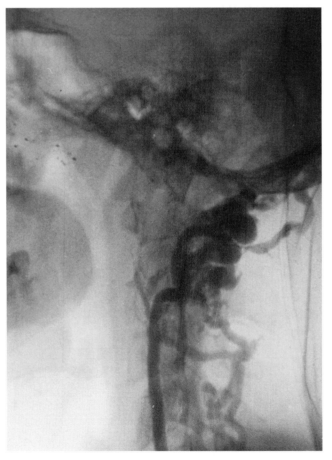

FIGURE 56.12. Arteriovenous aneurysm on the posterior arch of the atlas due to a gunshot lesion of the left VA.

at the atlanto-occipital membrane. The occluded left VA in the V2 segment can be seen on the postoperative angiogram (Figure 56.13a). The contralateral VA is normal (Figure 56.13b). No filling of arteriovenous fistulae from both VAs is seen on the postoperative angiograms.

The surgical repair of arteriovenous aneurysms of the VAs is much more demanding, particularly in the V3 segment, than elective reconstructive surgery. Intraoperative Doppler is very useful for assessing the completeness of the surgical repair, particularly in cases of congenital arteriovenous malformations. Intraoperative Doppler evaluation of the blood flow in the reconstructed blood vessel and graft and at the sites of anastomoses is necessary and sufficient in most cases. Very rarely intraoperative completion angiography is required.

The immediate (1 month) results of VA surgery are given in Table 56.6. The patients whose symptoms cleared or diminished were defined as improved; 94.5% of patients with atherosclerosis and 93.5% of patients with VA kinks improved postoperatively. In the group with VA anomalies, 49 (16.4%) patients were unchanged. This was due to diagnostic errors; in some cases surgical correction was not appropriate. Only 2 (0.7%) patients in this group worsened and 1 (0.3%) patient died due to a brain stem stroke.

Out of 1142 operations there were 11 deaths (1%). All but three deaths were in the group with atherosclerosis. Six patients died from ischemic vertebrobasilar stroke, 3 from myocardial infarction, 1 from hemorrhagic stroke, and 1 death was not related to the operation.

Other, nonmortal complications are presented in Table 56.7.

Permanent deficit resulting from complications was defined as a severe complication and occurred with an incidence 0.9%.

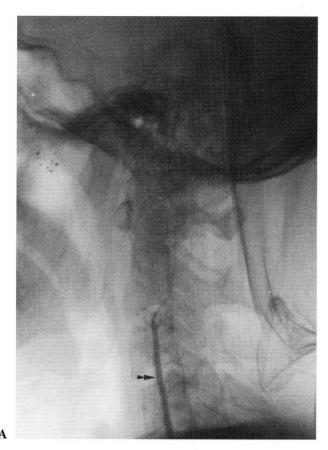

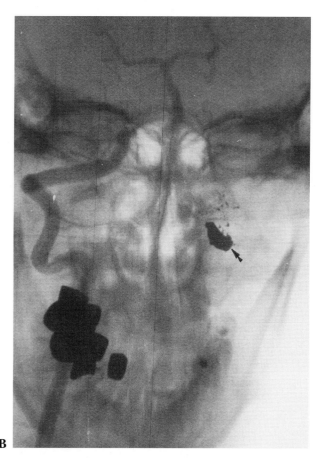

A   B

FIGURE 56.13. **A,** Postoperative angiogram of the ligated left VA (arrow). **B,** Postoperative angiogram of the right VA (anterioposterior view); arrow points to the bullet embedded at the base of the skull.

TABLE 56.6. Immediate postoperative results in 1099 patients with vertebrobasilar disease.

	Atherosclerotic ($n = 293$)	Coiling (kinking) ($n = 508$)	Anomalies ($n = 298$)	Total ($n = 1099$)
Improved	277 (94.5%)	475 (93.5%)	246 (82.6%)	998 (90.8%)
Unchanged	6 (2.0%)	27 (5.3%)	49 (16.4%)	82 (7.5%)
Worsened	2 (0.7%)	4 (0.8%)	2 (0.7%)	8 (0.7%)
Died	8 (2.7%)	2 (0.4%)	1 (0.3%)	11 (1%)

TABLE 56.7. Perioperative complications in 1112 patients who underwent surgery (1142 operations).

Type of complication	Number of operations	Percentage
Horner's syndrome	69	6.0
Temporary	64	5.6
Permanent	5	0.4
Phrenic nerve palsy	37	3.2
Temporary	35	3.1
Permanent	2	0.2
Brachial plexalgia	15	1.3
Inferior laryngeal nerve palsy	3	0.3
Lymphocele	1	0.1
Wound hematoma	6	0.5

Long-term Results

The long-term results of surgical repair of the VAs, according to their pathology, are presented in Figure 56.14. The cumulative survival rate at 10 years for VA anomalies was 97%. There were no stroke-related deaths in this group. The high survival rate in this group is a result of the young age of the patients. There was an 88% cumulative survival rate at 10 years for the group with VA kinks and coils. In this group, only two deaths were due to a stroke. The cumulative survival rate at 10 years for atherosclerotic patients was 53%. Most of the deaths were due to heart disease or cancer. Three deaths were due to vertebrobasilar stroke, and one was due to hemispheric stroke.

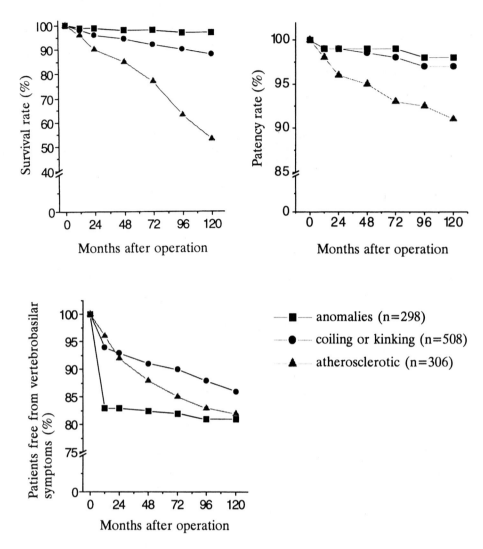

FIGURE 56.14. Cumulative analysis of long-term results: survival of operated patients, patency of repaired vertebral arteries, and patients free from vertebrobasilar symptoms.

The patency rate of repaired VAs at 10 years was 98% in the anomalies group, 97% in kinks and coils group, and 91% in atherosclerosis group.

The diminishing percentage of patients free from vertebrobasilar symptoms over subsequent years is very similar in for both the atherosclerosis and VA kinks groups; at 10 years it was 82% and 86%, respectively. Freedom from vertebrobasilar symptoms was lowest during the immediate postoperative period in the VA anomalies group due to the difficulties in evaluation of these patients and errors made in establishing the diagnosis and surgical repair. However, long-term results have been very good and stable in these patients during the 10 years of follow-up. Cumulative freedom from vertebrobasilar symptoms in this group was 81% at 10 years.

Our immediate and long-term results in the atherosclerosis and kinked VAs groups are similar to those published by Berguer[9] and Kieffer et al.[39]

Reconstruction of cervical VAs is a time-honored procedure in the surgical management of vertebrobasilar insufficiency. Indications for surgery and techniques of repair are well defined in atherosclerotic VA lesions. In cervical osteochondrosis, when the VAs are compressed in the osseous canal, the procedure of choice is revascularization of distal VA between the C1 and C2 transverse processes. The hemodynamic and clinical importance of VA kinks and coils are still underestimated by neurologists and vascular surgeons. Appreciation of the relation between hemodynamic disturbances, as assessed by duplex scanning and TCD, and clinical manifestations in these patients, as well as personal experience in surgical repair of these lesions, are needed by most vascular surgeons. The immediate and long-term results of surgical repair of kinked VAs support the expediency of surgery for this pathology.

We believe that there is a great future for surgery of VA anomalies. Extended experience, expertise, and dedication are necessary to evaluate these young patients. When the standard rules of operation[47] are adhered to, the operation is rewarding for both the patient and the physician.

References

1. Alpers BJ, Berry RG, Paddison RM. Anatomical studies of the circle of Willis in normal brain. *Arch Neurol Psychiatry.* 1959;11:409–418.
2. Archie JP Jr. Improved carotid hemodynamics with vertebral reconstruction. *Ann Vasc Surg.* 1992;6:138–141.
3. Barkauskas EM. Surgical correction of the lesions of the proximal part of vertebral arteries. *Khirurgia (Moscow).* 1977;5:17–21.
4. Barkauskas EM, Pauliukas PA. Surgical treatment of the anomalies of vertebral arteries. *Khirurgia (Moscow).* 1982; 9:20–22.
5. Benedetti-Valentini T Jr, Gossetti B, Irace L. Isolated symptomatic lesions of the vertebral artery: cure after surgical repair. *Ital J Surg Sciences.* 1985;15:299–303.
6. Berguer R. Distal vertebral bypass: technique the "occipital connection," potential uses. *J Vasc Surg.* 1985;2: 621–626.
7. Berguer R. Techniques for reconstruction of the vertebral artery. In: Chang, JB, ed. *Modern Vascular Surgery.* New York/Berlin/Heidelberg: Springer-Verlag; 1992:99–107.
8. Berguer R. Reconstruction of the branches of the aortic arch and the vertebral artery. In: Bernstein E, Callow A, Nicolaides A, et al, eds. *Cerebral Revascularization.* London/Los Angeles/Nicosia: Med-Orion; 1993:427–447.
9. Berguer R. Current methods of vertebral artery revascularization. In: Caplan L, Shifrin E, Nicolaides A, et al, eds. *Cerebrovascular Ischemia: Investigation and Management.* London/Los Angeles/Nicosia: Med-Orion; 1996:563–575.
10. Berguer R, Andaya LV, Bauer RB. Vertebral artery by-pass. *Arch Surg.* 1976;111:976–979.
11. Berguer R, Feldman AJ. Surgical reconstruction of the vertebral artery. *Surgery.* 1983;93:670–675.
12. Caplan LR, Shifrin EG. Natural history of vertebrobasilar arterial disease. In: Caplan L, Shifrin E, Nicolaides A, et al, eds. *Cerebrovascular Ischemia: Investigation and Management.* London/Los Angeles/Nicosia: Med-Orion; 1996:549–561.
13. Cate WR, Scott HW. Cerebral ischemia of central origin: relief by subclavian-vertebral artery thromboendarterectomy. *Surgery.* 1959;45:19–31.
14. Clark K, Perry MO. Carotid vertebral anastomosis: an alternative technique for repair of the subclavian steal syndrome. *Ann Surg.* 1966;163:414–416.
15. Comerota AJ, Maurer AH. Surgical correction and SPECT imaging of vertebrobasilar insufficiency due to unilateral vertebral artery stenosis. *Stroke.* 1992;23:602–606.
16. Contorni L. Il circolo collaterale vertebro-vertebrale nella obliterazione del' arteria subclavia alla sua origine. *Minerva Chirurgica.* 1960;15:268–271.
17. Crawford ES, De Bakey ME, Fields WS. Roentgenographic diagnosis and surgical treatment of basilar artery insufficiency. *JAMA.*1958;168:509–514.
18. Daseler EH, Anson BJ. Surgical anatomy of the subclavian artery and its branches. *Surg Gynecol Obstet.* 1959;108: 149–174.
19. Denny-Brown D. Basilar artery syndromes. *Bull N Engl Med Center.* 1953;15:53–60.
20. Deriu GP, Ballotta E, Franceshi L, et al. Surgical management of extracranial vertebral artery occlusive disease. *J Cardiovasc Surg.* 1991;32:413–419.
21. Deruty R, Soustiel JF, Pelisson-Guyotat I, et al. Extracranial surgery for vertebro-basilar ischemia. *Neurol Res.* 1991;13: 89–93.
22. Dmitriev AE, Dudkin BP, Iatsishin BS, et al. Characteristics of blood flow in the vertebral arteries in scalenus anticus syndrome. *Khirurgia (Moscow).* 1991;6:29–32.
23. Elkin DC, Harris MH. Arteriovenous aneurysm of the vertebral vessels: report of ten cases. *Ann Surg.* 1946;124: 934–951.
24. Giangola G, Imparato AM, Riles TS, et al. Vertebral artery angioplasty in patients younger than 55 years: long-term follow-up. *Ann Vasc Surg.* 1991;5:121–124.
25. Habozit B. Vertebral artery reconstruction: results in 106 patients. *Ann Vasc Surg.* 1991;5:61–65.
26. Hardin CA, Poser CM. Rotational obstruction of the vertebral artery due to redundancy and extraluminal fascial bands. *Ann Surg.* 1963;158:133–137.
27. Hennerici M, Klemm C, Rautenberg W. The subclavian steal phenomenon: a common vascular disorder with rare neurologic deficits. *Neurology.* 1988;38:669–673.
28. Hopkins LN, Martin NA, Hadley MN, et al. Vertebrobasilar insufficiency, II: microsurgical treatment of intracranial vertebrobasilar disease. *J Neurosurg.* 1987;66:662–674.
29. Husni EA, Bell HS, Storer J. Mechanical occlusion of the vertebral artery: a new clinical concept. *JAMA.* 1966;196: 475–478.
30. Husni EA, Storer J. The syndrome of mechanical occlusion of the vertebral artery: further observations. *Angiology.* 1967;18:106–116.
31. Hurvitz SA. Surgical treatment of partial extraluminal occlusion of the vertebral artery. *Surg Gynecol Obstet.* 1976; 143:257–262.
32. Hutchinson EC, Yates PO. Cervical portion of vertebral artery: clinico-pathological study. *Brain.* 1956;79:319–331.
33. Imparato AM. Vertebral arterial reconstruction: a nineteen-year experience. *J Vasc Surg.* 1985;2:626–633.
34. Imparato AM. Vertebral artery surgery—how I do it. In: Chang JB, ed. *Modern Vascular Surgery.* New York, NY: PMA Publishing Corporation; 1991:87–95.
35. Imparato AM, Lin JPT. Vertebral arterial reconstruction: internal plication and vein patch angioplasty. *Ann Surg.* 1967;166:213–221.
36. Jack CR, Boulos RS, Mechta BA, et al. Cerebral angiography in brainstem revascularization. *Am J Neuroradiol.* 1987; 8:211–219.
37. Kachel R. Percutaneous transluminal angioplasty (PTA) of supraaortic arteries, especially of the carotid and vertebral artery: an alternative to vascular surgery? *J Maladies Vasc.* 1993;18:254–257.
38. Kieffer E, Koskas F, Bahnini A, et al. Long term results after Reconstruction of the cervical vertebral artery. In: Caplan L, Shifrin E, Nicolaides A, et al, eds. *Cerebrovascular Ischemia: Investigation and Management.* London/Los Angeles/Nicosia: Med-Orion; 1996:617–625.
39. Kimura K, Yamaguchi T, Yasaka M, et al. Hemodynamics of the vertebral artery in subclavian steal syndrome and

subclavian steal phenomenon. *Rinsho-Shinkeigaku*. 1991;31: 970–973.

40. Kojima N, Tamaki W, Fujita K, et al. Vertebral artery occlusion at the narrowed scalenovertebral angle: mechanical vertebral occlusion in the distal first portion. *Neurosurgery*. 1985;16:672–674.

41. Nagashima C, Iwama K, Sakata A, et al. Effects of temporary occlusion of a vertebral artery on the human vestibular system. *J Neurosurg*. 1970;33:388–394.

42. Nicholls SC, Koutlas TC, Strandness DE. Clinical significance of retrograde flow in the vertebral artery. *Ann Vasc Surg*. 1991;5:331–336.

43. Nishijima M, Harada J, Nogami K, et al. Operative correction of kinking and coiling of the origin of vertebral artery and stellate ganglioectomy in patients with severe vertigo and dizziness. *No-Shinkei-Geka*. 1989;17:255–261.

44. Ogawa A, Sakurai Y, Kayama T, et al. Revascularization of vertebrobasilar occlusive disease. *No-Shinkei-Geka*. 1988;16: 149–155.

45. Ogawa A, Yoshimoto T, Sakurai Y. Treatment of proximal vertebral artery stenosis: Vertebral to subclavian transposition. *Acta Neurochirurgica*. 1991;112:13–18.

46. Pasch AR, Schuler JJ, De-Bord JR, et al. Subclavian steal despite ipsilateral vertebral occlusion. *J Vasc Surg*. 1985;2: 913–916.

47. Pauliukas PA, Barkauskas EM, Bickuviene JJ, et al. Surgical correction of vertebral artery anomalies causing vertebrobasilar insufficiency. In: Bernstein EF, Callow AD, Nicolaides AN, et al, eds. *Cerebral Revascularization*. Nicosia, Cyprus: Med-Orion; 1993:359–378.

48. Pauliukas PA, Barkauskas EM, Shifrin EF, et al. Experience with reconstructions of vertebral arteries. In: Caplan L, Shifrin E, Nicolaides A, et al, eds. *Cerebrovascular Ischemia: Investigation and Management*. London/Los Angeles/ Nicosia: Med-Orion; 1996:577–601.

49. Pauliukas PA, Streikus LK, Riapiachka AA. The anomalies of vertebral arteries: evaluation and surgical treatment. *Khirurgia (Moscow)*. 1990;11:10–15.

50. Powers SR, Drislane TM, Nevins S. Intermittent vertebral artery compression: a new syndrome. *Surgery*. 1961;9: 257–264.

51. Riggs HE, Rupp CH. Variation in form of circle of Willis. The relation of the variations to collateral circulation: anatomic analysis. *Arch Neurol*. 1963;8:8–14.

52. Senter HJ, Bittar SM, Long ET. Revascularisation of the extracranial vertebral artery at any level without cross-clamping. *J Neurosurg*. 1985;62:334–339.

53. Sheehan S, Bauer R, Meyer JS. Vertebral artery compression in cervical spondyliosis. *Neurology*. 1960;70:968–986.

54. Smith JM, Koury HJ, Hafner CD, et al. Subclavian steal syndrome. A review of 59 consecutive cases. *J Cardiovasc Surg*. 1994;35:11–14.

55. Spetzler RF, Hadley MN, Martin NA, et al. Vertebrobasilar insufficiency, I: microsurgical treatment of extracranial vertebrobasilar disease. *J Neurosurg*. 1987;66:648–661.

56. Stopford JSB. The arteries of the pons and medulla oblongata. *J Anat*. 1916;50:131–164.

57. Sundt TM, Whisnant JP, Piepgras DG, et al. Intracranial bypass grafts for vertebral-basilar ischemia. *Mayo Clin Proc*. 1978;53:12–18.

58. Thevenet A, Ruotolo C. Surgical repair of vertebral artery stenoses. *J Cardiovasc Surg*. 1984;25:101–110.

59. Tomita K. Another new etiology of vertebral artery insufficiency—a case of dynamic entrapment of vertebral artery by cervical nerve. *J Jpn Orthop Ass*. 1985;59:285–291.

60. Van Schill PE, Ackerstaff RG, Vermeulen FE, et al. Longterm clinical and duplex follow-up after proximal vertebral artery reconstruction. *Angiology*. 1992;43:961–968.

61. Wallenberg A. Acute bulbar affection. *Arch Psychiatr Nervenheilkd*. 1895;27:504–509.

62. Wesolowski AS, Gillie E, McMahon JS, et al. New arteriographic and surgical techniques for vertebral arteriopathies. *Circulation*. 1973;48(suppl III):211–219.

57

Traumatic Injuries to the Brachiocephalic Arteries

David G. Stanley

Traumatic injuries to the brachiocephalic arteries are rare, and consequently, their exact incidence is unknown. However, these injuries most often involve the carotid arteries, usually the common carotid arteries. Less commonly involved are the vertebrobasilar arteries and the thoracic outlet vessels. Traumatic injuries can be categorized as blunt trauma (from falls or a blunt instrument) or penetrating trauma (from gunshot and stab wounds).

Trauma to the Cervical Carotid Artery

Traumatic injuries to the carotid arteries are as old as the history of man, and the majority have a penetrating etiology. Gunshot wound injuries to the carotid artery are approximately three to four times as common as stab wound injuries to the carotid artery.[1]

The artery most often injured by penetrating gunshot wounds is the carotid artery, followed by the subclavian, vertebral, and innominate arteries. The most common artery injured by sharp penetrating injuries is the subclavian artery, followed by the common carotid artery. Blunt injuries, generally due to motor vehicle accidents, most commonly injure the subclavian or innominate arteries, with a lesser frequency of injury to the common carotid arteries and vertebral arteries.[2]

Apparently, the first ligation of the carotid artery for trauma was performed by David Fleming of the HMS Tonnant in October 1803.[3] During World Wars I and II the primary treatment of carotid artery injuries was ligation. American and British military surgeons reported a 44% mortality. Of those patients surviving carotid artery ligation, 29.6% had a permanent neurologic deficit. This high mortality and morbidity led Makins to advocate a nonoperative approach to carotid wounds.[4] During the Korean war, repair of carotid injuries, rather

than ligation, became common. Fogelman illustrated a 35% mortality in nonoperative injuries compared with a 10% mortality following carotid artery repair.[2]

During the Vietnam war, Bradley recognized that soldiers who presented with neurologic deficits had a high mortality from hemorrhagic cerebral infarction following carotid artery repair.[5] This experience resulted in recommendations against revascularization in patients presenting with coma or severe neurologic deficits with carotid artery injuries. Today, there continues to be debate concerning the appropriate management of patients with preoperative neurologic deficits with concomitant carotid trauma. The debate is in part a result of the very low incidence of patients presenting with carotid penetrating injuries and neurologic deficits. In the American Association for Surgery and Trauma study of 9 trauma centers, only 27 cervical carotid injuries with neurologic deficits were reported over a 5-year period, with an incidence of 0.5 patients per year per trauma center.[6]

Often, patients presenting with carotid injuries have associated wounds of the larynx, esophagus, trachea, jugular vein, and major nerves and muscles. They may also present with a large hematoma or significant bleeding. All of these factors are critical in the surgeon's decision concerning immediate exploration versus arteriography and other preoperative evaluations. If the patient is comatose and suspected of taking alcohol or drugs, it is difficult to evaluate the etiology of the neurologic deficit. It is generally agreed, however, that a comatose patient with a very high blood alcohol level may be treated by the surgeon in the same way as a patient with little or no neurologic deficit, particularly if there is no localizing neurologic deficit.

It is useful to divide patients with carotid injuries into three groups according to the presence or absence of neurologic deficits: (1) no neurologic deficit, (2) mild to moderate neurologic deficits, (3) severe neurologic deficits with hemiplegia or coma (Table 57.1). Fortu-

TABLE 57.1. Classification of patients with carotid injury by neurological deficit.

Group 1	None
Group 2	Mild to moderate
Group 3	Severe with hemiplegia or coma

nately, most patients with penetrating carotid injuries are in group 1.[7]

Several excellent studies support surgical repair of carotid artery injuries in all patients in groups 1 and 2. An exception may be patients with carotid artery occlusion and no neurologic symptoms. In these patients, careful noninvasive or arteriographic studies are indicated. Sometimes the study may show a very small residual channel, and successful repair may be anticipated. It is also important to determine if the patient has thrombus extending into the mid or distal internal carotid arteries or the middle cerebral arteries. In these patients, thrombectomy and repair may be very hazardous because inadequate removal of all thrombi may lead to embolus to the ipsilateral cerebral hemisphere.

All wounds that penetrate the skin, subcutaneous tissue, and sternocleidomastoid muscle should be explored. Cervical penetrating wounds have been categorized into three zones as described by Monson et al.[8] Zone 1 reaches from the arch of the aorta to 1 cm above the clavicle. Zone 2 extends from 1 cm above the clavicle to the angle of the mandible. Zone 3 extends from the angle of the mandible to the base of the skull (Figure 57.1). An arteriogram is very helpful in evaluating injuries in zones 1 and 3 because noninvasive evaluation and clinical examination are very difficult in these areas. Although some surgeons do preoperative arteriography in all stable patients, those patients with penetrating injuries in zone 2 with no neurologic deficit may be operated on without preoperative arteriography. All patients with evidence of neurologic deficit should have arteriographic study, including intracranial films, if they are stable. Prompt repair of the carotid artery in patients with no neurologic deficit results in excellent outcomes. The more extensive the neurologic deficit the higher the mortality. In Perry's series, of 49 patients in group 1, no mortality was reported. In contrast, in 8 group 2 patients a 12% mortality was reported, and in 15 group 3 patients a 33% mortality was noted.[9]

Operative Management

Preoperative arteriography is valuable in determining optimum placement of the incision. If the arterial injury has not been identified by arteriography, wide surgical exposure is needed to gain control of the proximal common carotid artery. The customary carotid incision for endarterectomy may generally be made. After the com-

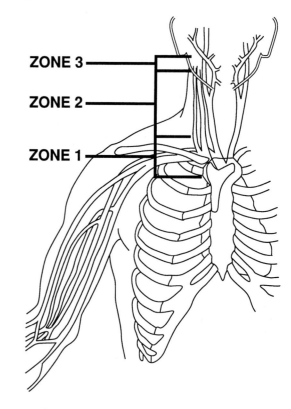

FIGURE 57.1. Zone categories of cervical penetrating wounds.

mon carotid artery is controlled, the area of injury may be dissected out and controlled by general pressure while exposing and controlling the internal and external carotid arteries. Injuries to the external carotid arteries may be repaired or the artery ligated, according to the preference of the surgeon. After gaining proximal control, the internal carotid artery backflow is quickly evaluated. If reverse flow is greater than 70 mm Hg, a shunt is not necessary. However, if it is less than 50 mm Hg, a shunt is recommended. A stab wound to the common carotid artery with little damage to the arterial wall may often be repaired primarily. However, internal carotid artery injuries are often difficult to repair and may require patch angioplasty or saphenous vein replacement of the injured artery. Of course, this type of repair should be done with a shunt in place. Heparin should be given during the period of carotid artery occlusion. Following repair, a small drain may be left in place for 12 hours if the surgeon is concerned about postoperative bleeding.

Postoperative Care

Patients should be carefully monitored in an intensive care unit for 12 to 24 hours following surgery. Any change in neurologic status should be quickly addressed and the patient evaluated by noninvasive ultrasound imaging or repeat arteriography. If postoperative evaluation reveals a problem with the repair or a postoperative thrombus, immediate return to the operating room is indicated. Patients in groups 1 and 2 should be followed carefully with continuous blood pressure and oxygen-saturation monitoring. Aggressive rehabilitation efforts are pursued in patients with neurologic deficits when the patient becomes stable. In most cases, recovery of these patients is directly related to the neurologic status prior to surgery.

Blunt Injuries to the Carotid Artery

Blunt injuries are relatively uncommon compared with penetrating injuries. Major damage to the carotid artery may occur either directly or through a stretch or rotational injury involving the cervical vertebra. Thrombosis may occur due to direct injury or from intimal dissection. The blunt injury may be associated with fractures of the mandible or cervical spine and may reveal abrasions or hematomas. Approximately one half of patients present with no observable evidence of neck injury.

Recently, a patient was referred to our practice by an otolaryngologist who noted a left carotid bruit at the time of evaluation for hearing loss. Duplex evaluation revealed an unusual finding. The left proximal common carotid artery appeared to have 90% or greater stenosis with a velocity of 232 cm/s in the area of stenosis. On close questioning, the patient recalled that she had fallen approximately 2 months earlier, hitting the left side of her neck on the bed post. The accident was forgotten until she was questioned following the duplex examination.

The patient had no true transient ischemic attack symptoms. Arteriograms revealed a weblike stenosis in the left common carotid artery (Figure 57.2). Exploration of the artery subsequently confirmed an intimal flap nearly occluding the common carotid artery. There was no evidence of atheroma. The flap was excised and the patient recovered satisfactorily. This case illustrates that many blunt injuries to the carotid artery are asymptomatic, and in fact, some are probably not ever identified. The occasional weblike stenosis found at the time of carotid surgery may be due to a chronic intimal flap from previous trauma.

Blunt carotid injuries in children may be due to falls with blunt objects in their mouths, leading to transpharyngeal trauma to the carotid artery. As in adults, these blunt injuries are often asymptomatic, and diagnosis is made only after arteriography. In other patients, a lucid interval is followed by neurologic deficits that occur hours to days after the trauma. Patients who present with a concomitant concussion or in a comatose condition from alcohol and/or drugs, make it difficult to obtain

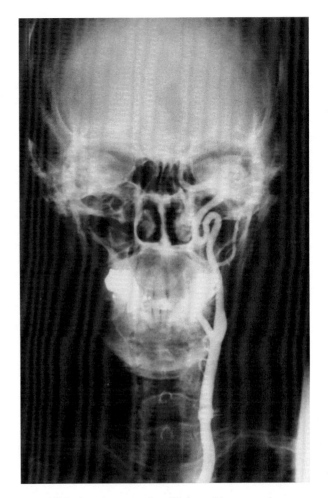

FIGURE 57.2. Arteriogram of an 82-year-old woman demonstrating a weblike stenosis and near occlusion of the common carotid secondary to blunt trauma.

information concerning the onset of symptoms. Delayed thrombosis or embolism may explain the lucid interval seen in some patients.

Symptoms may include ipsilateral neck pain or headaches, and oculosympathetic paresis may be present. Arteriography most commonly demonstrates occlusion of the distal carotid artery. However, dissection, intimal flaps, and pseudoaneurysms are sometimes seen.[10] In the majority of cases, diagnosis is made by either duplex ultrasound or arteriography.[11]

Arterial dissection can sometimes be effectively treated with heparin if it is not contraindicated by other injuries such as intracranial bleeding or pelvic fractures. The usual intensive treatment for stroke patients and specialized rehabilitation care may enable some of these patients to regain a reasonable degree of activity.

Vertebrobasilar Artery Injuries

The majority of vertebrobasilar artery injuries are nonpenetrating injuries. The occasional penetrating injury that results in laceration or disruption of the vertebral artery may be treated by ligation above and below the area of injury. If the contralateral vertebral artery is patent, the patient usually has a good recovery.

Most blunt injuries of the cervical vertebral arteries are due to contusion by sudden rotation and stretching between C1 and C2. A rotation–extension movement is the most common source of injury and is generally related to dissection of the artery from minor falls, vehicle accidents, sudden spontaneous rotation of the head, and other relatively minor activities. Arteriography typically reveals narrowing or occlusion with associated pseudoaneurysm. Rarely, spontaneous dissections from arteritis, fibromuscular dysplasia, and cystic medial degeneration are reported. The severity in the clinical course of the patient with vertebral artery dissection varies. Some patients have delayed or progressive infarction early after the injury. Anticoagulation may be helpful in selected patients. Spinal tap should be considered prior to anticoagulation in these patients to rule out intracranial bleeding.[12]

Intrathoracic Brachiocephalic Injuries

Intrathoracic injuries of the brachiocephalic arteries present one of the most difficult challenges for surgeons. Such an injury may be related to stab wounds to the base of the neck, gunshot wounds, or vehicle accidents, with fracture of the clavicle and first rib. Although occasionally a patient presents with neurologic deficits, most are seen with other findings, including shock, brachial plexus injuries, fractures to ribs and extremities, and concussions. Arterial disruption is frequently found on computed tomograph scans of the upper chest or on arteriogram. All stable patients should undergo arteriography to help plan the approach to repair of the injured vessel. Common carotid and subclavian injuries are more frequently seen[2] (Table 57.2).

Operative Management

Careful planning of the operative approach is necessary in order to gain control of the bleeding vessel. In some cases, control of the proximal vessel through placement

TABLE 57.2. Locations of arterial injuries.

Artery injured	Number
Subclavian	13
Common carotid	10
Innominate	3
Vertebral	2

From Abouljoud et al.[2]

of a intraluminal balloon, either after exposure of the distal artery or (in a subclavian artery) through the distal brachial artery, may be helpful. Injuries of the innominate and proximal common carotid arteries may require median sternotomy with extension up into the neck when indicated for common carotid exposure. The left subclavian artery is more difficult to expose and may be approached by transverse division of the sternum, extending the incision into the third rib interspace anteriorly on the left side of the chest. It is rarely necessary to divide or resect the median portion of the clavicle to improve exposure.

Primary repair of the vessels may be performed or, if destruction of the vessel is significant, the vessel can be replaced with a synthetic graft or a saphenous vein graft. If the patient survives the initial injury and surgical repair, long-term recovery is related primarily to the presenting neurologic deficits or brachial plexus injuries. Edema of the arm may result from subclavian injuries if the subclavian vein is sacrificed or thrombosed in the perioperative period. An attempt should be made to repair venous injuries whenever possible. Hematomas in the area of brachial plexus should be evacuated, and contaminated injuries irrigated thoroughly.

References

1. Perry MO. Carotid injuries. In: Veith F, ed. *Current Critical Problems in Vascular Surgery*. St Louis, Mo: Quality Medical Publishing; 1989:465–469.
2. Abouljoud M, Obied F, Horst H, et al. Arterial injuries of the thoracic outlet: a ten-year experience. *Am Surg*. 1993; 59:590–595.
3. Garrison EH. *History of Medicine*. Philadelphia, Pa: WB Saunders; 1929.
4. Rich N, Spencer FC. *Carotid and Vertebral Injuries. Vascular Trauma*. Philadelphia, Pa: WB Saunders; 1978:chap 11.
5. Bradley EL. Consequence of cerebral vascular injury. Management of penetrating carotid injuries. *J Trauma*. 1973; 13:49.
6. Richardson R, Obeid F, Richardson J, et al. Neurologic consequences of cerebrovascular injury. *J Trauma*. 1992; 32:755–760.
7. Thal ER, Snyder WH, Hayes RJ, et al. Management of carotid artery injuries. *Surgery*. 1974;76:955.
8. Monson DU, Saletta JD, Freeark RJ. Carotid vertebral trauma. *J Trauma*. 1969;9:987.
9. Perry MO. Management of specific arterial injuries. In: Nejarian JS, Delaney JP, eds. *Advances in Vascular Surgery*. Chicago, Ill: Yearbook Medical Publishers; 1983:170.
10. Pretre R, Reverdin A, Kalonji T, et al. Blunt carotid artery injury: difficult therapeutic approaches for an under recognized entity. *Surgery*. 1994;115:375–381.
11. Cogbill T, Moore E, Meissner M, et al. The spectrum of blunt injury to the carotid artery: a multicenter perspective. *J Trauma*. 1994;37:473–479.
12. Senter H, Sarwar M. Non-traumatic dissecting aneurysm of the vertebral artery. *J Neurosurg*. 1982;56:128.

58

Repair of Coarctation of the Aorta

Kazutomo Goh, Yoshihiko Kubo, and Tadahiro Sasajima

Coarctation of the aorta is a congenital narrowing of the aorta, with the narrowing usually located adjacent to the ductus arteriosus or ligamentum arteriosum. Less commonly, congenital narrowing of the aorta may be recognized anywhere in the aorta.

Repair of coarctation of the aorta in neonates and infants has been a challenge for surgeons, and the problem of recoarctation has not been solved completely. In this chapter we discuss the morphology and pathophysiology of the disease, and various methods of repair, and we describe and review the results of repair.

Coarctation of the Aorta

Morphology

Classically, coarctation of the aorta was classified as *infantile* or *preductal* type, and *adult* or *postductal* type (Figure 58.1). Although there is some merit to these classifications, coarctation of the aorta should be considered with respect to the anatomical and clinical spectrum—from discrete narrowing to diffuse hypoplasia, and from asymptomatic patients to critically ill neonates. Several types of obstructive lesions are observed: the shelf lesion, isthmic narrowing, the waist lesion, and combinations of these lesions in different degrees.[1]

Older children commonly present with isolated discrete coarctation. This discrete lesion consists of the localized waist or hourglass appearance outside, and the "shelf" inside. Infolding of the aortic media and hypertrophied intima opposite the ductus arteriosus form the shelf. Degenerative changes such as aneurysm formation, dissection, or compensatory change such as development of collateral circulation may be seen more frequently as the patient gets older.

In contrast, neonates or infants usually present with much more serious symptoms. In these patients, the waist and the shelf are less prominent. The ductus arteriosus and the descending aorta form a large and continuous lumen. But the isthmus and arch are often hypoplastic. The ductal tissue may be found in the aortic wall adjacent to the ductus arteriosus. Associated intracardiac anomalies are much more common in these patients.

Patent ductus arteriosus, interatrial communication, and hypoplasia of the isthmus and arch are common associated lesions. In fact, these may be considered a part of the anomaly in neonates and infants. The definition of aortic arch hypoplasia is difficult but we usually use Moulaert's criterion.[2] Association of left-sided obstructive lesions such as aortic stenosis at various levels, bicuspid aortic valve, and mitral stenosis is frequent. And association of abnormal interventricular or great vessel communication with diminished ascending aortic flow such as ventricular septal defect (VSD), with or without transposition of the great arteries, double outlet right ventricle, or aortopulmonary window, is also frequent.[3]

Pathophysiology

Pathophysiology, clinical course, and the management of the coarctation are determined by the degree of aortic obstruction, the patency of the ductus arteriosus, and the associated intracardiac anomalies.

The mildest form is a mild to moderate isolated coarctation with closed ductus arteriosus. There may be hypertension of the upper body and left ventricular hypertrophy, and a development of collateral circulation. These may be tolerated for a long period without significant symptoms. However, if the degree of obstruction is severe, left ventricular pressure overload and subsequent left ventricular failure and hypoperfusion of the lower body can develop.

If the ductus arteriosus is open, the lower body perfusion may be maintained by the blood flow from the right ventricle through the ductus arteriosus. The lower body blood pressure is still lower than that of the upper body, and the oxygen content of the lower body is lower than

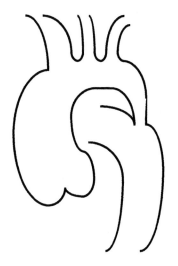 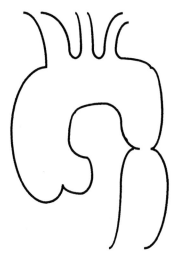

FIGURE 58.1. Infantile and adult type of coarctation.

"Infantile" or "preductal" type   "Adult" or "postductal" type

that of the upper. As the pulmonary vascular resistance becomes lower over the month after birth, and as the ductus arteriosus starts closing, the lower body perfusion becomes less, and the left ventricular afterload becomes larger. If this process of ductal closure occurs rapidly, it may not be tolerated; left ventricular failure and hypoperfusion of the lower body develop rapidly.

In the presence of VSD and patent ductus arteriosus, left-to-right shunting through the VSD and relatively higher pulmonary arterial pressure may favor the lower body perfusion through the ductus and the oxygen content in the blood to the lower body for a certain period after birth. However, as the pulmonary vascular resistance becomes lower and the ductus arteriosus starts closing, the left ventricular afterload becomes higher, and the left-to-right shunting increases. This leads to left ventricular volume overload and subsequent congestive heart failure. The lower body perfusion is also compromised as the ductal flow becomes less. The clinical presentation is congestive heart failure and hypoperfusion of the lower body. When more complex intracardiac anomalies are present, problems such as hypoxia or left-sided intracardiac obstruction complicate the hemodynamics further. Thus, the patients in the neonatal period or early infancy with coarctation and VSD or major associated intracardiac anomalies usually present with a critically ill state of congestive heart failure and significant lower body hypoperfusion.

Diagnosis and Management

Symptomatic Neonates and Infants

Symptomatic neonates and infants usually present with marked congestive heart failure and cardiovascular col-

lapse. The symptoms are tachycardia, tachypnea, and weak pulses. Oliguria, and metabolic acidosis may be noticed. Cardiomegaly, seen in chest x-ray films and as biventricular hypertrophy on electrocardiographs, is common. Echocardiography is useful in making the diagnosis of coarctation and in finding other associated intracardiac anomalies. Prompt resuscitation is necessary in these patients. Prostaglandin E_1 administration without delay is particularly important.[4] It may reopen the closing ductus arteriosus and may relieve the obstruction of coarctation itself. Mechanical ventilation with a muscle relaxant may be necessary in very sick patients. PO_2 and PCO_2 should be monitored and adjusted closely to control the pulmonary vascular resistance. FIO_2 should be minimal and PCO_2 should be above 45 mm Hg to control the pulmonary vascular resistance. If the left ventricular failure supervenes, catecholamines and vasodilators are administered. In the presence of acidosis and oliguria, sodium bicarbonate and diuretics are given. Operation should be scheduled within a day or a few days while the general condition is being stabilized. If the patient does not respond well to resuscitation, the operation should be performed without delay.

Older Patients

Mild to moderate isolated coarctation, without significant associated cardiovascular lesions, can be tolerated well without symptoms. Older patients in this state often present with hypertension or weak femoral pulses. Chest radiographs may show cardiomegaly and rib notching as the patient gets older. Electrocardiograms may be normal or may show left ventricular hypertrophy. Echocardiograms can show the anatomy of the coarctation and the pressure gradient across the coarctation. Computerized tomography, magnetic resonance imaging, and angiography are useful in visualizing the anatomy. Elective operation is usually indicated if a resting gradient across the coarctation is 30 mm Hg or greater, or the luminal diameter is 50% or less.

Surgical Techniques for Coarctation Repair

Several techniques for repairing coarctation have been proposed (Figure 58.2). No single technique is distinctly superior to the others.[5-8] One should be aware of the advantages and disadvantages of each technique and select the most appropriate procedure according to the anatomy, associated intracardiac anomalies, and the pathophysiology of the individual patient.[9,10]

Resection of the coarctation with end-to-end anastomosis has been preferred by many surgeons. The advantage of this technique is the potential to remove the ductal tissue that may be responsible for late recoarctation. With extended resection, it can be applied to the patients with isthmus and arch hypoplasia. The disadvantages are greater tension on the suture line, more extensive dissection, and the circumferential scar on the aorta. Development of more precise vascular anastomotic technique and application of monofilament absorbable sutures may overcome the disadvantages.[11-13] Experience from other cardiovascular procedures indicates that the circumferential suture line does grow if a monofilament absorbable suture is used appropriately.[14] Favorable results with this technique and its modification (extended resection and end-to-end anastomosis) for neonates and infants have been reported.[15-20]

After the initial poor experience with resection and end-to-end anastomosis for sick neonates and infants, the subclavian flap aortoplasty technique was adopted by many surgeons, and favorable results have been reported.[21-24] This technique does not require extensive dissection and is easy to perform. The suture line is not circumferential, and less tension is expected. Also, it can be accomplished without prosthetic material. On the other hand, it sacrifices the circulation to the left arm, it may leave the ductal tissue at the coarctation, and it cannot relieve the arch hypoplasia. A patch augmentation can be added to the procedure. Modification of the technique, for example, isthmus flap aortoplasty, has been described to preserve the left subclavian artery.[25]

Reversed subclavian flap aortoplasty is another option to relieve the obstruction of the aorta between the left subclavian and left carotid arteries.[26] It may be performed in combination with resection and end-to-end to end anastomosis technique.

Patch aortoplasty does not require extensive resection, it is easily performed in a relatively short time, and it does not sacrifice the left subclavian artery.[27] The higher

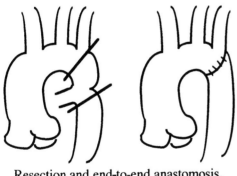
Resection and end-to-end anastomosis.

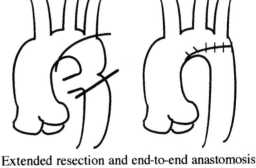
Extended resection and end-to-end anastomosis

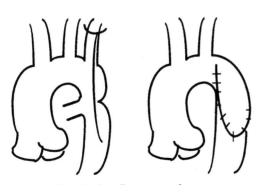
Subclavian flap aortoplasty

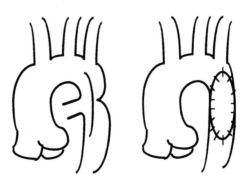
Patch aortoplasty

FIGURE 58.2. Common surgical techniques for coarctation repair.

incidence of late aneurysm formation on the aortic wall opposite the patch is the major disadvantage of this technique. It can be combined with resection and end-to-end anastomosis or subclavian flap aortoplasty when these techniques alone are inadequate for repair. It is useful for critically ill patients or for redo cases.[28,29]

In the presence of certain large VSDs or other associated intracardiac anomalies, coarctation repair may have to be combined with pulmonary artery banding. Some prefer to repair the coarctation and the associated intracardiac anomalies simultaneously on cardiopulmonary bypass through the midline sternotomy.[3,30] In fact, midline sternotomy and primary repair of the coarctation and associated lesion may be the treatment of choice in patients with aortic coarctation, VSD, and subaortic stenosis.[31]When the coarctation is repaired through the midline sternotomy, extended resection and end-to-end anastomosis or augmentation of the aortic arch by patching of the undersurface of the aorta are frequently utilized.[32]

With the development of interventional cardiology, the use of balloon dilatation for the coarctation has been reported. Complications such as aortic rupture, inadequate dilation, or femoral arterial troubles have been reported.[33,34] However, with more experience, the incidence of technique-related complications has decreased.[35] Although the long-term results and the incidence of aneurysm formation have to be further evaluated in the light of more experience,[36,37] this technique is useful for sick infants or for patients with recurrent coarctation and provides favorable results.[38,39]

Resection and End-to-End Anastomosis

After careful induction of anesthesia, the right radial artery is cannulated to monitor the perfusion pressure of the upper body or the innominate artery. Care is taken to keep the body temperature below 35°C. The patient is placed in the right lateral position. The chest is entered through the third or fourth intercostal space. If prominent collateral circulation is expected, the chest is entered through the rib bed. The left lung is retracted anteroinferiorly. The mediastinal pleura posterior to the descending aorta and along the left subclavian artery is incised longitudinally. Several sutures are placed on the anterior end of the pleura and are pulled up to provide a good operative field. The vagus nerve is identified and secured on the pleural side. The aortic arch beyond its junction with the left subclavian artery, the left subclavian artery, the isthmus, the ductus arteriosus, and the descending aorta to its second or third intercostal arteries are dissected and mobilized. The dissection plane should be kept close to the adventitia of the aorta so as not to damage the lymphatic vessels. Abbott's artery behind the junction of the left subclavian artery and the

aorta should not be compromised. If the body temperature is still high at this stage, cold saline may be poured into the thoracic cavity. Great care should be taken not to cool the heart directly. Steroid administration may also be beneficial to prevent spinal cord ischemia during aortic cross-clamping. The left lung is inflated and ventilated for a few minutes before aortic cross-clamping. The ductus arteriosus is doubly ligated and divided. A curved vascular clamp is placed across the isthmus or the aortic arch with the left subclavian artery. Another clamp is placed across the descending aorta well distal to the coarctation. The coarctation is then excised with care so as not to leave the ductal tissue near the ductal insertion. An incision into the undersurface of the arch or into the lateral wall of the left subclavian artery may be added if necessary. A 6-0 or 7-0 PDS or Maxon suture is used for anastomosis. The end-to-end anastomosis is started from the area most distal to the surgeon. Half of the posterior continuous sutures are placed with the aortic ends held apart. Then the rest of the suture is made with the aortic ends approximated together without tension. On completion of the anastomosis, the distal clamp is released to let the air flood out with the blood. The proximal clamp is gradually released with great care. If hypotension is encountered, the clamp may have to be reapplied. Fluid administration and catecholamine support may be necessary. The mediastinal pleura is roughly approximated, and a chest tube is left in the thoracic cavity before chest closure.

Extended Resection and End-to-End Anastomosis

In the presence of aortic arch hypoplasia, extended resection should be considered. The dissection along the arch is extended to its junction with the innominate artery or to the ascending aorta. Distal dissection is extended to the level of the third or fourth intercostal arteries. The proximal aortic clamp is placed across the left subclavian artery, left carotid artery, and the aortic arch between the innominate and left carotid arteries. We find it useful to apply one vascular clamp across the carotid artery and aortic arch and another clamp to the left subclavian artery for secure control of the proximal end. After the distal aortic clamp is placed, the coarctation is resected, and the undersurface of the arch is incised for a large anastomosis. The rest of the procedure is done in the same fashion as the conventional end-to-end anastomosis, with great care not to have undue tension on the suture line.

Subclavian Flap Aortoplasty

The dissection of the aorta, ductus arteriosus, and the coarctation is similar to that for resection and end-to-end anastomosis, but to a lesser extent. Dissection of the left subclavian artery is carried out so that the branches of the artery are identified. After ligation of the ductus arteriosus, the branches of the left subclavian artery are ligated. A vascular clamp is placed across the aortic arch between the left subclavian artery and left carotid artery. Another clamp is placed on the descending aorta well below the coarctation. An incision is made along the lateral wall of the left subclavian artery, across the coarctation, and into the descending aorta well below the coarctation. The left subclavian artery is then transected just proximal to its branches. The intimal shelf is excised very carefully so as not to damage the posterior wall of the aorta. The tip of the subclavian flap and the lower end of the aortic incision are approximated with a 6-0 or 7-0 polypropylene suture. The side wall of the flap and the aortic incision are anastomosed from the proximal end with a 6-0 or 7-0 polypropylene suture. The rest of the procedure is similar to that for resection and end-to-end anastomosis.

Reversed Subclavian Flap Aortoplasty

For reversed subclavian flap aortoplasty, proximal dissection of the aorta is extended to the arch proximal to the left carotid artery. The left carotid artery should be mobilized also. A curved vascular clamp is placed across the left carotid artery and the aortic arch between the left carotid and the innominate artery, leaving the left carotid artery several millimeters to the aortic side. Another clamp is placed across the descending aorta. The branches of the left subclavian arteries are ligated, and the left subclavian artery is incised just proximal to the branches. An incision is made along the medial wall of the left subclavian artery across the arch between the left subclavian and the left carotid artery, into the origin and the proximal segment of the left carotid artery. The subclavian flap is then approximated to the incision on the aortic arch and the left carotid artery. Anastomosis is performed with a continuous 6-0 or 7-0 suture. Great care should be taken not to allow any air into the left carotid artery when the vascular clamps are released. The rest of the procedure is as the same as for the previous techniques.

Patch Aortoplasty

Minimal dissection is necessary for patch aortoplasty. After dissection around the aorta adjacent to the coarctation and the ductus arteriosus, the ductus arteriosus is ligated. Vascular clamps are placed to exclude the narrowed segment. A longitudinal incision, well above and below the coarctation at its ends, is made on the aorta. A patch of Dacron or expanded polytetrafluoroethylene is anastomosed to the incision.

Operations for Recoarctation

Unfortunately, recoarctation is observed after any of these techniques. Reoperation is usually indicated if the pressure gradient is greater than 30 mm Hg.

With refined technique and the new balloons available, balloon dilatation has become the procedure of choice for recoarctations. Reports have suggested that it is effective in more than 70% of patients, and it can be performed with low mortality and morbidity.[33,34] Hijazi and associates have reported that the mean peak systolic pressure gradient decreased from 40.3 to 7.5 mm Hg.[34]

When balloon dilatation is not suitable for relief of the narrowing, operation should be done. When the initial operation is resection and end-to-end anastomosis or subclavian flap aortoplasty, patch artoplasty can be performed with low mortality and low morbidity. But late aneurysm formation is still a concern if it is the second operation. If dissection around the coarctation can be extended satisfactorily, resection and end-to-end anastomosis or subclavian flap aortoplasty should be considered. When the area of coarctation cannot be reached safely, bypass operation with a prosthetic graft is an option. For patients with aortic arch hypoplasia and recoarctation, patch augmentation of the arch and recoarctation through median sternotomy under cardiopulmonary bypass and deep hypothermic circulatory arrest should be considered.[40]

Results of Coarctation Repair

With the improvement of perioperative management, operative strategy, and operative technique, operative mortality in neonates and infants has decreased significantly. Isolated coarctation and coarctation with VSD can be treated with acceptable results. On the other hand, the operative results for patients with complex intracardiac anomalies are still poor. Table 58.1 shows the operative mortality of coarctation repair for infants by several authors.[6,8,13,17,41,45,46] Young age at operation, presence of aortic arch hypoplasia, and need for pulmonary artery banding are also associated with early mortality.[41-45]

Complications

Postoperative hypertension encountered after coarctation repair, known as paradoxical hypertension, is not uncommon. The mechanism of paradoxical hypertension has been investigated, and imbalance of neurological and humoral factors has been suggested.[36] Involvement of vasopressin, atrial natriuretic factor, the renin–angiotensin system, and aldosterone have been investigated.[46-49] Administration of sodium nitroprusside

TABLE 58.1. Operative mortality of repair of coarctation of the aorta for neonates and infants with or without associated cardiac lesions.

Author	Number of patients	Morality (%)			
		Overall	Isolated CoA	CoA with VSD	CoA with complex CHD
Harlan et al.[13]	47	32	18	11	44
Trinquet et al.[46]	178	20	8	11	37
Lacour-Gayet et al.[17]	66	14	13	0	28
Messmer et al.[8]	53	8	0	0	18
Rubay et al.[6]	146	6	0	4	22
Merrill et al.[45]	139	7	0	2	15
Demircin et al.[41]	75	9	2	17	27

CoA, coarctation of the aorta; VSD, ventricular septal defect; CHD, congenital heart disease.

is effective in most patients. However, there are some patients in whom treatment with nitroprusside is not effective. The protective effect of beta-blockade, as with propranolol, has been suggested.[50] Intestinal ischemia or postcoarctation syndrome observed after coarctation repair is manifested by mild to severe symptoms such as abdominal discomfort, tenderness, and ileus. The mechanism of this syndrome is not fully understood, but it may be related to the mechanism of paradoxical hypertension. This syndrome is relatively rare in patients under 2 years of age.

The most common postoperative complication is recoarctation. It is more common than previously thought.[42] Most authors define recoarctation as a stenosis with a resting pressure gradient of 20 mm Hg or greater, and reoperation is usually indicated when the pressure gradient is 30 mm Hg or greater. It is more common when the initial operation is performed in the neonatal period or early infancy.[51] The involvement of the ductal tissue may play some role in the development of recoarctation in the early postoperative period. There are many reports pointing out the superiority of one operative technique to another. But recoarctation does occur after any of the surgical techniques that have been described, and the incidence of recoarctation is not directly affected by any of these techniques. Table 58.2 shows the incidence of recoarctation after different techniques by different authors.[6,8,15,17,29,46]

Paraplegia is a serious problem once it occurs, although the incidence of postoperative paraplegia is low.[52] Hyperthermia during the operation and aberrant right subclavian artery are risk factors for this complication.[53] Hyperthermia should be avoided in any patients with coarctation. When there is any possibility of hypoperfusion due to inadequate collaterals to the lower body, or of spinal cord ischemia in relatively older patients, cardiopulmonary bypass, left heart bypass, and temporary shunting should be established before the aorta is cross-clamped.

Aneurysm formation in the late postoperative period is most commonly seen after initial patch aortoplasty.[54] The aneurysm is usually seen opposite the patch. Aortic arch hypoplasia may enhance aneurysm formation.[55] This complication is also seen after subclavian flap aortoplasty and balloon dilatation of the coarctation. Therefore, patch aortoplasty should be reserved for certain limited situations such as reoperation, coarctation repair in a very sick patient, and in combination with resection and end-to-end anastomosis or subclavian flap aortoplasty.

Persistent hypertension may be observed after successful operation. It is more evident when an exercise test is performed, and it is more often observed when the initial operation is performed in older age.[5] Structural changes of the upper aortic segment and the left ventricle, resetting of baroreceptors, and associated humoral response may contribute to this phenomenon.[56–58]

TABLE 58.2. Recoarctation after coarctation repair in neonates and infants.

Author	Number of patients	Overall incidence (%)	Initial procedure and incidence (%)				Parameters of evaluation
			RETE	ERETE	SFA	PA	
Cobanoglu et al.[15]	134	83	92	—	75	—	Freedom from reoperation at 5 yr
Yee et al.[28]	110	14	22	—	—	12	Incidence of recoarctation
Trinquet et al.[46]	178	85	81	86	89	—	Freedom from recoarctation at 5 yr
Lacour-Gayet et al.[17]	66	90	—	90	—	—	Freedom from recoarctation at 5 yr
Messmer et al.[8]	53	—	9	—	0	42	Incidence of recoarctation
Rubay et al.[6]	146	—	10	—	12	—	Incidence of recoarctation

RETE, resection and end-to-end anastomosis; ERETE, extended resection and end-to-end anastomosis; SFA, subclavian flap aortoplasty; PA, patch aortoplasty.

Atypical Coarctation

The narrowing of the aorta may be found in the lower thoracic or upper abdominal aorta in rare instances. It is usually a diffuse lesion with occasional association of adjacent arterial branch lesions. Histopathology of the lesion shows the dysplastic nature of the aortic wall. It is known as midaortic dysplastic syndrome, abdominal coarctation, or atypical coarctation.[59]

Patients present with hypertension, claudication of the lower extremities, or left ventricular hypertrophy in older age. Angiography, computerized tomography, and magnetic resonance imaging all confirm diagnosis of the disease.

The surgical treatment consists of placement of a bypass graft on the aorta over the narrowing, patch aortoplasty, and revascularization of the visceral vessels if there is any stenosis in these vessels. Operative results are usually good, and hypertension is cured in most of the patients.[60]

References

1. Pellegrino A, Deverall PB, Anderson RH, et al. Aortic coarctation in the first three months of life. *J Thorac Cardiovasc Surg.* 1985;89:121–127.
2. Moulaert AJ, Bruins CC, Oppenheimer-Dekker A. Anomalies of the aortic arch and ventricular septal defect. *Circulation.* 1976;53:1011–1015.
3. Pigott JD, Chin AJ, Weinberg PM, et al. Transposition of the great arteries with aortic arch obstruction. *J Thorac Cardiovasc Surg.* 1987;94:82–86.
4. Jones RD, Duncan AE, Mee RB. Perioperative management of neonatal aortic isthmic coarctation. *Anesthesia and Intensive Care.* 1985;13:311–318.
5. Kappetein AP, Guit GL, Bogers AJJC, et al. Noninvasive long-term follow-up after coarctation. *Ann Thorac Surg.* 1993;55:1153–1159.
6. Rubay JE, Sluysmans T, Alexandrescu V, et al. Surgical repair of coarctation of the aorta in infants under one year of age. Long-term results in 146 patients comparing subclavian flap angioplasty and modified end-to-end anastomosis. *J Cardiovasc Surg.* 1992;33:216–222.
7. Bertolini A, Dalmonte P, Tom P, et al. Goretex patch aortoplasty for coarctation in children: Nuclear magnetic resonance assessment. *J Cardiovasc Surg.* 1992;33:223–228.
8. Messmer BJ, Minale C, Muhler E. Surgical correction of coarctation in early infancy: does surgical technique influence the result? *Ann Thorac Surg.* 1991;52:594–603.
9. Zannini L, Gargiulo G, Albanese SB, et al. Aortic coarctation with hypoplastic arch in neonates: a spectrum of anatomic lesions requiring different surgical options. *Ann Thorac Surg.* 1993;56:288–284.
10. Amato JJ, Galdieri RJ, Cotroneo JV. Role of extended aortoplasty related to the definition of the aorta. *Ann Thorac Surg.* 1991;52:615–620.
11. Chiu I, Hung C, Chao S, et al. Growth of the aortic anastomosis in pigs. *J Thorac Cardiovasc Surg.* 1988;95:112–118.
12. Schmitz-Rixen T, Storck M, Erasmi H, et al. Vascular anastomoses with absorbable suture material: an experimental study. *Ann Vasc Surg.* 1991;5:257–264.
13. Harlan JL, Doty DB, Brandt B III, et al. Coarctation of the aorta in infants. *J Thorac Cardiovasc Surg.* 1984;88:1012–1019.
14. Contis JC, Heffron TG, Whitington PF, et al. Use of absorbable suture material in vascular anastomoses in pediatric liver transplantation. *Transplantation Proc.* 1993;25:1878–1880.
15. Cobanoglu A, Teply JF, Grunkemeier GL, et al. Coarctation of the aorta in patients younger than three months: a critique of the subclavian flap operation. *J Thorac Cardiovasc Surg.* 1985;89:128–135.
16. Korfer R, Meyer H, Kleikamp G, et al. Early and late results after resection and end-to-end anastomosis of coarctation of the thoreacic aorta in infancy. *J Thorac Cardiovasc Surg.* 1985;890:616–622.
17. Lacour-Gayet F, Bruniaux J, Serraf A, et al. Hypoplastic transverse arch and coarctation in neonates. *J Thorac Cardiovasc Surg.* 1990;100:808–816.
18. Lansman S, Shapiro AJ, Schiller MS, et al. Extended aortic arch anastomosis for repair of coarctation in infancy. *Circulation.* 1986;74:I37–I41.
19. Elliot MJ. Coarctation of the aorta with arch hypoplasia: Improvements on a new technique. *Ann Thorac Surg.* 1987;44:321–323.
20. van Son JAM, van Asten WNJC, van Lier HJJ, et al. A comparison of coarctation resection and subclavian flap angioplasty using ultrasonographically monitored postocclusive reactive hyperemia. *J Thorac Cardiovasc Surg.* 1990;100:817–829.
21. Myers JL, McConnell BA, Waldhausen JA. Coarctation of the aorta in infants: does the aortic arch grow after repair? *Ann Thorac Surg.* 1992;54:869–874.
22. Baudet E, al-Qudah A. Late results of the subclavian flap repair of coarctation in infancy. *J Cardiovasc Surg.* 1989;30:445–449.
23. Ziemer G, Jonas RA, Perry SB, et al. Surgery for the coarctation of the aorta in neonates. *Circulation.* 1986;74:I25–I31.
24. Kopf GS, Hallenbrand W, Kleinman C, et al. Repair of aortic coarctation in the first three months of life: immediate and long-term results. *Ann Thorac Surg.* 1986;41:425–430.
25. Brown JW, Fiore AC, King H. Isthmus flap aortoplasty: an alternative to subclavian flap aortoplasty for long-segment coarctation of the aorta in infants. *Ann Thorac Surg.* 1985;40:274–279.
26. Hart JL, Waldhausen JA. Reversed subclavian flap angioplasty for arch coarctation of the aorta. *Ann Thorac Surg.* 1983;36:715–717.
27. Rostad H, Abdelnoor M, Sorland S, et al. Coarctation of the aorta, early and late results of various surgical techniques. *J Cardiovasc Surg.* 1989;30:885–890.
28. Yee ES, Turley K, Soifer S, et al. Synthetic patchangioplasty. A simplified approach for coarctation in repairs during early infancy and thereafter. *Am J Surg.* 1984;148:240–243.
29. Yee ES, Soifer SJ, Turley K, et al. Infant coarctation: a spectrum in clinical presentation and treatment. *Ann Thorac Surg.* 1986;42:488–493.

30. Planche C, Serraf A, Comas JV, et al. Anatomic repair of transposition of great arteries with ventricular septal defect and aortic arch obstruction. *J Thorac Cardiovasc Surg.* 1993;105:925–933.

31. Bove EL, Munich LL, Pridjian AK, et al. The management of severe subaortic stenosis, ventricular septal defect, and aortic arch obstruction in neonates. *J Thorac Cardiovasc Surg.* 1993;105:289–296.

32. DeLeon SY, Downey FX, Baumgartner NE, et al. Transsternal repair of coarctation and associated cardiac defects. *Ann Thorac Surg.* 1994;58:179–184.

33. Hellenbrand WE, Allen HD, Golinko RJ, et al. Balloon angioplasty for recoarctation results of valvuloplasty and angioplasty of congenital anomalies registry. *Am J Cardiol.* 1990;65:793–797.

34. Hijazi ZM, Fahey JT, Kleinman CS, et al. Balloon angioplasty for recurrent coarctation of aorta. Immediate and long-term results. *Circulation.* 1991;84:1150–1156.

35. Fletcher SE, Nihill MR, Grifka RG, et al. Balloon angioplasty of native coarctation of the aorta: midterm follow-up and prognostic factors. *J Am Coll Cardiol.* 1995;25:730–734.

36. Rocchini AP, Rosental A, Barger AC. Pathogenesis of paradoxical hypertension after coarctation resection. *Circulation.* 1976;54:382–387.

37. De Lezo JS, Sancho M, Pan M, et al. Angiographic follow up after balloon angioplasty for cooarctation of the aorta. *J Am Coll Cardiol.* 1989;13:689–695.

38. Cooper RS, Ritter SB, Rothe WB, et al. Angioplasty for coarctation of the aorta: long-term results. *Circulation.* 1987;75:600–604.

39. Lock JE, Bass JL, Amplatz K, et al. Balloon dilation angioplasty of aortic coarctation in infants and children. *Circulation.* 1983;68:109–116.

40. Ralph-Edwards AC, Williams WG, Coles JC, et al. Reoperation for recurrent aortic coarctation. *Ann Thorac Surg.* 1995;60:1303–1307.

41. Demircin M, Arsan S, Pasaoglu I, et al. Coarctation of the aorta in infants and neonates: Results and assessment of prognostic vaiables. *J Cardiovasc Surg.* 1995;36:459–464.

42. Kappetein KP, Zwindeman AH, Bogers AJJC, et al. More than thirty-five years of coarctation repair. An unexpected high relapse rate. *J Thorac Cardiovasc Surg.* 1994;107:87–95.

43. Cohen M, Fuster V, Steele PM, et al. Coarctation of the aorta. *Circulation.* 1989;80:840–845.

44. Zehr KJ, Gillinov AM, Redmond JM, et al. Repair of coarctation of the aorta in neonates and infants: a thirty-year experience. *Ann Thorac Surg.* 1995;59:33–41.

45. Merrill WH, Hoff SJ, Stewart JR, et al. Operative risk factors and durability of repair of coarctation of the aorta in neonate. *Ann Thorac Surg.* 1994;58:399–403.

46. Trinquet F, Vouhe PR, Vernant F, et al. Coarctation of the aorta in infants: which operation? *Ann Thorac Surg.* 1988;45:186–191.

47. Stewart JM, Gewitz MH, Woolf PK, et al. Elevated arginine vasopressin and lowered atrial natriuretic factor associated with hypertension in coarctation of the aorta. *J Thorac Cardiovasc Surg.* 1995;110:900–908.

48. Parker FB Jr, Streeten DH, Farrell B, et al. Preoperative and postoperative renin levels in coarctation of the aorta. *Circulation.* 1982;66:513–514.

49. Sehested J, Kornerup HJ, Pedersen EB, et al. Effects of exercise on plasma renin, aldosterone and catecholamines before and after surgery for aortic coarctation. *Eur Heart J.* 1983;4:52–58.

50. Leenen FH, Balfe JA, Pelech AN, et al. Postoperative hypertension after repair of coarctation of aorta in children: protective effect of propranolol? *Am Heart J.* 1987;113:1164–1173.

51. Hopkins RA, Kostic I, Klages Armiru U, et al. Correction of of coarctation of the aorta in neonates and young infants. An individualized surgical approach. *Eur J Cardiothorac Surg.* 1988;2:296–304.

52. Brewer III LA, Fosburg RG, Mulder GA, et al. Spinal cord complications following surgery for coarctation of the aorta. *J Thorac Cardiovasc Surg.* 1972;64:368–381.

53. Crawford FA, Sade RM. Spinal cord injury associated with hyperthermia during aortic coarctation repair. *J Thorac Cardiovasc Surg.* 1984;87:616–618.

54. del Nido PJ, Williams WG, Wilson GJ, et al. Synthetic patch angioplasty for repair of the coarctation of the aorta: experience with aneurysm formation. *Circulation.* 1986;74:I32–I36.

55. Bogeart J, Gewillig M, Rademakers F, et al. Transverse arch hypoplasia predisposes to aneurysm formation at the repair site after patch angioplasty for coarctation of the aorta. *J Am Coll Cardiol.* 1995;26:521–527.

56. Leskinen M, Reinita A, Tarkka M, et al. Reversibility of hypertensive vascular changes after coarctation repair in dogs. *Pediatr Res.* 1992;31:297–299.

57. Pelech AN, Kartodihardjo W, Balfe JA, et al. Exercise in children before and after coarctectomy: hemodynamic, echocardiographic, and biochemical assessment. *Am Heart J.* 1986;112:1263–1270.

58. Kimball TR, Reynolds JM, Mays WA, et al. Persistent hyperdynamic cardiovascular state at rest and during exercise in children after successful repair of coarctation of the aorta. *J Am Coll Cardiol.* 1994;24:194–200.

59. Poulias GE, Skoutas B, Doundoulakis N, et al. The mid-aortic dysplastic syndrome. Surgical consideration with a 2 to18 year follow-up and selective histopathological study. *European Journal of Vascular Surgery.* 1990;4:75–82.

60. Bergamini TM, Bernard JD, Mavoudis C, et al. Coarctation of the abdominal aorta. *Ann Vasc Surg.* 1995;9:352–356.

59

Vascular Trauma

Raul Mattassi and Cesare Zorzoli

Vascular Trauma

The incidence of vascular trauma has increased considerably in the last 35 years, not only because of various military conflicts but also because of civilian trauma such as that resulting from urban violence, traffic accidents, and home accidents. Other important origins of vascular trauma are iatrogenic lesions.

Vascular trauma is an acute pathology that requires immediate management. It may be localized in any vessel of the body; because injuries of other tissues and organs often coexist, a multidisciplinary approach is frequently necessary. Best management is achieved in trauma centers organized especially to treat these often severe cases.

Historical Background

Battlefield wounds and hemorrhage with fatal outcome have been well known since the beginning of history. War surgeons were forced to try any possible treatment to avoid exsanguination. This necessity has stimulated great progress in surgical techniques. In ancient times Hippocrates and Galen knew that ligation of arteries would stop bleeding from a wound, and the Greek Archinogenes (A.D. 97) used this method in limb amputation.

During the Middle Ages, arterial ligation was not used, and treatment of hemorrhage consisted of applications of red-hot irons and boiling oil. In the fourteenth century Ambroise Paré, a French military surgeon in the army of King Francis I, rediscovered ligation of arteries in the treatment of bleeding wounds. In 1552 he treated a carotid artery injury in a duelist by ligation; the outcomes were aphasia and hemiplegia.[1] The first successful repair of an injured artery was by Hallowell in 1762; he repaired a brachial artery.[2] The Italian Paolo Assalini, a military surgeon in Napoleon's army, created a special device for arterial clamping in acute hemorrhage that can be considered the first hemostatic clamp (Figure 59.1).[3]

During the Balkan War (1912) Soubbotitch successfully repaired arteries and veins in Belgrade,[4] and the Germans Lexer[5] and Stich[6] successfully repaired injured vessels by vein transplants during World War I.

In spite of this pioneer work, reconstruction of injured vessels was not common because antibiotics and blood transfusions were not available. In World War II among 2471 acute arterial injuries in American soldiers in Europe, only 81 were repaired and all but 3 by lateral suture.[7]

Only during the Korean War, with the systematic repair of injured vessels and the consequent drop in amputation rate from about 50% to 13%, did modern reconstructive techniques become the standard treatment for vascular trauma.[8,9] The Vietnam experience and the data of the Vascular Registry with a casuistic of 1000 casualties were extremely important in clarifying management and long-term results of reconstructive surgery for vascular injuries.[10]

New conflicts in recent decades have brought about significant progress in the management of vascular trauma.[11–13] Routine use of temporary intraluminal shunting is one of the most significant advances in this area.[14,15]

Incidence

The incidence of trauma is high, and it is the leading cause of death in the United States in people under age 30.[16] Nevertheless, vascular injury is a relatively rare consequence of trauma. In World War II the incidence of vascular trauma was only about 2.5%.[17] Its incidence has increased considerably in civilians due to a rise in urban violence, traffic accidents, and diagnostic and therapeutic procedures. A German statistic for the period between 1953 and 1963 demonstrated an incidence of 0.3%,[18] and a North Carolina epidemiologic study of the period between 1988 and 1990 reported an incidence of vascular lesions in trauma of 3.6%.[19] The incidence of

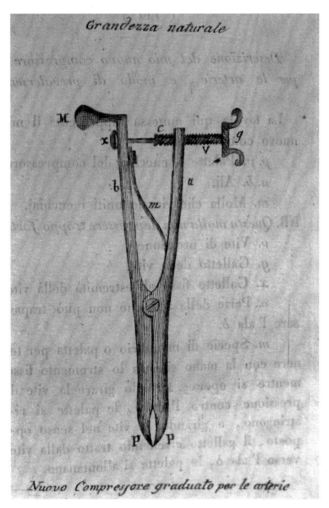

FIGURE 59.1. New graduated compressor for arteries: the first hemostatic clamp for arteries, invented by Paolo Assalini in 1812.

vascular trauma by civilian violence, including gunshot wounds, is highly variable but generally increasing (Table 59.1).

Etiology

Individuals may experience trauma in both military and civilian life. In war conditions, vascular trauma is due principally to the energy dissipated on impact by shrapnel (e.g., mines, bombs, rockets, and mortar shells) and by high- or low-velocity missiles. Bullets traveling at low velocity (<1000 m/s) produce relatively little damage and only a direct vascular lesion. A high-velocity missile (>1000 m/s) is able to destroy a large amount of tissue because of its great energy and cavitation phenomenon.[20] Impact with bone transfers energy to shell fragments that subsequently act as secondary missiles and thus increase destruction. The suction effect, with its introduction of dirt and clothing fragments, increases the risk of infection and necessitates extensive débridement.[21]

Civilian trauma is due to the following:

- Traffic accidents, which often cause severe, complex injuries[22]
- Urban violence, which may include stab wounds and missile injuries caused by handguns or even military-type rifles (these vascular lesions are now similar to military vascular injuries)[23]
- Accidents at work by machines in factories
- Sports accidents
- Iatrogenic trauma, which is increasing in incidence because of diagnostic and therapeutic endovascular procedures[24,25]

Different surgical procedures, including orthopedic[26] and cancer surgeries,[27] may also increase the incidence of vascular lesions.

Localization

The most common sites of vascular trauma are the limbs, with some differences between military and civilian trauma, as seen in Tables 59.2 and 59.3. Arterial trauma is often associated with other lesions of veins, nerves, and bones (Table 59.4).

Type of Lesions

According to the mechanism of trauma and the effect on the arterial wall, a distinction has been made between penetrating injury and blunt trauma (Figure 59.2). Penetrating injuries from stab and knife wounds usually en-

TABLE 59.1. Incidence of blunt and penetrating vascular trauma.

Author	Community	Total cases	Blunt trauma	Penetrating trauma
Sharma[92]	Bronx (US)	191	7 (4.3%)	184 (95.7%)
Weinmann[87]	Innsbruck (Austria)	36	25 (69%)	11 (31%)
Kurtogiu[90]	Istanbul (Turkey)	115	29 (25%)	86 (75%)
Padberg[92]	Newark (US)	69	34 (49%)	35 (51%)
Lazarides[94]	Athens (Greece)	18	12 (67%)	4 (33%)
Bongard[89]	Torrance (US)	37	26 (70%)	11 (30%)
Byone[91]	Columbia (US)	198	42 (21%)	156 (79%)
Mattassi[95]*	Milan (Italy)	99	80 (81%)	19 (19%)

*Author's casuistry.

TABLE 59.2. Localization of vascular injuries in military trauma.

Artery	Incidence (%)
Superficial femoral	34
Brachial	30.4
Popliteal	28
Common femoral	7.8
Axillary	6.5
Iliac	0.9
Subclavian	0.3

From Rich and Spencer.[28]

TABLE 59.3. Localization of vascular injuries in civilian trauma.

Artery	Incidence (%)
Forearm (ulnar or radial)	20
Brachial	18
Femoral	17
Subclavian	7
Popliteal	6
Thoracic aorta	5
Carotid	5
Axillary	5
Abdominal aorta	5
Other abdominal vessels	5
Iliac	4
Tibial	3

From Drapanas.[29]

TABLE 59.4. Incidence of combined injuries.

Artery (%)	Nerve injury (%)	Venous injury (%)	Bone injury (%)
Axillary	91.5	33	27.1
Brachial	71.3	19	33.9
Iliac	11.5	42.3	7.6
Common femoral	15.2	39.1	19.5
Superficial femoral	20	45.5	23.6
Popliteal	37.3	52	40

From Rich and Spencer.[28]

tail damage limited to the wound tract. The artery may be damaged only on its external layers without opening of the lumen. This kind of lesion is frequently not recognized and may manifest itself later by secondary rupture or aneurysm. More deep penetrating wounds may provoke a lateral arterial section with copious hemorrhage and false aneurysm (Figure 59.3). Because the arterial wall is not able to contract, hemostasis is rare.

Transfixion is a particular vascular trauma that may lead to traumatic arteriovenous fistulas. Complete arterial section may provoke massive hemorrhage in great vessels, such as the aorta, with early death by exsanguination. In smaller, muscular vessels (caliber <8 mm) spontaneous contraction of the arterial transected extremities may stop hemorrhage in a few minutes. Laceration of the arterial wall, often extended and with loss of a piece of vessel wall, is the most severe lesion.

The effect of blunt trauma or stretching (as in joint dislocation) on vessels depends on the different arterial layers' sensitivities to trauma, which decreases from the intima (the most sensitive) to the adventitia (the most resistant). Subadventitial disruption with intramural hema-

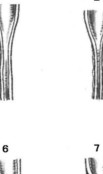
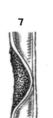
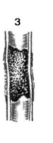
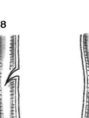
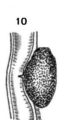
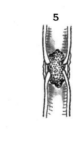

FIGURE 59.2. Different types of arterial injuries: **1**, spasm; **2**, spasm with external compression; **3**, endoluminal thrombosis; **4**, intimal tear with thrombosis; **5**, intimal laceration with occluding thrombus; **6**, intimal flap with occlusion; **7**, intramural hematoma occluding the lumen; **8**, laceration; **9**, lateral disruption; **10**, extramural hematoma occluding the lumen.

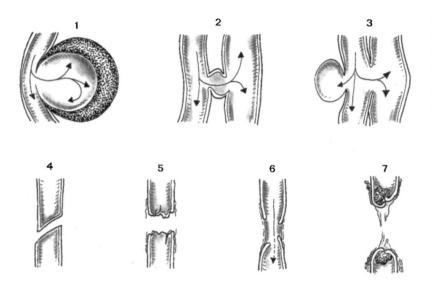

FIGURE 59.3. Different aspects of arterial lesions: **1,** false aneurysm; **2, 3,** arteriovenous fistulas; **4,** complete arterial transection; **5,** arterial dilaceration; **6,** intimal and media disruption with continuity maintained from the stronger adventitia; **7,** arterial disruption with thrombosis.

toma is a limited or circumferential laceration of intima and media with intact adventitia and thrombosis. It is the most common vascular lesion in blunt trauma (Figure 59.4). An intimal tear (Figure 59.5) may seem to be minor arterial damage, but it is considered a severe lesion because an intimal flap may progress to extensive dissection and delayed thrombosis. In arteriosclerotic patients vascular trauma may cause rupture or extensive detachment of sclerotic plaques (Figure 59.6). The incidence of arterial spasm, secondary to trauma, has probably been overestimated; it is considered extremely rare and is normally secondary to a small intimal tear.[17]

Pathophysiology of Traumatic Ischemia

Hemorrhage and thrombosis are the initial effects of vascular injury. Both thrombosis, with blood flow reduction, and hemorrhage, with shock and peripheral arterial vasoconstriction, reduce tissue blood perfusion. Muscular fibers are the most sensitive to ischemia, which produces edema. Growth of muscle volume in inextensible compartments of the limbs increases tissue pressure and thus occludes vessels that pass through the compartment. Complete circulatory arrest may cause thrombosis.[30,31]

Striated muscle tolerates total ischemia for about 6 hours before myonecrosis begins.[32] Beyond 8 hours the amputation rate is 86%,[33] and after 12 hours the limb is unsalvageable.[34] These statistical data are relative because limbs have different local collateral circulation, and sensitivity to ischemia may vary significantly.[31]

Necrosis of muscle tissue causes release of myoglobin into the blood, which is filtrated by the kidney and causes tubular necrosis in the kidney. Revascularization of an ischemic limb with diffuse myonecrosis may provoke a massive inflow of myoglobin into the main circulation and subsequent acute renal failure. Acid metabolites from tissue necrosis may cause acidosis and alterations in cardiac function. This clinical picture is known as postischemic or reperfusion syndrome.[35]

Clinical Manifestations

The clinical signs in a patient with vascular trauma are related to shock, hemorrhage, ischemia, and rarely arteriovenous fistulas with vascular bruits. The incidence of these signs is as follows[29]: shock, 50%; ischemia, 24%; hemorrhage, 13%; and vascular bruit, 8%.

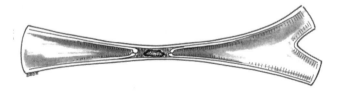

FIGURE 59.4. Effect of stretching on artery: intima and media are completely disrupted but adventitia (more elastic and resistant) maintains continuity.

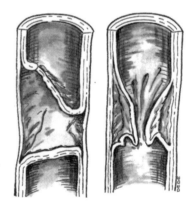

FIGURE 59.5 Anatomical–pathological aspect of intimal tear in an artery.

FIGURE 59.6. Traumatic dissection of atherosclerotic intima.

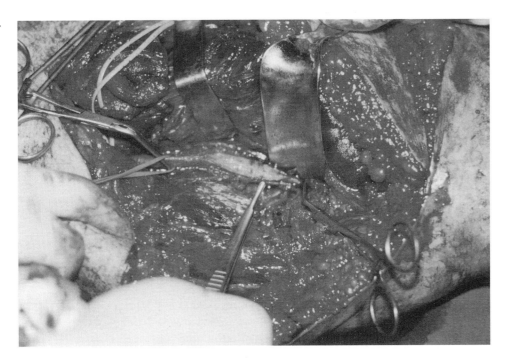

Shock, the most severe clinical manifestation, is due to internal hemorrhage caused by thoracic or abdominal trauma, external hemorrhage, or polytrauma. Ischemia may vary in severity according to the source of blood flow reduction. The clinical picture varies from slight ischemia to compartment ischemia to complete, severe ischemia due to acute occlusion of proximal main vessels.

External hemorrhage manifests itself with a visible jet of red blood through a skin injury, although a clot often stops hemorrhage temporarily because of first aid compression or low blood pressure. Venous hemorrhage may exist alone (5% in our experience) or be combined with arterial hemorrhage.

Hematomas are far more common than external bleeding. They may be variable in size, pulsating, and compress tissues, with subsequent aggravation of ischemia and neurological trauma. A vascular bruit or thrill audible at the site of trauma is often due to arteriovenous fistulas,[13,36] but incomplete arterial compression by a hematoma may also cause bruits.

Diagnosis

Prompt diagnosis of vascular trauma and early recognition of the level and etiology of a lesion are the goals in managing patients with this pathology. Obtaining a history of trauma and physical examination are the first and most important steps in diagnosis. In hemodynamically unstable patients history and physical examination may be the only diagnostic procedures if prompt surgical intervention is mandatory, as in the case of thoracic or abdominal injuries with heavy bleeding.

Signs of ischemia (pain, pallor, pulselessness, paresthesia, and paralysis) distal to the wounded area are highly predictive of arterial trauma. However, ischemia may not always be present immediately after trauma. An intimal tear or intramural hematoma may maintain blood flow for some time until thrombosis and subsequent acute ischemia develop. A pulse wave may even be transmitted through areas of limited fresh clot.[21] Distal pulses may be present in up to 20% of patients with surgically proven arterial injury.[29,37,38]

Detailed examination of a wound from penetrating trauma in which the direction of the penetrating object is established may be helpful in determining the presence of vascular trauma. Doppler measurement of the ankle–brachal index has been used as a screening technique, but inaccuracy remains.[39]

Arteriography has traditionally been the standard examination to diagnose vascular injuries.[40,41] It is a safe and precise examination with high sensitivity, specificity, and accuracy.[42] It may be performed by direct puncture or by use of an endovascular catheter.

The diagnostic efficacy of duplex ultrasonography in vascular trauma has been studied experimentally[43] and clinically[44] in recent years. Accuracy of diagnosis is equal or superior to angiography, and duplex ultrasonography is also able to detect venous injuries and the extent of hematomas; other advantages include that it is a noninvasive method and more cost-effective for screening than arteriography.[45] This diagnostic method may replace arteriography for initial diagnosis of vascular trauma.

Ordinary radiographs may be of some use, but accuracy is low. Computed tomographic (CT) scanning, especially with infusion of contrast medium, is accurate in the detection of hematomas and blood expansion outside of vessels. The main disadvantage is that the procedure takes time and may not be applicable in nonhemodynamically stable patients.

Principles of Treatment

Treatment is based on three principal points: resuscitation, control of hemorrhage, and vascular repair. The patient with polytrauma and symptoms of shock must be treated first to correct poor hemodynamic conditions. Airway maintenance and respiratory assistance are initiated. Adequate intravenous access lines are obtained for rapid fluid and blood replacement.[16] Because saphenous veins are often useful for vascular repair they should be preserved if possible.

Fluid and blood infusion should replace loss without exceeding 30% of the hematocrit value because excessive increases may unnecessarily raise blood viscosity.[21] Prophylactic antibiotics are considered appropriate, although real effectiveness has not been proved.

Hemorrhage from wounds is often effectively controlled temporarily by direct digit pressure or compressive bandage.[46] Because these bleeding wounds are often compressed by emergency workers, patients may arrive at the hospital without direct bleeding because of clot formation. The penetrating objects that remain imbedded should be removed only in the operating room to avoid sudden renewal of bleeding.

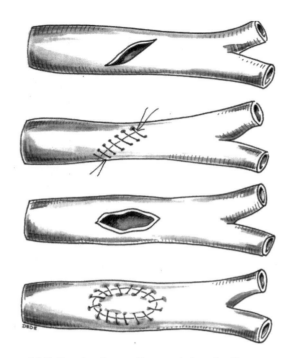

FIGURE 59.7. Repair of a small artery injury by direct suture or patch graft.

In chest or abdominal hemorrhage from main vessels, compression for bleeding control is normally not possible. The introduction of a balloon catheter, inflated on the rupture site, may be effective in temporarily stop-

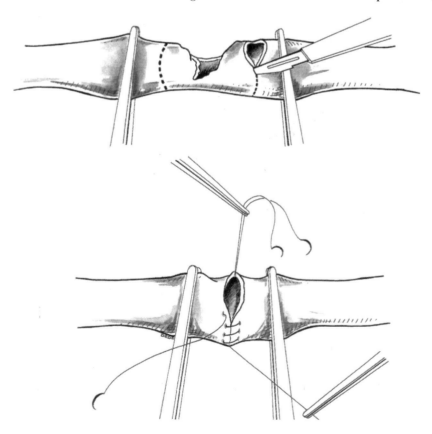

FIGURE 59.8. Arterial defect corrected with end-to-end anastomosis.

ping blood loss. The site of rupture can be quickly detected by duplex ultrasonography.

In a few selected cases arterial trauma has been treated by endovascular techniques with catheter-directed arterial embolization[47] or stent graft application.[48] Besides these limited cases, surgical treatment is the elective therapeutic approach to vascular trauma.

Arterial ligation should be limited to arteries with good collateral circulation such as the external carotid artery, individual arteries of celiac axis, hypogastric artery, radial artery, ulnar artery, or tibial artery. The profunda femoris artery is an important collateral vessel in age-related arteriosclerotic occlusions of the superficial femoral artery. For this reason we always try to reconstruct traumatic lesions of this vessel. The procedure of choice in vascular trauma is surgical reconstruction of injured vessels.

After deciding which vessels to treat, a good operatory field should be prepared. To obtain a vein graft from a noninjured area, a lower limb outside the traumatized area is prepared. The incision should be the traditionally used arterial approach with the possibility of extending in both directions. In case of active bleeding, proximal control with clamping reduces hemorrhage immediately.

After arterial exposition arteriotomy is performed to visualize injury. Injured arteries should be excised back to the area without injury. It is extremely important to recognize and resect all damaged vessel. Missed intimal tears may evolve to secondary thrombosis and increase amputation risk. Before injury repair, a distal thrombectomy is often performed with Fogarty catheter if no backflow is observed from the distal vascular bed. Extensive débridement of contaminated tissue is usually necessary.

Different techniques are available for vascular repair. Small puncture wounds are repaired with direct suture (Figure 59.7). If the margins of the lesion are damaged, they should be excised; vascular repair is performed with a vein patch to avoid stenosis (Figure 59.7).[29,49] End-to-end anastomosis is possible only if no excessive tension results (Figures 59.8 and 59.9).[50]

Interposition of a graft is the most frequent reconstruction technique (Figure 59.10 and 59.11); it was per-

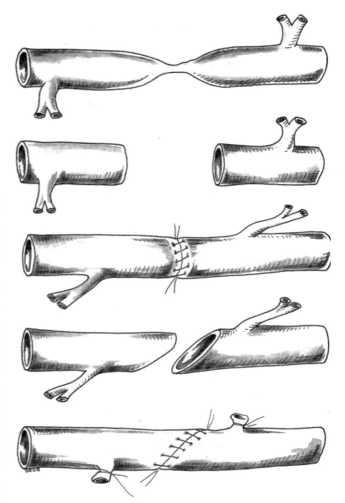

FIGURE 59.9. Arterial lesion repaired by transverse or oblique direct end-to-end anastomosis with section of the injured arterial wall and without excessive tension.

formed in 73 of 91 operations (80%) in our clinic. Saphenous vein is considered an excellent graft material.[51] Using a venous graft from a nontraumatized limb is preferred because otherwise the vein itself may be damaged or may sustain collateral circulation in case of posttraumatic deep venous thrombosis.

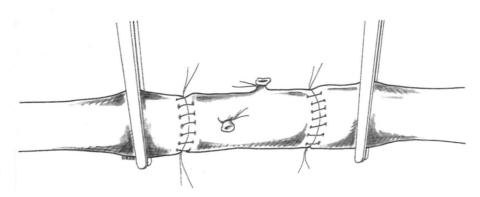

FIGURE 59.10. Arterial defect corrected with graft.

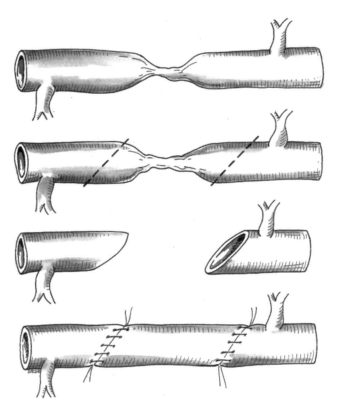

FIGURE 59.11. Repair of arterial lesion due to stretch mechanisms with graft using oblique anastomosis.

A polytetrafluoroethylene graft is used if veins are not available or in the repair of great vessels damaged by blunt trauma. In contaminated areas, such as in gut lesions or popliteal gunshot wounds, injured vessels are ligated and extra-anatomical bypasses are made through clean tissues.[52] Because of the reported high incidence of infection, secondary hemorrhage, and limb amputation with indiscriminate use of prosthetic grafts in combat wounds,[28] they should be avoided. If the caliber of donor vein is much smaller than that of the host vessel a panel compound graft with two segments of vein opened

longitudinally and sewn together side by side (Fig. 59.12)[53] or a spiral graft (Fig. 59.13) is prepared.[54]

The incidence of contemporary venous injuries is about 40%.[55] Venous bleeding may result in significant hemorrhage and should be controlled. Venous repair rather than ligation, as emphasized by many authors, should be the procedure of choice in main veins.[56,57] Significant arterial flow reduction after venous ligation has been demonstrated experimentally in canine models[58]; limb amputation after femoral or popliteal artery reconstruction with homonymous vein ligation has been reported.[59,60] In hemodynamically unstable patients with complex injuries, venous ligation is sometimes preferred because it avoids prolonged and intricate venous repair.[61,62]

Nerve injuries are common in limb trauma, especially trauma of the upper limbs (see Table 59.4). Controversy exists about whether immediate or delayed repair is preferable; delayed repair is most common. Bone fractures, which are often associated with blunt trauma, require orthopedic stabilization. Complex comminuted fractures may require complex and time-consuming procedures. External fixators are preferred.

Postoperative Treatment

In the postoperative period the vascular trauma patient is controlled at different levels. Hemodynamic stability is the first goal of treatment; vital parameters are followed to recognize and promptly correct any adverse changes. Postischemic syndrome with acidosis and myoglobinuria is a severe complication that may cause renal failure. Blood and urine samples should be collected and monitored daily. Infusion of hypertonic mannitol seems to reduce postischemic effects.[63] The viability of repaired vessels should also be monitored. Signs of thrombosis should be noted and promptly corrected. Necrosis of traumatized soft tissues in the postoperative period requires débridement and sometimes amputation in spite of a patent vascular repair.

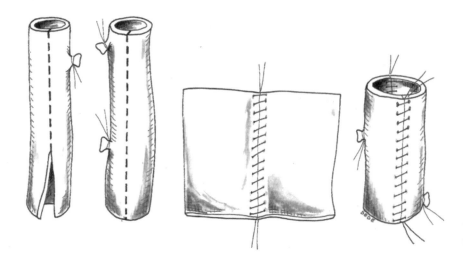

FIGURE 59.12. Panel compound graft realized with two longitudinally opened veins. A double-sized vessel is obtained from a smaller vein.

FIGURE 59.13. The spiral technique makes possible a venous graft of any needed size.

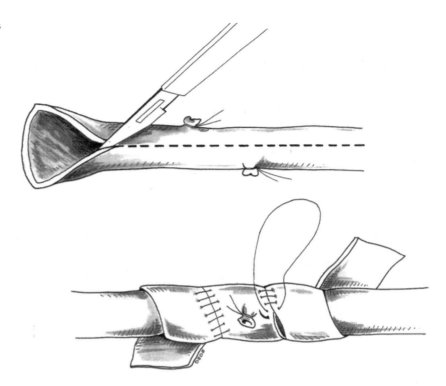

Thoracic Vascular Trauma

Thoracic vascular trauma refers to lesions of the aorta and its main branches, the epiaortic vessels in their intrathoracic tract, the pulmonary vessels, the superior and inferior venae cavae, the main veins in the thoracic inlet, the intercostal arteries, and the internal mammary arteries. Relatively rare, lesions of the thoracic vessels represent 9% of all vascular lesions reported in the emergency units of metropolitan areas.[64]

Thoracic vessel lesions from penetrating injuries are still prevalent (15%–20% of vascular lesions from penetrating injuries[65,66]), but an increase in vascular lesions from blunt thoracic trauma has been reported, particularly due to trauma from traffic accidents.[67] A penetrating or thorax perforating injury may affect vessels by any of the following means:

- Wall or intraluminal lesion, with subsequent thrombosis (due to blast effect or cavitation)
- Partial transection with bleeding in the pleural cavity, mediastinum, or extrapleural, suprapleural, or suprasternal areas that causes a contained, sometimes pulsatile hematoma, depending on whether the veins or the arteries are affected
- Total transection with free hemorrhage, including external hemorrhage
- Formation of an arteriovenous fistula, generally between the subclavian or innominate artery and the homologous vein

A patient may present as normotensive with a manifest injury in the supraclavicular or superior mediastinum area and normal chest x-ray results; proximity to the main vessels is assumed from the missile or stab track. The patient may be somewhat hypotensive with the same injuries and present clinically or exhibit on chest x-ray films a hematoma contained in the mediastinum or supraclavicular or suprasternal area. In both cases, a thoracic aortogram via a retrograde femoral approach is necessary to identify the lesion (aorta, artery, or vein) and plan the necessary surgery.

The patient in shock or with a mediastinum hematoma or an acute hemothorax must immediately undergo an emergency thoracotomy or sternotomy.[68] The approach is determined by injury location.

If the injury is located in the superior, suprasternal, or supraclavicular mediastinum an anterolateral thoracotomy in the third or fourth intercostal space should be performed. This approach may subsequently be extended to a contralateral thoracotomy or sternotomy. A left anterolateral thoracotomy must always be performed when the thorax descending aorta requires clamping.

After evacuation of the hemothorax, the injured vessel should be visualized and controlled by manual dissection. Using digital hemostasis or a vascular clamp, a lesion of the superior vena cava, the ascending aorta, or the pulmonary artery may be immediately repaired using a Prolene 4 - or 5-O suture.

In case of hemorrhage or an air leak from the lung, an aortic clamp must immediately be placed on all of the hilar structures before identification and repair of the lesion. Intrathoracic hemorrhage from an artery or subclavian vein lesion is controlled by manual compression or packing directly at the pleural apex in the thorax through the thoracotomy. Reanimatory maneuvers are fundamental and provide for the following:

- Security of the airway
- Catheterization of a vein, generally the great saphenous vein, for full flow infusions, provided complex trauma with a lesion of the abdominal vessels is not involved
- Control of hypothermia by warming the infused fluids and covering the abdomen and lower limbs with silver thermal blankets
- Immediate availability of blood for transfusion
- Recovery of hematic bleeding with autotransfusion
- Mechanical ventilation to maintain gas exchange and utilization of heated gas mixtures to prevent hypothermia

In elective or semiemergency surgery the approach depends on direct clinical examination of the location and direction of the penetrating injury, the track of the missile, or the angiogram of the injured vessels. A number of cervicothoracic incisions are possible.

Lesions of the innominate artery may be controlled by a median sternotomy (quite often the extension of an emergency thoracotomy) with mobilization of the upper left innominate vein. Lateral arterial suture is the favored technique even though a bypass graft between the ascending aorta and distal tract of the innominate artery is often needed.[69] Lesions of the innominate veins, particularly the left one, are managed by ligation.

The median sternotomy allows control of any lesions of the proximal common left carotid artery; for the distal tract, the incision is made along the anterior border of the sternocleidomastoid muscle. Rapid reconstruction of the carotid injury is critical, particularly for patients in the first stage of coma.[70,71] Prolonged ischemia offers a less favorable prognosis than ischemic infarcts evolving into hemorrhagic infarcts.[72]

If a lesion of the proximal right subclavian artery is suspected, in stabilized conditions, a median sternotomy with a right supraclavicular extension is recommended. Removal of the third clavicle median and transection of the scalenus anterior muscle allow good control of the three sections of artery.

Control of the less common injury of the proximal intrapleural tract of the left subclavian artery is obtained through a left anterolateral thoracotomy. If the injury affects both the left and right distal tracts, a supraclavicular approach by clavicle dissection (but not removal) is recommended. Subsequent reconstruction of the bone should not be difficult.

Special care should be given to preparing, clamping, and suturing because the artery is particularly fragile and tends to tear. Back bleeding of the lateral vessels of the subclavian artery (vertebral, internal mammary, and thyrocervical trunk) is abundant, and ligation of these vessels is often necessary.[73] Reconstruction of the subclavian artery is generally performed through end-to-end anastomosis after resection of the injured borders or through autogenous saphenous vein graft. The accompanying vein lesion should be reconstructed, usually through a lateral venous suture, but more complex reconstructions with autogenous vein grafts are also possible.

Large defects of the collateral venous supply caused by trauma do not allow for sufficient compensation for subclavian vein ligation,[74] and a large area of edema of the upper limb may result. Recently, success was reported in treatment of subclavian artery lesions by endovascular transluminal positioning of a stented graft. A distant vascular approach, reduced bleeding due to nondissection in an area affected by trauma, the possibility of treating almost inaccessible vessels and accompanying lesions, and a reduced need for anesthesia represent the main benefits of the intravascular technique.[75]

The incidence of blunt thoracic trauma causing lesions of the great vessel is increasing. Thoracic aorta rupture is responsible for 10% to 15% of deaths in traffic accidents.[76–79] In most cases drivers or passengers are involved, but thoracic aorta rupture is also seen in pedestrians who have been run down and people who have fallen from great heights. The most frequent site of injury is at the isthmus of the descending thoracic aorta, just under the left subclavian artery, near the ligamentum arteriosum.

The lesion consists of a limited tear (a few millimeters in length) of the intima and the media that tends to expand to the circumference of the aorta and causes a several-centimeter rupture of the two intimal ends with complete transection of the aorta. Survival depends mainly on the resistance of the adventitia, thanks to its collagen content, and the resistance of the mediastinum supportive tissue and pleura that interfere with intrapleural rupture and subsequent massive hemothorax. Lesions of the ascending aorta, slightly above the innominate artery, are most common. They constitute lethal lesions of intrapericardiac rupture and cardiac tamponade.

Various theories have been put forth to explain the pathogenic mechanism of lesions. In deceleration trauma, at the moment of impact the heart, the arch, and the ascending aorta continue in a forward or upward movement while the isthmus and the descending aorta are limited by their posterior insertions.[80] The aortic isthmus has been proven to be the weakest tract of the aorta.[81] A sudden rise in hydrostatic endoluminal pressure may also cause the aorta to rupture. Anatomically, we may distinguish the following:

- Complete ruptures, when all three arterial layers are involved; survival is rare
- Subadventitial ruptures that may expand the rupture in both retrograde and antegrade directions
- Intimal ruptures, which are generally isolated and difficult to diagnose; they tend to heal spontaneously

Forces responsible for isthmus rupture may include the following:

- Impact from falling
- Compression subsequent to frontal impact
- Sudden horizontal decelerations combined with chest compression
- Crush injuries

The mechanical factor responsible for isthmus rupture is the shear stress determined by the different speed of deceleration between the mobile aortic arch and the more fixed descending aorta. This brings about a rupture opposite the site of fixation of the insertion and accounts for the frontal localization of the descending aorta isthmus rupture.[74]

Lesions of the ascending aorta are brought about by bending stress that the heart, violently displaced caudally, bears suddenly on the aortic arch around a fulcrum represented by the hilar structures of the left lung. Torsion stress results from anteroposterior compression with a left movement of the heart on the aortic arch convexity combined with the stretching movements of the neck or rotation of the head that the patient instinctively makes to protect himself or herself from front impact. The innominate and subclavian arteries are thus torn. This mechanism explains the common carotid artery tear opposite the head rotation because the artery undergoes excessive stress.[69,82-84] Ruptures of the descending thoracic aorta, generally combined with fractures or dislocations of the lower thoracic vertebrae and ruptures of intercostal arteries from costal dislocated fractures, may result from blunt vascular trauma.

Diagnosis

Blunt thorax vascular trauma, especially involving the thoracic descending aorta, is clinically insidious. It must be suspected even without physical signs when examining victims of high-speed (60–65 km/h) traffic accidents or patients who have fallen from higher than 8 m.[85,86] Information about the circumstances of the accident (e.g., whether deaths occurred or whether seat belts were used) is also useful.[87-89] Combined fractures, including costal, sternum, or spine fractures, pulmonary contusion, cranial trauma, lesions of abdominal organs (e.g., kidneys, liver, and spleen), or maxillofacial lesions, are part of the clinical picture.

There is a significant relation between pelvic fractures and aortic lesions.[90] In a recent complete review of related literature in English,[91] the most common symptoms were reported to be thoracic pain (76%), dyspnea (56%), consciousness loss and coma (36.8%), and hypotension (25%).

Thorax contusion marks (such as the typical mark of the steering wheel on the anterior chest) are evident in only one third of patients.[92] No pathognomic physical signs exist, but intrascapular murmur, decreased femoral pulse, paraparesis, or paraplegia is indicative of descending aortic thoracic lesion.

Rare is the so-called syndrome of acute coarctation[93] characterized by a hypertension of the upper extremities with different pulse amplitudes in upper and lower extremities. Different amplitudes seem to be determined by dissection of an intimal flap or compression of the aortic lumen by the hematoma.

The first instrument of examination, around which the rest of the diagnosis revolves, is the chest radiography. The main radiological signs that suggest rupture of the thoracic descending aorta include the following:

- Widened superior mediastinum in orthostatism >8 cm
- Obscuration of the aortic knob and outline of the descending aorta
- Shifting to the right of the nasogastric tube
- Shifting to the right of the trachea
- Depression over 40 degrees of the left main stem bronchus
- Presence of a left-sided hemothorax
- Presence of a left pleural cap (sign of extrapleural hematoma)
- Fracture of the first or second rib
- Fracture of the sternum

Because the widened superior mediastinum may be interpreted differently even by expert radiologists and because elderly patients often have physiologic widening of the mediastinum,[94,95] the radiological signs most indicative of rupture of the isthmus thoracic descending aorta are a shifting to the right of the nasogastric tube (and thus the esophagus) and trachea and a downward deviation of the left main stem bronchus.[84] Patients with particularly sclerotic aortas exhibit a clear sign of rupture of the thoracic aorta: the "broken halo sign," a fractured calcified ring located laterally from the hematoma.[96] The most indicative signs of lesions of the innominate artery from blunt trauma are a widening of the superior mediastinum, a characteristic pointed appearance of the right edge of the hematoma, and a shift of the nasogastric tube to the left.[82]

Even if chest radiography is not always sensitive enough to identify an aortic lesion, it remains a useful screening test to determine which traumatized patients require further diagnostic procedures. The usefulness of a CT scan in the subsequent diagnostic procedure is debated. Because the CT scan allows for early recognition of a mediastinum hematoma or hemothorax but is unable to identify intimal lesions, it is not always useful.[97] Recent reports[98–100] confirm the importance of transesophageal echocardiography (TEE) in the diagnosis of aortic intimal lesions.

The main benefits of TEE are its sensitivity and specificity in identifying the aortic lesion; the prompt availability of the equipment in emergency, intensive care, and operating units; the opportunity to examine the patient while stabilizing him or her; and the speed of examination, which allows use of TEE even in critical patients. TEE makes it possible to determine which patients do not require angiography to identify intimal lesions that do not involve the media and the adventitia.[100] However, angiography is more specific in traumatic lesions of the atherosclerotic aorta because the atheromatous plaque protruding into the aortic lumen may offer a false-positive result with TEE. TEE disadvantages include that it is impossible to encompass the innominate and epiaortic vessels in the investigation and that its quality depends on the technician.

Particular attention should be paid to passive mobilization of the head in patients with skull or spine fractures. Angiography (digital subtraction intra-arterial angiography) remains the gold standard in the diagnosis of aortic lesions.[95,101,102] In emergency units, the decision to proceed with angiography is based solely on the knowledge of the circumstances of the trauma and on the findings of the chest radiography (fracture of the first rib and clavicle, displaced fracture of several ribs, bilateral costal fractures, costal fractures with frail chest, or dislocated fracture of the sternum). Angiography is performed via a retrograde femoral approach, provided an acute coarctation syndrome is not suspected. In such cases the right axillary artery is catheterized.

Angiography confirms the diagnosis of vessel rupture, defines its topography, and provides evidence of possible combined lesions of the thoracic and abdominal aorta or the main branches. The typical angiographic picture of aorta rupture is a fusiform aneurysm, generally expanded to the whole aorta circumference, due to a "sleeve" stretching of the adventitia. Intimal rupture is visualized as a linear, irregular shadow in the vessel. It is important to search for anterograde or retrograde dissections or aortic stenoses from an intimal flap.

Treatment

Generally, rupture of the thoracic descending aorta requires emergency surgery. Emergency intervention without prior angiography is advisable in patients at very high risk for hemodynamic instability, reinfusions notwithstanding, especially in the presence of left-sided he-

mothorax, pseudocoarctation, hemomediastinum, and supraclavicular hematoma.[103]

In such situations, a left thoracotomy is performed, and the results are more complex than with the technique described earlier of digital hemostasis of a penetrating injury to a vessel. In case of complete rupture of the vessel and a hemothorax, the proximal clamping of the vessel is complicated and unprompted.[104]

A surgery protocol is established for the various lesions of polytraumatized patients. In patients with stable aortic lesions, those that require immediate surgery are the extradural hematoma and the hemorrhagic abdominal lesions, both parenchymatous (kidney, spleen, and liver) and vascular (mesenterium or main retroperitoneal vessels). Skeletal or maxillofacial lesions are treated after the aorta.

In hemodynamically stable patients, angiography is performed immediately but surgical intervention may be postponed. All measures necessary for the complete hemodynamic monitoring of the patient must be implemented, including right radial artery catheterization for pressure control, introduction of a Swan–Ganz catheter, and selective bronchial intubation using the Carlens tube.

In case of thoracic descending aortic lesions at the isthmus, the standard approach is the left posterior lateral thoracotomy in the fourth or fifth intercostal space (Figure 59.14) with the patient lying on the right lateral decubitus with the left hip rotated outward to allow access to the abdomen and the left inguinal femoral vessels. Retracting the lung exposes the rupture. The aortic arch between the left common carotid and left subclavian arteries, the subclavian artery just after its origin, and the descending aorta just under the rupture are encircled with vascular tape one after the other. Dissection proceeds from distal to proximal to place the lower clamp nearest to the rupture.

The main problems associated with this surgical technique are related to aortic clamping. Proximal hypertension may affect the left ventricle and the brain, and distal ischemia may affect the more sensitive organs such as the kidney, intestine, and particularly spinal cord. Standard surgery techniques are reviewed in the following sections.

Clamp and Repair

The clamp and repair technique consists of clamping the thoracic descending aorta up and down the tear (usually clamps are placed on the aortic arch, proximal to the origin of the left subclavian artery, and on the distal tract of the descending aorta). Hypertension is controlled by administration of vasodilatative drugs (Fluothane, nitroprusside, nitro derivatives, and isoflurane). A transversal aortotomy exposes the lesion. Back

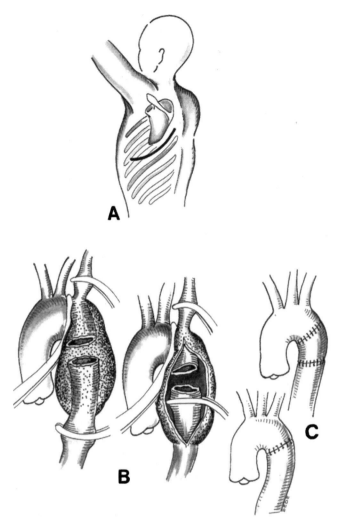

FIGURE 59.14. Surgical treatment of rupture of isthmic aorta. **A,** Posterolateral thoracotomy in the fourth to fifth intercostal space. **B,** Clamping and opening of mediastinal hematoma. **C,** Aortic reconstruction by direct anastomosis or prosthesis interposition.

hemorrhage from intercostal arteries is blocked by balloon catheters, Silastic loops, or ligation.

Partial tears that do not involve the whole circumference of the vessel are repaired by a 3- or 4-O polypropylene monofilament continuous suture after the proximal and distal segments of the vessel are mobilized and the injured segment is resected.[105] In case of a larger rupture (>2 cm), a woven Dacron graft (recommended because it does not require any preclotting) is inserted. The cross-clamp time must not exceed 30 minutes because of the high risk of spinal cord ischemia.[106–108]

Benefits, apart from the simplicity of the technique, are that no heparinization or extracorporeal circulation is required. An autotransfusion device is useful.

Graft of Sutureless Intraluminal Aortic Prosthesis

Through a lengthwise aortotomy, a woven Dacron prosthesis with a rigid ring at both ends is implanted and fixed to the vessel by an external ring while the aorta is clamped. Although theoretically the intervention may be performed rapidly, difficulty implanting, possible displacement, and mismeasurement of vessel and prosthesis diameters may prolong surgery.

If an adequate blood flow needs to be maintained and the time of surgery is prolonged, the following techniques could be utilized.

Temporary External Shunt

A temporary external shunt treated with a superficial coat of ammoniochloridate triclodecyl heparin eliminates the need for systemic heparinization of the patient. It is implanted upward (in the ascending aorta or arch) and downward (in the aortic or femoral aorta) in the excluded tract and allows for the perfusion of the inferior hemisomus.

The flow depends on both the location of the implant and the shunt diameter. A pressure of at least 60 mm Hg is necessary to prevent spinal cord lesion. Possible risks are the laceration of the vessel at the implant point, pseudoaneurysms, and hemorrhage. An inability to affect the flow rate is the drawback of this technique.

Extracorporeal Circulation

Left Atrium–Femoral Artery Partial Bypass

A left atrium–femoral artery bypass does not require an oxygenator, only a nontraumatic biomedical centrifugal pump that, without heparin, maintains a flow rate of 2 to 3.5 L/min. Encouraging results were reported in comparison with previous pumps, especially in the prevention of medullar ischemia.[109] The left atrium–femoral artery bypass has the same advantages as the external shunt but does not offer any guarantee in case of massive bleeding.

Right Atrium–Femoral Artery Partial Bypass

Blood is withdrawn from the right atrium through a femoral vein and, after oxygenation, is refused into the femoral artery. The main advantages of the right atrium–femoral artery partial bypass are maintenance of a valid medullar and renal perfusion in case of prolonged clamping, the possibility of massive infusion in case of copious hemorrhage, and the possibility of inducing hypothermia. However, this procedure requires systemic heparinization and thus increases the risk of hemorrhage, particularly when combined lesions are present.

Complete extracorporeal circulation with total bypass in-depth hypothermia is seldom recommended. In case

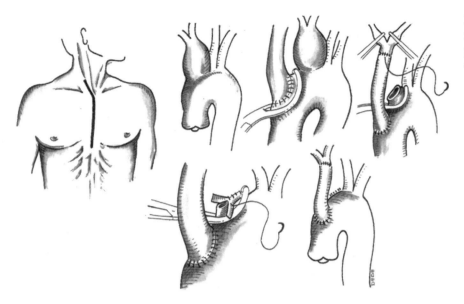

of traumatic lesions of the innominate artery (Figure 59.15) a median sternotomy with subsequent pericardiotomy is performed. The ascending aorta as well as the tract just after the origin of the innominate artery is exposed and the hematoma is controlled. If the aortic arch or common left carotid artery is not extensively damaged, the use of extracorporeal circulation or a temporary shunt is unnecessary.

In the first stage, a preclotted Dacron knitted prosthesis is sutured end to side to the ascending aorta by lateral clamping. Subsequently the innominate artery is dissected near its bifurcation and the tract proximal to the lesion.

Clamping is performed at these points, the innominate artery is completely dissected (the flow to the right carotid artery is maintained via the right subclavian artery), and the graft is placed end to end on the distal end of the innominate artery. The proximal end is oversewn.

Abdominal Vascular Trauma

Abdominal vascular trauma refers to lesions, caused by blunt or open trauma, that involve the abdominal aorta and the inferior vena cava, the celiac axis and the superior mesenteric artery and vein, the renal arteries and veins, the iliac arteries and veins, the portal vein, and the hepatic veins.

In the first casuistry reviews by American authors covering wartime, the incidence of abdominal vascular injuries was 2% (World War II),[110] 2.3% (Korean War),[111] and 2.9% (Vietnam).[112] This relatively low incidence, also confirmed by reports on more recent wars (in Croatian, Middle Eastern, and Gulf Wars),[113–115] depends on the high mortality rate due to the wounding power of

firearms combined with patients' delayed arrival in well-equipped clinics.

The experience in civilian practice is completely different. The 30-year Houston County Hospital[116] review reports that 33.8% of all cardiovascular injuries (5760 cases) involve abdominal vessels. Furthermore, vascular injury is present in 25% of the patients treated for abdominal penetrating wounds from firearms and in 10% of those treated for stab wounds.[117]

Data collected from rural areas are slightly different (16% of abdominal vascular lesions with 69% of penetrating wounds) and reflect the different activities of the population.[118,119] Vascular lesions from blunt abdominal trauma constitute an infrequent event: 5% to 10% of the x-ray screened or laparotomized patients.[120,121]

Pathophysiology

Pathophysiologic, diagnostic, and therapeutic aspects differ between penetrating wounds and blunt trauma. Penetrating abdominal wounds cause vascular lesions similar to those observed in the thorax or limbs, including lateral wall defect with free bleeding or pulsatile hematoma, partial or total transection of the vessel with hemorrhage or thrombosis, blast effect with intimal flaps and secondary thrombosis, and formation of an arteriovenous fistula (more frequently in the portal system and the hepatic, renal, and iliac vessels).

Blunt abdominal trauma produces vascular lesions through different mechanisms: deceleration or direct blow. Blunt trauma from deceleration may engender an avulsion of the main vessel branches; avulsions of the lateral branches of the superior mesenteric artery in the proximal and distal tracts are typical and correspond with the proximal tract of the jejunum and the cecum, points of postperitoneal fixation. Another defect caused by deceleration is the intimal tear with subsequent thrombosis, quite frequent at the level of the renal arteries, 2 to 3 cm from the origin.

Violent crush abdominal trauma or posterior blows to the spine may cause both a tear of the most exposed vessels (e.g., the left renal vein with massive postperitoneal hematoma or a partial tear of the subrenal aorta with production of a false aneurysm)[122-124] and an intimal lesion with flap and secondary thrombosis (e.g., of the infrarenal abdominal aorta,[125,126] mesenteric superior artery,[127] or iliac arteries[128,129]). A typical example of secondary thrombosis with intimal flap is the so-called seatbelt aorta.[130-132]

Diagnosis

A patient with a vascular lesion from a penetrating wound generally reaches the hospital alive only 10% to 15% of the time and presents with severe shock or more or less significant hypotension. The degree of hypotension depends on whether an active hemorrhage or a contained hematoma is present in the postperitoneal tamponments at the base of the mesenterium or hepatoduodenal ligament. Subsequent diagnostic–therapeutic interventions depend on the hemodynamic response to the first reanimation maneuvers.

Persistence of a severe collapse condition, notwithstanding rapid crystalloid infusion through a central venous line, calls for a high temporary hemostasis. In such an event, a left lateral thoracotomy must be performed in the emergency room[133] to clamp the descending aorta to sustain cardiac output and cerebral flow and stop intraabdominal bleeding.[134] This maneuver is effective in terms of promoting rapid hemostasis but requires a thoracic incision that may limit respiratory function. Temporary hemostasis may also be obtained by percutaneous insertion of an aortic occlusion balloon into the left humeral artery.[135,136] Once the hemodynamic condition has improved, a laparotomy may be performed to localize the bleeding.

If the patient responds to infusion therapy and remains stable, a clinical diagnostic evaluation is possible. Evaluating the wounds and obtaining a history of causes and circumstances of the trauma allow the area of injury to be determined.

Clinical signs that suggest a vascular lesion are rapid distension and tension of the abdomen with signs of peritoneal irritation, the presence of a bruit, and an asymmetry of femoral pulses. Paracentesis may also be effective for diagnosis of vascular lesions. Useful diagnostic investigations available in emergency units include the following:

- Chest radiography to evaluate combined associated thoracic lesions

- Abdominal radiography to view the peritoneal track, possible retention of the missile, or any sign of peritonism
- One-shot intravenous pyelogram to assess the regular functioning of both kidneys and ureters, critical information when a perirenal hematoma is found during laparotomy[137]
- Abdominal echography

If hemodynamic conditions remain stable, angiography and CT scanning with contrast may be used.

Vascular lesions from blunt abdominal trauma are difficult to diagnose. If a hemoperitoneum from complete avulsion of an artery is present, signs of peritoneal irritation associated with acute hypotension prevail in the clinical picture and a laparotomy is mandatory. The only signs that suggest a renal intimal lesion with secondary thrombosis are flank pain accompanied by microhematuria or macrohematuria. In case of microhematuria or macrohematuria in a clinically stable patient, contrast CT scanning may be used to assess renal morphology and functioning. The absence of renal enhancement and outflow and the presence of a cortical rim from collateral circulation reveal a thrombosis of the renal artery. In this case, angiography is unnecessary.

Angiography remains the fundamental investigation in the diagnosis of abdominal vascular lesions from blunt trauma to identify lesions of the pelvic arteries associated with pelvic fractures and the intimal or subadventitial tears of the subrenal aorta or iliac veins.

Treatment

In the hemodynamically stabilized patient a midlaparotomy is performed to remove clots, recover free blood for autotransfusion, localize the bleeding, or control hematoma. Control of active hemorrhage is a priority. In fact, at the opening, no packing effect is exerted by the wall and the temporary hemostasis is obtained by digital or by aortic compression at the level of the celiac aorta. Extremely useful and of rapid execution is clamping of the infradiaphragmatic aorta through the lesser omentum opening or blunt opening of the left crus of the diaphragm and preparation of the aorta for direct clamping (Figure 59.16).

Hemorrhage from parenchymatous organs (liver and spleen) is controlled by packing, clips, or resection. Aortic or main vessel perforation is controlled by proximal and distal clamping. Venous hemorrhage from the inferior vena cava or other main veins is controlled through vascular clamps or sponge stick compression.

After hemostasis intestinal lesions have to be immediately clamped to avoid further fecal contamination. Minor lesions can be immediately repaired by a polypropylene monolayer suture and then vessels can be reconstructed. Vascular reconstruction is a priority inter-

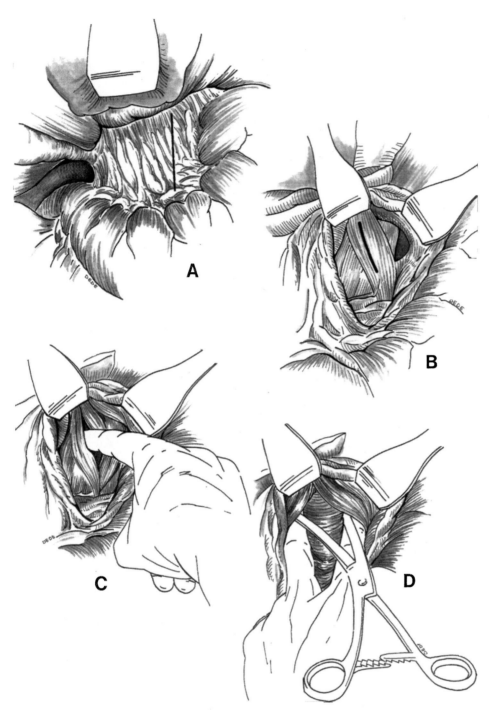

FIGURE 59.16. Proximal supraceliac infradiaphragmatic control of the aorta.
A. Exposure and opening of the
lesser omentum.
B. Incision of the left crus of diaphragm.
C. Blunt dissection.
D. Clamping.

vention to limit any possible contamination with bowel contents. The only exception is the contained retroperitoneal hematoma when it is possible to perform the intestinal lesion repair first and then proceed to vascular interventions, after irrigating the intraoperative area with antibiotic solution and changing gloves, drapes, and instruments.

There are two approaches in the management of abdominal vascular lesions. To control aorta, celiac axis, and superior mesenteric artery lesions, a left laterocolic approach (Figure 59.17) is adopted with medial rotation of the left colon, spleen, pancreas end, and gastric fundus that are progressively freed from their postperitoneal attachments by blunt and sharp dissection. Usually the left kidney is left in place because its medial rotation may cause ventral aorta distortion. In a few minutes, the aorta is completely exposed from hiatus to bifurcation.

To control the inferior vena cava, portal vein, and right renal pedunculus, a right laterocolic approach

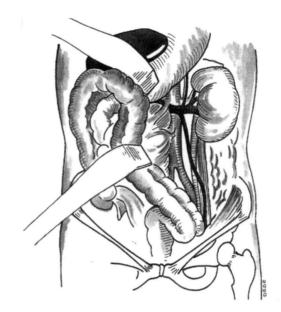

FIGURE 59.17. Left laterocolic approach.

(Figure 59.18) is adopted with blunt dissection of the right colon and medial mobilization of the hepatic flexure of colon; the inferior vena cava and subrenal aorta are exposed using a wide Kocher maneuver.

For practical purposes,[137] there are five typical locations of hematoma or hemorrhage from abdominal vascular lesions: supramesocolic midline, inframesocolic midline, lateral perirenal, lateral pelvic, and portal.

In the supramesocolic midline, hematoma or hemorrhage is caused by lesions of the suprarenal aorta, celiac axis, proximal tract of the superior mesenteric artery, or

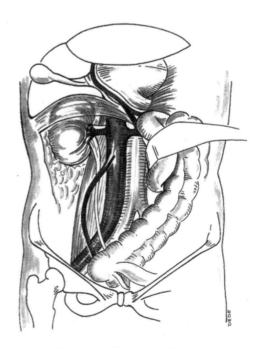

FIGURE 59.18. Right laterocolic approach.

renal arteries. Hemorrhage is rapidly controlled by clamping the descending thoracic aorta at the diaphragmatic hiatus, opening the lesser omentum longitudinally, retracting the stomach and esophagus to the left, bluntly dissecting the fibers of the left crus of the diaphragm, detaching the periaortic areolar tissue, guiding the vascular clamping over two fingers until the tips touch the vertical body behind the aorta, and occluding the aorta[138] (Figure 59.16).

Minor perforations of the suprarenal aorta are immediately repaired with a continuous Prolene 3- or 4-O suture, but larger perforations may require a polytetrafluoroethylene patch or rarely a prosthesis implant.[139] The survival rate with perforations is 36%,[140] but an associated lesion of the inferior vena cava carries a 100% mortality rate.

Ligation is acceptable treatment for lesions of the celiac axis because an abundant collateral circulation, mainly provided for by the gastroduodenal artery, ensures vascularization. The hepatic artery should be grafted only when a lesion distal to the origin of the gastroduodenal artery is present. Conversely, lesions of the superior mesenteric artery need to be reconstructed because collateral circulation may be insufficient.

The lesion (section or thrombosis) of the superior mesenteric artery is immediately identified at the celiotomy because of "black bowel." Revascularization is vital for lesions extending from the origin to the first branch, the left inferior pancreatic duodenal artery (first segment; generally associated with lesions of the head of the pancreas), and the left inferior pancreatic duodenal artery to the origin of the middle colic artery. Generally, an aortic mesenteric bypass, preferably in vein, with proximal anastomosis from the distal aorta, is recommended. The most common approach for lesions of the second segment is the left laterocolic with medial rotation of the bowels, eventually combined with a section of the pancreas head.

Perioperative angiography is important to control patency of the graft and to evaluate bowel reperfusion. A second-look intervention is mandatory to control the condition of the gut. Lesions in the tract immediately distal to the middle colic artery can be repaired with resection and end-to-end suture, whereas lesions of the jejunal arteries that present in emergency involve ligation of the artery and resection of the ischemic intestine.

Lesions of the superior mesenteric vein may occur either at the junction with the splenic vein at the origin of the portal vein, which requires transection of the pancreas head, or at the base of the mesenteric insertion. A lateral venous suture with 5-O polypropylene sutures is the standard repair. Survival rates after repair of the mesenteric artery and vein are 57% and 72%, respectively.[140,141]

Hematoma in the submesocolic midline originates from a lesion of the infrarenal abdominal aorta or the infrarenal inferior vena cava. For the aorta, the left latero-colic retroperitoneal or transperitoneal midline approach is suggested with the aorta clamped at the root of the mesentery; the survival rate after repair reaches 45%.[141]

Hematoma from injury of the inferior vena cava infiltrates the right paracolic cavity, shifts the ascending colon, and protrudes into the medial mesentery. The right laterocolic approach with left rotation of the bowels and with a wide Kocher maneuver is the best approach because it allows exposure of the vessel from the inferior rim of the liver to the iliac bifurcation. In case of perforation of the junction of the renal veins and the vena cava, an assistant manually compresses the infrarenal vena cava and the suprahepatic vein to allow the renal veins to be looped and clamped and the lesion to be repaired. When there is no time to dissect, medial mobilization of the right kidney allows for application of a clamp across the vena cava to the junction of the right renal vein. Such a maneuver is useful to treat posterior perforation of the suprarenal infrahepatic vena cava, and care is taken not to avulse the lumbar veins.[143]

A hemorrhage from the inferior vena cava may be controlled in all locations by inserting a Foley catheter balloon into the laceration. Hemorrhage is controlled first by sponge stick compression to control the leakage and assess the extension of the lesion. Once hemostasis is obtained and the hemodynamic condition is stabilized, the vessel is dissected upward and downward for clamping laterally with a Satinsky clamp if possible. Isolated anterior lesions are reconstructed by transverse venous suture using a 5-O polypropylene monofilament suture. Wider lesions are treated by venous patches, using a resected ovarian or mesenteric inferior vein. Posterior lesions can be repaired from inside the vena cava. Reconstruction with prosthetic material (externally supported polytetrafluoroethylene) is not recommended because of the high risk of sepsis and thrombosis.[142]

Lesions of the right iliac vein confluence are treated by separation of the overlying common iliac artery for venous reconstruction and subsequent arterial reanastomosis. Survival after reconstruction of lesions of the vena cava reaches 70% for the subhepatic area and 75% for the infrarenal area.[143]

A lateral perirenal hematoma suggests a lesion of the renal artery, renal vein, or kidney. When urography, CT scan, and selective renal arteriography results are normal, surgery is not recommended for the perirenal hematoma from blunt trauma. An urgent laparotomy is performed if positive findings of vascular and parenchymatous lesions are found in hemodynamically unstable patients or following penetrating wounds.

The first step consists of control of the renal artery and vein at their aortic and vena cava origin before entering the hematoma. When active hemorrhage is present, as with penetrating wounds, the most rapid maneu-ver is retroperitoneal mobilization of the kidney and visual clamping of the hilar structures.

Once the temporary hemostasis is performed, the general conditions of the patient, the presence of associated lesions, times of renal ischemia, and severity of the vascular ureteral and parenchymatous lesions should be assessed. Nephrectomy is the favored approach when there are associated lesions, the patient is hypotensive, and the right kidney is healthy and functioning (the pre-operation one-shot urography is thus important). It must also be taken into account that renal function is seriously altered after 6 hours of partial ischemia and 3 hours of total occlusion.[146]

Renal revascularization techniques provide for venous or prosthetic bypass from the aorta, reimplants or transposition of the hepatic artery to the right and of the splenic artery to the left, or, in particularly complicated cases, ex vivo reconstruction with reimplant in the iliac fossa. Lesions of the right renal vein always require reconstruction; otherwise nephrectomy is ineluctable. The left renal vein, because of the abundant collateral flow, can be ligated. The literature shows survival rates of 87%[141] and 94%[145] for renal artery injuries from penetrating wounds, whereas renal vein injury entails a survival rate of 42% to 88%[149] depending on the associated lesions.

An intimal tear of the renal artery with secondary thrombosis may result from deceleration trauma. The clinical picture, which is poorly suggestive (flank pain with microhematuria or macrohematuria), dramatically contrasts with the limited time available for revascularization (12–18 hours maximum).[144]

Clinical suspicion, supported by readily available investigations such as urography and CT scan, leads to a rapid diagnosis and intervention, taking into consideration that selective arteriography may cause an unjustified delay.[148] Furthermore, taking into account the low rate of recovery of renal functionality and the incidence of delayed nephrectomy (35%) due to complications following revascularization (particularly hypertension), the present surgery-oriented approach prevails only if concurrent lesions are present and revascularization is performed only within 12 hours of trauma.[147]

Revascularization outcome can be assessed after resolution of the acute tubular necrosis (6–8 weeks). Dean's recommendation[150] to always adopt a surgical approach in the management of intimal or subadventitial flaps of the renal arteries remains valid, although it is well known that few lesions evolve into total occlusion, false aneurysm, or arteriovenous fistula. The technique for lesion repair provides for wide mobilization of the artery, segmental dissection of the intimal disruption, or direct reanastomosis.

Hemorrhages and hematoma in the lateral pelvic area are caused by iliac vessel lesions and account for 20% of the abdominal vascular lesions. For vascular lesions from penetrating wounds, the clinical presentation is that of severe intraperitoneal or postperitoneal hemorrhage in a shocked patient who presents with subumbilical, inguinal, or back orifice; a tense abdomen, especially in the hypogastric area; a femoral hyposphygmic pulse; or pulselessness.

Immediate hemostasis is obtained through a midlaparotomy, clamping of the subrenal aorta and inferior vena cava, and clamping of the iliac external artery and vein or femoral common artery and vein to Scarpa's triangle.

Control of hypogastric artery outflow is usually obtained with a Fogarty catheter inserted through the vascular lesion. After removal of the hematoma, the lesions associated with the enteron, colon, and urinary system are assessed.

In the absence of potentially septic lesions, the arterial lesion is immediately repaired. Besides the current techniques of arterial reconstruction (continuous suture, resection and end-to-end suture, prosthetic vein graft, or autologous vein graft), an external iliac artery injured by an accident may be replaced with a graft of the ipsilateral internal iliac artery or transposition of the iliac artery on the contralateral side for lesions of the aortic bifurcation.[151] In case of intestinal contamination, prosthetic grafts should be avoided. The iliac artery is ligated and a crossover extra-anatomic femorofemoral bypass is performed to provide peripheral vascularization.

The venous lesion, particularly at the level of the common iliac vein and the external iliac vein, is repaired with a continuous suture, but ligation of these vessels is also acceptable. Rarely, blunt trauma associated with pelvic fractures injures the main vessels (1% of all pelvic fractures).[152,153] Iliac and femoral vessel lesions are described in association with fractures of the distal portion of the ilium, which constitutes the anterior component of the acetabulum.[154]

Hemorrhage is caused by lesions of the branches of the hypogastric artery and of the valveless venous plexus of bone and soft tissues. It occurs particularly when fractures involve the posterior ring of the pelvis.[155] Replacement of lost blood, stabilization of the internal and/or external fractures, and performance of a selective angiography to define the pelvic vascular damage and for embolization of the vessel are the first priorities.[154,156,157] The survival rate after hemostasis with embolization is 10% to 15% higher than with hypogastric ligation.[156]

Often, the complexity of the hypogastric plexus requires embolization of several branches of the two hypogastric arteries and subsequent aggravation of ischemia in already traumatized areas. Cases of ischemic lesions on the rectal mucosa have been reported.[157] Angiography and embolization should be performed on patients with unstable pelvic fractures that require transfu-

sion of 4 to 6 blood units and with persisting clinical hemodynamic instability.[158]

Hematoma or hemorrhage in the portal area suggests injury of the portal vein and/or hepatic artery with possibly concurrent lesion of the common biliary duct. The hepatoduodenal ligament and the left ligament of the liver are clamped (Pringle maneuver that excludes the vascular afference of the portal vein and hepatic artery).

An injury of the portal vein is generally repaired with 5-O polypropylene continuous sutures, whereas larger lesions require either transposition of the splenic vein or a bypass in the saphenous vein around the ligated portion. In hypothermic, acidotic patients with coagulopathy, the portal vein must be ligated to ensure survival.[159] Ligation is performed for lesions of the common hepatic artery and is generally well tolerated; selective ligations of the hepatic branches may require lobectomy, particularly because of necrosis of the hepatic parenchyma injured and already sutured.

Lesions of the hepatic veins or posthepatic vena cava from penetrating wounds and avulsions of the hepatic veins from blunt trauma are extremely dangerous. In hemodynamically stable patients without hemoperitoneum the trend is not to intervene on the hematoma.

In patients with severe hypotension and active hemorrhage from the suprahepatic area, a wide midlaparotomy with eventual sternotomy should be performed. Initial blood flow is controlled manually with packs, because exposure of the posthepatic vena cava and hepatic short and frail veins requires mobilization of the liver, a maneuver that increases bleeding.

In such cases[160,161] it is possible to proceed to liver vascular isolation by clamping the infradiaphragmatic aorta, occluding the subhepatic and infrahepatic vena cava, and using the Pringle maneuver. The lesion is exposed by dissecting the triangular ligament and the anterior and posterior coronary ligament. Reconstruction requires continuous suture or a patch, but a reinforced polytetrafluoroethylene prosthetic graft is rarely used because of the danger of infection or thrombogenicity. The main limitation of vascular isolation is the significant hemodynamic imbalance involved in cardiac preload.

Several surgical successes[162–164] with the aid of an atrium caval shunt, which allows backflow to the left atrium when the portion of the posthepatic vena cava is excluded, have been reported. Surgery consists of isolating the inferior intrapericardiac and supradiaphragmatic vena cava and the infrarenal inferior vena cava, loading them on a loop, and introducing a shunt (a no. 8 endotracheal tube) through the right atrium until the distal end is positioned under the renal vein. By fastening the loops of the shunt, hemostasis is achieved except in the retrohepatic area.

On the whole, patients with lesions of the portal vein have a survival rate of 50%, taking into account that lesions of the portal vein are almost always associated with other lesions. Patients with retrohepatic inferior vena cava lesions have a survival rate of 40% to 50%.[164]

Vascular Trauma of Extremities

Traumatic injuries of the limbs have changed significantly in the last 10 to 20 years because of the variety of causes. Urban violence is the main reason for the high incidence of penetrating injuries of the limbs by low-velocity missiles. Blunt trauma in traffic accidents with bone fracture and/or joint dislocation is another important cause of vascular trauma. Iatrogenic lesions from extensive use of arterial catheterization and intra-arterial drug injections[165] are new trauma mechanisms that entail specific management problems.

The extremities, by far the most frequent sites of vessel injuries, have an incidence of vascular trauma of more than 80%.[166] Lower limbs are more often involved than upper limbs, in a relation of about two thirds to one third (Table 59.5). All types of vascular lesions are possible in limbs, and all arteries may be affected by trauma, although the frequency varies (Table 59.6).

The effects of occlusion at different levels on distal flow are variable according to some critical points with poor collaterals, as demonstrated in a study by De Bakey and Simeone on casualties of World War II[170] (Table 59.7). The incidence of combined lesions, including venous injuries, nerve trauma, bone fracture, and soft tis-

TABLE 59.5. Incidence of upper and lower limb trauma.

Author	Number of cases	Upper limb	Lower limb
Bongard et al.[167]	37	15 (41%)	22 (59%)
Kurtoglu et al.[168]	115	30 (26%)	85 (74%)
Byone et al.[169]	198	101 (39%)	159 (61%)
Mattassi*	99	33 (33%)	66 (67%)

*Author's casuistry.

TABLE 59.6. Site of vascular injuries in the limbs*: Distribution of 99 cases.

Artery	Number
Superficial femoral	24
Popliteal	24
Brachial	19
Radial, ulnar	7
Common femoral	6
Tibial	6
Axillary	4
Subclavian	3
Iliac, external	1
Superficial femoral vein (only)	3
Popliteal vein (only)	2
Total	99

*Author's casuistry.

TABLE 59.7. Incidence of amputation after ligation of different arteries.

Artery	Amputation (%)
Aorta	100
Femoral, common	81
Popliteal	72
Tibial, both anterior and posterior	69
Brachial, proximal	55
Iliac, common	54
Femoral, superficial	50
Iliac, external	46
Axillary	43
Radial and ulnar together	39
Subclavian	28
Brachial, distal	25
Tibial, posterior	13
Tibial, anterior	8
Radial	5
Cubital	1

From Debakey and Simeone.[6]

sue damage, is high; such combined lesions may require amputation even if arterial reconstruction is successful.

Diagnosis

Clinical signs of vascular trauma have been divided into pathognomonic, or "hard signs" (distal ischemia with absent or diminished pulses, bruit, pulsatile hematoma, and arterial bleeding), and less specific, or "soft signs" (small stable hematoma, nerve injury, shock, and wound near a major vessel). Unfortunately one or more of these signs may not be present, and sure diagnosis becomes difficult. Missed prompt diagnosis of vascular trauma on extremities may lead to sudden secondary thrombosis or progressive worsening in peripheral perfusion that increases the risk of amputation.[171–173]

Arteriography is considered the most useful diagnostic method.[174,175] If it confirms diagnosis in cases with unclear clinical signs of vascular injury it is termed *exclusion arteriography*. Arteriography is performed preoperatively by classical techniques or in emergency situations by the manual injection, single-film method.[176] The technique consists of a single manual injection of 25 to 50 mL of contrast media and the execution of a single x-ray picture in the selected area of the limb with a portable x-ray machine. This method, which may be repeated intraoperatively, is preferred in emergency situations.

Duplex sonography has been claimed to have sensitivity (95%), specificity (99%), and overall accuracy (98%) similar to arteriography,[169] but the technique is not always available in emergency units and requires an experienced technician. Venography may be useful to determine the site and entity of venous trauma and venous thrombosis and the anatomy of collateral veins but can be used only in hemodynamically stable patients.[177,178]

Special Problems in Treatment

Limb vascular injuries often require resolution of special problems related to the sites and characteristics of trauma. Minimal intimal injuries without hemorrhage or arterial occlusion may have a benign course and should be treated conservatively,[179,180] but a more recent study[181] demonstrated a high incidence of long-term complications. Currently, aggressive treatment of intimal minor lesions with surgical repair is recommended until long-term benignity of these injuries is definitively demonstrated.

In hemodynamically unstable patients with concomitant peripheral vascular injuries, all efforts should first be directed toward correcting the life-threatening pathology. Even ligature of main arteries is allowed if this procedure may be lifesaving. The most appropriate surgical approach to vessels is one that ensures proper exposure. The best incisions are simple, directly on the explorable vessels, and with the possibility of proximal and distal extension.

In case of concomitant arterial and venous lesions the best sequence is to begin with venous reconstruction to provide better outflow for arteries.[182] Whether immediate vascular repair is more or less critical than preliminary orthopedic stabilization is controversial. Initial vascular repair reduces the time of ischemia, and the surgeon works more easily without an external fixator on the limb. However, orthopedic movements of the limb after vascular repair may damage the vascular suture. Vascular repair before orthopedic stabilization is usually the favored approach for ischemic limbs.[167,183] Indwelling shunt placement (Figure 59.19) in the early

stages of surgery[184,185] changes the conditions because the limb is immediately revascularized and the orthopedic surgeon is allowed to proceed before the vascular surgeon begins vascular reconstruction.[186] If artery and vein are injured, both are shunted. The shunt is currently used in selected cases rather than as a general measure.

Edema often occurs after revascularization of ischemic tissues, soft tissue trauma, or venous occlusion. Because muscles are located in inextensible compartments, local pressure rises. Local high pressure occludes vessels, damages nerves, and promotes muscle necrosis (Figure 59.20) due not only to general limb ischemia but especially to local hypertension.[187] The best treatment of this compartment syndrome is early decompression by fasciotomy. Prompt recognition of compartment syndrome is an important diagnostic challenge because omitted or delayed fasciotomy results in high amputation rates. Pain, compartment tension, and paralysis are significant clinical signs, but contemporary traumatic nervous injury may blur the clinical picture. Measure of compartment pressure is useful to establish whether fasciotomy is indicated and may also be executed before surgery if necessary. A pressure higher than 45 mm Hg is considered an indication for fasciotomy.[188]

Extensive muscle trauma may be an underestimated problem. In blunt trauma, swelling of traumatized muscles that may become necrotic is not easy to recognize (Figure 59.21). Often débridement is not complete, and successive necrosis with sepsis is the main cause of secondary amputation. A second-look procedure 24 to 48 hours after operation to control the spread of necrosis has been suggested[189] but is not popular. Vascular grafts

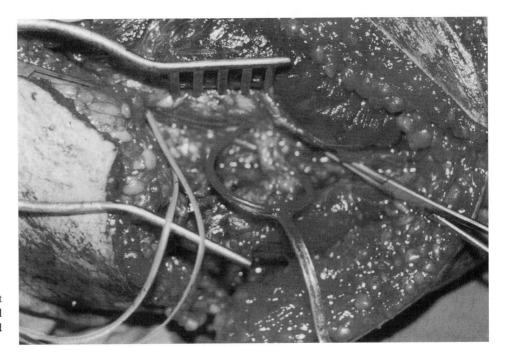

FIGURE 59.19. Indwelling shunt in a resected superficial femoral artery: femoral vein is intact and no shunt is needed.

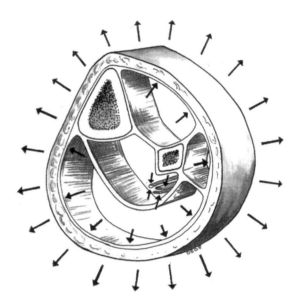

FIGURE 59.20. Schema of effects of pressure increase in compartment syndrome in the calf. Edematous muscles are not allowed to expand because of inextensible fascia.

should be covered with vital muscle or skin. This is sometimes possible by simple mobilization of adjacent tissue, but in larger wounds a transposed muscle flap[190] and a free tissue transfer,[191,192] local fasciocutaneous flaps,[193] or porcine skin xenografts and cadaver homografts have been used.[194]

Nerve injuries are frequently not repaired immediately, even if they are recognized during vascular operation.[167,195,196] Whether this decision depends on the advantages of a second operation or the unavailability of a neurosurgeon at primary operation is unclear. Malagon et al.[197] suggested early neurosurgery (within 7 days of injury) for traumatized brachial plexus because the dissection is easier and the results are more positive. Vollmar advocates immediate nerve reconstruction to avoid

a second operation with difficult recognition of nerve segments.[198] The technique requires a microsurgical method.[199,200]

The decision to perform a primary amputation is difficult. It is well known that an ischemic and anesthetic extremity with extensive soft tissue trauma and bone fracture with loss of osseous tissue is better treated by immediate amputation. Such a complex of negative signs is extremely rare; however, ischemia may not be irreversible, anesthesia may resolve quickly after revascularization and decompression, traumatized tissue may not extensively necrotize, and bone fractures may be repaired successfully. The difficulty in predicting outcome of a traumatized limb by initial observation explains why surgeons are reluctant to perform primary amputation. Different score methods to predict outcome of traumatized limbs are known, including the Mangled Extremity Syndrome Index,[201] the Limb Salvage Index,[202] the Predictive Salvage Index,[203] and the Mangled Extremity Severity Score.[204] A recent study performed with the purpose of investigating the applicability of these methods concluded that none was specific enough to permit primary amputation on that basis alone.[205] The best approach to this decision is individual evaluation of each patient in a multidisciplinary consultation and taking into account whether patients are young, healthy, and resistant to amputation.

A traumatic complete or incomplete amputation of a limb may be corrected by replantation.[206,207] Replantation is feasible if the duration of ischemia is short (5–10 hours for forearm and arm, 12 hours for hand, and 16–24 hours for fingers), the cut is clean (without extensive crushing of tissues), and contamination is not profound. The technique requires (1) débridement of necrotic tissue, (2) bone stabilization (perhaps with shortening), (3) vessel reconstruction, (4) nerve reconstruction, and (5) muscle and skin suture.[198] Results are

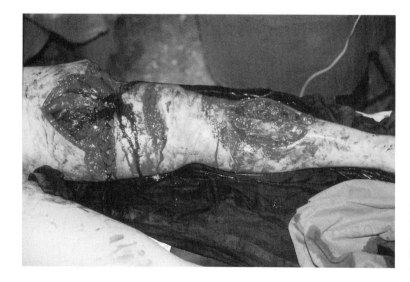

FIGURE 59.21. Severe multilevel trauma of the lower limb with multiple fractures and extensive muscle damage: in the first hours the difficulty differentiating viable from necrotic muscles makes complete débridement difficult.

better on distal (hand and fingers) than on proximal amputations (arm and forearm) because of incomplete nerve recovery.[208,209]

Management of Specific Vessels

Subclavian and Axillary Arteries

Injuries of subclavian and axillary arteries are relatively rare (7% in our casuistic) because of the protected anatomic location. Main causes are penetrating trauma[210] and blunt trauma with two main mechanisms: direct contusion of shoulder with piercing and shearing trauma on vessels by fractured bones and a brutal stretching trauma.[211–214] Anterior shoulder dislocation[215] (Figure 59.22) and proximal humeral fractures[216] may also cause vascular trauma. These injuries are considered severe because of their frequent association with lesions of the brachial plexus (that surrounds the axillary artery),

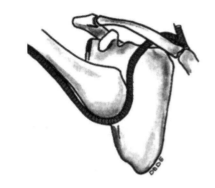

FIGURE 59.22. Mechanism of vascular trauma by shoulder dislocation.

which often causes the most disabling long-term sequelae.[217] Nerve injuries may be at a distal level on the brachial plexus or a proximal level with total avulsion of the plexus (Figure 59.23); in the latter case the neurological injury is irreparable.[218–221]

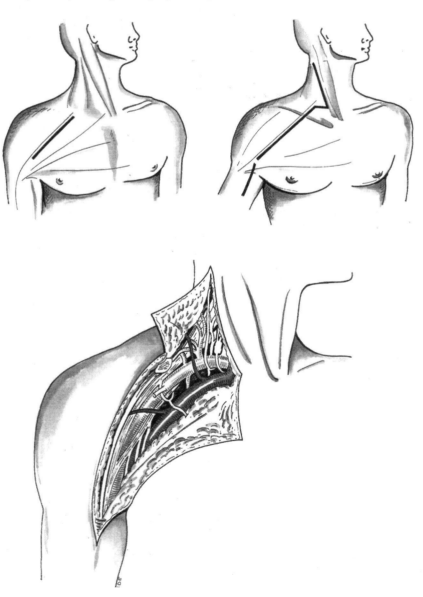

FIGURE 59.23. Anatomical aspect of subclavian and axillary arteries after resection of the clavicle. Notice the close relation with the brachial plexus, which explains the high frequency of associated nerve injuries.

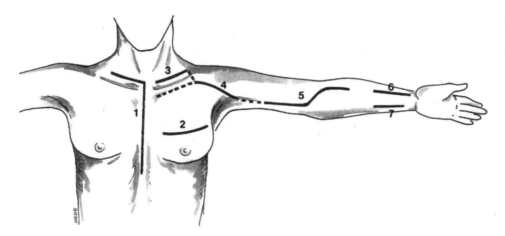

FIGURE 59.24. Incision lines for surgical approach to arteries of the upper limbs.

Collateral circulation is rich at this level; arterial occlusion with preserved distal pulses is reported in about 20% of patients.[222] The diagnostic approach should establish the site of arterial injury and the extent of neurological damage. Complete palsy of the upper extremity with muscle serratus major and homolateral Bernard–Horner syndrome suggests a medullary avulsion of the plexus.[218]

The surgical approach varies according to the vessel that must be reached (Figure 59.24). The right subclavian artery requires a median sternotomy with possible supraclavicular extension (Figure 59.24, incision 1), the left subclavian artery requires a third interspace left thoracotomy combined with a left supraclavicular incision (Figure 59.24, incisions 2 and 3), and the axillary artery requires a deltoid–pectoral approach with incision in the small pectoral muscle (Figure 59.24, incision 4). This last approach may be extended proximally by clavicular resection.[223]

Arterial reconstruction proceeds according to general principles (see the first section of this chapter). Venous reconstructions are preferred, although ligation is better tolerated in the upper limbs than in the lower limbs.[224]

If signs of neurological injury exist, the brachial plexus should be examined directly by surgical approach. With total avulsion of the plexus, the injury is irreparable and primary amputation should be considered. With a peripheral nervous lesion, immediate nerve repair with microsurgical technique and external saphenous nerve graft is possible; if a second correction is preferred, nerves should be marked by application of metal clips and positioned at a subcutaneous level.[218]

Brachial Artery

The brachial artery is one of the most commonly injured arteries.[166] Lesions are due to different causes: penetrating wounds, iatrogenic trauma after catheterization (Figure 59.25), supracondylar fractures of the humerus (Figure 59.26), and posterior elbow dislocation[225–227]; fractures of the humerus diaphysis rarely cause vascular injury.

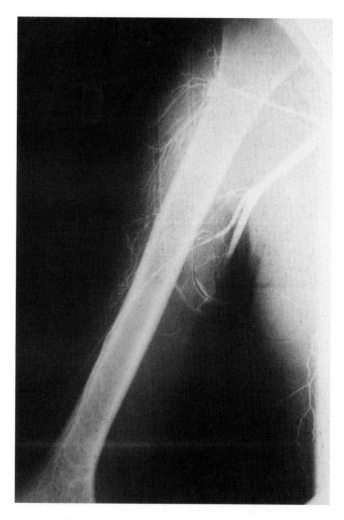

FIGURE 59.25. Traumatic occlusion of the brachial artery.

The deep brachial artery provides important collateral flow: in the experience during World War II the amputation rate was 55.7% for ligation above the deep brachial artery and only 25.8% for ligation below the artery.[170] The median nerve may sometimes be injured at the distal brachial artery at the point where it crosses the vessel.

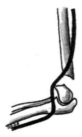

FIGURE 59.26. Mechanism of brachial artery lesion following fracture of the humerus.

Volkmann's ischemic retraction after only a short interruption of flow is reported in children; the mechanism of this complication is unclear.[228]

The brachial artery is exposed by a longitudinal incision on its course; an elbow incision should be bayonet shaped (Figure 59.24, incision 6). Vessel repair is made by end-to-end suture or graft interposition. Some authors avoid prosthetic material grafts because of the high occlusion rate found with their use.[229]

When extensive soft tissue damage makes covering the graft impossible, plastic surgery should be used (Figure 59.27). Skin may be taken from the thorax,[230] the great dorsal area,[231] or the contralateral forearm with vessel anastomosis.[232]

Forearm Arteries (Radial and Ulnar)

Although injuries of the radial and ulnar arteries are common,[166] excellent collateral circulation through the palmar arches makes ischemia extremely rare. Congenitally incomplete arches are infrequent[233] but if present may increase the risk of ischemia after forearm arterial injury.

Incision for radial artery exposure is made along a line that follows the medial border of the brachioradialis muscle to the radial depression on the wrist (Figure 59.24, incision 6). The ulnar artery is exposed along the line that connects epitrochlea to the lateral edge of the pisiform (Figure 59.24, incision 7).

Ligation is possible for single-artery injury without ischemia and good collateral flow. For injury of two arteries or ischemia after single-vessel thrombosis, repair with microsurgical techniques is required. If two vessels are injured, both should be repaired.

External Iliac and Common and Deep Femoral Arteries

The external iliac and common femoral arteries are rarely injured. Incidence was 1% for the external iliac artery and 6% for the common femoral artery in our experience, which reflects the frequency reported in other series.[170,182] Main causes are penetrating wounds or hip dislocation. Deep femoral artery trauma is extremely

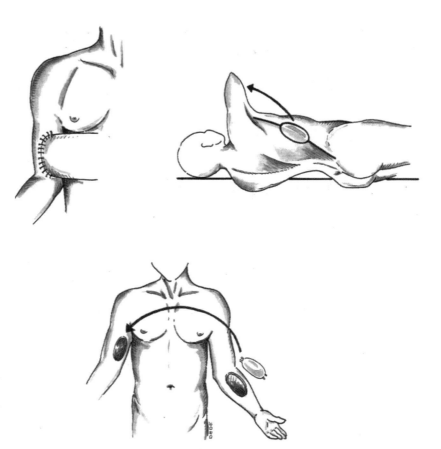

FIGURE 59.27. Different plastic surgery techniques to cover an open wound of the upper limb: anterothoracic skin graft, posterolateral thoracic cutaneomuscular graft, and contralateral forearm graft.

rare (no case in our casuistic). Occlusion of the external iliac and common femoral arteries is usually related to severe ischemia.[170] Deep femoral artery traumatic occlusion alone normally never causes ischemia.

The iliac artery is exposed by an abdominal lateral oblique incision with an extraperitoneal approach (Figure 59.28, incision 1). The external iliac artery just before the inguinal ligament is easily exposed by a short incision parallel to the ligament; this approach is useful only for proximal control of the artery for distal injury (Figure 59.28, incision 2). Better exposure of the external iliac artery with distal and proximal extension possibility is achieved by a vertical incision that crosses the inguinal ligament. The common femoral artery is exposed through a classic vertical incision in the groin (Figure 59.28, incision 3). The deep femoral artery is approached in the same way as the common femoral artery or by a middle crural approach with an incision along a line connecting the anterior–superior iliac spine with the medial edge of the patella (Figure 59.28, incision 4).[234]

Vascular repair is performed with described techniques. Profunda femoris injuries should be repaired because they have been associated with a high incidence of late arteriovenous fistulas or false aneurysms.[235]

Superficial Femoral Artery

The superficial femoral artery has a high incidence of traumatic lesions (24% in our casuistic). Trauma is

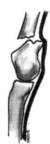

FIGURE 59.29. Superficial femoral artery injury following distal femoral fracture.

caused by penetrating injuries, but a high incidence of blunt trauma is also seen (Figure 59.29). The middle and distal thirds of the artery are most often involved.[229] Blunt trauma often causes extensive soft tissue damage with skin detachment, muscle loss, and potential necrotic areas. Neurological injuries are less frequent in the lower limb than in the upper limb (about 20%).[218]

The superficial femoral artery is exposed through a vertical incision along a line from the middle of the groin to the medial femoral condylus (Figure 59.28, incision 5). Direct suture is sometimes possible because proximal and distal segments can be mobilized with a gain of about 1 cm in length. Saphenous veins are the preferred conduits for interposition grafts. Because venous injuries are common and venous outflow may be disturbed, the saphenous vein should be taken from the contralateral side.[182]

Superficial femoral vein ligation is considered less damaging, but long-lasting edema may occur. Direct repair seems to be preferable. Because associated fractures are common, whether vascular repair or orthopedic stabilization should be the priority is questioned (Figure 59.30). In unclear cases, shunting of the vein and artery is the best way to solve the dilemma, because it allows the orthopedist to first stabilize the limb.[186]

Popliteal Artery

Popliteal artery injuries are frequent in civilian populations (24% in our casuistic). The main reported causes vary according to a population's social conditions and way of life. In some series penetrating wounds, mainly gunshot wounds, dominate,[237] whereas in others blunt trauma is the main cause of popliteal artery injuries.[236] The mean amputation rate is by far the highest among all peripheral vessel injuries (about 30%), although wide variations exist between different reports (from 0% to 61%).[187,189,237–240] Blunt trauma more often results in amputations, probably because of the concomitant soft tissue trauma and consequent obliteration of frail collateral arteries around the knee.[210] Traumatic dislocation of the knee often results in vascular compromise (up to 64% in complete dislocation)[241] (Figure 59.31).

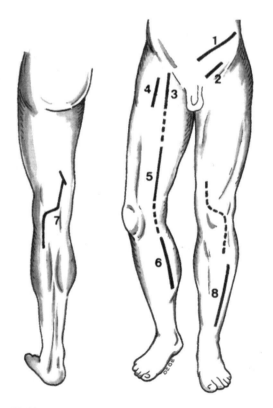

FIGURE 59.28. Incision lines for surgical approach to arteries of the lower limb.

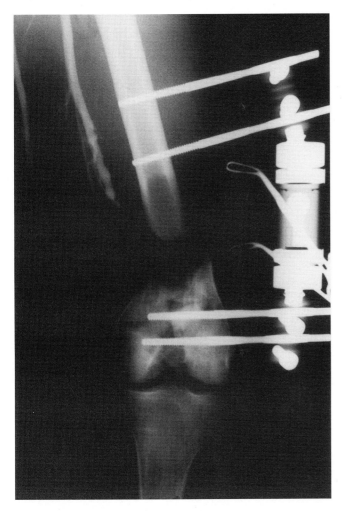

FIGURE 59.30. Tight distal trauma with superficial artery injury and large bone loss.

Cadaver experiments have demonstrated that rupture of the popliteal artery occurs at hyperextension of 50 degrees of the tibia.[242] All types of complete knee dislocations may cause vascular disruption, although anterior dislocation seems to be the most ominous injury.[243] A delay in revascularization of a popliteal occlusion increases the risk of irreversible damage: for delays longer than 8 hours, the amputation rate was 86% in Green and

Allen's study.[244] The importance of ischemic tolerance in popliteal occlusion is based on experimental work in animals. Limb salvage by revascularization after 6 hours of ischemia was 90%; after 12 to 18 hours 50%, and after 24 hours 20%.[245]

Although this study emphasizes the importance of avoiding delay in revascularization, the outcome of popliteal trauma also depends on many other factors, such as type of trauma, concomitant injuries, anatomical location, blood pressure, coagulopathy, and extent of interrupted collateral pathways.[236] Consequently, the outcome of patients with adequate collateral flow and delayed revascularization is less severe than for patients with acute ischemia.[183]

Angiography (Figure 59.32) is indicated particularly in patients with knee trauma and dislocation or fracture and compression injuries from car accidents. If clear clinical signs of ischemia are present, surgery should be performed without other examinations to save time. Intraoperative single-film hand-injected arteriography is possible when the condition is unclear. Fasciotomy (Figure 59.33), performed before revascularization if is-

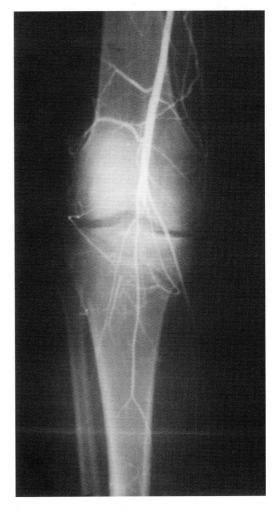

FIGURE 59.32. Occlusion of the popliteal artery due to knee dislocation from popliteal trauma.

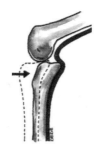

FIGURE 59.31. Mechanism of posterior knee dislocation in popliteal trauma.

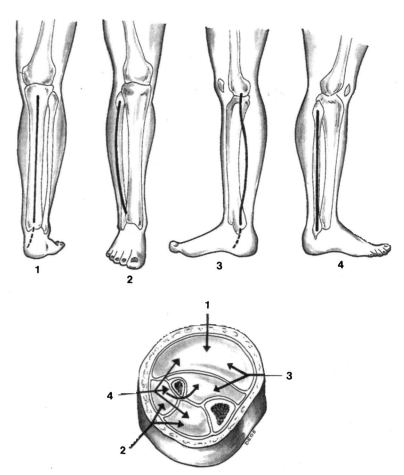

FIGURE 59.33. Techniques of fasciotomy in the calf: **1**, posterior access; **2**, anterolateral incision; **3**, medial access; **4**, perifibular approach to all compartments.

chemic signs and compartment syndrome are evident, enhances collateral flow during reconstruction.[239]

The popliteal artery is usually exposed by a medial approach because this incision can easily be extended proximally and distally and also because saphenous vein is easily obtained from a supine patient (Figure 59.28, incisions 5 and 6). For these reasons the posterior approach (Figure 59.28, incision 7) is rarely chosen.

In combined bone fractures and popliteal trauma, vascular reconstruction is generally performed before fracture reduction and fixation to shorten the duration of ischemia. In extremely unstable fractures with significant bone loss, the orthopedic procedure is performed first after insertion of an indwelling shunt.[237]

Saphenous graft interposition is the most common reconstruction method. Contemporary vein reconstruction is extremely important in popliteal trauma because it enhances arterial patency and significantly reduces secondary venous stasis.[246] In case of extensive soft tissue trauma on the vessel area with diffuse contamination and infection risk, a long, extra-anatomic vein bypass graft may be used (Figure 59.34).

Tibioperoneal Trunk and Tibial Vessels

Injuries of tibioperoneal trunk and tibial vessels have an incidence of about 5% in the civilian population[247,248]

(6% in our casuistry) and up to 20% in trauma from war.[182] In World War II ligation of two vessels resulted in an amputation rate of 69%.[170]

In civilian trauma amputation rates vary widely according to the type of trauma and vessels injured: blunt trauma and shotgun injuries are more dangerous for the peroneal trunk (with a 50% amputation rate), and in lesions of all three vessels the incidence was 60% in a series of 51 patients.[249] Crush injuries may increase amputation risk because of extensive vessel disruption and compartment syndrome.

Angiography for diagnosis is mandatory. Although indications for reconstruction are not clearly established, maintaining patency in at least two vessels is recommended.[249] Reversed saphenous vein bypass is preferred.

Anterior and posterior tibial arteries are exposed with vertical incisions according to the traditional technique (Figure 59.28, incisions 6 and 8). Fasciotomy is a routine procedure in these injuries and is mainly performed before vascular reconstruction. Because bypass procedure may be performed through the same fasciotomy incisions, covering the graft may be difficult. In these cases fasciotomy is better performed by a perifibular single anterolateral incision and bypass procedures by a medial approach. Sometimes blunt trauma to the calf may cause ischemia only because of compartment syndrome with-

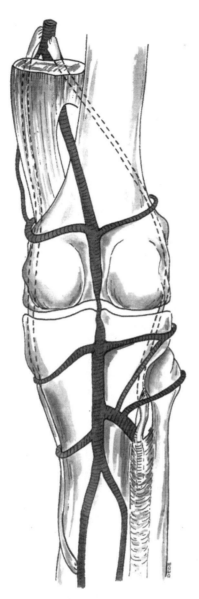

FIGURE 59.34. The possible extra-anatomic bypass to anterior and posterior tibial arteries in popliteal injuries with contamination of the popliteal area.

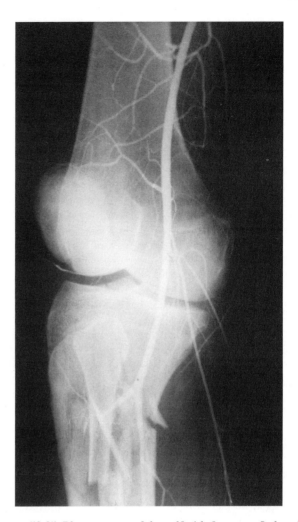

FIGURE 59.35. Blunt trauma of the calf with fractures. Ischemia and no distal pulse are present. There are clinical signs of compartment syndrome. Angiography shows occlusion of the anterior tibial artery but patent posterior tibial and peroneal arteries. Fasciotomy was performed with reappearance of distal pulses and complete recovery.

out significant vessel injury; fasciotomy alone is able to resolve acute symptoms (Figure 59.35).

Vascular Injuries of the Neck

Vascular trauma of the cephalic vessels is relatively rare. Carotid trauma is reported as occurring in less than 2 per 1000 patients with trauma that requires hospital admission.[250] Vertebral trauma is much more uncommon; because of less obvious clinical signs it often goes undetected.[251]

Carotid Artery

Injuries of the carotid artery are most often due to penetrating trauma, such as from knives or low-velocity bullets. Blunt trauma is much more uncommon,[251,252] although a recent multicenter study in a rural US state demonstrated an incidence of 33% of blunt trauma due mainly to motor vehicle accidents.[250] The common carotid artery is involved in about 50% of cases, with a slight prevalence of the left vessel.[253]

Different injuries are possible. In penetrating wounds pseudoaneurysm, carotid cavernous fistula, and occlusion are more common, whereas in blunt trauma intimal dissection is more often seen.[250] Injury mechanisms of blunt trauma include (1) hyperextension of the neck with contralateral rotation of the head, (2) direct cervical blow, (3) basilar skull fractures, and (4) blunt intraoral trauma.[254]

Because of the carotid site and neck anatomy, associated injuries are frequent (62%). Esophageal perforation, vertebral artery trauma, cranial nerve injuries, and internal jugular vein lesions are reported. Other associated injuries are thoracic injuries; extremity, facial, skull, and spinal fractures; abdominal injuries; and spinal cord trauma.[250]

Clinical manifestations of carotid trauma are associated with the characteristics of injury and brain circulatory conditions of the patient. Neurological symptoms are divided into three groups according to Thal and associates[255]:

Group 1: patients with no neurological deficit
Group 2: patients with mild neurological deficit
Group 3: patients with severe neurological deficit

Patients with minor intimal tears with no immediate carotid occlusion may initially be free of neurological symptoms, but the tears slowly progress until stroke due to thrombosis becomes evident.[252] This progression of symptoms may range from hours to several days. In other cases slight symptoms such as transient cerebral ischemic attacks, Bernard–Horner syndrome, monocular visual defects, and limb paresis in lucid patients are described.[256] Acute stroke and coma are manifested in the most severe cases.

Because the cervical fascia is a relatively strong structure, hematoma from carotid injury is contained deep in the neck, may compress airways, and thus may require emergency procedures. Injuries to cranial nerves may be manifested by vocal cord or diaphragm paresis. Shock is a severe clinical sign that was present in 28% of Ramadan and coworkers' patients.[250]

Clinical examination should begin with suspicion of carotid injury. A cervical bleeding wound with a history that describes the direction of injury is often helpful. A bruit on the carotid level and signs of cranial nerve injuries should be recognized. Arterial hemorrhage from a cervical penetrating injury that pierces the platysma muscle and signs of expanding hematoma are highly suspicious of carotid injury. Neurological examination to establish patient status and group classification according to Thal et al.[255] is mandatory for further management. Closed head trauma may hide the clinical picture.

Some authors suggest physical examination alone to diagnose carotid artery injury,[257,258] but the majority consider angiography the most helpful examination.[259–261] Angiography accurately diagnoses or excludes carotid artery injury and can be the basis of the management plan.

Recently duplex scanning has been used successfully for diagnosis in potential cervical vascular injury.[262] A comparative study established that duplex scanning is able to diagnose cervical vascular trauma as well as angiography,[263] but until now this examination was greatly underutilized. The unavailability of duplex scanning instruments at odd hours may have contributed to this underuse. Duplex scanning may have a far more important role in screening of these diseases in the future. Patients with unstable hemodynamic conditions often undergo surgery without angiogram.

The purpose of dividing the neck into three zones to evaluate penetrating wounds is for diagnosis and management. Zone I extends inferiorly from the clavicle to include the thoracic outlet, zone II extends from the clavicle to the angle of the mandible, and zone III includes the area between the angle of the mandible and the base of the skull.[263,264] It is often difficult to establish whether vascular injury exists in zones I and III. Angiograms are more often performed for trauma in these areas.

The decision to operate on a patient with carotid artery trauma must be carefully evaluated and depends on different data: occlusion of the injured carotid artery, neurological condition, and involved vessels. Thrombosed carotid arteries should not be revascularized because incomplete extraction of thrombotic debris may increase the risk of distal embolization.[259,265] All efforts should be made to establish definitively whether the carotid artery is completely occluded: in some cases partial permeability exists notwithstanding an angiographic indication of the opposite. Duplex scanner control after angiography may be helpful for accurate diagnosis. Complete occlusion of the carotid artery and severe stroke are contraindications for surgery because of associated high mortality rates.[259,265,266]

If the carotid artery is not occluded, neurological conditions determine whether to proceed with surgery. In patients without neurological deficit (group I) and with mild signs (group II) the vessel should be repaired surgically.[250,253,255,265] If the decision is made to operate, surgery should be undertaken as soon as possible to prevent secondary thrombosis of the vessel. This is particularly dangerous in injuries of the internal carotid artery because thrombosis may progress into the head and even embolize distally and result in severe and irreversible stroke. The importance of avoiding vascular reconstruction delay is supported by data that demonstrate that about two thirds of blunt carotid artery injuries are neurologically intact but more than half of the patients are discharged with significant neurological deficit.[250] A diagnostic delay, especially in blunt carotid artery trauma, is the main cause of late stroke.

Surgical revascularization in patients after complete stroke or in a comatose state with patent carotid arteries is controversial. During the Korean and Vietnam Wars revascularization appeared to lower mortality rates to 10%,[267] but other studies suggest that revascularization to lessen neurological deficits may convert anemic infarcts into hemorrhagic ones.[268,269] Some studies seem to indicate that neurological deterioration after vascular repair is not due to hemorrhagic infarction but rather to edema.[270,271] Moreover, it seems that observations in elderly patients who have undergone revascularization after atherosclerotic strokes may not be comparable to observations in a younger population after trauma.[250] The major cause of untoward outcome in stroke seems to be the ischemic insult itself rather than reperfusion hemorrhage.[270,271] Many believe that all injured and patent carotid arteries should be revascularized, regardless of the neurological conditions.[250,266,271–274] Even stroke and coma, although severe conditions, are not considered contraindications for surgery by some authors because the outcome in revascularized patients holds the advantage of limiting infarct size.[272] Not all authors agree with this strategy, and controversy remains.

Revascularization is performed by standard vascular techniques. Traditional exposure is through an incision along the anterior border of the sternocleidomastoid muscle. The injured external carotid artery is repaired or ligated. Injuries of common or internal carotid arteries are treated by clamping and repair. Use of systemic heparinization or shunt is controversial.[256] Some consider stump pressure above 60 mm Hg to be safe and no shunt is required.[275]

Repair is performed by lateral suture, resection and anastomosis, patch angioplasty, and interposition graft. Saphenous vein is the preferred graft, although cephalic vein may also be used.[276] In trauma of the internal carotid artery that requires resection and graft interposition, the external carotid artery can be used as graft.

Injuries of zone III may be difficult to expose. Section of the digastric muscle, excision of the styloid process, and subluxation of the mandible are useful maneuvers; the latter one is difficult and requires collaboration with a maxillofacial surgeon.[253] High inaccessible injuries, such as carotid cavernous fistulas and other high zone III internal carotid artery injuries are treated with detachable balloons or coil occlusions.[277]

Carotid artery ligation is rarely indicated and only as a lifesaving compromise in case of extensive irreparable damage or for complete carotid artery occlusion. Stroke incidence in these patients is about 50% because thrombosis progresses through the internal carotid artery.[253] Heparin may be helpful in preventing neurological damage.[275] Transcranial bypass from external carotid artery to intracranial vessels has been attempted to maintain adequate cerebral perfusion, but this technique is seldom used.[277]

Strict postoperative control is mandatory to recognize secondary bleeding that may cause acute respiratory difficulties and affect patency of the carotid artery. Surgical results depend on preoperative neurological status and treatment. Best results are in the group without neurological signs who undergo carotid artery revascularization. One advantage of revascularization was stressed in a recent study on different trauma centers: in patients without neurological signs stroke incidence was 8% after repair, 41% with no operation, and 50% after ligation.[250]

Vertebral Artery

Vertebral artery injuries are rare, perhaps because the vessel is protected in the bony canal. Sometimes this artery is injured along with the carotid artery by penetrating wounds. Bleeding may be continuous because of associated venous trauma. These injuries probably have often been missed in the past but, because preoperative angiography is now common, they are more often diagnosed.[278] Ligation is normally well tolerated and often is the therapy of choice. Only in specific patients with arteriovenous fistulas is surgical repair indicated. Exposure of the bony canal is possible but rarely indicated. Catheter occlusion with detachable balloon or coils, as described for carotid artery trauma, is also possible.

Acknowledgment

We acknowledge the contributions of Mrs. Renata Dedè for the drawings, and Mrs. Isabella Riva, Mrs. Nicoletta Piardi, and Mrs. Fanny Riva for the preparation of this manuscript.

References

1. Paré A. The Apologie and Treatise of Ambroise Paré Containing the Voyages Made in the Divers Places and Many Writings Upon Surgery. In: Key G, ed., Falcon Education Books; 1957.
2. Hallowell. Cited by Lambert in a letter to Dr. Hunter. *Med Observ Inq.* 1762; ch. 30, p. 360.
3. Assalini P. *Manuale di chirurgia del cavaliere Assalini.* Giacomo Pirola, ed. Milan: 1812.
4. Subbotitch. (1912). Cited by Rich in: Rich NM, Spencer FC. *Vascular Trauma.* Philadelphia, Pa: WB Saunders; 1978.
5. Lexer, E. Spätoperation einer arterio-venôsen Subclavia-Fistel nach Granatverletzung. *Münchener Medizinische Wochenschrift.* 1916;68:979.
6. Stich R, Fromme A. Die Verletzung der Blutgefäße und deren Folgezustände (Aneurysmen). *Ergebnisse der Chirurgie und Orthopädie.* 1921;13:144.
7. De Bakey ME, Simeone FA. Battle injuries of the arteries in World War II: an analysis of 2,471 cases. *Ann Surg.* 1946; 123:534–578.
8. Jahnke EJ Jr, Seeley SF. Acute vascular injuries in the Korean War. *Ann Surg.* 1953;138:158.
9. Hughes CW. Acute vascular trauma in Korean War casualties: an analysis of 180 cases. *Surg Gynecol Obstet.* 1954; 99:91.
10. Rich NM, Baugh JH, Hughes CW. Acute arterial traumas in Viet-Nam: 1,000 cases. *J Trauma.* 1970;10:359–369.

11. Fasol R, Irvine S, Zilla P. Vascular injuries caused by antipersonnel mines. *J Cardiovasc Surg*. 1989;30:467.

12. Radonic V, Baric D, Petricevic A, et al. Military injuries to the popliteal vessels in Croatia. *J Cardiovasc Surg*. 1994; 35:27.

13. Khoury G, Sfeir R, Nabbout G, et al. Traumatic arteriovenous fistulae: the Lebanese war experience. *Eur J Vasc Surg*. 1994;8:171.

14. Barros D'Sa A. The rationale for arterial and venous shunting in the management of limb vascular injuries. *Eur J Vasc Surg*. 1989;3:471.

15. Barros D'Sa A. Twenty five years of vascular trauma in Northern Ireland. *BMJ*. 1995;310:1.

16. Shires GT. *Principles of Trauma Care*. New York, NY: McGraw-Hill; 1985.

17. Barral X. *Les Urgences en Chirurgie Vasculaire*. Paris: Masson; 1988.

18. Vollmar J. *Rekonstruktive Chirurgie der Arterien*. Stuttgart: Georg Thieme Verlag; 1967.

19. Oller D, Rutledge R, Clancy T, et al. Vascular injuries in a rural state: a review of 978 patients from a state trauma registry. *J Trauma*.1992;32:740–746.

20. Krauss M. Studies in wound ballistics: temporary cavity effects in soft tissues. *Mil Med*. 1957;121:221–224.

21. Perry MO. Arterial injuries: general principles of management. In: Rutherford R, ed. *Vascular Surgery*. Philadelphia, Pa: WB Saunders; 1989:583–605.

22. Bongard FS, White GH, Klein SR. Management strategy of complex extremity injuries. *Am J Surg*. 1989;158:151.

23. Rich MN. Penetrating upper extremity vascular injuries. In: Greenhalgh MR, Kollier LH, eds. *Emergency Vascular Surgery*. London: WB Saunders; 1992:287–297.

24. Kresowik TF, Khourdy MD, Miller BV, et al. A prospective study of the incidence and natural history of femoral vascular complications after percutaneous transluminal coronary angioplasty. *J Vasc Surg*. 1991;13:328.

25. Bergentz SV, Bergqvist D. *Iatrogenic Vascular Injuries*. New York, NY: Springer-Verlag; 1989.

26. Lazarides MK, Arvanitis DP, Dayantas JN. Iatrogenic arterial trauma associated with hip joint surgery: an overview. *Eur J Vasc Surg*. 1991;5:549.

27. Myers SI, Harward TRS, Putnam JB, et al. Vascular trauma as a result of therapeutic procedures for the treatment of malignancy. *J Vasc Surg*. 1991;14:314.

28. Rich NM, Spencer FC. *Vascular Trauma*. Philadelphia, Pa: WB Saunders; 1978.

29. Drapanas T, Hewitt RL, Weichert RF. Civilian vascular injuries: a critical appraisal of three decades of management. *Ann Surg*. 1970;172:315.

30. Snyder WH, Watkins WL, Whidden LL, et al. Civilian popliteal artery trauma: an 11-year experience with 83 injuries. *Surgery*. 1974;85:101.

31. Barros D'Sa AAB. Shunting in complex lower limb vascular trauma. In: Greenhalgh RM, Hollier LH, eds. *Emergency Vascular Surgery*. London: WB Saunders; 1992;331–344.

32. Sanderson RA, Foley RK, McIvor GWD. Histological response on skeletal muscle to ischemia. *Clin Orthop*. 1975; 113:27.

33. Green NE, Allen BL. Vascular injuries associated with dislocation of the knee. *Am J Bone Joint Surg*. 1977;130:428.

34. Gorman JF. Combat wounds of the popliteal artery. *Ann Surg*. 1968;168:974.

35. Haimovici H. Metabolic syndrome secondary to acute arterial occlusions. In: Haimovici H, ed. *Vascular Emergencies*. New York, NY: Appleton Century Crofts; 1982:267–270.

36. Hewitt RL, Smith AD, Drapanas T. Acute traumatic arteriovenous fistulas. *J Trauma*. 1973;13:901.

37. Alberty RE, Goodfriend G, Boyden AM. Popliteal artery injury with fractural dislocations of the knee. *Am J Surg*. 1981;142:36.

38. Perry MO. *The Management of Acute Vascular Injuries*. Baltimore, Md: Williams & Wilkins; 1981.

39. Lynch K, Johansen K. Can Doppler pressure measurement replace "exclusion" arteriography in penetrating extremity trauma? *Ann Surg*. 1991;214:737.

40. Snyder WH, Thal ER, Bridges RA. The validity of normal arteriography in penetrating trauma. *Arch Surg*. 1978;113: 424.

41. Smith PL, Linn WN, Ferris EJ, et al. Emergency arteriography in extremity trauma: assessment of indications. *AJR Am J Roentgenol*. 1981;137:803.

42. Jebara VA, Haddad SN, Ghossain MA, et al. Emergency arteriography in the assessment of penetrating trauma of the lower limbs. *Angiology*. 1991;7:527.

43. Panetta TF, Sales CM, Marin ML, et al. Natural history, duplex characteristics, and histopathological correlation of arterial injuries in a canine model. *J Vasc Surg*. 1992; 16:867.

44. Byone RP, Miles WS, Bell RM, et al. Noninvasive diagnosis of vascular trauma by duplex ultrasonography. *J Vasc Surg*. 1991;14:346.

45. Fry WR, Smith RS, Sayers DV, et al. The success of duplex ultrasonographic scanning in diagnosis of extremity vascular proximity trauma. *Arch Surg*. 1993;128:1368.

46. Feliciano DV, Bitondo GC, Mattox KL, et al. Civilian trauma in the 1980s. *Ann Surg*. 1984;199:717.

47. Panetta TF, Sclafani SJA, Goldstein AS, et al. Percutaneous transcatheter embolization for arterial trauma. *J Vasc Surg*. 1985;25:54.

48. Marin ML, Veith FJ, Panetta TF, et al. Transluminally placed endovascular stented graft repair for arterial trauma. *J Vasc Surg*. 1994;20:466.

49. Barros D'Sa AAB. Management of vascular injuries of civil strife. *Injury*. 1982;14:51.

50. Patman RD, Poulos E, Shires GT. The management of civilian arterial injuries. *Surg Gynecol Obstet*. 1964;118: 725.

51. Moore WS, Swanson RJ, Campagna G, et al. The issue of fresh tissue arterial substitutes in infected fields. *J Surg Res*. 1975;18:229.

52. Daugherty ME, Sachatello CR, Ernst CB. Improved treatment of popliteal artery injuries. *Arch Surg*. 1978;113:1317.

53. Earle AS, Horsley GS, Villavicencio JL, et al. Replacement of venous defects by venous autografts. *Arch Surg*. 1960;80: 119.

54. Chu-Yeng Chiu R, Tersis J, MacRae ML. Replacement of superior vena cava with the spiral composite vein graft: a versatile technique. *Ann Thorac Surg*. 1974;17:555.

55. Rich NM. Principles and indications for primary venous repair. *Surgery*. 1982;91:492.

56. Gasper MR, Treiman RL. The management of injuries to major veins. *Am J Surg.* 1960;100:171.

57. Rich NM, Hughes CW. Vietnam vascular registry: a preliminary report. *Surgery.* 1969;65:218.

58. Hobson RW II, Howard EW, Wright CV, et al. Haemodynamics of canine femoral venous ligation: significance in combined arterial and venous injury. *Surgery.* 1973;74:824.

59. Rich NM, Hobson RW II, Collins GJ, et al. The effect of acute popliteal venous interruption. *Ann Surg.* 1976;183:365.

60. Phifer TJ, Gerlock AJ Jr, Vekovius WA, et al. Amputation risk factors in concomitant superficial femoral artery and vein injuries. *Ann Surg.* 1984;199:241.

61. Hardin WD, Adinolfi MF, O'Connell RC, et al. Management of traumatic peripheral vein injuries: primary repair or vein ligation? *Am J Surg.* 1982;144:235.

62. Timberlake GA, O'Connell RC, Kerstein MD. Venous injury: to repair or ligate? the dilemma. *J Vasc Surg.* 1986;4:553.

63. McCord JM. Defense against free radicals has therapeutic implications. *JAMA.* 1984;251:2187.

64. Bongard F, Dubrow T, Klein SR. Vascular injuries in the urban battleground: experience at a metropolitan trauma center. *Ann Vasc Surg.* 1990;4:415.

65. Fellciano DV, Bitondo CG, Mattox KL, et al. Civilian trauma in the 1980s: a 1-year experience with 456 vascular and cardiac injures. *Ann Surg.* 1984;199:177.

66. Mattox KL, Feliciano DV, Burch J, et al. Five thousand seven hundred sixty cardiovascular injuries in 4459 patients: epidemiologic evolution 1958 to 1987. *Ann Surg.* 1989;209:698.

67. Newman RJ, Rastagi S. Rupture of the thoracic aorta and its relationship to road traffic: accident characteristic. *Injury.* 1984;15:296.

68. Feliciano DV, Bitondo CG, Cruse PA, et al. Liberal use of emergency center thoracotomy. *Am J Surg.* 1986;152:654.

69. Johnston RH, Wall MJ, Mattox KL. Innominate arterial trauma: a thirty-year experience. *J Vasc Surg.* 1993;17:134.

70. Liekweg WG, Greefield LJ. Management of penetrating carotid arterial injury. *Ann Surg.* 1978;188:587.

71. Brown MF, Graham JM, Feliciano DV, et al. Carotid artery injuries. *Am J Surg.* 1982;144:748.

72. Ledgerwood AM, Mullins RJ, Lucas CE. Primary repair vs ligation for carotid artery injuries. *Arch Surg* 1980;115:488.

73. Feliciano DV, Mattox KL. Thoracic and abdominal vascular trauma. In: Veith FJ, Hobson RW, Williams RA, et al., eds. *Vascular Surgery: Principles and Practice.* 2nd ed. New York, NY: McGraw-Hill; 1994:947–966.

74. Bongard F. Thoracic and abdominal vascular trauma. In: Rutherford RB, ed. *Vascular Surgery.* 4th ed. Philadelphia, Pa: WB Saunders; 1995:681–704.

75. Marin ML, Veith FJ, Panetta TF, et al. Transluminally placed endovascular stented graft repair for arterial trauma. *J Vasc Surg.* 1994;20:466.

76. Parmley LF, Mattingly TW, Manion WC, et al. Non penetrating traumatic injury of the aorta. *Circulation.* 1958;18:1086.

77. Greendyke RM: Traumatic rupture of aorta: special reference to automobile accidents. *JAMA.* 1996;195:527.

78. Smith RS, Chang FC. Traumatic rupture of the aorta: still a lethal injury. *Am J Surg.* 1986;152:660.

79. Cicero J, Mattox KL. Epidemiology of chest trauma. *Surg Clin North Am* 1989;69:15.

80. Sevitt S. The mechanisms of traumatic rupture of the thoracic aorta. *Br J Surg.* 1977;64:166.

81. Lundevall J. The mechanism of traumatic rupture of the aorta. *Acta Pathological Microbiological Scandinavian.* 1964;62:34.

82. Graham JM, Feliciano DV, Mattox KL, et al. Innominate vascular injury. *J Trauma.* 1982;22:647.

83. Eller JI, Ziter MH. Avulsion of the innominate artery from the aortic arch: an evaluation of roentgenographic findings. *Radiology.* 1970;94:75.

84. Fischer RG, Hadlock F, Ben-Menachem Y. Laceration of the thoracic aorta and brachiocephalic arteries by blunt trauma: report of 54 cases and review of literature. *Radiol Clin North Am.* 1981;19:91.

85. Mattox KL. Approaches to trauma involving the major vessels of the thorax. *Surg Clin North Am.* 1989;69:77.

86. Mattox KL. Contemporary issues in thoracic aortic trauma. *Semin Thorac Cardiovasc Surg.* 1991;3:281.

87. Wexler L, Silverman J. Traumatic rupture of innominate artery: a seat belt injury. *N Engl J Med.* 1970;282:1186.

88. Woelfel FG, Moore EE, Cogbill TH, et al. Severe thoracic and abdominal injuries associated with lap-harness seatbelt. *J Trauma.* 1984;24:166.

89. Arajarvi E, Sartavinta S, Toloner J. Aortic ruptures in seatbelt wearers. *J Thorac Cardiovasc Surg.* 1989;98:355–361.

90. Ochsner MG, Hoffman AP, Di Pasquale D, et al. Associated aortic rupture–pelvic fracture: an alert for orthopedic and general surgeons. *J Trauma.* 1992;33:429.

91. Duhaylongsod FG, Glower DD, Wolfe WG. Acute traumatic aortic aneurysm: the Duke experience from 1970 to 1990. *J Vasc Surg.* 1992;15:331.

92. Sturm JT, Perry JF Jr, Olson FR, et al. Significance of symptoms and signs in patients with traumatic aortic rupture. *Ann Emerg Med.* 1984;13:867.

93. Symbas PN, Tyras DH, Ware RE, et al. Rupture of the aorta: a diagnostic triad. *Ann Thorac Surg.* 1973;15:405.

94. Ayella RJ, Hankins JR, Turney SZ, et al. Ruptured thoracic aorta due to blunt trauma. *J Trauma.* 1977;17:199.

95. Gundry SR, Williams S, Burney RE, et al. Indications for aortography. Radiography after blunt chest trauma: a reassessment of the radiographic findings associated with traumatic rupture of the aorta. *Invest Radiol.* 1983;18:230–237.

96. Perchinsky MJ, Long WB, Urman S, et al. "The broken halo sign": a fractured calcified ring as an unusual sign of traumatic rupture of the thoracic aorta. *Injury.* 1994;25:649–652.

97. Durham RM, Zuckerman D, Wolverson M, et al. Computed tomography as a screening exam in patients with suspected blunt aortic injury. *Ann Surg.* 1994;220:699–744.

98. Brooks SW, Young JC, Cmolik B, et al. The use of transesophageal echocardiography in the evaluation of chest trauma. *J Trauma.* 1992;32:761–768.

99. Kearney PA, Smith DW, Johnson SB, et al. Use of transesophageal echocardiography in the evaluation of traumatic aortic injury. *J Trauma.* 1993;34:696–703.

100. Smith MD, Cassidy JM, Souther S, et al. Transesophageal echocardiography in the diagnosis of traumatic rupture of the aorta. *N Engl J Med.* 1995;332:356–362.

101. Barcia TC, Livoni JP. Indications for angiography in blunt thoracic trauma. *Radiology.* 1983;147:15–19.

102. Hills MW, Thomas SG, McDougall PA, et al. Traumatic thoracic aortic rupture: investigation determines outcome. *Aust N Z J Surg.* 1994;64:312–318.

103. Clark DE, Zeiger MA, Wallace KL, et al. Blunt aortic trauma: signs of high risk. *J Trauma.* 1990;30:701.

104. Kieffer E. Traumatisme de l'aorte thoracique. In: Barral X, ed. *Les Urgences en Chirurgie Vasculaire.* Paris: Masson; 1988:224–246.

105. Orriager MB, Kirsh MM. Primary repair of acute traumatic aortic disruption. *Ann Thorac Surg.* 1983;35:586–591.

106. Mattox KL, Holman M, Pickard LR, et al. Clamp/repair: a safe technique for treatment of blunt injury to the descending thoracic aorta. *Ann Thorac Surg.* 1985;40:456.

107. DelRossi AJ, Cernaianu AC, Madden LD, et al. Traumatic disruptions of the thoracic aorta: treatment and outcome. *Surgery.* 1990;108:864.

108. Cowley RA, Turney SZ, Hankins JR, et al. Rupture of thoracic aorta caused by blunt trauma: a fifteen-year experience. *J Thorac Cardiovasc Surg.* 1990;100:652.

109. McCroskey BL, Moore FA, Moore EE, et al. A unified approach to the torn thoracic aorta. *Am J Surg.* 1991;1862:473.

110. De Bakey ME, Simeone FA. Battle injuries of the arteries in World War II: an analysis of 2471 cases. *Ann Surg.* 1946;123:534.

111. Hughes CW. Arterial repair during the Korean War. *Ann Surg.* 1958;147:555.

112. Rich NM, Baugh JH, Hughes CW. Acute arterial injuries in Vietnam: 1000 cases. *J Trauma.* 1970;10:539.

113. Luetic' V, Šoša I, Tonkovi I, et al. Military vascular injuries in Croatia. *Cardiovasc Surg.* 1993;1:3–6.

114. Lovric' Z. Reconstruction of major arteries of extremities after war injuries. *J Cardiovasc Surg.* 1993;24:33–37.

115. Bajec J, Gang RK, Lari AR. Post Gulf war explosive injuries in liberated Kuwait. *Injury.* 1993;24:517–520.

116. Mattox KL, Feliciano DV, Burch J, et al. Five thousand seven hundred sixty cardiovascular injuries in 4459 patients: epidemiologic evolution 1958 to 1987. *Ann Surg.* 1989;209:2698.

117. Feliciano DV, Burch JM, Spjut-Patrinely V, et al. Abdominal gunshot wounds: an urban trauma center's experience with 300 consecutive patients. *Ann Surg.* 1988;208:362.

118. Oller D, Rutledge R, Clancy T, et al: Vascular injuries in a rural state reported by Johnson G and Baker CC. *Penetrating Abdominal Vascular Injury.* In: Greenlagh RM, Holier LH, eds. *Emergency Vascular Surgery.* London: WB Saunders; 1992:217–227.

119. Humphrey PW, Nichols WK, Silver D. Rural vascular trauma: twenty year review. *Ann Vasc Surg.* 1994;8:179–185.

120. Fischer RP, Miller Crotchedd P, Reed RL. Gatrointestinal disruption: the hazards of nonoperative management in adults with blunt abdominal injury. *J Trauma.* 1988;28:1445.

121. Cox CF. Blunt abdominal trauma: a 5-year analysis of 870 patients requiring celiotomy. *Ann Surg.* 1984;199:467.

122. Feliciano DV. Abdominal vascular injuries. *Surg Clin North Am.* 1988;68:741.

123. Bass A, Papa M, Morag B, et al. Aortic false aneurysm following blunt trauma of the abdomen. *J Trauma.* 1983;23:1072.

124. Zahrani HH. False aneurysm of the abdominal aorta after blunt trauma. *Eur J Vasc Endovasc Surg.* 1991;5:685–687.

125. Lassonde J, Laureandeau F. Blunt injury of the abdominal aorta. *Ann Surg.* 1981;194:745–748.

126. Lock JS, Hoffman AD, Johnson RC. Blunt trauma of the abdominal aorta. *J Trauma.* 1987;27:647–677.

127. Pezzella AT, Griffen WO, Ernst CB. Superior mesenteric artery injury following blunt abdominal trauma: case report with successful primary repair. *J Trauma.* 1978;18:472.

128. Smejkal R, Izant R, Born C, et al. Pelvic crush injuries with occlusion of iliac artery. *J Trauma.* 1998;28:1479.

129. Buscaglia LC, Matolo N, Macbeth A. Common iliac artery injury from blunt trauma: case reports. *J Trauma.* 1989;29:697.

130. Clyne CAC, Ashbrooke EA. Seat-belt aorta: isolated abdominal aortic injury following blunt trauma. *Br J Surg.* 1985;72:239.

131. Warrian RK, Shoenut JP, Iannicello CM, et al. Seat-belt injury to the abdominal aorta. *J Trauma.* 1988;28:1505.

132. Randhawa MPS, Menzolan JO. Seat belt aorta. *Ann Vasc Surg.* 1990;4:370–377.

133. Baker CC, Thomas AN, Trunkey DD. The role of emergency room thoracotomy in trauma. *J Trauma.* 1980;20:848–854.

134. Lim RC, Miller SE. Management of acute civilian vascular injuries. *Surg Clin North Am.* 1982;62:113.

135. Wolf RK, Berry RE. Transaxillary intra-aortic balloon tamponade in trauma. *J Vasc Surg.* 1986;1:95–97.

136. Gupta BK, Khaneja SC, Flores L, et al. The role of intra-aortic occlusion in penetrating abdominal trauma. *Surg Gynecol Obstet.* 1989;143:249.

137. Feliciano DV. Approach to major abdominal vascular injury. *J Vasc Surg.* 1988;7:730–736.

138. Veith FJ, Gupta S, Daly V. Technique for occluding the supraceliac aorta through the abdomen. *Surg Gynecol Obstet.* 1980;151:426.

139. Accola KD, Feliciano DV, Mattox KL, et al. Management of injuries to the suprarenal area. *Am J Surg.* 1986;154:613.

140. Accola KD, Feliciano DV, Mattox KL, et al. Management and injuries to the superior mesenteric artery. *J Trauma.* 1986;26:313–319.

141. Feliciano DV, Burch JM, Graham JM. Abdominal vascular injury. In: Moore EE, Mattax KL, Feliciano DV, eds. *Trauma.* East Norwalk, Conn: Appleton & Lange: 1991:533–552.

142. Kretz JG. Traumatismes de la veine cave inferieure. In: Barral X, ed. *Les Urgences en Chirurgie Vasculaire.* Paris: Masson; 1988:184–190.

143. Burch JM, Feliciano DV, Mattox KL, et al. Injuries to the inferior vena cava. *Am J Surg.* 1988;156:548.

144. Barlow B, Gandhi R. Renal artery thrombosis following blunt trauma. *J Trauma.* 1980;20:614–617.

145. McAninch JW, Carroll PR, Klostermann PW, et al. Renal reconstruction after injury. *J Urol.* 1991;145:932–937.

146. Lohse JR, Shoe RM, Belzer FO. Acute renal artery occlusion. *Arch Surg.* 1982;117:801.

147. Spiraak SJA, Resnick MI. Revascularization of traumatic thrombosis of the renal artery. *Surg Gynecol Obstet.* 1987;164:22.

148. MacAninch JW, Carroll PR, Armenakas NA, et al. Renal gunshot wounds: methods of salvage and reconstruction. *J Trauma.* 1939;35:279–283.

149. Wiencek RG, Wilson RF. Abdominal venous injuries. *J Trauma.* 1986;26:771.

150. Dean RH. Management of renal artery trauma [editorial]. *J Vasc Surg.* 1988;8:89–90.

151. Landreneau RJ, Mitchum P, Fry WJ. Iliac artery transposition. *Arch Surg.* 1989;124:978.

152. Rothenberg DA, Fisher RP, Perry JF, et al. Major vascular injuries secondary to pelvic fractures: an unsolved clinical problem. *Am J Surg.* 1978;136:660–662.

153. Klein SR, Saroyan RM, Baumgartner F, et al. Management strategy of vascular injuries associated with pelvic fractures. *J Cardiovasc Surg.* 1992;33:349–357.

154. Frank JL, Reimer BL, Raves JJ. Traumatic iliofemoral artery injury: an association with high anterior acetabular fractures. *J Vasc Surg.* 1989;10:198–201.

155. Matalon T, Athanasoulis CH, Marcolies MN, et al. Hemorrhage with pelvis fractures: efficacy of transcatheter embolisation. *Am J Roentgenol.* 1979;133:859–864.

156. Mucha P, Welch TJ. Hemorrhage in major pelvic fractures. *Surg Clin North Am.* 1988;68:757.

157. Mucha P. Pelvic fractures. In: Moore EE, Mattax KL, Feliciano DV, eds. *Trauma.* East Norwalk, Conn: Appleton & Lange; 1991:553–569.

158. Petersen SR, Sheldon GF, Lim RC. Management of portal vein injuries. *J Trauma.* 1979;19:616–661.

159. Buetcher FJ, Sereda D, Gomez G, et al. Retrohepatic vein injuries: experience with 20 cases. *J Trauma.* 1989;29:1698.

160. Huguet C, Nordlinger B, Bahini A, et al. L'exclusion vasculaire du foie. In: Kieffer E. *Chirurgie de la Veine Cave Inferieure et des Branches.* Paris: ESF; 1985:57–68.

161. Kundsk KA, Sheldon GF, Lim RC. Atria caval shunting after trauma. *Surg Clin North Am.* 1972;52:699–710.

162. Rovito PF. Atrial caval shunting in blunt hepatic vascular injury. *Ann Surg.* 1987;205:318.

163. Burch JM, Feliciano DV, Mattox KL. The atriocaval shunt: facts and fiction. *Ann Surg.* 1988;207:555.

164. Kundks KA, Bongard F, Lim RC, et al. Determinants of survival after vena cava I injury: analysis of a 14 year experience. *Arch Surg.* 1984;119:1109.

165. Blair SD. Intra-arterial drug injection. In: Greenhalgh RM, Hollier LH, eds. *Emergency Vascular Surgery.* London: WB Saunders; 1992:377–385.

166. Drapanas T, Hewitt RL, Weichert RF, et al. Civilian vascular injuries: a critical appraisal of three decades of management. *Ann Surg.* 1970;172:315.

167. Bongard FS, White GH, Klein SR. Management strategy of complex extremity injuries. *Am J Surg.* 1989;158:151.

168. Kurtoglu M, Ertekin C, Bulut T, et al. Management of vascular injuries of the extremities. *Int Angiol.* 1991;10:95.

169. Byone RP, Miles WS, Bell RM, et al. Noninvasive diagnosis of vascular trauma by duplex ultrasonography. *J Vasc Surg.* 1991;14:346.

170. De Bakey ME, Simeone FA. Battle injuries of the arteries in World War II: an analysis of 2,471 cases. *Ann Surg.* 1946;123:534.

171. Smith RF, Szilagyi DE, Elliott JP. Fracture of long bones with arterial injury due to blunt trauma. *Arch Surg.* 1969;99:315.

172. Makin GS, Howard GM, Green RL. Arterial injuries complicating fractures or dislocations: the necessity of a more aggressive approach. *Surgery.* 1966;59:203.

173. Barral X. *Les Urgences en Chirurgie Vasculaire.* Paris: Masson; 1988.

174. MacDonald EJ, Goodman PC, Winestock DP. The clinical indications for arteriography in trauma to the extremity: a review of 114 cases. *Radiology.* 1975;116:45.

175. Saletta JD, Freeark RJ. The partially severed artery. *Arch Surg.* 1968;97:198.

176. O'Gorman RB, Feliciano DV, Bitondo CG. Emergency center arteriography in the evaluation of suspected peripheral vascular injuries. *Arch Surg.* 1984;119:568.

177. Gerlock AJ, Thal ER, Snyder WH III. Venography in penetrating injuries of the extremities. *AJR Am J Roentgenol.* 1976;126:1023.

178. Weber J, May R. *Funktionelle Phlebologie.* Stuttgart: Georg Thieme Verlag; 1990.

179. Dennis JW, Frykberg ER, Crump JM, et al. New perspectives on the management of penetrating trauma in proximity to major limb arteries. *J Vasc Surg.* 1990;11:84.

180. Frykberg ER, Crump JM, Dennis JW. Nonoperative observation of clinically occult arterial injuries: a prospective evaluation. *Surgery.* 1991;109:85.

181. Tufaro A, Arnold T, Rummel M, et al. Adverse outcome of nonoperative management of intimal injuries caused by penetrating trauma. *J Vasc Surg.* 1994;20:656.

182. Rich NM, Baugh JH, Hughes CW. Acute arterial injuries in Vietnam: 1000 cases. *J Trauma.* 1970;10:359.

183. Snyder WH, Watkins WL, Whiddon LL. Civilian popliteal artery trauma: an eleven year experience with 83 injuries. *Surgery.* 1979;85:101.

184. Eger M, Goleman L, Goldstein A, et al. The use of a temporary shunt in the management of arterial vascular injuries. *Surg Gynecol Obstet.* 1971;132:67.

185. Szuchmacher PH, Freed JS. Immediate revascularization of the popliteal artery and vein: report of a case. *J Trauma.* 1978;18:142.

186. Barros D'Sa AB. Shunting in lower limb vascular trauma. In: Greenhalgh RM, Hollier LH. *Emergency Vascular Surgery.* London: WB Saunders; 1992:331–344.

187. Matsen FA III. *Compartment Syndrome.* New York, NY: Grune & Stratton; 1980.

188. Matsen FA III, Winquist RA, Kruguire RB. Diagnosis and management of compartment syndrome. *J Bone Joint Surg Am.* 1980;62:286.

189. Lange RH, Bach AW, Hansen ST Jr. Open tibial fractures with associated vascular injuries: prognosis for limb salvage. *J Trauma.* 1985;25:203.

190. Strinden WD, Dibbell DG, Turnipseed WD, et al. Coverage of acute vascular injuries of the axilla and groin with

transposition muscle flaps: case report. *J Trauma.* 1989;
29:512.

191. Melissinos EG, Parks DH. Post trauma reconstruction
with free tissue transfer: analysis of 442 consecutive cases.
J Trauma. 1989;29:1095.

191. Khouri RK, Shaw WW. Reconstruction of the lower extremity with microvascular free flaps: a 10 year experience
with 304 consecutive cases. *J Trauma.* 1989;29:1086.

193. Hallock GG. Local fasciocutaneous flaps for cutaneous
coverage for lower extremity wounds. *J Trauma.* 1989;
29:1240.

194. Ledgerwood AM, Lucas CE. Biological dressings for exposed vascular grafts. *J Trauma.* 1975;15:567.

195. Flint LM, Richardson JD. Arterial injuries with lower extremity fractures. *Surgery.* 1983;93:5.

196. Meyer JP, Goldfaden D, Barrett J, et al. Subclavian and innominate artery trauma: a recent experience with nine
patients. *J Cardiovasc Surg.* 1988;29:283.

197. Malagon G, Bordeaux J, Legre R, et al. Emergency versus
delayed repair of severe brachial plexus injuries. *Clin Orthop.* 1988;237:32.

198. Vollmar J. *Rekonstruktive Chirurgie der Arterien.* Stuttgart:
Georg Thieme Verlag; 1985.

199. Edshage S. Peripheral nerve suture. *Acta Chir Scand.*
1964;331(suppl):221–228.

200. Millesi H. Looking back on nerve surgery. *International
Journal of Microsurgery.* 1980;2:143.

201. Gregory RT, Gould RJ, Peclet M. The mangled extremity
syndrome (M.E.S.): a severity grading system for multisystem injury of the extremity. *J Trauma.* 1985;25:1147–1150.

202. Russel WL, Sailors DM, Whittle TB, et al. Limb salvage
versus traumatic amputation: a decision based on a seven
part predictive index. *Ann Surg.* 1991;213:473–481.

203. Howe HR, Poole GV, Hansen KJ, et al. Salvage of lower
extremities following combined orthopedic and vascular
trauma: a predictive salvage index. *Am Surg.* 1987;53:205.

204. Johansen K, Daines M, Howey T, et al. Objective criteria
accurately predict amputation following lower extremity
trauma. *J Trauma.* 1990;30:568.

205. Lazarides MK, Arvanitis DP, Kopadis GC, et al. *Eur J Vasc
Endovasc Surg.* 1994;8:226–230.

206. Shaw RS. Treatment of the extremity suffering near or total severance with special considerations of the vascular
problem. *Clin Orthop.* 1963;29:56.

207. Williams GR, Carter DR, Frank GR, et al. Replantation of
amputated extremities. *Ann Surg.* 1966;163:788.

208. Chung-Wei C, Yun-Quing Q, Zhong-Jia Y. Extremity replantation. *World J Surg.* 1978;2:513.

209. Owen E. Replantation abgetrennter Extremitäten. *Langenbecks Arch Chir.* 1975;339:613.

210. Snyder WH, Thal ER, Perry MO. Vascular injuries of the
extremities. In: Rutherford RB. *Vascular Surgery.* Philadelphia, Pa: WB Saunders; 1989:613–646.

211. Kieffer E, Tricot JF, Marval M, et al. Traumatismes fermés
des troncss supra-aortiques. *J Chir.* 1979;116:333.

212. Costa MC, Robbs JV. Nonpenetrating subclavian artery
trauma. *J Vasc Surg.* 1988;8:71.

213. Mercier CI, Tuornigand P, Quilichini F, et al. Les prob-
lèmes posés par les traumatismes de l'artère sous-cavière
vus en urgence. *J Mal Vasc.* 1977;2:9.

214. Orek SL, Burgess A, Levine AM. Traumatic lateral displacement of the scapula: a radiographic sign of neurovascular disruption. *J Bone Joint Surg.* 1984;66A:758.

215. Berga C, Prat S, Ninot S, et al. The arterial complications
of closed injuries to the shoulder girdle. *Angiologia.* 1992;
44:139.

216. Laverick MD, Barros D'Sa AAB, Kirk SJ, et al. Management of blunt injuries of the axillary artery and the neck
of the humerus: case report. *J Trauma.* 1990;30:360.

217. Graham JM, Mattox KL, Feliciano DV, et al. Vascular injuries of the axilla. *Ann Surg.* 1982;195:232.

218. Barral, X. *Les Urgences en Chirurgie Vasculaire.* Paris: Masson; 1988.

219. Sampson LN, Britton JC, Eldrup-Jorgensen J, et al. The
neurovascular outcome of scapulothoracic dissociation. *J
Vasc Surg.* 1993;17:1083.

220. Tomaszek DE. Combined subclavian artery and brachial
plexus injuries from blunt upper-extremity trauma. *J
Trauma.* 1984;24:161.

221. Fitridge RA, Rapits S, Miller JH, et al. Upper extremity arterial injuries: experience at the Royal Adelaide Hospital,
1969 to 1991. *J Vasc Surg.* 1994;20:941.

222. Smith LL, Foran R, Gaspar MR. Acute arterial injuries of
the upper extremity. *Am J Surg.* 1963;106:144.

223. Cormier JM, Sutot J, Frileux CL, et al. *Nouveau Traité de
Technique Chirurgicale.* Paris: Masson; 1977.

224. Crady R, Procter D, Hyde G. Subclavian axillary vascular
trauma. *J Vasc Surg.* 1986;3:24.

225. Hofammann K, Moneim M, Omer G, et al. Brachial
artery disruption following closed posterior elbow dislocation in a child: assessment with intravenous digital angiography. A case report with review of the literature.
Clinical Orthopaedics and Related Research. 1984;184:
145–149.

226. Urse J, Auwers F, Posevitz L. Brachial artery transection
after closed elbow dislocation: a case report and review of
the literature. *Vasc Surg.* 1985;19:247–251.

227. Goldmann MH, Kent S, Schaumburg E. Brachial artery
injuries associated with posterior elbow dislocation. *Surg
Gynecol Obstet.* 1987;164:95.

228. Ottolenghi C. Prophilaxie du syndrome de Volkmann
dans les fractures supra-condyliennes du coude chez l'en-
fant. *Rev Chir Orthop Reparatrice Appar Mot.* 1971;57:517.

229. Bongard FS. Management strategy of combined orthopedic and vascular injuries. *Perspect Vasc Surg.* 1990;3:8.

230. Morelfatio D. Les lambeau plats. *EMC Techniques Chirurgi-
cales.* 4, 45080—1–13.

231. Mitz V. Le lambeau musculaire et musculocutané du
grand dorsal. In: Magalon G, Mitz V, eds. *Les Lambeau
Pédiculés Musculaires et Musculocutanés.* Paris: Masson;
1984.

232. Kevorkian B, Legre R, Magalon G, et al. Le lambeau anti
brachial à pédicule radial: a propos de 13 observations.
Ann Chir Plast Esthet. 1985;30:121.

233. Coleman SS, Anson BJ. Arterial patterns in the hand
based upon a study of 650 specimens. *Surg Gynecol Obstet.*
1961;113:409.

234. Gillot CL, Frileux C, Pillot-Bienayhe P, et al. Abord direct
pour pontage de l'artere femoral profonde, la voi sus-
medio-crurale. *J Chir.* 1975;110:45.

235. Saletta JD, Freeark RJ. Injuries to the profunda femoris artery. *J Trauma.* 1972;12:778.

236. Weimann S, San Nicolo M, Sandbichler P, et al. Civilian popliteal artery trauma. *J Cardiovasc Surg.* 1987;28:145.

237. Snyder WH. Vascular injuries near the knee: an updated series and overview of the problem. *Surgery.* 1982;91:502.

238. Shah DM, Naraynsingh V, Leather RP. Advances in the management of acute popliteal vascular injuries. *J Trauma.* 1985;25:793.

239. Lim LL, Michuda MS, Flanigan DP, et al. Popliteal artery trauma: 31 cases without amputation. *Arch Surg.* 1980;115:1307.

240. Padberg FT, Rubelowsky JJ, Hernandez-Maldonado JJ, et al. Infrapopliteal artery injury: prompt revascularization affords optimal limb salvage. *J Vasc Surg.* 1992;16:877.

241. Hoover NH. Injuries of the popliteal artery associated with fractures and dislocations. *Surg Clin North Am.* 1961;41:1099.

242. Kennedy JC. Complete dislocation of the knee joint. *J Bone Joint Surg Am.* 1969;45:889.

243. Jones RE, Smith EC, Bone GE. Vascular and orthopedic complications of knee dislocation. *Surg Gynecol Obstet.* 1979;149:554.

244. Green NE, Allen BL. Vascular injuries associated with dislocation of the knee. *J Bone Joint Surg.* 1977;59A:236.

245. Miller HH, Welch CS. Quantitative studies on the time factor in arterial injuries. *Ann Surg.* 1949;130:428.

246. Rich NM, Collins GJ, Andersen CA, et al. Autogenous venous interposition grafts in repair of major venous injuries. *J Trauma.* 1977;17:512.

247. Kelly G, Eiseman B. Civilian vascular injuries. *J Trauma.* 1975;15:507.

248. Perry MO, Thal ER, Shires GT. Management of arterial injuries. *Ann Surg.* 1971;173:403.

249. Keeley SB, Snyder WH, Weigelt JA. Arterial injuries below the knee: fifty-one patients with 82 injuries. *J Trauma.* 1983;23:285.

250. Ramadan F, Rutledge R, Oller D, et al. Carotid artery trauma: a review of contemporary trauma center experiences. *J Vasc Surg.* 1995;21:46.

251. David JW, Halbroch TL, Hoyt DB, et al. Blunt carotid artery dissection: Incidence, associated injuries, screening, and treatment. *J Trauma.* 1990;30:1514.

252. Perry MO, Snyder WH, Thal ER. Carotid artery injuries caused by blunt trauma. *Ann Surg.* 1980;192:74.

253. Bradley EL. Management of penetrating carotid injuries: an alternative approach. *J Trauma.* 1973;13:248.

254. Abad C, Diluch A, Espino J. Isolated blunt trauma of the common carotid artery. *J Cardiovasc Surg.* 1993;34:507.

255. Thal ER, Snyder WH, Hays RJ, et al. Management of carotid artery injuries. *Surgery.* 1974;76:955.

256. Jernigan WR, Gardner WC. Carotid artery injuries due to closed cervical trauma. *J Trauma.* 1971;11:429.

257. Rivers SP, Patel Y, Delany HM, et al. Limited role of arteriography in penetrating neck trauma. *J Vasc Surg.* 1988;8:112.

258. Frykberg ER, Vines FS, Alexander RH. The natural history of clinically occult arterial injuries: a prospective evaluation. *J Trauma.* 1989;29:577.

259. Yamada S, Kindt GW, Youmans JR. Carotid injuries due to nonpenetrating injury. *J Trauma.* 1967;7:333.

260. Scalfani SJA, Cavaliere G, Atweh N, et al. The role of angiography in penetrating neck trauma. *J Trauma.* 1986;31:557.

261. Weigelt JA, Thal ER, Snyder WH, et al. Diagnosis of penetrating cervical esophageal injuries. *Am J Surg.* 1987;154:619.

262. Fry WR, Dort JA, Smith RS, et al. Duplex scanning replaces arteriography and operative exploration in the diagnosis of potential cervical vascular injury. *Am J Surg.* 1994;168:693.

263. Monson DU, Saletta JD, Freeark RJ. Carotid vertebral trauma. *J Trauma.* 1969;9:987.

264. Roon AJ, Christensen N. Evaluation and treatment of penetrating carotid injuries. *J Trauma.* 1979;19:391.

265. Perry MO. Injuries of the brachiocephalic vessels. In: Rutherford RB, ed. *Vascular Surgery.* Philadelphia, Pa: WB Saunders; 1995:705–713.

266. Unger SW, Tucker WS, Mudeza MA, et al. Carotid arterial trauma. *Surgery.* 1980;87:477.

267. Rich N, Spencer FC. Carotid and vertebral injuries. In: Rich N, Spencer FC, eds. *Vascular Trauma.* Philadelphia, Pa: WB Saunders; 1978.

268. Wylie EJ, Hein MF, Adams JE. Intracranial hemorrhage following surgical revascularization for treatment of acute strokes. *J Neurosurg.* 1964;21:212.

269. Cohen CA, Brief D, Mathewson CJ. Carotid artery injuries: an analysis of eighty-five cases. *Am J Surg.* 1970;120:210.

270. Ledgerwood AM, Mullins RJ, Lucas CE. Primary repair versus ligation for carotid artery injuries. *Arch Surg.* 1980;115:488.

271. Weaver FA, Yellin AE, Wagner WH. The role of arterial reconstruction in penetrating carotid injuries. *Arch Surg.* 1988;123:1106.

272. Brown MF, Graham JM, Feliciano DV, et al. Carotid artery injuries. *Am J Surg.* 1982;144:748.

273. Fabian TC, George SM, Croce MA. Carotid artery trauma: management based on mechanism of injury. *J Trauma.* 1990;30:953.

274. Karlin RM, Marks C. Extracranial carotid artery injury: current surgical management. *Am J Surg.* 1983;146:225.

275. Ehrenfeld WK, Stoney RJ, Wylie EJ. Relation of carotid stump pressure to safety of carotid artery ligation. *Surgery.* 1983;93:299.

276. Schwarts JA, Turner D, Sheldon GF, et al. Penetrating trauma of the internal carotid artery at the base of the skull. *J Cardiovasc Surg (Torino).* 1987;28:542.

277. Gewertz B, Samson D, Ditmore QM, et al. Management of penetrating injuries of the internal carotid artery at the base of the skull utilizing extracranial-intracranial bypass. *J Trauma.* 1980;20:365.

278. Meier DE, Brink BE, Fry WJ. Vertebral artery trauma. *Arch Surg.* 1981;116:236.

Section 7
Aortoiliac Occlusive Disease

60

Aortoiliac Occlusive Disease

Erich Minar, Herbert Ehringer, and Peter Polterauer

Epidemiologic and Angiographic Data

Available data on the incidence of atherosclerosis of the lower limbs differ, depending on whether purely clinical observations were made or whether they were combined with noninvasive laboratory data. Using noninvasive tests, 11.7% of a population with a mean age of 66 years was found to have large-vessel occlusive disease, but less than one fifth of them experienced symptoms.[1] McDaniel and Cronenwett[2] conducted an extensive review of the literature and concluded that intermittent claudication was caused by aortoiliac occlusive disease in 53% of the patients younger than 40 years, whereas femoropopliteal disease usually was responsible for claudication in older patients. Aortoiliac disease seems to appear about 10 years earlier than femoropopliteal disease when the conditions are relatively isolated. In a report of 440 consecutive peripheral arteriograms—performed for vascular disease—femoropopliteal disease was three to five times more frequent than iliac disease.[3] Among patients with iliac disease, stenoses were three times more frequent than occlusions—a distribution that was reversed in the femoropopliteal region. The majority of lesions were short, 80% of iliac stenoses being 5 cm or less.[3] In a series of more than 900 patients investigated with angiography, Münster et al.[4] observed isolated obstructions of the iliac arteries in about 10%.

In 15% to 20% of patients with aortoiliac disease, the stenotic plaques are limited to the aortic bifurcation and the proximal portion of the common iliac artery. In 25% to 30% the atherosclerotic process extends downward to involve the external iliac artery, often with total occlusion of the internal iliac artery as well. In about 60% the aortoiliac disease extends down to involve the femoropopliteal segment. Stenosis or occlusion of the common iliac artery is found more often than stenosis or occlusion of the external iliac artery.[5] Progression of moderate stenosis to occlusion can be observed in 10% to 15% of patients within 5 years.[6]

Although atherosclerotic disease of the infrarenal aorta is very common, complete obstruction is rare and is usually in a severely atherosclerotic distal aorta. Occlusion of the distal aorta was first described by Leriche in 1923, and autopsy series reported a prevalence of about 0.15%.[7]

Etiology and Pathophysiology

Current theories of atherogenesis take into account such different factors as hemodynamic forces, endothelial damage, platelet function, thrombosis, migration and proliferation of smooth muscle cells, cholesterol levels, lipoprotein infiltration and modification, development of lipid-containing macrophage-derived foam cells, senescence, and inflammation. It seems likely that all these factors can promote the development of atherosclerosis and that it is a combination of these factors that may determine the extent and severity of plaque development and clinical sequelae.

Recent research revealed the cellular nature of atherosclerotic lesions and an active inflammatory component in the disease.[8] Oxygen radicals play an important role by leading to lipid peroxidation, and there is increasing evidence that oxidative modification of low-density lipoprotein (LDL) plays an important role in atherogenesis. The modification of LDL may lead to its unregulated uptake by macrophages through a scavenger receptor, and the macrophages may play a protective role against the cytotoxic effects of oxidized LDL. Oxidized LDL is a powerful chemoattractant for circulating human monocytes.[9] The monocyte has been accepted as the source of the lipid-laden macrophages. Monocytes and macrophages also produce chemotactic and growth factors for vascular smooth muscle cells.

A new feature emerging from analysis of the structure and cell composition of human atherosclerotic plaques is the involvement of the immune system in these lesions. Oxidized LDL is strongly immunogenic, and immune complexes taken up by macrophages are a putative factor possibly involved in atherogenesis. Plaque macrophages and T cells have been shown to produce specific cytokines that—by influencing cell proliferation and lipid accumulation—seem to be important for lesion progression. Furthermore, the expression of activation-dependent adhesion molecules is also likely to be important in the progression of atherosclerotic inflammation. In a review of the histology of atherosclerotic aortas and arteries, 92% showed some degree of adventitial inflammation.[8] Subclinical chronic periarteritis and periaortitis are common histological findings, and chronic periaortitis is thought to be a local complication of advanced atherosclerosis caused by an autoallergen such as oxidized LDL.

In the normal adult aorta, the media represents about 60% to 70% of the total aortic wall thickness, and the intima and adventitia represent about 15% and 20%, respectively. In patients with chronic periaortitis, histology reveals an intimal thickening similar to that in normal aortas but marked reduction of media and profound thickening of adventitia to about 10 mm.

The smooth muscle cell is the principle cell type in the media and also in intimal proliferation. The intimal smooth muscle cells proliferate in response to injury of many types and are considered responsible for the production of the extracellular matrix. Matrix proteins—such as elastin, collagen, and proteoglycans—play a vital role in maintaining the structural integrity of normal blood vessels, and there are quantitative and qualitative compositional alterations in atherosclerosis.[10] The major role of the interstitial collagens is to provide mechanical support to counter the forces exerted by blood under constant pressure. In the infrarenal aorta, collagen types I and III comprise the majority (>90%) of the six different collagens that have been identified in the vessel wall.[11]

Atherosclerosis is a systemic disease in which plaques develop primarily at branches in the arteries and in areas where the blood flow is slow and turbulent. Specific hemodynamic factors may be critical in atherosclerotic plaque localization in the aorta. Mechanical stresses associated with blood flow and pressure have been linked to the pathogenesis of atherosclerosis.[12] The artery wall is normally exposed to two major mechanical forces: (1) wall shear stress acting principally at the blood–endothelium interface and related directly to the flow velocity profile and (2) tensile stress acting across the vessel wall and related directly to pressure and radius. Regional differences in aortic atherosclerosis may be attributable to local flow pattern specific to each aortic segment.[13] In the aortoiliac region, flow is characteristi-

cally triphasic, with reversal of flow and shear stress direction in late systole. Elevated shear rates tend to protect against plaque formation. Concerning the carotid artery, at the flow divider where wall shear stress is highest the vessel tends to be spared. An analogous geometric situation prevails at the distal aortic bifurcation, where lateral locations—opposite the central flow divider at the origin of the common iliac arteries—are preferential sites of plaque formation and are regions of low wall shear stress. Evidence has demonstrated that regions of relatively low wall shear stress and oscillations in shear stress direction are also regions of increased endothelial permeability.[14] Furthermore, low flow velocity and reduced wall shear stress and oscillations in flow direction are also associated with increased near-wall particle residence time, thus resulting in prolonged exposure of the arterial wall to atherogenic particles, such as lipoproteins, and to cellular blood elements. All of these factors could be associated with plaque formation. In contrast, inhibition of plaque formation by high velocity and wall shear stress has been demonstrated.[15]

The possible complications of a plaque include plaque ulceration (Figure 60.1) or disruption, plaque hemor-

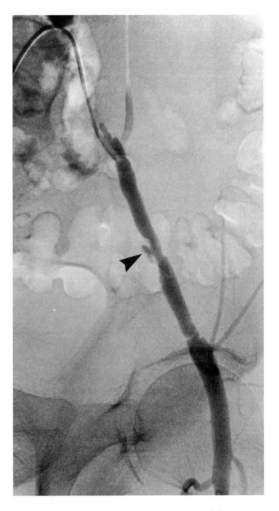

FIGURE 60.1. Ulcerated plaque in the external iliac artery.

rhage, and thrombus formation. Thrombosis is the usual link between an atherosclerotic plaque and the occurrence of clinical manifestations.

As in any organ, blood flow to the lower limbs depends on perfusion pressure and is inversely related to the resistance to flow. Under normal conditions the resistance to flow depends primarily on the degree of vasoconstriction in the microcirculation—the vascular tone—and on the characteristics of the blood itself. Studies in humans and experimental animals indicate that about 90% of the cross-sectional area of the aorta has to be encroached before distal pressure and flow are affected, whereas in smaller arteries such as iliac and femoral arteries the critical stenosis varies from 70% to 90%.[16,17] A reduction of the lumen cross-sectional area by 75% corresponds to a diameter reduction of 50%.

Resting blood flow may be normal as a result of compensatory decrease in peripheral vascular resistance. With advanced peripheral occlusive disease, the resting blood flow may be diminished despite maximal reduction in peripheral vascular resistance. The stress of exercise results in a fall in pressure due to peripheral vasodilation and limited inflow if there is significant arterial disease. The pressure drop across a given stenosis is proportional to the flow across the narrowing, which explains why relatively insignificant stenosis at rest may be associated with significant pressure gradients—and thus symptoms—with exercise. However, a few patients have disease of the arteries of supply (e.g., the internal iliac or deep femoral artery) but not of the arteries of conduction. These patients may have false-negative exercise tests.

Risk Factors

Research studies to date have found that although the risk factors for atherosclerosis are similar in all vascular beds, the dominant risk factor seems to vary by anatomical location. Several epidemiologic studies on the risk factors of vascular disease were initiated, but only a few have dealt with the specific risk factors for lower limb arterial disease. Analysis of the specific risk factors for aortoiliac disease is even more difficult because most of the large epidemiological studies have not assessed the location of lower limb involvement. The diagnosis of peripheral arterial occlusive disease in many epidemiological studies was made according to symptoms of intermittent claudication as determined by a standard questionnaire. However, the sensitivity of such questionnaires, particularly for larger vessels such as the aorta and iliac vessels, is low.[18]

Despite the difficulties of analysis because of the small number of studies available, it has been known for some time that patients—irrespective of their sex—with chronic aortoiliac disease due to atherosclerosis most often present with a typical risk profile that includes young age, smoking, hypercholesterolemia, and rarely diabetes.[19] Friedman et al.[20] compared in a prospective arteriographic study the risk factors in 43 patients with Leriche's syndrome and 66 patients with femoropopliteal obstruction. Patients with aortoiliac involvement were significantly younger (49 versus 61 years), more often had increased serum cholesterol levels (49% versus 23%), and less often had diabetes (9% versus 36%). A study by Stubbs[21] revealed similar data.

Smoking

Epidemiological studies point to cigarette smoking as the single most powerful risk factor for peripheral vascular disease.[22] Several clinical studies have confirmed the deleterious effects of tobacco on the peripheral arterial circulation.[23] Cigarette smoking is known to provoke morphological and functional changes in the endothelial cells and to have a negative influence on blood viscosity and lipid profile. Willems and Plair[24] reported in 1962—based on an autopsy study of 989 aortas—that atherosclerosis was found more often in the aortas, but not in the carotid, renal, or lower limb arteries, of smokers compared with nonsmokers. It was also demonstrated that the severity of atherosclerosis of the aorta was significantly more pronounced in smokers and that it increased proportionally with the intensity and duration of tobacco use.[25] Only one epidemiological study has focused on the relationship between tobacco and the site of atheroma.[26] The relative risk for developing aortoiliac atherosclerosis differed according to the degree of tobacco consumption. For patients who smoked one pack of cigarettes or more per day, the relative risk of developing aortoiliac atheroma was three to five times greater compared with the risk of developing distal lesions. A strong correlation was found between the number of cigarettes smoked daily and the intensity of aortoiliac lesions as seen on arteriographic studies.[27] Women with a history of smoking are particularly susceptible to aortoiliac disease.[28]

Postoperative results are improved significantly in patients who stop smoking.[29] The risk of occlusion of aortofemoral bypasses at 3- to 5-year follow-up is two to three times as high if patients continue to smoke.[30] Once arterial disease is present, continuation of smoking generally worsens the vascular prognosis. The risk of amputation has been found to be greater in smokers, occurs at a younger age, and is performed at a higher level on the limb.[29]

Dyslipidemia

At the aortoiliac level, hypercholesterolemia ranks immediately after tobacco consumption as a risk factor for atherosclerosis. Patients with familial hypercholesterolemia have a high tendency for atheroma in the aortoiliac vessels.[31] Lesions due to atheroma can partially reverse after correction of hypercholesterolemia. Hypertriglyceridemia presently is not considered an independent risk factor. However, it can promote the development of arterial thrombosis.

Diabetes

Subjects with diabetes exhibit severe atherosclerotic changes. Diabetes is frequently associated with leg arterial disease, and several mechanisms are proposed as possible links between diabetes and atherosclerotic lesions. During the course of diabetes, arterial lesions are predominant at the infrapopliteal level, whereas the aortoiliac location seems to be spared.[32]

Hypertension

An association between hypertension and leg arterial disease has been identified in several epidemiological and case-control studies. Data given by Vogt et al.[28] indicate that elevated systolic blood pressure is an independent correlate of disease in the aortoiliac and femoropopliteal segments.

Hyperhomocysteinemia

Hyperhomocysteinemia, a disorder in the metabolism of methionine induced by a congenital enzymatic deficit, has recently been reported to be an independent vascular risk factor. This factor also seems to promote aortoiliac lesions. Patients with hyperhomocysteinemia presented with aortoiliac involvement more often than those without this metabolic disorder.[33]

Hormones

Peripheral arterial occlusive disease in women may be related to premature menopause, which eliminates a protective estrogen effect. Weiss et al.[34] observed twice the expected frequency of premature menopause in women with aortoiliac disease. When matched for tobacco abuse, women with isolated aortoiliac involvement had premature menopause significantly more often. Others[35] reported a high percentage of oral contraceptive use by young women with aortoiliac disease.

Aortoiliac Hypoplastic Syndrome

The association of small aortas with early onset of aortoiliac occlusive disease has been described in women and men.[36,37] Several authors have attempted to characterize a particular anatomical shape of the aortic bifurcation that might promote aortoiliac atherosclerosis in women. This syndrome has been called female aortoiliac hypoplastic syndrome. The criteria for definition— according to Jernigan et al.[38]—are the following: a high bifurcation of the abdominal aorta, a straight course of the iliac arteries, an acute angle of the aortic bifurcation (about 20 to 30 degrees), an infrarenal aortic diameter of ≤14 mm, and an iliac artery diameter of ≤7 mm. (The normal infrarenal aortic diameter is about 19 mm in men and 17 mm in women.) Addiction to smoking in these patients who develop aortoiliac occlusive disease is paralleled only by that seen in patients with Buerger's disease.

Collateral Circulation

Stenotic processes of the abdominal aorta and iliac arteries usually occur slowly enough so that satisfactory collateral circulation develops, and some affected patients are almost asymptomatic. However, despite the development of prominent collateral blood vessels, the resistance of the collateral circuits is always greater than that of the original unobstructed artery. Plethysmographic measurements of reactive hyperemia at the calf after transitory circulatory arrest by tourniquet have demonstrated that the possibilities for compensation of a chronic occlusion decrease in the following order: common iliac artery—external iliac artery—superficial femoral artery (SFA)—popliteal artery—common femoral artery.[39] However, despite this higher reactive hyperemia, patients with chronic aortoiliac obstructions often have a lower pain-free walking capacity than patients with SFA occlusion.[40] This lower pain-free walking capacity can be explained by the greater muscle mass that has to be supplied by the collateral arteries in these patients compared to patients with SFA occlusion. The absolute transport capacity of the collateral vessels is higher in the aortoiliac than in the femoral group, but the relative capacity is not higher compared with the poststenotic tissue mass.

The clinical picture of patients with occlusive disease depends mainly on the possibilities of collateral circulation. The anatomical situation allows different collateral pathways for compensation of aortoiliac occlusive disease. These pathways can be divided into the following groups:

1. Epigastric system: subclavian artery—internal thoracic artery—superior epigastric artery—inferior epigastric artery—external iliac artery (so-called Winslow pathway)
2. Lumbar system: lumbar arteries—circumflex iliac artery—external iliac artery; or lumbar arteries—iliolumbar artery—internal iliac artery—external iliac artery

3. Mesenteric system (see Figure 60.2): superior mesenteric artery—middle colic artery—left colic artery—inferior mesenteric artery (so-called Riolan anastomosis); or inferior mesenteric artery—superior rectal artery—inferior rectal artery—inferior pudendal artery—internal iliac artery

4. Iliofemoral system (see Figure 60.3): deep femoral artery—medial circumflex femoral artery—obturator artery—superior gluteal artery—inferior gluteal artery—internal iliac artery

In patients with aortic obstruction distal to the inferior mesenteric artery, this artery serves as one of the main collateral arteries. The same collateral pathway develops in patients with occlusion of the left common iliac artery, whereas in right-sided occlusions other collateral arteries are of greater functional importance. Although the collateral pathway over the inferior mesenteric artery can often be demonstrated by angiography, the clinical picture of the so-called mesenteric steal syndrome is observed very rarely. This syndrome is characterized by abdominal pain induced by exercise (walking) and is caused by increased blood supply to the legs with concomitant critical reduction of blood supply to intestinal vessels of the inferior mesenteric artery. However, the possibilities for collateral compensation by other visceral arteries are responsible for the rareness of this clinical picture.

The collateral circulation from the subclavian artery via the internal thoracic artery to the external iliac

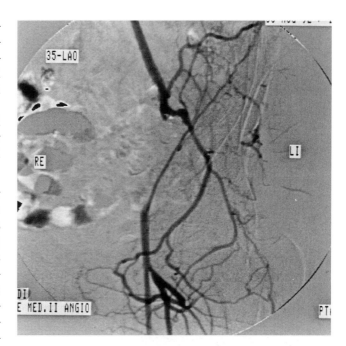

FIGURE 60.3. Digital subtraction angiogram demonstrating occlusion of the left external iliac artery and collateral circulation between the internal iliac and deep femoral arteries (iliofemoral system).

artery is often unrecognized. Patients with lower extremity vascular disease may suffer exacerbation of their symptoms if this collateral pathway is divided by abdominal incision. Furthermore, before using the internal thoracic artery for coronary bypass surgery, function of this vessel as a collateral to the lower extremities should be excluded.[41]

Isolated obstructions at the origin of the internal iliac artery do not limit blood inflow into the affected extremity. However, the internal iliac arteries act as a valuable source of collateral blood inflow into the lower extremities in patients with obstruction of the aortoiliac segment. In these patients internal iliac obstruction severely limits blood flow into the affected lower extremities.

Atheroembolism

Atheromatous disease affecting the arteries that supply the lower limbs usually causes failure of circulation due to stenosis and subsequent occlusion. However, such plaques may also cause recurrent emboli. The embolization of cholesterol-rich atheromatous debris in terminal arteries can produce livedo reticularis or local digital ischemia, the so-called blue toe syndrome (Figure 60.4). Blue toe syndrome may be associated with abdominal pain (by visceral ischemia) or renal atheroembolism that leads to decreased renal function and hypertension.

Although most arterial emboli originate from the heart, atheroemboli usually originate from an athero-

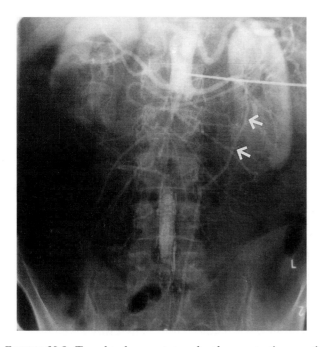

FIGURE 60.2. Translumbar aortography demonstrating aortic occlusion beginning just distal to the renal arteries. The main collateral pathway is the Riolan anastomosis (arrows). (A myelography had been done a few months before because of misinterpretation of the patient's symptoms.)

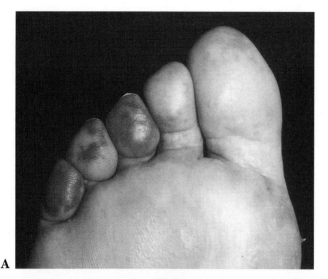

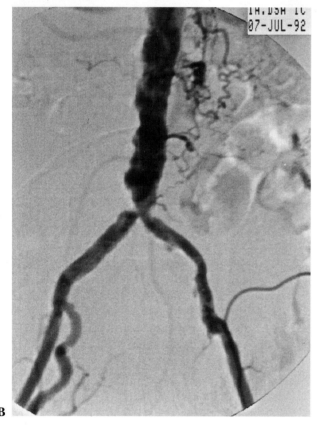

FIGURE 60.4. **A,** Blue toe syndrome: ischemia of the toes—the third toe is most severely affected—caused by distal embolization of thrombotic or atheromatous material. **B,** Digital subtraction angiography of the abdominal aorta and iliac arteries of this patient presenting with blue toe syndrome: severe, diffuse atherosclerotic changes of the abdominal aorta and bifurcation are the probable origin of the distal embolization.

sclerotic aorta or iliac artery.[42] Gagliardi et al.[43] reported that mural thrombi of the aorta were responsible for 5% of peripheral arterial emboli, and such thrombi ac-

counted for 3.8% of nonaneurysmal aortoiliac lesions operated on during a 9-year period in their series.

Multiple mural thrombi are frequent, and the ulcers often have undermined edges that probably account for recurrent embolic phenomena. Thick mural thrombi overlying zones of ulceration usually exhibit little organization. The frequency of ulceration and mural thrombosis in the abdominal aorta observed at autopsy suggests that emboli of thrombotic and atheromatous debris usually cause little disturbance clinically due to rapid clearance and sufficient collateral circulation. The incidence of atheroembolism in postmortem studies was reported to be between 0.8% and 4%, mostly in combination with severe atherosclerosis of the aorta.[44]

Biplanar aortoiliac arteriography with runoff views is the preferred method to detect areas of arterial irregularity as possible sources of such atheroembolism. No controlled trials have been undertaken to compare the efficacy of oral anticoagulant agents with antiplatelet therapy for prophylaxis in this situation.

Diagnosis

History

The main objective of the medical history in patients with cardiovascular diseases is to provide a comprehensive cardiovascular profile of an individual patient based on presenting symptoms, history of present illness, cardiovascular risk status, and prior cardiovascular diseases. Exact assessment of the vascular history concerning angina pectoris, myocardial infarction, transitory ischemic attack or stroke, claudication, and risk factors is necessary.

In the assessment of claudication, three factors must be defined because they are important for the further management of these patients: (1) the degree of disablement, (2) the progression of the disease with deterioration of symptoms, and (3) the duration of symptoms (e.g., in patients with a short history of a few weeks of claudication thrombolytic treatment may be helpful because the occlusive material will have little organization; the symptoms may improve because the collateral circulation has not had time to develop).

Chronic aortoiliac obstruction generally develops in the setting of progressive atherosclerotic occlusive disease. This process develops slowly enough that extensive collateral supply to the pelvis and lower extremities can develop. When complete occlusion finally occurs, the blood supply changes little. Therefore, patients with chronic aortoiliac occlusion regularly present with claudication and not with acute ischemic symptoms.

The patient with claudication characteristically complains of muscle cramping after a well-defined distance of walking, although the muscle discomfort may be variously described as fatigue, weakness, or numbness of the extremity. The patient with aortoiliac occlusive disease complains of pain in the thigh and buttock, sometimes spreading down into the calf muscles and occasionally up into the lower back. However, a history of buttock or hip claudication is not sufficiently reliable as an indicator of significant iliac disease because it was demonstrated that as many as 67% of patients with objective evidence of inflow disease had only calf claudication.[45] The patient who complains of symmetrical thigh and buttock pain—often associated with erectile impotence due to internal iliac insufficiency—is usually found to have an occlusion of the infrarenal aorta and/or aortic bifurcation (Leriche's syndrome). However, these patients may also report weakness and heaviness of the limbs rather than actual localized pains. The distance walked until appearance of claudication pain may vary depending on the patient's speed, the type of terrain, and the presence or absence of an incline. The typical exertional muscular pain of the patient with intermittent claudication disappears rapidly after effort ceases.

The symptoms of claudication are typical but may be mimicked as pain due to neurospinal or musculoskeletal conditions such as sciatic nerve entrapment, spinal canal stenosis, lumbar disk protrusion, or arthrosis of the hip or knee. The relation of the pain to the exercise and the time for recovery after exercise are helpful in the differential diagnosis. However, it may be clinically difficult to assess the relative contributions of two conditions to the patient's disability.

Sometimes patients with objectively documented arterial occlusive disease do not suffer from claudication. Lack of claudication may result from either a sedentary lifestyle without sufficient movement or limited tolerance because of other diseases.

Clinical Examination

The clinical examination of patients with peripheral arterial occlusive disease includes inspection of feet, palpation of pulse, and auscultation of vessels. Even in an era of advanced technology the physical examination remains the principle means of assessing patients with vascular disease. It provides confirmation not only of the presence but also of the location and severity of the occlusive disease. Clinical evaluation by an experienced examiner seems to be nearly equal to a noninvasive vascular laboratory evaluation in the diagnosis and judgment of the severity of peripheral vascular disease.[46] However, for aortoiliac disease—especially when multisegment disease is present—the clinical assessment can sometimes be difficult. The sensitivity of the physical examination to detect an arterial lesion in the aortoiliac segment depends on the thoroughness of the procedure (e.g.,

whether auscultation is carried out before and after exercise).

Bilateral palpation of the femoral pulse is necessary to assess the quality of the femoral pulse and to feel for a thrill. A palpable thrill suggests a severe stenosis (or an arteriovenous fistula). The critical clinical sign in the examination of the aortoiliac segment is the strength of the femoral pulse. The value of this sign has been tested against intra-arterial pressure measurements with conflicting results.[47,48] It is thus difficult to make therapeutic decisions based on this physical sign alone. In patients with absent groin pulses, one can find iliac or common femoral occlusions. If the femoral pulse is impalpable, the examiner should feel the pulse above the inguinal ligament in case the external iliac artery is patent. Occasionally patients with iliac occlusion have enough collateral circulation for a groin pulse to be felt with the patient at rest. Because multiple pathology is common in the elderly, absent or reduced pulses are not definite signs that arterial insufficiency is responsible for the patient's symptoms.

If symptoms suggest claudication and the physician finds normal peripheral pulses, claudication may be caused by proximal stenosis. Auscultation of the arteries from the navel to the groin at rest and after exercise is most useful in diagnosing aortoiliac stenosis. The differentiation of stenosis from occlusion is based mainly on the presence or absence of a vascular bruit. However, sometimes a bruit is due to collateral flow. A bruit immediately below the umbilicus on one side or the other suggests common iliac artery stenosis. If the bruit is maximal just above the inguinal ligament, stenosis of the external iliac artery can be suspected. However, a bruit only indicates turbulent flow but does not necessarily indicate a significant stenosis. For an experienced examiner, the characteristics of such a bruit are very helpful for judging the severity of a stenosis. Compared with functional bruits, pathological bruits are longer and may extend into the diastole. The intensity and duration of a bruit is markedly increased after exercise of the extremity, and the presence of a stenotic lesion might be unmasked only by auscultation after exercise. The increased flow following exercise results in increased turbulence and often an audible bruit by increasing velocity through and distal to the stenosis. Auscultation after exercise is thus very helpful in detecting and localizing milder stenotic lesions. An exercise test also reveals which patients are more limited by dyspnea or angina pectoris than by claudication on exercise.

Examination of the capillary and venous filling time are valuable tests for evaluation of the severity of peripheral arterial occlusive disease. However, when the atherosclerotic process is confined to the aortoiliac segment, these tests are often within normal limits.

Laboratory Tests

In most patients the diagnosis of aortoiliac disease can be made confidently on clinical grounds from a history of the site of claudication pain and a clearly reduced femoral pulse volume. However, quantitative objective documentation of arterial obstruction and its severity requires further tests in a vascular laboratory.

An estimated 65% of patients who require lower extremity revascularization have multilevel arterial occlusive disease.[49] In patients with combined inflow (aortoiliac) and outflow arterial disease it is most important to evaluate the hemodynamic effect of each lesion. Because the general surgical principle is to repair the proximal lesion first, it is necessary to determine whether the proximal lesion is severe enough to have a clinical impact. Unrecognized aortoiliac disease might cause failure of a femoropopliteal bypass graft.[50] Furthermore, it would be advantageous to decide in advance whether inflow revascularization will be sufficient to relieve the patient's symptoms or whether both inflow and outflow procedures will be required (individually or combined).[51] The goals of laboratory investigations are the following:

- To confirm objectively a clinically suspected arteriopathy
- To document the location of arterial lesions
- To localize and assess hemodynamically significant lesions
- To determine the severity of disease
- To contribute to etiological diagnosis
- To detect other arterial sites affected by atherosclerosis
- To monitor the natural history of the occlusive disease
- To confirm success or failure of a therapeutic intervention

Segmental Pressure Measurements

Segmental pressure measurements are a commonly used simple quantitative method for diagnosing and localizing arterial occlusive disease by noninvasive measurement of leg pressures with a sphygmomanometer and a Doppler velocity detector. The Doppler probe is placed over an ankle artery. The great advantage of Doppler-derived segmental pressure measurement is that it is easy to perform and the equipment is simple and inexpensive.

To adjust for differences in systemic pressure, the ratio of the leg pressure to the higher brachial pressure as the reference standard is used to calculate the thigh– or ankle–brachial index. Although the ankle–brachial index provides a summation of the effects of obstruction at all levels, the segmental pressures of the thigh, calf, and ankle are measured to locate the levels of significant disease. This multisegmental pressure profile is of particular value in patients with diffuse occlusive disease. Pressure gradients between adjacent cuffs or differences between the pressures in the two limbs at corresponding sites indicate the presence of occlusive disease in this segment. A gradient of 30 mm Hg between adjacent segments is considered abnormal. The optimal cuff size for recording blood pressure is essential, because the measurements are more accurate when the width of the cuff is about 20% greater than the diameter of the limb.

An obstructive lesion in the aortoiliac segment should result in a decreased pressure in the thigh. One technique for segmental pressure measurement uses a wide cuff (18 cm) for the thigh rather than the usual arm cuff (10–12 cm). A wide cuff permits only a single measure above the knee but theoretically provides a more accurate measurement of the absolute high thigh pressure, whereas narrower cuffs result in some artifactual elevation of measured pressure. Most laboratories consider the narrow cuff to overestimate pressure by about 30 mm Hg, but Heintz et al.[52] found a mean difference in thigh pressure of 55 mm Hg between measurements with the two types of cuffs. Despite the theoretical disadvantages, most laboratories use a four-cuff technique with proximal and distal narrow thigh cuffs to also obtain information regarding the presence of proximal or middle SFA disease.

Flanigan et al.,[53] who compared high thigh pressures obtained with both wide and narrow cuffs to intra-arterial pressure of the common femoral artery, reported poor accuracy for both the wide and narrow cuffs. Lynch et al.[54] reported a sensitivity for detection of significant aortoiliac disease of 97% but a low specificity of only 50%. They considered the presence of a hemodynamically significant lesion when the high thigh pressure was less than 30 mm Hg greater than the highest brachial pressure. Francfort et al.[55] reported that in the absence of SFA disease, sensitivity of segmental pressure measurements was 96% to detect significant aortoiliac disease, and they found no difference using the three- or four-cuff technique. However, in the presence of SFA disease, the four-cuff technique was significantly more sensitive (100%) and more specific (76%) than the three-cuff technique. The major disadvantage of this method of pressure measurement with cuffs in the thigh is that significant infrainguinal occlusive disease may produce false-positive results for aortoiliac occlusive disease. Therefore a normal high thigh pressure seems generally reliable in ruling out hemodynamically significant aortoiliac occlusive disease, whereas an abnormal pressure does not differentiate definitively between aortoiliac and SFA disease. Concerning the previously mentioned problems, some authors concluded, however, that the accuracy of the diagnosis of aortoiliac disease by thigh pressure measurement is unsatisfactory,[56,57] particularly in patients with SFA disease. Franzeck et al.[58] suggested that some of the errors of thigh pressure measurement may be related to the site at which Doppler signals are obtained. They recommend—especially in patients with multilevel disease—that any abnormal thigh pressures be confirmed by using the knee as a sensing site for the Doppler signals.

Some groups[59] have measured the common femoral artery pressure noninvasively with a flat pneumatic bladder that was held firmly in place by a clap. This bladder is used to compress the femoral artery against the pubic ramus and permits indirect pressure measurement at this level. The authors who used this method reported good results compared to the accuracy with thigh pressure measurements. However, this method is not in wide clinical use, and there are difficulties in obese patients and those with calcified arteries.

Some investigators have attempted to preoperatively calculate the anticipated hemodynamic response to lower extremity arterial reconstruction by use of segmental Doppler pressure measurements. Moneta[51] uses the following formula to predict the hemodynamic outcome of inflow reconstruction:

$$\text{Postoperative ankle–brachial index} =$$
$$1.1 \times \text{preoperative ankle–brachial index}/$$
$$\text{preoperative high thigh index.}$$

The value of the systolic ankle pressure is related to the degree of ischemia. Systolic ankle pressure is a very specific parameter, but sensitivity is suboptimal. Normally the systolic pressure in the ankle is 10 to 20 mm Hg higher than the systolic pressure in the brachial artery because of the reflected wave phenomenon. The ankle–brachial index is also useful for grading the degree of ischemia.

Intermittent claudication may be associated with normal pressures at rest if the arterial lesions are proximal. Therefore the sensitivity is greatly increased if pressure measurements are done after exercise or induced hyperemia.[60] A fall of pressure of 20% or more indicates the presence of significant arterial disease. The magnitude of the abnormal ankle pressure response to exercise is indicative of the severity of arterial occlusive disease. Furthermore, the time it takes to recover basal pressure after exercise (e.g., on a treadmill) allows an optimal functional assessment of arterial insufficiency. With a single lesion in the aortoiliac region, the recovery time may be between 5 and 15 minutes. Exercise tests are also useful for monitoring patients after vascular surgery, because significant residual or recurrent stenosis can be present even if the resting ankle pressure is normal.

Medial calcifications in some patients (such as diabetic or elderly patients) do not allow the measurement of systolic pressure because the arteries are incompressible. When the vessels are intensely calcified, cuff pressures as high as 300 mm Hg may fail to compress and occlude the arteries. The measurement of toe pressures by photoplethysmography has the advantage that incompressible vessels are seldom encountered in the toes.

Penile Blood Pressure

The measurement of penile blood pressure permits assessment of vasculogenic impotence. According to the ankle–brachial index, a penile–brachial pressure ratio can be used. A penile–brachial index of ≥ 0.8 is considered normal, and a value of < 0.6 is abnormal.[61]

Plethysmography

Plethysmography encompasses by definition all methods that record changes in limb volumes. Plethysmography permits recording of dimensional changes of digits or limb segments with each heartbeat or in response to temporary obstruction of venous return (occlusion plethysmography). Today mercury-in-rubber strain gauges are mostly used for recording such volume changes. The change in blood volume after transient circulatory arrest by a tourniquet against time represents the rate of blood flow. Such flow measurements by plethysmography are not required in routine clinical practice.

Pulse Volume Recording

The pulse volume recorder is a calibrated air plethysmograph that assesses the arterial circulation by measuring the expansion of a limb under a pneumatic cuff during the cardiac cycle. It uses arterial pulsatility as an index of vessel patency. Both the amplitude and configuration of the tracings—usually obtained from the thigh, calf, and ankle—are evaluated. These measurements are useful in evaluating the degree of arterial occlusive disease, estimating the collateral circulation, and localizing obstructive lesions.[62] Pulse volume recording is frequently used as a backup test when segmental pressures are impossible to measure because of noncompressible vessels. Because it is not necessary to occlude the arterial flow under the cuff as with pressure measurements, even stiff calcified arteries can be judged. However, pulse volume recording tracings from the thigh may suffer from the same limitations as thigh pressures taken with a wide cuff.

Some authors[63] have reported better results for detection of aortoiliac disease by combining pulse volume recording with pressure measurements. The combination of both achieved an overall accuracy of 97%.

Pulse volume recording is an adaptation of oscillography, which can provide the clinician with very useful information that is mainly of a qualitative order. The performance of the test is strongly augmented by recording oscillations after exercise such as knee bending or heel raising. Knee bending is the better exercise to detect iliac or proximal femoral artery disease. The time necessary for the oscillations to recover the normal amplitude is an indicator of the compensation.

Femoral Artery Flow Velocity Waveform Analysis

Characterization of the Doppler (continuous or pulsed wave) velocity waveform from the common femoral artery is widely used to detect aortoiliac occlusive disease. Interpretation of only the auditory signal is possible, but documentation should also be done in every patient. The simplest approach is based on visual interpretation of the overall shape of the curve. The normal flow velocity waveform pattern consists of a high systolic acceleration in combination with a negative velocity during early diastole and a low forward flow during late diastole (triphasic pattern), and the presence of proximal disease produces a series of qualitative changes in the shape of the femoral artery waveform (Figure 60.5).

Sometimes a signal has a relatively normal velocity waveform contour but still differs from the signal on the contralateral leg, indicating the possible presence of an obstructive lesion. Differences between Doppler spectra obtained from limbs with and without hemodynamically significant aortoiliac stenosis were more pronounced during reactive hyperemia than at rest.[64]

A dampened or absent reverse flow in early diastole—which refers to loss of the normal triphasic pattern—is highly suggestive of a flow-reducing proximal lesion. High accuracy using this simple technique was re-ported,[65] but Baker et al.[66] have observed a high false-positive rate with a specificity of only 62%. The finding of false-positive results, which can be due to technical errors in the position of the probe relative to the artery or scar tissue or hematoma between the probe and the vessel, is a major problem with this technique.

More objective quantitative methods have been studied to avoid the problem of false-positive results. Different parameters derived from the signal, such as pulsatility index, damping factor, transit time, pulse decay time, acceleration, and deceleration, that are capable of detecting significant aortoiliac disease have been developed. Except for the pulsatility index, none of these parameters is widely used. The determination of the pulsatility index (PI) is the simplest method of quantitative analysis. This index is defined as the ratio of the peak-to-peak velocity difference to the mean velocity over the cardiac cycle (Figure 60.6). It should be noted that the peak-to-peak PI is also independent of the probe-to-vessel angle. The normal PI for the common femoral artery is between 5.5 and 10. Johnston et al.[67] have found sensitivity and specificity of 95% in detecting significant inflow disease when using a value below 5.5 as abnormal. With advancing proximal stenosis, the systolic peak is blunted and the reverse component is lost, which results in a decrease in PI. With very severe stenosis, the

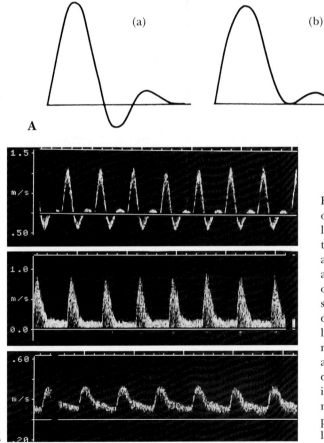

FIGURE 60.5. **A,** Schematic presentation of various shapes of common femoral artery flow velocity waveform: (a) normal with triphasic pattern (negative velocity during early diastole and low forward flow during late diastole); (b) absence of the reverse component (indicative of hemodynamically significant proximal stenosis); (c) strongly dampened waveform indicative of proximal obstruction with poor collateralization. **B,** Corresponding velocity recordings by pulsed Doppler with spectral analysis: (top) normal triphasic pattern; (middle) loss of reverse flow and spectral broadening according to turbulent flow; (bottom) monophasic curve with markedly depressed peak systolic velocity and increased diastolic velocity indicative of severe proximal obstruction.

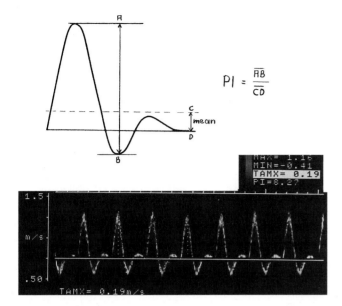

FIGURE 60.6. Schema demonstrating the calculation of the pulsatility index (PI). The PI calculated for the lower normal triphasic curve is 8.27.

PI drops to a range of 2 to 3. Flanigan et al.[68] found the PI to be closely related to the pressure gradient across the aortofemoral segment. The PI was also found to be sufficiently accurate for making decisions about the type of surgery to be performed.[68]

A problem with PI is that a number of patients' values fall into a gray zone (PI between 3 and 5.5). Furthermore, PI is not influenced only by inflow stenosis but also by advanced disease in the SFA. This leads to reduced specificity in patients with multisegmental disease. Thiele et al.[69] thus suggested that an additional method be used to assess the hemodynamic significance of proximal lesions in patients with SFA disease and a PI <4.0. Because the state of the peripheral circulation has a major effect on this measurement, in patients with rapid peripheral runoff the size of the reversed flow wave may be reduced, which falsely suggests the presence of aortoiliac disease.

Although the PI value cannot adequately identify different categories of severity of stenosis, for practical purposes this method can be used with sufficient reliability to determine whether a hemodynamically significant aortoiliac lesion is present. By combining Doppler flow velocity studies with multisegmental pressure measurements, Fronek et al.[70] were able to diagnose correctly 143 of 148 limbs with significant (≥50%) aortoiliac stenosis.

Duplex Sonography

Duplex scanning combines high-resolution B-mode ultrasound imaging with pulsed wave Doppler spectral analysis. The image is used primarily to locate the arter-

ies and is required for the detection of associated aneurysms and evaluation of the arterial wall. The estimate of degree of stenosis is based on the Doppler velocity data. Color flow duplex sonography combines real-time ultrasound imaging with semiquantitative color encoding of the Doppler information. The addition of color flow to modern duplex technology allows more rapid and accurate detection of stenotic areas by demonstrating an abnormal color flow pattern (Figure 60.7). A turbulent flow is characterized by a wide band of frequencies on the spectral analysis of the signal. It also enables the examiner to rapidly assess the areas of no flow that indicate total occlusion. However, flow information in a color Doppler image is only semiquantitative, and therefore accurate diagnosis and grading of stenosis depend on evaluation of the Doppler frequency spectrum and measurement of peak systolic velocity (Figure 60.8).

Duplex scanning is highly accurate compared with angiography in the detection of lesions that reduce vessel diameter by 50% or more. The most important diagnostic criterion for identifying such stenoses by duplex scanning is the percentage increase in peak systolic blood flow velocity (PSV) at the site of the lesion compared with the prestenotic or poststenotic PSV. A stenosis of >50% diameter reduction is indicated by the following criteria: (1) a doubling in PSV in the segment containing the lesion compared with the velocity in an adjacent normal segment, (2) a considerable widening of the spectral waveform (spectral broadening) in the presence of hemodynamically significant lesions where disturbed flow occurs around a stenosis, and (3) analysis of the femoral waveform that demonstrates a loss of reverse flow in early diastole distal to the lesion.

Many recent studies have demonstrated the reliability of duplex sonography for detection of significant lesions

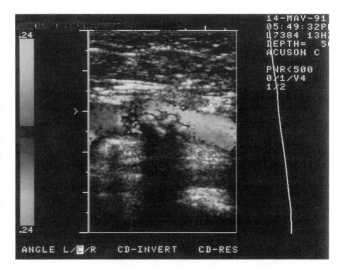

FIGURE 60.7. Color Doppler image of calcified plaque with significant stenosis as indicated by narrowing of the color band and change of the color Doppler signal, which indicates an increase in flow velocity.

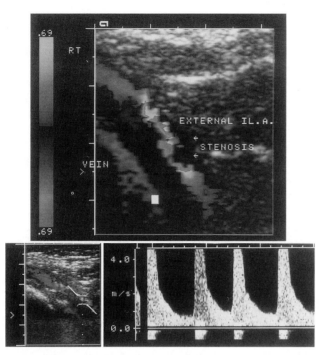

FIGURE 60.8. Color Doppler image of flow through an external iliac artery with severe stenosis. The Doppler spectral analysis (bottom) shows markedly increased peak systolic velocity (>4 m/s).

with generally excellent sensitivity and specificity in the iliac arteries as well.[71-74] Karacagil et al.[74] reported a sensitivity of 100%, a specificity of 85%, and a negative predictive value of 100% for detection of isolated aortoiliac disease. This high negative predictive value demonstrates the reliability of duplex imaging to virtually exclude significant occlusive disease. However, accuracy was lower in patients with multisegmental disease. Kohler et al.[71] observed a sensitivity of 89% and specificity of 90% in identification of >50% stenosis in the beginning of the duplex imaging era.

The percentage increase in PSV is directly related to the change in cross-sectional area of the vessel at the site of the stenosis and is independent of the total amount of flow. Therefore, some hemodynamically significant lesions cannot be detected by duplex scanning, because they become of hemodynamic importance only under conditions of increased flow. Legemate et al.[75] thus proposed the use of flow-related spectral analysis criteria such as the ΔPSV (= increase of PSV across the stenosis). They found a cutoff level for ΔPSV of 1.4 m/s to be best able to detect significant lesions in patients at rest.

There is also interest in the ability of duplex scanning to predict pressure gradients across an iliac artery stenosis, particularly when the stenosis is mild to moderate and therefore of uncertain hemodynamic significance. Some authors have used an adapted version of the

Bernoulli equation for calculation of the pressure gradient across stenoses from velocity parameters. The equation can be simplified to

$$\Delta P = 4 \ (Vmax^2),$$

where ΔP is the pressure drop across a stenosis and Vmax is the peak systolic velocity found by Doppler at the site of stenosis. To use this simplified equation, arteries should be straight, without significant side branches, and of large caliber so that flow is (at least theoretically) laminar; the lesions should be focal. Langsfeld et al.[72] reported that the duplex-derived pressure gradients calculated with this modified Bernoulli equation correlated well with the gradients measured during angiography ($r = 0.90$). Strauss et al.[76] reported that the correlation between intra-arterially measured iliac artery pressure gradients and those predicted by duplex scanning could be improved by focusing on mean rather than maximal pressure gradients (the correlation between mean duplex-determined gradients and nonsimultaneously obtained mean catheter gradients was 0.77). They found that the mean pressure gradients may allow more accurate determination by duplex scanning of mild to moderate iliac artery stenosis. Weber et al.[77] reported that Doppler gradients were usually higher than the manometer gradients. This finding may be explained by pressure recovery occurring in the relaminarized poststenotic region. Legemate et al.[75] observed that omission of the prestenotic or poststenotic PSV could lead to significant overestimation of the pressure gradient, especially in the range of hemodynamically borderline significant lesions. Therefore, they recommended the use of a modified version:

$$\Delta P = 4 \ (PSV_2^2 - PSV_1^2)$$

where ΔP = peak systolic pressure gradient, PSV_2 = peak systolic velocity in the stenosis, and PSV_1 = peak systolic velocity in the prestenotic or poststenotic region. However, Legemate et al. also reported that in some patients an accurate calculation of the pressure gradient could not be obtained by this method.

Because of technical aspects of duplex scanning and the hemodynamics of blood flow, duplex scanning may theoretically show considerable errors in the measurement of blood flow velocity.[78] Erroneous grading of stenosis is mainly due to difficulties in correct placement and sampling of pulsed wave Doppler with an angle of insonation less than 60 degrees, especially in deeper iliac vessels.

Unsuccessful duplex scanning could be the result of a gaseous abdomen (patients should fast overnight in preparation for the study) or ultrasonographic reflections from a severely calcified wall. In obese patients, it may not be possible to examine the full length of each iliac artery. Although some thin people can be examined with a 5-MHz probe, a lower frequency (3.5 MHz) is required for adequate penetration to examine the aortoiliac segment in many patients.

Despite some limitations of this technique, the ability of duplex scanning to distinguish high-grade stenosis from occlusion, to detect hemodynamically significant disease, and to localize disease accurately is unique among the noninvasive tests. Until recently, angiography and intra-arterial pressure measurements were the most widely used and reliable diagnostic modalities to evaluate the severity of stenosis in the aortoiliac arteries. Today duplex sonography is playing an increasing role in providing both anatomical and functional evidence of disease. With an experienced investigator—the duplex examination of the distal aorta and the iliac arteries requires considerable experience—duplex scanning can today replace arteriography as a screening tool for the identification of treatable aortoiliac lesions. Patients can also be selected for possible angioplasty before angiography. The question of whether duplex imaging can be used as the sole diagnostic method prior to surgery deserves more consideration in the future.

Intravascular Ultrasound Imaging

Intravascular ultrasound imaging is a diagnostic tool that works particularly well in the aortoiliac region.[79] The different ultrasonic properties of fat, connective tissue, and calcified tissue allow an exact evaluation of intimal plaque composition. Intravascular ultrasound imaging also allows for accurate measurement of residual lumen diameter or area for quantitative assessment of the severity of lesions. This method is clearly superior to contrast arteriography and transcutaneous ultrasound in terms of characterization and quantification of the extent of vessel wall disorders. The specific intraluminal and transluminal data offered by intravascular ultrasound imaging seem especially important for optimal selection of the recanalizing interventional procedure such as stent placement.

Intra-arterial Pressure Measurement

Some authors believe that an accurate hemodynamic evaluation of the aortoiliac system for the purpose of determining the need for an inflow procedure requires invasive pressure measurements.[80] Evaluation of the hemodynamic effect of a stenosis by measuring the resting arterial pressure gradient is a commonly used method. An important principle is that the hemodynamic effect of a given stenosis depends on the flow rate. The pressure gradient across a significant stenosis increases when the rate of blood flow is increased. Therefore, some iliac stenoses in patients with claudication may have no gradient at rest, but a gradient develops with an increase in

the rate of blood flow. Three methods may be used to increase blood flow: (1) exercise, (2) ischemia produced by inflation of a tourniquet (normally the fall in blood pressure after ischemia is less than 15 mm Hg), and (3) pharmacological vasodilation. This concept of induced vasodilation to evaluate arterial disease was first described by Sako et al.[81]

Different criteria have been proposed for determining the hemodynamic significance of aortoiliac disease using intra-arterial pressure measurements, and considerable disagreement exists as to what constitutes an acceptable pressure gradient in the aortoiliac system. Brewster et al.[45] used a femoral–brachial gradient of >5 mm Hg at rest or a 15% drop in femoral systolic pressure during hyperemia—after occlusion of leg blood flow with a pneumatic cuff on the thigh—as a criterion for an abnormal test. Flanigan et al.[82] reported that a 15% or greater decrease in the femoral–brachial ratio after intra-arterial administration of 30 mg papaverine gave the highest accuracy in the identification of proximal disease. They also reported that all patients with such a decrease in femoral–brachial pressure index improved clinically after aortoiliac revascularization. When using a lower dosage of papaverine—to avoid a possible transient drop in systemic pressure—it is important to verify any increase in blood flow. Moneta[51] recommends a systolic pressure gradient of >5 mm Hg at rest or >15 mm Hg with drug-induced hyperemia as criteria of hemodynamically significant proximal lesions.

Kikta et al.[83] determined that a resting femoral–brachial pressure index of more than 0.9 and a less than 15% decrease of this index after papaverine administration indicated an acceptable inflow for proceeding with distal bypass. Noer et al.[84] measured the systolic pressure gradients across the aortoiliac segment in patients with different kinds of obstructions. In patients with occlusion of both the aorta and the iliac arteries the pressure drop was about 60%, and in patients with iliac artery occlusion it was about 50%. However, pressure varied widely in patients with iliac stenosis, ranging from a minimal drop to a drop of about 60%. The degree of stenosis on the angiogram was significantly correlated with the pressure drop. No difference in pressure drop was observed between patients with visualization of rich or poor collateral networks.

Should intra-arterial pressure measurement always be done during angiography? The pressure gradient across a ≥75% diameter stenosis read by angiography is generally significant. Patients with an entirely normal arteriogram probably have no demonstrable pressure gradients. However, in patients with about 20% to 75% stenosis, the hemodynamic significance of their lesions cannot be predicted accurately by angiography and should be verified by pressure measurements (Figure 60.9).

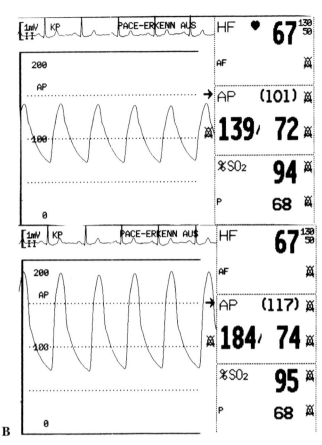

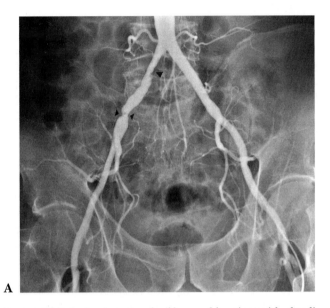

FIGURE 60.9. **A,** Angiogram of a 56-year-old patient with claudication in the right leg. The hemodynamic significance of the stenoses in the right common iliac artery cannot be judged on this angiogram. **B,** The intra-arterial pressure measurement demonstrates the hemodynamic importance by a significant gradient: (top) pressure curve in the external iliac artery; (bottom) pressure curve in the abdominal aorta.

Exercise Testing

None of the hemodynamic tests correlate well with the degree of exercise impairment or functional limitation in patients with claudication.[85] Furthermore, a number of medical treatments can improve treadmill exercise performance and functional status significantly without a change in ankle–brachial index or leg blood flow.[86] Consequently, therapeutic success in patients with claudication cannot be monitored only by changes in peripheral hemodynamics. Treadmill testing is designed to obtain objective data on the functional exercise capability of patients with claudication. Two different approaches—constant load testing and graded exercise testing—are in clinical use. The primary exercise outcome assessment in previous clinical trials of patients with claudication has been the change in walking distance or time on a constant load treadmill protocol. With this test the distance at which the patient first notices the onset of claudication pain is recorded, and the test is terminated when the patient reaches a maximum level of pain. Published guidelines have defined clinical success of claudi-

cation therapy as an increase in walking time or distance on a treadmill protocol set at 2 mph and 12% grade.[87] However, the use of a constant workload has several limitations, including significant within-subject and between-subjects variability.[88] Recently, the graded testing concepts developed for patients with cardiac disease have been extended to patients with peripheral arterial occlusive disease. Hiatt et al.[88] have recently summarized in an excellent review the advantages of a graded treadmill test—compared with a constant load treadmill test protocol—and have recommended the use of such graded treadmill protocols to assess the benefits of therapeutic interventions.

Especially in young patients laboratory tests of the aortoiliac segment may be less sensitive unless major stress such as ischemic exercise is applied. The main advantage of exercise testing is that it increases the sensitivity of other tests for smaller degrees of stenosis and therefore assesses adequacy of collateral circulation. Treadmill walking can be followed by repeated segmental blood pressure recordings or pulse volume recordings. The combination with postexercise ankle blood pressure measurement allows objective testing independent of the subjective symptoms of the patient.

Angiography

Angiography has remained until now the gold standard for providing anatomical information on which decisions regarding technical aspects of a planned surgical revascularization are made. It has been the gold standard despite being the most invasive modality. However, angiography provides only anatomical information and sometimes fails to detect hemodynamically less critical lesions, because these lesions are of hemodynamic significance only under conditions of increased flow and not in the resting state. It has become increasingly clear that the role of angiography should be to outline the anatomical distribution of arterial disease and not to guess its functional significance or even make the initial diagnosis.

Angiography can be misleading without multiple views. The main difficulty in angiographic evaluation of the aortoiliac segment arises from the fact that the majority of pelvic studies include only a single anteroposterior projection. Because most plaques have an asymmetric geometry with the bulk of the lesion on the posterior wall, in anteroposterior projection there may not be narrowing of the lateral wall until the plaque is in a very advanced stage. A posterior plaque can be suggested by a decrease in the density of the contrast column on the arteriogram, but this finding is easily overlooked. A single-plane arteriography is unreliable in the diagnosis of aortoiliac disease. Views obtained in the lateral and oblique planes increase the reliability of angiography. Angulation of up to 30 degrees between the right anterior oblique and left anterior oblique view is generally used for the iliac vessels. Markedly eccentric lesions such as those located at branching points and bifurcations should be visualized in at least two—preferably perpendicular—projections. However, even biplane angiograms cannot give the functional significance of borderline lesions. Ideally, before obtaining films, the technician should be informed of the possibility of aortoiliac stenosis and obtain proper oblique films and eventually also intraluminal pullback pressure gradients.

The conventional cut film technique or digital subtraction angiography can be used. The selection of the angiographic approach depends on the clinical problem, the results of noninvasive evaluation, and the status of the prospective puncture site. In diagnostic angiography, a retrograde transfemoral puncture is the preferred approach in the majority of patients. With the introduction of intravenous digital subtraction angiography, translumbar aortography has been completely replaced even in patients with occlusion of the aorta or both iliac arteries. Intravenous digital subtraction angiography is

the investigation of choice in this situation, but a transbrachial approach may also be used. The possibility of intravenous injection of the contrast medium also decreases the risk of local complications, but there are some important limitations with this technique. The quality of imaging is often poor because of less imaging resolution, especially in obese patients (Figure 60.10). Furthermore, with the required higher volumes of contrast medium, there is a risk of fluid overload in patients with cardiac insufficiency. In patients with long vascular occlusions and sparse development of collateral vessels, only intra-arterial digital subtraction angiography can demonstrate the runoff vessels including the trifurcation of the popliteal artery. Nonionic contrast media are increasingly used because they are less painful and cause less nephrotoxicity. However, they are more expensive.

The conventional angiography criterion is that a 50% reduction of diameter is critical. However, this criterion is imprecise because there can be difficulties with interpretation and because the effects of multiple areas of narrowing and blood flow are not considered. Furthermore, the measurement of diameter reduction is often inaccurate, and interobserver agreement is not optimal. These limitations of angiography can be overcome by measurement of intra-arterial pressure gradient during angiography (Figure 60.9). The problem of prediction of the hemodynamic significance of an arteriographically localized iliac lesion can also be managed by use of duplex sonography.

Angiography is the only method that provides sufficient information about collateral vessels in patients with aortoiliac occlusive disease. It is also very useful in determining the etiology of the occlusive disease.[89] The angiographic appearance of atherosclerotic disease varies greatly. The aorta and its primary branches may also be involved in Takayasu's arteritis. In patients with this disease—primarily young women <40 years—the abdominal visceral arteries are often involved by proximal stenotic lesions. These lesions are smooth and concentrically tapered. Sometimes aneurysmal changes are also found. In the acute phase of Takayasu's disease, the walls of the vessels may be thickened (which can be seen by duplex sonography). The classic angiographic appearance of fibromuscular dysplasia—mostly involving the renal arteries—is that of a string of beads. It may also be seen in the proximal external iliac artery. Some casuistic reports have noted cystic adventitial disease of this location. The angiographic pattern of ergotism is characterized by multiple focal stenoses or long segmental stenoses. We have observed a similar pattern in a young man with hyperhomocysteinemia (Figure 60.11). One form of ergot toxicity that leads to permanent arterial stenosis is caused by methysergide maleate. This substance induces a type of retroperitoneal fibrosis that encases the aorta and iliac arteries and can lead to occlu-

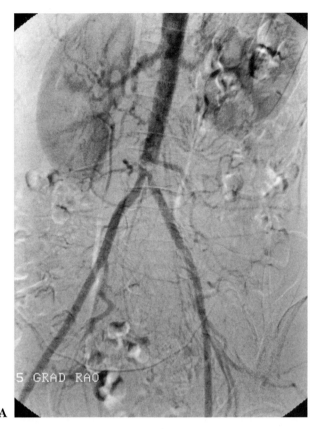

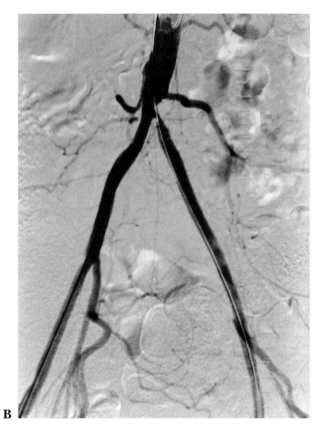

A   **B**

FIGURE 60.10. **A,** Intravenous digital subtraction angiography of the abdominal aorta and iliac arteries in a patient with left-sided claudication. There is suspicion of stenosis in the region of the aortic bifurcation, but a definitive diagnosis is not possi-ble. **B,** The corresponding intra-arterial digital subtraction an-giography of the same patient reveals the exact morphology of the lesions in the aortic bifurcation and left common iliac artery.

sion.[89] In patients with neurofibromatosis the abdominal aorta may be diffusely ectatic or narrowed, and the vas-cular abnormalities are centered around the origins of the visceral arteries. Radiation fibrosis, which must be considered in patients with specific histories of radiation therapy many years before examination, results in long segments of stenosis of the arteries in the field of radia-tion treatment.

Angioscopy

In contrast to angiography, angioscopy provides a more precise, three-dimensional color view of the vascular sur-face, thus enabling direct real-time examination of the vascular surface.[90] Technological progress, including the development of miniature video cameras, glass fiber op-tics, and effective lighting systems, has enabled clinical applications of percutaneous angioscopy, particularly in conjunction with surgical or interventional vascular pro-cedures. Angioscopy allows monitoring of the interven-tional therapy and qualitative assessment of the vascular surface pathology. The definitive role of angioscopy in routine clinical practice remains to be determined.

Spiral Computed Tomographic Angiography

Spiral computed tomographic angiography is a fast and minimally invasive technique for evaluating abdominal and pelvic vasculature.[91] It is quicker, less invasive, and provides less radiation exposure than conventional an-giography. An additional advantage is that once acquired the data can retrospectively be reconfigured into any possible projection, whereas conventional angiography requires an additional contrast injection and further ra-diation exposure for each additional view. By reducing examination time and contrast material, there is also a reduction of costs. Although conventional angiography allows optimal evaluation of the lumen of a vessel, it does not provide information about the qualitative or even quantitative changes of the vessel wall or surrounding tis-sue. However, computed tomographic angiography can demonstrate mural thrombi, atheromatous calcification, and additional perivascular abnormalities. The rare dis-ease entity of the so-called penetrating atherosclerotic ulcer of the aorta can be diagnosed by typical morphol-ogy on computed tomography.[92]

The main indication for aortic imaging by computed tomographic angiography is suspected aneurysmal dis-

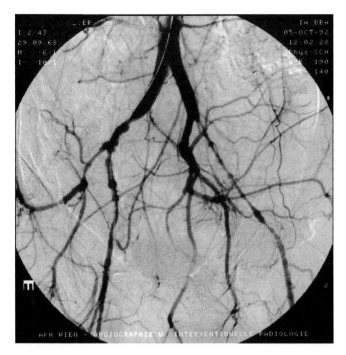

FIGURE 60.11. Intra-arterial digital subtraction angiography of the iliac arteries in a 24-year-old man with hyperhomocysteinemia. The angiogram demonstrates multiple focal and long segmental stenoses in both external iliac arteries. (Consecutive control studies by color flow duplex sonography demonstrated a rapidly changing pattern of these vasospasm-induced stenoses.)

ease or aortic dissection. However, in the near future computed tomographic angiography may also serve as a relatively inexpensive and noninvasive alternative to arteriography in evaluating aortoiliac occlusive disease.

Magnetic Resonance Angiography

Magnetic resonance angiography, which noninvasively images flowing blood, is a recent addition to the potential armamentarium of vascular imaging modalities. It has several advantages over conventional angiography in that it is safe and noninvasive and allows the calculation of many projections. The quality of magnetic resonance angiography has improved in recent years because of optimization of the pulse design and the examination protocol.[93] Contrast-enhanced turbo-FLASH (fast low-angle shot) magnetic resonance angiography has been demonstrated to be a useful imaging technique for patients with advanced aortoiliac disease.[94] Magnetic resonance angiography is not currently a routine examination, but it will likely become an accepted method for both preoperative evaluation and postoperative follow-up.

Other Diagnostic Tests

Various tests have a potential application for evaluating the severity of cutaneous ischemia. The clinical indica-

tion for these tests is the evaluation of the state of perfusion of the skin with special reference to skin viability.

Dynamic capillaroscopy makes it possible to record red blood cell velocity and flow rate. *Transcutaneous O_2* measurement in the skin can be used to assess the microcirculatory and tissue consequences of ischemia. This test is valuable for assessing the magnitude of ischemia and for predicting the healing potential of skin wounds or ulcers. The most useful application of this method is in optimizing the level of amputation.

The *laser Doppler* assesses microvascular perfusion by measuring the flux of red blood cells near the surface of the skin. The network of cutaneous microvessels is the target of laser light, and the resulting Doppler shifted signals are highly related to flow velocities in the cutaneous microcirculation. *Radioisotope methods* such as the isotope clearance method have been used to measure blood flow in the skin and subcutaneous tissue. These methods have no importance in the routine vascular laboratory assessment.

General Cardiovascular Risk

Atherosclerosis of the arteries of the lower limbs is one of the strongest indicators for atherosclerosis in other vessels of the body, such as coronary or brain vessels. Patients with mild symptoms of claudication are mostly treated conservatively. However, the consulted physician should also use this opportunity to exclude potentially fatal atheromatous disease involving other vessels. Reports concerning late survival in patients with peripheral occlusive disease have indicated that the 5- to 10-year mortality rate (about 30%–50%) is several times higher than the risk of amputation during the same interval.[95] The relative risk of mortality is elevated twofold to sevenfold in men and women with unisegmental and multisegmental disease that involves the aortoiliac and femoropopliteal segment.[28] Multisegmental disease is associated with higher morbidity and mortality rates.[96]

Ischemic Heart Disease

Assessment of the risk of ischemic heart disease is important, because this is the main prognostic factor in atherosclerotic patients. The approach to cardiac risk stratification of patients who undergo peripheral vascular surgery remains controversial. The success of algorithms using clinical risk factors to determine the cardiac risk has been inconsistent.[97] Intermittent claudication often interferes with performance of treadmill or bicycle exercise electrocardiograms; dipyridamole thallium imaging identifies high-risk patients before surgery for aortoiliac occlusive disease. Dipyridamole myocardial scintigraphy has been accepted as a sensitive noninvasive approach to risk stratification with excellent negative predictive value. However, low positive predictive value of abnormal scans is a shortcoming that contributes to extensive preoperative cardiac evaluation and intervention with associated high morbidity, mortality, and costs. Bry et al.[97] conclude that evaluation of cost-effectiveness does not justify general cardiac screening with myocardial scintigraphy.

About 40% of those with clinical indications of associated ischemic heart disease have been shown angiographically to be candidates for myocardial revascularization.[98] Some patients with symptomatic coronary disease who are at extremely high risk should undergo coronary revascularization before peripheral vascular reconstruction. Patients with moderate risk may need more intense intraoperative monitoring. Patients without evidence of cardiac ischemia with stress may undergo vascular surgery with a low risk of perioperative cardiac ischemia.

Cerebrovascular Disease

Stroke is a rare but devastating complication of aortoiliac reconstructions. The management of patients with planned aortoiliac reconstructions who also have advanced carotid artery disease remains controversial. The dilemma is with the management of patients who require such reconstructions but also have asymptomatic carotid artery stenosis. In most studies, no significant difference in perioperative neurological complications has been noted between patients with and without significant carotid artery disease.[99,100] However, some authors conclude that carotid endarterectomy in selected patients who require abdominal aortic reconstruction is safe and, when performed before distal reconstruction, reduces perioperative stroke rate and may improve long-term survival. They have thus proposed correcting high-grade asymptomatic carotid stenosis before reconstructing the aorta.[101]

Conservative Treatment

There are two aims of therapy: (1) to retard the rate of progression of atherosclerosis and (2) to diminish the arterial insufficiency and treat the symptoms. Severely affected patients with critical limb ischemia are candidates for lumen-opening procedures such as bypass or angioplasty to maintain limb viability. However, because the majority of patients with claudication are not at short-term risk of limb loss, the primary therapeutic goal is to improve exercise performance and functional status. The indications for treatment depend on the patient's requirements, lifestyle, and work.

Prophylactic Treatment

Risk Factor Modification

The treatment of all patients with peripheral arterial occlusive disease is initially directed at cardiovascular risk factor modification, because these individuals have a high risk of future cardiovascular mortality. Cessation of smoking improves the prognosis in patients with atherosclerotic disease.[102] Moreover, continued cigarette smoking after arterial reconstructive surgery adversely influences the patency rates of bypass grafts.[117] In addition to strongly advising the patient to quit smoking, the physician should consider supporting the use of nicotine chewing gum. Placebo-controlled studies have demonstrated that the addition of such a chewing gum increases the rate of smoking cessation.[103]

Patients who are treated for dyslipidemia have a decreased progression rate of angiographically assessed lesions.[104] The risk of amputation is increased by diabetes. However, it has not been demonstrated until now that the control of diabetes influences prognosis of diabetic macroangiopathy. Treatment of hypertension deserves special care, because normalization of blood pressure may aggravate ischemic symptoms.

Antithrombotic Therapy

Leg artery disease is a marker of generalized atherosclerosis and therefore an indicator associated with increased risk of premature death. Antithrombotic therapy with antiplatelet agents—especially aspirin—can modify the natural history of chronic lower extremity arterial insufficiency and lower the incidence of associated cardiovascular events.[105] Aspirin delays the progression of established arterial occlusive disease as assessed by serial angiography.[106] Furthermore, antiplatelet therapy reduces the risk of vascular occlusion after peripheral artery procedures.[107] The present recommendation of a daily dose of about 100 mg aspirin is based on findings that this dose is as clinically efficacious as and safer than higher doses.[108] Ticlopidine is a promising alternative in patients with aspirin intolerance.[109] A recently developed new substance—clopidogrel—seems promising for the future.

Physical Training

Exercise has been demonstrated to be a very effective means of improving claudication-limiting physical activity in patients with peripheral arterial disease. Several well-controlled studies have shown the favorable influence of regular exercise on intermittent claudication.[110,117] Regular exercise elicits well-established and clinically important changes in treadmill exercise performance and community-based walking ability. Most authors agree that supervised training is superior to home training. The most successful programs are likely to be those that combine regular supervised group sessions with daily home exercise programs. Regularity rather than intensity should be stressed by counseling physicians. Various types of exercise have been used in exercise conditioning programs. The exercise regimen should continue for at least 3 months and should be controlled by some objective test of walking ability such as on a treadmill. The patients should be informed about the importance of continuing with the exercises on their own and the risk of deterioration if they stop. Any exercise program must be practical and fit in with the patient's normal lifestyle.

Good results can be expected from physical training in patients with intermittent claudication independent of the location of the atherosclerotic process. Patients with aortoiliac occlusions seem to benefit as much as patients with femoropopliteal obstructions.[111,112] Ekroth et al.[111] reported that the mean increase in walking distance was 2.4 times the initial value, and this was independent of the location of the arterial occlusion. Jonason et al.[112] could not confirm earlier observations that patients with proximal arterial obstructions do not benefit from physical training.

Different mechanisms are discussed as possible explanations for the beneficial effects of physical training.[110] Exercise has been shown to reverse most of the hemorheological abnormalities seen in patients with peripheral arterial disease,[113] and it also favorably modifies risk factors. Weight reduction is an important part of the therapy because it lessens the load on the legs and reduces the need for blood supply.

Patients with mild rest pain have been shown to improve as much from exercise as those with intermittent claudication.[112] However, patients with critical limb ischemia should be excluded from exercise programs.

Drug Therapy

Compared with exercise, the place of drugs in the management of patients with intermittent claudication is less clear. Analysis of numerous publications on the demonstration of the efficacy of drug therapy with vasoactive substances has shown the existence of methodological errors and inaccuracies with regard to patient selection, investigative methods, and statistical evaluation.[87] These problems have prevented objective and rational evaluation, and the evidence for clinically significant benefit remains unconvincing. In any case, if a favorable effect exists, its amplitude seems to be quite limited.

Several so-called vasoactive drugs have been used, and a few positive double-blind studies of these drugs have been published. The studies indicate a favorable effect of the drugs acting on microcirculation or hemorheolog-

ical parameters.[114,115] In recent years there has been increasing recognition of the importance of rheological abnormalities—increased whole blood viscosity, increased red cell aggregation, reduced red cell deformability, and increased fibrinogen level—in patients with peripheral arterial disease. In some patients, increased viscosity appears to be a critical factor responsible for intermittent claudication.[116] This recognition of the contribution of rheological abnormalities has encouraged the research and development of rheologically active treatment. In the United States, pentoxifylline is the only hemorheological agent currently approved by the US Food and Drug Administration for treatment of intermittent claudication. A critical review of the pentoxifylline trials concluded that the actual improvement in walking distance attributable to pentoxifylline is often unpredictable, may not be clinically important compared with the effects of placebo, and does not justify the added expense for most patients.[117] The drug may have a role in a few patients with markedly reduced walking distance who cannot engage in exercise therapy. Vasodilators are of no value,[118] but metabolically active drugs such as L-carnitine—which improves ischemic skeletal muscle metabolism—seem promising.[119]

Hemodilution

Because of the dominant role of hematocrit on blood viscosity, hemodilution has been viewed as a possible therapy. Placebo-controlled studies have demonstrated a significant increase in pain-free walking distance for patients undergoing hemodilution therapy.[120] The hemodilution should be done hypervolemically or isovolemically, and the hematocrit values should be between 38% and 42%.[121]

Systemic Thrombolytic Therapy

Systemic thrombolytic therapy for the treatment of acute and chronic arterial occlusions of the limbs has been used in Europe for about three decades.[122] It is an attractive nonsurgical alternative in reopening chronically occluded aortoiliac occlusions (Figure 60.12). An ultra-high-dose regimen of streptokinase makes it possible to restore patency in almost two thirds of recently occluded arteries.[123] The treatment is more successful in patients with a short history of occluded arteries, but aortic occlusions with a history of about 1 year and iliac obstructions up to 6 months' duration can also be recanalized. Pilger et al.[124] reported a recanalization rate of 52% with no major complications. The recanalization rate did not vary for different thrombolytic drugs (streptokinase, urokinase, and recombinant tissue plasminogen activator). In cases of successful thrombolysis and residual obstruction, subsequent balloon angioplasty was done. Pil-

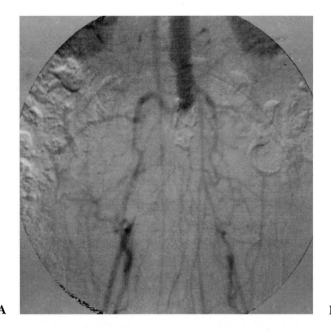

A

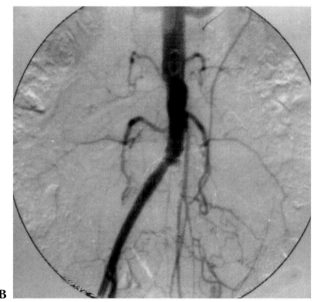

B

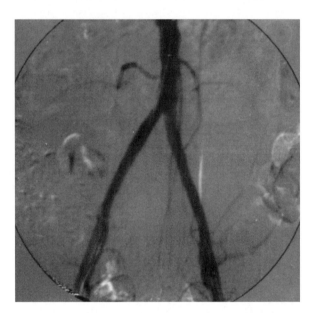

C

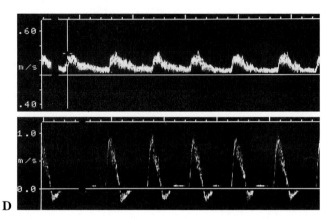

D

FIGURE 60.12. **A,** Occlusion of the distal abdominal aorta and both common iliac arteries in a 50-year-old woman with severe bilateral claudication. **B,** After systemic thrombolysis with ultra-high-dose streptokinase (9×10^6 units on 3 consecutive days): recanalization of the aorta and the right common iliac artery. **C,** After subsequent recanalization of the left common iliac artery by percutaneous transluminal angioplasty. **D,** Doppler spectral analysis of the flow velocity in the right common femoral artery: (top) before systemic thrombolysis; (bottom) after recanalization.

ger et al. concluded that thrombolytic therapy followed by percutaneous transluminal angioplasty seems to be an effective and safe treatment regimen for patients with chronic aortoiliac disease.

Systemic thrombolytic therapy might be more acceptable than surgical reconstruction to the patient with aortoiliac disease. However, the main disadvantages are an inability to predict successful thrombolysis and the risk of hemorrhage. Because of the possibility of serious bleeding complications, systemic infusion of thrombolytic agents was gradually abandoned for the treatment of aortoiliac disease and replaced with local application of thrombolytic agents whenever technically possible.

References

1. Criqui MH, Fronek A, Barrett-Connor E, et al. The prevalence of peripheral arterial disease in a defined population. *Circulation.* 1985;71:510–515.

2. McDaniel MD, Cronenwett JL. Basic data related to the natural history of intermittent claudication. *Ann Vasc Surg.* 1989;3:273–277.

3. Martin EC. Percutaneous therapy in the management of aortoiliac disease. *Semin Vasc Surg.* 1994;7:17–27.

4. Münster W, Wierny L, Porstmann W. Lokalisation und Häufigkeit arterieller Durchblutungsstörungen der unteren Extremitäten. *Dtsch Med Wochenschr.* 1966;91: 2073–2079.

5. Cachovan M. Aortoiliakale Arterienverschlüsse. In: Alexander K, ed. *Gefäß-Krankheiten.* Munich: Urban Schwarzenberg, 1994:507–508.

6. Schoop W. Spontanverlauf der peripheren stenosierenden Arteriosklerose und Einfluß von Katheterinterventionen. *Z Kardiol.* 1991;80(suppl 9):21–23.

7. Starer F, Sutton RJ. Aortic thrombosis. *BMJ.* 1958;1: 1255–1258.

8. Parums DV. Inflammation and atherosclerosis. In: Stehbens WE, Lie JT, eds. *Vascular Pathology.* London: Chapman & Hall; 1995:329–351.

9. Steinberg D, Witztum JL. Lipoproteins and atherogenesis. *JAMA.* 1990;264:3047–3052.

10. Stehbens WE. Atherosclerosis and degenerative diseases of blood vessels. In: Stehbens WE, Lie JT, eds. *Vascular Pathology.* London: Chapman & Hall; 1995:175–269.

11. Barnes MJ. Collagens of normal and diseased blood vessel wall. In: Nimni ME, ed. *Collagen.* Boca Raton, Fla: CRC Press; 1988:275–290.

12. Glagov S, Zarins CK, Giddens DP, et al. Mechanical factors in the pathogenesis, localization, and evolution of atherosclerotic plaques. In: Camillieri JP, Berry CL, Fiessinger JN, et al., eds. *Diseases of the Arterial Wall.* Berlin: Springer-Verlag; 1989:217–239.

13. Bassiouny HS, Zarins CK, Kadowaki MH, et al. Hemodynamic stress and experimental aortoiliac atherosclerosis. *J Vasc Surg.* 1994;19:426–434.

14. Caro GG, Fitz-Gerald JM, Schroter RC. Atheroma and arterial wall shear: observation, correlation, and proposal of a shear-dependent mass transfer mechanism for atherogenesis. *Proc R Soc Lond (B Biol Sci).* 1971;117:109–159.

15. Zarins CK, Bomberger RA, Glagov S. Local effects of stenosis: increased flow velocity inhibits atherogenesis. *Circulation.* 1981;64(suppl 2):221–227.

16. May AG, Van de Berg L, De Weese JA. Critical arterial stenosis. *Surgery.* 1963;54:250–259.

17. Schultz RD, Hokanson DE, Strandness DE Jr. Pressure-flow and stress-strain measurements of normal and diseased aortoiliac segments. *Surg Gynecol Obstet.* 1967;124: 1267–1276.

18. Criqui MH, Fronek A, Klauber MR, et al. The sensitivity, specificity, and predictive value of traditional clinical evaluation of peripheral arterial disease: results from noninvasive testing in a defined population. *Circulation.* 1985;71: 516–522.

19. Cacoub P, Godeau P. Risk factors for atherosclerotic aortoiliac occlusive disease. *Ann Vasc Surg.* 1993;7:394–405.

20. Friedman SA, Holling HE, Roberts B. Etiologic factors in aortoiliac and femoropopliteal vascular disease. *N Engl J Med.* 1964;271:1382–1385.

21. Stubbs DH, Kasulke R, Kapsch DN, et al. Populations with the Leriche syndrome. *Surgery.* 1981;83:612–616.

22. Levy LA. Smoking and peripheral vascular disease: epidemiology and podiatric perspective. *J Am Podiatr Med Assoc.* 1989;79:398–402.

23. Kannell WB, McGee DL. Update on some epidemiologic features of intermittent claudication: the Framingham Study. *J Am Geriatr Soc.* 1985;33:13–17.

24. Willems SL, Plair CM. Cigarette smoking and arteriosclerosis. *Science.* 1962;138:975–977.

25. Strong JP, Richards ML. Cigarette smoking and atherosclerosis in autopsied men. *Atherosclerosis.* 1976;23:451–476.

26. Weiss NS. Cigarette smoking and arteriosclerosis obliterans: an epidemiologic approach. *Am J Epidemiol.* 1971;95: 17–25.

27. Hughson WG, Mann JI, Garrod A. Intermittent claudication: prevalence and risk factors. *BMJ.* 1978;1:1379–1381.

28. Vogt MT, Wolfson SK, Kuller LH. Segmental arterial disease in the lower extremities: correlates of disease and relationship to mortality. *J Clin Epidemiol.* 1993;46: 1267–1276.

29. Silbert S, Zazeela H. Prognosis in arteriosclerotic peripheral vascular disease. *JAMA.* 1958;166:1816–1821.

30. Provan JL, Sojka SG, Murnaghan JJ, et al. The effect of cigarette smoking on the long-term success rates of aorto-femoral and femoropopliteal reconstructions. *Surg Gynecol Obstet.* 1987;165:49–52.

31. Rubba P, Riccardi G, Pauciullo P, et al. Different localization of early arterial lesions in insulin-dependent diabetes mellitus and in familial hypercholesterolemia. *Metabolism.* 1989;38:962–966.

32. Conrad MC. Large and small artery occlusion in diabetes and non diabetes with severe vascular disease. *Circulation.* 1967;36:83–91.

33. Boers GHJ, Smals AGH, Trijbels FJM, et al. Heterozygosity for homocystinuria in premature peripheral and cerebral occlusive arterial disease. *N Engl J Med.* 1985;313:709–715.

34. Weiss NS. Premature menopause and aortoiliac occlusive disease. *Journal of Chronic Diseases.* 1972;25:133–138.

35. Holmes DR, Burbank MK, Fulton RE, et al. Arteriosclerosis obliterans in young women. *Am J Med.* 1979;66: 997–1000.

36. Cronenwett JL, Davis JT, Gooch JB, et al. Aortoiliac occlusive disease in women. *Surgery.* 1980;88:775–784.

37. Palmaz JC, Carson SN, Hunter G, et al. Male hypoplastic infrarenal aorta and premature atherosclerosis. *Surgery.* 1983;94:91–94.

38. Jernigan WR, Fallat ME, Hatfield DR: Hypoplastic aortoiliac syndrome: an entity peculiar to women. *Surgery.* 1983;94:752–757.

39. Ehringer H. Die reaktive Hyperämie nach arterieller Sperre. In: Bollinger A, Brunner V, eds. *Meßmethoden bei arteriellen Durchblutungsstörungen.* Bern: Huber; 1971: 20–33.

40. Bollinger A, Schlumpf M, Buholzer F, et al. Ergometric performance and peripheral hemodynamics in patients with isolated occlusions of the iliac and femoral arteries. *Vasa.* 1973;2:228–232.

41. Farber A, Grunert JH, Ranke K, et al. The role of left internal thoracic artery in chronic iliac artery occlusion. *Vasa.* 1995;24:79–82.

42. Jenkins DM, Newton WD. Atheroembolism. *Am Surg.* 1991;57:588–590.

43. Gagliardi JM, Batt M, Khodja RH, et al. Mural thrombus of the aorta. *Ann Vasc Surg.* 1988;2:201–204.

44. Warren BA. Atheroembolism: clinical and experimental aspects. In: Stehbens WE, Lie JT, eds. *Vascular Pathology.* London: Chapman & Hall; 1995:415–435.

45. Brewster DC, Waltman AC, O'Hara PJ, et al. Femoral artery pressure measurement during arteriography. *Circulation.* 1979;60(suppl 1):120–124.

46. Campbell WB, Cole SE, Skidmore R, et al. The clinician and the vascular laboratory in the diagnosis of aortoiliac stenosis. *Br J Surg.* 1984;71:302–306.

47. Johnston KW, Demorais D, Colapinto RI. Difficulty in assessing the severity of aortoiliac disease by clinical and arteriographic methods. *Angiology.* 1981;32:609–614.

48. Sobinsky KR, Borozan PG, Gray B, et al. Is femoral pulse palpation accurate in assessing the hemodynamic significance of aortoiliac occlusive disease? *Am J Surg.* 1984;148:214–216.

49. Brewster DC, Perler BA, Robison JG, et al. Aortofemoral graft for multilevel occlusive disease: predictors of success and need for distal bypass. *Arch Surg.* 1982;117:1593–1600.

50. Charlesworth D, Harris PC, Cave FB, et al. Undiagnosed aorto-iliac insufficiency: a reason for early failure of saphenous vein bypass graft for obstruction of the superficial femoral artery. *Br J Surg.* 1975;62:567–570.

51. Moneta GL, Yeager RA, Taylor LM Jr, et al. Hemodynamic assessment of combined aortoiliac/femoropopliteal occlusive disease and selection of single or multilevel revascularization. *Semin Vasc Surg.* 1994;7:3–10.

52. Heintz SE, Bone GE, Slaymaker EE, et al. Value of arterial pressure measurements in the proximal and distal part of the thigh in arterial occlusive disease. *Surg Gynecol Obstet.* 1978;146:337–341.

53. Flanigan DP, Gray B, Schuler JJ, et al. Utility of wide and narrow blood pressure cuffs in the hemodynamic assessment of aortoiliac occlusive disease. *Surgery.* 1982;92:16–20.

54. Lynch TG, Hobson RW, Wright CB, et al. Interpretation of Doppler segmental pressures in peripheral vascular occlusive disease. *Arch Surg.* 1984;119:465–467.

55. Francfort JW, Bigelow PS, Davis JT, et al. Noninvasive techniques in the assessment of lower-extremity arterial occlusive disease: the advantages of proximal and distal thigh cuffs. *Arch Surg.* 1984;119:1145–1148.

56. Faris IB, Jamieson CW. The diagnosis of aortoiliac stenosis. *J Cardiovasc Surg.* 1975;16:597–601.

57. Flanigan DP, Gray B, Schuler JJ, et al. Comparison of Doppler-derived high thigh pressure and intraarterial pressure in the assessment of aorto-iliac occlusive disease. *Br J Surg.* 1981;68:423–425.

58. Franzeck UK, Bernstein EF, Fronek A. The effect of sensing site on the limb segmental blood pressure determination. *Arch Surg.* 1981;116:912–916.

59. Barringer M, Poole GV Jr, Shircliffe AC, et al. The diagnosis of aortoiliac disease: a noninvasive femoral cuff technique. *Ann Surg.* 1983;197:204–209.

60. Carter SA. Response of ankle systolic pressure to leg exercise in mild or questionable arterial disease. *N Engl J Med.* 1972;287:578–582.

61. Kempczinski RF. The role of the vascular diagnostic laboratory in the evaluation of male impotence. *Am J Surg.* 1979;138:278–282.

62. Raines JK. The pulse volume recorder in peripheral arterial disease. In: Bernstein EF, ed. *Noninvasive Diagnostic Techniques in Vascular Disease.* St Louis, Mo: Mosby;1982:360–369.

63. Rutherford RB, Lowenstein DH, Klein MF. Combining segmental systolic pressures and plethysmography to diagnose arterial occlusive disease of the legs. *Am J Surg.* 1979;138:211–218.

64. Van Asten WN, Beijneveld WJ, Pieters BR, et al. Assessment of aortoiliac obstructive disease by Doppler spectrum analysis of blood flow velocities in the common femoral artery at rest and during reactive hyperemia. *Surgery.* 1991;109:633–639.

65. Walton L, Martin TRP, Collins M. Prospective assessment of the aorto-iliac segment by visual interpretation of frequency analysed Doppler waveforms: a comparison with arteriography. *Ultrasound Med Biol.* 1984;10:27–32.

66. Baker JD, Machleder HI, Skidmore R. Analysis of femoral artery Doppler signals by LaPlace transform damping method. *J Vasc Surg.* 1984;1:520–524.

67. Johnston KW, Kassam M, Cobbold RS. Relationship between Doppler pulsatility index and direct femoral pressure measurements in the diagnosis of aortoiliac occlusive disease. *Ultrasound Med Biol.* 1983;9:271–281.

68. Flanigan DP, Collins JT, Goodreau JJ, et al. Femoral pulsatility index in the evaluation of aortoiliac occlusive disease. *J Surg Res.* 1981;32:392–399.

69. Thiele BL, Bandyk DF, Zierler RE, et al. A systematic approach to the assessment of aortoiliac disease. *Arch Surg.* 1983;118:477–481.

70. Fronek A, Coel M, Bernstein EF. The importance of combined multisegmental pressure and Doppler flow velocity studies in the diagnosis of peripheral arterial occlusive disease. *Surgery.* 1978;84:840–847.

71. Kohler TR, Nance DR, Cramer MM, et al. Duplex scanning for diagnosis of aortoiliac and femoropopliteal disease: a prospective study. *Circulation.* 1987;76:1074–1080.

72. Langsfeld M, Nepute J, Hershey FB, et al. The use of deep duplex scanning to predict hemodynamically significant aortoiliac stenoses. *J Vasc Surg.* 1988;7:395–399.

73. Moneta GL, Yeager RA, Antonovic R, et al. Accuracy of lower extremity arterial duplex mapping. *J Vasc Surg.* 1992;15:275–283.

74. Karacagil S, Lofberg AM, Almgren B, et al. Duplex ultrasound scanning for diagnosis of aortoiliac and femoropopliteal arterial disease. *Vasa.* 1994;23:325–329.

75. Legemate DA, Teeuwen C, Hoeneveld H, et al. How can the assessment of the hemodynamic significance of aortoiliac arterial stenosis by duplex scanning be improved? A

comparative study with intraarterial pressure measurement. *J Vasc Surg.* 1993;17:676–684.

76. Strauss AL, Roth FJ, Rieger H. Noninvasive assessment of pressure gradients across iliac artery stenoses: duplex and catheter correlative study. *J Ultrasound Med.* 1993;12:17–22.

77. Weber G, Strauss AL, Rieger H, et al. Validation of Doppler measurement of pressure gradients across peripheral model arterial stenosis. *J Vasc Surg.* 1992;16:10–16.

78. Gill RW: Measurement of blood flow by ultrasound: accuracy and sources of error. *Ultrasound Med Biol.* 1985;11:625–641.

79. Diethrich EB. Endovascular treatment of abdominal aortic occlusive disease: the impact of stents and intravascular ultrasound imaging. *Eur J Vasc Surg.* 1993;7:228–236.

80. Sawchuk AP, Flanigan DP, Tober JC, et al. A rapid, accurate, noninvasive technique for diagnosing critical and subcritical stenoses in aortoiliac arteries. *J Vasc Surg.* 1990;12:158–167.

81. Sako Y. Papaverine test in peripheral arterial disease. *Surg Forum.* 1966;17:141–143.

82. Flanigan DP, Williams LR, Schwartz JA, et al. Hemodynamic evaluation of the aortoiliac system based on pharmacologic vasodilatation. *Surgery.* 1983;93:709–714

83. Kikta MJ, Flanigan DP, Bishara RA, et al. Long-term follow-up of patients having infrainguinal bypass performed below stenotic but hemodynamically normal aortoiliac vessels. *J Vasc Surg.* 1987;5:319–328.

84. Noer I, Praestholm J, Tonnesen KH. Direct measured systolic pressure gradients across the aorto-iliac segment in multiple-level-obstruction arteriosclerosis. *Cardiovasc Intervent Radiol.* 1981;4:73–76.

85. Hiatt WR, Nawaz D, Regensteiner JG, et al. The evaluation of exercise performance in patients with peripheral vascular disease. *J Cardiopulm Rehabil.* 1988;12:525–532.

86. Dahllof A, Holm J, Schersten T, et al. Peripheral arterial insufficiency: effect of physical training on walking tolerance, calf blood flow, and blood flow resistance. *Scand J Rehabil Med.* 1976;8:19–26.

87. Heidrich H, Allenberg J, Cachovan M, et al. Guidelines for therapeutic studies on peripheral arterial occlusive disease in Fontaine stages II–IV. *Vasa.* 1992;21:339–343.

88. Hiatt WR, Hirsch AT, Regensteiner JG, et al. Clinical trials for claudication: assessment of exercise performance, functional status, and clinical end points. *Circulation.* 1995;92:614–621.

89. Stanson AW. Diagnostic angiography, imaging, and intervention. In: Stehbens WE, Lie JT, eds. *Vascular Pathology.* London: Chapman & Hall; 1995:699–728.

90. Gross CM, Biamino G. Peripheral angioscopy. In: Lanzer P, Rösch J, eds. *Vascular Diagnostics.* Berlin: Springer-Verlag; 1994:509–522.

91. Van Leeuwen MS, Polman LJ, Noordzij J, et al. Computed tomographic angiography. In: Lanzer P, Rösch J, eds. *Vascular Diagnostics.* Berlin: Springer-Verlag; 1994:454–462.

92. Sartoretti-Schefer S, Sartoretti C, Kotulek T, et al. Atherosclerotic penetrating ulcer of the aorta. Typical morphology on CT: a review of five cases. *Eur Radiol.* 1995;5:657–662.

93. Hartkamp MJ, Bakker CJG, Kouwenhoven M, et al. Peripheral vascular MR imaging. In: Lanzer P, Rösch J, eds. *Vascular Diagnostics.* Berlin: Springer-Verlag; 1994:421–440.

94. Sivananthan UM, Ridgway JP, Bann K, et al. Fast magnetic resonance angiography using turbo-FLASH sequences in advanced aortoiliac disease. *Br J Radiol.* 1993;66:1103–1110.

95. Dormandy J, Mahir M, Ascady G, et al. Fate of the patient with chronic leg ischemia. *J Cardiovasc Surg.* 1989;30:50–57.

96. Jonasen T, Ringquist I. Mortality and morbidity in patients with intermittent claudication in relation to the location of the occlusive atherosclerosis in the leg. *Angiology.* 1985;36:310–314.

97. Bry JD, Belkin M, O'Donnell TF Jr, et al. An assessment of the positive predictive value and cost-effectiveness of dipyridamole myocardial scintigraphy in patients undergoing vascular surgery. *J Vasc Surg.* 1994;19:112–121.

98. Hertzer NR. The natural history of peripheral vascular disease: implications for its management. *Circulation.* 1991; 83(suppl):I12–I19.

99. Turnipseed WD, Berkhoff HA, Belzer FD. Postoperative stroke in cardiac and peripheral vascular disease. *Ann Surg.* 1980;192:365–368.

100. Barnes RW, Liebman PR, Marszalek PB. The natural history of asymptomatic carotid disease in patients undergoing cardiovascular surgery. *Surgery.* 1981;90:1075–1083.

101. Bower TC, Merrell SW, Cherry KJ Jr, et al. Advanced carotid disease in patients requiring aortic reconstruction. *Am J Surg.* 1993;166:146–151.

102. Juergens JL, Barker NW, Hines EA. Atherosclerosis obliterans: review of 520 cases with special reference to pathogenic and prognostic factors. *Circulation.* 1960;21:188–195.

103. Tonnessen P, Fryd V, Hansen M, et al. Effect of nicotine chewing gum in combination with group counseling on the cessation of smoking. *N Engl J Med.* 1988;318:15–18.

104. Duffield RG, Miller NE, Brunt JN, et al. Treatment of hyperlipidemia retards progression of symptomatic femoral atherosclerosis. *Lancet.* 1983;2:639–642.

105. Antiplatelet Trialist's Collaboration. Collaborative overview of randomized trials of antiplatelet therapy, I: prevention of death, myocardial infarction, and stroke by prolonged antiplatelet therapy in various categories of patients. *BMJ.* 1994;308:81–106.

106. Hess H, Mietaschk A, Deichsel G. Drug-induced inhibition of platelet function delays progression of peripheral occlusive arterial disease: a prospective double-blind arteriographically controlled trial. *Lancet.* 1985;1:416–419.

107. Antiplatelet Trialist's Collaboration. Collaborative overview of randomized trials of antiplatelet therapy, II: maintenance of vascular graft or arterial patency by antiplatelet therapy. *BMJ.* 1994;308:159–168.

108. Clagett GP, Krupski WC. Antithrombotic therapy in peripheral arterial occlusive disease. *Chest.* 1995;108(suppl):431S–443S.

109. Boissel JP, Peyrieux JC, Destors JM. Is it possible to reduce the risk of cardiovascular events in subjects suffering from intermittent claudication of the lower limbs? *Thromb Haemost.* 1989;62:681–685.

110. Hiatt WR, Wolfel EE, Regensteiner JG. Exercise in the treatment of intermittent claudication due to peripheral arterial disease. *Vasc Med Rev.* 1991;2:61–70.

111. Ekroth R, Dahllöf G, Gundevall B, et al. Physical training of patients with intermittent claudication: indications, methods, and results. *Surgery.* 1978;84:640–643.

112. Jonason T, Jonzon B, Ringquist I, et al. Effect of physical training on different categories of patients with intermittent claudication. *Acta Medica Scandinavica.* 1979;206:253–258.

113. Ernst EE, Matrai A. Intermittent claudication, exercise, and blood rheology. *Circulation.* 1987;76:1110–1114.

114. Clissold SP, Lynch S, Sorkin EM. Buflomedil: a review of its pharmacodynamic and pharmacokinetic properties, and therapeutic efficacy in peripheral and cerebral vascular disease. *Drugs.* 1987;33:430–460.

115. Ward A, Clissold SP. Pentoxifylline: a review of its pharmacodynamic and pharmacokinetic properties and its therapeutic efficacy. *Drugs.* 1987;34:50–97.

116. Dormandy JA, Hoare E, Colley J, et al. Clinical, hemodynamic, rheological, and biochemical findings in 126 patients with intermittent claudication. *BMJ.* 1973;4:576–581.

117. Radack K, Wyderski RJ. Conservative management of intermittent claudication. *Ann Intern Med.* 1990;113:135–146.

118. Coffman JD. Vasodilator drugs in peripheral vascular disease. *N Engl J Med.* 1979;300:713–717.

119. Brevetti G, Chiariello M, Ferulano G, et al. Increase in walking distance in patients with peripheral vascular disease treated with L-carnitine: a double-blind crossover study. *Circulation.* 1988;77:767–773.

120. Ernst E, Matrai A, Kollar L. Placebo-controlled, double-blind study of hemodilution in peripheral arterial disease. *Lancet.* 1987;8548:1449–1451.

121. Kiesewetter H, Jung F, Erdlenbruch W, et al. Haemodilution in patients with peripheral arterial disease. *Int Angiol.* 1992;11:169–175.

122. Poliwoda H, Alexander K, Buhl V, et al. Treatment of chronic arterial occlusions with streptokinase. *N Engl J Med.* 1969;280:689–692.

123. Martin M, Fiebach O, eds. Fibrinolytische Behandlung peripherer Arterien-und Venenverschlüsse. Bern: Huber; 1994.

124. Pilger E, Decrinis M, Stark G, et al. Thrombolytic treatment and balloon angioplasty in chronic occlusion of the aortic bifurcation. *Ann Intern Med.* 1994;120:40–44.

61

Recanalization and Stent Placement in Iliac Artery Obstructions

Johannes Lammer and Siegfried Thurnher

High-grade iliac artery obstructions are primarily caused by atheromatous disease. However, thromboembolic disorders, posttraumatic or tumorous stenoses, vasculitis, radiation damage, and fibromuscular disease might be rare causes of iliac artery obstructions. Intermittent claudication and critical leg ischemia are the indications for revascularization procedures.

Since the pioneering work of Charles Dotter, Eberhard Zeitler, Andreas Grüntzig, Friedrich Olbert, and Charles Tegtmeyer, percutaneous transluminal angioplasty (PTA) has become an accepted modality for treatment of iliac artery obstructions.[1–5] Placement of an endovascular endoprosthesis has been experimentally tested by Dotter, Cragg, and Maass.[6,7] However, it was the pioneering work of Julio Palmaz that introduced stent placement to clinical practice.[8] The basic mechanism by which various intravascular stents work is opposition of elastic recoil of vascular stenoses by means of either self-expansion or assisted expansion on an angioplasty balloon. Stents and stent grafts have further expanded the indications for endovascular iliac artery revascularization.[9,10]

Indications for Iliac Artery PTA and Stent Placement

Clinical indications include lifestyle-limiting intermittent claudication, which was categorized by Fontaine into stages IIa and IIb (less than 250 m walking distance) and by Rutherford into the categories 1 (mild claudication, postexercise ankle pressure >50 mm Hg) to 3 (severe claudication, postexercise ankle pressure <50 mm Hg). Critical leg ischemia with rest pain (Fontaine III, Rutherford 4) and tissue loss with nonhealing ulcer or gangrene (Fontaine IV, Rutherford 5 and 6) are, of course, also indications for endovascular revascularization of iliac artery obstructions.[11] Furthermore, distal embolization from an iliac artery plaque with blue toe syndrome might be an indication for balloon dilatation or stent placement.[12,13]

Based on the angiographic demonstration of the aortoiliac and leg arteries, the Society of Cardiovascular and Interventional Radiology issued the following recommendations for PTA[14]:

Category 1 (PTA procedure of choice): stenoses <3 cm in length that are concentric and noncalcified
Category 2 (well suited for PTA): stenoses 3 to 5 cm in length; calcified or eccentric stenoses <3 cm in length
Category 3 (amenable to PTA with moderate chance of success): stenoses 5 to 10 cm in length; chronic occlusions <5 cm in length
Category 4 (limited role of PTA): stenoses >10 cm in length, chronic occlusions >5 cm in length; extensive bilateral aortoiliac disease, in combination with abdominal aortic aneurysm

Thus, PTA is the modality of choice for short (<5 cm) segmental stenoses of iliac arteries. Long, diffuse stenoses (>5 cm) and iliac artery occlusions of one segment (either the common or external iliac artery) are amenable to endoluminal therapy, which has been shown to produce reasonable long-term results, but its superiority to bypass surgery has not been proved so far. Long occlusions that include both segments of the iliac artery (common and external iliac artery) should be treated surgically, if surgery is not contraindicated otherwise.

Technique of PTA of Iliac Artery Stenoses

PTA of iliac artery stenoses can be performed using an ipsilateral retrograde approach, a contralateral antegrade approach using a crossover technique, or a transaxillary access route.[15] Most commonly, unilateral stenoses are treated by retrograde dilation, whereas bilateral stenoses are dilated from one common femoral artery puncture using a crossover technique (Figure

61.1). However, in bilateral stenoses of the origin of the common iliac artery that involve the distal aorta, a bilateral retrograde approach ("kissing balloon" technique) should be used (Figures 61.2 through 61.4).[16]

After percutaneous puncture of the common femoral artery, a catheter introducer sheath is inserted and the obstruction is recanalized by a straight or curved guide wire. Once the occlusion is passed, an angiogram (20 mL of contrast medium, 300 mg I/mL flow rate of 10 mL/s) and pressure monitoring in the aorta and common femoral artery should be performed. In lesions close to the hypogastric artery, oblique views (lateral anterior oblique 30° for the right, right anterior oblique 30° for the left iliac artery) are recommended. From the angiograms the appropriate size of the balloon can be estimated. Exact measurements of vessel dimensions and morphology may be obtained using intravascular ultrasound. In general, an 8- to 10-mm balloon is suitable for common iliac arteries, whereas a 7- to 8-mm balloon is used for external iliac arteries. Balloon dilatation at a pressure of 6 to 10 bar for 30 seconds is done at the point of stenosis. For long lesions, long balloons are preferable to overlapping dilatation with short balloons. After PTA a control angiogram and intravascular pressure monitoring must be performed. A residual stenosis of more than 30% and a resting residual mean pressure gradient of more than 10 mm Hg indicate that PTA was insufficient. Repeated PTA, if necessary with a larger balloon, or stent placement is indicated to improve the result.

Technique of Stent Placement in Iliac Arteries

Balloon-expandable and self-expandable stents were introduced into clinical practice in the late 1980s.[17] By means of continuous pressure to the arterial wall, stents prevent vascular recoil and remodeling. Thus, the initial result of endovascular recanalization is improved.[9,18–26] It has been accepted that stent placement is indicated if PTA alone does not sufficiently improve the arterial diameter and reduce the pressure gradient. Most stents can be inserted through a 7-F vascular sheath. "Road mapping" is very helpful for exact placement of stents. In both self-expanding and balloon-expandable stents, it is necessary to press the stent into the arterial wall to permit rapid endothelialization of the stent. This can be done by a high-pressure balloon at 10 to 12 atm. We and various groups recommend using flexible stents such as the Wallstent for long and tortuous iliac artery segments (Figures 61.3 and 61.5 through 61.9).[9] If exact placement is mandatory, as in obstructions at the aortic bifurcation or the iliac bifurcation, stents that have minimal shortening, such as the Palmaz stent, are recommended (Figures 61.1, 61.2, and 61.4).[18] If stenting at the aortic bifurcation is necessary, an overlap of the contralateral common iliac artery should be avoided because late thrombotic occlusions have been observed. Also, to avoid spontaneous thrombosis, the hypogastric artery should not be crossed by stents. Although long-term patency of side branches crossed by stents has been described experimentally and clinically, thrombotic occlusion was also found.

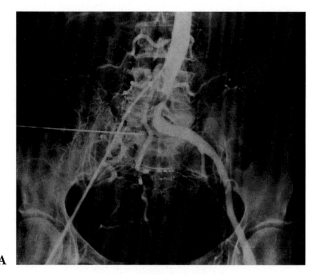

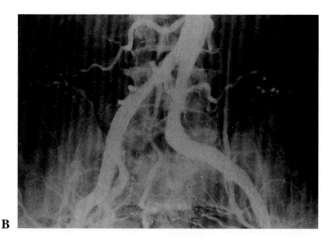

FIGURE 61.1. **A,** Complete occlusion of unknown extent of the right common iliac artery involving external iliac artery was traversed by a catheter and guide wire. Short-segment, eccentric, high-grade stenosis of the left common iliac artery was also present. **B,** After stent placement and percutaneous transluminal angioplasty (PTA) of the right iliac artery and PTA of the left iliac artery, full patency of the iliac arteries was restored.

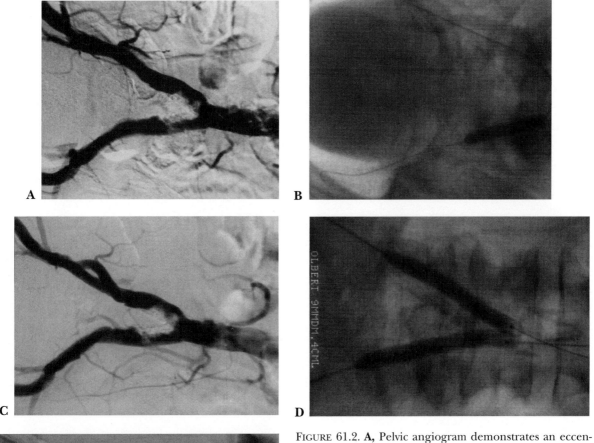

FIGURE 61.2. **A,** Pelvic angiogram demonstrates an eccentric, high-grade stenosis of the left and a moderate stenosis of the right common iliac artery. **B,** Balloon angioplasty was done in a crossover technique using an 8-mm balloon. **C,** Postangioplasty angiogram shows residual stenoses of both common iliac arteries. **D,** Two Palmaz stents were placed side by side in both common iliac arteries using the "kissing balloon" technique. **E,** After percutaneous transluminal angioplasty and stent placement, angiogram shows resolution of the stenoses, with full luminal patency and smooth contours.

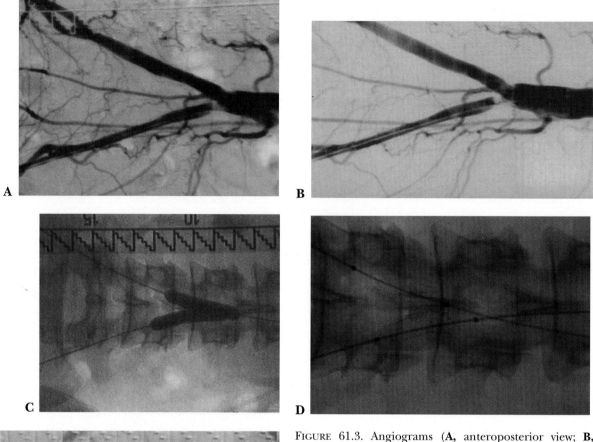

FIGURE 61.3. Angiograms (**A,** anteroposterior view; **B,** oblique view) demonstrate short-segment high-grade stenosis of the left common iliac artery close to the aortic bifurcation with a guide wire in place. **C,** Balloon angioplasty in "kissing balloon" technique. **D,** Placement of two Wallstents side by side in both proximal common iliac arteries, covering the iliac orifice. **E,** Angiogram shows free flow with good patency.

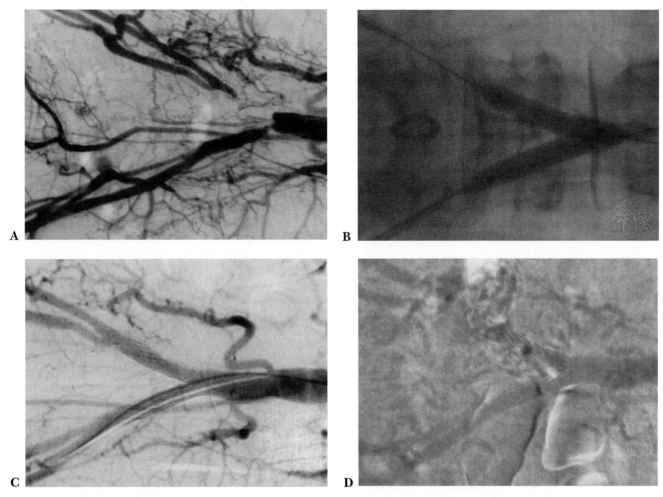

FIGURE 61.4. **A,** Diagnostic angiogram reveals a long segment of occlusion in the right common iliac artery and a high-grade stenosis at the origin of the left common iliac artery. **B,** After balloon dilatation in the "kissing balloon" technique and placement of two Palmaz stents, angiogram (**C**) shows excellent morphologic results. **D,** Intravenous angiogram at 1-year follow-up reveals free patency of stents.

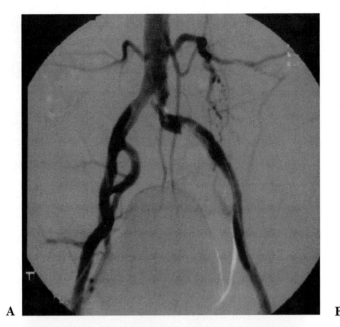

A

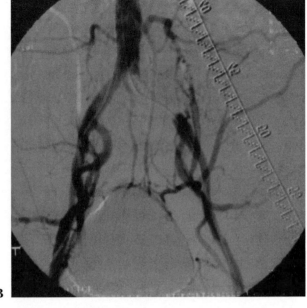

B

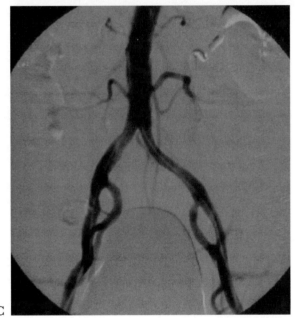

C

FIGURE 61.5. **A,** Angiogram discloses eccentric tandem stenoses of the left common iliac artery. **B,** The post-PTA angiogram reveals angioplasty dissection with abrupt vessel closure. **C,** Angiogram after placement of a Wallstent endoprosthesis shows a normal-appearing iliac artery.

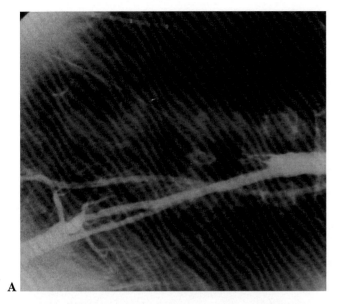

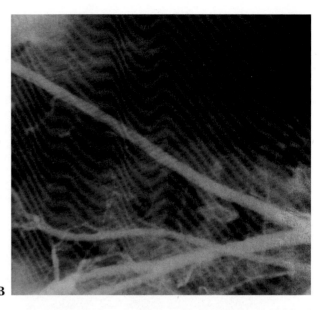

A B

FIGURE 61.6. Images of a patient with severe claudication on the right. **A,** Complete occlusion of the right common and external iliac arteries after retrograde catheterization. **B,** Angiogram obtained after placement of two Wallstents and PTA shows excellent morphologic result.

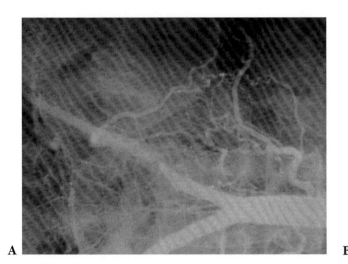

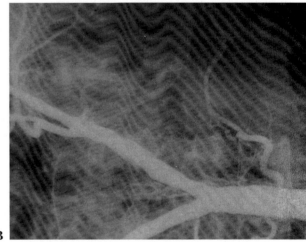

A B

FIGURE 61.7. **A,** High-grade stenosis of the distal right common iliac artery. **B,** After placement of a Wallstent endoprosthesis and subsequent balloon angioplasty, full patency and smooth contours are seen.

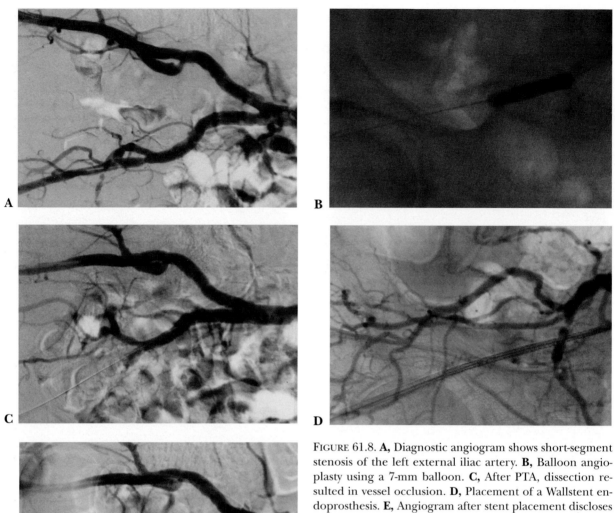

FIGURE 61.8. **A,** Diagnostic angiogram shows short-segment stenosis of the left external iliac artery. **B,** Balloon angioplasty using a 7-mm balloon. **C,** After PTA, dissection resulted in vessel occlusion. **D,** Placement of a Wallstent endoprosthesis. **E,** Angiogram after stent placement discloses a markedly improved lumen of the left external iliac artery.

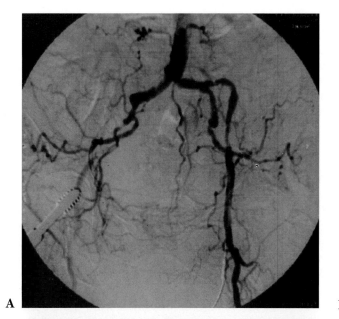

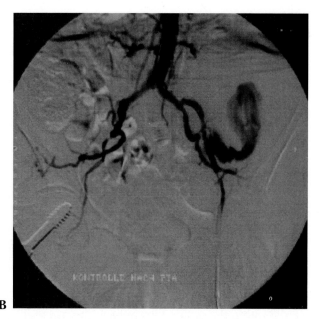

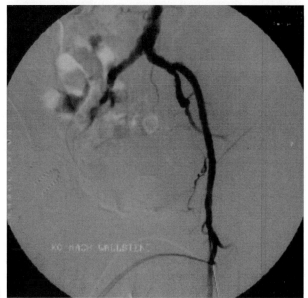

A

B

C

FIGURE 61.9. Major complication during treatment of severe atherosclerotic disease of the iliac arteries. **A,** Angiogram shows long-segment occlusion of the right external iliac artery and tandem stenoses of the left external iliac artery. **B,** After PTA of left external iliac artery using a 7-mm by 4-cm balloon, angiogram revealed local arterial rupture with extravasation of contrast medium. **C,** The leak was successfully treated by means of placement of a Wallstent endoprosthesis, as shown by angiogram. However, a large retroperitoneal hematoma, requiring surgery, was found on a computed tomography scan.

In aortoiliac plaques, which cannot be sufficiently treated by balloon angioplasty alone, bilateral stent placement is necessary. In these patients, both stents should be placed more proximally into the aortic lumen to cover the aortic part of the obstructing plaque. The success of stent placement should also be documented by angiography and pressure recording.

Technique of Recanalization of Iliac Artery Occlusions

Iliac artery occlusions were not recommended for PTA when stents were not available, because the immediate and long-term results were poor.[19-21] Distal emboliza-

tion or angioplasty-induced dissections were a common complication. The introduction of intra-arterial fibrinolysis and stent placement has changed the clinical results.[22-26] Thus, segmental obstructions of the common or external iliac artery should primarily undergo endoluminal recanalization and stent placement before any bypass technique is applied.

Whether intra-arterial fibrinolysis should be used first in every case is still under debate. Thrombi appropriate for lysis can be found within the iliac artery even 9 to 12 months after the thrombotic event. Two methods can be used for intra-arterial fibrinolysis:

1. Placement of a curved catheter, such as a sidewinder Simmons-1 or a single-curve catheter, proximal to the

obstruction and infusion of recombinant tissue plasminogen activator at a dose of 2.5 mg/h or urokinase in a dose of 60,000 U/h for 6 hours. Heparin should be infused in a dose of 1000 U/h after an initial bolus of 5000 units. Thrombin time, partial thromboplastin time, and fibrinogen level should be tested after 3 hours to determine systemic effects, if any.

2. Retrograde or antegrade crossover probing of the obstruction with a guide wire and insertion of a pulse spray catheter. The catheter should be placed exactly within the obstruction. Local pulse spray fibrinolysis is performed using 10 to 15 mg of recombinant tissue plasminogen activator for 90 minutes or 600,000 units of urokinase for 90 minutes. The pulse spray technique causes the thrombus to be fragmented, thus permitting a larger surface area of the thrombus to interact with the fibrinolytic agent.

The purpose of fibrinolysis is to dissolve the thrombus material within the artery. This reduces the risk of distal embolization. After successful fibrinolysis the stenosis that caused the obstruction can be demonstrated on angiography. Finally, a stent is placed within the obstruction to press the plaque material to the vessel wall. After balloon dilatation within the stent, a confirmatory angiogram of the obstruction and a peripheral runoff of arteries is performed.

Results of PTA

Definition of Success

Primary success is angiographically defined by a gain of more than 50% of stenosis diameter or less than 30% residual stenosis with antegrade flow. Hemodynamic success recorded by intra-arterial pressure measurements is defined by a transstenotic mean pressure gradient of <10 mm Hg at rest. Clinical success means an improvement by at least one clinical stage or category. The ankle—arm Doppler index should improve by at least 0.15.

Adjunctive Pharmacological Treatment

In general, 5000 units of heparin are given during the procedure and 500 to 1000 U/h of heparin are infused for 24 to 48 hours after successful PTA. The partial thromboplastin time should be prolonged to 1.5 or 2.0 times the normal value. Acetylsalicylic acid before and after PTA is recommended at a dose of 50 to 100 mg/d. If stents are placed, ticlopidine is recommended at a dose of 250 mg/d for at least 30 days. Because ticlopidine might cause leukopenia, continuation for more than 30 days should be prescribed only if the white blood cell count is monitored.

The German–Austrian Multicenter Study, which was a prospective, double-blind, randomized trial, revealed no statistical difference in terms of long-term patency between acetylsalicylic acid medication and placebo. Only the side effects were significantly higher (13.5% versus 7.3%, $P < .001$) in the acetylsalicylic acid group (unpublished data).

Long-Term Results

A large number of reports have documented the primary technical success rates and the long-term results of PTA and stent placement in iliac artery obstructions.[15,17,27–41] The primary technical success rate of PTA in iliac artery stenoses is about 95%. In iliac artery occlusions, recanalization is successful in 70% to 80% (Table 61.1). The primary long-term patency rate after balloon angioplasty of stenoses is 85% at 2 years and 65% at 5 years.[39] Becker et al.[15] compiled data from the literature about PTA, showing an average technical success rate of 92%, a 2-year patency rate of 81%, and a 5-year patency rate of 72% for 2679 procedures. After stent placement, the 2-year patency rate was 90% and the 5-year patency rate was 75%, regardless of the stent type used. For the Palmaz stent a multicenter trial that involved 486 patients revealed a technical success rate of 99%. Clinical patency at follow-up was 90% after 1 year and 84% after 2 years.[17] There has been only one prospective randomized trial comparing PTA and stent placement in the iliac arteries. After 2 years the restenosis rate was 27% for PTA and 14% for stent placement.[37] In iliac artery occlusions the primary 2-year patency rate was 83%, the 5-year patency rate was 55%, and the secondary or assisted 2-year and 5-year patency rates were 90% and 75%, respectively.[38] Stent patency rates were significantly higher in short versus long lesions (88% versus 63% at 3 years). At multivariate analysis, lesion length was the only predictive factor for long-term patency.[34]

Complications

Complications have been categorized as major and minor. Complications from the use of angioplasty or stent placement include dissection, occlusion, embolization, arterial rupture, and limb loss and death.[25,40,41] Death and limb loss due to endoluminal revascularization were observed in 0.2% of patients in each treatment group. Arterial rupture and arterial perforation are also rare events (0.2%) that are managed currently by placement of a polyester- or polytetrafluoroethylene-covered stent graft (Figure 61.9).[45] The most common major complication after PTA or stent placement in iliac arteries is thromboembolism. Embolization after stenting of iliac artery occlusions was reported by Vorwerk in 4.8% and by Strecker in 2.8% of patients.[34,38] The overall rate of

TABLE 61.1. Effects of local thrombolysis, percutaneous transluminal angioplasty, and/or stent implantation of iliac artery stenosis or occlusion.

Study	No. of lesions	Lysis	PTA	Stent placement	Primary recanalization rate*	No. of early reocclusions	Cumulative patency rate (%)	Mean follow-up (mo)†
Auster et al.[24]	8	8	7	0	7 of 8 (88)	0	100	8 (1–19)
Becker et al.[42]	64	0	50	0	50 of 64 (78)	0	78	NA (6–48)
Blum et al.[22]	667	0	667	0	67 of 82 (82)	0	58	36
Colapinto et al.[20]	15	9	12	12‡	12 of 15 (80)	1	92	7 (1–14)
Johnston[31]	68	0	0	48§	48 of 68 (71)	2	93	6 (1–22)
Kichikawa et al.[43]	5	5	5	5‖	5 of 5 (100)	0	100	10 (2–18)
Long et al.[39]	47	47	43	18‡	46 of 47 (98)	2	87	21 (3–53)
Long et al.[35]	12	0	12	12‡	NA	0	100	9.5(1–16.5)
Palmaz et al.[18]	171	0	171	171‡	NA	2	100	6 (1–24)
Rees et al.[44]	53	0	53	53§¶	NA	1	85.3	36
Sapoval et al.[41]	118	6	118	118‡§	NA	1	85	16 (3–36)
Stokes et al.[30]	70	0	70	0	66 of 70 (94)	3	66	(6–60)
Strunk et al.[40]	64	0	64	64¶	NA	4	81	(1–54)
Vorwerk and Günther[9]	118	0	118	118§	NA	3	88	24 (1–65)
Vorwerk et al.[38]	101	0	101	101§	NA	3	79.8	29 (1–78)

* Numbers in parentheses are percentages; † Numbers in parentheses are ranges. NA, not available; ‡ Palmaz stent; § Wallstent prosthesis; ‖ Gianturco stent; ¶ Strecker stent.

major complications is 3.9% to 6%; 2.5% to 3% require surgery. Minor complications such as a puncture-site hematoma or false aneurysm were reported in 4% to 5%. Thus, a total complication rate of about 10% may be expected.[15]

Conclusion

PTA for iliac artery obstruction has proved to be an effective and safe procedure. An initial success rate of 95% and a 2-year patency rate of 85% in combination with a mortality rate of only 0.2% justify the use of this method even in patients with lifestyle-limiting claudication.[15,34] Because of the short hospital stay of 48 hours, this method is also cost-effective. Therefore, hemodynamically significant and symptomatic stenoses as long as 5 cm should be treated by PTA. Whether stents will improve the result in all cases or should be used only if PTA fails remains unclear. The treatment of segmental iliac artery occlusions is currently under discussion. The use of intra-arterial fibrinolysis and stents has increased the success rate of endoluminal revascularization to 70% to 80%. The primary 2-year patency rate of stents in previously occluded iliac artery segments is 80% to 85%, and the secondary or assisted 2-year patency rate is 90%. These results are absolutely comparable to those of aortoiliofemoral reconstructive surgery, which is associated with a 1-year patency rate of 90%.[32] However, the morbidity is low in endovascular revascularization. Therefore, the European consensus document on chronic critical leg ischemia has proposed the following in recommendation number 23: "On a pragmatic basis, if the angiogram

shows a technically suitable lesion and an experienced interventional radiologist is available, a percutaneous catheter procedure should be tried as the first option, even though surgery may eventually be needed." However, recommendation number 22 emphasizes that "catheter procedures should be performed only by those appropriately trained in angiographic and angioplasty techniques."[32]

Long occlusions of the common and external iliac artery and bilateral occlusions have a lower chance of permanent patency, as analyzed by Strecker.[34] Therefore, patients with these lesions should primarily undergo surgical revascularization.

References

1. Dotter CT, Judkins MP. Transluminal treatment of arteriosclerotic obstructions: description of a new technique and a preliminary report of its application. *Circulation.* 1964;30:654–670.
2. Zeitler E, Schopp W, Zahnow W. The treatment of occlusive arterial disease by transluminal catheter angioplasty. *Radiology.* 1971;99:19.
3. Zeitler E. Percutaneous dilatation and recanalization of iliac and femoral arteries. *Cardiovasc Intervent Radiol.* 1980;3:207–212.
4. Grüntzig A, Hopff M. Perkutane rekanalisation chronischer arterieller Verschlüsse mit einem neuen Dilatationskatheter: Modifikation der Dotter-Technik. *Dtsch Med Wochenschr.* 1974;99:2502–2510.
5. Tegtmeyer CJ, Moore TS, Chandler JG, Wellons HA, Rudolf LE. Percutaneous transluminal dilatation of a complete block in the right iliac artery. *AJR Am J Roentgenol.* 1989;133:532–535.

6. Cragg A, Lund G, Rysavy J, Castaneda F, Castaneda-Zuniga W, Amplatz K. Nonsurgical placement of arterial endoprosthesis: a new technique using nitinol wire. *Radiology.* 1983;147:261–263.

7. Maass D, Kropf L, Zollikofer CL, et al. Transluminal implantations of intravascular "double helix" spiral prostheses: technical and biological considerations. *Proc Eur Soc Artif Organs.* 1982;9:252–256.

8. Palmaz JC, Richter GM, Noeldge G, et al. Intraluminal stents in atherosclerotic iliac artery stenosis: preliminary report of a multicenter study. *Radiology.* 1988;168:727–731.

9. Vorwerk D, Günther RW. Mechanical revascularization of occluded iliac arteries with use of self-expandable endoprostheses. *Radiology.* 1990;175:411–415.

10. Pernès JM, Auguste MA, Hovasse D, Ginier P, Lasry B, Lasry JL. Long iliac stenosis: initial clinical experience with the cragg endoluminal graft. *Radiology.* 1995;196:67–72.

11. Rutherford RB, Becker GJ. Standards for evaluating and reporting the results of surgical and percutaneous therapy for peripheral artery disease. *J Vasc Interv Radiol..* 1991;2:169–174.

12. Kumpe DA, Zwerdlinger S, Griffin DJ. Blue digit syndrome: treatment with percutaneous transluminal angioplasty. *Radiology.* 1988;166:37–44.

13. Brewer ML, Kinnison ML, Perler BA, White RI Jr. Blue toe syndrome: treatment with anticoagulants and delayed percutaneous transluminal angioplasty. *Radiology.* 1988;166:31–36.

14. Standards of Practice Committee of the Society of Cardiovascular and Interventional Radiology. Guidelines for percutaneous transluminal angioplasty. *Radiology.* 1990;177:619–626.

15. Becker GJ, Katzen BT, Dake MD. Noncoronary angioplasty. *Radiology.* 1989;170:921–940.

16. Tegtmeyer CJ, Kellum CD, Kron IL, Mentzer RM. Percutaneous transluminal angioplasty in the region of the aortic bifurcation: the two balloon technique with results and long-term follow-up study. *Radiology.* 1985;157:661–665.

17. Palmaz J, Laborde J, Rivera F, Encarnacion C, Lutz J, Moss J. Stenting of iliac arteries with the Palmaz stent: experience from a multicenter trial. *Cardiovasc Intervent Radiol.* 1992;15:291–297.

18. Palmaz JC, Garcia OJ, Schatz RA, et al. Placement of balloon-expandable intraluminal stents in iliac arteries: first 171 procedures. *Radiology.* 1990:174:969–975.

19. Ring E, Freiman D, McLean G, Schwarz W. Percutaneous recanalization of iliac artery occlusions: an unacceptable complication rate. *AJR Am J Roentgenol.* 1982;139:587–589.

20. Colapinto RF, Stronell RD, Johnston WK. Transluminal angioplasty of complete iliac obstructions. *AJR Am J Roentgenol.* 1986;146:859–862.

21. Rubinstein ZJ, Morag B, Peer A, Bass A, Schneiderman J. Percutaneous transluminal recanalization of common iliac artery occlusions. *Cardiovasc Intervent Radiol.* 1987;10:16–20.

22. Blum U, Gabelmann A, Redecker M, et al. Percutaneous recanalization of iliac artery occlusions: results of a prospective study. *Radiology.* 1993;189:536–540.

23. Hausegger KA, Lammer J, Klein G, et al. Perkutane Rekanalisation von Becken-arterienverschlüssen: Fibrinol-yse, PTA, Stents. *Rofo Fortschr Geb Rontgenstr Neuen Bildgeb Verfahr..* 1991;155:550–555.

24. Auster M, Kadir S, Mitchell S, et al. Iliac artery occlusion: management with intrathrombus streptokinase infusion and angioplasty. *Radiology.* 1984;153:385–388.

25. Hess H, Mietschak A, Brückl R. Peripheral arterial occlusions: a 6-year experience with local low-dose thrombolytic therapy. *Radiology.* 1987;163:753–758.

26. Poredos P, Keber D, Videcnik V. Late results of local thrombolytic treatment of peripheral arterial occlusions. *Angiology.* 1989;40:941–947.

27. Gallino A, Mahler F, Probst P, Nachbur B. Percutaneous transluminal angioplasty of the arteries of the lower limbs: 5-year follow-up. *Circulation.* 1984;70:619–623.

28. Van Andel GJ, van Erp WF, Krepel VM, Breslau PJ. Percutaneous transluminal dilatation of the iliac artery: long term results. *Radiology.* 1985;156:321–323.

29. Johnston KW, Rae M, Hogg-Johnston SA, et al. 5-year results of a prospective study of percutaneous transluminal angioplasty. *Ann Surg.* 1987;206:403–412.

30. Stokes KR, Strunk HM, Campbell DR, Gibbons GW, Wheeler HG, Clouse ME. Five-year results of iliac and femoropopliteal angioplasty in diabetic patients. *Radiology.* 1990;174:977–982.

31. Johnston KW. Iliac arteries: reanalysis of results of balloon angioplasty. *Radiology.* 1993;186:207–212.

32. Second European Consensus Document on Chronic Critical Leg Ischemia. *Circulation.* 1991;84(suppl):1–126.

33. Sapoval MR, Long AL, Pagny JY, et al. Outcome of percutaneous intervention in iliac artery stents. *Radiology.* 1996;198:481–486.

34. Strecker EP, Boos IBL, Hagen B. Flexible tantalum stents for the treatment of iliac artery lesions: long-term patency, complications, and risk factors. *Radiology.* 1996;199:641–647.

35. Long A, Sapoval M, Beyssen B, et al. Strecker stent implantation in iliac arteries: patencies and predictive factors for long-term success. *Radiology.* 1995;194:739–744.

36. Vorwerk D, Guenther R, Schürmann K, Wendt G, Peters I. Primary stent placement for chronic iliac artery occlusions: follow-up results in 103 patients. *Radiology.* 1995;194:745–749.

37. Richter G, Nöldge G, Roeren T, Brado M, Allenberg J, Kaufmann G. Further analysis of a randomized trial comparing primary iliac stenting and PTA. In: Liermann D, ed. *Stents: State of the Art and Future Developments.* Morin Heights, Canada: Polyscience; 1995:30–35.

38. Vorwerk D, Günther RW, Schürmann K, Wendt G. Aortic and iliac stenoses: follow-up results of stent placement after insufficient balloon angioplasty in 118 cases. *Radiology.* 1996;198:45–48.

39. Long AL, Page PE, Raynaud AC, et al. Percutaneous iliac artery stent: angiographic long-term follow-up. *Radiology.* 1991;180:771–778.

40. Strunk HM, Schild HH, Düber C, et al. Ergebnisse angiographischer Verlaufskontrollen nach perkutaner Stentimplantation in Beckenarterien mit Vergleich zwischen Wall- und Palmaz-Stent. *Rofo Fortschr Geb Rontgenstr Neuen Bildgeb Verfahr.* 1993;159:251–257.

41. Sapoval MR, Chatellier G, Long AL, et al. Self-expandable stents for the treatment of iliac artery obstructive lesions: long-term success and prognostic factors. *AJR Am J Roentgenol.* 1996;166:1173–1179.

42. Becker GJ, Palmaz JC, Rees CHR, et al. Angioplasty-induced dissections in human iliac arteries: management with Palmaz balloon-expandable intraluminal stents. *Radiology.* 1990;176:31–38.

43. Kichikawa K, Uchida H, Yoshioka T, et al. Iliac artery stenosis and occlusion: preliminary results of treatment with Gi-

anturco expandable metallic stents. *Radiology.* 1990; 177:799–802.

44. Rees CR, Palmaz JC, Garcia O, et al. Angioplasty and stenting of completely occluded iliac arteries. *Radiology.* 1989;172:953–959.

45. Gardiner JA Jr, Meyerovitz MF, Stokes KR, Clouse ME, Harrington DP, Bettman MA. Complications of transluminal angioplasty. *Radiology.* 1986;159:201–208.

62

Aortoiliac Occlusive Disease

Aurel Andercou

The terminal aorta and iliac arteries represent the most common location of atherosclerosis and therefore are of major surgical importance.

Surgical Anatomy

From an anatomico-topographical viewpoint, the terminal aortic region is situated above the promontory of the sacrum, having a triangular shape with the base downward. The triangle's base corresponds to the lumbosacral disk, situated at the level of the upper stricture of the pelvis. The triangle's point corresponds to the lower margin of the horizontal duodenum, and the two sides of the triangle correspond to the median margins of the psoas muscles. In a sagittal plane the base of the region is formed of the anterior part of the last lumbar vertebra and the intervertebral neighboring disks, covered by the anterior longitudinal ligament. The anterior side of the region is covered by the posterior parietal peritoneum and possibly by the sigmoid mesocolon.

The bifurcation of the terminal aorta into the two common iliac arteries is situated at the upper edge of the L4–L5 disk.[5] Most commonly it is found at about 6 cm from the promontory of the sacrum, above the bifurcation of the inferior vena cava. Three variants of aortic bifurcation may be distinguished:

1. Normal bifurcation, found in 71% of the cases, corresponding to the lower one third of the L4 vertebra
2. Low subduodenal bifurcation, corresponding to the upper half of the L5 vertebra
3. High retroduodenal bifurcation, corresponding to the upper one third of the L4 vertebra[5]

Stratigraphically, the region has three subperitoneal planes:

1. The anterior, nervous plane is formed of the upper hypogastric plexus, injury of which may cause sexual impotence. Lower mesenteric vessels, at the left of the aorta, are in this plane. In its lower part the region is covered by the sigmoid mesocolon.
2. The middle, arterial plane is formed of the terminal aorta and its bifurcation.
3. The deep, venous plane is formed of the origin of the inferior vena cava, situated at the level of the L4–L5 disk, at the lower right of the aortic bifurcation.

The middle sacral vessels, whose injury may cause severe hemorrhage, pass in the prevertebral plane.

The right common iliac artery, with a downward and sideways trajectory, is situated on an anterior plane in relation to the inferior vena cava. It crosses the origin of the left iliac vein at almost a right angle. When the bifurcation of the aorta is high, the right common iliac artery also covers the left edge of the inferior vena cava.

The left common iliac vein is situated in the fork of the common iliac arteries, inferior in relation to the homonymous artery. The iliac-arterial fork is higher than the iliac-venous fork and anterior to it and straddles the left common iliac vein.

In a healthy organism the dissection of the arterial from the venous plane is easy to perform because of the lax fibrous structures, but with atherosclerosis there are serious adhesions; sometimes the two structures are wrapped in a common fibrous sheath that makes dissection difficult and increases the risk of injuring the more delicate structures.

The relations of the terminal aorta are the following:

- Anterior: small intestine loops, parietal peritoneum, and mesentery
- Left: left ureter, left psoas muscle, left Toldt's coalescent fascia, and the root of the sigmoid mesocolon
- Right: venous bifurcation and the mesentery root
- Above: horizontal or third segment of the duodenum
- Below: the promontory of the sacrum
- Posterior: prevertebral plane, to which it is intimately attached, especially in the presence of atherosclerosis

The common iliac arteries are the terminal branches of the abdominal aorta. Each common iliac artery is wrapped in a connective–vascular sheath that continues the aortic sheath and then is continued by the sheaths of the external iliac and inferior epigastric arteries. The two external iliac arteries separate above the promontory at a 60- to 70-degree angle.

The common iliac arteries, 5 to 6 cm long, are directed downward, laterally, and slightly to the front. The left common iliac artery is more slanted, whereas the right one is 1.5 mm longer. Each common iliac artery is a passage artery that splits into two terminal branches: one posterointernal, the internal iliac (or inferior epigastric) artery, distributed to the pelvic organs and wall; and one lateral, the external iliac artery. The bifurcation of the common iliac artery is situated 4 to 5 cm from the median line, at the level of the sacral wing and the L5–S1 space. The distance between this bifurcation and the anterosuperior iliac spine may vary from 9 to 12 cm.

As the common iliac vessels pass along the middle margin of the iliac psoas muscle (psoas major), the latter becomes a satellite of the common iliac artery, up to the level of the sacroiliac joint, and then a satellite of the external iliac artery, up to the inguinal ligament. The relations of the common iliac artery are the following:

- *Anterior:* the origin is near the upper hypogastric plexus, which must be protected during dissection. On the left, the ureter crosses the left common iliac artery at 2.5 cm above the bifurcation. On the right, the ureter is at the level of the bifurcation. Regardless of the level of the common iliac artery bifurcation, this indicates its vicinity with the ureter, which must be protected. During coloparietal detachment the ureter is attached to the peritoneum. In the middle, the artery neighbors the following structures: middle sacral artery, upper hypogastric plexus, the prominent part of the promontory, internal iliac ganglia, the root of the sigmoid mesocolon, and the upper hemorrhoidal artery
- *Lateral:* internal iliac lymph nodes, genitofemoral nerve, ascending lumbar vein, genital vessels, and the psoas muscle. Genital vessels flank the common iliac artery and approach it without crossing it; farther below, they cross the external iliac artery

Etiopathogenesis of Atherosclerosis

By far the most frequent aortoiliac occlusive lesion is atherosclerosis. Other occlusions are exceptional, secondary to atherosclerotic lesions. Thus, a patient with atherosclerosis may develop thrombosis, which completes the occlusion. More rarely, embolization of cardiac myxoma or

vascular prostheses or fragments of prostheses may occur. Atherosclerosis is a chronic disease, of degenerative metabolic character, involving large- and medium-sized arteries of elastic or musculoelastic type; it is characterized by focal, disseminated deposits of lipids, carbohydrates, blood components, and calcium in the arterial intima, causing loss of elasticity and narrowing of the lumen.

In primary atherogenesis, in childhood and adolescence (the number of diagnosed patients under 35–40 years old is rather high), the genetic inheritance of membrane receptors plays an important role.[14,22] In adult atherogenesis other multiple risk factors are added, so that atherosclerosis has a "multifactorial determinism." Major risk factors include hyperlipoproteinemia, diabetes mellitus, arterial hypertension, and smoking.[14,38,46]

Hyperlipoproteinemia

The implication of hyperlipoproteinemia in atherogenesis is documented by experimental, histopathological, genetic, and epidemiological data.[57,79] Besides genetic disturbances, the lipoprotein metabolism disturbance is also induced by exogenous factors such as diet rich in saturated fatty acids or cholesterol, alcoholism, and oral contraceptive use.

The most important risk factors of atherogenesis are high levels of cholesterol (>220 mg/dL), triglycerides (>170 mg/dL), and lipids (>80 mg/dL).[79] Secondary hyperlipoproteinemia may also occur in patients with diabetes mellitus, nephrotic syndrome, chronic alcoholism, hyperthyroidism, and myelomatosis, the last indicating the possible intervention of immune mechanisms in lipoprotein metabolism regulation.[79] The increased circulating LDL level leads to endothelial damage and accumulation of cholesterol in the arterial wall; its accumulation in the smooth muscle cell and macrophage leads to cell proliferation, appearance of foam cells, necrosis, and proliferation of the connective matrix of the arterial wall.

Diabetes Mellitus

The atherogenic risk of diabetes mellitus is not directly related to the degree of hyperglycemia, treatment of which does not influence mortality by atherosclerosis. In diabetes mellitus, atherogenesis is favored by three converging mechanisms:

1. Damage of the adventitious vasa vasorum, with subsequent impairment of trophism and lipoid deposits
2. Enhancement of vascular injury because of the frequent association with arterial hypertension and obesity

3. Increase of thrombogenic risk, caused by impairment of erythrocytic plasticity following hemoglobin glycosilation by hyperlipemia and plasma concentration; the damage of the endothelium increases the risk of thrombosis, and parietal microthrombi favor lipoid deposit[38,79]

Secondary hyperlipidemia in diabetes mellitus leads to hypersynthesis of glycosaminoglycans in the arterial intima, which binds lipoproteins. Serum insulin and glucose, independent from lipoproteins, stimulate the proliferation of smooth muscle cells in the artery.

We have found that the association between peripheral atherosclerotic disease and diabetes mellitus is most harmful because it speeds the evolution of atherosclerosis, often causes early onset of gangrene, and negatively affects the response to surgical therapy.

Arterial Hypertension

After the age of 50, the importance of arterial hypertension in the development of atherosclerosis is greater than that of hypercholesterolemia, which points to the necessity of its early treatment. The role of hypertension in atherogenesis is manifested through the following mechanisms:

- Increase of mechanical pressure on the arterial walls favors the infiltration of lipoids in the walls
- High arterial pressure stimulates micromuscular proliferation and collagen synthesis in the vascular intima, increasing the number of fibrous plates in the arteries

Hereditary or induced (by aspirin or indomethacin) deficiency in the synthesis of prostaglandins PgA and PgE in the kidney allows the arterial pressure to increase, thus proving indirectly the involvement of prostaglandins in atherogenesis.[79]

Smoking

Smoking is incriminated in atherogenesis, especially when it exceeds 20 cigarettes per day. It has two adverse effects: it increases cardiac output and the myocardial contraction rate, and it increases peripheral resistance. The mechanisms of nicotine action are manyfold:

- Nicotine favors the release of catecholamines from the adrenals and sympathetic nervous system, causing peripheral vasospasm, mobilization of fatty acids, increase of adhesion, platelet aggregation, and degranulation
- Nicotine produces toxic microlesions and generates mitogenic factors

- Carbon monoxide increases the level of carboxyhemoglobin, leading to hypoxia and increased blood coagulation
- Nicotine negatively influences the stability of cell membrane receptors specific to lipoprotein metabolism

Secondary risk factors in the etiology of atherosclerosis are age, sex, diet, obesity, sedentary living, psychosomatic status, nervous or hepatic dysfunctions, and stress.

Pathogenesis of Atherosclerosis

The main pathogenetic hypotheses are each focused on one pathogenetic factor that may explain the onset of the disease:[14]

1. *The theory of endothelial defect* under the action of risk factors; selective endothelial continuity and permeability are altered, and platelet microaggregates that release macrophages in the intima and trigger the formation of the atherosclerotic plate are produced
2. *The theory of lipid infiltration,* according to which circulating lipids penetrate into the arterial wall either due to their high plasma concentration or under the action of arterial hypertension; their defective metabolization triggers the accumulation of foam cells and then formation of the atherosclerotic plate
3. *The hemodynamic theory,* by which blood flow disturbances represent a direct mechanical aggression that leads to the original endothelial injury
4. *The thromboatherogenetic theory,* according to which the original defect is also hemostatic disturbance, including an excess of factor XII fibrin stabilizer, with fibrin deposit in the intima; high cholesterol levels are associated with high plasma fibrinogen levels, which speed platelet aggregation and immobilization of monocytes, with subsequent formation of the atherosclerotic plate
5. *The lysosomal theory* considers as the primary factor the impairment of lysosomal activity in the smooth muscle cells, the lysosomes being incapable of metabolizing the lipids in the arterial wall
6. *The monoclonal theory,* by which the origin of intimal proliferation is represented by the existence of a unique and abnormal cell clone of smooth muscle cells, which occurs as a result of viral mutant factors; they proliferate similarly to benign tumoral cells

Each of these theories emphasizes one mechanism in the presence of a certain cluster of risk factors, but none of them can be held solely responsible for triggering the atherogenic process. The various initial aggressive factors eventually lead to the joining of the pathogenetic mechanisms, and therefore the evolution of atherosclerosis after onset is less controversial. The major role is attributed to lipoprotein metabolism disturbances, namely, cholesterol.

The pathogenetic events at a cellular level that cause the formation of the atherosclerotic plate may be summarized as follows. Normally, a small amount of lipoproteins, especially cholesterol, passes through the endothelium and is cleared by the scavenger cells. If the amount increases, the scavenger cells become overloaded and become foam cells. They lose the capacity of leaving the intima across the endothelium and become sclerosed. The necrotized debris attracts macrophages and smooth muscle cells of secretory phenotype into the intima. Together with the stimulated endothelial cells they realize a connective cellular system that tends to isolate the cell debris and represents the beginning of the atherosclerotic plate. The presence of minimal function proteins suggests the onset of a self-maintained inflammatory process.

If the triggering factors of the previously mentioned process persist, the atherosclerotic plate develops and tends to obstruct the vascular lumen. Complications appear, such as fissure, ulceration, calcification, local formation of thrombi, hemorrhage in the plate, and distal embolization of fragments detached from the atherosclerotic plate.

Bifurcation of the Aorta as the Preferred Site of Atheromatous Lesions

It has been statistically documented that the preferred site of atheromas is the bifurcation of the aorta (30%), followed by the iliac bifurcation (26%), which indicates the aortoiliac segment as the preferred site of atheromatous processes—56% of the total number of sites.

Mechanical factors that interfere with hemodynamics play a decisive role in this localization. At the bifurcation the vascular structure, with the circular and longitudinal arrangement of elastic and resistance elements, changes to achieve the bifurcation spur of the two iliac branches. The spur loses some elasticity to gain resistance, achieving a mechanical division of the linear flow, which is directed to the lateral wall of the common iliac arteries. The spur is subjected to constant microtrauma, and the laminar flow is transformed into a turbulent one.

The origin angle of the iliac arteries with the aorta is also important because it explains the various locations of the areas of maximal stress. Thus, in the case of a wide

angle the location of atheromas is predominantly on the lateral walls of the iliac arteries, whereas with a sharper angle the location is mostly on the bifurcation spur.

Atheromas alter the structure of the aortoiliac wall by inducing patches of parietal hardening that alternate with relatively supple areas. The variations in elasticity and flow resistance influence the blood flow and its velocity, which become uneven. At a constant peripheral resistance, diastolic output and pressure decrease with the rigidity of the aorta. Systolic pressure increases maximally. The output and pressure variations are maximal, which puts the aortic wall under increased strain.

Alteration of aortoiliac elasticity is accompanied by alterations of the segmental cross section through the atheromatous plate. By the synergic effect of these alterations, the blood flow pattern becomes irregular, the velocity being in reverse proportion to the cross section. Alteration of the vascular diameter makes the laminar blood flow turbulent. When the aortic wall loses its elasticity, the pressure variations may cause ruptures of the aortic wall tissue.

Humoral and enzymatic changes are added to the local mechanical changes. High cholesterol levels induce excessive incorporation of cholesterol in the endothelial cell membrane and decrease cellular flexibility. The stress at the bifurcation causes microlesions that result in retraction of the cells, enlargement of the intercellular space, and increased embedding of lipoproteins in the intima. The lesions progress and cause denudation of connective tissue areas and release of mitogenic factors that attract smooth muscle cells and macrophages to the intima. Reendothelization is thus stimulated, but the new endothelial cells secrete mitogenic factors whose action is synergic with that of the platelet factors, maintaining the atherogenic process.

It has been clinically confirmed that Leriche's syndrome begins at the level of the common iliac arteries. This occlusion syndrome of the bifurcation of the common iliac arteries reaches the aortic bifurcation at the mature stage.[33,34]

Pathomorphological changes of the aortoiliac segment are followed by hemodynamic alterations, in terms of blood flow velocity, pressure, and direction. Impaired circulation is accompanied by alteration of nonspecific elements of protection against intravascular coagulation, leading to conditions that favor thrombosis. This phenomenon, separate as a mechanism but closely related to the atheroma, represents the so-called thrombosis of completion of atheromatosis. Aortoiliac atherosclerotic occlusion, by impairing hemodynamics, establishes new pathways and directions of circulation in an attempt to compensate for the circulatory deficit of the lower limbs, achieving the collateral circulation that explains the "compensated" forms of chronic aortoiliac occlusion.

Clinical Picture of Aortoiliac Occlusion

The rich collateral circulation explains the relatively late onset of symptoms of peripheral disease in aortoiliac occlusion. The development of collateral circulation depends on the acute or chronic character of the occlusion, the level and extent of the segment involved, and the condition of the lower vascularization. Collateral circulation appears like natural functional bypasses on multiple levels. It develops in the following ways:

- Winslow's circulation system through the intercostal arteries—external iliac artery
- Upper and lower epigastric arteries—lower mesenteric artery—hemorrhoidal artery—deep branches of the inferior epigastric artery
- Lumbar arteries (especially the first two pairs)—iliolumbar arteries—upper gluteal arteries
- Intercostal arteries—lumbar arteries—deep circumflex iliac artery—iliolumbar artery—upper gluteal artery

The evolution of atherosclerotic occlusion is asymptomatic for a long time because of the slow pathomorphological process and the many possibilities of collateral circulation development on the pre-existent anastomoses.

In most cases the clinical picture takes the aspect of chronic peripheral ischemic syndrome. Aggravation of the chronic ischemia or superimposition of an acute obstructive episode leads to acute peripheral ischemic syndrome, which may lead to loss of the lower limb or even the patient's life.

The clinical picture of aortoiliac occlusion was first described by Leriche in 1940.[34,64] The mean age of the patients is between 44 and 46 years. The disease is predominant in men, with the sex ratio varying between 1:11 and 1:25. The case history should emphasize risk factors: smoking, diet rich in saturated fats and/or carbohydrates, arterial hypertension, and diabetes mellitus. Relevant family history should be noted.

Diagnosis of associated diseases is important because it can worsen the prognosis. Because atherosclerosis is a generalized disease, the patient should be considered from a more general viewpoint, and an overall assessment of the vascular status is necessary. In this respect, we could refer to "hard" and "soft" factors of the vascular condition.[41,42,47] Hard factors include the following:

1. Stroke, transient cerebral ischemia, amaurosis fugax
2. Angina, acute myocardial infarction
3. Intermittent claudication, nocturnal pain in the lower limbs
4. Heavy smoking
5. Abdominal pulsating mass

Soft factors include the following:

1. Tiredness
2. Subjective changes of body temperature, especially coldness
3. Edema
4. Alteration of the color of extremities
5. Muscular cramps

Subjective Alterations

Paresthesia consists of alterations that do not correspond to the real condition. Numbness is manifested as a feeling of heaviness in the affected limb. Prickling sensation is also perceived as itchiness, initially occurring in certain positions, then with heavy exercise, in the cold, and, finally, at rest. Hypesthesia refers to a decrease in sensitivity and occurs after the feeling of numbness. Hyperesthesia occurs at the light mechanical or thermal touch of the ischemic area and is manifested by pain.

Involuntary muscular contractions, fascicular or by muscular groups, originally with and after heavy physical exercise, end by painful contraction with a feeling of rupture and adaptation to painless positions. Hyperventilation, alkalosis, and hypocalcemia alter neuromuscular excitability and make this an early symptom experienced long before claudication appears.

The feeling of tiredness and decrease of muscular force have a progressive onset. The feeling of a cold limb, following impaired blood flow, causes discomfort. The extremity acquires the temperature of the environment.

Pain is the sign that attracts attention, and it occurs in 90% of patients. It is due to the presence of kinins, lactic and pyruvic acid, potassium, and acid catabolites in the circulation, inducing metabolic acidosis. The cause of metabolic acidosis is the shift of cell metabolism to anaerobic glycolysis, when partial pressure of oxygen in the interstitial fluid and cells decreases gradually to zero and the adenosine triphosphate reserve is quickly depleted. Regarding pain, the important factors are the intensity, rate of occurrence, triggering factor, form, character, site, duration, and time from physical exercise discontinuation until it subsides. Exercise-induced pain is called *intermittent claudication,* and rest pain is called *discontinuous pain.*

Intermittent claudication occurs as a deep cramp of the obstructed muscles, forcing the patient to stop until pain subsides. The claudication index, described as the distance walked by the patient on a flat surface until claudication appears, depends on the severity of the occlusion, the speed of its onset, and the development of collateral circulation. It occurs in the thigh, buttock, and hip. Its presence in the shank and foot indicates an associated femoropopliteal occlusion. In the beginning, pain occurs with heavy physical exercise, then with lighter exercise. It is due to insufficient blood flow at muscular effort (when blood flow increases 10 times more than at rest) and also to the lowering of pain threshold of the ischemic tissues. Later, pain occurs at rest, with warmth (by increased metabolism), and especially at night.

Sexual dynamic disturbances occur in about 10% of the patients and are due to impaired vascularization through the internal iliac arteries; they include an inability to have a stable erection.

Objective Alterations

The first signs of vascular distress are the following:

- Body bearing and weight, obesity, general morbidity, and dyspnea
- Psychiatric disposition, for the cerebrovascular status
- Aspect of fingers and tobacco smell
- Forms of hypercholesterolemia with xanthoma

General physical examination reveals an ill patient, with biological age exceeding the chronological age, with a pained, anxious facial expression. Objective signs appear late in the chronic ischemic syndrome, but they are early in acute ischemia.

Changes of the color of the integument appear late, with pallor first associated with physical exercise or exposure to cold, then becoming permanent. Cyanotic aspect occurs when slow venous circulation is present (venous thrombosis, heart failure). Moist gangrene is specific to mixed arterial and venous distress. Redness of extremities is due to anoxic capillary paralysis, with slowing of capillary arterial circulation, to which slow oxyhemoglobin decomposition at low temperatures is added, which maintains a higher oxygen level in the venous blood. Cyanotic petechiae alternating with the pale ones indicate extremely severe ischemia, which is generally irreversible, during acute venous thrombosis or lower limb ischemia.

Alterations of the skin and visible structures include thin, parchmentlike skin; falling hair; and deformed, thick nails with loss of shine and coarse surface. These changes are even more obvious when associated with dermatomycoses, which are prone to appear on ischemic areas.

Skin temperature is lower on the affected side, a difference of 2 to 4° being relevant. Trophic lesions are characterized by ulcerations, necrosis, and gangrene. Ulceration and necrosis are alterations of the skin and subcutaneous tissue, which occur more frequently in case of trauma.

They are patchy, necrobiotic lesions, located on the thighs or fingers, originally no more than a dot, then growing in size. The result is an atonic wound, grayish in aspect, often involving bones and joints. Gangrene may be dry, dehydrated, mummylike, or humid, when superinfection occurs, especially when associated with diabetes mellitus. Gangrenous zones are painful until the onset of necrosis, when the pain is felt only at the edges.

Edema complicates the course in the end stage of the disease; it is white or purple, indicating venous or lymphatic involvement. Examination of the abdomen may evidence symmetric or asymmetric deformity on the aortic tract, possibly synchronized with the heartbeats; abdominal aortic aneurysm may be suspected. Perspiration may also be affected. Anhydrosis indicates severe ischemia with cessation of sweat gland function, the leg being pale, dry, and cold.

Palpation of the arteries in the initial stages evidences decrease of amplitude. In the more advanced stages the pulse changes are obvious, down to lack of pulse in the posterior tibial, plantar, popliteal, and superficial femoral arteries, unilaterally or bilaterally. In cases of aortoiliac occlusion with developed collateral circulation, pulsations may be perceived in the abdomen, above the inguinal ligaments or in Scarpa's triangle, which must be not confounded with the femoral pulse. In case of relatively tight stenoses, palpation may evidence systolic vibrations that point above the site of the stenosis. Their amplitude may indicate the degree of stenosis.

Auscultation may detect murmurs that are more intense when the vessel is more superficial and stenosis is tighter. The presence of a murmur indicates greater than 70% stenosis. In abdominal aortic aneurysms, pulsating tumorlike masses are found in the abdomen, manifested at auscultation as a continuous murmur.

Examination of the body systems must be detailed, with special emphasis on the following:

- Overall vascular status (arterial hypertension, renovascular hypertension, abdominal angina)
- Heart condition, taking into account that coronary disease coexists in 18% to 35% of patients
- Neurological condition (ischemic vascular accidents, amaurosis fugax)

Clinical Tests

From the viewpoint of circulation, atheromatosis is a bidirectional disease: centrifugal and centripetal, because it goes "up" the large vessels, whose injury affects the flow in the peripheral vessels. Therefore, the assessment of peripheral circulation may provide information on the main vascular axes. The tests are easy to perform in any outpatient practice unit by the family doctor without special training in angiology. The Romanian school of surgery has made important contributions regarding these tests, some of which bear Romanian names.[64-66]

Cosacescu's test (named for a Romanian surgeon between the two world wars), or the dermographic sign. The affected limb is scratched longitudinally from top to bottom (a normal fork would do). In the area having blood flow, dermographism is positive, as marked by a hyperemic trace, whereas the area without blood flow is negative, the trace remaining pale.

Ion Jianu's test (named for a Romanian surgeon between the two world wars), or the iodine cutaneous test. The affected limb is swabbed with iodine tincture. After 24 hours the tincture is absorbed in the healthy areas, but not in the injured ones.

Posture test. The temperature of the environment should be below 20°C, and the patient should be calm, lying on the back. The skin color is noted, then the legs are raised to a vertical position. In aortoiliac occlusion the spontaneous onset of pallor is noted in the foot or whole leg because of hypoxia. The patient is then asked to sit on the side of the bed with legs hanging down. Normally, color is restored within 5 seconds, and the veins are refilled within 7 seconds. In the patient with occlusion of the terminal aorta, pallor involves the whole leg, reactive hyperemia reappears in 15 to 20 seconds, with a diffuse character, and venous refill takes 20 to 25 seconds. In the patient with extensive arterial occlusions, with deterioration of collateral circulation, arteriovenous anastomoses are open and venous refill occurs before reactive hyperemia, which indicates a poor prognosis. Reactive hyperemia does not occur in patients with arteriopathy who have undergone lumbar sympathectomy.

Moscovici's test. The affected limb is raised to a vertical position and wrapped with an Esmarch bandage. After 5 minutes the leg is put down on the floor and the bandage is removed. Blood will flow down to the limit of the affected area, recoloring the skin.

Hertei's cuff test. The cuff is applied to three limbs, one remaining uncuffed. Normally, arterial pressure increases by 50 to 60 mm Hg in the uncuffed limb. By rotation it may be established whether one of the lower limbs is affected, because the blood pressure in this limb increases significantly.

Paraclinical Examinations

Noninvasive Tests

Technological progress has made possible a number of noninvasive angiological tests, most of them providing information on the pathomorphology of the arterial system in atherosclerosis and especially on its function.

Oscillometry

Oscillometry, still performed in eastern Europe, is only for orientation and allows the assessment of permeability of the main arterial trunk. The oscillometric index depends on the cardiac output, arterial pressure, peripheral resistance, and vessel elasticity. This index cannot be compared in different patients and not even in the same patient in different examination conditions. A difference of more than 1 unit between one limb segment and the corresponding contralateral area is abnormal. Abnormal values do not indicate the extent of the lesions or of the peripheral and collateral blood flow.

For exercise oscillometry, measurements are taken before and then every 30 seconds during standard exercise. In the limb with occlusive injuries, both pressure and oscillometric index decrease with exercise.[65]

Ultrasound Examination

Ultrasound examination indicates the following:

- Blood flow velocity with Doppler ultrasound
- Direction of blood flow, both flux and reflux
- Size of arterial lumen and thickening of the arterial wall
- Permeability of the main arterial trunk, by measuring distal arterial pressure: the site and degree of arterial stenosis may be evidenced; arterial stenosis is indicated by a difference greater than 20 to 30 mm Hg between the segments of the same limb or between the two lower limbs; in aortic stenosis, systolic arterial pressure is consistently decreased in both limbs

Computed Tomography

Computed tomography allows examination of the aorta and iliac arteries, detection of true or false aneurysms and ruptured aneurysms, and detection of graft infection. By injection of contrast media, the presence of thrombi in an aneurysm lumen may be detected.[7,8,35]

Nuclear Magnetic Resonance Imaging

Modern devices allow the measurement of blood flow, because the flowing blood has a lower degree of magnetization than the vessel. The method is useful in establishing the diagnosis of aortic aneurysm (by visualizing multiple layers), rupture of the aorta, or suppuration of prostheses.

Thermometry and Thermography

Temperature differences are important. Infrared measurement allows delineation of areas with hypothermia due to impaired blood flow.

Transcutaneous PO_2 Monitoring

Determination of PO_2 indicates where to perform the amputation. A PO_2 pressure of 30 to 40 mm Hg in the arterial blood indicates blood flow at the limit of viability.[56]

Invasive Methods

Invasive methods evidence morphological changes of the arterial system. Direct measurement of arterial blood pressure is useful for the diagnosis of aortoiliac stenoses and in performing retrograde angioplasty of the iliac and femoral arteries.[35] Direct measurement of arterial blood flow provides information on the peripheral vascular bed of the limb. It may be performed electromagnetically or ultrasonographically. Rest pain occurs with more than 30% decrease of the normal arterial blood flow.[35]

Radioisotopic Methods

Radioisotropic methods investigate the rate of accumulation of the radioactive medium after its systemic administration. Isotopic clearance is the most frequently used method of assessment of blood flow in the skin and subcutaneous tissues. The study of the microcircuit by this method (technetium 99, iodine 131, and xenon 133) allows establishment of indications and contraindications of abdominal aorta reconstruction, the prognosis of surgery, and the selection of patients for amputation.[36]

Arteriography

Arteriography represents the recording of the full passage of the contrast media through the investigated arterial segment. Images are serial and may be monoplane or biplane. It may also be achieved by pulse teleradioscopy, radiocinematography in two planes, or recording on magnetic tape or diskette. Injection of the contrast medium is performed by electronic automatic injectors of high pressure. The approach and opacity of the aorta and its branches may be realized by various techniques.

Dos Santos arteriography may be performed by translumbar puncture of the aorta in the costal–vertebral angle, 9 to 13 cm left of the median line, with upward and median direction of the needle.

Seldinger's technique injects the opaque dye through a radiopaque catheter. The introduction may be retrograde, by transcutaneous puncture of the femoral artery, or anterograde, by route of the left axillary artery. With a radiopaque catheter that has performant curvatures, selective opacification of the abdominal branches of the aorta may be achieved, thus obtaining selective angiography. Seldinger's technique by femoral approach is indicated in iliofemoral, unilateral occlusions but is not used in patients with Leriche's syndrome, for which the anterograde approach is recommended.

For Vialett–Steinberg's intravenous aortography, a dose of 1 mL/kg body weight of contrast medium is injected fast in both arms, so that a radiopaque bolus is obtained. The time of exposure is determined in accordance with the circulation time from arm to tongue, which is the same as the circulation time from arm to upper lumbar aorta. The technique is useful when aortic aneurysm is suspected.

Digital subtraction angiography provides arterial images following intravenous or intra-arterial injection of the contrast medium. It has the advantage that smaller amounts of contrast medium are required than with classic aortography.

The principles of radiological semeiology are as follows:[64,65]

A. Morphological aspect

Atheromatous plate appears as a missing margin, irregular in shape and size, narrowing the arterial lumen asymmetrically

Stenosis becomes obvious when the lumen reduction is 50%

Stenosis may be preceded by a spindle-shaped dilatation

Occlusion appears radiologically as a defect of lumen filling over a segment or as a thrombosis completing a preexisting stenosis

Aortic aneurysms are frequently pervaded by clots and do not reveal their full shape and size on arteriography

In case of aortic rupture, aortography indicates the site and extent, the two channels, the communication orifices, and the damage of the emerging trunks

The volumetric aspect of the main vessels and their distribution to each sector is seen

Megadolichoartery is evidenced in large arteries that appear abnormally long, large, and sinuous, the origin of the trunks being displaced and distorted; the contrast medium progresses slowly

B. Dynamic aspect

Opacification normally takes place simultaneously in analog arterial territories

When there is a pressure gradient between two anastomotic systems, blood circulation direction is reversed

The filling circulation of the limbs is assessed in relation to the caliber and number of collateral vessels

The intensity of vascular bed opacity below the obstruction provides information on collateral circulation

The topographic aspect reflects the relation between organs and their distributive vessels[75]

Angioscopy

Angioscopy poses technical difficulties. It is useful in the long-term follow-up of patients with implanted intravascular stents or with arterectomy.[9]

Other Paraclinical Examinations

The assessment of the vascular status may be completed by eye fundus examination and determination of retinal central artery pressure.

The heart is examined clinically and functionally by electrocardiogram, x-ray, ultrasound and Doppler ultrasound, exercise tests, possibly cardiac catheterization, and possibly cineangiocardiography. The lung is examined clinically and paraclinically by spirometry, total lung and respiratory volume studies, measurements of circulation time and alveolar permeability, and simple chest x-ray examination. The liver is examined by hepatic tests: total direct and indirect bilirubin, thymol, alkaline phosphatase, and serum transaminase determinations. The kidney is assessed by urine tests: obervation of aspect and color; measurement of volume, specific density, pH, osmolarity, urea, creatine, creatinine, uric acid, glycosuria, and ketonic bodies; microscopic examination; urinary clearance test; urine culture; and urography.

Hematological examinations include typing of blood group and Rh factor, blood cell counts, and erythrocyte sedimentation rate. Serum examinations include total protein measurement, protein electrophoresis, and urea, creatine, and creatinine determinations. Carbohydrate and lipid metabolism are investigated by glucose tolerance test and measurement of blood sugar level, cholesterol, and triglycerides.

Hemostasis and fibrinolysis studies include determination of bleeding time, clot retraction, Howell's time, Quick's time (prothrombin time), plasma fibrinogen, coagulation factors, and thromboelastography. Acid–base balance is examined by the micro-Astrup method. Electrolyte examinations include measurement of Cl^-, Na^+, K^+, Ca^+, P^+, and Mg^-. Microbiological and parasitological examinations are carried out in the blood, pharynx, urine, and feces.

Positive and Differential Diagnosis

Positive Diagnosis

The following are taken into account for the diagnosis of atherosclerotic occlusion of the terminal aorta: family history, personal history, risk factors, history of the disease, clinical symptoms, and paraclinical examinations.

The history of the disease includes the following clinical elements: intermittent claudication in the lower limbs and buttocks, progressive atrophy of lower limb muscles, pale skin, broken nails, mycosis, decreased or absent pulse in the femoral arteries and distally to them, and sexual impotence in men.

The nature of atherosclerosis is evidenced by age over 40 years, involvement of large and medium vessels, other atherosclerotic sites, and presence of major risk factors. Distribution of the atherosclerotic damage is assessed by arterial pressure in arms and ankles, duplex ultrasound, and aortography.

The severity of the aortoiliac damage is assessed by aortography in two planes, duplex ultrasound, and digital subtraction angiography. The effect of the aortoiliac in-jury on the distal vascular bed is assessed by thermometry, thermography, plethysmography, Po_2 measurement, and radioisotopic techniques. For the diagnosis of aortic aneurysms, duplex ultrasound, computed tomography, and magnetic resonance imaging may be used.[57]

Differential Diagnosis

Differential diagnosis with thromboangiitis obliterans is based on the following: age between 20 and 40 years, predominantly found in men, involvement of large or medium vessels, and superficial thrombophlebitis migrans. Differential diagnosis of pain in the lower limbs includes the following:

Exercise pain of the following origins

Neurogenic: ischemia or horse tail compression, compression of the lower extremity nerves, Dejerine's disease

Locomotor: lumbar and pelvic arthropathies or arthropathies of the knees and metatarsal bones

Traumatic: musculoligament injuries, hematoma, tendinitis

Compressive syndromes: anterior lodge syndrome

Rest pain of the following origins

Neurogenic: peripheral venopathy, nerve compression, postinflammatory peripheral nerve sequelae, causalgia

Medullary benign and malignant tumors

Locomotor: rheumatoid polyarthritis, gout, popliteal synovial cysts, osteomyelitis, plantar arthropathy

Traumatic and polytraumatic injury

Other diseases: erythromelalgia, cellulitis, lipoma, benign and malignant bone tumors

Differential diagnosis of pain of vascular origin is established with the following:

- Deep or superficial phlebitis, where pain is less sharp and located in the venous tract
- Lymphangitis and lymphadenitis, which accompany infections
- Arterial embolism and thrombosis with sudden onset, violent pain, and signs of acute ischemic syndrome

In general, embolism occurs in a patient with the clinical picture of heart disease, whereas thrombosis occurs as a complication against an atheromatous background in a patient with intermittent claudication.

Classification of Aortoiliac Atherosclerotic Occlusion

Several criteria that may be used to classify aortoiliac atherosclerotic occlusion are described in the following sections.

Leriche and Fontaine's Classification by Clinical Stages

Stage I: paresthesia or short pains following prolonged walking or standing that subside at rest. The affected limb is pale and colder than normal. Pulse is diminished. Toes are sensitive to cold; the sensation of numb finger may occur.

Stage II: typical intermittent claudication located in the thigh or buttocks that subsides with difficulty even at rest. Skin is cold, dry, and thin and lacks elasticity. Distal pulsation is faint.

Stage III: ischemic pain occurs when the patient is resting and the legs are in a horizontal position. In a declive position, with the leg hanging, pain subsides. Disturbances of the touch sensation occur.

Stage IV: pain is intense and continuous and does not subside in a hanging position. Pretrophic or trophic (gangrene) disturbances occur.

World Health Organization Classification According to the Stage of Evolution

Stage I: characteristic pain with qualitatively normal pulses

Stage II: intermittent claudication pain and qualitatively normal pulses

Stage III: continuous pain during exercise and rest, subsiding when the leg is reclining; absent podiac or posterior tibial pulse

Stage IV: pain intensified in reclining position, absent pulse, with or without gangrene

Classification According to the Speed of Disease Evolution

Chronic Leriche's syndrome (classic): progressive, slow occlusion

Subacute Leriche's syndrome: a more severe evolution by early secondary thrombosis and less developed collateral circulation

Classification According to the Site of Aortoiliac Occlusion

High type: may include extension to the renal and mesenteric arteries

Medium type: obstruction at the aortic bifurcation

Low type: bilateral obstruction of the common iliac arteries and their branches

Diffuse type: aortoiliofemoral and popliteotibial lesion

Incomplete type: occlusion of one third or one half of the lumen, symmetrically, bilaterally, or unilaterally, with complete abolition of the axillofemoral shunt and bilateralization within a short period

Evolution and Prognosis

The average life expectancy of the patients with aortoiliac occlusion is clearly reduced by the evolution of the occlusion or the complications of atheromas in other sites.

Aggravation of the ischemia is due to the progression of the lesions, their extent above and below, and the appearance of stenoses and thromboses. Local trauma and infections, intercurrent pathological states, arterial hypotension, heart failure, and anemia may speed the evolution. Trophic ulcerations and gangrene occur, especially when diabetes mellitus is associated. Coronary lesions limit surgical therapy and increase operative risk; they reduce average life expectancy to half. The existence of other arterial injury (renal, mesenteric, or carotid) may induce the syndrome of "arterial steal" in the postoperative course. Association with gastric or duodenal ulcer prevents oral treatment with anticoagulants and vasodilators, influencing prognosis negatively.

Prognosis depends on the site and extent of the injury, the existence of other sites of atherosclerosis (coronary, cerebral, renal, or mesenteric), diabetes mellitus, duration of the disease, and intercurrent diseases. If there is no treatment from the beginning of the disease, prognosis may look like this: risk of extension of the injuries by thrombosis—10% within 5 years; risk of coronary disease or stroke—20% within 5 years; risk of amputation—20% within 10 years.[79] The cause of death is myocardial infarction, cerebrovascular accident, rupture of aneurysmal aorta, or sudden death.

Surgical Treatment

Nonsurgical therapy does not provide satisfactory results. In principle, it is recommended that any potentially lethal coronary artery lesion should be treated prior to surgical intervention on the abdominal aorta. Surgical treatment must be associated with prophylactic antibiotic therapy with second-generation cephalosporin before, during, and after the operation—for example, ceftriaxone, 1 to 2 g/d. Surgical therapy may be structured as follows:

Direct aortoiliac interventions:
    Operations to remove obstructions
    Reconstructive operations
Indirect interventions: sympathectomy
Amputations

Direct Surgery to Remove Obstructions

Angioplasty with an enlarging patch is a minimal operation frequently associated with other surgical techniques such as thromboendarterectomy, arterial bypass, and embolectomy. Because it is a minor intervention, it is suitable for limited atheromas in an artery with a permeable lumen below and without occlusion at other levels. The patch is made of synthetic material.[41,42,64-66]

Embolectomy is indicated in acute embolic ischemia. Direct embolectomy is more rarely used, being completed with Fogarty catheter control above and below the site. Indirect embolectomy using a Fogarty catheter achieves primary embolectomy and embolectomy in the reobstruction of the arterial axis and vascular prostheses.

Thromboendarterectomy

Thromboendarterectomy (TEA) removes the whole obstruction represented by the atheroma and completing thrombosis, together with the intima and part of the arterial tunica media. A cleavage plane must be found in the structure of the tunica media before the limiting external elastic lamella.[6,53] To achieve TEA the following must be taken into account:

- The lesions visualized by arteriography must be of limited extent.
- The vessel lumen must be completely cleaned of all debris of the intima or atheroma fragments.
- The distal section of the intima is sutured to the arterial wall to prevent the formation of a flap that may cause obstruction of the lumen and thrombosis.[23,37]

The most frequently used techniques of TEA are as follows:

- Semiclosed technique with stripper ring (Volmar)
- Semiclosed technique followed by the application of angioplasty with patch
- Open technique by longitudinal arteriotomy, for lesions of limited extent
- TEA by eversion of the artery, which makes possible maintenance of sexual potency in 80% of patients
- TEA with equipment that produces oscillations at a frequency of 8000 rpm, causing separation of the adventitia from the obstructive block
- Gaseous TEA; cleavage of the intima of the tunica media is obtained by pressure injection of CO_2
- TEA with cryocatheter makes the atheromatous plate adhere to the catheter suddenly brought to $-20°$ Celsius
- TEA with balloon catheter, used in elderly patients with many ailments and high surgical risk; balloon catheters are much more resistant than Fogarty catheters
- Laser TEA
- TEA by trituration with Le Ween's apparatus uses a mechanical device that breaks the atheromatous plates from outside the artery, which are then extracted by vigorous pull; after eversion of the intima, the fragments are removed by arteriotomy of the iliac artery[54,55]; however, one third of the patients are subjected to a more complex operation due to evolution of the disease.[54,55]

The advantages of TEA are that no postoperative infectious complications occur and collateral circulation is not affected. Disadvantages of TEA are that it cannot be used to treat extended lesions, it does not relieve obstructions of the inferior mesentery artery ostium, it may be complicated by aortic or iliac rupture, it includes the risk of an intimal flap, and it cannot be used when aortic aneurysms are present.[16,53,69]

Percutaneous Transluminal Angioplasty

Percutaneous transluminal angioplasty (PTA) accomplishes fragmentation of the intima and tunica media without loss of the artery's elastic properties. The technique is indicated in the primary stages of atherosclerotic arterial disease; the major indication is marked aortoiliac stenosis, which produces a transstenotic pressure gradient of 10 mm Hg. The best results are obtained in a solitary stenosis less than 4 cm long, and the indicated maximum length is 10 cm.

PTA may be applied in stenosis of the distal aorta or the aortic bifurcation by the kissing balloon technique, by which two catheters are introduced simultaneously by Seldinger's bilateral puncture, the risk of distal embolization thus being prevented.[2,45,78] Another variant is the crossover technique, in which in parallel with the deobstruction of the iliofemoral artery on the side on which the catheter is introduced, it is possible to achieve deobstruction of the contralateral iliac artery.[23]

Thrombosis of the vessel after PTA occurs more rarely than after other techniques, but long-term results are poorer than with reconstructive surgery.[30,44,46] In our experience (Surgical Clinic II of Cluj-Napoca, Romania), PTA was used in 11.3% of the patients, with good results for 11.8 ± 3.5 months; afterward, surgical treatment was required, which correlates with data reported in the literature.[46]

Percutaneous Laser Angioplasty

Lasers employed are of several types: argon in the visible spectrum, NaCl:YAC in infrared spectrum, and ultraviolet, functioning in a pulsating manner. At the level of the atheromatous plate, the luminous radiation is absorbed, which produces heat. The heat causes instantaneous evaporation of intracellular, extracellular, and some tissular water, achieving so-called photothermal ablation of the plate.[10,20,52] The technique is more difficult to use for calcified plates, which require 2000°C temperatures to be destroyed. However, by disintegration of the collagen and plate matrix, the latter may be easily extracted mechanically.[29,72]

Endovascular Stents

The use of stents is based on the introduction of mechanical devices with a centrifugal radial surface that dilates the vessel. Their first clinical use dates from 1987, by Sigwart and Rousseau,[9,81] who used a self-expanding steel mesh. It is introduced through an angioplasty catheter that is elongated until the moment of insertion and then springs to its original diameter and dilates the vessel.

Palmez[30] uses a semirigid stent placed through an angioplasty catheter, which, at the balloon's inflation, dilates both the stenotic site and the stent, the latter maintaining a conveniently open lumen. The newest stents are those "with memory," made of nitinol spiral wire (a nickel and titanium alloy), which have a calorically controlled memory of their shape.

Direct Reconstructive Surgery: Arterial Bypass

The idea of vascular bypass was first mentioned by Alexys Carell (1910)[65p530]; the first realization of the idea belongs to Jean Kunlin (1949).[65p545] The objective of the operation is to bring the arterial blood above the occlusion into the arterial axis below, irrigating the ischemic territory insufficiently supplied by collateral circulation.[17,28,59] Classification of bypasses is based on the following criteria:

A. Material used
    1. Biological (homologous) grafts
        a. Autografts
        b. Xenografts
    2. Artificial prostheses (allografts)
B. Topographical
    1. Anatomical bypass
    2. Extra-anatomical bypass

In aortoiliac surgery, only artificial prostheses are used because of the large vessel caliber. Today two types of synthetic materials are used to make artificial arterial prostheses: Dacron and expanded polytetrafluoroethylene.

Dacron prostheses are monothread, multithread, knitted, or woven. Elasticity is obtained by embossing. Porosity must be minimal at implantation and maximal at biological incorporation. Incorporation of the prosthesis after its mounting in the vascular axis takes place quickly by the formation of a 1-mm fibrin layer on the inner surface. The fibrin layer is then organized through the contribution of fibroblasts. These prostheses function well in areas with large-volume, high-velocity blood flow. They require anterior precoagulation.[68]

Polytetrafluoroethylene prostheses (commercial name: Gore-Tex) present, when analyzed by electron microscopy, very fine knots linked by fibers, producing a mesh structure with micropores of 4 to 110 μm. Having electronegative pores, the prosthesis presents a reduced risk of thrombosis; it requires anterior precoagulation. The disadvantage of clamping at the folding sites was eliminated by ring prostheses.[60-63]

The conditions required for proper functioning of a bypass are as follows:

- Good run-in and runoff (distal bed)
- Normal coagulation or hypocoagulation
- Sufficient arterial pressure to maintain normal flow through the bypass

Disadvantages of bypasses are as follows:

- Early and late risk of infection
- Appearance of false aneurysms
- Secondary occlusion

Anatomical Bypass

Aortobifemoral Bypass

Indications for aortobifemoral bypass are as follows:

- Occlusion of terminal infrarenal aorta
- Unilateral or bilateral occlusion of the iliac axis
- Abdominal aortic aneurysms

The operation may be preceded by percutaneous endoluminal angioplasty for the injuries limited to the iliac artery.

Aortofemoral bypass is performed transperitoneally by median xiphopubic laparotomy with the patient in Trendelenburg's position, using Y-shaped prostheses.[60-63] Abdominal aortic aneurysms longer than 7 cm are treated by applying an aortobifemoral bypass (or, only rarely, an aortounifemoral bypass), with optional cover of the prosthesis with a sheath formed of the remaining aneurysmal sac.[19,21,28,40]

Proximal anastomosis of the prosthesis may be end-to-end or end-to-side type.[50] I prefer the end-to-end type whenever possible, because it prevents, theoretically at least, hemodynamic disturbances such as whirls.[1] Distal anastomosis may also be end-to-end or end-to-side type.

Aortounifemoral Bypass

The indications for aortounifemoral bypass are much more limited than for other procedures and refer especially to extensive unilateral iliac atherosclerotic occlusions.[45,57]

Runoff is ensured by the superficial femoral artery. In case of its obstruction, distal anastomosis is performed on the deep femoral artery, taking into account that the output of the deep femoral artery may equal that of the external iliac artery, and it is enough to maintain the mobility of the leg.[76] The approach for the aortounifemoral bypass may be transperitoneal or retroperitoneal by pararectal incision.

Aortoiliac bypass is practically excluded from current surgical practice and has been replaced by PTA.[23]

Surgical Treatment of Multilevel Lesions

Single aortoiliac occlusion occurs in only one third of patients according to our experience (Surgical Clinic II, Cluj-Napoca, Romania); the other patients present multilevel lesions of the femoral or femoropopliteal segment. Collateral circulation allows a distal perfusion in 80% to 85% of patients, but in the remaining 15% to 20% distal revascularization is necessary, which can be achieved by long aortofemoropopliteal or distal aortofemoropopliteal bypasses.[18,25,33,34] Long bypasses down to the knee joint may be performed with artificial prostheses, whereas those below this level require internal saphenous vein grafts.

The lifetime of bypasses using artificial prostheses is in reversed proportion to the length of the tract, and therefore some technical contrivances are recommended:

- Bypasses with intermediate stops
- Sequential bypasses
- Composed bypasses

Long bypasses may be performed during one operation or over successive operations.[1,24,27]

An aortofemoropopliteal bypass with intermediate stop has a side-to-side anastomosis placed on the lower part of the common femoral artery, which revascularizes the thigh through the deep femoral artery. This anastomosis must be 2 to 3 cm long. Sequential bypasses include two separate bypasses, an aortofemoral bypass with a synthetic graft and a distal anastomosis on the upper part of the common femoral artery and another bypass with an internal saphenous vein graft that starts from the distal part of the common femoral artery and extends down to the level of the popliteal artery.[11,13,18,25] Composed bypasses are achieved by associating a proximal synthetic graft with an internal saphenous vein graft, with an end-to-end anastomosis in the middle or lower one third of the thigh.[1,18]

Extra-anatomical Bypass

An extra-anatomical bypass ensures a blood supply through pathways that do not follow the natural arterial tract. It is indicated when an anatomical bypass cannot be performed to save the affected extremity.[51,77] The major indications for extra-anatomical bypasses are as follows:

1. Very high risk of aortoiliac approach because of
   a. Adhesions following abdominal surgery or radiation
   b. Calcareous aorta
2. Extensive surgical interventions are ruled out because of
   a. Cardiorespiratory failure
   b. Renal failure
   c. Old age
3. Risk of anatomical grafts because of
   a. Suppurations of the implant zone (suppurative adenitis, bone tuberculosis, osteomyelitis, pelviperitonitis)

   b. Replacement of an anatomical bypass that shows suppurations or an anastomotic aneurysm manifested by hemorrhage[12,64–66,74]

To achieve an extra-anatomical bypass that passes the flexion areas that cause bending or folding of the graft, synthetic prostheses with rings or spirals are recommended.[11]

Bypasses used in aortoiliac surgery are axillofemoral, axillopopliteal, and thoracofemoral arteries.

Axillofemoral Bypass

In an axilliofemoral bypass, the graft is mounted proximally on the axillary artery side to end, then tunneled under the large pectoral muscle; it descends down the anterior axillary line to the iliac crest, then parallel to the crural arch to Scarpa's triangle, and is anastomosed distally end to side to the common femoral artery.[3] Axillofemoral bypass may be completed by a contralateral femorofemoral bypass, obtaining vascular prosthesis of both lower extremities.[12,31,65,66]

Axillopopliteal Bypass

An axillopopliteal bypass is used to revascularize the shank in the following cases:

- Failure of an aortofemoral or axillofemoral bypass
- Severe atherosclerosis that affects the superficial and deep femoral arteries, which cannot be used for revascularization
- Sepsis in the inguinal region due to infection of a previous vascular prosthesis[48,49]

Thoracic Artery–Femoral Artery Bypass

Thoracofemoral artery bypass is an alternative required when axillofemoral bypasses exhibit frequent thrombolization.[13,15,43,48,49] This bypass, using the thoracic artery as a source of inflow, has the following advantages:

- Decreased risk of infection because of deep positioning
- Shorter tract, closer to the physiological one, which ensures better hemodynamics

The operation is performed in disabled patients who have a history of multiple surgical interventions. It is performed through a retroperitoneal approach to the aorta, either without section of the diaphragm or with thoracophrenolaparotomy.[13,21,48,49] It may be completed with a femorofemoral crossover bypass.

Complications

Revascularization Syndrome

Revascularization syndrome consists of morphological and biochemical alterations, with local and general repercussions, occurring after reestablishment of arterial flow over a large segment with prolonged ischemia. The syndrome threatens the patient's life. Severe *metabolical changes* occur, starting from the revascularized musculature:

- Metabolic acidosis caused by anaerobic metabolism
- Decrease of blood pH in the ischemic area
- Decrease of P_{O_2} and increase of P_{CO_2} in peripheral venous blood
- Increase of serum K^+ in the venous flow in direct relationship with the degree and duration of arterial occlusion by alteration of cell membrane permeability
- Increase of azotemia and creatinine levels
- Progressive increase of creatinephosphokinase, documenting directly the lesions of the striated muscles; high levels indicate muscular necrosis
- Increase of LDH_4 and LDH_5 isoenzymes and transaminases
- Myoglobinemia and myoglobinuria, leading to alteration of cell membrane permeability, accumulation of acid radicals in the cell, and release of proteolytic enzymes that dissolve muscular proteins; myoglobin precipitates in the renal tubules and thus affects renal function
- Coagulation disturbances, caused by release of active tissular thromboplastin, which triggers intravascular coagulation that causes microembolism or severe pulmonary embolism

The clinical picture is typical. Locally, it is characterized by the following:

- Severe pain
- Marked tissular ischemia accompanied by coldness, pallor, cyanotic areas on the skin, and anesthesia
- Rigidity of the limb (rigor mortis)
- Massive edema of the extremity with tense, hard, wooden skin

Edema occurs because of the alteration of capillary membrane permeability in conditions of anoxia and by the effect of protein catabolism substances that penetrate into systemic circulation and influence coloidoosmotic pressure, finally resulting in fluid egress. Manifestations from other organs and systems are also present:

- The cardiovascular system responds by bradycardia and arterial hypotension.
- The respiratory system develops acute respiratory failure by microembolism.
- The kidney is affected because of myoglobin precipitation in the renal tubules, with onset of oliguria or acute renal failure with anuria. K^+ levels increase more markedly than urea.
- The digestive tract responds by ileus paralyticus.
- The nervous system develops postischemic encephalopathy with neuroplegia and anxiety.

The more extended and severe the lesions, the more severe the evolution of the syndrome. In the end, vascular collapse occurs, with acute renal failure, cardiac arrest, venous thrombosis, and local and general infections.

The prognosis for the leg is uncertain. Treatment consists of fasciotomy, largely open or semiclosed, using a fasciotome that sections the fascia subcutaneously. Sometimes the extremity must be amputated.[70]

Circulatory Disturbances by Arterial Steal Syndrome

Arterial steal syndrome is produced after good arterial flow is reestablished in a certain area, but a stenotic lesion exists in other segments or revascularization territories. The most common forms of arterial steal syndrome are as follows:

- Renal steal, after reconstruction of the renal aorta
- Mesenteric steal, after reconstruction of the lower aorta
- Iliofemoral steal, after contralateral aortoiliofemoral reconstruction

Treatment consists of a second surgical intervention to ensure adequate arterial flow in the ischemic area.

Cholesterol Embolism

Cholesterol embolism is a rare complication of aortic surgery or interventional radiology but has an 81% mortality rate.[39]

Early Infection of the Wound

Early infection is manifested by inflammatory signs of the wound and is favored by lymphorrhagia in Scarpa's triangle. The greatest danger of early infection is dehiscence of sutures. The arterial wall becomes brittle and macerated, allowing the suture to cut through it. The site of the infection at the level of the synthetic prosthesis may lead to permeability of the prosthesis, with onset of hemorrhage through the prosthesis and risk of septic embolism.[71,80]

Late Local Complications

Late Hemorrhage

The most common cause of late hemorrhage is infection. Its severity increases through the loss of circulating blood volume and the risk of septic embolism. Infection at the level of the prosthesis leads to local fibrinolysis, which prevents closure of the prosthesis mesh. Clinically, hemorrhage manifests itself by a fistulous tract with granulation tissue appearing on the bypass tract, most frequently in Scarpa's triangle.

Late hemorrhage at the level of the aortic anastomosis is severe and life-threatening. A retroperitoneal hematoma, mediastinal hematoma, or even hemoperitoneum may develop fast and can lead to hemorrhagic shock. Surgical treatment consists of an extra-anatomical bypass.

Pulsating Hematoma

Even minimal bleeding at the level of an arterial suture may cause formation of a pulsating hematoma, which may develop a fibrous capsule peripherally, borrowing the aspect of false aneurysm, which maintains communication with the artery. The false aneurysm may contain blood clots due to blood stasis, with a potential for thromboembolism. Pulsating hematoma may break and produce a diffuse hematoma or break into overt hemorrhage. Surgical treatment consists mostly of an extra-anatomical bypass, because hemostasis at the level of anastomoses is followed by hemorrhage recurrence or hematoma.

Arteriovenous Fistula

Arteriovenous fistula is due to a patent or dehisced suture that causes a hematoma that opens into a vein. The complication is more likely to occur if the venous segment was submitted to preparative surgical maneuvers during the operation. The redirection of arterial blood flow with decrease in arterial blood flow below the fistula determines variable ischemia, and increased pressure in the venous segment will interfere with venous return below the fistula. Treatment of arteriovenous fistula requires another operation of separate arterial and venous reconstruction.

Aortodigestive Fistula

Aortodigestive fistula is a severe, life-threatening complication. It is caused by a hematoma originating in the dehiscence of the proximal aorta–prosthesis anastomosis that results if the posterior parietal peritoneum has not been completely closed. Adherence of the hematoma occurs, with a tendency of encapsulation into the duodenum or an intestinal loop, followed by erosion of the gastrointestinal tract and upper gastrointestinal bleeding. Emergency surgery is required, because the condition may lead to the patient's exsanguination.

Late Arterial Thrombosis

The following are the main causes of late arterial thrombosis:

- Progression of atherosclerosis with decreased capacity to receive the distal vascular bed
- Intercurrent or chronic diseases favoring thrombosis, such as increased body temperatures, viral infections, diabetes mellitus, or prolonged arterial hypotension
- Patient does not continue anticoagulant therapy for a long enough time or does not avoid positions that clamp bypasses

The onset of thrombosis is slow and progressive, which allows collateral circulation to develop and leads to chronic ischemic syndrome that may be easily aggravated with exercise. Clinical symptoms of late arterial thrombosis are as follows:

- Disappearance of pulsations in the arterial axis or bypass
- Progressive decrease of skin temperature
- Waste of the muscular mass
- Alterations of skin, hair, and nails

Late thrombosis requires circulatory reassessment of the affected limb and study of the distal vascular bed to evaluate the necessity of another vascular reconstruction.[32]

Chronic Infection of Prostheses

Chronic infection of prostheses is a complication with a poor prognosis. The infection may occur immediately after the operation. Following an abundant lymphorrhagia, secretion becomes seropurulent, and a fistulous tract is maintained, through which hemorrhagic secretions are evacuated intermittently. In other cases the infection occurs months or even years after the operation, as a result of an inflammatory process or abscess, commonly in Scarpa's triangle. It is emptied through a spontaneous opening or incision.

At the level of the fistula, granulation is noted, and the discharge contains pus and sometimes blood. On instrumental examination of the wound the fistulous tract is found to follow the prosthesis. Sometimes the wound is enlarged because of marginal necrosis, and the prosthesis is exposed.[4]

The infection may cause dehiscence of the anastomosis with heavy external hemorrhage. Dehiscence occurs mostly at the level of the distal anastomosis, but it may also be found at the proximal aortic anastomosis when the infection involves the full prosthetic tract.

Besides the opening and drainage of the purulent secretion, surgical treatment consists of an extra-anatomical bypass that circumvents the septic area. In the case of suppurations in Scarpa's triangle, bypass through the obturating hole is a good solution.[58]

General Complications

Aortoiliac surgery is a serious operation that sometimes entails heavy blood loss and general complications.

Hemodynamic Complications

Hemodynamic complications occur because of blood storage by clamping and circulating blood loss, and they may or may not cause a state of shock.

Hemodynamic disturbances without shock occur with loss of 10% to 25% of the circulating blood volume. During aortic clamping, hemodynamic disturbances marked by arterial hypertension above the site and hypoperfusion below may occur. Arterial hypertension may lead to left ventricular insufficiency, acute pulmonary edema, or cerebrovascular accidents in elderly patients. Hemodynamic disturbances with shock may present under two clinical aspects:

1. *Hypovolemic shock* occurs when blood loss is more than 25% of the circulating volume. It is very important to take all available measures to limit blood loss, such as careful hemostasis during aortic approach, limitation to minimal blood purge during preparation of the aorta, good precoagulation of Dacron prostheses, and accurate performance of anastomoses.
2. *Cardiogenic shock* may be of distributive or obstructive type.

Cardiac Complications

Cardiac complications depend on the preoperative condition of the myocardium. Atherosclerosis also affects the coronary arteries. The most frequent cardiac complications are decompensated left cardiac insufficiency with pulmonary edema and cardiac arrest due to hypokalemia, acidosis, hypoxia, and catecholaminic stress.

Pulmonary Complications

Pulmonary complications consist of bronchopneumonia, atelectasis, and acute pulmonary edema. "Shock lung" is characterized by severe pulmonary failure due to fibrin microaggregates in pulmonary circulation. Microscopy evidences areas with atelectasis and hemorrhage as well as alveolar and interstitial edema. Microthrombi come from the hypoirrigated territory, where they are formed as the result of blood stasis, acidosis, and hypoxia. They penetrate circulation when the blood flow is reestablished and then stop in the pulmonary capillaries. Prognosis is often fatal.

Renal Complications

In surgery of the terminal aorta the kidney almost constantly suffers from low blood flow. In 3% of patients, acute renal failure occurs and results in death in 12%.[65]

Acute renal failure occurs after clamping of the suprarenal aorta, but it may also occur after subrenal clamping. It is explained by mobilization of microthrombi and cell or atheroma debris in the renal arteries, with destructive effects, and by intraoperative and postoperative hypotension. The characteristic anuria is explained by reduced glomerular filtration resulting from hypovolemia or arterial blockage; increased tubular backflow, with penetration of the tubular fluid into the renal interstitial space, edema, and compression of the tubules; and tubular obstruction by cell debris, cylinders, erythrocytes, and hemoglobin.

Acute renal failure is frequently associated with simultaneous embolism of the mesentery or lower limbs. Fistulae may be produced between the aortoiliac segment and the ureter, through a mechanism resembling aortoduodenal or aortojejunal fistulae, clinically manifested by hematuria.[73] Treatment consists of repeated sessions of kidney dialysis.

Neurological Complications

Neurological complications include those of the cerebrum and medulla. Cerebral complications are cerebrovascular accidents by two mechanisms: cerebral ischemia or arterial hypertension. They occur more frequently in patients with histories of cerebrovascular damage. Medullary complications occur after prolonged aortic clamping, especially suprarenal clamping, which sometimes causes medullary infarction by occlusion of radicular vessels, manifested by transient paresthesia or definitive senile paraplegia.[26]

References

1. Andercou A, Galea F, Ciuce C, et al. Long aorto-femoro-popliteal and ilio-femoro-popliteal bypasses. Paper presented at: Ninth Symposium of the Romanian Society of Angiology and Vascular Surgery; October 1–2,1992; Cluj-Napoca, Romania.
2. Andros G, Harris RW, Dulawa LB, Oblath RW, Salles-Cunha SX. Balloon angioplasty of iliac, femoral, and infrainguinal arteries. In: Bergan JJ, Yao JST, eds. *Techniques in Arterial Surgery*. Philadelphia, Pa: WB Saunders; 1990: 381–399.
3. Bacourt F. Le pontage axillo-femoral trente ans après. *J Chir (Paris)*. 1993;130:146–156.
4. Baird RN. Infective complications following reconstructive arterial surgery. In: Bell PRF, Jamieson CW, Ruckley CV, eds. *Surgical Management of Vascular Disease*. Philadelphia, Pa: WB Saunders; 1992:985–999.
5. Bareliuc N. Essentials of descriptive and topographical anatomy: angiology. In: Pop D, Popa I, eds. *Sistemul Aterial Artic [Aortic Arterial System]*. Vol 1. Bucharest, Romania: Ed. Medicala; 1982:23–313.
6. Bell PRF, Jamieson CW. Profundoplasty and iliac endarterectomy. In: Bell PRF, Jamieson CW, Ruckley CV, eds. *Surgical Management of Vascular Disease*. Philadelphia, Pa: WB Saunders; 1992:519–529.
7. Bergan JB. Vascular imaging. In: Najarian JS, Delaney JP, eds. *Progress in Vascular Surgery*. Chicago, Ill: Year Book Medical Publishers; 1988:47–55.
8. Bergan JJ, Yao JST. Operative correction of aortoiliac occlusions. In: Bell PRF, Jamieson CW, Ruckley CV, eds. *Surgical Management of Vascular Disease*. Philadelphia, Pa: WB Saunders; 1992:501–513.
9. Bergeron P, Rudondy P, Poyen V, Pinot JJ, Alessandri C, Martelet JP. Long-term peripheral stent evaluation using angioscopy. *Int Angiol*. 1991;3:182–186.
10. Berlien HP, Philipp C, Engel Murke F, Fuchs B. Laseran-

wendung in der Gefässchirurgie. *Zentralbl Chir.* 1993;118: 383–389.

11. Blaisdell FW. Extra-anatomical bypass grafts. In: Najarian JS, Delaney JP, eds. *Progress in Vascular Surgery.* Chicago, Ill: Year Book Medical Publishers; 1988:241–247.

12. Blaisdell FW. Axillofemoral and axillopopliteal grafts. In: Bergan JJ, Yao JST, eds. *Techniques in Arterial Surgery.* Philadelphia, Pa: WB Saunders; 1990:339–349.

13. Branchereau A, Espinoza H, Rudondy P, Magnan PE, Reboul J. Descending thoracic aorta as an inflow source for late occlusive failures following aortoiliac reconstruction. *Ann Vasc Surg.* 1991;5:8–15.

14. Caluser I. *Aterogeneza Primar [Primary Atherogenesis].* Bucharest, Romania: Ed. Medicala; 1988.

15. Canepa CS, Schubart PJ, Taylor RM Jr, Porter JM. Supraceliac aortofemoral bypass. *Surgery.* 1987;101:323–326.

16. Charlesworth D. The occluded aortic and aortofemoral graft. In: Bergan JJ, Yao JST, eds. *Reoperative Arterial Surgery.* Orlando, Fla.: Grune & Stratton; 1986:271–278.

17. Chervu A, Moore WS. Vascular grafts and sutures. In: Bell PRF, Jamieson CW, Ruckley CV, eds. *Surgical Management of Vascular Disease.* Philadelphia, Pa: WB Saunders; 1992: 367–381.

18. Cirafici I, Chapuis N, Merlini M. Revascularisation proximale et distale simultanee pour obstruction arterielle des membres inferieurs a deux niveaux: indications, techniques, et resultats. *Helv Chir Acta.* 1993;59:829–833.

19. Clark ET, Gewertz BL, Bassiouny HS, Zarins CK. Current results of elective aortic reconstruction for aneurysmal and occlusive disease. *J Cardiovasc Surg (Torino).* 1990;31: 438–441.

20. Connolly JE. Angioscopy and laser endarterectomy in vascular disease. In: Najarian JS, Delaney JP, eds. *Progress in Vascular Surgery.* Chicago, Ill: Year Book Medical Publishers; 1988:93–105.

21. Criado E, Johnson GJF Jr, Burnham S, Buehrer J, Keagy BA. Descending thoracic aorta-to-iliofemoral artery bypass as an alternative to aortoiliac reconstruction. *J Vasc Surg.* 1992;15:550–557.

22. Cucuianu M, Vonica A. Hyperlipoproteinemia and atherosclerosis. In: Cucuianu M, Rus HG, Niculescu FI, Vonica A, eds. *Biochimie: Aplicatii Clinice [Biochemistry: Clinical Applications].* Cluj-Napoca, Romania: Dacia; 1991:13–81.

23. Cumberland DC. Techniques in angioplasty. In: Bell PRF, Jamieson CW, Ruckley CV, eds. *Surgical Management of Vascular Disease.* Philadelphia, Pa: WB Saunders; 1992: 491–501.

24. Dalman RL, Taylor LM Jr, Moneta GL, Yeager RA, Porter JM. Simultaneous operative repair of multilevel lower extremity occlusive disease. *J Vasc Surg.* 1991;13:211–219.

25. Darke SG. Aortopopliteal and iliopopliteal bypass. In: Bell PRF, Jamieson CW, Ruckley CV, eds. *Surgical Management of Vascular Disease.* Philadelphia, Pa: WB Saunders; 1992: 537–545.

26. De Palma RG. Operations for impotence. In: Bell PRF, Jamieson CW, Ruckley CV, eds. *Surgical Management of Vascular Disease.* Philadelpia, Pa: WB Saunders; 1992:781–789.

27. Deriu GP, Grego F, Ballotta E, et al. Indications for revascularization procedures in patients with intermittent claudication. *Minerva Cardioangiol.* 1990;38:245–270.

28. De Weese JA. Surgery for aortoiliac occlusion. In: Bergan JJ, Yao JST, eds. *Techniques in Arterial Surgery.* Philadelphia, Pa: WB Saunders; 1990:17–27.

29. Dietrich ER. Surgical laser recanalization techniques. In: Sanborn TA, ed. *Laser Angioplasty.* New York, NY: Alan R. Liss; 1989:77–93.

30. Eikelboom BC, Odink HF, De Valois JC. Percutaneous transluminal angioplasty. In: Bell PRF, Jamieson CW, Ruckley CV, eds. *Surgical Management of Vascular Disease.* Philadelphia, Pa: WB Saunders; 1992:469–491.

31. El-Massry S, Saad E, Sauvage LR, et al. Axillo-femoral bypass with externally supported, knitted Dacron grafts: a follow-up through twelve years. *J Vasc Surg.* 1993;17: 107–114.

32. Enon R, Reigner R, Lescalie F, L'Hoste P, Peret M, Chevalier JM. In situ thrombolysis for late occlusion of suprafemoral prosthetic grafts. *Ann Vasc Surg.* 1993;7: 270–274.

33. Fagarasanu D. Aortoiliac obstructive syndrome (Leriche's syndrome). In: Pop D, Popa I, eds. *Sistemul Aterial Aortic [Aortic Arterial System].* Vol 2. Bucharest, Romania: Ed. Medicala; 1983:724–751.

34. Fagarasanu D, Pavelescu I, Pacescu M, Iliescu V. Aortoiliac obstructive syndrome. In: Proca E, ed. *Tratat de Patologie Chirurgical [Treatise of Surgical Pathology].* Vol 5, pt 2. Bucharest, Romania: Ed. Medicala; 1994:67–93.

35. Faris TB, McCollum P, Mantese V, Lusry R. Investigation of the patient with atheroma. In: Bell PRF, Jamieson CW, Ruckley CV, eds. *Surgical Management of Vascular Disease.* Philadelphia, Pa: WB Saunders; 1992:131–197.

36. Fozard JB, Wilkinson D, Parkin A, Kester RC. The application of isotope limb blood flow measurement to diagnostic problems in vascular surgery. *Ann R Coll Surg Engl.* 1990; 72:45–48.

37. Frisch M, Bour P, Berg P, Fieve G, Frisch R. Long-term results of thrombectomy for late occlusions of aortofemoral bypass. *Ann Vasc Surg.* 1991;5:16–20.

38. Hancu N, Cuparencu R, Dutu A. *Farmacoterapia Aterosclerozei [Drug Therapy of Atherosclerosis].* Bucharest, Romania: Ed. Medicala; 1988.

39. Hawthorn IE, Rochester J, Gaines PA, Morris-Jones W. Severe lower limb ischaemia with pulses: cholesterol embolisation—a little known complication of aortic surgery. *Eur J Vasc Surg.* 1993;7:470–474.

40. Hollier LH. Screening for aortic aneurysm. In: Bell PRF, Jamieson CW, Ruckley CV, eds. *Surgical Management of Vascular Disease.* Philadelphia, Pa: WB Saunders; 1992: 835–843.

41. Jamieson CW. Aortoiliac endarterectomy. In: Bell PRF, Jamieson CW, Ruckley CV, eds. *Surgical Management of Vascular Disease.* Philadelphia, Pa: WB Saunders; 1992: 513–519.

42. Jamieson CW. General vascular surgical technique. In: Bell PRF, Jamieson CW, Ruckley CV, eds. *Surgical Management of Vascular Disease.* Philadelphia, Pa: WB Saunders; 1992: 513–519.

43. Kalman PG, Johnston KW, Walker PM. Descending thoracic aortofemoral bypass as an alternative for aortoiliac revascularization. *J Cardiovasc Surg (Torino).* 1991;32: 443–446.

44. Kotb MM, Kadir S, Bennett JD, Beam CA. Aortoiliac angioplasty: is there a need for other types of percutaneous intervention? *J Vasc Interv Radiol.* 1992;3:67–71.

45. Kram HB, Gupta SK, Veith FJ, Wengerter KR. Unilateral aortofemoral bypass: a safe and effective option for the treatment of unilateral limb-threatening ischemia. *Am J Surg.* 1991;162:155–158.

46. Kwasnik EM, Siouffi SY, Jay ME, Khuri SF. Comparative results of angioplasty and aortofemoral bypass in patients with symptomatic iliac disease. *Arch Surg.* 1987;122: 288–291.

47. Marston A. Clinical evaluation of the patient with atheroma. In: Bell PRF, Jamieson CW, Ruckley CV, eds. *Surgical Management of Vascular Disease.* Philadelphia, Pa: WB Saunders; 1992:119–131.

48. McCarthy WJ, Flinn WR, Pearce WN, Yao JST, Bergan JJ. Thoracic aortofemoral bypass. In: Bergan JJ, Yao JST, eds. *Techniques in Arterial Surgery.* Philadelphia, Pa: WB Saunders; 1990:363–367.

49. McCarthy WJ, McGee G, Lin WW, Pearce WB, Flinn WR, Yao JST. Axillary-popliteal artery bypass provides successful limb salvage after removal of infected aortofemoral grafts. *Arch Surg.* 1992;127:974–978.

50. Melliere D, Labastie J, Becquemin JP, Kassab M, Paris E. Proximal anastomosis in aortobifemoral bypass: end-to-end or-end-to-side? *J Cardiovasc Surg (Torino).* 1980;31: 77–80.

51. Miller JH. Partial replacement of an infected arterial graft by a new prosthetic polytetrafluoroethylene segment: a new therapeutic option. *J Vasc Surg.* 1993;17:546–558.

52. Miyamoto A, Sakurada M, Arai T, et al. Efficacy of carbon monoxide laser in selectively intimal thermal welding: implications for laser balloon angioplasty. *Jpn Circ J.* 1993;57: 825–831.

53. Naylor AR, Ah-See AK, Engeset J. Aortoiliac endarterectomy: an 11-year review. *Br J Surg.* 1990;77:190–193.

54. Nevelsteen A, Boeckxstaens C, Smet G, Willekens FG, Suy R. Extensive aorto-ilio-femoral endarterectomy with LeVeen plaque cracker. *J Cardiovasc Surg (Torino).* 1988;29: 441–448.

55. Nevelsteen A, Wouters L, Suy R. Long-term patency of the aortofemoral Dacron graft: a graft limb related study over a 25-year period. *J Cardiovasc Surg (Torino).* 1991;32: 174–180.

56. Norwood SH, Nelson LD. Continuous monitoring of mixed venous oxygen saturation during aortofemoral bypass grafting. *Am Surg.* 1986;52:114–115.

57. Olin JW, Cressman MD, Joung JR, Hoogwerf BJ, Weinstein CE. Lipid and lipoprotein abnormalities in lower-extremity arteriosclerosis obliterans. *Cleve Clin J Med.* 1992;59: 491–497.

58. Olofsson P, Stomey RJ. Surgical management of chronic prosthetic aortic graft infection. In: Najarian JS, Delaney JP, eds. *Progress in Vascular Surgery.* Chicago, Ill: Year Book Medical Publishers; 1988:213–217.

59. Ota K. *An Atlas of Vascular Access.* Edinburgh, Scotland: Churchill Livingstone; 1987:73–79.

60. Polterauer P, Contreras F, Kretschmer G, et al. Die PTFE-Kunststoffprothese als arterieller Gefässersatz: Erfarung über 5 Jahre. *Wien Klin Wochenschr.* 1984;96:249–259.

61. Polterauer P, Kretschmer G, Wagner O, Waneck R, Piza F, Lechner G. Die PTFE-Bifurkationsprothese: Frühergebnisse. *Chirurg.* 1984;55:106–110.

62. Polterauer P, Prager M, Hölzenbein TH, Karner J, Kretschmer G, Schemper M. Dacron versus polytetrafluoroethylene for Y-aortic bifurcation grafts: a six-year prospective, randomized trial. *Surgery.* 1992;111:626–633.

63. Polterauer P, Wagner O, Kretschmer G, Piza F. The PTFE Y-graft: one year experience in twenty-one patients. A preliminary report. *Int J Artif Organs.* 1982;5:263–266.

64. Pop D, Popa T. Operative technique in arterial disease: direct surgery. In: Pop D, Popa T, eds. *Sistemul Arterial Aortic [Aortic Arterial System].* Vol 2. Bucharest, Romania: Ed. Medicala; 1983:298–350.

65. Pop D, Popa T. Arterial bypass. In: Proca E. *Tratat de Patologie Chirurgical [Treatise of Surgical Pathology].* Vol. 5, pt 2. Bucharest, Romania: Ed. Medicala; 1994:530–554.

66. Pop D, Popa T, Constantinescu M. Arterial stealing syndrome. In: Pop D, Popa T, eds. *Sistemul Arterial Aortic [Aortic Arterial System].* Vol 2. Bucharest, Romania: Ed. Medicala; 1983:67–97.

67. Poulias GE, Doundoulakis N, Prombonas E, et al. Aortofemoral bypass and determinants of early success and late favorable outcome. Experience with 1000 consecutive cases. *J Cardiovasc Surg (Torino).* 1992;33:664–678.

68. Prager M, Polterauer P, Huk I, Trubei W, Nanobashvili J, Claeys L. Should Dacron or PTFE be used for aorto-iliac reconstruction? In: Greenhalgh RM, Fowkes FGR, eds. *Trials and Tribulations of Vascular Surgery.* London: WB Saunders; 1996:313–324.

69. Pretre R, Katchatourian G, Bednarkiewicz M, Faidutti B. Aortoiliac endarterectomy: a 9-year experience. *Thorac Cardiovasc Surg.* 1992;40:152–154.

70. Robinson KP. Amputations in vascular patients. In: Bell PRF, Jamieson CW, Ruckley CV, eds. *Surgical Management of Vascular Disease.* Philadelphia, Pa: WB Saunders; 1992:609–637.

71. Schellack J, Stewart MT, Smith RB, Perdue GD, Salam A. Infected aortobifemoral prosthesis: a dreaded complication. *Am Surg.* 1988;54:137–141.

72. Seeger JM, Abela GS. Laser angioplasty of iliofemoral and distal arteries. In: Bergan JJ, Yao JST, eds. *Techniques in Arterial Surgery.* Philadelphia, Pa: WB Saunders; 1990: 399–406.

73. Simon G, Ballanger P, Midy D, Junes F, Baste JC, Boisieras P. Fistules arterielles ilio-ureterales après chirurgie reconstructive aorto-iliaque. *Prog Urol.* 1992;2:85–92.

74. Stanley JC, Burkel WE, Graham LM. Endothelial cell seeding of synthetic vascular prosthesis. In: Najarian JS, Delaney JP, eds. *Progress in Vascular Surgery.* Chicago, Ill: Year Book Medical Publishers; 1988:105–118.

75. Stefanovici B, David M, Nubert G. Abdominal aortography. In: Branzeu P, Gavrilescu S, eds. *Angiografia îm Practica Medical [Angiography in Medical Practice].* Timișoara, Romania: Ed. Facla; 1977:108–136.

76. Sterpetti AV, Feldhaus RJ, Schultz RD. Combined aortofemoral and extended deep femoral artery reconstruction: functional results and predictors of need for distal bypass. *Arch Surg.* 1988;123:1269–1273.

77. Stoney RJ, Quigley TM. Extra-anatomic bypass: a new look (opposing view). *Adv Surg.* 1993;26:151–162.

78. Van den Akker PJ, van Schilfgaarde R, Brand R, van Bockel JH, Terpstra JL. Long term success of aortoiliac operation for arteriosclerotic obstructive disease. *Surg Gynecol Obstet.* 1992;6:485–496.

79. Vlaicu R. Atherosclerosis. In: Paun R, ed. *Tratat de Medicină Internă. Bolile Cardiovasculare [Treatise of Internal Medicine. Cardiovascular Diseases].* Pt 3. Bucharest, Romania: Ed. Medicala; 1992:7–43.

80. Wakefield TW, Pierson CL, Schaberg DR, et al. Artery, periarterial adipose tissue, and blood microbiology during vascular reconstructive surgery: perioperative and early postoperative observations. *J Vasc Surg.* 1990;11:624–628.

81. Wolf YG, Schatz RA, Knowles HJ, Saeed M, Bernstein EF, Dilley RB. Initial experience with the Palmaz stent for aortoiliac stenoses. *Ann Vasc Surg.* 1993;7:254–261.

63

Radio Contrast Agents: History and Evolution

Mohammed A. Quader, Carol J. Sawmiller, and Bauer E. Sumpio

Radio contrast agents are the essential elements of investigative radiology. Small differences in tissue densities of the body do not allow optimal radiographic evaluation without contrast enhancement. Soon after the discovery of x-rays by Roentgen, enhancement of radiopacity was felt necessary to obtain better contrast of images. It became obvious that elements with high atomic numbers would enhance x-ray images. Bismuth, lead, and barium salts were used to develop the first angiogram of an amputated hand, experiments that were published in 1896 by Haschek and Lindenthal in Vienna.[1] However, these heavy metal salts were not safe enough to be used in living humans. For the last few decades, modifications in the structure of these contrast agents were continually sought in an effort to limit their toxicity; however, the search for the ideal contrast agent continues.

The discovery of iodine as a safe radio contrast agent was accidental. In the early 1920s, when iodine-containing compounds were used to treat syphilis, Osborne et al. observed that the urine of patients treated with iodine was radiopaque; they went on to perform the first successful clinical pyelogram in 1923 at the Mayo Clinic.[2] In the same year, Berberich and Hirsch successfully employed strontium bromide to perform a femoral angiogram.[3] In 1924 sodium iodide was used by Brooks to perform an angiogram.[4]

Development of Current Contrast Agents: An Evolution

In the 1920s, iodine was accepted as a radiopaque agent safe enough to be used for contrast studies in humans. Subsequently, several attempts were made to discover the ideal contrast agent. In the mid 1920s, Binz and Rath[5] synthesized several derivatives of iodopyridone to improve biological tolerance. From their work at the School of Agriculture in Berlin emerged two of the earliest contrast agents, Uroselectan and Diodrast, once used worldwide (Figure 63.1).

Meanwhile, Moniz[6] attempted to visualize the cerebral arteries of animals by using several salts of heavy metals, including iodine. He first performed a carotid angiogram in 1927 by using sodium iodide. Moniz then hypothesized that increasing the molecular size of a contrast agent could reduce the toxicity; he therefore used colloid thorium dioxide (Thorotrast), which became widely employed. However, its nonbiodegradable property and its association with the later development of malignancy limited the usefulness of Thorotrast.

Until 1933, all the iodinated radio contrast agents used were either the salts of iodine or the derivatives of monoiodinated or diiodinated pyridone, a five-carbon-ring molecule (Figure 63.2). With the knowledge that increasing the content of iodine in an agent led to greater radiopacity, researchers began attempts to incorporate more than two iodine atoms into a molecule. In 1933, the chemist Wallingford[7] noticed the nontoxic properties of para-aminohippuric acid, a six-carbon-ring compound; he went on to produce an iodine derivative of para-aminoiodohippuric acid that could incorporate up to three iodine atoms per molecule. With this discovery, truly modern contrast agents were born. Wallingford went on to increase the iodine content of benzene rings. He soon learned that the active derivative, the free amine, was toxic and substituted an acetyl group. The resulting compound was acetrizoate, the first true iodinated benzoic acid derivative (Figure 63.3). When given intra-arterially, however, these contrast agents caused significant pain, thought to be secondary to their viscosity and their ionic character. In 1953, two scientists[8] working at different institutions realized that a fully substituted triiodobenzoic acid was superior to acetrizoate; thus they produced diatrizoic acid, which is widely used as the sodium or meglumine salt. Iothalamate, an isomer of diatrizoate, was developed by Hoey[7] in the early 1960s to improve water solubility. Both of these contrast agents

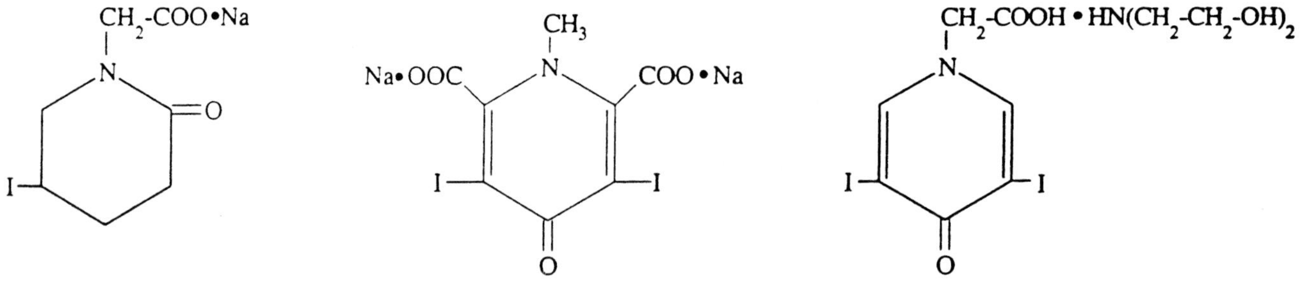

Uroselectan Uroselectan B Diodrast

Figure 63.1. Chemical structures of the earliest contrast agents, Uroselectan, Uroselectan B, and Diodrast, which were derivatives of iodopyridones.

are still widely used, with a current annual consumption of about 2000 metric tons.

Lasser et al.[6] extensively studied the mechanisms of adverse reactions to these contrast agents and ultimately concluded that the binding of contrast agents by hydrophobic bonds to biomacromolecules is the root cause of their toxicity. When a molecule of an ionic contrast agent dissolves in solution, it produces two particles, compared with only one with nonionic contrast agents. Subsequently, attempts were made to reduce the osmolality of contrast agents to improve tolerance. Chemists synthesized triiodinated benzoic acid compounds without a charge element (cation) by combining metrizoic acid and glucosamine to produce metrizamide, which is water soluble and has low osmolality. In addition, it was found to be an essentially painless angiographic medium. Whereas the vascular pain threshold falls somewhere between 600 and 700 mOsm, metrizamide's osmolality is only 485 mOsm. However, the use of metrizamide was limited secondary to its precipitation when subjected to high temperatures for sterilization purposes.

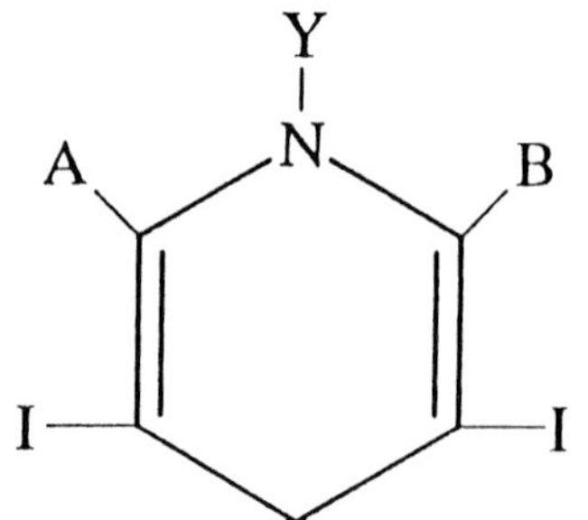

FIGURE 63.2. Chemical structure of diiodopyridone, a five-carbon-atom ring supporting attachment of two iodine atoms per molecule.

A

B

C

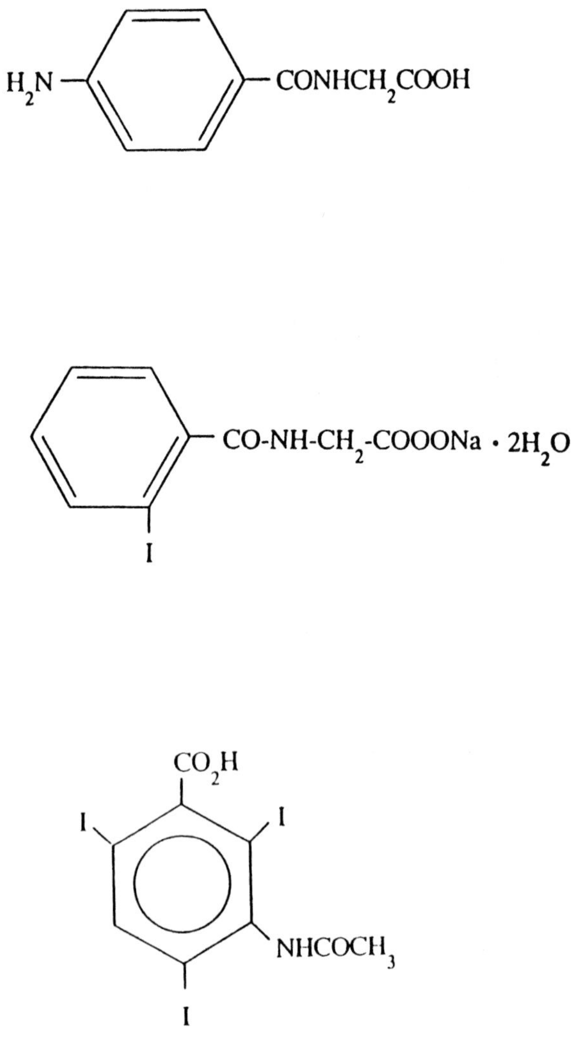

FIGURE 63.3. Chemical structure of aminohippuric acid (**A**), a six-carbon-atom ring, and its iodinated derivatives, sodium iodohippurate (**B**) and acetrizoic acid (**C**).

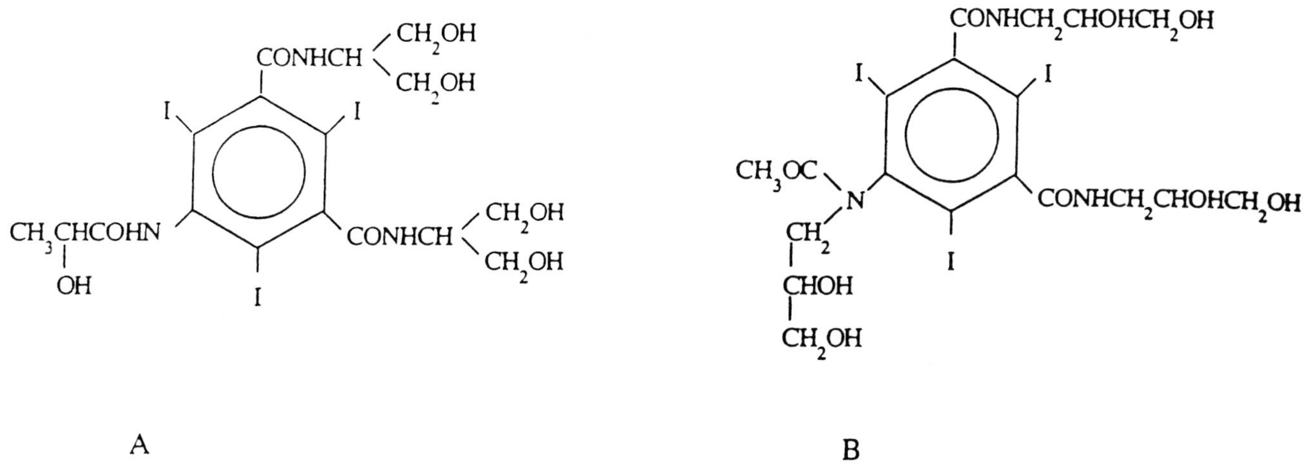

FIGURE 63.4. Chemical structures of iopamidol (A) and iohexol (B).

In the mid 1970s, further attempts were made to improve the water solubility of metrizamide. Improvements were made by replacing simple sugar moieties with other hydrophilic, water-solubilizing sugar moieties, stably distributed around the benzene ring. Iohexol and iopamidol were thus produced (Figure 63.4). These two agents have equivalent water solubilities and were superior to metrizamide in withstanding autoclaving, but they have high osmolality. Further development was needed. Successful attempts to combine two triiodobenzoic acid derivatives decreased the number of particles released in solution and concomitantly increased the iodine content of each molecule from three to six atoms in agents such as ioxaglic acid (Figure 63.5). However, these agents were more toxic than the parent compounds. Various nonionic dimers were produced, but none were widely accepted because they all had high viscosity.

Interest then turned once again toward developing monomers with osmolality lower than iohexol by introducing new radiopaque substitutes to anions to increase the iodine content while maintaining high water solubility. Unfortunately, the improvements have been mar-

ginal in manufacturing costs and in biological tolerance compared with the previous compounds.

In 1978, Sovak et al.[10] announced their findings that the osmolality of ionic molecules in solution increases linearly with concentration and that nonionic contrast agents behave differently. Nonionic contrast agents form complexes in solution, thereby decreasing osmolality. Recent refinement of this discovery has been made by Sovak et al.,[11] who developed a new class of nonionic contrast agents in 1990. These new agents are derived from a primary carboxamide that has an inherent but small hydrophilic group; because of its small size, two neighboring iodines are exposed to create a hydrophobic area, which causes the molecule to aggregate. These new compounds have low osmolality and low viscosity, and they hold promise for future use in contrast studies.

Synthesis of Contrast Agents

The introduction of iodine into benzene rings requires activation by amino groups. The starting material is nitrobenzoic acid or nitroisophthalic acid. The nitro com-

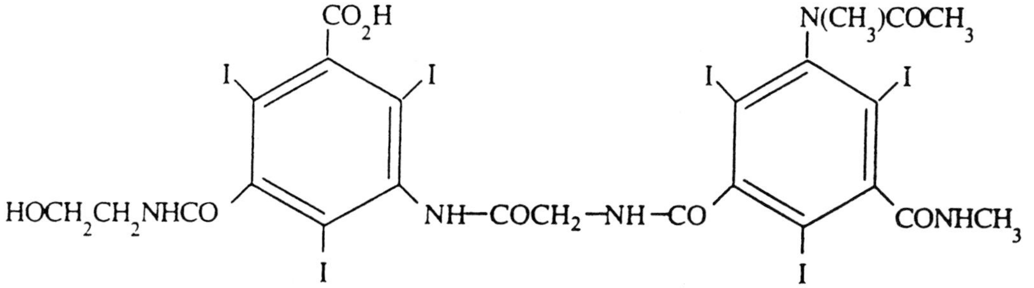

FIGURE 63.5. Chemical structure of a dimer, ioxaglic acid.

pounds are then reduced, and iodine is introduced as iodine chloride. The triiodinated compounds precipitate and are easily removed. The synthesis of ionic contrast agents is thus complete. After acylation of an anion group, the iodine is locked in the ring, making deiodination practically impossible. Steps for nonionic contrast agents are more elaborate, essentially consisting of desalination. In this process, all ionic by-products are removed using ion exchange resin, and new groups are attached in stepwise fashion as required by design.

Toxicity of Contrast Agents

Although contrast agents have revolutionized diagnostic activity in modern medicine, their associated adverse effects still compromise their utility. Intravascular injection of a contrast agent may be complicated by the occurrence of adverse effects, which can be systemic, such as pain, generalized weakness, nausea, vasodilatation, and hypotension,[12-14] or specific to a particular organ system, such as contrast-induced nephropathy (CIN). A generalized feeling of pain, nausea, and headache could also represent rapid fluid shifts secondary to the hyperosmolar nature of contrast agents, especially at the level of neurons. For example, this may occur in certain areas of the brain that are not protected by the blood–brain barrier, such as the chemoreceptor trigger zone in the area postrema. Along the same lines, in patients with brain metastasis, the breach in the blood–brain barrier could potentially place them at high risk for development of seizures. Up to 6% of patients with brain metastasis develop seizure following radio contrast studies. These reactions seem to occur more frequently after the administration of ionic as compared with nonionic contrast agents.[15]

Allergic Reactions

Severe anaphylactic reactions to contrast agent administration can occur in up to 0.022% of studies.[16] The incidence of allergic reactions to contrast agents is higher than expected in certain groups of patients, such as those with history of prior allergic reactions to contrast agents, those with allergies or asthma, and those who are elderly. The interactions between the hydrophobic groups on the contrast agents and biomacromolecules are the most likely mechanism for the adverse reactions.[9]

Hyperosmolarity and Viscosity

Contrast agents are 3 to 10 times the osmolarity of serum, with ionic agents typically having a higher osmolarity than nonionic agents. The hyperosmolar effects of contrast agents on vascular endothelium are well described in the literature. Previous studies have shown contrast agents to be directly toxic to the vascular endothelium.[17] After in vivo contrast exposure, intact segments of aorta demonstrated endothelial cell shrinkage, expansion of intracellular clefts, and areas where the endothelial layer had separated and lifted off the subendothelium.[18] The mechanism of these effects is unclear but has been postulated to be related to the hyperosmolar nature of contrast agents. Endothelial cells not only undergo acute injury, but their proliferation is markedly decreased for up to 7 days following brief exposure to contrast, indicating that the effect of contrast agents may last longer than previously believed.[19] However, cell viability remains intact, and widespread cell death does not appear to occur. At the level of the cell membrane, contrast-associated hyperosmotic cell shrinkage is a potent activator of Na^+–K^+–Cl^- cotransport and Na^+–H^+ cotransport exchange pumps in endothelial cells from peripheral vessels.[20] As protons are exchanged extracellularly, the intracellular compartment becomes alkalinized. Intracellular Ca^{++}–dependent reactions may be influenced by osmotically induced pH changes. This can lead to alterations in the release of vasoactive substances such as prostacyclin and endothelial-derived relaxation factor and may affect the cytoskeletal organization of endothelial cells, leading to the typical morphologic changes and cellular dysfunction seen after hyperosmolar exposure.[21]

The effect of contrast agents on endothelial cells cannot, however, be fully attributed to hyperosmolar cell injury. Some new ionic contrast agents with osmolalities equal to or less than those of nonionic agents exhibit greater toxicity in vivo and in vitro, and nonionic agents with the same osmolalities have been shown to have different cellular toxicity.[22]

Contrast agents directly affect vascular smooth muscle cell contractile function, with different effects from ionic and nonionic agents. Ionic contrast agents bind calcium, but nonionic contrast agents have minimal calcium-binding properties,[23] which may contribute to the different effects seen with these agents. Na^+–K^+ ATPase may be involved in smooth muscle cell relaxation, with alterations in Na^+–Ca^{++} and Na^+–H^+ exchange.[18] Vasoconstriction was due primarily to hyperosmolarity, whereas dilation was probably due to elevations of cyclic adenosine monophosphate or cyclic guanosine monophosphate.[18] The stabilizing compounds present in contrast agents, such as disodium edetate and sodium citrate, can chelate calcium and produce hypocalcemia. The hypocalcemia is transient and can manifest as generalized weakness or cramps. Hypocalcemia could also be responsible for the electrophysiologic changes on the cell membrane with their attendant adverse effects on neuromuscular cell functions.

TABLE 63.1. Incidence of contrast-induced nephropathy.

Reference year	Studies	Number studied	Cases of acute renal failure	
			Number	Percentage
Metys et al.[27]	Angiography	110	0	0
Reiss et al.[28]	Angiography	2710	8	0.29
Port et al.[29]	Angiography	7400	8	0.1
Older et al.[30]	Angiography	90	9	10
Swartz et al.[31]	Angiography	109	14	13
Byrd and Sherman[32]	IVP, Angiography,CAT, OCG	12,000	18	0.15
Krumlovasky et al.[33]	IVP, Angiography, CAT, OCG	712	8	0.11
Shusterman[34]	Angiography	266	45	17
Moore and Steinberg[35]	Angiography	929	160	17

IVP, intravenous pyelography; CAT, computerized axial tomography; OCG, oral cholelystography.
From Byrd and Sherman.[32]

The increased effects of ionic contrast agents on depolarization of the cell membrane, intracellular ion alterations, and effects on intracellular second messengers warrant further investigation for better understanding of their adverse effects.

Contrast-Induced Nephropathy

Contrast-induced nephropathy (CIN) is the most common potentially serious adverse reaction to radiocontrast agents. CIN manifests as increasing creatinine levels, with or without oliguria, in the 24 to 48 hours after administration of the contrast agent. Oliguria is more common in patients with preexisting renal insufficiency, and permanent renal failure may occur in up to 50% of these patients. A nephrogram that persists 24 hours after a contrast study is characteristic of CIN but not pathognomonic.[24] The degree of renal cortical attenuation on computed tomography scan obtained 24 hours after the patient received a contrast aortogram was also posited to be a marker of CIN.[25] Other distinct features of oliguric CIN include low urinary sodium levels and a fractional excretion of sodium of less than 1.[26]

Retrospective analysis of large series of patients has suggested that the incidence of CIN in the general population ranges from 0.1% to 13% (Table 63.1).[27-35] The more severe the preexisting renal insufficiency, the higher the incidence of CIN. VanZee et al. noted a CIN incidence of 1.4%, 9.2%, and 39% for patients with preprocedure creatinine levels of less than 1.5 mg/dL, between 1.5 and 4.5 mg/dL, and greater than 4.5 mg/dL, respectively. When the subgroups of patients with diabetes mellitus (DM) were analyzed, the incidence was 0%, 50%, and 100%, respectively, for these same serum creatinine levels (Table 63.2).[36] Age at onset and type of DM seemed to affect this predisposition towards CIN. For example, type I DM predisposed more toward the development of CIN than did type II DM.[37] Other less well-established risk factors in the development of CIN include congestive heart failure, advanced age, volume depletion, proteinuria, hyperuricemia, and preexisting use of other nephrotoxic agents (Table 63.3).

Pathogenesis

Although the pathogenesis of CIN has been studied extensively, the exact mechanism is still unknown. Many observations have been made, however, and many hypotheses postulated. These mechanisms can be divided into those that have a direct or indirect effect on renal function (Figure 63.6).

TABLE 63.2. Incidence of contrast-induced nephropathy in patients with renal insufficiency before the study.

Group	Creatine level < 1.5 mg/dL		Creatine level =1.5–4.5 mg/dL		Creatine level >4.5 mg/dL		Total	
	Number	Percentage	Number	Percentage	Number	Percentage	Number	Percentage
No preceding renal disease or dysfunction	1/169	0.6	—	—	—	—	1/169	0.6
Nondiabetic renal disease or dysfunction	3/95	3.2	2/66	3	5/16	31	10/77	5.6
Diabetic patients	0/19	0	5/10	50	2/2	100	7/31	23
All patients surveyed	4/283	1.4	7/76	9.2	7/18	39	18/377	4.8

From VanZee et al.[22]

TABLE 63.3. Risk factors for the development of contrast-induced nephropathy.

Established risk factors
- Existing renal insufficiency
- Diabetes mellitus

Possible risk factors
- Congestive heart failure
- Advanced age
- Volume depletion
- Atherosclerotic vascular disease
- Volume of contrast infused
- Use of concomitant nephrotoxic medications
- Multiple myeloma
- Proteinuria
- Hypercalcemia
- Uricosuria

Mechanisms That Have Direct Effects on Renal Function

1. *Tubular injury.* In the tubular injury theory, contrast material is directly toxic to the cells of the proximal tubular epithelium. Humes et al.[38] demonstrated the toxic effects of contrast agents in rabbit proximal renal tubular segments and noted that these effects are enhanced by hypoxia. Similarly, the renal mitochondrial oxygen consumption supported by succinate and pyruvate-malate was inhibited in a dose-dependent manner by Diatrizoate.[38] However, these changes are nonspecific and do not directly relate to development of renal toxicity.

2. *Intraluminal precipitation of proteins.* Another proposed mechanism of CIN involves the precipitation of proteins in the lumen of renal tubules. It has been postulated that intratubular precipitation of contrast agents with proteins might result in acute renal failure. In one study, there were significant differences in the severity of proteinuria of patients who developed CIN compared with those who did not develop CIN.[39]

However, it should be noted that proteinuria as a direct predisposing factor for CIN in patients with multiple myeloma is not universally accepted. In one study, no correlation was noted between urinary protein excretion and degree of renal impairment after contrast study in patients with multiple myeloma.[37]

Mechanisms That Have Indirect Effects on Renal Function

1. *Alterations in renal hemodynamics.* A number of investigators have proposed that contrast-induced changes in renal hemodynamics are significant contributors to CIN. Contrast agents can cause profound perturbations in renal hemodynamics, and these changes are exaggerated in diabetic patients. They cause initial transient vasodilatation followed by a period of prolonged vasoconstriction with concomitant decreases in renal blood flow.[40] Some of the altered renal hemodynamics observed after administration of contrast agents have been hypothesized to be secondary to changes in blood cells, such as acute increase in granulocyte count, presumed to be due to impaired granulocyte adhesion, and also an increase in red blood cell rigidity and clumping with resultant increase in blood viscosity.[41] Platelet activation and release of cytokines can herald activation of coagulation, complement, and thrombolytic cascades. The role of a potent endothelium-derived contracting factor, *endothelin,* in the development of CIN has been studied. Administration of a contrast agent can cause an increase in serum endothelin level.[42] The release of endothelin from cultured bovine endothelial cells was more pronounced with an ionic contrast agent (iothalmate) compared with a nonionic contrast agent (ioversol).[34] However, it is yet to be determined whether endothelin is a marker of cellular toxicity caused by contrast agents or a cause of nephrotoxicity. This hypothesis remains to be tested in human beings.

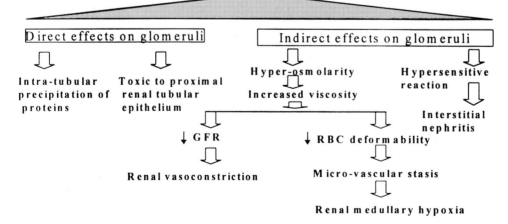

FIGURE 63.6. Pathogenesis of contrast-induced nephropathy. RBC, red blood cell; GFR, glomerular filtration rate.

2. *Uricosuria.* Contrast agents have been observed to result in increased uricosuria. The intratubular uric acid deposition has been postulated as another possible mechanism of CIN. However, evidence to support this increase in uricosuria as a cause of CIN is sparse.[43]

3. *Immunologic factors.* CIN could also represent a hypersensitivity reaction to a contrast agent.[44] Although rare, associated systemic manifestations of anaphylaxis can be seen in the setting of CIN. In addition, contrast agents are capable of activating the complement system, which might play a role in the CIN as seen in renal transplant patients.[45]

Ionicity and CIN

Because of their low osmolarity and expected benefits, nonionic contrast agents have been preferentially used, especially in patients with DM, chronic renal failure, or both. However, their high cost has limited the indications for their use. Few studies have addressed the beneficial effects of nonionic contrast agents. In one study it was observed that administration of nonionic contrast media resulted in significantly fewer nonrenal contrast media–related adverse effects compared with ionic contrast media (10.2% versus 31.6%). In addition, the adverse cardiac effects such as angina, hypertension, hypotension, arrhythmias, or myocardial infarction occurred more often with ionic contrast agents (7.2% versus 24.5%). The same study observed that New York Heart Association classification III or IV and serum creatinine of greater than 1.5 mg/dL predicted a higher incidence of adverse events as a result of contrast media alone.[46] These effects were postulated to be secondary to electrophysiologic changes caused by the ionic contrast agents—for example, by prolonging the action potential of the myocardial cell, prolonging the QT interval, or changing the ST segment and T-wave amplitude. These electrophysiologic changes have been well described in in vitro models.[47]

In another study, Lautin et al. compared the renal toxicity of low- and high-osmolarity contrast media in 303 patients undergoing lower extremity angiography. The study revealed a 7% versus 26% incidence of CIN when low- versus high-osmolarity contrast media were administered. When the data were analyzed for patients who had elevated serum creatinine levels before angiography, the incidence of CIN was 10% versus 41% for low-osmolarity contrast media versus high-osmolarity contrast media. Diabetic patients with existing renal insufficiency (serum creatinine level of >1.5 mg/dL) had a higher incidence of CIN with high-osmolarity contrast media than with low-osmolarity contrast media. This effect was not seen in patients without preexisting renal insufficiency.[48] It is important to emphasize, however, that these findings are not universally accepted, nor have they been unequivocally reproduced in other studies.

Role of Adjunct Interventions

Ongoing efforts have been made to prevent the morbidity associated with contrast agents. In addition to the judicious use of contrast agents, especially in high-risk patients, various adjunctive measures such as intravenous hydration, vasodilators, diuretic agents, calcium channel blockers, and theophylline have been tested.

Weisberg et al. evaluated the efficacy of concomitant administration of vasodilators (dopamine or atrial natriuretic peptide) or mannitol during cardiac catheterization in patients with preexisting chronic renal insufficiency. The incidence of CIN was 80% in the diabetic group versus 0% in the nondiabetic group. The authors concluded that the use of a vasodilator or mannitol is protective in nondiabetic patients with azotemia.[49] In contrast, the prophylactic use of nifedipine in the prevention of CIN has not been established.[50]

In another study, Solomon et al. compared the effect of preangiographic intravenous hydration with saline, saline with mannitol, and saline with the diuretic furosemide in 78 patients with chronic renal insufficiency. They noted an overall incidence of 26% of CIN but an incidence of 11%, 28%, and 40% in the saline, saline plus mannitol, and saline plus furosemide groups, respectively. However, one study demonstrated that simple hydration with 0.45% saline before a contrast study was more beneficial than hydration with concomitant diuretic or use of mannitol.[51]

References

1. Haschek E, Lindenthal O. A contribution to the practical use of photography according to Roentgen. *Wien Chir Wochenschr.* 1896;9:63.
2. Osborne E, Sortherland C, Sholl A, Roundtree L. Roentgenography of the urinary tract during excretion of sodium iodide. *JAMA.* 1923;80:368.
3. Berberich J, Hirsch S. Die roenthenographische Darstellung der Arterinn und Venen am Lebenden. *Munchen Klin Wschr.* 1923;49:2226.
4. Brooks B. Intraarterial injection of sodium iodide. *JAMA.* 1924;82:1016.
5. Binz A, Rath C. Uber Biochemische eig Enschaften von derivaten des Pyridins und Chinolins. *Biochem Z.* 1928;203:218.
6. Moniz E. *Die Cerebrale Arteriographie und Phlebographie.* Berlin: Springer-Verlag; 1940:413.
7. Hoey G. Organic iodide compounds as x-ray contrast media. In: Knoeffel PK, ed. *International Encyclopedia of Pharmacology and Therapeutics.* Oxford, England: Pergamon Press; 1971:23–132.
8. Sovak M. Contrast media: A journey almost sentimental. *Invest Radiol.* 1994;29(suppl)S4–S14.
9. Lasser E. Adverse systemic reactions to contrast media. In: Sovak M, ed. *Radio Contrast Agents: Hand Book of Experimental Pharmacology.* Vol 73. Berlin: Springer-Verlag; 1984:525–532.

10. Sovak M, Ranganathan R, Lang JH, Lasser EC. Concepts in design of improved intravascular contrast agents. *Ann Radiol.* 1978;21:283–289.

11. Sovak M, Terry RC, Douglass JG, Schweitzer L. Primary carboxamides: Nonionic isotonic monomers. *Invest Radiol.* 1991;26(suppl 1):S159–S161.

12. Keizur JJ, Das S. Current perspectives on intravascular contrast agents for radiological imaging studies. *J Urol.* 1994; 151:1470–1478.

13. Pugh ND, Griffith TM, Karlsson JO. Effects of iodinated contrast media on peripheral blood flow. *Acta Radiol Suppl.* 1995;399:155–163.

14. Shehadi W. Contrast media adverse reactions: occurrence, recurrence, and distribution pattern. *Radiology.* 1982;143: 11–17.

15. Barrett B, Prfery J, McDonald J, Hefferton D, Reddy E. Non-ionic low osmolality versus ionic high osmolality contrast material for intravenous use in patients perceived to be high risk: randomized trial. *Radiology.* 1992;183: 105–110.

16. Ansell G,Tweedie MC, West CR, Evans P, Couch L. The current status of reactions to intravenous contrast media. *Invest Radiol.* 1980;15(suppl 6):S32–S39.

17. Schneider KM, Ham K, Friedhuber A, Rand M. Functional and morphologic effects of ioxilan, iohexol, and deatrizoate on endothelial cells. *Invest Radiol.* 1988;23(suppl 1): S147–S149.

18. Schneider KM, Rand MJ. Vasodilatation and vasoconstriction in the rabbit isolated aorta: effect of ioxilan, iohexol, and diatrizoate. *Invest Radiol.* 1988;23(suppl 1): S150–S152.

19. Sawmiller C, Powell RJ, Quader MA, Dudrick SJ, Sumpio BE. The differential effect of contrast agents on endothelial cell and smooth muscle cell growth in vitro. *J Vasc Surg.* 1998;27:1128–1140.

20. Vigne P, Lopez Farre A, Frelin C. Na⁺–K⁺–Cl⁻ cotransporter of brain capillary endothelial cells: properties and regulation by endothelins, hyperosmolar solutions, calyculin A, and interleukin-1. *J Biol Chem.* 1994;269:19925–19930.

21. Escobales N, Longo E, Cragoe E. Osmotic activation of Na⁺–H⁺ exchange in human endothelial cells. *Am J Physiol.* 1990;259(4 Pt 1):C640–C646.

22. Beynon HL, Walport M, Dawson P. Vascular endothelial injury by intravascular contrast agents. *Invest Radiol.* 1994;29(suppl 2):S195–S197.

23. Karstoft J, Baath L, Jansen I, Edvinsson L. Calcium antagonistic effect of an angiographic contrast medium in vitro: a comparison of the effects of iohexol with the effects of nifedipine in isolated arteries. *Invest Radiol.* 1995;30: 21–27.

24. Older R, Korobkin M, Cleeve DM, Schaaf R, Thompson W. Contrast-induced acute renal failure: persistent nephrogram as clue to early detection. *Am J Roentgenol.* 1980; 134:339–342.

25. Love L, Johnson MS, Bresler M, et al. The persistent computed tomography nephrogram: its significance in the diagnosis of contrast-associated nephrotoxicity. *Br J Radiol.* 1994;67:951–957.

26. Fang LST, Sirota RA, Ebert TH, Lichtenstein NS. Low fractional excretion of sodium with contrast media–induced acute renal failure. *Arch Intern Med.* 1980;140:531–533.

27. Metys R, Hornych A, Burianova B, Jirka J. Influence of triiodinated contrast media on renal function. *Nephron.* 1971;8:559–565.

28. Reiss MD, Bookstein JJ, Bleifer KH. Radiologic aspects of renovascular hypertension. *JAMA.* 1973;221:375–378.

29. Port FK, Wagoner RD, Fulton RE. Acute renal failure after angiography. *Am J Roentgenol.* 1974;121:544–550.

30. Older RA, Miller JP, Jackson DC, Johnsrude IS, Thompson WM. Angiographically induced renal failure and its radiographic detection. *Am J Roentgenol.* 1976;126:1039–1045.

31. Swartz R, Rubin J, Leening B, Silva P. Renal failure following major angiography. *Am J. Med.* 1978;65:31–37.

32. Byrd L, Sherman RL. Radiocontrast induced acute renal failure: A clinical and pathophysiologic review. *Medicine.* 1979;58:270–279.

33. Krumlovsky FA, Simon N, Santhanam S, del Greco F, Roxe D, Pomaranc MM. Acute renal failure associated with administration of radiographic contrast material. *JAMA* 1978;239:125–127.

34. Shusterman N. Risk factor and outcome of hospital acquired renal failure. *Am J Med.* 1987;83:65–71.

35. Moore RD, Steinberg EP. Nephrotoxicity of high osmolarity versus low osmolarity contrast media: Randomized clinical trial. *Radiology.* 1992;182:649–655.

36. VanZee BE, Hoy W, Talley T, Jaenike J. Renal injury associated with intravenous pyelography in nondiabetic and diabetic patients. *Ann Intern Med.* 1978;89:51–54.

37. Harkonen S, Kjellstrand C. Exacerbation of diabetic renal failure following intravenous pyelography. *Am J Med.* 1977;63:939–946.

38. Humes DH, Hunt DA, White MD. Direct toxic effects of the radiocontrast agent diatrizoate on renal proximal tubule cells. *Am J Physiol.* 1987;252(suppl F):F246–F255.

39. Shafi T, Yin Chou S, Porush J, Shapiro W. Infusion intravenous pyelography and renal function: effects in patients with chronic renal insufficiency. *Arch Intern Med.* 1978; 138:1218–1221.

40. Larson TS, Hudson J, Mertz J, Romero L, Knox G. Renal vasoconstrictive response to contrast medium: the role of sodium balance and the renin–angiotensin system. *J Lab Clin Med.* 1983;101:385–391.

41. Dean RE, Andrew JH, Read RC. The red cell factor in renal damage from angiographic media. *JAMA.* 1964;187: 27–31.

42. Heyman SN, Clark L, Cantley L, Spokes K. Effect of Ioversol versus Iothalamate on endothelin release and radiocontrast nephropathy. *Invest Radiol.* 1993;28:313–318.

43. Harkonen S, Kjellstrand C. Contrast nephropathy: editorial review. *Am J Nephrol.* 1981;1:69–77.

44. Kleinknecht D, Deloux J, Hornberg J. Acute renal failure after intravenous urography: detection of antibodies against contrast media. *Clin Nephrol.* 1974;2:116–119.

45. Heideman M, Claes G, Nilson AE. The risk of renal allograft rejection following angiography. *Transplantation.* 1976;21:289–293.

46. Hill JA, Winneford M, Cohen MB, et al. Multicenter trial of ionic versus nonionic contrast media for cardiac angiography: the Iohexol Cooperative Study. *Am J Cardiol.* 1993; 72:770–775.

47. Maytin O, Castillo C, Castellanos A. The genesis of QRS changes produced by selective coronary arteriography. *Circulation.* 1970;41:247–255.

48. Lautin ME, Freeman N, Belizon I. Radiocontrast-associated renal dysfunction: a comparison of lower-osmolarity and conventional high-osmolarity contrast media. *AJR Am J Roentgenol.* 1991;157:59–65.

49. Weisberg LS, Kurnik PB, Kurnik BR. Risk of radiocontrast nephropathy in patients with and without diabetes mellitus. *Kidney Int.* 1994;45:259–265.

50. Khoury Z, Schlicht JR, Como J, Karschner JK. The effect of prophylactic nifedipine in renal function in patients administered contrast media. *Pharmacotherapy.* 1995;15: 59–65.

51. Solomon R, Werner C, Mann D, D'Ella J, Silva P. Effects of saline, mannitol, and furosemide to prevent acute decreases in renal function induced by radiocontrast agents. *N Engl J Med.* 1994;331:1416–1420.

Section 8
Femoropopliteal Occlusive Disease

64

The Pathogenesis of Vascular Disease

Richard M. Fleming

The prevalence of vascular disease has increased in both the United States and Europe since the end of World War II. The pathogenesis of vascular disease has been directly linked to changes in dietary habits and lifestyle practices and the discovery of penicillin by Sir Alexander Fleming in 1928, which led to a reduction in deaths secondary to bacterial infections. Multiple theories have evolved regarding the various factors associated with an increased risk of vascular disease. It is important to realize, however, that the study of the pathogenesis and subsequent treatment of vascular disease requires a "bigger picture" approach rather than consideration of just one or two factors. In this chapter, we review the contributions made by many investigators who have looked at one or more of these issues. We discuss the relationship (Fleming's Unified Theory of Vascular Disease[1]) between these factors (Figure 64.1) and their overall role in the pathogenesis of vascular disease, including coronary artery disease, carotid artery disease, and peripheral vascular disease. We also review the importance and benefit of looking at each of these contributing factors when evaluating and treating an individual with vascular disease.

Sources of Endothelial Injury

The initiation of vascular disease begins with injury to the endothelial wall. This process can begin as soon as stretching of the endothelium occurs, which is while the child is within the mother's uterus and blood is pulsing through the arteries and veins. This pulsation of blood is necessary for survival, but it initiates the stretching of endothelial cells and the potentiation for injury. Clearly the human organism is designed to deal with this phenomenon or it would be incompatible with life itself. It is also clear from human history that longevity is not related to medical science, in that Muhammad lived for 62 years, Gandhi for 79 years, Buddha for 80 years, and Methuselah for 969 years.

It is now clear that endothelial injury can occur from many causes. Such injuries can be caused by rupture of endothelial plaques after the formation of foam cells. This endothelial rupture may or may not expose collagen or other connective tissue, which can then precipitate the clotting cascade that is discussed later. Other causes include trauma to the blood vessel, free radical (e.g., oxygen) formation, bacterial invasion of the vessel, and formation of a thrombus, with subsequent activation of growth factors, inflammatory mediators, and vasoconstrictors and potential lumen occlusion.

Once the endothelial cells are damaged, the phospholipoproteins that are released include phosphatidylinositol 4,5-biphosphate (PIP_2) and phosphatidylcholine (PC). Both undergo a series of changes and ultimately become a 20-carbon polyunsaturated fat known as arachidonic acid (AA), which is then released from the endothelial cell. Regardless of the cause of endothelial injury, the overall process is as shown in Figures 64.1 and 64.2.

The presence of fatty streaks, which has been documented in children[2] as young as 10 years, gives way to fibroproliferative infiltration by smooth muscle cells from the media. The mechanism for fibroproliferative infiltration is the release of such substances as platelet-derived growth factor (PDGF) and will be discussed later. Once the endothelium is injured or denuded, there is an increased receptiveness to immunoglobulin G and a vasospastic responsive to 5-hydroxytryptamine in the presence of thromboxane A_2 (discussed later). The vasodilative response to 5-hydroxytryptamine is inhibited in the presence of dysfunctional endothelium. The increased uptake of immunoglobulin G[3] is correlated with an increased replication of endothelium necessary to repair and replace damaged endothelium.

The Fleming Unified Theory of Vascular Disease was developed by Dr. Fleming in June 1997.

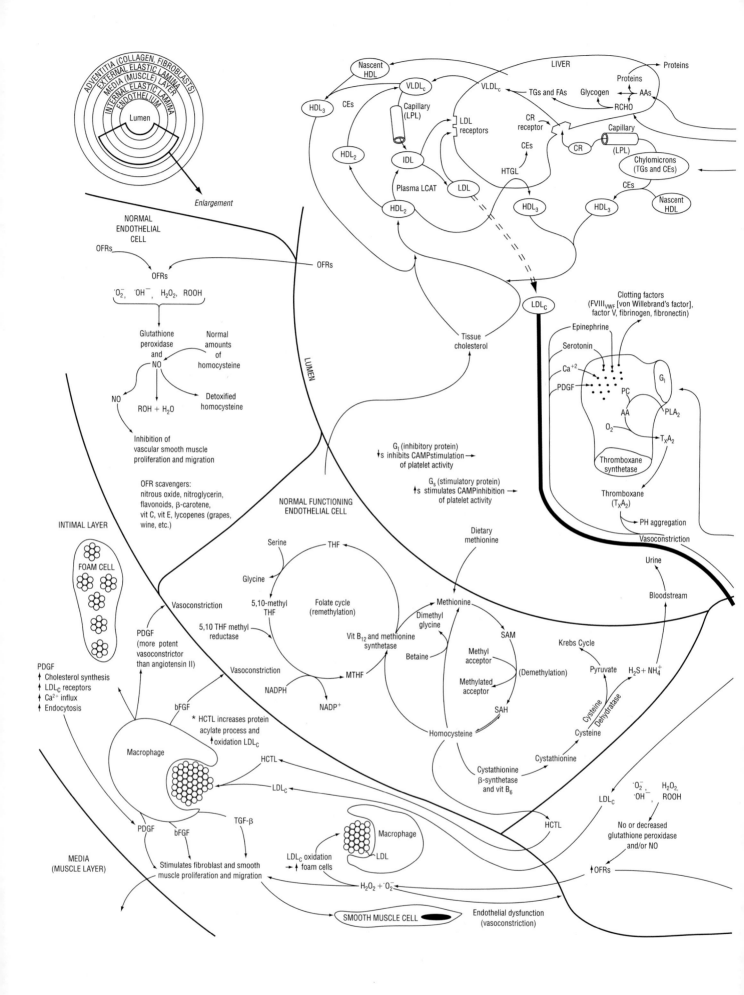

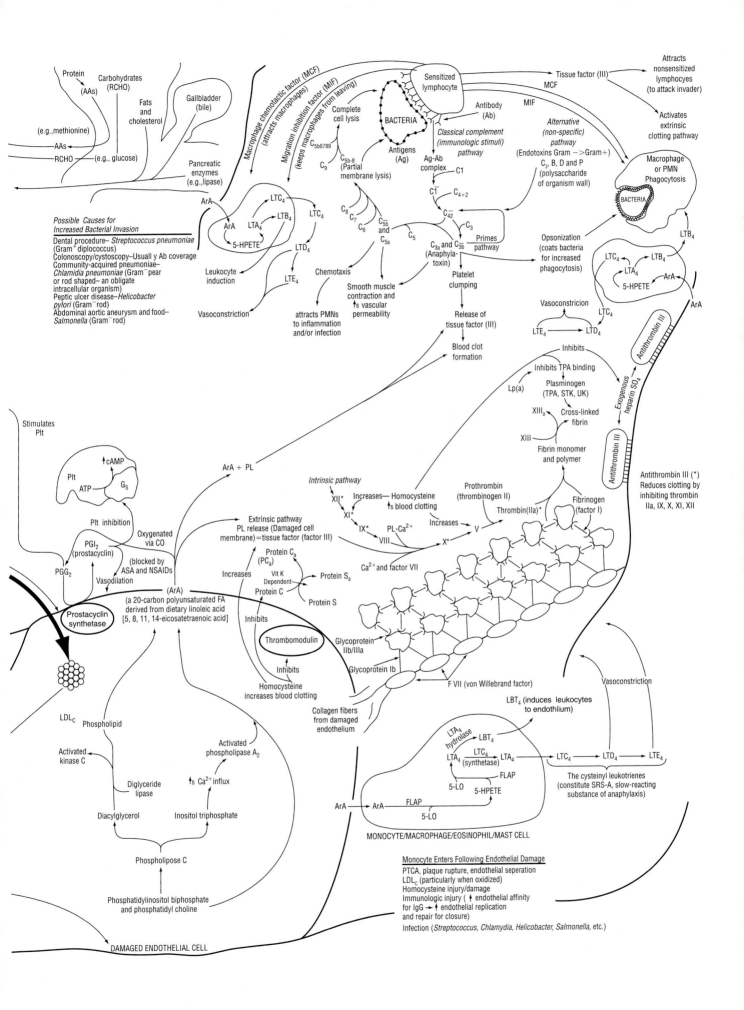

FIGURE 64.1. The Fleming Unified Theory of Vascular Disease. The interrelatedness of each of the various (eight) groups of factors is shown in this schematic of an artery. The artery represents any artery within the body, including coronary, carotid, and peripheral arteries. See text for details. AA, amino acid; ArA, arachidonic acid; bFGF, basic fibroblastic growth factor; CEs, cholesterol esters; CO, cyclooxygenase; CR, chylomicron remnant; FAs, fatty acids; FLAP, 5-lipoxygenase-activating pro- tein; HCTL, homocysteine thiolactone; 5-HPETE, 5-hydroper- oxyeicostetranoic acid; HTGL, hepatic triglyceride lipase; LCAT, lecithin-cholesterol acyltransferase; 5-LO, 5-lipoxyge- nase; MTHF, 5-methyl tetrahydrofolate; NO, nitrous oxide; OFRs, oxygen free radicals; PDGF, platelet-derived growth fac- tor; Plt, platelets; PL, phospholipoprotein; SAH, *S*-adenosyl ho- mocysteine; SAM, *S*-adenosyl methionine; TGF-β, tissue growth factor β; TGs, triglycerides; THF, tetrahydrofolate.

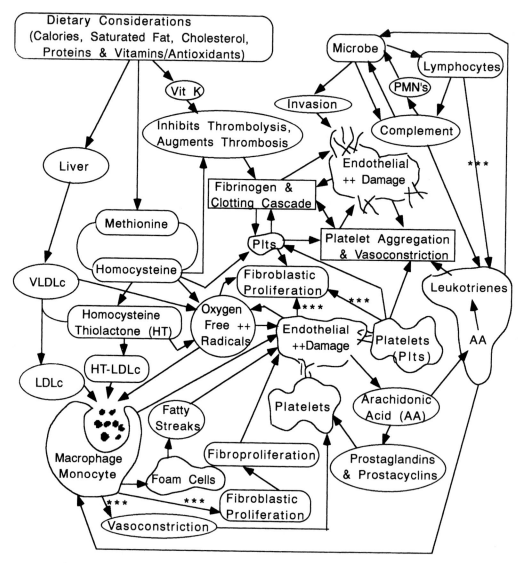

FIGURE 64.2. Simplified model of Fleming's Unified Theory of Vascular Disease. Eight groups of factors are fitted together in the overall explanation of vascular disease. These include di- etary concerns, which generate very-low-density lipoprotein cholesterol (VLDLc) and low-density lipoprotein cholesterol (LDLc). These are phagocytized by macrophages along with homocysteine thiolactone ([HT]-LDLc), which results from the metabolic catabolism of the amino acid methionine. En- dothelial damage results in activation of prostacyclins, prostaglandins, and leukotrienes. Bacterial invasion precipi- tates both inflammatory and complement activation as the body makes an effort to remove the offending organisms. The initiation of fibroproliferation results in advanced atheroscle- rotic plaques that produce further endothelial problems, pro- moting further disease. ***, growth factors or other chemical mediators; ++, other interactions not shown here (but dis- cussed in text); endothelial damage, endothelial damage and dysfunction. PMNs-polymorphonuclear leukocytes.

Dietary Factors Involved in Vascular Disease: The First Group of Factors

Numerous factors must be considered when looking at the dietary changes[4-6] required to reduce lipids. These changes include five major issues. The first is *caloric consumption*. It is now known that rats that consume twice the recommended number of calories necessary for survival demonstrate a decreased lifespan, with greater health problems, whereas rats that consume 70% of the recommended number of calories live twice as long as the average rat, with fewer health problems. There is no reason to believe this is different for humans.

Regardless of whether consumed calories begin as protein, carbohydrate, fat, or alcohol, excess caloric consumption is stored primarily as triglycerides or fats. This has been shown in the Tarahumara Indians, who have virtually no coronary artery disease despite relatively low levels of high-density lipoprotein cholesterol. When the Tarahumarans were placed on hypercaloric diets, they demonstrated a significant increase in plasma lipids[7] as well as weight. These fats eventually accumulate by way of production of very-low-density lipoprotein cholesterol and, subsequently, low-density lipoprotein cholesterol (LDLc), which is deposited in the subendothelial region of blood vessels. This is an excellent source of fatty acids, which are the primary energy source for organs such as the heart; however, excess accumulation results in monocyte and macrophage phagocytization and the initial development of fatty streaks.

Monocytes exit the lumina of blood vessels and become tissue macrophages that engulf the LDLc in an effort to remove the extracellular material. Eventually this phagocytized LDLc results in the macrophages' becoming foam cells. These macrophages release a number of chemical mediators, including PDGF, which causes vasoconstriction of the blood vessel. PDGF is in fact a more potent vasoconstrictor than angiotensin II. Also released is basic fibroblastic growth factor (bFGF), which enhances fibroblast formation in the medial layer and migration into the subendothelial region; this results in the more advanced stages of atherosclerotic disease (namely, fibroproliferation). The release of basic fibroblastic growth factor[8] from arteries after trauma or intervention (e.g., catheter-induced deendothelialization) increases intimal smooth muscle proliferation along with restenosis. Additionally, TGFb is released, which also promotes fibroproliferation.

Probably more important than any other factor is the role of excessive dietary fat, particularly the *saturated fats*. It has been shown that dietary fat consumption is extremely important for two reasons: (1) fat has 9 calories per gram and (2) saturated fats, which pervade the diets in most industrialized countries today, is artherogenic. The residents of these countries are plagued with vascular disease, cancer, and other related health problems. Regardless of the study considered, successful attempts at reducing cholesterol levels have required simultaneous reductions in dietary saturated fat intake. However, some quantity of dietary fat is necessary (essential fatty acids) for the healthy survival of the human species. The essential fatty acids are polyunsaturated fats (fatty acids) and include linoleic acid (9,12-octadecadienoic), linolenic acid (9,12,15-octadecatrienoic), and AA (5,8,11,14-eicosatetraenoic). AA can be synthesized in the body from linolenic acid. Studies in the 1970s and 1980s saw people lowering fat intake to less than 10% of their total caloric intake. When fat consumption is less than 8% of the daily total caloric intake, significant health issues arise, including immunologic problems.

In the 1940s and 1950s, the ability to preserve food increased as a result of our ability to hydrogenate food. This process of saturating a fat (*trans*-fat) was good for extending the shelf life of food, but not the "shelf life" of people. Saturated fats are particularly problematic, and even a single high-fat meal[9] has been shown to inhibit normal endothelial function by way of oxidative injury. The overall goal, therefore, is not to eliminate all fat from the diet but to reduce the amount of saturated fat and reduce the percentage of calories consumed as fat to approximately 15% of the total caloric intake, assuming the correct amount of calories[4-6] is being eaten daily.

The third dietary factor is *cholesterol intake*. Obviously, the ingestion of cholesterol is of concern because of the relationship between dietary cholesterol and very-low-density lipoprotein cholesterol production by the liver. There is also a relationship[10] between cholesterol levels, heart disease, and systolic blood pressure. However, the major contributing factor would appear to be not the amount of cholesterol in the diet but the amount of saturated fats found in foods that are also relatively high in cholesterol content. Of the cholesterol consumed daily, approximately 10% is absorbed across the gastrointestinal tract. Because the daily American diet includes an average of 250 to 500 mg of cholesterol, 25 to 50 mg are absorbed daily. However, the liver makes an average of 1000 mg of cholesterol daily. This explains why changes in dietary cholesterol intake *alone* may or may not be associated with changes in serum cholesterol levels and, subsequently, with the severity of atherosclerotic disease. This was first emphasized by Ancel Keys, who discussed the benefits of the Mediterranean diet. Dietary changes that do not take into account caloric and saturated fat intake, in addition to cholesterol, may demonstrate initial improvements but are unable to maintain control or reversal of vascular disease. This is the principal problem behind vegetarian diets, when *both* caloric and fat intake are not controlled.

A fourth dietary concern is protein and subsequently *homocysteine,* which is discussed in the next section as an independent risk factor. It is important to note here, however, that elevations in homocysteine result in increased phagocytosis of LDLc and LDLc–homocysteine–thiolactone complexes. This complex results in an increased oxidative load and further endothelial and subendothelial injury.

Finally, the role of *antioxidants* must be taken into consideration. Whether the oxygen free radicals (OFRs) are produced by way of damaged endothelium, excessive homocysteine, or responses to inflammatory or infectious agents, the effect of OFRs is the same. These extremely toxic compounds cause endothelial damage and dysfunction, resulting in vasoconstriction in addition to fibroblastic proliferation, increased phagocytosis of LDLc by macrophages, and further endothelial damage. Therefore, the ingestion of vitamins C and E, carotenoids such as beta carotene and lycopene, flavonoids (found in grape juice), selenium, flaxseed, or soy protein and the use of medications such as nitroglycerin have a positive (e.g., vasodilative) effect by reducing the levels of OFRs.[9,11] Other vitamins such as vitamin K must also be considered because of the effect on the extrinsic clotting pathway, particularly in individuals who take warfarin or related medications.

The Role of Homocysteine: The Second Group of Factors

Homocysteine has been recognized as a risk factor[12–16] for vascular disease ever since researchers looked at the prevalence of elevated homocysteine levels in younger individuals who were thought to have premature coronary artery disease. The enzymatic pathway of homocysteine shows it to be a metabolic product of the essential dietary amino acid methionine. Some endothelial cells have been shown[17] to have less cystathionine β-synthase activity, which could potentially increase their risk of endothelial damage. Excessive accumulation of homocysteine results in several vascular responses. The first is an overwhelming of the endothelial tissue's ability to detoxify the OFRs generated from the homocysteine. The OFRs not only use up the nitrous oxide that would have a vasodilative effect but actually cause endothelial dysfunction and vasoconstriction.

The OFRs also stimulate fibroblast[18,19] and smooth muscle proliferation and migration to the subendothelial region, thereby enhancing the progression of vascular disease. Homocysteine is also metabolized to homocysteine thiolactone,[20,21] which increases the harmful acylate process and oxidative process of LDLc, thereby increasing phagocytosis of LDLc and LDLc–homocysteine–

thiolactone complexes by macrophages with the subsequent development of foam cells and fatty streaks.

Homocysteine increases the formation of thrombi and blood clots by interfering with heparin sulfate's activation of antithrombin III and decreasing antithrombin III levels. Homocysteine has also been shown to inhibit thrombomodulin expression, induce the expression of tissue factor, and reduce the binding of tissue plasminogen activator (TPA) to its endothelial receptor. Homocysteine also increases factors XI and V, decreases protein C activation, and increases the expression of thromboxane A_2 (TxA2). Homocysteine subsequently promotes a hypercoagulable state that has been shown to increase the risk for multiple vascular problems,[22–26] including myocardial infarction, cerebrovascular accidents, deep venous thrombosis, and peripheral vascular disease, particularly when coupled with stenotic lesions[27,28] where changes in entry *(a)* and exit *(w)* angles to and from a narrowed vessel will further promote thrombus formation.

The Role of Hyperfibrinogenemia and Hypercoagulability: The Third Group of Factors

Damage to the endothelium of a blood vessel may occur from rupture of a plaque, cracking, fissuring, de-endothelialization (e.g., angioplasty), stretching of endothelial cells (advanced atherosclerosis), inflammatory or immunologic reactions (e.g., lupus anticoagulant), or surgical interventions. Once this has occurred with membrane phospholipid release (phosphatidylinositol 4,5-biphosphate and phosphatidyl choline), the connective tissue components are exposed. Paramount in this process is the release of AA and the exposure of collagen and von Willebrand's factor necessary for initiation of thrombus formation. However, as mentioned previously,[27] narrowed entry *(a)* and exit *(w)* angles also promote thrombus formation.

Once von Willebrand's factor and collagen are exposed, platelets are attracted to the area, where they bind to the damaged subendothelium (von Willebrand's factor–collagen complexes or polymers) and attach by means of platelet glycoproteins (glycoprotein Ib). When there is inadequate release of von Willebrand's factor (type I defect) or defective von Willebrand's factor (type II defect) is released, bleeding disorders (von Willebrand's disease) occur. When the platelets have no glycoprotein Ib (Bernard–Soulier syndrome), bleeding problems also occur. When there are no homeostatic abnormalities, the attachment of platelets to von Willebrand's factor–collagen complex occurs, with subsequent attraction of additional platelets that bind to each other by way of another glycoprotein known as glycoprotein IIb/IIIa. This glycoprotein is absent in individuals with Glanzmann's thrombasthenia, who also have bleeding disorders.

As shown in Figures 64.1 and 64.2, the release of AA leads to the production of antagonistic pathways (namely, prostacyclins and prostaglandins) that have opposing effects on platelet activation and vasomotor function. The AA also enters the monocyte/macrophage cells (mononuclear phagocytic/reticuloendothelial system), which is discussed later. The damaged endothelium (extrinsic pathway) also releases tissue thromboplastin (tissue factor), and the simultaneous disruption of blood flow (e.g., narrowed vessel, exposed subendothelium) initiates the intrinsic pathway for blood coagulation. Any factor that increases blood viscosity will also increase the tendency for blood clot formation. Such factors include cancer, inflammatory states, and hyperfibrinogenemia.

The extrinsic and intrinsic pathways converge where prothrombin/thrombinogen (factor II) is converted to thrombin (factor IIa), which is responsible for converting fibrinogen into fibrin monomers and subsequently fibrin polymers. Excessive fibrinogen augments this reaction and promotes thrombus formation. A pronounced effect of homocysteine is the promotion of a hypercoagulable state by increasing certain factors and inhibiting others. Likewise, lipoprotein(a), which has a molecular structure similar to those of LDLc and plasminogen,[29] impairs tissue plasminogen activation of plasminogen while inhibiting the binding of tissue plasminogen activator to the endothelial receptor for tissue plasminogen activator. This last effect is similar to one of the hypercoagulable properties of homocysteine.

One of the frequently unaddressed benefits of exercise is the beneficial impact on clotting factors. It has been demonstrated[30] that lower fibrinogen levels are seen in individuals who exercise regularly. Multiple factors that increase the potential for thrombus formation are reduced with exercise, including thromboxane A_2.[31]

The Role of Antioxidants: The Fourth Group of Factors

OFRs are extremely toxic for all living things. This includes not only the lytic effect on bacteria, which are phagocytized by polymorphonuclear leukocytes and monocytes/macrophages, but also the damage that can occur to the body itself. Multiple enzymatic pathways exist within the body to reduce these toxic products.

OFRs are reduced in endothelial cells (and elsewhere) by means of the enzyme glutathione peroxidase. If this enzyme is missing (as in hyperhomocysteinemia) or overwhelmed, the OFRs accumulate and cause endothelial damage. This oxidative stress has been shown to be associated with coronary artery disease[32–35] as well as cancer,[36] diabetes,[37] and even cardiac failure.[38] Whereas

high-density lipoprotein cholesterol serves as a scavenger mechanism for moving LDLc/cholesterol esters, antioxidants serve as free radical scavengers. Unlike high-density lipoprotein cholesterol, antioxidants do not merely move the offending agent around but catabolize the offending molecules.

Increased OFRs not only cause endothelial injury, but they also initiate a series of events including the oxidation of LDLc, which results in an increased propensity for phagocytosis of LDLc by macrophages. Increased levels of homocysteine also result (discussed previously) in the formation of LDLc–homocysteine–thiolactone complexes, which are also phagocytized by macrophages. These macrophages then release several substances (growth factors), to be discussed later. They include PDGF, basic fibroblastic growth factor, and tissue growth factor β. OFRs also cause endothelial dysfunction with subsequent vasoconstriction, which not only decreases blood flow but also enhances the potential for thrombosis.

In the presence of normally functioning endothelium, nitrous oxide, like nitroglycerin, results in inhibition of vascular smooth muscle (vasodilation) and decreases the proliferation and migration of fibroblasts and smooth muscle cells from the media (muscular) layer of the vessel into the subintimal layer. As the levels of OFRs increase, nitrous oxide (NO) is consumed, resulting in enhanced OFR effect without antagonism. Antioxidants have been shown to scavenge the OFRs and reduce the effects of vascular disease[39,40] independent of other risk potentiators or risk factors.

Endothelial and Other Growth Factors: The Fifth Group of Factors

The basic role of the vascular system is to maintain the integrity of blood flow throughout the body. To do this, when damage occurs in one part of the vascular system, the affected area must take action to reduce the overall risk to the rest of the body. An underlying theme to living organisms is the use of a limited number of chemical reactions and mediators to produce various effects throughout the body. These chemical mediators are released from different cells of the body in an effort to carry out their individual tasks and communicate with other cells. Chemical mediators (factors) that have one effect in the vascular system have different effects in other parts of the body. For example, activation of smooth muscles in blood vessel walls results in vasoconstriction, whereas activation of smooth muscles in bronchial endothelium results in bronchospasm, even though the same chemical substances are being released.

When the endothelium is injured, collagen fibers are exposed and tissue factor is released. Both of these events stimulate the formation of blood clotting and fibrin development. The damaged endothelium releases AA, which stimulates prostaglandin, prostacyclin, and thromboxane A_2 formation. The AA also activates the leukotriene pathways, which are discussed in greater detail later. Platelets are activated by the formation of a fibrin clot (discussed previously), elevations in homocysteine levels, and prostaglandin synthesis. The platelets release PDGF, epinephrine, and additional thromboxane A_2. The thromboxane A_2 attracts more platelets, and the epinephrine increases platelet aggregation and promotes vasoconstriction. The PDGF, which is also released from macrophages that phagocytize cholesterol, causes vasoconstriction.

Once released, PDGF stimulates fibroblast and smooth muscle proliferation and migration from the media to the intimal layer, where fatty streaks are converted to fibrous plaques.[41,42] As a result of PDGF, macrophages exhibit an increase in LDLc receptors (increased uptake of LDLc) and an increased influx of calcium into the macrophage. The increased phagocytosis of LDLc is associated with an increase in cholesterol synthesis.

Another factor released after endothelial injury is basic fibroblastic growth factor, which is angiogenic and has been found in greater than normal quantities in atherosclerotic vessels[43] and damaged[44] vessels. Although basic fibroblastic growth factor has been shown to be associated with collateralization of blood vessels, it has also been shown[8] to produce vasoconstriction and is released from macrophages. After angioplasty, vasoconstriction routinely occurs[45] in both distal and control regions[46] of the vessel. The three primary mitogenic effects of basic fibroblastic growth factor are smooth muscle and fibroblastic proliferation, as noted previously, and endothelial cell proliferation. Endothelial cell proliferation occurs by means of two mechanisms, the first being a direct effect and the second by upregulation[47,48] of vascular endothelial growth factor, thereby promoting angiogenesis. An additional function for heparin has been postulated[49] based on early research.

Tissue growth factor β is also released from macrophages and stimulates the proliferation and migration of fibroblasts and smooth muscle cells into the intimal layer, further promoting the advancement of fatty streaks to fibrous plaque formation. Other chemical mediators have been shown to be involved in other aspects of vascular disease. These are discussed independently in the following sections.

The Role of Leukotrienes: The Sixth Group of Factors

The release of AA from damaged endothelial cells has been shown to lead to the production of prostaglandins and prostacyclins, which are antagonistic pathways that have added to the understanding of the molecular mechanisms involved in thrombogenesis. Their actual role, although chemically complex, is rather limited in the overall unified theory of vascular disease. More important in the overall regulation and control are the chemical substances known as leukotrienes. These potent chemical mediators have been largely unrecognized until recently. The development of leukotriene inhibitors has resulted in a better understanding of decompression-induced pulmonary injury[50] and treatment options for bronchospastic disease,[51,52] which is the pulmonary equivalent of vasospastic problems.

Once AA is released, it can enter the leukotriene pathway in monocytes/macrophages, eosinophils, or mast cells. Leukotriene production occurs within these cells and gives rise to two pathways free of antagonists. The first is the production of leukotriene B4 (LTB4), which attracts more leukocytes to the region, including the site of damaged endothelium and, as we shall see later, sites of bacterial invasion. The second pathway results in the production of three chemical mediators known as leukotriene C4 (LTC4), leukotriene D4, (LTD4) and leukotriene E4 (LTE4). These three substances are known as cysteinyl leukotrienes and constitute what was formerly called slow-reacting substance of anaphylaxis. Both leukotriene D4 and leukotriene E4 cause vasoconstriction and are activated not only by endothelial injury but also by activated lymphocytes.

The Role of the Complement Cascade (Classic and Alternative Pathways): The Seventh Group of Factors

Although frequently forgotten in the investigation of vascular disease, the complement cascade cannot be ignored. Like all reactions in the body, the role of complement is not limited to certain regions of the body and, as such, should be expected to have a potential role in either the cause of or response to vascular disease. There are two major pathways to the complement system that represent a humoral response to infectious processes. In conjunction with lymphocytes, antibodies, macrophages, and polymorphonuclear leukocytes, these two pathways defend the body and vascular system against foreign invasion. In the next section we discuss the issue of bacterial involvement in vascular disease.

The introduction of bacteria into the vascular space and into the intimal region of a blood vessel would result in activation of the complement pathways as it does elsewhere in the body. Sensitized lymphocytes produce antibody (Ab) to the bacterial antigen (Ag). The antigen–antibody complexes (immunologic stimulus) activate the first component (C1) of the "classic" pathway, which leads to a series of reactions that produce several important components, including C3b, which results in opsonization (coating of the microbe to optimize phagocytosis), and C3a and C5a, which are anaphylatoxins that result in smooth (vascular) muscle contraction and an increase in vascular permeability. C5a also serves as a chemotactic or attractant for leukocytes. The classic pathway terminates as C5b–C6–C7–C8–C9, which results in bacteriolysis.

The alternative pathway is activated in the presence of endotoxins or shock resulting from the polysaccharide of the microbial wall. This is more prominent for gram-negative organisms but can occur with gram-positive microbes. The alternative pathway is also primed by the C3b produced by way of the classic pathway.

Once the lymphocyte recognizes the microbe and produces an antigen–antibody complex (interaction), the lymphocyte is sensitized. The sensitized lymphocyte releases three major chemical mediators: *transfer factor*, which attracts nonsensitized lymphocytes to the region where they become sensitized; *macrophage chemotactic factor* (MCF), which attracts macrophages to the region for phagocytosis and lysis of microbes (particularly after opsonization); and *migration inhibition factor* (MIF), which keeps the macrophages present and inhibits their leaving.

The Role of Bacterial Involvement: The Eighth Group of Factors

The presence of bacterial infections is not a new problem, and recent work has shown that *Helicobacter pylori* is a major causative agent for gastric ulcers. Atherectomy specimens from coronary plaques in our laboratory and others have demonstrated bacterial agents in some of the lesions. Evidence to date demonstrates microbes not only in coronary plaques[53–56] but also in carotid artery stenosis,[57] which may lead to cerebrovascular accidents. These findings are not surprising, because it has long been recognized that disease in other vascular beds of the body has associated bacterial involvement (e.g., salmonella with abdominal aortic aneurysms).

The bacterial pathogens currently implicated are *Streptococcus pneumoniae, Chlamydia pneumoniae,* and *Helicobacter pylori.* The high prevalence of these bacterial pathogens probably accounts for their detection in atherosclerotic plaques and does not exclude other pathogens. Like rheumatic heart disease and valvular diseases that require prophylactic antibiotic coverage, individuals with vascular disease should be considered for prophylactic antibiotic coverage if there is any question about further vascular injury.

The presence of bacterial invasion in an atheromatous plaque may precipitate further problems by means of an inflammatory reaction, which may include either the complement or leukotriene pathway. The generation of OFRs may bring further problems as a result of the oxidative stress, as discussed previously.

Putting It All Together: The Eight Groups of Factors

To date, research in several different areas of vascular disease has progressed independent of research in other areas. This limitation has allowed investigators to concentrate on specific areas of interest. However, it has also limited our understanding of the interrelatedness (Figure 64.3) of each of the different factors involved.

Significant research has demonstrated the presence of atheromatous plaques in both animal models and human subjects. Diet-induced hypercholesterolemia has demonstrated fatty plaques within 1 to 2 weeks in nonhuman primates. Monocytic involvement is seen early in the process, with the formation of fatty streaks. This has also been seen in children as young as 10 years. We have seen data with progression of disease in adults in as little as 104 days,[58] which suggests that once change has begun, it can progress quite rapidly. These changes are consistent with abrupt changes in coronary blood flow[4,5] that occur too suddenly to be accounted for by changes in LDLc levels alone. Such changes can be accounted for by changes in fibrinogen or viscosity[27,28] and require that these factors also be taken into account. Likewise, improvement in serum lipids has not always been associated with clinical improvement,[59,60] despite reductions in serum lipids. We do know, however, that total serum cholesterol levels should be reduced to below 150 mg/dL, triglycerides to below 150 mg/dL, and LDLc to less than 100 mg/dL to substantially reduce the risk and progression of vascular disease. Despite the frequent testing of cholesterol, this is too often ignored or left untreated.[61]

Several factors must be taken into account when evaluating a person for vascular disease, regardless of whether one is concerned about coronary artery disease, carotid disease, deep venous thrombosis, or other problems. First, you must determine the severity of LDLc and triglyceride levels to determine the load already present, which stimulates fatty streaks, calcium deposition, and fibroproliferation. We know that dietary changes, primarily reduction in calories and the amount of saturated fats, are the primary pivotal points around which reduction of this risk factor occurs. Cholesterol intake, too, must be addressed, but it is more related to foods with high saturated fat and caloric loads. In appropriate indi-

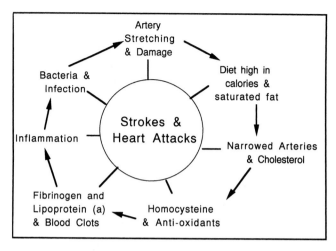

FIGURE 64.3. Damage to an artery from one group of factors may predispose the artery to further damage from other factors.

viduals, medications may in fact be necessary, but their benefit is significantly blunted without the necessary dietary changes. However, cholesterol is not the only detrimental factor affecting blood vessels. To complete the puzzle, the other pieces of the Fleming Unified Theory of Vascular Disease must be considered.

The presence of elevated homocysteine levels would suggest any of a number of other health issues (e.g., chronic renal failure, psoriasis, nitrous oxide and other medications) that need to be addressed directly, in addition to correcting nutritional factors. Treatment includes reducing contributing factors[62] and providing appropriate vitamin supplementation (vitamins B_{12} and B_6 and folate) while monitoring plasma homocysteine levels in an attempt to reduce homocysteine to the normal range of 5 to 15 mmol/L. The oxidative stress that results from hyperhomocysteinemia not only produces endothelial injury but may also be a sign of an already taxed endothelial system. The resultant OFRs along with the homocysteine can promote vasoconstriction, macrophage phagocytosis of LDLc or LDLc–homocysteine–thiolactone complexes, and stimulation and migration of fibroblasts and smooth muscle cells into the subendothelial (intimal) region, where fibrous plaque formation progresses in the presence of fatty streaks. Homocysteine additionally increases the coagulability of blood, which can be particularly problematic in vessels that have stenotic lesions or in individuals who are otherwise predisposed to clotting tendencies. These problems can be addressed nutritionally and pharmacologically but only after they are considered.

Regardless of the etiology of endothelial injury, the release of AA leads to multiple pathways, each of which must be considered, as noted previously. Although research in the arena of prostaglandins and prostacyclins

has yielded much useful information, these are pathways that antagonize each other. Attempts to manipulate one has led to the blockage or the unrestrained expression of the other. However, the leukotriene pathway, when activated, has only one noted effect on blood vessels, that being the promotion of vasoconstriction and further inflammatory response. Although helpful in the bleeding scenario, this effect becomes nonproductive in vascular disease, where limitations in blood flow are the issue. Control of these cysteinyl leukotrienes has demonstrated promise in other disease states and suggests great potential for vascular disease. Recent work confirms another component of the Fleming Unified Theory hypothesis: that leukotrienes play a role in diseased coronary arteries. Like nitrous oxide, interleukins produce vasospasm in diseased arteries while leaving no effect on nonatherosclerotic coronary arteries.[63]

A review of most cardiology textbooks reveals the prevalence of cardiovascular disease problems in individuals with inflammatory and connective tissue diseases, whereas there is a paucity of such problems reported for individuals in immunodeficient states. Activation of these inflammatory pathways attracts leukocytes to the region where complement and bacterial involvement may have already been initiated. Several studies have implicated bacterial involvement in individuals who already exhibit vascular problems. Results suggest that the damaged vessel is predisposed to bacterial invasion, which must be considered and treated. Inflammation and damage to the endothelium would appear to be necessary for bacterial involvement to occur. However, once it has occurred, the presence of both complement and cellular responses to the invasion would be no different here than elsewhere in the body, and the importance of this inflammatory and infectious process has only recently been recognized.

The Fleming Unified Theory of Vascular Disease takes information not only from our laboratory but from throughout the world and recognizes the importance of various contributions made by many investigators. It is apparent that each group of factors should somehow be linked together if the studies reported to date are correct. The models shown in Figures 64.2 and 64.3 are simplified versions of how these eight groups of factors fit together. During a patient's initial screening for vascular disease, all eight groups of factors should be checked and treated when abnormal. Periodic reassessment of the patient's response to treatment should include rechecking the abnormal factors as well as diagnostic assessment of change, including nuclear imaging; ultrasound; ·O₂max evaluation; and, when indicated, angiography. The task before us now is to take this broader working model and apply it to the screening and treatment of vascular disease in each individual.

References

1. Fleming RM. Determining the outcome of risk factor modification using positron emission tomography (PET) imaging. Paper presented at: International College of Angiology 4th World Congress; June 29, 1998; Lisbon, Portugal.

2. Stary HC, et al. Evolution of atherosclerotic plaques in the coronary arteries of young adults [abstract]. *Arteriosclerosis.* 1983;2:471.

3. Hansson GK, et al. Ultrastructural studies on nonatherosclerotic rabbits. *Exp Mol Pathol.* 1980;33:301.

4. Fleming RM, Ketchum K, Fleming DM, Gaede R. Treating hyperlipidemia in the elderly. *Angiology.* 1995;46:1075–1083.

5. Fleming RM, Ketchum K, Fleming DM, Gaede R. Assessing the independent effect of dietary counseling and hypolipidemic medications on serum lipids. *Angiology.* 1996;47:831–840.

6. Fleming RM. *How to Bypass Your Bypass: What Your Doctor Doesn't Tell You About Cholesterol and Your Diet.* Bethel, Conn: Rutledge Books; 1997.

7. McMurry MP, Cerqueira MT, Connor SL, Connor WE. Changes in lipid and lipoprotein levels and body weight in Tarahumara Indians after consumption of an affluent diet. *N Engl J Med.* 1991;325:1704–1708.

8. Staab ME, Simari RD, Srivatsa SS, et al. Enhanced angiogenesis and unfavorable remodeling in injured porcine coronary artery lesions: effects of local basic fibroblast growth factor delivery. *Angiology.* 1997;48:753–760.

9. Plotnick GD, Corretti MC, Vogel RA. Effect of antioxidant vitamins on the transient impairment of endothelium-dependent brachial artery vasoactivity following a single high-fat meal. *JAMA.* 1997;278:1682–1686.

10. Newman WP, Freedman DS, Voors AW, Freedman DS, Voors AW. Relation of serum lipoprotein levels and systolic blood pressure to early atherosclerosis. The Bogalusa Heart Study. *N Engl J Med.* 1986;314:138–144.

11. Prasad K, Kalra J. Oxygen free radicals and hypercholesterolemic atherosclerosis: effect of vitamin E. *Am Heart J.* 1993;125:958–973.

12. McCully KS, Wilson RB. Homocysteine theory of arteriosclerosis. *Atherosclerosis.* 1975;22:215–227.

13. Verhoef P, Hennekens CH, Malinow MR, Willett WC, Stampfer MJ. A prospective study of plasma homocyst(e)ine and risk of ischemic stroke. *Stroke.* 1994;25:1924–1930.

14. Alfthan G, Pekkanen J, Jauhianen M, et al. Relation of serum homocysteine and lipoprotein(a) concentrations to atherosclerotic disease in a prospective Finnish population based study. *Atherosclerosis.* 1994;106:9–19.

15. Selhub J, Jacques PF, Bostom AG, et al. Association between plasma homocysteine concentrations and extracranial carotid-artery stenosis. *N Engl J Med.* 1995;332:286–291.

16. Perry IJ, Refsum H, Morris RW, Ebrahim SB, Ueland PM, Shaper AG. Prospective study of serum total homocysteine concentration and risk of stroke in middle-aged British men. *Lancet.* 1995;346:1395–1398.

17. Jacobsen DW, Savon SR, Stewart RW, et al. Limited capacity for homocysteine catabolism in vascular cells and tissues: a pathophysiologic mechanism for arterial damage in hyperhomocysteinemia [abstract]. *Circulation* 1995;92(suppl 1):104.

18. Tsai J-C, Perella MA, Yoshizumi M, et al. Promotion of vascular smooth muscle growth by homocysteine: a link to atherosclerosis. *Proc Natl Acad Sci U S A.* 1994;91:6369–6373.

19. Lentz SR, Sobey CG, Piegors DJ, et al. Vascular dysfunction in monkeys with diet-induced hyperhomocyst(e)inemia. *J Clin Invest.* 1996;98:24–29.

20. Parthasarathy S. Oxidation of low-density lipoproteins by thiol compounds leads to its recognition by the acetyl LDL receptor. *Biochim Biophys Acta.* 1987;917:337–340.

21. Olszewski AJ, McCully KS. Homocysteine metabolism and the oxidative modification of proteins and lipids. *Free Radic Biol Med.* 1993;14:683–693.

22. Pancharuniti N, Lewis CA, Sauberlich HE, et al. Plasma homocyst(e)ine, folate, and vitamin B-12 concentrations and risk for early-onset coronary artery disease. *Am J Clin Nutr.* 1994;59:940–948.

23. Mayer EM, Jacobsen DW, Robinson K. Homocysteine and coronary atherosclerosis. *J Am Coll Cardiol.* 1996;27:517–527.

24. Graham IM, Daly LE, Refsum HM, et al. Plasma homocysteine as a risk factor for vascular disease. The European Concerted Action Project. *JAMA.* 1997;277:1775–1781.

25. Tawakol A, Omland T, Gerhard M, Wu JT, Creager MA. Hyperhomocysteinemia is associated with impaired endothelial-dependent vasodilation in humans. *Circ J Am Heart Assoc.* 1997;95:1191–1121.

26. Kottke Marchant K, Green R, Jacobsen DW, et al. High plasma homocysteine: a risk factor for arterial and venous thrombosis in patients with normal hypercoagulation profiles. *Clin Appl Thromb Hemost.* In press.

27. Fleming RM, Harrington GM, Gibbs HR, Swafford J. Quantitative coronary arteriography and its assessment of atherosclerosis. Part I. Examining the independent variables. *Angiology.* 1994;45:829–833.

28. Fleming RM, Harrington GM. Quantitative coronary arteriography and its assessment of atherosclerosis. Part II. Calculating stenosis flow reserve from percent diameter stenosis. *Angiology.* 1994;45:835–840.

29. Eaton DL, Fless GM, Kohr WJ, et al. Partial amino acid sequence of apolipoprotein(a) shows that it is homologous to plasminogen. *Proc Natl Acad Sci U S A.* 1987;84:3224–3228.

30. Elwood PC, Yarnell JW, Pickering J, Fehily AM, O'Brien JR. Exercise, fibrinogen, and other risk factors for ischaemic heart disease. Caerphilly Prospective Heart Disease Study. *Br Heart J.* 1993;69:183–187.

31. Rauramaa R, Salonen JT, Kukkonen-Harjula K, et al. Effects of mild physical exercise on serum lipoproteins and metabolites of arachidonic acid: a controlled randomised trial in middle-aged men. *BMJ (Clin Res Ed).* 1984;288:603–606.

32. Stephens NG, Parsons A, Schofield PM, Kelly F, Cheeseman K, Mitchinson MJ. Randomized controlled trial of vitamin E in patients with coronary disease. Cambridge Heart Antioxidant Study (CHAOS). *Lancet.* 1996;347:781–786.

33. Kushi LH, Folsom AR, Prineas RJ, Mink PJ, Wu Y, Bostick RM. Dietary antioxidant vitamins and death from coronary artery disease in postmenopausal women. *N Engl J Med.* 1996;334:1156–1162.

34. Kardinaal AF, Kok FJ, Ringstad J, et al. Antioxidants in adipose tissue and risk of myocardial infarction: the EURAMIC study. *Lancet.* 1993;342:1379–1384.

35. Rimm EB, Stampfer MJ, Ascherio A, Giovannucci E, Colditz GA, Willett WC. Vitamin E consumption and the risk of coronary heart disease in men. *N Engl J Med*. 1993; 328:1450–1456.

36. Omenn GS, Goodman GE, Thornquist MD, et al. Effects of a combination of beta carotene and vitamin A on lung cancer and cardiovascular disease. *N Engl J Med*. 1996; 334:1150–1155.

37. Baker DE, Campbell RK. Vitamin and mineral supplementation in patients with diabetes mellitus. *Diabetes Educ*. 1992;18:420–427.

38. Prasad K, Gupta JB, Kalra J, Lee P, Mantha SV, Bharadwaj B. Oxidative stress as a mechanism of cardiac failure in chronic volume overload in canine model. *J Mol Cell Cardiol*. 1996;28:375–385.

39. Kushi LH, Folsom AR, Prineas RJ, et al. Dietary antioxidant vitamins and death from coronary heart disease in postmenopausal women. *N Engl J Med*. 1996;334:1156–1162.

40. Hertog MG, Feskens EJ, Hollman PC, Katan MB, Kromhout D. Dietary antioxidant flavonoids and risk of coronary heart disease: the Zutphen Elderly Study. *Lancet*. 1993;342:1007–1011.

41. Faggiotto A, Ross R, Harker L. Studies of hypercholesterolemia in the nonhuman primate. I. Changes that lead to fatty streak formation. *Arteriosclerosis*. 1984;4:323.

42. Faggiotto A, Ross R. Studies of hypercholesterolemia in the nonhuman primate II: Fatty streak conversion to fibrous plaque. *Arteriosclerosis*. 1984;4:341.

43. Hughes SE, Crossman D, Hall PA. Expression of basic and acidic fibroblast growth factors and their receptor in normal and atherosclerotic human arteries. *Cardiovasc Res*. 1993;27:1214–1219.

44. More RS, Brack MJ, Underwood MJ, Gershlick AH. Growth factor persistence after vessel wall injury in a rabbit angioplasty model. *Am J Cardiol*. 1994;73:1031–1032.

45. Fischell TA, Derby G, Tse TM, Stadius ML. Coronary artery vasoconstriction routinely occurs after percutaneous transluminal coronary angioplasty: a quantitative arteriographic analysis. *Circ J Am Heart Assoc*. 1988;78:1323–1334.

46. Altstidl R, Goth C, Lehmkuhl H, Bachmann K. Quantitative angiographic analysis of PTCA-induced coronary vasoconstriction in single-vessel coronary artery disease. *Angiology*. 1997;48:863–869.

47. Brogi E, Wu T, Namiki A, Isner JM. Indirect angiogenic cytokines upregulate VEGF and bFGF gene expression in vascular smooth muscle cells, whereas hypoxia upregulates VEGF expression only. *Circ J Am Heart Assoc*. 1994;90: 649–652.

48. Stavri GT, Zachary IC, Baskerville PA, Martin JF, Erusalimsky JD. Basic fibroblast growth factor upregulates the expression of vascular endothelial growth factor in vascular smooth muscle cells. *Circ J Am Heart Assoc*. 1995;92:11–14.

49. Bombardini T, Picano E. The coronary angiogenetic effect of heparin: experimental basis and clinical evidence. *Angiology*. 1997;48:969–976.

50. Little TM, Butler BD. Dibutyryl cAMP effects on thromboxane and leukotriene production in decompression-induced lung injury. *Undersea Hyperb Med*. 1997;24: 185–191.

51. Tan RA, Spector SL. Antileukotriene agents: finding their place in asthma therapy. *Contemp Int Med*. 1997;9:46–53.

52. O'Byrne PM, Israel E, Drazen JM. Antileukotrienes in the treatment of asthma. *Ann Int Med*. 1997;127:472–480.

53. Muhlestein JB, Hammond EH, Carlquist JF, et al. Increased incidence of *Chlamydia* species within the coronary arteries of patients with symptomatic atherosclerotic versus other forms of cardiovascular disease. *J Am Coll Cardiol*. 1996;27:1555–1561.

54. Voie AL. Infections may cause secondary CVD events. *Medical Tribune*. Internist & Cardiologist Edition. August 14, 1997:1.

55. Jancin B. Antimicrobial prevention of MIs tested in trials. *Internal Medicine News*. October 1, 1997:8.

56. Boschert S. Severe periodontitis worsens diabetes, CAD. *Internal Medicine News*. November 15, 1997:10.

57. Maass M, Krause E, Engel PM, Kruger S. Endovascular presence of *Chlamydia pneumoniae* in patients with hemodynamically effective carotid artery stenosis. *Angiology*. 1997;48:699–706.

58. Fleming RM. The natural progression of atherosclerosis in an untreated patient with hyperlipidemia: assessment via cardiac PET. *Int J Angiol*. Submitted.

59. Fleming RM. The clinical importance of risk factor modification: looking at both myocardial viability (MV) and myocardial perfusion imaging (MPI). *Int J Angiol*. Submitted.

60. Fleming RM. The importance of physiologic information from cardiac PET in assessing coronary artery disease in people with "normal" coronary angiograms. *Int J Angiol*. Submitted.

61. Boschert S. Cholesterol often measured, but seldom treated. *Internal Medicine News*. September 1, 1997:40.

62. Modica P. Coffee drinking increases plasma homocysteine, possible CVD risk. *Medical Tribune*. Internist & Cardiologist Edition. February 6, 1997:2.

63. Allen S, Dashwood M, Morrison K, Yacoub M. Different leukotriene constrictor response in human atherosclerotic coronary arteries. *Circulation*. 1998;97:2406–2413.

65

The Role of Angioscopy in Vascular Reconstructive Surgery of the Lower Extremities

Peter M. Sanfelippo

The traditional mainstay in structural vascular diagnosis has been contrast-enhanced angiography. The availability of small-diameter angioscopes has opened an era of intraluminal vascular assessment.

In this review I examine the history of vascular endoscopy, the structure and function of angioscopes, the indications for angioscopy, the techniques and complications of angioscopy, and the results of experience with angioscopy in lower extremity revascularization.

Background Review

History of Vascular Endoscopy

Vascular endoscopy began in 1913 when Rhea and Walker[1] introduced the concept of intraoperative visualization of the cardiac chambers at thoracotomy with the use of a lighted rigid tube. Subsequent investigators introduced modifications.

True vascular endoscopy had its first clinical applications in 1966 by Greenstone et al.,[2], who employed choledochoscopes. Towne and Bernhard[3] employed rigid choledochoscopes, arthroscopes, and flexible endoscopes in 91 vascular reconstructions. Based on that experience, the authors advocated vascular endoscopy as an alternative to operative arteriography for postreconstruction evaluation.

Beginning in the 1980s, the capability to manufacture small-diameter flexible scopes permitted a wide range of intravascular applications. Grundfest et al.[4] reported the use of intraoperative video angioscopy in patients undergoing peripheral and coronary arterial surgery. They reported significant findings in 26% of their patients. White et al.[5] compared intraoperative video angioscopy and conventional arteriography in peripheral vascular operations. They observed disparity between angioscopy and arteriography in 20% of these cases.

Structure and Function of Angioscopes

Basic to understanding angioscopes is an understanding of light transmission by fine glass fibers. When light is propagated at steep angles to the axis of a glass fiber, a portion escapes to the outside. Light traveling at shallow angles is bounced back within the fiber and is retained for transmission. Optically, the greater the optical index of refraction, the larger the range of angles permitted for total internal reflection and therefore transmission of light and images. The use of optical fibers for light transmission with a larger range of angles is possible if a thin coating or cladding of lower index of refraction is applied to the fiber surface.

Image transmission by optical fiber bundles involves the following process. The object viewed—the token image—is captured by the convex input lens, and the image is refocused (point for point) on the array of fibers in the optical bundle. The fibers are arranged coherently, and therefore the image at the distal end of the fiber-optic bundle is the same as the token image. The fiber bundle is only of the magnitude of 1 mm and therefore presents an image too small for appreciation by the unaided eye. This limitation can be solved by a magnifying lens or projection of the image onto the image converter—the retina—of a video camera.

The components of the angioscopic system are as follows. The viewing bundle, illumination fibers from a high-intensity light source, to carry light, must be of very high intensity because of the limited size of illumination fibers—0.2 mm. This is coupled to the observer by means of a magnifying lens or input to a chip video output. Some systems include a working channel of 0.4 mm and, if steering capability is desired, cables along the inner surfaces to deflect the tip.

The function of an angioscopic system is to permit endovascular visualization. The function is limited by the outer diameter of the scope and the ability to provide a clear field ahead of the scope.

Indications for Angioscopy

There are three indications for angioscopy. First, angioscopy is indicated to monitor a vascular procedure—to access an anastomosis or result of endarterectomy, thromboembolectomy, laser angioplasty, atherectomy, or valve destruction. Second, angioscopy is indicated to facilitate surgical decisions—to access the target vessel to determine the optimal site for anastomosis and the extent of disease and to view the quality of a vein graft, the completeness of valve destruction, or the location of tributaries. Third, angioscopy is indicated for obtaining data for clinical and endovascular pathological correlations.

Techniques of Angioscopy

Two considerations are key to successful angioscopy, regardless of the vessel being inspected. First, a clear field ahead of the scope is obtained by irrigation with a balanced salt solution and elimination of antegrade flow in the vessel being examined. Second, the optimal scope is selected based on the size of the vessel to be examined, the presence or absence of the need for a working channel, and steering ability.

In preparation of in situ vein grafts, the scope is positioned in the proximal vein. Irrigation through the scope clears tributary flow and closes valves. The valvulotomes can then be passed from a distal position, and the valve leaflets are engaged and cut. On withdrawal of the scope after valve lysis, tributaries can be identified for closure.

In assessing lower extremity arterial anastomoses, a scope smaller than the vessel lumen is essential to avoid vessel spasm. Irrigation through the scope or through a parallel catheter and control of inflow and collateral flow with vascular clamping, Silastic looping, or external compression optimize visualization. When monitoring intraluminal procedures, such as thrombectomy, atherectomy, or laser angioplasty, the scope is passed with the therapeutic device.

Complications

The complications of lower extremity arterial angioscopy are systemic and local. The systemic complications include the potential introduction of bacteria and excessive fluid administration. A closed irrigation system and video monitoring should minimize introduction of bacteria. Excessive fluid administration can be minimized by vascular control to minimize blood in the viewing field, an expeditious examination—the longer the procedure, the larger the volume of fluid needed—and coordination with the anesthesia providers. Local vascular complications include perforation, intimal damage, and vessel spasm. These complications can be minimized by avoiding too large a scope and by advancing the scope only when the lumen is visualized.

Results With Angioscopy

The utility of vascular endoscopy was examined by Towne and Bernhard[3] in their article titled "Vascular Endoscopy: Useful Tool or Interesting Toy?" In lower extremity revascularization, angioscopy has been employed in three aspects: completion assessment of grafts and anastomoses, preparation of in situ grafts, and thromboembolectomies of native vessels and prosthetic grafts.

Mehigan and Olcott[6] and Seeger and Abela[7] reported on lower extremity revascularizations and found a high yield of detail that is precise and readily applicable in vascular reconstructions. The results of angioscopy in 86 peripheral vascular procedures were reported by Grundfest et al.[8] in 1988. They found that the angioscopic findings resulted in changes in the operative management in 14% of anastomoses. They also found potential causes of graft occlusion in 30% of the angioscopies.

In a prospective study of the findings of completion arteriography and angioscopy, Baxter et al.[9] found that angioscopy was measurably more accurate in detecting technical problems. Harward et al.,[10] in a series of 50 patients, demonstrated improved early graft patency in the angioscopy patients compared with the patients assessed by arteriography. In the selection of saphenous vein grafts for lower extremity revascularization, angioscopy reveals abnormal vein segments and permits careful valve destruction and tributary identification.[11–13]

The benefits of angioscopic thromboembolectomy include increased accuracy of detection and localization of embolus and thrombus, ability to control balloon inflation and avoidance of overinflation, ability to assess for residual thrombus, and ability to guide manipulation of the balloon catheter in selected vessels. These results have been reported from several centers.[14–16]

I have observed the following in my own work. In the preparation of in situ grafts, complete valve incompetence and tributary identification were accomplished with angiography in 100% of patients with the addition of a mean of 7 minutes of operating time. In the assessment of anastomoses without angiography, success was achieved in 60% with the addition of a mean of 5 minutes of operating time. Angioscopy was 100% successful in facilitating and assessing extraction of thromboembolic material with the addition of a mean of 13 minutes of operating time.

In summary, angioscopy is technically simple, requires minimal additional time, and is safely applicable to lower extremity arterial reconstructions. Angioscopy simplifies and facilitates performance of in situ vein bypasses. It provides endoluminal data during endovascular procedures and is a tool for quality control.

References

1. Rhea L, Walker IC, Cutler EC. The surgical treatment of mitral stenosis. *Arch Surg.* 1924;9:689–690.
2. Greenstone SM, Shore LM, Herringman EC, Massell TB. Arterial endoscopy. *Arch Surg.* 1966;93:811–813.
3. Towne JB, Bernhard VM. Vascular endoscopy: useful tool or interesting toy? *Surgery.* 1977;82:415–r19.
4. Grundfest WS, Litvack F, Sherman T, et al. Delineation of peripheral and coronary detail by intraoperative angioscopy. *Ann Surg.* 1985;202:394–400.
5. White GH, White RA, Kopchok GE, et al. Intraoperative video angioscopy compared with arteriography during peripheral vascular operations. *J Vasc Surg.* 1987;6:488–495.
6. Mehigan JT, Olcott C. Video angioscopy as an alternative to intraoperative arteriography. *Am J Surg.* 1986;152: 139–143.
7. Seeger JM, Abela GS. Angioscopy as an adjunct to arterial reconstructive surgery. *J Vasc Surg.* 1986;4:315–320.
8. Grundfest WS, Litvack F, Glick D, et al. Intraoperative decisions based on angioscopy in peripheral vascular surgery. *Circ J Am Heart Assoc.* 1988;78(suppl I):I14–I17.
9. Baxter BT, Rizzo RJ, Flinn WR, et al. A comparative study of intraoperative angioscopy and completion arteriography following femorodistal bypass. *Arch Surg.* 1990;125: 997–1002.
10. Harward TRS, Govostis DM, Rosenthal GJ, et al. Impact of angioscopy on infrainguinal graft patency. *Am J Surg.* 1994; 168:107–110.
11. Miller A, Stonebridge PA, Tsoukas AI, et al. Angioscopically directed valvulotomy. *J Vasc Surg.* 1991;13:813–821.
12. Gilbertson JJ, Walsh DB, Zwolak RM, et al. A blinded comparison of angiography, angioscopy, and duplex scanning in the intraoperative evaluation of in situ saphenous vein bypass grafts. *J Vasc Surg.* 1992;15:121–127.
13. Sales CM, Goldsmith J, Veith FJ. Prospective study of the value of prebypass saphenous vein angioscopy. *Am J Surg.* 1995;170:106–108.
14. White GH, White RA, Kopchok GE, et al. Angioscopic thromboembolectomy. *J Vasc Surg.* 1988;7:318–323.
15. Segalowitz J, Grundfest WS, Treiman RL, et al. Angioscopy for intraoperative management of thromboembolectomy. *Arch Surg.* 1990;125:1357–1361.
16. LaMuraglia GM, Brewster DC, Moncure AC, et al. Angioscopic evaluation of unilateral aortic graft limb thrombectomy. *J Vasc Surg.* 1993;17:1069–1074.

66

Preoperative Cardiac Risk Evaluation and Management in the Patient with Peripheral Vascular Disease: The Surgeon's Perspective

*Munier M. Nazzal, Timothy F. Kresowik, Jamal J. Hoballah, William J. Sharp,
Beth A. Ballinger, and John D. Corson*

Perioperative cardiac events secondary to atherosclerotic coronary artery disease (CAD) remain a major cause of clinical concern.[1-3] Although mortality rates are now quite low in patients undergoing peripheral vascular surgical procedures, associated deaths related to cardiac causes range from 33.4% to 100%.[3-12] In addition, a perioperative myocardial infarction may be associated with significant morbidity. The prevalence of CAD in patients who have peripheral vascular disease (PVD) has been clearly demonstrated.[11,13] Hertzer et al. found that among 1000 patients with PVD, severe correctable CAD was present in 25% and severe inoperable CAD in 6%. Only 8% of the patients had no angiographic evidence of CAD.[11] The need for and importance of preoperatively identifying and stratifying the severity of CAD in patients undergoing peripheral vascular surgery is self-evident. The mere intensification of medical therapy based on preoperative risk assessment can reduce the risk of perioperative cardiac events.[14] In addition, myocardial revascularization can provide both short- and long-term survival advantages in selected patients at high risk of CAD.[11,15-17]

Techniques for preoperative cardiac assessment are quite variable. The use may range from routine[11,18,19] to selective use only.[20-22] Goldman's Cardiac Risk Index was the first systematic use of preoperative stratification of CAD.[4] Different strategies have since emerged to predict perioperative cardiac events. However, the best approach to decrease the risk of perioperative cardiac events in all patients at risk is yet to be determined. The ideal test should be very sensitive and highly specific and should provide risk stratification at low cost with minimal mortality and morbidity.

Another problem lies in determining the optimal management after identifying CAD before a general vascular surgical procedure. Although coronary revascularization may be protective to the myocardium, it can carry a significant risk to life, particularly in elderly patients.[23-25]

In this chapter we review the various methods of cardiac risk assessment and suggest a practical approach to the care of the vascular patient with CAD. Valvular heart disease is also an important issue but will not be discussed in this chapter.

CAD in Patients with PVD: Extent of the Problem

In the Cleveland Clinic Study reported by Hertzer et al.,[11] patients were stratified by their PVD problem. Severe correctable coronary ischemia was present in 36% of patients with abdominal aortic aneurysm, 32% of patients with cerebrovascular disease, and 28% of patients with lower extremity ischemia. Normal coronary arteries were identified in only 6%, 9%, and 10%, respectively. Patients aged 55 to 69 years with intermittent claudication had a 14-fold increase in the incidence of myocardial infarction and a 2-fold increase in the incidence of cardiac deaths over a 10-year follow-up in comparison with an age-matched group without PVD.[26] In an earlier study it was found that 39% sustained a nonfatal myocardial infarction or stroke within 10 years of the onset of extremity symptoms.[27] Only 22% of patients remained alive 15 years after the onset of intermittent claudication. PVD is also an independent predictor of late mortality in patients with stable CAD, with a 25% greater likelihood of mortality at any time.[16]

The reported incidence of postoperative myocardial complications after peripheral vascular surgery varies widely among different reports (Tables 66.1 through 66.3). This variation may be due in part to different methods used for diagnosing cardiac events and to the

TABLE 66.1. Incidence of perioperative myocardial infarction after aortic surgery.

Year	Reference	Patients (n)	Incidence (%)
1986	Johnson et al. [109]	459	2.0
1986	Szyalagi et al [110]	1748	5.0
1988	Bernstein et al. [111]	123	0.8
1989	Wilson et al. [112]	126	1.6
1990	Cappeler et al. [113]	349	2.9
1990	Clark et al. [114]	200	1.5
1990	Maon et al. [115]	144	4.2
1990	McEnroe et al. [19]	95	5.2
1990	Golden et al. [17]	500	3.0
1991	Shah et al. [116]	280	2.5
1992	Bunt [28]	156	0
		Total: 4180	Average: 3.6

Modified from Bunt.[28]

TABLE 66.2. Incidence of perioperative myocardial infarction with femoropopliteal and femorotibial bypass.

Year	Reference	Patients (n)	Incidence (%)
Femoropopliteal bypass			
1986	Taylor et al. [117]	239	1.7
1988	Parker et al. [118]	223	2.0
1989	Whittemore et al. [119]	300	3.0
1990	Petrovic et al. [120]	132	2.3
1991	Towne et al. [121]	361	2.2
1992	Bunt [28]	72	1.4
		Total: 1327	Average: 2.2
Femorotibial bypass			
1984	Rutherford et al. [122]	156	3.2
1988	Andros et al. [123]	224	5.4
1988	Ascer et al. [124]	24	8.3
1990	Kalmer et al. [125]	65	4.6
1992	Bunt [28]	90	3.3
		Total: 559	Average: 4.5

Modified from Bunt.[28]

TABLE 66.3. Incidence of perioperative myocardial infarction with carotid surgery.

Year	Reference	Patients (n)	Incidence (%)
1981	Hertzer and Lee [126]	355	1.6
1983	O'Donnell et al. [127]	531	2.5
1989	Kirschner et al. [128]	1035	0.2
1989	Yeager et al. [129]	249	4.0
1989	Edwards et al. [130]	3028	0.7
1990	Salenius et al. [131]	331	0
1992	Bunt [28]	114	0
		Total: 5643	Average: 0.9

Modified from Bunt.[28]

variability of the surgical procedures. Prospective studies with frequent postoperative screening for myocardial ischemia are expected to have a higher incidence of cardiac events than retrospective studies.[28]

Methods of Evaluation of Cardiac Risk

Various approaches to the preoperative assessment of cardiac risk in patients with PVD have been advocated. These approaches include the use of clinical risk factors and electrocardiogram (ECG), ventricular function and ejection fraction determination, echocardiography, exercise stress testing, pharmacological stress testing, and coronary arteriography. Descriptions of these methods and their limitations follow.

Clinical Risk Factors and ECG

Clinical risk factors were initially used in conjunction with ECG to evaluate preoperative cardiac risk status by Goldman.[4] Later, the combination of clinical risk factors and ECG abnormalities was used to screen for cardiac catheterization.[12,29] The factors evaluated were age, prior myocardial infarction, congestive heart failure, arrhythmias, hypertension, diabetes mellitus, Q wave on the ECG, and history of angina, smoking, valvular heart disease, ventricular ectopy, or stroke.[11,21,22,30,31] In general, these clinical risk factors were considered minimally useful predictors of cardiac events.[19,32,33] Angiographic evidence of CAD has been identified in only 55.4% to 68% of patients with positive clinical risk factors.[10,11,21] In one of these studies, the incidence of severe, angiographically confirmed CAD was 15% in patients with no clinical evidence of CAD and 44% in patients with clinical evidence of CAD. Of note, normal coronary arteries were present in only 14% of patients without clinical evidence of CAD and 4% of patients with clinical evidence of CAD.[11]

An abnormal ECG has been associated with a three-fold increase in the risk of perioperative cardiac events.[34,35] Even in the absence of a previous myocardial infarction, an abnormal ECG carries an increased risk of perioperative cardiac events. P-wave abnormalities and a preoperative dysrhythmia on ECG have been found to be independent predictors of postoperative cardiac events. They were found in 76.5% of patients before major vascular operations compared with 49.3% before major general surgery procedures.[36] However, a normal ECG failed to predict the presence of CAD in 32% to 45% of the patients with PVD who underwent coronary

Table 66.4: Goldman variables arranged by point value.

Variable	Point value
Third heart sound or jugular venous distention	11
Recent myocardial infarction	10
Nonsinus rhythm or premature atrial contractions on electrocardiogram	7
More than five premature ventricular contractions	7
Age >70 years	5
Emergency surgery	4
Poor general medical condition	3
Intraperitoneal, intrathoracic, or aortic surgery	3
Important valvular aortic stenosis	3

Data from Goldman et al.[4]

TABLE 66.5. Goldman predictive classes.

Class	Point range	Cardiac complications (%)
I	0–5	1
II	6–12	7
III	13–25	14
IV	>26	78

Data from Goldman et al.[4]

angiography.[10,11] In their initial report, Goldman et al.[4] assigned points to different risk factors (Table 66.4). They further stratified the risks into classes (Table 66.5) based on the sum of points from all factors. The use of this classification failed to accurately predict the outcome in patients undergoing abdominal aortic surgery. An extended form of the Goldman criteria also failed to predict deaths 50% of the time in patients after elective abdominal aortic procedures.[37] In a prospective study of patients undergoing elective abdominal aortic surgery, the use of the same Goldman criteria failed to differentiate between Goldman classes with respect to the incidence of myocardial events or cardiac deaths.[19] Other investigators have suggested different clinical criteria as the most important predictors of cardiac events. These criteria include ventricular ectopy,[21] congestive heart failure,[12] stroke,[21] and myocardial infarction.[30] Singly, however, each criterion failed to identify CAD in 30% to 85% of the cases.[10,11] The specificity of the clinical criteria can be improved by increasing the number of criteria assessed. However, greater specificity is achieved at the expense of sensitivity. Thus, clinical criteria alone are not sufficiently accurate to be used for cardiac screening before major vascular surgical procedures.[21]

Ambulatory ECG Monitoring (Holter Monitor)

Continuous ambulatory ECG monitoring has been successful in detecting ST-segment changes in patients with CAD.[38,39] An ambulatory ECG can identify ischemic ST-segment shifts, indicative of subendocardial ischemia, which are highly suggestive of myocardial perfusion abnormalities.[40,41] These abnormalities are often asymptomatic and cannot be detected by clinical risk analysis or resting ECG. Hence, this test is a relatively simple method of detecting silent myocardial ischemia.[40-43] The criteria of a positive ambulatory study, which suggests a high risk of adverse perioperative cardiac outcome, include ischemia for 60 minutes or longer, 2 mm or greater ST-segment depression, and six or more ischemic episodes per day.[44] Ambulatory ECG studies are particularly important in patients with PVD, of whom 40% to 75% are estimated to have silent ischemia.[42,43] The applicability of this screening method is hampered by the limited ambulatory capacity of most patients with PVD. Patients with underlying cardiac problems such as left ventricular hypertrophy, those medicated with digitalis, and those with conduction defects also present a challenge in the interpretation of Holter monitor tracings. Cost is another prohibitive factor preventing this technique from being used to screen every asymptomatic patient under consideration for a vascular surgery procedure. An ambulatory ECG provides a high false-positive result in asymptomatic patients with few clinical risk factors.[41] An argument can be made to limit Holter monitor screening to patients with multiple risk factors who are also able to ambulate satisfactorily. Men over age 40 and women over age 55 with two or more CAD risk factors and patients with multiple-organ PVD are appropriate candidates for ambulatory ECG monitoring.

Ejection Fraction

The ejection fraction (EF) reflects left ventricular function. It has been used as another means of preoperative cardiac risk assessment in patients who plan to undergo a vascular surgical procedure.[45,46] It can be measured by B-mode echocardiography, contrast cineangiography, or radionuclide angiography, and the measurement has been found to be reproducible, irrespective of the technique used.[47] The multigated acquisition scan is one of the most widely used techniques for EF measurement. It has a low radiation exposure, and in addition to determining the EF, a multigated acquisition scan can show myocardial wall motion abnormalities as well as left ventricular systolic and diastolic function at rest and during exercise. Values found at the peak of exercise have been suggested to be of more significance than other exercise changes.[48] However, in contrast, resting studies have been reported by others to be more useful than those obtained during exercise.[49]

The use of EF is of controversial value in predicting preoperative cardiac risk. Several reports have suggested that the EF is able to predict a perioperative myocardial infarction.[45,46,50] In one study, no perioperative myocardial infarctions occurred in patients with an EF greater than 56%. However, 70% and 80% of the patients with an EF less than 30% sustained cardiac events after lower extremity and aortic vascular procedures, respectively.[47,48] In another study, an EF below 20% indicated a high surgical risk, and values between 20% and 35% indicated a moderate surgical risk, whereas an EF of 35% to 45% predicted a mild surgical risk for cardiac complications after major vascular procedures.[51] Other investigators have found no clear relationship between the EF and CAD when predicting perioperative cardiac morbidity.[19,52] The controversy regarding usefulness of the EF to predict perioperative myocardial events is not surprising, because it is a measure of the function of the left ventricle at one point in time and mostly in a nonstressed heart.[17,50] A normal EF does not indicate the absence of coronary artery disease or identify the extent of myocardium at risk for infarction during the perioperative period. Many patients undergoing coronary artery bypass graft (CABG) surgery have a normal EF preoperatively despite significant, correctable CAD.[53] Prior infarction and scarring of the myocardial muscle, rather than active ischemia, may reduce the EF. To be of more predictive value, EF results should be interpreted in the context of other more specific tests of heart function.

Stress Testing

The cardiac responses to the physiological changes of surgery are effectively evaluated only by measuring cardiac function under stress. The induction of cardiac stress can be achieved by exercise or by a number of pharmacological substances. Pharmacological testing is especially useful in patients who cannot adequately exercise, as is true for a large proportion of patients with PVD. The most widely used pharmacological agents are vasodilator drugs (dipyridamole and adenosine) or inotropic agents (dobutamine). The reaction to stress can be measured by electrocardiography, echocardiography, or radionuclide imaging using substances such as technetium or thallium.

Electrocardiographic Exercise Treadmill Testing

In electrocardiographic exercise treadmill testing, exercise increases the work of the heart and myocardial oxygen demand, thus mimicking the stress of a major surgical procedure. The exercise performed may include isometric hand gripping, stationary cycling, or treadmill testing. Exercise treadmill testing should only be done under the supervision of a cardiologist. Throughout the test, the heart rate and blood pressure are continuously monitored. The patient is observed closely for development of cardiac ischemic symptoms, which occur in about 3% of patients.[54] The test is negative if the patient can achieve the age- and sex-predicted goal without cardiac ischemic symptoms or evidence of ST-segment depression. However, exercise as a means of inducing cardiac stress in the patient with PVD is frequently hindered by the patient's inability to exercise because of lower extremity ischemic symptoms. Exercise stress testing is useful only when the patient can achieve at least 85% of the predicted maximal heart rate. This cannot be reached in as many as 70% of patients with PVD, resulting in a marked reduction in sensitivity.[55-57] The specificity of exercise testing ranges from 51% to 82% and its sensitivity from 74% to 88%.[54,58] Although considered by some investigators to be the best kind of stress to detect myocardial ischemia,[51] exercise testing has been found to have a false-positive result for significant CAD in 40% and a false-negative result in 15% of patients.[59] In the Coronary Artery Surgery Study (CASS), in patients with a history of angina pectoris, results of exercise testing were normal in two thirds of men and one third of women with angiographically demonstrated CAD.[60]

Stress Echocardiography

Echocardiography after stressing the heart with dobutamine or dipyridamole has been used to detect significant CAD. Dobutamine stress echocardiography (DSE) has been widely investigated.[30,51,61] Intravenous dobutamine administration increases myocardial contractility, resulting in the enhancement of existing myocardial wall motion abnormalities.[62] Dobutamine is a synthetic catecholamine with β_1, β_2, and α_1 receptor stimulating properties. At low doses it is a potent positive inotrope, whereas at high doses it has chronotropic effects that result in increased myocardial oxygen demands.[63] It produces ischemia by elevating myocardial oxygen demand out of proportion to supply; however, it did not severely reduce coronary perfusion during the study.[62] Dobutamine is infused intravenously beginning with a small dose of 2.5 μg/kg per minute, which is then increased to 5 μg/kg per minute and then gradually, by increments of 5 μg/kg per minute, to a dose of 30 to 50 μg/kg per minute. The infusion is terminated if the patient develops any of the following: a new regional wall motion abnormality or thickening in two or more wall segments, a 2-mm or more ST-segment depression, symptoms of angina, decline of more than 15 mm Hg in systolic blood pressure from baseline, or other significant arrhythmias or side effects (e.g., nausea or headache). DSE is not always tolerated by patients because of minor side effects such as nausea, vomiting, and insignificant arrhythmias (12%). Arrhythmias not requiring termination of the test occur in 3.3%. Serious, life-threatening complications) may occur in 0.5% of cases. If none of the previously mentioned end points are reached, the infusion is terminated at 85% of the patient's maximal sex- and age-predicted heart rate or after reaching the maximal dose.[64,65] After dobutamine infusion, transthoracic echocardiography is used to identify cardiac wall motion responses and thus patients at high risk of developing future myocardial events.[30] In a study of the use of DSE for risk stratification in patients undergoing aortic surgery, 29% of patients with an abnormal DSE had cardiac events compared with only 4.6% of those with a normal DSE. The test was found to have a sensitivity of 92% and negative predictive value of 95% in contrast to a specificity of 44% and positive predictive value of 29% for cardiac complications after aortic surgery.[30]

It is useful to compare the efficacy of DSE with the efficacy of other modalities. In patients undergoing both DSE and coronary angiography, DSE had a sensitivity of 71%.[66] In the same study, Afridi et al. examined the ability of DSE to predict perioperative cardiac events and found a sensitivity of 85%.[66] In this study, which compared exercise, dobutamine, and dipyridamole stress echocardiography, all performed in the same group of patients, dobutamine had an intermediate sensitivity, being inferior to exercise. Its specificity was inferior to those of the other two tests. Furthermore, dobutamine had a higher incidence of side effects (11%) compared with exercise echocardiography (3%) and dipyridamole stress echocardiography (1%).[54] Other studies, however, suggest that DSE carries a similar range and incidence of side effects in comparison with exercise, and much fewer side effects than dipyridamole.[67,68]

In addition to transthoracic echocardiography, dobutamine can be used with transesophageal echocardiography in an attempt to improve accuracy. This has resulted in a sensitivity of 90% and specificity of 94%. This improved sensitivity was even higher in patients with previous CABG surgery (100%), although the specificity was lower (75%).[69] The test can be done in a portable fashion in the intensive or coronary care unit and can be adjusted and tailored according to the patient's medications.[70]

One limitation of DSE is an image quality in 5% of the patients that is insufficient to allow accurate analysis.[51] Dobutamine should not be used in patients with severe aortic stenosis, severe hypertension, unstable angina, recent myocardial infarction, tachyarrhythmias, or poor left ventricular function.

Radionuclide Cardiac Imaging

Myocardial perfusion can be assessed by a number of diffusible radionuclides such as potassium 43 and its analogs such as thallium 201 (Tl 201) and technetium 99

metastable (Tc 99m) agents. The uptake of these agents depends on myocardial perfusion, myocardial mass, and myocardial cellular integrity. Thallium 201, one of the most widely used agents in the United States, is used in 70% of the myocardial perfusion studies.[71] The uptake of Tl 201 by the myocardium is linearly related to blood flow within the physiological range.[72] The first pass extraction of Tl 201 by the myocardium is 88%.[73] The proportion of the injected Tl 201 dose that localizes to the myocardium increases from 3.5% at rest to 8% to 10% after dipyridamole administration. Thallium 201 should be injected at the peak levels of coronary artery blood flow induced by exercise or pharmacological agents such as dipyridamole, adenosine, or dobutamine. Images are taken immediately and 4 hours later. Several views of the ventricles are examined. Areas with diminished uptake of Tl 201 reflect decreased blood flow in the myocardium. If the defect in Tl 201 uptake persists 4 hours later, it is called a *fixed defect*. However, if Tl 201 redistributes to that area, it is called a *reversible defect*. A fixed defect represents an area of scarred myocardium or infarct; a reversible defect represents an area of ischemic myocardium that may be improved by revascularization. Reversibility and redistribution are explained by two facts. First, the myocardial washout half-life of Tl 201 is 4 to 6 hours. Second, the presence of regional ischemia decreases the rate of washout, providing substrate for redistribution. Severe coronary artery stenosis may even result in a persistent defect on delayed images.[74] Reinjection of Tl 201 before redistribution imaging might improve the sensitivity of the test for identifying severely ischemic but viable myocardium.

The interpretation of the Tl 201 scan, as mentioned before, depends on the differential uptake of Tl 201 by normal and ischemic myocardium. Thus, the presence of global ischemia may result in uniform but delayed uptake of Tl 201. This will result in a scan falsely interpreted as normal. Also, a false-positive scan for ischemia may be caused by left ventricular hypertrophy, variations in the coronary anatomy, or soft tissue attenuation by breast tissue.

The problems noted with Tl 201 led to the search for alternative perfusion agents. Two Tc 99m agents have been used, namely, Tc 99m sestamibi and Tc 99m teboroxime. Tc 99m sestamibi is primarily cleared by the hepatobiliary system. This clearance takes more than an hour, thus allowing images within that hour and the possibility of repeating a technically unsatisfactory scan without the need for reinjection. This quality represents an advantage of Tc 99m sestamibi over Tl 201, which redistributes after injection.[75]

Another radiopharmaceutical agent used to evaluate myocardial perfusion is Tc 99m teboroxime. Following intravenous injection, Tc 99m teboroxime is taken up by the myocardium in direct proportion to blood flow. The clearance of Tc 99m teboroxime is also by the hepatobiliary system and is a rapid process. Because of rapid clearance, images can be obtained 10 minutes after injection. Similarly, the myocardial washout is rapid, with an early biological half-life of 6 minutes, again allowing for more rapid imaging.[76]

These and other imaging agents have been used in different protocols to evaluate heart perfusion and function. No one protocol is ideal for all clinical scenarios.[71] The choice of the imaging agent depends on the questions to be answered. Both Tl 201 and Tc 99m sestamibi can be used for the detection of CAD. However, because of its more widespread use and familiarity, Tl 201 is better used for risk stratification. In obese patients, Tc 99m sestamibi is the agent of choice because of the soft tissue attenuation seen with Tl 201 in patients weighing more than 200 pounds.[71]

Dipyridamole Thallium Scan

Dipyridamole inhibits reuptake and transport of endogenously produced adenosine, which is a potent vasodilator that accumulates in the interstitium and produces coronary vasodilatation. The intravenous administration of dipyridamole produces a degree of coronary vasodilatation greater than that produced by exercise, without the associated increase in myocardial oxygen consumption. This results in an increase of coronary blood flow to three to five times its resting value.[77,78] The vasodilatation induced by dipyridamole is more pronounced in nonstenotic vessels than stenotic vessels. Side effects have been reported in up to 50% of patients who receive intravenous dipyridamole. These include light-headedness, headache, chest pain, shortness of breath, flushing, blurred vision, hypotension, nausea, and vomiting. Of the patients who receive intravenous dipyridamole, 28% experience chest pain and 16% develop ST-segment depression. Interestingly, the chest pain that develops during a dipyridamole thallium scan (DTS) is not a reliable predictor of CAD unless associated with ST-segment depression. The side effects of dipyridamole can be reversed with administration of theophylline.[72]

An initial report on the assessment of the cardiac status of patients before surgery with DTS showed a good negative predictive value and a poor positive predictive value.[79] Subsequent studies validated the correlation between thallium redistribution and perioperative cardiac events.[18-20,22] In a comparison with the EF as determined by B-mode echocardiography, DTS was found to have a higher sensitivity (96% versus 73%) for the evaluation of cardiac morbidity before abdominal aneurysm surgery.[19] In general, the test has been found to be oversensitive in predicting perioperative complications, reducing its positive predictive value.[21,43,80] In three of these studies, patients had a 4% to 9% incidence of perioperative cardiac

events.[18,19,21] At our institution, a study was done routinely screening 394 preoperative vascular patients with a DTS irrespective of the patient's cardiac history or symptomatology. Thirty-eight percent had normal studies, 19% had fixed defects, and 43% had reversible defects. The incidence of redistribution was not significantly different between patients with clinical evidence of CAD and those without clinical evidence of CAD. However, a fixed defect was more common in patients with known coronary disease. After vascular procedures, cardiac mortality was higher in patients with fixed and redistribution myocardial defects when compared with those with a normal DTS. There was no difference in survival between patients with fixed and reversible defects.[81] Similar results have been noted in another prospective blinded study where no correlation could be found between the presence of a redistribution defect and poor cardiac outcome.[82] Interestingly, in another study, clinical symptoms of CAD and age were found to be more significant predictors of adverse cardiac outcome than a positive DTS.[83] Our study showed a fixed defect was associated with an increased incidence of myocardial complications.[81] Similarly, Cutler et al. and Kiat et al. showed that the presence of a fixed defect was not a benign condition.[72,84] Further similar results were obtained in another study in which a fixed defect in patients undergoing abdominal aortic aneurysm replacement was accompanied by a 47% incidence of a cardiac event, whereas presence of a redistribution defect was associated with a 25% incidence of a cardiac event.[85] To increase the complexity of this issue, reperfusion of previously fixed-appearing defects after extended periods of imaging or upon reinjection has been noted.[84,86] Furthermore, some "fixed defects" may appear normally perfused after myocardial revascularization.[87] Finally, fixed defects have been identified as one of the strongest predictors of late cardiac events, but not perioperative events.[88] This suggests less utility in the short term, but allows prognostication in the long term. It has been suggested that DTS accuracy and efficacy can be improved if results of imaging are combined with clinical parameters of cardiac disease and quantitative assessment of the number of defects.[21,22,32,81]

Adenosine Thallium Scan

Adenosine thallium scan (ATS) and DTS are governed by the same principles for the evaluation of the myocardium.[70] Adenosine induces increased coronary blood flow by directly acting on the myocardium. It has a shorter half-life (<10 seconds) than dipyridamole (30 minutes).[70] The side effects of adenosine are closely related to those of dipyridamole except they are more short-lived and tend to occur more frequently. These side effects are also reversed by aminophylline. In one study using adenosine infusion to evaluate cardiac status, the infusion protocol was completed in 80% of the patients, required a dose reduction in 13%, and was terminated early in 7%. Although minor and well-tolerated side effects were reported in 81.1% of patients, only 0.8% required aminophylline to alleviate side effects. A transient AV block occurred in less than 10% of patients, especially those over 70 years of age.[89] Adenosine and dipyridamole are both contraindicated in patients with severe bronchospasm and asthma, a history of allergic reaction to either agent or to aminophylline, and, finally, hypotension or atrioventricular type II heart block.

Dobutamine Thallium Scan

Dobutamine thallium scanning is based on the same principles as dipyridamole thallium scanning. It has been found reliable to screen patients for redistribution defects.[31] The incidence of ischemic events after major vascular procedures in one study was 1.8% in patients with normal dobutamine thallium studies and 11% in those with fixed defects. Patients with reversible defects who underwent CABG surgery had 0% incidence of perioperative ischemic events compared with 50% in a group with a reversible defect and no antecedent CABG surgery.[31] Further studies using this methodology are awaited.

Coronary Angiography

Coronary angiography has been the traditional gold standard for the evaluation of patients thought to have CAD. Although routine cardiac catheterization has been advocated by some[11,90,91] to evaluate preoperative cardiac risk, the expense cannot justify such nonselective use. Furthermore, it is an invasive procedure, with up to a 3% incidence of associated vascular complications.[92] The ability of coronary catheterization to accurately map disease in the coronary vessels is not disputed. However, the relationship between the degree of coronary stenosis and its physiological significance is still unclear. One study showed that the absence of an angiographic stenosis did not correlate with myocardial functional capacity.[93] In addition, the presence of a stenotic artery on angiography may be insignificant if it supplies a scarred area or if the resulting decreased flow is offset by good collateral circulation. Of note, patients with angiographically documented, severe, nonreconstructable CAD have been shown to tolerate aortic reconstruction without mortality.[21] Pursuing coronary angiography is not free of significant risk, as 1.7% of patients have been reported to die in the process of preoperative screening or treatment for CAD.[18]

Advocates of an aggressive preoperative approach consisting of routine coronary angiography in the detection of CAD base this stance on the assumption that perioperative risk might be reduced and long-term survival improved after myocardial revascularization. Selective coronary angiography, when initial cardiac screening is revealing, provides a more acceptable, cost-effective approach than performing angiography on all patients, which would be prohibitively expensive. Coronary angiography should be reserved for patients who are legitimate candidates for myocardial revascularization on its own merits or for those vascular surgical patients where the choice of vascular surgical procedure would be influenced by the coronary angiographic findings.

Role of Myocardial Revascularization Before Vascular Surgery

The role of myocardial revascularization in patients with CAD has been extensively evaluated. There is not uniform agreement on the value of coronary artery bypass preceding another major operative intervention.[60,94] One study has suggested that coronary revascularization before vascular surgery is associated with mortality lower than that of aggressive medical therapy (with delay of surgery when necessary), especially in high- and medium-risk patients with stable CAD.[95] In low-risk patients, the limited data in the same study showed an insignificant trend toward greater mortality with medical therapy when compared with coronary revascularization.[95] The CASS data showed that perioperative mortality after noncardiac operations in patients without CAD was 0.5%, compared with 0.9% in patients with CAD who underwent preliminary CABG surgery. Mortality increased to 2.4% when patients were given only medical therapy for their CAD.[60] Similar results were reported previously in patients undergoing carotid endarterectomy, with a reduction in mortality from 12.9% to 2.6% after CABG surgery.[96] The largest series of patients with PVD studied by coronary angiography was from the Cleveland Clinic.[11] All patients underwent coronary catheterization before undergoing a planned vascular reconstruction. This policy resulted in a 21.6% coronary artery bypass rate before the vascular intervention. The 5-year survival of patients with PVD who underwent CABG surgery was 72%, compared with 43% for those with CAD who refused CABG surgery, and 22% for patients with severe, noncorrectable CAD.[11] The timing of coronary revascularization in relation to the peripheral vascular procedure is another important factor. In a review of 1093 patients who underwent peripheral vascular and CABG procedures, the greatest benefit conferred by myocardial revascularization was seen when it was done before a vascular procedure. Better results were obtained when the patient was discharged after coronary revascularization with later elective scheduling of the vascular procedure as opposed to simultaneous or same-admission vascular surgical procedures.[97] An early mortality of 0.2% (none due to cardiac deaths) was reported in the first group, as compared with 4% in each of the other two groups (60% and 70% of the mortality was due to cardiac death in each of the latter groups, respectively).

The prevalence of CAD in patients with PVD increases with age.[26] The assumption that detecting and treating CAD in these aging patients will reduce perioperative cardiac complications after vascular reconstructive procedures may not be true. If the mortality and morbidity of coronary angiography and bypass were negligible, this might be an ideal approach. In the Cleveland Clinic study, 5.2% of all patients died after a CABG procedure.[11] Another study has reported a 16.7% mortality after CABG surgery.[18] The CASS data also showed that mortality after CABG surgery in patients over 65 (most patients with PVD fall in this age category) was 5.2%, and in those older than 75 the mortality jumped to 9.5%.[25] In still another study, the mortality rate of coronary bypass surgery in patients over 80 with PVD increased four times when compared with those with no vascular disease.[98]

Percutaneous transluminal angioplasty (PTCA) is more benign than CABG surgery. However, it is also not without complications and, unfortunately, is not applicable to many patients with PVD. Cardiac morbidities of 5.6% to 11%, with a mortality of 1.9%, have been reported after PTCA.[99,100] In the period from 1987 to 1990, in the United States, the in-hospital mortality after PTCA ranged from 2.5% to 3.9%. Furthermore, CABG surgery was required after PTCA in 2.8% to 5.3% of patients.[101] The mortality from CABG surgery is doubled when done within 6 hours of PTCA.[102] In the frequently cited Cleveland Clinic study, the operative mortality for coronary revascularization in patients with PVD was 5.2% compared with a mortality rate of 1.2% for elective coronary surgery in non-PVD patients.[11] The combined morbidity and mortality of coronary revascularization and a major vascular procedure may even exceed that of a peripheral vascular reconstruction alone when performed with aggressive preoperative and perioperative medical therapy and careful invasive hemodynamic monitoring.

The role of myocardial revascularization before a major peripheral vascular reconstructive procedure remains unresolved. However, the high incidence of CAD in patients with PVD is well documented, and it is the leading cause of morbidity and mortality in patients after a major vascular reconstructive procedure. Further, one fifth of patients leaving the hospital after a noncardiac vascular operation have been noted to have a cardiac event within 2 years.[103] Cardiac-related mortality has been found in 20% of patients with PVD over an 11-year follow-up.[104] Unfortunately, many studies supporting the prophylactic role of myocardial revascularization are nonrandomized and noncontrolled.[11,34,96,97,105] Furthermore, most such studies excluded complications of coronary angiography and myocardial revascularization from their data. Thus, there are no prospective randomized studies available to critically examine the role of myocardial revascularization on the perioperative morbidity and mortality rates after peripheral vascular procedures. Nor are there any studies to examine the effect of the timing of coronary revascularization as it relates to long-term patient survival after peripheral vascular procedures. In a meta-analysis of published data, Mason et al.[106] attempted to address some of these problems. Interestingly, they concluded that vascular surgery without preliminary cardiac catheterization and coronary revascularization should produce better clinical results. The authors attributed these findings to the additional morbidity risks associated with cardiac catheterization and revascularization. In a more recent study of patients undergoing abdominal aortic aneurysm repair, however, there was no difference in complications or cardiac mortality rates between patients with preoperative cardiac evaluation and those without preoperative cardiac evaluation.[107]

Issues

A review of cardiac screening modalities and a description of the controversies in cardiac risk assessment has been provided. In describing a management strategy, three issues must be briefly revisited. The first of these is, "Whom do we screen?" The two extremes, screening everybody and screening nobody, are not logical. The bulk of evidence in the literature suggests that patients with clinical indicators (e.g., age >70, a history of angina pectoris, a Q wave on ECG, a history of ventricular ectopic activity, and diabetes mellitus) are optimal candidates to screen.[20] However, the increased incidence of silent CAD in patients with PVD makes this approach not entirely reliable.

The second issue should address the choice of the ideal cardiac screening method. Each proposed screening method has its own inherent limitations. The most aggressive approach, namely, cardiac catheterization of every patient, is prohibitively costly and too invasive. Cardiac stressors can be used as predictors of perioperative cardiac complications. These tests help stratify patients into risk groups and can be used to help determine the need for cardiac catheterization. However, problems with the interpretation of these tests, as explained earlier, have been encountered. These problems may be, in

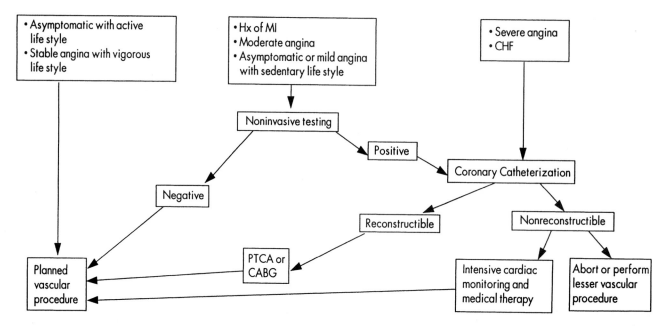

FIGURE 66.1. Cardiac evaluation of patients with peripheral vascular disease. Hx, history; MI, myocardial infarction; CHF, congestive heart failure.

part, responsible for the controversies that have evolved on the subject of cardiac risk assessment. A variety of reasonable stress tests can be chosen depending on the patient's condition and ability to exercise, as well as the institutional facilities.

A final unresolved problem relates to the appropriate management of CAD after it is identified in the patient with PVD. A practical approach would be individualized and dictated by each patient's unique condition. Our proposed management algorithm is outlined in Figure 66.1. Patients with a history and symptoms of severe myocardial disease may need coronary angiography and possible myocardial revascularization. Patients without a history or current symptoms of CAD who are leading an active lifestyle require special consideration. They may have no evidence of cardiac disease by ECG or chest x-ray examination and no need for further cardiac evaluation before vascular intervention either. However, if major vascular intervention is planned in these good risk, often younger patients, detection and treatment of significant symptomatic CAD is worthwhile. A third group of patients with stigmata of heart disease and a sedentary lifestyle may benefit from stress testing and possible further myocardial evaluation, as dictated by the results of stress testing. In those patients with reconstructable CAD and an acceptable surgical risk, myocardial revascularization can be done. In contrast, in the presence of nonreconstructable CAD or for a poor-risk patient, an aborted or a lesser vascular procedure than that previously proposed may be chosen in light of the cardiac investigation findings. Aggressive perioperative monitoring and medical therapy are invaluable in such poor risk patients. In

the presence of less compelling indications for elective vascular surgery such as asymptomatic carotid artery disease, a small aortic aneurysm, or nonthreatening limb ischemia, selective cardiac evaluation in the absence of stigmata of CAD might be indicated. In such patients the benefit of peripheral vascular surgery is related to long-term survival. This in turn is a function of cardiac status and optimal treatment of existing CAD.[108] Close consultation and cooperation between the vascular surgeon, cardiologist, and anesthesiologist will assure optimal surgical results and improved long-term cardiac health.

References

1. Saphir O, Priest WS, Hamburger WW, et al. Coronary arteriosclerosis, coronary thrombosis, and the resulting myocardial changes. *Am Heart J.* 1935;10:567, 762.
2. Wilson LB. Fatal postoperative embolism. *Ann Surg.* 1912; 56:809–818.
3. Master AM, Dack S, Jaffe HI: Postoperative coronary artery occlusion. *JAMA.* 1938;110:1415–1418.
4. Goldman L, Caldera DL, Nussbaum SR, et al. Multifactorial index of cardiac risk in noncardiac surgical procedures. *N Engl J Med.* 1977;297:845–850.
5. Szilagyi DE, Smith RF, DeRusso FJ, Elliott JP, Sherrin FW. Contribution of abdominal aortic aneurysmectomy to prolongation of life. *Ann Surg.* 1966;164:678–699.
6. Hertzer NR. Myocardial ischemia. *Surgery.* 1983;93: 97–101.
7. Thompson JE, Hollier LH, Patman RD, Persson AV. Surgical management of abdominal aortic aneurysms: factors influencing morbidity and mortality; A 20-year experience. *Ann Surg.* 1975;181:654–661.

8. Young AE, Sandberg GW, Couch NB. The reduction of mortality of abdominal aortic aneurysm resection. *Am J Surg.* 1977;134:585–590.

9. Yeager RA, Weigel RM, Murphy ES, McConnell DB, Sasaki TM, Vetto RM. Application of clinically valid risk factors to aortic aneurysm surgery, *Arch Surg.* 1986;121:278–281.

10. Taylor LM, Yeager RA, Moneta GL, McConnell DB, Porter JM. The incidence of perioperative myocardial infarction in general vascular surgery. *J Vasc Surg.* 1991;15:52–61.

11. Hertzer NR, Beven EG, Young JR, et al. Coronary artery disease in peripheral vascular patients: a classification of 1000 coronary angiograms and results of surgical management. *Ann Surg.* 1984;199:223–233.

12. DeBakey ME, Lawrie GM. Combined coronary artery and peripheral vascular disease: recognition and treatment. *J Vasc Surg.* 1984;1:605–607.

13. Tomatis LA, Fierens EE, Verbrugg GP. Evaluation of surgical risk in peripheral vascular disease by coronary arteriography: a series of 100 cases. *Surgery.* 1972;71:429–435.

14. Andrews TC, Goldman L, Creager MA, et al. Identification and treatment of myocardial ischemia in patients undergoing peripheral vascular surgery. *J Vasc Med Biol.* 1994;5:8-15.

15. Rihal CS, Eagle KA, Mickel MC, Foster ED, Sopko G, Gersh BJ. Surgical therapy for coronary artery disease among patients with combined coronary artery and peripheral vascular disease. *Circ J Am Heart Assoc.* 1995;91: 46–53.

16. Eagle KA, Rihal CS, Foster ED, Mickel MC, Gersch BJ. Long term survival in patients with coronary artery disease: importance of peripheral vascular disease. *J Am Coll Cardiol.* 1994;23:1091–1095.

17. Golden MA, Whittemore AD, Donaldson MC, Mannick JA. Selective evaluation and management of coronary artery disease in patients undergoing repair of abdominal aortic aneurysm. A 16-year experience. The Coronary Artery Surgery Study (CASS) investigators. *Ann Surg.* 1990;212: 415–420.

18. Cutler BS, Leppo JA. Dipyridamole thallium 201 scintigraphy to detect coronary artery disease before abdominal aortic surgery. *J Vasc Surg.* 1987;5:91–100.

19. McEnroe CS, O'Donnell TF Jr, Yeager A, Konstam M, Mackey WC. Comparison of ejection fraction and Goldman risk factor analysis to dipyridamole-thallium 201 studies in the evaluation of cardiac morbidity after aortic aneurysm surgery. *J Vasc Surg.* 1990;11:497–504.

20. Eagle KA, Singer DE, Brewster DC, Darling RC, Mulley AG, Boucher CA. Dipyridamole-thallium scanning in patients undergoing vascular surgery: Optimizing preoperative evaluation of cardiac risk. *JAMA.* 1987;257:2185–2189.

21. Cambria RP, Brewster DC, Abbott WM, et al. The impact of selective use of dipyridamole-thallium scans and surgical factors on the current morbidity of aortic surgery. *J Vasc Surg.* 1992;15:43–51.

22. Eagle KA, Coley CM, Newell JB, et al. Combining clinical and thallium data optimizes preoperative assessment of cardiac risk before major vascular surgery. *Ann Intern Med.* 1989;110:859–866.

23. Kennedy JW, Kaisar GC, Fisher LD, et al. Multivariate discriminant analysis of the clinical and angiographic predictors of operative mortality from the Collaborative Study in Coronary Artery Surgery (CASS). *J Thorac Cardiovasc Surg.* 1980;80:876–887.

24. Kennedy JW, Kaiser GC, Fisher LD, et al. Clinical and angiographic predictors of operative mortality from collaborative study in coronary artery surgery (CASS). *Circulation.* 1981;63:793–802.

25. Gersh BJ, Kronmal RA, Frye RL, et al. Coronary arteriography and coronary artery bypass surgery: morbidity and mortality in patients ages 65 years or older. A report from the Coronary Artery Surgery Study. *Circulation.* 1983;67: 483–491.

26. Kallero KS. Mortality and morbidity in patients with intermittent claudication as defined by venous occlusion plethysmography. A ten-year follow-up study. *J Chronic Dis.* 1981;34:455–462.

27. Boyd AM. The natural course of arteriosclerosis of lower extremities. *Angiology.* 1960;11:10–18.

28. Bunt TJ. The role of a defined protocol for cardiac risk assessment in decreasing perioperative myocardial infarction in vascular surgery. *J Vasc Surg.* 1992;15:626–634.

29. Brown OW, Hollier LH, Pairolero PC, Kazmier FJ, McCready RA. Abdominal aortic aneurysm and coronary artery disease. A reassessment. *Arch Surg.* 1981;116:1484–1488.

30. Lalka SG, Sawada SG, Dalsing MC, et al. Dobutamine stress echocardiography as a predictor of cardiac events associated with aortic surgery. *J Vasc Surg.* 1992;15:831–840.

31. Elliott BM, Robison JG, Zellner JL, Hendrix GH. Dobutamine-201TI imaging . Assessing cardiac risks associated with vascular surgery. *Circulation.* 1991;84(5 suppl): III54–III60.

32. Lette J, Waters D, Lassonde J, et al. Postoperative myocardial infarction and cardiac death. *Ann Surg.* 1990;211: 84–90.

33. Agati L, Voci P, Biltta F, et al. Dipyridamole myocardial contrast echocardiography in patients with single-vessel coronary artery disease: perfusion, anatomic and functional correlates. *Am Heart J.* 1994;128:28–35.

34. Cooperman M, Pflug B, Maritin EW, et al. Cardiovascular risk factors in patients with peripheral vascular disease. *Surgery.* 1978;84:505–509.

35. Velanovich V. The value of routine preoperative testing in predicting postoperative complications: a multivariate analysis. *Surgery.* 1991;109:236–243.

36. Velanovich V. Preoperative screening electrocardiography: predictive value for postoperative cardiac complications. *South Med J.* 1994;87:431–434.

37. Johnston KW. Multicenter prospective study of nonruptured abdominal aortic aneurysm. Part II: Variables predicting morbidity and mortality. *J Vasc Surg.* 1989;9: 437–447.

38. Coy KM, Imperim GA, Lambert CR, et al. Silent myocardial ischemia during daily activities in asymptomatic men with positive exercise test response. *Am J Cardiol.* 1987;59: 45–49.

39. Rocco MB, Barry J, Campbell S, et al. Circadian variation of transient myocardial ischemia in patients with coronary artery disease. *Circulation.* 1987;75:395–400.

40. Mangnano DT, Browner WS, Hollenberg M, et al. Association of perioperative myocardial ischemia with cardiac morbidity and mortality in men undergoing noncardiac surgery. *N Engl J Med.* 1991;323:1781–1787.

41. Crawford MH, Mendoza CA, O'Rourke RA, White DH, Boucher CA, Gorwit J. Limitations of continuous ambulatory electrocardiogram monitoring for detecting coronary artery disease. *Ann Intern Med.* 1978;89:1–5.

42. Pasternack PF, Grossi EA, Baumann FG, et al. The value of silent myocardial ischemia monitoring in the prediction of perioperative myocardial infarction in patients undergoing peripheral vascular surgery. *J Vasc Surg.* 1989;10: 617–625.

43. Raby KE, Goldman L, Creager MA, et al. Correlation between preoperative ischemia and major cardiac events under peripheral vascular surgery. *N Engl J Med.* 1989;321: 1296–1300.

44. Miller DD. Clinical risk factor analysis and electrocardiographic evaluation modalities. *Semin Vasc Surg.* 1991;4: 67–76.

45. Pasternack PF, Imparato AM, Riles TS, et al. The value of the radionuclide angiogram in the prediction of perioperative myocardial infarction in patients undergoing lower extremity revascularization procedures. *Circulation.* 1985; 72(3 Pt 2):II13–II17.

46. Pasternack PF, Imparato AM, Bear G, et al. The value of radionuclide angiography as a predictor of perioperative myocardial infarction in patients undergoing abdominal aortic aneurysm resection. *J Vasc Surg.* 1984;1:320–325.

47. Starling MR, Crawford MH, Sorensen SG, et al. Comparative accuracy of apical biplane cross-sectional echocardiography and gated equilibrium radionuclide angiography for estimating left ventricular size and performance. *Circulation.* 1981;63:1075–1084.

48. Giboons RJ, Lee KL, Cobb FR, Coleman RE, Jones RH. Ejection fraction response to exercise in patients with chest pain, coronary artery disease and normal resting ventricular function. *Circulation.* 1982;66:643–648.

49. Crawford MH, Peter MA, Amon KW, et al. Comparative value of 2-dimensional echocardiography and radionuclide angiography for quantitative changes in left ventricular performance during exercise limited by anginal pectoris. *Am J Cardiol.* 1984;53:42–46.

50. Kazmers A, Cerqueira MD, Zierler RE. The role of preoperative radionuclide ejection fraction in direct abdominal aortic repair. *J Vasc Surg.* 1988;8:128–136.

51. Crawford MH. The preoperative cardiac evaluation of the patient with vascular disease: Ejection fraction and stress echocardiography. *Semin Vasc Surg.* 1991;4:77–82.

52. Franco CD, Goldsmith J, Veith FJ, et al. Resting gated blood pool ejection fraction: a poor predictor of perioperative myocardial infarction in patients undergoing vascular surgery for infrainguinal bypass grafting. *J Vasc Surg.* 1989;10:650–661.

53. Moraski RE, Russel RO, Smith M, et al. Left ventricular function in patients with and without myocardial infarction and one, two, or three vessel coronary artery disease. *Am J Cardiol.* 1975;35:1–9.

54. Beleslin BD, Ostojic M, Stepanovic J, et al. Stress echocardiography in the detection of myocardial ischemia: head-to-head comparison of exercise, dobutamine, and dipyridamole tests. *Circulation.* 1994;90:1168–1176.

55. McPhail NV, Ruddy TD, Calvin JE, Davies RA, Barber GG. A comparison of dipyridamole-thallium imaging and exer-

56. Mc Phail NV, Calvin JE, Shariatmader A, Barber GG, Scobie TK. The use of preoperative exercise testing to predict cardiac complications after arterial reconstruction. *J Vasc Surg.* 1988;7:60–68.

57. Cutler BS, Wheeler HB, Paraskos JA, Cardullo PA. Applicability and interpretation of electrocardiographic stress testing in patients with peripheral vascular disease. *Am J Surg.* 1981;141:501–506.

58. Severi S, Picano E, Michelassi C, et al. Diagnostic and prognostic value of dipyridamole echocardiography in patients with suspected coronary artery disease: comparison with exercise electrocardiography. *Circulation.* 1994;89: 1160–1173.

59. Gage AA, Bhayana JN, Balu V, et al. Assessment of cardiac risk in surgical patients. *Arch Surg.* 1977;112;1488–1474.

60. Foster ED, Davis KB, Carpenter JA, Abele S, Fray D. Risk of noncardiac operation in patients with defined coronary disease: the Coronary Artery Surgery Study (CASS) registry experience. *Ann Thorac Surg.* 1986;41:42–50.

61. Berthe C, Pierard LA, Hiernaux M, et al. Predicting the extent and location of coronary artery disease in acute myocardial infarction by echocardiography during dobutamine infusion. *Am J Cardiol.* 1986;48:1167–72.

62. Fung AY, Gallagher KP, Buda AJ. The physiologic basis of dobutamine as compared with dipyridamole stress interventions in the assessment of critical coronary stenosis. *Circulation.* 1987;76:943–951.

63. McGillem MJ, De Boe SF, Friedman HZ, et al. The effects of dopamine and dobutamine on regional function in the presence of rigid coronary stenosis and subcritical impairment of reactive hyperemia. *Am Heart J.* 1988;115: 970–977.

64. Upton MT, Rerych SK, Newman GE, Port S, Cobb FR, Jones RH. Detecting abnormalities in left ventricular function during exercise before angina and ST-segment depression. *Circulation.* 1980;62:341–349.

65. Picano E, Mathias W Jr, Pingitore A, Bigi R, Previtali M. Safety and tolerability of dobutamine-atropine stress echocardiography: a prospective, multicentre study. ECHO Dobutamine International Comparative Study Group. *Lancet.* 1994;344:1190–1194.

66. Afridi I, Quinines MA, Zighbi WA, Cheirif J. Dobutamine stress echocardiography: sensitivity, specificity, and predictive value for future cardiac events. *Am Heart J.* 1994;127: 1510–1515.

67. Salustki A, Fioretti PM, Pozzoli, MMA, et al. A comparison of dobutamine and high dose dipyridamole stress echocardiography in the diagnosis of coronary artery disease [abstract]. *Circulation.* 1990;82:193.

68. Mazeika RK, Nadazdin A, Oakley CM. Diagnostic accuracy of dobutamine stress echocardiography in coronary artery disease [abstract]. *Circulation.* 1990;82:193.

69. Prince CR, Stoddard MF, Morris GT, et al. Dobutamine two-dimensional transesophageal echocardiographic stress testing for detection of coronary artery disease. *Am Heart J.* 1994;128:36–41.

70. Ramadan FM, Keagy BA, Johnson G Jr. Preoperative evaluation of cardiac risk. *Adv Surg.* 1995;28:301–315.

71. Wackers FJ. The maze of myocardial perfusion imaging protocols in 1994. *J Nucl Cardiol.* 1994;1:180–188.
72. Cutler BS. Interpretation and results of intravenous dipyridamole thallium scintigraphy. *Semin Vasc Surg.* 1991;4: 83–89.
73. Mueller TM, Marcus ML, Ehrhardt JC, Chaudhuri T, Abboud FM. Limitations of thallium-201 myocardial perfusion scintigrams. *Circulation.* 1976;54:640–646.
74. Gould KL, Lipscomb K, Hamilton GW. Physiological basis for assessing critical coronary artery stenosis: instantaneous flow response and regional distribution during coronary hyperemia as measures of coronary flow reserve. *Am J Cardiol.* 1974;33:87–94.
75. Iskandarian AS, Heo J, Kong B, Lyons E, Marsch S. Use of technetium-99m isonitrile (RP-30A) in assessing left ventricular perfusion and function at rest and during exercise in coronary artery disease, and comparison with coronary arteriography and exercise thallium-201 SPECT imaging. *Am J Cardiol.* 1989;64:270–5.
76. Stewart RE, Aschwaiger M, Hutchins GD, Chiao PC, et al. Myocardial clearance kinetics of technetium-99m-SQ30217: a marker of regional myocardial blood flow. *J Nucl Med.* 1990;31:1183–1190.
77. Feldman FM, Nichols WW, Pepire CJ, et al. Acute effect of intravenous dipyridamole on regional coronary hemodynamics and metabolism. *Circulation.* 1981;64:333–344.
78. Wilson RF, Laughlin DE, Ackell PH, et al. Transluminal, subselective measurement of coronary artery blood flow velocity and vasodilator reserve in man. *Circulation.* 1985; 72: 82–92.
79. Boucher CA, Brewster DC, Darling RC, Okada RD, Strauss HW, Pohost GM. Determination of cardiac risk by dipyridamole-thallium imaging before peripheral vascular surgery. *N Engl J Med.* 1985;312:389–394.
80. Mc Cann RL, Clements FM. Silent myocardial ischemia in patients undergoing peripheral vascular surgery: incidence of association with perioperative cardiac morbidity and mortality. *J Vasc Surg.* 1989;9:583–587.
81. Schueppert MT, Kresowik TF, Corry DC, et al. Selection of patients for cardiac evaluation before peripheral vascular operation. *J Vasc Surg.* 1996;23:802–809.
82. Mangano DT, London MJ, Tabau JF, et al. Dipyridamole-thallium 201 scintigraphy as a preoperative test: a reexamination of its predictive potential. *Circulation.* 1991;84:493–502.
83. Baron JF, Mundler O, Vicaut E et al. Dipyridamole-thallium scintigraphy and gated radionuclide angiography to assess cardiac risks before abdominal aortic surgery. *N Engl J Med.* 1994;10:663–669.
84. Kiat H, Berman DS, Maddahi J, et al. Late reversibility of tomographic myocardial thallium-201 defect: an accurate marker of myocardial viability. *J Am Coll Cardiol.* 1988;12:1456–1463.
85. O'Donnell TF. Dipyridamole-thallium scanning for elective aortic aneurysms: its influence on patient management in relationship to contemporary clinical noninvasive cardiac screening. *Semin Vasc Surg.* 1991;4:90–99.
86. Dilsizian V, Rocco TP, Freedman NM, Leon MB, Bonow RO. Enhanced detection of ischemic but viable myocardium by the reinjection of thallium after stress-redistribution imaging. *N Engl J Med.* 1990;323:141–146.
87. Liu P, Kiess MC, Okada RD, et al. The persistence defect on exercise thallium imaging and its fate after myocardial revascularization: does it represent scar or ischemia? *Am Heart J.* 1985;110:996–1001.
88. Cutler BS, Hendel RC, Leppo JA. Dipyridamole-thallium scintigraphy predicts perioperative and long-term survival after major vascular surgery. *J Vasc Surg.* 1992;15:972–979.
89. Cerqueira MD, Verani MS, Schwaiger M, et al. Safety profile of adenosine stress perfusion imaging: Results from the adenosine multicenter trial registry. *J Am Coll Cardiol.* 1994;23:384–389.
90. Hertzer NR, Young JR, Beven EG, et al. Late results of coronary bypass in patients with infrarenal aortic aneurysm: the Cleveland Clinic study. *Ann Surg.* 1987;205: 360–367.
91. Hertzer NR, Young JR, Beven EG, et al. Late results of coronary bypass in patients presenting with lower extremity ischemia: the Cleveland Clinic study. *Ann Vasc Surg.* 1986;1:411–420.
92. Ricci MA, Trevisani GT, Picher DB. Vascular complications of vascular catheterization. *Am J Surg.* 1994;167:375–378.
93. Folland ED, Vogel RA, Hartigan P, et al. Relation between coronary artery stenosis assessed by visual caliper and computer methods and exercise capacity in patients with single–vessel coronary artery disease. *Circulation.* 1994;89: 2005–2014.
94. McCollum CH, Garcia-Rinaldi R, Graham JM, DeBakey ME. Myocardial revascularization prior to subsequent major surgery in patients with coronary artery disease. *Surgery.* 1977;81:302–304.
95. Yusuf S, Zucker D, Peduzzi P et al. Effect of coronary artery bypass graft surgery on survival: overview of 10-year results from randomized trials by the Coronary Artery Bypass Graft Surgery Trialists Collaboration. *Lancet.* 1994; 344:563–570.
96. Ennix CL Jr, Lawrie GM, Morris GC Jr, et al. Improved results of carotid endarterectomy in patients with symptomatic coronary disease: an analysis of 1,546 consecutive carotid operations. *Stroke.* 1979;10:122–125.
97. Reul GJ Jr, Cooley DA, Duncan JM, et al. The effect of coronary bypass on the outcome of peripheral vascular operations in 1093 patients. *J Vasc Surg.* 1986;3:788–798.
98. Mullany CJ, Darling GE, Pluth JR, et al. Early and late results after isolated coronary artery bypass surgery in 159 patients aged 80 years and older. *Circulation.* 1990;82(5 suppl):IV229–IV236.
99. Allen JR, Helling TS, Harzler GO. Operative procedures not involving the heart after percutaneous transluminal coronary angioplasty. *Surg Gynecol Obstet.* 1991;173: 285–288.
100. Huber KC, Evans MA, Bresnaham JF, et al. Outcome of noncardiac operations in patients with severe coronary artery disease successfully treated preoperatively with coronary angioplasty. *Mayo Clin Proc.* 1992;67:15–21.
101. Jollis JG, Peterson ED, DeLong ER, et al. The relationship between the volume of coronary angioplasty procedures at hospitals treating Medicare beneficiaries and short term mortality. *N Engl J Med.* 1994;331:1625–1629.
102. Clark RE. The Society of Thoracic Surgeons National Database status report. *Ann Thorac Surg.* 1994;57:12–19.

103. Landesberg G, Luria MH, Cotev S, et al. Importance of long-duration postoperative ST-segment depression in cardiac morbidity after vascular surgery. *Lancet.* 1993;341: 715–719.

104. Pobyk DK. Cardiac evaluation and risk reduction in patients undergoing major vascular operation. *West J Med.* 1994;161:50–56.

105. Yeager RA. Basic data related to cardiac testing and cardiac risk associated with vascular surgery. *Ann Vasc Surg.* 1990;4:193–197.

106. Mason JJ, Owens DK, Harris RA, et al. The role of coronary angiography and coronary revascularization before noncardiac vascular surgery. *JAMA.* 1995;273:1919–1925.

107. D'Angelo AJ, Puppala D, Farber A, et al. Is preoperative cardiac evaluation for abdominal aortic aneurysm repair necessary? *J Vasc Surg.* 1997;25:152–156.

108. Kresowik TF, Hoballah JJ, Sharp WJ, Corson JD. Cardiac screening tests prior to lower extremity revascularization: Routine versus selective application. *Semin Vasc Surg.* 1997;10:55–60.

109. Johnson JN, McLoughlin GA, Wake PN, Hlesby CR. Contribution of extraperitoneal and transperitoneal methods of aortoiliac reconstructions: a twenty–year experience. *J Cardiovasc Surg.* 1986;27:561–565.

110. Szyalagi DE, Elliott JP, Smith RE, Reddy DJ, McPharlin M. A thirty-year survey of reconstructive therapy of aortoiliac occlusive disease. *J Vasc Surg.* 1986;3:421–429.

111. Bernstein EF, Dilley RB, Randolph H. The improving outlook for patients over seventy years of age undergoing abdominal aortic aneurysmoraphy. *Ann Surg.* 1988;207: 318–324.

112. Wilson SE, Wolf GL, Cross AP. Percutaneous transluminal angioplasty vs. operation for peripheral atherosclerosis. *J Vasc Surg.* 1989;9:1–9.

113. Cappeler WA, Ramirez H, Kartmann H. Abdominal aortic aneurysm: risk factors and complications and their influences on indication for operation. *J Cardiovasc Surg.* 1990; 30:572–578.

114. Clark ET, Gewertz BL, Bassionay HS, Zarins CK. Current results of elective aortic reconstruction for aneurysmal and occlusive disease. *J Cardiovasc Surg.* 1990;31:438–441.

115. Maon RA, Newton GB, Cassel W, Maksha F, Giron F. Combined epidural and general anesthesia in aortic surgery. *J Cardiovasc Surg.* 1990;31:442–448.

116. Shah DM, Chang BB, Paty PSK, et al. Treatment of abdominal aortic aneurysm by exclusion and bypass: an analysis of outcome. *J Vasc Surg.* 1991;13:15–21.

117. Taylor LM, Phinney EG, Porter JM. Present status of reversed vein bypass for lower extremity revascularization. *J Vasc Surg.* 1986;3:288–291.

118. Parker HJ, Fell G, Devine TJ, King RB. Femoropopliteal bypass using autogenous vein or modified human umbilical vein. *J Cardiovasc Surg.* 1988;29:727–730.

119. Whittemore AD, Kent KC, Donaldson MC, Couch NP, Mannick JA. What is the proper role of PTFE grafts in infrainguinal reconstruction? *J Vasc Surg.* 1989;10:299–305.

120. Petrovic P, Lotina S, Djorjuic D, et al. Results of 132 PTFE bifurcated graft implantations. *J Cardiovasc Surg.* 1990;30: 898–901.

121. Towne JB, Bandyk DF, Seabrook GR, Schmitt DO. Experience with in situ saphenous vein bypass during 1981–1989: determinant factors of long term patency. *J Vasc Surg.* 1991;13:137–149.

122. Rutherford RB, Jones DN, Bergentz SE, et al. The efficacy of dextran 40 in preventing early postoperative thrombosis following difficult low extremity bypass. *J Vasc Surg.* 1984;1:765–770.

123. Andros G, Harris RW, Salles-Cunha SX, et al. Bypass grafts to the ankle and foot. *J Vasc Surg.* 1988;7:785–790.

124. Ascer E, Veith FJ, Gupta SK. Bypass to plantar arteries and other tibial branches: an extended approach to limb salvage. *J Vasc Surg.* 1988;8:434–438.

125. Kalmer TW, Lambert GE, Richardson JD, Banis JC, Garrison RN. Utility of inframalleolar arterial bypass grafting. *J Vasc Surg.* 1990;11:164–168.

126. Hertzer RN, Lee CD. Fatal myocardial infarction following carotid endarterectomy: 355 patients followed six to eleven years after operation. *Ann Surg.* 1981;194:212–218.

127. O'Donnell TF, Callow AB, Willet C, Payne D, Richard J. The impact of coronary artery disease on carotid endarterectomy. *Ann Surg.* 1983;198:705–712.

128. Kirschner DL, O'Brien MS, Ricotta JJ. Risk factors in a community experience with carotid endarterectomy. *J Vasc Surg.* 1989;10:178–186.

129. Yeager RA, Moneta GL, McConnell DB, et al. Analysis of risk factors for myocardial infarction following carotid endarterectomy. *Arch Surg.* 1989;124:1142–1145.

130. Edwards WH, Edwards WH Jr, Jenkin JM, Mulherin JL. Analysis of a decade of carotid reconstructive operations. *J Cardiovasc Surg.* 1989;30:424–430.

131. Salenius JP, Harju E, Riekkinnen H. Early cerebral complications in carotid endarterectomy: risk factors. *J Cardiovasc Surg.* 1990;31:162–166, 1990.

67

Popliteal Artery Entrapment Syndrome

Sibu P. Saha

Popliteal artery entrapment syndrome is a rare clinical entity. Stuart,[15] a medical student at the University of Edinburgh in 1879, was the first to describe an anomalous course of the popliteal artery in an amputated leg of a 60-year-old man who developed gangrene of the foot as a result of a large popliteal aneurysm. Haming[7] reported the first successful treatment of popliteal artery entrapment syndrome in a 12-year-old boy who developed claudication and was found to have an anomalous course of the popliteal artery. The term *popliteal artery entrapment syndrome* was first coined by Love and Whelan[9] in 1965. Extrinsic compression of the popliteal artery, which is the basis of this syndrome, results from either an abnormal course of the popliteal vessels or an aberrant attachment of the gastrocnemius muscle or plantaris muscle over the normally positioned vessels. On the basis of this finding at the popliteal fossa, Insua et al.[8] have classified these variants into four groups. In patients with type I popliteal artery entrapment syndrome,[5] the most commonly found abnormality, the popliteal artery deviates medially to the normally placed medial head of the gastrocnemius muscle. In type II there is an abnormal attachment of the medial deviation of the popliteal artery. The popliteal artery is compressed by a muscle band of the medial head of the gastrocnemius muscle in type III. In type IV a fibrous band of the popliteal muscle causes compression of this artery. Rich and his associates[12] described compression of both artery and vein, which is now classified as type V.

There are reports of unusual cases of popliteal entrapment syndrome, such as tibial nerve entrapment[11] and popliteal artery thrombosis as a result of bony exostosis[10] at the popliteal fossa. Brener et al.[2] reported a case of arterial entrapment of the femoropopliteal saphenous vein bypass graft by the gastrocnemius muscle. This syndrome has also been reported in athletes as a result of muscular hyperdevelopment; no other abnormalities could be found. The patient develops symptoms of intermittent claudication only while running. In view of this finding, the term *functional popliteal entrapment syndrome*[13] has been added to this clinical condition. Recurrent pathologic findings vary from premature atherosclerosis to stenosis, thrombosis,[4] embolization, and aneurysm[6] formation in the popliteal artery.

Diagnosis

Calf claudication in young patients between 20 and 30 years of age is indicative of popliteal artery entrapment syndrome. About 90% of the patients are men, and approximately 20% of the patients have bilateral disease. Clinically, they may have a normal, reduced, or absent pulse. Plantar flexion may diminish or occlude the pulse. The duplex scan[3] measures decreased flow with plantar flexion. The angiogram shows middle popliteal artery compression, particularly with plantar flexion or abnormal course of the artery. Occasionally, the angiogram shows segmental occlusion of the popliteal artery (Figure 67.1) or poststenotic dilatation.

Differential diagnoses include Buerger's disease, adductor canal syndrome, compartment syndrome,[1] cystic disease of the adventitia of the popliteal artery, and others.

Treatment

Surgery is the treatment of choice for popliteal artery entrapment syndrome. Most often division of the medial head of the gastrocnemius muscle or the abnormal fibrous band would be sufficient to release the compression of the popliteal artery. Occasionally, bypass may be necessary, particularly in cases of stenosis, occlusion, or aneurysm formation. The ideal conduit is the saphenous vein. Intra-arterial thrombolytic therapy may be of some benefit in unusual cases of distal embolization with acute ischemia. Steurer et al.[14] reported successful re-

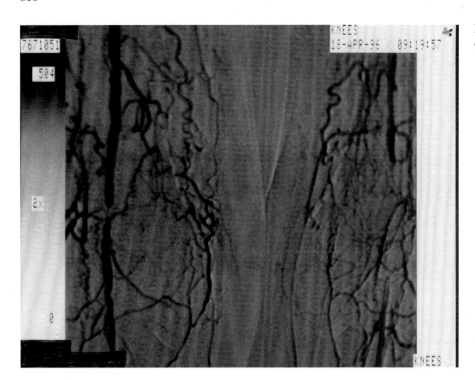

FIGURE 67.1. Angiogram showing occlusion of the middle popliteal artery.

sults with a catheter-based procedure, namely percutaneous transluminal thromboembolectomy, thrombolysis, and angioplasty, in three patients with thromboembolic complication of the popliteal artery entrapment syndrome. These patients later underwent division of the aberrant muscles. With this approach they were able to avoid arterial reconstruction. Early diagnosis and prompt surgical intervention provide long-term satisfactory results and prevent limb loss.

Acknowledgment

I gratefully acknowledge the assistance of Ms. Connie Powell in the preparation of this manuscript.

References

1. Allen MJ, Barnes MR, Bell PR, Bolia A, Hartshorne TC. Popliteal entrapment syndrome misdiagnosed as a compartment syndrome. *Eur J Vasc Endovasc Surg.* 1993;7: 342–345.

2. Brener BJ, Alpert J, Brief DK, Parsonnet V. Iatrogenic entrapment of femoropopliteal saphenous vein bypass grafts by the gastrocnemius muscle. *Surgery.* 1975;78:668–674.

3. Chernoff DM, Walker AT, Khorasani R, Polak JF, Jolesz FA. Asymptomatic functional popliteal artery entrapment: demonstration at MR imaging. *Radiology.* 1995;195: 176–180.

4. Gaines VD, Ramchandani P, Soulen RL. Popliteal entrapment syndrome. *Cardiovasc Int Radiol.* 1985;8:156–159.

5. Gibson MH, Mills JG, Johnson GE, et al. Popliteal artery entrapment syndrome. *Ann Surg.* 1977;185:341–348.

6. Gyftokostas D, Koutsoumbelis C, Mattheou T, Bouhoustos J. Post stenotic aneurysm in popliteal artery entrapment syndrome. *J Cardiovasc Surg.* 1991;32:350–352.

7. Haming JJ. Intermittent claudication at an early age due to an anomalous course of the popliteal artery. *Angiology.* 1959;10:369–371.

8. Insua JA, Young JR, Humphries AW. Popliteal artery entrapment syndrome. *Arch Surg.* 1970;101:771.

9. Love JW, Whelan TJ. Popliteal artery entrapment syndrome. *Am J Surg.* 1965;109:620–624.

10. Lowell B, Carl-Magnus R, Pavel L, Erik GL. Popliteal artery thrombosis in a young woman, secondary to exostosis. *J Cardiovasc Surg.* 1979;20:193–196.

11. Podore PC. Popliteal entrapment syndrome: a report of tibial nerve entrapment. *J Vasc Surg.* 1985;2:335–336.

12. Rich NM, Collins GJ, McDonald PT, et al. Popliteal vascular entrapment: its increasing interest. *Arch Surg.* 1979; 114:1377–1384.

13. Rignault DP, Pailler J, Lunel F. The functional popliteal entrapment syndrome. *Int Angiol.* 1985;4:341–343.

14. Steurer J, Hoffman U, Schneider E, Bollinger A. A new therapeutic approach to popliteal artery entrapment syndrome. *Eur J Vasc Endovasc Surg.* 1995;10:243–247.

15. Stuart TPA. A note on a variation in the course of the popliteal artery. *J Anat Physiol.* 1879;13:162.

68

Diabetic Vascular Disease: Biochemical and Molecular Perspectives

Khurram Kamal, Robert Chang, and Bauer E. Sumpio

The discovery of insulin in 1921 heralded a major change in the natural history of diabetes mellitus. Chronic complications of diabetes mellitus, relatively uncommon before this time, began to emerge as a main source of mortality and morbidity in diabetic patients. Diabetes mellitus imparts end-organ damage in many tissues including kidney, skin, nerve, retina, and heart.[1] Vascular disease is a characteristic pathological feature of diabetes associated with all of the major chronic complications of diabetes mellitus. The development of diabetic angiopathy is a slow process exacerbated by chronic hyperglycemia and many other metabolic abnormalities in patients with diabetes.

Diabetes mellitus is a worldwide health problem. It afflicts 6% of the general population and is the eighth leading cause of death in the United States.[2] Diabetes-induced chronic complications including vascular disease, nephropathy, retinopathy, and neuropathy are the principal causes of increased morbidity in diabetic patients.[3] Epidemiological studies have established the importance of better glycemic control in the prevention of chronic complications of diabetes.[4] This finding provided a strong impetus for investigational studies to further understand the biochemical abnormalities involved in diabetic vascular disease.

Abnormalities in Basic Biochemical Mechanisms

The last two decades have witnessed a gradual evolution in our knowledge of key biochemical pathways that are important in the pathogenesis of diabetic vascular disease. Despite tremendous advancement in our understanding, there is still no single framework or unified theory available to explain the complex pathophysiology of diabetic vascular disease. Only by understanding these biochemical pathways will we be able to develop strategies to prevent and treat diabetic vascular disease.

Polyol Pathway

The polyol pathway utilizes an enzyme, aldose reductase, to convert glucose into sorbitol. Sorbitol is then further oxidized by sorbitol dehydrogenase to fructose using nicotinamide adenine dinucleotide (NAD) as a cofactor (Figure 68.1). Sorbitol consumption is a slow process, and the six-carbon sugar alcohol may accumulate in the cell during hyperglycemia.[5] Hyperglycemia-induced sorbitol oxidation causes an increased ratio of reduced NAD (NADH) to oxidized NAD (NAD^+) that may lead to redox potential alterations. The term *hyperglycemic pseudohypoxia* has been coined to describe this state, associated with changes in free radicals and prostaglandins.[6] The same group suggested that an increased NADH/NAD^+ ratio might be involved in vascular dysfunction because the use of pyruvate appears to normalize these vascular abnormalities.

Activation of the polyol pathway results in intracellular depletion of myoinositol, a precursor of phosphatidylinositol. Both elevated glucose and sorbitol concentrations have been implicated in the diminished uptake of myoinositol by the cells that results in disturbed inositol signaling.[5] Recent studies have also suggested that decreased intracellular myoinositol levels can impair Na^+, K^+–adenosine triphosphatase activity. This raises the intracellular Na^+ levels, which affects the nodal depolarization process and in turn slows nerve conduction velocity.[7] Finally, the increased utilization of reduced nicotinamide-adenine dinucleotide phosphate (NADPH) in the polyol pathway leaves the cells more susceptible to oxidative stress.[8,9]

Although the polyol pathway affects many intracellular processes, its significance has not been firmly established in vascular tissue.[10] In one study, endothelial cell cultures supplemented with myoinositol failed to prevent the replicative delay induced by glucose.[11] However, encouraging data that establish the effect of aldose reductase inhibitors on vascular wall responsiveness have recently been published.[12] Tesfamariam and colleagues[13]

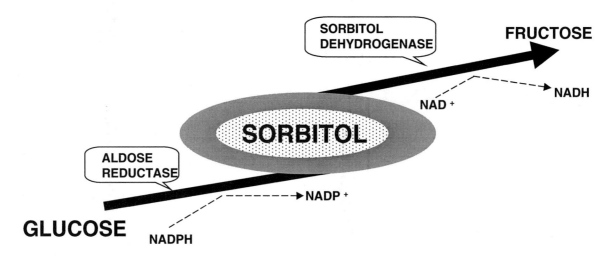

FIGURE 68.1. Polyol pathway. Glucose is converted by aldose reductase to sorbitol, which is then metabolized by sorbitol dehydrogenase to fructose. Hyperglycemia leads to increased levels of sorbitol in the cell. NADH, reduced nicotinamide adenine dinucleotide; NAD+, oxidized nicotinamide adenine dinucleotide; NADP+, oxidized nicotinamide-adenine dinucleotide phosphate; NADPH, reduced nicotinamide-adenine dinucleotide phosphate.

have shown that abnormal endothelial-dependent relaxation in normal arteries exposed to high glucose levels can be prevented if the arteries are pretreated with sorbinil, an aldose reductase inhibitor.

Diacylglycerol–Protein Kinase C Pathway

Protein kinase C (PKC) is a large family of enzymes with multiple isoforms that participates in diverse intracellular signal transduction pathways.[14] Hyperglycemia increases diacylglycerol (DAG) and PKC levels in different tissues, including retina,[15] aorta,[16] renal glomeruli,[17] and cultured vascular smooth cells.[18] Subsequent studies showed that hyperglycemia causes preferential elevation of the PKC β-II isoform.[16]

PKC is primarily regulated by DAG, an intermediate in phospholipid metabolism (Figure 68.2). Activation of PKC results in translocation of kinase from a cytosolic pool to a membranous pool. The hydrolysis of membranous phospholipids produces DAG in the cell.[14] However, glycolytic intermediates can also synthesize DAG after sequential conversion to phosphatidic acid (de

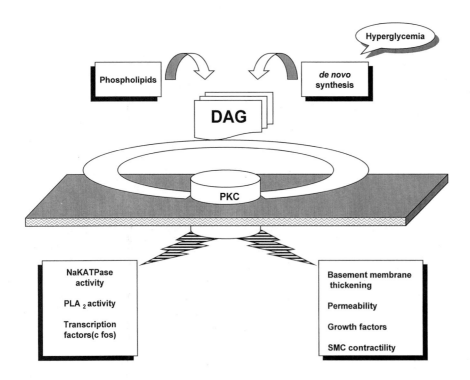

FIGURE 68.2. Protein kinase C–diacylglycerol pathway. Activity of intracellular protein kinase C (PKC) is regulated by diacylglycerol (DAG) levels. Diabetes stimulates the PKC activity by increasing de novo synthesis of DAG from glycolytic intermediates without altering the inositol phosphate levels. Activated PKC affects the activation of cytosolic or calcium-sensitive phospholipase A_2 (PLA$_2$), inhibition of Na+,K+–adenosine triphosphatase, and activity of transcription factor (c-*fos*). These cellular alterations are thought to cause increased basement thickening and increased vascular permeability and to affect smooth muscle cell (SMC) contractility and growth factor functions.

novo synthesis).[19] Lee[20] has demonstrated that hyperglycemia results in increased de novo synthesis, but no changes were observed in inositol phosphate levels.

Hyperglycemia-induced activation of the PKC–DAG pathway causes both intracellular biochemical changes and functional alterations in various tissues. Intracellular changes, for example, include activation of phospholipase A_2, inhibition of Na^+,K^+–adenosine triphosphatase, increase in prostaglandin E_2, and increase in messenger RNA (mRNA) levels of c-*fos* and c-*jun*.[21,22] Similarly, functional studies using diabetic animals and granulation tissue models have documented changes in vascular permeability and contractility as the result of PKC activation.[21]

New synthetic PKC inhibitors have been shown to improve the diabetic-induced vascular dysfunction in two recent animal studies.[23] At present, there is no PKC inhibitor available for systemic use in humans. However, *d*-alpha tocopherol (vitamin E) can prevent the increase in DAG and PKC activities in cultured rat aortic smooth cells and diabetic rats.[24] This may have important implications in the management of diabetes and its complications for the future.

Nonenzymatic Glycation

The process of advanced glycation entails nonenzymatic reactions of glucose and reactive amino groups. The initial glycation process produces reversible early glycation products that are also known as Schiff bases and Amadori products. These adducts undergo a series of chemical rearrangements to form irreversible advanced glycation end products (AGEs).[25] AGEs have not been structurally characterized completely, but the major AGEs include carboxymethyllysine, pentosidine, and pyrroline[25] (Figure 68.3).

AGEs modulate cellular function through receptors that have recently been characterized on endothelium, mononuclear phagocytes, mesangial cells, and smooth muscle cells.[26,27] The process of AGE turnover is incompletely understood at present. However, receptor-mediated uptake followed by intracellular degradation results in low molecular weight AGE-rich peptide formation; these products are released in circulation and excreted by the kidneys.[25,28] Interestingly, one recent study showed an eightfold increase in low molecular weight AGE levels in diabetic patients with renal failure, and both hemodialysis

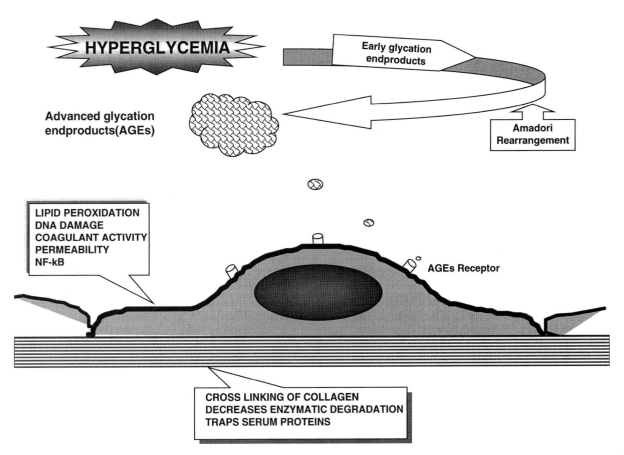

FIGURE 68.3. Formation of advanced glycation end products (AGEs). Glucose interacts with proteins to form early glycation end products. These early products undergo slow chemical rearrangement that leads to AGEs. AGEs interfere with multiple cellular and matrix functions.

and peritoneal dialysis were ineffective in removing low molecular weight AGEs.[29]

AGEs have been shown to affect the cellular activities in a variety of ways. Several studies have shown that AGEs induce lipid oxidation,[30] DNA damage,[25] heme oxygenase, and activation of transcription factor NF-kB.[31] Activation of NF-kB causes transcriptional activation of cytokines and adhesion molecules that play an important role in atherogenesis.[32,33] In the endothelium, AGEs enhance procoagulant activity and permeability across the monolayer.[34] Similarly, in monocytes/macrophages AGEs induce chemotaxis, synthesis of growth factors such as the platelet-derived growth factor (PDGF),[35] and production of tumor necrosis factor α and interleukin 1α.[36] These cytokines in turn perturb the function of mesenchymal and endothelial cells.

AGE formation on extracellular matrix results in the cross-linking of collagen[37] and decreased enzymatic degradation.[38] Glycated collagen traps a variety of serum proteins such as low-density lipoproteins (LDL)[39] and immunoglobulins.[40] These proteins also serve as sites for continued AGE formation. An important recent development is the pharmacological use of aminoguanidine to intervene in AGE formation. In animal studies, aminoguanidine has been shown to ameliorate diabetic retinopathy[41] and nephropathy.[42]

Free Radicals (Oxidative Stress)

Free radicals are atoms or molecules that contain one or more unpaired electrons. Many different types of free radicals have been identified in the body. Major ones include superoxide ($\cdot O_2^-$), hydrogen peroxide (H_2O_2), and hydroxyl radical ($\cdot OH$). Free radicals show variable reactivity and have extremely short lifetimes. They have

been shown to cause lipid peroxidation of cell membrane, damage proteins, and can attack DNA. The human body has evolved intricate defense systems to protect against free radical damage. The antioxidant defense system is composed of enzymes (superoxide dismutase catalase) and substances such as vitamin E (alpha tocopherol).[43,44]

Several mechanisms through which hyperglycemia facilitates free radical formation in the body have been proposed (Figure 68.4). For instance, glucose has an ability to undergo autoxidation and reduce molecular oxygen, which in turn produces free radicals.[45] Similarly, formation of AGEs and activated polyol pathways have been implicated as the cause of oxidative stress in patients with diabetes mellitus.[46] Few studies have examined the effects of hyperglycemia on antioxidant defenses, and they have resulted in conflicting reports.[46]

The adverse effects of increased free radical formation secondary to hyperglycemia are still not completely understood. It has been shown that superoxide anion can inactivate nitric oxide (NO) in a reaction that produces peroxynitrite ($ONOO^-$), an oxidizing agent.[47] This agent may impair vasodilative responses, as suggested by another report that showed restoration of impaired aortic ring relaxation in the presence of free radical scavengers.[48] Furthermore, antioxidants have been shown to restore endothelial dysfunction in many in vitro studies. For example, antioxidants can prevent impaired endothelial proliferation observed in patients with elevated glucose levels and normalize elevated glucose-dependent increases in PDGF production by human endothelial cells.[49,50]

Although human studies in diabetic patients have detected increased levels of malondialdehyde, a marker for lipid peroxidation, many aspects of diabetes-induced ox-

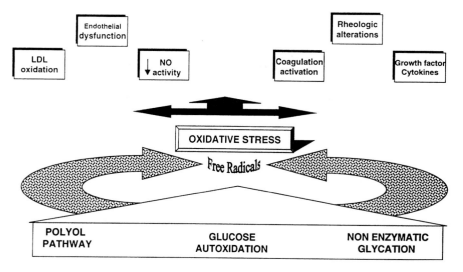

FIGURE 68.4. Glucose autoxidation, activated polyol pathway, and nonenzymatic glycation lead to the formation of free radicals. The resultant oxidative stress impairs multiple molecular mechanisms. LDL, low-density lipoprotein; NO, nitric oxide.

idative stress are still not clear.[46] Further studies are required to determine the significance of free radicals in complex diabetic angiopathy.

Manifestations of Diabetic Vascular Disease

The changes in biochemical pathways over time tend to cause diverse changes in vascular structure and function. An increased susceptibility of certain vascular beds to sustain damage suggests the importance of the local biochemical milieu of tissues in determining the site of tissue damage. This finding led to the concept of microvascular and macrovascular disease in patients with diabetes mellitus. However, these descriptive distinctions are not always obvious. Some biochemical abnormalities can lead to large and small vessel dysfunction. Thus, the heterogeneity in endothelium and matrix organization are the key factors in tissue-specific damage.

Atherosclerosis

The term *diabetic macroangiopathy* is often used to describe an accelerated atherosclerosis and its manifestations in diabetic patients. Many believe that this term should also encompass the nonatherosclerotic changes frequently observed in large vessels such as deposition of material positive for periodic acid–Schiff's reagent and calcium deposition.[51] Atherosclerosis is more prevalent, accelerated, and extensive in patients with diabetes mellitus.[52,53] At the microscopic level, atherosclerosis in diabetic patients is indistinguishable from the lesions seen in nondiabetic patients.[54]

Epidemiological studies have clearly established an association between diabetes and atherosclerosis. Studies have shown in increased mortality rate due to coronary artery disease in diabetic patients as compared with nondiabetic patients. Similarly, the stroke rate and prevalence of peripheral vascular disease are increased in patients with diabetes.[55,56]

Predisposing Factors

The abnormalities in lipid and lipoprotein metabolism are known to affect the initiation and progression of atherosclerosis. A wide variety of alterations in composition and concentration of various lipoproteins are present in diabetes mellitus. Predominant changes in the lipid profile are hypertriglyceridemia, low levels of high-density lipoprotein, and increased chylomicron remnants.[57,58] LDL levels range from low to mildly elevated in diabetes and improve with glycemic control.[59] Similarly, compositional changes are multiple; increases in apolipoproteins B and E, the cholesterol/lecithin ratio, and small dense particles have been described.[59,60] The level of lipoprotein(a), an LDL-like protein with apolipoprotein B-100 and apolipoprotein(a) components, has been shown to be elevated in patients with insulin-dependent diabetes mellitus.[61]

Hypertension is approximately twice as common in diabetic patients as in the general population. There is an increased prevalence of hypertension in patients with diabetes independent of age, renal disease, and obesity factors.[62,63] The degree and duration of hyperglycemia are not major factors in the development of macrovascular complications, as demonstrated by the World Health Organization multinational study and subsequently by a London cohort study.[64,65]

Several prospective studies have attempted to determine the role of hyperinsulinemia as an independent risk factor for the development of atherosclerosis.[66–68] In the San Antonio heart study, Ferranini[69] noted a state of insulin resistance (hyperinsulinemia) in subjects with obesity, non–insulin-dependent diabetes mellitus, hypertension, impaired glucose tolerance, and hypertriglyceridemia. However, in this study it is not certain whether insulin resistance is the result of these conditions or is the basic cellular defect responsible for these abnormalities. At present, due to conflicting epidemiological data and limited experimental evidence, the status of hyperinsulinemia as a major independent risk factor is not firmly established.

Hyperhomocysteinemia has been described as an independent risk factor in the development of atherosclerosis and occlusive arterial disease.[70] In a recent study, hyperhomocysteinemia, after a standard methionine loading, was found in 21% of coronary artery disease patients, 32% of patients with peripheral arterial disease, and 2% of control subjects.[71] Higher levels of homocysteine are present in patients with diabetes than in age-matched control subjects, and an association with macrovascular disease was also noticed.[72,73] Further studies are required to determine the underlying mechanisms and clinical significance of hyperhomocysteinemia in diabetic vascular disease.

Smoking is another well-known risk factor for cardiovascular disease. Smoking enhances the risk of myocardial infarction[74] and peripheral vascular disease[75] in patients with diabetes. The postulated mechanisms are enhanced endothelial damage,[76] abnormalities of the clotting system,[77] and adverse changes in lipoprotein metabolism.[78]

Mechanisms of Atherosclerosis

Atherosclerosis is a complex process that evolves as the result of numerous abnormalities in cellular and noncellular regulatory mechanisms. Many recent reviews have discussed in detail the pathological mechanisms of atherosclerosis.[79–81] Our objective is to present a brief synopsis of the mechanisms that are unique to diabetes. Diabetes mellitus is known to induce two major modifications—oxidation and glycation—of the lipoproteins.

Chronic hyperglycemia results in enhanced glycation of the apolipoproteins present in different types of circulating lipoprotein.[82] Although LDL levels are not usually high in diabetes, the condition is thought to cause LDL glycation.[83] Glycation of LDL results in impaired binding of the glycated LDL to the LDL receptor, which may contribute to the hyperlipidemia observed in diabetic patients.[84] Furthermore, glycated LDL can enhance cholesteryl ester formation and accumulation in human macrophages. It offers a possible mechanism by which glycation of LDL may lead to the formation of the foam cells characteristic of early atheromatous lesions.[85] Glycation of HDL accelerates its plasma clearance[86] and diminishes its ability to cause cholesterol efflux into the cells.[87]

The second chemical modification encompasses the enhanced oxidation of lipoproteins as a result of increased formation of free radicals in diabetes mellitus. LDL isolated from diabetic patients is more susceptible to oxidation than that from nondiabetic patients.[88] Oxidized LDL is a chemotaxin for monocytes.[89] It can potentiate the adherence of monocytes to endothelial cells[90] and promote the expression of certain adhesion molecules, such as vascular cell adhesion molecule and endothelium–leukocyte adhesion molecule.[91] Furthermore, compositional alterations in LDL lead to the formation of small, dense LDL particles that are more prone to oxidation.[92]

The mechanisms by which these diabetes-induced modifications in lipoprotein promote atherosclerosis are still not completely known. Investigators have implicated activation of the immune system as resulting from these modifications in lipoproteins.[93] Most studies have focused on immune mechanisms related to modified LDLs. Substantial evidence suggests that modified LDLs (oxidized or glycated LDLs) are immunogenic and trigger the autoantibody production that in turn promotes formation of immune complexes.[94,95] LDL-containing immune complex induces intracellular accumulation of cholesteryl ester formation in macrophages.[96] The uptake of LDL-containing immune complexes also results in the release of cytokines such as tumor necrosis factor α and interleukin 1 from macrophages, which are known to influence the behavior of smooth muscle cells and the endothelium.[97]

Diabetes induces a host of chemical modifications in lipoproteins that culminate in accelerated atherosclerosis. However, diabetes also causes many other structural and functional changes in different components of the vascular system. Although the term *diabetic microangiopathy* has been used frequently in the literature, we review the studies systematically to ensure clarity.

Endothelium

A large body of evidence suggests that diabetes or elevated glucose levels result in endothelial dysfunction. High concentrations of glucose have been shown to be toxic to the endothelium and inhibit endothelial proliferation.[98] Our in vitro studies have also shown that elevated glucose levels inhibit the proliferation of immortalized human dermal microvascular endothelial cells.[99] Conversely, increased thymidine incorporation has been demonstrated in retinal endothelial cells from streptozocin-induced diabetic rats.[100] This finding may represent differences among various microvascular beds.[101] High glucose levels can also induce DNA damage in the form of increased single-strand breaks along with increased DNA repair.[102] This putative nuclear derangement can interfere with gene expression and proliferation. For instance, endothelial cells cultured in high concentrations of glucose exhibit increased levels of mRNA for fibronectin, laminin, and collagen type IV.[103] Furthermore, elevated glucose levels impair endothelial cell migration and increase integrin expression, as shown by two recent in vitro studies.[104,105]

Insulin and insulinlike growth factor I (IGF-I) receptors have been identified on the endothelial cell surface.[106] These apically located receptors on the endothelium transport insulin in a unidirectional manner by receptor-mediated transcytosis.[107] Insulin and IGF-I have also been found to stimulate the growth of retinal endothelial cells.[108] At present, more information is needed to further understand the effects of elevated glucose levels on endothelium.

Basement Membrane

The interface between endothelium and interstitial space harbors an electron-dense mesh network that constitutes the basement membrane. It is composed of collagen type IV and glycoproteins such as fibronectin, laminin, and proteoglycans.[109,110] A thickened basement membrane is a distinctive feature of diabetic microangiopathy.[111,112] Several studies in diabetic patients have reported alterations in the macromolecular composition of the basement membrane including increases in hydroxylysine and glucose disaccharide content.[112] Similarly, other investigators have shown decreases in the proteoglycans, heparan sulfate, and laminin.[113,114] The major structural component, collagen type IV, is also increased in the basement membrane in patients with diabetes.[115,116]

Several mechanisms have been advocated to explain these alterations in basement membrane.[111] Formation of AGEs in diabetes mellitus is associated with basement membrane dysfunction,[117] and the administration of aminoguanidine has been reported to ameliorate the increase in glomerular basement membrane.[118] Although the polyol pathway has been implicated, a recent study failed to demonstrate any beneficial effect of aldose reductase inhibition on basement membrane thickening despite the suppression of the polyol pathway.[119] The extent and precise role of the PKC–DAG pathway in basement membrane thickening is still unknown. However, elevated glucose levels are shown to increase the synthesis of matrix proteins in mesangial cell cultures.[120] The treatment of mesangial cells with PKC–DAG analogs also increases the matrix protein transcription approximately twofold.[17]

Smooth Muscle Cells and Contractility

Abnormalities in vascular smooth muscle cell (VSMC) physiology contribute to the development of atherosclerosis and hypertension.[81,121] Despite advances in smooth muscle physiology,[122] the role of VSMCs in diabetic vascular disease is not firmly established. Many studies have examined VSMC proliferation as a potential marker for aberrant VSMC behavior in patients with diabetes. VSMCs exhibit increased growth when exposed to high glucose concentrations in vitro.[123] Similarly, animal studies have shown increased thymidine incorporation and proliferation of aortic smooth muscle cells in diabetic animals as compared to nondiabetic control animals.[124] Interestingly, insulin has also been reported to stimulate the proliferation of rat VSMCs.[125]

Functional studies have focused on the contractile responses of VSMCs in diabetes mellitus. Human studies have demonstrated an increase in blood pressure responses to angiotensin II and norepinephrine in patients with diabetes.[126,127] However, Vierhapper [128] failed to show an acute interaction between insulin and angiotensin II pressor responses, although he could not exclude a chronic effect. Yagi et al.[129] have reported an inhibitory effect of insulin on norepinephrine- and angiotensin II–induced contraction of isolated rabbit femoral arteries and veins.

The underlying mechanisms responsible for these abnormal contractile responses in diabetes are obscure. Current evidence suggests the possible role of intracellular calcium, endothelin, and NO for abnormal smooth muscle cell contractility. Standley et al.[130] and Saito et al.[131] have reported that the agonist-induced transient rise (Ca^{2+}) in cultured smooth muscle cells is reduced in the presence of insulin. Abdominal aorta isolated from diabetic animals exhibits abnormal endothelial-dependent relaxation to acetylcholine and adenosine diphosphate.[132] This hyperglycemia-induced impaired relaxation of smooth muscle cells is reversible by PKC inhibitors[133] and cyclooxygenase inhibitors.[134]

Endothelin 1, a vasoactive polypeptide, binds to specific receptors and thus activates the inositol signal cas-

cade. It causes vasoconstriction and has a strong mitogenic effect on smooth muscle cells and endothelium.[135] In a recent study, endothelin levels have been found to be elevated in diabetic patients.[136] In vitro studies have also shown that hyperglycemia and insulin stimulate endothelin 1 secretion by endothelium.[137,138] Oliver et al.[139] have further demonstrated enhanced endothelin 1 gene transcription in cultured bovine endothelial cells exposed to insulin.

NO, a ubiquitous bioregulatory mediator, is known to modulate vascular tone, platelet function, and immune reactions.[140] A number of studies have reported interesting findings about abnormalities in NO metabolism in diabetes. Human studies, in general, have failed to demonstrate an increase in NO synthesis in diabetic patients.[141] However, elevated glucose concentrations were shown to stimulate basal rate L-arginine transport and NO synthesis in human endothelial cells in a recent in vitro study.[142] Many investigators have also described NO as a mediator of the vasodilative effect of insulin.[141,143] However, these studies did not clarify the underlying mechanisms and significance of these findings in diabetic vascular disease.

The abnormal activation of chemical pathways such as formation of AGEs and free radicals has been implicated in the attenuation of NO activity.[141] Bucala et al.[144] recently demonstrated the quenching of NO by glycated albumin. Aminoguanidine, which interferes with the formation of glycation end products, inhibited cytokine-induced NO production in an animal model.[145] The aforementioned studies undoubtedly identify abnormal smooth muscle cell mitogenic activity and impaired contractility but fail to explain the entire picture of altered hemodynamics observed in diabetic patients.

Permeability

The delicate balance of vessel wall permeability is normally maintained by hemodynamic factors and the structural integrity of wall components. Diabetes-induced changes in wall permeability have been studied in various tissues, such as retina,[146] glomeruli,[147] and myocardium.[148] Studies with different tracers have shown increased vascular permeability in diabetic hearts, which may have a role in cardiomyopathy.[148,149] Similarly, increased leakage of fluorescein from retinal capillaries of diabetic patients has been demonstrated.[150] Few in vitro studies have been conducted to examine the direct effect of high glucose concentration on transendothelial permeability. In the Boyden chamber model, exposure to elevated glucose concentrations increases albumin permeability across the endothelial monolayer.[151]

The increased permeability of the vessel wall in diabetes has been attributed to activation of the polyol pathway,[152,153] to the formation of advanced glycation end products,[154,155] and to the activation of the PKC pathway.[156] Recent studies have also proposed a possible link between glucose-induced production of vascular endothelial growth factor (VEGF) and increased vascular permeability.[157] However, the significance of these factors has not been established, and their interaction with other factors remains unclear.

Impaired Hemodynamics

Microvascular circulation is known to adapt to hemodynamic alterations by structural and functional changes. It has been shown that capillary blood flow and pressure are increased in different microvascular beds early in the course of diabetes.[158,159] Studies using laser Doppler flowmetry have provided evidence of impaired hyperemic responses in the foot skin of diabetic patients.[160] These initial changes are followed by a loss of autoregulation in various microvascular beds.[158,161] Sandemann et al.[162] recently demonstrated a fall in raised capillary pressure with better glycemic control.

The proponents of the hemodynamic hypothesis believe strongly that the mentioned changes expose microvessels to hemodynamic stresses and may cause basement membrane thickening and increased wall permeability. The precise mechanisms responsible for hemodynamic abnormalities have not been fully determined. Abnormalities in NO production in patients with diabetes mellitus may contribute to these hemodynamic abnormalities. Pharmacological manipulation of microvascular function is a relatively novel idea and has a potential role in limiting end-organ damage by restoring the abnormal flow parameters. In this respect, Tooke[163] has recently demonstrated normalization of the elevated nailfold capillary pressure after treatment with an angiotensin-converting enzyme inhibitor.

Hemorheology

The role of rheological factors in cardiovascular diseases has recently been highlighted by several epidemiological studies.[164–166] Rheological factors may promote atherosclerosis, thrombosis, and obstruction of microcirculatory flow distal to atherosclerotic stenosis.[165] The Edinburgh Artery Study has elucidated the association of rheological factors with the severity of atherosclerosis in an older population and with the presence of leg ischemia for a given degree of peripheral vascular disease.[167]

Many investigators have associated hemorheological abnormalities in diabetes mellitus with diabetic vascular disease, but their precise role remains uncertain. For instance, plasma and blood viscosity have been found to be increased from 10% to 50% in patients with diabetes.[168–170] Diabetic patients with multiple chronic complications have elevated plasma and blood viscosity levels.[171] It has been proposed that alterations in the plasma protein profile[172,173] and disturbances in erythrocyte behavior[174] may be responsible for the hemorheological abnormalities observed in diabetic patients.

In diabetic patients, erythrocytes exhibit reduced deformability[175,176] and are predisposed to increased aggregation.[177,178] Many defects identified in the erythrocyte membrane may contribute to the abnormal behavior of erythrocytes in patients with diabetes. Hyperglycemia has been found to alter the physiochemical properties of proteins in the erythrocyte membrane, which may involve nonenzymatic glycation of these proteins.[179] Similarly, there is decreased sialylation of glycophorin A, a major glycoprotein of the erythrocyte membrane, which may further interfere with the surface charge of erythrocytes. The resultant decrease in repulsion force provides a possible explanation for the increased erythrocyte aggregation characteristic of diabetes.[180] These effects at the tissue level can be further exacerbated by malfunction of other enzyme systems in erythrocytes. For instance, glutathione metabolism in erythrocytes is impaired in patients with diabetes and can predispose erythrocytes to an oxidative stress.[181]

Coagulation

Hemostatic imbalances in diabetes mellitus encompass a spectrum of abnormalities ranging from defects in the coagulation cascade to alterations in cellular interactions. An endothelial contribution to hemostasis is well established.[182] Hyperglycemia induces a decrease in prostacyclin synthesis[183] and an increase in tissue factor synthesis by endothelium.[184] Similarly, increased plasma levels of von Willebrand's factor, a complex glycoprotein released by the endothelium, has been reported in diabetic patients.[185] The elevated level of von Willebrand's factor was found to correlate with the deterioration in diabetic neuropathy in one recent study.[186]

Various abnormalities in the coagulation cascade have been identified in diabetic patients (Figure 68.5). Substantial evidence indicates clear increases in plasma levels of multiple coagulation factors, such as fibrinogen,[187] factor VII,[188] and factor VIII.[189,190] In fact, plasma fibrinogen level correlates with glycemic control[191] and improves with insulin therapy.[192] Hyperglycemia reduces the biological activity of antithrombin III[193] and results in a drop in thrombin–antithrombin complex levels.[194] Protein C and S levels are also depressed.[195]

The fibrinolytic system promotes the lysis of fibrin, which is of paramount importance for maintenance of vascular patency. Elevated levels of insulin in patients with non–insulin-dependent diabetes mellitus are associated with elevated plasminogen activator inhibitor levels,[196] whereas levels of plasminogen activator inhibitor

FIGURE 68.5. Abnormalities of the hemostatic system in diabetes. t-PA, tissue-type plasminogen activator.

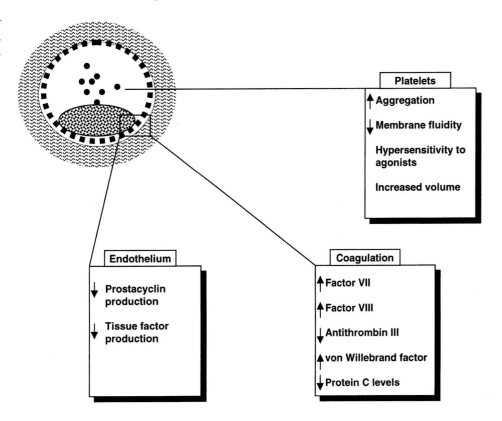

Platelets
↑ Aggregation
↓ Membrane fluidity
Hypersensitivity to agonists
Increased volume

Endothelium
↓ Prostacyclin production
↓ Tissue factor production

Coagulation
↑ Factor VII
↑ Factor VIII
↓ Antithrombin III
↑ von Willebrand factor
↓ Protein C levels

are normal or slightly elevated in patients with insulin-dependent diabetes mellitus.[197] A recent in vitro study demonstrated an increase in plasminogen activator inhibitor production by endothelium when incubated with very-low-density lipoproteins from hyperglycemic patients.[198] There is a trend in diabetes toward a state of depressed fibrinolysis accompanied by an accelerated procoagulant state.

The megakaryocyte–platelet system, a cornerstone in hemostasis, is activated in diabetes. Diverse studies have confirmed platelet hypersensitivity in diabetes to aggregating agents, such as adenosine diphosphate, collagen, arachidonic acid, and thrombin.[199–201] The functional hyperactivity results in an increased release of the contents of α granules, namely platelet factor 4 and β-thromboglobulin.[202] Diabetic patients with angiopathy are prone to an increased number of activated large platelets in their circulation[203] (Table 68.2).

The underlying mechanisms to explain the state of thrombophilia in diabetes are not well established. Nonenzymatic glycation may decrease the activity of antithrombin III,[204] heparin cofactor II, and fibrin.[205] Moreover, glycation of the platelet membrane reduces its fluidity[206] and may be an important factor in increased platelet hypersensitivity.[207] Glucose autoxidation leads to the formation of free radicals, which have been shown to cause the activation of coagulation.[208]

Growth Factors

Growth factors represent a large family of polypeptides that influence cellular activity through specific receptors; activation of signal transduction pathways is the result. Growth factors stimulate cellular proliferation, angiogenesis, and chemotaxis and regulate protein production. We present a succinct review of recent studies that have unraveled a potential role of various growth factors in diabetic vascular disease.

Transforming growth factor β (TGF-β) is a family of homodimeric peptides shown to affect endothelial and smooth muscle cell growth and migration and is a potent modulator of extracellular matrix.[209] It has three isoforms and binds to three main membrane receptors that are serine–threonine kinases. TGF-β has been associated with diabetic nephropathy and proliferative diabetic retinopathy.[210] It enhances matrix protein accumulation in diabetic nephropathy. Defective extracellular matrix remodeling by TGF-β has been implicated in diabetic vascular disease.[211] Furthermore, in one recent study increased levels of circulating TGF-β were detected in *Streptozocin*-diabetic rats.[212] Elevated glucose concentration in vitro induces increases in TGF-β production by endothelial and smooth muscle cells.[213]

VEGFs are homodimeric glycoproteins with multiple isoforms that bind to high-affinity receptors with tyrosine kinase activity. They are potent mitogens and chemoattractants for endothelial cells.[214] Several studies have shown elevated levels of VEGFs in the vitreous and aqueous of the eye in patients with proliferative diabetic retinopathy. Conversely, patients with nonproliferative diabetic retinopathy do not have high VEGF levels.[215] The mechanism of elevated VEGF levels in diabetes is not known. Oxidative stress secondary to an activated polyol pathway may be responsible for increased production of VEGFs by endothelium.[216]

The fibroblast growth factor (FGF) family is composed of nine structurally related polypeptides including prototypes FGF-1 (acidic) and FGF-2 (basic) that show strong affinity to heparin.[217] FGF is a potent mitogen for endothelium and vascular smooth muscle cells. Diabetic patients with proliferative retinopathy have high levels of bFGF in their eyes. Elevated glucose concentration increases mRNA of bFGF in various tissues of diabetic animals and in smooth muscle cell cultures.[210] Furthermore, one recent study in humans detected increased levels of a bFGF-like substance in the plasma of middle-aged diabetic patients.[218] It is thought that an activated PKC pathway may contribute to an increase in bFGF concentration under hyperglycemic conditions.[210]

PDGF is a dimeric molecule comprising two polypeptide chains and a strong stimulant for smooth muscle cell proliferation. PDGF levels in diabetic patients have been measured by various investigators in an attempt to establish a direct correlation between PDGF levels and diabetic angiopathy. At present, results are inconclusive because both elevated PDGF and normal PDGF levels were found in different studies.[219,220] Hyperglycemia-induced increase in smooth muscle cell proliferation may result from an increased expression of PDGF receptors on smooth muscle cells, as shown in one study.[221] Similarly, in another in vitro study, an elevated ambient glucose concentration was shown to increase PDGF production in vascular endothelium.[222]

IGF-I belongs to the peptide family that has a structural homology to insulin and circulates by binding to specific binding proteins. Its actions are mediated by receptors that have tyrosine kinase activity.[223] Although IGF-I has been implicated in the regulation of atherosclerosis and angiogenesis, its precise contribution in diabetic angiopathy is not entirely understood. Numerous studies have detected abnormalities of IGF-I levels or function in both diabetic nephropathy and proliferative diabetic retinopathy.[210] Similarly, decreased IGF mRNA levels were reported in the heart and aorta of diabetic animals.[125] In non–insulin-dependent diabetes mellitus, IGF-I treatment results in decreased levels of triglycerides, very-low-density lipoprotein triglycerides, and LDL cholesterol. However, systemic IGF-I therapy is also known to cause potentially serious adverse effects in diabetic patients.[224]

The underlying mechanisms responsible for alterations in growth factor production and function are not completely known. Activation of biochemical pathways secondary to chronic hyperglycemia may explain some of these alterations. For instance, an activated PKC pathway promotes the secretion of bFGF and TGF-β.[210] Similarly, formation of AGEs has been shown to stimulate the production of PGDF and IGF-I.[210,225]

New Developments

The Diabetes Control and Complication Trial has verified the significance of intensive diabetic therapy in the development and progression of chronic complications of diabetes mellitus.[226] However, insulin therapy alone may not be sufficient to prevent or reverse all of the chronic complications. This finding provides strong incentive to develop alternate methods aimed at the specific biochemical abnormalities responsible for chronic complications.

Initial efforts were directed toward improving the present methods of controlling chronic hyperglycemia because it has a direct association with chronic complications. All of the present therapeutic regimens require intermittent insulin administration, which is not only nonphysiological but also requires active patient participation. Mechanized insulin delivery systems and glucose sensors lessen the patient burden. A glucose sensor is a device that uses various physicochemical principles to detect changes in blood glucose levels.[227] It is available as an independent monitoring system or can be incorporated into an insulin delivery system.[190] Although various experimental models have been developed, efforts are now being directed toward developing implantable miniature devices.[228]

New insulin delivery systems were essentially developed to circumvent the problem of erratic insulin absorption after subcutaneous administration.[229] The new insulin delivery systems include continuous intraperitoneal,[230] nasal,[231] rectal,[232] and transdermal[233] insulin infusion. Among these, the intraperitoneal insulin infusion has been studied most extensively; it results in less systemic hyperinsulinemia compared with the subcutaneous route.[234] The intraperitoneal delivery system has an implantable, programmable pump that offers reliable delivery and peritoneal absorption of insulin.[235]

The progress in artificial systems to control blood glucose level was accompanied by the landmark development of pancreatic transplantation as an endogenous source of insulin supply in diabetic patients.[236] Most pancreatic transplantation operations can be performed as a combined pancreatic and kidney transplant or solitary pancreatic transplant.[237] Pancreatic transplantation results in favorable glucose metabolism, decreases hypoglycemic episodes, and normalizes the glycosylated hemoglobin levels.[238] However, the effects of pancreatic transplantation on the chronic complications of diabetes such as retinopathy,[239] neuropathy,[240] and peripheral microcirculation[241] are not well established. Stratta et al.[242] emphasized the importance of early pancreatic transplantation in a recent study that showed better results, acceptable complication rates, and facilitated rehabilitation in diabetic patients. At present, the use of isolated pancreatic islet transplantation is still at investigative stages.[243]

The alternate novel approach to prevent end-organ damage in diabetes is the development of new chemical agents that specifically intervene in the activation of biochemical pathways. A number of studies have been conducted on how aldose reductase inhibitors, aminoguanidine, PKC inhibitors, and antioxidants affect the development of chronic complications. Both in vitro and animal studies have produced encouraging results using these agents. However, only a few agents have been used in humans, with variable results. Further studies are required to confirm the role of other agents.

Because many abnormalities of growth factors have been identified in diabetic vascular disease, modulation of growth factor imbalances may be a feasible alternative treatment.[244] Specific targeting of growth factors is being studied in relation to various diabetic complications. For instance, octreotide, a somatostatin analog, has been shown to decrease serum and renal IGF-I levels and to reduce renal hyperfiltration.[245] Furthermore, it inhibits IGF-I–induced growth of retinal endothelial cells and stabilizes proliferative diabetic retinopathy.[244] Similarly, decorin, which is a TGF-β inhibitor, has been shown to prevent matrix accumulation in the glomeruli.[246] Many studies have also reported beneficial effects of angiotensin-converting enzyme inhibitors and calcium antagonists on growth factor–induced smooth muscle cell proliferation.[244] Further studies are required to explore more specific therapeutic options to manipulate growth factors.

Conclusion

Biochemical approaches to understanding diabetic vascular disease have clearly enhanced our basic comprehension of the disease process. Studies portrayed in this chapter confirm the complexity of the biochemical events involved in the pathogenesis of diabetic vascular disease. Diabetes mellitus results in a spectrum of changes in multiple molecular pathways. These biochemical alterations of diabetes affect diverse structural components that engender major functional abnormalities of the vascular system. Several vascular beds show predilection toward diabetes-induced damage. Diabetic angiopathy has a central role in the development of almost all of the major complications of diabetes mellitus. Conventional therapeutic interventions have failed to produce optimal control over the progression of diabetic complications. As a result, alternative approaches including innovative insulin delivery systems, pancreas transplantation, suppression of biochemical pathways, and growth factor modulation are being formulated.

References

1. Nathan DM. Long term complications of diabetes mellitus. *N Engl J Med*. 1993;328:1676–1684.
2. Harris M, Hadden WC, Knowles WC, Bennett PH. Prevalence of diabetes and impaired glucose tolerance and glucose levels in the US population aged 20–40 years. *Diabetes*. 1987;36:523–534.
3. Krolewski AS, Warram JH, Freire MBS. Epidemiology of late diabetic complications: a basis for development and evaluation of preventive programs. *Endocrinol Metab Clin North Am*. 1996;25:217–242.
4. Skyler JS. Diabetic complications: the importance of glucose control. *Endocrinol Metab Clin North Am*. 1996;25:243–254.
5. Greene DA, Lattimer SA, Sima AAF. Sorbitol, phosphoinositides, and sodium-potassium-ATPase in the pathogenesis of diabetic complications. *N Engl J Med*. 1987;316:599–606.
6. Williamson JR, Chang K, Frangos M. Hyperglycemic pseudohypoxia and diabetic complications. *Diabetes*. 1993;42:801–813.
7. Greene DA, Sima AFA, Stevens MJ, Feldman EL, Lattimer SA. Complications: neuropathy, pathogenetic considerations. *Diabetes Care*. 1992;15:1902–1925.
8. Barnett PA, Gonzalez RG, Chylack LT, Chen H-M. The effect of oxidation on sorbitol pathway kinetics. *Diabetes*. 1986;35:426–432.
9. Asahine T, Kashiwagi A, Nishio Y, et al. Impaired activation of glucose oxidation and NADPH supply in human endothelial cells exposed to H_2O_2 in high glucose medium. *Diabetes*. 1995;44:520–526.
10. Hawthrone GC, Bartlett K, Hetherington CS, Alberti KGMM. The effect of high glucose on the polyol pathway activity and myoinositol metabolism in cultured endothelial cells. *Diabetologia*. 1989;32:163–166.
11. Lorenzi M, Toledo S. Myoinositol enhances the proliferation of human endothelial cells in culture but fails to prevent the delay induced by high glucose. *Metabolism*. 1986;35:824–829.
12. Wakasugi M, Noguchi T, Inoue M, Tawata M, Shindo H, Onaya T. Effect of aldose reductase inhibitors on prostacyclin synthesis by aortic ring from rats with streptozotocin-induced diabetes. *Prostaglandins Leukot Essent Fatty Acids*. 1991;44:233–236.
13. Tesfamariam B, Cohen R. Role of sorbitol and myoinositol in the endothelial cell dysfunction caused by elevated glucose [abstract]. *Federation Proceedings*. 1990;4.
14. Nishizuka Y. Protein kinase C and lipid signaling for sustained cellular responses. *FASEB J*. 1995;9:484–496.

15. Shiba T, Inoguchi T, Sportman JR, Heath WF, Bursell S, King GL. Correlation of diacylglycerol level and protein kinase C activity in rat retina to retinal circulation. *Am J Physiol.* 1993;265(suppl):E783–E793.

16. Inoguchi T, Batten R, Handler E, Sportman JR, Heath W, King GL. Preferential elevation of protein kinase C isoform beta II and diacylglycerol levels in the aorta and heart of diabetic rats: differential reversibility to glycemic control by islet cell transplantation. *Proc Natl Acad Sci U S A.* 1992;89:11059–11063.

17. Ayo SH, Radnik R, Garoni JA, Troyer DA, Kriesberg JI. High glucose increases diacylglycerol mass and activates protein kinase C in mesangial cell culture. *Am J Physiol.* 1992;261(suppl):F571–F577.

18. Williams B, Schrier RW. Characterization of glucose-induced in situ protein kinase C activity in cultured vascular smooth muscle cells. *Diabetes.* 1993;41:1464–1472.

19. Dunlop M, Larkins RG. Pancreatic islet synthesize phospholipid de novo from glucose via acyldihydroxy acetone phosphate. *Biochem Biophys Res Commun.* 1985;132:467–473.

20. Lee TS, Saltman KA, Ohashi H, King GL. Activation of protein kinase C by elevation of glucose concentration: proposal for a mechanism in the diabetic vascular complications. *Proc Natl Acad Sci U S A.* 1989;86:5141–5145.

21. King GL, Kunisaki M, Nisho Y, Inoguchi T, Shiba T, Xia P. Biochemical and molecular mechanisms in the development of diabetic complications. *Diabetes.* 1996;45(suppl 3):S105–S108.

22. Kreisberg JI, Garoni J, Radnik R, Ayo S. High glucose and TGF beta 1 stimulate fibronectin gene expression through a cAMP response element. *Kidney Int.* 1994;46:1019–1024.

23. Ishii H, Jirousek MR, Koya D, et al. Amelioration of vascular dysfunction in diabetic rats by an oral PKC beta inhibitor. *Science.* 1996;272:728–731.

24. Kunisaki M, Bursell S, Umeda F, Nawata H, King GL. Normalization of diacylglycerol-protein kinase c activation by vitamin E in aorta of diabetic rats and cultured rat smooth muscle cells exposed to elevated glucose. *Diabetes.* 1994;43:1372–1377.

25. Vlassara H, Bucala R. Advanced glycation and diabetes complications: an update. In: Marshall SM, Home PD, Rizza RA, eds. *The Diabetes Annual.* 9th ed. Amsterdam: Elsevier Science; 1995:227–244.

26. Vlassara H, Brownlee M, Cerami A. Novel macrophage receptor for glucose-modified protein is distinct from previously described scavenger receptors. *J Exp Med.* 1986;164:1301–1309.

27. Brett J, Schmitt AM, Zou YS, et al. Tissue distribution of the receptor for advanced glycation end products (RAGE): expression in smooth muscle, cardiac myocyte, and neural tissue in addition to vascular tissue. *Am J Pathol.* 1993;143:1699–1712.

28. Vlassara H, Bucala R. Recent progress in advanced glycation and diabetic vascular disease: role of advanced glycation end product receptors. *Diabetes.* 1996;45(suppl 3):S65–S66.

29. Makita Z, Bucala R, Rayfield EJ, et al. Diabetic-uremic serum advanced glycosylation end products are chemically reactive and resistant to dialysis therapy. *Lancet.* 1994;343:1519–1522.

30. Bucala R, Makita Z, Koschinsky T, Cerami A, Vlassara H. Lipid advanced glycosylation: pathway for lipid oxidation in vivo. *Proc Natl Acad Sci U S A.* 1993;90:6434–6438.

31. Yan S-D, Schmidt A-M, Anderson GM, et al. Enhanced cellular oxidant stress by the interaction of advanced glycation end products with their receptors/binding proteins. *J Biol Chem.* 1994;269:9889–9897.

32. Collins T. Endothelial nuclear factor kB and initiation of atherosclerosis. *Lab Invest.* 1993;68:499–508.

33. Schmidt A-M, Hori O, Chen JX, et al. Advanced glycation endproducts interacting with their receptors induce expression of vascular cell adhesion molecule-1 (VCAM-I) in cultured human endothelial cells and in mice: a potential mechanism for the accelerated vasculopathy in diabetes. *J Clin Invest.* 1995;96:1395–1403.

34. Esposito C, Gerlach H, Brett J, Stern D, Vlassara H. Endothelial receptor-mediated binding of glucose-modified albumin is associated with increased monolayer permeability and modulation of cell surface coagulant properties. *J Exp Med.* 1989;170:1387–1407.

35. Kirstein M, Brett J, Radoff S, Ogawa S, Stern D, Vlassara H. Advanced glycosylation induces the transendothelial human monocyte chemotaxis and secretion of PDGF: role in vascular disease in diabetes and aging. *Proc Natl Acad Sci U S A.* 1990;87:9010–9014.

36. Vlassara H, Brownlee M, Manogue KR, Dinarello CA, Pasagian A. Cachectin/TNF and IL-I induced by glucose modified proteins: role in normal tissue remodeling. *Science.* 1988;240:1546–1548.

37. Kent MJC, Light ND, Bailey AJ. Evidence for glucose-mediated covalent cross-linking of collagen after glycosylation. *Biochem J.* 1985;225:745–752.

38. Lubec G, Pollak A. Reduced susceptibility of non enzymatically glucosylated glomerular basement membrane to protease: is thickening of glomerular membrane due to reduced proteolytic degradation? *Renal Physiol.* 1980;3:4–8.

39. Brownlee M, Vlassara H, Cerami A. Non enzymatic glycosylation products on collagen covalently trap low-density lipoprotein. *Diabetes.* 1985;34:938–941.

40. Brownlee M, Ponger S, Cerami A. Covalent attachment of soluble protein by non enzymatically glycosylated collagen: a role in the in situ formation of immune complex. *J Exp Med.* 1983;158:1739.

41. Hammes H-P, Martin S, Federlin K, Geisen K, Brownlee M. Aminoguanidine treatment inhibits the development of experimental diabetic retinopathy. *Proc Natl Acad Sci U S A.* 1991;88:11555–11558.

42. Soulis-Liparota T, Cooper M, Papazoglou D, Clark B, Jerum G. Retardation by aminoguanidine of development of albuminuria, mesangial expansion, and tissue fluorescence in streptozotocin-induced diabetic rats. *Diabetes.* 1991;40:1328–1334.

43. Halliwell B. Free radical, antioxidant, and human disease: curiosity, cause, or consequence? *Lancet.* 1994;344:721–724.

44. Cheeseman KH, Slater TF. An introduction to free radical biochemistry. *Br Med Bull.* 1991;49:481–493.

45. Hunt JV, Dean DT, Wolff SP. Hydroxyl radical production and autoxidative glycosylation: glucose autoxidation as the cause of protein damage in the experimental glycation model of diabetes mellitus and aging. *Biochem J.* 1988;256: 205–212.

46. Giugliano D, Paolisso G, Ceriello A. Oxidative stress and diabetic vascular disease. *Diabetes Care.* 1996;19: 257–267.

47. Beckman JS, Beckman TW, Chen J, Marshall PA, Freeman BA. Apparent hydroxyl radical production by peroxynitrite: implication for endothelial injury from nitric oxide and superoxide. *Proc Natl Acad Sci U S A.* 1990;87:1620–1624.

48. Tesfamariam B, Cohen RA. Free radical mediate endothelial dysfunction caused by elevated glucose. *Am J Physiol.* 1992;263(suppl):H321–H326.

49. Curcio F, Ceriello A. Decreased cultured endothelial proliferation in high glucose medium is reversed by antioxidants: new insights on the pathophysiological mechanisms of diabetic vascular complications. *In Vitro Cell Dev Biol.* 1992;28:787–790.

50. Curcio F, Pegoraro I, Dello Russo P, Falleti E, Perella F, Ceriello A. Sod and GSH inhibit the high glucose-induced oxidative damage and the PDGF increased secretion in cultured human endothelial cells. *Thromb Haemost.* 1995; 74:969–973.

51. Andersen JL, Rasmussen LM, Ledet T. Diabetic angiopathy and atherosclerosis. *Diabetes.* 1996;45(suppl 3):S91–S94.

52. Pyorala K, Laasko M, Uusitupa M. Diabetes and atherosclerosis: an epidemiologic view. *Diabetes Metab Rev.* 1987; 3:463–524.

53. Jarret RJ. Cardiovascular disease and hypertension in diabetes mellitus. *Diabetes Metab Rev.* 1989;5:547–558.

54. Gensler SW, Haimovici H, Hoffert P, Steinman C, Beneventano TC. Study of vascular lesion in diabetic and non diabetic patients. *Arch Surg.* 1965;91:617–622.

55. Barret-Connor E, Khow KT. Diabetes mellitus: an independent risk factor for stroke? *Am J Epidemiol.* 1988;128: 116–123.

56. Beach KW, Bedford GR, Bergelin RO, et al. Progression of lower-extremity arterial occlusive disease in type II diabetes mellitus. *Diabetes Care.* 1988;11:464–472.

57. Kim DK, Escalante DA, Garber AJ. Prevention of atherosclerosis in diabetes: emphasis on treatment for the abnormal lipoprotein metabolism. *Clin Ther.* 1993;15:766–778.

58. Laakso M. Epidemiology of diabetic dyslipidaemia. *Diabetes Rev.* 1995;3:408–422.

59. Chait A, Brunzell JD. Diabetes, lipids, and atherosclerosis. In: LeRoith D, Taylor SI, Olefsky JM, eds. *Diabetes Mellitus.* Philadelphia, Pa: Lippincott-Raven Publishers; 1996:772–780.

60. Barakat HA, Carpenter JW, Mclendon VD, et al. Influence of obesity, impaired glucose tolerance, and NIDDM on LDL structure and composition: possible link between hyperinsulinemia and atherosclerosis. *Diabetes.* 1990;39: 1527–1533.

61. Haffner SM. Lipoprotein(a) and diabetes: an update. *Diabetes Care.* 1993;6:835–840.

62. Chriestlieb AR, Warram JH, Krolewski AS, et al. Hypertension, the major risk factor in juvenile-onset insulin dependent diabetes. *Diabetes.* 1981;30(suppl 2):90–96.

63. Brazilay J, Warram JH, Bak M, Laffel LM, Canessa M, Krolewski AS. Predisposition to hypertension: a risk factor for nephropathy and hypertension. *Kidney Int.* 1992;41: 723–730.

64. West KM, Ahuja MMS, Bennett PH, et al. The role of circulating glucose and triglyceride concentration and their interaction with other "risk factors" as determinant of arterial disease in nine population samples from WHO multinational study. *Diabetes Care.* 1983;6:361–369.

65. Morrish NJ, Stevens LK, Head J, Fuller JH, Jarrett RJ, Keen H. A prospective study of mortality among middle-aged diabetic patients. The London cohort of the WHO multinational study of vascular disease in diabetics, II: associated risk factors. *Diabetologia.* 1990;33:542–548.

66. Fontbonne A, Charles MA, Thibult N, et al. Hyperinsulinemia as a predictor of coronary heart disease mortality in a healthy population: the Paris prospective study, 15-year follow-up. *Diabetologia.* 1991;34:356–361.

67. Modan M, Or J, Karasik A, et al. Hyperinsulinemia, sex, and risk of atherosclerotic cardiovascular disease. *Circulation.* 1991;84:1165–1175.

68. Ferrara A, Barret-Connor E, Edelstein SL. Hyperinsulinemia does not increase the risk of fatal cardiovascular disease in elderly men or women without diabetes: the Rancho Bernardo study, 1984 to 1991. *Am J Epidemiol.* 1994; 140:857–869.

69. Ferrannini E, Haffner SM, Mitchell BD, Stern MP. Hyperinsulinemia: the key feature of a cardiovascular and metabolic syndrome. *Diabetologia.* 1991;34:416–422.

70. Clarke R, Daly L, Robinson K, et al. Hyperhomocysteinemia: an independent risk factor for vascular disease. *N Engl J Med.* 1991;324:1149–1155.

71. Boers GHJ. Hyperhomocysteinemia as a risk factor for arterial and venous disease: a review of evidence and relevance. *Thromb. Haemost.* 1997;78:520–522.

72. Munshi MN, Stone A, Fink L, Fonseca V. Hyperhomocysteinemia following a methionine load in patients with non-insulin dependent diabetes mellitus and macrovascular disease. *Metabolism.* 1996;45:133–135.

73. Araki A, Sako Y, Ito H. Plasma homocysteine concentration in Japanese patients with non-insulin dependent diabetes mellitus: effect of parental methylcobalamin treatment. *Atherosclerosis.* 1993;103:149–157.

74. LaCroix AZ, Lang J, Scherr P, et al. Smoking and mortality among older men and women in three populations. *N Engl J Med.* 1991;324:1619–1625.

75. Palumbo PJ, O'Fallen WM, Osmundson PJ, Zimmerman BR, Langworthy AL, Kazmier FJ. Progression of peripheral occlusive arterial disease in diabetes mellitus: what factors are predictive? *Arch Intern Med.* 1991;151:717–721.

76. Blann AD, McCollum CN. Adverse influence of cigarette smoking on the endothelium. *Thromb Haemost.* 1993;70: 707–711.

77. Kimura S, Nishinaga M, Ozawa T, Schimada K. Thrombin generation as an acute effect of cigarette smoking. *Am Heart J.* 1994;28:7–11.

78. Freeman DJ, Griffin BA, Murray E, et al. Smoking and plasma lipoproteins in man: effects on low density lipoprotein cholesterol levels and high density lipoprotein subfraction distribution. *Eur J Clin Invest.* 1993;23:630–640.

79. Clinton K, Libby P. Cytokinins and growth factors in atherogenesis. *Arch Pathol Lab Med.* 1992;116:1292–1300.

80. Basha JB, Sower JR. Atherosclerosis: an update. *Am Heart J.* 1995;131:1192–1202.

81. Ross R. The pathogenesis of atherosclerosis: a perspective for the 1990s. *Nature.* 1993;362:801–809.

82. Curtiss LK, Witzum JL. Plasma apolipoproteins AI, AII, B, CI, and C are glycosylated in hyperglycemic diabetic patients. *Diabetes.* 1985;34:452–461.

83. Bucala R, Makita Z, Vega G, et al. Modification of low density lipoprotein by advanced glycation end products contribute to the dyslipidemia of diabetes and renal insufficiency. *Proc Natl Acad Sci U S A.* 1994;263:2893–2898.

84. Ginsberg HN. Lipoprotein physiology in non diabetic and diabetic states: relationship to atherogenesis. *Diabetes Care.* 1991;14:839–855.

85. Lopes-Virella MF, Klein RL, Lyon TJ, Stevenson HC, Witztum JL. Glycosylation of low density lipoprotein enhances cholesteryl ester synthesis in human monocyte-derived macrophage. *Diabetes.* 1988;37:550–557.

86. Witzum JL, Fisher M, Pietro T, Steinbrecher UP, Elam RL. Non enzymatic glycosylation of high density lipoprotein accelerates its catabolism in guinea pigs. *Diabetes.* 1982;31:1029–1032.

87. Duell PB, Oram JF, Beirman EL. Non enzymatic glycosylation of HDL and impaired HDL-receptor-mediated cholesterol efflux. *Diabetes.* 1991;40:377–384.

88. Tsai EC, Hirsch IB, Brunzell JD, Chait A. Reduced peroxyl radical trapping capacity and increased susceptibility of LDL to oxidation in poorly controlled IDDM. *Diabetes.* 1994;43:1010–1014.

89. Cushing SD, Berliner JA, Valente AJ, et al. Minimal modified low density lipoprotein induces monocyte chemotactic protein I in human endothelial cells and smooth muscle cells. *Proc Natl Acad Sci U S A.* 1987;84:2955–2958.

90. Berliner JA, Territo MC, Sevanian A, et al. Minimally modified low density lipoprotein stimulates monocyte-endothelial interactions. *J Clin Invest.* 1990;85:1260–1266.

91. Drake TA, Hannani K, Fei HH, Lavi S, Berliner JA. Minimally oxidized LDL induces tissue factor expression in cultured human endothelial cells. *Am J Pathol.* 1991;138:601–607.

92. Chait A, Brazg RL, Tribble DL, Krauss RM. Susceptibility of small, dense low density lipoprotein to oxidative modification in subjects with the atherogenic lipoprotein phenotype, pattern B. *Am J Med.* 1993;94:350–356.

93. Lopes-Virella MF, Virella G. Cytokines, modified lipoproteins, and arteriosclerosis in diabetes. *Diabetes.* 1996;45(suppl 3):S40–S45.

94. Witztum JL, Steinbrecher UP, Kesaniemi YA, Fisher M. Autoantibody to glycosylated protein in the plasma of patient with diabetes mellitus. *Proc Natl Acad Sci U S A.* 1984;81:3204–3208.

95. Lopes-Virella M, Virella G. Immune mechanisms of atherosclerosis in diabetes mellitus. *Diabetes.* 1992;41(suppl 2):86–91.

96. Gisinger C, Virella GT, Lopes-Virella M. Erythrocyte-bound low density lipoprotein (LDL) immune complex leads to cholesteryl ester accumulation in human monocyte derived macrophage. *Clin Immunol Immunopathol.* 1991;59:37–52.

97. Virella G, Munoz JF, Galbraith GM, Gissinger C, Chassereau C, Lopes-Virella MF. Activation of human monocyte-derived macrophage by immune complex containing low density lipoprotein. *Clin Immunol Immunopathol.* 1995;75:179–189.

98. Lorenzi M, Cagleiro E, Toledo S. Glucose toxicity for human endothelial cells in culture. *Diabetes.* 1985;34:621–627.

99. Kamal K, Mills I, Sumpio BE. Proliferation of immortalized human dermal microvascular endothelial cells is inhibited by elevated glucose. *FASEB J.* 1995;9:A872.

100. Sharma NK, Gardiner TA, Archer DB. A morphologic and autoradiographic study of cell death and regeneration in the retinal microvasculature of normal and diabetic rats. *Am J Ophthalmol.* 1985;100:51–60.

101. Lorenzi M, Cagliero E. Pathobiology of endothelial and other vascular cells in diabetes mellitus. *Diabetes.* 1991;40:653–659.

102. Lorenzi M, Monstisano DF, Toledo S, Barrieux A. High glucose induced DNA damage in cultured human endothelial cells. *J Clin Invest.* 1986;77:322–325.

103. Cagliero E, Roth T, Roys S, Lorenzi M. Characteristics and mechanisms of high glucose induced overexpression of basement membrane component in cultured human endothelial cells. *Diabetes.* 1991;40:102–110.

104. Mascardo RN. The effect of hyperglycemia on the directed migration of wounded endothelial cell monolayer. *Metabolism.* 1988;37:102–110.

105. Roth T, Podesta F, Stepp MA, Boeri D, Lorenzi M. Integrin overexpression induced by high glucose and human diabetes: potential pathway to cell dysfunction in diabetic angiopathy. *Proc Natl Acad Sci U S A.* 1993;90:9640–9644.

106. Jialal I, Crettaz M, Hachiya HL, et al. Characterization of the receptors for insulin and insulin-like growth factors on micro- and macrovascular tissue. *Endocrinolgy.* 1985;117:1222–1229.

107. Wallum BJ, Taborsky GJ Jr, Porte D Jr. Cerebrospinal fluid insulin levels increase during intravenous insulin infusions in man. *J Clin Invest.* 1987;64:190–194.

108. King GL, Goodman AD, Bunzey S, Moses A, Kahn CR. Receptors and growth-promoting effect of insulin and insulin-like growth factor on cells from bovine retinal capillaries and aorta. *J Clin Invest.* 1985;75:1028–1036.

109. Sages H. Collagens of basement membranes. *J Invest Dermatol.* 1982;79(suppl 1):51S–59S.

110. Faucet DW. *A Textbook of Histology.* 12th ed. New York, NY: Chapman & Hall; 1994.

111. Reddi AS. The basement membrane in diabetes. In: Marshall SM, Home PD, Rizza RA, eds. *The Diabetes Annual.* Amsterdam: Elsevier Science; 1995:245–263.

112. William JR, Tilton RG, Chang K, Kilo C. Basement membrane abnormalities in diabetes mellitus: relationship to clinical microangiopathy. *Diabetes Metab Rev.* 1988;4:339–370.

113. Vernier RL, Steffes MW, Sisson-Ross S, Mauer SM. Heparan sulfate proteoglycan in the glomerular basement membrane in type I diabetes mellitus. *Kidney Int.* 1992;41: 1070–1080.

114. Shimomura H, Spiro RG. Studies on macromolecular component of human glomerular basement membrane and alteration in diabetes: decreased levels of heparan sulfate proteoglycan and laminin. *Diabetes.* 1987;36:374–381.

115. Ziyadeh FN. Renal tubular basement membrane and collagen type IV in diabetes mellitus. *Kidney Int.* 1993;43: 114–120.

116. Rasmussen LM, Ledet T. Aortic collagen alteration in human diabetes mellitus: changes in basement membrane collagen content and susceptibility to total collagen to cyanogen bromide solubilization. *Diabetologia.* 1993;36: 445–453.

117. Brownlee M, Cerami A, Vlassara H. Advanced glycosylation end products in tissue and the biochemical basis of diabetic complications. *N Engl J Med.* 1988;318:1315–1321.

118. Ellis EN, Good BH. Prevention of glomerular basement membrane thickening by aminoguanidine in experimental diabetes mellitus. *Metabolism.* 1991;40:1016–1019.

119. Engerman RL, Kern TS, Garment MB. Capillary basement membrane in retina, kidney, and muscle of diabetic dogs and galactosemic dogs and its response to 5 years of aldose reductase inhibition. *J Diabetes Complications.* 1993; 7:241–245.

120. Ayo SH, Radnick RA, Glass WF, et al. Increased extracellular matrix synthesis and mRNA in mesangial cells grown in high glucose medium. *Am J Physiol.* 1991;260(suppl): F185–F191.

121. Pauletto P, Sarzani R, Rappelli A, Chiavegato A, Pessina AC, Sartore S. Differentiation and growth of vascular smooth muscle in experimental hypertension. *Am J Hypertens.* 1994;121:4–11.

122. Somlyo AP, Somlyo AV. Signal transduction and regulation in smooth muscle. *Nature.* 1994;327:231–226.

123. Natarajan R, Gonzalez N, Xu L, Nadler JL. Vascular smooth muscle cell exhibit increased growth in response to elevated glucose. *Biochem Biophys Res Commun.* 1992; 187:552–560.

124. Alipui C, Ramos K, Tenner TE Jr. Alteration of rabbit aortic smooth muscle cell proliferation in diabetes mellitus. *Cardiovasc Res.* 1993;27:1229–1232.

125. Bornfeldt KE, Arnqvist HJ, Capron L. In vivo proliferation of rat vascular smooth muscle in relation to diabetes mellitus, insulin-like growth factor-I, and insulin. *Diabetologia.* 1992;35:104–108.

126. Weidmann P, Beretta-Piccoli C, Trost BN. Pressor factors and responsiveness in hypertension accompanying diabetes mellitus. *Hypertension.* 1985;7(suppl 7):II33–II42.

127. Drury PL, Smith GM, Ferris JB. Increased vasopressor responsiveness to angiotensin II in type I (insulin-dependent) diabetic patients without complications. *Diabetologia.* 1983;27:174–179.

128. Veirhapper H. Effect of exogenous insulin on blood pressure regulation in healthy diabetic subjects. *Hypertension.* 1985;7(suppl 2):II49–II53.

129. Yagi S, Takata S, Kiyokawa H. Effect of insulin on vasoconstrictive response to norepinephrine and angiotensin II in rabbit femoral artery and vein. *Diabetes.* 1988;37:1064–1067.

130. Standley PR, Zhang F, Ram JL, Zemel MB, Sower JR. Insulin attenuates vasopressin induced calcium transients and a voltage-dependent calcium response in rat vascular smooth muscle cells. *J Clin Invest.* 1991;88:1230–1236.

131. Saito F, Hori MT, Fittengoff M, Hino T, Tuck ML. Insulin attenuates agonist-mediated calcium mobilization in cultured rat smooth muscle cells. *J Clin Invest.* 1993;92: 1161–1167.

132. Tesfamariam B, Brown ML, Deykin D, Cohen RA. Elevated glucose promotes generation of endothelial-derived vasoconstrictor prostanoid in rabbit aorta. *J Clin Invest.* 1990;85:929–932.

133. Tesfamariam B, Brown ML, Cohen RA. Elevated glucose impairs the endothelium-dependent relaxation by activating protein kinase C. *J Clin Invest.* 1991;87:1643–1648.

134. Tesfamariam B, Jakubowski JA, Cohen RA. Contraction of diabetic rabbit aorta caused by endothelium-derived PGH$_2$-TxA$_2$. *Am J Physiol.* 1989;26(suppl):H1327–H1333.

135. McMillen MA, Sumpio BE. Endothelins: polyfunctional cytokines. *J Am Coll Surg.* 1995;180:621–637.

136. Takahashi K, Ghatei MA, Lam H-C, O' Halloran DJ, Bloom SR. Elevated plasma endothelin in patients with diabetes mellitus. *Diabetologia.* 1990;33:306–310.

137. Yamauchi T, Ohnaka K, Takayanagi R, Umeda F, Nawata H. Enhanced secretion of endothelin-I by elevated glucose levels from cultured bovine aortic endothelial cells. *FEBS Lett.* 1990;267:16–18.

138. Hu R-M, Levin ER, Pedram A, Frank HJL. Insulin stimulates production and secretion of endothelin from bovine endothelial cells. *Diabetes.* 1993;42:351–358.

139. Oliver FJ, deRubia G, Feener EP, et al. Stimulation of endothelin-I gene expression by insulin in endothelial cells. *J Biol Chem.* 1991;266:23251–23256.

140. Moncada S, Higgs A. The L-arginine-nitric oxide pathway. *N Engl J Med.* 1993;329:2002–2012.

141. Sobrevia L, Mann GE. Dysfunction of the endothelial nitric oxide signalling pathway in diabetes and hyperglycemia. *Exp Physiol.* 1997;82:432–452.

142. Sobrevia L, Nadal A, Yudilevich DL, Mann GE. Activation of L-arginine transport (system y+) and nitric oxide synthetase by elevated glucose and insulin in human endothelial cells. *J Physiol.* 1996;490:775–781.

143. Scherrer U, Randin D, Vollenweider P, Nicod P. Nitric oxide release account for insulin's vascular effect in humans. *J Clin Invest.* 1994;94:2511–2515.

144. Bucala R, Tracey KJ, Cerami A. Advanced glycosylation products quench nitric oxide and mediate defective endothelium-dependent vasodilation in experimental diabetes. *J Clin Invest.* 1991;87:432–438.

145. Corbett JA, Tilton RG, Chang K, et al. Aminoguanidine, a novel inhibitor of nitric oxide formation, prevents diabetic vascular dysfunction. *Diabetes.* 1992;41:552–556.

146. Cunha-Vaz J, De Abreu JRE, Compos AJ, Figo GM. Early breakdown of the blood-brain barrier in diabetes. *Br J Ophthalmol.* 1975;59:649–656.

147. Mogenesen CE. Microalbuminuria predicts clinical proteinuria and early mortality in maturity-onset diabetes. *N Engl J Med*. 1984;310:356–360.

148. Yamaji T, Fukuhara T, Kinoshita M. Increased capillary permeability to albuminuria in diabetic rat myocardium. *Circ Res*. 1993;72:947–957.

149. Kubota I, Fukuhara T, Kinoshita M. Permeability of small coronary arteries and myocardial injury in hypertensive diabetic rats. *Int J Cardiol*. 1990;29:349–355.

150. White NH, Waltman SR, Krupin T, Santiago JV. Reversal of abnormalities in ocular fluorophotometry in insulin-dependent diabetes after five to nine months of improved metabolic control. *Diabetes*. 1982;31:80–85.

151. Yamashita T, Mimura K, Umeda F, Kobayashi K, Hashimoto T, Nawata H. Increased transendothelial permeation of albumin by high glucose concentration. *Metabolism*. 1995;6:739–744.

152. Chakrabarti S, Prasher S, Sima AA. Augmented polyol pathway activity and retinal pigmented epithelial permeability in the diabetic BB rats. *Diabetes Res Clin Pract*. 1990; 8:1–11.

153. Williamson JR, Chang K, Rowold E, et al. Sorbinol prevents diabetes-induced increases in vascular permeability but does not alter collagen cross-linking. *Diabetes*. 1985; 34:703–705.

154. Daniels BS, Hauser EB. Glycation of albumin, not glomerular basement membrane, alters permeability in an in vitro model. *Diabetes*. 1992;41:1415–1421.

155. Vlassara H, Fuh H, Makita Z, Krungkrai S, Cerami A, Bucala R. Exogenous advanced glycosylation end products induce complex vascular dysfunction in normal animals: a model for diabetic and aging complication. *Proc Natl Acad Sci U S A*. 1992;89:12043–12047.

156. Lynch JJ, Ferro TJ, Blumenstock FA, Brockenauer AM, Malik AB. Increased endothelial albumin permeability mediated by protein kinase C activation. *J Clin Invest*. 1990;85:1991–1998.

157. Williams B. Factors regulating the expression of vascular permeability/vascular endothelial growth factor by human vascular tissue. *Diabetologia*. 1997;40(suppl):S118–S120.

158. Tooke JE. Microvascular function in human diabetes. *Diabetes*. 1995;44:721–726.

159. Parving H-H, Viberti GC, Keen H, Christiansen JS, Lassen NA. Hemodynamic factor in the genesis of diabetic microangiopathy. *Metabolism Clinical and Experimental*. 1983; 32:943–949.

160. Rayman G, Williams SA, Spencer PD, Smaje LH, Wise PH, Tooke JE. Impaired microvascular hyperaemic response to minor skin trauma in type I diabetes. *BMJ*. 1986;292:1295–1298.

161. Parving H-H, Kastrup H, Smidt UM, Andersen AR, Feldt-Rasmussen B, Christiansen JS. Impaired autoregulation of glomerular filtration rate in type I (insulin-dependent) diabetic patients with nephropathy. *Diabetologia*. 1984; 27:247–252.

162. Sandeman DD, Shore AC, Tooke JE. Relation of skin capillary pressure in patients with insulin-dependent diabetes mellitus to complications and metabolic control. *N Engl J Med*. 1992;327:760–764.

163. Tooke JE, Sandeman DD, Shore AC. Microvascular hemodynamics in hypertension and diabetes. *J Cardiovasc Pharmacol*. 1991;18(suppl 2):S51–S53.

164. Lowe GDO. Blood viscosity and cardiovascular disease. *Thromb Haemost*. 1992;67:494–498.

165. Fowkes FGR, Pell JP, Donnan PT, et al. Sex difference in susceptibility to etiologic factors for peripheral atherosclerosis: importance of plasma fibrinogen and blood viscosity. *Arterioscler Thromb*. 1994;14:862–868.

166. Smith WC, Lowe GDO, Lee AJ, Tunstall-Pedoe H. Rheological determinant of blood pressure in a Scottish adult population. *J Hypertens*. 1992;10:467–472.

167. Lowe GDO, Fowkes FGR, Dawes J, Donnan PT, Lennie SE, Housley E. Blood viscosity, fibrinogen, and activation of coagulation and leukocyte in peripheral arterial disease and the normal population in the Edinburgh Artery Study. *Circulation*. 1993;87:1915–1920.

168. Memeh CU. Difference between plasma viscosity and protein of type I and type II diabetic Africans in early phases of diabetes. *Horm Metab Res*. 1993;25:21–23.

169. Zioupos P, Barbenel JC, Lowe GDO, MacRury S. Foot microcirculation and blood rheology in diabetes. *J Biomed Eng*. 1993;15:155–158.

170. Brown CD, Zhao Z-H, Berweck S, Chan S, Friedman EA. Effect of alloxan-induced diabetes in hemorheology in rabbits. *Horm Metab Res*. 1992;24:254–257.

171. Schut NH, Van Arkel EC, Hardeman MR, Bilo HJ, Michels RP, Vreeken J. Blood and plasma viscosity in diabetes: possible contribution to late organ complications? *Diabetes Res*. 1992;19:31–35.

172. McMillian DE. Plasma protein changes, blood viscosity, and diabetic microangiopathy. *Diabetes*. 1976;25:858–864.

173. Reid HL, Memeh CU. Abnormal serum protein profile in African diabetics. *Med Sci Res*. 1990;18:321–322.

174. MacRury SM, Lowe GDO. Blood rheology in diabetes mellitus. *Diabetes Med*. 1990;7:285–291.

175. McMillian DE, Utterback NG, LaPuma J. Reduced erythrocyte deformability in diabetes. *Diabetes*. 1978;27:895–901.

176. MacRury SM, Small M, Andersen J, MacCuish AC, Lowe GD. Evaluation of red cell deformability by a filtration method in type I and type II diabetes with and without vascular complications. *Diabetes Res*. 1990;13:61–65.

177. Le Devehat C, Vimeux M, Bondoux G, Khodabandehlov T. Red blood cell aggregation in diabetes mellitus. *Int Angiol*. 1990;9:11–15.

178. Ziegler O, Guerci B, Muller S, et al. Increased erythrocyte aggregation in insulin-dependent diabetes mellitus and its relationship to plasma factors: a multivariate analysis. *Metabolism*. 1994;43:1182–1186.

179. Watala C. Hyperglycemia alters the physio-chemical properties of proteins in erythrocyte membrane in diabetic patients. *Int J Biochem*. 1992;24:1755–1761.

180. Roger ME, Williams DT, Niththyananthan R, Rampling MW, Heslop KE, Johnston DG. Decrease in erythrocyte glycophorin sialic acid content is associated with increased aggregation in human diabetes. *Clin Sci*. 1992;82:309–313.

181. Murakami K, Kondo T, Ohtsuka Y, Fujiwara Y, Shimada M, Kawakami Y. Impairment of glutathione metabolism in erythrocyte from patients with diabetes mellitus. *Metabolism.* 1989;38:753–758.

182. Bombeli T, Mueller M, Haeberli A. Anticoagulant properties of the vascular endothelium. *Thromb Haemost.* 1997; 77:408–423.

183. Ono H, Umeda F, Inoguchi T, Ibayashi H. Glucose inhibits the prostacyclin production by cultured aortic endothelial cells. *Thromb Haemost.* 1988;60:174–177.

184. Boeri D, Almus FE, Maiello M, Cagliero E, Rao LV, Lorenzi M. Modification of tissue-factor mRNA and protein response to thrombin and interleukin-I by high glucose in cultured human endothelial growth. *Diabetes.* 1989;38:212–218.

185. Porta M, LeSelva M, Molinatti PA. von Willebrand factor and endothelial abnormalities in diabetic microangiopathy. *Diabetes Care.* 1991;14(suppl 1):167–172.

186. Plater ME, Ford I, Dent MT, Preston FE, Ward JE. Elevated von Willebrand factor antigen predicts deterioration in diabetic peripheral nerve function. *Diabetologia.* 1996;39:336–343.

187. Ganda OP, Arkin CF. Hyperfibrinogenemia: an important risk factor for vascular complications in diabetes. *Diabetes Care.* 1992;15:1245–1250.

188. Ceriello A, Giugliano D, Quatraro A, DelloRusso P, Torella R. Blood glucose may condition factor VII levels in diabetic and normal subjects. *Diabetologia.* 1988;31: 889–891.

189. Khawand CE, Jamart J, Doonckier J, et al. Hemostasis variable in type I diabetic patient without demonstrable vascular complication. *Diabetes Care.* 1993;16:1137–1145.

190. Reach G. Continuous glucose monitoring with a subcutaneous sensor: rationale, requirement and achievement, and prospects. In: Marshall SM, Homes PD, Alberti KGMM, Krall LP, eds. *The Diabetes Annual.* 7th ed. Amsterdam: Elsevier Science; 1993:332–348.

191. Ostermann H, Vandeloo J. Factors of hemostatic system in diabetic patients: a survey of controlled studies. *Haemostasis.* 1986;16:386–416.

192. DeFeo P, Gaisano MG, Haymond MW. Differential effect of insulin deficiency on albumin and fibrinogen synthesis in humans. *J Clin Invest.* 1991;88:833–840.

193. Ceriello A, Giugliano D, Quatraro A, et al. Daily rapid blood glucose variation may condition antithrombin III biological activity but not its plasma concentration in insulin-dependent diabetes. *Diabetes Metab.* 1987;13:16–19.

194. Ceriello A, Giugliano D, Quatraro A, Marchi E, Barbanti M, Lefebure P. Evidence for a hyperglycemia-dependent decrease of antithrombin III-thrombin complex formation in humans. *Diabetologia.* 1990;33:163–167.

195. Ceriello A, Quatraro A, Della Russo P, et al. Protein C deficiency in insulin-dependent diabetes: a hyperglycemia-related phenomenon. *Thromb Haemost.* 1990;64:104–107.

196. Gough SCL, Grant PJ. The fibrinolytic system in diabetes mellitus. *Diabet Med.* 1991;8:898–905.

197. Walmsley D, Hampton KK, Grant PJ. Contrasting fibrinolytic responses in type I (insulin-dependent) and type II (non-insulin-dependent) diabetes. *Diabet Med.* 1991;8: 954–959.

198. Stiko-Rahm A, Wiman B, Hamsten A, Nilsson J. Secretion of plasminogen activator inhibitor I from cultured umbilical vein endothelial cells is induced by very low density lipoprotein. *Arteriosclerosis.* 1990;10:1067–1073.

199. Davis JW, Hartman CR, Davis RF, Kyner JL, Lewis HDJ, Phillips PE. Platelet aggregate ratio in diabetes mellitus. *Acta Haematol.* 1982;67:222–224.

200. Winocour PD. The role of platelet in the pathogenesis of diabetic vascular disease. In: Draznin B, Melmed S, LeRoith D, eds. *Complications of Diabetes Mellitus.* New York, NY: Alan R. Liss, Inc; 1989:37–42.

201. Winocour PD, Perry DW, Kinlough-Rathbone RL. Hypersensitivity to ADP of platelet from diabetic rats associated with enhanced fibrinogen binding. *Eur J Clin Invest.* 1992; 22:19–23.

202. Winocour PD, Halushka PV, Colwell JA. Platelet involvement in diabetes mellitus. In: Longenecker GL, ed. *The Platelet: Physiology and Pharmacology.* New York, NY: Academic Press; 1985:341–366.

203. Tschoepe D, Roesen P, Schwippert B, Gries FA. Platelet in diabetes: the role in hemostatic regulation in atherosclerosis. *Semin Thromb Hemost.* 1993;19:122–128.

204. Villanueva GB, Allen N. Demonstration of altered antithrombin III activity due to non enzymatic glycosylation at glucose concentration expected to be encountered in severely diabetic patients. *Diabetes.* 1988;37: 1103–1107.

205. Ceriello A, Marchi E, Barbanti M, et al. Non-enzymatic glycation reduces heparin cofactor II antithrombin activity. *Diabetologia.* 1990;33:205–207.

206. Winocour PD, Watala C, Perry DW, Kinlough-Rathbone RL. Decreased platelet membrane fluidity due to glycation or acetylation of membrane proteins. *Thromb Haemost.* 1992;68:557–582.

207. Cohen I, Burk D, Fullerton RJ, Veis A, Green D. Non enzymatic glycation of human blood platelet proteins. *Thromb Res.* 1989;55:341–349.

208. Collier A, Rumley AG, Patterson JR, Leach JP, Lowe GD, Small M. Free radical activity and hemostatic factor in NIDDM patients with and without microalbuminuria. *Diabetes.* 1992;41:909–913.

209. Border WA, Noble NA. Transforming growth factor beta in tissue fibrosis. *N Engl J Med.* 1994;331:1286–1292.

210. Pfeiffer A, Schatz H. Diabetic microvascular complications and growth factors. *Exp Clin Endocrinol.* 1995;103: 7–14.

211. Yokoyama H, Deckert T. Central role of TGF-beta in the pathogenesis of diabetic nephropathy and macrovascular complications: a hypothesis. *Diabetes Med.* 1996;13:313–320.

212. Bollineni JS, Reddi AS. Transforming growth factor-beta 1 enhances glomerular collagen synthesis in diabetic rats. *Diabetes.* 1993;42:1673–1677.

213. Morishita R, Nakamura S, Nakamura Y, et al. Potential role of an endothelium-specific growth factor, hepatocyte growth factor, on endothelial damage. *Diabetes.* 1997; 46:138–142.

214. Ferrara N, Davis-Smith T. The biology of vascular endothelial growth factor. *Endocr Rev.* 1997;18:4–25.

215. Aiello LP, Avery R, Arrigg R, et al. Vascular endothelial growth factor in ocular fluid of patients with diabetic retinopathy and other retinal disorders. *N Engl J Med.* 1994;331:1480–1487.

216. Tilton RG, Kawamura T, Chang KC, et al. Vascular dysfunction induced by elevated glucose levels in rats is mediated by vascular endothelial growth factor. *J Clin Invest.* 1997;99:2192–2202.

217. Friesel RE, Maciag T. Molecular mechanisms of angiogenesis: fibroblast growth factor signal transduction. *FASEB J.* 1995;9:919–925.

218. Zimering MB, Eng J. Increased basic fibroblast growth factor-like substance in plasma from a subset of middle-aged or elderly male diabetic patients with microalbuminuria or proteinuria. *J Clin Endocrinol Metab.* 1996;81:4446–4452.

219. Harrison AA, Dunbar PR, Neale TJ. Immunoassay of platelet-derived growth factor in the blood of patients with diabetes mellitus. *Diabetologia.* 1994;37:1142–1146.

220. Lev-Ran A, Hwang DL. Epidermal growth factor and platelet-derived growth factor in blood in diabetes mellitus. *Acta Endocrinologica.* 1990;123:326–330.

221. Kawano M, Koshikawa T, Kanzaki T, Morisaki N, Saito Y, Yoshida S. Diabetes mellitus induces accelerated growth of aortic smooth muscle cells: association with overexpression of PDGF beta-receptor. *Eur J Clin Invest.* 1993;23:84–90.

222. Okuda Y, Adrogue HJ, Nakajima T, et al. Increased production of PDGF by angiotensin and high glucose in human vascular endothelium. *Life Sci.* 1996;59:1455–1461.

223. Delafontaine P. Insulin-like growth factors and its binding proteins in the cardiovascular system. *Cardiovasc Res.* 1995;30:825–834.

224. Borg WP, Sherwin RS. Metabolic effects of insulin-like growth factor 1. In: Marshall SM, Home PD, Rizza RA, eds. *The Diabetes Annual.* Amsterdam: Elsevier Science; 1995:57–69.

225. Kirstein M, Astom C, Hintz R, Vlassara H. Receptor specific induction of insulin like growth factor I in human monocyte by advanced glycosylation end products: modified proteins. *J Clin Invest.* 1992;90:439–446.

226. Diabetes Control and Complication Trial Research Group. The effect of intensive treatment of diabetes on development and progression of long-term complications in insulin-dependent diabetes mellitus. *N Engl J Med.* 1993;329:977–986.

227. Kaufman FR. Glucose sensors in the mid-1990s. In: Marshall SM, Home PD, Rizza RA, eds. *The Diabetes Annual.* 10th ed. Amsterdam: Elsevier Science; 1996:252–257.

228. Zier H, Kerner W, Bruckel J, Pfeiffer EF. Glucosensor Unitec Ulm: a portable continuously measuring glucose sensor and monitor. *Biomed Technik.* 1990;35:2–4.

229. Pickup JC, William G. *Textbook of Diabetes.* 2nd ed. Oxford, England: Blackwell Science Ltd; 1997.

230. Salem J, Charles MA. Devices for insulin administration. *Diabetes Care.* 1990;13:955–979.

231. Illum L, Davis SS. Intranasal insulin: clinical pharmacokinetics. *Clin Pharmacokinet.* 1992;23:30–41.

232. Kennedy FB. Recent developments in insulin delivery techniques: current status and future potential. *Drugs.* 1991;42:213–227.

233. Tachibana K, Tachibana S. Transdermal delivery of insulin by ultrasonic vibration. *J Pharm Pharmacol.* 1991;43:270–271.

234. Duckworth WC, Saudek CD, Henry RR. Why intraperitoneal delivery of insulin with implantable pumps in NIDDM? *Diabetes.* 1992;41:657–661.

235. Wredling R, Liu D, Lins PE, Adamson U. Variation of insulin absorption during subcutaneous and peritoneal infusion in insulin-dependent diabetic patients with unsatisfactory long-term glycemic response to continuous subcutaneous insulin therapy. *Diabetes Metab.* 1991;17:456–459.

236. Larsen JL, Stratta RJ. Pancreas transplantation: a treatment option for insulin-dependent diabetes mellitus. *Diabetes Metab.* 1996;22:139–146.

237. Sutherland DER. Pancreatic transplantation: an update. *Diabetes Metab Rev.* 1993;1:152–165.

238. Morel P, Chau C, Brayman K, et al. Quality of metabolic control at 2 to 12 years after a pancreas transplant. *Transplant Proc.* 1992;24:835–838.

239. Scheider A, Meyer-Schwickerath E, Nusser J, Land W, Landgraf R. Diabetic retinopathy and pancreas transplantation: a 3-year follow-up. *Diabetologia.* 1991;34(suppl 1):S95–S99.

240. Muller-Felber W, Landgraf R, Wagner S, et al. Follow-up study of sensory-motor polyneuropathy in type I (insulin-dependent) diabetic subjects after simultaneous pancreas and kidney transplantation and after graft rejection. *Diabetologia.* 1991;34(suppl 1):113–117.

241. Abendroth A, Schmand J, Landgraf R, Illner WD, Land W. Diabetic microangiopathy in type I (insulin-dependent) diabetic patients after successful pancreatic and kidney or solitary kidney transplantation. *Diabetologia.* 1991;34(suppl 1):131–134.

242. Stratta RJ, Taylor RJ, Bynon JS, et al. Surgical treatment of diabetes mellitus with pancreatic transplantation. *Ann Surg.* 1994;220:809–817.

243. Pipeleers D, Keymeulen B, Korburt G. Islet transplantation. In: Marshall SM, Home PD, eds. *The Diabetes Annual.* Amsterdam: Elsevier Science; 1994:299–330.

244. Serri O, Renier G. Intervention in diabetic vascular disease by modulation of growth factors. *Metabolism.* 1995;44:83–90.

245. Serri O, Beauregard H, Brazeau P, et al. Somatostatin analog, octreotide, reduces increased glomerular filtration rate and kidney size in insulin-dependent diabetes. *JAMA.* 1991;265:888–892.

246. Border WA, Noble NA, Yamamoto T, et al. Natural inhibitor of transforming growth factor-beta protects against scarring in experimental kidney disease. *Nature.* 1992;360:361–364.

69

Composite Grafts for Limb Salvage

John B. Chang and Theodore A. Stein

Progressive peripheral arterial occlusive disease of the lower extremity leads to inadequate blood flow for the delivery of nutrients to the distal leg. If left untreated, ulceration and gangrene can occur. Limbs are amputated to prevent sepsis and the loss of life. Revascularization of the occluded arterial system can provide sufficient blood flow to salvage limbs destined for failure. After arterial reconstruction, nearly one half of these patients feel better and return to a near normal level of activity.[1]

Preservation of the lower extremity requires identifying the sites of occlusion, determining the adequacy of distal perfusion, and planning arterial reconstruction. To bypass the occluded segment, various materials have been used for grafts to increase blood flow to patent vessels. Autogenous veins, synthetic materials such as polytetrafluoroethylene (PTFE), and composites of vein and PTFE have been used for femoropopliteal and femorotibial bypass grafts.[2-5]

The greater saphenous vein is considered by most to be the best conduit for distal lower extremity arterial revascularization to prevent loss of the limb.[6-9] The greater saphenous vein is also our first choice for the bypass conduit, but it is often unavailable or inadequate for a graft. In many patients, it has been used for other lower extremity bypasses or coronary bypasses, and the remaining length is insufficient for the graft. It is considered inadequate if the luminal diameter is too small (<3.0 mm) or if there is gross evidence of fibrosis. We prefer to use the proximal portion of the vein for graft construction, because the lumen is larger.

When the greater saphenous vein cannot be used for the entire length, another source must be found. We have used either PTFE grafts or composite grafts composed of a segment of the greater saphenous vein and PTFE. Other choices of the vein segment to combine with a prosthetic graft to form a composite graft are the lesser saphenous, cephalic, basilic, jugular, and in situ deep leg veins, such as the tibial vein. Most of our composite grafts have a proximal portion of PTFE anastomosed to a distal portion of greater saphenous vein segment. When multiple levels of occlusion prevent the conventional technique for a single inflow and single outflow of femoropopliteal or femorotibial bypasses, multiple bypasses or a sequential bypass with dual outflows can restore adequate blood flow.[10] Composites of two different vein segments can also be used to construct grafts. Patients with combined disease in the aortoiliac arterial system can be treated before or after femoropopliteal or femorotibial bypass.

Patients who have multiple graft failures are difficult to manage, and many eventually require limb amputation. To restore adequate blood flow in these patients and save the limb, it is necessary to perform the bypass with attention to detail and technical precision and to choose the best graft for these patients. Although the greater saphenous vein graft is clearly the best choice, it is usually unavailable. When a prosthetic graft or a graft of an autogenous vein other than the greater saphenous vein is used, the long-term outcome of the repeat bypass after graft failure has been only minimally satisfactory.[11-14] The poorer results with prosthetic grafts for long bypasses with below-knee outflow indicate that these grafts are not a good choice to achieve long-term patency.[11-15] In our experience, composite grafts are a better option. The graft patency and limb salvage rates have been shown to be better with composites of vein and PTFE for popliteal and infrapopliteal bypass procedures.[4,16,17] Patency rates for composite grafts have been reported to be 65% at 1 and 2 years after femorotibial bypasses[18] and have ranged from 28% to 53% at 5 years.[3,19]

Bypass Graft Procedures

We have determined the long-term efficacy of composite grafts, autogenous vein grafts, and PTFE grafts for limb salvage. Between 1975 and July 1996, 781 patients had 1025 arterial revascularization procedures, with the proximal anastomosis at the femoral artery level and the distal anastomosis below the knee. Patients were followed from 0 to 16 years. More than one bypass was performed in 19.7% of the patients. There were 52 femoropopliteal composite graft bypasses in 50 patients, 279 femoropopliteal greater saphenous vein graft bypasses in 258 patients, and 186 femoropopliteal PTFE graft bypasses in 165 patients. There were also 135 femorotibial composite graft bypasses in 113 patients, 337 femorotibial greater saphenous vein graft bypasses in 313 patients, and 36 femorotibial PTFE graft bypasses in 36 patients. In most patients, the greater saphenous vein was used for initial bypasses.[20] When the vein could not be used, PTFE grafts were the second choice for femoropopliteal bypasses and composite grafts were the second choice for femorotibial bypasses. Patients who required multiple bypasses had composite sequential bypass grafts to bridge occlusions.

All patients had ischemic rest pain and some also had gangrene and/or ischemic ulcers. Claudication only was not considered an indication for a bypass procedure. Surgery was indicated by limb-threatening ischemia and was determined by the criteria of the Society for Vascular Surgery and the International Society for Cardiovascular Surgery.[21] Before operation, patients had Doppler spectral images determined at all levels, pulse volume recordings, and segmental pressure measurements to determine the site of occlusion. The mean ankle/brachial systolic pressure index was <0.4. Some diabetic patients had incompressible arteries, and metatarsal and toe pressures and pulse volume recordings were obtained to determine the severity of disease. The coexistence of other vascular diseases, such as carotid artery disease, aortoiliac disease, and aneurysmal disease, was determined by Doppler and duplex scans. Conventional angiography or digital subtraction angiography was used to determine the distal runoff to the foot. Magnetic resonance angiography has also been suggested for the preoperative evaluation of these patients.[22]

Femoropopliteal Artery Bypass

The first choice for a graft was the greater saphenous vein. Reversed greater saphenous vein segments were used for most (72%) vein femoropopliteal procedures and the in situ greater saphenous vein for others. After the location of the occlusion is determined, the superficial femoral artery and deep femoral artery should be evaluated for the inflow source. The common femoral artery should be considered when these arteries are inadequate, and the iliac artery may even be used if necessary. The greater saphenous vein was anastomosed to the donor artery end-to-side in pure vein grafts and with composite grafts. PTFE was used for femoropopliteal bypasses only when distal runoff was good. The size of the

PTFE graft was selected on the basis of the distal runoff and the size of the donor and receiving arteries. Although PTFE sizes ranged from 6 to 10 mm, the most common size was 8 mm. A tunnel was made along Hunter's canal, and the graft was pulled through to be anastomosed to the popliteal artery below the knee. Patients with occlusive disease in the superficial femoral artery with limited runoff at the remaining popliteal segment from thrombosis had a thrombectomy and thrombolysis therapy with urokinase or streptokinase before completion of the bypass procedure.

Femorotibial Artery Bypass

The best choice for the femorotibial bypass graft is also the autogenous greater saphenous vein. The in situ greater saphenous vein was used for most (68%) of our vein femorotibial grafts. An end-to-side anastomosis was made between the graft and the best inflow artery. The conventional femorotibial bypass graft was usually passed through a subcutaneous tunnel and the distal graft anastomosed to a tibial artery with good runoff. For these long distal bypasses, the greater saphenous vein is frequently unavailable for the entire length, and a composite graft is constructed of a proximal segment of the greater saphenous vein to a distal segment of PTFE. Femorotibial bypasses with PTFE alone were performed only as a last resort to prevent amputation, because these grafts have had poor long-term results.[5]

Angioplasty

While doing femoropopliteal or femorotibial bypasses, it is often necessary to perform an additional procedure. Some patients with multiple stenoses of the runoff vessels require an endarterectomy, angioplasty, or transluminal balloon dilation to improve distal blood flow. Grafts occlude if blood flow is <50 mL/min in PTFE grafts and <10 mL/min in vein grafts.[23]

Repeat Arterial Bypasses

Some patients experience graft failure and a repeat revascularization procedure is required to prevent loss of limb. For femoropopliteal bypasses, the autogenous vein is used in most cases for an initial bypass and was available for most first repeat bypasses.[20] Most patients who required second or more repeat femoropopliteal bypasses lacked sufficient autogenous vein for another graft, and composite and PTFE grafts were used in 80% of these procedures. For femorotibial procedures, the autogenous vein was again used for most initial bypasses but was available in only 20% of first repeat bypasses, 10% of second repeat bypasses, and no higher repeat procedures. Composite grafts were used for most repeat femorotibial bypasses using a single outflow for limbs with good distal runoff and dual outflows to either bridge occlusions or increase blood flow to the distal runoff beds.

Composite Graft

The principle for using the composite graft is that the distal vein segment is able to absorb some of the energy from the pulsatile flow and minimize flow disturbances. The composite graft is ideal for patients with multiple occlusions, because revascularization of the distal leg requires bridging occluded segments.[24] Whenever possible, we try to use the PTFE segment between a proximal artery and the patent portion of an occluded distal artery to increase flow distally (Figure 69.1). Then the proximal end of the vein graft is anastomosed to this distal artery below the insertion of the PTFE graft, and the distal end of the vein graft is inserted into a more distal artery, which has the best runoff. If the patent portion of the occluded artery is too short to accommodate two anastomoses for both the PTFE and vein grafts, the distal end of the prosthetic graft is anastomosed to the artery and the proximal end of the vein is anastomosed to the distal portion of the PTFE graft (Figure 69.2).

When a single distal anastomosis is required for revascularization (Figure 69.3), the autogenous vein graft is

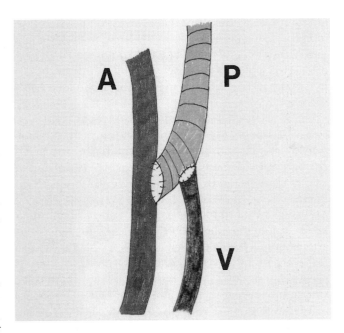

FIGURE 69.2. Composite graft with the proximal polytetrafluoroethylene graft (P) anastomosed to a short, patent segment of an artery (A) and the distal vein graft (V) anastomosed to the distal portion of the polytetrafluoroethylene graft.

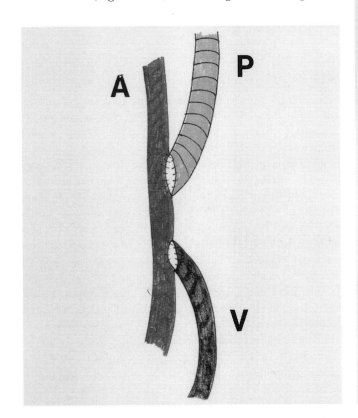

FIGURE 69.1. Composite graft with the patent segment of an artery (A) interposed between the proximal polytetrafluoroethylene graft (P) and the distal vein graft (V).

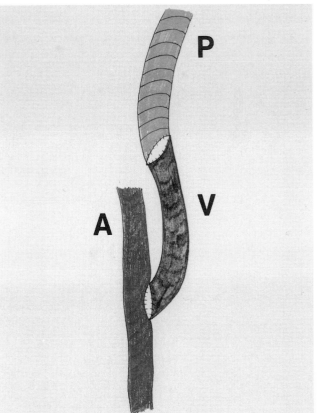

FIGURE 69.3. Composite graft with a single distal anastomosis into the artery (A). The proximal polytetrafluoroethylene graft (P) is anastomosed end-to-end to the vein graft (V).

anastomosed to the distal artery in an end-to-side fashion. Then an anastomosis is made between the proximal end of the vein graft and the distal end of the PTFE graft by careful spatulation of the vein end to match the orifice of the PTFE graft with the PTFE graft situated below the vein.

When the greater saphenous vein is not available and revascularization to a tibial artery is required, the adjacent tibial vein can be used as a conduit to the artery (Figure 69.4). The vein is ligated proximal to the end-to-side anastomosis with the PTFE graft and distal to the side-to-side anastomosis with the tibial artery to increase perfusion of the distal beds. If the runoff of the tibial artery is poor, the tibial vein is not ligated to allow for an arteriovenous fistula to decrease the peripheral vascular resistance in the artery. At other times it is convenient to use a small distal saphenous vein remnant, which is left in situ. In Figure 69.5, such a remnant has been used for a composite graft after a valvotomy and ligation of any branches. The PTFE graft is anastomosed end-to-side to the vein remnant, which is then anastomosed side-to-side to a tibial artery.

When a patient has extensive occlusive disease of the femorotibial arterial system with poor runoff from the tibial arteries, a single distal bypass graft is inadequate to support perfusion of the distal beds. To increase distal blood flow, small segments of the three tibial arteries are used to form a multiple sequential bypass with the com-

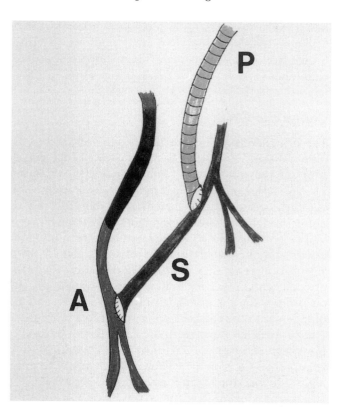

FIGURE 69.5. Composite graft utilizing an in situ segment of a saphenous vein remnant (S) to receive the proximal polytetrafluoroethylene graft (P) and for a distal end-to-side anastomosis with a tibial artery (A).

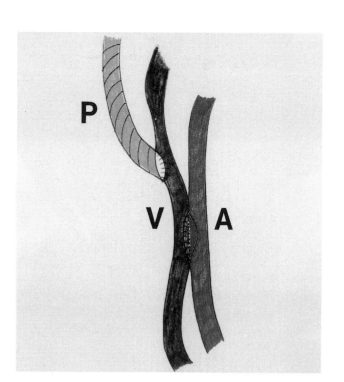

FIGURE 69.4. Composite graft with a proximal polytetrafluoroethylene graft (P) anastomosed end-to-side to a tibial vein (V); distally the vein is anastomosed side-to-side to the tibial artery (A).

posite graft (Figure 69.6). The proximal end of a reversed segment of the greater saphenous vein is anastomosed end-to-side to the tibial artery (i.e., posterior tibial artery) with the best runoff. Then a side-to-side anastomosis of the vein graft is made with the anterior wall of the middle tibial artery (i.e., peroneal artery). Next the distal end of the vein graft is anastomosed to the third tibial artery (i.e., anterior tibial artery). Then the distal end of the PTFE graft is anastomosed end-to-side to the proximal portion of the reversed vein segment next to the tibial artery with best runoff (in this case the posterior tibial artery). The priority for the sequence of the anastomoses arrangement should always be the anastomosis to the artery that has the best runoff.

In the absence of an adequate superficial vein for the construction of a composite graft to a single tibial artery that has extremely poor runoff, we have used a limited section of a tibial vein (Figure 69.7). Longitudinal incisions are made in the walls of the tibial vein and artery and an anastomosis is made to form a posterior wall. Then the end of the PTFE graft is anastomosed to the vein and artery to form an anterior wall. This type of anastomosis is a combination of a composite graft and an arteriovenous fistula.

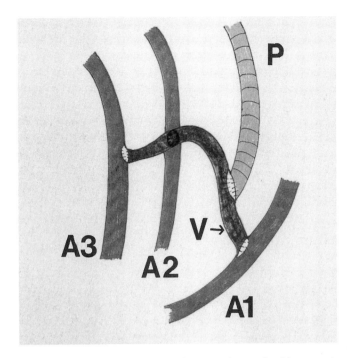

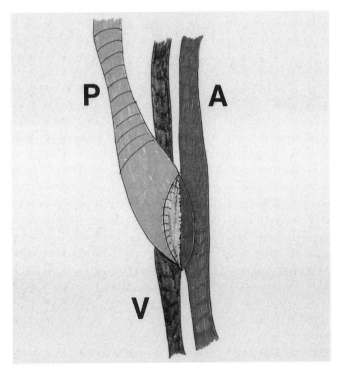

FIGURE 69.6. Multiple sequential composite graft with a proximal polytetrafluoroethylene graft (P) anastomosed end-to-side to a vein graft (V) that has the proximal end anastomosed to the posterior tibial artery (A1), the middle segment anastomosed side-to-side to the peroneal artery (A2), and the distal end anastomosed to the side of the anterior tibial artery (A3).

FIGURE 69.7. Composite graft with the proximal polytetrafluoroethylene graft (P) comprising the anterior wall of the anastomosis with the tibial artery (A) and the tibial vein (V) and a side-to-side anastomosis between the posterior walls of the artery and vein.

In another patient with multilevel occlusive disease, the deep femoral artery, the superficial femoral artery, and all tibial arteries were occluded and a multiple sequential bypass was required to bridge the occlusions to prevent impending ischemia and gangrene (Figure 69.8). Only a small segment of the popliteal artery and two segments of the tibial arteries were patent. The proximal end of a PTFE graft was anastomosed to the common femoral artery, a side-to-side anastomosis was done between the PTFE graft and a patent portion of the distal deep femoral artery, and a side-to-side anastomosis was made between the PTFE graft and the popliteal artery. Then a small segment of autogenous vein was anastomosed between two tibial arteries in an end-to-

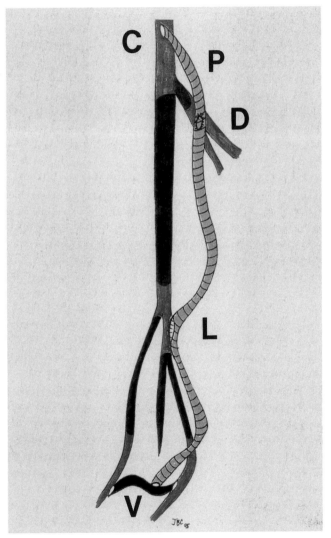

FIGURE 69.8. Multiple sequential composite graft with the polytetrafluoroethylene graft (P) having a proximal anastomosis with the common femoral artery (C), a side-to-side anastomosis with the deep femoral artery (D), a side-to-side anastomosis with the distal popliteal artery (L), and a terminal end-to-side anastomosis with a short segment of vein graft (V).

side fashion, and the distal end of the PTFE graft was inserted end-to-side into the vein graft.

Often an endarterectomy is required before completing a bypass. In these cases, a small segment of autogenous vein can be used to form a composite graft and the angioplasty. A patient who had limb-threatening ischemia from extensive occlusion of the distal arteries with the exception of a small portion of the popliteal artery had an extended endarterectomy of the popliteal–tibial artery segment (Figure 69.9). After performing the vein patch angioplasty, the distal end of the PTFE graft was anastomosed to the proximal end of the vein patch. This technique has been used for extensive occlusive disease including the distal popliteal artery and the proximal portion of the tibial arteries when the length of the vein graft is limited (Figure 69.10). The distal end of the PTFE graft is anastomosed end-to-end to the proximal end of the available length of autogenous vein graft. After an extended endarterectomy of the distal popliteal–tibial artery segment, the distal end of the autogenous vein graft is used to form the angioplasty.

In another patient, an endarterectomy was done from the popliteal artery to the proximal posterior tibial artery (Figure 69.11). A short PTFE graft was placed between the common femoral artery and the deep femoral artery, using an end-to-side anastomosis. Then a vein graft was anastomosed to the distal deep femoral artery just distal to the PTFE anastomosis. Occasionally a patient with severe distal ischemia has proximal occlusion of a previous bypass graft and occlusion of the distal su-

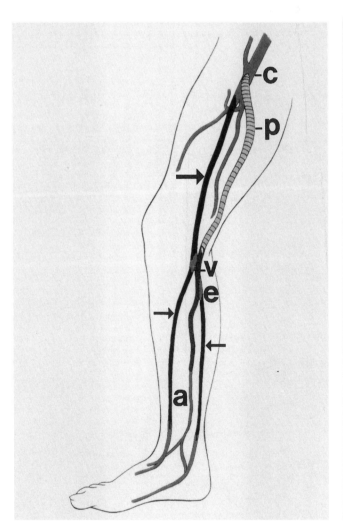

FIGURE 69.9. Diagram showing the presence of occlusions (arrows) in the arterial system and location of the composite bypass graft. A polytetrafluoroethylene graft (p) extends from the common femoral artery (c) and is anastomosed end to end to a vein graft (v) that has been used to form an angioplasty graft after an extended endarterectomy (e) of the popliteal artery, tibioperoneal trunk, and peroneal artery (a).

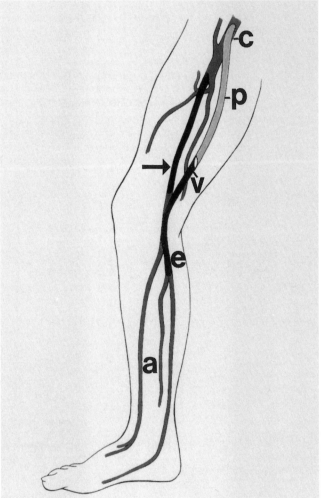

FIGURE 69.10. Diagram showing the presence of occlusion (arrow) in the arterial system and location of the composite bypass graft. The distal end of a polytetrafluoroethylene graft (p) extends from the common femoral artery (c) and is anastomosed end-to-end to the proximal end of a vein graft (v) whose distal end has been used for an angioplasty patch after an extended endarterectomy (e) to the proximal tibial arteries (a).

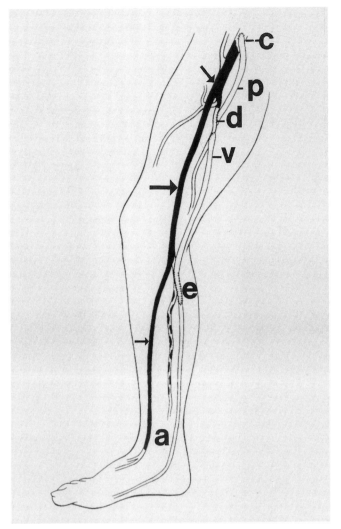

FIGURE 69.11. Diagram showing the presence of occlusions (arrows) in the arterial system and location of the composite bypass graft. A polytetrafluoroethylene graft (p) extends from the common femoral artery (c) and is anastomosed end-to-side to the deep femoral artery (d). A vein graft (v) extends from the deep femoral artery to form an angioplasty graft after an extended endarterectomy (e) of the popliteal artery, tibioperoneal trunk, and posterior tibial artery (a).

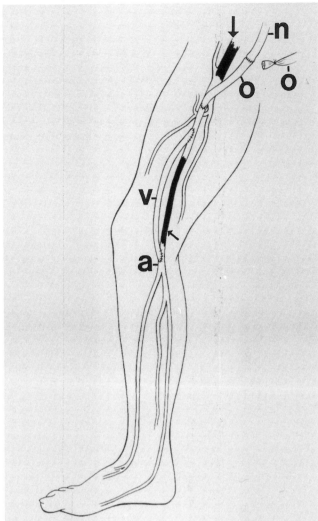

FIGURE 69.12. Diagram showing the presence of occlusions (arrows) in the arterial system and location of the composite bypass graft. An occluded graft (o) is ligated and divided, and a new graft (n) is anastomosed to the thrombectomized end of the old graft. A vein graft (v) is then anastomosed proximally to the patent portion of the superficial femoral artery and distally to the distal portion of the popliteal artery (a).

perficial femoral artery (Figure 69.12). If conventional thromboembolectomy is not feasible because the donor artery is occluded, the graft is ligated and divided. The distal end of the graft can be thrombectomized, and another bypass procedure is done with a graft anastomosed to the distal portion of the old graft. This approach was used to perfuse the patent segment of the femoral artery system by utilizing the terminal portion of the previously attached graft. Once the proximal femoral arterial system is revascularized, a small segment of a vein graft is extended from the proximal superficial femoral artery system to the distal popliteal artery. In another situation with a previous bypass graft occluded (Figure 69.13), the

graft is ligated and divided, and the terminal portion of the old graft is thrombectomized and anastomosed to a new bypass graft. If the femoral artery system cannot be revascularized, a vein graft is inserted into the distal popliteal artery.

In patients with extensive obstructive disease (Figure 69.14), a PTFE graft is anastomosed to the distal deep femoral artery to revascularize this arterial system so that a vein segment can be anastomosed to the artery for distal perfusion of the tibial arteries. This type of multiple sequential composite bypass conserves the length of the vein segment needed for a graft. Another vein-conserving procedure is to extend a PTFE graft from the patent por-

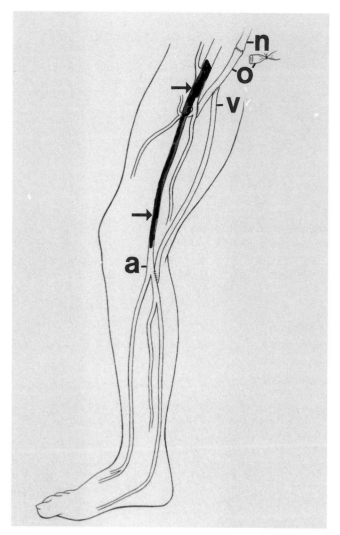

FIGURE 69.13. Diagram showing the presence of occlusions (arrows) in the arterial system and location of the composite bypass graft. An occluded graft (o) is ligated and divided. A new graft (n) is anastomosed to the thrombectomized end of the old graft. A vein graft (v) is then anastomosed proximally to the distal portion of the graft and distally to the distal portion of the popliteal artery (a).

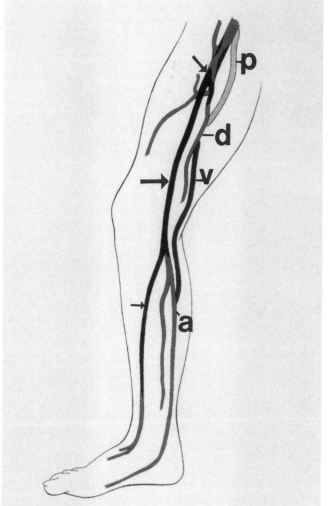

FIGURE 69.14. Diagram showing the presence of occlusions (arrows) in the arterial system and location of the composite bypass graft. A polytetrafluoroethylene graft (p) is anastomosed to the deep femoral artery (d), and a vein graft (v) extends from the deep femoral artery to the posterior tibial artery (a).

tion of the superficial femoral artery to the level of the ankle (Figure 69.15). After anastomosing the proximal end of a short vein graft to the peroneal artery and the distal end to the anterior tibial artery, the PTFE graft is anastomosed end-to-side to the vein graft.

Postoperative Follow-Up

Patients who had an initial bypass with autogenous vein were given aspirin (325 mg/d) and Persantine (25 mg four times daily). Patients who had other grafts or a repeat bypass received Coumadin to increase clotting time to 1.5 times that of the control and Persantine (25 mg

four times daily) to prevent graft occlusion. Patients who smoke cigarettes must be encouraged to stop, because graft failure is more common in those who smoke.[25]

Continual surveillance is necessary to detect complications and prevent graft failures.[26,27] Our patients are routinely seen 3, 6, and 12 months after the bypass procedure and then at 1-year intervals. At each visit, a detailed history for symptoms of claudication, rest pain, or ischemia is taken, and pedal pulses are determined. Segmental pressures and blood flow by Doppler ultrasonography are determined at each visit, following guidelines of the Intersocietal Commission for the Accreditation of Vascular Laboratories. Graft occlusion is determined from the ankle/brachial pressure index, duplex scan-

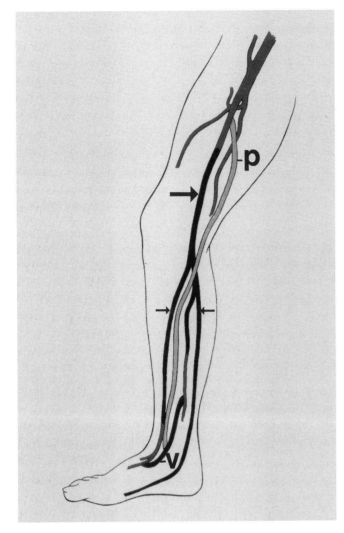

FIGURE 69.15. Diagram showing the presence of occlusions (arrows) in the arterial system and location of the composite bypass graft. A polytetrafluoroethylene graft (p) is anastomosed proximally to the superficial femoral artery and distally end-to-side to a short vein graft that has its proximal end anastomosed to the peroneal artery and its distal end to the anterior tibial artery.

ning, continuous wave Doppler waveforms, and plethysmographic waveforms. When the ankle/brachial pressure index is decreased by more than 15%, the midgraft peak systolic velocity is less than 35 cm/s, and duplex scanning indicates a greater than 50% stenosis,[28] patients should be monitored closely to determine the appropriate treatment. Conventional or digital angiography was performed on patients who might require surgical revascularization.

We evaluated the outcome of the bypass procedures in our patients by statistical analysis of the life-tables.[29] The results of the grafts with in situ vein are combined with those of the reversed vein segments, because these grafts

have a similar low incidence of restenosis.[30] The incidence of graft occlusion or failure is higher with PTFE grafts than with composite grafts and greater saphenous vein grafts. At 10 years, the primary patency rates for femoropopliteal bypasses with PTFE, composites, and vein grafts were 28%, 52%, and 56%, respectively. In situ greater saphenous vein grafts yield slightly better results than reversed vein segments.[20] Graft failure occurs in many patients within 30 days of operation and occurs most frequently after repeat bypass procedures.

Early recognition of thrombosis and early treatment by thrombectomy, thromboendarterectomy, or thrombolysis will salvage many of these grafts.[31] These grafts can remain functional for many years and prevent loss of a limb. Even PTFE, with which the secondary patency rate at 3 years is 84%,[32] remains a better option than amputation.[33] At 10 years, our secondary patency rates for PTFE, composite, and vein grafts are 32%, 64%, and 59%, respectively. When revascularization fails, limbs become gangrenous and amputation is necessary. Our limb salvage rates are 68% in patients with PTFE grafts, 78% in patients with femoropopliteal composite grafts, and 82% in patients with vein grafts. Most deaths are due to cardiac complications. Ten-year survival rates are 50% for patients with vein grafts, 37% for those with PTFE, and 34% for those with composite grafts. Because patients who had vein grafts were several years younger than those with composite grafts, the adjusted mortality rates are similar. Age appears to have little effect on mortality and patency rates.[34]

Femorotibial bypasses present a special problem, because blood is transported in a long graft to arteries of smaller diameter. In our experience graft occlusion and failure are highest with the PTFE grafts, which were associated with a primary patency rate of only 16% at 5 years. Others have reported a 5-year patency rate of 28%.[33] When these grafts fail, the thrombus can be removed or another graft type can be used to revascularize the distal leg to prevent amputation. These grafts probably should be reserved for patients who have no autogenous veins, including the saphenous, basilic, and cephalic veins, that could be used either alone or in a composite graft. The in situ greater saphenous vein grafts provide the best primary patency rate.[20] The 5- and 10-year primary patency rates with greater saphenous vein grafts were 75% and 68%, respectively. Although grafts of the greater saphenous vein appear to be ideal, the decision to use a long length of the vein should be considered in relation to the cardiac health of the patient. In many patients, a composite graft may be a reasonable compromise. The 5- and 10-year patency rates with composite grafts were 45% and 16%, respectively. Many patients can have sequential bypass grafts (femoropopliteotibial) with dual outflow to improve distal blood flow. Our 10-year secondary patency rates were 78% with vein grafts and 38% with composite grafts. The limb salvage rates were 87%

for femorotibial vein grafts, 60% for composite grafts, and 37% for PTFE grafts.

Autogenous vein grafts are superior to prosthetic grafts for infrapopliteal arterial reconstruction.[6–8,15,35] At 4 years the primary patency rate of autogenous vein grafts has been reported to be 80% and the limb salvage rate 70%.[36] We have achieved good long-term patency rates and limb salvage with the greater saphenous vein bypass grafts and feel it is the conduit of choice for both femoropopliteal and femorotibial bypasses. When the greater saphenous vein is unavailable for a graft, our second choice is a composite graft composed of a distal segment of the greater saphenous vein and a proximal segment of PTFE. Other veins, such as the cephalic and basilic veins, have been used for femoropopliteal and femorotibial bypass, but patency rates have been lower and more revisions are necessary.[37,38] We now use composites grafts to salvage the lower extremity after PTFE grafts have failed and after most multiple graft failures. However, these grafts have the highest early primary graft failure rates.[20,36]

During the early recovery period after a repeat bypass, patients need to be followed closely to maintain the graft. Primary graft occlusion after repeat femoropopliteal bypasses is increased for all graft types. Five-year patency rates after repeat bypasses have ranged from <30% to 57% and limb salvage rates are low.[11,14,16,39–42] These results suggest that composite grafts can be used to achieve a reasonable outcome for femoropopliteal revascularizations even when the greater saphenous vein is unavailable. With long distal bypass procedures, femorotibial composite grafts can also preserve the lower extremity. The 5-year patency rates are 63% with autogenous vein grafts and range from 28% to 45% with composite grafts.[4,16,20] We believe that our results with femorotibial composite grafts have been good because we used double outflow sequential grafts to decrease the peripheral vascular resistance and increase blood flow to the distal runoff bed when blood flow to these beds was poor. Composite grafts with a single outflow were used when distal runoff was good. Early recognition of thrombosis and treatment by thromboendarterectomy or thrombectomy, which will salvage many of these femorotibial grafts, are important. Thus, composite grafts should be an option for these patients.

An attempt should be made to preserve the lower extremity. If arterial testing indicates that collateral circulation is marginal and it is likely that the bypass will improve distal perfusion, amputation should be not performed in patients who have had multiple graft failures. After amputation many patients become nonambulatory, their health and spirit decline progressively, and they die.[19,43] Meticulous attention must be taken in the creation of the composite graft and in the technical placement of this graft with particular concern for the outflow. If complications are detected early and managed expeditiously, composite grafts for distal revascularization can successfully preserve the lower limb for an extended time.

References

1. Gibbons GW, Burgess AM, Guadagnoli E, et al. Return to well-being and function after infrainguinal revascularization. *J Vasc Surg.* 1995;21:35–45.
2. El-Masery S, Saad E, Sauvage LR, et al. Femoropopliteal bypass with externally supported knitted Dacron grafts: a follow-up of 200 grafts for one to twelve years. *J Vasc Surg.* 1994;19:487–494.
3. Quinones WJ, Colburn MD, Ahn SS, et al. Very distal bypass for salvage of the severely ischemic extremity. *Am J Surg.* 1993;166:117–123.
4. Raithel D. Role of PTFE grafts in infrainguinal arterial reconstruction: a ten year experience. In: Wang ZB, Becker H-M, Mishima Y, Chang JB, eds. *The Proceedings of the International Conference on Vascular Surgery.* Vol 1. New York, NY: International Academy Publisher; 1993:205–214.
5. Whittemore AD, Kent KC, Donaldson MC, et al. What is the proper role of polytetrafluoroethylene grafts in infrainguinal reconstruction? *J Vasc Surg.* 1989;10:299–305.
6. Taylor LM, Edwards JM, Porter JM. Present status of reversed vein bypass grafting: five-year results of a modern series. *J Vasc Surg.* 1990;11:193–206.
7. Veith FJ, Gupta SK, Ascer E, et al. Six year prospective multicenter randomized comparison of autologous saphenous vein and expanded polytetrafluoroethylene graft in infrainguinal arterial reconstruction. *J Vasc Surg.* 1986;3:104–114.
8. Belkin M, Conte MS, Donaldson MC, Mannick JA, Whittemore AD. Preferred strategies for secondary infrainguinal bypass: lessons learned in 300 consecutive reoperations. *J Vasc Surg.* 1995;21:282–293.
9. Archie JP Jr. Femoropopliteal bypass with either adequate ipsilateral reversed saphenous vein or obligatory polytetrafluoroethylene. *Ann Vasc Surg.* 1994;8:475–484.
10. Jarrett F, Berkoff HA, Crummy AB. Sequential femorotibial bypass: clinical results. *Can J Surg.* 1980;23:1–8.
11. Ascer E, Collier P, Gupta SK, et al. Reoperation for polytetrafluoroethylene bypass failure: the importance of distal outflow site and operative technique in determining outcome. *J Vasc Surg.* 1987;5:298–310.
12. Dennis JW, Littooy FN, Greisler HP, et al. Secondary vascular procedures with polytetrafluoroethylene grafts for lower extremity ischemia in a male veteran population. *J Vasc Surg.* 1988;8:137–142.
13. Green RM, Ouriel K, Ricotta JJ, et al. Revision of failed infrainguinal bypass graft: principles of management. *Surgery.* 1986;100:646–653.
14. Whittemore AD, Clowes AW, Couch NP, et al. Secondary femoropopliteal reconstruction. *Ann Surg.* 1981;193:35–42.
15. Veterans Administration Cooperative Study Group 141. Comparative evaluation of prosthetic, reversed, and in situ bypass grafts in distal popliteal and tibial-peroneal revascularization. *Arch Surg.* 1988;123:434–438.

16. Londrey GL, Ramsey DE, Hodgson KJ, et al. Infrapopliteal bypass for severe ischemia: comparison of autogenous vein, composite, and prosthetic grafts. *J Vasc Surg*. 1991;13: 631–636.

17. Bottger TC, Jonas J, Maier M, Junginger T. Risks and follow-up after crural vascular reconstruction in the extremity at risk for ischemia. *Zentralbl Chir*. 1995;120:221–227.

18. Britton JP, Leveson SH. Distal arterial bypass by composite grafting. *Br J Surg*. 1987;74:249–251.

19. Little JM. Successful amputation—by whose standards? *Am Heart J*. 1975;90:806–807.

20. Chang JB, Stein TA. The long-term value of composite grafts for limb salvage. *J Vasc Surg*. 1995;22:25–31.

21. Ad Hoc Committee on Reporting Standards, Society for Vascular Surgery, and the International Society for Cardiovascular Surgery. Standards for reports dealing with lower extremity ischemia. *J Vasc Surg* 1986;4:80–94.

22. Hoch JR, Tullis MJ, Kennell TW, McDermott JM, Acher CW, Turnipseed WD. Use of magnetic resonance angiography for the preoperative evaluation of patients with infrainguinal arterial occlusive disease. *J Vasc Surg*. 1996;23: 792–801.

23. Stirnemann P, Ris HB, Do D, Hammerli R. Intraoperative flow measurement of distal runoff: a valid predictor of outcome of infrainguinal bypass surgery. *Eur J Surg*. 1994;160: 431–436.

24. Chang JB. Popliteal and tibial artery revascularization. In: Chang JBC, ed. *Vascular Surgery*. New York, NY: Spectrum Publications; 1985:194–229.

25. Sayers RD, Thompson MM, Dunlop P, London NJ, Bell PR. The fate of infrainguinal PTFE grafts and an analysis of factors affecting outcome. *Eur J Vasc Surg*. 1994;8: 607–610.

26. Erickson CA, Towne JB, Seabrook GR, Freischlag JA, Cambria RA. Ongoing vascular laboratory surveillance is essential to maximize long-term in situ saphenous vein bypass patency. *J Vasc Surg*. 1996;23:18–27.

27. Bergamini TM, George SM, Massey HT, et al. Intensive surveillance of femoropopliteal-tibial autogenous vein bypasses improves long-term graft patency and limb salvage. *Ann Surg*. 1995;221:507–515.

28. Dalsing MC, Cikrit DF, Lalka SG, Sawchuk AP, Schulz C. Femorodistal vein grafts: the utility of graft surveillance criteria. *J Vasc Surg*. 1995;21:127–134.

29. Lagakos SW. Statistical analysis of survival data. In: Bailar JC III, Mosteller F, eds. *Medical Uses of Statistics*. 2nd ed.

Boston, Ma: New England Journal of Medicine Books; 1992:281–291.

30. Mills JL, Bandyk DF, Gahtan V, Esses GE. The origin of infrainguinal vein graft stenosis: a prospective study based on duplex surveillance. *J Vasc Surg*. 1995;21:16–25.

31. Ikeda Y, Rummel MC, Bhatnagar PK, et al. Thrombolysis therapy in patients with femoropopliteal synthetic graft occlusions. *Am J Surg*. 1996;171:251–254.

32. Sanchez LA, Suggs WD, Marin ML, Lyon RT, Parsons RE, Veith FJ. The merit of polytetrafluoroethylene extensions and interposition grafts to salvage failing infrainguinal vein bypasses. *J Vasc Surg*. 1996;23:329–335.

33. Parsons RE, Suggs WD, Veith FJ, et al. Polytetrafluoroethylene bypasses to infrapopliteal arteries without cuffs or patches: a better option than amputation in patients without autologous vein. *J Vasc Surg*. 1996;23:347–356.

34. Gouny P, Bertrand P, Decaix B, et al. Distal bypass for limb salvage: comparative study in patients below and above 80 years of age. *J Cardiovasc Surg (Torino)*. 1994;35:419–424.

35. Michaels JM. Choice of materials for above-knee femoropopliteal bypass graft. *Br J Surg*. 1989;76:7–14.

36. De Frang RD, Edwards JM, Moneta GL, et al. Repeat leg bypass after multiple prior bypass failures. *J Vasc Surg*. 1994;19:268–277.

37. Gentile AT, Lee RW, Moneta GL, Taylor LM Jr, Edwards JM, Porter JM. Results of bypass to the popliteal and tibial arteries with alternative sources of autogenous vein. *J Vasc Surg*. 1996;23:272–280.

38. Hölzenbein TJ, Pomposelli FB, Miller A, et al. Results of a policy with arm veins used as the first alternative to an unavailable ipsilateral infrainguinal bypass. *J Vasc Surg*. 1996; 23:130–140.

39. Burnham SJ, Flanigan DP, Goodreau JJ, et al. Nonvein bypass in below-knee reoperation for lower limb ischemia. *Surgery*. 1978;84:417–424.

40. Painton JF, Avellone JC, Plecha FR. Effectiveness of reoperation after late failure of femoropopliteal reconstruction. *Am J Surg*. 1978;135:235–237.

41. Tyson RR, Grosh JD, Reichle FA. Redo surgery for graft failure. *Am J Surg*. 1978;136:165–170.

42. Edwards JM, Taylor LM Jr, Porter JM. Treatment of failed lower extremity bypass grafts with new autogenous vein bypass grafting. *J Vasc Surg*. 1990;11:136–145.

43. Whittemore AD, Donaldson MC, Mannick JA. Infrainguinal reconstruction for patients with chronic renal insufficiency. *J Vasc Surg*. 1993;17:32–41.

70

The Diabetic Foot

Travis J. Phifer

Diabetes mellitus is the most common human endocrine disease, occurring with a frequency in the United States population of between 1% and 5%.[1,2] The eye, kidney, and cardiovascular system are usual end-organ targets, with substantial consequent morbidity related to blindness, renal failure, and limb ischemia. Although only about 2% of diabetic patients reportedly require amputation, this figure represents at least 50% of the total number of amputations performed for reasons other than trauma.[2,3] The financial impact on the health care system just for amputations related to diabetes is thus substantial.[4,5] Also, reported mortality after amputation of a leg approaches 70% at 5 years.[6] Further study of the problem is thus warranted.

Loss of the lower extremity in a diabetic patient is generally consequent to some combination of neuropathy and ischemia complicated by infection. In one study, as many as 80% of diabetic patients presenting with serious pedal infections had signs of peripheral neuropathy.[7] Also, more than 50% of diabetic patients have some evidence of arterial occlusive disease after 10 to 15 years.[8] This combination of neuropathy and ischemia then potentiates tissue loss and infection. Only the most aggressive therapeutic efforts, based on pathophysiologic principles, salvage such extremities. In this chapter I address pathophysiologic processes common to the diabetic patient, limiting the discussion to issues relevant to the foot and emphasizing both preventative and therapeutic modalities directed toward limb preservation.

Neuropathy

Most patients with diabetes for more than a decade,[9] and up to 90% of diabetic patients with foot lesions,[4] have manifestations of peripheral neuropathy. Manifestations of such neuropathy vary widely to include paresthesia, dysesthesia, and even hypersensitivity. Some become completely insensate, with increased risk of injury to the plantar surface during barefoot ambulation. Autonomic dysfunction produces dry, scaly skin predisposed to cracking, and the loss of vasomotor tone results in the formation of edema.[10] Motor neuropathy also occurs.

As a consequence of the motor neuropathy, atrophy of the intrinsic muscles occurs and the normal bony architecture of the foot shifts; claw toe deformities and maldistribution of forces to the metatarsal heads result.[5,11] The neuropathic ulcer is a direct consequence of these mechanical factors, which potentiate trauma on weight bearing in a foot already impaired by sensory neuropathy. Neuropathic ulcers occur most commonly at the level of the first, second, or fifth metatarsal head, although any deformity in architecture of the foot that results in abnormal distribution of pressure to areas not normally protected by padding but subjected to repetitive insults potentiates development of a neuropathic ulcer. Hypertrophic skin changes develop at pressure points and produce further increases in pressure by as much as 26% as a direct consequence of the callus formation alone.[12] What often appears as only a relatively minor dermal ulcer is frequently deceiving, with much more extensive tissue loss below the surface that may involve muscles, tendons, and joint capsules. Although certainly potentiated by ischemia, the neuropathic ulcer occurs independently of arterial occlusive disease.

Prevention is the best treatment for neuropathic ulcers. Essential to this end, after diagnosis, is recognition and avoidance of the major factors (Table 70.1) that predispose a limb to ulceration.[13] The monofilament test is an inexpensive and simple, yet highly reliable, diagnostic tool for assessment of the peripheral sensory neuropathy associated with diabetes mellitus.[14,15] A positive test mandates institution of preventive measures to always include diligent surveillance by daily inspection of the feet by another individual or by the affected individual using a mirror; special shoes and foot padding may sometimes be necessary. Meticulous care of the nails and any callus formation and strict control of serum glucose levels and

TABLE 70.1. Clinical findings predicting areas of high plantar pressure.[13]

History
Prior ulceration
Prior surgery involving the metatarsal bones
Physical finding
Callus*
Hemorrhagic callus*
Blister or macerated skin*
Limited hallux dorsiflexion (<30 degrees)
Prominent metatarsal heads inadequately covered with soft tissue†
Other plantar bony prominences
Radiograph finding: Charcot's fracture

*High pressure or shear capable of injuring soft tissue is being generated.

†Detected by gently stroking a finger across the plantar surface of the forefoot.

abstinence from all tobacco products are essential. In compressive neuropathy, as contrasted to progressive distal axonopathy, decompression of the nerve at the point of entrapment is also of potential therapeutic benefit.[16] The contribution to this process of metabolic derangements is not completely clear, although some reports indicate stabilization or improvement of the neuropathy after administration of either prostaglandin E_1 or the prostaglandin precursor linolenic acid.[17,18]

If preventive measures fail, basic treatment of a formed ulcer first requires correction of any pressure derangements to the plantar surface. Complete and prolonged bed rest is perhaps ideal for healing of such wounds, although it is certainly not practical and is often dangerous to general health. Redistribution of abnormal pressure is a reasonable and practical compromise. With simple, shallow lesions, padding of the shoe and minor débridement are adequate. Larger and deeper ulcers require more extensive soft tissue débridement, sometimes extending to bone and involving tendon sheaths, tendons, periarticular ligaments, and even the joint capsule. Healing of these more extensive wounds also requires elimination of the pressure. Short of bed rest, the full contact cast is perhaps the best method to achieve this goal.[19–21] Such casts, popularized for treatment of the neuropathic soft tissue lesions of patients with leprosy, utilize minimal padding and molding to the shape of the foot and leg with the addition of a walking heel. These casts redistribute pressure to the entire surface of the foot and lower leg, thus sparing the ulcer. Such casts are also of some practical value in care of the ulcer, because the cast is usually changed on a weekly basis after initial removal of the cast for assessment of fit after 24 to 48 hours. Conversion back to a shoe is gradual, with interim use of a thick sandal with a pliant sole. Care of the ulcer itself after débridement is by standard wound care technique that depends on the stage of wound healing.

Ischemia

Arterial occlusive disease is substantially more prevalent and more rapidly progressive in diabetic patients than in the general population.[22] More than 50% of those with diabetes diagnosed for 10 to 15 years have evidence of arterial occlusive disease.[8] In one study of a population over 40 years of age with non-insulin-dependent diabetes treated by diet alone compared to a control population without diabetes, the prevalence of arterial occlusive disease increased by 10-fold as measured by noninvasive parameters.[23] In the Framingham Study, the age-adjusted incidence of lower extremity claudication in diabetic patients was 12.6% in men and 8.4% in women versus an incidence in nondiabetic patients of 3.3% and 1.3%, respectively.[24] Even in diabetic patients diagnosed for less than 1 year, some data show vascular calcification apparent on plain radiographs in as many as 22%, with absence of one or more ankle pulses in 13%.[5] Ankle/brachial arterial pressure ratios also are abnormal in 22% of patients with type II diabetes versus 3% of control subjects,[22] which suggests an increased incidence of occult arterial occlusive disease. Furthermore, arterial insufficiency is also a pathogenic factor in some 62% of diabetic patients with nonhealing dermal ulcers and in 46% of those who undergo major amputation.[25]

A diabetic patient with arterial occlusive disease requires the same evaluation and treatment as a nondiabetic patient with this problem. Indications for evaluation and treatment of lower extremity arterial occlusive disease are the clinical manifestations of ischemia—claudication, rest pain, and tissue loss. Simple functional claudication is the weakest of these indications. In fact, claudication alone often responds to medical regimens that thus negate the need for invasive procedures.[26] Disabling claudication that prevents gainful employment or meaningful existence is of more importance. Also, claudication that originates from aortoiliac occlusive disease generally receives more attention than claudication that originates from infrainguinal occlusion. The traditional justification for this approach relates to proven durability of aortoiliac reconstructive procedures, as well as the potentially catastrophic nature of complications associated with aortoiliac occlusive disease. Rest pain and tissue loss are solid indications for evaluation and treatment of arterial occlusive disease at any level in any patient population.

Pertinent to the discussion at the beginning of this chapter, the indication of tissue loss is of particular importance to the diabetic patient. Diabetic patients often present with ischemia and/or infection of the feet or toes. Such problems are all too often ascribed to small-vessel disease of diabetes. Absence of a palpable and normal ankle pulse, or abnormal noninvasive tests, mandates prompt and aggressive evaluation of the lower extremity arterial system in such patients to include arteriography.[27] The measurement of ankle pressures is sometimes helpful in this situation. A pressure of less than 80 mm Hg in either the anterior or posterior tibial artery at the ankle level is a general indication for further evaluation.[28] In the diabetic patient, however, such pressure measurement by noninvasive techniques is prone to error, primarily because of loss of compliance of the arterial wall related to medial calcinosis of the arteries. The consequent lack of compression of such vessels results in a falsely high recording of pressures and a false sense of security in the presence of significant arterial occlusive disease. Other noninvasive modalities useful in evaluation of lower extremity arterial perfusion include the recording of analog waveforms and pulse volume recordings, as well as direct imaging and interrogation of flow characteristics with duplex ultrasonography. The best and most economical screening test is simple palpation of the lower extremity pulses, although medial calcinosis sometimes also complicates this examination by making palpation of even a normal pulse difficult.

Femoral and popliteal arterial occlusive disease occurs with a similar incidence in the diabetic and nondiabetic populations. Multisegmental occlusive disease below the popliteal artery in the tibial vessels, however, is more common in the diabetic population. Despite involvement of infrageniculate arteries between the knee and ankle, foot vessels in the diabetic patient are not commonly involved in the arteriosclerotic process. In fact, there is sparing of the dorsalis pedis artery in about 70% of diabetic patients.[29,30]

The issue of microvascular disease in the diabetic patient deserves special mention. Traditional teaching attributes many problems of tissue loss and infection in the diabetic patient to supposed small-vessel disease. This common misconception dates to a report by Goldenberg et al. in 1959 of periodic acid Schiff–positive material in the arterioles supposedly specific for diabetes.[31] Subsequent work[29] using the same technique employed by Goldenberg, however, failed to demonstrate such lesions specific to the diabetic patient. Likewise, no evidence exists for the endothelial proliferation reported by Goldenberg.[32] Thickening of the basement membrane does occur, but with increased capillary luminal diameter.[32,33] Also, this intimal thickening in the basement membrane occurs in some 23% of nondiabetic patients.[32] Abnormalities of the microcirculation in the diabetic patient are thus of a nonocclusive nature, and besides thickening of the basement membrane include an increased transcapillary escape rate of albumin[34] with decreased microcirculatory volume as well as decreased erythrocyte velocity.[35]

Despite such microcirculatory derangements, measurements of the transcutaneous partial pressure of oxygen in the ulcerated diabetic foot are often elevated,[36] suggesting no impairment of oxygen diffusion across the capillary membrane. Elevation of venous oxygen saturation in the diabetic foot associated with increased total resting blood flow, however, implicates arteriovenous shunting.[37] Also, a form of metabolic tissue hypoxia termed *hyperglycemia-induced pseudohypoxia*[30,38,39] exists in the diabetic patient related to hyperglycemia. During periods of hyperglycemia existing for more than 4 hours, oxygen utilization decreases because of shunting of glucose through the sorbitol pathway rather than the glycolytic pathway. This results in decreased mitochondrial pyruvate utilization and a reduction in energy production, with accumulation not only of sorbitol and fructose but also lactate. These metabolic derangements correlate with skeletal and smooth muscle dysfunction as well as neural impairment and increased capillary permeability, and help explain the disproportionate degree of tissue loss in diabetic patients after relatively mild periods of ischemia. Of note, however, inhibitors of key enzymes of the sorbitol pathway (e.g., aldose reductase) limit these problems in animal models.[38,39]

Reconstruction of vascular obstructive lesions at the aortoiliac level in diabetic patients is no different than in nondiabetic patients. Endovascular procedures, including balloon angioplasty and stent placement, are sometimes effective in the treatment of selected lesions. Treatment of more diffuse disease and more complex lesions is generally with surgical bypass procedures using standard techniques established for placement of vascular grafts from the aorta to the femoral vessels. Such grafts, usually fabricated of Dacron and frequently bifurcated in design, are of proven durability, with patency rates in excess of 70% at 15 years.[40]

Autogenous saphenous vein is generally the conduit of choice for arterial reconstruction at the infrainguinal level. Patency of polytetrafluoroethylene as well as autogenous saphenous vein, however, is similar at 2 years.[41] Beyond 2 years, there is a trend toward superior patency of autogenous saphenous vein over polytetrafluoroethylene in the above-knee location and a statistically significant difference at the below-knee level. At all time intervals in the infrageniculate circulation, the durability of autogenous saphenous vein clearly exceeds that of the prosthetic graft. Some thus favor utilization of polytetrafluoroethylene for above-knee reconstructions and save autogenous vein for later, more complex procedures such as below-knee distal reconstruction or coronary artery bypass grafting.[42] Because of substantially reduced patency, there is little if any reason to use prosthetic grafts in below-knee reconstructions. An exception is perhaps when a lower extremity ulcer or minor amputation site in an ischemic limb requires healing and no autogenous vein is available for graft construction. With need for graft patency in this scenario sometimes limited to the time required for wound healing, the use of a substantially less durable polytetrafluoroethylene graft at the below-knee level is perhaps justified.[41]

Utilization of autogenous saphenous vein in the infrainguinal arterial circulation is either as a translocated (reversed or nonreversed) or nontranslocated (in situ) graft. Each technique has a unique set of technical nuances and touted advantages. Critical evaluation of these autogenous venous grafts, however, shows very acceptable durability with little discernible difference between the translocated and nontranslocated techniques.[43]

Despite historical opinion to the contrary,[44,45] the risk of revascularization and success of vascular reconstruction are similar in both diabetic and nondiabetic populations.[46,47] Preoperative studies[47] show a 40% versus 41% incidence, respectively, of prior myocardial infarction and a 13% versus 11% incidence, respectively, of prior cerebral infarction. In regards to graft durability, several series summarized in Table 70.2 show similar graft patency in both diabetic and nondiabetic populations. The data reported by Hurley et al. actually show more favorable outcomes for diabetic patients, with 65% graft patency at 5 years in contrast to 52% in the nondiabetic cohort,[47] although the use of vein in 94% of the diabetic patients and in only 76% of the nondiabetic patients probably contributes to this discrepancy. Both Shah[48] and Rosenblatt,[49] however, reported similar vein graft patency for diabetic as well as nondiabetic patients. The primary graft patency reported by Rosenblatt et al. at 1 and 4 years of 95% and 89%, respectively, in a group of diabetic patients and 85% and 80%, respectfully, in an equal cohort of nondiabetic patients is particularly notable, with some 80% of these grafts to a target below the knee and with significantly more grafts in the diabetic patients to tibial and pedal vessels.[49] Another study reported overall primary graft patency at 3 years of 58%, with no statistically significant difference between insulin-controlled and non–insulin-controlled diabetic and nondiabetic patients.[46] Of some concern, however, a recent study reporting results of an aggressive revascularization policy in patients with juvenile-onset diabetes showed a 16% actuarial mortality rate during the 24-month period of study and actuarial primary vein graft patency of 66% at 2 years.[50]

In the diabetic population with arterial occlusive disease sometimes primarily limited to tibial vessels with sparing of foot vessels and normal inflow, questions that address the propriety of the site of graft origin and destination are reasonable. Although the traditional infrainguinal graft originates at the common femoral level, the profunda femoris, popliteal, and tibial arteries are also appropriate sites for graft origin under these circumstances. The durability of such short grafts is acceptable.[51–55] Also, graft targets even into the arch of the foot are attainable using modern techniques of revascularization.[56]

Infection

Besides neuropathy and ischemia, infection is the third major consideration in pathology of the diabetic foot. Infection of the foot is a particularly common problem for the diabetic patient and is one of the most frequent reasons for hospitalization. Hospitalization is expensive in such patients, with an average hospital stay in excess of 1 month in 89% and in excess of 3 months in 44%.[57] Such foot infections result by some estimates in an estimated annual expenditure for medical and surgical treatment of approximately $200 million.[58]

The typical diabetic patient with lower extremity infection is obese and in the fifth decade of life with a history of type II diabetes lasting for approximately 18 years.[7] Such patients frequently have impaired arterial blood supply or neuropathy. Both of these processes potentiate an infectious process.

Any diabetic patient who presents with lower extremity infection thus warrants early and careful evaluation of arterial perfusion to the foot, with appropriate and timed vascular reconstruction. Simply attributing infection associated with even minor tissue loss to small-vessel disease of diabetes is common yet inappropriate. Limb salvage is highly unlikely in such cases unless the treatment regimen includes successful restoration of arterial perfusion to the extremity.

Education of both the patient and family is necessary to prevent infection and preserve the limb. Wearing properly fitting shoes, avoiding unprotected ambulation, and observing good personal foot hygiene are extremely important. Equally important is frequent and meticulous self-inspection of the entire foot with particular attention to the sole and intertriginous spaces, a task

TABLE 70.2. Primary patency rates of infrainguinal bypass grafting for diabetic and nondiabetic patients.

Reference	Year	Nondiabetic patients (%)			Diabetic patients (%)		
		1 yr	4 yr	5 yr	1 yr	4 yr	5 yr
Hurley et al.[47]	1987	—	—	52	—	—	62
Shah et al.[48]	1988	90	—	76	91	—	74
Rosenblatt et al.[49]	1990	85	80	—	95	89	—

often complicated by impaired vision in the patient with diabetes. Many of the infectious problems common to the diabetic patient can be prevented, which is the goal.

As discussed and referenced in the section of this chapter related to neuropathic ulcers, peripheral neuropathy common to diabetes mellitus alters the foot by several different mechanisms. Mechanical disadvantages produced by muscle atrophy and the subsequent changes of foot architecture predispose a patient to neurotrophic ulcer. The neurotrophic ulcer, then, often becomes secondarily infected. Impairment of arterial perfusion only worsens this process. Loss of sensation and autonomic denervation further potentiate an infectious process in the foot of the diabetic patient. Significant trauma, from both repetitive blunt or abrasive injury and penetration with sharp objects, often goes unnoticed by the unwary diabetic patient affected by this type of neuropathy. Dry and scaly skin associated with autonomic denervation results in cracking and thus provides a port of entry for microorganisms. Accumulation of moisture in the interdigital spaces and the excess buildup of keratin and other debris around the nail plates results in bacterial overgrowth and also potentiates infection. Foot infections in the diabetic patient often begin around the nail plate (30%), in the interdigital web space (60%), and less commonly (10%) from penetrating injury.[59] These local infections then spread to the deep compartments of the foot through the tendons and lumbricals of the involved toes. Diabetic foot infections thus range from minor fungal infections and simple cellulitis to major bacterial infections and necrotizing fasciitis associ-

ated with systemic manifestations that endanger both limb and life. The deep ascending infections are those most responsible for subsequent major amputation[60] and as such deserve special attention to the mechanism of development, the organisms involved, and the methods of treatment.

Figure 70.1[5] shows the anatomic compartments of the deep plantar space involved in infectious processes. These compartments are the central, medial, and lateral compartments.[5,60] An intermuscular septum that extends from the medial calcaneal tuberosity to the head of the first metatarsal head separates the central compartment from the medial compartment. Similarly, a lateral intermuscular septum that extends from the calcaneus to the fifth metatarsal head separates the central compartment from the lateral compartment. The roof of each compartment consists of the metatarsal bones and interosseus fascia. The floor of each compartment consists of the rigid plantar fascia. These septa separate intrinsic muscles of the great toe and fifth digit from the soft tissue structures of the medial compartment (plantar arch vessels, medial and lateral plantar nerves, extrinsic flexor tendons of the toes, and intrinsic muscles of the second through fourth toes). The rigid fascial components at the boundaries of these compartments help contain infectious processes within the compartment of origination (generally the central compartment), with deceptively few if any dorsal or plantar anatomic abnormalities apparent. Also, edema associated with an infection sometimes produces necrosis of intracompartmental soft tissue consequent to elevation of pressure within

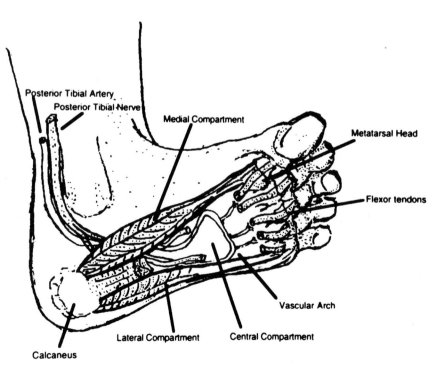

FIGURE 70.1. Plantar compartments of the foot: beneath the plantar surface are the three compartments of the foot. The medial compartment contains the intrinsic muscles of the great toe. The central compartment contains the intrinsic muscles of the middle toes, extrinsic flexor tendons, the vascular arch, and the plantar nerves. Infections can ascend into the lower leg along the flexor tendons and neurovascular bundles.[5]

these tight fascial compartments. In advanced cases, spread of infection between compartments occurs either at the proximal calcaneal convergence of the septa or by direct septal perforation. Also, advanced infections in the deep plantar compartments sometimes spread to the dorsum of the foot or along tendon sheaths to the ankle and lower leg regions. Related both to elevated intracompartmental pressures and small-vessel thrombosis associated with advanced infection, tissue ischemia and muscle necrosis progress. Bullous lesions on the plantar surface are a late sign of this process indicative of loss of plantar arch patency and associated with massive plantar tissue necrosis.

The clinical presentation of deep infections of the foot is often quite subtle. Fever, chills, and leukocytosis may be absent even with limb-threatening infection. Pain and tenderness are often minimal. With containment of the infectious process to the plantar compartments, foot architecture changes very little. Although a loss of plantar surface contour occurs, dorsal foot swelling is variable. A presentation of only mild swelling of the foot but toxic symptoms thus requires careful investigation for a deep infection. The appearance of bullous lesions on the dorsum of the foot is a late sign indicative of significant tissue necrosis. Systemic symptoms and signs, such as malaise and nausea with spiking fever and the development of ketoacidosis, often herald significant deep infection perhaps associated with necrotizing cellulitis or fasciitis. Hyperglycemia is often a sign of limb- or life-threatening infection. The radiographic appearance of soft tissue gas is also generally a negative prognostic sign. Gas develops in the soft tissues either from the pumping action associated with an open wound and continued ambulation or from gas-producing organisms such as certain gram-negative and clostridial species. True gas gangrene, usually caused by infection with *Clostridium perfringens,* is less common but associated with an extremely toxic and rapidly progressive clinical course. Infections caused by gas-producing gram-negative organisms and other clostridial species, however, are generally much less virulent. Differentiation, usually possible using clinical criteria and a gram stain of any exudate or tissue from the wound, is critical for prompt delivery of appropriate antibiotic therapy and choice of the correct type and extent of surgical intervention.

The differential diagnosis of an acutely inflamed foot in a diabetic patient includes soft tissue infections, sometimes associated with underlying osteomyelitis, acute gouty arthritis, and Charcot's joint. The incidence of Charcot's joint in diabetic patients ranges between approximately 0.5% and 2.2%[61] and is related to repetitive trauma of an insensate foot. Joints typically involved in this process are the interphalangeal, metatarsophalangeal, metatarsotarsal, and intertarsal joints. Although the area is inflamed and may be associated with edema and effusions, a simple Charcot's joint is not toxic and the affected patient has a normal leukocyte count and erythrocyte sedimentation rate. In acute gout, in contrast, the great toe is most commonly involved at the level of the first metatarsophalangeal joint. Affected patients usually lack symptoms of systemic toxicity but often have increased serum uric acid levels and elevated erythrocyte sedimentation rates. The finding of uric acid crystals in fluid aspirated from an acutely inflamed joint is of more significance, however, in the diagnosis of acute gout.

Osteomyelitis commonly occurs in the foot of the diabetic patient (68% of cases with chronic ulceration) but often remains undiagnosed. A high index of suspicion is appropriate, particularly with chronically inflamed wounds, although osteomyelitis also occurs in uninflamed ulcers.[62] The diagnosis is problematic, because differentiating between osteomyelitis and diabetic osteoarthropathy is difficult. Cultures of bone obtained by percutaneous biopsy or from surgical excision provide proof. However, obtaining such specimens through a route not involved by the ulcer is often impractical or unreasonable. Plain radiographs for diagnosis of osteomyelitis are neither sensitive nor specific.[62-64] Radioactive isotope bone scans are very sensitive[65] but sometimes lack specificity. Combinations of scans increase accuracy, with a sensitivity of 100% and a specificity of 81% reported after a three-phase technetium 99 methylene diphosphate bone scan combined with an indium 111 oxine leukocyte scan.[66] The role of computed tomography and magnetic resonance imaging scans are particularly useful in determining the extent of soft tissue involvement, although their role in the diagnosis of osteomyelitis is less certain.[67] Computed tomography scans are useful, however, in detecting bony sequestra associated with osteomyelitis. Some recommend simply probing for bone in chronic wounds as a highly specific but much less sensitive test for osteomyelitis.[13] Gently probing in an attempt to reach bone with a sterile instrument, combined with interpretation of plain radiographs repeated after 2 weeks if initially negative, is perhaps a reasonable approach. Also, recurrent infection in a chronic wound deserves further consideration and raises suspicion of undiagnosed underlying occult osteomyelitis.

Diabetic foot infections are usually polymicrobial.[68,69] Organisms commonly associated with these infections include gram-positive cocci (*Staphylococcus aureus* and groups D and B streptococci), enteric aerobic gram-negative rods (*Escherichia coli, Klebsiella* species, *Enterobacter aerogenes, Proteus mirabilis,* and *Pseudomonas aeruginosa*), and anaerobes (*Bacteroides fragilis, Peptostreptococci* species, and clostridial species). Anaerobes sometimes outnumber aerobes by 10-fold. The organisms most commonly associated with bacteremia are *Bacteroides fragilis* and *Staphylococcus aureus.*

Accurate determination of the organism or organisms responsible for infection of the foot in a diabetic host is often difficult. Surface cultures obtained by simple swabs of an ulcer are of little value, because they are usually contaminated by a multiplicity of organisms that colonize the wound and the offending pathogen that has caused the infection. More reliable results come from cultures of curettage obtained from the base of a wound after débridement or from needle aspirates.[68–70] In the case of osteomyelitis, the most accurate cultures of bone specimens are obtained by percutaneous biopsy or surgical excision through approaches that do not traverse the infected field.

Prompt initiation of antibiotic therapy, after collection of cultures, is imperative. The issue of outpatient oral therapy versus inpatient intravenous therapy remains controversial. Much depends on the extent of infection, temporal progression of the infectious process, condition of the host both in terms of ability to resist infection and capability of understanding the problem and complying with treatment regimens, and the presence or absence of symptoms and signs of systemic toxicity. The choice of antibiotic depends on the organism presumed responsible for the infection (perhaps based on gram stain results prior to availability of culture results) and assessment of the severity of the infection. A convenient classification of severity of infections of this type for choosing an empirical antibiotic regimen is on the basis of whether the infection is limb threatening, life threatening, or neither. Table 70.3[13] offers a reasonable guideline for initial choice of empirical antibiotic therapy. Alteration of the antibiotic regimen is then appropriate depending on the response to the empirical regimen and the results of cultures. In general, aminoglycosides are probably best avoided in the diabetic host in favor of less nephrotoxic regimens. Fluoroquinolones are best used with other agents as empirical therapy in these infections because of their inadequate activity against gram-positive and anaerobic organisms. Single drug therapy with cefoxitin or ceftizoxine,[58] however, is sometimes adequate.

Selection of optimal surgical therapy for the infected diabetic foot is contingent on the coexistence of abscess formation and the extent of tissue necrosis. Simple infections that manifest primarily as cellulitis generally require no surgical intervention and are best treated by placing the extremity at rest and in an elevated position with the concomitant administration of either oral or parenteral antibiotics. In cases of life-threatening infection, however, primary guillotine amputation is necessary for control of sepsis.[71]

Wide drainage of all abscesses is imperative. Drainage with simple needle aspiration or percutaneous drains is inadequate. Figures 70.2 and 70.3[5] show optimal sites for incisions to drain abscesses. Careful choice of the inci-

TABLE 70.3. Selected empirical antimicrobial regimens for foot infections in patients with diabetes mellitus.*

Non–limb-threatening infection
Oral regimen
    Cephalexin
    Clindamycin
    Dicloxacillin
    Amoxicillin/clavulanate
Parenteral regimen
    Cefazolin
    Oxacillin or nafcillin
    Clindamycin

Limb-threatening infection
Oral regimen: fluoroquinolone and clindamycin
Parenteral regimen
    Ampicillin/sulbactam
    Ticarcillin/clavulanate
    Cefoxitin or cefotetan
    Fluoroquinolone and clindamycin

Life-threatening infection
Parenteral regimen
    Imipenem/cilastatin
    Vancomycin, metronidazole, and aztreonam
    Ampicillin/sulbactam and an aminoglycoside

*These regimens may require adjustment if the patient has a history of allergies or if there are clinical or epidemiological factors that suggest unusual pathogens. doses would be commensurate with the severity of infection, with adjustment for renal dysfunction when indicated.
From Caputo et al.[17]

sion site optimizes the potential for healing and minimizes morbidity of the surgical scar. Drainage of abscesses of the pulp space of the toes is best through lateral incisions placed parallel to the neurovascular bundles. Transverse pulp incisions often result in painful scars on the weight-bearing surface. Drainage of web space abscesses is best through diamond-shaped incisions at either the plantar or dorsal aspect of the web space, depending on the exact site of abscess formation and the degree of dorsal tracking. Incisions in the interdigital portion of the web space are slow in healing and thus best avoided. Similarly, drainage of the uncommon abscess of the heel pad is best through an incision placed at either the medial or lateral aspect of the heel pad that thus avoids the weight-bearing surface. Drainage of deep plantar abscesses in the medial and central compartments is through a medial incision just above the plantar surface of the forefoot. Drainage of abscesses that involve the lateral compartment is through a similar incision on the lateral aspect of the forefoot.

Necrotic tissue in all such wounds, particularly in association with major infection, requires adequate débridement. With extensive infection, initial débridement and control of sepsis are generally necessary even prior to reconstruction of the arterial supply to the limb.[72] Adequate débridement means removal of all involved soft tis-

FIGURE 70.2. Plantar incisions: diamond-shaped incisions are placed in the lower portion of the web space. Heel, medial, and central compartments are drained above the plantar surface. The toe pulp is drained in a longitudinal direction.[5]

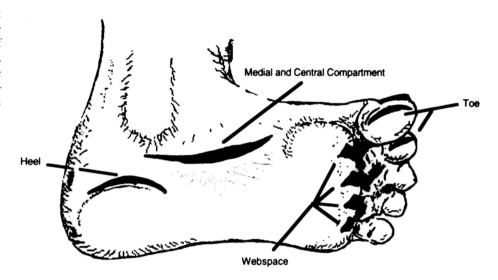

sue, including necrotic muscle, fascia, tendons, and cartilage. With associated osteomyelitis, traditional treatment involves aggressive surgical débridement, sometimes with limited amputation of the infected bone, followed by a prolonged course of antibiotic therapy that extends perhaps 4 to 6 weeks. Removal of an infected bony prominence also helps in elimination of the cause of the tissue necrosis.[73] Multiple débridement procedures are often necessary. Careful daily inspection with serial débridement is particularly valuable in the case of neurotrophic ulcers. Accurate assessment of the extent of tissue necrosis in such wounds is often difficult at ini-

tial inspection. As an adjunct to surgical débridement of major areas of tissue necrosis, wet-to-dry dressings performed with saline-moistened fine mesh gauze are helpful in removing any remaining necrotic tissue without damaging viable tissue by too radical débridement. Heat soaks and whirlpool therapy may damage tissue and promote infection.[13] Topical hyperbaric oxygen therapy is of unproven benefit,[74] yet its use remains controversial. After removing most of the necrotic tissue, and particularly after the wound begins granulation, maintenance of a moist environment with either a moistened gauze or a bio-occlusive dressing is necessary to optimize wound

FIGURE 70.3. Dorsal incisions: dorsal web space diamond-shaped incisions are used to drain web space abscesses. Dorsal forefoot incisions are placed to avoid the venous arcade. Lateral compartment and heel incisions are placed above the plantar surface.[5]

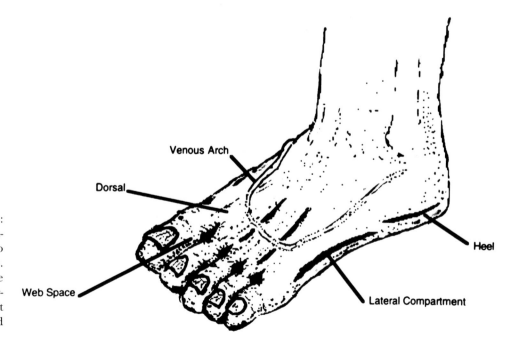

healing. Placement of a split thickness skin graft also sometimes facilitates closure of a clean granulating wound.

If other measures fail, amputation becomes necessary. Amputation of only a digit or ray is optimal. Major amputation of the extremity, however, is sometimes required. Preservation of as much viable skin as possible is desirable in these situations rather than strict adherence to classic amputation lines. Such practice, along with the liberal use of open wound care techniques with subsequent skin grafting, facilitates closure of these difficult wounds.

References

1. Foster DW. Diabetes mellitus. In: Wilson JD, Braunwald E, Isselbacher KJ, et al., eds. *Harrison's Principles of Internal Medicine.* 12th ed. New York, NY: McGraw-Hill; 1991:1739.

2. Stemmer EA. Influence of diabetes mellitus on the patterns of vascular occlusive disease. In: Moore WS, ed. *Vascular Surgery: A Comprehensive Review.* 3rd ed. Orlando, Fla: Grune & Stratton; 1991:390.

3. Warren R, Kihn RB. A survey of lower extremity amputations for ischemia. *Surgery.* 1968;63:107–120.

4. Boulton AJM. The diabetic foot: neuropathic in etiology? *Diabetes Med.* 1990;7:852–858.

5. Bridges RM Jr, Deitch EA. Diabetic foot infections: pathophysiology and treatment. *Surg Clin North Am.* 1994;74: 537–555.

6. O'Neal LW. Surgical pathology of the foot and clinicopathologic evaluations. In: Levin ME, O'Neal LW, eds. *The Diabetic Foot.* 3rd ed. St. Louis, Mo: Mosby; 1983:162.

7. Leichter SB, Allweiss P, Harley J, et al. Clinical characteristics of diabetic patients with serious pedal infections. *Metabolism.* 1988;37(suppl 1):22–24.

8. Brandman O, Redisch W. Incidence of peripheral vascular changes in diabetes mellitus. *Diabetes.* 1953;2:194–198.

9. Penn I. The impact of diabetes mellitus on extremity ischemia. In: Kempczinski RF, ed. *The Ischemic Leg.* Chicago, Ill: Year Book Medical Publishers; 1985:1–69.

10. Bouton AJM. Detecting the patient at risk for diabetic foot ulcers. *Practical Cardiology.* 1983;9:135–145.

11. Harrison MJ, Faris IB. The neuropathic factor in the etiology of diabetic foot ulcers. *J Neurol Sci.* 1976;28:217–223.

12. Young MJ, Cavanagh PR, Thomas G, et al. The effect of callus removal on dynamic plantar foot pressures in diabetic patients. *Diabetes Med.* 1992;9:55–57.

13. Caputo GM, Cavanagh PR, Ulbrecht JS, et al. Assessment and management of foot disease in patients with diabetes. *N Engl J Med.* 1994;331:854–860.

14. Birke JA, Sims DS. Plantar sensory threshold in the ulcerative foot. *Leper Rev.* 1986;57:261–267.

15. Sosenko JM, Kato M, Soto R, et al. Comparison of quantitative sensory-threshold measures for their association with foot ulceration in diabetic patients. *Diabetes Care.* 1990;13:1057–1061.

16. Dellon AL. Treatment of symptomatic diabetic neuropathy by surgical decompression of multiple peripheral nerves. *Plast Reconstr Surg.* 1992;89:689–697.

17. Hoshi K, Mizushima Y, Kiyokawa S, et al. Prostaglandin E$_1$ incorporated in lipid microspheres in the treatment of peripheral vascular diseases and diabetic neuropathy. *Drugs Exp Clin Res.* 1986;12:681–685.

18. Keen H, Payan J, Allawi J, et al. Treatment of diabetic neuropathy with gamma-linolenic acid. *Diabetes Care.* 1993; 16:8–15.

19. Novick A, Birke JA, Graham SL, et al. Effect of a walking splint and total contact casts on plantar forces. *Journal of Prosthetics and Orthotics.* 1991;3:168–178.

20. Mueller MJ, Diamond JE, Sinacore DR, et al. Total contact casting in treatment of diabetic plantar ulcers: controlled clinical trial. *Diabetes Care.* 1989;12:384–388.

21. Skolnick AA. Foot care program for patients with leprosy also may prevent amputations in persons with diabetes. *JAMA.* 1992;267:2288.

22. Beach KW, Bedford GR, Berglin RO, et al. Progression of lower-extremity arterial occlusive disease in type 2 diabetes mellitus. *Diabetes Care.* 1988;11:464–472.

23. Beach KW, Brunzell JD, Strandness DE. Prevalence of severe arteriosclerosis obliterans in patients with diabetes mellitus. *Arteriosclerosis.* 1982;2:275–281.

24. Kannel WB, McGee DL. Diabetes and cardiovascular disease: the Framingham Study. *JAMA.* 1979;241:2035–2038.

25. Pecoraro RE, Reiber GE, Burgess EM. Pathways to diabetic limb amputation: basis for prevention. *Diabetes Care.* 1990; 13:513–521.

26. Fuchs JCA. Atherogenesis and medical management of artherosclerosis. In: Rutherford RB, ed. *Vascular Surgery.* 3rd ed. Philadelphia, Pa: WB Saunders; 1989:194.

27. LoGerfo FW, Gibbons GW, Pomposelli FB Jr, et al. Trends in the care of the diabetic foot. *Arch Surg.* 1992;127: 617–621.

28. Chang BB, Shah DM, Darling RC III, et al. Treatment of the diabetic foot from a vascular surgeon's viewpoint. *Clin Orthop.* 1993;296:27–30.

29. Strandness DE Jr, Priest RE, Gibbons GE. Combined clinical and pathologic study of diabetic and nondiabetic peripheral arterial disease. *Diabetes.* 1964;13:366–372.

30. Menzoian JO, LaMorte WW, Paniszyn CC, et al. Symptomatology and anatomic patterns of peripheral vascular disease: differing impact of smoking and diabetes. *Ann Vasc Surg.* 1989;3:224–228.

31. Goldenberg SG, Alex M, Joshi RA, et al. Nonatheromatous peripheral vascular disease of the lower extremity in diabetes mellitus. *Diabetes.* 1959;8:261–273.

32. Banson BB, Lacy PE. Diabetic microangiopathy in human toes: with emphasis on the ultrastructural changes in dermal capillaries. *Am J Pathol.* 1964;45:41–58.

33. Britland ST, Young RJ, Sharma AK, et al. Relationship of endoneural capillary abnormalities to type and severity of diabetic polyneuropathy. *Diabetes.* 1990;39:909–913.

34. Parving HH, Rasmussen SM. Transcapillary escape rate of albumin and plasma volume in short- and long-term juvenile diabetes. *Scand J Clin Lab Invest.* 1973;32:81–87.

35. Rendall M, Bergman T, O'Donnell G, et al. Microvascular blood flow, volume, and velocity measured by laser Doppler techniques in IDD. *Diabetes.* 1989;38:819–824.

36. Wyss CR, Matsen FA, Simmons CW, et al. Transcutaneous oxygen tension measurements on limbs of diabetic and non-diabetic peripheral vascular disease. *Surgery.* 1984;95: 339–345.

37. Irwin ST, Gilmore J, McGrann S, et al. Blood flow in diabetics with foot lesions due to "small vessel disease." *Br J Surg.* 1988;75:1201–1206.

38. Cameron NE, Cotter MA. Dissociation between biochemical and functional effects of the aldose reductase inhibitor, ponalrestat, on peripheral nerve in diabetic rats. *Br J Pharmacol.* 1992;107:939–944.

39. Cameron NE, Cotter MA. Impaired contraction and relaxation in aorta from streptozotocin-diabetic rats: role of polyol pathway. *Diabetologia.* 1992;35:1011–1019.

40. Szilagyi DE, Elliott JP Jr, Smith RF, et al. A thirty year survey of the reconstructive surgical treatment of aortoiliac occlusive disease. *J Vasc Surg.* 1986;3:421–436.

41. Veith FJ, Gupta SK, Ascer E, et al. Six year multicenter randomized comparison of autogenous saphenous vein and expanded polytetrafluoroethylene grafts in infrainguinal reconstructions. *J Vasc Surg.* 1986;3:104–114.

42. Quinones-Baldrich WJ, Martin-Paredero V, Baker JD, et al. Polytetrafluoroethylene grafts as the first-choice arterial substitute in femoropopliteal revascularization. *Arch Surg.* 1984;119:1238–1243.

43. Harris PL, How TV, Jones DR. Prospective randomized clinical trial to compare in situ and reversed saphenous vein grafts for femoropopliteal bypass. *Br J Surg.* 1987; 74:252–255.

44. Moore WS, Malon JM. Vascular reconstruction in the diabetic patient. *Angiology.* 1978;29:741–747.

45. Barker WF. Peripheral vascular disease in diabetes: diagnosis and management. *Med Clin North Am.* 1971;55: 1045–1055.

46. Jensen LP, Schroeder TV, Lorentzen JE. In situ saphenous vein bypass surgery in diabetic patients. *European Journal of Vascular Surgery.* 1992;6:533–539.

47. Hurley JJ, Auer AI, Hershey FB, et al. Distal arterial reconstruction: patency and limb salvage in diabetics. *J Vasc Surg.* 1987;5:796–802.

48. Shah DM, Chang BB, Fitzgerald KM, et al. Durability of tibial artery bypass in diabetic patients. *Am J Surg.* 1988;156:133–135.

49. Rosenblatt MS, Quist WC, Sidawy AN, et al. Results of vein graft reconstruction of the lower extremity in diabetic and nondiabetic patients. *Surgery Gynecology and Obstetrics.* 1990;171:331–335.

50. Kwolek CJ, Pomposelli FB, Tannenbaum GA, et al. Peripheral vascular bypass in juvenile-onset diabetes mellitus: are aggressive revascularization attempts justified? *J Vasc Surg.* 1992;15:394–401.

51. Pomposelli FB Jr, Jepsen SJ, Gibbons GW, et al. Efficacy of the dorsal pedal bypass for limb salvage in diabetic patients: short-term observations. *J Vasc Surg.* 1990;11: 745–752.

52. Andros G, Harris RW, Salles-Cunha SX, et al. Bypass grafts to the ankle and foot. *J Vasc Surg.* 1988;7:785–794.

53. Klammer TW, Lambert GE, Richardson JD, et al. Utility of inframalleolar artery bypass grafting. *J Vasc Surg.* 1990; 11:164–170.

54. Shah DM, Darling RC III, Chang BB, et al. Is long vein bypass from groin to ankle a durable procedure? An analysis of a ten-year experience. *J Vasc Surg.* 1992;15:402–408.

55. Harrington EB, Harrington ME, Schanzer H, et al. The dorsalis pedis bypass: moderate success in difficult situations. *J Vasc Surg.* 1992;15:409–416.

56. Andros G, Harris RW, Saller-Cuhna SX, Dulawa LB, Oblath RW. Lateral plantar artery bypass grafting: defining the limits of foot revascularization. *J Vasc Surg.* 1989; 10:511–521.

57. Larsson U, Andersson GBJ. Partial amputation of the foot for diabetic or arteriosclerotic gangrene: results and factors of prognostic value. *J Bone Joint Surg.* 1978;60: 126–130.

58. Hughes CE, Johnson CC, Bamberger DM, et al. Treatment and long-term follow-up of foot infections in patients with diabetes or ischemia: a randomized, prospective, double blind comparison of cefoxitin and ceftizoxime. *Clin Ther.* 1987;10(suppl A):36–49.

59. Bose K. A surgical approach for the infected diabetic foot. *Int Orthop.* 1979;3:177–181.

60. Goldman FD. Deep space infections in the diabetic patient. *J Am Podiatr Med Assoc.* 1987;77:431–443.

61. Sinha S, Munichoodappa I, Kozak GP. Neuro-arthropathy (Charcot joints) in diabetes mellitus (clinical study of 101 cases). *Medicine.* 1972;51:191–210.

62. Newman LG, Waller J, Palestro CJ, et al. Unsuspected osteomyelitis in diabetic foot ulcers: diagnosis and monitoring by leukocyte scanning with indium 111 oxyquinoline. *JAMA.* 1991;266:1246–1251.

63. Keenan AM, Tindel NL, Alavi A. Diagnosis of pedal osteomyelitis in diabetic patients using current scintigraphic techniques. *Arch Intern Med.* 1989;149:2262–2266.

64. Park HM, Wheat J, Siddiqui AR, et al. Scintigraphic evaluation of diabetic osteomyelitis: concise communication. *J Nucl Med.* 1982;23:569–573.

65. Sachs W, Kanat IO. Radionucleotide scanning in osteomyelitis. *J Foot Surg.* 1986;25:311–314.

66. Eisenberg B, Wrege SS, Altman MI, et al. Bone scan: indium-WBC correlation in the diagnosis of osteomyelitis of the foot. *J Foot Surg.* 1989;28:532–536.

67. Erdman WA, Tamburro F, Jayson HT, et al. Osteomyelitis: characteristics and pitfalls of diagnosis with MR imaging. *Radiology.* 1991;180:533–539.

68. Sapico FL, Witte JL, Canawati HN, et al. The infected foot of the diabetic patient: quantitative microbiology and analysis of clinical features. *Reviews of Infectious Diseases.* 1984;6:S171–S176.

69. Wheat LJ, Allen SD, Henry M, et al. Diabetic foot infections: bacteriologic analysis. *Arch Intern Med.* 1986;146: 1935–1940.

70. Lipsky BA, Pecoraro RE, Larson SA, et al. Outpatient management of uncomplicated lower-extremity infections in diabetic patients. *Arch Intern Med.* 1990;150:790–797.

71. McIntyre KE Jr, Bailey SA, Malone JM, et al. Guillotine amputation in the treatment of nonsalvageable lower-extremity infections. *Arch Surg.* 1984;119:450–453.

72. McIntyre KE Jr, Bailey SA, Malone JM, et al. Toe and foot amputations. In: Ernst SB, Stanley JC, eds. *Current Therapy in Vascular Surgery.* 2nd ed. Philadelphia, Pa: BC Decker; 1991:694.

73. Tillo TH, Giurini JM, Habershaw GM, et al. Review of metatarsal osteotomies for the treatment of neuropathic ulcerations. *J Am Podiatr Med Assoc.* 1990;80:211–217.

74. Leslie CA, Sapico FL, Ginunas VJ, et al. Randomized controlled trial of topical hyperbaric oxygen for treatment of diabetic foot ulcers. *Diabetes Care.* 1988;11:111–115.

Section 9
Carotid Occlusive Disease

71

Noninvasive Evaluation of Carotid Artery Disease

David G. Stanley

Accurate, reliable, noninvasive vascular diagnostic laboratory tests are fundamental in evaluating patients with suspected carotid artery disease. After the initial evaluation, including a complete history and physical examination, the skilled clinician can accurately diagnose symptomatic carotid or vertebral artery disease. However, physical examination for carotid artery disease is limited primarily to listening for bruits over the carotid bifurcation and subclavian areas, palpating internal and external carotid pulses, and evaluating the patient for unequal radial pulses or brachial blood pressures. Thus, a noninvasive ultrasound test is generally the next diagnostic step in patients with suspected disease.

Historical Background

In the past, the presence of a carotid bruit was used to alert the clinician to possible carotid artery stenosis. Bruits are the result of turbulent flow through irregular, tortuous, or stenotic arteries. In the general population, asymptomatic carotid bruits occur in approximately 4% of the population over age 45. Carotid bruits are reported in about 8% of the population over age 75.[1-3]

Elderly hypertensive patients have been found to have as high as a 19% incidence of subclavicular or carotid bruits.[4] Female patients with hypertension, diabetes, or symptomatic vascular disease have a higher incidence of bruits. In patients with previous endarterectomy, asymptomatic bruits are found on the contralateral side in 25% to 40% of cases. Patients referred to specialists for aortoiliac or coronary artery disease have asymptomatic bruits 15% to 30% of the time.[5]

Some early studies suggested that carotid endarterectomy was not an efficacious procedure for stroke prevention because the annual stroke rate in patients with asymptomatic bruits is only 1% to 2%.[3,6] In retrospect the relatively low stroke rate is not surprising, because in a high-risk population, only approximately 50% of bruits correlate with significant (>75% diameter) arterial stenosis. In a recent study in Finland investigators found that bruits were 59% accurate in detecting moderate to significant (50% to 70% diameter) stenoses.[7] The sensitivity of bruits as a screening examination decreases as the degree of stenosis increases. In the Finnish study only 22% of patients with significant (88% to 100% diameter) stenosis had a bruit present.

Bruits are best viewed as a helpful indicator of turbulent flow that may or may not be atherosclerotic in etiology. The turbulent flow can also occur due to tortuous or kinked carotid arteries, hypertension, tachycardia, thyrotoxicosis, fibromuscular hyperplasia, atrioventricular malformations, and high output states such as found in patients with anemia. The detection of a bruit often varies among examiners. As illustrated in the Finnish study, some very highly stenotic and occluded arteries have insufficient flow and may not create enough turbulence for a bruit to be found. A number of patients with embolic transient ischemic attacks, and in particular Hollenhorst plaques, do not have flow-reducing stenosis.[8] Despite the unreliability of using bruits for the diagnosis of significant carotid stenosis, the asymptomatic bruit is certainly a clue for possible significant carotid artery disease and should be investigated by the examining physician.

In the early 1960s, with the advent of carotid endarterectomy, surgeons relied on arteriograms for confirmation of suspected carotid stenosis. Arteriography was introduced by Dos Santos and colleagues in 1931, when Dr. Dos Santos, clearly a self-confident man, injected contrast media into his own vessels and found that the arteries were visualized.[9] Since that time, selective carotid angiography has been the most accurate means of evaluating the carotid arteries. However, the mortality, morbidity, and expense associated with selective carotid angiography has limited its usefulness as a diagnostic screening test. Another noninvasive, accurate, reproducible test was needed as a screening test and for serial follow-up of patients.

Great enthusiasm greeted the advent of intravenous digital subtraction angiography. Because it is less invasive, it can be performed safely as an outpatient procedure. However, renal complications, dye allergy problems, and a high number of technically inadequate images have limited its usefulness. Few surgeons feel comfortable using only an intravenous digital subtraction angiography to make their treatment decisions.

In 1954 the ultrasonic Doppler technique was first reported for evaluation of the carotid artery.[10] In 1964 Goldberg reported the clinical use of velocity measurements for detection of carotid artery disease,[11] and in 1969 Brockenbrough popularized the Doppler flowmeter for detection of carotid stenosis and periorbital techniques for evaluating carotid collateral flow.[12] In 1974 Gee et al. developed ocular pneumoplethysmography for detection of decreased distal internal carotid artery and ophthalmic artery flow secondary to proximal carotid stenosis.[13] In addition, by the early 1970s, many surgeons used the handheld Doppler instrument to perform periorbital evaluations in their offices. This noninvasive study was used as an additional examination to determine which patients needed angiography.

In 1982 Kartchner and colleagues developed the carotid phonoangiograph.[14] The carotid phonoangiograph recorded the bruit sound wave patterns heard by the technician and displayed patterns that could be permanently recorded on Polaroid film. Also in 1982, color-coded echo flow images were possible by analyzing the Doppler frequency shift and representing various velocities as a color-coded flow within a diagram of the artery. The color-coded arterial map depicted high-velocity signals as blue, moderately increased velocity signals as yellow, and normal-velocity signals as red. These two studies were helpful for a time. The continued evolution and refinement of ultrasound imaging and blood flow measurement by Doppler imaging has now rendered these studies archaic and rarely used in the modern diagnostic laboratory.

Modern Duplex Ultrasound Evaluation

In 1969 Olinger was able to use ultrasound technology to view the carotid arteries. Subsequently, the development of high-resolution imaging rapidly accelerated.[15] Ultrasound imaging alone was soon found inadequate to accurately diagnose carotid stenosis. Areas of calcification caused sonic shadowing and an inability to view the entire artery. Zones of hemorrhage or thrombus were echo free and had the same appearance as intra-arterial blood. Therefore, in 1974, a Doppler velocity device was added to the image system to provide more accurate evaluation of stenosis and the ability to distinguish soft plaque or thrombus from pulsatile blood by velocity measurements.[16]

Continuous wave and pulsed wave Doppler systems are used for noninvasive blood flow velocity measurements. Continuous wave detectors are the simplest, with two separate crystals on the probe, one transmitting and one receiving simultaneously. Continuous wave detectors interrogate all velocities in the path of the sound beam and may include more than one vessel. Pulse-gated Doppler systems use one crystal that alternately transmits a short burst of high-frequency sound waves followed by a period in which the crystal is in a receiving mode. The pulse-gated Doppler uses a small sample volume that can be placed in the center of the blood vessel. This reveals information about the amount of turbulence in the flow, called spectral broadening. By using the ultrasound image to direct the Doppler sample volume placement, the technician can examine the area of the suspected stenosis. Thus, a more accurate peak frequency or velocity measurement is obtained. The examiner not only hears the audio signal but also visualizes the spectral analysis displayed as a sonogram frequency on a time graph. The accuracy of the peak frequency or velocity depends greatly on the angle of measurement. Velocity should be measured at an angle of 60 degrees (or, if not possible, at an angle of less than 60 degrees) to avoid misleading data. Spectral broadening of the waveform can also be used as an indicator of turbulence in the vessel.

Modern duplex ultrasound systems combine real-time B-mode scanning with pulsed wave Doppler spectrum analysis. Duplex instruments can demonstrate high-quality gray-scale images of plaques and color flow images that are coded to the velocity of the arterial blood stream. Doppler sample volume can be precisely placed. The sample can come from as small as 1 mm³ of area within the stenosed vessel. Images can be obtained in the transverse and sagittal dimension as well as anterior, lateral, and posterior views from the clavicle to the angle of the mandible. This evaluation is now the mainstay of the modern vascular laboratory.

In addition to duplex ultrasound, transcranial Doppler ultrasonography now allows the ultrasound technician to evaluate the intracranial arteries and the circle of Willis. Transcranial Doppler uses low-frequency (2-MHz) pulsed wave Doppler through various thin bone areas of the skull such as the temporal bone, foramen magnum, and orbit. The Doppler signal is evaluated by color flow image and spectral analysis. This technique allows the physician to gather more information concerning collateral flow distal to an internal carotid artery occlusion and intracranial stenoses. Some surgeons also report using transcranial Doppler to monitor patients' cerebral blood flow during carotid endarterectomy and to help determine which patients may benefit from intraoperative shunts. Transcranial Doppler with color flow imaging can be useful in revealing large, non-thrombosed cerebral aneurysms through its ability to show blood flow patterns.[17] It is also helpful in visualizing and determining the hemodynamic status of carotid–cavernous sinus fistulas.[18]

Transcranial testing is not considered a necessary component of a complete cerebrovascular examination. A significant number of technically inadequate studies have contributed to its lack of acceptance. Otis and colleagues at Scripps Clinic report that using a galactose/palmitic acid-based microbubble contrast agent increases the technical adequacy of the transcranial ultrasound significantly.[19] Transcranial Doppler with color flow imaging is an emerging technique that provides interesting information of limited clinical significance.

Various nuclear brain scanning techniques were used over the years as an aid in evaluating carotid artery stenosis. In the 1960s, some patients were suspected of having carotid artery stenosis or occlusion when one cerebral hemisphere had a delayed image on the scan compared with the contralateral hemisphere. Computed tomography scanning has proven useful for documenting possible infarcts secondary to emboli and for ruling out aneurysms, brain tumors, and other intracranial pathology.

Magnetic resonance angiography is emerging as an accurate way to evaluate arterial flow in carotid and vertebral arteries and the circle of Willis. Blakely and others recently published extensive reviews of the literature that demonstrated that magnetic resonance angiography is not more accurate than carotid duplex in predicting occlusion or >70% stenosis of the carotid arteries.[20,21]

Carotid Testing in the Vascular Laboratory

The purpose of noninvasive carotid evaluation is to detect significant carotid disease and to provide the clinician with accurate information regarding (1) the degree of stenosis, (2) the morphology of the plaque (soft, fibrous, calcific, subintimal hemorrhage, and presence or absence of ulceration), and (3) the occlusion of the internal carotid artery at the bifurcation or distally. No one diagnostic test is capable of consistently giving such detailed information, so a variety of tests have been developed for use by the vascular diagnostician.

Indirect Methods of Detecting Carotid Artery Stenosis

Indirect methods of detecting carotid artery stenosis measure changes in distal pressures, distal internal carotid artery pressures, and peripheral arterial blood flow. Two widely used methods are ocular pneumoplethysmography and periorbital Doppler examination. In our laboratory, the periorbital Doppler examination is performed along with direct spectrum analysis of the ophthalmic artery. Unfortunately, indirect techniques are helpful only in lesions that reduce distal blood pressure. Even with proximal stenosis, if the patient has a widely patent circle of Willis, the distal pressure may not be reduced, which results in a false-negative examination. However, in patients with proximal stenoses and positive indirect studies, it can be assumed that collateral flow may not be completely compensating for the proximal stenoses. These types of noninvasive studies are helpful to the vascular surgeon in evaluating which patients are most likely to be at risk of stroke from a carotid occlusion and whether a shunt may be helpful during carotid endarterectomy. If the cervical carotid artery examination is negative and the indirect study is positive, the patient may have a carotid siphon stenosis. Indirect studies cannot reliably differentiate between occlusion and high-grade stenosis of the proximal internal carotid artery.

Ocular pneumoplethysmography evaluates the ophthalmic artery pressure by a suction device placed on the eyeball and ophthalmodynamometry. Although there may be slight discomfort to the patient, this test is generally used and is relatively simple to perform and interpret. In addition to detecting proximal occlusion or stenosis of the internal carotid artery, it can also be used to evaluate collateral flow to the ipsilateral internal carotid artery by measuring the ophthalmic artery pressure before and after externally occluding the ipsilateral common carotid artery. The limitations of this procedure are that it cannot be used in patients with severe cataracts or severe hypertension in which the systolic end point cannot be measured. Unfortunately, hypertension and cataracts are fairly common in the patient age group that requires this study.

Ocular plethysmography measures the arrival time of the ocular pulse wave in each eye and compares one ocular pulse with the arrival time of the contralateral side. The relatively simple test is not limited by severe hypertension; however, interpretation by evaluating the pulse wave curves can be complex. Digital pulse timing with ocular plethysmography uses a system with suction cups applied to the cornea that evaluates the ocular pulse, and photo-sealed detectors on the earlobes detect pulses from the external carotid system. The time differential between upstrokes of the pulse waves is measured in milliseconds. A 30-ms delay in ear-to-ear pulses indicates stenosis of the ipsilateral external carotid artery, and a delay greater than 10 ms in eye-to-eye pulses indicates stenosis of the ipsilateral internal carotid artery. A 30-ms delay in both eye-to-ear pulses suggests bilateral internal carotid stenosis or occlusion. A 30-ms delay in ear-to-eye pulse bilaterally indicates bilateral external carotid artery stenosis or occlusion.

Periorbital Doppler examination evaluates the velocity and direction of blood flow in branches of the ophthalmic artery. Flow should proceed outward from the orbit. When the external carotid circulation is compressed there should be a slight increase or no change in flow in the ophthalmic artery branches on the ipsilateral side.

If the ipsilateral internal carotid artery is occluded or significantly stenotic antegrade flow through the ophthalmic artery into the periorbital arteries is reduced. Occasionally, reverse flow is noted in a patient with proximal internal carotid artery stenosis and may decrease or cease with compression maneuvers. A directional Doppler instrument is necessary for this study. The best results are obtained by compressing multiple collateral vessels such as the temporal and supraorbital vessels concomitantly. This technique increases the accuracy to approximately 85% to 99%.[22] This test is relatively simple to perform and interpret but depends on the technician's experience and care in performing the study.

Duplex and Color Flow Examination

The most commonly used and accepted direct noninvasive methods of carotid evaluation are duplex gray-scale and Doppler color flow imaging (DCFI). These duplex instruments commonly image at 5.0 to 10.0 MHz with pulse-gated, angle-corrected Doppler transducer operating at 3.0 to 5.0 MHz. Carotid scanning generally is performed at 5.0 to 7.5 MHz. The transducer should be small enough to allow access to the small areas of the neck. Another important feature is a Doppler angle correction that electronically calculates for changes in Doppler beam angles. The technician and interpreter must be familiar with the principles of Doppler ultrasound because both duplex and DCFI have limitations and certain artifacts that can cause false readings. Extensive plaque calcification and deep or tortuous vessels may result in inadequate studies. The limitations on the maximum Doppler shift frequency can be measured at different depths of tissue. High velocities can result in frequencies that are in excess of the Nyquist limit, which results in an aliasing of the spectral waveform. The primary purpose of the gray-scale image is to (1) detect the area of disease, (2) evaluate the composition of the plaque, and (3) determine whether ulceration is present.

The degree of stenosis is better evaluated by Doppler spectral analysis than by image alone. Doppler spectral analysis measures the peak frequency or velocity of the arterial flow. As the carotid artery narrows, the volume of flow is maintained by increasing the velocity through the stenosed portion of the artery. Throughout the artery,

the flow is essentially normal up to a diameter narrowing of approximately 60% diameter or 70% to 80% area. A 40% to 60% diameter stenosis results in increased velocities to maintain the volume of flow. Hemodynamically significant effects begin at >60% diameter or >84% area stenosis as flow volume decreases.

Protocol for Noninvasive Cerebrovascular Examination

For consistently accurate tests, specific procedures must be followed by the vascular technician. The technician should obtain a brief, pertinent cerebrovascular history including indications for the tests (Table 71.1). Technicians obtain bilateral brachial blood pressures and auscultate for aortic, subclavian, and carotid bruits. All examinations are previewed and then recorded for review by the interpreter and for future reference if necessary. The preview should include the vessel portrayed in the anterior, lateral, and posterior longitudinal approaches as well as cross-sectional images. The clearest views are then recorded. The longitudinal examination is begun as proximal as possible in the common carotid artery. The technician proceeds cephalad and comments on the vessel wall characteristics.

The technician measures and comments on the location and characteristics of the plaque seen on the vessel walls. The suspected presence of subintimal hemorrhage and/or ulceration and plaque is carefully documented. A Doppler sample is obtained with the pulsed wave

TABLE 71.1. Indications for cerebrovascular examination.

Symptoms
Visual disturbances (amaurosis fugax, blurred vision, diplopia, Hollenhorst plaque, or sparkles)
Unilateral hemiplegia
Sensory or motor deficits
Speech disturbance (slurred or aphasia)

Asymptomatic carotid bruit

History of nonspecific transient ischemic attack symptoms

Known arteriosclerotic cardiovascular disease (e.g., coronary, aortoiliac, or extremity disease)

Risk factors
Strong family history of cardiovascular disease or strokes
Diabetes mellitus
Hypertension
Hypercholesterolemia
Smoking history

Preoperative examination for older patients who are to undergo major surgery

Follow-up of patients with known disease for possible progression of plaque

Endarterectomy (intraoperative assessment and postoperative follow-up)

High risk for carotid angiography, (e.g. allergy to dye)

Doppler transducer in the common carotid artery, carotid bulb, proximal and distal internal carotid arteries, external carotid artery, and vertebral artery. In examinations with no observed plaque, a representative sample of each artery is sufficient. If plaque is seen in the vessel, a Doppler sample is obtained proximal to the stenosis, within the stenosis, and distal to the stenosis.

A transverse image is obtained beginning as proximal as possible in the common carotid. (An image of the innominate and subclavian arteries is also included whenever possible.) The examination proceeds cephalad to the carotid bulb and internal and external carotid arteries. If plaque is present, the diameter of the vessel and the patent area remaining are measured when possible (i.e., 3.5-mm patent area in an 8-mm bulb).

Plaque Identification

Evaluation of plaque includes a description of the plaque as seen during carotid imaging. The composition, character, and extent of the plaque are noted. Plaque composition is described as soft, fibrous, calcific, or subintimal hemorrhage. Soft plaque is seen as soft gray echoes with a color lighter than that of the vessel wall. Fibrous plaque is seen as being densely echogenic and brighter than or equal to the image of the vessel walls. Calcific plaque, which causes acoustic shadowing and subintimal hemorrhage due to its lack of echogenicity, is seen as an anechoic area.

The character of the plaque is described as smooth, irregular, or ulcerated. The extent is measured by the following grades: grade 1 (0%–20%), grade 2 (20%–75%), grade 3 (75%–90%), grade 4 (90%–99%), and occluded. Ulcers must be measured and recorded in the longitudinal and transverse planes. Other observed data (i.e., tortuous vessels, thyroid cyst, aneurysm, and lymphadenopathy) are noted on the patient's worksheet. Each vessel is noted on the ultrasound imaging worksheet, with the predominant component listed first.

Plaque Morphology

Carotid-origin transient ischemic attacks and strokes are primarily the result of emboli from unstable carotid bifurcation plaques rather than from decreased flow due to high-grade stenosis or occlusion.[23] Soft plaques are the most frequent cause of emboli of carotid origin and may be composed of soft cholesterol material, platelets, or more frequently blood clots secondary to subintimal hemorrhage.[24] Following subintimal hemorrhage, the plaque may either increase greatly in size with secondary stenosis or occlusion or erode through a thin intima to form an ulceration with subsequent embolization of the

TABLE 71.2. Risk of cerebrovascular events in asymptomatic patients over 5 years' observation by plaque composition and stenosis.

Type of plaque	Area stenosis (%)	Patients	Events	Event (%)
Calcified	> 75	37	4	11
Dense	> 75	42	27	64
Soft	< 75	47	14	31
Soft	> 75	42	42	100

Adapted with permission from O'Holleran et al.[29]

thrombus.[25] Carotid angiography is nonspecific, and findings are unrelated to intramural thrombus. Duplex scanning is the test of choice in detecting intraplaque hemorrhage.[26]

Several authors have published articles that demonstrate the high risk of stroke in patients with these unstable plaques.[22,27–28] Dr. J. M. Johnson followed asymptomatic patients with soft, dense, and calcific plaques for 5 years. He found that plaque composition was an excellent predictor of cerebrovascular events. Patients with asymptomatic calcific plaques (>75% area stenosis) followed for 5 years had an 11% incidence of neurological events, primarily transient ischemic attacks. Patients with asymptomatic dense or fibrous plaques with more than 75% area of stenosis had a 60% incidence of transient ischemic attacks or strokes. Patients with soft plaques with 75% or greater stenosis had a 100% incidence of neurological events after 4 years (Table 71.2). Two of these patients had strokes while undergoing carotid angiography.[29] In our experience, the majority of the soft plaques found on ultrasound imaging are related to subintimal hemorrhage.

Vertebral and Subclavian Artery Investigation

After a thorough investigation of the carotid arteries, the vertebral and subclavian arteries are viewed longitudinally. Stenosis of these vessels most often occurs at their origin. A Doppler signal is obtained at the vessel's origin, if possible, and the anteroposterior diameter of the vertebral artery is measured. Recordings should be as concise as possible. Spectral waveforms are recorded and hard copies are obtained using a suitable printer. Indirect tests such as ocular pneumoplethysmography or ophthalmic and periorbital Doppler signals are performed when indicated.

If a subclavian artery stenosis is noted, the patient is also evaluated for subclavian steal. Indications for subclavian steal evaluation include abnormal subclavian artery peak systolic frequency or velocity, asymmetrical brachial blood pressures (>10 mm Hg blood pressure differential), arm ischemia symptoms, and posterior circulation symptoms.

The subclavian artery signal is located bilaterally, and peak systolic frequency or velocity is recorded. A blood pressure cuff is applied to the affected arm (taking either the arm with lower pressure or the arm with higher subclavian frequency). The ipsilateral vertebral artery is located and direction of blood flow is determined. If the flow is reversed, a continuous steal is present and no further evaluation is needed. If an intermittent or transient steal is suspected, the blood pressure cuff is inflated approximately 20 mm Hg higher than the systolic pressure in the affected arm while the technician observes the vertebral artery waveform. After 3 minutes, the cuff is deflated rapidly and any change in characteristic of the vertebral artery waveform is noted. The waveform is frozen on the analyzer screen and the results printed.

Continuous steal results show a reverse in the vertebral artery signal before blood pressure cuff inflation. In transient steal, flow in the vertebral artery is antegrade in systole and reversed in diastole before the cuff is inflated. On cuff release, flow is reversed only. In addition, there may be augmentation of the signal. Latent steal abnormalities show an immediate decrease in the systolic peak of the vertebral artery on cuff release.

Noninvasive cerebrovascular studies must be of high quality and accurate for proper interpretation. Ideally, the interpreting physician should have clinical experience in the diagnosis and treatment of vascular disease to make interpretation of the studies clinically relevant. One advantage of vascular specialists interpreting the study results is that the pathology seen during the duplex studies is visualized again in the operating room. Of course, physician interpreters should have training in evaluating and interpreting carotid studies and should be monitored by more experienced physicians early on.

Interpretation of Carotid Studies

The primary motivation of the medical director and other interpreting physicians of a vascular laboratory must be to provide clinically relevant information of importance to the referring physician. The medical director must ensure that all interpreting physicians have adequate initial interpretive training and participate in postgraduate courses and quality assurance meetings. The interpreting physicians should be compensated, but monetary gain should not be the primary reason for interpreting studies. The physician should know the capabilities and limitations of the technicians and the equipment used for examinations. The medical director is responsible for overseeing the clinical operation of the laboratory, for regular dialogue and meetings with the technical and medical staff, and for quality assurance via correlation of the studies with contrast angiograms and specimens found at surgery. Statistics should be kept on

the accuracy of the testing, and discrepancies should be investigated. All interpreting physicians, and particularly the medical director, must supervise the technicians who perform the studies and encourage them to become certified in their field of noninvasive testing, give them frequent feedback directly and through regularly scheduled quality assurance meetings, and ensure that they regularly attend continuing medical education programs on a national level. Each vascular laboratory must have rules for interpretation to provide consistency among the interpreting physicians. The interpretation format should also be followed by all physicians.

At our noninvasive laboratory, cerebrovascular imaging includes a brief record of the patient's age, risk factors, and symptoms. The instrumentation for and quality of the test are recorded. The common internal and external carotid arteries, including longitudinal and transverse views with specific references to the location of the plaque and its characteristics, are described. Plaque characteristics noted include whether the plaque is homogeneous or heterogeneous and whether the components are soft, fibrous, calcific, soft with subintimal hemorrhage, or ulcerated. Ulcerations are described by depth, as illustrated in Table 71.3. Carotid occlusion is recognized by the indications noted in Table 71.4.

Technicians routinely measure the peak systolic and end-diastolic velocities. Peak systolic velocity is documented at the area of most severe stenosis, with care taken to obtain a proper Doppler angle. End-diastolic velocity is again documented at the area of greatest stenosis in the carotid artery and measured at the end of diastole.

TABLE 71.3. Ulcerations described by depth.

Ulceration	Depth (mm)
Type I	1–2
Type II	3–4
Type III	> 4

TABLE 71.4. Characteristics of carotid occulusions.

- Speckled, heterogeneous, weakly echogenic material within the lumen
- Lack of lateral pulsations in the internal carotid artery on B-mode image
- Vertical pulsations in the occluded artery or the artery immediately proximal to the occlusion
- Absent Doppler flow sounds in the area of occlusion
- Drumbeat sound proximal to the occlusion
- Observation on spectrum analysis of flow dropping to zero during diastole in the common carotid artery proximal to the occlusion
- Contralateral common carotid artery has increased peak frequency (asymmetry of the common carotid artery complexes)
- Increased peak frequency in the ipsilateral external carotid artery, especially during diastole

The technician must obtain accurate velocity measurements. When angle is corrected, the velocity measurements are more consistently accurate for degree of stenosis than either Doppler imaging or arteriography.

Depending on the preferences of the interpreter and technician and the machine used, frequency shift values rather than blood velocity measurements may be computed. Each is equally accurate assuming that the same transducer is used and proper sampling technique is followed. Frequency shift values in kilohertz can be readily converted to velocity measurements in meters per second using the following formula:

$$\text{Velocity (m/s)} = (0.78) \, [\text{frequency shift (KHz)}] / [\text{transducer frequency (MHz)}] \, (\text{cosine of the Doppler angle}).$$

Doppler waveform spectral broadening is distal to the stenosis in the area of maximum turbulence. Spectral broadening can be of particular assistance to the interpreter when stenosis is >70% or when sonic shadowing from a calcified plaque does not allow accurate velocity measurements at the site of maximum stenosis.

TABLE 71.5. Grading system for internal carotid artery stenosis.

Grade	Area stenosis
1	0%–20%
2	20%–75%
3	75%–90%
4	90%–99%
5	Occluded

Internal carotid artery stenosis is graded as noted in Table 71.5. Some interpreters give the degree of stenosis in diameter reduction and others in area reduction. Physician interpreters and technicians should use a single standard within a given laboratory. Arteriograms most frequently express stenoses as diameter reduction, and ultrasounds most often express them as area reduction. Generally, it is better to express stenoses as area reduction because it more accurately portrays the hemodynamic consequences. Figure 71.1, which assumes a circumferential plaque, graphically demonstrates on an *x–y* scatter chart the relationship between diameter and area reduction. Some plaques, of course, are not cir-

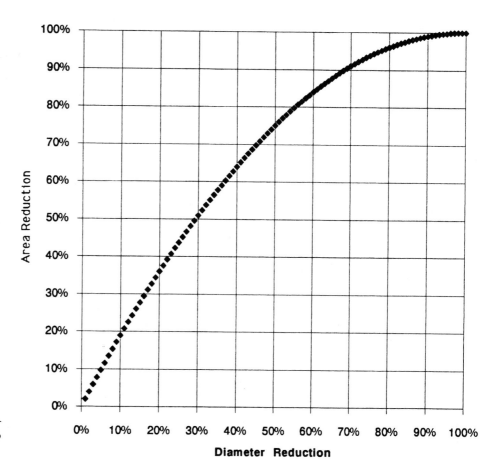

FIGURE 71.1. Conversion of percentage reduction in diameter to percentage reduction in area.

cumferential and present an interpretive problem in arteriography given its inherent two-dimensional nature.

DCFI Interpretation Criteria

DCFI requires slightly different interpretive skills. DCFI machines may use transducers of different megahertz and offer more sophisticated software and processing techniques than machines that provide only gray-scale images. DCFI offers both color and gray-scale images. The colorized blood flow image can be helpful in diagnosing areas of high turbulence, where the color patterns become mixed. It is also useful in differentiating occlusion from high-grade stenosis, where a small string of color seen through the stenosis may help distinguish between the two. If the DCFI does not reveal a patent artery, an arteriogram is recommended to distinguish between high-grade stenosis and occlusion. DCFI is helpful, but interpreters should be wary of relying too heavily on the color images because aliasing, technician error, and machine maladjustments can result in inaccurate color images. The interpretive criteria summarized in Table 71.6 are widely used for the categorization of carotid artery disease. Figures 71.2 through 71.5 show varying degrees of stenosis as demonstrated by representative spectral waveforms. Figures 71.6 through 71.12 show representative gray-scale and DCFI images.

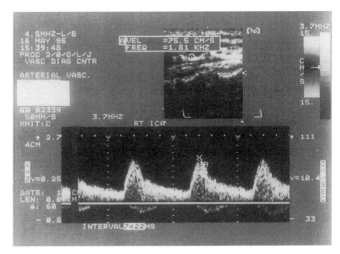

FIGURE 71.3. Moderately diseased internal carotid artery waveform with spectral broadening.

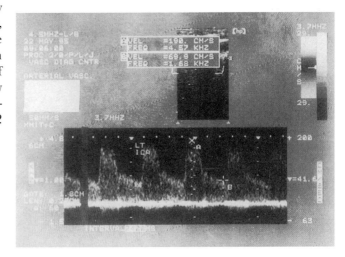

FIGURE 71.4. Severely diseased internal carotid artery waveform.

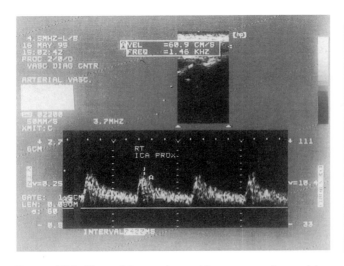

FIGURE 71.2. Normal internal carotid artery waveform with a clear spectral window.

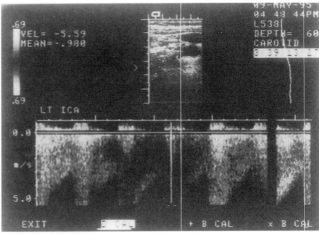

FIGURE 71.5. Critically diseased internal carotid artery waveform.

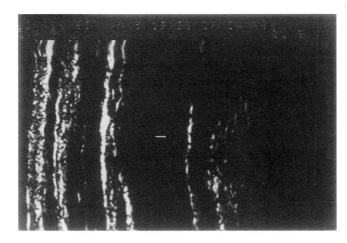

FIGURE 71.6. Essentially normal internal carotid artery and carotid bulb on gray-scale imaging.

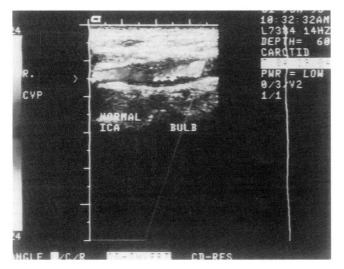

FIGURE 71.7. Longitudinal normal internal carotid artery and bulb on Doppler color flow imaging.

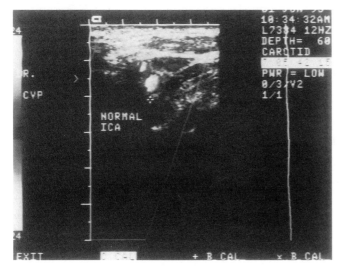

FIGURE 71.8. Transverse normal internal carotid artery and bulb on Doppler color flow imaging.

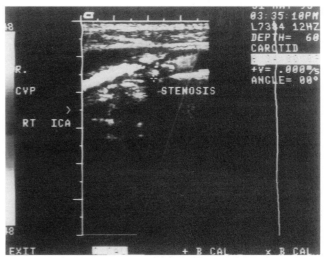

FIGURE 71.9. Longitudinal significantly diseased internal carotid artery and bulb on Doppler color flow imaging.

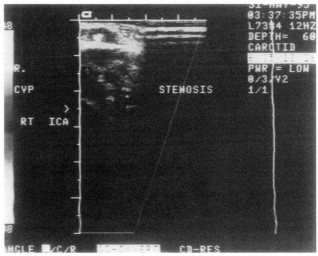

FIGURE 71.10. Transverse significantly diseased internal carotid artery and bulb on Doppler color flow imaging.

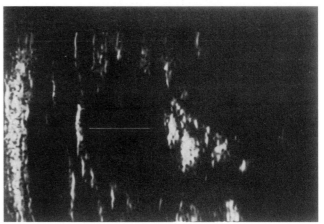

FIGURE 71.11. Internal carotid artery with irregular plaque and ulceration on gray-scale imaging.

TABLE 71.6. Diagnostic criteria for categories of carotid artery disease.

Grade	ICA peak systolic		Waveform description	Image description
	Velocity (cm/sec)	Frequency (Hz)		
Normal/mild 0%–20% area reduction	< 125	< 4000	Peak systolic window clear Minimal or no spectral broadening	Minimal plaque may or may not be visualized
Moderate 20%–75% area reduction	< 125	< 4,000	Decreased or no window Spectral broadening	Plaque characteristics visualized
Severe 75%–90% area reduction	>125	>5000	Diastolic flow increased Diffuse spectral broadening	Plaque characteristics visualized
Critical 90%–99% area reduction	>140	>9000	Diastolic flow increased Marked spectral broadening	Plaque characteristics visualized
Occluded	No signal	No signal	CCA: no flow or reversed ICA: not applicable	No flow seen

CCA, common artoid artery; ICA, internal cartoid artery.

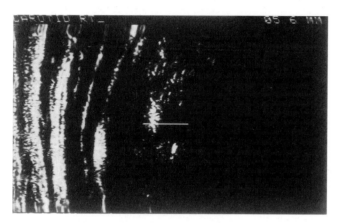

FIGURE 71.12. Carotid bulb with sonic shadowing.

Interpretation Summary

The interpreting physician should always try to make the conclusions as clinically relevant as possible. The common, external, and internal carotid arteries should each be mentioned, particularly noting the approximate percent stenosis. If known, the plaque surface characteristics and the type of plaque should be described. The status of the subclavian and vertebral arteries should be noted and characterized as either normal, mildly diseased, moderately diseased, significantly diseased (flow reducing), or occluded. If a subclavian steal is found it should be mentioned and categorized as latent, transient, or continuous. The equipment used and whether the image was unsatisfactory, poor, fair, good, or excellent should be noted. The physician should also mention whether the study results are limited due to technical difficulty.

Sometimes a physician interpreter's comments are helpful. If findings are inconclusive, the interpreter may recommend an arteriogram, magnetic resonance angiogram, or repeat ultrasound (at no charge). He or she may also suggest when a follow-up study could be ordered and the reason why further workup may be necessary. If the study is not the original study, the interpreter and technician should have the previous study available for comparison and comment on any progression or changes in the plaque.

Correlations of Noninvasive Carotid Studies

Noninvasive cerebrovascular studies offer patients a comfortable, convenient, low-cost method for determining carotid artery pathology without mortality and morbidity risks. Arteriograms are often four times as expensive as noninvasive ultrasound studies (Figure 71.13). Arteriograms also produce stroke in 1.2% of patients according to the Asymptomatic Carotid Atherosclerosis Study.[30] Because of these factors and the emergence of noninvasive carotid ultrasound as a highly accurate modality, there is a growing trend to perform carotid endarterectomy on the basis of the noninvasive ultrasound examination only.[31–34] When duplex scanning is used by the vascular surgeon to replace arteriography, several issues should be addressed.

The most important requirement is that the vascular laboratory that performs the tests have a rigorous and ongoing quality assurance program. The vascular laboratory must be able to supply this information. If the laboratory is affiliated with a hospital, it should also participate in that institution's quality assurance program and Joint Commission on Accreditation of Hospitals proceedings.

Knowing the accuracy of the noninvasive testing available in each facility is thus critical. Monitoring the qual-

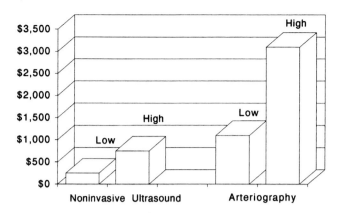

FIGURE 71.13. Cost comparison of cerebrovascular studies.

ity and accuracy of carotid artery testing is required in modern noninvasive vascular laboratories. Indeed, rigorous and statistically valid quality assurance is essential for accreditation by the Intersocietal Commission for the Accreditation of Vascular Laboratories (ICAVL). A specific quality assurance plan that includes a list of specific duties and the persons responsible for them, written statistical methods, and a schedule for meetings and methods by which the information is disseminated to all affected parties is necessary.

Quality Assurance of Carotid Artery Investigations

Careful prospective studies in our laboratory that compare the noninvasive test data to arteriograms and to findings at surgery have convinced us that, in many cases, patient treatment, whether medical or surgical, can be determined on the basis of noninvasive studies. In our laboratory, carotid artery evaluation reports that contain the results of arteriography and/or noninvasive testing and the operating room carotid artery plaque measurements and findings are compiled each month. During regularly scheduled quality assurance meetings, the medical and technical staff review the monthly results and carefully evaluate false-positive and false-negative studies to determine the cause of the error and, if possible, to formulate strategies to avoid similar problems in the future. The noninvasive study reports, noninvasive videotapes, arteriography reports, arteriography films, and operative reports are available for review. Discussion focuses on whether the correct clinical decision was made as a result of the carotid ultrasound study.

Following the quality assurance meetings, the data are compiled for statistical analysis as outlined in a later section. The methodology offers precise and statistically valid measurement. The quality assurance reports are reviewed to collect data for the number of true-positive,

false-positive, false-negative, and true-negative results using two separate gold standards. The first gold standard is arteriography, to which the duplex on the operative and nonoperative sides are separately compared. The second gold standard (on the operative side) is the operating room measurement of the plaque specimen by graded dilators and calipers at the time of removal, to which the duplex and arteriography are separately compared.

To be considered a positive finding, the test has to reveal clinically significant stenosis of >75%. To be considered a negative finding the test has to reveal stenosis of <75%. To be considered a false-positive result, the test has to be read as >75% stenosis and be >+10% off the gold standard measurement. To be considered a false-negative result, the test has to be read as <75% stenosis and be <−10% off the gold standard measurement. For valid comparison, the noninvasive and arteriographic studies must be performed within 3 months of each other (except for 99% stenosis versus occlusion, which must be performed within 1 month).

The data are then displayed in 2 × 2 dichotomous diagnostic decision matrices for ease of manipulation. This yields four matrices. Then the sensitivity, specificity, positive predictive value, negative predictive value, and overall accuracy of the different methodologies are calculated. Sensitivity indicates the percentage of tests that correctly diagnose that disease is present. Specificity indicates the percentage of tests that correctly diagnose that disease is not present. The positive predictive value indicates how likely it is that disease is present with a positive test result. The negative predictive value indicates how likely it is that disease is not present with a negative test result. Table 71.7 shows sample 2 × 2 decision matrices and sensitivity, specificity, and positive and negative predictive values.

Each carotid study is also reviewed to compare the exact correlation with arteriogram findings within four treatment categories. The four treatment categories are as follows: 0% to 25% stenosis (not significant), 25% to 75% stenosis (moderate), 75% to 99% stenosis (significant), and occluded. The exact correlation percentage, P_o, and the kappa statistic, κ, are then calculated. The kappa statistic is a measure of how well the test correlates with the gold standard and indicates its individual predictive value. Table 71.8 shows an example of an exact correlation matrix.

When Is Arteriography Needed?

Arteriograms are valuable in assessing brachiocephalic artery pathology in patients where ultrasound evaluation is suboptimal due to the anatomical location of the artery or technically inadequate images. Patients with

TABLE 71.7. Accuracy of noninvasive studies and arteriogram reports versus surgical specimen.

Gold standard arteriogram

		≥ 75% stenosis	< 75% stenosis
NIV (operative)	Positive	True positive 271	False positive 15
	Negative	False negative 18	True negative 18

Sensitivity	93.77%
Specificity	54.55%
Positive predictive value	94.76%
Negative predictive value	50.00%
Overall accuracy	89.75%

Gold standard arteriogram

		≥ 75% stenosis	< 75% stenosis
NIV (nonoperative)	Positive	True positive 84	False positive 18
	Negative	False negative 8	True negative 112

Sensitivity	91.30%
Specificity	86.15%
Positive predictive value	82.35%
Negative predictive value	93.33%
Overall accuracy	88.29%

Gold standard surgery specimen

		≥ 75% stenosis	< 75% stenosis
Arteriogram	Positive	True positive 309	False positive 4
	Negative	False negative 16	True negative 9

Sensitivity	95.08%
Specificity	69.23%
Positive predictive value	98.72%
Negative predictive value	36.00%
Overall accuracy	94.08%

Gold standard surgery specimen

		≥ 75% stenosis	< 75% stenosis
NIV	Positive	True positive 596	False positive 2
	Negative	False negative 25	True negative 12

Sensitivity	95.97%
Specificity	85.71%
Positive predictive value	99.67%
Negative predictive value	32.43%
Overall accuracy	95.75%

From Vascular Diagnostics Center of Oak Ridge, Oak Ridge, Tenn. Used with permission.
NIV, noninvasive

atypical neurological symptoms may require thoracic or intracranial evaluation by arteriograms. Examples where arteriograms are especially helpful include the following:

1. Aortic arch and intrathoracic carotid and vertebral artery disease are addressed by use of arteriography for patients with symptoms but without significant cervical carotid artery disease and those with noninvasive findings of subclavian, vertebral, or distal internal carotid artery disease.
2. Arteriograms are no longer ordered specifically to look for carotid siphon disease or tandem lesions. Reviews of patients with tandem lesions have demonstrated that the risk of carotid endarterectomy is not significantly increased and in the vast majority of patients symptoms are relieved.[35,36]
3. Concern that patients may have intracranial tumors, cerebral aneurysms, or other vascular malformations has been found to be of little importance. Akers et al. reported on 1000 arteriograms obtained in patients with suspected cerebral vascular pathology. Significant information revealed by the arteriography was more than discounted by the higher morbidity from the arteriograms.[37] Still, it is prudent to combine computed tomography scans and noninvasive studies in selected patients for a more complete intracranial workup. This approach is most commonly indicated in patients with previous strokes or atypical symptoms or complaints.
4. Controversy continues regarding the diagnosis of ulcerations in arteriography versus duplex imaging. The accuracy of the studies depends on the dedication of the ultrasound technician or the radiologist in obtaining multiple views and looking diligently for ulceration. Goodson et al. reported sensitivity for detecting ulcers as 90% with duplex technique and 54% for arteriography.[38] In a series of patients, O'Donnell et al. reported that 87% of ulcers were identified by ultrasound whereas arteriography diagnosed only 59%.[27] Senkowsky reported on 21 patients with tran-

TABLE 71.8. 1991–1994 correlation of cartoid duplex studies.

Gold standard angiogram categories

Carotid scan categories	0–25% (t_1)	25–75% (t_2)	75–99% (t_3)	Occluded (t_4)
0–25% (m_1)	8			
25–75% (m_2)		116	22	1
75–99% (m_3)	1	29	274	
Occluded (m_4)			3	35

$a_1 =$ 8
$a_2 =$ 116
$a_3 =$ 274
$a_4 =$ 35
$\Sigma a_1{:}a_4 =$ 433

$P_o = \Sigma a_1{:}a_4 / n =$ 0.88548

$m_1 =$ 8
$m_2 =$ 139
$m_3 =$ 304
$m_4 =$ 38
$n = \Sigma m_1{:}m_4 =$ 489

$P_c = \Sigma m_1 * t_1{:}m_4 * t_4 / n{\char`\^}2 =$ 0.470435

Kappa $= P_o - P_c / 1 - P_c =$ 0.783748

This kappa value indicates that the carotid duplex scans have some individual predictive value.

$t_1 =$ 9
$t_2 =$ 145
$t_3 =$ 299
$t_4 =$ 36

From Vascular Diagnostics Center of Oak Ridge, Oak Ridge, Tenn. Used with permission.

sient ischemic attacks who had normal arteriograms; B-mode ultrasound subsequently identified ulcerative plaques. These patients were found to have 20% to 50% stenosis and ulceration at the time of surgery.[39]

Moore et al. have demonstrated in two retrospective studies that medium and large ulcerative plaques carry a high stroke risk.[40] Dixon et al. reported that patients with large ulcerations develop stroke at rates of 7.5% per year when followed after initial diagnosis.[41] Senkowsky's report identified 21 patients with transient ischemic attacks and normal arteriograms with ulcerative lesions identified on duplex imaging. At the time of surgery, all patients had ulcers and 20% to 30% stenosis.[40] Johnson and colleagues followed 184 patients with ulcerative plaques by duplex imaging for 1 year. During that year, all patients with ulcers less than 2 mm in depth were asymptomatic. Patients with ulcerative plaques 2 to 4 mm deep were symptomatic 30% of the time. All patients in the study with 4 mm or greater ulceration were symptomatic at the time of initial evaluation and had prompt surgery.[42] The diagnosis of carotid ulcers is important, and B-mode ultrasound is at least as accurate as arteriography in evaluating ulceration.

5. In the patient diagnosed with occlusion of the internal carotid artery on duplex imaging, a high-grade stenosis may be called an occlusion because Doppler techniques are not sensitive to flow velocities below 6 cm/s. Although patients with occluded internal carotid arteries are not operable, missing the opportunity to perform an endarterectomy in a patient with high-grade stenosis incorrectly diagnosed as occlusion is unfortunate. Thus, it is a prudent policy to order arteriography for patients who have had symptoms within a month and appear to have occlusion on ultrasound imaging. It is also possible to occasionally diagnose a patent internal carotid artery with ultrasound in patients who have been reported to have occlusion on arteriography. Arteriography or duplex imaging alone should not be relied on for symptomatic patients with reported ipsilateral carotid artery occlusion.

6. In addition to the preceding indications for arteriography, it is appropriate to order arteriography for patients with suboptimal duplex imaging such as calcification with sonic shadowing, patients with thick necks or poor ultrasound penetration, and patients with very high bifurcations and when ultrasound images do not correlate with spectral analysis.

When Are Follow-Up Noninvasive Vascular Examinations Needed?

Noninvasive vascular duplex testing plays an increasingly prevalent role in the long-term care of patients with significant carotid vascular disease. Several factors, including the progressive nature of atherosclerosis, the test's accuracy, its noninvasive nature, and the importance of early intervention for stroke prevention, have propelled this trend. This trend has naturally brought up a cost–benefit issue because although duplex testing is relatively inexpensive compared with arteriography, long-term surveillance and repeat testing can be costly.

However, it has been demonstrated to the satisfaction of Medicare and the vascular surgery community that appropriate duplex ultrasound follow-up is cost-effective when all factors are considered. Evidence is now emerging that supports the use of long-term follow-up in patients with moderate (50%–79%) stenosis.[43] Still, the question of what constitutes appropriate guidelines for follow-up studies remains. In an effort to address this question an ad hoc committee of the Western Vascular Surgery Society developed guidelines to help practitioners and third-party payers.[44] Table 71.9 shows the Western Vascular Surgical Society's and the author's practice guidelines.

TABLE 71.9. Guidelines for the long-term follow-up of carotid artery disease.

Patient status	Author guidelines*	Western Vascular Surgical Society†
Postoperative	4, 10 mo, annual if symptoms or >70% blockage, or at 3 yr without symptoms	6 wk, 6 mo, 12 mo, and annually thereafter
Nonoperative		
20%–50% stenosis	No follow-up generally recommended	Annual
50%–79% stenosis	Generally annual examination if >70% occluded	Every 6 mo

* The author's patients are called by the vascular technician and asked a series of questions that determine patient status.

† From Ad Hoc Committee of the Western Vascular Surgical Society.[44]

Business Administration of the Noninvasive Vascular Laboratory

Carotid artery noninvasive testing is the mainstay of the vascular surgeon's diagnosis and treatment decisions in the prevention of carotid-origin stroke. As vascular testing moved out of the laboratory and into the clinical setting in the early 1970s, vascular surgeons, due to their training and the large number of patients whom they treat in their specialty area, were generally the first to recognize the value and potential of these services. Historically, it has been common for specialists to provide and to invest financially in these services or to have a compensatory relationship for interpretive or oversight services. Initially, many hospitals and radiologists were not sufficiently interested to invest the time and money to establish this type of service. Therefore, many vascular diagnostic laboratories were established by vascular surgeons as part of their offices or as freestanding facilities. As the advantages of duplex scanning became more obvious, the number of vascular laboratories increased dramatically in the 1980s. The number of tests, as well as some examples of abuse by those entering the market primarily for profit, increased as well. As third-party payers (particularly the federal government in the Medicare program) became aware of the frequent use of noninvasive vascular tests, restrictions on reimbursement and guidelines on test indications were established.

Concurrent with new restrictions on the indications and reimbursements for the studies, the cost of providing vascular laboratory services also began to increase. Perhaps the greatest single factor that increased costs was color flow duplex technology, requiring equipment that is approximately twice as expensive as the gray-scale equipment and requiring a more costly service contract. Contributing to this inflationary cycle is the necessity for emergency, night, and weekend testing. Other factors include an increasing bureaucratic workload that requires the aid of a large clerical staff with high administrative overhead costs.

Additionally, vascular laboratory reimbursement decreased in the 1980s when Medicare established diagnosis-related groups. Under diagnosis-related groups the technical component of inpatient vascular studies was considered to be part of the overall hospitalization cost and no additional payment was provided. Unless the medical director or administrator of the vascular laboratory was able to obtain reimbursement from the hospital for the service, only the physician component could be billed to Medicare.

Initially, outpatient services were reimbursed as usual, customary, and reasonable charges. This approach led to a wide difference in payments for vascular studies across the country and, at times, even in the same community. To further control rising Medicare costs in 1989, Congress mandated the resource-based relative value scale, which established baseline reimbursement in the American Medical Association's current procedure terminology listing. This adversely affected reimbursement for vascular laboratories because payments for duplex scanning were drastically cut. The average reimbursement for carotid duplex scanning was cut from $238 in 1991 to $148 under 1992 resource-based relative value scale reimbursement. Reimbursement thus dropped 38% and provided $32 less per test than the average cost of a duplex scan to the laboratory (including the physician's time in interpreting). Since 1992 reimbursement has increased slightly to $160, which is still less than the average cost of performing the test. Because many carriers have adopted the resource-based relative value scale methodology, it is becoming increasingly more difficult to mitigate Medicare deficits by charging higher fees to private insurance carriers.

Recent changes that threaten the financial viability of the vascular laboratory include managed care contracts for providing health care. Health care providers offer discounted rates to health maintenance organizations, point-of-service plans, and preferred provider organizations to obtain the contracts. A vascular laboratory can lose a substantial market share if the facility in which it is based does not obtain a managed care contract.

Recently Medicare and commercial insurance companies have begun to develop global pricing and capitated payment programs to pay for specific operative procedures. Medicare's initial favorable experience with global pricing for coronary artery bypass grafts has led to consideration of expanding the program to other areas. Vascular laboratories will likely see a fixed reimbursement contract expanded to carotid endarterectomies in the future. In this situation, carotid studies would be part of the contract and could not be billed separately.

Most recently, the capitation model has been expanded by third-party payers to include multiple procedures or diagnoses. In this model, a group of vascular surgeons might contract to provide all vascular care for patients, including the service of the vascular diagnostic laboratory, at a fixed fee per patient per month. If the cost of the services exceeds the payments, the contracting group absorbs the loss. Both the health maintenance organization and capitation models provide a strong disincentive to order noninvasive studies. Fortunately, in some cases, the noninvasive tests replace a more expensive arteriogram, digital subtraction angiogram, or magnetic resonance angiogram.

Vascular surgeons who provide noninvasive testing must be astute businesspeople and negotiators as well as physicians. Federal fraud and abuse regulations have begun to affect the vascular laboratory. Due to concerns about possible overutilization and financial conflicts of interest, compensation and ownership arrangements, commonly termed self-referral, have come under professional and government scrutiny. Self-referral of patients becomes a conflict of interest when it leads to unnecessary care or medical testing purely for financial gain. In contrast to other professions, medicine has traditionally refrained from incorporating explicit rules on financial conflicts of interest in its ethical codes.[45] Due to public and government pressure, however, the American Medical Association's Council on Ethical and Judicial Affairs issued self-referral guidelines in 1986 and 1989.[46,47] In 1992 the council revisited this issue and concluded that "in general, physicians should not refer patients to a health care facility outside their office practice at which they do not directly provide care or services when they have an investment interest in the facility. Physicians may invest in and refer to an outside facility if there is a demonstrated need in the community for the facility and alternative financing is not available."[48]

The American Medical Association's report was necessitated by several studies that explored physician ownership of medical services and focused on the utilization, cost, and service characteristics of facilities and physicians with compensation arrangements versus facilities and physicians without financial incentives. The studies demonstrated generally higher utilization and costs in facilities that had a financial arrangement with the referring physician.[49–51]

The potential problems associated with self-referral are more than an esoteric exercise for vascular surgeons. These studies have been used by federal and state lawmakers to pass legislation that prohibits self-referral of Medicare and Medicaid patients. The federal effort is embodied in the Stark I and Stark II laws, named for Representative Pete Stark, a Democrat from California. Since 1995 the Stark law has covered 11 common service categories, including clinical laboratory services, physical therapy, occupational therapy, radiology, radiation therapy, durable medical equipment, ambulances, parenteral and enteral nutrition, outpatient prescription drugs, home infusion therapy, and inpatient and outpatient hospital services. Narrowly defined safe harbors are included in the Stark law that allow for certain exemptions, but the self-referral laws remain poorly defined. For example, regulations for the Stark I law enacted in 1989 had not yet been released at the time of this writing. In spite of this lack of regulatory law, it appears that most compensatory relationships within the defined services in which the physician does not directly provide or supervise care or services are suspect. Although the Stark law has been passed and presumably will be enforced, the pace of this enforcement may be slow due to the recent change in Congress and strident opposition from the American Medical Association, the American Hospital Association, and other industry groups.[52]

The basic flaw of the existing studies in the literature and the Stark law is that both ignore the unique nature of medicine and its inherent conflicts of interest. This is true in both the health maintenance organization or capitated setting in which physicians are rewarded for restricting care and self-referral situations in which the reverse may be true. The guiding principle for physicians has always been that they must do what is medically necessary and in the best interest of the patient. Unfortunately, the Stark laws and the existing literature make little or no reference to the medical necessity of testing and instead define abuse merely as a financial relationship.

To better understand the effect of financial relationships in our practice and to focus attention on the medical necessity of testing, we performed a retrospective study in our laboratory. Medical necessity was used to classify tests ordered by physicians with financial relationships versus those ordered by physicians without financial ties.

We analyzed a random representation of carotid artery duplex studies from 1993 and 1994. The ordering symptom was noted, and the degree of stenosis found was categorized by hemodynamic significance: 0% to 25%, insignificant; 25% to 75%, moderate; 75% to 100%, significant. Lastly, the patient outcome was sorted into three categories: no duplex follow-up, duplex follow-up, and surgery.

Of the 400 carotid tests abstracted, 80%, or 320, were ordered by physicians without any compensatory relationship with the laboratory, and 20%, or 80, were ordered by vascular surgeons who had a compensatory relationship. The physicians without compensatory relationships represented a wide spectrum of surgical, medical subspecialty, and family practice training. Differences in ordering symptoms between the two groups were unrevealing. The uncompensated physicians ordered more tests with essentially normal findings, 41.25% versus 22.50% ($P = .002$), and compensated physicians ordered more tests with clinically significant stenoses of >75% (38.75% versus 12.81%; $P = .0001$). Results showed 88.3% of the uncompensated physicians' patients in the no follow-up category (stenosis <50%) compared with 50% of the compensated physicians' patients ($P = .0001$). Moreover, 23.75% of compensated physicians' patients had follow-up (stenosis >50%) compared with only 3.44% of the uncompensated physicians' patients ($P = .0001$); 26.5% of the compensated physicians' patients underwent surgery compared with 7.81% of the uncompensated physicians' patients ($P = .0001$). Indications for surgery were the same in both groups.

Issues of disease prevalence and specialty training must be considered, but the study suggests that the compensated group ordered testing more appropriately and efficiently than the uncompensated group. In the black-and-white world of the Stark law, our limited study suggests that it may be appropriate to repeal or reform current laws based on utilization alone and instead focus on medical appropriateness as the basis for controlling fraud.

Intersocietal Commission for the Accreditation of Vascular Laboratories

The ICAVL was formed in the late 1980s to provide a means for accrediting vascular laboratories in response to the interdisciplinary concern about the variability in quality among vascular laboratories in the United States, Canada, and Puerto Rico. The ICAVL is a nonprofit organization established to review facilities that perform comprehensive testing for vascular disease with noninvasive testing modalities. Accreditation by the ICAVL means that the vascular diagnostics center has been intensively reviewed and judged to meet the commission's strict standards. The comprehensive review scrutinizes the laboratory's policies, testing techniques, equipment, and staff credentials. Before accreditation, the ICAVL may also conduct on-site inspections, with final approval coming from the ICAVL board of directors.

The ICAVL is unique among medical accreditation organizations in that it originated from 11 sponsoring societies that represent the medical specialties of radiology, ultrasonography, vascular surgery, neurology, cardiology, neurosurgery, and internal medicine. This unusual interdisciplinary perspective led to nonbiased accreditation criteria and an especially exhaustive accreditation process. ICAVL accreditation is important because it provides peer recognition of the thoroughness and quality of the vascular laboratory. Perhaps the most important benefit of ICAVL accreditation is the introspective

process that it forces the laboratory's entire staff to pursue. Weak and strong areas in training, education, staffing, equipment, testing protocols, quality assurance, and procedures become (sometimes painfully) apparent and can thus be recognized. ICAVL accreditation may eventually be linked to reimbursement.

Despite the multiple pressures on vascular laboratories, noninvasive testing will continue to play an important role in the diagnosis and treatment of carotid disease. Physicians and administrators of vascular laboratories must now have a clear understanding of the costs of providing these tests and be very active in negotiations for reimbursement that is high enough to allow the laboratory to remain in business.

References

1. Heyman A, Wilkinson WE, Heyden S, et al. Risk of stroke in asymptomatic persons with cervical arterial bruits: a population study in Evans County, Georgia. *N Engl J Med.* 1980;302:838–842.
2. Sandok BA, Whisnant JP, Furlan AJ, et al. Carotid artery bruits: prevalence survey and differential diagnosis. *Mayo Clin Proc.* 1982;57:227–230.
3. Wolf PA, Kannel WB, Sorlie P, et al. Asymptomatic bruit and the risk of stroke. *JAMA.* 1981;245:1442–1445.
4. Sutton KC, Dai WS, Kuller LH. Asymptomatic carotid artery bruits in a population of elderly adults with isolated systolic hypertension. *Stroke.* 1985;16:781–784.
5. Lefkowitz D. Asymptomatic carotid artery disease in the elderly. *Clin Geriatr Med.* 1991;7:417–428.
6. Chambers BR, Norris JW. Outcome in patients with asymptomatic neck bruits. *N Engl J Med.* 1986;315:860–865.
7. Leopjarvi M, Kallanranta T, Siniluoto T, Tolonen U. Bruit and stenosis of the internal carotid artery. *Surgical Research Comm.* 1990;7:173–181.
8. Buck TJ. The clinical significance of the asymptomatic Hollenhorst plaque. *J Vasc Surg.* 1986;4:559–562.
9. Dos Santos R, Lanas AC, Caldough JP. *Arteriographie des Membres et de L'aorta Abdominale.* Paris: Massomet Cie; 1931, 1992.
10. Miyazaki N, Cato K. Measurement of cerebral bloodflow by ultrasonic Doppler technique: hemodynamic comparison of the right and left carotid artery in patients with hemoplasia. *Jpn Circ J.* 1954:329–383.
11. Goldberg RD. Doppler physics and preliminary report for a test for carotid insufficiency. In: Goldberg RD, Saris LD, eds. *Ultrasonics in Ophthalmology: Diagnostic and Therapeutic Applications.* Philadelphia, Pa: WB Saunders; 1967:199.
12. Brockenbrough EC. Screening for the prevention of stroke: use of a Doppler flowmeter. Alaska/Washington Regional Medical Program; 1969.
13. Gee W, Smith CA, Henson CE, et al. Ocular pneumoplethysmography in carotid artery disease. *Medical Instrumentation.* 1974;8:244–248.
14. Kartchner MM, McRae LP, Morrisson FD. Noninvasive detection in evaluation of carotid occlusive disease. *Arch Surg* 1973;106:528–535.

15. Olinger CP. Ultrasonic carotid echo arteriography. *American Journal of Roentgenology and Radium Therapy.* 1969; 106:282.

16. Barber FE, Baker DW, Nation AWC, et al. Ultrasonic duplex echo-Doppler scanner. *IEEE Trans Biomed Eng.* 1974; 81:109.

17. Baumgartner RW, Mattle HP, Kothbauer K, Schroth G. Transcranial color-coded duplex sonography in cerebral aneurysms. *Stroke.* 1994;12:2429–2434.

18. Lin SK, Ryu SJ, Chu NS. Carotid duplex and transcranial color-coded sonography in evaluation of carotid-cavernous sinus fistulas. *J Ultrasound Med.* 1994;7:557–564.

19. Otis S, Rush M, Boyajian R. Contrast-enhanced transcranial imaging: results of an American phase-two study. *Stroke.* 1995;2:203–209.

20. Blakely DD, Oddone EZ, Hasselblad V, et al. Noninvasive carotid artery testing: a meta-analytic review. *Ann Intern Med.* 1995;122:360–367.

21. Kerrie IC, Murphy KP, Jones AJ, et al. Magnetic resonance angiography or AIDSA for diagnosis of carotid pseudo occlusion? *Eur J Vasc Surg.* 1994;8:562–566.

22. AbuRahma AF. Methods of noninvasive cerebrovascular techniques. In: AbuRahma AF, Diethrich EB, eds. *Current Noninvasive Vascular Diagnosis.* Littleton, Mass: PSG Publishing Co; 1988:51.

23. Bundt TJ, Haynes JL. Carotid endarterectomy: one solution to the stroke problem. *Am Surg.* 1985;51:61–69.

24. Moore WS, Borne C, Malone JM, et al. Immediate and long term results after prophylactic endarterectomy. *Am J Surg.* 1984;138:228–233.

25. Steffen CM, Gray-Wale AC, Byrne KE, et al. Carotid artery disease: plaque ultrasound characteristics in symptomatic and asymptomatic vessels. *Stroke.* 1986;11:17.

26. Maiuri S, Gallicchio B, Laconetta G, et al. Intraplaque hemorrhage of the carotid arteries: diagnosis by duplex scanning. *J Neurosurg Sci.* 1994;38:87–92.

27. O'Donnell TF, Erdos L, Mackey WC, et al. Correlation of B-mode ultrasound imaging and arteriography with pathological findings at carotid endarterectomy. *Arch Surg.* 1985;120:443–449.

28. Johnson JM, Kennelly M, O'Holleran L, et al. A comparison of angiography and ultrasound in the diagnosis of carotid artery disease. *Contemporary Surgery.* 1985;26: 31–36.

29. O'Holleran LW, Kennelly MM, McClurken M, Johnson JM. Natural history of asymptomatic carotid plaque. *Am J Surg.* 1987;154:659–662.

30. Executive Committee for the Asymptomatic Carotid Atherosclerosis Study. Endarterectomy for asymptomatic carotid artery stenosis. *JAMA.* 1995;273:1421–1428.

31. Jackson JM, Kennelly M, O'Holleran L, et al. A comparison of angiography and ultrasound in the diagnosis of carotid disease. *Contemporary Surgery.* 1985;26:31–36.

32. Thomas GI, Jones TW, Stavney LS, et al. Carotid endarterectomy after Doppler ultrasonic examination without angiography. *Am J Surg.* 1986;151:616–619.

33. Crew JR, Dean M, Johnson JM, et al. Carotid surgery without angiography. *Am J Surg.* 1985;148:18–23.

34. Boyle MJ, Wilensky AP, Grimly RP. Accuracy of duplex versus angiography in patients undergoing carotid surgery. *J R Soc Med.* 1995;88:20–23.

35. Roederer GO, Langlois YE, Chan ARW, et al. Is syphon disease important in predicting outcome of carotid endarterectomy? *Arch Surg.* 1983;118:1177–1181.

36. Shular JJ, Flanagin DM, Lim LT, et al. The effect of carotid syphon stenosis on stroke rate, death, and relief of symptoms following elective carotid endarterectomy. *Surgery.* 1982;92:1058–1067.

37. Akers DL, Bell WH, Kirstein MD. Does intracranial dye study contribute to evaluation of carotid disease? *Am J Surg.* 1988;156:87–90.

38. Goodson SF, Flannigan DP, Bishara RA, et al. Can carotid duplex scanning supplant arteriography in patients with focal carotid territory symptoms? *J Vasc Surg.* 1987;5: 551–557.

39. Senkowsky J, Bell WH, Kirstein MD. Normal angiograms in carotid pathology. *Am Surg.* 1990;56:726–729.

40. Moore WS, Boran C, Malone JM, et al. The natural history of non-stenotic asymptomatic ulcerative lesions of the carotid artery. *Arch Surg.* 1978;113:1352–1359.

41. Dixon S, Pais OS, Raviola C, et al. Natural history of non-stenotic asymptomatic ulcerative lesions of the carotid artery: a further analysis. *Arch Surg.* 1982;117:1493.

42. Johnson JM, Ansel AL, Morgan S, et al. Ultrasonographic screening for evaluation followup of carotid artery ulceration: a new basis for assessing risk. *Am J Surg.* 1983;146: 188–193.

43. Mansour MA, Mattos MA, Faught WE, et al. The natural history of moderate (50–79%) internal carotid artery stenosis in symptomatic, nonhemispheric, and asymptomatic patients. *J Vasc Surg.* 1995;21:346–356.

44. Ad Hoc Committee of the Western Vascular Surgery Society. Vascular laboratory utilization and payment: report of the Ad Hoc Committee of the Western Vascular Society. *J Vasc Surg.* 1992;16:163–170.

45. Rodwin MA. The organized American medical profession's response to financial conflicts of interest: 1890–1992. *Milbank Q.* 1992;70:703–741.

46. Council on Ethical and Judicial Affairs. Conflicts of interest. In: *Proceedings of the House of Delegates, 40th Interim Meeting, American Medical Association;* December 7–10, 1986; Chicago, Ill.

47. Council on Ethical and Judicial Affairs, American Medical Association. Conflicts of interest: update. In: *Proceedings of the House of Delegates, 138th Annual Meeting;* June 18–22, 1989; Chicago, Ill: 188–189.

48. Council on Ethical and Judicial Affairs, American Medical Association. Conflicts of interest: physician ownership of medical facilities: council report. *JAMA.* 1992;267:2366.

49. Office of Inspector General. *Financial Arrangements Between Physicians and Health Care Businesses.* Washington, DC: Department of Health and Human Services; 1989.

50. Health Care Cost Containment Board. *Joint Ventures Among Health Care Providers in Florida. Draft Report.* Tallahassee: State of Florida; 1991:2.

51. Hillman BJ, Joseph CA, Mabry MR, et al. Frequency and costs of diagnostic imaging in office practice: a comparison of self-referring and radiologist-referring physicians. *N Engl J Med.* 1990;323:1604–1608.

52. Johnsson J. Enforcement of self-referral ban delayed. *American Medical News.* http://www.ama-assn.org/public/ journals. Week 3, 1995.

72

Long-Term Benefit of Carotid Endarterectomy With Vein Patch Graft

John B. Chang and Theodore A. Stein

Carotid artery disease is a manifestation of progressive atherosclerosis. Its prevalency increases with age, cigarette smoking, and hyperlipemia.[1] Etiological factors associated with the risk for atherosclerosis, such as heredity, obesity, diabetes mellitus, anxiety, and stress, may also influence the progression of carotid artery disease. It frequently coexists with other peripheral arterial diseases. Almost 50% of patients who have significant carotid artery disease also have coronary artery disease.[2] Arterial occlusive disease of the lower extremity frequently coexists with carotid artery disease and has been reported to occur in 60% of patients.[3,4] Abdominal aortic aneurysms are also present in 20% of patients with carotid artery disease.[5] Carotid artery disease occurs in 10% of patients with abdominal aortic aneurysms.[6,7]

In the early stage of the disease atheromatous plaque forms on the intima, and a moderate progressive growth occurs in 60% of patients.[8] Necrosis of the interior of the plaque occurs when oxygen and nutrients are unable to reach the center of the atheroma; subintimal hemorrhage increases necrosis. The shear force of the turbulent blood flow may erode the plaque overlying the necrotic center, embolic plaque material may be released into the artery, emboli may be deposited in a distant artery, and ischemic events, such as a stroke, transient ischemic attack, or amaurosis fugax, may be consequences.

Multicenter collaborative studies in North America and Europe have been conducted to determine the benefit of carotid endarterectomy. These studies have concluded that carotid endarterectomy reduces the risk of ipsilateral carotid territory ischemic stroke in patients with symptomatic carotid artery disease of 70% to 99% stenosis.[9,10] A recent review of the reported risks of stroke and death after more than 17,000 carotid endarterectomies for symptomatic disease indicates that the 30-day perioperative mortality rate is 1.6% and the risk of fatal stroke is 0.9%.[11] The combined risk of any stroke and/or death is 5.6%.[11] These perioperative mortality and morbidity rates are acceptably low, and most patients with symptomatic carotid artery disease benefit from carotid endarterectomy. It is particularly beneficial for patients with recent hemispheric and retinal transient ischemic attacks or nondisabling strokes.[9] Many patients with asymptomatic carotid stenosis also appear to have a reduced risk for stroke after endarterectomy.[12–14] Further studies on these patients are necessary to determine when the benefit of endarterectomy outweighs the risk for complications.

The type of arteriotomy closure may also influence the long-term efficacy of carotid endarterectomy. We are reporting our results on the long-term benefit of vein patch angioplasty and primary closure of the arteriotomy in our patients.

Methods

Indications for carotid endarterectomy include (1) symptomatic lesions, (2) unilateral stenosis exceeding 70% in diameter, (3) bilateral stenoses exceeding 50% in diameter, (4) unilateral stenosis exceeding 50% in diameter and contralateral occlusion, (5) rapid progressive stenosis greater than 50%, and (6) a markedly ulcerated plaque. Our preoperative evaluation includes obtaining a detailed medical history and complete physical assessment of the patient. Each patient undergoes a carotid duplex scan, a computed axial tomography scan, and/or a magnetic resonance imaging study of the head to rule out infarction and nonvascular pathology; a cardiac evaluation; and a study of the aortic arch by either extracranial and intracranial arteriography or magnetic resonance angiography.

Patients are given antibiotics prophylactically. Before carotid endarterectomy the radial artery is catheterized for intraoperative and postoperative monitoring.

General anesthesia is administered via an endotracheal tube, and the patient is maintained in a normotensive and normocarbic state. The carotid artery is shunted. Electroencephalographic (EEG) monitoring has been used in the past. The patient is placed in a semi-Fowler position with the neck extended and rotated to the contralateral side.[15] Betadine solution is placed on the neck, chest, and leg when a vein graft will be used. A semivertical incision is made on the neck along the anterior border of the sternocleidomastoid muscle. In younger female patients, a transverse incision is occasionally made under the mandible at the level of the bifurcation. Sharp and blunt dissection is used, and electrocoagulation and ligatures control hemostasis. The sternocleidomastoid muscle is freed and retracted laterally.

The facial branch of the internal jugular vein should be located, because the carotid artery usually bifurcates below this vein. The vein is freed, ligated, and divided, and the carotid sheath is carefully opened. The common carotid artery is freed, and further dissection exposes the carotid artery bifurcation. Then 0.5 to 1.0 mL of a 0.5% marcaine solution is infiltrated into the carotid body. The first branch of the external carotid artery is next identified by careful dissection. The proximal external carotid artery is then freed and encircled with a vessel loop. The internal carotid artery is located and dissected distally. Frequently the ansa hypoglossi nerve, running anteriorly and medially or occasionally laterally and joining with the hypoglossal nerve, can be identified. The hypoglossal nerve should be identified and preserved intact.

When the lesion is high, with high bifurcation, the "sling vessels" are carefully freed, ligated, and divided and the hypoglossal nerve is further freed distally. In select cases, the ansa hypoglossal can be divided to facilitate mobilization of the hypoglossal nerve. The digastric muscle can also be divided to gain additional distal exposure, but care must be taken to avoid injury to the glossopharyngeal nerve. Mandible joint subluxation or dislocation has been used in redo procedures for patients with high distal lesions.

The type of carotid endarterectomy closure is determined on a patient-by-patient basis. Primary closure is routinely used for internal carotid arteries ≥5 mm in diameter. When the arteriotomy does not extend beyond the bulb, primary closure is also suitable.[16] The greater saphenous vein patch is used for arteries <5 mm in diameter, after restenosis, and for female patients. In the repair of a carotid endarterectomy the scarred media should be excised and the vein graft anastomosed to healthy tissue.[17]

In suitable patients, a 2.5- to 3.0-in length of proximal greater saphenous vein is harvested and divided at the line of branches. We recommend that the vein graft be taken only above the knee to obtain a diameter of greater than 3.5 mm and avoid a possible rupture of the vein patch.[16,18,19] However, rupture has occurred early in 0.7% of vein grafts and rarely with grafts taken from the groin.[20]

Systemic heparinization, usually 6000 to 7000 units, is then initiated. The common, internal, and external carotid arteries are cross-clamped using atraumatic vascular clamps. A longitudinal arteriotomy is made that extends from the proximal common carotid artery to a point distal from the plaque in the internal carotid artery. Then a T-shaped indwelling shunt catheter is introduced into the common and internal carotid arteries. Extreme care is taken to evacuate all air and clots from the shunt and arterial system before the shunt is opened. During this maneuver, intraoperative EEG recording can be helpful in monitoring the technique of cross-clamping and shunting. However, after evaluating 300 patients with EEG monitoring, we have found that EEG monitoring is not cost-effective. Carotid endarterectomy with routine shunting can be done safely without EEG monitoring. When the lesion is critically stenotic and a single arteriotomy is difficult to perform, two separate arteriotomies, one on the proximal common carotid artery and one on the distal internal carotid artery, are done. The arteriotomies are connected after the shunt is inserted and cerebral circulation is restored through the shunt.

The endarterectomy is begun opposite from the origin of the external carotid artery and extends down to the proximal common carotid artery with the aid of a dissection spatula. A detailed description of the technique has been provided elsewhere.[15] At the point of normal intima, sharp dissection is used to cut the intima to the opposite side of the common carotid artery. Then dissection is extended distally toward the external carotid artery to free up the proximal portion of the plaque. Next the distal plaque is freed by extending the dissection distal from the common carotid artery to normal intima above the plaque in the internal carotid artery. Dissection is continued down the internal carotid artery to the origin of the external carotid artery. Careful blunt dissection into the external carotid artery may extend beyond the first branch and continues along the medial border of the plaque. The plaque specimen can now be removed in one piece, completing the endarterectomy procedure.

If the end point of the internal carotid artery dissection is not clean, the normal intima is tacked down with interrupted 6-O Prolene sutures to prevent possible distal dissection. If the end point is clean, no tack-down sutures are necessary. The arterial lumen is irrigated with a copious amount of heparinized solution. All possible debris should be removed from the arterial lumen. Then the arteriotomy is repaired using the greater saphenous vein graft or by primary closure. The patch graft should extend proximally beyond the cut margin of the intima of the common carotid artery and distally beyond the end point. Any kinking of the internal carotid artery is corrected by shortening the segment by plication. Transverse sutures of 6-O Prolene are placed in the redundant portion of the segment to cause eversion of the redundant part. When the vein patch is placed at the arteriotomy after eversion suturing, the carotid arterial system becomes straighter. With primary closure the angle of the branching of the carotid bifurcation remains unchanged.

Most perioperative strokes, believed to be related to technical errors made during the endarterectomy and/or reconstruction of the carotid artery, are related to ischemia during cross-clamping, postoperative thrombosis and embolism, intracerebral hemorrhage, and other surgical problems.[21] Thus the indwelling shunt catheter is removed before completing closure of the arteriotomy, and all air and clots are removed from the arterial system. Circulation is restored first to the external carotid artery and then to the internal carotid artery in a sequential manner. If there is no major problem or bleeding from the anastomosis, heparin is neutralized with Protamine in about a 3:4 ratio. The wound spaces are irrigated with an antibiotic solution of kanamycin sulfate. The incisions are closed using 2-O Vicryl or Dexon sutures and 4-O absorbable sutures to the skin in a subcuticular fashion. A sterile dressing is applied to the wound. On the neck, a gentle pressure dressing is applied using 4-in. × 8-in. gauze pads. Using a sterile towel, a gentle collar is made around the neck incision dressing.

The patient is allowed to recover from general anesthesia while on the operating table and is asked to move all extremities on command. Once neurologically intact, the patient can be extubated and transferred to the recovery room. Until the patient's neurological assessment is completed, the surgical instruments remain uncontaminated in the operating room.

In the recovery room, cardiac and neurological evaluations are made periodically. For the first night the patient either remains in the recovery room or is moved to the intensive care unit for observation. On the first postoperative day, the dressing is removed, and the patient is allowed to ambulate and eat a regular diet. The patient can usually be discharged from the hospital on the first or second postoperative day, unless there are specific reasons to keep the patient longer. Patients are instructed to take an antiplatelet agent, buffered aspirin, and/or Persantine. Noninvasive vascular studies including duplex scanning are performed for follow-up evaluation.

We have followed 551 patients who had 644 carotid endarterectomies for symptomatic carotid artery disease between 1974 and 1996. Primary closure of the arteriotomy was done in 106 carotid endarterectomies in 86 patients. In 465 patients, a greater saphenous vein patch was used to close 538 arteriotomies after carotid endarterectomy. The mean follow-up time for patients with primary closure was 3.8 years and for patients with vein patch 3.6 years. One fifth of the patients were followed for more than 10 years. Carotid duplex scans were used to determine the patency of the internal carotid artery and vein patch.

The long-term benefit of carotid endarterectomy with vein patch angioplasty or primary closure of the arteriotomy has been determined. Mortality, morbidity from stroke or transient ischemic attack, and restenosis rates were calculated. The freedom from significant restenosis was defined as a greater than 50% narrowing of the diameter of the lumen.

Results and Comments

In our 551 patients with 644 carotid endarterectomies, six (0.9%) patients had perioperative strokes on the ipsilateral side within 30 postoperative days. After 106 primary closures of the arteriotomies, three (2.8%) patients had perioperative strokes, and all were fatal. After 538 vein patch grafts, three patients (0.6%) had perioperative strokes, and one of these was fatal (0.2%). Another study found a perioperative stroke rate of 4.6% with vein patches and 2.3% with prosthetic patches.[22] In a larger series of more than 3000 carotid endarterectomies, the overall perioperative stroke rate was 2.2%.[21] Others have reported an operative mortality rate of 1.1% to 1.4% and a operative stroke rate of 1.4% to 1.5%.[23,24] The perioperative mortality rate has been reported to be 1.3% for asymptomatic stenoses and 1.8% for symptomatic stenoses.[11] Asymptomatic patients also have a lower perioperative stroke rate than symptomatic patients; after a prior stroke the rate was 7.1%.[25] The Asymptomatic Carotid Atherosclerosis Study found a combined risk for perioperative stroke and death of 1.5%.[12] When the contralateral carotid artery is occluded, the risk of perioperative stroke is increased.[26] Many perioperative strokes can be prevented by minimizing the cross-clamping time and ischemia and avoiding technical errors that lead to postoperative thrombosis, embolism, and intracerebral hemorrhage.

After 30 days, 4 (3.8%) of our patients with primary closure of the arteriotomy had strokes and 10 (1.9%) patients who had vein patches for repair of the arteriotomy had strokes. The overall mortality rates were 25.6% for patients with primary closure and 15.1% for patients with vein patch. Most deaths were from cardiac complications, and the lower ($P < .005$) mortality rate with the vein patch grafts was not stroke related (Table 72.1). We experienced no graft ruptures in our study. One-year survival rates were lower ($P < .04$) after primary closure

TABLE 72.1. Life table survival for primary closure and vein grafts.

Closure	Time (yr)	At risk	Died	Lost	Survival	SE
Primary	0–1	86	8	30	0.8873	0.0375
	1–2	48	1	5	0.8678	0.0415
	2–3	42	3	5	0.8019	0.0530
	3–4	34	1	3	0.7772	0.0568
	4–5	30	0	3	0.7772	0.0568
	5–6	27	1	6	0.7449	0.0630
	6–7	20	2	1	0.6685	0.0763
	7–8	17	0	0	0.6685	0.0763
	8–9	17	0	0	0.6685	0.0763
	9–10	17	1	1	0.6279	0.0817
	10–11	15	0	2	0.6279	0.0817
	11–12	13	2	2	0.5233	0.0959
Vein	0–1	465	9	128	0.9776	0.0074
	1–2	328	19	46	0.9167	0.0152
	2–3	263	9	45	0.8824	0.0184
	3–4	209	8	38	0.8452	0.0218
	4–5	163	5	28	0.8168	0.0245
	5–6	130	4	23	0.7893	0.0273
	6–7	103	5	14	0.7482	0.0315
	7–8	84	2	14	0.7287	0.0335
	8–9	68	0	16	0.7287	0.0335
	9–10	52	4	13	0.6647	0.0432
	10–11	35	4	11	0.5745	0.0561
	11–12	20	0	10	0.5745	0.0561

than after vein patch graft (88.7% versus 97.8%). The rates then fell in a nearly parallel fashion. The respective 5-year, 10-year, and 14-year rates were 77.7%, 62.8%, and 38.5% for patients with primary closure and 81.7%, 66.5%, and 57.5% for patients with vein patch graft.

Stroke-free survival was also better ($P < .02$) in patients with vein patch graft (Table 72.2). One-year stroke-free survival rates were lower ($P < .025$) for primary closure than for vein patch graft (86.1% versus 96.8%). The rates then fell in a nearly parallel fashion. The respective 5-year, 10-year, and 14-year rates were 75.4%, 60.9%, and 37.3% for patients with primary closure and 80.3%, 66.5%, and 57.2% for patients with vein patch graft. Even when the contralateral carotid artery was occluded, the 5-year stroke-free survival rate was 74%.[27] Although we believe that vein patch angioplasty is more beneficial than primary closure, others have not found the same results.[28]

Following endarterectomy, restenosis (>50%) of the carotid artery occurs in some patients. It occurs disproportionally in women, cigarette smokers, patients 70 years or older, those with smaller (<4.0-mm diameter) arteries, those with ulcerated lesions, and patients who have undergone primary closure of arteriotomies in small arteries.[29–32] In our patients, the incidence of freedom from restenosis (<50% stenosis) with vein patch grafts was 94.1% at 5 years and 90.8% at 10 years. After primary closure the incidence of freedom from restenosis was 89.3% at 5 years and 89.3% at 10 years. Restenosis was more frequent ($P = .06$) with primary closures; at 13

years, it was 17.9% and 32.0% with vein patch grafts and primary closures, respectively. In another study, the cumulative incidence of restenosis after carotid endarterectomy has been reported to be 31% at 7 years.[31]

Several other studies have also demonstrated that vein patch angioplasty reduces the incidence of restenosis.[1,19,23,33,34] Women appear to benefit from vein grafts more than men.[35] Other studies have found that Dacron patch angioplasty also lowers the incidence of restenosis.[23,32] Still other studies have found that the occurrence of restenosis is similar for primary closure of the arteriotomy and vein patch grafts.[36,37] One study indicated that vein patch angioplasty increased restenosis rates.[38] Most stenoses, however, were 25% to 50% diameter reductions, and the vein was taken distally near the medial malleolus.[38]

Because most stenoses of <50% are clinically insignificant, restenosis has been defined as >50% stenosis. Many primary closures of the arteriotomy result in thickening of the arterial wall and narrowing of the lumen, which can cause increased flow and turbulence. A well-constructed vein patch, however, slightly increases the diameter of the lumen and straightens the arterial tree. Although some studies have indicated that approximately 10% to 15.5% of vein patches will became aneurysmal,[39,40] we have not found dilations of proximal greater saphenous vein grafts to be aneurysmal. Others prefer a prosthetic patch because dilations occur less often.[40,41] We use the greater saphenous vein patch to

TABLE 72.2. Stroke-free rates for primary closure and vein grafts.

Closure	Time (yr)	At risk	Stroke	Lost	Stroke free	SE
Primary	0–1	86	10	28	0.8611	0.0408
	1–2	48	1	5	0.8422	0.0440
	2–3	42	3	5	0.7782	0.0540
	3–4	34	1	3	0.7543	0.0574
	4–5	30	0	3	0.7543	0.0574
	5–6	27	1	6	0.7228	0.0630
	6–7	20	2	1	0.6487	0.0753
	7–8	17	0	0	0.6487	0.0753
	8–9	17	0	0	0.6487	0.0753
	9–10	17	1	1	0.6094	0.0803
	10–11	15	0	2	0.6094	0.0803
	11–12	13	2	2	0.5078	0.0937
Vein	0–1	465	13	127	0.9676	0.0088
	1–2	325	20	46	0.9035	0.0161
	2–3	259	9	45	0.8692	0.0192
	3–4	205	8	37	0.8319	0.0224
	4–5	160	5	27	0.8035	0.0250
	5–6	128	4	23	0.7759	0.0277
	6–7	101	5	14	0.7346	0.0318
	7–8	82	2	14	0.7150	0.0338
	8–9	66	0	16	0.7150	0.0338
	9–10	50	3	13	0.6657	0.0418
	10–11	34	4	11	0.5723	0.0563
	11–12	19	0	10	0.5723	0.0563

close the arteriotomy for most patients, because restenosis, mortality, and morbidity rates are low.

References

1. Salonen R, Salonen JT. Progression of carotid atherosclerosis and its determinants: a population-based ultrasonography study. *Atherosclerosis.* 1990.81:33–40.

2. Rihal CS, Gersh BJ, Whisnant JP, et al. Influence of coronary heart disease on morbidity and mortality after carotid endarterectomy: a population-based study in Olmstead County, Minnesota (1970–1988). *J Am Coll Cardiol.* 1992; 19:1254–1260.

3. Salasidis GC, Latter DA, Steinmetz OK, Blair J-F, Graham AM. Carotid artery duplex scanning in preoperative assessment for coronary artery revascularization: the association between peripheral vascular disease, carotid artery stenosis, and stroke. *J Vasc Surg.* 1995;21:154–162.

4. Alexandrova NA, Gibson WC, Norris JW, Maggisano R. Carotid artery stenosis in peripheral vascular disease. *J Vasc Surg.* 1996;23:645–649.

5. Karanjia PN, Madden KP, Lobner S. Coexistence of abdominal aortic aneurysm in patients with carotid stenosis. *Stroke.* 1994;25:627–630.

6. Cabellon S Jr, Moncrief CL, Pierre DR, Cavanaugh DG. Incidence of abdominal aortic aneurysm in patients with atheromatous arterial disease. *Am J Surg.* 1983;146: 575–576.

7. Allardice JT, Allright GJ, Wafula JMC, Wyatt AP. High prevalence of abdominal aortic aneurysm in men with peripheral vascular disease: screening by ultrasonography. *Br J Surg.* 1988;75:240–242.

8. Javid H, Ostermiller WE, Hengesh JW, et al. Natural history of carotid bifurcation atheroma. *Surgery.* 1970;67: 80–86.

9. North American Symptomatic Carotid Endarterectomy Trial Collaborators. Beneficial effect of carotid endarterectomy in symptomatic patients with high-grade stenosis. *N Engl J Med.* 1991;325:445–453.

10. European Carotid Surgery Trialists' Collaborative Group. MRC European carotid surgery trial: interim results for symptomatic patients with severe (70–99%) or with mild (0–29%) carotid stenosis. *Lancet.* 1991;337:1235–1243.

11. Rothwell PM, Slattery J, Warlow CP. A systematic review of the risks of stroke and death due to endarterectomy for symptomatic carotid stenosis. *Stroke.* 1996;27:260–265.

12. Executive Committee for the Asymptomatic Carotid Atherosclerosis Study. Endarterectomy for asymptomatic carotid artery stenosis. *JAMA.* 1995;273:1421–1428.

13. European Carotid Surgery Trialists' Collaborative Group. The risk of stroke in the distribution of an asymptomatic carotid artery. *Lancet.* 1995;345:209–212.

14. Hobson RW II, Weiss DG, Fields WS, et al. Efficacy of carotid endarterectomy for asymptomatic carotid stenosis. *N Engl J Med.* 1993;328:221–227.

15. Chang JB. Carotid endarterectomy (how I do it, a safe approach). In: Chang JB, ed. *Modern Vascular Surgery.* Vol 5. New York, NY: Springer-Verlag; 1992:52–85.

16. Archie JP Jr. Carotid endarterectomy with reconstruction techniques tailored to operative findings. *J Vasc Surg* 1993;17:141–149.

17. Meyer FB, Piepgras DG, Fode NC. Surgical treatment of recurrent carotid artery stenosis. *J Neurosurg* 1994;80: 781–787.

18. O'Hara PJ, Hertzer NR, Krajewski LP, Beven EG. Saphenous vein patch rupture after carotid endarterectomy. *J Vasc Surg* 1992;15:504–509.

19. Katz MM, Jones GT, Degenhardt J, Gunn B, Wilson J, Katz S. The use of patch angioplasty to alter the incidence of carotid restenosis following thromboendarterectomy. *J Cardiovasc Surg.* 1987;28:2–8.

20. Tawes RL Jr, Treiman RL. Vein patch rupture after carotid endarterectomy: a survey of the Western Vascular Society members. *Ann Vasc Surg.* 1991;5:71–73.

21. Riles TS, Imparato AM, Jacobowitz GR, et al. The cause of perioperative stroke after carotid endarterectomy. *J Vasc Surg.* 1994;19:206–216.

22. Treiman RL, Foran RF, Wagner WH, Cossman DV, Levin PM, Cohen JL. Does routine patch angioplasty after carotid endarterectomy lessen the risk of perioperative stroke? *Ann Vasc Surg.* 1993;7:317–319.

23. Goldman KA, Su WT, Riles TS, Adelman MA, Landis R. A comparative study of saphenous vein, internal jugular vein, and knitted Dacron patches for carotid artery endarterectomy. *Ann Vasc Surg.* 1995;9:71–79.

24. Bernstein EF, Torem S, Dilley RB. Does carotid restenosis predict an increased risk of late symptoms, stroke, or death? *Ann Surg.* 1990;212:629–636.

25. Mattos MA, Hodgson KJ, Londrey GL, et al. Carotid endarterectomy: operative risks, recurrent stenosis, and long-term stroke rates in a modern series. *J Cardiovasc Surg.* 1992;33:387–400.

26. Gasecki AP, Eliasziw M, Ferguson GG, Hachinski V, Barnett HJ. Long-term prognosis and effect of endarterectomy in patients with symptomatic severe carotid stenosis and contralateral carotid stenosis or occlusion: results from NASCET. *J Neurosurg.* 1995;83:778–782.

27. Jacobowitz GR, Adelman MA, Riles TS, Lamparello PJ, Imparato AM. Long-term follow-up of patients undergoing carotid endarterectomy in the presence of a contralateral occlusion. *Am J Surg.* 1995;170:165–167.

28. Myers SI, Valentine RJ, Chervu A, Bowers BL, Clagett GP. Saphenous vein patch versus primary closure for carotid endarterectomy: long-term assessment of a randomized prospective study. *J Vasc Surg.* 1994;19:15–22.

29. Maki HS, Kruger RA, Kuehner ME. The problem of recurrent stenosis following carotid endarterectomy. *Wis Med J.* 1991;90:583–585.

30. Clagett GP, Rich NM, McDonald PT, et al. Etiologic factors for recurrent carotid artery stenosis. *Surgery.* 1983;93:313–318.

31. Healy DA, Zierler RE, Nicholls SC, et al. Long-term follow-up and clinical outcome of carotid restenosis. *J Vasc Surg.* 1989;10:662–669.

32. Ouriel K, Green RM. Clinical and technical factors influencing recurrent carotid stenosis and occlusion after endarterectomy. *J Vasc Surg.* 1987;5:702–706.

33. Ten Holter JBM, Ackerstaff RGA, Thoe Schwartzenberg GWS, Eikelboom BC, Vermeulen FEE, Van Den Berg ECJM. The impact of vein patch angioplasty on long-term surgical outcome after carotid endarterectomy: a prospective follow-up study with serial duplex scanning. *J Cardiovasc Surg.* 1990;31:58–65.

34. Rosenthal D, Archie JP Jr, Garcia-Rinaldi R, et al. Carotid patch angioplasty: immediate and long-term results. *J Vasc Surg.* 1990;12:326–333.

35. De Letter JA, Moll FL, Welten RJ, et al. Benefits of carotid patching: a prospective randomized study with long-term follow-up. *Ann Vasc Surg.* 1994;8:54–58.

36. Curley S, Edwards WS, Jacob TP. Recurrent carotid stenosis after autologous tissue patching. *J Vasc Surg.* 1987;6:350–354.

37. Fabiani J-N, Julia P, Chemla E, et al. Is the incidence of recurrent carotid artery stenosis influenced by the choice of the surgical technique? Carotid endarterectomy versus saphenous vein bypass. *J Vasc Surg.* 1994;20:821–825.

38. Clagett GP, Patterson CB, Fisher DF Jr, et al. Vein patch versus primary closure for carotid endarterectomy: a randomized prospective study in a selected group of patients. *J Vasc Surg.* 1989;9:213–223.

39. Gonzalez-Fajardo JA, Perez JL, Mateo AM. Saphenous vein patch versus polytetrafluoroethylene patch after carotid endarterectomy. *J Cardiovasc Surg (Torino).* 1994;35:523–528.

40. Ricco JB, Saliou C, Dubreuil F, Boin-Pineau MH. Value of the prosthetic patch after carotid endarterectomy. *J Mal Vasc.* 1994;19(suppl A):10–17.

41. Lord RSA, Raj TB, Stary DL, Nash PA, Graham AR, Goh KH. Comparison of saphenous vein patch, polytetrafluoroethylene patch, and direct arteriotomy closure after carotid endarterectomy, I: perioperative results. *J Vasc Surg.* 1989;9:591–599.

73

Eversion Endarterectomy of the Carotid Artery

D. Raithel

In 1970 Etheredge described an eversion endarterectomy (EEA) of the carotid bifurcation that he applied in 72 cases.[1] EEA by transection of the common carotid artery was first mentioned by DeBakey et al. in 1959.[2] After transection of the common carotid artery (CCA) he performed an EEA at the bifurcation of the internal and external carotid artery. Thevenet reimplanted the divided internal carotid artery (ICA) into the CCA in patients with kinking or tortuosity of the ICA.[3] Jones mentioned the anatomic results of the EEA.[4]

Kieny was the first to perform EEA of the ICA, and he and his colleagues published their results in 1988 and 1989.[5,6] They analyzed the results of 212 EEAs of the ICA associated with reimplantation performed between January 1985 and July 1990 in 206 patients.[5] We started using this technique in 1987 and published our results in 1990.[7] From mid-1987 until mid-1995 we performed more than 6000 reconstructions of the carotid artery with this technique. The reason for the application of this new method was the high rate of restenosis after conventional carotid endarterectomy and some technical problems in correcting the elongated ICA (Figure 73.1). With increasing frequency of carotid reconstructions we found restenoses at the distal end of the arteriotomy or of the patch angioplasty.

The difference between the operative technique of the EEA of the ICA and the technique of conventional carotid endarterectomy is that an elongated ICA can be optimally and easily reconstructed by EEA.[8] The operative principle is based on the following (Figure 73.2 through 73.6):

- Oblique transection of the ICA from the CCA
- EEA of the ICA
- Endarterectomy of the carotid bifurcation and external carotid artery
- Reimplantation of the ICA into the CCA
- Intraoperative angioscopy

This operative technique allows for optimal correction of the elongated ICAs, and an angioscopy after carotid endarterectomy is an alternative or an adjunct to angiography or ultrasonography.

EEA allows an optimal correction of elongated ICAs by shortening the ICA after endarterectomy or by reimplanting the ICA a little further into the CCA. When endarterectomizing the ICA the endarterectomy is carried out solely by eversion in the cranial direction, mostly in the layer of the external elastic membrane. Pulling at the specimen should be avoided; the endarterectomy is performed solely by eversion (Figure 73.4). After dilatation by bombines (maximum 4.5–5 mm) the ICA is reimplanted into the CCA after endarterectomy of the latter and after endarterectomy of the external carotid artery (ECA) in the typical way with a 6.0 or 7.0 suture in continuous technique. The elongation of the ICA is thus corrected.

After EEA of the ICA intraoperative quality control must be maintained to exclude a distal intimal flap in the ICA, which could lead to thrombosis and ultimately stroke (Figure 73.6). For angioscopic control we use a flexible and controllable angioscope (Olympus Optical, Ltd, Tokyo) with an outer diameter of 2.2 to 3.6 mm and an irrigation channel. This angioscope is connected to a video camera with a recorder for photo documentation.

If angioscopy shows a dissected intimal cylinder or plaque that reaches very far in the cranial direction and if we suspect that this plaque might not be safely removed in the channel direction, we have to evert the ICA once again and correct this finding. If we find an intimal dissection, it is better to transect the ICA in a highly oblique way and to interpose a 6-mm polytetrafluoroethylene graft or a segment of the greater saphenous vein in carotido-carotidal position (Figure 73.7).

The most popular technique is still the conventional endarterectomy of the carotid bifurcation through a longitudinal arteriotomy followed by direct suture or patch

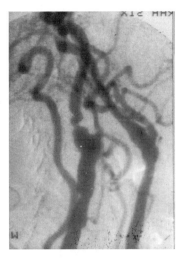
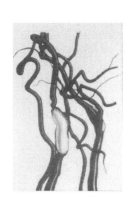

FIGURE 73.1. ICA restenosis after cartoid endarterectomy with patch angioplasty.

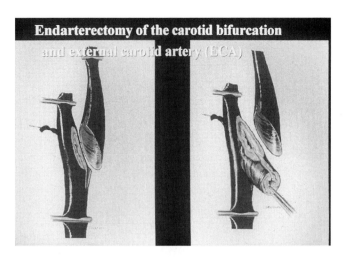

FIGURE 73.4. Endarterectomy of the CCA and ECA.

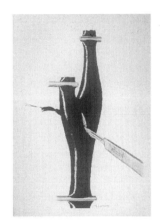
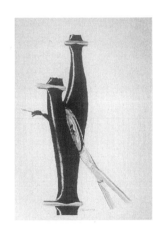

FIGURE 73.2. Technique of eversion endarterectomy. Oblique transsection of the ICA from the CCA.

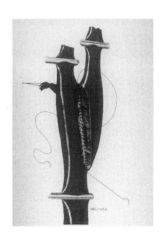
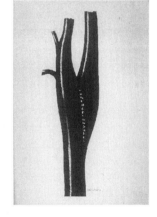

FIGURE 73.5. Reimplantation of the ICA into the CCA.

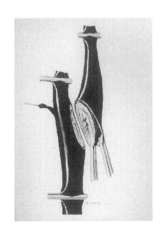
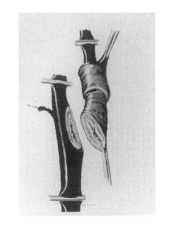

FIGURE 73.3. Eversion endarterectomy of the ICA after transsection of the ICA from the CCA.

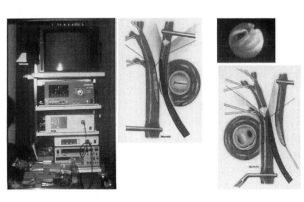

FIGURE 73.6. Intraoperative angioscopic control of the ICA and ECA after eversion endarterectomy.

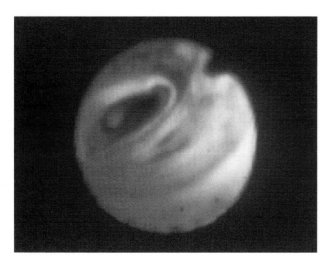

FIGURE 73.7. Angioscopic control of the ICA: intimal flap/dissection—redo by graft interposition.

angioplasty.[10,11] With increasing frequency of carotid reconstructions we are more frequently confronted with the problem of recurrent stenoses. The rate of restenosis reported in the literature ranges from 1.2% to 23.9%, depending on the study method.[7] Several clinical and technical factors influence the development of recurrent carotid stenoses, but in some cases the etiology remains unclear. Although a variety of causal factors for recurrent carotid stenoses have been proposed, technical failure more frequently results in restenoses than systemic factors. Technical failures include clamp traumas, intimal and medial flaps, strictures at the distal end of the arteriotomy, and inadequate resection of the ICA. In a series of approximately 6000 carotid endarterectomies performed at the Nuremberg Medical Center between August 1984 and July 1991 we found 66 patients with carotid restenosis. In this group the cause for restenosis was inadequate resection of the elongated ICA in 27 patients (Figure 73.1). Due to this high rate of restenosis after conventional carotid endarterectomy and some technical problems in correcting the elongated ICA we were searching for new methods to perform carotid endarterectomy. In accordance with Kieny's recommendation we now also recommend EEA of the ICA, a technique we began using in 1987. This procedure allows for easier correction of an elongated or kinked ICA. In our patient population we found carotid lesions in combination with kinking in 37%.[7,8]

Comparing conventional endarterectomy with EEA, we had a combined morbidity and mortality rate in the first group of 3.8% and in the second group of 2.5%. This difference was not statistically significant.[7] The mean clamping time in the group of patients undergoing carotid endarterectomy was 17.2 minutes (9–63 minutes); in the group undergoing EEA it totaled 14 minutes (8–24 minutes). In an initial series of 122 patients who were followed up we found a restenosis rate of 1.9% after a mean follow-up period of 28 months.[7,8]

Intraoperative quality control—preferably by angioscopy—is necessary.[9] In a consecutive series of 196 patients undergoing carotid surgery we found abnormalities in the ICA in 32%; 29% of these were thrombi and small remaining debris and suture irregularities and 3% intimal flaps or dissection.[9] In 13% of the pathological findings no correction was necessary. In 16% the remaining thrombi or irregularities could be removed by endoscopic procedures and by flushing out the thrombi with saline solution. Intimal flaps and dissection were corrected by graft interposition (Figure 73.7).

Angioscopic control of the carotid artery is of great value in perioperative quality control and allows immediate revision before completion of the anastomosis. Another advantage of carotid angioscopy is that it is performed while the vessel is clamped, which means visibility is not influenced by collateral blood. Due to our excellent results with EEA in the carotid artery we now use this new technique exclusively (except in redo surgery, aneurysms, and dissections).

References

1. Etheredge SN. A simple technique for carotid endarterectomy. *Ann Surg.* 1970;120:275–278.
2. DeBakey ME, Crawford ES, Cooley DA, et al. Surgical considerations of occlusive disease of innominate, carotid, subclavian, and vertebral arteries. *Ann Surg.* 1959;149:690–710.
3. Thevenet A. Chirurgie des Lésions non athéromateuses carotidiennes. In: Kieffer E, Natali J, eds. *Aspects Techniques de la Chirurgie Carotidienne.* Paris: AERCV; 1987:219–239.
4. Jones CE. Carotid eversion endarterectomy revisited. *Am J Surg.* 1989;157:323–328.
5. Kieny R, Mantz F, Kurtz TH, et al. Les resténoses carotidiennes après endartériectomie. In: Kieffer E, Bousser MG, eds. *Indications et Résultats de la Chirurgie Carotidienne.* Paris: AERCV; 1998:77–100.
6. Kieny R, Hirsch D, Seiller MD, et al. Does carotid eversion endarterectomy and reimplantation reduce the risk of restenosis? *Ann Vasc Surg.* 1993;7:407–413.
7. Raithel D. New techniques in the surgical management of carotid-artery lesions. *Surgical Rounds.* 1990;13:53–60.
8. Raithel D. Choice of graft material in carotid surgery: vein versus PTFE. In: Veith FJ, ed. *Current Critical Problems in Vascular Surgery.* Vol 6. St Louis, Mo: Quality Medical Publishing; 1994:259–263.
9. Raithel D, Kasprzak P. Angioscopy after carotid endarterectomy. In: Greenhalgh RM, ed. *Vascular Imaging for Surgeons.* London: WB Saunders; 1995:141–146.
10. Vanmaele R, Van Schil P, De Measneer M. Closure of the internal carotid artery after endarterectomy: the advantages of patch angioplasty without its disadvantages. *Ann Vasc Surg.* 1990;4:81–84.
11. Vanmaele RG. Surgery for carotid stenosis: the quest for the ideal technique. *Eur J Vasc Surg.* 1993;7:361–363.

74

Surgically Excised Carotid Bifurcation Plaque

Anthony M. Imparato

The recently reported results of a number of prospective randomized clinical trials of the effects of carotid endarterectomy in decreasing the incidence of strokes in the presence of carotid artery bifurcation atherosclerosis[1-4] have emphasized the need to better understand the pathologic changes that occur at the bifurcation and how they relate to strokes.[5] The common denominator for selection of patients for randomization in four of the most recently reported studies, two for symptomatic[1,2] and two for asymptomatic patients,[3,4] was an estimation of carotid stenosis. In spite of the similarity of favorable clinical outcomes in surgical patients, the degree of stenosis considered to be critical for selection for operation varied among the groups from 50% to 70%. The techniques for measuring stenosis varied so much in the various study groups that even more differences were introduced.[6-8]

Clearly, then, the critical factors of carotid pathology that place patients at risk for suffering ischemic strokes cannot be accurately assessed from measurements of carotid stenosis alone.[5,9-13] Additionally, estimation of carotid stenosis from angiograms, even biplane studies, is inherently inaccurate however measured, because of the eccentric rather than uniformly concentric nature of the lesions (Figure 74.1). Estimates based on flow characteristics determined with Doppler probes similarly share inherent inaccuracy, because the determinations are highly technician dependent, and standardization of the technique is by comparison with angiograms. Ultimately an estimated range of stenosis rather than a precise figure is reported for each test. Furthermore, patients with less than a critical degree of carotid stenosis are not immune from suffering strokes. Though not yet shown to be helped by surgical intervention, they nevertheless harbor risk factors in their lesions unrelated to the degree of stenosis.[1-4]

What is the nature of the carotid plaque as determined from study of surgical arterial specimens both in situ and after removal by carotid endarterectomy in both symptomatic and asymptomatic patients deemed to be surgical candidates? Do the surgical findings confirm the traditional ideas[14] regarding the pathogenesis of atherosclerosis?

Carotid Bifurcation Plaque Materials and Methods

Surgeons who participated in the Joint Study of Extracranial Arterial Occlusions (1962–1972)[15] who performed carotid endarterectomies and met semiannually at regional workshops gave markedly different descriptions of the appearances of carotid bifurcation plaques as they saw them during surgery. Very early in our experience with carotid endarterectomy, we noted that the descriptive reports of our own pathologists, based on gross and microscopic inspection of fixed carotid endarterectomy specimens, were at variance, in descriptions and interpretations of findings, from our own observations of plaques in situ during surgery. I therefore decided to photograph carotid plaques in situ during surgery in all surgical patients and submit these records to the pathologist to assist him in the reconstruction of the plaques when viewing the gross surgical specimens and in interpreting the findings of microscopic examination.[9]

The specimens studied were then photographed in situ immediately after performing a long longitudinal arteriotomy after gentle saline irrigation to remove fresh (red, liquid) blood and then photographed again shortly after excision in the operating room before fixation. They were then immersed in 10% formalin and sent to the pathologist for processing. Virtually all specimens were removed in one piece.

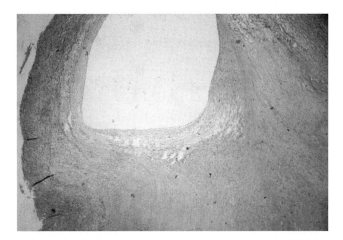

FIGURE 74.1. Eccentric as opposed to uniformly concentric configurations of carotid plaques that make it difficult to obtain accurate measurements of stenosis on biplane angiograms.

Carotid Plaque Spectrum

Although carotid bifurcation plaques found in surgical patients at operation on gross inspection differ markedly in appearance and composition from patient to patient, they share certain characteristics. Longitudinally they extend from the common carotid artery at approximately the level of the omohyoid muscle, across the carotid bulb, to involve the proximal 1 to 3 cm of the internal carotid artery. There the lesions gradually, eccentrically taper to a thin intima and only very rarely extend to the level of the digastric muscle (Figure 74.2). Release of the hypoglossal cranial nerve (XII N) by severing the sternocleidomastoid artery and vein and the descending hypoglossal branch almost invariably permits access to uninvolved areas of the internal carotid artery beyond visible plaque and beyond frequently occurring redundancy and kinking of the internal carotid artery (Figure 74.3). The bulkiest segment of plaque is almost invariably at the lateral wall of the carotid bulb and proximal 1 cm of the internal carotid artery opposite of the ostium of the external carotid artery, regardless of the varied composition of the plaque. Gross inspection reveals the spectrum of complexity of the lesions, which range from smooth, glistening white eccentric fibrous elevations of the luminal surfaces of the involved vessels (Figure 74.4) to completely encysted, localized collections of relatively fresh blood clot (Figure 74.5) to collections of toothpastelike consistency, yellow amorphous debris (Figure 74.6). Between these two extremes are various combinations of fresh and old blood and yellow atheromatous debris (Figure 74.7).

Breaks or fissures of the fibrous cases that cover the encysted material, either blood or atheromatous debris, occur to various degrees. The most extensive breaks appear as large, ulcerated areas with overhanging edges,

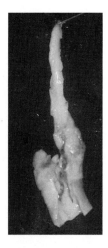

FIGURE 74.2. The longitudinal extent of a carotid bifurcation plaque is illustrated by an excised specimen. The distal extent almost always terminates in normal intima. Proximally, in the common carotid artery, the intima is frequently thick though smooth on its luminal aspect and requires tack-down sutures following carotid endarterectomy.

the bases of which may contain the remains of any of the previously described encysted materials. There may or may not be laminated salmon-colored flow thrombi at sites of ulceration. Ulcerations may have smooth or even sloping edges with smooth, otherwise clean bases. Smooth pits, sometimes multiple, are seen at sites where encysted blood, atheromatous debris, and surface breaks usually occur; they resemble healed ulcers (Figure 74.8).

Irregularly occurring yellow streaks (fatty streaks) are often seen. Their distribution, however, does not conform to the sites of most advanced pathologic changes but rather they appear to be irregularly scattered throughout the intima (Figure 74.9).

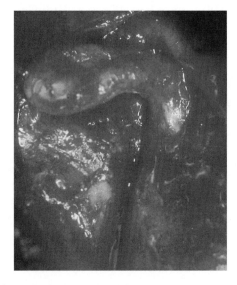

FIGURE 74.3. Redundancy and kinking of the distal internal carotid artery that, if not corrected after carotid endarterectomy, may lead to operative site thrombosis.

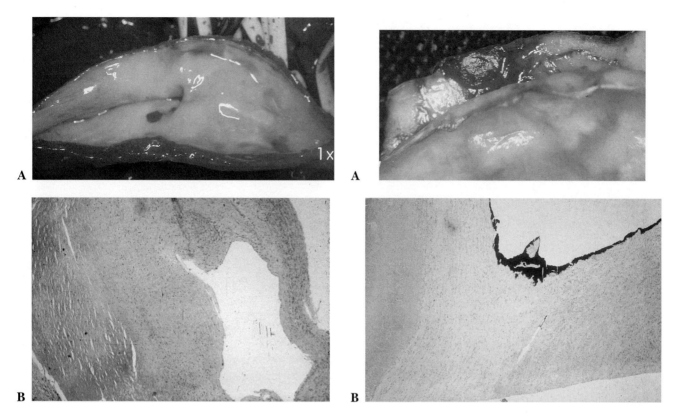

FIGURE 74.4. **A,** Gross appearance of a smooth, glistening, simple fibrous plaque at the carotid bifurcation. **B,** Microscopic appearance of a typical simple fibrous plaque producing marked luminal stenosis.

FIGURE 74.5. **A,** Recent bleeding into a simple fibrous plaque that raises a cap of fibrotic plaque to produce stenosis. **B,** Microscopic appearance of the hematoma produced within the wall of the fibrotic plaque by the recent hemorrhage shown.

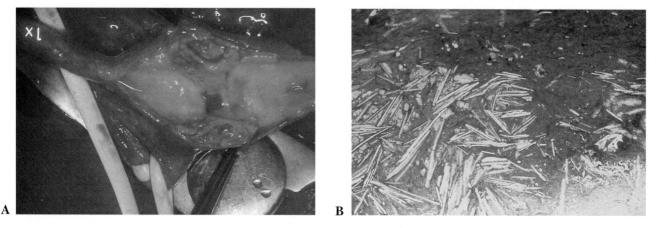

FIGURE 74.6. **A,** Gross appearance of encysted amorphous atheromatous debris producing a cholesterol abscess. **B,** Microscopic appearance of a cholesterol abscess with numerous cholesterol crystals.

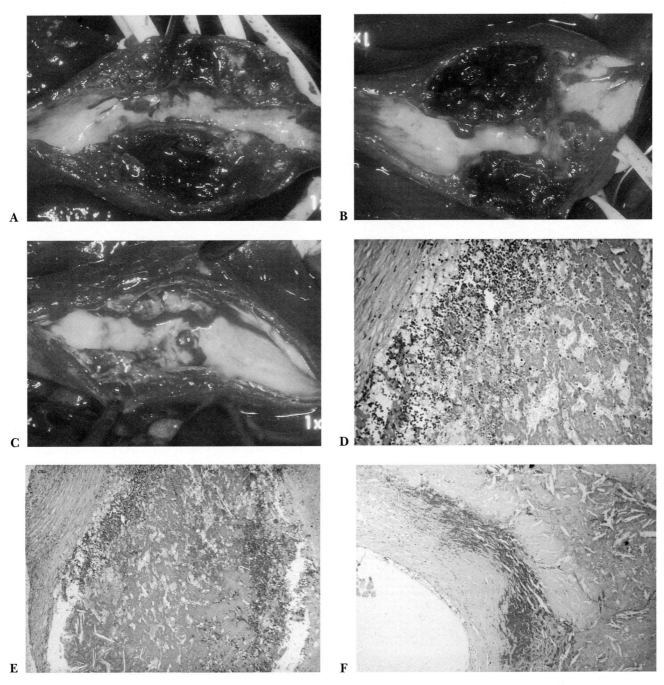

FIGURE 74.7. **A, B, C,** Gross appearances of blood of various ages totally encysted within fibrous plaques. The colors of the hematomas, ranging from maroon to chocolate brown, and their occurring in association with amorphous atheromatous debris attest to their gradual degradation to cholesterol ab-scesses. **D, E, F,** Microscopic appearances of plaque hematomas showing various stages of degradation from easily recognized formed blood elements to amorphous material to cholesterol clefts.

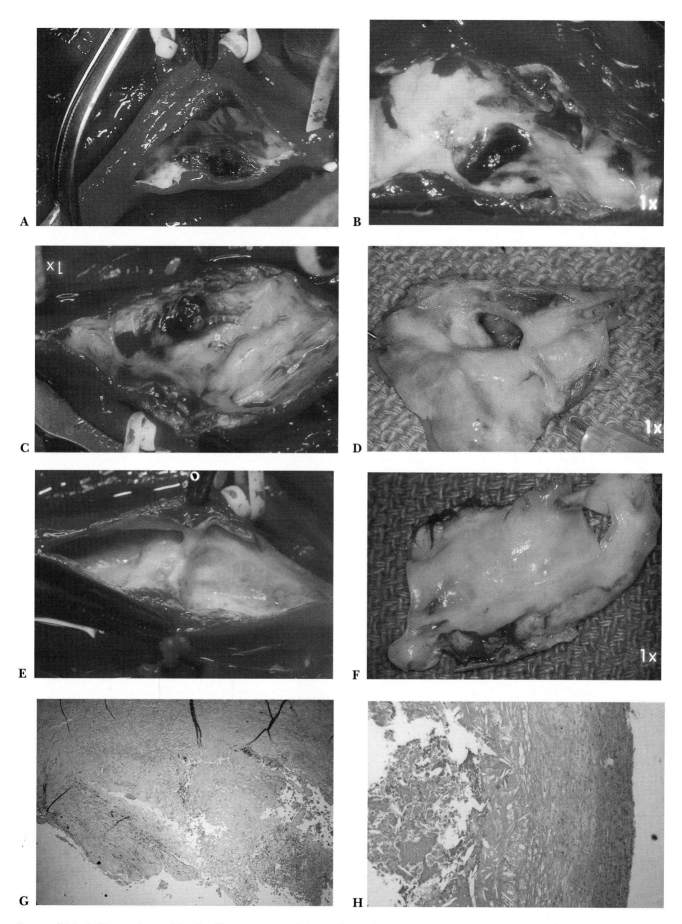

FIGURE 74.8. **A,** Fissure formed in the fibrous cap overlying a plaque hematoma. **B,** Unroofed plaque hematoma that has been
(Continued on page 890)

partially evacuated. **C,** Clear-cut, sharply demarcated ulcer resulting from evacuation of a plaque hematoma into the arterial lumen. **D,** Plaque ulcer with rounded edges and an area of apparent healing. **E,** "Pits" in a carotid plaque that appear to be healed ulcers. **F,** Thinned-out areas in a carotid plaque at sites of pits. **G,** Microscopic section of recently formed ulcer showing the edge of the disrupted fibrous cap that recently covered the underlying hematoma. **H,** Ulcer with atheromatous debris at its base and overlying thrombus that formed at the site of ulceration. **I,** Microscopic appearance of a healed ulcer.

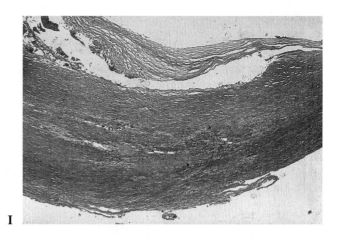

I

Stenosis of even marked degree may be due to bulging of encysted blood, of encysted atheromatous debris, or from simple (confirmed by microscopic examination) eccentric masses of fibrous tissue. In each instance stenosis is caused by bulging of the lateral wall of the carotid sinus and proximal internal carotid artery into the lumen.

Microscopically, the gross findings are almost always confirmed. Areas of stenosis that form a smooth, firm bulge into the arterial lumen microscopically consist of fibrotic tissue and resemble the myointimal proliferative lesions produced in experimental animals by altering blood vessel geometry to create abnormal flow patterns.[16-19] The areas that appear to be blood clots are seen as evenly dispersed localized collections of blood elements without lamination and are characteristic of hematoma or fresh stasis clot. Toothpastelike material consists of amorphous debris. Various stages of degradation of blood are encountered, including formation of cholesterol crystals and amorphous debris. Finally, hemosiderin is present. The simplest plaque, then, is entirely fibrotic; devoid of lipids, macrophages, and foam cells; and may be so advanced in development as to cause severe fibrotic stenosis.

Next in order of complexity appears to be the localized collections of evenly dispersed red blood cells, completely surrounded by fibrous plaque, isolated from the arterial lumen by an unbroken fibrous cap, and sometimes associated with neovascularity of the fibrous matrix. Of somewhat greater complexity are plaques that contain blood of apparently different ages as deduced from the state of preservation of the red blood cells, which eventually harbor among them clefts characteristic of cholesterol crystals. Of even greater complexity are encysted collections of atheromatous debris with or without associated recent and old hemorrhages, sometimes only hemosiderin.

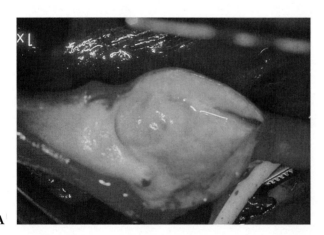

A

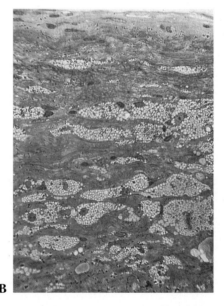

B

FIGURE 74.9. **A,** Gross appearance of fatty streaks that are irregularly dispersed at sites of intimal thickening, not closely related to sites of maximally developed carotid plaques nor to the sites where hemorrhage, cholesterol abscesses, ulceration, or thrombosis is found. **B,** Microscopic section of fatty streak showing foam cells within the media. The overlying fibrous intimal cap exhibits none of the characteristics of typical atherosclerosis.

Ulceration appears to occur when the fibrous cap overlying either hematoma or atheromatous debris ruptures and liberates part or all of the contents of the cavities. The remaining cavities (ulcers) with overhanging edges then serve as foci for deposition of flow thrombus, which may lead to thrombosis of the vessel or an ulcer site that eventually heals without thrombosis, resulting in smooth, clear-cut depressions or pits. Fatty streaks and lipid-laden macrophages do not appear to participate in this type of plaque evolution.

Total occlusions of the internal carotid artery (Figure 74.9) typically consist of an either markedly stenotic or ulcerated plaque at the origin of the internal carotid artery. Adherent laminated salmon-colored flow thrombus is found at the origin, beyond which red stasis clot loosely adherent to the intima extends various distances along the internal carotid artery. In late occlusions, the internal carotid artery contains loosely adherent fibrous strands.

Pathogenesis of Carotid Bifurcation Plaque

Surgical specimens viewed in situ in vivo indicate a stereotyped distribution of plaques related to the geometry of the involved arteries, which strongly suggests a primary hemodynamic etiology.[16,21] Indeed, the distal extent of plaque in the internal carotid artery correlates with the acuteness of the bifurcation angle of the two main branches of the common carotid artery so that a more acute angle indicates a longer extension of plaque in the internal carotid artery, and a more obtuse angle is associated with a shorter internal carotid plaque (A.M.I., unpublished data, 1975). Of the various hemodynamic conditions that have been cited as causative in the development of these plaques—increased shear stress,[22] decreased shear stress, [23,24] turbulence,[25,26] boundary layer separation,[27] and diminished lateral pressure (Bernoulli)[20]—none appears able to explain the entire spectrum of their distribution even in a site as localized as the carotid bifurcation. The common denominator, if one exists, is hidden in the various geometric configurations of arteries that predispose patients to atherosclerosis.[28]

Carotid Plaque Evolution Versus Traditional View of Pathogenesis of Atherosclerosis

A number of traditional views of atherosclerosis in general[30] and carotid lesions in particular[3] have in common the concept that lipid deposition in arterial walls (media) results in lipid-laden macrophages that ultimately rupture and invoke fibrous intimal proliferation through the discharge of free fats. The resulting "cholesterol" abscess may develop hemorrhage within it[22] or rupture, or its overlying fibrous cap may act as the nidus for thrombosis. Encysted blood within plaque may be from incorporation of luminal thrombus into the plaque by fibrous overgrowth, by fissuring of the fibrous cap overlying cholesterol abscesses and dissection of blood into the plaque, or from hemorrhage with fatty plaques from the revascularity sometimes encountered.

The findings in surgical specimens of carotid bifurcation plaques, however, would seem to favor two different sequences of events, starting with intimal fibrous (probably from transformed smooth muscle cells[29]) proliferation followed by intrafibrous plaque hemorrhage, secondary to intimal neovascularity.[33] Degradation of plaque hematoma leads to localized collections of atheromatous material. Embolization and thrombosis follow rupture of the fibrous cap,[34] which when intact contains the intraplaque hemorrhages and cholesterol abscesses.

Significance of Pathologic Findings at the Carotid Bifurcation

In an analysis of the gross and microscopic findings at the carotid bifurcation it was found that of the focal symptoms, known to be premonitory to stroke in a large percentage of patients, intraplaque hemorrhage was a major finding.[9,10,13] Additionally, secondary changes beyond mere fibrous intimal thickening, consisting of gross intraplaque hemorrhages, cholesterol abscesses, and subocclusive thromboses, were more frequent as the degree of stenosis became greater.[10] Severe stenosis, then, as a major criterion for selection of patients for operation, is reasonable though not precise, because it includes patients with hard fibrous plaques in whom the risk of stroke is less and excludes patients with advanced stroke-provoking pathologic changes in whom the degree of stenosis may be measured as less than critical: (70% or greater, North American Symptomatic Carotid Endarterectomy Trial [NASCET] and European Carotid Endaterectomy Trial [ECET]; 60% Asymptomatic Carotid Atherosclerosis Study [ACAS]; 50% Department of Veterans Affairs Cooperative Studies Program #167: Asymptomatic Carotid Artery Stenosis [VA Asympt]).

Efforts to delineate the specific pathologic components in carotid plaques (ultrasound,[35] nuclear magnetic resonance,[37] and computed tomography[37,38]) and the earliest manifestations of cerebral embolization producing subclinical silent infarcts[39,40] (computed tomography and nuclear magnetic resonance of brain; transcranial Doppler) are more recent developments. They merit ex-

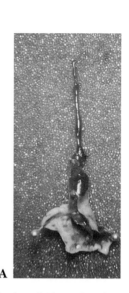

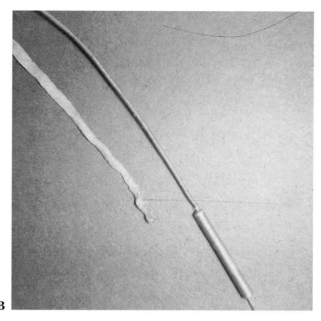

A   **B**

FIGURE 74.10. **A,** Total occlusion of an internal carotid artery showing salmon-colored flow thrombus that formed at the site of maximal stenosis and possibly ulceration. A maroon stasis clot is seen distal to the flow thrombus and may extend to the level of the first major branch of the internal carotid artery intracranially at the carotid siphon. **B,** Stasis clot in the internal carotid artery eventually becomes converted to a fibrous cord.

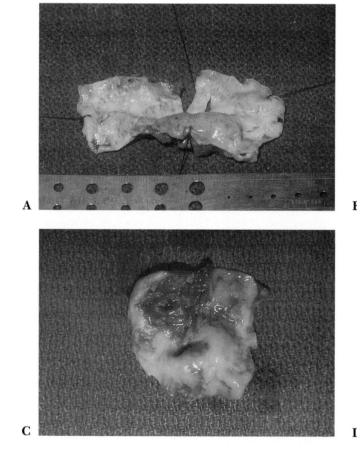

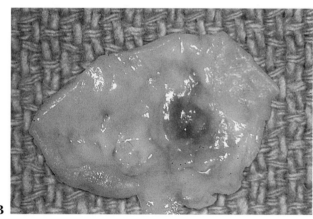

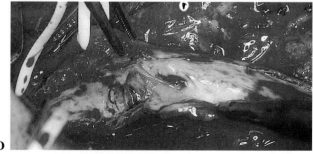

FIGURE 74.11. **A,** Gross appearance of a subneointimal hematoma in a recurrent fibrous plaque 5 years after carotid endarterectomy. **B,** Recurrent complex carotid plaque 7 years after carotid endarterectomy. The original plaque removed at operation is shown for comparison. **C,** Compound, ulcerated, atherosclerotic, recurrent plaque 12 years after carotid endarterectomy.

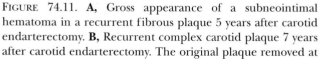

tensive investigation to confirm the facts that patients with soft, nonechogenic plaques and those with evidence of silent cerebral embolization should undergo surgery even when they exhibit less than critical stenoses.

Recurrent Carotid Stenosis After Endarterectomy

After carotid endarterectomy both early and late stenosis has become a major clinical entity, in part because of the long-term survival of many of the patients who undergo the procedure. Early recurrent stenosis must be differentiated from residual plaque from incomplete endarterectomy. Early stenosis[41] is the term applied to fibrous neointimal proliferation detected within the first 2 years after endarterectomy. It usually has a smooth, glistening white luminal surface that resembles the spontaneously occurring simple bifurcation plaques.[42-44] The distribution of areas of stenosis is variable and may involve either the entire or a part of the endarterectomized segment of carotid artery.

In our own series of carotid endarterectomies in which venous roof patch angioplasties were performed, although diffuse stenosis has rarely been encountered, focal stenoses, when seen, characteristically are at the tapered distal end of the angioplasty site or less often at the site where the common carotid artery's relatively thick but not stenotic intima was transected, an observation that has led to routine tacking of that transected intima. Late recurrent lesions (Figure 74.10) at the endarterectomy site closely resemble spontaneously occurring complex plaques and range from subneointimal encysted hematoma to ulcerated compound plaques, encountered as long as 20 years after carotid endarterectomy (A.M.I., unpublished data, 1998). As with the original plaques, both simple fibrous and complex recurrent plaques can be removed by endarterectomy[45] (Figure 74.11).

References

1. North American Symptomatic Carotid Endarterectomy Trial Collaborators. Beneficial effect of carotid endarterectomy in symptomatic patients with high-grade carotid stenosis. *N Engl J Med.* 1991;325:445–453.
2. European Carotid Surgery Trialists' Collaborative Group. MCA European carotid surgery trial: interim results for patients with severe (70% to 99%) or with mild (0% to 29%) carotid stenosis. *Lancet.* 1991;337:1235–1243.
3. Executive Committee for the Asymptomatic Carotid Atherosclerosis Study. Endarterectomy for asymptomatic carotid stenosis. *JAMA.* 1995;273:1421–1428.
4. Hobson RW II, Weiss DG, Fields WS, et al. Efficacy of carotid endarterectomy for symptomatic carotid stenosis. *N Engl J Med.* 1993;328:221–227.
5. Fisher CM, Ojemann RG. A clinico-pathologic study of carotid endarterectomy plaques. *Rev Neurol (Paris).* 1986; 142:573–589.
6. Rothwell PM, Gibson RJ, Slattery J, Sellar R, Warlaw CP, for the European Carotid Surgery Trialists' Collaborative Group. Equivalence of measurements of carotid stenosis: a comparison of three methods on 1001 angiograms. *Stroke.* 1994;25:435–439.
7. Rothwell PM, Gibson RJ, Slattery J, Warlaw C. Prognostic value and reproducibility of measurements of carotid stenosis: a comparison of three methods on 1001 angiograms. *Stroke.* 1994;25:2440–2444.
8. Eliasziw M, Smith RF, Singh N, Holsworth DW, Fox AJ, Barnett HJM, for North American Symptomatic Carotid Endarterectomy Trial Group. Further comments on the measurement of carotid stenosis from angiograms. *Stroke.* 1994;25:2445–2449.
9. Imparato AM, Riles TS, Gorstein F. The carotid bifurcation plaque: pathologic findings associated with cerebral ischemia. *Stroke.* 1979;10:238–245.
10. Imparato AM, Riles TS, Mintzer R, Baumann G. The importance of hemorrhage in the relationship between gross morphologic characteristics and cerebral symptoms in 376 carotid artery plaques. *Ann Surg.* 1983;197:195–203.
11. Lusby RJ, Ferrell LD, Ehrenfeld WK, et al. Carotid plaque hemorrhage: its role in the production of cerebral ischemia. *Arch Surg.* 1982;117:1479–1488.
12. Ammar AD, Ernst RL, Lin JJ, et al. The influence of repeated carotid plaque hemorrhages on the production of cerebrovascular symptoms. *J Vasc Surg.* 1986;3:857–859.
13. Gomez CR. Carotid plaque morphology and risk for stroke: current concepts of cardiovascular disease and stroke. *Stroke.* 1989;24:25–29.
14. Imparato AM. The carotid bifurcation plaque: a model for the study of atherosclerosis. *J Vasc Surg.* 1986;3:249–255.
15. Blaisdell FW, Clauss RH, Galbraith JG, et al. Joint study of extracranial arterial occlusion: a review of surgical considerations. *JAMA.* 1969;209:1889–1895.
16. Imparato AM, Baumann FG. Consequences of hemodynamic alterations of the arterial wall after revascularization. In: Towne JB, Bernhard VM, eds. *Complications in Vascular Surgery.* New York, NY: Grune & Stratton; 1980: 107–121.
17. Nathan IM, Imparato AM. Vibration analysis in experimental models of atherosclerosis. *Bull N Y Acad Med.* 1977; 58:849–868.
18. Imparato AM, Baumann FG. Electron-microscopic studies of fibromuscular arterial lesions experimentally produced in the dog renal arteries. *Surgery Gynecology and Obstetrics.* 1974;139:497–504.
19. Baumann FG, Imparato AM, Kim GE, et al. A study of the evolution of early fibromuscular lesions hemodynamically induced in the dog renal artery, II: scanning and correlative transmission electron microscopy. *Artery.* 1978;4: 67–99.
20. Texon M, Imparato AM, Lord J Jr. Hemodynamic concept of atherosclerosis. *Arch Surg.* 1960;80:47–53.
21. Imparato AM, Texon M, Helpern M, Lord J Jr. Experimental production of atherosclerosis by alteration of blood vessel configuration. *Surgical Forum of the American College of Surgeons.* 1961;12:245.
22. Ross J, Glomset FA. Pathogenesis of arteriosclerosis. *N Engl J Med.* 1976;295:369–377.
23. Caro CG, Fitzgerald JM, Schroter RC. Arterial wall shear and distribution of early atheroma in man. *Nature (London).* 1964;223:1159–1165.

24. Zarins CK, Giddens DB, Bharadavaj BK, et al. Carotid bifurcation atherosclerosis: quantitative correlation of plaque localization with flow velocity profiles and shear stress. *Circ Res.* 1983;53:502–508.

25. Sakata N, Takebayashi S. Localization of atherosclerotic lesions in curving sites of human internal carotid arteries. *Biorheology.* 1988;25:567–574.

26. Schwartz CJ, Mitchell JRP. Observations on localization of arterial plaques. *Circ Res.* 1962;11:63–73.

27. LoGerfo FW, Novak MD, Quist WC, et al. Flow studies in a model carotid bifurcation. *Arteriosclerosis.* 1981;1:235–242.

28. Texon M. The hemodynamic basis of atherosclerosis: further observations: the ostial lesion. *Bull N Y Acad Med.* 1972;48:733–740.

29. Ross R. The pathogenesis of atherosclerosis: an update. *N Engl J Med.* 1986;314:448–455.

30. Winternitz MC, Thomas RM, LeComte PM. Studies in the pathology of vascular disease. *Am Heart J.* 1937;14:399–404.

31. Solberg LA, Eggen DA. Localization and sequence development of atherosclerotic lesions in the carotid and vertebral arteries. *Circulation.* 1971;43:711–724.

32. Moon HD, Rinehart JF. Histogenesis of coronary arteriosclerosis. *Circulation.* 1952;6:481–488.

33. Fryer JA, Myers PC, Appleberg M. Carotid intraplaque hemorrhage: the significance of neovascularity. *J Vasc Surg.* 1987;6:341–345.

34. Ogata J, Masuda J, Yutani C, Yamaguchi T. Rupture of atheromatous plaque as a cause of thrombotic occlusion of stenotic internal carotid artery. *Stroke.* 1990;21:1740–1745.

35. Hatsukami TS, Thackray BD, Primozich JF, et al. Echolucent regions in carotid plaque: preliminary analysis comparing three-dimensional histologic reconstruction to sonographic findings. *Ultrasound Med Biol.* 1994;20:743–749

36. Kim D, Orron DE. *Peripheral Imaging and Intervention.* St Louis, Mo: Mosby–Year Book; 1992.

37. Castillo M, Wilson JD. CT angiography of the common carotid artery bifurcation: comparison between two techniques and conventional angiography. *Neuroradiology.* 1994;36:602–604.

38. Young GR, Humphrey PRD, Shaw MDM, et al. Comparison of magnetic resonance angiography, duplex ultrasound, and digital subtraction angiography in assessment of extracranial internal carotid artery stenosis. *J Neurol Neurosurg Psychiatry.* 1994;57:1466–1478.

39. Berguer R, Sieggreen MY, Lazo A, Hodakowaki GT. The silent brain infarct in carotid surgery. *J Vasc Surg.* 1986;3:442–447.

40. Zukowski AJ, Nicolaides AN, Lewis RT, et al. The correlation between carotid plaque ulceration and cerebral infarction seen on CT scan. *J Vasc Surg.* 1984;1:782–786.

41. Stoney BJ, String ST. Recurrent carotid stenosis. *Surgery.* 1976;80:705–710.

42. Clagett GP, Robinowitz M, Youkey JR, et al. Morphogenesis and clinicopathologic characteristics of recurrent carotid artery disease. *J Vasc Surg.* 1986;3:10–23.

43. Imparato AM, Weinstein GS. Clinicopathologic correlation in postendarterectomy recurrent stenosis. *J Vasc Surg.* 1986;3:657–666.

44. Schwarcz TH, Yates GN, Ghobrial M, Baker WH. Pathologic characteristics of recurrent carotid artery stenosis. *J Vasc Surg.* 1987;5:280–288.

45. Imparato AM. In discussion of: Stoney RJ, String ST. Recurrent carotid stenosis. *Surgery.* 1976;80:709–710.

75

Stroke

Maurice W. Nicholson and Sandra E. Ritz

Stroke, or cerebrovascular accident, is the sudden development of a nonconvulsive, focal neurological deficit due to a local disturbance in the cerebral circulation. It is most often caused by occlusion of an artery secondary to thrombosis or embolism. Less frequently, the etiology is rupture of an artery into the brain or subarachnoid space.

Stroke incidence and mortality rates have decreased in recent years, but stroke remains a major public health problem. Few stroke survivors ever completely return to their prior health status or functional capacity. Recent significant advances in acute stroke treatment can improve outcome and have led to rapidly changing recommendations for stroke prevention and treatment. Stroke is a medical emergency, and rapid intervention may prevent loss of brain tissue. In this chapter we review stroke epidemiology, prevention, pathophysiology, risk factors, clinical features and their basis, clinical assessment and diagnostic studies, imaging, medical treatment, surgical treatment, and rehabilitation.

Epidemiology

Stroke ranks as the third major cause of death in the United States after heart disease and cancer, with 150,000 deaths attributable to stroke annually.[1] A stroke strikes every minute in the United States and is the leading cause of adult disability in Americans. About 550,000 Americans, 50,000 Canadians, and 32,000 Mexicans experience a new or recurrent stroke each year.[2]

Worldwide stroke incidence rates are difficult to quantify, because measures depend on the accurate identification of all cases of first stroke, assessment of the underlying population at risk, and the age distribution of the study population. The average age-adjusted incidence of first strokes has been reported to be 114 per 100,000,[3] but estimates of new strokes worldwide range from 81 to 200 per 100,000 in different studies, with the stroke rate in developing countries as high as that in developed countries.[4,5]

The incidence of stroke increases with age, and men have 30% to 80% higher rates of stroke than women.[6] Stroke incidence and mortality rates are elevated in susceptible racial and ethnic groups (e.g., the 1992 death rate from stroke in African Americans was 45.0 per 100,000,[7] in contrast to the overall 1992 US rate of 26.6).[1] There are also regional differences: a southeastern area of the United States is known as the "stroke belt" because it has a 10% higher stroke rate than the rest of the country.[8]

First-ever strokes account for approximately 75% of acute events.[3] The recurrence rate is 7% to 10% per year and is highest in the first year after the initial stroke. Approximately one half of initial stroke victims live for 3 or more years and more than one third live for 10 years.[5] Mortality rates for intracerebral hemorrhages are much higher than those for infarction; in the 1984 Rochester, Minnesota, study, the 30-day case fatality rate was 48% for intracerebral hemorrhage compared with 17% for all strokes.[6]

Approximately 3.8 million individuals survive strokes annually in the United States.[1] The effects of strokes can be devastating, and the economic cost is enormous, because only about 10% of stroke survivors ever return to their prestroke health status, 48% are hemiparetic, 22% are unable to walk, 24% to 53% have complete or partial dependence, 12% to 18% are aphasic, and 32% are clinically depressed.[9] Many stroke survivors are unable to return to work, have significant disability, and often develop other health problems.

Strokes have profound social, psychological, and economic effects on stroke survivors and their families, friends, employers, and community. Between 1991 and 1992, 1 million Americans had disabilities that resulted from stroke and 71% of them had at least some limitations in vocational capacity.[1] By 1996 this number had tripled to 3 million Americans who were permanently disabled because of stroke; one third had mild impairments, one third had moderate impairments, and one third had severe impairments.[2]

The annual cost of stroke in the United States for direct health care costs and lost productivity ranges from $23.2 billion[1] to $40 billion.[2,9] This figure includes physician and nursing services, hospital and nursing home services, the cost of medications, and lost productivity that results from disability.

Previously, stroke was considered a hopeless disease with no effective treatment. With the improved recognition and treatment of associated risk factors, along with antihypertensive, anticoagulant, and antiplatelet drugs, the incidence of stroke and stroke mortality has decreased in recent years in the United States and other developed countries. The US death rate from stroke declined dramatically from 88.8% in 1950 to 26.6% in 1992.[1] The average annual incidence of stroke in the Rochester, Minnesota, area declined by 46%, from 213 per 100,000 between 1950 and 1954 to 115 per 100,000 between 1975 and 1979.[6] This decline of stroke in Rochester began at approximately the same time as control of hypertension improved in the community.[10] A subsequent 17% increase in incidence of stroke in that same area between 1980 and 1984 coincided with the introduction of computed tomography (CT), which appeared to increase the detection of less severe strokes.

Improved understanding of cerebral autoregulation and better management of hyperglycemia and hypertension have contributed to an improved outcome after acute stroke. The development and improvement of antibiotics and treatment protocols for acute stroke are now decreasing the morbidity and mortality rates from secondary complications of stroke.

Prevention

Stroke prevention has recently been given high priority as a public health strategy in the United States and has been targeted for cost containment by managed care health systems and other insurers.[11] The key to reducing the economic burden of stroke appears to rest in either preventing its occurrence or further reducing stroke mortality and improving the functioning and quality of life of stroke survivors.[12]

The US Public Health Service in conjunction with the National Health Promotion and Disease Prevention Objectives has set a goal to reduce stroke deaths to 20 per 100,000 by the target year 2000.[7] The National Institute for Neurological Disease and Stroke (NINDS), part of the National Institutes of Health, and national organizations such as the American Heart Association and the National Stroke Association have launched an educational campaign to regard stroke as an emergency. The goal is to educate health professionals and the public

that stroke needs to receive the same priority as myocardial infarction (MI).[13] The term *brain attack,* purposely used to resemble the term *heart attack,* has been coined to describe the recent move to treat stroke as a medical emergency.[14]

In the past, therapy was primarily aimed at preventing recurrence or progression of stroke. Recent research and therapeutic advances in the treatment of acute stroke have been developed, and the recommendations for stroke treatment and prevention are changing rapidly. Acute therapy initiated within a few hours of onset of stroke and aimed at limiting ischemic brain injury makes the rapid and accurate diagnosis of stroke, or brain attack, vitally important. At the 1996 National Symposium on Rapid Identification and Treatment of Acute Stroke, guidelines along the "chain of recovery" were developed for multiple time-critical steps for acute stroke care.[13]

Public awareness about stroke is minimal, and most stroke patients fail to present for medical attention within the short period in which early intervention may be effective in salvaging at-risk brain tissue. A comprehensive educational effort, aimed at both clinicians and the public, has begun to bring patients with brain attacks to specialized attention within the same time frame that the heart attack patient is handled.[1,2,15] The warning signs of brain attack now being publicized in the United States are presented in Table 75.1.

Education of clinicians on appropriate therapy for treatment and prevention of stroke, which rests on accurate evaluation of the stroke patient and identification of the responsible vascular lesion, includes new findings and recommendations on decisions regarding endarterectomy, anticoagulation therapy, antiplatelet agents, cerebrovascular angioplasty, immunosuppressant agents, and thrombolysis.[16]

Any delay in starting therapy after an acute stroke can result in progressive, irreversible loss of brain tissue. Just as emergency treatment in cardiac arrest aims at resuscitating the heart, all strokes should receive immediate attention aimed at saving the brain.[17] Educational efforts are now aimed at helping clinicians remember that for a stroke patient, time is brain tissue.[18]

Stroke teams, protocols, and programs are being developed within existing medical and community re-

TABLE 75.1. Warning signs of a brain attack

Sudden *weakness or numbness* of the face, arm, or leg on one side of the body
Sudden *dimness or loss of vision,* particularly in one eye
Sudden *difficulty speaking* or trouble understanding speech
Sudden *severe headache* with no known cause
Unexplained *dizziness, unsteadiness, or sudden falls,* especially with any of the other signs

From National Institute of Neurological Brain Disorders and Stroke (NINDS).[15]

sources to provide an organized approach to education, early intervention, and avoidance of mismanagement of stroke care. Although no single model for stroke care meets the needs of all institutions, a comprehensive stroke program approach has been reported to reduce costs and improve outcome for many important measures of stroke care across the spectrum from primary prevention through acute care and rehabilitation.[19,20]

Pathophysiology

The two major categories of brain damage in stroke are ischemia and hemorrhage: 61% to 81% of first strokes represent infarctions, 8% to 16% intracerebral hemorrhages, and 4% to 8% subarachnoid hemorrhages.[6] Ischemic strokes can occur through three different mechanisms: thrombosis, embolism, or hypoperfusion.

Ischemia

Cerebral ischemia is most often caused by an interruption of arterial blood flow to the brain. Reductions in cerebral blood flow below critical levels set into motion complex processes that involve cell depolarization, ionic dyshomeostasis, release of multiple neurotransmitters, massive entry of calcium into neurons, activation of second messenger systems, production of oxygen radicals, development of marked tissue acidosis, release of cytokines, activation of neutrophils, and altered gene expression.[21] The multiple effects of decreased cerebral blood flow lead to infarction of tissue and, if sustained, cause irreversible cell injury and death of brain tissue. Recent advances in the acute treatment of stroke have uncovered a narrow therapeutic "window of opportunity" of only a few hours in which ischemic brain tissue may sometimes be salvaged with reperfusion.[22–24] There is also ongoing research in the development of neuroprotective agents to counteract the chemical changes that occur with cerebral ischemia and cause more extensive tissue damage along the margin of the ischemic area.

Focal damage to brain tissue caused by diminished or absent blood flow to a focal area is termed *cerebral infarct* or *cerebral infarction*. The extent of damage depends on the location and duration of the poor perfusion, the ability of collateral vessels to perfuse the tissues at risk, and the effects of subsequent swelling and edema. Ischemic infarction may be the consequence of either thrombosis or embolism.

Thrombosis

Ischemic strokes are most commonly caused by thrombosis. Thrombosis occurs by obstructing blood flow from a localized occlusive process within one or more blood vessels. The narrowed cerebral vessels are commonly associated with hypertension, diabetes mellitus, atherosclerosis, and hyperlipidemia. Thrombotic strokes have a slow, stuttering, and more indolent onset. They are frequently preceded by minor signs or one or more transient attacks of focal neurological dysfunction. A history of prodromal episodes supports the diagnosis of cerebral thrombosis, because embolism or cerebral hemorrhage is rarely preceded by a transient neurological disorder.

Regardless of whether prior transient attacks have been seen, a thrombotic stroke usually occurs in a single attack that evolves over several hours. Other presentations of cerebral thrombosis include a stuttering and intermittent progression that extends over several hours or days; a partial stroke that occurs, recedes, and then recurs with rapid progression to a completed stroke; or a slow stroke that gradually evolves over 1 to 2 weeks.

Transient Ischemic Attack

A transient ischemic attack (TIA) is a transient focal neurological deficit of ischemic origin that completely resolves within 24 hours. It is usually linked to atherosclerotic thrombosis and is a warning sign of risk for future stroke and MI. TIAs are of sudden onset, limited severity, and usual duration of from 2 to 15 minutes. Individual attacks tend to involve either the eye or the brain, with the initial attacks being ocular and the later ones hemispheric.

TIAs are similar to angina pectoris, because both have a symptom complex of short duration; are caused by focal ischemia; are of variable severity, duration, and frequency; warn of impending infarction; may cause focal damage even though symptoms disappear; and share similar risk factors. TIAs and angina pectoris are both warning signs of impending ischemia and necessitate treatment to prevent brain attack and/or heart attack. A TIA lasting more than 30 minutes is uncommon,[25] and if it has not resolved almost completely within 4 hours, that event is a stroke 99% of the time.[18]

Embolism

Embolic strokes are due to the migration of material from a distant source to the central nervous system blood vessels that causes vascular occlusion. Embolic strokes tend to occur suddenly and are commonly associated with cardiac disease. Patients with atrial fibrillation (AF) have a 33% increased risk of developing cerebral infarcts that may be of embolic origin.[26] Two common sources of brain embolism are the left-sided chambers of the heart and the origin of the internal carotid artery (ICA).

Cardiac sources of brain embolism include heart valves, endocardium, and either clot or tumor within the atrial or ventricular cavities.[27] The mitral and aortic valves can be the sites of vegetation formation in patients in hypercoagulable states.

Artery-to-artery emboli are composed of clot, platelet clumps, or plaque fragments that break off from proximal vessels. They frequently result from the detachment of mural thrombi from the ICA at the site of an ulcerated atheromatous plaque.[28] The bright yellow cholesterol crystals in this type of embolic material can sometimes be visualized through examination of the retina soon after the embolic episode.

Emboli within the cerebral hemispheres are mostly distributed in the territory of the middle cerebral artery (MCA), which is the main and most direct branch of the ICA. These emboli commonly lodge at the junction between cortex and white matter and usually involve the bottom of the sulcus rather than the crest of the gyrus. A common feature of embolic infarcts is their relatively small size of less than 2.0 cm in diameter and their multiplicity within a single arterial territory.

A process termed *paradoxical embolism* involves clots that originate in systemic veins and travel to the brain through cardiac defects such as an atrial septal defect or a patent foramen ovale.[29] Air, fat, plaque material, particulate matter from injected drugs, bacteria, and tumor cells are other substances that can enter the vascular system and appear to embolize to cerebral vessels.

Hypoperfusion

Hypoperfusion can occur from cardiac arrest, abrupt drops in systemic blood pressure, shock, and cardiac dysrhythmias. The brain is affected diffusely. The extent of the brain injury is influenced by the duration and severity of the ischemic event, which is measured by blood pressure level on recovery. Outcome is also influenced by the patient's age (younger patients tolerate ischemia for longer periods), body temperature (hypothermia protects neurons), and serum glucose level (hypoglycemia at the time of the event has a protective effect because it limits the production rate of lactic acid).[28]

Hemorrhage

Intracranial hemorrhage is an injury from extravasation of blood into brain tissue or the subarachnoid space. It has a dramatic presentation of headache and sudden severe neurological deficits. The most frequent cause of spontaneous intracerebral hemorrhage is hypertensive vasculopathy, and the most common sites of this type of hemorrhage are the basal ganglia and the thalamus.[30] Spontaneous brain hemorrhage may also occur due to microaneurysms, arteriovenous malformations, vasculitis, and bleeding into a tumor. Rarely, an abscess may lead to intraparenchymal bleeding. Patients who take anticoagulant medications for treatment of coronary heart disease or prior TIAs may develop spontaneous intracerebral hemorrhages.

Endogenous coagulopathies, especially those caused by leukemia in the pediatric age group, may be an etiology of intraparenchymal hemorrhage.[31] A higher incidence of intracranial hemorrhages is seen in individuals who use exogenous agents such as cocaine, amphetamine, and phenylpropanolamine. Often, in spite of extensive diagnostic studies, no source of hemorrhage can be identified.

The initial clinical effects from brain hemorrhage are secondary to direct destruction and displacement of local tissues. Serial studies have shown that rebleeding may be more frequent than previously suspected.[32] Recent studies that used serial head CT scans found that recurrent intracerebral hemorrhage is a common complication, seen most frequently within the first few hours after the initial hemorrhage, although it can occur up to 24 hours after onset and is often associated with clinical worsening.[33] Secondary effects occur from edema and ischemic necrosis around the lesion. Local cerebral blood flow is decreased, with disautoregulation and blood–brain barrier disruption. Resorption of the hematoma occurs over a course of months. The process is slow, because macrophage activity occurs only along the edge of the mass.

Intracerebral hemorrhage is caused by the rupture of a blood vessel, generally the small arterioles in the basal ganglia, thalamus, cerebellum, or brain stem. It is often associated with long-term hypertension and usually presents with sudden onset of hemiparesis. Direct pressure on brain tissue or from compression of blood vessels produces ischemia in the surrounding tissues and, depending on the size of the hematoma, may cause a mass effect with compression of ventricles or midline shift.

Lobar hematoma is an intracerebral hematoma that extends to the surface of the brain. Surgical intervention may be indicated when a lobar hematoma is identified on CT scan, depending on the neurological status of the patient and the degree of intraventricular and intracerebral hemorrhage present.

Hemorrhagic stroke occurs when an ischemic cerebral infarct undergoes hemorrhagic transformation. The initial event is the occlusion of a blood vessel, most often of embolic origin, but over time red blood cells enter necrotic tissue. Hemorrhagic transformations, often fatal, are a risk of thrombolytic therapy.

Subarachnoid hemorrhage (SAH) is a hemorrhage into the subarachnoid space where the blood comes in direct contact with the cerebrospinal fluid. Nontraumatic SAH is most often caused by a ruptured intracranial aneurysm. A CT scan usually shows subarachnoid or intraventricular hyperintensity consistent with the presence of blood. If the CT scan is normal and a SAH is still suspected clinically, then a lumbar puncture should be performed to determine whether there has been bleeding into the subarachnoid space. Rebleeding and vasospasm are the major complications of SAH. Vasospasm can lead to ischemia and cerebral infarction.

Stroke Risk Factors

A substantial benefit in stroke prevention comes from primary prevention and health promotion efforts to identify those at increased risk and to reduce modifiable risk factors. The major modifiable risk factors for stroke include hypertension, cardiac disease (particularly AF), diabetes, hypercholesterolemia, cigarette smoking, asymptomatic carotid stenosis, and TIAs. Risk factors that cannot be modified have been referred to by Sacco as risk markers.[9] Stroke risk markers include age, gender, heredity, and race and ethnicity.

Risk Markers

Age

Stroke incidence rises exponentially with age, nearly doubling each decade after age 55.[5] Seventy-two percent of strokes occur in people 65 years or older. The number of stroke patients will inevitably increase as the population ages and life expectancy lengthens.

Gender

Stroke incidence has been reported to range from 30% to 80% higher in men than in women,[5] but stroke prevalence and stroke deaths are higher in women because of their longer average life expectancy.

Heredity

A family history of stroke among first-degree relatives has been identified as a determinant of stroke risk even after adjusting for other stroke risk factors.[34]

Race and Ethnicity

African Americans have a disproportionately higher stroke incidence and mortality rate than the US Caucasian population, even after adjustment for age, hypertension, and diabetes mellitus.[35,36] Stroke rates are 50% higher in African American men and 130% higher in African American women.[37] About one third of the increased stroke risk in African Americans is attributable to cardiovascular risk factors, another one third is attributable to factors related to family income, and a final one third is unexplained.[5]

Heterogeneity of the group hinders broad comparisons on data accumulated on Hispanic stroke rates.[9] Mexican Americans, who comprise the largest subgroup of US Hispanics, have similar stroke mortality rates as Caucasians in the 45- to 64-year-old age group and lower rates than Caucasians >65 years of age.[38] The estimated crude prevalence of stroke for Mexican Americans is 1.1% for men and 0.8% for women.[1] Hispanics in New York City who were predominantly from the Dominican Republic had an overall age-adjusted 1-year stroke incidence 1.6 times that of Caucasians.[9]

Asians, particularly Chinese and Japanese, have a very high stroke incidence that is higher than their rate of heart disease.[9] Infarction accounts for two thirds of stroke events in the Japanese who live in Japan or Hawaii. Stroke was a leading cause of death among US Native Americans in 1990 but was lower than in Caucasians.

The reasons for racial and ethnic differences in stroke are unclear, although some studies have suggested that a different distribution and prevalence of stroke risk factors may account for some but not all of these variations.[35] State health departments in the stroke belt, which has a 10% higher stroke rate than the rest of the United States, have developed prevention strategies (with attention to high blood pressure and smoking) specifically targeted at African Americans.[8]

Risk Factors

Hypertension

Hypertension is the strongest and most consistent risk factor for ischemic and hemorrhagic stroke[39] and is considered the most important treatable risk factor.[40] The relative risk of stroke among hypertensive persons is approximately three to four times greater than for nonhypertensive persons, and even borderline hypertension is associated with a relative stroke risk 1.5 times greater than that of normotensive persons.[11] The risk of stroke rises proportionately with increasing blood pressure and is especially strong for levels above 160/95 mm Hg.[5] Elevations of both diastolic and systolic pressures are associated with an increased probability of stroke. Isolated systolic hypertension, after controlling for age and diastolic pressure, also increases the risk of stroke.[41]

Health promotion aimed at even a modest improvement in the control of hypertension can result in a substantial reduction in stroke incidence. Factors that influence the effectiveness of blood pressure control are known. Age and ethnic origin are important determinants of response to specific antihypertensive agents.[42] Antihypertensive therapy can adversely affect perceived quality of life and result in medication noncompliance.[43]

Epidemiological studies of hypertension identify groups that require intensive focus for health promotion and antihypertensive treatment to prevent stroke. African Americans, Puerto Ricans, Cuban Americans, and Mexican Americans are more likely to suffer from high blood pressure.[1] Both African Americans and Caucasians in the US stroke belt have a greater prevalence of high blood pressure and higher stroke death rates than the rest of the country.

In Hispanic populations, hypertension is found in 22.8% of Cuban American men and 15.5% of women; 16.8% of Mexican American men and 14.1% of women; and 15.6% Puerto Rican men and 11.5% of women.[1] Among Asian/Pacific Islanders, 9.7% of men and 8.4% of women have hypertension, and 10.3% of American Indian/Alaskan Native men and 13.8% of women have hypertension.

Cardiac Disease

Ischemic heart disease, AF, valvular heart disease, MI, congestive heart failure, and left ventricular hypertrophy are each independent predictors of ischemic stroke.[11,40] New data suggest that patent foramen ovale, atrial septal aneurysm, mitral valve strands, and aortic arch atheroma may also be associated with stroke.[9] A recent prospective study from France found that an aortic arch wall ≥4 mm due to atherosclerotic plaques is a significant predictor of recurrent stroke or other vascular events.[44]

Cardiac conditions are a risk for stroke. Acute MIs, especially transmural and anterior wall infarcts, are associated with stroke. The risk of stroke is almost double with prior coronary artery disease, triple with left ventricular hypertrophy, and nearly quadruple with heart failure.[9] Measures that can effectively reduce the incidence of myocardial disease could lead to a substantial reduction in stroke incidence.

Valvular conditions that may lead to stroke include mitral stenosis, endocarditis, and prosthetic heart valves. In contrast to earlier studies that suggested an association of mitral valve prolapse to stroke, recent investigations have found that stroke was infrequent in persons with mitral valve prolapse unless they also had other risk factors.[45]

Nonvalvular AF is a significant independent risk factor for stroke even after adjusting for other factors such as age, hypertension, and other heart diseases.[46] Patients with AF were found to have a 33% increased risk of developing brain infarcts presumed to be of embolic origin. Nearly 15% of strokes in the Framingham Study have been attributed to AF.[47] AF affects more than 2 million Americans, and the incidence nearly doubles for each advancing decade of age.[9] Although the overall prevalence of AF is approximately 1%, it is close to 6% in those over age 65; the risk of stroke from AF increases significantly with age. Recent findings suggest that in those with nonrheumatic AF, therapy with warfarin was more than 85% effective in stroke prevention when the international normalized ratio prolongation was in the therapeutic range (2.0–3.0).[48]

The Honolulu Heart Program found that resting electrocardiogram abnormalities are independent predictors of stroke.[49] Men with major ST-segment depression, left ventricular strain, left ventricular hypertrophy, and major T-wave inversion had a considerably higher (2.5 to 5.4 times) incidence of both thromboembolic and hemorrhagic stroke than those with normal baseline electrocardiogram results.

Diabetes Mellitus

Diabetes mellitus is a significant risk factor for both cerebral infarction and ischemic heart disease in men and women.[9,50] The Honolulu Heart Program found that diabetes mellitus, independent of other risk factors, conferred a twofold increased risk of thromboembolic stroke on Japanese men living in Hawaii.[51] Although the impact of impaired glucose tolerance on stroke risk was found to be most substantial in older women in the Framingham Study,[40] few studies have been able to demonstrate an association between better control of hyperglycemia and decreased stroke risk.

Hypercholesterolemia

Increased lipid levels have been found to be associated with carotid artery disease, but the relationship between blood cholesterol level and atherosclerotic stroke was not found to be as strong as it was between blood cholesterol level and ischemic heart disease.[52] Recent studies have suggested that lipid-lowering agents of the 3-hydroxy-3-methylglutaryl coenzyme A reductase inhibitor class lower the relative risk of stroke about as much as they lower the risk of ischemic heart disease, particularly among patients with a history of heart disease.[53]

Findings from the Honolulu Heart Program suggest that an elevated serum cholesterol level should be considered a primary risk factor for thromboembolic stroke, presumably through its effect on both coronary and cerebrovascular atherosclerosis.[54] In contrast, low serum cholesterol levels have been found in Hawaiian, Japanese, and other populations despite an increased incidence of cerebral hemorrhage.[55]

Smoking

Cigarette smoking is an independent risk factor for stroke with adjusted relative risks of 2.5 for men and 3.1 for women.[9] Stroke risk increases in a dose–response manner: the more one smokes, the greater the risk of stroke.[11] In the Nurses' Health Study, the relative risk for smokers of subarachnoid hemorrhage was twice as great as for thromboembolic stroke.[56] Stopping smoking reduces stroke risk by more than half,[57] and stroke risk may reverse approximately 5 years after cessation.[58]

Alcohol Use

The effect of alcohol as a risk factor for ischemic stroke is controversial. Small to moderate amounts of alcohol may be protective whereas larger amounts may be deleterious. Light to moderate drinking can increase high-density lipoprotein cholesterol levels and reduce the risk of coronary artery disease, but chronic heavy drinking and acute intoxication in young adults was found to be associated with ischemic infarction.[9] In the Honolulu Heart Program, no significant relationships were noted between alcohol and thromboembolic stroke, but the risk of hemorrhagic stroke more than doubled for light drinkers and nearly tripled for those considered to be heavy drinkers.[59]

Transient Ischemic Attack

Estimates vary greatly on stroke risk following TIA because of differences in definitions of event, populations, and types of study design. The annual stroke risk after a TIA ranges from 1% to 15%, with an average risk around 4%.[9] The overall 5-year risk of stroke following TIA is approximately 33%, and patients with transient monocular blindness (amaurosis fugax) have a better outcome than those with transient cerebral ischemic events.[60] TIA caused by carotid atherosclerosis is a predictor not only of cerebral infarction but also of MI.[25] The average annual risk of stroke, MI, or death was 7.5% after TIA among hospital-referred patients.[61]

Asymptomatic Carotid Artery Stenosis

Asymptomatic carotid artery stenosis is frequent, and its incidence increases with age. Stroke risk is worse with severe stenosis. Stenosis >75% is associated with an annual stroke rate of 3.3%, and stenosis <75% has a rate of 1.3%.[62] In patients undergoing coronary artery bypass evaluated preoperatively for asymptomatic carotid artery stenosis, the presence of >75% stenosis in patients over age 60 was associated with stroke in 15%.[63] Carotid artery stenosis and carotid endarterectomy are further reviewed in Chapter 74, "Surgically Excised Carotid Bifurcation Plaque."

Exercise

The Honolulu Heart Program found that physical activity may be important in reducing the risk of stroke, particularly among nonsmoking men in older middle age.[64]

Obesity

Persons who are obese have higher levels of blood pressure, blood glucose, and atherogenic serum lipids, which alone could increase the incidence of stroke.[48] In nonsmoking men in older middle age who are free of commonly observed conditions related to cardiovascular disease, elevated body mass is associated with an increased risk of thromboembolic stroke.[65]

Oral Contraceptive Use

An increased stroke risk was reported in women over 35 years of age who used oral contraceptives, particularly in those who smoked cigarettes and had hypertension.[66] Stroke risk was highest in women taking oral contraceptives with higher levels of estrogen. The lower levels of estrogen in newer oral contraceptives appear to reduce the stroke risk, and there seems to be no increased risk of stroke in former oral contraceptive users.[67]

Drug Abuse

Cerebral complications of endocarditis or embolization of foreign material can occur in parenteral drug abusers. Cocaine-associated stroke, primarily in young adults, can follow cocaine administration by any route and may be caused directly by the drug itself.[68] It is frequently associated with vascular malformations and presents with intracranial hemorrhage more commonly than cerebral infarction. Parenteral cocaine and heroin administration can lead to infectious endocarditis and cerebral emboli.[69] Heroin abusers may also suffer hemorrhagic stroke secondary to infectious diseases or clotting disorders.

Barbiturates and other sedatives and tranquilizers can cause cerebral infarction in association with overdose and diffusely decreased brain perfusion. Amphetamine-induced intracranial hemorrhages may be secondary to acute hypertension and/or cerebral vasculitis associated with stimulant abuse. Phenylpropanolamine, ephedrine, and pseudoephedrine, which are all available in over-the-counter preparations such as decongestants and diet pills, have been associated with hemorrhagic stroke.[69]

Associated Medical Conditions

Autoimmune disease and collagen vascular disease are associated with increased risk of stroke.[70] Patients with systemic lupus erythematosus have an elevated stroke risk. Vasculopathy, hypercoagulable states, and hematological disorders may contribute to the risk of stroke.

An estimated 3% of cerebral infarctions occur in young adults (15 to 45 years).[25] Predisposing factors in young adults include coagulopathies, antiphospholipid antibodies, ethanol intoxication, migraine, drug use, carotid intimal dissection, patent foramen ovale, and human immunodeficiency virus.[71]

Stroke may be a complication of thrombolysis for MI, coronary angioplasty, and cardiac surgery.[72] Sickle cell anemia is an important cause of stroke in African American children, with acute hemiplegia as the most common manifestation.[25]

Stroke Risk Profile

A stroke risk profile based on the Framingham Study data was developed to help determine a patient's probability of stroke.[73] Probability of stroke compared with an average person of the same age and sex is determined by a point system using (1) age, (2) systolic blood pressure,

(3) antihypertensive therapy use, (4) presence of diabetes, (5) cigarette smoking, (6) history of cardiovascular disease, and (7) electrocardiogram abnormalities.

Clinical Features and Their Basis

Accurate diagnosis and treatment of stroke require a basic understanding of cerebrovascular anatomy. Clinical determination of whether a stroke is ischemic or hemorrhagic is occasionally difficult. Neuroimaging studies localize hemorrhages readily, but acute infarcts are not usually visualized on initial scans. Clinical findings help localize infarcts, and a knowledge of the major neurovascular syndromes described in the following sections is necessary.

Anterior Circulation

Approximately 80% to 85% of all ischemic strokes involve occlusion of vessels in the anterior circulation,[18] which includes the right and left ICAs and their major branches—the MCA and the anterior cerebral artery.

Anterior circulation ischemia from either an ICA or MCA occlusion often causes hemiparesis, sensory loss, and visual symptoms on the body side contralateral to the brain lesion.[16] Aphasia can occur with dominant hemisphere stroke, whereas nondominant hemisphere stroke often presents with a "neglect syndrome" in which patients are unaware of their deficit.

Internal Carotid Artery

The carotid system consists of three major arteries—the common carotid, internal carotid, and external carotid. Common carotid artery occlusion accounts for less than 1% of carotid artery syndromes, with the remainder being due to disease of the ICA itself.[25] The ICA can become stenosed because it is at a bifurcation where plaque can build up.

When a stenosis in the carotid artery is present, a bruit can often be heard with a stethoscope at the angle of the jaw or lower in the neck. Palpation may also reveal reduced or absent pulse in the common carotid artery in the neck, in the external carotid artery in the front of the ear, and in the ICA in the lateral wall of the pharynx.

The clinical manifestations of atherosclerotic thrombotic disease of the ICA are the most variable of any cerebrovascular syndrome. An occlusion of the anterior and middle cerebral arteries may occur from an embolus or propagating thrombus and cause an infarct in all or part of the middle cerebral territory.

Transient monocular blindness (amaurosis fugax) occurs before onset of stroke in approximately 25% of patients with symptomatic carotid occlusion.[25] The distal zone of the sylvian region is most vulnerable in TIAs with stenosis of the carotid artery, usually presenting with weakness or paresthesias of the arm.

Rare signs of carotid occlusion may include faintness in arising from a horizontal position or recurrent loss of consciousness when walking; headache and occasional ocular, retro-orbital, and neck pain; unilateral visual loss or dimness of vision with exercise, after exposure to bright light, or on assuming an upright position; premature cataracts; retinal atrophy and pigmentation; atrophy of the iris; leukomas; peripapillary arteriovenous anastomoses in the retinae; optic atrophy; claudication of jaw muscles; perforation of the nasal septum; saddle nose deformity; facial atrophy (unilateral or bilateral); indolent infections of the face; abnormal facial pigmentation; and loss of hair.[25]

Middle Cerebral Artery

The MCA supplies the lateral part of the cerebral hemisphere. In contrast to carotid occlusions, which are usually thrombotic, MCA occlusions are usually due to embolism.

The anterior circulation symptom complex is incomplete with occlusion in one of the branches of the MCA. An embolus that lodges in the superior division of the MCA presents with sensorimotor deficit in the contralateral face, arm, and leg and ipsilateral deviation of the head and eyes. Slow improvement occurs over time, often with increased leg function, but severe motor deficits of the arm and face remain. Sensory deficits may be profound initially and then partially improve. Global aphasia often occurs initially with left-sided lesions, with some improvement over time.

Occlusion of the inferior division of the MCA is usually due to cardiogenic embolism. Left-sided lesions result in aphasia, with improvement often noted over several months. Homonymous hemianopia occurs with either right- or left-sided lesions. Right-sided lesions can lead to left visual neglect.

Anterior Cerebral Artery

Occlusion of one anterior cerebral artery often presents with contralateral weakness, with the leg being most severely affected. Equal involvement of the arm, leg, and face usually represents an occlusion of the MCA. Total occlusion of one anterior cerebral artery distal to the anterior communicating artery presents with contralateral weakness—a sensorimotor deficit of the opposite foot and leg with lesser deficit in the arm and sparing of the face. The head and eyes may deviate to the side of the lesion. Motor aphasia, agraphia, and mild behavior changes can sometimes occur.

Posterior Circulation Ischemia

Posterior circulation, which includes the two vertebral arteries and the basilar artery, supplies the entire brain stem. Infarction of posterior circulation can begin with vertigo, nystagmus, and vomiting. Brain stem stroke often progresses to bilateral motor and sensory signs in varied presentations and can present with altered consciousness, diplopia, slurred speech, anisocoria, hiccup, visual disturbance, memory loss, loss of vertical gaze, and convergence.[16] Occlusion of the basilar artery is often fatal or results in a "locked-in" state—conscious, mute, quadriplegic, and permanently unable to respond except by blinking and eye movement.

Cerebellar stroke due to occlusion of the superior cerebellar artery, anterior inferior cerebellar artery, and posterior inferior cerebellar artery presents with ataxia of gait, dysmetria, vertigo, nausea, and emesis.[16] Decompressive cerebellar surgery may be required when cerebellar edema causes obstructive hydrocephalus or brain stem compression.

Brain stem involvement often presents with a crossed cranial nerve and long-tract sensory or motor deficit. Determination of the site of the lesion in brain stem syndromes requires thorough evaluation of presenting findings (i.e., cranial nerve deficits, motor signs, and patterns of sensory disturbances) because they relate to anatomy of the brain stem.

Posterior Cerebral Artery

The posterior cerebral artery supplies the upper brain stem and the temporal and occipital lobes, and an occlusion can have a variety of presentations.

In *anterior and proximal syndromes,* infarction of the sensory relay nuclei in the thalamus presents with hemiparesis and severe sensory loss of the opposite side of the body. As partial sensation returns, pain and paresthesia may develop and can persist for years (Dejerine–Roussy syndrome). Central midbrain and subthalmic syndromes include oculomotor palsy with contralateral hemiplegia, paralysis of vertical gaze (Parinaud's syndrome), stupor or coma, and hemiballism. Anteromedial–inferior thalamic syndromes present with an extrapyramidal movement disorder and may also include sensory loss and hemiataxia.

In *unilateral cortical syndromes,* temporal and occipital lobe occlusions present with homonymous hemianopia. Color dysnomia and aphasia may also occur, along with some memory loss. *Bilateral cortical syndromes* cause total cortical blindness, including a homonymous hemianopia and occasionally unformed visual hallucinations (Anton's syndrome). Bilateral lesions of the temporal lobes can cause severe memory deficits.

Posterior Inferior Cerebellar Artery

A posterior inferior cerebellar artery occlusion causes lateral medullary syndrome (Wallenberg's syndrome). This syndrome causes contralateral impairment of pain and thermal sense over half the body, ipsilateral Horner's syndrome, ipsilateral paralysis of the palate and vocal cord with diminished gag reflex, vertigo, ipsilateral face pain and sensory deficit, and loss of sense of taste.

Basilar Artery

Basilar artery occlusion involves many structures and presents with a syndrome composed of bilateral long-tract signs with cerebellar and cranial nerve abnormalties. Basilar artery syndrome can include paralysis or weakness of all extremities with intact sensation, diplopia, blindness or impaired vision, and cerebellar ataxia. The patient may be in a comatose or locked-in state.

Occlusion of branches at the bifurcation of the basilar artery can cause memory deficits, hallucinations, ocular movement disorders, confusion, and somnolence. Occlusion of the superior cerebellar artery presents with ipsilateral cerebellar ataxia, nausea and vomiting, slurred speech, and partial sensory deficits on the opposite side of the body.

Some of the main findings with occlusion of the anterior inferior cerebellar artery are vertigo, nausea, vomiting, nystagmus, tinnitus, facial weakness, ipsilateral cerebellar ataxia, ipsilateral Horner's syndrome, and contralateral loss of pain and temperature sense of the arm, trunk, and leg.

Lacunar State

The lacunar state is due to the occlusion of small arteries. It is highly correlated with hypertension and atherosclerosis and is also associated with diabetes mellitus. Lacunes, the cavities formed by the infarctions, range from 3 to 15 mm in diameter.[25] Symptoms may or may not occur depending on location of the lacunes. Diagnosis of lacunar infarction depends on the presentation of a stroke syndrome of limited proportions in combination with a CT scan that is either negative or shows a deep, small area of hypodensity.

Clinical Assessment and Diagnostic Studies

The presenting neurological deficits help localize the site of the infarct or hemorrhage. The severity of the symptoms may be an indication of the stroke magnitude. Approximately 80% of strokes or TIAs occur in the anterior circulation in the territory of the carotid artery. When a patient presents with hemiparesis and no classic vertebrobasilar signs, the ischemic event is most likely in the territory of the carotid artery.[18] Stroke mechanism guides treatment. Treatment strategies, outcome, and likelihood of recurrent stroke differ markedly by type of stroke. The delay in treatment of acute stroke may result in progressive, irreversible loss of brain tissue, so the diagnosis of stroke subtype and initiation of treatment must occur rapidly.

TOAST Classification

Because the etiology of ischemic stroke affects prognosis, outcome, and management, a system for categorization of subtypes of ischemic stroke mainly based on etiology was developed for the Trial of Org 10172 in Acute Stroke Treatment (TOAST).[74] Diagnoses of subtypes are based on clinical features and on data collected by imaging tests and laboratory assessments for prothrombotic states. In the present rapidly changing environment of acute treatment of stroke, this classification system provides a standardized approach to report responses to treatment.

The TOAST classification denotes five subtypes of ischemic stroke: (1) large-artery atherosclerosis, (2) cardioembolism, (3) small-vessel occlusion, (4) stroke of other determined etiology, and (5) stroke of undetermined etiology (see Table 75.2).

1. *Large-artery atherosclerosis.* In this category, the patients have clinical and brain imaging findings of either significant (>50%) stenosis or occlusion of a major brain artery or branch cortical artery.[74] Clinically, cortical impairment with aphasia, restricted motor involvement, neglect, and so forth or cerebellar dysfunction is seen. This clinical diagnosis is supported by eliciting a history of TIAs in the same vascular territory or carotid bruit. On CT or magnetic resonance imaging (MRI) scans, cortical or cerebellar lesions and brain stem or subcortical hemispheric infarcts greater than 1.5 cm in diameter may be of large-artery atherosclerotic origin. Inclusion in this category is not made if duplex or arteriographic studies are normal or show only minimal changes or if cardiogenic embolism cannot be excluded.

2. *Cardioembolism.* At least one cardiac source of an embolus must be identified for a possible or probable diagnosis of cardioembolic stroke. The TOAST classification divides cardiac sources into high- and medium-risk groups. High-risk sources include mechanical prosthetic valve, AF, mitral stenosis with AF, left atrial or atrial appendage thrombus, sick sinus syndrome, recent MI (<4 weeks), left ventricular thrombus, dilated cardiomyopathy, akinetic left ventricular segment, atrial myxoma, and infective endocarditis. Medium-risk sources include mitral valve prolapse, mitral annulus calcification, mitral stenosis without AF, left atrial turbulence, atrial septal aneurysm, patent foramen ovale, atrial flutter, lone AF, bioprosthetic cardiac valve, nonbacterial thrombotic endocarditis, congestive heart failure, hypokinetic left ventricular segment, and MI (<6 months). Clinical findings and results of brain imaging are similar to those in the category of large-artery atherosclerosis. Diagnosis of cardiogenic stroke is supported by history of a previous TIA or stroke in more than one vascular territory or systemic embolism.

3. *Small-artery occlusion (lacune).* This category includes patients who have one of the traditional clinical lacunar syndromes and show no evidence of cerebral cortical dysfunction. History of hypertension or diabetes mellitus, normal CT or MRI, or a brain stem or subcortical hemispheric lesion <1.5 cm in diameter supports inclusion in this category.[74] Potential cardiac sources of embolism are absent, and there is no or <50% stenosis of extracranial ICA.

4. *Acute stroke of other determined etiology.* This classification involves rare causes of stroke, including nonatherosclerotic vasculopathies, hypercoagulable states, or hematologic disorders. CT or MRI scans reveal an

TABLE 75.2. Features of subtypes of ischemic stroke based on Trial of Org 10172 in Acute Stroke Treatment classification.

Features	Type	Large-artery atherosclerosis	Cardioembolism	Small-artery occlusion	Other cause
Clinical	Cortical or cerebellar dysfunction	+	+	-	+/-
	Lacunar syndrome	-	-	+	+/-
Prior history		TIA same vascular area; carotid bruit; diminished pulses	TIA or stroke in >1 vascular area; systemic embolism	Diabetes; hypertension	Vasculopathy; hypercoagulable states; hematologic disorders
Imaging	Cortical, cerebellar, brain stem, or subcortical infarct >1.5 cm	+	+	-	+/-
	Subcortical or brain stem infarct <1.5 cm	-	-	+/-	+/-
Tests	Stenosis of extracranial ICA	+	-	-	-
	Cardiac source of emboli	-	+	-	-
	Other test abnormality	-	-	-	+

TIA, transient ischemic attack; ICA, internal cartoid artery.
Adapted from TOAST investigators.[74]

acute ischemic stroke. Other diagnostic studies rule out cardioembolism and large-artery atherosclerosis and reveal one of the unusual causes of stroke.

5. *Stroke of undetermined etiology.* This category includes strokes that cannot be determined with any degree of confidence and also includes those with two or more potential causes, which prohibits a final diagnosis.

Clinical Evaluation

Rapid and accurate clinical diagnosis of stroke is critical and depends on a combination of history, physical examination, neuroimaging, and laboratory and other diagnostic studies. Clinical assessment is also valuable in defining prognosis. Level of consciousness is the strongest predictor of short-term survival, and gross motor performance (especially the ability to walk) is most predictive of functional disability on discharge.[75]

Conditions That Mimic Stroke

In a 2-year study of 411 patients initially diagnosed with stroke on presentation to the emergency department, 78 (19%) were later diagnosed with other neurological conditions.[76] Four major conditions that were found to mimic stroke include unrecognized seizures with postictal deficits, systemic infections, brain tumors, and toxic–metabolic disturbances (hypoglycemia). Decreased level of consciousness and normal eye movement were associated with the likelihood of encephalopathy. Abnormal visual fields, diastolic blood pressure >90 mm Hg, AF, and history of angina were found in strokes. Multivariate analysis revealed that decreased consciousness independently predicted a nonvascular condition, and history of angina independently predicted true stroke.

History

History is gathered from the patient, family, friends, and paramedics. Accurate timing of onset of symptoms is essential if thrombolytic therapy is being considered. If someone observed the onset or the patient is communicative, exact timing can often be determined. Otherwise, the last time the patient was seen in his or her normal state is often used as an estimated time of onset. The medical history should include identification of stroke risk factors. Recent TIAs suggest an unstable situation similar to that of unstable angina; immediate preventive therapy is thus required.

The pattern of stroke onset, including types and progression of symptoms, should also be evaluated. A common description is that the patient was having breakfast and talking normally and then had sudden slurring of speech ("his speech got a little funny") and started to drop things. Assessment of symptoms will help localize the lesion and guide decisions about treatment.

If comatose on arrival, prognosis is poor and the patient is probably not a candidate for thrombolytic therapy. Intracranial hemorrhage should be considered if the history reveals sudden onset of severe headache, vomiting, therapy with anticoagulant agents, loss of consciousness, systolic blood pressure >200 mm Hg, and blood glucose level >9.4 mmol/L (170 mg/dL) in a nondiabetic patient.[77]

Physical Examination

Neurological findings help identify the anatomical location of the lesion and guide treatment decisions. Acute stroke patients are frequently quite ill on presentation, so some aspects of the general physical examination may need to be abbreviated. However, neurological examination must be sufficient and accurate to guide decisions on potentially hazardous therapeutic interventions.

Clinical trials routinely use similar stroke scales to compare baseline characteristics and predict outcome of treatment groups. Stroke scales include the National Institutes of Health Stroke Scale (NIHSS),[78] the European Stroke Scale,[79] the Canadian Neurological Scale,[80] and the Scandinavian Stroke Scale.[81] The 15-item NIHSS has high interrater reliability and validity,[82] is valid for predicting lesion size on brain CT,[83] and most accurately predicted outcome at 3 months in a comparative study of three stroke scales.[84] The modified NIHSS was reproducible among neurologists, emergency medicine physicians, house officers, and stroke research nurses and has shown improved reliability with video training.[85] This clinical examination scale for measurement of acute cerebral infarction can be performed in approximately 6.5 minutes[79] and has been utilized in pilot studies of recombinant tissue plasminogen activator (rtPA).[86-88] A summary of the modified NIHHS is provided in Table 75.3.

Frequently missed signs of brain dysfunction involve abnormalities of higher cortical function, level of alertness, the visual and oculomotor systems, and gait.[89,90] Testing of higher cortical function should include evaluation of language function, particularly if there are right visual field or right limb deficits. With left visual field or left limb deficits, evaluation should include testing for visual–spatial dysfunction and left neglect. The most common eye-movement abnormality in stroke patients is a conjugate-gaze paralysis, which usually indicates a frontal or deep hemispheral lesion in the hemisphere opposite to the gaze palsy or a lesion in the pons on the same side as the gaze palsy.[90] Nystagmus or dysconjugate palsies may indicate a vertebrobasilar lesion.

Family, friends, and care providers can provide insight into changes in level of awareness and behavior, which may indicate brain stem lesions or be a sign of increased intracranial pressure. Memory should be tested, because it can be affected by a focal central nervous system lesion.

TABLE 75.3. The modified National Institutes of Health stroke scale summary.

Neurological component	Scale definition	Grade
1a. Levels of consciousness (LOC)	Alert	0
	Not alert, but can be aroused to obey	1
	Not alert, obtunded	2
	Unresponsive	3
1b. LOC questions (month and age)	Answers both questions correctly	0
	Answers only one correctly	1
	Answers neither correctly	2
1c. LOC commands (open/close eyes, grip/release hand)	Performs both tasks correctly	0
	One task only	1
	Performs neither task	2
2. Gaze	Normal	0
	Partial gaze palsy	1
	Total gaze palsy	2
3. Visual field	No visual field loss	0
	Partial hemianopsia	1
	Complete hemianopsia	2
	Bilateral hemianopsia	3
4. Facial palsy	Normal	0
	Minor paralysis (asymmetric smile)	1
	Partial paralysis	2
	Complete paralysis	3
5. Motor arm	No drift	0
a. Left	Drift before 10 s	1
b. Right	Falls before 10 s	2
	No effort against gravity	3
	No movement	4
6. Motor leg	No drift	0
a. Left	Drift before 10 s	1
b. Right	Falls before 10 s	2
	No effort against gravity	3
	No movement	4
7. Ataxia	Absent	0
	One limb	1
	Two limbs	2
8. Sensory	Normal	0
	Mild loss	1
	Severe loss	2
9. Language	Normal	0
	Mild aphasia	1
	Severe aphasia	2
	Mute or global aphasia	3
10. Dysarthria	Normal	0
	Mild	1
	Severe	2
11. Extinction/inattention	Normal	0
	Mild	1
	Severe	2

Summary of modified National Institutes of Health Stroke Scale. Complete scale with instructions can be obtained from the National Institute of Neurological Disorders and Stroke.

Vital Signs

An immediate assessment of blood pressure and oxygenation is essential in all stroke patients because hypotension and hypoxia can exacerbate ischemic injury. Respiration may be compromised and respiratory failure can occur. Blood pressure must be closely monitored, because hypertension is common in stroke patients.

Diagnostic Studies

Baseline Studies

An electrocardiogram should be performed on all patients who have experienced stroke or TIA. MI is one of the major causes of death among acute stroke patients and is the leading cause of death in the 30 days after a TIA.[18] Cardiac monitoring for at least 24 hours after an acute stroke frequently reveals cardiac arrhythmias. If AF is present, it should be controlled with digitalis so that hypotension does not occur.

Pneumonia is a common cause of death among stroke patients, so a baseline chest x-ray study is recommended. Lumbar puncture may sometimes be necessary to rule out subarachnoid hemorrhage.

Laboratory Studies

Stroke protocols include guidelines for specific laboratory studies on suspected stroke patients on arrival to the emergency department. Glucose level should be checked immediately by finger stick because focal deficits may occur in patients with hypoglycemia.

Initial blood studies routinely performed include immediate complete blood cell count with differential, electrolytes, prothrombin time and partial thromboplastin time, and full chemistry panel. Urinalysis, along with urine culture if there are symptoms of a urinary tract infection, are also ordered. If stroke occurs in a young patient, he or she should be screened for collagen vascular disease and hypercoagulable states. History and examination may also indicate the need for toxic drug screening.

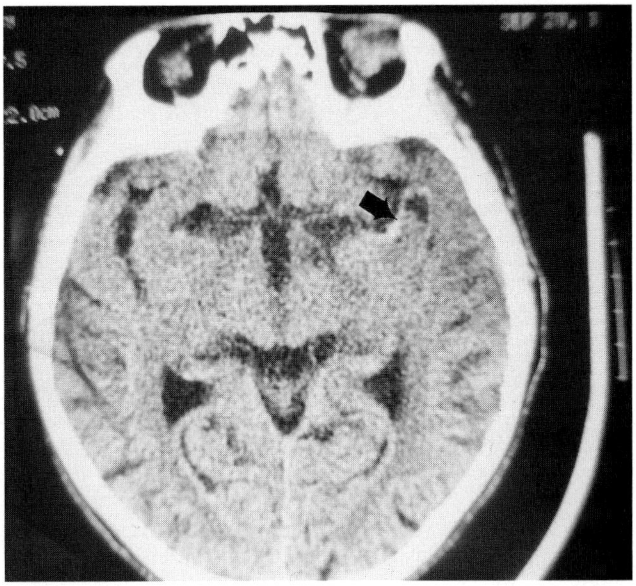

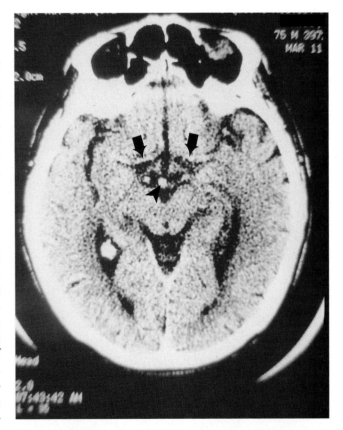

FIGURE 75.1. Axial noncontrast computed tomography scan demonstrating dense left middle cerebral artery sign (arrow) and subtle left temporal lobe lucency.

Imaging of Stroke

The following will initially focus on the imaging findings on CT and MRI in the acute ischemic stroke within the first 24 to 48 hours. The findings vary with time, extent of infarct, and type of imaging modality used. A brief discussion of intracerebral hemorrhage, subarachnoid hemorrhage, and venous occlusion will follow. Numerous examples are provided, with emphasis on MRI because of the expanding use of MRI in imaging the stroke syndrome.

Computed Tomography

CT is currently the most common imaging modality used in patients with a suspected acute stroke, but 50% to 60% of the scans are normal within the first 12 hours.[91] The major purpose of using CT is to exclude hemorrhage. Several early findings in confirming an ischemic stroke, however, are important, including visualizing a clot-filled artery and recognizing an area where there is loss of gray–white matter differentiation or sulcal effacement. Acute intraluminal thrombi are most commonly visualized in the MCA distribution (dense MCA sign) and have been reported in 25% to 50% of patients with MCA infarcts[92–94] (Figure 75.1). This finding needs to be interpreted with caution with the current high-resolution CT scanners, which allow better visualization of normal slightly dense vessels (Figure 75.2). Loss of gray–white

FIGURE 75.2. Axial noncontrast computed tomography scan demonstrating symmetrically relatively dense anterior and middle cerebral arteries bilaterally (arrows) and dense distal basilar artery (arrowhead).

matter differentiation may be the easiest to detect when there is obscuration of the lentiform nucleus or along the lateral insula (insular ribbon sign)[95] (Figure 75.3). Localized mass effect can be appreciated by comparing the two hemispheres and looking for subtle sulcal effacement (Figure 75.4). After the first 24 to 48 hours, many infarcts are seen as wedge-shaped areas of low density involving the cortex or gray matter and adjacent white matter. They may be in a vascular distribution if secondary to a branch occlusion or between major vascular distributions if secondary to hypoperfusion (Figure 75.5).

Magnetic Resonance Imaging and Magnetic Resonance Angiography

MRI, combined with magnetic resonance angiography, is an excellent method of imaging the acute stroke and more reliable than CT scans.[96] In addition to being more sensitive, MRI is more specific and may be necessary to distinguish between stroke and tumor in clinically confusing situations (Figure 75.6). Up to 80% of acute strokes are visible within the first 24 hours,[91] and, as might be expected, the earliest MRI findings are related to vascular abnormalities. These abnormalities include loss of the normally present flow void (Figure 75.7) and intravascular enhancement (Figure 75.8),[97] both of which occur immediately. The use of magnetic resonance angiography is superior to routine spin–echo sequences in detecting vascular occlusion and underlying stenosis. The entire carotid and vertebral systems can be imaged from below the cervical bifurcation to above the circle of Willis using a combination of two- and three-dimensional time-of-flight sequences (Figure 75.9).

The earliest morphologic findings are often seen on the T_1 sequences, especially gradient echo volume acquisitions (Figure 75.10). MRI is more sensitive than CT for identifying loss of gray–white matter interfaces and sulcal effacement. Abnormal T_2 hyperintensity occurs later, usually after 8 hours[98] (Figures 75.8B and 75.11). Parenchymal enhancement takes 1 to 3 days to develop, may take several different patterns, and may persist for weeks (Figure 75.12). Localized meningeal enhancement often occurs earlier but is seen less often. MRI sensitivity increases with the use of diffusion-weighted imaging.

Diffusion-weighted imaging, which is sensitive to the microscopic motion of water, may detect acute ischemia within minutes of its occurrence.[99] Other MRI advances such as perfusion techniques, spectroscopy, and imaging physiologic parameters with echoplanar imaging are currently being evaluated. The goal of all of these rapidly progressive MRI techniques is to define an ischemic process early enough to allow use of salvage therapies that limit damage or help preserve the at-risk penumbra.

Some centers are performing angiography in the hyperacute stage in anticipation of using fibrolytic therapy. The most specific and common angiographic finding (about 50%) is arterial occlusion.[100] Less common findings include retrograde arterial filling of cortical branches, slow antegrade flow, luxury perfusion, arteriovenous shunting (Figure 75.13), or mass effect.[101]

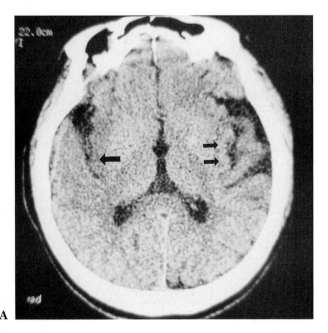
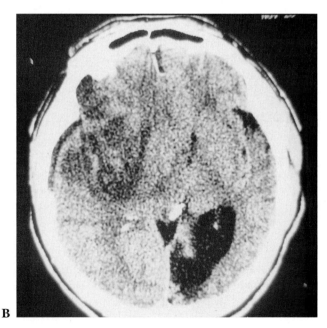

A   **B**

FIGURE 75.3. **A,** Axial noncontrast computed tomography scan demonstrating normal left insular cortex (double arrow) but loss of the right insular cortex (arrow), the insular ribbon sign. **B,** Follow-up scan several days later confirms extensive right middle cerebral artery distribution of partially hemorrhagic infarct with mass effect.

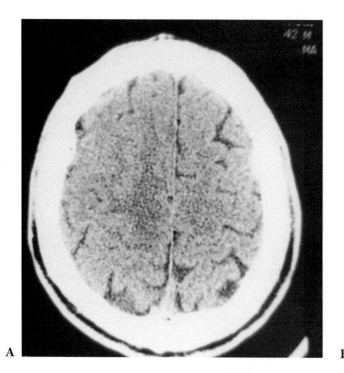

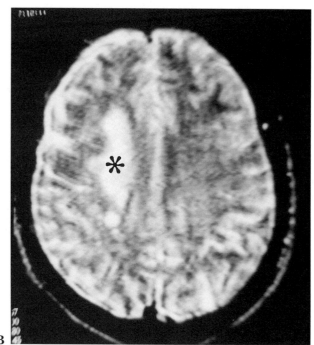

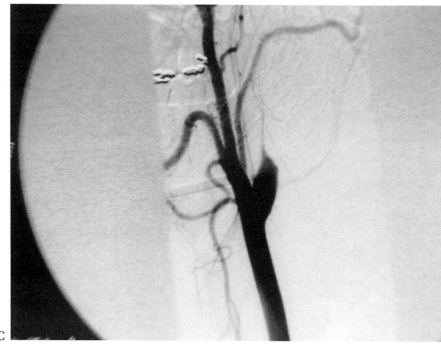

FIGURE 75.4. **A,** Axial noncontrast computed tomography scan demonstrates right convexity mass effect with loss of ipsilateral sulci and subtle white matter lucency. **B,** Follow-up magnetic resonance imaging scan confirms white matter ischemia (*) in this 42-year-old man. **C,** Arteriography confirms spontaneous right internal carotid dissection.

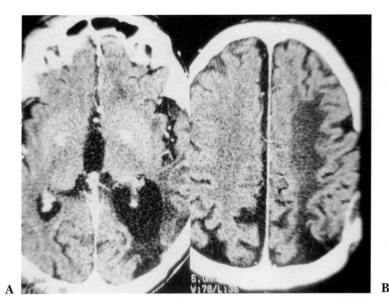

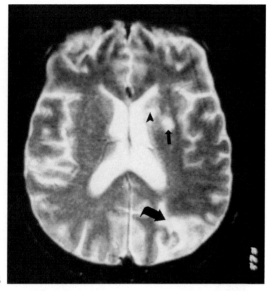

FIGURE 75.5. **A,** Axial computed tomography scan demonstrating extensive old left hemispheric watershed stroke. **B,** Axial T$_2$ magnetic resonance imaging scan in a different patient demonstrating watershed infarcts involving left parietal occipital region (large arrow), caudate nucleus (arrowhead), and corona radiata (small arrow).

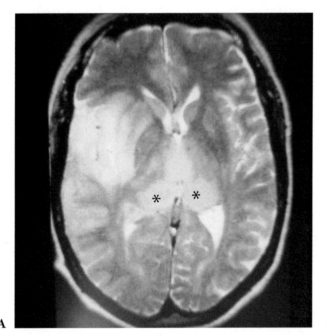

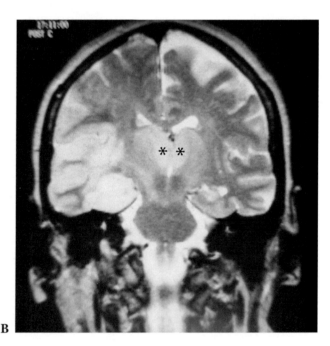

FIGURE 75.6. **A,** Axial T$_2$ magnetic resonance imaging scan demonstrating high intensity in the right temporal lobe, which was initially felt to be an ischemic middle cerebral artery infarct on computed tomography scanning because of the primary cortical involvement. Note the involvement of both thalami also in this magnetic resonance imaging scan (*). **B,** Coronal T$_2$ magnetic resonance imaging scan shows hyperintensity involving the right temporal lobe with prominent cortical and bithalamic involvement. This was an extensively infiltrating glioma that spread to the right thalamus and then left thalamus through the massa intermedia (*).

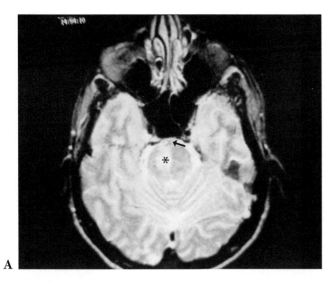

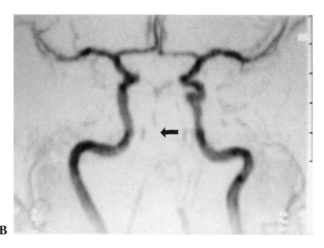

FIGURE 75.7. **A,** Axial T_2 magnetic resonance imaging scan demonstrating right pons infarct (*), and loss of the basilar artery flow void (arrow). Contrast this with Figure 75.14B, which has a normal basilar flow void. **B,** Intracranial magnetic resonance angiogram in same patient demonstrating nearly complete occlusion of the basilar artery (arrow).

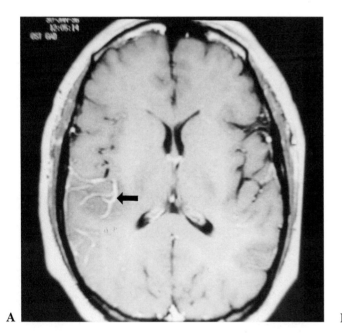

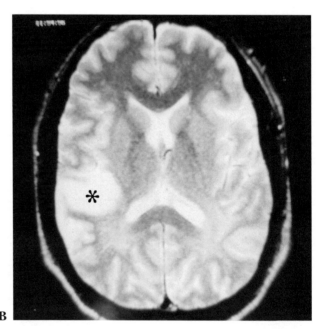

FIGURE 75.8. **A,** Axial contrast-enhanced T_1 magnetic resonance imaging scan demonstrating right posterior branch middle cerebral artery intravascular enhancement, manifestation of slow flow in the artery (arrow). **B,** Follow-up T_2 magnetic resonance imaging scan shows high-intensity infarct in the same distribution (*).

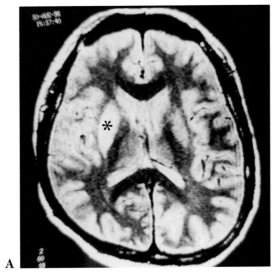

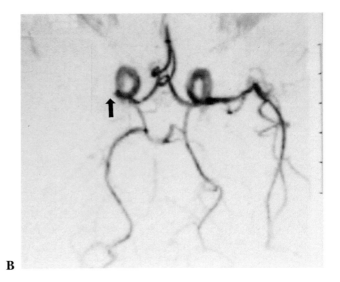

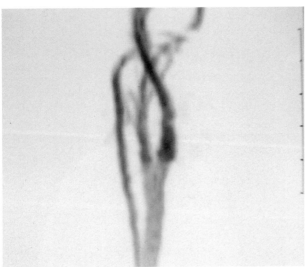

FIGURE 75.9. **A,** Axial proton density magnetic resonance imaging scan demonstrating high signal in the right lentiform nucleus (*) and insular cortex, consistent with ischemic stroke. **B,** Intracranial magnetic resonance angiogram (three-dimensional time of flight technique) shows right M_1 occlusion (arrow). **C,** Cervical carotid magnetic resonance angiogram (two-dimensional time of flight technique) is unremarkable.

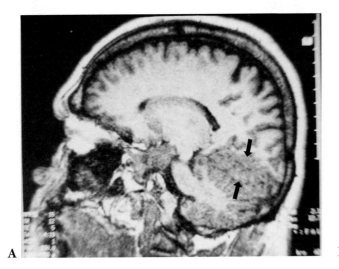

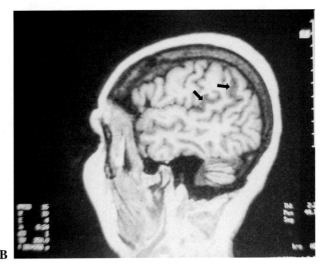

FIGURE 75.10. **A,** Sagittal T_1 gradient echo volume acquisition reveals loss of gray–white matter differentiation in the occipital lobe (arrows). **B,** A different patient demonstrates localized gray matter swelling (arrows) in the posterior parietal lobe, at the site of more limited cortical ischemia.

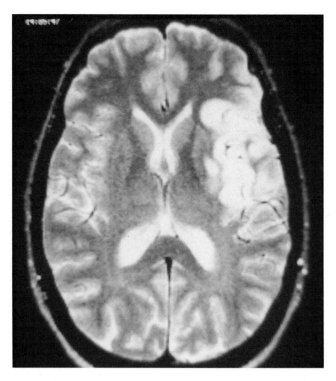

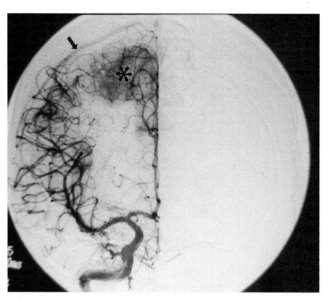

FIGURE 75.13. Right carotid injection in a 50-year-old man with a right convexity stroke reveals luxury perfusion in the infarct (*) and an early draining vein (arrow).

FIGURE 75.11. Axial T$_2$ magnetic resonance imaging scan demonstrates high intensity in the left middle cerebral artery distribution and subtle mass effect, consistent with a subacute infarct.

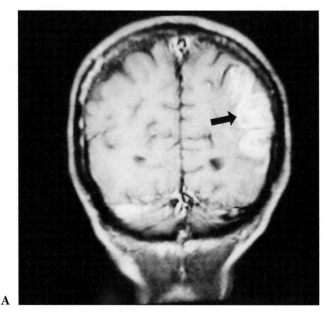

A

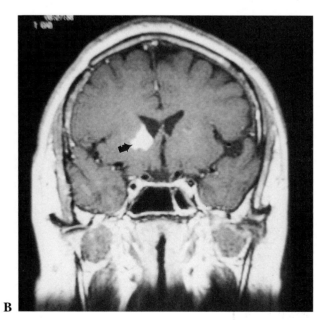

B

FIGURE 75.12. **A,** Left posterior parietal gyriform enhancement in a 7-day-old ischemia stroke (arrow). **B,** Localized homogeneous enhancement (arrow) in a 3-week-old caudate infarct.

Note the mild ipsilateral ventricular dilatation as a manifestation of early regional atrophy.

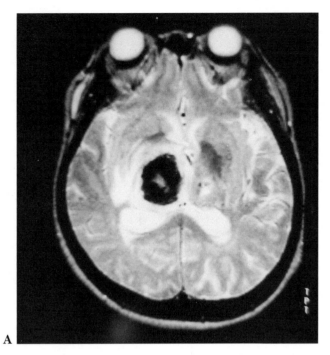

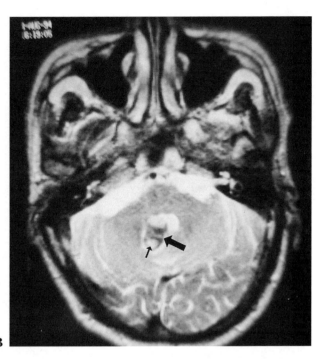

A   **B**

FIGURE 75.14. **A,** Axial T$_2$ magnetic resonance imaging scan showing a large subacute right thalamic hematoma. The low T$_2$ intensity is consistent with deoxyhemoglobin. The surrounding high signal is edema. **B,** Axial T$_2$ magnetic resonance imaging scan demonstrating a small right dentate nucleus hematoma (large arrow). The intensity is more heterogeneous, consistent with evolving blood products. The darker areas are deoxyhemoglobin, and the brighter areas are methemoglobin (small arrow).

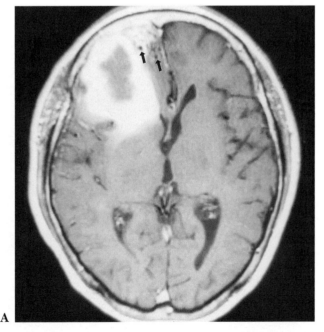

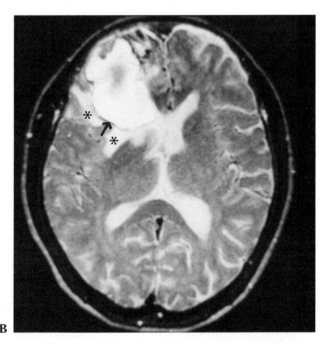

A   **B**

FIGURE 75.15. **A,** Axial noncontrast T$_1$ magnetic resonance imaging scan demonstrating large right frontal lobe hematoma. The high signal areas are methemoglobin. Note several punctate areas of signal void (arrow) medial to the ante- rior portion of the hematoma. These are flow voids of a small arteriovenous malformation. **B,** Axial T$_2$ magnetic resonance imaging scan on the same patient shows the surrounding edema (*) distinct from the hematoma (arrow).

Hemorrhage

In the acute stroke syndrome, the most useful information is the ability to detect an acute hemorrhage. CT is currently the most commonly used imaging device that allows rapid assessment of the location and type of hemorrhage and associated complications, but MRI use is increasing and allows better visualization of more subtle hemorrhages, especially those in the posterior fossa. Certain patterns, coupled with the clinical history, can limit the differentials, which facilitates the diagnostic workup. Hypertensive intracerebral hemorrhage often occurs in typical locations such as the putamen, external capsule, thalamus, pons, and dentate nucleus of the cerebellum[102] (Figure 75.14). Two thirds of the hemorrhages occur in basal ganglia. Lobar white matter hemorrhages can be due to either hypertension or other causes such as amyloid angiopathy or arteriovenous malformations. These hemorrhages are often large and may be associated with rapidly developing edema (Figure 75.15).[103] Other nontraumatic causes of intracranial hemorrhage include mycotic aneurysms, embolic infarction with reperfusion, coagulopathies, blood dyscrasias, drug abuse, tumor, venous infarction, vasculitis, and encephalitis. Subarachnoid hemorrhage has a typical CT pattern (Figure 75.16) and is often due to an underlying aneurysm in 80% to 90% of patients.[104] The pattern of the hemorrhage may predict the site of rupture, which is

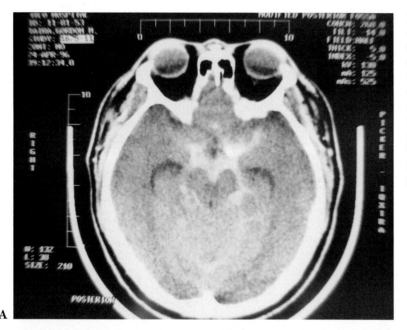

A

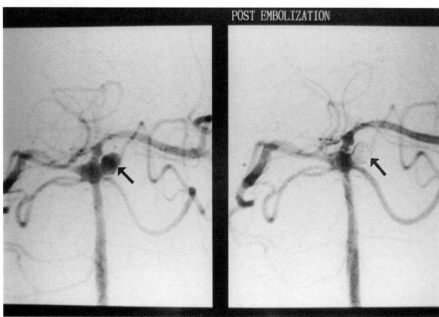

B

FIGURE 75.16. **A,** Axial noncontrast CT showing diffuse subarachnoid hemorrhage (high-density blood in the basal cisterns) and early hydrocephalus (dilated temporal horns). Hydrocephalus may develop within hours of the subarachnoid hemorrhage. **B,** Basilar arteriogram in the same patient demonstrates a left aneurysm (arrow) protruding between the superior cerebellar and posterior cerebral arteries. Left photo shows preembolization. Right photo is after endovascular obliteration using platinum coils (arrow).

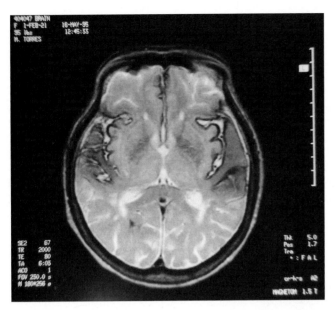

FIGURE 75.17. Axial T_2 magnetic resonance imaging scan with linear peripheral low signal consistent with hemosiderin staining of the pia in this patient who has had several subarachnoid hemorrhages.

usually the circle of Willis or middle cerebral bifurcation but unfortunately is often diffuse and therefore nonspecific as to location of the potential aneurysm. If subarachnoid blood is suspected, then CT imaging is the modality of choice because acute oxygenated blood is difficult to visualize on MRI scans. Repeated subarachnoid hemorrhages may be seen on MRI scans as low signal on the pial surfaces, referred to as superficial siderosis (Figure 75.17).

Venous Occlusion

Venous occlusions, uncommon causes of stroke syndromes (1%), are often misdiagnosed.[105] The superior sagittal sinus is the most commonly occluded sinus. Parasagittal hemorrhages or hemorrhagic infarcts in unusual locations may be the presenting CT or MRI finding, and these hemorrhages and infarcts may be unilateral (Figure 75.18) or bilateral (Figure 75.19). Venous occlusions must be confirmed relatively quickly because of spontaneous recanalization. Numerous CT and MRI findings have been described, but all change with time. Therefore, it is essential to maintain a high index of suspicion and understand the diverse imaging findings. Primary findings on CT or MRI scans include visualization of the dense clot within the sinus on noncontrast examinations (Figure 75.20) or recognition of the clot-filled sinus after contrast administration (the "empty delta sign" on CT scans) (Figure 75.21).[106] In chronic cases, secondary findings can include intense and irregular tentorial and falcine enhancement, presumably secondary to collateral veins.

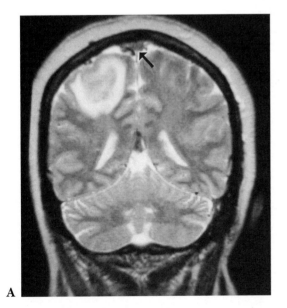

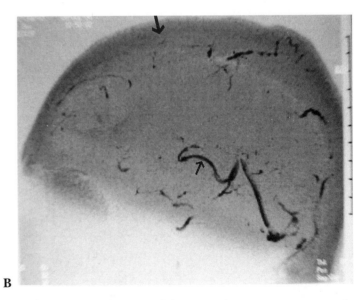

A   **B**

FIGURE 75.18. **A,** Coronal T_2 magnetic resonance imaging scan demonstrating right parasagittal partially hemorrhagic infarct and soft tissue clot in the superior sagittal sinus (arrow). Contrast this with the normal triangular shape flow void in the posterior aspect of the superior sagittal sinus in Figures 75.17 and 75.15B. **B,** Lateral view of the magnetic resonance venogram in the same patient, which reveals a normal internal cerebral vein (small arrow) and straight sinus but complete occlusion of the superior sagittal sinus (large arrow). Compare this with Figure 75.19A and B.

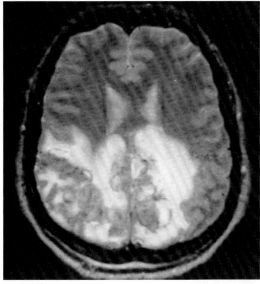

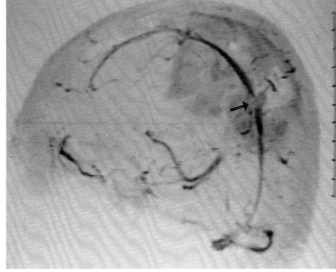

A   **B**

FIGURE 75.19. **A,** Axial T_2 magnetic resonance imaging scan with bilateral extensive partially hemorrhagic infarcts, which were secondary to superior sagittal sinus occlusion that occurred during removal of a high falx meningioma. **B,** Oblique view magnetic resonance venogram on the same patient performed several days after surgery confirms recanalization of most of the superior sagittal sinus, except for a persistent localized clot (arrow).

Other Diagnostic Studies

When CT and MRI studies are normal or equivocal, other tests of brain function, metabolism, and blood flow may be helpful in localizing the abnormality in the brain: positron emission tomography scanning, single photon emission CT, xenon-enhanced CT, and electroencephalogram. Transesophageal echocardiography or transthoracic echocardiography may help identify cardiogenic embolism.[107] Carotid and transcranial Doppler sonography systems are utilized in stroke to measure blood velocity, evaluate changes in blood flow patterns, detect severe stenosis or occlusion of cerebral arteries, and assess patients with subarachnoid hemorrhage for vasospasm.[108,109]

Medical Treatment

Acute stroke and TIAs should be treated as medical emergencies. TIAs, which are of limited severity and du-

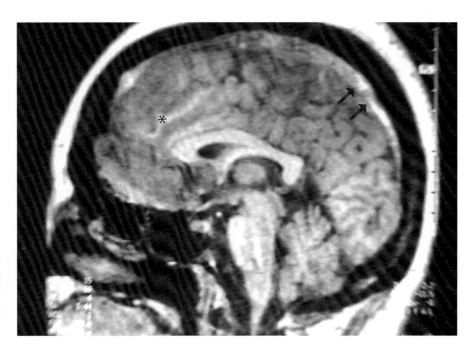

FIGURE 75.20. Sagittal T_1 magnetic resonance imaging scan showing high-intensity clot within the superior sagittal sinus (arrows) and blood (methemoglobin) in several anterior para falcine sulci (*).

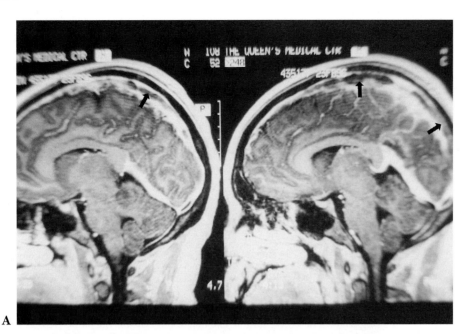

FIGURE 75.21. **A,** Sagittal post–contrast T_1 magnetic resonance imaging scan showing numerous filling defects in the enhancing superior sagittal sinus (arrows). **B,** Axial post–contrast CT demonstrating the empty delta sign of a clot-filled superior sagittal sinus (arrow).

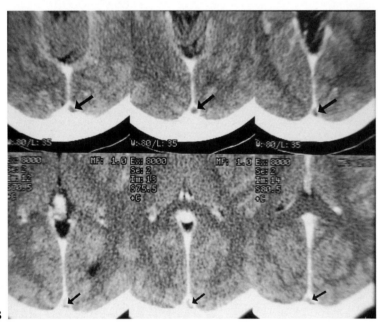

ration, are differentiated from stroke only after the symptoms have faded. In the acute symptomatic phase, the approach is that of the acute stroke, because TIA is a warning sign of impending ischemia and necessitates emergency treatment.

Unfortunately, the public's knowledge about stroke is inadequate, and many stroke patients do not seek medical care in a timely fashion. Early intervention is critical, but delays in hospital admission occur for the majority of stroke patients. Greater delays in admission are associated with referral patterns, patients with ischemic stroke, and stroke onset that occurs during the weekend or night.[110] Medical mismanagement is another problem in stroke care, because stroke patients often do not receive

indicated therapies and are sometimes given inappropriate treatments.[19] A recent study suggests that care given by neurologists costs more but results in better outcomes.[11] The 90-day mortality rates for stroke patients treated by neurologists were significantly lower than those treated by other specialists.

Acute Treatment of Stroke

A coordinated, multidisciplinary approach to stroke care through the use of stroke teams and protocols can improve outcome and reduce costs.[19] Widespread professional and public education is needed to reduce delays in symptom recognition, referrals, admission, and timely therapies. Stroke needs to receive the same priority as MI, and immediate stroke care begins with the stabilization of vital signs.

Emergent Supportive Intervention

Rapid medical assessment to ensure adequate oxygenation and cardiovascular stability is required for all stroke patients because hypotension and hypoxia exacerbate an acute ischemic neurological deficit. Supplemental oxygen should be provided if there is evidence of decreased oxygen saturation by pulse oximetry or blood gas determination.[112] Some stroke patients with inadequate ventilation may require acute intubation to improve oxygenation in a patient with asthma or other chronic respiratory problem or if the CT scan shows much edema in the cerebral hemispheres as a reaction to an infarction or hemorrhage. Intubation and hyperventilation are generally not used in basilar artery strokes because they rarely improve the outcome.

Most patients presenting with ischemic stroke have elevated blood pressure that usually returns to normal in a few days. The majority of initially hypertensive patients do not need any antihypertensive treatment. The treatment of hypertension in acute ischemic stroke patients remains an area of controversy, because elevated blood pressure has to be decreased within certain parameters, but hypotension must be avoided to prevent further ischemia and worsening of the neurological deficit. Conditions in acute stroke that warrant antihypertensive therapy include malignant hypertension and hypertensive encephalopathy, acute MI, aortic dissection, and blood pressure above the upper limits of autoregulation (>220/>120 mm Hg, which should be lowered by approximately 20% or until both are within the autoregulatory range).[113] Antihypertensive therapy in acute stroke must be individualized and agents selected that are easily titrated and will not cause increases in intracranial pressure or precipitous falls in arterial blood pressure.

Because hyperthermia may exacerbate ischemic injury, antipyretic agents should be administered to febrile stroke patients while the cause of the fever is investigated.[112] Significant hypoglycemia should be corrected immediately with intravenous glucose administration. Hypotension secondary to decreased cardiac output or hypovolemia (usually due to dehydration) requires intravenous administration of fluids or therapeutic interventions to optimize cardiac output.

Thrombolytic Therapy

Successful use of thrombolytic therapy for acute stroke depends on rapid assessment to exclude patients with hemorrhagic stroke or those at risk of hemorrhagic complications.[114] Thrombolytic therapy can provide rapid recanalization of occluded cerebral vessels, leading to improvement or resolution of neurological deficit. Intravenous rtPA is an effective therapy for reducing long-term neurological morbidity from acute ischemic stroke and has been approved by the US Food and Drug Administration for stroke treatment. In an acute ischemic stroke within 3 hours of symptom onset, intravenous rtPA administered at 0.9 mg/kg (with a maximum total dose of 90 mg) is recommended if the patient meets specific selection criteria.[112]

In the NINDS rt-PA Stroke Study, patients treated with tissue-type plasminogen activator intravenously were significantly more likely to have minimal or no disability at 3-month follow-up compared with patients treated with placebo.[23] Symptomatic hemorrhage was more common in patients with severe strokes (NIHSS score >22).[115]

Approximately 3% of stroke patients treated with rtPA died as a result of intracerebral hemorrhage in the European Cooperative Acute Stroke Study [22] and the NINDS studies.[23] Patients in the European Cooperative Acute Stroke Study and NINDS studies were rigorously selected, and whether patients with acute ischemic stroke treated with rtPA in routine clinical practice may actually be at greatest risk of intracerebral hemorrhage with rtPA use is questioned.[116] Most of the thousands of patients screened for the NINDS study were determined to be ineligible, usually because of presentation beyond 3 hours from stroke onset. Strict inclusion and exclusion guidelines for thrombolytic treatment with rtPA therapy and posttreatment management have been developed based on the NINDS study and are provided in Table 75.4.

The Multicenter Acute Stroke Trial—Europe[117] and the Australian Streptokinase Trial[118] were terminated prematurely because of an increased incidence of adverse outcomes in streptokinase-treated patients. Streptokinase was associated with significantly increased mortality rates in 10 days in the Multicentre Acute Stroke Trial—Italy,[119] so this third large, randomized study was also stopped prematurely. Streptokinase has not been found to be effective in the treatment of acute ischemic stroke.

Intra-Arterial Thrombolysis

Experience with intra-arterial thrombolysis for treatment of acute ischemic stroke has demonstrated dramatic clinical improvement; however, only a limited number of uncontrolled case studies have been undertaken.[112] The requirement of angiography usually results in significant treatment delays, so the role of intra-arterial thrombolysis for acute stroke treatment requires further investigation.

Neuroprotective Agents

Neuroprotective agents are being developed to interfere in the destructive cascade reaction initiated by stroke-in-

TABLE 75.4. Patient selection and treatment guidelines for recombinant tissue plasminogen activator therapy.

Inclusion criteria
Clinically significant neurological deficit
Signs and symptoms compatible with ischemic stroke: acute hemiparesis (face, arm, and possibly leg) or language difficulty
Well-established time of acute symptom onset within 3 h of initiation of treatment
Age 18 y or older (risks of therapy may be increased in patients >77 y)

Exclusion criteria
Computed tomography scan evidence of early infarction: significant hypodensity or edema, especially if more than one third of the middle
     cerebral artery territory is involved, hemorrhage, or tumor
Systolic blood pressure >185 mm Hg or diastolic blood pressure >110 mm Hg before treatment (medication may be required to consider
     inclusion)
Clinical presentation suggests subarachnoid hemorrhage or history of intracranial hemorrhage, arteriovenous malformation, aneurysm, or
     cerebral neoplasm
Oral anticoagulant use with elevated prothrombin time (aspirin is okay)
Heparin use with elevated partial thromboplastin time (or recent heparin use <48 h)
Major surgery within past 14 d (or intracranial or spinal surgery in past 2 mo)
Rapidly improving neurological deficit or minor symptoms only
Serum glucose <40 or >400 mg/dL
Platelet count <100,000/mm^3
Seizure at time of stroke onset or uncontrolled chronic seizure disorder
Gastrointestinal or genitourinary bleeding in the past 21 d, esophageal varices, or gastrointestinal ulcer
Recent myocardial infarction
Significant bleeding diathesis or other risk factor for systemic hemorrhage
     (abnormal prothrombin, partial thromboplastin, and coagulation times)
Arterial puncture at noncompressible site within 1 w
Prior stroke (within the past 3 mo) or recent serious head injury
Pregnancy
Coma or severe obtundation

Treatment guideline
Intravenous recombinant tissue plasminogen activator administered at 0.9 mg/kg (with a maximum total dose of 90 mg) within 3 h of symptom
     onset is recommended if the patient meets specific selection criteria

Selected posttreatment guidelines
Maintain blood pressure <180/110 mm Hg (but avoid hypotension)
No antiplatelet or anticoagulant treatment within the first 24 h
Close neurological observation with frequent monitoring of vital signs for at least 36 h
Standing protocol for urgent evaluation and treatment of intracranial hemorrhage
No invasive procedures (i.e., arterial or central venous punctures and nasogastric tube placement) during the first 24 h
No initiation of additional peripheral lines or insertion of urinary catheters <30 min after completion of recombinant tissue plasminogen
     activator infusion

Adapted from National Institute of Neurological Disorders and Stroke rt-PA Study Group[23] and Albers.[112]

duced ischemia. Clinical trials are under way on a wide array of potentially neuroprotective drugs. These agents target different sites in the ischemic cell death cascade. A combination therapy of neuroprotective drugs and thrombolytic agents may rescue more brain tissue than either treatment alone.[120] The role of neuroprotective agents in the routine management of ischemic stroke depends on the results of controlled clinical trials.

Acute Antithrombotic Therapy

Despite the surprisingly few adequate clinical trials to address their safety and efficacy, anticoagulant and antiplatelet agents are the most commonly used medications for treatment of acute ischemic stroke. Because of its immediate action, most neurologists use heparin in selected ischemic stroke patients.[121] Intravenous heparin

is most frequently administered for patients with progressive stroke, particularly in the vertebrobasilar circulation, and is also used for prevention of recurrent cardioembolic stroke. Therapeutic levels of heparin can be reached earlier if a bolus dose is given, but the dosing regimen must be balanced with bleeding risk. Heparin should be avoided or used with great caution in patients with large infarcts or uncontrolled hypertension and excessive prolongation of partial thromboplastin time because of their association with an increased risk of intracranial hemorrhage.[112]

A recent Hong Kong study found that nadroparin, a low molecular weight form of heparin, was effective for treatment of acute ischemic stroke within 48 hours of symptom onset.[122] Clinical trials of nadroparin and another low molecular weight heparin (Org 10172) are under way in the United States. Low-dose subcutaneous heparin (approximately 5000 U twice a day) can reduce the risk of deep venous thrombosis and is appropriate for immobilized stroke patients who are not treated with intravenous heparin or an oral anticoagulant.

The therapeutic effect of warfarin is delayed, so heparin is generally used if immediate anticoagulation is needed for the acute stroke patient. Warfarin is indicated for prevention of cardiogenic emboli and can be started when the patient stabilizes. Frequent monitoring of prothrombin time in the early stages of therapy is necessary due to the risk of hemorrhage.

Antiplatelet Agents

Oral aspirin therapy (160–325 mg daily) is recommended for the treatment of acute ischemic stroke patients who are not receiving heparin or rtPA.[112] The optimal dose of aspirin for prevention of stroke has not been established. Pending the outcome of several ongoing antiplatelet trials, the lowest dose of aspirin (75 mg/d) shown effective in the prevention of stroke and death in patients with ischemic cerebrovascular disease has been recommended.[123]

Ticlopidine is more effective than aspirin in secondary stroke prevention[124] and is more effective in women.[125] The high cost and possibility of severe neutropenia are disadvantages to ticlopidine therapy. Combinations of anticoagulant and antiplatelet agents in stroke treatment have not yet been studied.

Surgical Treatment

Therapies to halt or reverse ischemic neurological damage are currently limited. Prophylactic surgical treatment of stroke is primarily carotid endarterectomy for stenosis. Acute intervention surgery is primarily evacuation of certain specific intracerebral hemorrhages.

Carotid Endarterectomy

Carotid endarterectomy is discussed in Chapter 74. The Asymptomatic Carotid Artery Study has demonstrated the efficacy of carotid endarterectomy in stroke prevention among patients with carotid stenosis of >60% with no symptoms ipsilateral to the stenosis.[126]

The extracranial to intracranial bypass has been evaluated for treatment of carotid stenosis. The initial results of performing an anastomosis between the superficial temporal artery and a branch of the MCA looked promising. Extracranial to intracranial bypass was used in patients with severe stenosis proximal to the MCA in an area that was not amenable to surgery. A detailed and controversial trial of extracranial to intracranial bypass procedures found no evidence that these patients did better than patients treated medically.[127]

Surgery for Intracerebral Hemorrhage

The first successful operation for an intracerebral hematoma was performed in 1883 by MacEwan.[128] The advent of CT and MRI has revolutionized the management of patients with intracerebral hemorrhage. However, numerous series of medically and surgically treated patients with parenchymal hemorrhages have not been able to establish clear indications for surgery. A variety of surgical procedures, from open craniotomy with clot evacuation to stereotactic aspiration, have been used. The results of surgical evacuation of deep putamen hemorrhages have been very poor, and the procedure is rarely indicated.

Indications for Surgery

Parenchymal Hematoma

If a parenchymal hematoma is life-threatening and it is not a deep putamen or basal ganglion hemorrhage, especially in a young person, surgical evaluation may be reasonable. Surgical evaluation is especially recommended if a period of stabilization is followed by clinical deterioration.

Cerebellar Hemorrhage

Cerebellar hemorrhage is a special management problem, because a hematoma in the cerebellum, which is adjacent to the brain stem, can cause rapid and irreversible deterioration without warning. Surgical evacuation of cerebellar hematomas is associated with a low morbidity rate, and surgery is recommended for all lesions greater than 3 cm in diameter. Smaller lesions usually have a benign course and can be treated medically with close observation.

Hemorrhages Secondary to Aneurysms, Arteriovenous Malformations, or Tumor

Patients who are not moribund on presentation and are diagnosed preoperatively via MRI scan or angiography are often candidates for evacuation of the hematoma and treatment of the underlying problem. If a patient is moribund, the results of surgery are usually so poor that it is generally best to manage the patient medically to see whether he or she will stabilize and survive.

Subarachnoid Hemorrhage

The most frequent cause of subarachnoid hemorrhage, excluding trauma, is a ruptured aneurysm. With the advent of modern anesthesia and microsurgical techniques, the surgical treatment of aneurysms has evolved. Vasospasm secondary to SAH can be treated more aggressively. Emergent aneurysm clipping is necessary to prevent rebleeding. Nimodipine, a calcium channel blocker administered at the onset of SAH, has also decreased the incidence of vasospasm.

Surgical Techniques

The four surgical techniques for evacuation of intracerebral hemorrhages are (1) craniotomy with evacuation of hematoma, (2) stereotactic aspiration, (3) endoscopic clot aspiration, and (4) ventriculostomy.

1. *Craniotomy with evacuation of hematoma.* It is usually necessary to perform a craniotomy with direct exposure of the hematoma to adequately remove the clot. The cortical incision must be performed in an area that will produce as minimal a neurological defect as possible. The anterior superior temporal gyrus can be incised for temporal or putaminal lesions, the superior parietal lobule for parietal occipital lesions, and the superior frontal gyrus anterior to the motor strip for frontal lesions. For cerebellar lesions, a vermian or paramedian approach can be used, depending on the location of the lesion. It is advantageous to remove most of the hematoma, but the last adherent bits may be left behind to avoid injury and bleeding from the cavity wall. A biopsy should be taken of any tissue suspicious for an angioma or tumor.
2. *Stereotactic aspiration.* Stereotactic aspiration was first suggested by Backlund and von Holst,[129] and there have been many reports, especially from Japan, indicating good results. Reports from Germany and Japan in which thrombolytic agents were used at the time of stereotactic aspiration have been encouraging.[130,131]
3. *Endoscopic clot aspiration.* Endoscopic clot aspiration is a variation of stereotactic aspiration. This method uses interoperative ultrasound to locate the hematoma and an endoscope to visualize and evacuate. This technique is not widely used but appears to be gaining in popularity.[132]
4. *Ventriculostomy.* Ventricular drainage is often warranted when hydrocephalus or intraventricular hemorrhage is symptomatic. A standard ventricular drain is placed through a frontal burr hole, usually on the nondominant side. Continuous drainage through a closed sterile system is used. Often this drainage is only necessary for a few days, but on occasion a ventriculoperitoneal shunt may be necessary. Serial CT scans and trial clamping of the drainage usually help determine whether the drainage should be stopped or a permanent shunt should be placed.

Surgical Treatment of Specific Hemorrhage Locations

Putaminal Hemorrhage

Patients with putaminal hemorrhage can usually be divided into three groups.[133] In the first group, patients present in coma and have a massive hemorrhage and poor prognosis. Patients in the second group are alert but have significant neurological deficits and moderate-sized hematomas. Some make acceptable recoveries, but most are left with a substantial deficit. In the third group, mild deficits are found in relation to small hemorrhages; these patients generally make a good recovery. Patients with small- or moderate-sized hematomas in the putamen often make a good recovery, either spontaneously or with medical management. When hematomas are larger than 3 cm in diameter, the initial treatment is usually medical, but if the patient develops progressive neurological deficit or drowsiness despite medical treatment, early surgical removal of the hematoma may be considered. However, recent controlled studies of surgical evacuation of putaminal hemorrhages have demonstrated no clear benefit from surgical removal.[134]

Thalamus Hemorrhage

The usual presentation of thalamus hemorrhage is a hemisensory deficit and motor weakness if the internal capsule has been involved. Extension into the upper brain stem commonly leads to vertical gaze palsy, retraction, nystagmus, and skewed deviation with ptosis, myosis, and isochromia or unreactive pupils. A high mortality rate is associated with hemorrhage into the thalamus, especially if the hematoma is larger than 3.3 cm as seen on the CT scan. Patients recovering with smaller thalamic hemorrhages usually have significant disability. I do not operate on thalamic hemorrhages but sometimes place a ventricular shunt if there is acute hydrocephalus.

Lobar Hemorrhage

Hemorrhages may occur in the occipital lobe, frontal lobe, and, on occasion, temporal lobe. The clinical presentation varies with the location of the hemorrhage. There is a high incidence of associated abnormalities such as an arteriovenous malformation, metastatic tumor, and angiopathy. Angiography is usually indicated when a hemorrhage presents in one of these areas to adequately evaluate a possible etiology other than hypertension or arteriosclerosis. Most patients with spontaneous or hypertensive lobar hemorrhages make a good recovery with medical treatment. If the patient shows signs of a progressive neurological deficit despite medical treatment, surgical removal of the hematoma is indicated.[135]

Intraventricular Hemorrhage

Intraventricular hemorrhage is diagnosed easily on a CT or MRI scan and usually occurs secondary to a rupture of a parenchymal hematoma into the ventricular system. Rarely, a primary intraventricular hemorrhage can occur. The incidence of associated disorders such as hypertension, intracranial aneurysm, arteriovenous malformation, tumor, and coagulopathy is high. Ventriculostomy can be lifesaving and is indicated for neurological deterioration secondary to acute hydrocephalus. If the patient survives the acute phase, a ventricular peritoneal shunt may be necessary.

Cerebellar Hemorrhage

The onset of intracerebellar hemorrhage is usually sudden, with nausea, vomiting, and an inability to stand. Headache is present in a high percentage of patients. A diagnosis can usually be made easily on clinical examination, which reveals ataxia in the majority of patients. Facial palsy is present in 60%, and an ipsilateral gaze palsy is present in approximately half of these patients.[133] Cerebellar hemorrhage is an acute surgical emergency, because deterioration secondary to brain stem compression can occur quickly with very little warning. Evacuation of a cerebellar hematoma, even in patients who are deeply comatose, can result in good recovery if the time interval between the development of the comatose state and the surgery is short. A hematoma smaller than 3 cm usually does not require surgical removal. However, these patients must be carefully monitored, and if there is any evidence of brain stem compression, surgery should be performed immediately. In addition to removing the hematoma, it is often necessary to perform a ventricular drainage because hydrocephalus occurs secondary to obstruction.

Mesencephalic Hemorrhage

Mesencephalic hemorrhages may occur secondary to an arteriovenous malformation or hypertension. Successful evacuation of these hematomas has been reported, but the prognosis is usually poor and surgery is not indicated.

Pontine Hemorrhage

Pontine hemorrhage is the least treatable of all brain hemorrhages. A small hemorrhage into the pons is a traumatic event that often leads to immediate coma; rapid quadriplegia with pinpoint, barely reactive pupils; and extraocular movement disturbances. The prognosis is very poor, and most patients do not survive the acute phase.

Medullary Hemorrhage

Medullary hemorrhage is almost always fatal. Microsurgical removal of a small hematoma from the medulla has been reported, but this is an extremely uncommon surgical procedure.

Medical Conditions Associated With Brain Hemorrhage

Several medical conditions are associated with an increased incidence of intracranial hemorrhage and influence decisions about surgical treatment.

Occult Vascular Lesions

The histology of occult vascular lesions includes arteriovenous malformation, cavernous angioma, telangiectases, venous angioma, and tumor. Lesions may occur in childhood. The diagnosis may be suspected on the basis of CT and MRI findings, but histology is required for a specific diagnosis.

Anticoagulant Therapy

The increased use of anticoagulant agents has resulted in more patients with brain hemorrhage. Treatment consists of immediate transfusion with fresh-frozen plasma and administration of vitamin K to restore normal coagulation. Sometimes surgery is indicated because of neurological deterioration; it can be performed safely after administration of vitamin K.

Hemophilia

Usually hemophilia patients are deficient in factor VII, although some are deficient in factor IX or XI. Mild head trauma may produce a brain hemorrhage that can be a subdural hematoma or an intracerebral hematoma. Replacement therapy must be initiated immediately when a hemorrhage has been diagnosed and must be continued until after surgery.

Thrombocytopenia

A platelet count lower than $80,000/mm^3$ is diagnostic of thrombocytopenia. Intracerebral or subdural hemorrhages can occur secondary to minor head trauma or can occur spontaneously. Immediate platelet transfusion and corticosteroid therapy are necessary. Surgery can be performed if indicated.

Amyloid Angiopathy

Spontaneous lobar hemorrhage may be associated with amyloid angiopathy.[136,137] This condition is usually seen in patients over age 60 and may present with multiple hemorrhages. Patients with amyloid angiopathy often do poorly with surgery because of the difficulty in controlling intraoperative bleeding and the frequency of hemorrhage subsequent to surgery.[138]

Drug-Related Hemorrhage

Use of intravenous methamphetamines, cocaine abuse, and phenylpropanolamine ingestions have been associated with intracerebral hemorrhages. The surgical approach is the same, but drug withdrawal may complicate postoperative medical management.

Angiitis

Spontaneous hemorrhage may occur with inflammatory angiitis. Angiography usually establishes the diagnosis because the arteries have a beaded appearance. Surgical evacuation can be done if clinically indicated.

Medical Management and Rehabilitation

Stroke rehabilitation should begin as soon as the diagnosis of stroke is established and life-threatening problems are under control. Improvement of neurological deficit usually occurs if the patient survives, but the longer the delay in onset of recovery, the poorer the prognosis.[25] Stroke rehabilitation aims to hasten and maximize recovery from stroke by treating the disabilities caused by the stroke. The coordinated, multidisciplinary approach of an acute stroke program can significantly improve outcome, decrease length of hospital stay, and reduce costs.[19,20] Highest priorities for medical management and early rehabilitation of acute stroke are to prevent secondary complications from the present stroke, stabilize medical comorbidities, prevent recurrent stroke, and mobilize the patient as soon as medically feasible.

Secondary Complications of Stroke

Approximately 31% of people who have a stroke die within a year, with a higher percentage among people older than age 65.[14] Stroke survivors account for half of all patients hospitalized in the United States for acute neurological disease. Prevention, early recognition, and aggressive treatment of secondary complications of stroke can maximize neurological and functional recovery.

Neurological Complications

Severe brain edema occurs in about 15% of ischemic stroke patients, with maximal severity reached 72 to 96 hours after stroke onset.[112] Osmotic diuretics and hyperventilation to lower intracranial pressure may be useful for patients with neurological deterioration caused by cerebral edema. Corticosteroids are not recommended for reducing brain edema caused by ischemic stroke.

Temporal lobe tentorial herniation occurs when the medial part of the temporal lobe is displaced contralaterally and then forced into the oval-shaped tentorial opening through which the midbrain passes. This condition can be fatal if not revised by immediately treating the edema or evacuating the hematoma.

Seizures complicate less than 10% of all strokes,[139,140] so prophylactic administration of anticonvulsant agents is not recommended for patients who have not suffered seizures. Antiepileptic agents should be used only for prevention of *recurrent* seizures in acute ischemic stroke.

Recurrent Stroke

The stroke recurrence rate is 7% to 10% per year and is highest in the first year after an initial stroke.[5] In the Framingham Study, recurrence was found to be particularly common for thrombotic stroke and more frequent in men.[141] Therapy choice depends on determination of the etiology of the stroke. Anticoagulation with warfarin has been shown to decrease cardioembolic events and mortality rates in patients with nonvalvular AF in five randomized clinical trials.[142-146] Heparin is widely used for treatment of cardiovascular abnormalities and progressive ischemic stroke despite the lack of evidence for its benefits.[147] Antiplatelet agents are indicated to reduce stroke risk in patients with TIA or minor stroke.

Cardiac Disease

Approximately 75% of stroke patients have cardiac disease, which may have caused the stroke and may impact stroke recovery.[148] Cardiac disease is the second leading cause of early mortality and leading cause of late mortality after stroke.[149] In stroke patients, 66% have coronary artery disease, 50% have dysrhythmias, and 20% have congestive heart failure. Clinicians can assume that most or all elderly stroke patients have some significant cardiovascular disease and should be monitored appropriately.

Respiratory Complications

Pneumonia is the third major cause of death in the first 30 days after stroke and causes 7% to 34% of deaths in stroke patients.[149] Pneumonia incidence with all strokes is 32% but is higher in patients with subarachnoid hemorrhage and those in a comatose state. Risk factors for pneumonia in stroke patients include aspiration, poor expiratory muscle strength, decreased chest wall compliance, depressed immune response, and general debility. Symptoms of pneumonia may be difficult to recognize because they may present only with subtle changes. Significant alterations in an acute stroke patient's breathing pattern may indicate a large area of brain damage or brain stem dysfunction.

Thromboembolic Disease

Deep venous thrombosis and pulmonary embolism are frequent complications of stroke and are the fourth most common cause of death in the first 30 days after stroke.[150,151] Time of greatest risk is 4 to 5 days after stroke, with incidence of deep venous thrombosis after stroke reported as 40% to 50% and of pulmonary embolism as 9% to 15%.[149]

Predisposing factors for deep venous thrombosis and pulmonary embolism include venous stasis, hypercoagulability, and endothelial injury. Prophylactic subcutaneous heparin is widely used for nonhemorrhagic stroke. Stroke patients should be mobilized as soon as their clinical condition allows, with frequent monitoring for any changes attributable to pulmonary embolism. Warfarin, intermittent pneumatic compression, and elastic stockings are also effective preventive measures. Heparin is contraindicated in patients with hemorrhagic stroke, but other prophylactic treatments include placement of a blood filter in the inferior vena cava and kinetic therapy (rotational bed).[152]

Bowel and Bladder Dysfunction

Problems with bladder control and incontinence are common early in the hospital course after stroke, but they resolve in most patients. In cases in which a catheter is inserted during the acute phase, it should be removed as soon as possible, because indwelling catheters increase the risk of urinary tract infection. Persistent bladder incontinence may indicate a poor long-term prognosis for functional recovery.[5] Bowel management programs should be implemented in patients with persistent constipation or bowel incontinence.

Skin Problems

Skin breakdown is more likely in stroke patients with incontinence, infections, and limited mobility. Preventive measures including daily examination of the skin over pressure point areas; egg crate mattresses are important because approximately 15% of stroke patients develop decubitus ulcers.[149]

Pain

Central pain is quite uncommon after stroke and may be due more to peripheral mechanisms of spasticity and contracture than to brain injury. Neurogenic pain may occur weeks or months after strokes that affect the thalamus and usually involves the contralateral half of the body (Dejerine–Roussy syndrome). Pain perception and response may be influenced by aphasia, alteration in sensation, other medical conditions, depression, and anxiety.

Swallowing Disorders (Dysphagia)

Deficits can occur in any phase of swallowing, from the oral preparatory phase to the esophageal phase. Early as-

sessment and treatment help to prevent aspiration and dehydration or malnutrition from inadequate oral intake.

Depression and Mental Disorders

Depression occurs in 30% to 50% of poststroke patients and can impair functional outcome.[153] Assessment may be difficult in patients with aphasia or comprehension deficits. Other emotional or behavioral disturbances such as anxiety, mania, or outbursts of uncontrolled behavior may also occur in stroke patients but are much less common than depression.[5] Ischemic stroke has been found to increase the long-term risk of developing dementia among stroke patients initially found to be without dementia.[154]

Comorbid Diseases

Comorbid diseases are common in stroke patients. They may affect recovery from a stroke and limit or contraindicate specific treatments or rehabilitation. Important concurrent conditions that must be addressed in stroke care and may affect specific functional outcomes are cardiovascular diseases, chronic pulmonary diseases, diabetes mellitus, cancer, musculoskeletal diseases, severe psychiatric diseases, and neurological diseases. A recent study found that hypoxic–ischemic disorders related to comorbid medical conditions may be a significant independent risk factor for new dementia after stroke, even after adjustment for other recognized predictors of cognitive decline.[155] Because activity levels, nutritional intake, and metabolic demands change during recovery, many of these comorbid illnesses require frequent reevaluation.

Stroke Rehabilitation

Stroke rehabilitation is effective in reducing poststroke mortality rates by 28% at 3 months and 21% at 1 year when compared with best medical therapy.[156] It involves a multidisciplinary team approach that addresses all facets of a patient's life affected by disability after stroke. Disablement has been conceptualized by the World Health Organization in terms of impairment (organ dysfunction), disability (difficulty with tasks), and handicap (social disadvantage).[5] Stroke rehabilitation is a restorative and learning process that seeks to hasten and maximize recovery from stroke by treating the resultant impairments, disabilities, and handicaps.

Screening for poststroke rehabilitation is performed when the patient is medically and neurologically stable. The patient may be referred to a multidisciplinary inpatient or outpatient rehabilitation program. Periodic reassessment during rehabilitation documents progress and provides information to adjust treatment and plan for discharge or transfer.

Stroke rehabilitation begins with early mobilization of the patient and is based on four principles: (1) prevention of secondary complications, (2) remediation or treatment to reduce neurological impairments, (3) compensation for and adaptation to residual disabilities, and (4) maintenance of function over the long term.[5]

Assessment of Impairments

Hemiparesis is a presenting finding in three quarters of stroke patients. Acute neurological impairments frequently resolve spontaneously, but persisting disabilities lead to partial or total dependence in activities of daily living in 25% to 50% of stroke survivors.[5] Neurological findings that most strongly influence rehabilitation decisions include altered level of consciousness, cognitive deficits, motor deficits, disturbances in balance and coordination, somatosensory deficits, disorders of vision, unilateral neglect, speech and language deficits, dysphagia, affective disorders, and pain.

Assessment of Functional Health Patterns

Assessment and continuous monitoring of basic health functions are important throughout stroke rehabilitation to prevent complications and additional disability. Attention should be directed to vital signs, swallowing disorders, nutrition and hydration, bowel and bladder function, skin integrity, physical activity endurance, and sleep patterns.

Quality of Life Issues

Quality of life includes the ability to engage in life's activities, the satisfaction derived from them, and overall perceptions of health status and well-being.[5] Because depression, social support, and functional status have been identified as predictors of quality of life, stroke survivors require assistance in coping and in maintaining their support systems.[157] Contextual factors, especially family structure and functioning, become particularly critical during discharge planning and after return to a community living environment.[5] The ability to resume valued activities (e.g., return to work or vocational status, leisure and recreation activities, sexuality, and driving) should be addressed.

The risk of stroke recurrence and complications remains high, especially in severely disabled people with limited mobility. Continued health promotion efforts to prevent recurrent strokes and control risk factors should be pursued. Strong social support has been shown to improve outcomes, especially in patients with severe strokes.[158] Social support beyond the immediate family can wane over time after an acute stroke, so community resources become increasingly important for the long-term positive adaptation to disability. Information on the National Stroke Association, American Heart Association, Stroke Clubs International, National Aphasia Association, and many other national and regional organizations available to support stroke patients and their families should be provided.

Conclusion

Stroke is a complex disorder. The recent research and therapeutic advances in the treatment of acute stroke make the rapid and accurate diagnosis of brain attack essential. A comprehensive educational effort to improve awareness and action within the short window of opportunity is effective in salvaging at-risk brain tissue. A coordinated, multidisciplinary approach that uses established protocols for assessment and treatment can reduce costs and improve outcome in stroke prevention, acute care, and rehabilitation.

Acknowledgment
We thank Stephen Michael Holmes, MD, Neuroradiologist at Queens Medical Center in Honolulu, Hawaii, for his assistance and invaluable contributions on neuroimaging, and Jeffrey Liu, MD, Neurologist at Queens Medical Center, for his editorial assistance.

References

1. American Heart Association. *Heart and Stroke Facts: 1996 Statistical Supplement.* Dallas, Tex: American Heart Association; 1995.
2. National Stroke Association. Stroke facts. Available at: http://www.stroke.org. Accessed October 9, 1996.
3. Terent A. Stroke morbidity. In: Whisnant J, ed. *Stroke: Populations, Cohorts, and Clinical Trials.* Oxford, England: Butterworth-Heineman; 1993.
4. Viriyavejakul A. Stroke in Asia: an epidemiological consideration. *Clin Neuropharmacol.* 1990;13(suppl 3):S26–S33.
5. Gresham GE, Duncan PW, Stason WB, et al. *Clinical Practice Guideline Number 16: Post-Stroke Rehabilitation.* Rockville, Md: US Department of Health and Human Services, Public Health Service, Agency for Health Care Policy and Research; 1995. AHCPR publication 95-0662.
6. Broderick JP, Phillips SJ, Whisnant JP, O'Fallon WM, Bergstralh EJ. Incidence rates of stroke in the eighties: the end of the decline in stroke. *Stroke.* 1989;20:577–582.
7. National Center for Health Statistics. *Healthy People 2000 Review 1994.* Hyattsville, Md: Public Health Service; 1995.
8. *For a Healthy Nation: Returns on Investment in Public Health.* Washington, DC: US Department of Health and Human Services; 1994.
9. Sacco RL. Stroke epidemiology and risk factors. In: Sacco RL, ed. *New Approaches to the Treatment of Ischemic Stroke.* Vol 1. Belle Mead, NJ: Excerpta Medica; 1996:3–10.

10. Garraway WM, Whisnant JP, Drury I. The continuing decline in the incidence of stroke. *Mayo Clin Proc.* 1983; 58:520–523.

11. Gorelick PB. Stroke prevention. *Arch Neurol.* 1995;52: 347–355.

12. Taylor TN, Davis PH, Torner JC, Holmes J, Meyer JW, Jacobson M. Lifetime cost of stroke in the United States. *Stroke.* 1996;27:1459–1466.

13. NINDS symposium produces national plan for rapid stroke treatment [press release]. National Institute of Neurological Disorders and Stroke. Accessed December 1996. Available at: http://www.ninds.nih.gov/WHATSNEW/PRESSWHN/1996/strokepress.htm.

14. American Heart Association. Brain attack: home, health, and family heart and stroke A–Z guide. 1996. Available at: http://www.amhrt.org/hs96/battack.html.

15. Brain attack. [National Institute of Neurological Disorders and Stroke Web site]. Available at: http/www.ninds. nih. gov/healinfo/disorder/stroke/strokews/htm. Accessed March 5, 1997.

16. Koroshetz WJ, Ay H. Diagnosis and evaluation of stroke. In: Sacco RL, ed. *New Approaches to the Treatment of Ischemic Stroke.* Vol 1. Belle Mead, NJ: Excerpta Medica; 1996: 18–23.

17. Starkman S. Acute stroke and emergency medicine: the physician's perspective. *Current Approaches to Acute Stroke Management.* 1996;1:6–8.

18. Futrell N, Millikan CH. Stroke is an emergency. *Dis Mon.* 1996;42:199–264.

19. Brass LM. Stroke teams. *Current Approaches to Acute Stroke Management.* 1996;2:3–6.

20. Wentworth DA, Atkinson RP. Implementation of an acute stroke program decreases hospitalization costs and length of stay. *Stroke.* 1996;27:1040–1043.

21. Ginsberg MD. Pathophysiology and mechanisms of ischemic brain injury. In Sacco R, ed. *New Approaches to the Treatment of Ischemic Stroke.* Vol 1. Belle Mead, NJ: Excerpta Medica; 1996:11-17.

22. Hacke W, Kaste M, Fieschi C, et al. Intravenous thrombolysis with recombinant tissue plasminogen activator for acute hemispheric stroke: the European Cooperative Acute Stroke Study (ECASS). *JAMA.* 1995;274:1017–1025.

23. National Institute of Neurological Disorders and Stroke rt-PA Stroke Study Group. Tissue plasminogen activator for acute ischemic stroke. *N Engl J Med.* 1995;333:1581–1587.

24. NIH announces emergency treatment for stroke [press release] [National Institute of Neurological Disorders and Stroke Web site]. Available at: http://www.nih.gov/ninds/. Accessed December 1995.

25. Adams RC, Victor M. *Principles of Neurology.* 5th ed. New York, NY: McGraw-Hill; 1993.

26. Wolf PA, Dawser RT, Thomas HE Jr, et al. Epidemiologic assessment of chronic atrial fibrillation and risk of stroke: the Framingham Study. *Neurology.* 1978;28:973.

27. Caplan LR, Hier DB, D'Cruz I. Cerebral embolism in the Michael Reese stroke registry. *Stroke.* 1983;14:530–536.

28. Garcia JH, Ho KL, Caccamo DV. Pathology of stroke. In Barnett HJM, Stein B, Mohr JP, Yatsu FM, eds. *Stroke: Pathophysiology, Diagnosis, and Management.* 2nd ed. New York, NY: Churchill Livingstone; 1992:125-145.

29. Jones H, Caplan LR, Come P, et al. Paradoxical cerebral emboli: an occult cause of stroke. *Ann Neurol.* 1983;13: 314–319.

30. Camarata PJ, Heros RC, Latchaw RE. Brain attack: the rationale for treating stroke as a medical emergency. *Neurosurgery.* 1994;34:144–158.

31. Almani WS, Awid AS. Spontaneous intracranial bleeding in hemorrhagic diatheses. *Surg Neurol.* 1982;17:137.

32. Herbstein DS, Schaumberg HH. Hypertensive intracerebral hematoma: an investigation of the initial hemorrhage and re-bleeding using chromium CR51-labeled arthyrosites. *Arch Neurol.* 1974;30:412.

33. Kazui S, Naritomi H, Yamamoto H, Sawada T, Yamaguchi T. Enlargement of spontaneous intracerebral hemorrhage: incidence and time course. *Stroke.* 1996;27: 1783–1787.

34. Kiely DK, Wolf PA, Cupples LA, et al. Familial aggregation of stroke: the Framingham Study. *Stroke.* 1993;24: 1366–1371.

35. Kittner SJ, White LR, Losonczy KG, et al. Black-white differences in stroke incidence in a national sample. *JAMA.* 1990;264:1267–1270.

36. Gaines K, Burke G. Ethnic differences in stroke: black-white differences in the United States population: SECORDS Investigators (Southeastern Consortium on Racial Differences in Stroke). *Neuroepidemiology.* 1995;14: 209–239.

37. Gillum RF. Strokes in blacks. *Stroke.* 1988;19:1–6.

38. Gillum RF. Epidemiology of stroke in Hispanic Americans. *Stroke.* 1995;26:1707–1712.

39. Yano K, Popper JS, Kaga A, Chyou PH, Grove JS. Epidemiology of stroke among Japanese men in Hawaii during 24 years of follow-up: the Honolulu Heart Program. *Health Rep.* 1994;6.

40. Wolf PA, Belanger AJ, D'Agostino RB. Management of risk factors. *Neurol Clin.* 1992;10:177–191.

41. SHEP Cooperative Research Group. Prevention of stroke by antihypertensive drug treatment in older persons with isolated systolic hypertension. *JAMA.* 1991;265: 3255–3264.

42. Materson BJ, Reda DJ, Cushman WC, et al. Single-drug therapy for hypertension in men. *N Engl J Med.* 1993;328: 914–921.

43. Testa MA, Anderson RB, Nackley JF, et al. Quality of life and antihypertensive therapy in men. *N Engl J Med.* 1993; 328:907–913.

44. Diener HC. The French study of aortic plaques in stroke group. *N Engl J Med.* 1996;334:1216–1221.

45. Orencia AJ, Petty GW, Khandheria BK, et al. Risk of stroke with mitral valve prolapse in population-based cohort study. *Stroke.* 1995;26:7–13.

46. Wolf PA, Abbot RD, Kannel WB. Atrial fibrillation as an independent risk factor for stoke: the Framingham Study. *Stroke.* 1991;22:983–988.

47. Wolf PA, Abbott RD, Kannel WB. Atrial fibrillation: a major contributor to stroke in the elderly: the Framingham Study. *Arch Intern Med.* 1987;147:1561–1564.

48. Wolf PA, Cobb JL, D'Agostino RB. Epidemiology of stroke. In: Barnett HJM, Stein BM, Mohr JP, Yatsu FM, eds. *Stroke Pathophysiology, Diagnosis, and Management.* 2nd ed. New York, NY: Churchill Livingstone; 1992:3–27.

49. Knutsen R, Knutsen SF, Curb JD, Reed DM, Kautz JA, Yano K. Predictive value of resting electrocardiogram for 12-year incidence of stroke in the Honolulu Heart Program. *Stroke.* 1988;19:555–559.

50. Fujishima M, Kiyohara Y, Kato I, et al. Diabetes and cardiovascular disease in a prospective population survey in Japan: the Hisayama study. *Diabetes.* 1996;45(suppl 3): S14–S16.

51. Abbot RD, Donahue RP, MacMahon SW, et al. Diabetes and the risk of stroke: the Honolulu Heart Program. *JAMA.* 1987;257:949.

52. Jacobs DR. The relationship between cholesterol and stroke. *Health Rep.* 1994;6:73–77.

53. Bosworth, T. No longer a question: lowering lipids can reduce the risk of stroke. *Neurol Rev.* 1997;5:20.

54. Benfante R, Yano K, Hwang LJ, Curb JD, Kagan A, Ross W. Elevated serum cholesterol is a risk factor for both coronary heart disease and thromboembolic stroke in Hawaiian Japanese men: implications of shared risk. *Stroke.* 1994;25:814–820.

55. Yano K, Reed DM, MacLean CJ. Serum cholesterol and hemorrhagic stroke in Honolulu Heart Program. *Stroke.* 1989;20:1460–1464.

56. Colditz GA, Bonita R, Stampfer MA, et al. Cigarette smoking and risk of stroke in middle-aged women. *N Engl J Med.* 1988;318:937.

57. Abbott RD, Yin Yin MA, Reed DM, Yano K. Risk of stroke in male cigarette smokers. *N Engl J Med.* 1986;315: 717–720.

58. Wolf PA, D'Agostino RB, Kannel WB, Bonita R, Belanger AJ. Cigarette smoking as a risk factor for stroke: the Framingham Study. *JAMA.* 1988;259:1025–1029.

59. Donahue RP, Abbot RD, Reed DM, Yano K. Alcohol and hemorrhagic stroke: the Honolulu Heart Program. *JAMA.* 1986;255:2311–2314.

60. Biller J, Saver JL. Transient ischemic attacks: populations and prognosis. *Mayo Clin Proc.* 1994;69:493–494.

61. Howard G, Evans GW, Crouse JR, et al. A prospective reevaluation of TIA as a risk factor for death and fatal or nonfatal cardiovascular events. *Stroke.* 1993;25:342–345.

62. Norris JW, Zhu CZ, Bornstein NM, Chambers BR. Vascular risks of asymptomatic carotid stenosis. *Stroke.* 1991;22: 1485–1490.

63. Faggioli GL, Curl GR, Ricotta JJ. The role of carotid screening before coronary artery bypass. *J Vasc Surg.* 1990; 12:724–729.

64. Abbott RD, Rodriguez BL, Burchfiel CM, Curb JD. Physical activity in older middle-age men and reduced risk of stroke: the Honolulu Heart Program. *Am J Epidemiol.* 1994; 139:881–893.

65. Abbott RD, Behrens GR, Sharp DS, et al. Body mass index and thromboembolic stroke in nonsmoking men in older middle age: the Honolulu Heart Program. *Stroke.* 1994;25: 2370–2376.

66. Stadel BV. Oral contraceptives and cardiovascular disease. *N Engl J Med.* 1981;288:672.

67. Stampfer MJ, Colditz GA, Willett WC, et al. Prospective study of past use of oral contraceptive agents and risk of cardiovascular diseases. *N Engl J Med.* 1988;319:1988.

68. Klonoff DC, Andres BT, Obana WG. Stroke associated with cocaine use. *Arch Neurol.* 1989;46:989–993.

69. Brust JCM. Stroke and substance abuse. In: Barnett HJM, Stein BM, Mohr JP, Yatsu FM, eds. *Stroke Pathophysiology, Diagnosis, and Management.* 2nd ed. New York, NY: Churchill Livingstone; 1992:875–993.

70. Olsen ML. Autoimmune disease and stroke. *Stroke, Clinical Updates.* 1992;3:13–16.

71. Mitiguy J. Ischemic stroke in young adults: conditions, behaviors, risks. *Headlines.* 1993;4:2–8.

72. Maggioni AP, Franzosi MG, Santoro E. The risk of stroke in patients with acute myocardial infarction after thrombolytic and antithrombotic treatment. *N Engl J Med.* 1992;327:1–6.

73. Wolf PA, D'Agostino RB, Belanger AJ, Kannel W. Probability of stroke: a risk profile from the Framingham Study. *Stroke.* 1991;22:312.

74. Adams HP, Bendixen BH, Kappelle LJ, et al. Classification of subtype of acute ischemic stroke. *Stroke.* 1993;24:35–41.

75. Goldstein LB, Matchar DB. Clinical assessment of stroke. *JAMA.* 1994;271:1114–1120.

76. Libman RB, Wirkowski E, Alvir J, Rao H. Conditions that mimic stroke in the emergency department: implications for acute stroke trials. *Arch Neurol.* 1995;52:1119–1122.

77. Panzer RJ, Feibel JH, Barker WH, Griner PF. Predicting the likelihood of hemorrhage in patients with stroke. *Arch Intern Med.* 1985;145:1800–1803.

78. Brott T, Adams HP, Elinger CP, et al. Measurements of acute cerebral infarction: a clinical examination scale. *Stroke.* 1989;29:864–870.

79. Hantson L, De Weerdt W, De Keyser J, et al. The European stroke scale. *Stroke.* 1994;25:2215–2219.

80. Cote R, Hachinski VC, Shurvell BL, Norris JW, Wolfson C. The Canadian neurological scale: a preliminary study in acute stroke. *Stroke.* 1986;17:731–737.

81. Scandinavian Stroke Study Group. Multicenter trial of hemodilution in ischemic stroke: background and study protocol. *Stroke.* 1985;16:885–890.

82. Goldstein LB, Bertels C, Davis JN. Interrater reliability of the NIH stroke scale. *Arch Neurol.* 1989;46:660–662.

83. Brott T, Marler JR, Olinger CP, et al. Measurements of acute cerebral infarction: lesion size by computerized tomography. *Stroke.* 1989;20:871–875.

84. Muir KW, Weir CJ, Murray GD, Povey C, Lees KR. Comparison of neurological scales and scoring systems for acute stroke prognosis. *Stroke.* 1996;27:1817–1820.

85. Lyden P, Brott T, Tilley B, et al. Improved reliability of the NIH stroke scale using video training. *Stroke.* 1994;25: 2220–2226.

86. Brott TG, Haley EC Jr, Levy DE, et al. Urgent therapy for stroke, I: pilot study of tissue plasminogen activator administered within 90 minutes. *Stroke.* 1992;23:632–640.

87. Haley EC Jr, Levy DE, Brott TG, et al. Urgent therapy for stroke, II: pilot study of tissue plasminogen activator administered 91–180 minutes from onset. *Stroke.* 1992;23: 641–645.

88. Haley ED, Brott TG, Sheppard GL, et al. Pilot randomized trial of tissue plasminogen activator in acute ischemic stroke. *Stroke.* 1993;24:1000–1004.

89. Caplan LR. *The Effective Clinical Neurologist.* Boston, Mass: Blackwell; 1990.

90. Caplan LR. *Stroke: A Clinical Approach.* 2nd ed. Boston, Mass: Butterworth-Heinemann; 1993.

91. Bryan RN, Levy LM, Whitlow WD, et al. Diagnoses of acute cerebral infarction: comparison of CT and MR imaging. *AJNR Am J Neuroradiol.* 1991;12:611–620.

92. Bastianello S, Pierallini A, Colonnese C, et al. Hyperdense middle cerebral artery sign. *Neuroradiology.* 1991;33:202–211.

93. Leys D, Pruvo JP, Godefroy O, et al. Prevalence and significance of hyperdense middle cerebral artery in acute stroke. *Stroke.* 1992;23:317–324.

94. Tomsick T, Brott T, Barsan W, et al. Thrombus Localization with emergency cerebral CT. *AJNR Am J Neuroradiol.* 1992;13:257–263.

95. Truwit CL, Barkovich AJ, Gean A, et al. Loss of the insular ribbon: another CT sign of acute middle cerebral infarction. *Radiology.* 1990;176:801–806.

96. Shuaib A, Lee D, Pelz D, et al. The impact of MRI on the management of acute ischemic stroke. *Neurology.* 1992;42:816–818.

97. Mueller DP, Yuh WTC, Fisher DJ, et al. Arterial enhancement in acute cerebral ischemia: clinical and angiographic correlation. *AJNR Am J Neuroradiol.* 1993;14:661–668.

98. Yuh WTC, Crain MR, Loes DJ, et al. MR imaging of cerebral ischemia: findings in the first 24 hours. *AJNR Am J Neuroradiol.* 1991;12:621–629.

99. Chen D, Kwong KK, Gress DR, et al. MR diffusion imaging of cerebral infarction in humans. *AJNR Am J Neuroradiol.* 1992;13:1097–1102.

100. Horowitz SH, Zito TL, Donnaru MMAR, et al. CT-angiographic findings within the first five hours of cerebral infarction. *Stroke.* 1991;22:1245–1253.

101. Osborn AG. *Handbook of Neuroradiology.* St Louis, Mo: Mosby–Yearbook; 1991.

102. Okazaki H. Cerebral vascular disease. In: *Fundamentals of Neuropathology.* New York, NY: Szaku-Shoin; 1989:27–93.

103. Laissy JP, Normand G, Monroc M, et al. Spontaneous intracerebral hematomas from vascular causes. *Neuroradiology* 1991;33:291–295.

104. Volpe JJ. Value of MR in definition of neuropathology of cerebral palsy in vivo. *AJNR Am J Neuroradiol.* 1992;13:79–83.

105. Zimmerman RD, Ernst RJ. Neuroimaging of cerebrovenous thrombosis. *Neuroimaging Clin N Am.* 1992;2:463–485.

106. Virapongse C, Cazenave C, Quisling R, et al. The empty delta sign: frequency and significance in 76 cases of dural sums thrombosis. *Radiology.* 1987;162:779–785.

107. Husain AM, Alter M. Transesophageal echocardiography in diagnosing cardioembolic stroke. *Clin Cardiol.* 1995;18:705–708.

108. Caplan LR, Brass LM, DeWitt LD, et al. Transcranial Doppler ultrasound: present status. *Neurology.* 1990;40:696–700.

109. Delcker A, Diener HC. Use of transcranial Doppler in stroke: yes or no? *Current Approaches to Acute Stroke Management.* 1996;2:7–10.

110. Fogelholm R, Murros K, Rissanen A, Ilmavirta M. Factors delaying hospital admission after acute stroke. *Stroke.* 1996;27:398–400.

111. Mitchell JB, Ballard DJ, Whisnant JP, Ammering BS, Samsa GP, Matchar DB. What role do neurologists play in determining the costs and outcomes of stroke patients? *Stroke.* 1996;27:1937–1943.

112. Albers GW. Medical treatment for acute ischemic stroke. In: Sacco R, ed. *New Approaches to the Treatment of Ischemic Stroke.* Vol 2. Belle Mead, NJ: Excerpta Medica; 1996:3–9.

113. Alberts MJ. Management of hypertension in acute ischemic stroke. *Current Approaches to Acute Stroke Management.* 1996;1:12–14.

114. Hacke W, Grotta J, Diener HC. Thrombolytic therapy in ischemic stroke. *Current Approaches to Acute Stroke Management.* 1996;1:8–11.

115. Brott T. Thrombolysis for stroke. *Arch Neurol.* 1996;53:1305–1306.

116. Riggs JE. Tissue-type plasminogen activator should not be used in acute ischemic stroke. *Arch Neurol.* 1996;53:1306–1308.

117. Multicenter Acute Stroke Trial—Europe Study Group. Thrombolytic therapy with streptokinase in acute ischemic stroke. *N Engl J Med.* 1996;335:145–150.

118. Donnan GA, Davis SM, Chambers BR, et al. Trials of streptokinase in acute ischemic stroke. *Lancet.* 1995;345:578–579.

119. Multicentre Acute Stroke Trial—Italy (Mast-I) Group. Randomized controlled trial of streptokinase, aspirin, and combination of both in acute ischemic stroke. *Lancet.* 1995;346:1509–1514.

120. De Keyser J. Opportunities for neuroprotection. *Current Approaches to Acute Stroke Management.* 1996;2:11–15.

121. Marsh EE, Adams HP, Biller J, et al. Use of antithrombotic drugs in the treatment of acute ischemic stroke: a survey of neurologists in practice in the United States. *Neurology.* 1989;39:1631–1634.

122. Kay R, Wong K, Yu Y, et al. Low-molecular-weight heparin for the treatment of acute ischemic stroke. *N Engl J Med.* 1995;333:1588–1593.

123. Patrono C, Roth GJ. Aspirin in ischemic cerebrovascular disease: how strong is the case for a different dosing regimen? *Stroke.* 1996;27:756–760.

124. Gent M, Easton JD, Hachinski VC, et al. The Canadian American ticlopidine study (CATS) in thromboembolic stroke. *Lancet.* 1989;1215–1220.

125. Hershey L. Stroke prevention in women: role of aspirin vs. ticlopidine. *Am J Med.* 1991;91:288–292.

126. Toole JF. ACAS recommendations for carotid endarterectomy. ACAS Executive Committee. *Lancet.* 1996;347:212.

127. EC/IC Bypass Study Group. Failure of extracranial-intracranial arterial bypass to reduce the risk of ischemic stroke. *N Engl J Med.* 1985;313:1191–1200.

128. MacEwan W. An address on the surgery of the brain and spinal cord. *BMJ.* 1888;2:302.

129. Backlund EQ, von Holst H. Controlled subtotal evacuation of intracerebral hematomas by stereotactic technique. *Surg Neurol.* 1978;9:99–101.

130. Mohadjer M, Eggert R, May J, Mayfrank L. CT-guided stereotactic fibrinolysis of spontaneous and hypertensive cerebellar hemorrhage: long term results. *J Neurosurgery.* 1990;73:217.

131. Yoshida H, Komai N, Nakai E, et al. Stereotactic evacuation of hypertensive cerebellar hemorrhage using plasminogen activator. *No Shinkei Geka.* 1989;17:421.

132. Rubin JM, Dohrmann GJ. Use of ultrasonically guided probes and catheters in neurosurgery. *Surg Neurol.* 1982; 18:143.

133. Crowell RM, Ojemann G, Ogilvy CS. Spontaneous brain hemorrhage: surgical considerations. In: Barnett HJM, Stein B, Mohr JP, Yatsu FM, eds. *Stroke: Pathophysiology, Diagnosis, and Management.* 2nd ed. New York, NY: Churchill Livingstone; 1992:1169–1187.

134. Batjer HH, Reisch JS, Allen BC, Plaizier JL, Su CJ. Failure of surgery to improve outcome in hypertensive putaminal hemorrhage: a prospective randomized trial. *Arch Neurol.* 1990;47:1103–1106.

135. Yashon D, Kosnik EG. Chronic intracerebral hematoma. *Neurosurgery.* 1978;2:103.

136. Okazaki H, Regan R, Campbell RJ. Clinicopathologic studies of primary cerebral amyloid angiopathy. *Mayo Clin Proc.* 1979;54:22.

137. Wattendorf AR, Bots GT, Wendt LN, et al. Familial cerebral amyloid angiopathy presenting as a recurrent cerebral hemorrhage. *J Neurol Surg.* 1982;55:121.

138. Tyler KL, Poletti CE, Heros RC. Cerebral amyloid angiopathy with multiple intracerebral hemorrhages. *J Neurosurg.* 1982;57:286–289.

139. Olsen TS, Hogenhaven H, Thage O. Epilepsy after stroke. *Neurology.* 1987;37:1209–1211.

140. Weibe-Valazquez S, Blume WT. Seizures. In: Teasell RW, ed. *Long-term Consequences of Stroke. Physical Medicine and Rehabilitation: State-of-the-Art Reviews.* Vol 7. Philadelphia: Hanley & Belfus Inc. 1993;73–87.

141. Sacco RL, Wolf PA, Kannel WB, McNamara PM. Survival and recurrence following stroke: the Framingham Study. *Stroke.* 1982;13:290–295.

142. Boston Area Anticoagulation Trial for Atrial Fibrillation. The effect of low-dose warfarin on the risk of stroke in patients with non-rheumatic atrial fibrillation. *N Engl J Med.* 1990;323:1504–1511.

143. Connolly SJ, Laupacis A, Gent M, Roberts RS, Cairns JA, Joyner C. Canadian atrial fibrillation anticoagulant (CAFA) study. *J Am Coll Cardiol.* 1991;18:349–355.

144. Peterson P, Boysen G, Godtfredsen J, Andersen ED, Andersen B. Placebo-controlled, randomized trial of warfarin and aspirin for prevention of thromboembolic complications in chronic atrial fibrillation. *Lancet.* 1989;1: 175–178.

145. Ezekowitz MD, Bridgers SE, James KE, et al. Warfarin in the prevention of stroke associated with nonrheumatic atrial fibrillation. *N Engl J Med.* 1992;327:1406–1412.

146. Stroke Prevention in Atrial Fibrillation (SPAF) Investigators. Stroke prevention in atrial fibrillation study final results. *Circulation.* 1991;84:527–539.

147. Adams HP, Brott TG, Crowell RM, et al., eds. *Management of Patients With Acute Ischemic Stroke.* Dallas, Tex: American Heart Association; 1994.

148. Roth EJ. Heart disease in patients with stroke. *Arch Phys Med Rehabil.* 1993;74:752–760; 75:94–101.

149. Sandin KJ, Mason KD. *Manual of Stroke Rehabilitation.* Boston, Mass: Butterworth-Heinemann; 1996.

150. Warlow C, Ogston D, Doublas AS. Deep venous thrombosis of the legs and after strokes. *BMJ.* 1976;1: 1178–1183.

151. Brandstater ME, Roth EJ, Siebens HC. Venous thromboembolism in stroke: literature review and implications for clinical practice. *Arch Phys Med Rehabil.* 1992;73 (suppl):379–391.

152. Keeley RE, Bell LK, Mason RL. Cost analysis of kinetic therapy in the prevention of complications of stroke. *South Med J.* 1990;83;433–434.

153. Alexander DN. Approaches to rehabilitation of ischemic stroke. In: Sacco R, ed. New Approaches to the Treatment of Ischemic Stroke. Vol 2. Belle Mead, NJ: Excerpta Medica; 1996:16–20.

154. Tatemichi TK, Paik M, Bagiella E, et al. Risk of dementia after stroke in a hospitalized cohort: results of a longitudinal study. *Neurology.* 1994;44:1885–1891.

155. Moroney JT, Bagiella MS, Desmond DW, Paik MC, Stern Y, Tatemichi TK. Risk factors for incident dementia after stroke: role of hypoxic and ischemic disorders. *Stroke.* 1996;27:1283–1289.

156. Langhorne P, Williams BO, Gilchrist W, Howie K. Do stroke units save lives? *Lancet.* 1993;342:395–398.

157. King RB. Quality of life after stroke. *Stroke.* 1996;27: 1467–1472.

158. Glass TA, Matchar DB, Belyea M, Feussner JR. Impact of social support on outcome in first stroke. *Stroke.* 1993;24: 64–70.

Section 10
Other Vascular Diseases

76

Vasculitis

Shigeyuki Sasaki and Keishu Yasuda

Atherosclerosis is the primary underlying disease in more than 90% of those with vascular disorders. However, many patients suffer from other vascular disorders including inflammatory vasculitis or noninflammatory illnesses. Although vasculitis has a simple definition—inflammation, often associated with necrosis and occlusive changes of the blood vessels—its clinical manifestations vary and are complex.[65] Vasculitis may appear in systemic or localized blood vessels and may occur as a primary disorder of the blood vessels (primary vasculitis) or may be associated with a wide variety of different underlying diseases (secondary vasculitis).[48,65] The clinical approach to vasculitis has been developed since the first detailed description of polyarteritis nodosa (PAN) by Kussmaul and Maier in the nineteenth century. Since then our understanding of the immune mechanisms responsible for vasculitis, pathologic spectrum of the disorders, and therapeutic approach to fatal complications has improved. Numerous forms of vasculitis including Wegener's granulomatosis (WG), hypersensitivity vasculitis, temporal arteritis, and Takayasu's arteritis have been separated from PAN and established as individual disease entities with a variety of clinical manifestations through different mechanisms. Although these diseases have different pathogenesis, they were encompassed by the term *vasculitis syndrome* in the 1980s due to their similar systemic symptoms.

In this chapter we review current understanding of the classification, pathophysiology, etiology, clinical features, and diagnostic and therapeutic approaches to vasculitis.

Classification

Numerous attempts have been made to establish useful criteria to classify systemic vasculitis for diagnosis since the first descriptions of necrotizing vasculitis in the nineteenth century.[65,71,98,110] However, no distinctive criteria to classify the many different types of vasculitis have been established because of the wide variety of clinical manifestations, distribution of involved vessels, and poorly understood pathogenic mechanisms.[87]

One of the practical classifications that seems clinically useful is that reported by Fauci and associates in 1978.[38] They proposed a classification of vasculitis based on an admixture of clinical, pathologic, immunologic, and therapeutic variables. This classification with several modifications is shown in Table 76.1. Diseases are classified under several headings that may serve as points of differential diagnosis and determine the diagnostic and therapeutic approach.

Another practical classification is that based on the predominant type and size of the involved blood vessels. This classification (shown in Table 76.2) provides guidelines for clinicians about what to suspect and expect in the histologic diagnosis of vasculitis. Some vasculitides are focal and segmental in their distribution, and thus examination of serial sections of a biopsy is often required to specify histologic markers of the vasculitis. Involvement of veins can be an important discriminator, such as superficial phlebitis in thromboangiitis obliterans (Buerger's disease). Although a classification of vasculitis can be made based on the predominant type and size of the involved blood vessels, overlapping among the major types of vasculitis often occurs.[83] In addition, various sizes of blood vessels may be involved in an individual disease entity. The type of inflammatory cells that infiltrate in vasculitis is independent of the size of the involved blood vessels, and a mixed-cell infiltrate is commonly found for most vasculitides.

The American College of Rheumatology proposed criteria for vasculitis in 1990 for the following seven subtypes of systemic vasculitis: (1) PAN, (2) allergic granulomatosis (Churg–Strauss syndrome), (3) WG, (4) hypersensitivity vasculitis, (5) Henoch–Schönlein purpura,

TABLE 76.1. Classification of vasculitis based on an admixture of clinical, pathologic, immunologic, and therapeutic variables.

Polyarteritis nodosa group of systemic necrotizing vasculitis
Classic polyarteritis nodosa
Allergic granulomatosis (Churg–Strauss syndrome)
Overlap syndrome
Microscopic polyarteritis

Hypersensitivity vasculitis group
True hypersensitivity vasculitis
Henoch–Schönlein purpura
Essential mixed cryoglobulinemia with vasculitis
Vasculitis associated with malignancies (e.g., chronic lymphocytic
    leukemia, lymphoma, Hodgkin's disease, and multiple myeloma)
Vasculitis associated with connective tissue disease (e.g., systemic lupus
    erythematosus, rheumatoid arthritis, relapsing polychondritis,
    Reiter's syndrome, and Sjögren's syndrome)
Hypocomplementemic vasculitis (urticarial vasculitis)
Vasculitis associated with other primary disorders

Wegener's granulomatosis group

Giant cell arteritis
Takayasu's arteritis
Temporal arteritis

Angiocentric immunoproliferative disorders
Lymphomatoid granulomatosis
Benign lymphocytic angiitis
Angiocentric lymphoma

Behçet's disease

Thromboangiitis obliterans (Buerger's disease)

Mucocutaneous lymph node syndrome (Kawasaki's syndrome)

Miscellaneous vasculitides

TABLE 76.2. Classification of vasculitis based on the predominant type and size of the involved blood vessels.

Infectious angiitis
Spirochetal (syphilis)
Mycobacterial
Pyogenic bacterial or fungal
Rickettsial
Viral or mycoplasmal
Protozoal

Noninfectious angiitis

Involving large, medium, and small blood vessels
    Takayasu's arteritis
    Granulomatous (giant cell) arteritis
        Cranial (temporal) arteritis and extracranial giant cell arteritis
        Disseminated visceral granulomatous angiitis
        Granulomatous angiitis of the central nervous system
    Arteritis of rheumatic diseases and spondyloarthropathies

Involving predominantly medium and small blood vessels
Thromboangiitis obliterans (Buerger's disease)
Polyarteritis (periarteritis) nodosa
    Classic polyarteritis nodosa
    Microscopic polyarteritis
    Infantile polyarteritis
    Mucocutaneous lymph node syndrome (Kawasaki's syndrome)
Allergic granulomatosis and angiitis
    Wegener's granulomatosis
    Churg–Strauss syndrome
    Necrotizing sarcoid granulomatosis
Vasculitis of collagen–vascular disease
    Rheumatic fever
    Rheumatoid arthritis
    Spondyloarthropathies
    Systemic lupus erythematosus
    Dermatomyositis and polymyositis
    Relapsing polychondritis
    Systemic sclerosis
    Sjögren's syndrome
    Behçet's disease
    Cogan's syndrome

Involving predominantly small blood vessels (hypersensitivity angiitis)
Serum sickness
Schönlein–Henoch purpura
Drug-induced vasculitis
Mixed cryoglobulinemia
Hypocomplementemia
Familial Mediterranean fever
Vasculitis associated with malignancies
Retroperitoneal fibrosis
Inflammatory bowel disease
Primary biliary cirrhosis
Goodpasture's syndrome
Vasculitis associated with organ transplantation

(6) giant cell arteritis, and (7) Takayasu's arteritis.[88] The classification described by Fauci and associates seems to have greatly affected this grouping.[38] Each of these major categories has its own histopathologic features. Before describing each subtype of vasculitis, we discuss some proposed mechanisms responsible for the development of vasculitic diseases.

Pathophysiology

Significant progress has been made in the understanding of inflammation of the blood vessels over the past decade. Before the 1980s, immune complexes played the most important role in accounting for most pathogenic mechanisms of systemic vasculitis. However, intensive research has proved that at least the following four independent mechanisms are responsible for development of vasculitic diseases: (1) immune complexes, (2) antibody-mediated diseases, (3) cell-mediated/endothelial focus diseases, and (4) immunoproliferative disorders.

Immune Complexes

The diseases in the hypersensitivity vasculitis group have the strongest support for the immune complex mechanism.[54] True hypersensitivity vasculitis, which is generally preceded by exposure to antigenic triggers, is apparently mediated by immune complexes. Hepatitis B and hepatitis C are currently thought to mediate vascular inflammatory disease, because hepatitis viral antigens, specific antibodies, and immune complexes have been identified in both the circulation and tissue in inflammatory responses.[27,28,54] Most cases of mixed cryoglobulinemia have also been linked to hepatitis C.[1,28] In these conditions, vasculitis in small vessels follows exposure to discrete antigens by about 7 days and is often associated with activation of the complement and accumulation of immunoglobulin or complement in involved tissues. There is strong evidence of immune complex–mediated mechanisms in the development of Henoch–Schönlein purpura, urticarial vasculitis, and PAN in some patients.[54]

Antibody-Mediated Disease

Interest in the area of antibody-mediated disease has increased since the discovery of antineutrophil cytoplasmic antibodies (ANCAs). ANCAs are autoantibodies specific for protein antigens in the granules of neutrophils and the peroxidase-positive lysosomes of monocytes, which were first identified by Davis and his associates in 1982 with an immunofluorescent technique in patients with necrotizing glomerulonephritis (GN) and vasculitis.[31] The following research has demonstrated that ANCAs were frequently present in patients with WG and often appeared in patients with several conditions including crescentic GN, microscopic polyarteritis, and Churg–Strauss syndrome and in subsets of patients with PAN.[18,49,70] In addition, ANCAs often appear to correlate with the activity of these diseases.[49]

ANCAs include two major subsets by immunofluorescent observations: cytoplasmic pattern (C-ANCA) and perinuclear pattern (P-ANCA). The antigens responsible for the ANCA reaction include proteinase-3 in C-ANCA and myeloperoxidase in P-ANCA.[37] C-ANCA and P-ANCA account for more than 80% of ANCAs in patients with vasculitis; however, several minor specificities such as snow-drift pattern have been reported.

ANCA-associated small-vessel vasculitides are immunohistologically characterized by the absence of vascular deposits of immunoglobulin. This feature allows them to be distinguished from histologically identical small-vessel vasculitis with vascular immune deposits, such as mixed cryoglobulinemia, Henoch–Schönlein purpura, or serum sickness vasculitis. In addition, the ANCA-associated vasculitides can be subdivided based on the presence or absence of other clinical and pathologic features. The presence of necrotizing granulomatous inflammation in the absence of eosinophilia or asthma indicates a diagnosis of WG, whereas the presence of eosinophilia or asthma indicates a diagnosis of Churg–Strauss syndrome. The absence of granulomatous inflammation, eosinophilia, and asthma highly supports a diagnosis of microscopic polyarteritis. C-ANCAs are more frequent than P-ANCAs in patients with WG, whereas P-ANCAs are more frequent than C-ANCAs in patients with microscopic polyarteritis, Churg–Strauss syndrome, or ANCA-associated GN. ANCA-associated GN is the most common type of necrotizing GN and accounts for more than 50% of all patients with rapidly progressive GN.

Cell-Mediated/Endothelial Focal Disease

Several types of vasculitis, including giant cell arteritis and Takayasu's disease, have little evidence for immune complex or specific antibodies, and their pathophysiology is more suggestive of cell-mediated mechanisms. Activated endothelial cells may serve as antigen-presenting cells and sources of cytokine production, which suggests their ability to interact with immunocompetent cells. Endothelial cells may also promote expression of multiple adhesion molecules and may be the targets for cell-mediated immune damage including cytotoxic T cells and natural killer cells.

Immunoproliferative Disorders

Several types of vascular inflammatory disorders including the syndromes of benign lymphocytic angiitis and lymphomatoid granulomatosis demonstrate potent evidence of lymphoproliferative disorders. These conditions are angiocentric and predominantly T cell in nature with little tendency for vessel necrosis; they are often followed by the development of angiocentric lymphoma.

One of these representative mechanisms responsible for the development of vasculitic diseases, however, cannot account for the pathophysiology of each vasculitis in most cases. Most vasculitic syndromes represent admixtures of these proposed mechanisms. For example, patients with Kawasaki's syndrome demonstrate strong evidence of endothelial activation and cytokine production but also are associated with ANCAs. Further investigation for clearer understanding of pathophysiologic mechanisms will contribute to more advanced therapies.

In the remainder of this chapter we discuss the clinical and pathophysiologic features of main categories of vasculitic syndromes and provide a diagnostic and therapeutic approach to their treatment. Recent topics on Behçet's disease and inflammatory abdominal aortic aneurysms (IAAA) are also discussed in this chapter.

Polyarteritis Nodosa

Clinical Features and Their Basis

Keys to diagnosis:[88]

1. Twice or three times as common in men, particularly in the fourth and fifth decades

2. Multisystem disorders with symptoms and signs of systemic inflammation including weight loss, livedo reticularis, myalgias, testicular pain or tenderness, purpura, subcutaneous tender nodules, a symmetric polyarthritis, diastolic hypertension, or elevation of serum creatinine and blood urea nitrogen levels

3. Organ involvement of any combination of renal, gastrointestinal, central and peripheral nervous system, and skin organs; lung involvement is uncommon

4. Arteriogram showing aneurysms or occlusions of the visceral (including renal) arteries

5. Approximately 30% of PAN patients have hepatitis B surface antigenemia

6. Histologic changes showing the presence of granulocytes or mononuclear leukocytes in the small- or medium-sized artery wall

Since the first detailed description by Kussmaul and Maier in 1866, the terms *polyarteritis* and *periarteritis* have also been applied to other vasculitis syndromes including WG, rheumatic fever, syphilis, and hypersensitivity vasculitis. All of these cases had common clinical features of a general sparing of lung tissues and the microscopic features involving muscular arteries. Classic PAN is a focal necrotizing vasculitis mainly caused by immune complex–induced injury that involves the medium and small arteries. A focal and segmental inflammatory infiltrate by polymorphonuclear cells exists in all layers, and thus a fibrointimal proliferation may occur that induces occlusion of vessels. The aneurysmal formation can result from necrosis in the arterial medial layer.

Although the incidence of PAN is not precisely determined, it is generally considered to be quite rare, affecting approximately 5 to 10 individuals per million. Regarding a sex predilection, PAN is twice or three times as common in men as in women. PAN has been recognized to develop in persons of all ages but appears to have a peak onset in the fourth and fifth decades.[25,26,52]

The most common clinical signs found in PAN patients result from its devastating multisystem inflammatory nature.[86] Systemic complaints of fever, weight loss, myalgias, fatigue, and arthralgias are present in most PAN patients. Other clinical findings depend on the pattern and distribution of the target organ involvement. Digital cutaneous ischemic lesions and skin lesions including livedo reticularis, subcutaneous inflammatory nodules, and purpura develop in approximately 20% to 40% of all PAN patients. PAN patients may develop a symmetric polyarthritis mimicking rheumatoid arthritis. Muscle involvement may appear as simple myalgias or a proximal myopathy resembling polymyositis.[43] Severe proximal muscle weakness is rare in patients with PAN.

The kidneys are estimated to be affected in 75% to 85% of PAN patients. The renal manifestations of PAN may consist of GN, renal vasculitis, or aneurysmal formation of the renal vascular systems.[25,26,129] These manifestations may cause hematuria or renin-mediated hypertension. Renal failure is responsible for death in more than half of the patients with PAN.[25,26] Central nervous system disorders manifested by strokes, seizures, hemorrhage, mental status alterations, or cognitive deterioration are found in 25% of PAN patients.[25,26,101,102] Peripheral nerve damage is seen in nearly half of the patients with PAN, mainly due to mononeuritis multiplex.[103,116] Symmetric sensory involvement may be present as the glove and stocking neuropathy. Inflammation can also occur in the vertebral, carotid, and meningeal vessels. Cardiac involvement is commonly seen (in up to 80% of patients) and is second to renal disorders in causing death.[25,26,44] The vasculitic process of PAN may involve all cardiac areas including the endocardium, myocardium, or pericardium, but these complications are often difficult to detect until clinical manifestations such as coronary artery stenosis or infarction, pericarditis, or congestive heart failure develop.

Gastrointestinal involvement appears in nearly half of all PAN patients and results from ischemia of the mucosa, submucosa, or entire thickness of the bowel or from vasculitis in the splanchnic vessels.[25,26,52] These underlying causes can lead to typical symptoms of intestinal angina, visceral infarction, hemorrhage, or cholecystitis. The most catastrophic complication is visceral perforation, because it generally occurs when the underlying disease is uncontrolled and thus requires immunosuppressive therapy, whereas the subsequent septic process requires enhancement of host immune defenses.

Ocular involvement is seen in 10% to 15% of patients and is manifested by hemorrhages, conjunctivitis, or retinal detachment. Testicular involvement has been considered a source of diagnostic material. Orchitis may be present in 10% to 15% of male patients. Lung involvement is uncommon in patients with PAN, and its presence may suggest another type of vasculitis such as WG.[25,26,52]

Diagnostic Tests

There is no specific laboratory test for definitive diagnosis of PAN.[22] Anemia, leukocytosis, thrombocytosis, hypocomplementemia, and elevated erythrocyte sedimentation rate (ESR) and C-reactive protein (CRP) levels may be present.[25,26] Rheumatoid factor is found in a number of PAN patients. Approximately 30% of PAN patients have hepatitis B surface antigenemia. Either C-ANCA or P-ANCA is present in less than 50%. Factor VIII–related antigen levels may be a useful marker for medical therapy.

Biopsy is a useful diagnostic method to identify the presence and degree of PAN. Biopsy of involved organs or tissues that shows a necrotizing vasculitis can support the diagnosis of PAN. Adequate biopsy sites include skin, muscle, kidney, calf nerve, or testis, all of which should be selected based on involvement of the disease. In addition to biopsy, angiography is useful in diagnosing PAN. Selective arteriography of major abdominal branches including the celiac artery, superior mesenteric artery, or renal arteries reveals small arterial aneurysms in 70% to 80% of PAN patients.[127] Aneurysms can be seen in the cerebral, pulmonary, intercostal, and lumbar arteries. Because the hepatitis B virus is considered to be responsible for some cases of PAN, patients with hepatitis B surface antigenemia should undergo selective visceral arteriography.

The differential diagnosis of PAN is often problematic and requires excluding any other necrotizing vasculitis that is not consistent with patients' symptoms. When involvement of obvious target organs is not recognized, the renal, superior mesenteric, or celiac arteries should be examined first. When peripheral neurogenic symptoms are present, a sural nerve biopsy is of value.[130] Blind biopsies of the tissue in the absence of clinical symptoms of involvement are rarely helpful in diagnosing PAN.

Diagnostic criteria for PAN suggested by the American College of Rheumatology in 1990 are summarized in Table 76.3.[88] Patients who are suspected of having PAN should have at least 3 of these 10 criteria for diagnosis; the criteria have a sensitivity of 82.2% and a specificity of 86.6%.

Medical Treatment

The 5-year survival rate for untreated PAN patients ranges from 10% to 15%.[22,24] In general, steroids, cyclophosphamide, and azathioprine are used to control inflammation in PAN patients. With the use of corticosteroids, the 5-year survival rate improves to approximately 50%. The use of combination therapy with cyclophosphamide (1–2 mg/kg per day) and high-dose steroids (prednisone at 1 mg/kg per day) has been reported to ameliorate the 5-year survival rate to 80%. Patients without renal, central nervous system, or pulmonary involvement can be treated with steroids alone. Total control of PAN may require several years. In cases associated with hepatitis B, combination therapy with corticosteroids, plasma exchange, and antiviral agents such as vidarabine or interferon-α may be required.[54]

Surgical Treatment

Surgical treatment is usually not helpful for PAN patients, because revascularization of involved vessels is not reasonable due to the size of the vessels. However, a surgical approach might be indicated for patients with ruptured abdominal PAN aneurysms.[119]

The most common cause of death is renal failure, which causes approximately 50% of all deaths due to PAN. The second most common cause of death is central nervous system disorders.

Allergic Granulomatous Angiitis and Allergic Granulomatosis (Churg–Strauss Syndrome)

Clinical Features and Their Basis

Keys to diagnosis:

1. Predominant involvement of the pulmonary artery
2. A history of adult-onset bronchial asthma, usually developing 2 years before the onset of vasculitis
3. Peripheral eosinophilia, generally exceeding 1500 cells/mm³

In 1951 Churg and Strauss reported on 13 patients with systemic necrotizing vasculitis who had different

TABLE 76.3. Criteria for the diagnosis of polyarteritis nodosa.

Criterion	Definition
Weight loss > 4 kg	Loss of 4 kg or more of body weight since onset of illness, not due to dieting or other factors
Livedo reticularis	Mottled reticular pattern over the skin of portions of the extremities or torso
Testicular pain or tenderness	Pain or tenderness of the testicles not due to infection, trauma, or other causes
Myalgias, weakness, or leg tenderness	Diffuse myalgias (excluding shoulder and hip girdle) or weakness of muscles or tenderness of leg muscles
Mononeuropathy or polyneuropathy	Development of mononeuropathy, multiple mononeuropathies, or polyneuropathy
Diastolic BP >90 mm Hg	Development of hypertension with the diastolic BP higher than 90 mm Hg
Elevated BUN or creatinine level	Elevation of BUN level above 40 mg/dL or creatinine level above 1.5 mg/dL not due to dehydration or obstruction
Hepatitis B virus	Presence of hepatitis B surface antigen or antibody in serum
Arteriographic abnormality	Arteriogram showing aneurysms or occlusions of the visceral arteries not due to arteriosclerosis, fibromuscular dysplasia, or other noninflammatory causes
Biopsy of small or medium artery containing PMN	Histologic changes showing the presence of granulocytes or mononuclear leukocytes in the artery wall

BP, blood pressure; BUN, blood urea nitrogen; PMN, polymorphonuclear neutrophils.

features from classic PAN.[20] Clinical features of these patients included predominant involvement of the pulmonary artery, a history of bronchial asthma, and peripheral eosinophilia.[17,86] These patients had similar organ involvement as that found in classic PAN, with the exception of pulmonary involvement. According to the largest series reported by the Mayo Clinic, the incidence of this syndrome is clinically rare and is twice as common in men. The mean age of patients is approximately 47 years, but this syndrome has been reported to develop in both children and the elderly.[19]

In contrast to PAN, the lungs are commonly involved, with x-ray film changes in more than 90% of patients with this syndrome. Skin involvement manifested by purpura or nodules is noted in 60% to 70% of patients. The most common involvement of peripheral neuropathy is mononeuritis multiplex as seen in classic PAN patients.[91] Gastrointestinal, cardiac, or renal involvement is also frequently observed.[19,46]

Diagnostic Tests

Peripheral eosinophilia, generally exceeding 1500 cells/mm^3, and elevation of immunoglobulin E levels have been reported to be beneficial in distinguishing PAN.[17,70] Involved vessels usually include medium- and small-sized muscular arteries. Eosinophil infiltration is usually seen in and around these involved arteries. A striking history of asthma, usually developing 2 years before the onset of vasculitis, is noted in most patients.

Medical and Surgical Treatment

Because of the size of involved vessels, surgical treatment of these patients is not clinically advantageous. The initial treatment is generally a medical treatment that consists of administration of high-dose corticosteroids. Immunosuppressive therapy such as the use of cyclophosphamide may be useful for patients who fail to respond to high-dose corticosteroids.[25,26] The prognosis of patients with this disease is not clear but is considered similar to that of PAN.

Hypersensitivity Vasculitis

Clinical Features and Their Basis

Keys to diagnosis:

1. Patients over age 16 with palpable purpura or maculopapular rash
2. History of connective tissue disease, cryoglobulins, malignancies, or exposure to exogenous antigens such as drugs or toxins

3. Biopsy showing polymorphonuclear cells or eosinophils in the small- or medium-sized vessel wall

Hypersensitivity vasculitis is defined as an immune complex disease with deposition of antigen–antibody complexes into the small vessels such as arterioles, venules, or capillaries, usually of the dermis. The concept of hypersensitivity vasculitis was first described by Zeek, Smith, and Weeter in 1948.[134] The distinguishing features of hypersensitivity vasculitis include prominent involvement of the skin, the tendency toward small-vessel involvement, leukocytoclasis, and the frequent precipitation by a drug or serum. Early on, exposure to an exogenous antigen such as drugs, toxins, serum, or infection was thought to be responsible for development of hypersensitivity vasculitis (true hypersensitivity vasculitis).[14,95] However, it has been recognized that many patients could develop the same clinical and pathologic features without exposure to toxins or drugs. In addition, a wide variety of diseases including connective tissue disease, Henoch–Schönlein purpura, certain malignancies, and mixed cryoglobulinemia have been noted to cause the same clinical and pathologic features.[58,104] The current understanding of the term *hypersensitivity vasculitis* encompasses all of these disorders with the clinical and pathologic features previously described.[16] Any disease or condition (listed in Table 76.1) accompanied by circulating antigens can cause hypersensitivity vasculitis.

Hypersensitivity vasculitis, which comprises about 25% of vasculitis cases, frequently occurs in patients over age 16. Patients usually have a history of connective tissue disease, cryoglobulins, malignancies, or exposure to exogenous antigens such as drugs or toxins.[14] Polymorphonuclear cells or eosinophils commonly appear in vessel walls. Almost all patients (more than 95%) demonstrate purpura or other dermatologic findings including ulcerations, bullae, urticaria, livedo reticularis, or erythema multiforme. Other organ involvement includes arthritis, pulmonary infiltrates, neuropathy, and GN. Vasculitis of mesenteric circulation can cause bowel ischemia, which may lead to infarction, ischemic perforation, or hemorrhage.

True hypersensitivity vasculitis is the most common syndrome in the hypersensitivity vasculitis group. This syndrome is caused by exposure to an exogenous antigen such as drugs or toxins. The antigenic exposures reported to be responsible for this syndrome are listed in Table 76.4. In the typical case of true hypersensitivity vasculitis, vasculitis occurs 7 to 10 days after initial exposure to the antigen. In most patients the initial manifestation of this disease is the characteristic rash. Although a variety of cutaneous lesions can be seen in patients with true hypersensitivity vasculitis, the most common rash is palpable purpura. Other manifestations include fever, malaise, and weight loss. At times more significant organ

TABLE 76.4. Incriminate antigens associated with hypersensitivity vasculitis.

Drugs
Sulfa, penicillin, quinidine, tetracyclines, iodides, allopurinol, phenacetin, griseofulvin, phenothiazine, phenylbutazone, methyldopa, hydralazine, and so forth

Infections
Streptococcus, staphylococcus, meningococcus, leprosy, tuberculosis, malaria, subacute bacterial endocarditis, hepatitis B, human immunodeficiency virus, Epstein–Barr virus, cytomegalovirus, and so forth

Chemicals
Herbicides and insecticides

Immunizations
Influenza and allergy

Others
Foreign protein, insect bites, and so forth

---

involvement may be present including of the muscle, renal, pulmonary, or central nervous system. These manifestations are often chronic or recurrent. Histopathologic examinations in the biopsy specimen usually show the presence of polymorphonuclear leukocytes and associated leukocytoclasis. The prognosis for patients with true hypersensitivity vasculitis depends on the severity of disease, especially on target organ involvement. If the initiating antigen can be removed, the prognosis is generally good.

Henoch–Schönlein purpura is a syndrome clinically characterized by the following triad: palpable purpura, varying degrees of gastrointestinal ischemia, and GN.[124] Typically, the lesions of this disease may be identical to those of true hypersensitivity vasculitis.[99] Henoch–Schönlein purpura usually occurs in individuals under age 18, most often in the spring, and frequently includes gastrointestinal involvement such as gastrointestinal bleeding and colicky abdominal pain.

Henoch–Schönlein purpura can be distinguished by the deposition of immune complexes that contain immunoglobulin A (IgA) in the vasculitic tissues and the presence of IgA-containing circulating immune complexes.[58] An IgA-associated GN can be identified in about 50% of patients with Henoch–Schönlein purpura.

Cryoglobulinemic vasculitis implies the presence of serum immunoglobulins and other proteins that precipitate at temperatures below 37°C. Cryoglobulins are classified as follows: Type I cryoglobulins are monoclonal and usually identified in patients with hematologic malignancies. Type II cryoglobulins contain both mixed and monoclonal components, which are rarely identified in patients with connective tissue disease or malignancies. Most type II cryoglobulins were classified as idiopathic or essential until recently, but an association of type II cryoglobulins with hepatitis C has been established.[27,28] Type III cryoglobulins are polyclonal, in general represent immune complexes, and are found in patients with connective tissue disease, chronic infections, or inflammatory disorders.

The clinical manifestations in patients with cryoglobulinemia vary with the quantity and type of cryoglobulins and with organ involvement. Profound coldness may induce a variety of symptoms due to limb ischemia in patients with extremely elevated levels of cryoglobulins, generally type I or II. Patients with type III cryoglobulins usually show small-vessel vasculitis that reflects the underlying disorders. Among the three types of cryoglobulins, clinical features in most patients with type II cryoglobulins are distinctive. The skin, peripheral nerves, joints, liver, and kidneys are frequently involved. Renal involvement appears in 30% to 50% of patients and can be associated with hypertension, azotemia, or nephrosis. Renal involvement is considered a poor prognostic marker with a 5-year survival rate of approximately 60%. Causes of death in patients with type II cryoglobulins include cardiovascular, cerebrovascular, infectious, and vasculitic complications.

Hypersensitivity vasculitis associated with connective tissue disease or malignancy usually affects the small vessels. Patients with rheumatoid arthritis, systemic lupus erythematosus, or Sjögren's syndrome may exhibit cutaneous vasculitic involvement including palpable purpura. However, these disorders may be associated with large-vessel diseases such as systemic necrotizing vasculitis. The definite diagnosis for hypersensitivity vasculitis associated with connective tissue disease is generally based on clinical and serologic findings.

Malignancies may be associated with a variety of vascular disorders including deep venous thrombosis, arterial thromboembolism, and leukocytoclastic vasculitis. Malignancies most frequently associated with hypersensitivity vasculitis are lymphoproliferative or myeloproliferative disorders. The most common manifestations include palpable purpura, maculopapular rashes, and ulcers. In the majority of patients with an underlying malignancy, the vasculitis antedates the malignancy by many months. In general, these manifestations are poorly responsive to therapy but may remit with the treatment of underlying malignancies.

Urticarial vasculitis, or hypocomplementemic vasculitis, is a syndrome predominantly associated with urticaria that upon biopsy reveals leukocytoclastic vasculitis.[95,105,135] Patients with this syndrome suffer from attacks of urticaria that frequently last for longer than 24 hours at a time. Low-grade fever and arthralgias are characteristic features. Angioneurotic edema of the face and bowel may occasionally be observed. Kidneys are not generally involved, but membranoproliferative GN and pseudotumor cerebri have been reported in six patients. Because urticaria can also be observed in a variety of other immune complex conditions such as serum sickness, Henoch–Schönlein purpura, connective tissue disease, and hepatitis B, diagnosis for urticarial vasculitis depends on exclusion of these other immune complex conditions and adequate documentation by biopsy.

Diagnostic Tests

The sedimentation rate and acute phase reactants are usually elevated in patients with hypersensitivity vasculitis. Patients with urticarial vasculitis frequently demonstrate hypocomplementemia with marked depression of C1 through C3 complements. Leukocytosis and decreased serum complement levels may be noted, but no specific test is available for a definite diagnosis of hypersensitivity vasculitis. The most informative test is a biopsy of the affected dermis to determine whether leukocytoclastic vasculitis is present.

Medical and Surgical Treatment

Because of the size of involved vessels, surgical treatment for patients with hypersensitivity vasculitis is not clinically advantageous. In general, nonsteroidal and antihistamine therapy may suffice. For patients with true hypersensitivity vasculitis, treatment should focus on removal of the inciting antigen. For most patients with cryoglobulinemic vasculitis (generally type I or III), treatment is first directed at the underlying disorder, such as malignancies or connective tissue disease. Antiviral drugs (e.g., interferon-α) are indicated for patients with type II cryoglobulin, but relapse is common after cessation of the therapy. For more persistent cases or those associated with chronic rheumatologic disease or severe complications including renal, pulmonary, or mesenteric involvement, corticosteroids or cytotoxic drugs should be administered for immunosuppression.[15] In fulminant hypersensitivity vasculitis triggered by an exogenous antigen, plasma exchange has been reported to be beneficial.

Wegener's Granulomatosis

Clinical Features and Their Basis

Keys to diagnosis:[35,84]

1. Men and women are affected with almost equal frequency, and the disorder commonly occurs in the fifth decade
2. Triad: granulomatous vasculitis involving the respiratory system, GN, and hypersensitivity vasculitis in the small vessels
3. Presence of ANCA, highly specific to WG, is identified in 60% to 70% of patients

WG is a systemic, granulomatous inflammatory disease of unknown etiology.[11,35,131] WG affects small- and medium-sized blood vessels with major manifestations in the upper respiratory tract, lungs, and kidneys. WG affects men and women with almost equal frequency and occurs most commonly in the fifth decade.[3,62,80] There appear to be no linkages or associations with human leukocyte antigens (HLAs).[23,40,109] The most likely candidates for etiology are autoimmunity and infection.[40,56] Typically three organs are involved at onset or soon thereafter in classical WG, but the disease may take several years to develop in some cases. In addition to the typical three-organ involvement, WG may display other clinical manifestations including breast mass, prostatic nodule, gastrointestinal hemorrhage, diarrhea, palpable purpura, cranial nerve palsies, or erosive arthritis.[35]

Upper airway involvement occurs in 90% of patients and is the sole initial site of disease in 12%.[3,29,62] Perforation of the nasal septum and subsequent collapse of the nose may result in the typical saddle-nose deformity. Chronic sinusitis is frequently observed, and otitis media may develop through middle ear involvement. Inner ear involvement may result in sensorineural hearing loss. In addition, vertigo may occur due to vasculitic involvement of the endolymphatic sac vessels.

The lungs, which are affected in 85% of patients with WG, are the only initial site of disease in approximately 10%.[3,62] Patients with pulmonary involvement usually develop symptoms highly suggestive of pneumonia such as fever, cough, and occasionally chest pain but demonstrate normal flora in sputum cultures.[34] Chest x-ray examinations typically show nodules or infiltrates, often bilaterally. Patients with WG occasionally develop massive hemoptysis that results from diffuse alveolar hemorrhage.

Renal involvement is found in 77% of patients.[62,89] Patients whose upper airways and lungs are affected but who show no renal symptoms are referred to as having limited WG. Renal symptoms are those of rapidly progressive GN, including general malaise, edema, proteinuria, and rising serum creatinine levels.[11]

Arthritis and other symptoms found in rheumatic disease are observed with a high frequency (approximately 67%), but symptoms are usually mild.[62] Development of erosive arthritis is rare. Skin involvement is found in 46% of patients during their course, and occasionally skin involvement is among the initial manifestations.[62] Ocular involvement has been reported in 28% to 64% of patients.[62,93,112] Potential eye manifestations include pain, conjunctivitis, scleritis, diplopia, ptosis, proptosis, and retinal or optic nerve vasculitis. Orbital pseudotumors have been reported in approximately 15% of patients with WG.[93] The central nervous system, including cerebral infarction or diffuse cerebritis, is affected in 8% of patients. Mononeuritis multiplex may be associated with approximately 15% of WG patients.[93,101,102] Multiple cranial nerve palsies have also been described. Gastrointestinal and cardiovascular involvement is less common in WG than in other types of necrotizing arteritis, but the symptoms may be severe when they occur.[4,45,50,51,62,82,121]

Diagnostic Tests

WG is suspected in patients with fever, malaise, and multisystem disorders with prominent lung and upper airway manifestations.[35] Anemia, leukocytosis, thrombocytosis, hypergammaglobulinemia, and elevated acute-phase reactants are commonly found. Complement levels are usually normal. ANCAs, which are highly specific to WG, are identified in 60% to 70% of patients.[18] C-ANCAs are more common than P-ANCAs and have become a useful differentiating marker.[9]

Confirmation of the diagnosis of WG requires biopsy, and the lung is the best site to prove definitive histopathologic changes in WG.[84,92] The histopathologic changes of WG are characterized by granuloma formation and necrotizing vasculitis of small- and medium-sized arteries. Biopsy of the kidney may not be useful for definitive diagnosis, even in patients with severe renal disease.

Medical Treatment

Because the use of corticosteroids alone is generally ineffective in the long-term management of WG, several immunosuppressive agents should be combined.[2,12,39,114] The preferred regimen is 100 to 150 mg/d of oral cyclophosphamide for 1 year, with or without low-dose prednisone, followed by tapering of the daily dose. The combination of trimethoprim and sulfamethoxazole has also been shown to be effective for patients with WG.[122] The usual course of treatment is 160 mg/d of trimethoprim and 800 mg/d of sulfamethoxazole. In addition, methotrexate (MTX) has been reported to be effective for patients who do not respond to cyclophosphamide or experience relapses.[63] The use of MTX may cause significant side effects, including *Pneumocystis carinii* pneumonia, MTX pneumonitis, oral ulcers, or rash. Therefore the weekly dose of MTX should not exceed 15 mg.[63] High-dose corticosteroid therapy may be indicated for orbital pseudotumors that cause severe pain.

Surgical Treatment

Because of the size of involved vessels, surgical treatment of vascular lesions is rarely indicated for patients with WG. Subglottic stenosis is a troublesome complication of upper airway involvement that may require surgical correction.[29,85] For patients with orbital pseudotumors, sur-

gical decompression may be required because of excruciating pain, but it is technically difficult to avoid further loss of vision. Intensive plasma exchange may be undertaken for patients with severe active GN, but plasma exchange is not a widely accepted treatment at present.

Giant Cell Arteritis

Giant cell arteritis is the term commonly used for granulomatous arteritis of unknown origin that involves mainly large arteries with destruction of the internal elastic lamina.[66,72,76] Giant cell arteritis includes two syndromes, Takayasu's arteritis and temporal arteritis. The major differences between the two syndromes are the age at onset, severity and distribution of vascular involvement, racial distribution, and prognosis.

Takayasu's Arteritis

Clinical Features and Their Basis

Keys to diagnosis:[5]

1. Onset of claudication, pulse deficits, bruits, blood pressure discrepancies, or hypertension in patients less than 35 years of age that results from widespread and severe vascular involvement
2. Arterial stenosis or dilatation limited to the aorta or its major branches

Takayasu's arteritis is an idiopathic, systemic inflammatory disease that primarily involves elastic arteries such as the aorta, proximal parts of its major branches, and the pulmonary artery trunk.[55,61,75,126] Takayasu's arteritis predominates in women of reproductive age (less than 35 years of age) and is more prevalent in Asian populations, whereas temporal arteritis predominates in white populations. The incidence of Takayasu's arteritis in the United States is 2.6 per million. Vascular involvement may appear as arterial stenosis, occlusion, dilatation, and/or aneurysms. Takayasu's arteritis is also referred to as pulseless disease, nonspecific aortoarteritis, atypical aortic coarctation, and middle aorta syndrome. The cause of the disease is unknown, but it is thought to be an autoimmune phenomenon; chronic infection is considered to be one of the triggering mechanisms.

In the acute phase of Takayasu's arteritis, nonspecific symptoms such as fever, malaise, anorexia, weight loss, arthralgia, and myalgias can be present. However, these symptoms are generally transient. The symptoms in the chronic phase of Takayasu's arteritis depend on the vessels involved and may occur several years after the onset of disease. The most common site of vascular involvement is the aortic arch and its branches (Figure 76.1A). The second most common site is the proximal abdomi-

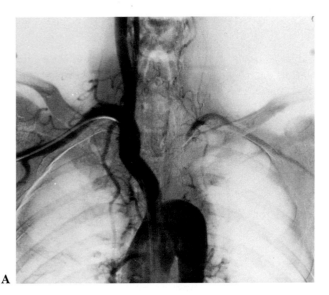

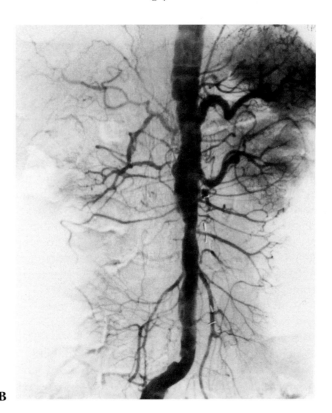

A   **B**

FIGURE 76.1. Angiograms in the thoracic (A) and abdominal (B) lesions in a patient with Takayasu's arteritis. **A,** The angiogram shows proximal obstruction of the left common carotid artery and left subclavian artery. The distal subclavian artery is visualized by the collateral arteries. **B,** An abdominal arteriogram in the same patient demonstrates a diffuse narrowing of the abdominal aorta and proximal obstruction of the right renal artery. Proximal occlusion of the left common iliac artery is recognized as well.

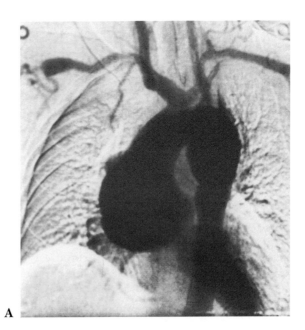

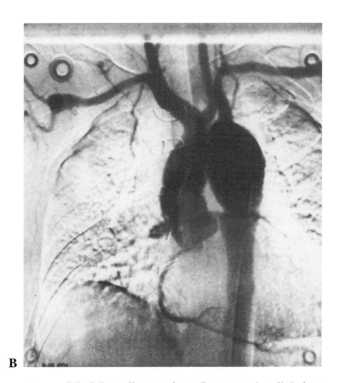

A   **B**

FIGURE 76.2. Preoperative (A) and postoperative (B) angiogram of the thoracic aorta in a patient with Takayasu's arteritis complicating annuloaortic ectasia (AAE) who underwent a modified Bentall procedure. Postoperative digital angiography showed a good runoff of the coronary arteries and no anastomotic stenosis or leakage.

nal aorta (Figure 76.1B) and its branches, including the visceral and renal arteries, but any branches of the aorta can be involved. The distribution of vascular involvement according to 191 autopsy cases in Japan is summarized in Table 76.5. Stenotic lesions are most common, but dilative or aneurysmal lesions are also observed in some cases (Figure 76.2). The most common sites of dilative lesions include the aorta (23%), brachiocephalic arteries (7%), and subclavian arteries (5%).

Clinical manifestations in the chronic phase include hypertension, cerebrovascular symptoms, claudication, and/or impotence. During the course of Takayasu's arteritis, 32% to 93% of patients develop hypertension, often regardless of disease activity. The coronary arteries have been considered to be rarely affected, but the incidence of coronary artery involvement has gradually increased. The pulmonary artery is involved radiographically in nearly half of all patients with Takayasu's arteritis, although most of these patients are asymptomatic. In the advanced stage, absent peripheral pulses, bruits, blood pressure asymmetry, retinal arteriovenous anastomoses, visual field deficits, or congestive heart failure may be present, depending on the location and extent of the vascular involvement.

The 5-year mortality rate for Takayasu's arteritis has been estimated to be 2% to 35%, depending on the severity of associated complications.[61,75,78] The most determinant factor for prognosis is the presence of heart failure, which may result from persistent hypertension or aortic insufficiency. Other causes of death related to Takayasu's arteritis include ischemic or hemorrhagic strokes and renal failure.

Diagnostic Tests

Histopathologic examination is the most common method for definite diagnosis in other types of vasculitis, but biopsy is not practical for diagnosing Takayasu's arteritis because of the size of the affected vessels. Angiography is the most reliable study to establish a diagnosis of Takayasu's arteritis. The characteristic pattern of arterial stenosis distributing in the aorta and its branches (Fig-

TABLE 76.5. Distribution of vascular lesions according to 191 autopsy cases in Japan.

Arteries	1958–1973 (%)	1975–1984 (%)
Ascending aorta	78	73
Coronary artery	11	45
Aortic arch	86	74
Brachiocephalic artery	82	57
Right subclavian artery	75	45
Right common carotid artery	82	50
Left common carotid artery	87	62
Left subclavian artery	88	57
Thoracic aorta	71	81
Abdominal aorta	59	67
Celiac artery	13	9
Superior mesenteric artery	15	5
Renal artery	24	40
Inferior mesenteric artery	8	2
Common iliac artery	3	27
Pulmonary artery trunk	45	35
Intrapulmonary branches	28	17

From Hotchi.[64]

ures 76.1 and 76.2) in a young person, often associated with pulmonary artery involvement, suffices for the diagnosis. In routine laboratory tests, anemia can be seen in approximately half of the patients. ESR and CRP levels are common and useful markers for evaluating the degree of inflammation.[55] Left ventricular hypertrophy and left atrial enlargement may result from hypertension. More than half of the patients exhibit cardiomegaly or an abnormal aortic contour in the chest roentgenogram.

Takayasu's arteritis can resemble a variety of congenital or acquired cardiovascular diseases. Clinical features of these diseases for differentiation are summarized in Table 76.6.[5]

Medical Treatment

Takayasu's arteritis may be medically treated with nonsteroidal anti-inflammatory drugs, corticosteroids, or other immunosuppressive agents such as cyclophos-

TABLE 76.6. Diseases that require differential diagnosis from Takayasu's arteritis.

Differential diagnosis	Clinical features for differentiation from Takayasu's arteritis
Marfan's syndrome	Aortic root dilatation, often associated with aortic dissection
Ehlers–Danlos syndrome	Aneurysms, frail nature of the blood vessels, Meischer's elastoma
Spondyloarthropathies	Aortic root dilatation (uncommon)
Fibromuscular dysplasia	Noninflammatory, stenosis > dilatative
Tuberculous, mycotic, or syphilitic arteritis	Aneurysms, stenoses rare
Sarcoid vasculopathy	Aneurysms and stenoses in vessels of any size
Other vasculitides:	
Behçet's disease	A sudden onset of pseudoaneurysms in vessels of any size, thrombophlebitis
Kawasaki's syndrome	Primarily affects infants and children; cardiac involvement (pericardial effusion, myocarditis, and coronary artery aneurysms)
Temporal arteritis	Mainly affects women over the age of 50; cardiac manifestations are rare, medical therapy attenuates vascular lesions

TABLE 76.7. Indications for surgical repair or angioplasty in patients with Takayasu's arteritis.

Renovascular stenosis causing significant hypertension
Coronary artery stenosis leading to myocardial ischemia
Extremity claudication induced by routine activity
Cerebral ischemia and/or critical stenosis of three or more cerebral vessels
Aortic regurgitation, often associated with dilatation of the aortic root
Thoracic or abdominal aortic aneurysms larger than 5 cm in diameter

phamide and/or cyclosporine. Treatment protocols for the active phase of Takayasu's arteritis, characterized by the presence of fever, pain of vascular origin, and an elevated ESR or CRP level, include daily prednisone in doses of 1 mg/kg for 1 to 3 months, followed by tapering if active Takayasu's arteritis has remitted. If corticosteroid tapering is not successful and leads to relapse of disease, the patient should be treated with daily cyclophosphamide 2 mg/kg or weekly MTX 0.15 to 0.3 mg/kg. Immunosuppressive therapy may improve vascular patency in some patients whose inflammatory lesions have occurred recently; however, in contrast to vascular lesions that occur in temporal arteritis, such reversibility is not common in most patients with Takayasu's arteritis.

In addition to treatment of vascular lesions, medical therapy for associated hypertension and heart failure is essential to improve prognosis. Because of the frequent presence of subclavian artery stenosis, blood pressure measured at an upper extremity may not be reliable in some cases. The most common cause of hypertension is high-renin hypertension due to renal artery stenosis; however, suprarenal aortic stenosis can cause the same sequence of events. Recognizing the distribution and severity of vascular lesions is essential for adequate management.

Surgical Treatment

Critical vascular lesions should be treated by angioplasty or surgical revascularization.[81,115,129] Indications for surgical repair or angioplasty are listed in Table 76.7. Generally, reconstructive surgery for Takayasu's arteritis is successful, but anastomotic insufficiency or relapse of pseudoaneurysms at the anastomotic sites has been reported in some cases. These interventions should be undertaken during periods of remission to achieve optimal results.[115]

Temporal Arteritis

Clinical Features and Their Basis

Keys to diagnosis:

1. Visual disturbances and persistent headache associated with systemic symptoms of fever, myalgias, or weight loss

2. Individuals over age 50, mainly women
3. Possible abnormal palpation of temporal arteries
4. Elevated ESR, diminished pulses with claudication in extremity involvement
5. Bilateral, symmetric tapering stenoses with collateral arteries and poststenotic dilatation

Temporal arteritis is the most common syndrome in giant cell arteritis and mainly affects women over age 50.[76,94] It is 10 times more common than Takayasu's arteritis, and its incidence is still increasing annually. Temporal arteritis is frequently associated with polymyalgia rheumatica, but the background for this association has not been elucidated.[21,32] Temporal arteritis is also identified in up to 15% of elderly patients with fever of unknown origin. Classic symptoms of temporal arteritis include visual disturbances and persistent headaches, often in the temporal areas, that usually occur after the onset of nonspecific systemic manifestations such as fever, headache, and myalgias.[59,94] Partial or complete visual loss is the most frequent complication, and other ischemic manifestations including necrosis of the tongue, multiple cranial nerve palsies, and hearing loss may occur in the head and neck region. The visual manifestations may result from retrobulbar neuritis, ischemic optic neuritis, ophthalmic arteritis, and/or occlusion of the central retinal vessels. The temporal arteries may be abnormal by palpation and are often associated with tenderness and swelling. If the patient has polymyalgia rheumatica, active motion of limb or pelvic girdle muscles is usually painful. Other sites that may be involved in patients with temporal arteritis include the visceral, renal, vertebral, and coronary arteries.

Diagnostic Tests

The only helpful laboratory test is of ESR, which is usually markedly elevated. Although some cases of typical temporal arteritis with normal ESR have been noted, the presence of a normal ESR strongly suggests other diagnostic possibilities such as diabetes mellitus or malignancies. However, it remains controversial whether ESR may serve as a marker for evaluating the effect of treatment or relapse.[94] Angiography may be undertaken for patients with visual disturbances or limb claudication. Bilateral, often symmetric, tapering stenoses with numerous collateral arteries and poststenotic dilatation may be revealed in the head and neck area.

The characteristic pathologic findings in temporal arteritis are granulomatous inflammation of the arterial wall associated with destruction of the internal elastic lamina and giant cell formation. Fragmentation of the elastic fiber may be found, and the giant cells may contain fragments of elastin, which are often in direct contact with the elastic lamina. Although biopsy of the temporal artery is the gold standard for the diagnosis of temporal arteritis, it is not necessary in all suspected cases. In patients with temporal artery involvement, characteristic angiogram, elevated ESR, and a typical history may suffice for the diagnosis if an appropriate biopsy site is not available.

Medical Treatment

Steroid therapy remains the preferred treatment.[32] Once the diagnosis of temporal arteritis is suspected, a high-dose regimen of prednisone (60–100 mg/d) should be instituted without delay to prevent catastrophic ocular complications. The dose of prednisone is tapered slowly after the systemic symptoms are resolved and the ESR reaches a normal level. Once the disease is controlled, the required dose of prednisone (<10 mg/d) is generally low enough to avoid serious side effects in most patients.

The relapse rate after discontinuing prednisone is relatively high at approximately 50%. Reported mean durations of steroid therapy ranged from 2 to 6 years. The mortality rate in patients with temporal arteritis is equal to that of age-matched controls, but the incidence of blindness is estimated to be 20% of patients. Early recognition and appropriate management are essential to avoid devastating ocular complications.

Surgical Treatment

Surgical intervention is generally limited to diagnostic biopsy.[72] Because vascular lesions in temporal arteritis generally respond well to medical therapy, revascularization is usually unnecessary. In contrast to Takayasu's arteritis, other complications that require surgical repair, such as aortic regurgitation, dissection, or aortic aneurysms, are rarely observed.

Behçet's Disease

Clinical Features and Their Basis

Keys to diagnosis:[67]

1. Recurrent aphthous stomatitis at least three times a year, along with two or more of the following: genital ulcerations; ocular inflammation, most commonly uveitis; skin lesions including erythema nodosum or pustules; meningoencephalitis and synovitis; and positive pathergy test
2. Vascular complications, including venous thrombosis, arterial occlusion, or aneurysm formation
3. Gastrointestinal or neurotic manifestations may appear in addition to the classic symptom triad

Behçet's disease is characterized by a chronic, systemic inflammatory disease of unknown etiology that involves mucocutaneous, ocular, articular, neurological, cardio-

vascular, and gastrointestinal systems.[7,68,69,90] Clinical manifestations in the classic form of Behçet's disease include recurrent aphthous stomatitis at least three times a year, along with two or more of the following: genital ulcerations; ocular inflammation, most commonly uveitis; skin lesions including erythema nodosum or pustules; and meningoencephalitis and synovitis.[67,90] Behçet's disease is found most often in young men between the ages of 20 and 40 in the Mediterranean, Middle East, and Japanese populations. The incidence of Behçet's disease in the United States is estimated to be about 1 in 20,000. The reported etiologic possibilities are infectious, autoimmune, and genetic. Histocompatibility of HLA-DRw52 and HLA-B51 has been reported to be associated with Behçet's disease in the Japanese. Although the etiology of Behçet's disease is unknown, vascular inflammation of the vasa vasorum that causes medial fragmentation and rupture is thought to be an important part of the underlying pathology.[6,132]

Vascular lesions can occur in both the arterial and venous systems and are often the main source of mortality.[74,77] Behçet's disease affects veins more often than arteries. The most frequent vascular lesions are venous occlusions and superficial thrombophlebitis in the extremities, which occur in approximately 30% of patients. The second most common complication is thrombosis of either vena cava, which often causes Budd–Chiari syndrome. Arterial vascular complications occur in about 10% of patients, including aneurysms in the larger arterial trunks or occlusions of the limb arteries.[6] These vascular manifestations occasionally appear very rapidly, presenting a sudden onset of rupture of pseudoaneurysms. Arterial lesions that may be affected by Behçet's disease are those located in the aorta and the subclavian, carotid (Figure 76.3), renal, splenic, iliofemoral (Figure 76.4), and pulmonary arteries. Rupture of arterial aneurysms may be the most common source of mortality.

A variety of gastrointestinal manifestations are present in approximately half of the patients with Behçet's disease (enteral Behçet's disease). Ulcerations in the ileocecal area occur in 75% of patients with enteral Behçet's disease, and perforation may occur in 40% of those patients. Intestinal perforation is the second most common cause of death in patients with Behçet's disease. Neural Behçet's disease is found in about 10% of patients with Behçet's disease; those affected present with clinical manifestations including meningoencephalitis, sensory and/or motor, and psychiatric symptoms. Respiratory involvement is not common, but hemoptysis may occur in patients with pulmonary artery involvement. Skin lesions such as erythema nodosum, pseudofolliculitis, or papulopustules are found in most patients (about 80%) and reflect small-vessel involvement in the skin. Synovitis and arthralgias, seen in about half of the patients, are charac-

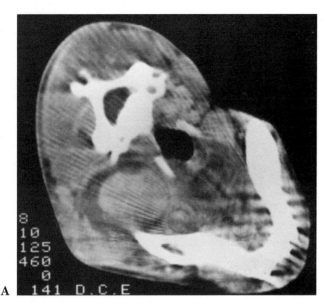

FIGURE 76.3. Preoperative computed tomography (A) and angiogram (B) scans in a 16-year-old male patient with a pseudoaneurysm of the common carotid artery. The patient underwent a patch closure of the ruptured arterial wall. Macroscopic findings at operation demonstrated a pseudoaneurysm with a punched-out perforated hole of 50 by 20 mm located in the common carotid artery.

teristic of joint involvement in those with Behçet's disease. The most commonly affected site is the knee joint.

The overall mortality rate for patients with Behçet's disease ranges from 3% to 4%, and death is usually due to rupture of aneurysms, intestinal perforation, or severe central nervous system disorders. The risk of blindness from ocular lesions is still high, ranging from 50% to 80%.

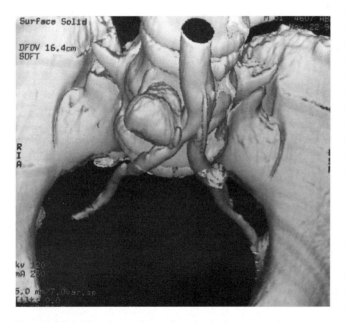

FIGURE 76.4. The three-dimensional spiral computed tomography scan of a patient with a pseudoaneurysm of the common iliac artery. The size of the pseudoaneurysm and the site of rupture are obvious.

Diagnostic Tests

There is no specific finding in routine laboratory tests for definitive diagnosis of Behçet's disease. The pathergy test is beneficial for determination of Behçet's disease involvement. In this test, the subject's skin is pricked with a needle, and a sterile pustule forms within 24 hours in positive cases. A positive pathergy test suggests involvement of one organ system in the diagnostic criteria.[67] The evaluation of vascular involvement is essential for diagnosis of vascular Behçet's disease and its treatment; however, a conventional arteriogram is not recommended for patients suspected of having Behçet's disease because of the increased risk of thrombosis during angiogram and pseudoaneurysm formation at the puncture site. In patients who require evaluation of vascular involvement for surgical intervention, transvenous digital subtraction angiogram should be used instead of the conventional arteriogram.

Medical Treatment

Corticosteroids are generally used to reduce inflammation. Immunosuppressive agents including chlorambucil, cyclophosphamide, azathioprine, and cyclosporine can be used for patients with more serious and life-threatening complications, such as severe eye inflammation, central nervous system involvement, or major arterial aneurysms.[133] Anticoagulation therapy may be indicated for patients with venous thrombotic complications, but anticoagulant agents should be avoided in patients who present with hemoptysis or pulmonary artery involvement.

Surgical Treatment

Behçet's disease often causes arterial pseudoaneurysms that may rupture suddenly. Surgical treatment is undertaken to save the patient's life, but revascularization of the arterial system is associated with a number of difficulties.[79] There is a high frequency of anastomotic dehiscence in the later period, and patency rates are substandard.[79] Choice of uninvolved anastomotic sites and reinforcement of the suture have been described as options for avoiding anastomotic dehiscence; however, an effective strategy for revascularization has not been established.

Buerger's Disease (Thromboangiitis Obliterans)

Clinical Features and Their Basis

Keys to diagnosis:

1. Ischemic signs and symptoms of the distal upper or lower extremities (beyond the knee or elbow) in smokers and usually adult men between the ages of 35 and 50
2. Absent distal pulses associated with preserved proximal pulses not due to atherosclerosis
3. Migratory superficial phlebitis
4. Preservation of the vessel wall structures in association with intraluminal and perivascular fibrous transformation

Buerger's disease (thromboangiitis obliterans, or TAO) is an inflammatory vasculitis that involves the medium and small arteries in the extremities.[13,73,96,107,108,120] The age at onset usually ranges from 35 to 50 years, and TAO is more frequently found in men. TAO is regarded as a disease of smokers only, and smoking is recognized as an accelerating factor of this disease.[73,107,108] Although the actual mechanism of TAO is unknown, some immunological mechanisms are thought to account for development of the disease.[36]

The earliest complaints of patients with TAO are usually rest pain in the feet or hands, painful digital ulcerations, or gangrene. Patients may also complain of Raynaud's symptoms or claudication that is usually limited to the foot. Limb involvement generally occurs in two or more extremities, predominantly in the lower limbs. The digits are usually cold, and tender, dry ulcers may be present in the tips of the toes or fingers. Ulceration is not present in 25% of patients but is recurrent in 45%. Migratory superficial phlebitis occurs in 30% of patients

and is often recurrent. The arterial pulses in the extremities depend on the extent of disease. The proximal pulses (femoral and axillary) in the extremities are usually normal, and the distal pulses including those at the radial, ulnar, posterior tibial, and dorsalis pedis arteries may be absent.[106] These distal pulses may also be normal in some patients, which is associated with the absence of more peripheral pulses distal to these arteries.

Histologically, the vessel wall structures are mostly preserved throughout the acute and chronic phases of this disease. In the acutely involved vessels, unorganized thrombus associated with multinuclear giant cells is present. The thrombi may contain microabscesses with neutrophils surrounded by epithelioid cells. Intraluminal and perivascular fibrous transformation are present in the chronic phase of TAO.[106] The survival rate of patients with TAO is considered to be the same as that of the general population. This is probably because the coronary, cerebral, and viscerorenal arteries are not involved in TAO patients.

Diagnostic Tests

In patients with TAO, routine laboratory tests are usually normal. If other diseases are suspected, more detailed tests including ESR or CRP, antinuclear antibody, rheumatoid factor, protein C and S, antithrombin III, or anticardiolipin antibodies should be examined. These tests are performed to exclude other vascular disorders, such as atherosclerosis, hypercoagulability, or other primary and secondary vasculitides. Arteriograms or measurements of arterial Doppler pressure are essential for definitive diagnosis. Patients with TAO usually exhibit distal arterial occlusion with normal proximal arteries in the extremities. Angiographic findings include tapering, abrupt occlusions, and tortuosity of affected vessels. The collateral arteries may have a corkscrew or tree root appearance (Figure 76.5).

The diagnostic criteria of TAO consist of an early age at onset before 45 to 50 years; a history of smoking; no risk factors for atherosclerosis such as diabetes mellitus, hyperlipidemia, and hypertension; no other vasculopathy; and distal occlusive disease only. Distribution of occlusive lesions should be identified by arteriography or segmental measurements of arterial Doppler pressures. Migratory superficial phlebitis is a helpful symptom for diagnosis but is not included in the diagnostic criteria.

Medical Treatment

Disease progression and major limb loss usually depend on whether the patient successfully quits smoking. In addition, local wound care and avoidance of trauma are important to prevent further progression of the disease. Prostaglandins have been reported to be effective for im-

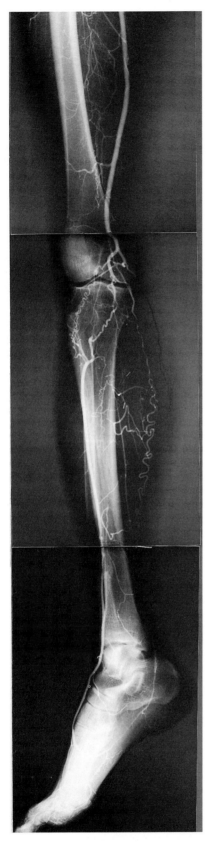

FIGURE 76.5. Arteriogram of the right lower extremity in a patient with thromboangiitis obliterans. Proximal obstruction of the popliteal artery and revisualization of the anterior and posterior tibial arteries by the collateral arteries are identified.

proving ulcerations in some cases, but discontinuance of the drug causes relapse of ulcers. Numerous other medications such as antiplatelet, vasodilator, and anticoagulant agents have been studied; however, results vary with reports, and no standard protocol has been established to inhibit progression of the disease.

Surgical Treatment

Surgical revascularization is indicated for only ≤10% of patients, mostly due to the lack of distal anastomotic sites available for outflow vessels.[100,125] The autosaphenous vein is generally used for a bypass graft, but the patency rate in patients with TAO is lower than that in atherosclerotic patients.[100,125] Sympathectomy may be effective against recurrent ulcers or rest pain in some patients.

Although the survival rate of patients with TAO is equal to that of the general population, toe or forefoot amputation is required during the course of disease in 20% of patients with leg involvement. In addition, another 20% undergo major limb amputation. In patients with upper extremity involvement, major amputation is rare, and digital amputation is required for less than 10% of patients.

Inflammatory Abdominal Aortic Aneurysms

Clinical Features and Their Basis

Keys to diagnosis:

1. Presence of abdominal aortic aneurysm associated with significant symptoms such as abdominal or back pain, weight loss, fever, and ESR elevation
2. A characteristic radiological finding of mantle core sign shown on the abdominal computed tomography scan
3. Fibrous extension to the adjacent retroperitoneum, which often causes hydronephrosis, and rigid adherence of adjacent structures to the aneurysmal wall

The concept of IAAA was first described by Walker et al. in 1972;[128] it was pathologically characterized by marked thickening of the aneurysmal wall with fibrous extension into the adjacent retroperitoneum and rigid adherence of adjacent structures to the aneurysmal wall.[8,33,111,113,123] IAAA comprises about 5% of abdominal aortic aneurysms and is also termed *perianeurysmal fibrosis* or *chronic periaortitis*.[10,33,60,123] Patients with IAAA usually show distinct clinical features including abdominal, back, or flank pain and may have laboratory findings that suggest the presence of active inflammation such as elevated ESR and CRP levels.[60] The etiology of IAAA is considered different from that of abdominal aortic aneurysms due to atherosclerosis, and possible mechanisms responsible for development of the disease include autoimmunity and periaortic lymphatic congestion.[47,111] The prognosis of patients with IAAA is generally the same as for abdominal aortic aneurysms, but some points should be noted in terms of diagnosis and surgical strategy.

Diagnostic Tests

In the routine laboratory tests, inflammatory responses including an elevated ESR, positive CRP, and leukocytosis are often seen in patients with IAAA.[111] Other serological studies usually demonstrate no specific results. In imaging studies, angiographic findings in patients with IAAA are the same as those with abdominal aortic aneurysms. The most distinguished finding is a characteristic mantle core sign, a thickened wall lying outside the lucent rim of the intima and subintima,[42] shown on the abdominal computed tomography scan (Figure 76.6). Generally, the mantle core sign tends to be thicker in the anterior and lateral wall of the aneurysm than in the posterior wall. In addition, the mantle core sign is usually limited to the periaortic wall and does not extend over the psoas muscles. Pyelography often demonstrates hydronephrosis, stenosis, occlusion, or median deviation of the ureter, which may be enough to suspect of the presence of IAAA.[113] Currently, the diagnosis of IAAA before operation can be made in 30% of patients with IAAA, and early recognition of IAAA may greatly contribute to allowing for an adequate operative strategy.

Medical Treatment

Surgical repair with prosthetic replacement of the aorta is the principal treatment. However, steroid therapy may be indicated as an option for some patients who exhibit the following criteria: (1) small aneurysms (<5 cm in diameter) with severe pain or weight loss; (2) presence of severe hydronephrosis; and (3) severe periaortic fibrosis and the rigid adherence of adjacent structures, which suggest great difficulty in surgical repair.[117] In general, prednisolone was administered to these patients at an initial dose of 30 mg/d, which was tapered to a maintenance dose of 5 mg/d depending on improvement of clinical manifestations and inflammatory findings. The efficacy of steroid therapy in the management of IAAA is, however, controversial.[57,117] In our experience, 6 out of 16 patients with IAAA have received steroid therapy during the last decade. Inflammation disappeared, based on laboratory test results, in all 6 patients, and 3 out of the 6 patients demonstrated a decrease in the size of the aneurysm. However, one patient underwent emergency operation because of a rapid increase in the size of the aneurysm. Steroid therapy should not be used as a substitute for surgery but may be used in patients who are unfit for surgery to decrease the mass and thus facili-

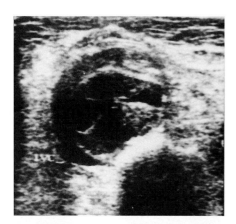

A

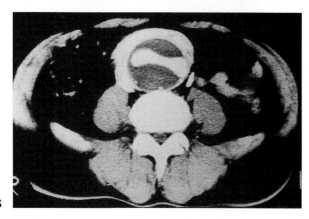

B

FIGURE 76.6. The transaxial view of ultrasonography (A) and mantle core sign, a thickened wall lying outside the lucent rim of the intima and subintima shown on the abdominal computed tomography scan (B) in a patient with inflammatory abdominal aortic aneurysms.

tate surgery;[57] the possible increased risk of rupture must be considered, however.

Surgical Treatment

Prosthetic replacement of the aorta with minimal exposure and incisions is essential to avoid unexpected injuries of the ureter or other surrounding tissues.[10,24,30] A retroperitoneal approach is recommended for patients with severe periaortic adhesion to the duodenum.[30,41,97] The severity of inflammatory changes and adhesions is generally greater in the anterior wall than in the lateral wall. If these inflammatory responses are too severe to expose the proximal aortic cross-clamping site in infrarenal IAAA cases, cross-clamping at the suprarenal or supravisceral sites should be considered. Operative mortality and long-term survival rates in patients with IAAA are almost the same as those with abdominal aortic aneurysms.[118]

References

1. Abel G, Zhang QX, Agnello V, et al. Hepatitis C virus in type II mixed cryoglobulinemia. *Arthritis Rheum.* 1993;10: 1341–1349.

2. Allen NB, Caldwell DS, Rice JR, et al. Cyclosporin A therapy for Wegener's granulomatosis. *Adv Exp Med Biol.* 1993;336: 473–476.

3. Anderson G, Coles ET, Crane M, et al. Wegener's granuloma: a series of 265 British cases seen between 1975 and 1985. A report by a sub-committee of the British Thoracic Society Research Committee. *Q J Med.* 1992;83:427–438.

4. Aoki N, Soma K, Owada T, et al. Wegener's granulomatosis complicated by arterial aneurysm. Intern Med. 1995;34: 790–793.

5. Arend WP, Michel BA, Bloch DA, et al. The American College of Rheumatology 1990 criteria for the classification of Takayasu arteritis. *Arthritis Rheum.* 1990;33:1129–1134.

6. Bartlett ST, McCarthy WJ 3d, Palmer AS, et al. Multiple aneurysms in Behçet's disease. *Arch Surg.* 1988;123: 1004–1008.

7. Behçet H. Ueber rezidivierende, Aphtoese, durch ein virus verursachte Geschwuere am Mund, am, Auge und an den Genitalien. *Dermatologische Monatsschrift* 1937;105: 1152–1157.

8. Boontje AH, van den Dungen JJ, Blanksma C, et al. Inflammatory abdominal aortic aneurysms. *J Cardiovasc Surg (Torino).* 1990;31:611–616.

9. Bosch X, Marquez A. c-ANCA as a marker of Wegener's disease [letter]. *Lancet.* 1996;347:117–118.

10. Braxton J, Salander JM, Gomez ER, et al. Inflammatory abdominal aortic aneurysm masquerading as occlusion of the inferior vena cava. *J Vasc Surg.* 1990;12:527–530.

11. Briedigkeit L, Kettritz R, Gobel U, et al. Prognostic factors in Wegener's granulomatosis. *Postgrad Med J.* 1993;69:856–861.

12. Briedigkeit L, Ulmer M, Gobel U, et al. Treatment of Wegener's granulomatosis. *Adv Exp Med Biol.* 1993;491–495.

13. Buerger L. Thromboangiitis obliterans: a study of the vascular lesions leading to presenile spontaneous gangrene. *Am J Med Sci.* 1908;136:567–580.

14. Calabrese LH, Duna G. Drug-induced vasculitis. *Curr Opin Rheumatol.* 1996;8:34–40.

15. Calabrese LH, Hoffman GS, Guillevin L. Therapy of treatment resistant systemic necrotizing vasculitis: polyarteritis, Churg-Strauss syndrome, Wegener's granulomatosis, and hypersensitivity vasculitis group disorders. *Rheum Dis Clin North Am.* 1995;21:41–57.

16. Calabrese LH, Michel BA, Bloch DA, et al. The American College of Rheumatology 1990 criteria for the classification of hypersensitivity vasculitis. *Arthritis Rheum.* 1990;33: 1108–1113.

17. Capewell S, Chapman BJ, Alexander F, et al. Pulmonary eosinophilia with systemic features: therapy and prognosis. *Respir Med.* 1992;86:485–490.

18. Carrie S, Hughes KB, Watson MG, et al. Negative ANCA in Wegener's granulomatosis. *J Laryngol Otol.* 1994;108: 420–422.

19. Chumbley LC, Harrison EG, DeRemee RA. Allergic granulomatosis and allergic angiitis (Churg-Strauss syndrome): report and analysis of 30 cases. *Mayo Clin Proc.* 1977;52:477–484.

20. Churg J, Strauss L. Allergic granulomatosis, allergic angiitis, and periarteritis nodosa. *Am J Pathol.* 1951;27: 277–301.

21. Cid MC, Ercilla G, Vilaseca J, et al. Polymyalgia rheumatica: a syndrome associated with HLA-DR4 antigen. *Arthritis Rheum.* 1988;31:678–682.

22. Conn DL. Polyarteritis. *Rheum Dis Clin North Am.* 1990; 16:341–362.

23. Cotch MF, Fauci AS, Hoffman GS. HLA typing in patients with Wegener granulomatosis [letter]. *Ann Intern Med.* 1995;122:635.

24. Crawford JL, Stower CL, Safi JH, et al. Inflammatory aneurysms of the aorta. *J Vasc Surg.* 1985;2:113–124.

25. Cupps TR, Fauci AS. The vasculitides. *Major Prob Intern Med.* 1981;21:1–211.

26. Cupps TR, Fauci AS. The vasculitic syndromes. *Adv Intern Med.* 1982;27:315–344.

27. Daoud MS, Gibson LE, Daoud S, et al. Chronic hepatitis C and skin diseases: a review. *Mayo Clin Proc.* 1995;70: 559–564.

28. Daoud M, Gibson LE, Lutz ME, et al. Chronic hepatitis C, cryoglobulinemia, and cutaneous necrotizing vasculitis: clinical, pathologic, and immunopathologic study of twelve patients. *J Am Acad Dermatol.* 1996;34:219–223.

29. Daum TE, Specks U, Colby TV, et al. Tracheobronchial involvement in Wegener's granulomatosis. *Am J Respir Crit Care Med.* 1995;522–526.

30. Davidson B, Gardham R. Left retroperitoneal approach for inflammatory abdominal aortic aneurysms. *Surgery.* 1992;111:719–720.

31. Davis DJ, Moran JE, Niall JF, Ryan GB. Segmental necrotizing glomerulonephritis with antineutrophil antibody: possible arbovirus aetiology? *BMJ.* 1982;285:606.

32. Delecoeuillerie G, Joly P, Cohen de Lara A, et al. Polymyalgia rheumatica and temporal arteritis: a retrospective analysis of prognostic features and different corticosteroid regimens (11 year survey of 210 patients). *Ann Rheum Dis.* 1988;47:733–739.

33. Downs A, Lye C. Inflammatory abdominal aortic aneurysm. *Can J Surg.* 1986;29:50–53.

34. Drucker Y, Mathur RS. Clinical images: Wegener's granulomatosis of the lungs. *Arthritis Rheum.* 1996;39:615.

35. Duna GF, Galperin C, Hoffman GS. Wegener's granulomatosis. *Rheum Dis Clin North Am.* 1995;21:949–986.

36. Eichhorn J, Sima D, Lindschau C, et al. Antiendothelial cell antibodies in thromboangiitis obliterans. *Am J Med Sci.* 1998;315:17–23.

37. Falk R, Jeannette JC. Anti-neutrophil cytoplasmic antibodies with specificity for myeloperoxidase in patients with systemic vasculitis and idiopathic necrotizing and crescentic glomerulonephritis. *N Engl J Med.* 1988;318:1651–1657.

38. Fauci AS, Haynes B, Katz P. The spectrum of vasculitis: clinical pathologic, immunologic, and therapeutic considerations. *Ann Intern Med.* 1978;89:660–676.

39. Fauci AS, Haynes BF, Katz P. Wegener's granulomatosis: prospective clinical and therapeutic experience with 85 patients for 21 years. *Ann Intern Med.* 1983;98:76–85.

40. Ferraro G, Meroni PL, Tincani A, et al. Anti-endothelial cell antibodies in patients with Wegener's granulomatosis and micro-polyarteritis. *Clin Exp Immunol.* 1990;79:47–53.

41. Fiorani P, et al. Extraperitoneal approach for repair of inflammatory abdominal aortic aneurysm. *J Vasc Surg.* 1991;13:692–697.

42. Fitzgerald EJ, Blackett RL. 'Inflammatory' abdominal aortic aneurysms. *Clin Radiol.* 1988;39:247–251.

43. Fort JG, Griffin R, Tahmoush A, et al. Muscle involvement in polyarteritis nodosa: report of a patient presenting clinically as polymyositis and review of the literature. *J Rheumatol.* 1994;21:945–948.

44. Fortin PR, Larson MG, Watters AK, et al. Prognostic factors in systemic necrotizing vasculitis of the polyarteritis nodosa group: a review of 45 cases. *J Rheumatol.* 1995; 22:78–84.

45. Fox AD, Robbins SE. Aortic valvulitis complicating Wegener's granulomatosis. *Thorax.* 1994;49:1176–1177.

46. Fraioli P, Barberis M, Rizzato G, et al. Gastrointestinal presentation of Churg Strauss syndrome. *Sarcoidosis.* 1994; 11:42–45.

47. Gaylis H. Etiology of abdominal aortic "inflammatory" aneurysms: hypothesis [letter]. *J Vasc Surg.* 1985;2:643.

48. Gibson LE, Su WP. Cutaneous vasculitis. *Rheum Dis Clin North Am.* 1995;21:1097–1113.

49. Goeken JA. Antineutrophil cytoplasmic antibody: a useful serological marker for vasculitis. *J Clin Immunol.* 1991; 11:161–174.

50. Goodfield NE, Bhandari S, Plant WD, et al. Cardiac involvement in Wegener's granulomatosis. *Br Heart J.* 1995;73:110–115.

51. Grant SC, Levy RD, Venning MC, et al. Wegener's granulomatosis and the heart. *Br Heart J.* 1994;71:82–86.

52. Guillevin L, Le Thi Huong Du, Godeau P, et al. Clinical findings and prognosis of polyarteritis nodosa and Churg-Strauss angiitis: a study of 165 patients. *Br J Rheumatol.* 1988;27:258–264.

53. Guillevin L, Lhote F, Sauvaget F, et al. Treatment of polyarteritis nodosa related to HBV with interferon alpha and plasma exchanges: results in 6 patients. *Ann Rheum Dis.* 1994;53:334–337.

54. Guillevin L, Ronco P, Verroust P, et al. Circulating immune complexes in systemic necrotizing vasculitis of the polyarteritis nodosa group. Comparison of HBV-related polyarteritis nodosa and Churg Strauss angiitis. *J Autoimmun.* 1990;3:789–792.

55. Hall SH, Buchbinder R. Takayasu's arteritis. *Rheum Dis Clin North Am.* 1990;16:411–422.

56. Haller H, Eichhorn J, Pieper K, et al. Circulating leukocyte integrin expression in Wegener's granulomatosis. *J Am Soc Nephrol.* 1996;7:40–48.

57. Hedges AR, Bentley PG. Resection of inflammatory aneurysm after steroid therapy. *Br J Surg.* 1986;73:374.

58. Helander SD, De Castro FR, Gibson LE. Henoch-Schönlein purpura: clinico-pathologic correlation of cutaneous vascular IgA deposits and the relationship to leukocytoclastic vasculitis. *Acta Derm Venereol.* 1995;75:125–129.

59. Henriet JP, Marin J, Gosselin J, et al. The history of temporal arteritis or ten centuries of fascinating adventure. *J Mal Vasc.* 1989;14(suppl C):93–97.

60. Hill J, Charlesworth D. Inflammatory abdominal aortic aneurysms: a report of thirty-seven cases. *Ann Vasc Surg.* 1988;2:352–357.

61. Hoffman GS. Treatment of resistant Takayasu's arteritis. *Rheum Dis Clin North Am.* 1995;21:73–80.

62. Hoffman GS, Kerr GS, Leavitt RY, et al. Wegener granulomatosis: an analysis of 158 patients. *Ann Intern Med.* 1992;116:488–498.

63. Hoffman GS, Leavitt RY, Kerr GS, et al. The treatment of Wegener's granulomatosis with glucocorticoids and methotrexate. *Arthritis Rheum.* 1992;35:1322–1329.

64. Hotchi M. Pathology of Takayasu's arteritis. In: Tanabe T, ed. *Intractable Vasculitis.* Sapporo: Hokkaido University Press; 1993:85–92.

65. Hunder GG. Vasculitis: diagnosis and therapy. *Am J Med.* 1996;100(suppl 2A):37S–45S.

66. Hunder GG, Bloch DA, Michel BA, et al. The American College of Rheumatology 1990 criteria for the classification of giant cell arteritis. *Arthritis Rheum.* 1990;33: 1122–1128.

67. International Study Group for Behçet's Disease. Criteria for diagnosis of Behçet's disease. *Lancet.* 1990;335: 1078–1080.

68. James DG. Behçet's syndrome. *N Engl J Med.* 1979;301: 431–432.

69. James DG, Spiteri MA. Behçet's disease. *Ophthalmology.* 1982;89:1279–1284.

70. Jennette JC, Falk R. Antineutrophil cytoplasmic autoantibodies and associated diseases: a review. *Am J Kidney Dis.* 1990;15:517–529.

71. Jorizzo J. Classification of vasculitis. *J Invest Dermatol.* 1993; 100:106S.

72. Joyce JW. The giant cell arteritides: diagnosis and the role of surgery. *J Vasc Surg.* 1986;3:827–833.

73. Joyce JW. Buerger's disease (thromboangiitis obliterans). *Rheum Dis Clin N Am.* 1990;16:463–470.

74. Kabbaj N, Benjelloun G, Gueddari FZ, et al. Vascular involvements in Behcet disease: based on 40 patient records. *J Radiol.* 1993;74:649–656.

75. Kerr GS, Hallahan CW, Giordano J, et al. Takayasu's arteritis. *Ann Intern Med.* 1994;120:919–929.

76. Klein RG, Hunder GG, Stanson AW, et al. Large artery involvement in giant cell (temporal) arteritis. *Ann Intern Med.* 1975;83:806–812.

77. Koç Y, Gullu I, Akpek G, et al. Vascular involvement in Behçet's disease. *J Rheumatol.* 1992;19:402–410.

78. Koide K. Takayasu's arteritis in Japan. *Heart Vessels.* 1992; 7(suppl):48–54.

79. Koike S, Matsumoto K, Kokubo M. A case of aorto-enteric fistula after reconstruction of abdominal aortic aneurysm associated with Behçet's disease and reference to reported 95 cases in Japan. *Jpn J Surg.* 1988;89:945–951.

80. Krafcik SS, Covin RB, Lynch JP 3rd, et al. Wegener's granulomatosis in the elderly. *Chest.* 1996;109:430–437.

81. Lagneau P, Michel JB, Vuong BD. Surgical treatment of Takayasu's disease. *Ann Surg.* 1987;205:157–166.

82. Lawson TM, Williams BD. Silent myocardial infarction in Wegener's granulomatosis. *Br J Rheumatol.* 1996;35: 188–191.

83. Leavitt RY, Fauci AS. Polyangiitis overlap syndrome. *Am J Med.* 1986;81:79–85.

84. Leavitt RY, Fauci AS, Bloch DA, et al. The American College of Rheumatology 1990 criteria for the classification of

Wegener's granulomatosis. *Arthritis Rheum.* 1990;33: 1101–1107.

85. Lebovics RS, Hoffman GS, Leavitt RY, et al. The management of subglottic stenosis in patients with Wegener's granulomatosis. *Laryngoscope.* 1992;102:1341–1345.

86. Lhote F, Guillevin L. Polyarteritis nodosa, microscopic polyangiitis, and Churg-Strauss syndrome: clinical aspects and treatment. *Rheum Dis Clin North Am.* 1995;21: 911–947.

87. Lie J. Histopathologic specificity of systemic vasculitis. *Rheum Dis Clin North Am.* 1995;21:883–909.

88. Lightfoot RW, Michel BA, Bloch DA, et al. The American College of Rheumatology 1990 criteria for the classification of polyarteritis nodosa. *Arthritis Rheum.* 1990;33: 1088–1093.

89. Luqmani RA, Bacon PA, Beaman M, et al. Classical versus non-renal Wegener's granulomatosis. *Q J Med.* 1994;87: 161–167.

90. Mangelsdorf H, White WL, Jorizzo JL. Behcet's disease: report of twenty-five patients from the United States with prominent mucocutaneous involvement. *J Am Acad Dermatol.* 1996;34:745–750.

91. Marazzi R, Pareyson D, Boiardi A, et al. Peripheral nerve involvement in Churg-Strauss syndrome. *J Neurol.* 1992; 239:317–321.

92. Mark EJ, Matsubara O, Tan-Liu NS, et al. The pulmonary biopsy in the early diagnosis of Wegener's (pathergic) granulomatosis: a study based on 35 open lung biopsies. *Hum Pathol.* 1988;19:1065–1071.

93. McDonald TJ, DeRemee RA. Head and neck involvement in Wegener's granulomatosis (WG). *Adv Exp Med Biol.* 1993;336:309–313.

94. McDonnell PJ, Moore GW, Miller NR, et al. Temporal arteritis: a clinico-pathologic study. *Ophthalmology.* 1986;83: 518–530.

95. McDuffie FC, Sams WM Jr, Maldonado JE, et al. Hypocomplementemia with cutaneous vasculitis and arthritis: possible immune complex syndrome. *Mayo Clin Proc.* 1973; 48:340–348.

96. McKusick VA, Harris WS, Ottsen OE, et al. Buerger's disease: a distinct clinical and pathological entity. *JAMA.* 1962;181:5–12.

97. Metcalf RK, Rutherford RB. Inflammatory abdominal aortic aneurysm: an indication for the retroperitoneal approach [see comments]. *Surgery.* 1991;109:555–557.

98. Michel BA. Classification of vasculitis. *Curr Opin Rheumatol.* 1992;4:3–8.

99. Michel BA, Hunder GG, Bloch DA, et al. Hypersensitivity vasculitis and Henoch-Schönlein purpura: a comparison between the 2 disorders. *J Rheumatol.* 1992;19:721–728.

100. Mills JL, Porter JM. Buerger's disease. *Semin Vasc Surg.* 1993;6:14–23.

101. Moore PM. Neurological manifestation of vasculitis: update on immunopathogenic mechanisms and clinical features. *Ann Neurol.* 1995;37(suppl 1):S131–S141.

102. Moore PM, Calabrese L. Neurologic manifestations of systemic vasculitides. *Semin Neurol.* 1994;14:300–306.

103. Moore PM, Fauci AS: Neurologic manifestations of systemic necrotizing vasculitis: a retrospective and prospective analysis of the clinical pathologic features and re-

sponses to therapy in 25 patients. *Am J Med.* 1981; 71:517–524.

104. Naschitz JE, Yeshurun D, Eldar S, et al. Diagnosis of cancer-associated vascular disorders. *Cancer.* 1996;77: 1759–1767.

105. O'Donnell B, Black A. Urticarial vasculitis. *Int Angiol.* 1995;14:166–174.

106. Ohta T, Shionoya S. Fate of the ischemic limb in Buerger's disease. *Br J Surg.* 1988;75:259–262.

107. Olin JW. Thromboangiitis obliterans. *Curr Opin Rheum.* 1994;6:44–49.

108. Olin JW, Young JR, Graor RA, Ruschhaupt WF, Bartholomew JR. The changing clinical spectrum of thromboangiitis obliterans (Buerger's disease). *Circulation.* 1990;82:(suppl IV):IV3–IV8.

109. Papiha SS, Murty GE, Ad'Hia A, et al. Association of Wegener's granulomatosis with HLA antigens and other genetic markers. *Ann Rheum Dis.* 1992;51:246–248.

110. Parums DV. The arteritides. *Histopathology.* 1994;25:1–20.

111. Pennell R, Hollier L, Lie J, et al. Inflammatory abdominal aortic aneurysms: a thirty-year review. *J Vasc Surg.* 1985; 2:859–869.

112. Power WJ, Rodriguez A, Neves RA, et al. Disease relapse in patients with ocular manifestations of Wegener granulomatosis. *Ophthalmology.* 1995;102:154–160.

113. Radomski S, Ameli FM, Jewett MA. Inflammatory abdominal aortic aneurysms and ureteric obstruction. *Can J Surg.* 1990;33:49–52.

114. Reinhold KE, Kekow J, Schnabel A, et al. Effectiveness of cyclophosphamide pulse treatment in Wegener's granulomatosis. *Adv Exp Med Biol.* 1993;:483–486.

115. Robbs JV, Human RR, Rajaruthnam P, et al. Operative treatment of nonspecific aortoarteritis (Takayasu's arteritis). *J Vasc Surg.* 1986;3:605–616.

116. Said G. Peripheral neuropathy in polyarteritis nodosa. *Springer Semin Immunopathol.* 1996;18:75–84.

117. Sasaki S, Sakuma M, Kunihara T, et al. Efficacy of steroid therapy in treatment of the inflammatory abdominal aortic aneurysms. *Int J Angiol.* 1997;6:234–236.

118. Sasaki S, Yasuda K, Takigami K, et al. Inflammatory abdominal aneurysms and atherosclerotic abdominal aortic aneurysms: comparisons of clinical features and long-term results. *Jpn Circ J.* 1997;61:231–235.

119. Selke FW, Williams GB, Donovan DL, et al. Management of intraabdominal aneurysms associated with periarteritis nodosa. *J Vasc Surg.* 1986;4:294–298.

120. Shionoya S. Buerger's disease: diagnosis and management. *Cardiovasc Surg.* 1993;1:207–214.

121. Spiera RF, Filippa DA, Bains MS, et al. Esophageal involvement in Wegener's granulomatosis. *Arthritis Rheum.* 1994;37:1404–1407.

122. Stegeman CA, Cohen TJ, Kallengerg CG, et al. Trimethoprim-sulfamethoxazole (co-trimoxazole) for the prevention of relapses of Wegener's granulomatosis. Dutch Co-Trimoxazole Wegener Study Group. *N Engl J Med.* 1996; 335:16–20.

123. Sterpetti AV, Hunter WJ, Feldhaus RJ. Inflammatory aneurysms of the abdominal aorta: incidence, pathologic, and etiologic considerations. *J Vasc Surg.* 1989;9:643–649.

124. Szer IS. Henoch-Schönlein purpura. *Curr Opin Rheumatol.* 1994;6:25–31.

125. Tada, Y. Surgical treatment of intractable vasculitis syndromes: with special reference to Buerger disease, Takayasu arteritis, and so-called inflammatory abdominal aortic aneurysm. *Nippon Rinsho.* 1994;52:2192–2202.

126. Takayasu U. A case with unusual changes of the central vessels of the retina. *Acta Soc Ophthalmol Jpn.* 1908;12:554–563.

127. Travers RL, Allison DJ, Brettle RP, et al. Polyarteritis nodosa: a clinical angiographic analysis of 17 cases. *Semin Arthritis Rheum.* 1979;8:184–199.

128. Walker DI. Inflammatory aneurysms of the abdominal aorta. *Br J Surg.* 1972;59:609–619.

129. Weaver FA, Yellin AE, Campen DH, et al. Surgical procedures in the management of Takayasu's arteritis. *J Vasc Surg.* 1990;12:429–437.

130. Wees SJ, Sunwoo IN, Oh SJ. Sural nerve biopsy in systemic necrotizing vasculitis. *Am J Med.* 1981;71:525–532.

131. Wegener F. Über eine eigenartige rhinogene Granulomatose mit besonderer Beteiligung des arteriensystems und der Nieren. *Beitrage zur Pathologischen Anatomie und zur Allgemeinen Pathologie.* 1939; 102:36–68.

132. Yamana K, Kosuga K, Kinoshita H, et al. Vasculo-Behçet's disease: immunologic study of the formation of aneurysm. *J Cardiovasc Surg.* 1988;29:751–755.

133. Yazici H, Pazarli H, Barnes CG, et al. A controlled trial of azathioprine in Behçet's syndrome. *N Engl J Med.* 1990; 322:281–285.

134. Zeek PM, Smith C, Weeter J. Studies on periarteritis nodosa, III: the differentiation between the vascular lesions of periarteritis nodosa and of hypersensitivity. *Am J Pathol.* 1948;24:889–918.

135. Zeiss CR, Burch FX, Marder RJ, et al. A hypocomplementemic vasculitic urticarial syndrome: report of four new cases and definition of the disease. *Am J Med.* 1980; 68:867–875.

77

Occlusive Vascular Disease in Cancer

Jochanan E. Naschitz, Daniel Yeshurun, and Jack Abrahamson

Paraneoplastic disorders are complications of cancer that occur at a distance from the primary tumor or metastases and are induced by the cancer through hormones, immune globulins, or other humoral mediators.[1] In 1865 Trousseau was the first to report an increased incidence of venous thrombosis in patients with cancer. The venous thrombosis was often migratory, and the cancer was occult and difficult to diagnose.[2] A variety of paraneoplastic thromboembolic disorders, confined to veins, arteries, or both, have been described and termed *Trousseau's syndrome*.[3-6] Thrombosis is the most frequent complication of cancer and the second cause of death in patients with overt malignant disease.[7,8]

In recent years, new variants of Trousseau's syndrome have been described and added to the extraordinary pleomorphism of manifestations previously recognized in this disorder. The new variants are an accelerated course of peripheral vascular disease[9] and enhancement of ischemic heart disease by occult cancer.[10]

Thrombotic episodes may precede the diagnosis of cancer by months or years and thus represent a potential marker for occult malignancy.[2,3,11-16] However, the value of thrombosis as an indication for cancer has been disputed.[14-18] Clues that support the presence of occult neoplasia in thromboembolic disorders have been published.[19] The observation that abnormalities in the blood coagulation system are associated with malignant disease[20-24] led to investigations into the existence of procoagulants in neoplastic tissue. A cysteine proteinase procoagulant, called *cancer procoagulant (CP)*, has been identified in malignant but not normal cells.[25-28] Preliminary data suggest that the CP assay has potential as an aid in diagnosing early-stage malignancies and thereby may significantly improve the survival rate of cancer patients.[29-31]

Thromboembolism (TE) associated with cancer may be devastating but is infrequently so. Hence, the pace of the thromboembolic disorder should dictate the intensity of anticoagulant treatment in each case.[3-5,8] The validated strategy is to administer intravenous heparin. New therapies such as long-term administration of low molecular weight heparin or insertion of an umbrella into the inferior vena cava as a substitute for anticoagulant therapy are currently being evaluated.[32-35] Thrombotic side effects of anticancer therapy have been appreciable,[36-40] and anticoagulant management has been highly effective in their prevention.[40,41]

Finally, a direct pathogenetic role of clotting activation in the progression of malignancy has been repeatedly proposed based on studies with anticoagulation or fibrinolytic treatment in experimental animals, selected clinical malignancies, and genetically modified animal models.[42-44]

Pathophysiology

The clinical, histological, and pharmacological evidence associating clotting and cancer has been reviewed.[4,45-48] There is increasing awareness of cancer cells being involved not only in activation of blood coagulation but also in causing injury to the endothelial lining of blood vessels and activation of platelets. In the following sections we describe the threefold role of cancer cells in the causation of TE.

Tumor Interaction With the Vascular Endothelium

In 1972 Warren and Vales [49] studied tumor cell adhesion to vessel walls. Two patterns were described. In the first, platelet–tumor aggregates appeared around intact endothelium. Separation of endothelial cell intercellular junctions was observed and later attributed to a vascular permeability factor secreted by the tumor. This separation gives tumor cells access to a highly thrombogenic subendothelial surface. In the second type, in which the endothelial lining was mechanically injured before tumor injection, the malignant cells were embedded in a monolayer of platelets and fibrin adherent to the subendothelium. Both patterns indicate a complex interaction among tumor cells and the vascular endothelium, platelets, and the coagulation system. Recent observations documented the capacity of bloodborne tumor cells to adhere to the endothelial lining and to cause injury to the endothelial cells. Platelets, which aggregate around tumor cells through an intrinsic property of the tumor, are activated by the latter and release materials that cause additional damage to the endothelial cells and attract more platelets. Activation of coagulation at a distance by the cancer cells and in situ where the endothelial lining is denuded perpetuates the thrombosis.[45,47] The following functions of the endothelial cell may be of importance in the pathogenesis of paraneoplastic TE: production of anticoagulant and fibrinolytic factors; synthesis of prostacyclin, which has platelet anti-aggregant action; synthesis of endothelium-derived relaxing factor; and inactivation of serotonin and catecholamines. Removal of, or damage to, the endothelium, which would prevent the release of vasodilators, platelet antiaggregants, and anticoagulants, is a likely mechanism of vasospasm and thrombosis.[50-52]

Damaged Endothelial Lining of Arteries

Fissuring and rupture of atherosclerotic plaques and subsequent thrombosis in situ play a major role in acute ischemic syndromes.[53,54] If a coexistent disorder at a distance from the ruptured atherosclerotic plaque causes activation of platelets or the clotting cascade, the tendency of thrombus formation at the site of the plaque is enhanced.[54] This is illustrated by the effects of smoking, increased circulating catecholamines,[54] coagulation factors,[55,56] fibrinogen,[57,58] leukocytes, blood viscosity,[59] and autoimmune phenomena[60] on the course of ischemic heart disease. Precipitation of the ischemic coronary and peripheral vascular syndromes by cancer could be mediated by similar mechanisms.[10]

Platelet Activation by Cancer Cells

Thrombocytopenia, abnormal platelet functions, and evidence for in vivo activation of platelets have been reported to occur with increased frequency in patients with cancer. Of the mechanisms that have been proposed to explain the process of tumor cell–induced platelet aggregation, more experimental support is needed for those related to generation of thrombin. Tumor microvesicles may also play a role in the interaction of platelets, tumor cells, and vascular subendothelium.[46,61]

Activation of Clotting

Cleavage of fibrinogen into fibrin and fibrinopeptides is induced by cancer cells, either directly or through mediator cells (namely macrophages). Many types of neoplastic cells have membrane-bound tissue factor molecules. If these molecules are released into the circulation, they bind factor VII and initiate the extrinsic clotting pathway.[4,47] Tissue factor is also generated by mononuclear cells when the latter are activated by the tumor cells.[62] Activation of monocyte/macrophages may occur in patients with cancer because of stimulation by tumor-specific antigens, immune complexes, or proteases. The T cell has been shown to play a central role in regulating monocyte procoagulant generation.

Tumor cells produce a cysteine protease, called *cancer procoagulant*, that directly activates factor X to set off coagulation.[29-31] Additional tumor-associated procoagulants are a membrane glycoprotein that binds coagulation factor VII,[28] a poorly characterized factor found in the plasma of patients with non–small-cell lung cancer that was temporarily called thrombosis-inducing activity,[63] and tumor putative factor V receptor, a tumor membrane phospholipid that favors the assembly of the prothrombin complex.[64]

Hyperviscosity due to an increase in immunoglobulin levels or in cellular elements of the blood,[8] antiphospholipid antibodies in a minority of cancer patients (particularly with lymphoma[65]), cytokine release, acute phase reactants, and neovascularization may contribute to clotting activation in the general population[56] and particularly in cancer patients.[66]

Inadequacy of Natural Anticoagulant and Fibrinolytic Systems

Reduction of antithrombin III levels in cancer patients may be the result of increased intravascular generation of thrombin that leads to increased consumption of antithrombin III.[67] Increased inhibition of thrombin has been observed.[68] This may account for the failure of response to heparin treatment.

The level of thrombomodulin, a key cofactor of the protein C anticoagulant pathway, is decreased in some patients with cancer. Tumor necrosis factor leads to internalization and degradation of the thrombomodulin molecule[69] and thus could have a role in the pathogenesis of thrombosis.

Thromboembolic Risk Further Enhanced by Chemotherapy

The main mechanisms of thrombogenesis associated with chemotherapeutic agents are a toxic effect directed toward the vascular endothelium, release of procoagulants and cytokines from tumor cells damaged by cell-targeted treatment, and decrease of naturally occurring anticoagulants partially due to hepatotoxicity.[66,70]

Clinical Features and Their Basis

The consequences of the hemostatic disorders in cancer are various: disseminated intravascular coagulation, either subclinical or overt; thrombosis and embolism; platelet aggregation and dislodgment; vasospasm; and hemorrhage caused by consumption of clotting factors. The clinical pleomorphism of paraneoplastic TE results from the variable association of venous, arterial, small-vessel, and endocardial lesions.[3-6] The manifestations of Trousseau's syndrome include venous thrombosis (either localized or recurrent and migratory); nonbacterial thrombotic endocarditis, often in conjunction with arterial embolization (to cerebral, renal, mesenteric, splenic, or peripheral arteries); and arterial thrombosis.

Specific Clinical Events

Migratory superficial thrombophlebitis, an uncommon but characteristic finding in patients with cancer, may affect superficial veins in unusual sites such as the upper extremities or chest wall. It is most often associated with pancreatic or gastrointestinal cancer.[8,12,13]

Deep venous thrombosis is by far the most frequent thromboembolic complication of cancer. The diagnosis is often difficult: enlarged pelvic nodes may cause extrinsic compression of large veins with subsequent swelling of an extremity. Clinical examination cannot distinguish this situation from intrinsic occlusion of a vein.[71,72] Among the tests aimed at confirming the clinical suspicion of venous thrombosis, several invasive and noninvasive techniques (plethysmographic procedures, continuous wave Doppler ultrasound, blood-pool radionuclide venography) fail to distinguish pseudothrombophlebitis caused by compression of a vein from true venous thrombosis.[73,74] The advantages of B-mode ultrasonography and duplex scanning compared with other tests for the diagnosis of deep venous thrombosis are their high sensitivity and the concomitant imaging of the surrounding soft tissues. Tumoral masses in close relation to the major veins are readily revealed.[72,75] Because probe compression of the pelvic veins is not possible, those veins should be explored with the aid of a duplex or color Doppler instrument. Computed tomography with contrast media and magnetic resonance imaging also provide useful data in the diagnosis of soft tissue masses and venous clots.[76]

Pulmonary embolism in cancer patients needs to be distinguished from tumor embolism, a difficult task because the clinical background, presenting symptoms, laboratory values, and roentgenographic findings do not vary greatly between patients with thrombotic embolism and those with tumor embolism.[77]

Upper extremity vein thrombosis may be paraneoplastic in nature or may result from obstruction of the venous outflow by Pancoast's tumor or an axillary tumor. In addition, long-term use of indwelling central catheters and infusion of chemotherapeutic agents are associated with catheter-related mural thrombi. On postmortem examination the distribution of intraluminal lesions was 38% in catheterized central veins, 9.2% in contralateral veins, and 5.6% in the right atrium; 5.6% of individuals showed instances of nonbacterial thrombotic endocarditis.[78]

Superior vena cava syndrome is usually seen in cases of lung cancer or lymphoma that result in external compression of the superior vena cava, with or without thrombosis.[79] Current management stresses the importance of accurate diagnosis of the underlying etiology before treatment.

Inferior vena caval and intracardiac thromboses secondary to renal and adrenal tumors need to be distinguished from malignant renal or adrenal tumors that infiltrate along the caval lumen until they reach the right atrium.[80]

Hepatic vein thrombosis and portal vein thrombosis are most often seen in patients with myeloproliferative disorders[81] or lymphoma.[82]

Splanchnic vein thrombosis is an often unsuspected complication of cancer. Portal hypertension and variceal hemorrhage may be the presenting symptoms. Death cannot usually be attributed to splanchnic vein thrombosis alone.[83]

Retinal vein thrombosis is a rare manifestation of hypercoagulability associated with cancer.[84]

Paradoxical embolism often complicates unsuspected venous thrombosis. The high prevalence of silent venous thrombosis in cancer patients and the presence of patent foramen ovale in up to 35% of the general population suggest that paradoxical emboli may be the cause of peripheral thromboembolic occlusion and stroke more often than presently believed.[85]

Stroke in cancer patients has been considered to have a different spectrum from that of the general population. Most of the studies have been autopsy based. A recent study that addressed this issue from a clinical perspective concluded that stroke seems not to occur more frequently in adult oncological than in nononcological populations.[86]

Digital gangrene occasionally preceded by Raynaud's phenomenon is an infrequent paraneoplastic disorder.[87,88]

Microvascular arterial thrombosis is more often seen in patients with myeloproliferative disorders. Cerebral microvascular occlusion may result in nonspecific neurological symptoms such as headache or dizziness, whereas microvascular thrombosis of the digits may manifest as erythromelalgia.[89]

Acute disseminated intravascular coagulation manifesting as widespread thrombotic and/or bleeding lesions and a severe consumptive deficiency of platelets and clotting proteins is rare in cancer patients in general but common in patients with acute promyelocytic leukemia. In the latter, the disorder may intensify when chemotherapy is administered.[90]

Paraneoplastic vasculitis disorders are currently not listed among variants of Trousseau's syndrome. However, this exclusion might be artificial, because thrombosis and endothelial injury induced by cancer via humoral mediators are common to both entities.[91]

Nonbacterial thrombotic endocarditis is most often seen in patients with mucin-producing adenocarcinoma. Clinical manifestations are caused by systemic emboli.[92] Echocardiographic scrutiny reveals valvular vegetations in only a few patients. This finding is consistent with the variable size of the vegetations, from microscopic to several centimeters in diameter.[93] Multifocal small cerebral emboli may manifest as disorders of consciousness and may be confused with metabolic encephalopathy.[94] Multiple emboli to skeletal muscles may cause muscular pain and weakness, which may be confused with myositis.[95]

An accelerated course of peripheral vascular and ischemic heart disease has been reported in association with Trousseau's syndrome. The cancer-associated claudication was characterized by a more accelerated course and often required vascular surgery, and the lasting relief of claudication depended on the efficiency of cancer therapy. Ischemia progressed rapidly and frequently required vascular surgery for limb salvage and a high incidence of graft occlusion.[9] In another study, the hypothesis was tested that cancer, by virtue of being a thrombotic diathesis, may enhance ischemic heart disease. A statistically significant increase in coronary instability indices was observed in all groups of patients with cancer in the 2-year period before cancer diagnosis compared with control subjects. Patients with colorectal cancer had the highest indices in the 2 years preceding cancer diagnosis; the lowest indices among patients with cancer were recorded in those with prostatic and bladder cancer. Other possible etiologic factors, particularly the known coronary risk factors and anemia, were not statistically related to an increased risk of coronary events in the 2-year period prior to cancer diagnosis.[10]

Incidence

The incidence of clinical episodes of TE in patients with cancer has varied from 1% to 11%.[1] Mucin-secreting adenocarcinomas of the gastrointestinal tract most often have been reported to be associated with TE phenomena, but lung, breast, ovarian, and other tumors are also associated with them.[1,3] The incidence of TE increases during the course of chemotherapy[96-98]; in one series, every second patient had one or several episodes of TE.[6] Severe thrombotic complications may occur in the early phase following high-dose chemoradiotherapy and bone marrow transplantation.[99,100] During or immediately following L-asparaginase therapy especially, intracranial thromboembolic complications have been observed.[101,102] Thromboemboli are found most often on postmortem examination of patients who died of cancer.[103]

It has also been questioned whether the reverse association is present: is TE associated with an increased rate of occult malignancy? A prospective study of Olmsted County, Minnesota, residents failed to provide evidence of an association between venous TE and occult malignancy,[16] but three recent prospective studies have established such evidence.[104-106] The incidence of TE at first presentation of cancer is unknown. In the medical population from a regional hospital, the incidence of occult cancer among patients with venous, arterial, or arterial and venous TE was 11.9%.[107]

Diagnostic Tests

It would be diagnostically important if occult cancer could be predicted on the basis of thromboembolic complications, which may present as the initial clinical symptomatology. Deep venous thrombosis is associated with a significantly higher frequency of malignancy during the first 6 months after diagnosis. Malignancies can be found with simple clinical and diagnostic methods. Extensive screening of 1383 patients with deep venous thrombosis would have resulted in beneficial earlier diagnosis in only two patients.[106] Hence, solitary idiopathic lower limb thrombosis merits a search for cancer only if there are abnormalities on physical examination, blood count, erythrocyte sedimentation rate, or chest x-ray film.[15-18,106-109] A recent study defined the "clues suggesting the paraneoplastic nature" of a thromboembolic disorder. These factors are age older than 50 years, multiple sites of venous thrombosis, associated venous and arterial TE, TE resistant to warfarin therapy, or the presence of associated paraneoplastic syndromes.[19] These six criteria were prevalent in several series of patients with paraneoplastic TE.[48]

Coagulation tests play a limited role in the diagnosis of the paraneoplastic nature of a TE disorder. Ancillary coagulation tests and recent more sensitive assays merely demonstrate the presence of overactive coagulation. A prospective analysis of routine clotting tests in cancer patients[110,111] demonstrated that at diagnosis, before treatment, only 8% of patients had elevated fibrinogen/fibrin degradation product levels, 14% had abnormal prothrombin times, 36% had thrombocytosis, and 48% had elevated fibrinogen levels. Although the incidence of the same alterations rose as the disease progressed, the mean values 1 month prior to death were not statistically different from the mean values at the time of entry into the study.[112,113] Sensitive tests for the detection of the hypercoagulable state in cancer are now available[114]:

1. Assays for detecting by-products of clotting reactions have become established means of identification of activation of blood coagulation. They include sensitive and specific assays for fibrinogen/fibrin derivatives (D-dimer, fibrinopeptide A, fibrin fragment Bfl), assays for the detection of activated peptides (prothrombin fragments 1 and 2, the protein C activation peptide), and assays for proteinase-inhibitor complexes (thrombin–antithrombin III complex).
2. Measurement of the proteins of the fibrinolytic system include the platelet survival test, spontaneous platelet aggregation, release of platelet factor 4 and β-thromboglobulin, and measurement of specific glycoproteins on the platelet membrane for the detection of activated platelets in vivo.
3. Measurement of proteins of the fibrinolytic system include plasminogen, antiplasmins, plasmin–antiplasmin complexes, and plasminogen activator inhibitors.
4. Measurement of the physiological coagulation inhibitors include antithrombin III, protein C, and protein S.

Studies utilizing one or more of these new tests suggest that virtually all patients with leukemia or solid tumors have laboratory signs of clotting activation prior to therapy.[113] The new coagulation tests might permit evaluation of the individual risk to develop thromboembolic events following cancer surgery.[114,115] Studies of plasma levels of D-dimer and fibrinopeptide A have indicated a possible use of these tests as markers of disease progression and response to therapy.[113,116]

Although there have been many advances in characterization and clinical applications of tumor markers, their clinical impact has been limited because the current markers do not detect early-stage disease. Cancer is potentially curable if discovered while the tumor burden is small and before metastasis occurs. Preliminary data with an antigen specific to tumor tissue, the "cancer procoagulant" (CP), suggests its possible role as a tumor marker and the ability to detect early-stage cancer.[1,30] The sensitivity for all samples analyzed from cancer patients was 80%, and the specificity was 83% for those with benign disease and 82% for those without cancer. The test was able to detect ovarian, colon, and kidney cancer at a sensitivity greater than 85% and stage I, II, and III small-cell lung carcinoma in 100% of samples. The CP assay did not perform as well for leukemia. Early-stage cancers were detected effectively regardless of site.

Sensitivity decreased as the stage of cancer progressed, which suggests that there was an anti-CP immunoglobulin G (IgG) with the forming of a CP–IgG complex.[29] Hence, screening patients with TE for the presence of CP could significantly affect early-stage diagnosis of malignant disease.

Medical Treatment and Invasive Endovascular Treatment

Sack et al.[3] found definite improvement of TE in 65% of patients treated with heparin but in only 19% of those treated with warfarin. Thirty-three percent of patients who experienced no improvement in their condition with warfarin treatment had a positive response to heparin therapy. Recurrence of TE after discontinuation of heparin therapy (in 53% of patients) also supports the role of heparin treatment in the control of paraneoplastic TE. Heparin treatment has also been effective in abolition of the chemotherapy-induced hypercoagulable state.[117]

In clinical practice it is important to establish the tempo of the disseminated intravascular coagulation.[1] If the latter is acute and life-threatening or chronic but debilitating, the validated strategy is to administer intravenous heparin; once heparin treatment has been started, repletion of platelets and coagulation factors is possible.[1,3-5] Intensive treatment of the cancer is vital in the care of patients with paraneoplastic TE. Response of the malignancy to treatment is often associated with regression of disseminated intravascular coagulation.[3-5]

The observation that therapy with warfarin is usually ineffective in patients with paraneoplastic TE[3,5] has been challenged. A suitable strategy[8] is based on administering heparin for 5 to 7 days followed by warfarin to maintain the international normalized ratio between 2.0 and 3.0 as long as the cancer is active. Maintenance of drug levels within the therapeutic range permits the safe use of anticoagulants even in patients with central nervous system metastases.[118] Recently, low molecular weight heparin has been introduced in the treatment of TE in general and in patients with cancer in particular; its use has resulted in significantly fewer bleeding complications and reduced mortality rates.[32,33] If low molecular weight heparin could replace standard heparin, many patients with TE could be treated at home.[119]

In recent years, the placement of a Greenfield filter in the inferior vena cava has been proposed as an alternative to heparin treatment in patients with cancer who have proximal vein thrombosis or pulmonary embolism. Although only nonrandomized studies addressing this method have been published, the results show that placement of a caval filter is as safe as anticoagulation for this particular group of patients.[34,35,118,120] Newer treatments include fibrinolytics and interventional radiologic techniques. Chemotherapy-induced veno-occlusive disease of the liver was successfully treated with intravenous urokinase,[82] and superior vena cava syndrome caused by mediastinal lymphoma was successfully treated by placement of expandable stents.[79] The use of ε-aminocaproic acid may be dangerous and is not indicated in patients with paraneoplastic TE.[121]

Primary prevention of TE in cancer patients during the time of increased risk associated with cancer therapy is achieved with various regimens. Hospitalized patients on bed rest or undergoing surgery are usually administered subcutaneous heparin and wear gradient-deterrent or pulsatile stockings.[8] Low molecular weight heparins[122,123] were effective in the prevention of postoperative TE in cancer patients. Long-term administration of very-low-dose warfarin was safe and effective for prevention of TE in patients with metastatic breast cancer.[124] The clinical relevance of the latter observation, if further confirmed, could be remarkable.

The multitude of classic manifestations of paraneoplastic TE is extended by recognition of new categories. That unexplained TE may serve as a hint for the presence of a hidden tumor may gain importance by testing the patients' sera for CP, an evolving test for early-stage cancer. Novel approaches for prevention of paraneoplastic TE at periods of elevated risk and for treatment of established TE have been proposed.

References

1. Bunn PA Jr. Paraneoplastic syndromes. In: DeVita VT Jr, Hellman S, Rosenberg SA, eds. *Cancer: Principles and Practice of Oncology.* Philadelphia, Pa: JB Lippincott; 1982; 1476–1517.

2. Trousseau A. *Phlegmasia Alba Dolens. Clinique Medicale de l'Hotel-Dieu de Paris.* Vol 3. London: New Sydenham Society; 1865:695–727.

3. Sack GH Jr, Levin J, Bell WR. Trousseau's syndrome and other manifestations of chronic disseminated coagulopathy in patients with neoplasms: clinical, pathophysiologic, and therapeutic features. *Medicine (Baltimore).* 1977; 56:1–37.

4. Rickles FR, Edward RL, Barb C, Cronlund M. Abnormalities of blood coagulation in patients with cancer. *Cancer.* 1983;51:301–307.

5. Bell WR, Starksen NF, Portfield JK. Trousseau's syndrome: devastating coagulopathy in the absence of heparin. *Am J Med.* 1985;79:423–430.

6. Goldsmith GH Jr. Hemostatic disorders associated with neoplasia. In: Forbes CD, Ratnoff OD, eds. *Disorders of Hemostasis.* Philadelphia, Pa: Grune & Stratton; 1984: 351–366.

7. Donati MB. Cancer and thrombosis. *Haemostasis.* 1994; 24:128–131.

8. Bona RD, Dhami MS. Thrombosis in patients with cancer. *Postgrad Med.* 1993;93:131–140.

9. Naschitz JE, Schechter L, Chang JB. Intermittent claudication associated with cancer: case studies. *Angiology.* 1987; 9:696–704.

10. Naschitz JE, Yeshurun D, Abrahamson J, et al. Ischemic heart disease precipitated by occult cancer. *Cancer.* 1992; 69:2712–2720.

11. Edwards EA. Migratory thrombophlebitis associated with carcinoma. *N Engl J Med.* 1949;240:1031–1034.

12. Lieberman JS, Borrero J, Urrdeaneta E, Wright IS. Thrombophlebitis and cancer. *JAMA.* 1961;177:542–545.

13. Nussbacher J. Migratory venous thrombosis of legs. *N Y State J Med.* 1964;64:2166–2173.

14. Gore JM, Appelbaum JS, Greene HL, Dexter L, Dalen JE. Occult cancer in patients with deep venous thrombosis. *Arch Intern Med.* 1987;147:556–560.

15. Goldberg RJ, Seneff M, Gore JM. Occult malignant neoplasm in patients with deep venous thrombosis. *Arch Intern Med.* 1987;147:251–253.

16. Griffin MR, Stanson AW, Brown ML, et al. Deep venous thrombosis and pulmonary embolism: risk of subsequent malignant neoplasia. *Arch Intern Med.* 1987;147: 1907–1911.

17. Kakkar VV, Howe CT, Nicolaides AN, Renny JTG, Clarke MB. Deep vein thrombosis of legs: is there a high-risk population? *Am J Surg.* 1970;120:527–530.

18. O'Connor NTJ, Cederholm-Williams SA, Fletcher EW, Allington M, Sharp AA. Significance of idiopathic deep venous thrombosis. *Postgrad Med.* 1984;60:275–277.

19. Naschitz JE, Yeshurun D, Abrahamson J. Thromboembolism: clues for the presence of occult neoplasia. *Int Angiol.* 1989;8:200–205.

20. Francis JL. Haemostasis and cancer. *Med Lab Sci.* 1989; 46:331–346.

21. Messmore H, Nand S. Hemostasis in malignancy. *Am J Hematol.* 1990;35:45–55.

22. Edwards RL, Rickles FR. Activation of blood coagulation in cancer: Trousseau's syndrome revisited. *Blood.* 1983; 62:14–31.

23. Gore JM, Appelbaum JS, Greene HL, Dexter JE. Occult cancer in patients with acute pulmonary embolism. *Ann Intern Med.* 1982;96:556–560.

24. Helin H. Macrophage procoagulant factors: mediators of inflammatory and neoplastic tissue lesions. *Med Biol.* 1986;64:167–176.

25. Pacchiarini L, Melloni F, Zucchella M, et al. Proaggregating and procoagulant activities of human mesothelioma tumor cells at different stages of "in vitro" culture. *Haematologica.* 1991;76:392–397.

26. Grignani G, Jamieson GA. Platelets in tumor metastasis: generation of adenosine diphosphate by tumor cells is specific but unrelated to metastatic potential. *Blood.* 1988; 71:855–849.

27. Grignani G, Pacchiarini L, Ricetti MM, et al. Mechanisms of platelet activation by cultured human cancer cells and cells freshly isolated from tumor tissues. *Invasion Metastasis.* 1989;9:298–309.

28. Zucchella M, Dezza L, Pacchiarini L, et al. Human tumor cells cultured "in vitro" activate platelet functions by producing ADP or thrombin. *Haematologica.* 1989;74:541–545.

29. Kozwich DL, Kramer LC, Mielicki WP, Fotopulos SS, Gor-

don SG. Application of cancer procoagulant as an early detection tumor marker. *Cancer.* 1994;74:1367–1376.

30. Cross BA, Gordon SG. An enzyme-linked immunosorbent assay for cancer procoagulant and its potential as a new tumor marker. *Cancer Res.* 1990;50:6229–6234.

31. Benson BA, Gordon SG. Analysis of serum cancer procoagulant activity and its possible use as a tumor marker. *Thromb Res.* 1989;56:431–440.

32. Hull RD, Rascob GE, Pineo GF, Green D, Trowbridge AA, Elliott CG. A randomized double-blind trial of low-molecular-weight heparin in the initial treatment of proximal vein thrombosis. *Thromb Haemost.* 1991;65(suppl):872–879.

33. Prandoni P, Lensing AWA, Buller HR, et al. Comparison of subcutaneous low-molecular-weight heparin with intravenous standard heparin in proximal vein thrombosis. *Lancet.* 1992;339:441–445.

34. Calligaro KD, Bergen WS, Haut MJ, Savares RP, Laurentis DA. Thromboembolic complications in patients with advanced cancer: anticoagulation versus Greenfield filter placement. *Ann Vasc Surg.* 1991;5:186–189.

35. Cohen JR, Tenenbaum N, Citron M. Greenfield filter as primary therapy of deep venous thrombosis and/or pulmonary embolism in patients with cancer. *Surgery.* 1991;109:12–15.

36. Rickles FR, Levine MN, Edwards RI. Hemostatic alterations in cancer patients. *Cancer Metastasis Rev.* 1992; 11:237–248.

37. Levine MN, Gent M, Hirsh J, et al. The thrombogenic effect of anti-cancer drug therapy in women with stage II breast cancer. *N Engl J Med.* 1988;318:404–407.

38. Barbui T, Finazzi G, Donati MB, Falanga A. Antiblastic therapy and thrombosis. In: *Thrombosis: An Update.* Florence: Scientific Press; 1992:305–314.

39. Rahr HB, Sorensen JV. Venous thromboembolism and cancer. *Blood Coagul Fibrinolysis.* 1992;3:451–460.

40. Shapiro AD, Clarke SL, Christian JM, Odom LF, Hatheway WE. Thrombosis in children receiving L-asparaginase: determining patients at risk. *Am J Pediatr Hematol Oncol.* 1993;15:400–405.

41. Levine M, Hirsh J, Gent M, et al. Double-blind randomised trial of very-low-dose warfarin for prevention of thromboembolism in stage IV breast cancer. *Lancet.* 1994;343:886–889.

42. Poggi A, Stella M, Donati MB. The importance of blood cell–vessel wall interactions in tumor metastasis. *Baillieres Clin Haematol.* 1993;6:731–752.

43. Zacharski RL, Donati MB, Rickles FR. Registry of clinical trials of antithrombotic drugs in cancer: second report. *Thromb Haemost.* 1993;70:357–360.

44. Poggi A, Blielli E, Castelli MP. Fibrinolysis and metastasis: the role of plasminogen activator inhibitor-1 (PAI-1) in a model of transgenic mice [abstract]. *Thromb Haemost.* 1993;69:775.

45. Al-Mondhiry H, McGarvey V. Tumor interaction with vascular endothelium. *Haemostasis.* 1987;17:245–253.

46. Bastida E, Ordinas A. Platelet contribution to the formation of metastatic foci: the role of cancer cell–induced platelet activation. *Haemostasis.* 1988;18:29–36.

47. Moake JL. Hypercoagulable states. *Adv Intern Med.* 1990;35:235–248.

48. Naschitz JE, Yeshurun D, Lev LM. Thromboembolism in cancer: changing trends. *Cancer.* 1993;71:1384–1390.

49. Vales O, Warren B. The adhesion of thromboplastic tumor emboli to vessel wall in vitro. *Br J Exp Pathol.* 1972;53:301–313.

50. Higgs EA, Moncada S. Prostacyclin: physiology and clinical uses. *Gen Pharmacol.* 1983;14:7–11.

51. Mendelsohn ME, Loscalzo JL. The endotheliopathies. In: Loscalzo JL, Creager MA, Dzau VJ, eds. *Vascular Medicine: A Textbook of Vascular Biology and Diseases.* Boston, Mass: Little, Brown; 1992:279–305.

52. Conger JD. Endothelial regulation of vascular tone. *Hosp Pract.* 1994:117–126.

53. Falk E. Plaque rupture with severe pre-existing stenosis precipitating coronary thrombosis: characteristics of coronary atherosclerotic plaques underlying fatal occlusive thrombi. *Br Heart J.* 1985;53:127–132.

54. Fuster V, Badimon L, Cohen M, Ambrose JA, Badimon JJ, Chesebro J. Insights into the pathogenesis of acute ischemic syndromes. *Circulation.* 1988;77:1213–1220.

55. Balleisen L, Schulte H, Assman G, Epping PH, Van De Loo J. Coagulation factors and the progress of coronary heart disease. *Lancet.* 1987;1:462–467.

56. Hamsten A. Hemostatic function and coronary artery disease. *N Engl J Med.* 1995;332:677–678.

57. Meade TW, Mellows S, Brozovic M, et al. Haemostatic function and ischemic heart disease: principle results of the Northwick Park Health Study. *Lancet.* 1986;2:533–537.

58. Wilhelmsen L, Svardsud K, Korsan-Bengsten K, Larsson B, Tibblin G. Fibrinogen as a cardiovascular risk factor for stroke and myocardial infarction. *N Engl J Med.* 1984;311:501–505.

59. Yarnell JWG, Baker JA, Sweetnam PM, Bainton O, O'Brien JR, Whitehead PJ. Fibrinogen, viscosity, and white blood cell count are major risk factors for ischemic heart disease. *Circulation.* 1991;83:836–844.

60. Wissler RW. Update on the pathogenesis of atherosclerosis. *Am J Med.* 1991;9(suppl):3–9.

61. Gasic GJ, Catalfamo JL, Gasic TB, Advalovic N. In vitro mechanism of platelet aggregation by purified plasma membrane vesicles shed by mouse 15091 A tumor cells. In: Donati I, ed. *Malignancy and the Haemostatic System.* New York, NY: Raven Press; 1981:27–33.

62. Edwards RL, Rickles FR, Cronlund M. Abnormalities of blood coagulation in patients with cancer: mononuclear cell tissue factor generation. *J Lab Clin Med.* 1981;98:917–928.

63. Maruyama M, Yagawa K, Hayashi S, et al. Presence of thrombosis-inducing activity in plasma from patients with lung cancer. *Am Rev Resp Dis.* 1989;140:778–781.

64. Van de Water L, Tracy PB, Aranson D, Mann KG, Dvorak F. Tumor cell generation of thrombin via prothrombinase assembly. *Cancer Res.* 1985;45:5521–5525.

65. Hill VA, Whittaker SJ, Hunt BJ, Liddell K, Spittle MF, Smith NP. Cutaneous necrosis associated with antiphospholipid syndrome and mycosis fungoides. *Br J Dermatol.* 1994;130:92–96.

66. Donati MB. Cancer and thrombosis. *Haemostasis.* 1994;24:128–131.

67. Damus PS, Wallace GA. Immunologic measurement of antithrombin III, heparin cofactor, and alpha-2 macroglobu-

lin in disseminated intravascular coagulation and hepatic failure coagulopathy. *Thromb Res.* 1976;5:27–38.

68. Falanga A, Ofosu FA, Cortelazzo S, et al. Preliminary study to identify cancer patients at risk of venous thrombosis following major surgery. *Br J Haematol.* 1993;85:745–750.

69. Moore KL, Esmon CT, Esmon H. Tumor necrosis factor leads to internalization and degradation of thrombomodulin from the surface of bovine aortic endothelial cells in culture. *Blood.* 1989;73:159–165.

70. Nachman RL, Silverstein R. Hypercoagulable states. *Ann Intern Med.* 1993;119:819–827.

71. Katherdahl DA. Calf pain mimicking thrombophlebitis. *Postgrad Med J.* 1980;68:107–115.

72. Naschitz JE, Yeshurun D, Gaitini D. Deep venous leg thrombosis and its differential diagnosis: the case for B-mode ultrasonography. *International Journal of Angiology.* 1993;1:218–224.

73. Zorba J, Schrier D, Posmituck G. Clinical value of blood pool radionuclide venography. *AJR AM J Roentgenol.* 1985;146:1051–1055.

74. Koopman MMW, Beek EJR, ten Cate JW. Diagnosis of deep vein thrombosis. *Prog Cardivasc Dis.* 1994;37:1–12.

75. Cronan JJ. Ultrasound evaluation of deep venous thrombosis. *Semin Roentgenol.* 1992;27:39–52.

76. Evans AJ, Sostman HD, Knelson MH, et al. Detection of deep venous thrombosis: prospective comparison of MR imaging with contrast venography. *AJR Am J Roentgenol.* 1993;161:131–139.

77. Goldhaber CZ, Dricker E, Buring JE, et al. Clinical suspicion of autopsy-proven thrombotic and tumor embolism in cancer patients. *Am Heart J.* 1987;114:1432–1436.

78. Raad II, Luna M, Khalil AM, Costerton JW, Lam C, Bodey GP. The relationship between the thrombotic and infectious complications of central venous catheters. *JAMA.* 1994;271:1014–1016.

79. Escalante CP. Causes and management of superior vena cava syndrome. *Oncology (Huntingt).* 1993;7:61–68.

80. Galli R, Parlapiano M, Pace Napoleone C, Pierangelli A. Neoplastic caval and intracardiac thrombosis secondary to reno-adrenal tumors: one-stage surgical treatment in deep hypothermia and cardiocirculatory arrest. *Minerva Urol Nephrol.* 1994;46:105–111.

81. Mitchell MC, Boitnott JK, Kaufman S, Cameron JL, Maddrey WC. Budd-Chiari syndrome: etiology, diagnosis, and management. *Medicine (Baltimore).* 1982;61:199–218.

82. Fogteloo AJ, Smid WM, Kok T, Van-Der-Meer J, Van-Imhoff GW, Daenen S. Successful treatment of veno-occlusive disease of the liver with urokinase in a patient with non-Hodgkin lymphoma. *Leukemia.* 1993;7:760–763.

83. Gollin G, Ward B, Meier GH, Sumpio BE, Gusberg RJ. Central splanchnic vein thrombosis: often unsuspected, usually uncomplicated. *J Clin Gastroenterol.* 1994;18:109–113.

84. Ronchetto F. Occlusion of a branch of the central retinal vein as a manifestation of hypercoagulability in a patient with lung cancer: a possible paraneoplastic event. *Recenti Prog Med.* 1994;85:108–112.

85. Chaikoff EL, Campbell BE, Smith RB 3d. Paradoxical embolism and acute arterial occlusion: rare or unsuspected? *J Vasc Surg.* 1994;20:377–384.

86. Chaturvedi S, Ansell J, Recht L. Should cerebral ischemic events in cancer patients be considered a manifestation of hypercoagulability? *Stroke.* 1994;25:1215–1218.

87. DeCross AJ, Sahasrabudhe DM. Paraneoplastic Raynaud's phenomenon. *Am J Med.* 1992;92:570–572.

88. Taylor LM, Hauty MG, Edwards JM. Digital ischemia as a manifestation of malignancy. *Ann Surg.* 1983;206:62–68.

89. Kurzrock R, Cohen PR. Erythromelalgia and myeloproliferative disorders. *Arch Intern Med.* 1989;149:105–109.

90. Tallman MS, Hakimian D, Kwaan HC, Rickles FR. New insights into the pathogenesis of coagulation dysfunction in acute promyelocytic leukemia. *Leuk Lymphoma.* 1993;11:27–36.

91. Naschitz JE, Rosner I, Rozenbaum M, Eilas N, Yeshurun D. Cancer-associated rheumatic disorders: clues to occult neoplasia. *Semin Arthritis Rheum.* 1995;24:231–241.

92. Min KW, Gyorkey F, Sato C. Mucin-producing adenocarcinomas and nonbacterial thrombotic endocarditis: pathogenetic role of tumor mucin. *Cancer.* 1980;45:2374–2382.

93. Lopez JA, Ross RS, Fishbein MC, Siegel R. Nonbacterial thrombotic endocarditis: a review. *Am Heart J.* 1987;113:773–780.

94. Collins RC, Al-Mondhiri H, Chernik NL. Neurologic manifestations of intravascular coagulation in cancer: a clinicopathologic analysis of 12 cases. *Neurology.* 1975;25:795–805.

95. Heffner RR Jr. Myopathy of embolic origin in patients with carcinoma. *Neurology.* 1971;21:840–843.

96. Weiss B, Tormey DC, Holland JF, Weinberg VE. Venous thrombosis during multimodal treatment of primary breast carcinoma. *Cancer Treat Rep.* 1981;65:677–679.

97. Levine MN, Gent M, Hirsh J. The thrombogenic effect of anticancer drug therapy in women with stage II breast cancer. *N Engl J Med.* 1988;318:404–408.

98. Clahsen PC, van-de-Velde CJ, Julien JP, Floiras JL, Mignolet FY. Thromboembolic complications after perioperative chemotherapy in women with early breast cancer: a European Organization for Research and Treatment of Cancer, Breast Cancer Cooperative Study Group Study. *J Clin Oncol.* 1994;12:1266–1271.

99. Catani L, Gugliotta L, Mattioli Belmonte M, et al. Hypercoagulability in patients undergoing autologous or allogeneic BMT for hematological malignancies. *Bone Marrow Transplant.* 1993;12:253–259.

100. Faioni EM, Krachmalnicoff A, Bearman SI, et al. Naturally occurring anticoagulants and bone marrow transplantation: plasma protein C predicts the development of venoclusive disease of the liver. *Blood.* 1993;81:3458–3462.

101. Fleischhack G, Solymosi L, Reiter A, Bender Gotze C, Eberl W, Bode U. Imaging methods in diagnosis of cerebrovascular complications with L-asparaginase therapy. *Klin Pediatr.* 1994;206:334–341.

102. Shapiro AD, Clarke SL, Christian JM, Odom LF, Hatheway WE. Thrombosis in children receiving L-asparaginase: determining patients at risk. *Am J Pediatr Hematol Oncol.* 1993;15:400–405.

103. Ambrus JL, Ambrus CM, Mink IB, Pickren JW. Causes of death in patients with cancer. *J Med.* 1975;6:61–64.

104. Aderka D, Brown A, Zelikovski A, Pinkhas J. Idiopathic deep vein thrombosis in an apparently healthy patient as

a premonitory sign of occult cancer. *Cancer.* 1986;57: 1846–1849.

105. Prandoni P, Lensing AWA, Buller HR, et al. Deep-vein thrombosis and the incidence of subsequent symptomatic cancer. *N Engl J Med.* 1992;327:1128–1233.

106. Nordstrom M, Lindblad B, Anderson H, Bergquist D, Kjellstrom T. Deep venous thrombosis and occult malignancy: an epidemiological study. *BMJ.* 1994;308:891–894.

107. Naschitz JE, Yeshurun D, Abrahamson J. Incidence and diagnostic significance of paraneoplastic thromboembolic disorders. *Int Angiol.* 1989;8:28–31.

108. McKenna MT. Deep venous thrombosis and the risk of cancer. *Arch Intern Med.* 1989;149:966–967.

109. O'Connor N. Venous thrombosis and cancer [letter]. *N Engl J Med.* 1993;328:886–889.

110. Zacharski LR, Henderson WG, Rickles FR, et al. Effect of warfarin on survival in carcinoma of the lung, colon, head and neck, and prostate. *Cancer.* 1984;53:2046–2052.

111. Zacharski LR, Moritz TE, Baczek LA, et al. Effect of Mopidamol on survival of carcinoma of the lung and colon: final report of Veterans Administration Cooperative Study No 188. *J Natl Cancer Inst.* 1988;80:90–97.

112. Edwards RL, Rickles FR, Moritz TE, et al. Abnormalities of blood coagulation tests in patients with cancer. *Am J Clin Pathol.* 1987;88:596–602.

113. Rickles FR, Levine MN, Edwards RL. Hemostatic alterations in cancer patients. *Cancer Metastasis Rev.* 1992;1: 241–260.

114. Falanga A, Barbui T, Rickles FR, Levine MN. Guidelines for clotting studies in cancer patients. *Thromb Haemost.* 1993;70:540–542.

115. Falanga A, Ofosu FA, Cortelazzo S, et al. Preliminary study to identify cancer patients at risk of venous thrombosis following major surgery. *Br J Haematol.* 1993;85: 745–750.

116. Gaddiucci A, Baicchi U, del Bravo B, Marrai R, Vispi M, Fioretti P. The assessment of the hemostasis system in patients with ovarian and cervical carcinoma. *Cancer.* 1991; 4:183–187.

117. Edwards RL, Klaus M, Matthews E, McCullen C, Bona RD, Rickles FR. Heparin abolishes the chemotherapy-induced increase in plasma fibrinopeptide A levels. *Am J Med.* 1990;89:25–38.

118. Schiff D, DeAngelis LM. Therapy of venous thromboembolism in patients with brain metastases. *Cancer.* 1994;73: 493–498.

119. Hirsh J, Levine MN. Low-molecular-weight heparin. *Blood.* 1992;79:1–17.

120. Hubbard KP, Roehm JO Jr, Abbruzzese JL. The bird's nest filter (1194): an alternative to long term oral anticoagulation in patients with advanced malignancies. *Am J Clin Oncol.* 1997;17:115–117.

121. Kazmler FJ, Bowle EJW, Hagedorn AB, Owen CA. Treatment of intravascular coagulation and fibrinolysis syndrome. *Mayo Clin Proc.* 1974;49:665–672.

122. Gallus A, Cade J, Ockelford P, et al. Organon (Org 10172) or heparin for the prevention of venous thrombosis after elective surgery for malignant disease? A double-blind, randomized, multicentre comparison. ANZ-Organon Investigators' Group. *Thromb Haemost.* 1993;70: 562–567.

123. Marassi A, Balzano G, Mari G, et al. Prevention of postoperative deep vein thrombosis in cancer patients: a randomized trial with low molecular weight heparin (CY 216). *Int Surg.* 1993;78:166–170.

124. Levine M, Hirsh J, Gent M, et al. Double-blind randomised trial of very-low-dose warfarin for prevention of thromboembolism in stage IV breast cancer. *Lancet.* 1994; 343:886–889.

78

Behçet's Disease

Hiroshi Inada and Tatsuki Katsumura

Behçet's disease is an inflammatory disease that affects multiple organs. It is an intractable disease that shows remission and regression alternately over the long term. It occurs frequently in southern Europe, the Middle East, China, and Japan. In Japan in 1991 it was estimated that 18,300 patients were affected by the disease (14.9 per 100,000 population), and the male to female ratio was 1:0.96.[1]

Genetic, immunological, bacterial, and environmental factors have been proposed as causative agents for Behçet's disease. According to several studies, an increased incidence of HLA-B51 and an abnormality of $\gamma\delta$ +T cells have been observed in Behçet's disease patients, but its etiology is not yet definite.[1,2]

In the clinical manifestation, there are four major symptoms: recurrent oral aphtosis, skin lesions (e.g., erythema nodosum, pseudofolliculitis, papulopustular lesions, acneiform nodules, and superficial thrombophlebitis), eye lesions (e.g., anterior uveitis, posterior uveitis, and retinal vasculitis), and recurrent genital ulcers. Arthritis, epididymitis, gastrointestinal lesions (e.g., ulcers of the terminal ileum and cecum), neurological lesions, and cardiovascular lesions are proposed as minor symptoms.

Various diagnostic criteria had been proposed in each country, but international diagnostic criteria were suggested by the International Study Group for Behçet's Disease in 1990 (Table 78.1).[3]

The frequency of major symptoms is as follows: oral aphtosis, 94.0%; skin lesions, 80.6%; eye lesions, 60.8%; and genital ulcers, 64.6%. The frequency of minor symptoms is as follows: arthritis, 51.2%; gastrointestinal lesions, 12.4%; epididymitis, 5.0%; vascular lesions, 6.6%; and neurological lesions, 10.1%.[4] Major symptoms occur frequently and may cause serious organ dysfunction, but minor symptoms, such as gastrointestinal, vascular, and neurological lesions, may be fatal. In the following section we discuss vascular involvement in Behçet's disease (i.e., vascular Behçet's disease).

Pathophysiology

Acute or chronic nonspecific inflammation is found in diseased vessels. In the aorta or muscular-type arteries, inflammation is found in all layers of the vessel, whereas in elastic-type arteries, there is hypertrophy of the intima, destruction of the media, or hypertrophy of the adventitia. Occlusive lesions or aneurysms are formed in the artery and thrombophlebitis in the vein.

TABLE 78.1. International diagnostic criteria for Behçet's disease.*

Recurrent oral ulceration	Minor aphthous, major aphthous, or herpetiform ulceration observed by physician or patient that recurred at least three times in one 12-mo period
Plus 2 of	
Recurrent genital ulceration	Aphthous ulceration or scarring observed by physician or patient
Eye lesions	Anterior uveitis, posterior uveitis, or cells in vitreous on slit lamp examination or rential vasculitis observed by ophthalmologist
Skin lesions	Erythema nodosum observed by physician or patient, pseudofolliculitis, or papulopustular lesions; or acneiform nodules observed by physician in postadolescent patients not on corticosteroid treatment
Positive pathergy test	Read by physician at 24–48 h

*Findings applicable only in absence of other clinical explanations.
From International Study Group for Behçet's Disease.[3]

Clinical Features

Subcutaneous thrombophlebitis is the most frequently seen feature among patients with vascular involvement (15.8% of patients with Behçet's disease[1]). Skin lesions are the major symptom, and prognosis is good.

Except in patients with subcutaneous thrombophlebitis, occlusive lesions occur in veins and occlusive or aneurysmal lesions in arteries. According to the statistical data from Japan,[4] there were 56 cases of venous occlusion, 22 cases of arterial occlusion, and 25 cases of arterial aneurysm in a total of 90 patients with vascular Behçet's disease who show some vascular involvement other than subcutaneous thrombophlebitis.

Arterial occlusive lesions involve the branches of the aorta, peripheral arteries, or pulmonary arteries and cause varying degrees of ischemia in the related organ. Arterial aneurysm involves the aorta, branch of the aorta, peripheral artery, or pulmonary artery and may eventually cause rupture. The involvement of a pulmonary artery may cause hemoptysis, chest pain, or dyspnea. Venous occlusive lesions involve the vena cava, visceral vein, or peripheral vein and may cause superior vena cava syndrome, Budd–Chiari syndrome, or swelling of a lower limb.

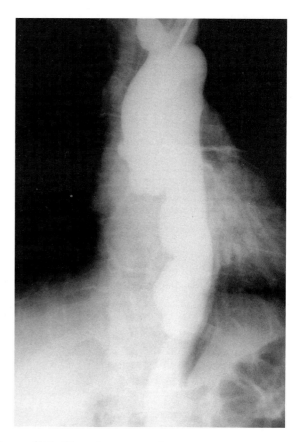

FIGURE 78.1. Thoracic aortography.

Diagnostic Tests

A pathergy test performed by insertion of a small needle into the skin is a simple and reliable test for Behçet's disease that shows high positive results. The increased inflammatory reaction is shown by erythrocyte sedimentation rate, C-reactive protein level, and white blood cell count. Higher positive rates of HLA-B51 are seen in patients with Behçet's disease than those without the disease. Serum immunoglobulin levels may be increased. Computed tomography, magnetic resonance imaging, radioisotope examination, ultrasonic echography, and angiography are used to determine vascular involvement.

Medical Treatment

Because Behçet's disease is a type of vasculitis, the inflammation should be suppressed with nonsteroidal antiinflammatory or corticosteroid drugs during the active phase of the disease. If inflammation is not sufficiently suppressed, immunosuppressive drugs, such as cyclosporine, may be added to the regimen. Antiplatelet or anticoagulant agents are administered to treat occlusion of arteries or veins. When the thrombus is fresh, a fibrinolytic drug such as urokinase is administered.

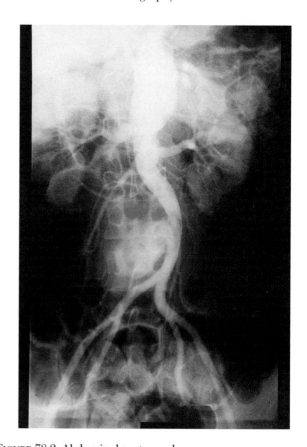

FIGURE 78.2. Abdominal aortography.

Surgical Treatment

In principle, a bypass operation is performed to treat arterial occlusion and a graft replacement is used to treat aneurysm. Thrombectomy is used to treat veno-occlusive lesions in some patients. Especially with surgical treatment of arterial lesions, disruption or rupture at the site of anastomosis is frequent, and care must be taken to anastomose the graft far enough from the lesion, to reinforce the anastomotic site (e.g., by wrapping it), and to suppress the inflammation medically as much as possible before and after the operation.

Case Reports

Patient 1

A 30-year-old man was hospitalized on an urgent basis for severe abdominal pain. For 5 years he had been treated for Behçet's disease with oral aphtosis, skin lesions, eye lesions, and genital ulcers. On physical examination, an 8- by 6-cm pulsatile abdominal mass was palpated, and hematological examination showed a white blood cell count of 9500 and C-reactive protein level of 4(+). Aortography, performed on the day after admission, demonstrated three saccular aneurysms in the thoracic aorta and fusiform dilatation of the innominate artery (Figure 78.1). The suprarenal abdominal aorta showed fusiform dilatation, and the infrarenal abdominal aorta had large saccular aneurysms that protruded into its right side (Figure 78.2). Emergency surgery was done to remove the saccular infrarenal abdominal aortic aneurysm soon after the aortography. During operation, a 9- by 6.5-cm pulsatile mass was found on the right side adjacent to the aorta (Figure 78.3A) and a 1.7- by 2-cm punched-out opening was found on the right lateral wall of the aorta (Figure 78.3B). The infrarenal abdominal aorta was replaced by a knitted Dacron Y graft, and each anastomotic site was reinforced by wrapping with mesh (Figure 78.4). Hypertrophy of the intima, destruction of the medial elastic lamina, and infiltration of nonspecific inflammatory cells, mainly lymphocytes, were shown by histopathological examination of the aortic wall (Figure 78.5). The postoperative course was good, and the patient was discharged.

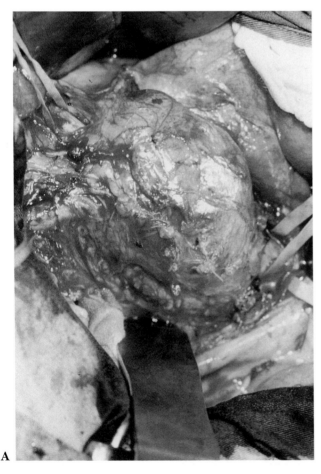

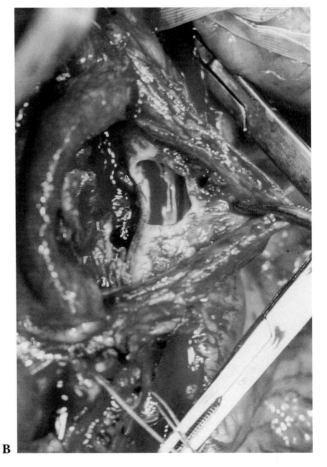

A
B

FIGURE 78.3. Operative finding of the abdominal aorta. **A,** Retroperitoneum was approached and the saccular aneurysm of the abdominal aorta was shown. **B,** The wall of the aneurysm was excised and the punched-out opening of the abdominal aorta was shown.

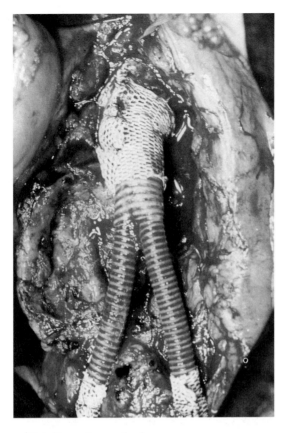

FIGURE 78.4. Operative method.

Patient 2

A 65-year-old woman, diagnosed with Behçet's disease with oral aphtosis and skin lesions, was admitted for treatment of the pulsatile mass on the back of her left hand. On physical examination, a pulsatile mass 3 cm in diameter was found on the back of her hand between the first and second fingers. Hematological examination showed a white blood cell count of 6000, an erythrocyte sedimentation rate of 67 mm/h, and a C-reactive protein level of 2.7 mg/dL. A radiograph showed a fusiform aneurysm at the peripheral left radial artery (Figure 78.6). At operation, a 2.3- by 2.0-cm fusiform aneurysm with thrombi (Figure 78.7) was ligated and extirpated, because of the patient's patent palmar arch. The histopathological finding of aneurysm showed destruction of medial elastic lamina and infiltration of neutrophils and plasma cells into the vessel wall. No ischemic symptoms were seen postoperatively, and the patient was discharged.

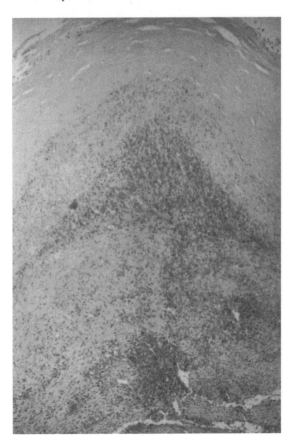

FIGURE 78.5. Histopathological finding of the aortic wall.

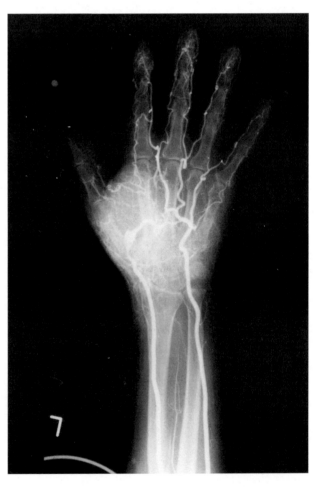

FIGURE 78.6. Angiography of left upper extremity.

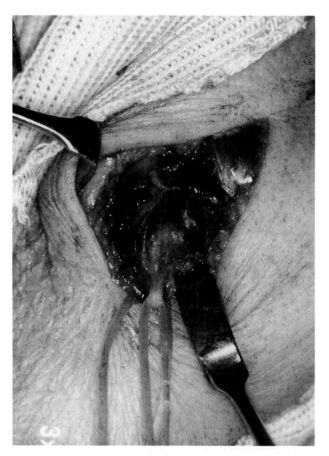

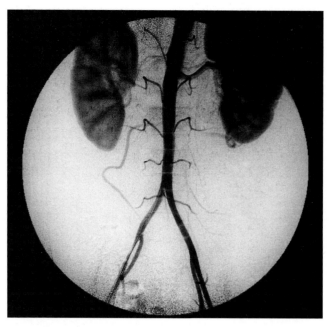

FIGURE 78.8. Abdominal aortography.

FIGURE 78.7. Operative finding of aneurysm on the back of left hand.

Patient 3

A 53-year-old man, diagnosed with Behçet's disease with oral aphtosis, skin lesions, and genital ulcers, was admitted for treatment of a varicose vein on his left leg. Besides the varicose vein, the bilateral dorsalis pedis artery was found to be pulseless. A white blood cell count of 7700, an erythrocyte sedimentation rate of 10 mm/h, and a C-reactive protein level of 0.3 mg/dL were shown hematologically. No deep vein thrombosis was seen on venography, but arteriography showed occlusion of the inferior mesenteric artery and right external iliac artery (Figure 78.8) in addition to an occlusive lesion on the bilateral leg and foot. The patient was discharged and followed medically, because he exhibited slight ischemic symptoms of the lower limb.

Patient 4

A 24-year-old man with Behçet's disease with oral aphtosis and skin lesions was admitted for treatment of a painful pulsatile mass on the right side of his neck. A pulsatile mass 2 cm in diameter was found in the right submandibular area, and hematological examination showed a white blood cell count of 11,200, a C-reactive protein level of 7.1 mg/dL, and an erythrocyte sedimentation rate of 16 mm/h. A fusiform aneurysm that contained thrombi was found in the right common carotid artery by computed tomographic examination (Figure 78.9). Arteriography showed a fusiform aneurysm at the origin of the right internal carotid artery (Figure 78.10). At operation, because the aneurysm was extended from the junction of the internal and external carotid arteries proximally to the internal carotid artery distally, end-to-side anastomosis of two reversed saphenous vein grafts to the proximal right common carotid artery was performed by side clamp and then end-to-end anastomosis of each graft to the right internal and external carotid arteries by cross-clamping, confirming that the stump pressure of the internal carotid artery was 70/50 mm Hg. Next, the right common carotid artery was ligated just below the aneurysm and then resected (Figure 78.11). Histopathologically, intimal fibrous hypertrophy, partial disappearance of the medial layer, and infiltration of lymphocytes and plasma cells into vessel wall were seen. Each graft to the right internal and external carotid arteries was shown to be patent by postoperative arteriography (Figure 78.12).

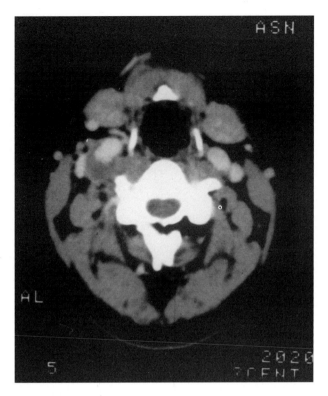

FIGURE 78.9. Enhanced computed tomographic scan of the neck.

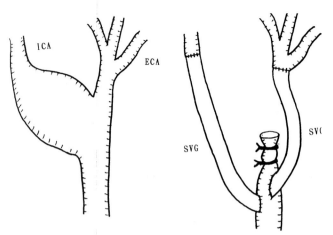

FIGURE 78.11. Schematic representation of the operative method. ICA, internal carotid artery; ECA, external carotid artery; SVG, saphenous vein graft.

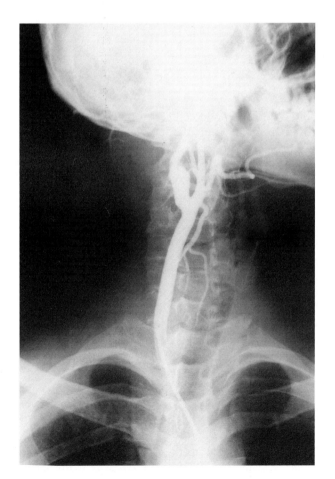

FIGURE 78.10. Angiography of the right carotid artery.

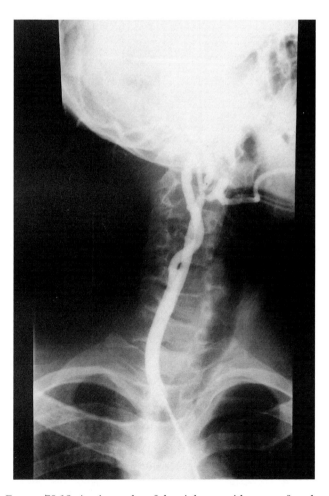

FIGURE 78.12. Angiography of the right carotid artery after the first operation.

During follow-up at an outpatient clinic, the patient was readmitted for a transient ischemic attack 3 months after discharge. In the arteriography, the graft to the right external carotid artery was patent, but the graft to the right internal carotid artery was occluded (Figure 78.13). Because there were no other remarkable neurological symptoms, the patient was discharged.

About 6 years and 5 months after the first operation, the patient noticed a pulsatile right cervical mass, after falling down, and was admitted to our hospital for the third time. An aneurysm was found at the site of proximal anastomosis of the graft to the right external carotid artery (Figure 78.14); therefore the right common carotid artery proximal to the aneurysm and the graft were ligated distally and a bypass was made from the right subclavian artery to the right external carotid artery with a knit Dacron graft. The right common carotid artery was occluded near its origin, and a bypass graft was patent postoperatively (Figure 78.15).

Four months after the second operation, a bypass graft was exposed at the upper neck and infected, and the graft was extirpated. No neurological symptoms ap-

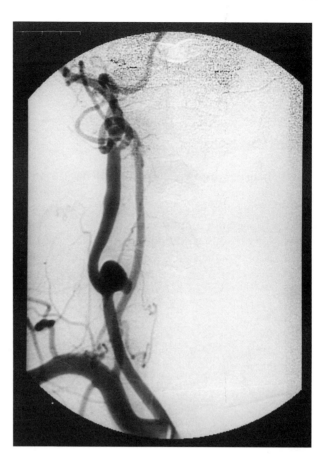

FIGURE 78.14. Angiography of the right carotid artery before the second operation.

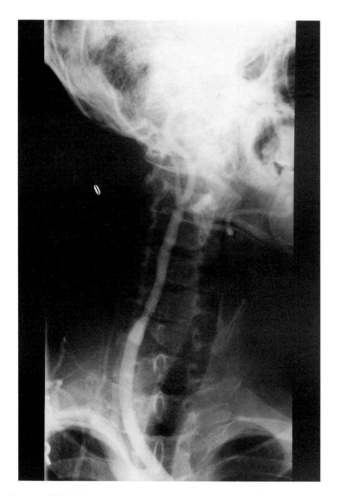

FIGURE 78.13. Angiography of the right carotid artery 3 months after the first operation.

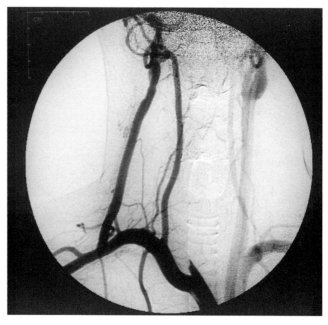

FIGURE 78.15. Angiography of the right carotid artery after the second operation.

peared after the operation, and the patient was discharged. This patient experienced many problems, but the inflammatory reaction was controlled in the normal range by corticosteroids, aspirin, and colchicine following the patient's initial admission.

Conclusion

Vascular Behçet's disease can be diagnosed relatively easily, because some of the major symptoms are almost exclusively associated with it. In surgical treatment, it is necessary to keep in mind that vascular Behçet's disease is a type of vasculitis and that disruption or rupture at the site of anastomosis may take place. To prevent these complications, inflammation must be controlled medically and the contrivance of surgical method (e.g., to anastomose the graft far enough from the lesion and to reinforce the anastomotic site) must be done.

References

1. Sakane T, Nishikawa M. Behçet's disease. *Nippon Rinsho.* 1993;51(suppl):596–610.
2. Takeuchi A, Ose T, Yoshino Y. Progress on diagnosis of Behçet's syndrome. *Nippon Naika Gakkai Zasshi.* 1991;80: 1736–1741.
3. International Study Group for Behçet's Disease. Criteria for diagnosis of Behçet's disease. *Lancet.* 1990;335:1078–1080.
4. Inada K, Hirose M. *Peripheral Vascular Disease.* Tokyo, Japan: Kanehara Shuppan; 1987:453–455.

79

Budd–Chiari Syndrome: Physiopathology, Diagnosis, and Treatment

Zhong Gao Wang

Budd–Chiari syndrome (BCS) refers to a variety of disorders caused by complete or incomplete obstruction of the hepatic veins (HVs), the suprahepatic inferior vena cava (IVC), or both; it is characterized by the clinical manifestations of portal hypertension with or without IVC hypertension. This chapter is based on my experience over the last 15 years with about 500 patients with BCS.

Physiopathology

The central veins of the liver receive blood from the hepatic sinusoids and drain it into the HVs, which empty their blood into the IVC. The venous system in the lower body also empties blood through the IVC. This explains the importance of location for both the suprahepatic IVC segment and the orifices of the HVs in the pathogenesis of BCS. Interestingly, in some regions of the world, such as China, Japan, Korea, India, and South Africa, occlusion of the suprahepatic IVC is relatively common and most often appears as a membrane or web of the IVC.

The main physiopathological factor that leads to BCS is an outflow blockage of the hepatic sinusoidal beds with characteristics of dilatation and congestion of the central veins and sinusoidal areas of the liver that result in progressive portal and IVC hypertension if the suprahepatic IVC is also involved. When blood constantly enters into the liver through the hepatic artery and the portal vein, the main hepatic venous outflow point is blocked, a high hydrostatic pressure in the hepatic sinusoids is created, and the plasma is extravasated into Disse's space and the lymphatics. The excessive formation of lymphatic fluid causes diffuse distribution of many small white vesicles on the surface of the liver and produces lymphatic leakage from the overloaded hepatic lymph vessels into the peritoneal cavity through Glisson's capsule. This leakage can often be seen during

laparotomy of patients with BCS as a "weeping liver," which is one of the main reasons the ascites are usually intractable (Figure 79.1). Moreover, pleural effusion occurred in 14% of patients in a series of 250.[1]

The left HV is an embryologically venous duct–related vessel. It drains blood into the IVC at a level slightly above the membrane of the IVC and thus is not as important as the right HV in the pathogenesis of BCS. The caudate lobe is usually exempt from hepatic venous occlusive lesions in patients with BCS; the venous flow of that area is increased for compensation and lobe hypertrophies. A distinctively enlarged caudate lobe may compress the retrohepatic IVC and thus produce a vicious cycle of caval obstruction that may worsen the disease.

Hepatomegaly and varices of the esophagus and gastric fundus develop, but splenomegaly is usually moderate. Hypersplenism is occasionally seen. IVC occlusion can cause renal dysfunction because of renal congestion.

Marked varicosities on the thoracoabdominal wall, especially those presenting on the loin or back but rarely on the umbilicus, called the captus medusa (0.2% in my series), remarkably differ from those caused by cirrhosis. Edema, pigmentation, and ulcer of the lower limbs are bilateral. In late stages of the disease, the skin of the distal lower limbs may appear similar to the bark of an old tree.

Venous congestion in the lower body sharply reduces venous return, which diminishes heart size. The patient usually has a small heart visible on x-ray radiograph and always has compromised heart function due to low cardiac output that causes palpitation and shortness of breath on slight exertion. The blood in the stagnated IVC is rheologically hypercoagulable and hyperviscous.[2] End-stage patients, due to dysfunctional digestive systems, impaired protein production, and constant albumin loss after repeated abdominoparacentesis, inevitably enter into a state of severe nutritional depletion and debilitation; they have cachexialike appearances with sticklike limbs and distended abdomens. Patients usually die

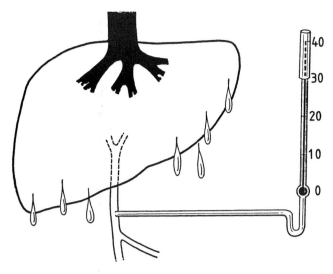

FIGURE 79.1. Pathogenesis of Budd–Chiari syndrome: occlusion of the inferior vena cava, hepatic veins, and their junction; "weeping liver"; and increased portal pressure.

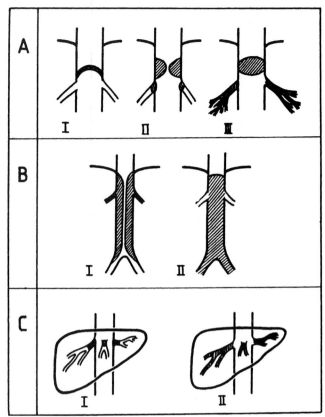

FIGURE 79.2. Classifications for Budd–Chiari syndrome.

of massive hematemesis because of ruptured varices of the esophagus, cardiac fundus of the stomach, cachexia due to intractable ascites or extreme malnutrition and emaciation, or hepatorenal failure.

I recommend the BCS classification shown in Figure 79.2 for localized, diffuse, and intrahepatic lesions.[3] In addition, a few patients (4%) have presented with accompanying occlusion of the superior vena cava.[1]

During 39 radical surgical procedures, I have found that the membranes are whitish, smooth, and glistening on both surfaces with a thickness of a few millimeters. They are tough, elastic, with or without fenestration, and may coexist with a localized constriction of the IVC or thrombus distal to the lesion.

The etiology of BCS varies. It includes membranous occlusion in about 40% of patients, thrombosis of unknown origin (perhaps mostly due to the web) in about 30%, and hypercoagulable status, polycythemia rubra vera, paroxysmal nocturnal hemoglobinuria, oral contraceptive use, pregnancy, postpartum status, hepatocellular carcinoma, endophlebitis of the IVC, external compression, Behçet's syndrome, myeloproliferative disease, leiomyoma of the IVC, pericarditis, hyperlipidemia, and trauma.

The etiology of BCS in Western countries is usually thrombosis or hypercoagulable states, and the lesions are always intrahepatic. In South Africa, China, India, Korea, and Japan, membranous obstruction of the IVC is rather common and usually is seen in the suprahepatic IVC.

The predisposing factors can be divided into (1) congenital malformation, (2) hypercoagulability, (3) poisoning material, (4) intraluminal nonthrombotic occlusion, (5) external compression, (6) lesions in the vessel wall,

and (7) miscellaneous factors, such as sickle cell anemia, protein-losing enteropathy, lipid nephrosis, protein C deficiency, and connective tissue disease.

Diagnosis

Keeping BCS in mind is the key to prompt diagnosis because of its typical clinical features. For patients with clues of portal hypertension with or without IVC hypertension, portal hypertension that accompanies relatively normal liver function, or varices on the thoracoabdominal wall (especially on the loins and lower limbs), the diagnosis of BCS should be highly suspected.

A chest radiograph always reveals small hearts in patients with advanced BCS and enlarged azygous shadows in about half of all patients. Technetium 99 and gallium 67 hepatic scintiscan may identify the characteristic area of central uptake in the hypertrophied caudate lobe, usually with apparent marked diminution or even absence of tracer uptake over the right and left hepatic lobes.

Radionuclide inferior vena cavography that reveals at least two of the following criteria is diagnostic of BCS: (1) a delay of more than 4 seconds in visualizing the heart; (2) sharply truncated IVC with marked collection of isotope activity, presenting an appearance of a shadow hang-up; and (3) extensive collateral circulation.

Computed tomography, magnetic resonance imaging, and single photon emission computed tomography may help in diagnosing BCS. Selective hepatovenography via a transfemoral, transjugular, or percutaneous transhepatic approach involves cannulating and imaging the HVs. Superior mesenteric arterial portography or splenoportography is able to clarify the portal system and its runoff.

B-mode ultrasonography, duplex sonography, and echocardiography can be used for screening patients with BCS. They are simple, reliable, and convenient noninvasive methods of diagnosis and have a correct diagnosis rate of more than 90% when compared with cavography.

Percutaneous transhepatic venography is used when selective intubation fails during cavography or during the process of liver biopsy, which gives further information about the patency status of the intrahepatic veins and the IVC and their collaterals. Cavography has been the best means for diagnosis of BCS. A catheter is introduced into the IVC through the femoral vein by a Seldinger technique, and if necessary another catheter is placed in the supradiaphragmatic IVC via the brachial or jugular vein. While the contrast is injected simultaneously from both directions, the occlusive lesion, location, extent, and collateral status can be visualized. Figure 79.3 shows a web of the IVC. IVC pressure can be measured during cavography. For those patients in whom BCS is caused by systemic disorders, tests should be added to define related etiology, such as paroxysmal nocturnal hemoglobinuria, polycytosis rubra vera, hypercoagulable status, autoimmunosuppressive diseases, antithrombin III deficiency, and so on.[2]

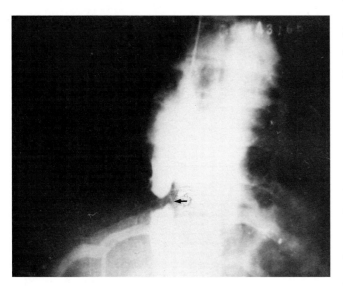

FIGURE 79.3. Cavography showing a web of the inferior vena cava (arrow).

Treatment

Conservative Therapy

The medical management of BCS consists of administration of diuretic, anticoagulation, and thrombolytic agents, Chinese herbs, and symptomatic treatment only for patients in the acute stage. Medical management is largely ineffective and offers only little hope for successful treatment of the majority of patients in the chronic stage.

Interventional Management

The main interventional methods for BCS include percutaneous transluminal angioplasty, laser-assisted angioplasty, and intraluminal stent. Percutaneous transluminal angioplasty has been used in the treatment of BCS, but its use is limited to the vena caval web or other localized occlusive lesions of the IVC. This method is simple and effective in some instances. But the possibility of life-threatening complications, such as cardiac tamponade, penetration of the vessel wall, fracture of the catheter, and pulmonary embolism, should be kept in mind whenever this procedure is carried out. Percutaneous transluminal angioplasty should first be used for localized lesions, but it is not indicated for those with fresh thrombus distal to the lesion. Transluminal laser-assisted angioplasty is used for more difficult cases.

Percutaneous transhepatic recanalization and dilatation have recently been reported as possible treatments for BCS, and I have used the technique successfully in two patients. I have also used balloon dilatation combined with placement of a self-expandable metallic stent; 48 patients were treated with the stenting technique, and 10 were treated with a transcardiac and femoral approach (Figure 79.4) or radical corrective approach.[4]

Surgery

The surgical management of BCS can be divided into four categories:

1. Indirect decompression: minor procedures (peritoneovenous shunts, thoracic duct–internal jugular vein reanastomosis); disconnection procedures for preventing bleeding from the esophageal varices; and promotion of collateral procedures such as splenopneumopexy
2. Decompression: all kinds of shunting procedures
3. Direct procedures: endovascular intervention (percutaneous transluminal angioplasty and stenting) and radical corrective procedures
4. Liver transplantation

Although I have used 19 different approaches, I describe only the most commonly used procedures in the following sections.[2,5]

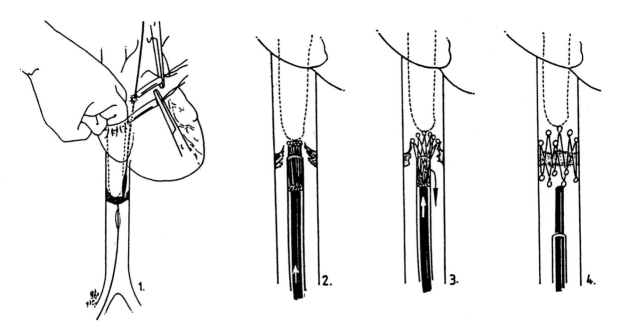

FIGURE 79.4. Combined transcardiac and transfemoral approaches to penetrate and dilate the membrane and deploy a stent.

Transcardiac Membranotomy

Transcardiac membranotomy, comparable to commissurotomy, is a relatively simple procedure. A right anterior thoracotomy through the fourth intercostal space or a median sternotomy is employed, the pericardium is incised, and the right atrium is exposed. A purse-string suture using 4-O Prolene is prepared on the atrium. A proper size side-wall clamp is applied on the right atrium as close as possible to its bottom without compressing the opening of the inlet of the SVC, the right coronary artery, and the sino-atrial node. A purse-string suture with a size allowing finger insertion using 4-O Prolene is prepared on the clamped part of the atrial wall. Two ends of the suture after detachment of needles are trapped into a vascular keeper (a segment of rubber catheter). The atrial wall encircled by the suture is properly opened without damaging the string-suture. The surgeon inserts his or her left index finger (covered with a finger glove with balloon as shown in Figure 79.5)[5] into the right atrium while the clamp is withdrawing and the vascular keeper is properly tightening to prevent bleeding. The surgeon advances the fingertip and touches a membranous obstruction that feels like a layer of strong cloth with fairly good elasticity that prevents the membrane from being broken. Penetrating maneuvers are repeated until the membrane is fractured. The full finger is then inserted into the IVC, and a dilatation manipulation is repeatedly exerted with the aid of balloon inflation and deflation if a localized stenosis of the IVC also exists. The orifices of the HVs can be perceived

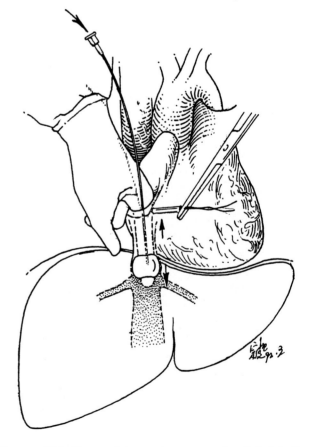

FIGURE 79.5. Transatrial membranotomy by digital balloon technique.

and accompanying membranous obstructions of the HVs, if present, can be penetrated and dilated by fingertip. Sometimes a dilatation maneuver is assisted by a large (>2 cm internal diameter) balloon catheter inserted from the femoral vein. Rarely, after a successful membranotomy, immediate reocclusion is perceived. In those cases, other operative alternatives should be adopted. The disadvantage of this procedure is that even after a successful membranotomy, the broken and irregular residual membrane still exists. The coexisting stenosis of the IVC may also remain, and the external compression may not be changed. One year after membranotomy, the patency curve seems stable .[5]

Cavoatrial Shunt

When a membrane cannot be disrupted, a cavoatrial shunt[6] should be constructed during surgery. It is indicated for those with localized unpenetrated obstructive lesions of the IVC and patency of the HVs. The high failure rate of venous prosthesis due to thrombosis is an obvious disadvantage. I used this procedure, aside from the patient's critical status, because (1) under some circumstances, large-caliber grafts are better than small-caliber grafts in preventing thrombus formation; (2) the pressure gradient between the IVC and the right atrium was significant; (3) the pressure in the abdominal cavity was positive, whereas it was negative in the thoracic cavity; and (4) the venous flow in the cavoatrial graft was accelerated during regular inspiration, which enhances the intrathoracic negative pressure due to the expansion of the thoracic cage. All of these factors contribute to the initiation of one-way blood flow in the shunting graft.

I advocate use of a 14- or 16-mm–internal diameter external ring-supported prosthesis for this purpose and use the anterior approach. A midline abdominal or right paramedian incision is made. The IVC can be isolated through three approaches, the right and left to the mesenteric approaches and a Kocher approach, but usually dissecting the retroperitoneum from the right to the upper part of the mesentery root. Part of the IVC is isolated from beneath and below the transverse portion of the duodenum, and the transverse colon is constantly elevated and the intestine pushed to the left. Preparation of a segment of the IVC (more than 4 cm long) is necessary for anastomosis. For those with many ascites, a median sternotomy is recommended; otherwise a right anterior thoracotomy at the fourth intercostal space is selected. The pericardium is incised and retracted for better exposure and manipulation. To provide passage of the graft a hole is made in the diaphragm at the proper position if a thoracotomy is employed. The graft is properly preclotted (if required). The end of the graft is tailored into a cobra shape. A suitable-sized Satinski clamp is applied on the IVC. An end-to-side prosthesis to IVC anastomosis is completed using 5-O Prolene sutures

in an eversion running fashion. The graft is usually brought to the thoracic cavity or mediastinum posterior to the transverse colon and anterior to the stomach and liver. The upper end of the graft is tailored and a graft-to-atrium end-to-side anastomosis is completed. Then two needles are inserted into the graft, the distal one for installing the heparin normal saline solution (10u/mL) and the proximal one for evacuating the air trapped in the graft. The clamps applied on the IVC and atrium are withdrawn in that order. The patency of a graft is confirmed by immediate relief of hepatosplenomegaly and reduction of the portal pressure if the HVs are patent to the IVC. A thoracic drainage tube is installed, bleeding is stopped, and incisions are closed in layers.

Mesoatrial Shunt

When occlusion of the IVC involves most or all of the IVC, a mesoatrial rather than cavoatrial shunt is indicated. Candidates for this operation usually are in poorer general condition, have a higher risk for surgery, and have more clinical manifestations of portal hypertension. Surgical manipulation is also more difficult. The upper midline abdominal incision is made, viscera explored, ascites aspirated, portal pressure measured, liver biopsy performed, and the superior mesenteric vein (SMV) isolated at the base of the mesocolon through the retroperitoneum right to Treitz's ligament. A dissection of the SMV at least 4 cm long below the pancreatic body is required. The right atrium is exposed using the previously mentioned method. A graft of 14 mm ID with external rings is used to make a bypass between the SMV and right atrium using end-to-side fashion (Figure 79.6).[6] After establishment of blood flow through the graft, more rapid and effective relief of hepatosplenomegaly can be noticed. The remarkably size-reduced spleen also can be easily felt, and a reduction of 40% to 50% of the portal pressure is usually revealed.

Splenoatrial Shunt

A splenoatrial shunt serves as an alternative when the SMV is unavailable.

Mesojugular Shunt

During the management of patients in the most severe condition with distinct malnutrition and massive ascites, aggressive pleural effusion with one to three thoraco-paracentesis procedures a week is required. No major procedures can be tolerated. I have developed a meso-jugular shunt that does not require a thoracotomy or median sternotomy (Figure 79.7). Only an upper midline abdominal incision and a small low transverse neck collar incision are required. The SMV is isolated first, followed by the right internal jugular vein; then the ex-

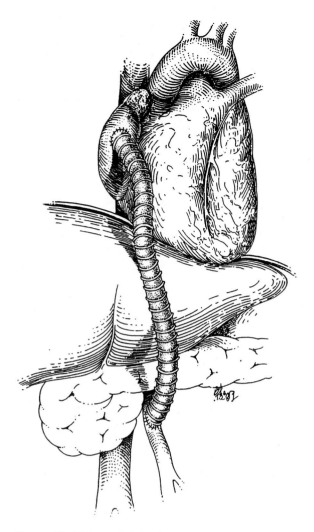

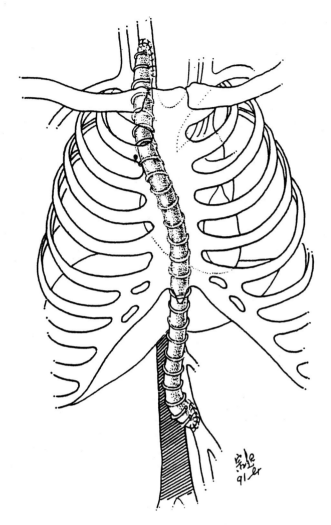

FIGURE 79.6. Mesoatrial shunt.

FIGURE 79.7. Retrosternal mesojugular shunt.

ternally ring-enforced graft of 14- or 16-mm inner diameter is brought into the neck incision retrosternally and the graft SMV and graft jugular vein end-to-side anastomoses are constructed. After establishment of blood flow, a portal decompressive effect is also immediately achieved. The ascites and pleural effusion disappear about 3 weeks postoperatively in all cases. More than 20 such procedures[3] that have been carried out resulted in an 80% survival rate, with half of survivors returning to normal work. It appears that the constant pumping mechanism produced by cardiac action intermittently compresses the ring-enforced graft with good elasticity to put pressure on the sternum and thus propel the blood flow in an upward direction because of a significant pressure gradient between the portal and jugular veins. This operative approach has now been used successfully even by other general surgeons who are not familiar with cardiac surgery to decrease portal hypertension in patients who are not in a critical state.[7]

Portosystemic Shunt

Mesocaval, portocaval, and splenorenal shunts are indicated for those with classic BCS (i.e., intrahepatic venous occlusion and patency of the IVC and a type III lesion).[6] This treatment resembles that for portal hypertension caused by cirrhosis.

Radical Corrective Procedure

None of the previously mentioned methods correct the original lesions found in the IVC and HVs. Senning reported a radical resection in 1983[8] through the anterior approach. I mostly used a lateral approach (Figure 79.8), and 37 such procedures have been carried out. Hypothermia and circulatory arrest or extracorporeal circulation with normal temperature or indigenous internal shunt with occluding balloon were used separately. The lesion and a small part of liver tissue surrounding

FIGURE 79.8. Radical resection with patch graft. G, graft; M, mediastinum; L, lung; A, atrium.

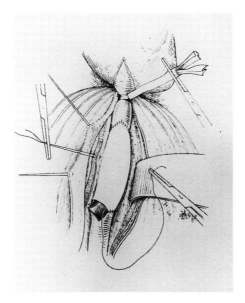

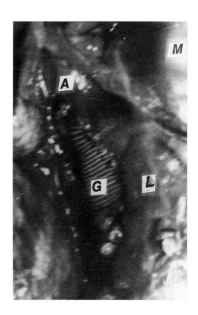

the IVC can be resected through the lumen to widen it if necessary, and a patch graft is sometimes applied. However, recurrence is still a problem.[9]

Liver Transplantation

In 1976 Putnam et al. reported the first successful liver transplant for a patient with end-stage liver failure due to localized stenosis of the suprahepatic IVC.[10] Campbell et al. reported 19 hepatic transplants done for 17 patients with BCS.[11] Their first patient did not receive anticoagulant therapy during the postoperative period, and recurrent thrombosis of the HVs in the newly transplanted liver rapidly developed. Sixteen patients who subsequently underwent transplantation were managed using early postoperative anticoagulant treatment when feasible. These results encouraged adoption of liver transplantation as a means for managing BCS. Ozawa and colleagues successfully completed a living donated (mother) liver transplantation for a 3-year-old child with BCS at Kyoto University of Japan in 1990.

Surgical Outcome

We surgically treated 380 patients before 1995. Good results were achieved in 67.6% of patients and fair in 10.5%; surgery was thus effective in 78.1% of patients.[6] The 5-year patency rates of the mesoatrial shunt, cavoatrial shunt, and membranotomy were 71.4%, 50.0%, and 66.7%, respectively, with exclusion of mortality. The patency was mostly confirmed by ultrasonography.[5] Long-term follow-up has not been completed, but a 10-year patency has been obtained in five patients, including three with mesoatrial shunts, transcardiac membranotomy, and mesocaval C shunt in each end.

Postoperative Complications

In a series of 380 patients treated surgically before 1995, 21 patients died within 30 days of surgery, which was an operative mortality rate of 5.5%. The postoperative complications were cardiac insufficiency (14.2%); encephalopathy (4.1%); pleural effusion (5.6%); chylous ascites (2.8%); hemothorax (2.5%); chylous thorax (1.4%); hydromediastinum, arrhythmia, stress ulcer, and pulmonary abscess (0.8%); and hepatitis B and cardiac tamponade (0.5%).[5]

Summary

BCS is not as rare as originally believed. A geographical prevalence is found in some areas of China, India, Korea, Japan, and South Africa. IVC webs are congenital and comprise the main cause of BCS in some geographical regions of the world. The diagnosis of BCS should be suspected in anyone who develops massive ascites or superficial varicosity and edema of the bilateral lower extremities. The diagnosis is not difficult as long as the physician keeps this somewhat uncommon syndrome in mind. It can be quickly confirmed by B-mode ultrasonography and cavography. Conservative therapy can be attempted first if the syndrome occurs acutely. Surgical approaches, which should be tailored to the individual patient's underlying physiopathological status, are as follows:

1. Balloon dilatation is the initial approach for those with IVC webs or localized stenosis or occlusion but without fresh thrombus distal to the lesion.
2. If a recoil is found, intraluminal stent is suggested.
3. If it fails, a transcardiac membranotomy or combined transfemoral balloon dilatation and stenting technique are employed.

4. A cavoatrial shunt is used for those with suprahepatic IVC occlusion and HV patency to the IVC.

5. A mesoatrial shunt is indicated for those with diffuse stenosis or occlusion of the IVC and HVs, usually including patients with serious BCS.

6. A mesojugular shunt is suitable for those with intractable ascites, pleural effusion, and high operative risk.

7. A radical corrective procedure is most indicated for those whose lesions require resection.

8. Liver transplantation should be considered in those with fulminant hepatic failure or end-stage disease.

The sooner the corrective techniques are used, the better the chance that patients will recover from BCS.

References

1. Wang ZG. Recognition and management of Budd-Chiari syndrome in 250 cases. *Bulletin of Heart Lung and Blood Vessel Diseases.* 1991;10:175–181.

2. Wang ZG, Jones S. Budd-Chiari syndrome. *Curr Probl Surg.* 1996;33:81–220.

3. Wang ZG, Wang SH, Wu JD, et al. Mesojugular shunt as means of managing severe Budd-Chiari syndrome. *Chin J Surg.* 1994;32:611–614.

4. Wang ZG, Wang SH, Wu JD, et al. Treating Budd-Chiari syndrome with balloon dilatation and intraluminal stent. *Natl Med J China* .1995;75:35–39.

5. Wang ZG. Budd-Chiari syndrome (How do I treat?). In: Chang JB, ed. *Modern Vascular Surgery.* Vol 5. New York, NY: Springer-Verlag; 1992:464–506.

6. Wang ZG. Budd-Chiari syndrome: experience from 430 cases. *Asian J Surg.* 1996;19:23–30.

7. Xiu PQ, Lu XP, Zhao RS, et al. Budd-Chiari syndrome. *Proceedings of the 3rd Chinese Vascular Society Conference.* Tianjin, China, May 1995;52.

8. Senning A. Transcaval posterocranial resection of the liver as treatment of the Budd-Chiari syndrome. *World J Surg.* 1983;7:632–640.

9. Wang ZG, Wang SH, Wu JD, et al. Radical resection for Budd-Chiari syndrome. *Chinese Journal of Thoracic and Cardiovascular Surgery.* 1995;75:35–39.

10. Putnam CW, Porter KH, Weil R, et al. Liver transplantation for Budd-Chiari syndrome. *JAMA.* 1976;236:1142–1143.

11. Campbell DA, Rolles K, Jamieson N, et al. Hepatic transplantation with perioperative and long term anticoagulation as treatment of Budd-Chiari syndrome. *Surg Gynecol Obstet.* 1988;166:511–517.

80

Vasospastic Syndrome

Shigeyuki Sasaki and Keishu Yasuda

Vasospastic diseases are peripheral vascular disorders caused by vasospasm, which means a reversible localized or diffuse vasoconstriction of arteries or smaller blood vessels. Vasospastic syndromes include Raynaud's disease, acrocyanosis, and livedo reticularis. Because the vasospasm is generally a temporary disorder, the ischemia is reversible. In this case, patients with vasospasm may suffer vasospastic attacks without organic devastating changes in the digits. However, the vasospasm can occur as a prolonged disorder with ischemia, which may lead to organic tissue damage. Raynaud's disease, acrocyanosis, and livedo reticularis each occur in a primary form or secondary to underlying diseases.[13–16] Primary cases are usually benign, and patients suffer little permanent ischemic damage, whereas those who experience the disorders secondary to underlying diseases tend to suffer extreme ischemic damage. Any disease or persistent vasoconstrictive stimulus that produces injuries in the blood vessels may elicit a vasospastic syndrome.

Primary Raynaud's Disease

Pathophysiology

A few studies on the pathology of primary Raynaud's disease have been undertaken. The digital arteries are probably normal in the early phase of the disease. Human digits generally contain many physiological arteriovenous shunts in addition to the capillary circulation. To regulate the body's core temperature, these shunts allow a large amount of blood to pass through the digits when an individual is warm and to close during exposure to cold temperatures. Pharmacological analysis with the use of agonists and antagonists has shown that α_1-adrenoreceptors and α_2-adrenoreceptors are present in arteries of the hand.[33] The major mechanism that regulates the physiological arteriovenous shunt flow is controlled by the sympathetic nervous system through the α_2-adrenoreceptors.[87,114] The α_2-adrenoreceptors play the most important role during reflex sympathetic vasoconstriction induced by cold exposure.[33,48] In healthy subjects, cold exposure has been reported to increase cyclic guanosine monophosphate, but not in those with Raynaud's phenomenon.[76]

In addition to the peripheral adrenergic system, digital blood flow through the arteriovenous anastomoses is also regulated by the central nervous system, including the hypothalamus and cerebral cortex.[87] Somatic afferent nerves, baroreceptors, and chemoreceptors also influence the vasomotor centers in the medulla oblongata. Serotonin may also be important in reflex sympathetic vasoconstriction.[35,36,99] Several pharmacological studies have shown that 5-hydroxytryptamine (5-HT)$_2$ receptors are present in arteries and veins of the hand. Intra-arterial 5-HT leads to a dose-dependent decrease in the digital blood flow, which is inhibited by the 5-HT$_2$ antagonist ketanserin.[35,99] Ketanserin also produces a large increase in digital blood flow during reflex sympathetic vasoconstriction, which is not related to an α_1-adrenoreceptor- or α_2-adrenoreceptor-mediated mechanism. The enhancement of cholinergic vasodilation has also been reported in Raynaud's phenomenon.[68,102]

Regarding the relationship between temperature and blood flow in the hands of patients with primary Raynaud's disease, the blood flow of the hand is decreased in a 20°C room with the hand in 32°C water, but the rate of flow returns to a normal level with the hand in 42°C water. Capillary blood flow in the finger in both warm and cool conditions in patients with Raynaud's disease is less than that in subjects without Raynaud's disease.[55] The cause of the decreased blood flow or vasospastic attacks of the fingers in patients with Raynaud's disease is not yet understood.[26,27,101] Recent reports have shown that endothelin 1 levels are increased in patients with Raynaud's disease.[116] However, later reports did not support this result and the physiological importance of endothelin in Raynaud's disease is unknown.[23,24,72]

Traditionally, two possible mechanisms have been proposed for Raynaud's disease: (1) a local fault theory, which is an abnormality at the level of the digital artery, and (2) a sympathetic overactivity theory.[12,32,33] A greater vasoconstrictive response to an α_2-adrenoreceptor agonist is found in patients with primary Raynaud's disease compared with subjects without Raynaud's disease; in addition, cooling can enhance this vasoconstrictive response.[33,48] However, emotional stress can induce attacks that could be explained by the sympathetic overactivity theory but not by the local fault theory. The local fault theory seems to be logical but has not yet been elucidated.[11,21,73,101]

Clinical Features and Their Basis

Primary Raynaud's disease is about four times as common in women, and the onset is usually between the second and fourth decades.[13-16,92] The incidence of Raynaud's disease in the general population of the United States is estimated as 5% to 20% but is higher in cool climates than in warm climates.[73,94] About 80% to 90% of patients with Raynaud's disease have primary Raynaud's disease and 10% to 20% secondary Raynaud's disease.[13-16,22,94] Familial aggregation of primary Raynaud's disease has also been reported.[49]

Most patients have vasospastic attacks only in the fingers, and a few patients have attacks only in the toes. Less than 50% of patients have both finger and toe involvement. Other areas including the nose, ears, lips, face, and chest may be affected in some patients. Generally, only one or two fingers are affected at the onset of the disease, and more fingers and toes are affected later.

Classic Raynaud's disease includes the typical three-phase color change. When blood flow stops, the fingers turn white and numb but the hands are not affected. When slow blood flow is subsequently restored, the digits turn blue because of desaturation of the hemoglobin in blood. If the digital blood flow is fully restored, the digits turn red because of reactive hyperemia, which is often associated with a throbbing pain. The typical three-phase color changes have been reported to occur in 4% to 65% of patients; the first phase (pallor) is often the only symptom in patients. More advanced symptoms including ulcerations, scarring, chronic paronychia, and necrosis have been reported in 13% of patients. Sclerodactyly is seen in approximately 10% of patients.

Diagnostic Tests

In general, patient history remains the most reliable method of diagnosis.[27,34] However, the assessment of Raynaud's phenomenon severity is often difficult, for the vasospastic attacks are not easily induced under experimental conditions.[74] The Raynaud's disease patient's physical examination is generally normal except for cool fingers. Measurement of finger systolic blood pressure during ischemia associated with local cooling is a useful diagnostic test. This test cools fingers by circulating water through a cuff around the proximal finger at 20°C, 15°C, 10°C, and 5°C for 5-minute intervals. Patients with Raynaud's disease usually show a decrease in finger systolic pressure, but differential diagnosis between primary and secondary Raynaud's disease cannot be achieved with this test.[34] Recently, the value of nail-fold capillary microscopy has been introduced as a noninvasive technique for the examination of the cutaneous microcirculation in vivo.[86,106] This technique may enable the identification of patients with no evidence of underlying disease who could be at risk of developing connective tissue disease.[79]

No specific laboratory test is available for definitive diagnosis of primary Raynaud's disease. Because the majority of patients with Raynaud's disease have the primary type, patients with no other systemic manifestations and normal physical examination usually undergo a minimum laboratory test. Elevated erythrocyte sedimentation rate or positive antinuclear antibodies may suggest the presence of underlying causes responsible for Raynaud's disease. Recently, von Willebrand factor and, to a lesser extent, thromboxane and tissue plasminogen activator antigen have been reported to be associated with disease severity in patients with Raynaud's phenomenon.[57] Anticollagen antibodies in primary Raynaud's phenomenon have also been investigated.[93] Further prospective studies are required to establish if these parameters can serve as markers of disease progression.

Medical and Surgical Treatment

General therapeutic methods include keeping warm, avoiding cold exposure, and stopping smoking.[2,115] Most patients respond well to conservative management of Raynaud's disease. Drug treatment is indicated for severe cases.[2,112] Nifedipine is currently considered the drug of first choice.[38,53,70,95,103,112] The initial daily dose is usually 10 to 20 mg for adults, increasing to as high as 60 to 90 mg/d to balance relief of symptoms with side effects. Some randomized studies have demonstrated the effect of nifedipine on reducing the frequency, duration, and severity of the disease.

Other therapeutic agents that inhibit peripheral vasoconstriction may give some relief of symptoms.[3,25,28,40,105] These drugs include reserpine, prazosin, angiotensin converting enzyme (ACE) inhibitors, glyceryl trinitrate, and guanethidine. Daily dosages and side effects of these drugs are summarized in Table 80.1. However, because few of these agents are backed by adequate placebo-controlled studies,[113] they should not be the first choice but can be used when nifedipine causes intolerable side

TABLE 80.1. Drug therapy for patients with Raynaud's phenomenon.

Drug	Type	Daily dosage (mg)	Remarks	Side effects
Nifedipine	Calcium channel blocker	60–90	Drug of first choice; effective for 70%	Headache, flushing, palpitations, etc.
Diltiazem	Calcium channel blocker	100–300	Fewer side effects than with nifedipine	Headache, dizziness, flushing, etc.
Reserpine	Peripheral sympathetic nerve inhibitor	0.125–0.5	No placebo-controlled study	Bradycardia, depression, edema, etc.
Guanethidine	Peripheral sympathetic nerve inhibitor	10–50	Suitable for patients with depression	Diarrhea, postural hypotension, impotence, etc.
Prazosin	α1-adrenoceptor antagonist	2–8	Effective for 70% but offers only temporary relief	Nausea, headache, palpitation, rash, diarrhea, dyspnea, etc.
Methyldopa	Central inhibitory α-adrenoceptor	1000–2000	No placebo-controlled study	Edema, drowsiness, headache, fever, hemolytic anemia, etc.
Ketanserin	5-HT$_2$ antagonist	80–120	Decreases the frequency of attacks	Dizziness, sedation, dry mouth, etc.
Prostaglandins	Direct peripheral vaso relaxant	Vary with analog	PGE$_1$ is not effective; PGI and its analog are under research	Hypotension, diarrhea, flushing, headache, etc.

5-HT; serotonin; PGE, prostaglandin E$_1$; PGI, PGI$_2$, prostacyclin.

effects. Ketanserin, a selective 5-HT$_2$ antagonist, may be the most promising therapeutic agent.[35,61,99]

Plasmapheresis and conditioning and biofeedback have been reported to be beneficial in some patients but are expensive and time-consuming. Thus, these therapies are not considered standard therapies for patients with Raynaud's disease. Sympathectomy is the only surgical treatment that has been undertaken for patients with Raynaud's disease. Thoracic sympathectomy for digital vasospasm may be effective for 50% to 60% of patients, but vasospastic attacks may recur within 6 to 24 months.[98] Lumbar sympathectomy for toe symptoms has provided better results and is effective for approximately 80% of patients. However, current therapeutic strategies for Raynaud's disease do not include thoracic or lumbar sympathectomy because of the high rate of recurrence that results from unknown mechanisms.

Secondary Causes of Raynaud's Disease

About 10% to 20% of patients with Raynaud's disease have the secondary type.[58] The underlying causes of secondary Raynaud's disease include drug use, exposure to chemicals, connective tissue diseases, neoplasms, compression of nerves or blood vessels, obstruction of blood vessels, vasculitis, and endocrine disorders.[5,8,17,31,39,43,50, 54,60,71,75] Among these causes, drugs and connective tissue diseases are the most common.[8,17,20,54,63–66,69,91, 97,107,109] Fifty percent of patients with suspected Raynaud's phenomenon have been reported to develop a connective tissue disease in approximately 8 years.[77] Clinical manifestations observed in these patients vary with primary cause, but tissue damage in the fingers from secondary Raynaud's disease tends to be more extreme than that from primary Raynaud's disease.[8,30] Nail-fold capillaroscopy has been reported to distinguish between primary and secondary Raynaud's phenomenon and may be used to identify patients presenting no evidence of underlying disease who could develop connective tissue disease.[79,80] Therapeutic strategies for secondary Raynaud's disease are in principle the same as those for primary Raynaud's disease, but treatment of

TABLE 80.2. Secondary causes of Raynaud's phenomenon.

Cause	Reported incidence (%)
Arteriovenous fistula	>50
Carpal tunnel syndrome	Common
Chemicals	
Vinyl chloride	Common
Heavy metals	
Connective tissue diseases	
Scleroderma	90
Systemic lupus erythematosus	10–44
Rheumatoid arthritis	
Sjögren's syndrome	
Polymyositis and dermatomyositis	30–40
Mixed connective tissue disease	70–85
Cryoproteinemia, cold agglutinins, polycythemia	3–10
Drugs	
ß-adrenoceptor antagonists	4–40
Ergot	0.01
Interferon	
Vinblastine and bleomycin	2.6–37
Methysergide	3
Hypothenar hammer syndrome	
Hypothyroidism	20–25
Neoplasms	
Obstructive arterial diseases	
Arteriosclerotic obliterans	
Thromboangiitis obliterans (Buerger's disease)	57
Primary biliary cirrhosis	
Primary pulmonary hypertension	10–30
Renal disease	
Thoracic outlet syndromes	
Hyperabduction syndrome	38.6
Cervical ribs	10
Other types	5.3
Trauma	
Vasculitis	

the underlying disease is more essential for these patients. Table 80.2 summarizes the causes and their incidence in patients with secondary Raynaud's disease.

Acrocyanosis

Pathophysiology and Clinical Features

Patients with acrocyanosis have persistent cyanosis and coldness in the fingers, hands, and toes; sometimes the distal arms and face are involved.[18,21] The cyanotic color is enhanced by coldness and relieved by warming. The incidence of acrocyanosis is unknown. The age range reported in the literature is 20 to 45 years, with no gender predominance. Familial aggregation of acrocyanosis and palmoplantar keratoderma has also been reported.[85] Devastating symptoms such as severe pain, ulceration, and contracture do not occur. The cause of idiopathic acrocyanosis is not understood. Pathologic findings of skin biopsies indicate only nonspecific thickening of the medial layers of the arterioles. Idiopathic acrocyanosis is a benign disease that may be only a cosmetic problem to patients.[18] Physical examination and laboratory tests are normal. Acrocyanosis may occur secondary to underlying diseases such as connective tissue diseases or any diseases that elicit central cyanosis (e.g., right-to-left shunt), or as a drug side effect.[4,19] Plasma levels of endothelin-1 have been reported to be enhanced in patients with essential acrocyanosis and further increased by cooling until 90 minutes after cold challenge.[78] This rise in plasma endothelin-1 may contribute to potentiating and prolonging cold-induced vasoconstriction/vasospasm and/or could be a marker for endothelial damage in essential acrocyanosis.

Diagnostic Tests

No specific laboratory tests are available for definitive diagnosis of idiopathic acrocyanosis. The differential diagnoses are Raynaud's disease, connective tissue disease, and central cyanosis. However, differentiation is not difficult if the pattern of vasospastic attacks, history, physical examination (including the skin temperature), and measurements of arterial oxygen saturation are reviewed carefully.[19,21,29,41]

Medical and Surgical Treatment

Treatment is usually unnecessary for patients with idiopathic acrocyanosis because it is a benign disease. For the few patients who request therapy for cosmetic or other reasons, small doses of guanethidine or reserpine may provide some relief. For patients with secondary acrocyanosis, treatment of the underlying disease is es-

sential.[83] Electrical neuromuscular stimulation has been tried for some cases refractory to usual treatment.[81,108]

Livedo Reticularis

Pathophysiology and Clinical Features

There are three types of livedo reticularis: (1) benign livedo reticularis (idiopathic livedo reticularis), (2) livedo reticularis with ulceration (livedo vasculitis, atrophie blanche), and (3) secondary livedo reticularis. The clinical sign of livedo reticularis derives from stasis of blood in the superficial venous drainage systems of the skin. Many factors can delay the flow of deoxygenated blood away from the skin, especially hyperviscosity of the blood and obstruction due to disease affecting dermal arteries, capillaries, or venules.[37]

Benign Livedo Reticularis

Patients with benign livedo reticularis show a mottled discoloration of the extremities in a reticular, or lacelike, pattern that is enhanced by cold exposure and relieved by warming. Pathologic findings are nonspecific but are often associated with widespread dilation of capillaries. Because the reticular pattern on the skin is reversible, it is believed to result from vasospasm of small arterioles in the dermis. The red to blue color is derived from deoxygenated blood in the surrounding venous plexus.

The incidence of this disease is rare; it affects women more often than men and usually during the second to fifth decades. Except for the mottled discoloration and coldness of the extremities, physical examination in patients with this form is normal.

Livedo Reticularis With Ulceration

Patients with livedo reticularis with ulceration usually show the same skin pattern as those with benign livedo reticularis, but the pattern does not disappear with warming.[46,118] In contrast to the pathologic findings in the benign form, the middle dermal vessels are often affected by segmental hyalinization. Skin infarction caused by occlusion of arterioles may be present. Patients with livedo reticularis with ulceration develop purpuric cutaneous nodules that can progress to ulcers. The ulcers are usually very painful and take months to heal.[118] Most ulcers occur on the feet, ankles, and calves. Healed ulcers leave smooth, white atrophic skin with surrounding hyperpigmentation, which may account for the name *atrophie blanche*.

Secondary Livedo Reticularis

Secondary livedo reticularis occurs with diseases that cause a significant decrease in skin blood flow, such as connective tissue disease, hyperviscosity states, thrombocythemia, diabetes mellitus, or obstructive arterial diseases.[1,6,9,10,45,47,51,52,56,67,84,90,104,111] In addition, amantadine hydrochloride causes livedo reticularis similar to the benign form, which can be relieved by warming.[88,89,100] Both legs are usually affected, and the disease is often associated with pedal edema. Cessation of medication is not necessary for patients with Parkinson's disease if livedo reticularis appears. Livedo reticularis associated with cerebrovascular lesions is known as Sneddon's syndrome.[42,62,96]

Diagnostic Tests

No specific tests are available for diagnosis of the benign form of livedo reticularis or livedo reticularis with ulcerations. In patients with secondary livedo reticularis, laboratory tests reflect the underlying diseases, including elevated anticardiolipin antibody levels[7,45,47,52,82,110,117]

Medical and Surgical Treatment

Treatment is unnecessary for patients with benign livedo reticularis because they have only cosmetic problems. Antiplatelet therapy with the use of aspirin, ticlopidine, or dipyridamole may give some relief to patients with painful ulcerations.[44,59] Most other therapies that have been tried for patients with ulceration are unsuccessful, but some patients who do not respond to any therapy show spontaneous remission. Amputations have been performed rarely for patients with deep, painful, and nonhealing ulcers. For patients with secondary livedo reticularis, treatment is for the underlying disease.

Bibliography

1. Abrahamian LM, Berke A, Van Voorhees A. Type 1 diabetes mellitus associated with livedo reticularis: case report and review of the literature. *Pediatr Dermatol.* 1991;8: 46–50.
2. Adee AC. Managing Raynaud's phenomenon: a practical approach. *Am Fam Physician.* 1993;47:823–829.
3. Aikimbaev KS, Oguz M, Ozbek S, Demirtas M, Birand A, Batyraliev T. Comparative assessment of the effects of vasodilators on peripheral vascular reactivity in patients with systemic scleroderma and Raynaud's phenomenon: color Doppler flow imaging study. *Angiology.* 1996;47:475–480.
4. Anderson RP, Morris BA. Acrocyanosis due to imipramine. *Arch Dis Child.* 1988;63:204–205.
5. Arpaia G, Cimminiello C, Bellone M, Aloisio M, Rossi F, Bonfardeci G. Need to expand microvascular investigation of patients with Raynaud's phenomenon of different etiology: clinical patterns of 106 consecutive patients. *Int Angiol.* 1994;13:15–18.
6. Asherson RA, D'Cruz D, Hughes GR. Cryoglobulins, anticardiolipin antibodies, and livedo reticularis. *J Rheumatol.* 1992;19:826.
7. Asherson RA, Mayou SC, Merry P, Black MM, Hughes GR. The spectrum of livedo reticularis and anticardiolipin antibodies. *Br J Dermatol.* 1989;120:215–221.
8. Bachmeyer C, Farge D, Gluckman E, Miclea JM, Aractingi S. Raynaud's phenomenon and digital necrosis induced by interferon-alpha. *Br J Dermatol.* 1996;135:481–483.
9. Baethge BA, Sanusi ID, Landreneau MD, Rohr MS, McDonald JC. Livedo reticularis and peripheral gangrene associated with primary hyperoxaluria. *Arthritis Rheum.* 1988; 31:1199–1203.
10. Baguley E, Asherson RA, Hughes GR. Anticardiolipin antibodies, livedo reticularis, and cerebrovascular accidents in SLE. *Ann Rheum Dis.* 1988;47:702–703.
11. Bartelink ML, Wollersheim H, Vemer H, Thomas CM, de Boo T, Thien T. The effects of single oral doses of 17 beta-oestradiol and progesterone on finger skin circulation in healthy women and in women with primary Raynaud's phenomenon. *Eur J Clin Pharmacol.* 1994;46:557–560.
12. Bedarida G, Kim D, Blaschke TF, Hoffman BB. Venodilation in Raynaud's disease [see comments]. *Lancet.* 1993; 342:1451–1454.
13. Belch JJ. Raynaud's phenomenon. *Curr Opin Rheumatol.* 1989;1:490–498.
14. Belch JJ. Raynaud's phenomenon. *Curr Opin Rheumatol.* 1990;2:937–941.
15. Belch JJ. Raynaud's phenomenon. *Curr Opin Rheumatol.* 1991;3:960–966.
16. Belch JJ. Raynaud's phenomenon: its relevance to scleroderma. *Ann Rheum Dis.* 1991;50(suppl 4):839–845.
17. Berger CC, Bokemeyer C, Schneider M, Kuczyk MA, Schmoll HJ. Secondary Raynaud's phenomenon and other late vascular complications following chemotherapy for testicular cancer. *Eur J Cancer.* 1995;31A(13–14): 2229–2238.
18. Bigby M, McCoy K. Reddish-blue hands and feet: acrocyanosis with atrophy. *Arch Dermatol.* 1988;124:265–268.
19. Blockmans D, Beyens G, Verhaeghe R. Predictive value of nailfold capillaroscopy in the diagnosis of connective tissue diseases. *Clin Rheumatol.* 1996;15:148–153.
20. Blockmans D, Vermylen J, Bobbaers H. Nailfold capillaroscopy in connective tissue disorders and in Raynaud's phenomenon. *Acta Clin Belg.* 1993;48:30–41.
21. Bollinger A. Function of the precapillary vessels in peripheral vascular disease. *J Cardiovasc Pharmacol.* 1985;7(suppl 3):S147–S151.
22. Bolster MB, Maricq HR, Leff RL. Office evaluation and treatment of Raynaud's phenomenon. *Cleve Clin J Med.* 1995;62:51–61.
23. Bottomley W, Goodfield M. A pathogenic role for endothelin in Raynaud's phenomenon? *Acta Derm Venereol.* 1994;74:433–434.
24. Bunker CB, Goldsmith PC, Leslie TA, Hayes N, Foreman JC, Dowd PM. Calcitonin gene–related peptide, endothelin-1, the cutaneous microvasculature, and Raynaud's phenomenon. *Br J Dermatol.* 1996;134:399–406.
25. Bunker CB, Reavley C, O'Shaughnessy DJ, Dowd PM. Calcitonin gene–related peptide in treatment of severe peripheral vascular insufficiency in Raynaud's phenomenon. *Lancet.* 1993;342:80–83.
26. Campbell PM, LeRoy EC. Raynaud phenomenon. *Semin Arthritis Rheum.* 1986;16:92–103.

27. Cardelli MB, Kleinsmith DM. Raynaud's phenomenon and disease. *Med Clin North Am.* 1989;73:1127–1141.

28. Challenor VF. Angiotensin converting enzyme inhibitors in Raynaud's phenomenon. *Drugs.* 1994;48:864–867.

29. Cimminiello C, Arpaia G, Milani M, Uberti T, Rocchini GM, Motta A, Cristoforetti G, Curri SB. Platelet function in patients with acrocyanosis. *Vasa.* 1987;16:12–15.

30. Cimminiello C, Arpaia G, Toschi V, Rossi F, Aloisio M, Motta A, Bonfardeci G. Plasma levels of tumor necrosis factor and endothelial response in patients with chronic arterial obstructive disease or Raynaud's phenomenon. *Angiology.* 1994;45:1015–1022.

31. Clements PJ. Raynaud's phenomenon, scleroderma, overlap syndromes, and other fibrosing syndromes [editorial]. *Curr Opin Rheumatol.* 1993;5:749–752.

32. Coffman JD. Pathogenesis and treatment of Raynaud's phenomenon. *Cardiovasc Drugs Ther.* 1990;4 (suppl 1):45–51.

33. Coffman JD. Raynaud's phenomenon: an update. *Hypertension.* 1991;17:593–602.

34. Coffman JD. The diagnosis of Raynaud's phenomenon. *Clin Dermatol.* 1994;12:283–289.

35. Coffman JD, Cohen RA. Serotonergic vasoconstriction in human fingers during reflex sympathetic response to cooling. *Am J Physiol.* 1988;254:H889–893.

36. Coffman JD, Cohen RA. Plasma levels of 5-hydroxytryptamine during sympathetic stimulation and in Raynaud's phenomenon. *Clin Sci (Colch).* 1994;86:269–273.

37. Copeman PW. Livedo reticularis: signs in the skin of disturbance of blood viscosity and of blood flow. *Br J Dermatol.* 1975;93:519–529.

38. Corbin DO, Wood DA, Macintyre CC, Housley E. A randomized double blind cross-over trial of nifedipine in the treatment of primary Raynaud's phenomenon. *Eur Heart J.* 1986;7:165–170.

39. Creutzig A, Caspary L, Freund M. The Raynaud phenomenon and interferon therapy. *Ann Intern Med.* 1996;125:423.

40. Creutzig A, Freund M. Double-blind, placebo-controlled study of intravenous prostacyclin on hemodynamics in severe Raynaud's phenomenon: the acute vasodilatory effect is not sustained. *J Cardiovasc Pharmacol.* 1995;26:388–393.

41. Davis E. Oscillometry of radial artery in acrocyanosis and cold sensitivity. *J Mal Vasc.* 1992;17:214–217.

42. Devos J, Bulcke J, Degreef H, Michielsen B. Sneddon's syndrome: generalized livedo reticularis and cerebrovascular disease: importance of hemostatic screening. *Dermatology.* 1992;185:296–299.

43. Doria A, Ghirardello A, Boscaro M, Viero ML, Vaccaro E, Patrassi GM, Gambari PF. Fibrinolysis and coagulation abnormalities in systemic lupus erythematosus: relationship with Raynaud's phenomenon, disease activity, inflammatory indices, anticardiolipin antibodies, and corticosteroid therapy. *Rheumatol Int.* 1995;14:207–211.

44. Drucker CR, Duncan WC. Antiplatelet therapy in atrophie blanche and livedo vasculitis. *J Am Acad Dermatol.* 1982;7:359–363.

45. Englert HJ, Loizou S, Derue GG, Walport MJ, Hughes GR. Clinical and immunologic features of livedo reticularis in lupus: a case-control study. *Am J Med.* 1989;87:408–410.

46. Feldaker M, Hines EA Jr, Kierland RR. Livedo reticularis with ulcerations. *Circulation.* 1956;13:196–216.

47. Fleischer AJ, Resnick SD. Livedo reticularis. *Dermatol Clin.* 1990;8:347–354.

48. Freedman RR, Baer RP, Mayes MD. Blockade of vasospastic attacks by alpha 2-adrenergic but not alpha 1-adrenergic antagonists in idiopathic Raynaud's disease. *Circulation.* 1995;92:1448–1451.

49. Freedman RR, Mayes MD. Familial aggregation of primary Raynaud's disease. *Arthritis Rheum.* 1996;39:1189–1191.

50. Friedman EI, Taylor LJ, Porter JM. Late-onset Raynaud's syndrome: diagnostic and therapeutic considerations. *Geriatrics.* 1988;43:59–63.

51. Genovese A, Spadaro G, Marone G. Livedo reticularis and congenital hypogammaglobulinemia. *J Med.* 1992;23:78–80.

52. Genovese A, Spadaro G, Marone G. Livedo reticularis in a patient with systemic lupus erythematosus and anticardiolipin antibodies. *Clin Exp Dermatol.* 1993;18:159–161.

53. Gjorup T, Kelbaek H, Hartling OJ, Nielsen SL. Controlled double-blind trial of the clinical effect of nifedipine in the treatment of idiopathic Raynaud's phenomenon. *Am Heart J.* 1986;111:742–745.

54. Grassi W, Blasetti P, Core P, Cervini C. Raynaud's phenomenon in rheumatoid arthritis. *Br J Rheumatol.* 1994;33:139–141.

55. Greenstein D, Gupta NK, Martin P, Walker DR, Kester RC. Impaired thermoregulation in Raynaud's phenomenon. *Angiology.* 1995;46:603–611.

56. Gross AS, Thompson FL, Arzubiaga MC, Graber SE, Hammer RD, Schulman G, Ellis DL, King LJ. Heparin-associated thrombocytopenia and thrombosis (HATT) presenting with livedo reticularis. *Int J Dermatol.* 1993;32:276–279.

57. Herrick AL, Illingworth K, Blann A, Hay CR, Hollis S, Jayson MI. Von Willebrand factor, thrombomodulin, thromboxane, beta-thromboglobulin, and markers of fibrinolysis in primary Raynaud's phenomenon and systemic sclerosis. *Ann Rheum Dis.* 1996;55:122–127.

58. Hirschl M, Kundi M. Initial prevalence and incidence of secondary Raynaud's phenomenon in patients with Raynaud's symptomatology. *J Rheumatol.* 1996;23:302–309.

59. Hoogenberg K, Tupker RA, van Essen LH, Smit AJ, Kallenberg CG. Successful treatment of ulcerating livedo reticularis with infusions of prostacyclin. *Br J Dermatol.* 1992;127:64–66.

60. Ishikawa M, Okada J, Shibuya A, Kondo H. CRST syndrome (calcinosis cutis, Raynaud's phenomenon, sclerodactyly, and telangiectasia) associated with autoimmune hepatitis. *Intern Med.* 1995;34:6–9.

61. Jaffe IA. Serotonin reuptake inhibitors in Raynaud's phenomenon. *Lancet.* 1995;345:1378.

62. Jura E, Palasik W, Meurer M, Palester CM, Czlonkowska A. Sneddon's syndrome (livedo reticularis and cerebrovascular lesions) with antiphospholipid antibodies and severe dementia in young men: a case report. *Acta Neurol Scand.* 1994;89:143–146.

63. Kahaleh B, Matucci CM. Raynaud's phenomenon and scleroderma: dysregulated neuroendothelial control of vascular tone. *Arthritis Rheum.* 1995;38:1–4.

64. Kahaleh MB. Raynaud's phenomenon, scleroderma, overlap syndromes, and other fibrosing syndromes. *Curr Opin Rheumatol.* 1994;6:603–606.

65. Kallenberg CG. Early detection of connective tissue disease in patients with Raynaud's phenomenon. *Rheum Dis Clin North Am.* 1990;16:11–30.

66. Kallenberg CG. Connective tissue disease in patients presenting with Raynaud's phenomenon alone. *Ann Rheum Dis.* 1991;50:666–667.

67. Kalter DC, Rudolph A, McGavran M. Livedo reticularis due to multiple cholesterol emboli. *J Am Acad Dermatol.* 1985;13:235–242.

68. Khan F, Coffman JD. Enhanced cholinergic cutaneous vasodilation in Raynaud's phenomenon. *Circulation.* 1994; 89:1183–1188.

69. Kingma K, Wollersheim H, Thien T. Raynaud's phenomenon and the vascular disease in scleroderma. *Curr Opin Rheumatol.* 1995;7:529–534.

70. Kiowski W, Erne P, Buhler FR. Use of nifedipine in hypertension and Raynaud's phenomenon. *Cardiovasc Drugs Ther.* 1990;4(suppl 5):935–940.

71. Kohli M, Bennett RM. Raynaud's phenomenon as a presenting sign of ovarian adenocarcinoma. *J Rheumatol.* 1995;22:1393–1394.

72. La Civita L, Giuggioli D, Del Chicca M, Longombardo G, Pasero G, Ferri C. Effect of isradipine on endothelin-1 plasma concentrations in patients with Raynaud's phenomenon. *Ann Rheum Dis.* 1996;55:331–332.

73. Lally EV. Raynaud's phenomenon. *Curr Opin Rheumatol.* 1992;4:825–836.

74. Lau CS, Khan F, Brown R, McCallum P, Belch JJ. Digital blood flow response to body warming, cooling, and rewarming in patients with Raynaud's phenomenon. *Angiology.* 1995;46:1–10.

75. Lavras CL, Valente CA. Primary biliary cirrhosis (PBC)–CREST (calcinosis, Raynaud's phenomenon, esophageal dysfunction, sclerodactyly, and telangiectasia) overlap syndrome complicated by Sjogren's syndrome and arthritis. *Intern Med.* 1995;34:451–454.

76. Leppert J, Ringqvist A, Ahlner J, Myrdal U, Sorensen S, Ringqvist I. Cold exposure increases cyclic guanosine monophosphate in healthy women but not in women with Raynaud's phenomenon. *J Intern Med.* 1995;237:493–498.

77. Luggen M, Belhorn L, Evans T, Fitzgerald O, Spencer GG. The evolution of Raynaud's phenomenon: a longterm prospective study. *J Rheumatol.* 1995;22:2226–2232.

78. Mangiafico RA, Malatino LS, Santonocito M, Spada RS, Tamburino G. Plasma endothelin-1 concentrations during cold exposure in essential acrocyanosis. *Angiology.* 1996;47: 1033–1038.

79. Mannarino E, Pasqualini L, Fedeli F, Scricciolo V, Innocente S. Nailfold capillaroscopy in the screening and diagnosis of Raynaud's phenomenon. *Angiology.* 1994;45: 37–42.

80. Maricq HR. Capillary abnormalities, Raynaud's phenomenon, and systemic sclerosis in patients with localized scleroderma. *Arch Dermatol.* 1992;128:630–632.

81. Martinez R, Saponaro A, Russo R, Dragagna G, Leopardi N, Santoro L, Martelli E. Effects of sympathetic stimulation on microcirculatory dynamics in patients with essential acrocyanosis: a study using mental stress. *Panminerva Med.* 1993;35:9–11.

82. McHugh NJ, Maymo J, Skinner RP, James I, Maddison PJ. Anticardiolipin antibodies, livedo reticularis, and major cerebrovascular and renal disease in systemic lupus erythematosus. *Ann Rheum Dis.* 1988;47:110–115.

83. Michiels JJ, Abels J, Steketee J, van Vliet H, Vuzevski VD. Erythromelalgia caused by platelet-mediated arteriolar inflammation and thrombosis in thrombocythemia. *Ann Intern Med.* 1985;102:466–471.

84. Naldi L, Marchesi L, Locati F, Berti E, Cainelli T. Unusual manifestations of primary cutaneous amyloidosis in association with Raynaud's phenomenon and livedo reticularis. *Clin Exp Dermatol.* 1992;17:117–120.

85. Nielsen PG. Diffuse palmoplantar keratoderma associated with acrocyanosis: a family study. *Acta Derm Venereol.* 1989; 69:156–161.

86. Ohtsuka T, Yamakage A, Tamura T. Image analysis of nail fold capillaries in patients with Raynaud's phenomenon. *Cutis.* 1995;56:215–218.

87. Olsen N. Centrally and locally mediated vasomotor activities in Raynaud's phenomenon. *Scand J Work Environ Health.* 1987;13:309–312.

88. Paulson GW, Brandt JT. Amantadine, livedo reticularis, and antiphospholipid antibodies. *Clin Neuropharmacol.* 1995;18:466–467.

89. Pearce LA, Waterbury LD, Green HD. Amantadine hydrochloride: alteration in peripheral circulation. *Neurology.* 1974;24:46–48.

90. Picascia DD, Pellegrini JR. Livedo reticularis. *Cutis.* 1987; 39:429–432.

91. Pistorius MA, Planchon B. Raynaud's phenomenon in systemic lupus erythematosus. *Rev Rhum Engl Ed.* 1995;62:349–353.

92. Planchon B, Pistorius MA, Beurrier P, De Faucal P. Primary Raynaud's phenomenon: age of onset and pathogenesis in a prospective study of 424 patients. *Angiology.* 1994; 45:677–686.

93. Riente L, Marchini B, Dolcher MP, Puccetti A, Bombardieri S, Migliorini P. Anti-collagen antibodies in systemic sclerosis and in primary Raynaud's phenomenon. *Clin Exp Immunol.* 1995;102:354–359.

94. Riera G, Vilardell M, Vaque J, Fonollosa V, Bermejo B. Prevalence of Raynaud's phenomenon in a healthy Spanish population. *J Rheumatol.* 1993;20:66–69.

95. Roath S. Management of Raynaud's phenomenon: focus on newer treatments. *Drugs.* 1989;37:700–712.

96. Rumpl E, Neuhofer J, Pallua A, Willeit J, Vogl G, Stampfel G, Platz T. Cerebrovascular lesions and livedo reticularis (Sneddon's syndrome): a progressive cerebrovascular disorder? *J Neurol.* 1985;231:324–330.

97. Saraux A, Allain J, Guedes C, Baron D, Youinou P, Le Goff P. Raynaud's phenomenon in rheumatoid arthritis. *Br J Rheumatol.* 1996;35:752–754.

98. Sayers RD, Jenner RE, Barrie WW. Transthoracic endoscopic sympathectomy for hyperhidrosis and Raynaud's phenomenon. *Eur J Vasc Endovasc Surg.* 1994;8:627–631.

99. Seibold JR. Serotonin and Raynaud's phenomenon. *J Cardiovasc Pharmacol.* 1985;7(suppl 7):S95–S98.

100. Shealy CN, Weeth JB, Mercier D. Livedo reticularis in patients with Parkinsonism receiving amantadine. *JAMA.* 1970;212:1522–1523.

101. Shepherd RF, Shepherd JT. Raynaud's phenomenon. *Int Angiol.* 1992;11:41–45.

102. Singh S, De Trafford J, Baskerville PA, Martin JF. Response of digital arteries to endothelium dependent and independent vasodilators in patients with Raynaud's phenomenon. *Eur J Clin Invest.* 1995;25:182–185.

103. Smith CR, Rodeheffer RJ. Raynaud's phenomenon: pathophysiologic features and treatment with calcium-channel blockers. *Am J Cardiol.* 1985;55:154B–157B.

104. Speight EL, Lawrence CM. Reticulate purpura, cryoglobulinaemia, and livedo reticularis. *Br J Dermatol.* 1993;129:319–323.

105. Teh LS, Manning J, Moore T, Tully MP, O'Reilly D, Jayson MI. Sustained-release transdermal glyceryl trinitrate patches as a treatment for primary and secondary Raynaud's phenomenon. *Br J Rheumatol.* 1995;34:636–641.

106. ter Borg E, Piersma WG, Smit AJ, Kallenberg CG, Wouda AA. Serial nailfold capillary microscopy in primary Raynaud's phenomenon and scleroderma. *Semin Arthritis Rheum.* 1994;24:40–47.

107. Toumbis IE, Cohen PR. Chemotherapy-induced Raynaud's phenomenon. *Cleve Clin J Med.* 1994;61:195–199.

108. Twist DJ. Acrocyanosis in a spinal cord injured patient—effects of computer-controlled neuromuscular electrical stimulation: a case report. *Phys Ther.* 1990;70:45–49.

109. Vayssairat M, Baudot N, Gaitz JP. Raynaud's phenomenon together with antinuclear antibodies: a common subset of incomplete connective tissue disease. *J Am Acad Dermatol.* 1995;35:747–749.

110. Weinstein C, Miller MH, Axtens R, Buchanan R, Littlejohn GO. Livedo reticularis associated with increased titers of anticardiolipin antibodies in systemic lupus erythematosus. *Arch Dermatol.* 1987;123:596–600.

111. Weir NU, Snowden JA, Greaves M, Davies JG. Livedo reticularis associated with hereditary protein C deficiency and recurrent thromboembolism. *Br J Dermatol.* 1995;132:283–285.

112. Wesseling H. Drug treatment in Raynaud's phenomenon. *Vasa Suppl.* 1987;18:48–53.

113. Wigley FM, Wise RA, Seibold JR, McCloskey DA, Kujala G, Medsger TJ, et al. Intravenous iloprost infusion in patients with Raynaud phenomenon secondary to systemic sclerosis: a multicenter, placebo-controlled, double-blind study. *Ann Intern Med.* 1994;120:199–206.

114. Wollersheim H, Cleophas T, Thien T. The role of the sympathetic nervous system in the pathophysiology and therapy of Raynaud's phenomenon. *Vasa Suppl.* 1987;18:54–63.

115. Wollersheim H, van Zwieten P. Treatment of Raynaud's phenomenon. *Eur Heart J.* 1993;14:147–149.

116. Yamane K. Endothelin and collagen vascular disease: a review with special reference to Raynaud's phenomenon and systemic sclerosis. *Intern Med.* 1994;33:579–582.

117. Yancey WJ, Edwards NL, Williams RJ. Cryoglobulins in a patient with SLE, livedo reticularis, and elevated level of anticardiolipin antibodies. *Am J Med.* 1990;88:699.

118. Young PC, Cuozzo DW, Seidman AJ, Benson PM, Sau P, James WD. Widespread livedo reticularis with painful ulcerations. *Arch Dermatol.* 1995;131:786–788.

Section 11
Chronic Venous Insufficiency Disease

81

Classification of Venous Insufficiency: Diagnosis and Treatment

Shunichi Hoshino and Hirono Satokawa

Venous insufficiency usually occurs in veins of the lower extremities and consists of mechanical problems of reflux, obstruction, or a combination of the two. The clinical process is usually slow, recurrent, and chronic. Therefore, we refer to the condition as *chronic venous insufficiency*. These lesions cause local venous hypertension, which results in venous stasis symptoms such as skin exanthema, pigmentation, lipodermatosclerosis, and stasis ulcers (Figures 81.1 and 81.2). The venous system consists of superficial veins, including the saphenous system, the deep vein system, and perforating veins. Reflux lesions may spread not only to the superficial venous system but also to multisegmental veins. Primary varicose veins, with reflux of superficial veins, are most often encountered clinically. Reflux flow in the deep vein system may be due to congenital valvular absences, prolapse of valves (floppy valves, primary deep vein insufficiency), dilation of valvular annuli, or postthrombotic syndrome.[5] In a vein lumen occluded with thrombi, the valve cusps become fixed and are unable to function properly. If thrombolysis occurs, recanalization results in a vessel without valves. However, most obstructive disorders are caused by deep vein thrombosis due to incomplete recanalization and the onset of acute deep vein thrombosis. Sakaguchi et al.[37] reported that 80% of obstructive diseases can be improved by recanalization within 2 years, but reflux may increase. These two components, reflux and obstruction, maintain the balance of a mixed condition, but the reflux component proved superior after 10 years.

Regarding the causes of deep vein insufficiency, radiological imaging showed that as few as 36% of limbs with severe chronic venous insufficiency were associated with postphlebitic changes.[47] The other two thirds were derived from vein valve prolapse.[4] Venous insufficiency from perforating veins alone is not as common but does play a role in combination with deep vein reflux. Recently it was reported that many patients with primary varicose veins had deep vein reflux.[10,36] The difference between deep vein reflux of primary varicose veins and primary deep vein insufficiency is controversial, and some offer a counterargument for the real significance of deep vein reconstruction.[10] However, because the aim of surgery for valvular reflux is segmental prevention of lower limb venous pressure, those with deep vein insufficiency may be candidates for surgical reconstruction.

Classification

Reporting Standards in Venous Disease provided by the ad hoc committee of the Society for Vascular Surgery[34] have been available since 1988. The classification by clinical severity is expressed on a scale of 0 to 3:

Class 0 Asymptomatic
Class 1 Mild insufficiency with signs and symptoms including mild to moderate ankle swelling, mild discomfort, and local or generalized dilatation of subcutaneous veins
Class 2 Moderate insufficiency including hyperpigmentation of the skin in the gaiter area, moderate brawny edema, and subcutaneous fibrosis
Class 3 Severe insufficiency, chronic distal leg pain associated with ulcerative or preulcerative skin changes, eczematous changes, and severe edema

This classification has contributed to uniform diagnosis and reporting of treatment results. However, advances in the understanding of chronic venous diseases have created a need to expand definitions to cover many other aspects including anatomy, pathophysiology, and etiology. A document entitled "Classification and Grading of Chronic Venous Disease in the Lower Limbs: A Consensus Statement (CEAP Classification)" was presented by the ad hoc committee of the American Venous Forum in 1994.[3] The classification is as follows:

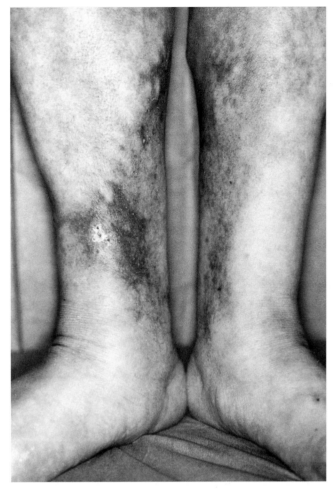

FIGURE 81.1. Ulcer scar and pigmentation of chronic venous insufficiency.

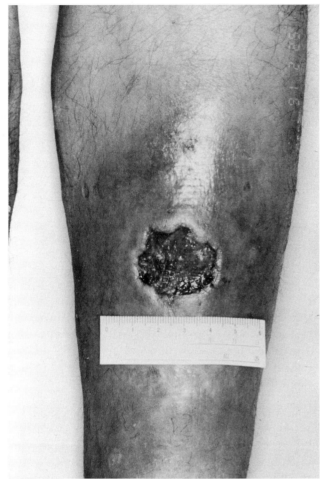

FIGURE 81.2. Venous stasis ulcer.

C Clinical signs (grade 0–6), supplemented by *A* for asymptomatic and *S* for symptomatic presentation
E Etiologic classification (congenital [Ec], primary [Ep], or secondary [Es])
A Anatomical distribution (superficial [As], deep [AD], or perforator [Ap], alone or in combination)
P Pathophysiologic dysfunction (reflux [PR] or obstruction [Po], alone or in combination)

Limbs in higher categories have more severe manifestations of chronic venous disease and may have some or all of the findings associated with less severe categories. Clinical classification is as follows:

Class 0 No visible or palpable signs of venous disease
Class 1 Telangiectases or reticular veins
Class 2 Varicose veins
Class 3 Edema
Class 4 Skin changes ascribed to venous disease (pigmentation, venous eczema, lipodermatosclerosis)
Class 5 Skin changes as defined previously with healed ulceration

Class 6 Skin changes as defined previously with present ulceration

The anatomical parts were subdivided into 18 segments. This classification is useful not only for case presentation but also for follow-up after surgery. The scoring system consists of an anatomical score, clinical score, and disability score. For scoring after surgery, because the procedures affect the anatomical score, we used the clinical score plus the disability score for follow-up.

Diagnosis

Clinical Examination

The first step of diagnosis is clinical examination including inquiring about the patient's history. A careful clinical history is an essential part of the investigation of venous disease and differential diagnoses. It is important to inquire about symptoms such as pain, swelling, and unsightliness, as well as type of work, lifestyle, labor history, and family history. History of limb swelling with redness and pain may be related to deep vein thrombosis. Patients often complain of fatigue occurring easily and swelling of the lower extremities that becomes worse during periods of standing and working.

In severe venous stasis, skin eczema, pigmentation, sclerotic skin changes, lipodermatosclerosis with inflammatory changes, and stasis ulcers may occur. Because these skin features may change rapidly, their size, location, shape, and depth should be recorded precisely. There is no difference between the swelling of deep vein thrombosis and that of chronic venous insufficiency. The size and tension of the veins can easily be assessed with the examiner's fingertips. The presence of thrills and bruits indicates arteriovenous fistulas. Tourniquet tests, such as the Brodie–Trendelenburg test, Perthes test, and retrograde leg milking test, are useful in determining blood flow. Tourniquet tests are useful in patients with chronic venous insufficiency, especially those with varicose veins. Although venous disorders are usually diagnosed by the Doppler method or duplex scanning, these bedside tests have recently come into more widespread use because they are simple and useful for screening in the outpatient clinic.

Plethysmography

Plethysmography is used to measure blood volume or volume change with an attachment probe. It is easy to measure general lower limb blood flow, and the results are useful in evaluating the treatment effects and follow-up.[1] Photoplethysmography measures the blood volume in the capillaries within the skin by reflected light. It is used to detect blood volume change, such as the venous refilling time after exercise, in either standing or sitting positions. Photoplethysmography and the tourniquet method are simple techniques to diagnose the reflux of superficial veins. However, quantitative evaluation is impossible because of the difficulty in calibration, and whole limb blood flow is not always reflected.

Strain-gauge plethysmography is the technique of measuring calf circumference and calculating its volume (Figure 81.3).[38] Strain-gauge plethysmography enables the measurement of volume change and calf pump function. Parameters such as venous volume and maximum venous outflow are measured by occlusion with a cuff; other parameters such as expelled volume and refilling time are measured using tip-toe movement techniques. Strain-gauge plethysmography shows the volume change only within a cross section, which is not equal to the whole volume of the calf.

Air plethysmography measures calf volume change using a long tubular air chamber that surrounds the entire limb from knee to ankle (Figure 81.4). Using air plethysmography, it is possible to detect whole limb volume changes as a result of exercise and postural change.[31] A

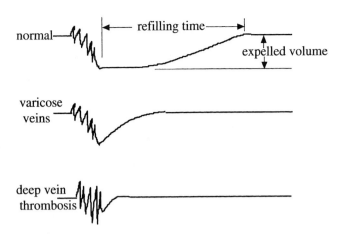

FIGURE 81.3. Tracing of strain-gauge plethysmography: (top) normal pattern; (middle) varicose vein with decreased refilling time; (bottom) deep vein thrombosis with decreased expelled volume and refilling time.

good linear correlation has been reported between residual volume fraction of air plethysmography and ambulatory venous pressure after exercise. Air plethysmography has been used to study the efficacy of the calf muscle pump and the effects of therapies such as surgery and sclerotherapy.

Ultrasound

Doppler Ultrasound

Doppler flow depends on changes in the reflected frequency of transmitted ultrasound from movement of red blood cells. Probes with 5- or 10-MHz frequencies placed in the inguinal and popliteal regions to detect blood flow are commonly used.[8] In phasic blood flow, respiratory changes in the groin show iliac and femoral vein patency and allow diagnosis of an obstruction by distal manual compression. The reflux wave is usually detected in the standing position. Retrograde flow shows the reflux using Valsalva's maneuver or calf milking. If retrograde flow at the groin, shown by decompression of the calf, is present, there is reflux in either the femoral vein or great saphenous vein. If the flow disappears during tourniquet or finger compression, the reflux is in the superficial vein. However, although Doppler ultrasound is useful in diagnosing venous insufficiency and patency of veins, the diagnosis is not precise because of possible detection of signals that may be reflected from a target other than the intended area.

B-Mode Ultrasound Imaging

For B-mode ultrasound imaging, the probes are usually of linear type and either 7.5 or 10 MHz for diagnosis of the lower limb. Change of vessel diameter using Valsalva's maneuver and compression using the probe re-

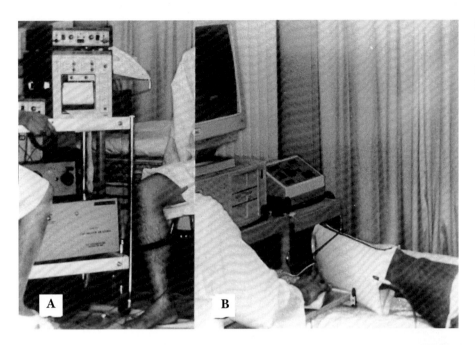

FIGURE 81.4. Measurement of calf volume changes by strain-gauge plethysmography and photoplethysmography (left) and using a cuff for air plethysmography (right).

veals abnormal images. Thrombus is recognized by abnormal echogenicity and because the vessel does not collapse when compressed. The echogenicity of venous thrombi changes over time, and its character is important to differential diagnosis of acute and chronic thrombi. Sullivan et al.[44] reported several criteria of patency of veins as follows: absence of intraluminal thrombus, compressibility of the vein by ultrasound probe, visualization of venous blood flow or valve motion, visualization of changes in vein diameter with quiet respiration or Valsalva's maneuver, and normal venous Doppler signals (spontaneous, phasic, and augmented). The iliac veins may not be seen clearly because of colon gas shadows. More than 90% of accurate diagnoses result from both ultrasound imaging and the compression technique.[30] It is important to become skillful in these methods because the diagnosis success rate using these techniques is highly dependent on the skill of the technician.

Duplex Ultrasonography

Duplex ultrasonography is a combination of B-mode ultrasonography and Doppler examination from which it is possible to measure blood flow at the B-mode imaging level (Figure 81.5). This method is more precise than and superior to B-mode imaging alone because it provides a three-dimensional image. Recently, color flow Doppler imaging has become a tool for diagnosis.[25] Color flow imaging displays a color image of the blood flow signal in the entire section and may decrease overall examination time while also making the echogenicity diagnosis more accurate. It is impossible to measure blood flow in the whole limb, but evaluation of individual vein blood flow enables the calculation of flow speed, reflux time, and reflux volume, which allow quantitative evalua-

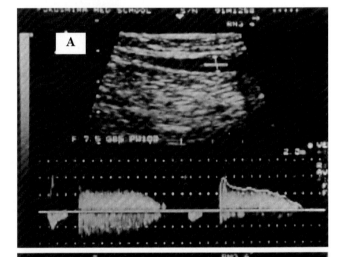

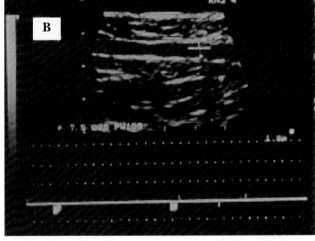

FIGURE 81.5. Reflux measurement by duplex scanning in a great saphenous vein treated with valvuloplasty: **A,** Reflux wave at the great saphenous vein. **B,** The reflux disappeared after valvuloplasty.

tion of the degree of reflux. The parameters of reflux are reported as valve closure time,[50] venous reflux index,[2] and velocity at peak reflux,[49] but, even with this information, limitations remain. Ultrasonography has become a popular diagnostic technique.

Venous Pressure and Phlebography

Ambulatory Venous Pressure

Local venous hypertension causes chronic venous insufficiency; therefore, measurement of venous pressure is considered a gold standard in diagnosing venous insufficiency.[24,32] Pressure is measured by puncture of the dorsal foot vein using either a butterfly or plastic needle; the venous line is then connected to a condenser and the pressure curve is recorded after lower limb exercise in a standing or sitting position. The same procedure, with the addition of a tourniquet, is then performed. The pressure read in the standing position is referred to as the ambulatory venous pressure; the value, which is high in severe outflow obstruction or deep vein insufficiency, is a useful index.

Limitations of this procedure include that it is invasive, not repeatable, and not available for screening. As mentioned previously, good linear correlation has been reported between the residual volume fraction of air plethysmography and ambulatory venous pressure after exercise. Air plethysmography is available for venous disease screening and may become a more common diagnostic tool than ambulatory venous pressure measurements.

Ascending Phlebography

Ascending phlebography indicates that the contrast medium is injected peripherally and passes proximally toward the heart. Because of the popularity of duplex ultrasonography, ascending phlebography has become less significant.[3] In the past, phlebography was conducted to diagnose deep vein competence and conditions of varicose veins and was done as dynamic phlebography.[26] We recently performed ascending phlebography to diagnose incompetent perforating veins in the standing position caused by operation or varicography of vulval varices; however, use of the technique is limited.

Descending Phlebography

Descending phlebography is used to diagnose reflux. Usually, with the patient in the supine position, the femoral vein is punctured by a plastic needle and contrast medium is then injected while performing Valsalva's maneuver in a semiupright position.[12] The amount of reflux toward the peripheral side is evaluated (Figure 81.6). There is no routine method for this procedure concerning whether to use Valsalva's maneuver and the supine or standing position. Retrograde phlebography is a modification of this technique.[45] An introducer system is used to puncture the arm vein through which a catheter is inserted and then passed through the heart to the femoral vein. The catheter may also be placed at the head of the femur and a contrast medium injected. The reflux is commonly evaluated by Herman and Kistner's grading scale[12,19] as follows:

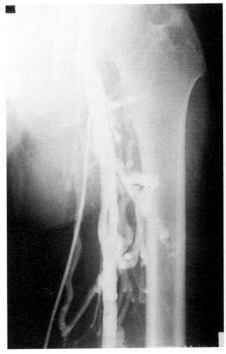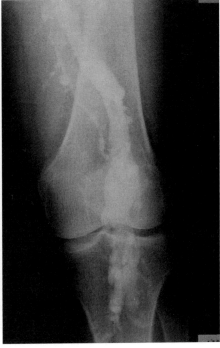

FIGURE 81.6. Descending phlebography: femoral vein is punctured at the groin (left), and the contrast medium passes into the calf (right); reflux is diagnosed as Kistner's grade 3.

0 No reflux
1 Reflux beyond the uppermost valve in the femoral
   vein but not beyond the proximal aspect of the thigh
2 Reflux into the femoral vein to the level of the knee
3 Reflux down to a level just below the knee
4 Reflux into the paired calf veins to the level of the
   ankle

Lea Thomas[27] reported that descending phlebography, using Valsalva's maneuver in the supine position, is useful because of the controlled standardization of Valsalva's maneuver compared with the standing position. However, the possible underestimation of reflux is a concern in the supine position. The reflux is an interaction between gravity in the standing position and venous insufficiency. There may be a leakage between cusps in instances when Valsalva's maneuver is not used. Given these conditions, we perform descending phlebography in the standing position using Valsalva's maneuver. Standardization of Valsalva's maneuver is exercised with a pressure monitor through a punctured line and while maintaining a pressure of more than 40 mm Hg for 10 seconds. Patients with reflux grade 3 or 4 require deep vein reconstruction[19]; however, strength of contrast media and reflux time are not considered for this grading. Therefore, we record the descending phlebography into a video system and measure the arrival time of the contrast medium to the popliteal region. Descending phlebography is useful in considering the indication and selection of surgical procedures; it is routinely performed if deep vein insufficiency is suspected.

Angioscopy

Until now, even with the clear images provided by ultrasonography, detailed intraluminal and valvular shape views have not been possible. Therefore, we used angioscopy intraoperatively for observation and diagnosis[13,39] (Figure 81.7). An angioscopic system, Olympus OES, was used with an AF type 28C, 2.8-mm diameter, together with another specially made type with 60-degree angles. The angioscope is inserted through a branch of the vein and guided into the deep venous system manually; the valves are then observed in retrograde. The angioscopic images are recorded with a video system. Blood is flushed from the lumen with a saline solution with heparin through the angioscope. Because of the restrictions of manipulation, it is difficult to observe remote points, and we routinely use the angioscope intraoperatively. Angioscope allows observation of obstructive changes and characteristics of thrombi in obstructive disorders, as well as evaluation of valvular incompetence in reflux disorders. It is easier to achieve a bloodless field in the venous system than the arterial system because of intraluminal pressure. Observation is more difficult in wider vessels, such as iliac veins and central veins, be-

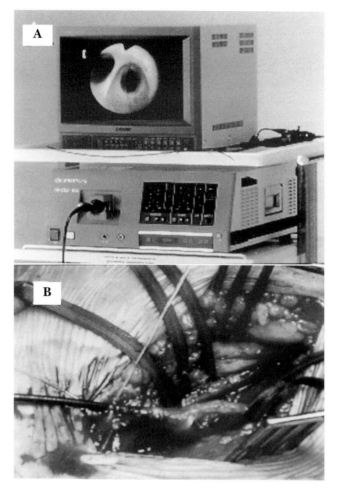

FIGURE 81.7. Angioscopic system: angioscopic images are recorded with a video system (top). An angioscope is inserted through a branch of the great saphenous vein (bottom).

cause of collateral blood flow and the angled shape of the vessels. The classification of angioscopic morphology of incompetent valves is as follows:

Type I   Valves with elongated and prolapsed cusps
Type II   Valves with expanded and depressed commissures, with cusp changes
Type III Valve cusps with other deformities
          (Figure 81.8)

In our series, the majority of severely deformed valves classified as types II and III were in the superficial venous system. Most incompetent valves were type 1 in the deep vein system, except for a few cases of type III valves due to postthrombotic syndrome.

Other Techniques for Investigation

Thermography

Thermography can detect differences in skin temperature. The typical signs are increases in temperature of

FIGURE 81.8. Angioscopic classification of incompetent valves.

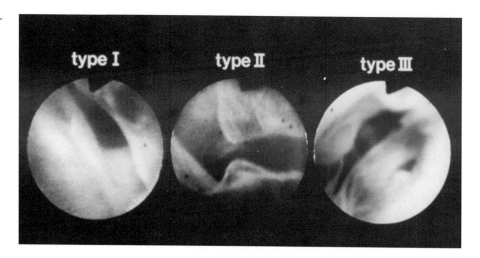

the overlying skin in deep vein thrombosis, varicose veins showing irregular lines in the standing position, and a "hot" pattern of incompetent perforating veins. We often apply a modified method of thermography for detecting the perforating veins. One method is to detect hot areas through incompetent perforating veins after cooling the skin of the leg with cold towels.[6] Another method is to detect cold areas by injecting cold saline into the dorsal foot veins with ankle tourniquet ligation. The accuracy of these methods is about 80%.

Computed Tomography and Magnetic Resonance Imaging

Computed tomography and magnetic resonance imaging are practical techniques for diagnosis. Helical computed tomography and magnetic resonance angiography are especially useful because of their superior three-dimensional imaging from any direction. Magnetic resonance angiography provides imaging of blood flow and is useful for diagnosis of deep vein thrombosis caused by anatomical disorders (Figure 81.9).

Diagram of Diagnosis

During evaluation of patients with chronic venous insufficiency, the history and clinical examination indicate the patients' conditions and clinical characteristics. If there is suspicion of venous disorders, plethysmography shows the blood flow of the limb and confirms the presence of obstruction or reflux diseases. Examinations with a Doppler flowmeter and duplex ultrasonography

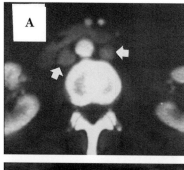

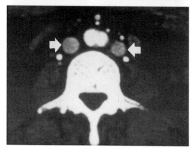

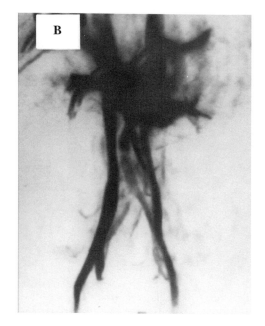

FIGURE 81.9. Vena cava duplication: **A,** Computed tomography reveals duplicated vena cava at the bilateral side of the aorta. **B,** Magnetic resonance angiography shows the course of the duplicated cava.

clearly show individual vein conditions. If sclerotherapy or surgical therapies are planned, phlebography is performed to confirm the presence of venous disease. Because diagnosis of the pelvic region by ultrasonography is difficult due to intestinal gas, computed tomography or magnetic resonance imaging is necessary for diagnosis. During surgery, angioscopy should be used to diagnose valvular insufficiency so that the proper surgical procedure can be selected.

Treatment

Treatment and management of venous insufficiency consist of conservative therapy, surgical therapy, and sclerotherapy. Clinically, various combined therapies are used based on the patient's lifestyle and circumstances. The appropriate method of management should be determined according to the potential benefits and problems of each therapy.

Lifestyle Instruction and Compression Therapy

Patients with venous insufficiency should be instructed to avoid standing for long periods of time, routinely rest, and wear support stockings[18] when standing or doing step-related exercises. If edema or skin changes are present, the limb must be kept clean and protected. Patients

with ulcers must rest with the limb elevated, wear compression bandages, and apply ointment locally to the affected areas. The condition of venous stasis ulcers will improve with this series of treatments, and management of the cause of the ulcers can then be planned. Compression therapy is provided by elastic bandage, elastic stocking, and air massage. The benefit of compression bandages varies according to skill and degree of wrapping, but they are useful for edematous limbs and after surgery because the degree of compression may be easily changed. Elastic stockings regulate the compression effect to the size of the limbs, and moderate-pressure stockings (20–30 mm Hg) are usually worn. Patients often find it difficult to wear elastic stockings for a long time, but it is an important part of management and must be strongly encouraged. Air massage equipment for lymphedema and prophylaxis of deep vein thrombosis is now available in portable models.

Surgical Treatment

For obstructive diseases, femorofemoral crossover bypass (Palma operation),[33] saphenopopliteal bypass (May–Husni operation) [14] (Figure 81.10), and reconstructive surgery using artificial grafts are performed. Long-term patency is difficult to maintain despite the creation of arteriovenous fistulas and many collateral vessels in chronic cases; surgical options for patients with severe symptoms are limited. However, surgical treatment is

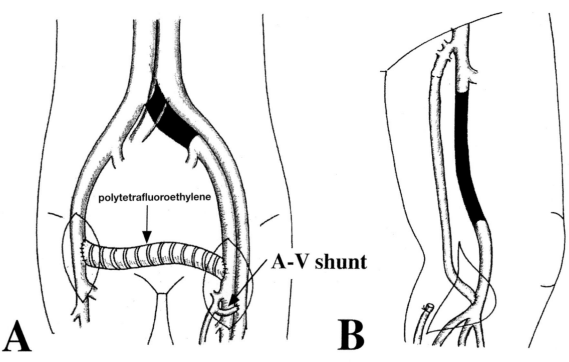

FIGURE 81.10. Schema of bypass surgery for deep vein obstruction: **A,** Femorofemoral vein crossover bypass using polytetrafluoroethylene. A-V, arteriovenous. **B,** Saphenopopliteal bypass (May–Husni operation).

necessary for individual veins such as superficial veins, deep veins, and perforating veins.

Treatment of the Superficial Vein System

Stripping surgery of the great and small saphenous veins has been performed using a stripper.[15] Recently, many varying techniques of vein removal have been used such as selective stripping of only the area with reflux[24] and an inversion method that prevents nerve injury.[48] High ligation of the saphenofemoral junction or the sapheno-popliteal junction is often combined with sclerotherapy. Reflux at the groin level recurred in many, which indicates failure to completely flush the saphenous vein and failure to remove tributaries. Complete removal of tributaries is important to prevent recurrence of varicose veins. A new option is valvuloplasty to preserve the great saphenous vein.[41] We have performed angioscopic valvuloplasty of the great saphenous vein in 59 limbs since 1989. Of the 59 limbs, 2 later showed occlusion and 2 showed recurrent varicose veins (3%). Our results were better than other reported results, but more data and prospective clinical trials are needed.

Deep Vein Reconstruction

Reconstructive surgery is indicated for patients with severe pigmentation and stasis ulcers, limitations on previous lifestyle, and reflux grading higher than grade 3.[19]

Some reports have shown deep vein reconstruction to be contraindicated for patients with primary deep vein insufficiency, because the reflux decision depended on nonstandard descending phlebography and unreliable improvement of the limb blood flow parameters. In our series, 12.5% of patients had damaged cusps, which might be caused by postthrombotic changes; the remaining cases were due to primary deep vein failure. We considered primary deep vein insufficiency a major factor in chronic venous insufficiency. If the reflux is significant and the patient suffers from venous stasis symptoms, the deep vein reflux should be corrected.

Valvuloplasty

There are two techniques of valvuloplasty: internal valvuloplasty with direct incision of the vein wall and external valvuloplasty in which repair is made from outside of the vein. Internal valvuloplasty was first reported in 1968 by Kistner, who made a longitudinal incision at the commissure line, repaired the cusps, and shortened the cusps with interrupted monofilament sutures.[19,21] Modifications of this valvuloplasty technique include one by Raju,[35,36] with transverse venotomy, and another by Sottiurai,[43] with transverse and vertical incisions (Figure 81.11). The basic valvular changes of primary venous insufficiency are elongation and prolapse of the cusps. The aim of these techniques is to elevate and shorten elongated cusps. One benefit of internal valvuloplasty is

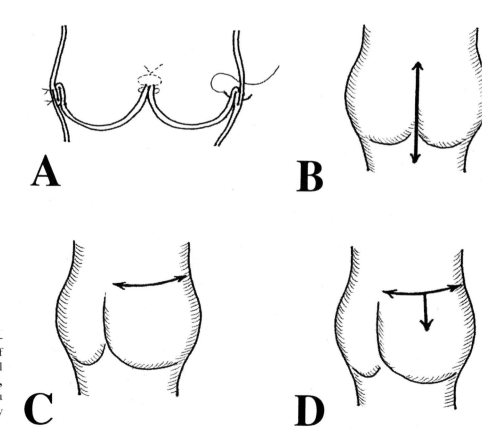

FIGURE 81.11. Technique of external valvuloplasty: **A,** Schema of external technique. **B,** Vertical incision by Kistner method. **C,** Horizontal incision by Raju method. **D,** T-shaped incision by Sottiurai method.

the ability to accurately repair with direct observation; results as good as 63% to 80% are reported after more than 4 years of follow-up.[7,29,36] The internal method is reliable, but anticoagulant agents are necessary; because of the venous incision, bleeding after simultaneous performance of surgical procedures such as stripping should be monitored. Because external valvuloplasty is done without venotomy, anticoagulants such as heparin and warfarin are unnecessary.

Some techniques for external repairs were reported recently. Kistner reported an external valve repair method.[20] It consists of a series of interrupted sutures placed along the decussation of the line of valve insertion. Jones and Kerstein[17] described a procedure of valve ring plication. Their technique was not precisely external valvuloplasty because the longitudinal venotomy was placed midway between the commissures and venotomy closure by a series of interrupted sutures. The wrapping method is used with a venocuff, consisting of a Silastic cuff and cutting kit, devised by Lane.[16] Gloviczki et al.[9] reported angioscopic valve repair under direct sight. Our technique is angioscopic valvuloplasty, which also includes intraoperative diagnosis, guiding of valvuloplasty, and evaluation of surgical results. Angioscopic external valvuloplasty not only makes direct venotomy unnecessary but also eliminates the need for coagulant therapy. Our technique consists of total valve ring plication by sutures and wrapping (techniques 1 and 2) and plication of the commissure (technique 3) (Figures 81.12 and 81.13).[13,39]

The suture and wrapping technique corrects reflux by enabling closure between the cusps, which results in an increase of valve profile and narrowing of the sinus. In technique 3, a needle is placed in both the commissure

and elongated cusps. The plication is performed by horizontal mattress suture with pledgets for reinforcement. We usually select the wrapping method for slightly elongated cusps and the commissure plication technique for severely prolapsed valves. The results of this external repair series are 63% to 100% successful at 2- to 8-year follow-up.[36,39] The criteria and results are still under investigation.

Venous Transplantation and Venous Segmentation Transposition

Valves involved in postthrombotic syndrome exhibit severely deformed cusps, which suggests no indication of valvuloplasty as a reconstructive surgery, and venous valve transplantation or segment transposition is chosen for these cases. As mentioned previously, one third of the patients experienced postthrombotic syndrome. Raju[36] reported that in 20% of patients, valvuloplasty failed and transplantation was performed instead. Good clinical results of venous transplantation were first reported by Taheri et al.[46] A brachial vein valve segment is usually attached to the popliteal or femoral vein. Valvular incompetence due to subsequent dilation has been reported; to avoid this problem, the transplanted segment is encased in an artificial graft.[36] The popliteal vein is in a better location than the femoral vein for transplantation of the brachial vein valve. Contributing factors include the similar diameter of the popliteal and brachial veins; the popliteal vein location stops reflux at the knee level as a gatekeeper.[42] Venous segment transposition is a technique of transposing one venous segment that has no repairable proximal valve to an adjacent segment that has a normal proximal valve. This procedure was re-

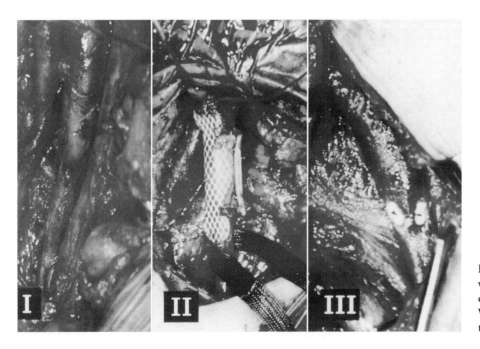

FIGURE 81.12. Angioscopic external valvuloplasty: **A,** Total valve ring plication with polypropylene sutures. **B,** Wrapping with Silastic cuff. **C,** Plication of the commissure.

FIGURE 81.13. Angioscopic view of technique 3 external valvuloplasty: **A,** The valve is a type I incompetent valve. **B, C,** A needle penetrates the cusps and vein wall. **D,** Adaptation line and plication of the commissure are visible.

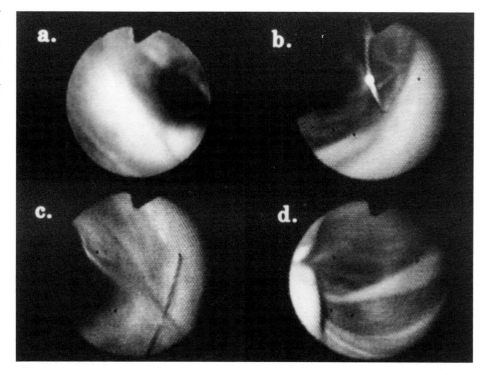

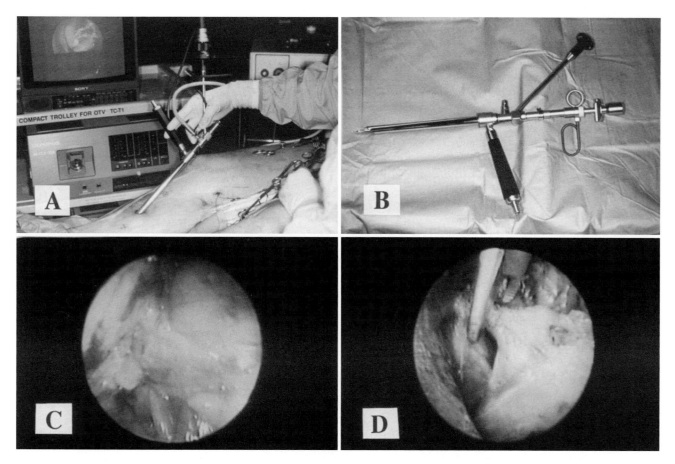

FIGURE 81.14. Endoscopic subfascial dissection of perforating veins: **A, B,** Endoscopic subfascial dissection system and surgical scene. **C, D,** A perforating vein is separated and cut after electrical coagulation.

ported by Kistner in 1979.[22] Three vessels, the great saphenous vein, the superficial femoral vein, and the deep femoral vein, offer multiple possibilities of arrangement. In chronic venous insufficiency, there may be reflux at the great saphenous vein, but the vein may not correlate with the host vessel. The transposition is simple and often useful in combination with valvuloplasty. Results of transposition varied from 17% to 78% 24 to 66 months after surgery and transplantation was successful 57% to 90% of the time.[21,36] However, valvuloplasty is superior to other reconstruction techniques and should be used if possible.[35]

Management of Incompetent Perforating Veins

In patients with chronic venous insufficiency, incompetent perforating veins often affect venous stasis and should be treated. The classic medical subfascial approach by Linton's operation is well known[28] but has the disadvantage of direct incision of the thickened skin with intense subcutaneous liposclerosis. Because it has become easier to detect the site of perforating veins by duplex ultrasonography, the approaches to surgical management of incompetent perforating veins have recently changed. For patients with early grade C2–3 (CEAP classification) venous insufficiency the incompetent perforating veins may be interrupted suprafascially through a small incision by preoperative echogenicity mapping. In contrast, patients with grade C4–6 venous insufficiency may be treated by a subfascial approach such as endoscopic subfascial dissection.[11] Our equipment for endoscopic subfascial dissection is a single endoscopic system with a lumen-dividing forceps, electrical coagulator, or scissors forceps (Figure 81.14).[40] This technique enables the surgeon to accurately and atraumatically perform a subfascial dissection from a small skin incision remote from the point of trophic disturbance. Endoscopic subfascial dissection is one of the best methods for endoscopic surgery and is minimally invasive.

Conclusion

Surgical reconstruction for patients with chronic venous insufficiency has been performed for more than two decades, and various results have been accumulated and reported. Presently, new options for treatment such as angioscopic external valvuloplasty, endoscopic dissection of perforating veins, and a combination of surgical techniques and sclerotherapy are available, and more satisfactory results are anticipated. However, because disorders of chronic venous insufficiency are not the only factor, systematic diagnosis using various investigation methods should enable proper management. Improving the quality of treatment and providing sufficient follow-up care for patients is critical.

References

1. Abramowitz HB, Queral LA, Flinn WR, et al. The use of photoplethysmography in the assessment of venous insufficiency: a comparison to venous pressure measurements. *Surgery.* 1979;86:434–441.
2. Beckwith TC, Richardson G, Sheldon M, Clarke GH. A correlation between blood flow volume and ultrasonic Doppler wave forms in the study of valve efficiency. *Phlebology.* 1993;8:12–16.
3. Beebe HG, Bergan JJ, Bergqvist D, et al. Classification and grading of chronic venous disease in the lower limbs: a consensus statement. *Int Angiol.* 1995;14:197–201.
4. Bergan JJ. Primary vs. secondary cause. *Straub Foundation Proceedings.* 1993;57:28–29.
5. Browse NL, Burnand KG, Lea Thomas ML. Primary (nonthrombotic) deep vein incompetence. In *Diseases of the Veins: Pathology, Diagnosis, and Treatment.* London: Edward Arnold; 1988:253–269.
6. Elem B, Shorey BA, Lloyd Williams K. Comparison between thermography and fluorescein test in the detection of incompetent perforating veins. *BMJ.* 1971;4:651–652.
7. Ferris EB, Kistner RL. Femoral vein reconstruction in the management of chronic venous insufficiency. *Arch Surg.* 1982;117:1571–1579.
8. Folse R, Alexander RH. Directional flow detection for localizing venous valvular incompetency. *Surgery.* 1970;67:114–121.
9. Gloviczki P, Marrell SM, Bower TC. Femoral vein valve repair under direct vision without venotomy: a modified technique with use of angioscopy. *J Vasc Surg.* 1991;14:645–648.
10. Hanrahan LM, Kechejian GJ, Cordts PR. Patterns of venous insufficiency in patients with varicose veins. *Arch Surg.* 1991;126:687–691.
11. Hauer G, Barkun J, Wisser I. Endoscopic subfascial dissection of perforating veins. *Surg Endosc.* 1988;2:5–12.
12. Herman RJ, Neiman HL, Yao JST, Egan TJ, Bergan JJ, Malave SR. Descending venography: a method of evaluating lower extremity venous valvular function. *Radiology.* 1980;137:63–69.
13. Hoshino S, Satokawa H, Iwaya F, Igari T, Ono T, Takase S. Valvuloplastie externe sous controle angioscopique preoperatoire. *Phlebologie.* 1993;46:521–530.
14. Husni EA. In situ saphenopopliteal bypass graft for incompetence of the femoral and popliteal veins. *Surg Gynecol Obstet.* 1970;120:279–284.
15. Jacobsen BH. The value of different forms of treatment for varicose veins. *Br J Surg.* 1979;66:182–184.
16. Jessup G, Lane RJ. Repair of incompetent venous valves: a new technique. *J Vasc Surg.* 1988;8:569–575.
17. Jones JW, Kerstein MD. Triangular venous valvuloplasty. *Arch Surg.* 1982;11:1250–1251.
18. Jones NAG, Webb PK, Rees RI, Kakkar VV. A physiological study of elastic compression stockings in venous disorders of the leg. *Br J Surg.* 1980;67:569–572.
19. Kistner RL. Surgical repair of the incompetent femoral vein valve. *Arch Surg.* 1975;110:1136–1342.
20. Kistner RL. Surgical technique of external venous valve repair. *Straub Foundation Proceedings.* 1990;55:15–16.

21. Kistner RL. Valve repair and segment transposition in primary valvular insufficiency. In: Bergan JJ, Yao JST, eds. *Venous Disorders*. Philadelphia, Pa: WB Saunders; 1991: 261–272.

22. Kistner RL, Sparkuhl MD. Surgery in acute and chronic venous disease. *Surgery*. 1979;85:31–43.

23. Koyano K, Sakaguchi S. Selective stripping operation based on Doppler ultrasonic findings for primary varicose veins of the lower extremities. *Surgery*. 1988;103:615–619.

24. Kriessmann A. Ambulatory venous pressure. In: Nicolaides AN, ed. *Investigation of Vascular Disorders*. London: Churchill Livingstone; 1981:461–477.

25. Labropoulos N, Leon M, Nicolaides AN, et al. Venous reflux in patients with previous deep venous thrombosis: correlation with ulceration and other symptoms. *J Vasc Surg*. 1994;20:20–26.

26. Lea Thomas M, Keeling FP. Varicography in the management of recurrent varicose veins. *Angiology*. 1986;37: 570–575.

27. Lea Thomas M, Keeling FP, Ackroyd J. Descending phlebography: a comparison of three methods and an assessment of the normal range of deep vein reflux. *J Cardiovasc Surg*. 1986;27:27–30.

28. Linton R. The postthrombotic ulceration of the lower extremity: its etiology and surgical treatment. *Ann Surg*. 1953;138:415–426.

29. Masuda EM, Kistner RL. Long-term results of venous valve reconstruction: a four- to twenty-one-year follow-up. *J Vasc Surg*. 1994;19:391–403.

30. Monreal M, Montserrat E, Salvador R, et al. Real-time ultrasound for diagnosis of symptomatic venous thrombosis and for screening of patients at risk: correlation with ascending conventional venography. *Angiology*. 1989;6: 527–533.

31. Nicolaides AN, Christopoulos DC. Methods of quantification of chronic venous insufficiency. In: Bergan JJ, Yao JST, eds. *Venous Disorders*. Philadelphia, Pa: WB Saunders; 1991:77–90.

32. Nicolaides AN, Zukowski AJ. The value of dynamic venous pressure measurements. *World J Surg*. 1986;10:919–924.

33. Palma EC, Esperon R. Vein transplants and grafts in surgical treatment of the postphlebitic syndrome. *J Cardiovasc Surg*. 1960;1:94–107.

34. Porter JM, Rutherford RB, Clagett GP, et al. Reporting standards in venous disease. *J Vasc Surg*. 1988;8:172–181.

35. Raju S. Venous insufficiency of the lower limb and stasis ulceration: changing concepts and management. *Ann Surg*. 1982;6:688–697.

36. Raju S, Fredericks R. Valve reconstruction procedures for nonobstructive venous insufficiency: rationale, techniques, and results in 107 procedures with two- to eight-year follow-up. *J Vasc Surg*. 1988;7:301–310.

37. Sakaguchi S. Phlebothrombosis and its sequelae: pathophysiology and surgical treatment. *J Cardiovasc Surg*. 1973; (suppl):576.

38. Sakaguchi S, Ishitobi K, Kameda T. Functional segmental plethysmography with mercury strain gauge. *Angiology*. 1972;23:127–135.

39. Satokawa H, Hoshino S, Ogawa T, et al. Venous valve angioscopic reconstruction: techniques and long-term results. *Japanese Journal of Phlebology*. 1996;7:63–70.

40. Satokawa H, Iwaya F, Igari T, et al. Endoscopic venous surgery [in Japanese]. *Jpn J Vasc Surg*. 1994;3:613–618.

41. Schanzer H, Skladany M. Varicose vein surgery with preservation of the saphenous vein: a comparison between high ligation–avulsion versus saphenofemoral banding valvuloplasty–avulsion. *J Vasc Surg*. 1994;20:684–687.

42. Shull KC, Nicolaides AN, Fernandes JF, et al. Significance of popliteal reflux in relation to ambulatory venous pressure and ulceration. *Arch Surg*. 1979;114:1304–1306.

43. Sottiurai VS. Surgical correction of recurrent venous ulcer. *J Cardiovasc Surg*. 1991;32:104–109.

43. Sullivan ED, Peter DJ, Cranley JJ. Real-time B-mode venous ultrasound. *J Vasc Surg*. 1984;1:465–471.

45. Taheri SA, Elias S. Descending phlebography. *Angiology*. 1983;3:299–305.

46. Taheri SA, Lazar L, Elias S, Marchand P, Hefner R. Surgical treatment of postphlebitic syndrome with vein valve transplant. *Am J Surg*. 1982;144:221–224.

47. Train JS, Schanzer H, Pierce EC, Dan SJ, Mitty HA. Radiologic evaluation of the chronic venous stasis syndrome. *JAMA*. 1987;258:941–944.

48. Van der Stricht J. Ambulatory stripping. *Phlebologie*. Paris: John Eurotext; 1992:1064–1066.

49. Vasdekis SN, Clarke GH, Nicolaides AN. Quantification of venous reflux by means of duplex scanning. *J Vasc Surg*. 1989;10:670–677.

50. Welch HJ, Faliakou EC, McLaughlin RL, Umphley SE, Belkin M, O'Donnell TF. Comparison of descending phlebography with quantitative photoplethysmography, air plethysmography, and duplex quantitative valve closure time in assessing deep venous reflux. *J Vasc Surg*. 1992; 16:13–20.

82

Physiology and Pathophysiology of Venous Return From the Lower Leg

Carl C. Arnoldi

Veins of the Lower Extremity

For practical clinical purposes and for understanding the physiology and pathophysiology of venous return from the lower limb, particularly the ankle and calf, it is convenient to distinguish between three major venous systems in the leg (Figure 82.1): (1) the veins deep to the fascia cruris, (2) the superficial veins in the subcutis (i.e., the saphenous veins and their tributaries), and (3) the communicating veins connecting the superficial veins to the deep venous system.

It is generally assumed that the deep venous system carries about 90% of the blood from the lower limb, and the superficial veins account for the remaining 10%. Although the blood stream is always directed toward the heart in the deep veins—at rest and during exercise—the blood in the superficial veins is drawn toward the deep veins through the communicating veins during exercise.

Physiology and Pathophysiology

Venous Flow in the Relaxed Lower Limb

The function of the veins is to convey blood from the periphery toward the heart. In the relaxed condition with complete inactivity of the muscles of the lower extremity—whether the subject is lying or standing—the veins of the lower limb may be regarded as a low pressure system compared with the arteries. In this state the pressure pushing the blood toward the heart is generally less than 10 mm Hg. This propulsive power is the remnant of the arterial blood pressure engendered by the left ventricle of the heart and is known as the *vis-a-tergo*. In a completely relaxed leg, with the subject in the upright position, this pressure drives the blood upward through the deep veins with a linear flow velocity of a few centimeters per second,[1] an indication of the remarkable difference between the cross-sectional area of the leg veins and arteries.

Venous Pump of the Calf

The transition from rest to rhythmic exercise in the upright position, such as walking, is accompanied by dramatic changes in pressure (Figure 82.2) and flow in the veins of the lower limb, especially the lower leg. Muscular exercise, which is accompanied by increased arterial inflow, at the same time ensures equal venous outflow under conditions favorable to the capillary circulation. This is made possible by the valves of the veins and by a series of correlated musculovenous pumps along the whole length of the limb.

The valves in the veins of the lower limb are unevenly distributed. In the deep veins inside the segments of the pump system valves are much more numerous than in the collecting veins and superficial system (Figure 82.1).[2] Their main functions are to alleviate the hydrostatic pressure by sectioning the column of blood reaching toward heart level and to prevent a flow of blood toward the periphery under the varying environmental conditions imposed by muscular activity. In the communicating veins, the valves permit flow from the superficial to the deep veins.

The pump unit[1] is a muscle, or a group of muscles with a common fascial sheath, with a synchronous effect on joint movement. Supplied by the same artery, these muscles are drained by densely valved veins emptying proximally into a sparsely valved collecting vein, generally placed in loose connective tissue.[1] The lower leg contains three units. The posterior unit, comprising the musculus triceps surae and the deep flexor muscles, is drained by the posterior tibial and gastrocnemial veins. The anterior unit containing the anterior tibial muscle is drained by the anterior tibial veins, and the lateral unit with the peroneal muscles is drained by the peroneal

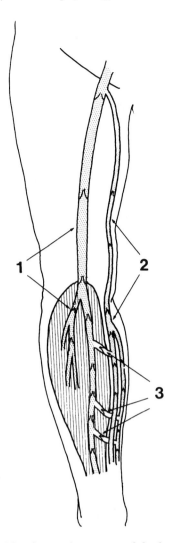

FIGURE 82.1. The three vein systems of the lower extremity involved in the drainage of the posterior section of the venous pump of the calf. 1, 2, and 3 represent the deep, superficial, and communicating veins, respectively. The communicating veins in the input area of the pump section are generally known as the ankle perforating veins.

veins. During walking the contractions of these muscle groups and the expulsion of blood from the pump units into the common collecting vein (popliteal vein) alternate rhythmically. The deep veins of the posterior unit (the calf) were chosen for measurements of deep vein pressure variations.

Methods of Investigation

Dynamic Intraosseous Phlebography

Dynamic intraosseous phlebography was devised by Arnoldi and Bauer[3] as a radiological test of the function of the venous pump of the calf during rhythmic activity. This method was chosen as a procedure that does not interfere with flow during exercise.

The procedure is as follows.[4] The subject is placed horizontally on a tiltable x-ray table. The skin of the lateral aspect of the os calcis is carefully rinsed and painted with a solution of iodine. Local anesthesia is applied to the skin and periosteum at the site of injection. One minute later a wide-calibered cannula is introduced through the compacta into the substantia spongiosa of the calcaneus. When the cannula is in situ, 5 mL of local anesthesia are injected slowly into the bone marrow. At this point the patient usually feels a stab of pain, but this is the only painful incident during the procedure.

The subject is then tilted into a nearly erect position. The leg to be examined rests lightly on a pedal and is rotated inward 30 degrees while the whole weight of the patient rests firmly on the other leg. A suitable contrast medium (10 mL) is injected into the bone marrow after 3 minutes of complete relaxation. The injection is performed as quickly as possible (45–60 seconds), and the first exposure is made immediately on completion.

The pedal is balanced to a considerable weight (12 kg), and moving it requires powerful contraction of the calf muscles. After the first exposure the patient is asked to force the pedal down as far as possible. This powerful contraction is repeated three times, and the second film is exposed immediately after completion of the third contraction. Only anteroposterior exposures are neces-

FIGURE 82.2. Pressures in the popliteal vein and in the deep and superficial veins at the level of the greatest circumference of the calf before, during, and after rhythmic muscular contractions in the nearly erect position. Tramp force on the pedal is given in kilograms. Vein pressures as lateral pressure at the point of measurement (left scale) and as pressure refer to the level of the angulus sterni (heart level).

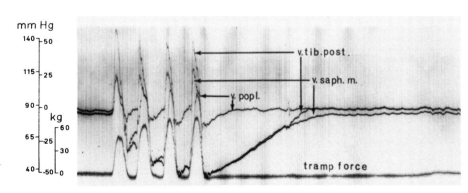

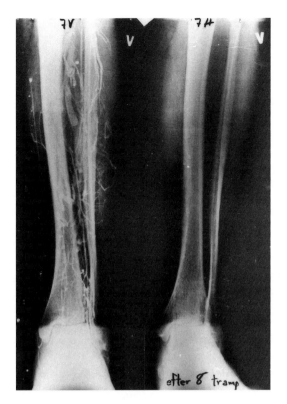

FIGURE 82.3. Dynamic intraosseous phlebographs from patient with simple varicose veins (group I). In this group the phlebographs are mostly indistinguishable from those obtained from healthy subjects.

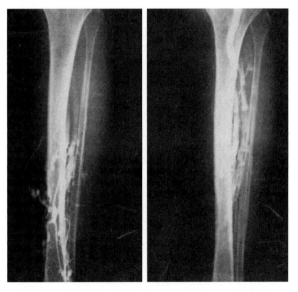

FIGURE 82.4. Dynamic intraosseous phlebographs from patient of group II (varicose veins and dilated and incompetent ankle perforating veins). In the first exposure the contrast medium had filled the deep veins of the ankle and has reached the superficial veins via the incompetent ankle perforating veins. After standard exercise the ankle veins are empty and the contrast medium has disappeared from ankle perforating and subcutaneous veins. Instead, it has filled the deep veins in the calf pump proper, where the valves are seen to be normal.

sary because the subcutaneous veins rarely disturb the picture of the deep veins and the ankle perforating veins.

Volunteers without venous insufficiency were examined for control data. The number of contractions chosen for standard exercise was the lowest number required to empty the veins of the lower leg of contrast material in all healthy subjects. The number necessary varies with the resistance of the individual pedal, and standard exercise had to be redetermined if the pedal was changed. Complete emptying of contrast under the conditions described was defined as normal function of the venous pump of the calf.

Findings in Patients With Chronic Venous Insufficiency

Patients with chronic venous insufficiency of the lower limb may be divided into five groups according to the findings by dynamic intraosseous phlebography.[1] Typical phlebographs from the five groups are shown in Figures 82.3 through 82.7.

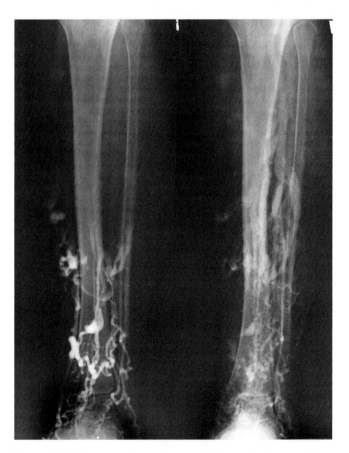

FIGURE 82.5. Dynamic intraosseous phlebographs from patient with postthrombotic syndrome (group III). Contrast medium is seen in the irregular deep veins, perforating veins, and superficial varicosities. Standard exercise had no effect on the contrast medium in the ankle region. In fact, the contrast-mixed blood has moved toward the heart at the same speed as if the patient had been standing quietly between the two exposures.

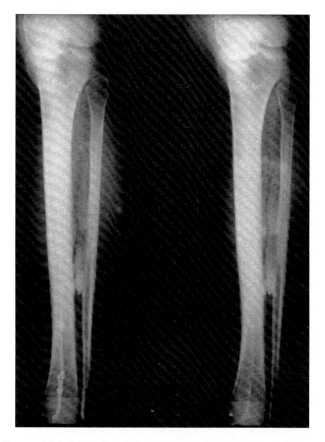

FIGURE 82.6. Dynamic intraosseous phlebographs from woman with cruralgia orthostatica (group IV). Exercise has had no effect on the distribution of contrast medium. The rate of flow appears to be the same as in the postthrombotic leg (Figure 82.5). Note the normal looking valves in the wide deep veins.

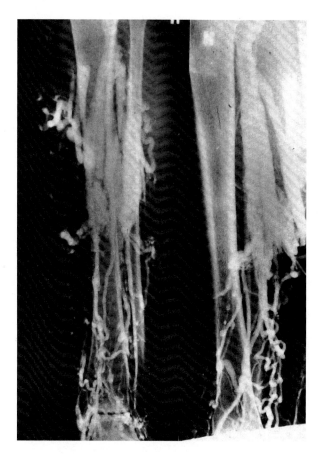

FIGURE 82.7. Dynamic intraosseous phlebographs from patient of group V. This woman has varicose veins and incompetent and dilated ankle perforating veins. The caliber of the deep veins of the calf is especially noticeable in the second (lateral) exposure. Standard exercise has no effect on the distribution of contrast medium (compare Figure 82.4).

Group I

Patients with simple varicose veins but normal communicating veins in the ankle region (ankle perforating veins) and normal deep veins of the calf made up group I. At the second exposure the injected contrast material had completely disappeared, which indicates normal function of the venous pump of the calf (Figure 82.8).

Group II

Group II included patients with varicose superficial veins and incompetent and dilated ankle perforating veins. The deep veins of the calf were usually normal, and the valves in the popliteal vein were always normal. The first exposure showed contrast medium in the deep veins of the ankle region (the input area of the calf pump), in the incompetent ankle perforating veins, and in the adjacent superficial varicosities. After muscular exercise the deep veins of the ankle and the superficial veins were usually empty, but contrast medium was now observed in the ankle perforating veins and in the deep veins inside the calf pump proper and in the thigh,

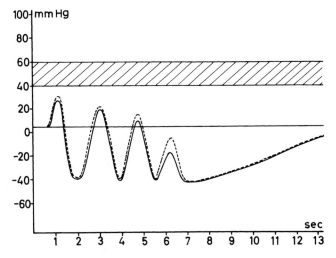

FIGURE 82.8. Mean pressure variations in the internal saphenous vein at the ankle. Pressures from healthy subjects (unbroken line) compared with mean values from patients of group I (dotted line). The hatched area (40–60 mm Hg) represents the range of arteriolar pressure in the skin and subcutis of the ankle region.

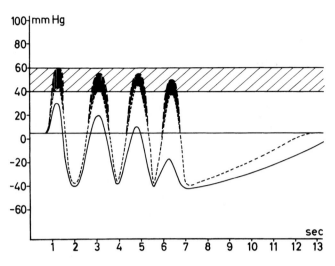

FIGURE 82.9. Mean pressure values from the internal saphenous vein at the ankle in healthy subjects (unbroken line) compared with mean pressure values in the internal saphenous and posterior tibial veins at the same level from patients of group II. The black areas between these latter graphs represent the pressure in the ankle perforating veins during systole. Other symbols as in Figure 82.8.

which indicates impaired calf pump function (Figure 82.9).

Group III

Group III included patients with postthrombotic syndrome (i.e., destruction of the valves in the superficial veins, the communicating veins, and the deep veins of the calf and thigh). Exercise had no effect on the distribution of contrast medium, and in the ankle region the

first and second exposures were practically identical. The second exposure showed that the contrast-mixed blood had flowed upward toward the heart with the same velocity as observed in the completely relaxed leg (i.e., with a speed of 1–2 cm/s), which indicates total incompetence of the calf pump (Figure 82.10).

Group IV

Group IV included women with cruralgia orthostatica or idiopathic dysfunction of the venous pump of the calf.[5-7] The ankle perforating veins were normal. Exercise had no effect on the distribution of contrast. The valves of the deep, superficial, and communicating veins were morphologically normal, but the deep intermuscular and intramuscular veins were unusually wide, which indicates total incompetence of the calf pump (Figure 82.11).

Group V

Group V included women with symptoms typical of cruralgia orthostatica. In contrast to group IV, group V patients showed superficial varicose veins and dilated and incompetent ankle perforating veins. Morphologically, they closely resembled the patients of group II, but exercise had no effect on the distribution of contrast medium. The deep intermuscular and intramuscular veins had the same wide caliber as seen in group IV. Symptoms indicate total incompetence of the calf pump (Figure 82.12).

Pressure Measurements in the Veins of the Lower Limb and in the Calcaneus

The general procedure is as follows.[8-12] Polyethylene tubes were introduced into both posterior tibial veins

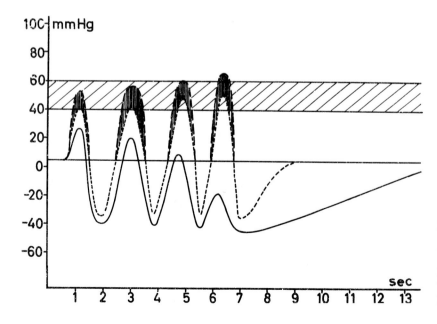

FIGURE 82.10. Mean pressure values from the internal saphenous vein at the ankle in healthy volunteers compared with mean pressure values from superficial and deep veins at the same level in patients of group III. Symbols as in Figure 82.9.

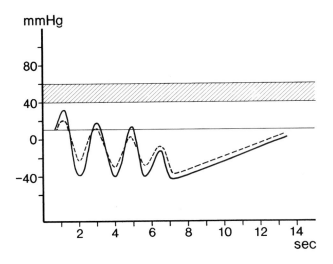

FIGURE 82.11. Mean pressure in the internal saphenous vein at the ankle in healthy volunteers and in patients of group IV. Symbols as in Figure 82.8.

and into the internal saphenous vein. The position of the tips of the tubes (points of measurement) was varied according to a standardized schedule, and simultaneous measurements were performed in the deep and superficial veins at the level of the upper border of the patella (popliteal vein), at the level of the greatest circumference of the calf, and in the ankle region. Simultaneous measurements were also made at different levels in the deep venous system (popliteal vein and proximal part of the posterior tibial vein or proximal and distal parts of the posterior tibial vein). Calcanean pressure was mea-

sured simultaneously with pressures at various levels in the deep and superficial veins.

Intraosseous pressure of the calcaneus was determined through a metal cannula with an outside diameter of 2 mm and a lumen of 1.40 mm. The introduction of the cannula into the bone marrow was performed as described under the section of this chapter on intraosseous phlebography. When the cannula was in situ it was connected to a polyethylene tube. The tubes in the veins of the lower limb and the one attached to the cannula in the calcaneus were connected to a set of manometers placed on the tiltable table. The pressures recorded were made with the subject lying horizontally and standing at angles 34 and 78 degrees to the horizontal plane.

Pressures were measured before, during, and after a series of rhythmic muscular contractions. At the beginning of the experiment the leg to be examined was kept relaxed and motionless for a prolonged period. In the semiupright and almost upright positions the whole weight of the body was supported by the other leg. A series of four short, powerful tramps that involved contractions of the muscles involved in plantar flexion of the ankle joint were then performed with intervening brief periods of relaxation. The powerful contractions involved a tramp force that corresponded to about 56% of maximum effort. The four tramps were timed to last 5 to 6 seconds. During the contractions, the forefoot (i.e., the region of the metatarsal heads) was pressed against a pelotte, 5 cm in diameter, on a rigid foot pedal. Plantar flexion in the ankle joint was avoided. After the last tramp the leg was kept in a state of relaxation until the pressure at all points of measurement had returned to the initial stable pressure level.

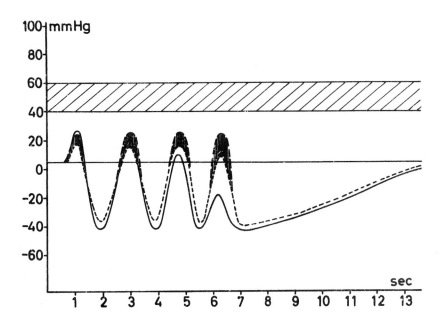

FIGURE 82.12. Mean pressure values from the internal saphenous vein at ankle level (unbroken line) in healthy volunteers compared with mean pressures in superficial and deep veins at the same level in patients of group V. Symbols as in Figures 82.9 and 82.10.

Pressure Recordings: Apparatus and Technique

Up to four pressures were recorded simultaneously. The pressure reference level for all manometers was the water level of a pressure reference system (Figure 82.13). The water level (2) was well defined in relation to the subject under investigation, at an average 56.9 cm (range 48–66 cm) below the angulus sterni in the nearly erect position. Using three-way stopcocks (4 and 5) the manometer (8) could be connected to the pressure reference system and at the same time disconnected from the venous tube (6) by means of a third three-way stopcock (7), which then allowed saline (3) to flow slowly through the tube into the vein or the calcaneus.

A standard pressure above or below the reference level was obtained by means of a three-way stopcock (4) that connected the manometer to a pressure system with a water level (1) usually 68 cm (corresponding to 50 mm Hg) above that of the reference level. The use of these pressure references, common to all manometers, enabled accurate pressure determinations independent of the position of the manometer.

The manometer recording system was found to be linear within the range of measurements. Standard and reference pressures were recorded immediately before and after each measurement of venous and intraosseous pressure, which lasted approximately 1 to 2 minutes. The tube manometer system was tested with a sine wave pressure of varying frequency. The amplitude was correctly recorded to approximately 15 cm/s. The error of measurement on the recorded graph corresponded to a pressure in the order of 1 mm Hg (range) or less.

The standard error of a single determination of pressure at rest in the nearly erect position was calculated from duplicate measurements made during the course of experiments on eight subjects. The standard error varied between 0.4 and 1.0 mm Hg for the pressures at the different points of measurement.

The angulus sterni was chosen as a convenient point of reference near the heart. The pressures observed were listed as pressures referred to the level of the angulus sterni or as lateral (transmural) pressure at the point of measurement.

Tramp Force Measurements

The foot pedal on the tiltable table was supported by a steel bar to which strain gauges were attached and connected to form a Wheatstone bridge. Deformation of the steel bar by pressure on the pedal changes the strain gauge resistances. Imbalance of the bridge was detected by an amplifier and recorded by an Elema klinik galvanometer together with blood and intraosseous pressures. There was a linear relationship between the force applied and the deflections of the galvanometer, and the tramp force could be estimated to the nearest kilopascal (kilogram in figures).

Intravenous and Intraosseous Pressure Recordings in the Nearly Erect Position

Pressures at Rest

The pressure at all points of measurement in healthy subjects was roughly equal to the calculated hydrostatic pressure of a column of blood reaching from the level of measurement to the level of the angulus sterni. However, pressures referred to this level showed slight but significant differences. The pressure in the calcaneus was always higher than the pressure in the posterior tibial vein in the ankle (mean difference plus 4.2 mm Hg) and in the internal saphenous vein at the same level (mean difference plus 5.8 mm Hg). Measured at the same vertical distance from the heart level, the deep venous pressure was also constantly 1 to 1.5 mm Hg higher than the subcutaneous pressure. The pulsatile waves of calcanean pressure synchronized with the arterial pulsations.

Effect of Rhythmic Muscle Contractions on Pressure in the Calcaneus and Veins of the Lower Limb

The first muscular contraction after a period of complete rest was always accompanied by a rise of pressure at all points of measurement in healthy subjects. The systolic pressure increase during the first contraction was

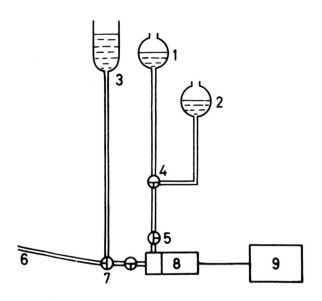

FIGURE 82.13. Pressure recording apparatus. A pressure reference (2) reservoir was maintained at a constant level and was joined by a stopcock (4) to a saline reservoir (1) to adjust pressure. Another saline reservoir (3) was connected to a stopcock (7) to fill the venous tube (6) or to the calcaneus. Using the three-way stopcocks, the pressures can be measured and compared to pressure of the reference system by opening the system to the manometer (8) and recorder (9).

FIGURE 82.14. Pressure tracings from the bone marrow of the calcaneus and posterior tibial vein at ankle level. Measurements performed before, during, and after four vigorous contractions of the calf muscles in a healthy volunteer in the nearly erect position. Pressures are in mm Hg and tramp force in kg.

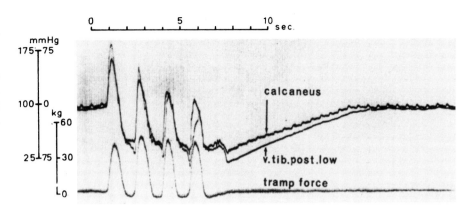

highest in the calcaneus and the ankle region of the posterior tibial veins (Figure 82.14), somewhat lower in the proximal part (Figure 82.15), and much lower in the popliteal vein (Figure 82.16). At the ankle the pressure rise in the internal saphenous vein during the first contraction reached an average of one third of the concurrent pressure rise in the posterior tibial vein (Figure 82.17).

On relaxation after contraction the pressure fell below the pressure at rest at all points of measurement. The pressure trough was deepest in the calcaneus and the deep veins of the calf and insignificant in the popliteal vein. The fall of pressure in the internal saphenous vein was significantly less than the simultaneous fall of pressure in the posterior tibial vein (Figure 82.17).

Continued Rhythmic Exercise

The pressure recordings from the popliteal vein showed only modest variations (Figure 82.16). In the posterior tibial vein in the calf (inside the pump unit), systolic pressure peaks remained high and stable (Figures 82.15 and 82.16). In the posterior tibial vein in the ankle (the input area of the calf pump), repeated contractions reduced the height of the pressure peaks significantly and deepened the diastolic pressure troughs (Figures 82.14, 82.15, and 82.17). In the internal saphenous vein at the ankle, the pressure graph was similar to that from the lower posterior tibial vein, except that the systolic peaks were lower and the diastolic pressure troughs more shallow than in the deep vein (Figure 82.17). In the calcaneus, intraosseous pressure closely followed the pres-

FIGURE 82.15. Pressure tracings from the posterior tibial vein inside the calf pump (high) and at the ankle (low). Methods and scales as in Figure 82.14. Note the sustained high systolic pressures in the proximal part of the vein and the gradually decreasing systolic pressures in the input area.

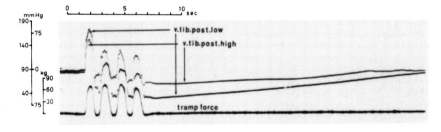

FIGURE 82.16. Pressure tracings from the posterior tibial vein in the proximal part of the calf (inside the pump unit) and popliteal vein proximal to the unit. Distance between points of measurement is 13 cm. Methods and scales as in Figure 82.14.

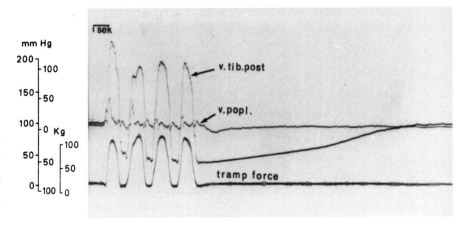

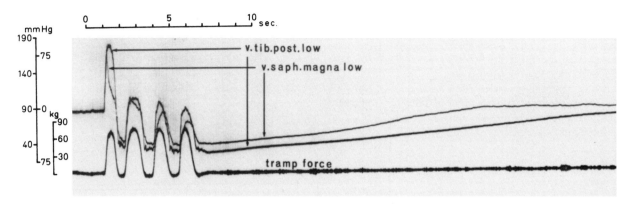

FIGURE 82.17. Pressure measurements from the posterior tibial and internal saphenous veins at the ankle. Methods and scales as in Figure 82.14.

sure in the posterior tibial vein in the ankle (Figure 82.14).

Results of Exercise

The calcaneus intraosseous and lower limb venous pressures were lowest on relaxation after muscular exercise. While the leg was hanging motionless and relaxed after the fourth tramp, the pressure rose at all points of measurement until it reached the stable level of the initial resting condition (Figures 82.14–82.17). In the calcaneus and posterior tibial vein in the ankle this pressure recovery period lasted, on average, about 35 seconds in men and 8 seconds in women and in the internal saphenous vein at the ankle about 25 seconds in men and 9 seconds in women.

Thus, calf muscle exercise lowered both ankle vein and calcanean pressures from resting values near the estimated hydrostatic pressure (72–100 mm Hg) to transmural (lateral) pressures between 30 and 40 mm Hg for a considerable period. The pressure variations in the calcanean bone marrow depended almost entirely on the pressure variations in the veins draining the bone.

The veins of the lower leg are converted to a high pressure system by muscular action in the upright position. Figure 82.18 shows pressure variations in the upper posterior tibial and internal saphenous veins and in the popliteal vein of a subject in the horizontal supine position at rest and during rhythmic muscular contractions.

The differences in resting pressures are clearly seen. Pressure variations during rhythmic contractions of the calf muscles are modest in the posterior tibial vein and insignificant at the other points of measurement. The relations remain constant; that is, the valves allow flow from the periphery toward the heart during all phases of the experiment. The pump unit in the calf does not act as a pump under such conditions, and the veins of the lower leg are a low pressure system when compared with the concomitant arterial pressures.

Figure 82.2 shows pressures from the same points of measurement after the subject had been raised to a nearly erect position. The pressures at rest all correspond to the calculated hydrostatic pressures. The modest difference between the posterior tibial and popliteal veins represents the *vis-a-tergo*. In this condition the veins of the lower limb are still a low pressure system.

However, rhythmic contractions of the calf muscles and the structure of the pump unit produce systolic and diastolic pressure variations of more than 100 mm Hg, and systolic pressure increases of more than 200 mm Hg have been recorded in healthy volunteers and in patients of groups I and III.

Figures 82.18 and 82.2 also show that, in the upright position, muscular exercise alters the relations between the venous pressures at different points of measurement in a regular pattern. Thus, during systole the pressure in the posterior tibial vein rises far above the pressure in both the popliteal and saphenous veins. At all points of

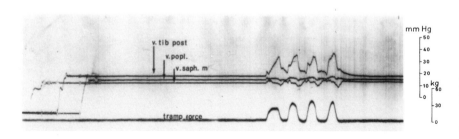

FIGURE 82.18. Pressure tracings from healthy subject in the horizontal position. Same patient and points of measurement as in Figure 82.14.

measurement the flow is directed toward the heart. Competent valves in the ankle perforating veins prevent flow from the deep to the superficial veins. During diastole the relations are reversed. The pressures in the popliteal and saphenous veins are now higher than those in the deep veins of the calf, with competent valves in the popliteal vein preventing a distal flow from the femur. The pressure difference indicates a flow through the ankle perforating veins from the superficial to the deep system.

Thus, in the upright position the action of the pump unit of the lower leg changes the veins inside the pump from a low to a high pressure system. However, under normal conditions the pump action lowers the venous pressure in the structures of the filling or input area (the ankle region) to mean values well below those of the resting phase. This is only possible as long as the structure of the pump is intact.

Pressure Variations in Deep and Superficial Veins and Calcaneus in Patients With Chronic Venous Insufficiency

Figures 82.8, 82.9, 82.10, 82.11, and 82.12 show characteristic dynamic phlebographs from the five groups of patients with different forms and degrees of chronic venous insufficiency, together with the mean pressure values in the ankle veins during rhythmic muscular exer-

cise. Figure 82.19 shows the mean pressure values in the calcaneus during rhythmic exercise in the five groups.

Differences Between Groups

Pressures at Rest
In the relaxed erect position the pressure at all points was approximately equal to the calculated hydrostatic pressure reaching from the point of measurement to the level of the angulus sterni (heart level). There were no demonstrable differences between the five groups or between patients and control subjects.

Pressure Variations During Rhythmic Muscular Exercise Compared With Dynamic Intraosseous Phlebography Results
In group I (simple varicose veins) the action of the venous pump of the calf induced a considerable fall in systolic and diastolic pressures at all points of measurement in the ankle and calcaneus. These results were similar to those from control subjects, and the second phlebographic exposure showed the veins in the lower leg to be almost or totally empty of contrast medium, which is also similar to control subjects. Thus, both methods of investigation indicated normal function of the musculovenous pump, and symptoms of chronic venous insufficiency were slight (Figures 82.3 and 82.8).

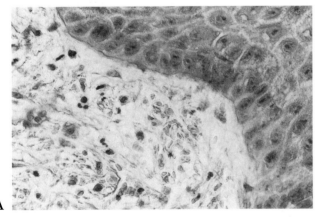

A

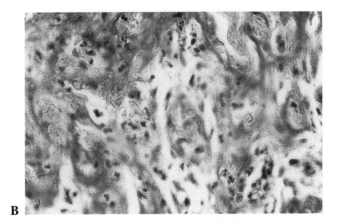

B

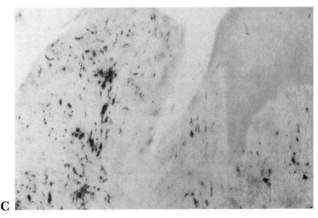

C

FIGURE 82.19. **A,** Border region epidermis–derma from patient with venous leg ulcer (group II). Note edema and extravascular erythrocytes (yellow) in derma (Martius scarlet blue × 400). **B,** Richly vascularized section of derma from patient with venous leg ulcer (group II). Dilated vessels with erythrocyte aggregations and agglutinations in edematous stroma (Martius scarlet blue × 400). **C,** Border of chronic leg ulcer (group III), stained for hemosiderin deposits. Hemosiderin confined to the derma (Perls' Prussian blue × 100).

TABLE 82.1. Consequences of continuous and intermittent hypertension.

	Constant hypertension	Intermittent hypertension
Macroscopic observations	Edema and faint redness of the skin	Edema and intense redness of the skin
	Venous dilation	Venous dilation
	Petechial bleedings (few)	Petechial bleedings (multiple)
		Ecchymoses
		Epidermal atrophy
		Depigmentation
		Necrosis
		Ulcer
Vital microscopic findings	Capillary dilation	Capillary dilation
	Dilated venules	Dilated venules
	Bleeding by diapedesis	Bleeding by diapedesis
	Hemoconcentration	Stasis
		Necrosis
Physiological results	Increased flow of lymph with low protein content	Increased flow of lymph with high protein content

In group II patients (with varicose veins, incompetent and dilated ankle perforating veins, and normal valves in the deep veins), the gradual fall in systolic pressure seen in healthy subjects and those in group I did not occur or was negligible. The depths of diastolic troughs and the duration of the period of pressure recovery did not differ significantly from normal findings. Both pressure recordings and phlebography showed the function of the venous pump to be severely impaired (Figures 82.4 and 82.9). The signs of chronic venous insufficiency were moderate to severe.

In group III patients (with postthrombotic syndrome [i.e., valvular incompetence in all three venous systems of the lower limb], occasionally combined with local obstructions of the deep veins), the systolic pressures remained high, and in the veins of the ankle region they increased from the first to the fourth contraction. The period of pressure recovery was significantly shorter than in any other group. Phlebography indicated complete absence of calf pump function, which is in keeping with the pressure pattern (Figures 82.5 and 82.10). The signs of chronic venous insufficiency were severe.

In group IV patients (women with cruralgia orthostatica with or without simple varicose veins, normal ankle perforating veins, and abnormally wide deep veins with morphologically intact valves), the phlebographic and pressure recording results gave widely different indications of the calf pump function. Rhythmic exercise had no effect on the distribution of contrast material in the veins of the lower limb, but the pressure graphs showed that the function of the muscle pump did lower the ankle vein pressures to values not significantly different from normal. The low pressure peak during the first contraction was characteristic. Special characteristics from this group are discussed later in this chapter (Figures 82.6 and 82.11). Clinically the characteristic symptom was orthostatic pain in the calf and a nonpitting edema of most of the lower leg.

In group V patients (women with varicose veins, incompetent and dilated ankle perforating veins, and ab-

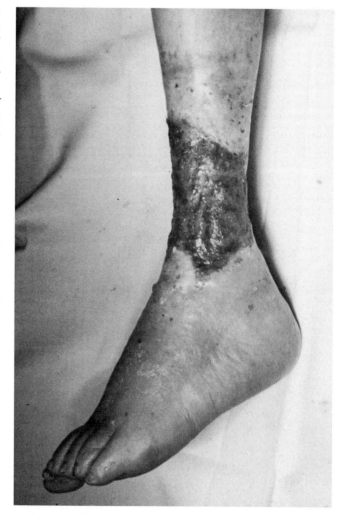

FIGURE 82.20. Long-standing (12 years) postthrombotic venous leg ulcer in a woman age 63. The ulcer encircles the ankle, which is fixed in equino position. The edema present during the first years after the thrombotic incident has disappeared, leaving a leathery induration of the subcutis (scarry fibrosis). Note the brownish staining of the skin of the ankle and foot (hemosiderin).

normally wide deep veins with normal looking valves), the action of the calf muscles had no influence on the distribution of contrast material in either the deep or superficial veins of the lower leg. The pressure curves and anatomical features were similar to those of group II. However, the systolic pressure peaks were substantially lower in group V than in group II patients. (Figures 82.7 and 82.12, cf. Figures 82.4 and 82.9). Clinically, the typical symptom was orthostatic pain in the calf and a—mostly—nonpitting edema of most of the lower leg.

Effects of Systolic Ambulatory Venous and Intraosseous Hypertension at the Ankle in Soft Tissues

Pathogenesis of Venous Leg Ulcer

From the previously mentioned results we may conclude the following:

1. Subcutaneous induration and venous leg ulcers may (groups II and III) or may not (group V) occur in the presence of incompetent and dilated ankle perforating veins.
2. These trophic changes may occur in the presence of a normal (group II) or shortened (group III) period of pressure recovery.
3. Leg ulcers occur when, during repeated calf muscle contractions, systolic pressure increases are sustained

at a level approximately 40 to 60 mm Hg above resting level in the subcutaneous veins of the ankle (groups II and III).

Patients with only moderately increased systolic pressure after repeated contractions (group V) may have edema, but induration and ulceration are never observed. Thus, high systolic pressure in the superficial veins of the ankle during exercise such as walking appears to be the main factor in the pathomechanism of the trophic changes in the soft tissues of the ankle region.[17]

The importance of this intermittent venous hypertension was further elucidated by the results of a series of experiments by Boersma and van Limborgh.[13] They examined and compared the effects of continuous versus intermittent venous hypertension in the lower limbs of frogs. The differences are shown in Table 82.1.

By means of vital capillary microscopy, Fagrell[14-16] demonstrated capillary dilation with perivascular edema and deoxygenated blood in the small veins and venules in the skin of the ankle region in patients corresponding to groups II and III.

The histological sections from normal ankle skin (Figure 82.21) and from the borders of a venous leg ulcer (Figure 82.19) further illustrate the microcirculatory changes characteristic of the skin and subcutis of the ankle in patients with severe chronic venous insufficiency.

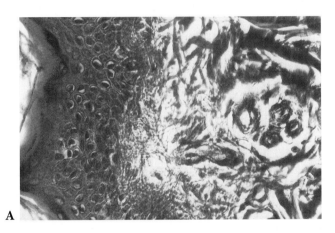

A

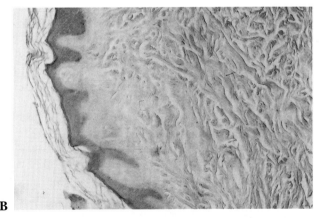

B

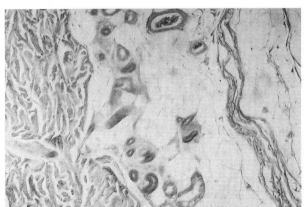

C

FIGURE 82.21. **A,** Epidermis and derma from normal skin of the ankle region. Vessels in lower center are empty (Martius scarlet blue × 400). **B,** Epidermis and dermis from normal skin of the ankle region, stained for hemosiderin deposits (Perls' Prussian blue × 100). **C,** Derma and subcutis stained for hemosiderin deposits. Note the arterioles and venules of the subcutis. Most of them are empty (Perls' Prussian blue × 100).

Thus, the pathomechanism of the trophic changes in the soft tissues of the ankle region observed in the patients of groups II and III may be summarized as follows: a decrease in the arteriovenous pressure difference of approximately 50 mm Hg during a period of walking retards the blood flow through the capillary bed and results in a relative hypoxia. Dilation of the capillaries due to increased resistance to flow and high pressure, as well as hypoxia, causes increased permeability of the capillary wall and edema. Proteins escape easily into the interstitial fluid,[18] and after prolonged hypoxemia even erythrocytes may penetrate the capillary wall.[19] These observations explain the high protein content of the interstitial fluid in patients with leg ulcers[20] and in frog limbs exposed to intermittent venous hypertension,[13] as well as the discoloration of the skin of the ankle by hemosiderin that is an almost constant finding in these patients (Figure 82.20).

The end results are subcutaneous fibrosis (induration), devitalization, and ulceration in the region where systolic hypertension in the superficial ankle veins is highest (i.e., the site of the incompetent and dilated ankle perforating veins). In the previously mentioned experiments on frogs the leg ulcer always appeared at the site of the only perforating vein in the lower limb.

Skeletal Changes at the Ankle Associated With Chronic Venous Insufficiency

Gilje and Andresen[21] observed periosteal apposition of bone and osteosclerotic changes in cancellous bone in the skeleton of the lower leg in more than 50% of patients with venous leg ulcers. They assumed that these changes were caused by the same circulatory disorder responsible for development of leg ulcers.

As seen from Figure 82.14 the intraosseous pressure of the calcaneus closely reflects the pressure in the deep veins of the ankle in both healthy subjects and the various groups of patients with chronic venous insufficiency.[11,12,22] Systolic venous hypertension is thus always accompanied by systolic intramedullary hypertension in this region. The pressure patterns noted in the calcaneus are identical to those observed in the distal parts of the tibia and fibula. The possible correlation between ambulatory systolic intraosseous hypertension and skeletal changes at the ankle was investigated by Arnoldi, Linderholm, and Vinnerberg.[22]

Material: Selection and Grouping

For this study, 92 patients (68 women and 24 men) with various forms of chronic venous insufficiency were examined. Only patients with clinical and phlebographi-

cally unilateral varicosis or calf pump dysfunction were included. All patients underwent bilateral phlebographic examination.

Two methods were used: (1) ascending intravenous phlebography[23] to evaluate the morphology of the entire lower limb and (2) dynamic intraosseous phlebography as described earlier to assess the function of the venous pump of the calf. Dynamic phlebography facilitated the division of patients into five groups as already described.

Methods

The patients selected were examined as discussed in the following sections.

Clinical Examination

Each patient underwent thorough clinical examination for trophic soft tissue lesions of the lower limb. The presence or absence of edema, eczema, induration, and leg ulcer was noted.

X-Ray Examinations

Frontal and lateral exposures of the lower leg were made bilaterally. The examinations included the bones, soft tissues, and ankle joint. Using the sound limb as a control, the radiographs of the affected limb were studied and the presence or absence of the following changes from normal was noted:

1. Abnormal calcification of soft tissues, including phleboliths and diffuse subcutaneous calcification
2. Structural changes of bone, including periosteal apposition of bone and structural changes of cancellous bone
3. Signs of degenerative osteoarthritis of the ankle joint

Measurements of Intramedullary Calcanean Pressure

The calcanean pressure was measured on the affected side with the patient in a nearly erect position on a tiltable table. The procedure was described earlier.

Statistical Calculations

Differences between pressure means in the groups were evaluated with Student's t test. The statistical significance of the difference in frequency of various signs of tissue changes between the groups was evaluated with the χ^2 test or, in the case of low expected frequencies, with the Fisher exact probability test.[24]

Correlation between intramedullary pressure, y (mm Hg), and each of the various signs of tissue changes in groups I through III and in groups IV and V (x_1 through x_9) were evaluated from product moment correlation coefficients (point serial r) [25]; $x = 1$ was used to indicate absence of sign, and $x = 2$ was used to indicate presence of sign.

The contingency coefficient was used as a measure of the extent of association between the signs. χ^2 was calculated by the aid of 2×2 contingency tables, incorporating a correction for continuity. The statistical significance of the value of the contingency coefficient to indicate an association between the two variables was evaluated from the χ^2 value.[24]

Multiple regression analysis was made according to the method of least squares. The linear regression equation calculations were made on a digital computer. The program used computed a sequence of multiple linear regression equations in a stepwise manner. At each step one variable was added to the regression equation. The variable added was the one that made the greatest reduction in the error sum of squares. The Kolmogorov–Smirnow test as described by Liliefors[26] was used to test normality of distribution of y values and residuals.

Results

Clinical Examination

There were four signs of special significance: edema, eczema, subcutaneous induration, and leg ulcers. Although edema of the lower leg was seen in less than one third of patients in group I, it was present in almost 100% of the patients in other groups. In groups I, II, and III edema was pitting, circumscribed, and located in the lower half of the lower leg. In group IV the edema was of the nonpitting type, and in both groups IV and V it was distributed fairly evenly over the entire lower leg. Eczema was observed fairly frequently in groups II and III but rarely in the others. Subcutaneous induration and leg ulcers were seen only in groups II and III. Leg ulcers were approximately twice as common in group III as

in group II. The distribution of soft tissue changes is shown in Table 82.2.

X-Ray Examination

Calcification of soft tissue structures and structural changes of bone were noted in a large number of patients with chronic venous insufficiency.

Phleboliths in the vein walls were often observed. The subcutaneous veins of the ankle region were most often affected, the subcutaneous veins of the proximal calf less often, and the deep veins of the lower leg rarely (Figure 82.22).

Diffuse subcutaneous calcification was observed in a few patients, all with severe and long-standing chronic venous insufficiency (group III). This type of calcification appeared as irregular patches of fine nodules without definite relation to the larger veins (Figure 82.23).

Periosteal new bone apposition was seen in groups II and III as irregular sawtooth projections from cortical bone or as duplication of the cortex of the shaft of the fibula and tibia (Figure 82.24 and 82.25). In the vicinity of the ankle joint the periosteal changes took on the appearance of osteophytes (Figure 82.25). Periosteal apposition was never observed in groups I, IV, and V.

Structural changes of cancellous bone were best observed in the juxtaarticular ankle region. The x-ray changes varied. Coarsening of trabeculae, thickening of cortex, and rarefied subcortical zones were the most common observations. These structural changes were only observed in patients of groups II and (especially) III.

There were unilateral x-ray indications of *degenerative osteoarthritis of the ankle joint* in five patients in group III. The x-ray changes were moderate, consisting of slight subchondral sclerosis and marginal and subchondral osteophytes. Signs of more severe cartilage degeneration

TABLE 82.2. Maximum contraction pressure during the fourth tramp minus pressure in the resting state (y, in mm Hg) and the number and percentage frequency of observed presence of signs (x_1 through x_9) in the five groups of patients examined.

	y (mm Hg) M Md	SD (Range)	x_1 n_2 $f\%$	x_2 n_2 $f\%$	x_3 n_2 $f\%$	x_4 n_2 $f\%$	x_5 n_2 $f\%$	x_6 n_2 $f\%$	x_7 n_2 $f\%$	x_8 n_2 $f\%$
Group I	0	10.6	4	0	0	0	0	0	0	0
$n = 15$	4	(−18–14)	27	0	0	0	0	0	0	0
Group II	33	14.1	21	10	17	10	10	0	8	5
$n = 23$	29	(16–62)	92	44	74	44	44	0	35	22
Group III	58	13.2	20	7	19	17	14	5	13	13
$n = 20$	62	(30–77)	100	35	95	85	70	25	65	65
Group IV	−12	8.8	17	0	0	0	0	0	0	0
$n = 17$	−13	(−28–3)	100	0	0	0	0	0	0	0
Group V	17	6.1	17	2	0	0	1	0	0	0
$n = 17$	18	(5–26)	100	12	0	0	6	0	0	0

n, number of patients; M, arithmetic mean; Md, median; SD, standard deviation; x_1, edema; x_2, eczema; x_3, induration; x_4, leg ulcer; x_5, phleboliths; x_6, diffuse subcutaneous calcification; x_7, periosteal apposition of bone; x_8, structural changes of cancellous bone; n_2, number of positive findings; $f\%$, percentage frequency of positive findings.

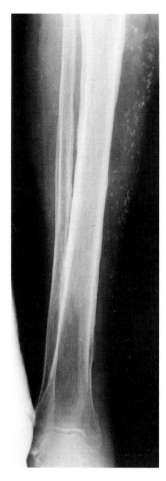

FIGURE 82.22. Phleboliths in the subcutaneous veins of the calf. Duplication of cortex on the distal medial side of the tibia. Patient from group II.

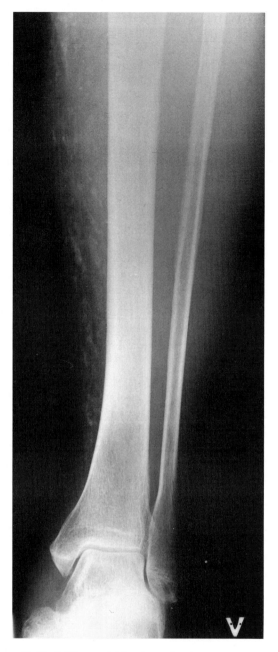

FIGURE 82.23. Diffuse calcification of soft tissue. Patient from group III.

with decreased joint space were apparent in only two patients. Table 82.2 shows the distributions of pathologic x-ray changes in the different groups.

Calcanean Pressure Measurements

Mean calcanean pressures taken with the subjects in the nearly erect position were measured in the five groups before, during, and after four contractions of the calf muscles (Figure 82.26). In each group the pressure was compared with data from healthy subjects. Figure 82.27 shows the mean difference between maximum contraction pressure during the fourth contraction and the resting pressure. In groups II and III these were approximately 30 and 60 mm Hg, respectively. In group V it was less pronounced (approximately 17 mm Hg), and in groups I and IV the pressure differences were low or negative. Intergroup differences for intracalcanean pressure minus resting pressure are given in Table 82.2.

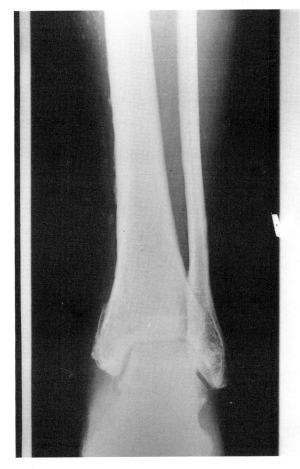

FIGURE 82.24. Sawtooth apposition of new bone on the tibial cortex and malleoli. Patient from group III.

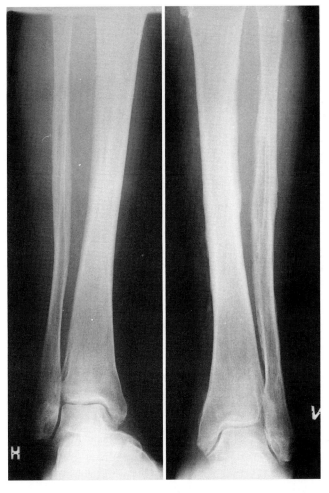

FIGURE 82.25. Unilateral apposition of new bone on fibula and tibia. Medial narrowing of ankle joint space. Patient from group III.

Tissue Changes Related to Intracalcanean Pressure

The relationship between tissue changes and the mean intracalcanean pressure at the fourth contraction is shown for groups I through V (Figure 82.27 and Table 82.3). Table 82.3 gives the numbers in each group, the tissue changes, the percentage frequency, and the mean systolic intracalcanean pressure at the fourth contraction related to resting pressure. Table 82.2 shows the statistical significance of the intergroup differences. The pressure differences between groups I and II, and particularly between groups I and III, are statistically significant, as are the differences in almost all tissue changes. In group III the pressure was on average higher, and most of the tissue changes were more frequent than in group II. Between groups IV and V and group I, the only differences were pressure and the presence of edema.

Superficial varicose veins and incompetent and dilated ankle perforating veins were characteristic of both groups II and V, but the groups differed in systolic pressure during the fourth tramp and in the percentage frequency of several of the tissue changes.

The results from groups II and III show that high systolic intraosseous pressures, sustained during repeated muscle contractions, are associated with a high frequency of both soft tissue and skeletal changes. Patients in whom the systolic pressure peaks decrease normally on rhythmic exercise (groups I and IV) or remain at a moderate level (group V) show few such changes.

Groups I, II, and III may be regarded as belonging to the same nosological entity. They represent different degrees of pathological changes in the veins (especially the valves) of the lower limb.

In groups IV and V the deep veins of the calf were abnormally wide, but the valves were morphologically nor-

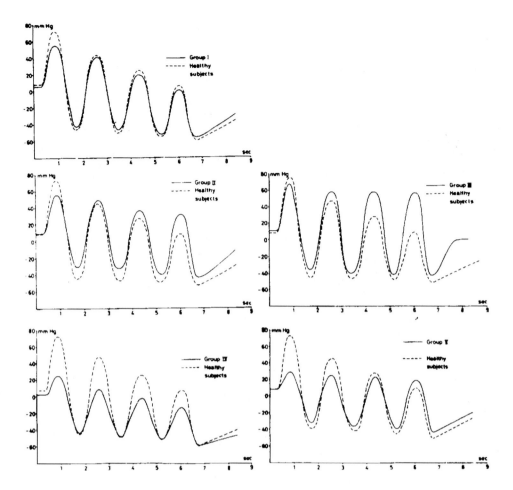

FIGURE 82.26. Mean calcanean pressures before, during, and after four short powerful contractions of the calf muscles in groups I through V. Data from the five groups of patients (unbroken line) are compared with data from healthy subjects (dotted line). The average force of contraction of the calf muscles (tramp force) was approximately the same during the four contractions and equal in all groups (no statistically significant differences).

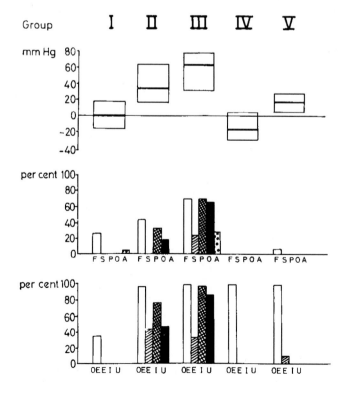

FIGURE 82.27. Pathological changes of soft tissues and bones of the lower leg and their relation to intramedullary pressure of the calcaneus during the fourth muscular contraction of the calf muscles. Data from 92 patients with various forms of unilateral dysfunction of the venous pump of the calf.

The upper part of the figure shows mean maximum systolic calcanean pressure during the fourth contraction and range in each group in millimeters of mercury. (This pressure was, on average, 4–9 mm Hg higher than the mean difference between the contraction pressure during the fourth systole and the pressure at rest; cf. Table 82.3).

The middle part of the figure represents percentage frequency in groups I through V of abnormal x-ray findings in subcutis and bones of the lower leg and ankle joint. F, phleboliths; S, diffuse subcutaneous calcification; P, periosteal apposition of new bone; O, structural changes of cancellous bone; A, roentgenological signs of degenerative osteoarthritis of the ankle joint.

The lower part of the figure represents percentage frequency in groups I through V of trophical changes of the skin and subcutis of the lower leg. OE, edema; E, eczema; I, induration of subcutis; U, venous leg ulcer.

TABLE 82.3. Differences between groups (see Table 82.2 and Figure 82.27) in maximum contraction pressure during the fourth tramp minus pressure in the resting state (Dy, mm Hg, expressed as differences between means) and differences in the frequency of signs of tissue changes ($Dx_1 - Dx_9$, expressed as differences of percentage frequencies).

Group	D_y	Dx_1	Dx_2	Dx_3	Dx_4	Dx_5	Dx_6	Dx_7	Dx_8
I–II	−32.4***	−65***	−44*	−74***	−44**	−44**	0	−35**	−2
I–III	−57.9***	−73***	−35***	−95***	−85***	−70***	−25*	−65***	−6
I–IV	+11.9**	−73***	0	0	0	0	0	0	
I–V	−16.8***	−73***	−12	0	0	−6	0	0	
II–III	−25.5***	−8	−19	−21	−41*	−26	−25*	−30	−4
II–V	+15.6***	−8	32	74***	44**	38*	0	35*	2

*, $.01 < P < .05$; **, $.001 < P < .01$; ***, $P < .001$. P is the probability that a difference is caused by chance.

mal. In these groups other mechanisms seem to play an important role in the dysfunction of the venous pump of the calf.

If groups I, II, and III are treated as one group ($n = 58$) we obtain the product moment correlation coefficients between pressure and tissue changes given in Table 82.4. They show that there is a close positive correlation between the intracalcanean pressure at the fourth contraction minus the resting pressure and most of the tissue changes observed (i.e., edema, induration, leg ulcer, phleboliths, periosteal apposition of bone, structural changes of cancellous bone, and osteoarthritis of the ankle joint). Subcutaneous calcification and eczema appear to have a low positive correlation to intracalcanean pressure.

Groups IV and V, treated as one group ($n = 34$), showed no statistically significant correlation between the systolic intracalcanean pressure and tissue changes in spite of a range of pressures of the same magnitude as groups I, II, and III together, although at a lower level.

Table 82.5 shows contingency coefficients for the association between the different signs and their statistical significance in groups I, II, and III together. Several signs are evidently closely associated, particularly edema, but osteoarthritis of the ankle joint is also closely associated with most of the other observed signs (i.e., there is a marked association between soft tissue and skeletal changes).

In groups IV and V together the presence of edema is associated with absence of most other evidence of tissue

TABLE 82.4. Product moment correlation coefficients (point biserial r)[25] between maximum contraction pressure during the fourth tramp minus pressure in the resting state (y) and various pathological tissue changes ($x_1 - x_9$) in groups I + II + III, $n = 58$.

Using the Kolmogorov–Smirnow test the probability that the deviation of the distribution of y values was caused by random factors was found to be $> .05$ (i.e., the y values did not deviate statistically significantly from a normal distribution).

Sign	Correlation coefficient (r)
x_1 edema	.68**
x_2 eczema	.26*
x_3 induration	.73**
x_4 leg ulcer	.66**
x_5 phleboliths	.61**
x_6 diffuse subcutaneous calcification	.21
x_7 periosteal apposition of bone	.70**
x_8 structural changes of cancellous bone	.73**
x_9 osteoarthritis of ankle joint	.40**

*, $.01 < P < .05$ (correlation coefficient $> .26$); **, $P < .01$ (correlation coefficient $> .34$).

changes (cf. Table 82.2). Multiple regression analysis was used to assess how closely the intracalcanean pressure could be predicted from the observed tissue changes in groups I, II, and III together. The signs x_1, x_2 . . . x_9 were considered to be independent variables, and the intracalcanean pressure during the fourth tramp related to resting pressure (y) was considered the dependent variable of a linear regression equation. The results are given in Table 82.6. The coefficients of signs

TABLE 82.5. Contingency coefficients indicating the association between the different signs in the patient groups I + II + III ($n = 58$).

	x_1	x_2	x_3	x_4	x_5	x_6	x_7	x_8	x_9
x_1 edema	—								
x_2 eczema	.42***	—							
x_3 induration	.15	.30***	—						
x_4 leg ulcer	.29**	.16	.14	—					
x_5 phleboliths	.33***	.11	.19*	.04	—				
x_6 diffuse subcutaneous calcification	.57***	.23**	.48***	.37***	.33***	—			
x_7 periosteal apposition of bone	.37***	.05	.23**	.09	.04	.30***	—		
x_8 structural changes of cancellous bone	.41***	.00	.28**	.14	.09	.25**	.04	—	
x_9 osteoarthritis of ankle joint	.54***	.19*	.45***	.33***	.30***	.03	.26**	.20*	—

*, $.01 < P < .05$; **, $.001 < P < .01$; ***, $P < .001$. P is the probability that an association between variables is caused by chance.

TABLE 82.6. Coefficients of regression (b_k), constants (a), residual standard deviations (RSD), and the squares of the coefficients of multiple correlation (R^2) in different multiple regression equations with the intracalcanean pressure as the dependent variable, calculated for the groups I + II + III ($n = 58$). Equations 1, 2, and 3 were obtained from the second, fourth, and ninth step, respectively, in the calculation of the sequence of multiple regression equations.

Equation number	b_1	b_2	b_3	b_4	b_5	b_6	b_7	b_8	b_9	a	RSD	R^2
1			27***					27***		−47	±13	0.19
2	19***		16**					23***	14**	−73	±12	0.28
3	±18***	−8	+10	+10*	+9*	+1	+2	+17***	+15**	−76	±10	0.47

The subscripts of the coefficients of regression indicate the association with the variables x_1 through x_9 (see Tables 82.4 and 84.5). Significance symbols as in Table 82.5. Using the Kolmogorov–Smirnow test the probability that the deviation of the residuals from a normal distribution was caused by random factors was found to be 0.2 (i.e., the distribution of the residuals did not deviate statistically significantly from a normal distribution).

such as induration and structural changes of cancellous bone were statistically significant. Thus, the presence of induration and structural changes of cancellous bone are highly predictive of intraosseous hypertension, and the same is true of edema and osteoarthritis of the ankle joint. As much as 87% of the variation in y might be explained by the observed presence or absence of the nine signs, and the residual standard variation was approximately 10% of the total variation in y. Combining groups IV and V and performing a similar multiple regression analysis did not result in any statistically significant coefficients.

Pathomechanism of Systolic Venous and Intraosseous Hypertension in the Ankle Region

In groups II and III mean pressures at rest and during the first calf muscle contraction and diastolic pressure immediately after muscle contraction (diastole), as well as possible directions of flow during these phases, are summarized in the schematic drawings of Figures 82.28 through 82.32.[27]

Healthy Subjects

Functioning valves in the slender ankle perforating veins of healthy subjects (Figures 82.27, 82.28, 82.29, and 82.30) keep the systolic pressure in the subcutaneous veins at a relatively low level (about one third of the concurrent systolic pressure in the deep veins of the ankle). During diastole, when the pressure relations are reversed, competent valves in the saphenous system prevent distally directed flow in these veins and excessive filling of the deep veins of the input area. Reduced blood volume thus diminishes the effect on ankle vein pressure during the following systole (cf. Figure 82.17).

Group I

Competent valves in the ankle perforators prevent excessive filling of the deep veins of the ankle, and the pressures in this area remain normal (cf. Figure 82.8).

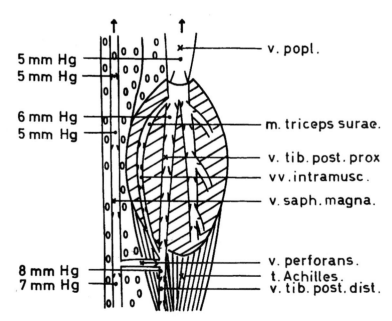

FIGURE 82.28. Mean vein pressures and flow direction in the lower leg in healthy volunteers in the relaxed nearly erect position.

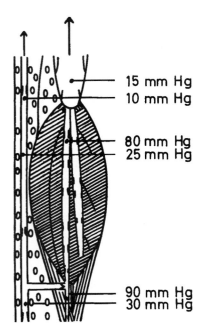

FIGURE 82.29. Mean venous blood pressures during contraction of the calf muscles (systole) in healthy subjects.

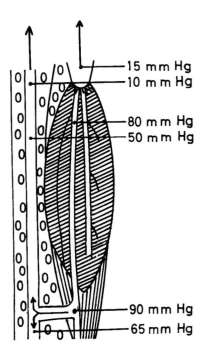

FIGURE 82.31. Mean systolic pressures and direction of flow during systole in patients from group III.

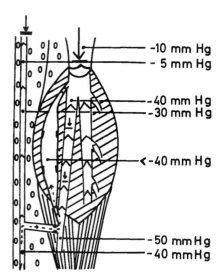

FIGURE 82.30. Mean venous blood pressures and possible flow direction during the period of relaxation immediately after muscle contraction (diastole) in healthy volunteers.

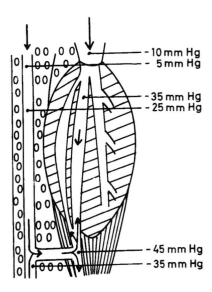

FIGURE 82.32. Mean pressures and direction of flow during diastole in patients from group III.

Group II

Dilated ankle perforating veins with incompetent valves in group II patients (Figure 82.9) permit the high systolic pressure to be transmitted to the subcutaneous veins at the ankle, where it reaches a level of approximately two thirds of the deep pressure. This also happens in group III and is illustrated in Figure 82.31. During diastole the incompetent valves in the varicose (dilated) saphenous system allow a rapid distal flow through these veins and the dilated ankle perforating veins to the veins of the input area of the calf pump. This distal flow is illustrated by Trendelenburg's test and was quantified by Bjordal.[28,29] During the following systole the contraction acts on a blood volume much larger than normal, and the pressure remains high (cf. Figure 82.9).

Group III

In group III (Figures 82.10, 82.31, and 82.32) the diastolic filling of the veins of the ankle region follows the pattern of group II but is enhanced by additional distally directed blood flow through the deep channels. This is reflected in the steadily rising systolic pressures, the brief period of pressure recovery, and the more shallow diastolic pressure troughs (Figure 82.10).

Conclusion

In the ankle region, the input area of the musculovenous pump of the calf, dysfunction or incompetence of the pump due to valvular insufficiency in the varicose superficial veins, the ankle perforating veins, and in group III the deep veins under the fascia cruris results in intermittent systolic venous and intraosseous hypertension responsible for soft tissue damage and skeletal changes. The ultimate cause of these tissue changes seems to be interference with capillary blood flow due to high resistance on the venous side of the capillary bed. (All patients examined in these studies had normal arterial circulation in the lower limbs.)

The pressure graphs represent the effect of rhythmic contraction and relaxation of the muscles of the posterior pump unit alone. The three units of the lower leg may work independently,[1] but during normal activity such as walking the contractions of the muscles of the three segments follow each other in a regular pattern. The period of high systolic pressure in the subcutaneous veins of the ankle lasts from 50% to 70% of the duration of walking time.[30]

Pain and Venous Distension

Quiet motionless sitting or standing may cause discomfort in the lower leg even in completely healthy subjects. This discomfort is generally described as a sense of heaviness and tiredness or sometimes as restlessness. Women seem to suffer from these complaints more often than men and may have actual pain during the premenstrual period. Rest with the legs raised brings relief, and elastic support stockings may prevent more serious discomfort.

In groups I and II these slight to moderate symptoms were common, and when pain was present it was usually located along the dilated varicose veins. Severe pain, however, was not characteristic in these groups. In group III (postthrombotic syndrome) severe diffuse pain in the calf was fairly common, and in groups IV and V it was the dominating symptom.

Idiopathic Dysfunction of the Venous Pump of the Calf (Cruralgia Orthostatica)

Clinical Features

Cruralgia orthostatica was first described by Arnoldi.[1,5,7] It is almost exclusively confined to women of fertile age. Although the etiology is unknown, that it is confined to women, that more than 70% of these patients have their menarche at age 15 or later, and that the symptoms, as a rule, disappear gradually after menopause may indicate that hormonal factors play a pathogenetic role.

Two thirds of the 317 patients examined by Arnoldi[5] presented with varicose veins and incompetent ankle perforating veins (group V). Of the remainder some had varicose veins, but none had incompetent ankle perforating veins (group IV). None suffered from thrombosis of the deep veins.

Symptoms and Signs

For patients with cruralgia orthostatica, the typical pain is felt deep in the calf and usually described as a bursting ache. It is most pronounced after prolonged standing, sitting, and walking and disappears relatively quickly when the feet are rested above the level of the heart or when a sufficiently strong compression bandage or stocking is applied to the lower leg. Orthostatic pain may be slight, moderate, or severe, and some patients have even asked for amputation "if nothing else can be done."

Edema of the lower leg is a constant finding. In group IV the edema is not of the pitting type but evenly distributed from the ankle to the knee. The leg appears thick rather than swollen. In group V the thick leg might show additional pitting edema at the ankle. When patients have been standing for some time the skin of the foot and ankle may take on a reddish-blue color. This cyanotic discoloration can become pronounced, but it is not a constant finding in these women. More than half of the women in groups IV and V had noticed a marked tendency to subcutaneous ecchymoses.

Paraclinical Examinations

Results obtained by dynamic intraosseous phlebography were described previously (Figures 82.6 and 82.7) Typical for groups IV and V were the abnormally wide intermuscular and intramuscular veins of the calf with normal looking valves and the total retention of contrast medium after standard exercise.

Although the phlebographic evidence indicated total incompetence of the venous pump (by definition) in groups IV and V, the results of venous pressure measurements showed that the action of the musculovenous pump reduced the pressure in the deep and superficial veins of the ankle region in the patients of group IV (Figure 82.11). This also occurs during exercise of long duration (5 minutes), when the blood flow is likely to be fast. Consequently, the pump functions efficiently at high flow rates.[6] The phlebographic evidence indicates, however, that the calf pump works with a larger than normal systolic residual blood volume.

A characteristic feature in groups IV and V was the low systolic pressure during the first contraction after a period of complete rest. In healthy subjects and in patients of groups I, II, and III the pressure rise in the posterior tibial veins was approximately 1 mm Hg per kg applied tramp force, but in groups IV and V the pressure rise per kg applied force was only about 50% of normal values.[17]

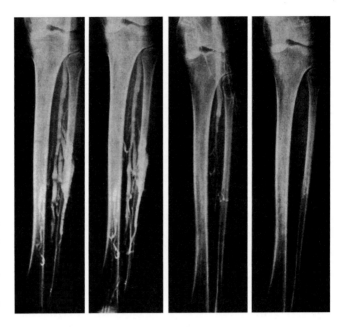

FIGURE 82.33. Dynamic intraosseous phlebographs from a woman of group IV (idiopathic dysfunction of the venous pump of the calf or cruralgia orthostatica): (left) without and (right) with elastic compression.

Possible Causes of Idiopathic Calf Pump Dysfunction and Cruralgia Orthostatica

Present evidence points to lax mesenchymal structures, such as muscle fascias, perhaps particularly laxness of the soleus arch, and ineffective compression of the veins during muscle contraction as causes of idiopathic calf pump dysfunction and cruralgia orthostatica. This leaves the deep veins of the standing or walking patient in a state of constant overdistension. The typical bursting ache felt deep in the calf could be due to activation of pain receptors in the vein wall that react on distension. This conception is strengthened by the images in Figure 82.33, which show the effect on the phlebographic pattern when a compression bandage is applied, and by the clinical experience that such bandages provide effective pain relief.

Final Conclusions

The clinical and experimental observations reported in this chapter allow us to come to some fairly well-founded conclusions and raise some questions that, as yet, cannot be answered. Pain (cruralgia orthostatica) may be found in conjunction with high venous pressures, as in some of the postthrombotic patients of group III. However, this type of pain is more closely correlated to venous disten-

sion, which is mostly associated with abnormally low systolic venous pressures.

Degenerative soft tissue and skeletal changes are undoubtedly correlated with high ambulatory venous pressures in the ankle region. The main area of investigation included the musculovenous pump proper (i.e., the calf proximal to the transition of the musculus gastrocnemius into the Achilles tendon) and the filling (input) area distal to the pump (i.e., the ankle region). It is in the latter area that sustained high systolic venous and intraosseous pressure have the greatest effect on the various tissues—skin, subcutis, fascia, muscles, tendons, and bone. However, although venous hypertension must be effective in changing the microcirculation in all these components, they react very differently.

The loose subcutaneous tissue of the whole ankle region and the skin in the area of the highest systolic pressures in the vicinity of the incompetent ankle perforating veins seem to be the most vulnerable structures. Most of the tissue changes are located here. The skeleton of the ankle is also affected, but the time factor differs considerably. Large areas of induration and persistent leg ulcers may have been present for years before the first roentgenologic signs of skeletal reaction become apparent. Another remarkable factor is the very different reaction to systolic venous hypertension superficial to and beneath the fascia cruris. In most cases, when incising through the scarred or necrotic tissues of the ulcer area and continuing through the fascia, the surgeon encounters apparently unaffected structures.

Mostly the tendons and a few muscles of the region appear normal. Only in rare cases of severe and long-standing postthrombotic syndromes do the muscles show signs of degenerative change; the tendons never show such signs. The reason for this diversity of reaction is not yet known.

Pathophysiology in Relation to Treatment

During the voyage to Troy, King Philoctetes developed a leg ulcer that soon became so noisome that his shipmates could not stand the smell. They therefore put him ashore on the island Lemnos, where the local physicians tended to his wound—not very successfully—for 9 years. Philoctetes was a great archer and had inherited his bow and arrows from Heracles.

In the 10th year of the siege of Troy an oracle revealed that the city could not be conquered without these magic weapons. So Machaon, the most famous surgeon and one of the Asclepiads, was sent to Lemnos and the cure was finally effected. Machaon "cut away the decaying flesh from the wound, applied healing herbs and the serpentine stone."[31] (Translated into the language of present-day textbooks it means that surgery was followed by the application of a pressure bandage with maximum compression on the tortuous posterior arch vein and ankle perforating veins.)

In those days the cure was considered no mean feat and in fact a miracle. Philoctetes and his weapons joined the battle with the well-known result. Machaon was made an Honorary FICA (Fellow of the International College of Asclepiads), and a temple was built in his honor in the Peloponese. Interspecialty jealousy was, however, also rampant in those days, and a few physicians spread the rumor that not Machaon, but his timorous brother Podaleirius, the dermatologist, was in charge of the case.

Modern Conservative Treatment

Bed Rest

Although treatment of leg ulcers by compression bandages was described in texts from the Old Kingdom of ancient Egypt and (re)introduced in Europe during the seventeenth century, these ulcers were still described as a *crux medicorum* during the first decades of our century, when the most effective treatment seemed to be rest in bed with the affected leg elevated. Because this treatment eliminates the pathologically high systolic venous pressures in the ankle region of patients of groups II and III, the results were generally good. However, continued bed rest is both expensive and dangerous, especially for elderly people. Further, the ulcers tended to recur as soon as the patient resumed an active ambulatory life.

Ambulatory Compression

Ambulatory treatment by means of compression bandages or stockings is now the basis of purely conservative treatment for trophic soft tissue changes and pain, especially of the cruralgia orthostatica type, and is equally important in treatment based on sclerotherapy or surgery. The effects of ambulatory compression of the lower leg may be summarized thus:

- Compression of the subcutaneous varicosities, especially of the posterior arch vein, interrupts or reduces the distally directed flow through these veins during diastole. Thus, filling of the deep veins through the incompetent and dilated ankle perforating veins during this phase is minimized. In group II patients the volume of blood in the deep veins of the input area and the height of systolic pressures are thus normalized. In patients of group III compression has the same effect. However, reflux from the deep veins proximal to the ankle region during diastole is still possible.
- Walking with compression reduces existing edema by a massage action, and the mechanism referred to earlier and the heightened subcutaneous tissue pressure minimize the tendency to continued edema.
- Distension of deep and subcutaneous veins is reduced. Compression is thus a very effective remedy for orthostatic pain.

Sclerotherapy and Surgical Treatment

Unfortunately, the beneficial effects of compression disappear when the treatment is discontinued. The aim of both sclerotherapy and surgical treatment of chronic venous insufficiency is, apart from cosmetic improvement, to normalize physiological conditions in the lower leg permanently, either by closing the varicose veins and ankle perforating veins (sclerotherapy) or by extraction and ligation (surgery). The methods are often combined.

In expert hands both sclerotherapy and surgery give excellent cosmetic results, especially if the methods are combined. In patients of groups II and (to a lesser degree) III with severe soft tissue changes at the ankle, a high percentage of permanent cure can be achieved if the principles mentioned earlier are adhered to. Thus, in a series of 1147 leg ulcers, Arnoldi and Hæger,[32] using surgical methods, obtained healing in 97% of group II and 84% of group III patients. However, most patients of the latter group had to continue to wear moderate-compression stockings.

Surgery and sclerotherapy have no place in the treatment of group IV patients (except for cosmetic reasons in those who also suffer from varicose veins). The same holds true in patients of group V. The orthostatic pain characteristic of these groups demands continued use of compression stockings. Today every angiologist (phlebologist) who knows what he or she is doing and why should be able to "do a Machaon."

References

1. Arnoldi CC. The venous return from the lower leg in health and in chronic venous insufficiency. A synthesis. *Acta Orthop Scand Suppl.* 1964;64:7–75.

2. Dodd H, Cockett F. *The Pathology and Surgery of the Veins of the Lower Limb.* Edinburgh: Churchill Livingstone, Ltd; 1956:424–447.

3. Arnoldi CC, Bauer G. Intraosseous phlebography. *Angiology.* 1960;11:44–51.

4. Arnoldi CC. Venous pressure in the legs of healthy human subjects at rest and during muscular exercise in the nearly erect position. *Acta Chir Scand.* 1965;130:570–583.

5. Arnoldi CC. Idiopatisk dysfunktion av vadens venpump. *Läkartidningen.* 1970;67:6055–6063.

6. Arnoldi CC, Linderholm H. Venous blood pressures in the lower limb at rest and during exercise in patients with idiopathic dysfunction of the venous pump of the calf. *Acta Chir Scand.* 1969;135:601–609.

7. Arnoldi CC. Pain in the lower leg in patients with chronic venous insufficiency (cruralgia orthostatica). *Acta Chir Scand.* 1965;129:57–65.

8. Arnoldi CC. The influence of posture upon the pressure in the veins of the normal human leg at rest and during rhythmic muscular exercise. *Acta Chir Scand.* 1966;131; 423–429.

9. Arnoldi CC. Venous pressures in patients with valvular incompetence of the veins of the lower limb. *Acta Chir Scand.* 1966;132:628–645.

10. Arnoldi CC, Greitz T, Linderholm H. Variations in cross-sectional area and pressure in the veins of the normal lower leg during rhythmic muscular exercise *Acta Chir Scand.* 1966;132:507–522.

11. Arnoldi CC, Linderholm H. Intraosseous pressure of the calcaneus and venous pressure in the calf of healthy human subjects in the erect position. *Acta Chir Scand.* 1966; 132:646–662.

12. Arnoldi CC, Linderholm H. Intracalcanean pressures in patients with different forms of dysfunction of the venous pump of the calf. *Acta Chir Scand.* 1971;137:21–27.

13. Boersma W, van Limborgh J. Experimental investigations on the development of the ulcus cruris venosum in the frog. *Folia Angiologica.* 1967;9:48–63.

14. Fagrell B. Microcirculatory changes of the skin in venous disorders of the leg, studied by vital capillaroscopy. In:

15. Schneider KW, ed. *Die Venöse Insuffizienz.* Baden-Baden, Germany: Verlag Gerhard Witztorck; 1972:202–212.

16. Fagrell B. Vital microscopy in the pathophysiology of deep venous insufficiency. In: Eklöf B, Gjöres JE, Thulesius O, Bergquist D, eds. *Controversies in the Management of Venous Disorders.* London: Butterworths; 1989:243–248.

17. Fagrell B. Clinical evaluation of the microcirculation in health and disease. *J Physiol Pharmacol.* 1993;44(suppl 2): 103–119.

18. Arnoldi CC, Linderholm H. On the pathogenesis of the venous leg ulcer. *Acta Chir Scand.* 1968;134:427–440.

19. Landis EM. Capillary pressure and capillary permeability. *Physiol Rev.* 1934;14;404–465.

20. Zweifach BW. The structural basis of permeability and other functions of blood capillaries (Cold Spring Harbor Symposia). *Quant Biol.* 1940;8:216–223.

21. Haxthausen H. Om Pathogenesen ved Ulcus Cruris Varicosum. *Nord Med.* 1936;12:1665–1672.

22. Gilje O, Andresen I. Osseous x-ray findings in ulcus cruris. *Acta Derm Venereol (Stockh).* 1956;36:294–299.

23. Arnoldi CC, Linderholm H, Vinnerberg A. Skeletal and soft tissue changes in the lower leg in patients with intracalcanean hypertension. *Acta Chir Scand.* 1972;138:25–37.

24. Greitz T. The technique of ascending phlebography of the lower limb. *Acta Radiol.* 1954;42:421–429.

25. Siegel S. *Nonparametric Statistics for Behavioral Sciences.* New York, NY: McGraw-Hill; 1956.

26. Garret H. *Statistics in Psychology and Education.* 5th ed. New York, NY: Longmans, Green & Co; 1960.

27. Lilliefors HW. On the Kolmogorov-Smirnow test for normality with mean and variance unknown. *J Am Stat Assoc.* 1967;62:399–402.

28. Arnoldi CC. Physiology and pathophysiology of the venous pump of the calf. In: Eklöf B, Gjöres JE, Thulesius O, Bergquist D, eds. *Controversies in the Management of Venous Disorders.* London: Butterworths; 1989:6–23.

29. Bjordal RI. *Blood Circulation in Varicose Veins of the Lower Extremities* [Ph.D. diss]. Oslo, Norway: Universitetsforlaget; 1973.

30. Bjordal RI. Pressure and flow measurements in venous insufficiency of the legs. In: Eklöf B, Gjöres JE, Thulesius O, Bergquist D, eds. *Controversies in the Management of Venous Disorders.* London: Butterworths; 1989:24–35.

31. Fegan WS, Fitzgerald DE, Milliken JC. The results of simultaneous pressure recordings from the superficial and deep veins of the leg. *Irish J Med Sci.* 1964;62:363–378.

32. Graves R. *The Greek Myths.* Vol 2. London: Penguin Books; 1959:326.

33. Arnoldi CC, Hæger K. Ulcus cruris venosum: crux medicorum? *Läkartidningen.* 1967;64:2149–2157.

83

Microvascular Aspects of Degenerative Joint Diseases

Carl C. Arnoldi

This chapter describes vascular disturbances in chronic joint disorders of the hip and knee with emphasis on early and late osteoarthritis, late rheumatoid arthritis, and osteonecrosis. The central theme is the effects of intermittently and chronically increased resistance to venous drainage from soft tissues, especially the synovium, and from juxtachondral bone marrow. I attempt to show a correlation between the vascular changes and the signs and symptoms of degenerative joint disease.

My interest in these aspects of circulatory pathology, not commonly discussed among angiologists, was awakened in the 1960s and early 1970s during studies of the pathophysiology of the venous return from the lower limb, briefly summarized in Chapter 82. The main inspiration was the finding that intraosseous pressure was more closely related to the pressure in the veins draining the bone than to the arterial pressure and that intermittently increased resistance to venous blood flow could be responsible for localized severe degenerative soft tissue changes (induration and leg ulcers) and visible changes in the regional bones.

In this chapter I confine myself to discussing vascular changes and their probable or possible effects on joint structure and function. Readers with special orthopedic or rheumatologic interests may refer to the references.

Osteoarthritis of the Human Hip and Knee

Investigations of Juxtachondral Bone Marrow

Until the 1950s it was a widely held opinion that the degenerative changes observed in joint-bearing bone were the results of failure of arterial supply.[1] In 1953 Harrison et al.[2] found hyperplasia of the intraosseous arteries of the femoral head and signs of venous stasis and interstitial lymphedema. Their conclusion was that the arterial supply to the bone marrow was increased rather than de-

creased, a conclusion that has not been seriously challenged since. Later investigations gave evidence of disturbed venous outflow from the femoral head and neck in osteoarthritis of the hip, disturbed venous outflow from the distal part of the femur in patients with osteoarthritis of the knee,[3-6] and increased intramedullary pressure.[7]

These early observations have been confirmed by others, and the current consensus seems to be that vascular changes in joint-bearing bone are characteristic features of manifest osteoarthritis. However, opinions have differed widely as to the importance and place of circulatory changes in the pathogenesis of the disorders. Are they late secondary phenomena (as most orthopedic surgeons and rheumatologists think), or could they be early phenomena and of primary importance? I examine the evidence at hand.

Intraosseous and Intravenous Pressure and Flow Measurements

Methods

Measurements were performed with the patient in a horizontal or nearly horizontal position.[8] In most series a polyethylene tube was introduced into the internal saphenous vein at the ankle and the tip placed at the same distance from the heart and heart level as the points of measurement in the bones. The midaxillary plane at the level of the first costal insertion at the sternum was chosen to indicate heart level, and this was the reference level for all pressures measured. The extraosseous venous pressure was used as a control or reference for the pressure measured in the bone marrow. Intraosseous pressure depends on and varies with the pressure in the veins draining the bone.[9-11] The pressure recording system used is described in Chapter 82.

TABLE 83.1. Pulse pressure amplitude, intraosseous pressure in femoral neck, and femoral vein pressure (mm Hg) in 15 patients with unilateral osteoarthritis (series 1).

Site of measurement	Unaffected hip joint (15 cases) mean and range	Standard deviation	Arthritic hip joint (15 cases) mean and range	Standard deviation	Difference between arthritic and unaffected hip
Intramedullary pulse pressure amplitude	4 (2–11)	2.9	6.8 (2–18)	5.2	2.8**
Neck pressure	18.7 (13.5–25.3)	3.6	48.4 (27.8–74.8)	16.3	29.7***
Femoral vein pressure	11.9 (6.5–15.6)	2.5	11.9 (6.5–15.6)	2.5	
Mean difference between intramedullary neck pressure and femoral vein pressure in unaffected hips = 6.8 mm Hg ($P < .001$)					

*, $.01 < P .05$; **, $.001 < P < .01$; ***, $P < .001$; P is the possibility that the difference is caused by chance.

Statistical Methods

Conventional statistical methods were employed. P values were obtained from the tables of Fisher and Yates.[9] The arithmetical mean and median of the groups were compared, and agreement between them was taken to indicate an approximately normal distribution.

Material

Two series of patients with painful primary osteoarthritis of the hip joint were examined.[8] The first series consisted of 15 patients with unilateral osteoarthritis in whom the intraosseous pressure of the femoral neck was measured on both sides at the same time as the pressure in the femoral vein. (Bilateral intraosseous phlebography was performed immediately after these measurements.)

The second series measured the intraosseous pressure in the femoral head and neck on one side only in 15 patients undergoing operation for severe painful osteoarthritis; venous pressures were not determined. The first series examined differences between healthy and affected hips, whereas in the second series measurements were taken to determine possible pressure differences between the femoral head and neck.

Results, First Series

Femoral Vein

In the first five patients examined the femoral venous pressure was measured on both sides. However, these results showed that the pressures from the healthy and affected sides were equal. Therefore, in the other 10 patients the pressure in the femoral vein was measured on one side only, in the unaffected limb in 6 patients and on the arthritic side in 4 patients. The pressures ranged between 6.5 and 16 mm Hg, with a mean pressure of 12 mm Hg (Table 83.1).

Femoral Neck

The pressure tracings were always pulsatile, and the pulse pressure was higher on the arthritic side than on the nonarthritic side (Figure 83.1 and Table 83.1). The

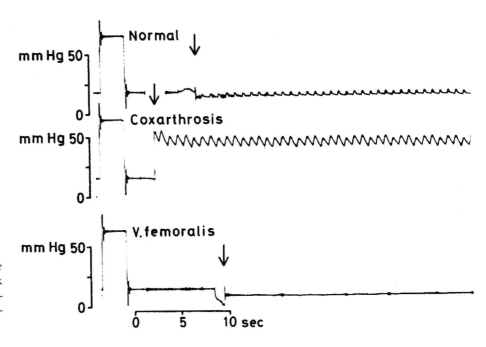

FIGURE 83.1. Bilateral pressure recordings from femoral neck and left femoral vein from a patient with unilateral osteoarthritis of the hip joint.

TABLE 83.2. Intramedullary pressures (mm Hg) of the femoral head and neck measured simultaneously in patients with osteoarthritis (series 2).

	Number of patients	Femoral head mean and range	Standard deviation	Femoral neck mean and range	Standard deviation	Difference
Intramedullary pulse pressure	15	5.8 (1–29)	7.3	4.4 (1–17)	4.2	1.4
Intramedullary pressure	15	32.3 (30.9–88.7)	16.6	43.1 (23–66.7)	13.9	10.8***

***, $P < .001$.

intraosseous pressure was always higher than the femoral venous pressure. In the healthy hips the difference between intramedullary and venous pressures ranged between 2.3 and 17 mm Hg (Table 83.1). The intraosseous pressure of the arthritic hip was higher than that of the healthy hip. There was a relatively wide variation in the differences (12–59 mm Hg), with a mean difference of 30 mm Hg.

Results, Second Series

Pulsatile pressure graphs were always obtained from both points of measurement. The average pulse pressure in the femoral head was somewhat greater than in the neck (Table 83.2), but the difference was not statistically significant in this series. The intraosseous pressure of the femoral neck was similar to that observed in the arthritic joints of the first series. The pressure in the femoral head was always higher than that in the neck.

Intraosseous Pressure and Flow in Healthy and Osteoarthritic Femoral Heads During Loading and Passive Joint Movements

The effect of intermittent calf muscle contractions on intracalcanean pressure is mentioned in Chapter 82. Pressure measurements during joint loading and movements were first reported by Arnoldi et al.[12] and Bünger et al.[13] in horses and puppies, respectively. In humans, pressure measurements during loading were published by Hejgaard and Arnoldi[14] and Arnoldi,[15] who examined pressures in the patella and femoral and tibial condyles in pain-free knees and knees with patellar pain (PP) syndromes.

Material

Six patients, four women and two men, with a median age of 69 years (58–79 years) were examined bilaterally.[16] Eight hips had moderate to severe osteoarthritis and significantly increased uptake of ^{99m}Tc-polyphosphate.

Four hips were without symptoms, were radiographically normal, and had neutral isotope uptake.

Methods

Pressure Measurements

The patients were examined on the operating table, prior to alloplasty, lying supine under general anesthesia. The cannula for pressure measurement was placed with the tip in the center of the femoral head under guidance of an image intensifier. The general procedure for measurements followed that described earlier. The tube in the extraosseous vein, when used, was placed with the tip at the junction of the internal saphenous and superficial femoral veins.

Pressure Recording

The cannulae for pressure measurements were connected to Bentley transducers (American Edwards Laboratories, Santa Ana, Calif., USA) that in turn were connected to a 4 Press 8041 measuring system (Simonsen & Weel, Copenhagen, Denmark) with a six-channel printer (BBC SE 460, Austria). The pressure (and flow) tracings were controlled visually during the measurements on a quadriscope (Simonsen & Weel).

Laser Doppler Flowmetry

Laser Doppler flowmetry (LDF) is based on the Doppler shift of a monochromatic beam of light from a 2-mV helium–neon laser source reflected from moving blood cells in the tissue. This shift of wavelength is converted into an electronic signal and is presented digitally in millivolts. LDF can provide continuous, real-time monitoring of changes in local perfusion and an estimate of the relative blood flow in different tissue regions (e.g., the bone marrow of the femoral head).

The laser Doppler flowmeter produces an output signal that is linear over the entire measured range and is proportional to the microvasular blood cell perfusion of the target tissue. The perfusion value is the product of the number of cells moving in the measured volume and the mean velocity of these cells but is independent of the direction of the movement of the blood cells. The measured area is approximately 1.5 to 2 mm², and the maximum penetration depths in trabecular and cortical bone are approximately 3.5 and 2.9 mm, respectively. The reproducibility error of the perfusion recorded with this method is approximately 7%.[17]

The LDF output signal is strictly relative in nature, and a calibration standard to convert the signal into an absolute quantitative index of blood flow in various organs and different individuals is not possible because of the spatial variation in the vascular bed. However, LDF is useful for monitoring dynamic responses of the microvasculature to various physiological stimuli at a single site or to demonstrate regional distribution of perfusion in a specific organ.[18,19]

In animals, LDF has proven useful in measuring perfusion in cancellous bone after regulation of the systemic blood pressure.[20] More recently, the blood perfusion of the femoral head was monitored by LDF after selective occlusion of the blood supply to the femoral head[21] and after introduction of intracapsular hyperpressure.[22] The LDF signal was obtained through either the cartilage of the femoral head[20] or a drill hole in the bone.[21] However, Swiontkowski et al.[23] found a close correlation between measurements through articular cartilage and those obtained intraosseously through a drill hole. Animal studies have shown undisturbed blood flow after bone cannulation for pressure measurements.[24,25]

LDF in Author's Investigations

In my investigations,[16,26] a cannula identical to that used for pressure measurement was inserted parallel to the pressure cannula. The tips of the two cannulae were always placed at the same level in the femoral head at a distance of 1 to 1.5 cm. After removal of the trocar, the cannula was flushed with a heparin–saline solution and a 15-cm-long LDF probe ensheathed in metal and with a diameter of 2.2 mm was inserted into the cannula. The tip of this probe reached just beyond the tip of the cannula and was placed lightly against the bone marrow tissue. The probe was connected to the laser Doppler flowmeter (Periflux PF 3, Perimed, Stockholm, Sweden), and the output signal, measured in millivolts, was recorded on the same strip chart as the pressure tracing. The time constant selector could be set to 0.02 seconds to observe whether the flow was pulsatile or to 0.2 seconds for average and more comparable readings. All tracings (pressure and flow) in the figures should be read from right to left.

The first measurements were performed with the hip in the neutral position. After measurements at rest, an assistant put pressure on the straight leg with the patient's foot pressed to the flat surface of a weight-recording device on the chest of the assistant. Several brief periods of pressure were then applied to the patient's foot, and the force used was recorded. Total immobility was attempted between each period of loading. With the patient's limb still straight, two to three brief periods of external and internal rotation of the femur were performed. The force used during these movements, which were rapid and powerful, was not measured numerically. The next set of maneuvers, comprising external and internal rotation of the femur and flexion beyond 70 degrees, was performed with the hip at 70-degree flexion and the knee at 90-degree flexion.

Results

Pressure and Flow at Rest

In healthy hips the pressure in the center of the femoral head was low, with a median pressure of 18 mm Hg (15–22 mm Hg). The corresponding flow was 180 mV (150–200 mV). In osteoarthritis the median pressure was 44 mm Hg (32–56 mm Hg), and the flow was 130 mV (80–160 mV).

Pressure and Flow During Loading

Healthy Hips

In healthy hips the pressure in the femoral head rose steeply to a moderately high pulsatile plateau and depended on the load applied. The flow showed very moderate changes, with a small increase during the initial phase, followed by a slight decrease during continued loading, and ending with a moderate increase when the load was released (Figure 83.2). After repeated periods of loading, the flow showed a slightly higher velocity than in the pre-exercise period.

Osteoarthritic Hips

Two different patterns were observed in osteoarthritic hips. Type 1 (Figure 83.3) resembled the pressure graphs from healthy femoral heads, and type 2 showed an initial brief rise of pressure followed by a fall below the pressure level at rest (Figure 83.4). It was characteristic that the pulse amplitudes increased slightly during loading in type 1, whereas they decreased during the pressure fall in type 2.

A comparison between pressure tracings and radiographic findings showed that the two type 1 curves came from joints with femoral heads showing but moderate radiographic changes, whereas the type 2 pattern joints showed severe changes, especially deformity and lateral displacement of the femoral head.

Flow charts during loading were obtained only from femoral heads with type 2 pressure patterns (Figure 83.4). Essentially, they showed the same flow variations as observed in healthy femoral heads, but the difference between high and low flow rates was accentuated.

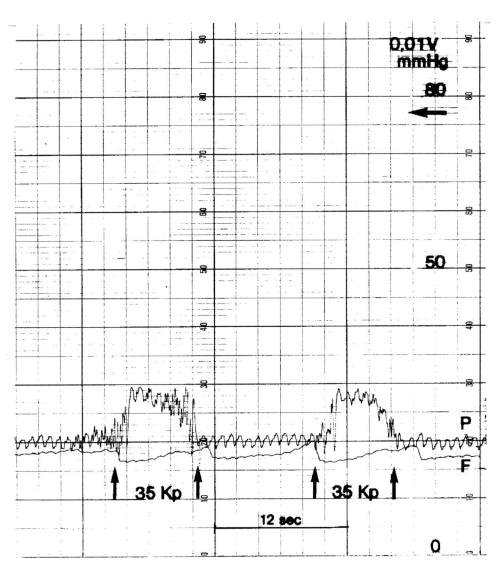

FIGURE 83.2. Pressure (P) and flow (F) chart from center of healthy femoral head during and after two periods of joint loading. Kp, kilopascals.

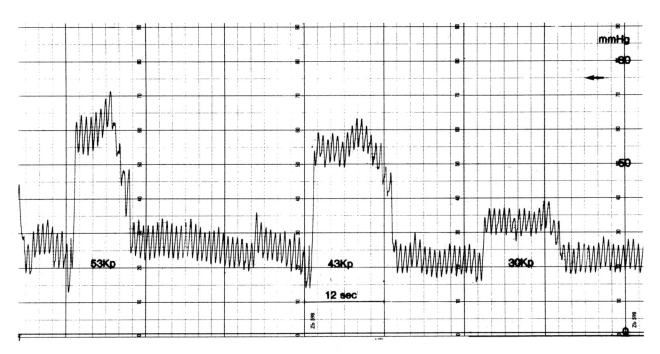

FIGURE 83.3. Pressure tracing from osteoarthritic femoral head in the neutral position before, during, and after three periods of joint loading (type 1 pattern).

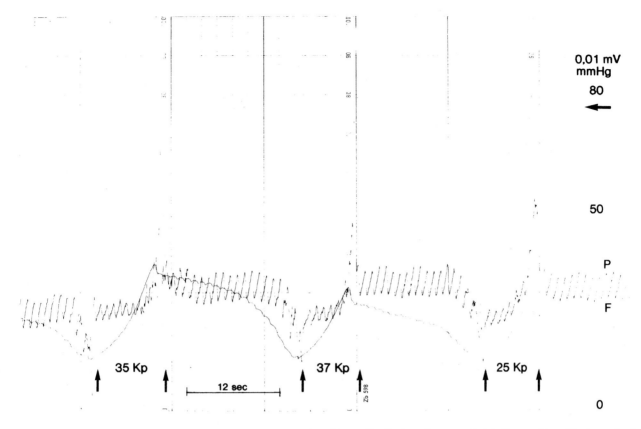

0,01 mV
mmHg

80
←

50

P

F

35 Kp   37 Kp   25 Kp

12 sec

0

FIGURE 83.4. Pressure and flow chart from severely deformed and laterally displaced osteoarthritic femoral head before, during, and after three periods of joint loading (type 2 pattern).

Pressure and Flow During Joint Movements

Healthy Femoral Head in Neutral Position

The pressure and flow charts from the femoral heads of healthy hips were fairly uniform (Figure 83.5). The pressure at the center of the head was hardly affected by the maneuvers, whereas the flow velocity increased steeply during the movement to maximal rotation but showed a decrease as inward rotation was sustained.

Healthy Femoral Head at 70-Degree Flexion

Figure 83.6 shows essentially the same characteristic minimal pressure reaction for the femoral head at 70-degree flexion as in the neutral position. A considerable increase of flow was observed as long as inward rotation in flexion was maintained.

Osteoarthritic Femoral Head in Neutral Position

In osteoarthritic femoral heads internal rotation produced pressure and flow charts similar to those observed in type 2 charts on loading.

Osteoarthritic Femoral Head at 70-Degree Flexion

The considerable initial rise in pressure at the beginning of the maneuver was followed by a relatively quick return to resting level. A gradual and moderate increase of flow velocity during the period of rotation was followed by a steep increase as the hip was brought back to a neutral position in flexion (compare Figure 83.7 with Figure 83.5, which shows pressure and flow in the contralateral healthy femoral head during the same maneuver).

Conclusion

The experiments clearly show that osteoarthritis of the hip affects both pressure and flow in the femoral head during loading and joint movements. When considering the changes observed during the loading experiments, it should be remembered that the compression forces applied to the hip joint were very modest compared with the forces at play during, for example, standing and walking. The rotation maneuvers, however, were performed forcefully and rapidly and can be assumed to correspond more closely to real-life conditions.

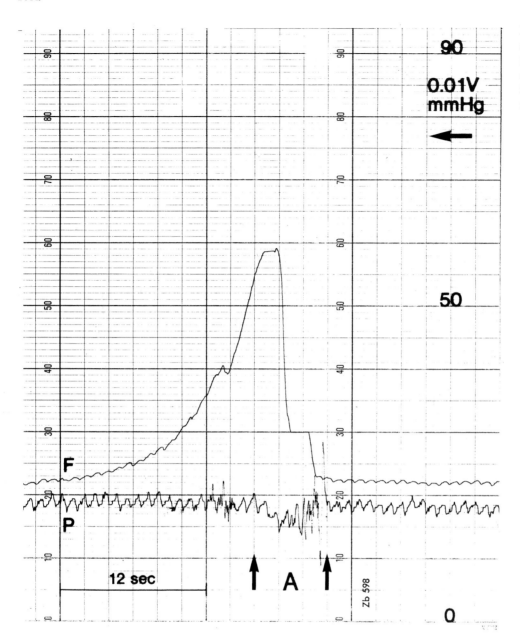

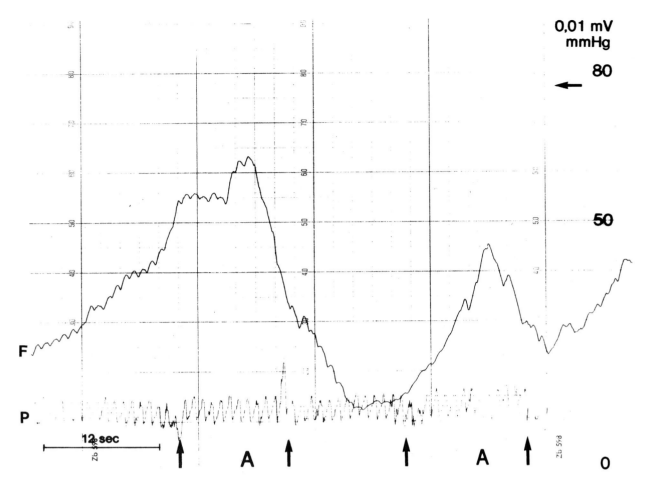

FIGURE 83.6. Pressure (P) and flow (F) chart from healthy femoral head before, during, and after forceful internal rotations (A) with the hip joint in 70-degree flexion.

The overall results indicate a free flow from the healthy bone marrow of the femoral head and, consequently, modest pressure variations. In osteoarthritis the evidence suggests increased resistance to flow, and the maneuvers add periods of very high intermittent pressure peaks to the chronic intraosseous hypertension observed at rest.

Intraosseous Phlebography

Intraosseous phlebography was used to determine (1) changes from normal in the direction of venous blood flow from juxtachondral bone marrow, (2) morphological changes of the intraosseous and extraosseous drainage system, and (3) changes in the speed of drainage from bone marrow (serial phlebography). This information required an investigation of unilateral joint disorders.[8,27,28]

Local anesthesia of the skin and periosteum was used in my first intraosseous phlebography experiments. Later, because no difference in the results could be de-

tected, general anesthesia was preferred. However, the first series provided useful subjective information about the character and site of pain during injection of contrast medium (raising intramedullary pressure). In general, the irradiation and distribution of pain were toward the knee.

Specially constructed 15- or 17-cm conical needles (AB Stille-Werner, Stockholm), each with an external diameter of 4.55 mm at the tip and a lumen measuring 2.60 mm, were used for the larger joints (hip and knee). Shorter needles were found more practical for the ankle joint, vertebrae, patella, and smaller bones.

The position of the tip of the cannula was controlled by image intensification. If gentle suction with a syringe produced a flow of blood, then the tip was in the bone marrow.

Various types of contrast material have been used over the years, and the amount of contrast injected has varied according to the size of the bone: 8 mL has been the standard injection in the hip and knee, and 1 or 2 mL has been the standard in the small joints and the patella.

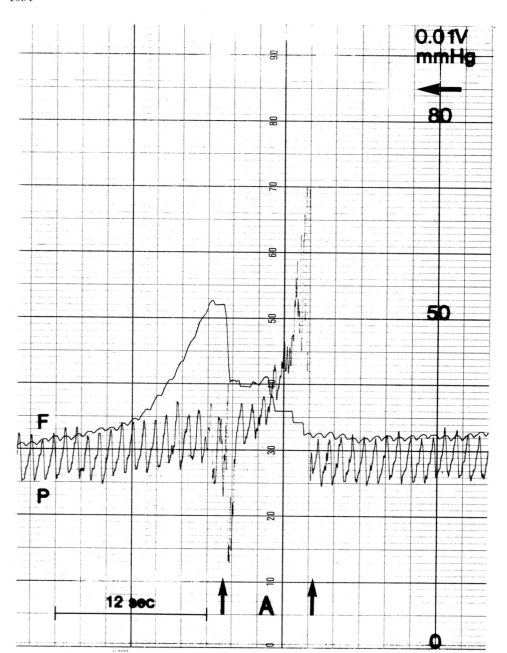

FIGURE 83.7. Pressure (P) and flow (F) chart from osteoarthritic femoral head before, during, and after one forceful internal rotation (A) of the femur.

Serial phlebography[8] was performed in some studies, the first exposure being taken during the injection of contrast material, with subsequent exposures at 30 seconds and 1, 3, 6, 12, 20, and 30 minutes. Occasionally, a final exposure was made after 50 to 60 minutes. In analyzing these phlebographic series the evacuation time was taken as the number of minutes between the injection of contrast and the first contrast-free exposure. More than 800 examinations were performed, and no complications were encountered.

Material

The patients examined were identical to the first of the two series described under the section on pressure measurements.

Results

Healthy Hip

The veins that drain the femoral head and neck usually follow the same path as the arteries. Blood leaves the bone marrow through superior and inferior retinacular vessels that drain to the medial circumflex and gluteal veins. The distal part of the femoral neck drains into the lateral circumflex veins that usually empty into the deep femoral vein, but connections to the obturator veins are not uncommon. No veins leaving the femoral head via the femoral head ligament were observed in this series.

In healthy hips the injected contrast material leaves the intramedullary space within 3 to 6 minutes. The extraosseous veins are thus well filled, and details such as valves are clearly seen (Figure 83.8). Filling of intramedullary vessels was observed only in a small, cir-

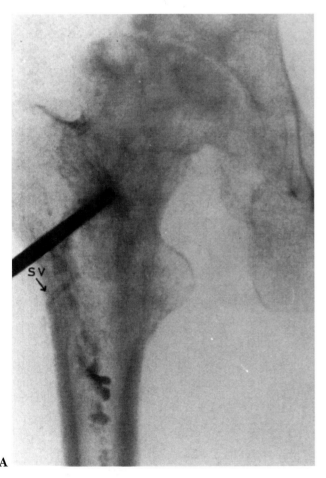

A

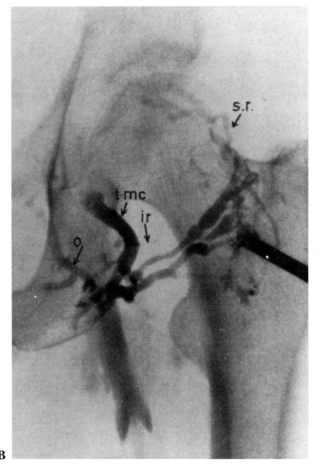

B

FIGURE 83.8. Intraosseous phlebographs from right hip with severe painful osteoarthritis (A) and healthy left hip (B) exposed simultaneously 30 seconds after injection of contrast material. In the healthy hip the contrast-mixed blood leaves the intraosseous space without noticeable filling of intraosseous vessels. Drainage takes place through superior retinacular (sr) veins to gluteal veins and via two medial circumflex (tmc) veins to femoral and obturator (o) veins, as well as through inferior retinacular (ir) veins emptying into the trunk of the medial circumflex vein.

These extraosseous veins are well filled, and the arrangement of valves is clearly visible. In the right hip (A) the contrast material is collected in enlarged, tortuous intraosseous vessels that extend from the base of the neck to the border between the upper and middle thirds of the diaphysis. The only visible connection between intraosseous and extraosseous veins are slender vessels at the lateral aspect of the proximal part of the diaphysis that drain contrast-mixed blood to superficial veins (sv).

cumscribed area around the tip of the cannula. The intraosseous channels of this area formed a fine-meshed network of minute vessels. In all cases the contrast medium had disappeared from the intramedullary and extraosseous veins within 6 minutes, except for occasional retention of contrast in the valvular sinuses of the extraosseous veins.

Osteoarthritic Hip

Generally, the phlebographs from osteoarthritic hips were characterized by partial or complete absence of extraosseous veins that normally drain the femoral head and neck (Figures 83.8 and 83.9). Foveolar veins were never observed. The retinacular vessels had often disappeared completely, and in most cases the medial circumflex veins were narrowed or missing. The filling of the remaining extraosseous veins was generally poor.

The area of small intraosseous vessels around the tip of the cannula was enlarged. The vessels of this area were generally wider and more irregular than the corresponding vessels on the unaffected side. In all cases tortuous intraosseous vessels filled with contrast medium were seen extending from the region of the injection site toward or into the diaphysis. In many cases drainage from the femoral head and neck occurred solely through these descending intramedullary vessels to slender perforating veins that emerged from the proximal half of the femoral shaft to join branches of the deep femoral vein or superficial veins on the lateral aspect.

As a rule, the extraosseous veins were empty of contrast material within a few minutes of injection. However, compared with the healthy side, the drainage of contrast material from the intramedullary vessels was delayed. The intraosseous veins often remained filled with contrast material throughout the observation period (Figure 83.9).

Osteoarthritic Knee

Examinations of flow by means of LDF have not been performed for the knee as yet. In principle, the phlebo-

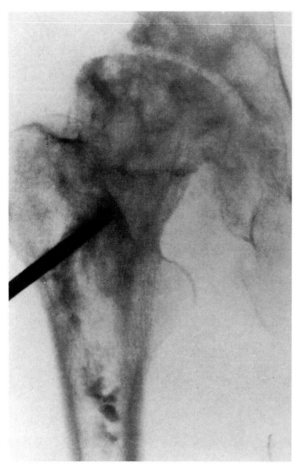

A

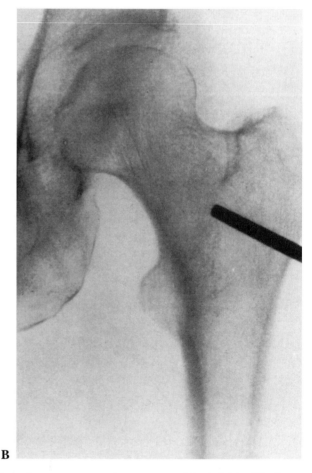

B

FIGURE 83.9. Intraosseous phlebographs from the same patient as in Figure 83.8 exposed simultaneously 30 minutes after injection of contrast material. In the osteoarthritic hip (A), large quantities of contrast remain in the intraosseous space. No filling of extraosseous veins was seen. The left hip (B) shows no sign of contrast material in extraosseous or intraosseous veins (complete evacuation was noted 3 minutes after the injection).

graphic examinations and pressure measurements showed the same difference between healthy and osteoarthritic knees as described previously for hip joints. Further reference to conditions in the knee joint is found in the section titled "Intraosseous Engorgement–Pain Syndrome."

99mTc-Phosphate Scintigraphy

Clinical experience shows that in painful osteoarthritic joints the uptake of bone-seeking agents is increased (Figure 83.10), even at a very early stage. The uptake is also increased in knee and hip joints with intraosseous engorgement–pain syndromes, probably preosteoarthritic states (see section on this syndrome and radiographically silent osteoarthritis), in the early stages of osteonecrosis,[29] and generally in all inflammatory joint diseases. However, the physiological basis for the binding of the tracer to skeletal tissue and the cause of increased uptake are still subjects of discussion. It is generally accepted, however, that perfusion of blood through bone is essential for the uptake of bone-seeking isotopes. In the absence of perfusion, as in infarction and sequestration of bone, this area appears in the scintigram as a "cold" spot.[30] Inversely, we may conclude that increased

uptake means the area is supplied with arterial blood. In all examinations of joints with osteoarthritis and intraosseous engorgement–pain syndromes the pressure tracings from juxtachondral bone marrow showing increased tracer uptake have been pulsatile.

Christensen[31] found convincing evidence that in skeletal tissue the tracer is located particularly in formative areas and in the resorptive surfaces in Howship's lacunae (i.e., areas with increased bone metabolism, anabolic as well as catabolic, both dependent on blood supply).

Methods

Most of the scintigraphic examinations of the hip and knee described here were made during the period between 1972 and 1979. The technique used was as follows: 12 mCi of 99mTc-polyphosphate were administered 2 hours before the patient was examined with a 5-in, dual probe, whole body rectilinear scanner. The collimators used had an almost depth-independent response over the range of 7 to 12 cm, and joint regions were examined in positions symmetrical to the collimators. Scintigrams were assessed visually from photorecordings and corresponding video display processing. The positive result from these series was an increased osseous tracer uptake in the joint region based on visual assessment of the scintigram. In patients with unilateral positive scintigraphic findings, visual observation was supplemented by numerical assessment.

Material and Results

Ten patients with osteoarthritis of the hip or knee who suffered from severe rest pain were assessed using intraosseous pressures, phlebography, and 99mTc-polyphosphate scintigraphy (Figure 83.10 and Table 83.3).[27] Severe painful osteoarthritis in the hip or knee was always accompanied by intramedullary venous stasis (Figure 83.11). In the knee joint the signs of venous retention were more often found in the femur than in the tibia.

The pressure measurements showed the same differences as previously between healthy and affected joints, and these differences were similar to those of the earlier series. Again, high intramedullary pressure was found more often in the distal femur than in the proximal tibia. Finally, the investigation showed that high intraosseous pressure and abnormal distribution and retention of contrast material always coincided with a high uptake of 99mTc-polyphosphate in the region (Figure 83.10 and Table 83.3).

Conclusions

The examinations of pressure and flow, the state of the venous drainage from juxtachondral bone, and the es-

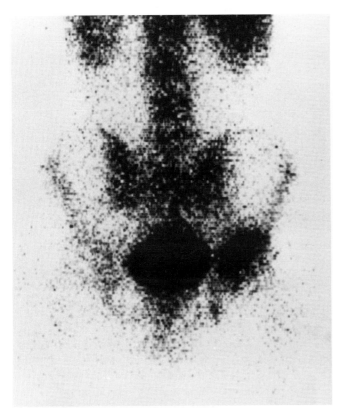

FIGURE 83.10. 99mTc-polyphosphate scintigraph from a patient with osteoarthritis of the left hip.

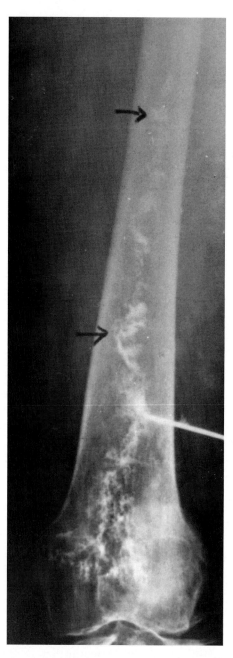

FIGURE 83.11. Intraosseous phlebograph exposed 30 minutes after injection of contrast material.

sentially metabolic studies by means of ^{99m}Tc-polyphosphate scintigraphy clearly indicate that in manifest and painful osteoarthritis of the hip and knee joints the venous drainage from juxtachondral bone is impaired. The increased resistance to outflow, in combination with intact arterial inflow, causes a significant chronic intraosseous hypertension to which is added an intermittent further pressure increase during the daily activities of normal life. Intact, maybe increased,[2] arterial inflow is indicated by the high pressure level with pulsatile pressure graphs, and increased metabolic activity, anabolic and/or catabolic, is indicated by the increased uptake of isotopes.

Synovial Membrane in Osteoarthritis and Rheumatoid Arthritis

Seen with the naked eye the internal surface of healthy synovial membrane is smooth, moist, glistening, and pink. Villi are few and small. Microscopic examination reveals an inner layer of synovial lining cells (synoviocytes) that cover a mostly loose fibrous stroma that contains nerves, blood vessels, and lymphatics. The vessels in the stroma are not a dominant feature (Figure 83.12).

Vascular Changes in the Synovial Membrane

In the literature on osteoarthritis the microscopic changes in the synovial membrane are usually compared with those taking place in patients with rheumatoid arthritis. Although the etiology and pathogenesis of these joint diseases are different, we continue to discuss them together, especially because this comparison may be of importance for future studies on osteoarthritis.

Twenty-four osteoarthritic joints were observed.[32] Gross inspection of the synovial membrane showed various degrees of hyperemia, edema, fibrosis, and hypertrophy of the villi. Contrary to the findings in joints with rheumatoid arthritis, surface fibrin deposits were never present.

In the osteoarthritic patients synovial changes fell into two relatively distinct groups: one predominantly proliferative and the other predominantly fibrous. Proliferative synovitis is characterized by bulky volume, the edematous tissue often resembling bunches of small, juicy grapes (Figure 83.13). In these cases the amount of synovial fluid is always increased. In fibrous synovitis the joint is usually dry. Most of the grapelike protuberances have disappeared and been replaced by patches of stringy bands of fibrous tissue (Figure 83.14). For patients with proliferative and fibrous synovitis the average duration of symptoms was 4 and 8 years, respectively.

Microvascular Changes in the Synovium

It has been suggested that the vascular changes in the synovium are caused by a vasculitis localized to venules and capillaries; however, electron microscopic examinations in patients with rheumatoid arthritis[33] and osteoarthritis[34,35] have shown that the capillary structure is normal but that the transcapillary migration of circulating blood cells is greatly increased. This finding is in agreement with the electron microscopic findings in my study[32] (Figure 83.15).

TABLE 83.3. Findings in 10 patients with rest pain and osteoarthritis of the hip or knee, examined by bilateral intraosseous phlebography, intraosseous pressure measurements, and technetium 99 m polyphosphate scintigraphy.

	A. Patients with unilateral pain and osteoarthritis	B. Patients with bilateral pain and osteoarthritis
n	6	4
Age (mean and range)	54.3 (30–68)	52.5 (34–61)
Men	4	2
Women	2	2
Hip	2	0
Knee	4	4
Phlegogram		
Affected joint norm/abn	0/6	0/8
Normal joint norm/abn	6/0	—
Intraosseous pressure (mm Hg) mean and range		
Affected joint	* 44.0 (33–80)	41.4 (42–50)
Normal joint	* 14.6 (3–24)	—
Scintigraphy		
Affected joint norm/inc	0/6	0/8
Normal joint norm/inc	6/0	—

n, number of patients; norm, normal; abn, abnormal; inc, increased. *One set of measurements was excluded due to technical faults. Thus, the pressure values represent measurements from five patients.

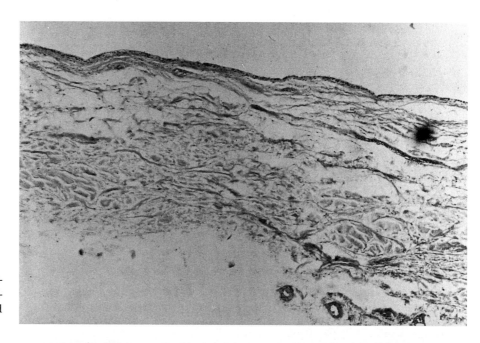

FIGURE 83.12. Healthy synovium removed from the hip joint of an elderly patient (hematoxylin and eosin × 5).

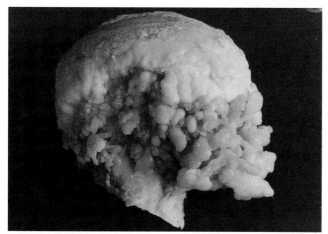

FIGURE 83.13. Femoral head from a 71-year-old woman with osteoarthritis: proliferative synovitis.

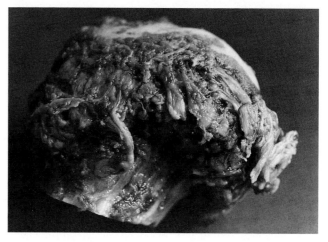

FIGURE 83.14. Femoral head from a 71-year-old man with osteoarthritis: fibrous synovitis.

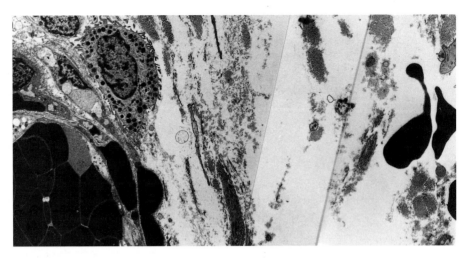

FIGURE 83.15. Survey electron microscopy of synovial membrane from a 65-year-old woman with osteoarthritis that shows dilation of venule engorged with erythrocytes (to the upper right), edema of interstitial tissue, free erythrocytes (left), and bundles of collagen fibers (magnification 4000×).

Microvascular disturbance is an essential factor in most mesenchymal diseases, and it is generally agreed that vascular changes in rheumatoid synovium are part of an inflammatory process. Goldie[35] found that, although less intense in osteoarthritic synovium, vascular changes in both types of synovium have the same pattern, and, in his opinion, the changes in osteoarthritis are also caused by an inflammatory process.

Material

Synovial biopsies from 10 healthy joints, 21 osteoarthritic joints, and 14 rheumatoid joints were examined by light microscopy.[32] Both hip and knee joints were included (Table 83.4).

Methods

The following staining methods were used in all cases:

1. Hematoxylin and eosin stain was used to show general cellular components.
2. Martius scarlet blue (MSB) stain was used to visualize erythrocytes in the interstitial tissues, intravascular erythrocyte stasis, agglutination, and fibrin thrombi of various ages. By this method erythrocytes are stained a bright yellow, as are recently formed fibrin thrombi. Later, these thrombi are stained scarlet, and old thrombi are stained a deep blue. MSB is also an excellent stain for collagen (blue).
3. Perls' Prussian blue stain demonstrated hemosiderin deposits.
4. von Kossa's method visualized calcium deposits in the synovium.

Results

The overall results of the investigation are summarized in Table 83.4. In this context only the findings directly connected to changes in vessels and their contents in os-

TABLE 83.4. Histological findings in normal, osteoarthritic, and rheumatoid synovium from hip and knee joints.

	Normal	Osteoarthritic	Rheumatoid
Total number of biopsies	10	21	14
Surface fibrin	0	0	8
Rows of Synoviocytes			
1	5	3	0
2–3	4	15	6
>3	1	2	8
Vascularization of synovial membrane			
Poor	7	4	0
Moderate	2	5	2
Rich	1	12	12
Vascularization of stroma			
Poor	9	3	0
Moderate	1	10	6
Rich	0	8	8
Stroma			
Edematous	2	14	10
Fibrous	0	6	4
Neutral	8	1	0
Vessels			
Stasis	1	19	14
Unstructured agglutination of erythrocytes	0	14	10
Fibrin thrombi	0	11	11
Free erythrocytes in stroma	0	11	12
Interstitial bleeding	0	1	3
Hemosiderin deposits			
None	10	2	1
Scattered	0	11	8
Many	0	2	2
Masses	0	6	3
Inflammation cells			
None	9	4	0
Scattered	1	5	2
Masses	0	12	12
Calcium deposits			
None	0	16	2
Scattered	1	5	11
Masses	0	0	1

teoarthritic and rheumatoid arthritic synovium are dealt with in more detail.

Number and Caliber of Vessels

Compared with healthy synovium (Figure 83.12), the osteoarthritic (Figure 83.16) and rheumatoid synovium were characterized by a rich network of mostly dilated vessels.

Intravascular Erythrocytes

More than 80% of smaller veins were tightly packed with erythrocytes, still distinguishable as separate blood corpuscles. Many vessels showed gradual changes, often inside the same vessel, the aggregations of erythrocytes becoming structureless agglutinations; transition from this stage into fibrin thrombi was a frequent finding (Figures 83.16 and 83.17). These changes were common to both joint disorders.

Vessel Wall Permeability

Permeability to formed blood elements was increased, as judged by the amounts of single, free erythrocytes in extravascular stroma (Figures 83.17 and 83.18). Their number, as well as the degree of edema, seemed greater in rheumatoid than in osteoarthritic synovium.

Interstitial Hemosiderin Deposits

Hemosiderin crystals lying free in interstitial tissue or engulfed by macrophages were common in both disorders. In osteoarthritis the free crystals were more frequent in the late fibrous stages of synovitis than in the early proliferative stage, and the juxtaposition to massive strands of collagen was notable in both osteoarthritis and rheumatoid arthritis (Figure 83.18).

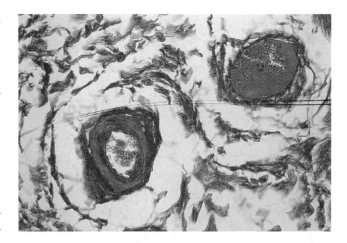

FIGURE 83.17. Arteriole and venule in rheumatoid synovium. Venule clogged by recently formed fibrin thrombus. The vessels are placed in edematous stroma with free extravascular erythrocytes (Martius scarlet blue × 400).

Calcium Deposits

Calcium deposits were noted in 5 of 6 osteoarthritic specimens with fibrous synovitis and in 12 of 14 with rheumatoid arthritis, with proliferative as well as fibrous synovitis.

Comment

My investigations thus showed that dilation, stasis, and thrombotic occlusion of synovial vessels, particularly smaller veins and venules, are prominent features in both osteoarthritis and rheumatoid arthritis. The vascular changes in rheumatoid synovium are initiated by an inflammatory process, but the same changes were observed in osteoarthritic synovium where the histological signs of inflammation were absent or slight.

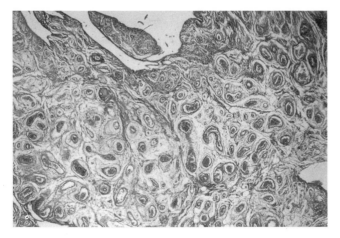

FIGURE 83.16. Synovial membrane from osteoarthritic hip joint: dilated venules with erythrocyte stasis and agglutination in edematous interstitial tissue; proliferative synovitis (Martius scarlet blue × 25).

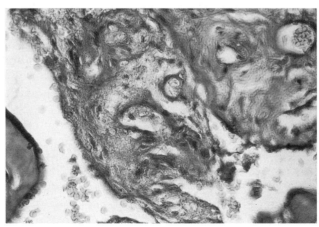

FIGURE 83.18. Osteoarthritic synovium. Villi with vessels and free extravascular erythrocytes and traces of fibrin thrombi (Martius scarlet blue × 400).

The vascular changes observed indicate chronic venous stasis. In the hip, and to a lesser degree the knee, with their tough and rigid fibrous capsules, an increase in synovial fluid and the bulk of the synovium is accompanied by a rise in intraarticular pressure.[36] A pressure rise of 10 mm Hg, which leaves the arterial inflow to the synovium intact, would be enough to compress the thin-walled intraarticular veins and create a blockage to venous drainage; chronic stasis is probably one of the factors mainly responsible for the remarkable tendency to chronic blockage (thrombosis) of synovial and subsynovial veins.

The effect on mesenchymal tissue of long-standing intermittent high pressure on the venous side of the capillary (e.g., edema, induration, or ulceration) is well known from patients with severe chronic venous insufficiency of the lower limb (see Chapter 82). My gross inspection and histological findings combined with the changes in the amount of intraarticular fluid indicate that chronic venous stasis and hypertension lead to a similar development in osteoarthritic synovium, with proliferative synovitis as the early stage of a process that gradually leads to fibrous transformation of the synovial membrane. The similarity of vascular changes in osteoarthritic and rheumatoid synovium and the clinical appearance of the joints in the late stages of rheumatoid joint disease indicate that the same mechanism is influential in rheumatoid joints.

Synovial Fluid in Advanced Osteoarthritis of the Hip Joint

It has long been known that in osteoarthritis the synovial fluid shows increased protein concentration[37] and an abnormal protein pattern, probably due to the permeability of the synovial membrane to plasma proteins.[38-40]

Material and Methods

By means of bilateral arthropuncture, synovial fluid from the hip joints of 46 patients with unilateral osteoarthritis was obtained during total hip replacement.[41] Blood samples were taken simultaneously. From 34 of the 46 osteoarthritic hips it was possible to obtain fluid samples ranging from a few drops to a maximum of 10 mL. However, because blood was present in 5 of the samples, only 29 were suitable for analysis. One to two drops of synovial fluid were obtained from 26 of the 46 healthy hips, but three samples were omitted because blood was present. Extraction of synovial fluid from both hips was only possible in eight patients.

Quantitative estimation of four nonimmunoglobin proteins was performed. The proteins studied were orosomucoid, MW 44,000d; transferrin, MW 74,000d; ceruloplasmin, MW 160,000d; and α_2-macroglobulin,

MW 820,000d. The simultaneously aspirated synovial fluids and sera were analyzed by electroimmunoassay according to Laurell's technique.[42] Synovial fluid and serum from the same patient were analyzed within the same run and performed as double determination. Analytical variations between each run were 5%.

The proteins studied were chosen because they have different molecular weights and because all are synthesized in the liver. Local synthesis and destruction have never been demonstrated.[38] Biopsies of synovial membrane from osteoarthritic hips and from hips with femoral neck fractures (for control data) were obtained and prepared as described previously.

Results

Histochemistry

The ratios of synovial fluid concentration to serum concentration (SF/S) from the osteoarthritic group were higher than those from healthy joints (Tables 83.5 and 83.6). Average ratios for the four proteins related to molecular weight are illustrated in Figure 83.19 (total material). Log SF/S against log MW indicated an almost straight curve, steeper for the healthy than for the osteoarthritic group, which indicates increasing difference with increasing molecular weight. In the eight patients from whom synovial fluid was obtained in both hips the difference between diseased and healthy joints was significant for α_2-macroglobulin and ceruloplasmin (Table 83.6).

Histology

Light microscopic examination of synovial membranes from the 29 osteoarthritic hips where fluid extraction was successful showed all to have slight to moderate inflammatory changes compared with healthy hips. As described previously, I distinguished between two types of synovial changes in the osteoarthritic hip joint: proliferative and fibrous synovitis. The proliferative synovitis appears to be an earlier state and is characterized by obvious dilation and frequently blockage of venules and capillaries and marked edema of the interstitial tissue with free erythrocytes and deposits of hemosiderin. Proliferative synovitis was always accompanied by increased fluid in the joint. Fibrous synovitis showed the same features except that the interstitial edema was more or less masked by fibrous scar tissue and more massive hemosiderin deposits and the joint usually contained very little fluid.

Correlation

Proliferative synovitis showed higher SF/S ratios than the fibrous type. The difference was significant for α_2-macroglobulin and ceruloplasmin (Table 83.7). Only characteristic cases were included, and all transitional

FIGURE 83.19. Log/log plot of ratio of synovial fluid concentration to serum concentration and molecular weight from hip joints with osteoarthritis (black circles) and from healthy hip joints (open circles). Ratios determined for the four nonimmunoglobin proteins represent the mean SD of 29 and 23 samples, respectively.

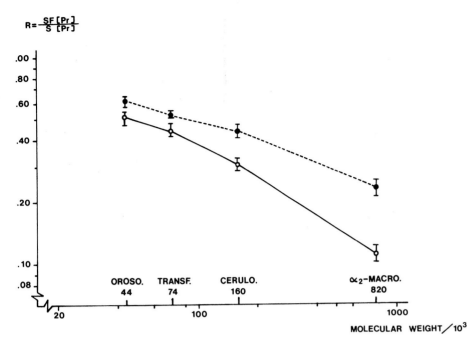

TABLE 83.5. Synovial fluid concentrations of proteins compared to serum concentrations.

SF/S Concentration	Orosomucoid	Transferrin	Ceruloplasmin	α_2_Macroglobulin
Osteoarthritis (29)	0.61 ± 0.14	0.53 ± 0.11	0.44 ± 0.14	0.23 ± 0.10
Normal (23)	0.51 ± 0.16	0.45 ± 0.12	0.30 ± 0.09	0.11 ± 0.04
Statistical significance	$P < .05$	$P < .05$	$P < .001$	$P < .001$

Data are ratios of protein concentration in synovial fluid to serum, the denominator. Statistical analysis was performed using Mann–Whitney's rank sum.

TABLE 83.6. Intraindividual comparison of synovial fluid concentrations of proteins compared to serum concentrations.

SF/S Concentration	Orosomucoid	Transferrin	Ceruloplasmin	α_2_Macroglobulin
Osteoarthritis (8)	0.57 ± 0.17	0.55 ± 0.08	0.44 ± 0.04	0.23 ± 0.06
Normal (8)	0.54 ± 0.09	0.49 ± 0.14	0.30 ± 0.09	0.13 ± 0.05
Statistical significance	NS	NS	$P < .01$	$P = .001$

Data are ratios of protein concentration in synovial fluid to serum, the denominator; NS, not significant.

TABLE 83.7. Correlation between histologic type and synovial fluid/serum ratios (SD).

	Orosomucoid		Transferrin		Ceruloplasmin		α_2_Macroglobulin	
Histologic Type	Ratio	No.	Ratio	No.	Ratio	No.	Ratio	No.
Proliferative	0.60 ± 0.16	12	0.53 ± 0.12	10	0.47 ± 0.16	11	0.27 ± 0.12	13
Fibrous	0.57 ± 0.10	8	0.47 ± 0.10	7	0.37 ± 0.10	8	0.16 ± 0.07	8
Statistical significance	NS		NS		$P < .05$		$P < .01$	

NS, not significant.

types were excluded. A comparison between Tables 83.4 and 83.6 gives the impression that the permeability of the four proteins did not differ significantly in fibrous synovitis and healthy synovium.

Comments

In this study I have correlated ratios to molecular weight. However, Stokes' radius, a function of molecular weight, volume, and shape, is a more appropriate expression of protein size than molecular weight alone.[43] Thus, the fact that fibrinogen, which has a lower molecular weight than α_2-macroglobulin, is rarely seen as fibrin on the surface of synovium from osteoarthritic as opposed to rheumatoid joints may be because fibrinogen, being thread shaped, has a very large Stokes' radius, considerably larger than that of α_2-macroglobulin. Stokes' radius for the four proteins investigated here has been determined[43-45] and correlates roughly with the proteins' molecular weights.

Kushner and Somerville,[38] using the criteria of average total protein concentration and average serum C-reactive protein, compared their relationship quantitatively to inflammation and found that increased synovial inflammation corresponded to higher SF/S ratios; the larger the molecule, the greater the increase. On comparing different joint diseases it was found that osteoarthritic patients had the least evidence of inflammation. The findings (Table 83.7) that proliferative synovitis had the highest ratios and that the largest molecules showed the greatest increase indicate that increased permeability of the synovial membrane to plasma proteins is due to transcapillary migration. This finding is also confirmed histologically. The slight inflammatory signs in the synovium suggest that simple mechanical factors (stasis and intravascular hypertension due to increased resistance to venous drainage) are predominantly responsible for the increased capillary permeability in osteoarthritis. The histological changes in the microvasculature in rheumatoid arthritis suggest that this mechanism also plays a role in rheumatoid joint disease (and probably all forms of exudative synovitis). (See also the section on pain and the effects of neuropeptides.)

Microvascular Changes in Juxtachondral Bone Marrow in Late Stages of Osteoarthritis and Rheumatoid Arthritis

Material and Methods

Seven femoral heads from osteoarthritic hips, median age 71 years (58–78 years), and five from hips with late stages of rheumatoid arthritis, median age 62 years (55–72 years), were examined by light microscopy.[16] All femoral heads were removed during hip alloplasty. The decalcified specimens were stained with hematoxylin and eosin, MSB, safranin O, and Perls' Prussian blue stain. Only the findings relating to the microvasculature of the bone marrow are discussed here.

Results

Osteoarthritic Bone Marrow

Generally, the cell contents and structure appeared normal for the age of patients with osteoarthritic bone marrow. Fat vacuoles were abundant. Small vessels (sinusoids and venules) often showed erythrocyte aggregation and agglutination. Free erythrocytes and hemosiderin deposits were frequently noted. Over considerable areas the bone marrow was replaced by other mesenchymal tissues, mostly fibrous tissue and occasionally fibrocartilage. In the trabeculae the bone structure varied between laminar and woven, and areas of both bone destruction and new bone formation were common. The vessels in the haversian canals were usually open, but areas of erythrocyte agglutination and fibrin thrombi were not uncommon.

Bone Marrow in Rheumatoid Arthritis

Generally, the changes found in rheumatoid bone marrow resembled those found in osteoarthritis, except for substantial aggregations of mononuclear inflammatory cells, often adjacent to vessels clogged with erythrocyte agglutinations (Figure 83.20) or thrombi. Replacement of bone marrow cells with vascularized fibrous tissue was observed in all specimens.

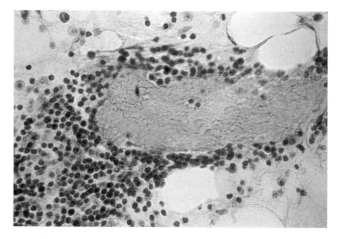

FIGURE 83.20. Rheumatoid arthritis, femoral head. Venule in bone marrow blocked by erythrocyte agglutination. Nodule of inflammatory mononuclear cells and fat vacuoles (hematoxylin and eosin × 400).

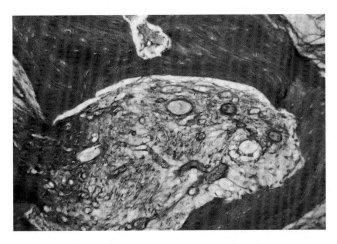

FIGURE 83.21. Well-vascularized invasive tissues in bone marrow of osteoarthritic femoral head. Erythrocyte agglutinations in many vessels (Martius scarlet blue × 100).

Comments

In both groups of patients considerable areas showed changes with substitution of bone marrow tissue by more primitive mesenchymal tissues, mostly well-vascularized fibrous tissue interspersed with patches of fibrocartilage. Blockage of small vessels (venules, sinusoids, and very rarely small arteries) by erythrocyte agglutinations and thrombi was highly characteristic of both disorders (Figures 83.20 and 83.21). Although the vessels in the haversian canals quite often showed the same picture, such findings were far less common than in nontraumatic femoral head necrosis. The overall impression of microvascular conditions in the bone marrow and synovial membrane was a state of impaired venous drainage.

Intraosseous Engorgement–Pain Syndromes and Radiographically Silent Osteoarthritis

One of the cardinal symptoms of osteoarthritis is pain in the joint region at rest, often irradiating from the hip downward toward the knee and from the knee to the calf. It may occur early or late in the course of the disease and is usually aggravated by previous activity; prolonged rest may bring relief. In its most severe form, rest pain is constant. The pain is described as deep, aching, or boring. Osteotomy or fenestration of juxtachondral bone is usually accompanied by an immediate fall of intraosseous pressure and relieves pain within 24 hours.[46]

This type of hip or knee pain is often found in those without visible radiographic joint changes, and, conversely, instead of sclerosis, joint-bearing bone often displays a (transient) osteopenia. Synovitic effusion can be demonstrated in most of the painful joints. Patients usually belong to the 35- to 55-year age group. The painful state may last for months or even years and may disappear spontaneously or after conservative or surgical (fenestration) therapy. However, preliminary information indicates that a high percentage of such patients (at present about 35%) develop manifest osteoarthritis in the same joint at a later stage (C.C.A., unpublished data). Rest pain is often accompanied by more or less severe restriction of movement in these joints.

The term *intraosseous engorgement–pain syndrome*[47] defines a syndrome characterized by rest pain in a radiographically nonarthritic joint with juxtachondral bone marrow engorgement, as observed by intraosseous phlebography, and increased uptake of bone-seeking isotopes. In unilateral cases the intraosseous pressure is most often, but not invariably, higher on the painful than on the unaffected side. Rest pain, especially in the knee region in the patellar pain syndromes[14,15] and in the hip region in the first stages of nontraumatic femoral head necrosis,[48] creates diagnostic problems.

Intraosseous Engorgement–Pain Syndromes

I[49] investigated whether pain at rest in the knee is associated with increased intraosseous pressure.

Material

I examined 36 men and 17 women admitted to the hospital for disorders such as suspected lesions of the semilunar cartilages or loose bodies in the knee. All patients underwent surgery, prior radiographs of the knees having been taken in the standing position. At arthrotomy the state of the articular cartilage in the medial, lateral, and patellofemoral compartments was assessed by eye. The presence of erosion was taken as evidence of osteoarthritis.

Before operation, the type of pain was fully assessed. Almost all patients had typical episodes of locking of the knee with acute pain. Some had pain on movement or weight bearing. Others complained of rest pain. The presence or absence of rest pain and osteoarthritis allowed for the creation of four groups (Table 83.8).

Methods

The methods for measuring intraosseous and intravenous pressures have been described previously. In this investigation the points of measurement were in the most distal part of the femur and the most proximal part of the tibia. The pressure in the internal saphenous vein was measured at the level of the knee joint. The patients were examined lying supine in the horizontal position.

TABLE 83.8. Mean pressure (SD range, in mm Hg) in the saphenous vein and intramedullary pressure in the proximal tibial and distal femoral metaphyses from knee joints with and without pain at rest and osteoarthritis, respectively.

Group	Number of patients	P vein	P tibia	P femur	DP	P of maximal pressure in tibia or femur	Number of patients with maximal pressure in	
							Tibia	Femur
Without osteoarthritis								
A—without pain	16	10.1 ± 1.3 (3.8–22.3)	9.8 ± 2.1 (1.1–30.0)	8.6 ± 1.8 (0–19.8)	1.2 ± 1.6	11.6 ± 2.1 (1.1–30.0)	10	6
B—with pain	17	11.0 ± 1.7 (1.0–29.1)	31.9 ± 5.0 (5.1–78.9)	28.4 ± 4.1 (4.1–59.1)	3.5 ± 5.4	39.5 ± 4.3 (5.4–78.9)	10	7
With osteoarthritis								
C—without pain	11	11.3 ± 1.6 (5.9–24.7)	13.1 ± 3.1 (0.3–38.2)	13.4 ± 3.0 (0.3–28.9)	−0.3 ± 3.7	17.9 ± 3.3 (1.7–38.2)	5	6
D—with pain	9	12.1 ± 1.8 (3.1–23.3)	12.5 ± 4.0 (0–35.2)	24.7 ± 4.7 2.9–46.4)	−12.2 + 7.6	30.3 ± 3.2 (16.2–46.4)	2	7

P, mean pressure; SE, standard error of the mean; DP, mean pressure difference between tibia and femur. Ranges are given within brackets—all pressures are given in millimeters of mercury.

Results

Venous Pressure

The pressure in the saphenous vein was within the expected range, and there were no intergroup differences (Table 83.8).

Intraosseous Pressure

Of the 16 patients with no osteoarthritis and no rest pain (group A), 14 had normal intraosseous pressures measured in cancellous bone, 2 to 12 mm Hg above the pressure in the adjacent extraosseous vein.[50] Similar normal values were found in 6 of 11 patients with osteoarthritis but no rest pain (group C). In 7 of 9 with osteoarthritis and rest pain (group D) low pressures were found in the tibia, but in 6 of these 7 abnormally high pressures were recorded in the femur. In contrast, high pressures were found in either or both the tibia and femur in 15 of 17 patients with no osteoarthritis but with rest pain (group B). Of this group, 5 had anatomically normal knees with neither meniscus injury nor loose bodies. See Tables 83.8 and 83.9.

In group D (rest pain and osteoarthritis) the highest pressure was usually found in the femur, but in group B (rest pain but no osteoarthritis) it was equally distributed between the tibia and femur. In group D the pressure difference between the tibia and femur was not significant. Thus, in this series increased intraosseous pressure seemed to be more closely associated with the symptom of rest pain than with radiographic signs of osteoarthritis.

Intraosseous Phlebography and ^{99m}Tc-Polyphosphate Scintigraphy

Intraosseous phlebography and ^{99m}Tc-polyphosphate scintigraphy examinations were performed on a series of patients with rest pain but without radiographic signs of osteoarthritis of the knee and hip joints.[27] The techniques were as described previously, including those for serial phlebography, where an evacuation time of up to 6 minutes was regarded as normal.

TABLE 83.9. Mean differences of intraosseous pressures in tibia and femur, mean differences of maximal pressures in tibia and femur between the groups specified in Table 83.8, and P values.

Groups	Tibia		Femur		Maximal pressure	
					Tibia–Femur	
B and A	+22.1	P<.001	+19.8	P<.001	+27.9	P <.001
D and A	+2.7	NS	+16.1	P<.001	+18.7	P<.001
C and A	+3.3	NS	+4.8	NS	+6.3	NS
D and C	+0.6	NS	−11.3	P.05	−12.4	.01<P<.02
B and D	+19.4	.01<P<.02	+3.7	NS	+9.2	NS
B and C	+18.8	.001<P<.01	+15.0	.01<P<.02	+21.6	P<.001

P, probability that the difference is caused by chance; NS, not significant.

FIGURE 83.22. **A, B,** Bilateral intraosseous phlebographs from the tibiae of a patient with intraosseous engorgement–pain syndrome of the left knee. **B,** Exposed 30 minutes after contrast injection.

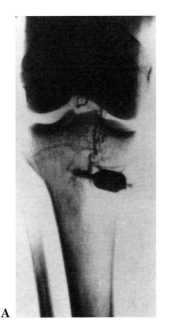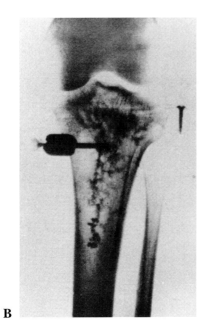

A   B

Results

Intraosseous Phlebography

The intraosseous engorgement–pain syndrome results were similar to those obtained from patients with manifest painful osteoarthritis (cf. Tables 83.1 and 83.9). The bone marrow on the painful side always showed prolonged evacuation time, often in conjunction with intraosseous hypertension (Figures 83.22 and 83.23).

99mTc-Polyphosphate Scintigraphy

With one exception, the scintigrams from the joints with intraosseous engorgement–pain syndrome all showed increased tracer uptake (Table 83.10).

Radiographically Silent Osteoarthritis of the Hip Joint

In patients with intraosseous engorgement–pain syndromes of the hip and knee joints, routine radiography is by definition negative; that is, they show none of the accepted changes of osteoarthritis: narrowing of the joint space, subchondral cysts, or osteosclerosis. On the contrary, the joint-bearing bone is often osteopenic compared with the bone farther from the affected joint.[47] Occasionally, osteophytes may be observed, but if all other parameters are negative, I have not considered this proof of osteoarthritis.[51]

FIGURE 83.23. Simultaneous bilateral pressure measurements from femoral condyles and internal saphenous vein of a patient with intraosseous engorgement–pain syndrome of the right knee.

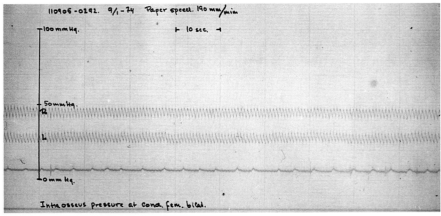

TABLE 83.10. Findings in seven patients with intraosseous engorgement–pain syndrome of the hip or knee, examined by means of bilateral intraosseous phlebography, intraosseous pressure measurements, and technetium 99m polyphosphate scintigraphy.

	A. Patients with unilateral pain and osteoarthritis	B. Patients with bilateral pain and osteoarthritis
n	4	3
Age (mean and range)	49.0 (33–69)	46.7 (25–58)
Men	3	1
Women	1	2
Hip	0	1
Knee	4	2
Phlegogram		
Affected joint norm/abn	0/4	**1/5
Normal joint norm/abn	*3/1	—
Intraosseous pressure (mm Hg) mean and range		
Affected joint	40.3 (25–59)	41.3 (32–47)
Normal joint	16.0 (13–19)	—
Scintigraphy		
Affected joint norm/inc	0/4	1/5
Normal joint norm/inc	4/0	—

n, number of patients; norm, normal; abn, abnormal; inc, increased. *Clearance time >6 min, distribution of contrast normal. **Clearance time <6 min, distribution of contrast normal.

Although routine radiography of the hips did not suggest the presence of osteoarthritis, the subjective symptoms of the group dealt with here were largely identical with those of patients with manifest and painful osteoarthritis. Thus, pain at rest and on loading was always present, and most patients with long-standing subjective complaints in the hip also showed more or less severe restriction of joint movement, typically initiated by increasing pain as the joint was moved into extreme internal rotation or extreme flexion.

In most cases intraosseous engorgement–pain syndromes disappear spontaneously or after conservative treatment for synovitis. In rare cases pain and restriction of function may become so severe that operative treatment is indicated. Fenestration (core decompression) has been useful in many cases, and total alloplasty is rarely necessary.

We have performed this operation in a number of radiographically negative joints of patients with persistent and intractable rest pain; I have thus had the opportunity to study the changes in the different structures of these joints.[16]

Material

Between 1975 and 1989 severe intraosseous engorgement–pain syndrome led to total alloplasty of 11 hip joints in 9 patients. Scintigraphy, but not intraosseous phlebography or pressure measurements, was performed on this group.

The median age was 51 years (36–72 years). In 10 of 11 hips one or several abnormalities were observed that are usually regarded as disposing a patient to osteoarthritis. ^{99m}Tc-polyphosphate scintigraphy showed increased uptake in all affected hips but of varying loca-

tion, the most common configuration being a ring encircling the femoral head at the border between the cartilage of the femoral head and the femoral neck. Proliferative synovitis was present in all hip joints, and inspection of the femoral head and acetabulum showed localized, symmetrical, and usually modest areas of slight cartilage degeneration; the three main areas were the cartilagenous border of the femoral head, the area around the fovea, and restricted sections of the weight-bearing area of the femoral head and acetabulum.

Light Microscopic Examination

Methods

The following stains were used: hematoxylin and eosin, MSB, safranin O, Perls' Prussian blue, and von Kossa's stain.

Results

Synovium

In all examined hips the synovium was edematous and showed increased vascularity of the peripheral layer. In 2 of the 11 patients isolated aggregations of mononuclear inflammatory cells were observed near the surface of the synovium. MSB staining demonstrated numerous dilated veins and venules and a few thick-walled arterioles near the synovial surface. Scattered erythrocytes were observed in interstitial tissue in 8 of 11 specimens, and in 10 of 11 specimens intravascular erythrocyte agglutinations and fibrin thrombi were numerous. Perls' Prussian blue, von Kossa's, and safranin O staining failed to show deposits of hemosiderin, calcium, or synovial inclusions of cartilage particles.

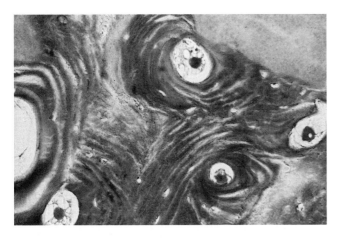

FIGURE 83.24. Haversian canals in woven bone in osteochondral end plate. Radiographically silent osteoarthritis. Fibrin thrombi in four canals (Martius scarlet blue × 250).

Cancellous Bone

All specimens were characterized by osteopenia of the joint-bearing cancellous bone. The bone structure was mostly laminar, but in 4 of 11 hips circumscribed areas of woven bone were observed. Fibrin thrombi, some clearly intravascular, in haversian canals were not uncommon (Figure 83.24). They were usually found in woven bone and surrounded by empty lacunae.

Bone Marrow Vessels

Over large areas the cellular contents of the bone marrow appeared normal, but most of the marrow vessels, including a few arterioles, showed erythrocyte aggregations. Agglutinations and fibrin thrombi of different ages were common in veins and venules. Most sinusoids appeared of normal width. Invasion of vascularized fibrous tissue was not as dominant as in manifest osteoarthritis or rheumatoid arthritis but had the same character.

Comments

This group of patients with intraosseous engorgement–pain syndrome showed the early proliferative form of synovitis, and the vascular changes here and in the bone marrow were largely identical with those described in connection with osteoarthritis. The lack of hemosiderin and calcium deposits may also suggest an early stage of the disorder.

Thus, the evidence collected indicates that although intraosseous engorgement–pain syndrome is usually reversible, it is a potential precursor to osteoarthritis. It also shows that the characteristic microvascular changes are phenomena that appear quite early in the development of human osteoarthritis.

Experimental Osteoarthritis: Vascular Changes

Degenerative osteoarthritis is generally divided into two groups: primary and secondary. *Primary* indicates that the etiology is unknown; *secondary* indicates that some earlier event or joint disorder has started the process. The range of tissue reactions in the mesenchymal joint tissues appears limited, because the final stages of primary osteoarthritis, rheumatoid arthritis, osteonecrosis, and traumatic and infectious sequelae show a similar morphology: cartilage destruction, deformation or destruction of juxtachondral bone, and fibrous transformation of the synovium. *Osteoarthrosis* is a suitable name for this common end state.

In human joints the earliest stages of osteoarthritis are rarely available for studies of the kind reported in this chapter. Even the group of patients described with radiographically silent osteoarthritis had shown increasingly severe symptoms 1 to 8 years before the time of operation. For the early joint processes we must refer to studies of experimental osteoarthritis in animals. Most of these experiments have been performed on dog and rabbit knees and have given valuable and sometimes surprising results.

Osteoarthritis is generally supposed to be the result of cartilage wear and tear and is age dependent. Consequently, most experimental studies have been performed on joints in which this wear-and-tear process has been promoted by making the joints unstable by surgical methods. However, other methods have been used by other authors, and in this section I describe the vascular changes seen in two completely different models: the artificially unstable and the artificially immobilized knee.

Unstable Knee

McDevitt et al.[52] induced experimental osteoarthritis in the knees of adult dogs by sectioning the anterior cruciate ligament, the contralateral knee serving as control. The dogs were kept postoperatively mobile until killed 1 to 48 weeks after operation.

Microscopic Changes in the Synovium

Vascular proliferation in the synovial membrane was seen at 1 week. Generally, vascularity intensified over the first 12 weeks, persisted for 24 weeks, and then subsided. Increased thickness of the synovium with yellowish discoloration, villous folds, and adhesions were also noted after 2 or more weeks. Fibrosis of the subintimal layers of the synovial membrane was noted from 3 to 4 weeks and was especially pronounced in dogs killed after 12 to 24 weeks.

Perfusion Changes in the Synovial Membrane

To evaluate the time relationship between the synovial reaction and the development of osteoarthritis, Christensen et al.[53] used rabbits in which one knee was made unstable by cutting the cruciate ligaments, excising the medial collateral ligament, and extirpating the medial meniscus.[54]

The relationship was evaluated by calculating the ratio between the washout rates of [133]xenon injected intraarticularly into both knees. Radioactive xenon is an inert, lipophilic gas that readily crosses cell membranes and is rapidly exhaled after one circulation through the lungs.[55]

In healthy joints, Phelps et al.[56] found a biexponential washout curve after intraarticular injection of [133]xenon. Analysis of its location in joint tissue during the fast and slow phases of the washout curve revealed that the initial rapid phase was explicable by washout to the blood vessels across the synovial membrane, whereas the subsequent slower phase was from articular fat. Christensen et al.,[53] in a 1-year follow-up of six rabbits, found biexponential washout curves, and the initial washout proved faster on the osteoarthritic side throughout the period (Figure 83.25).

Scintigraphy of the knee region of rabbits given ^{99m}Tc-microspheres intracardially showed a marked increase in the flow to the knee region on the osteoarthritic side, thus supporting the xenon measurements.

Comment

These studies showed a considerable increase in the synovial blood flow during the very early stages of experimental osteoarthritis. The flow increase partly reflects a major surgical trauma, but the continued effects (followed up to 1 year) are more likely due to traumatic synovitis caused by instability of the knee. In other words, the model incorporates a synovial reaction of considerable duration in the early stages of osteoarthritis.

Synovial Fluid Changes in Experimental Osteoarthritis

Kofoed[57] used the method of Hulth et al.[54] to produce unilateral osteoarthritis of the right knees of six rabbits. Three weeks after the operation, when synovitis was well established in the unstable knees, he performed in vivo measurements of PO_2 and PCO_2, using mass spectrometry, and pH by means of a monocrystalline antimony pH electrode.[58]

Results

Notable hypoxia, hypercapnia, and acidity were demonstrated in synovial fluid and subchondral bone marrow in the joints with synovitis (Table 83.11). Kofoed concluded that these signs are probably due to regional venous congestion. His findings and conclusions agree well with the findings of Grønlund et al.,[59] who observed that acute simulated effusion into a joint resulted in decreased regional blood flow and hypoxia.[60-62]

Early Reactions of Bone and Cartilage

Bone

Microscopically, osteophytes were observed as early as 1 week postoperatively[63] and could be observed with the

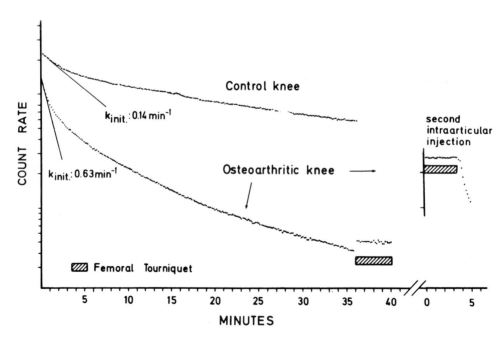

FIGURE 83.25. [133]Xenon washout curves from the knee joints of rabbits 23 weeks postoperatively. Biexponential curve and constant count rate after circulatory arrest are seen in both the later slow phase and the initial phase of the washout curve.

TABLE 83.11. PO_2, PCO_2, and pH values in synovial fluid from rabbits with unilateral experimentally produced knee-joint synovitis. From Kofoed. [57]

	Normal joint cavity				Joint with synovitis			
Animal	Rel.Ar	PO_2	PCO_2	pH	Rel.Ar	PO_2	PCO_2	pH
1	0.78	69.7	32.7	7.53	0.76	17.3	55.4	7.32
2	0.81	19.7	44.7	7.47	0.73	16.7	51.8	7.36
3	0.56	45.9	56.0	7.36	0.59	22.0	76.6	6.92
4	1.17	20.0	31.2	7.45	0.75	11.8	54.7	7.26
5	0.66	45.3	58.2	7.47	0.60	15.3	79.5	7.03
6	0.77	35.9	45.4	7.32	0.74	22.9	53.3	7.03
Mean	0.79	39.4	44.7	7.43	0.70	17.7	61.9	7.15
SE	0.21	18.8	11.3	0.07	0.08	4.2	12.6	0.17

Arterial values during the experiments

	PO_2	PCO_2	pH	PO_2	PCO_2	pH		
Mean	100.1	31.9	7.41	100.8	31.4	7.39		
SE	25.2	5.4	0.02	20.2	4.2	0.04		

Paired t test, $PO_2 < .05$, $PCO_2 < .001$, $pH < 0.001$.

naked eye 2 weeks after operation.[52] The high early (4–12 weeks after operation) uptake of ^{99m}Tc-phosphate could be located to the osteophytes, but increased subchondral uptake in the weight-bearing part of the knee joint was not seen until osteoarthritis was advanced.

Cartilage

Reimann et al.,[64] 1 to 26 and 18 to 24 months postoperatively, examined 42 rabbits, 6 in each group, in which one knee was destabilized by the method of Hulth et al.[54] They observed a generalized temporary depletion of the sulfated glycosaminoglycan content of the cartilage as early as 1 week postoperatively, rapidly increasing from the cartilage surface toward the deeper layers, reaching a maximum after 4 weeks and thereafter slowly decreasing. They concluded that it is reasonable to relate the early generalized glycosaminoglycan depletion to the simultaneous severe posttraumatic synovitis demonstrated, for example, by the xenon washout experiments.[53]

Experimental Osteoarthritis Caused by Immobilization of the Knee Joint

Finsterbush and Friedman[65] immobilized the right lower extremity of 28 rabbits in plaster of paris. The animals were divided into five groups (four mobile knees served as controls). After 2, 4, 6, and 8 weeks of immobilization the animals were killed and the joints examined.

Gross Findings

Two weeks postoperatively periarticular muscle atrophy and hyperemia were noted. Inside the joint the synovium appeared hyperemic, and the amount of synovial fluid had increased. The articular cartilage seemed normal. In joints immobilized for 4 weeks the synovium had proliferated and was hyperemic. The cartilage had lost its luster and was soft. The appearance of the joints after 6 weeks did not differ from those immobilized for 4 weeks, except for increased thickening of the capsule and ulceration of cartilage in the contact areas of most joints. After 8 weeks the joints showed less hyperemia and more thickening of the soft tissues than those immobilized for shorter periods.

Microscopic Findings

After 2 weeks of immobilization there was proliferation of blood capillaries in the subsynovial region and no articular cartilage changes. Joints immobilized for 4 weeks showed synovial hyperplasia, formation of villi, and proliferation of cells in the superficial layer. Capillaries surrounded by young fibrous tissue were observed perforating both the subchondral bone and the calcified cartilage. After 6 weeks the changes in the articular cartilage were a combination of destruction and repair. The synovium was less hyperemic and the subsynovial layer more fibrotic. Joints immobilized for 8 weeks also showed segments of bone denuded of overlying articular cartilage.

Finsterbush and Friedman[65] stress that the vascular changes were observed before signs of cartilage degeneration appeared. They further note the possibility that a lack in function of the venous pump system might be influential in early tissue hyperemia.

Langenskïold et al.[66] used this model in their studies on experimental osteoarthritis, and Shu-zheng et al.[67] recently performed intraosseous phlebography, intraosseous pressure measurements, and microvascular casting followed by scanning electron microscopy in rabbits that had one knee immobilized in extension with a plastic splint for 5 weeks.

Radiography showed the characteristic features of osteoarthritis in the immobilized knees. The intraosseous pressure was significantly higher in immobilized than in control knees ($P < .001$), and phlebography showed venous engorgement of subchondral and medullary vessels. The microvascular morphology, studied after casting by scanning electron microscopy, showed especially that the sinusoids changed shape, were dilated, and tended to leak casting material.

Comments

Although apparently completely different, both methods of producing experimental osteoarthritis (instability and immobilization) seem to lead to the same result. In both models hyperemia, particularly of the synovial membrane, is a very early phenomenon, as is excess of synovial fluid of abnormal oxygenation and acidity. The work by Shu-zheng et al.[67] places changes in intraosseous microvasculature and intraosseous hypertension at or very near the beginning of the process leading to osteoarthritis.

Nontraumatic Osteonecrosis

Idiopathic, Alcohol-Induced, and Steroid-Induced Femoral Head Necrosis

In nontraumatic femoral head necrosis the anterosuperior portion of the femoral head becomes infarcted and the precise cause or causes of this infarction are uncertain. Following death of bone tissue, spontaneous repair does occur but appears to be arrested, again by unknown factors. Subchondral fractures, impaction, collapse, and fragmentation of the sequestered part of the femoral head result in secondary disabling osteoarthritis.

Nontraumatic femoral head necrosis is known to be associated with alcoholism, steroid therapy, dysbaric phenomena, sickle cell anemia, and several rarer diseases. In many cases, however, no such connections can be demonstrated (idiopathic femoral head necrosis). My own experience is restricted to idiopathic and alcohol- and steroid-induced osteonecrosis.

Clinical Picture

The clinical picture is very similar to that of osteoarthritis. The patient complains of pain in the groin and trochanteric region, frequently irradiating to the thigh and knee. Pain at rest is often experienced very early on, and pain is accentuated by loading of the hip joint and joint movements, especially inward rotation. Limping and restricted mobility are other typical signs. The disorder may begin suddenly[68] or insidiously, sometimes related to minor physical exertion.[69]

Paraclinical Examinations

The patients' radiographs are often negative. A narrow translucent zone, the "crescent sign," near the osteochondral junction may be the first sign of developing necrosis. In later stages, radiography shows large defects in the contour of the femoral head or cyst formation in the bone marrow.

Scintimetry or scintigraphy reveals high uptake of bone-seeking radionuclides in the femoral head.[69,70] In the early stages this uptake is evenly distributed in the femoral head, indicating a generally increased bone metabolism. Later, the necrotic part of the head may lose its ability to bind bone-seeking isotopes and appears as an empty area surrounded by bone with high isotope uptake (the "cold-in-hot spot"). In these stages the increased isotope uptake is especially marked in the border zone between the necrosis and more healthy bone marrow.[70]

Pertrochanteric intraosseous phlebography shows a delay in venous drainage very similar to the drainage disturbances in osteoarthritis,[71-73] and intraosseous pressure measurements reveal even higher pressure in the femoral neck than observed in osteoarthritis.[48,74-76] The articular cartilage generally remains unaffected for a long time (in contrast to osteoarthritis), and the joint space is of normal height until narrowed by secondary osteoarthritis. The final diagnosis is still made by histological examination (e.g., core biopsy). No specific pathological differences between idiopathic and alcohol- or steroid-induced femoral head necrosis have been recorded.[77]

Interpretation of Paraclinical and Histological Findings

The most widely accepted interpretation of paraclinical and histological findings is that for some unknown reason blood supply via the retinacular arteries to the proximal part of the femoral head is interrupted.[69,78,79] The site and character of the vascular blockage is uncertain, and many believe that arterioles and capillaries are more prone than larger vessels to blood supply interruption.[78,80,81] Invasion of granulation tissue into the necrotic marrow space has been noted, as has the hyperemic character of the living bone marrow outside the necrotic zone.[68]

This explanation of the etiology and progress of nontraumatic femoral head necrosis as the result of interrupted arterial blood supply may seem attractive to some. However, it takes no account of the universal findings of generally increased femoral head metabolism during the early stages (scintigraphy) and the high pulsatile intraosseous pressure observed through all stages, and it is by no means universally accepted. Thus Jacqueline and Rutishauser[82] agree that the primary abnormality is vascular but suggest that it is caused by venous stasis giving rise to a gradually worsening ischemia followed by resorption of bone and fibrous replacement.

Kahlstrom et al.[83] suggested that bone necrosis might result from fat embolism, and this theory has been accepted by Jones and several others. Clinical evidence of fat embolism has been reported in many of the conditions associated with nontraumatic necrosis,[84] including sickle cell anemia, decompression sickness, pancreatitis, alcoholism, and hypercortisonism. Since 1971 Jones and his coworkers have demonstrated fat globules that appear to be intravascular in the subchondral haversian canals of necrotic femoral heads from alcoholic patients and patients taking high doses of steroids. His conception of the role of fat embolism was summarized in 1985.[85] Among those critical of his histological findings are Catto[77] and Glimcher and Kenzora.[86] The pathogenesis of femoral head necrosis is discussed in greater detail later in this chapter.

Intraosseous Flow and Pressure in the Femoral Head in Late-Stage Nontraumatic Femoral Head Necrosis

Several authors have shown intraosseous pressure in the bone marrow of the femoral neck to be elevated in nontraumatic femoral head necrosis and that the pressure generally reached values above those found in osteoarthritis.[29,76,87–89]

Intraosseous Pressure and Flow Measurements

Until recently no method has allowed direct measurement of blood flow in human bone, and simultaneous measurements of intraosseous pressure and blood flow have not been previously reported. My investigations[16,26,90] were performed to examine regional intraosseous pressure and blood flow at various levels in the healthy and osteonecrotic femoral heads and to compare the findings with histological observations.

Material

The 15 patients—8 men and 7 women with a mean age of 43 years (34–67 years)—were classed according to whether they had idiopathic, alcohol-induced, or steroid-induced osteonecrosis. Further, the examinations were performed only on advanced cases (ARCO stages 3 and 4).[91] For comparison, pressure and flow were measured in six hips in two men and four women, with a mean age of 50 years (28–63 years), without any clinical, radiographic, or scintigraphic evidence of hip disorders. These patients were undergoing surgery of the contralateral hip.

Methods

Intraosseous pressure and LDF in the bone marrow were measured simultaneously, prior to surgery, with the patients lying supine on the operating table under general anesthetic. The procedures and apparatuses for measurements of pressure and flow have been described previously.

Intraosseous Pressure and Flow Measurements at Different Levels in the Femoral Head

Procedure

After achieving a steady state, intraosseous pressure and LDF values were recorded in three different places in the proximal part of the femur: (1) in the intertrochanteric region, (2) immediately distal to the rim of the necrotic segment, and (3) in the osseous part of the necrotic area. In the healthy femoral heads the points of measurement were the trochanteric area and the center of the femoral head.

Results

The results of the flow measurements are given as the average of four measurements in each region. For statistical evaluation, Wilcoxon's test for paired data and Spearman's test for correlation were used, with a significance level of .05. In all cases and at all points of measurement both intraosseous pressure and LDF tracings showed pulsatile excursions synchronic with the patients' electrocardiograms.

In six healthy femoral heads intraosseous pressure in the trochanteric area was 21 ± 7 mm Hg and in the center 19 ± 3 mm Hg. The corresponding LDF values were 221 ± 63 mV and 224 ± 75 mV, respectively.

In eight patients with osteonecrosis, measurements were obtained from all three selected areas, intertrochanteric, rim zone, and sequester (Figure 83.26). The mean intraosseous pressure in the trochanteric region was 38 ± 7 mm Hg compared with 61 ± 9 mm Hg in the rim zone and 55 ± 9 mm Hg in the necrotic area. The corresponding mean LDF values were 165 ± 16 mV in the trochanteric area, 430 ± 77 mV at the rim, and 36 ± 6 mV inside the sequester. The differences in flow values between the various zones were significant at the .05 level. The differences in intraosseous pressure between the rim zone and the trochanteric region and between this area and the sequester were statistically significant,

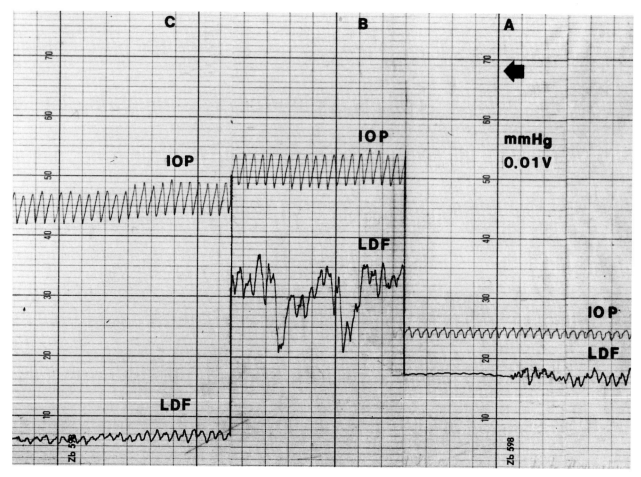

FIGURE 83.26. Intraosseous pressure (IOP) in millimeters of mercury and laser Doppler flow (LDF) measured in the trochanteric region (A), at the rim of the necrosis (B), and in-side the sequester (C). Patient with idiopathic nontraumatic femoral head necrosis.

whereas the difference between the rim zone and the sequester was not.

Measurements During Simulated Joint Loading and Passive Movements

In measurements during simulated joint loading and passive movements, the tips of the cannulae were placed in the center of the femoral head; in patients with osteonecrosis they were placed outside the sequester.

Results

Healthy Femoral Heads

The results from healthy femoral heads corresponded to the results from previous examinations, referred to under the section on osteoarthritis (Figures 83.2 and 83.5).

Osteonecrotic Femoral Heads During Loading

As in healthy femoral heads the pressure rise during loading depended on the load applied. The flow variations were modest. A characteristic difference between affected and healthy femoral heads was the pressure level, which was considerably higher in the femoral heads with osteonecrosis. Figure 83.27 is a typical pressure and flow chart from an osteonecrotic femoral head.

Osteonecrotic Femoral Heads During External and Internal Rotation

In general, the intraosseous pressure was considerably higher than the already high level at rest during external and internal rotation, and the intraosseous flow was hardly affected (Figure 83.28). Flexion of the hip joint

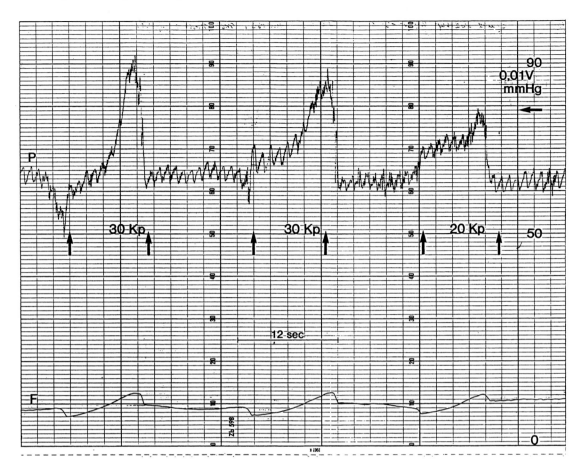

FIGURE 83.27. Intraosseous pressure (P) and flow (F) tracings before, during, and after three periods of loading. Osteonecrotic femoral head. Point of measurement: center of femoral head (outside necrotic area).

did not affect the results of these maneuvers. In this relatively small number of subjects, the striking differences in pressure and flow reactions to joint movements between healthy and osteonecrotic femoral heads were similar in all patients examined and probably characteristic of a larger group.

Comment

I interpret the low pressures and high flow rates at rest and during joint movements as signs of free drainage (intraosseous and extraosseous) from the healthy bone marrow. Conversely, the very high pressure and slow flow at rest and the marked pressure increases together with unaltered slow flow during joint maneuvers indicate severe impairment of drainage from bone marrow in nontraumatic femoral head necrosis.

Histology in Advanced Stages of Femoral Head Necrosis

Methods

The staining methods used in this series[16] were the same as those used in examinations of osteoarthritis.

Results

Synovium

The three types of nontraumatic osteonecrosis showed similar synovial changes. The stroma beneath the lining cells was mostly edematous. In the deeper layers of the thickened membrane, fibrosis was dominant. The vascularity of the membrane varied widely from a density of vessels reminiscent of osteoarthritic synovium to fibrous areas with very few vessels. In the more densely vascular-

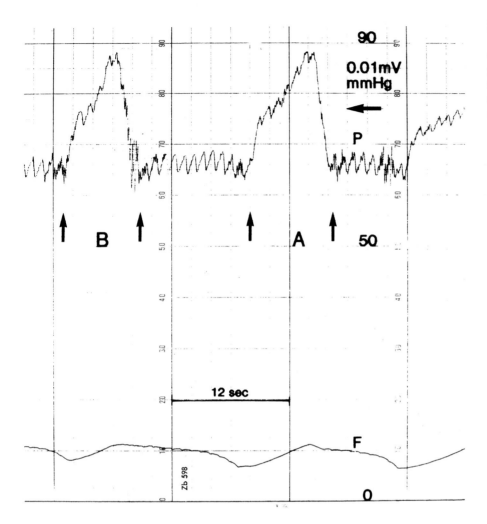

FIGURE 83.28. Intraosseous pressure (P) and flow (F) chart from center of the femoral head (outside necrotic area). Steroid-induced osteonecrosis: **A,** Period of external rotation. **B,** Period of internal rotation.

ized zones erythrocyte aggregations and agglutinations were common, as were extravascular erythrocytes.

Bone Marrow and Soft Tissues

In the necrotic area the characteristic finding in all three types of femoral head necrosis was displacement of healthy soft tissue by masses of more or less primitive mesenchymal tissue and fibrocartilage (Figure 83.29). These primitive invasive tissues were generally well vascularized, and their vessels showed numerous areas with intravascular erythrocyte aggregations, agglutinations, and newly formed or older fibrin thrombi (Figure 83.30). Free erythrocytes in the interstitial space were common. In the rim zone distal to the necrosis the soft tissue of the more normal looking marrow was also well vascularized with the same signs of intravascular stasis or blockage in many vessels, especially veins and venules. The arteries and arterioles of these areas were generally inconspicuous.[92] These findings were also apparent in areas some distance from the border of the necrosis. Particularly in the subchondral necrosis area, the invasive primitive but

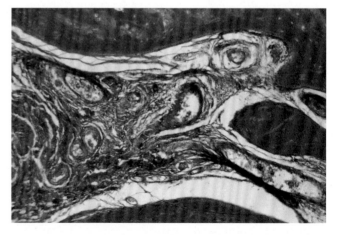

FIGURE 83.29. Osteonecrotic bone marrow. Invasive, vascularized primitive tissues between trabeculae (Martius scarlet blue × 100).

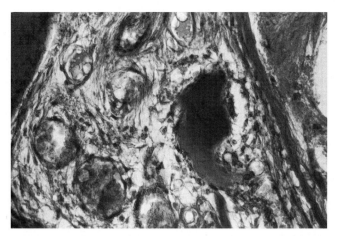

FIGURE 83.30. Vessels in invasive bone marrow tissue. Erythrocyte aggregations, agglutinations, and an old fibrin thrombus (Martius scarlet blue × 250).

recognizable tissues gave way to zones of completely unstructured and nonvascularized debris.

Bone Marrow and Trabeculae

Visibly dead trabeculae, often with fractures and without any osteoblastic or osteoclastic activity, were common in the center of the necrosis. In the apparently intact trabeculae of the rim zone on both the necrotic and intact side, fibrin thrombi in the haversian canals or blockage by fibrous tissue was characteristic with MSB staining (Figure 83.31).

Comment

The light microscopy findings go a long way in explaining the very high pulsatile intraosseous pressure and the

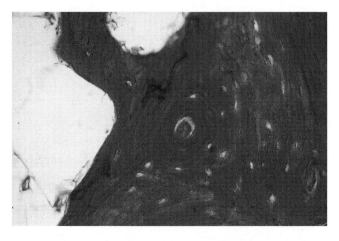

FIGURE 83.31. Two haversian canals in trabecula with blockage of canals by tissue, probably old thrombi in vessel surrounded by or transformed into collagen. (See Starklint et al.[92])

slow but still pulsatile flow. Especially important are the changes in microvasculature, with largely unaffected arteries and arterioles but dilated veins and venules often blocked by erythrocyte agglutinations or fibrin thrombi.

The microscopic examinations were of patients with late-stage osteonecrosis and secondary synovitis. The signs of blockage in the vascularized zones in the synovium described earlier may play an additional role in the obvious drainage difficulties in nontraumatic femoral head necrosis (see the section on osteoarthritis), but the findings cited here indicate that intraosseous venous blockage is of importance (and that these phenomena may be due to an abnormal local tendency to thrombosis).

General Discussion

Known and Suspected Causes of Increased Pressure in Juxtachondral Bone Marrow

All my investigations indicate that increased intraosseous pressure is due to increased flow resistance in veins that drain joint-bearing bone marrow. Intraosseous hypertension may be intermittent, chronic, or a combination of both, with chronically high pressure increasing periodically.

Further, these investigations have shown that the cause of abnormally high resistance to venous flow from the bone marrow is to be found proximal to the joint structures (i.e., between the joint and the heart), in the joint, or in the bone marrow.[16]

Supraarticular Causes of Increased Intravenous Pressure

The results of pathologic changes in supraarticular drainage are best known from ankle conditions in those suffering from severe and long-standing venous insufficiency[11] (see Chapter 82).

Articular and Intraosseous Changes Influencing Pressure in Joint-Bearing Bone

Figure 83.32 shows in schematic form the known and suspected factors influencing bone marrow pressure:

1. Intraarticular blockage of veins that drain juxtaarticular bone
2. Compression of the draining veins by structural stretching or torsion as they pass through the fibrous capsule
3. Compression deformation of closed or semiclosed intraosseous compartments
4. Intravascular or extravascular blockage of intraosseous venous circulation

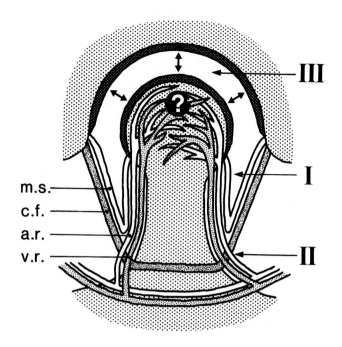

FIGURE 83.32. The relations between retinacular vessels and synovial and fibrous capsules of the hip joint. m.s., synovial membrane; c.f., fibrous capsule; a.r., retinacular artery; v.r., retinacular vein. Roman numerals and question mark refer to known and suspected causes of vascular disturbances in the synovium and femoral head bone marrow.

Intraarticular Blockage of Veins That Drain Juxtaarticular Bone

Anatomical studies and measurements of venous pressure have shown that in osteoarthritis the extracapsular veins in the hip and knee regions are normal with normal pressure.[28,48] The hindrance to venous drainage must therefore be sought deep to, or in, the fibrous capsule of the joint.

Most of the investigations described in the following were conducted on the joints proximal and distal to the femur. Both joints are characterized by a subsynovial course of arteries and veins, and the most important drainage from the femoral head and neck and from a large part of the femoral condyles is via these subsynovial channels.

Vascular synovitis is a characteristic early manifestation in both types of experimental osteoarthritis described earlier in the intraosseous engorgement–pain syndromes, including radiographically silent osteoarthritis, and is also observed in manifest osteoarthritis, primary as well as secondary, and in rheumatoid arthritis.

Thus, increased intraarticular volume gives rise to increased intraarticular pressure, the rise in pressure depending on the degree of volume increase and the strength of the fibrous capsule and its resistance to stretching.[36] In addition to compression by extravascular

forces, my histological examinations showed that intravascular blockage by erythrocyte agglutinations and fibrin thrombi is extremely common in the vessels, mostly venules, of osteoarthritic and rheumatoid arthritic synovium, further increasing the resistance to venous flow.

Experimental Tests

The possibility that intraarticular effusion may influence the pressure in juxtachondral bone marrow was tested in experiments on rabbits.[60] In the rabbit knee the femoral condyles are ensheathed by large synovial joint recesses, and the vessels supplying and draining this region have the same subsynovial course as those in human hips and knee joints.

Material and Methods

Five adult rabbits were used. Experiments were performed with the rabbits under intravenous anesthesia. Blood pressure, intraarticular pressure of the knee joint, and intraosseous pressure of the lateral femoral condyle were measured simultaneously (Figure 83.33).

On the seven knees investigated, 30 experiments were performed. At five different values of intraarticular pressure, from a few millimeters of mercury to above the blood pressure level, corresponding intraosseous pressures were recorded simultaneously.

Results

A rise of intraarticular pressure resulted in a significant pressure rise in the juxtaarticular bone marrow ($P < .001$) (Figure 83.34). The rise in intraosseous pressure diminished as the level of systemic blood pressure was approached, and a rise above this level did not result in a further rise of bone marrow pressure. The rapid rise of intraarticular pressure induced by infusion of saline was followed by a much slower rise of intraosseous pressure. Lowering of the pressure in the joint was followed by a slower reduction of bone marrow pressure.

Comments

Pressure in the marrow of joint-bearing bone is clearly influenced by that in the joint cavity. These experimental results have been subsequently confirmed and enlarged upon by Bünger et al.[13,61,62] and Lucht.[93] The increase in intraosseous pressure when joint pressure is elevated is probably due to compression of the veins that drain the bone marrow. This contention is supported by the observation that an abrupt rise of joint pressure is followed by a gradual increase of intraosseous pressure. This indicates a gradual filling of the semiclosed intraosseous space by initially unimpeded arterial inflow. The maximum intraosseous pressures observed in this study

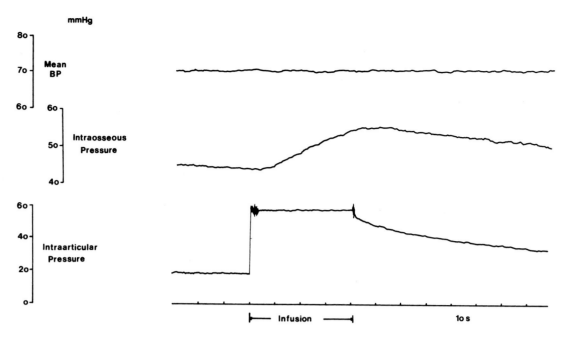

FIGURE 83.33. Tracing of intraosseous pressure increase induced by joint infusion of saline. Simultaneous pressure curves from a single experiment on a rabbit knee.

reached a level somewhat below the mean systemic blood pressure. These results corresponded to the highest intraosseous pressures observed at rest in painful osteoarthritis, intraosseous engorgement–pain syndromes, and other disorders with synovitic effusion.

Clinical Observations in Fractures of the Femoral Neck: Joint Tamponade by Hemarthrosis and Synovitis

In fractures of the femoral neck, Soto-Hall et al.[94] suggested hip joint tamponade as a contributory etiological mechanism in posttraumatic osteonecrosis of the femoral head.

Computed tomography has proved valuable in diagnosing hip joint effusion.[95,96] Egund et al.[95] performed computed tomography on 34 femoral neck fractures 1 to 32 days after internal fixation. All except one showed an increased distance between the femoral neck and the anterior aspect of the joint capsule compared with the intact side, indicating varying degrees of hip joint hemarthrosis and/or synovitis. Hip joint aspiration in 11 patients revealed increased intracapsular pressure varying between 10 and 112 mm Hg and volumes of aspirated fluid up to 23 mL. The authors concluded that increased intracapsular pressure may contribute to decreased femoral head vitality.

These investigations may also explain the high pressure in the femoral head found in many of Arnoldi and Linderholm's patients.[97] Sustained increase of intracapsular pressure at levels no higher than 40 mm Hg can produce hypoxia and ischemic changes in the femoral

head of the rabbit.[23,98,99] Recently, Kristensen et al.[100] showed restoration of blood flow after aspiration of hemarthrosis in undisplaced fractures, and Harper et al.[101] showed that aspiration of the hip joint in intracapsular fractures produced a significant decrease in intraosseous pressure and an increase in pulse pressure within the femoral head.

Comment

These experiments and observations strongly indicate that compression of the subsynovial drainage veins from juxtaarticular bone (suggested by *I* in Figure 83.32) is a valid explanation of the chronic intraosseous stasis and hypertension characteristic of joints with chronic vascular synovitis discussed here.

Compression of Draining Veins During Their Transcapsular Course

In rheumatoid arthritis of the knee joint the intraarticular pressure is least in the lightly flexed position, and further flexion produces extremely high pressure.[36,102] In most hip joints the first sign of synovitic effusion is pain provoked or accentuated by inward rotation. The mechanism provoking this effect is probably related to increased resistance to outflow, intact arterial inflow, and movement-associated increase in intraosseous pressure. To determine whether capsular stretching and/or torsion in joints without effusion may influence the pressure in juxtaarticular bone marrow, experiments were conducted on healthy fetlock joints in horses.[12]

Material and Methods

Six adult horses were used for experiments performed under halothane anesthesia. Following the principles mentioned earlier, blood pressure was measured in an artery of the hind leg and simultaneous pressure measurements were taken inside the fetlock joint and the bone marrow proximal to it. Radiographs of the joints were normal. In the standing position the fetlock joint in the horse is loaded in slight hyperextension.

Results

Figure 83.34 shows intraosseous pressures at different degrees of flexion in six joints without infusion of saline. There was a rise in intraosseous pressure with flexion beyond 40 degrees. At 60 degrees of flexion the rise was significant ($P < .05$), and from 60 to 80 degrees it was highly significant ($P < .001$). Intraosseous pressure was only rarely above the level of systemic blood pressure.

Comments

The equine fetlock, like the human hip and knee and rabbit knee joints, has large synovial recesses that cover the entry and exit of the vessels to and from juxtachondral bone marrow. Equine experiments with injection of saline also confirmed the earlier experiments on rabbits. However, in this context the most interesting result was the effect on intraosseous pressure of movements in a healthy joint per se. One reasonable explanation for at least part of the steep rise in pressure on flexion beyond a certain degree is strangulation of the draining veins during their transcapsular course, as suggested by *II* in Figure 83.32.

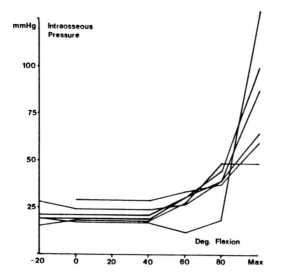

FIGURE 83.34. Experiments on horses. Relation between degree of flexion and intraosseous pressure in juxtaarticular bone marrow in the six fetlock joints examined.

Observations on Human Joints

Capsular Stretching or Torsion: Venous and Arterial Compression

The experiments performed with pressure measurements in the femoral head during forceful internal rotation of the deformed and laterally displaced osteoarthritic head showed some unusual and perhaps characteristic changes (Figure 83.4). After a brief but significant increase the pressure fell to a level below that recorded before the maneuver, and during this phase the pressure might reach a very low level. At the same time the pulse amplitudes were reduced but did not disappear completely.

These changes could be a result of increased tension in the fibrous joint capsule. The thin-walled veins with low intraluminar pressure are compressed, causing the brief intraosseous pressure increase. As the tension in the capsule increases, the thick-walled arteries passing through the capsule are also partly compressed, resulting in reduction of arterial pressure and pulse amplitude, as well as intraosseous flow. At cessation of capsular stretching the intraosseous pressure, pulse amplitude, and flow rapidly return to the initial levels. These are the only cases in which I have noted an influence of joint movement on arterial pressure.

Comment

This evidence from animal and human experiments may support the mechanism referred to as *II* in Figure 83.32. However, because the maneuvers used often included an element of compression deformation it is difficult to be certain.

Compression Deformation

Compression deformation occurs when a joint is under load, and pressure variations have been studied in both the femoral head (part of a tubular bone) and the patella (a short bone).[15,16]

Tubular Bone

Healthy Femoral Head

Femoral head pressure was measured for series of brief periods of loading in anesthetized supine patients. Loading the joint was accompanied by a steep but moderate rise of pressure and an increase of flow rate. The pressure rise depended on the loading force applied. Unloading was followed by a steep drop in pressure below the initial stable level that, however, reestablished itself almost immediately.

Osteoarthritic Femoral Head

In the femoral heads from osteoarthritic joints the level of loading pressure appeared to depend on the rest pressure level, the degree of deformation and displacement of the femoral head, and the site of measurement: high rest pressure induced high loading pressures, and these pressures were higher in the immediate subchondral zone than in the center of the femoral neck.

Femoral Neck in Nontraumatic Femoral Head Necrosis

Pressure rises during loading depended on the force applied; because the resting level was much higher than in healthy joints and considerably higher than in osteoarthritis, the loading pressure peaks reached values above the levels noted in healthy and osteoarthritic joints. At these high levels the pressure tracings could become, but seldom were, apulsative. It should be noted, however, that the forces applied during the loading experiments (maximum 50–55 kg) fell far short of the forces assumed to develop during ordinary standing or walking. No measurements have been made on conscious subjects during normal activity.

Short Bone Compared With Tubular Bone

Increased but relatively moderate pressure levels were thus reached in the femoral head from healthy to osteonecrotic joints during loading (compression). Although loading pressures measured in the femoral head were characterized by mostly pulsatile pressure tracings and, with the forces applied, relatively modest pressure increases, measurements from the patella during loading in flexion showed somewhat different results.

In these experiments pressures were recorded simultaneously in the patella and the femoral and tibial condyles.[14,15] The measurements were made on pain-free knees and those with patellar pain (PP) syndromes. At rest and in the horizontal position, the measurements generally showed a somewhat higher pressure in the patella than in the femur and tibia in both pain-free control knees and PP knees. Loading during sustained knee flexion accentuated these pressure differences. In both pain-free and PP knees the initial peak pressures in the patella during flexion reached values far exceeding 100 mm Hg. In PP knees the patellar pressure remained at a high level near the diastolic blood pressure during sustained flexion, and the pressure tracings were nonpulsatile. The pressure increases in the femoral and tibial condyles were modest, and the pressure curves were always pulsatile.

The results of the various experiments and maneuvers performed during those investigations, together with the histological findings,[14–16] indicate that the differences in pressure variations between the patella and the femoral and tibial condyles are due mainly to the following circumstances: (1) difference in bone structure and (2) different conditions for venous drainage in the three areas of measurement.

Anatomy and Conditions for Venous Drainage

The patella belongs to the group of short bones. It consists of a normally densely woven cancellous network surrounded on all sides by a solid but still elastic cortical shell, and, in the age groups with which I was concerned in PP syndromes, it is highly vascularized. In contrast, the femoral and tibial condyles are part of tubular bones, and their cancellous bone marrow merges into loosely structured diaphyseal bone marrow extending far beyond the knee region and the points of measurement used in my studies. The anatomical structure of tubular bone ensures that an increase in intramedullary pressure provoked by bone compression and deformation may disperse over a large area, from the marrow of the condyles upward through the femur and distally through the tibia. In the enclosed marrow of the patella dispersion is negligible. Release of intraosseous pressure is only possible through drainage to extraosseous veins, not, as in the two other areas of measurement, through both intraosseous and extraosseous channels.

Primary Intravascular Blockage of Venous Microcirculation Inside the Bone Marrow of the Femoral Head

Investigations on nontraumatic femoral head necrosis are still hampered by the fact that a satisfactory animal test model has not yet been found. Measurements of pressure and flow, as well as histological observations, show a severe blockage of venous drainage from the femoral head marrow. The large number of blocks in small veins and venules, including the haversian vessels and those in the invasive primitive tissues, indicates an etiology that includes a remarkable local tendency to venous thrombosis. The suspected causes of the vascular disturbances, referred to as ? in Figure 83.32, are further discussed elsewhere in this chapter.

General Comment

A brief attempt has been made to isolate some of the factors that influence intraosseous pressure and flow in joint-bearing bone by raising resistance to venous drainage. However, the only pathologic factor that is wholly independent in this respect is supraarticularly induced intermittent hypertension of chronic venous insufficiency. The other intraarticular and intraosseous blocking mechanisms are apparently interdependent and, in various degrees, influential in the pathogenesis of pain and degenerative changes of the various disorders.

Changes in Capillary Flow: Edema

Ultimately, the basic pathophysiology of these joint disorders is concerned with changes in conditions of capillary flow and their effects on cellular environment. Under normal conditions the capillary membrane is permeable to such hydrophilic solutes as ions but to a lesser degree to colloid solutes (e.g., plasma proteins). The transfer of water, electrolytes, and other substances between plasma and interstitial fluid is controlled by the relative hydrostatic and osmotic pressure gradients between the two compartments. Water, electrolytes, and nonelectrolytes are filtered through the capillary membrane at the arteriolar end by hydrostatic pressure. A certain protein osmotic effect is present in the interstitial fluid.

The effective hydrostatic and osmotic pressures are, respectively, higher and lower at the arteriolar end of the capillary than at the venous end, and a small fraction of the plasma fluid with its contents leaves the capillary at the arteriolar end and returns to it at the venous end (approximately 1%). Thus, interstitial fluid is a plasma ultrafiltrate. The normal dynamic balance between intracellular and extracellular fluid and plasma, and thus the cellular environment, depends primarily on the capillary membrane function as described earlier.

Immediate Cause of Localized Edema

The immediate cause of edema is an imbalance between the transudation of water and electrolytes leaving the circulation through the capillary wall into the interstitial fluid and their return to circulation. The factors controlling these processes are (1) capillary hydrostatic pressure, (2) concentration of serum protein, (3) concentration of protein in the interstitial fluid, (4) tissue tension, and (5) lymph flow. Change in any of these forces is followed by the establishment of a new balance by the counteraction of the other forces (i.e., edema tends to be self-limiting). With the establishment of a new balance, water and electrolyte exchange may be normal, although the volume of interstitial fluid is increased. It follows, therefore, that this development is only observed in vascularized tissues. Studies referred to in this chapter furnish certain information about the local effects of changes in factors 1, 3, and 4 cited earlier.

Changes in Capillary Hydrostatic Pressure

The disorders under consideration are all characterized by chronic or intermittent high resistance to local ve-

nous drainage or chronically high resistance intermittently increased. High resistance to venous flow results in increased hydrostatic pressure at the venous end of the capillary with increased capillary distension. This has a double effect: the increase in capillary blood pressure augments the transudation of water, electrolytes, and serum proteins into the interstitial fluid compartment, and the decrease in the effective osmotic pressure of plasma. Capillary and venule walls become permeable to even very large protein molecules, and the permeation thus increases at edema formation, as observed in synovia of osteoarthritic joints and the subcutis in chronic venous insufficiency of the lower limb. Intermittent venous hypertension is especially prone to increase the permeability of large protein molecules[103] and of such formed elements as erythrocytes.[104]

Tissue Tension

Burch and Sodeman[105] defined *tissue tension* as the pressure with which tissue structures resist changes in their anatomical relations. Such pressure varies considerably from tissue to tissue. Thus, subcutaneous is always lower than intramuscular tissue tension in the lower leg, and among these muscles those with a tight fascia show a higher tissue tension than those with loose fascial coverings, both at rest and during muscle contraction.[106] Apart from the structure of the muscle fascia, muscular tissue tension was found to depend on the amount of extravascular fluid and the filling of its vessels. No measurements of tissue tension in bone and cartilage have been performed, except measurements of intraosseous pressure.

Influence of Tissue Tension on Blood Flow

Edema increases tissue tension, which, it is generally agreed, tends to reduce blood flow. The cause may be arteriolar closure at high extravascular pressure[107] or a reduction of local arteriovenous pressure difference and hence blood flow as local venous pressure increases equal to the rise in the surrounding tissue pressure.[108]

In studies of patellar pressure under various experimental conditions[15] it was noted that in this limited and noncompliant bone marrow space, increasing intraosseous pressure (tissue tension) affected the pulsatile excursions on the pressure tracings from the marrow. Under the circumstances of the experiments, an increase of intraosseous pressure to 40 to 60 mm Hg enlarged the pulse waves. However, if the pressure increased further the tracings became nonpulsatile. In the osteoarthritic femoral head I found significantly higher pressures and pulse excursions immediately below the cartilage than in the femoral head but never apulsative pressure tracings.

Nielsen,[109] in experiments on soft tissue arteries of the lower limb, observed that the precapillary vessels collapsed with cessation of blood flow when the (effective) transmural arterial pressure was reduced to zero. Sejrsen stated: "When the tissue pressure reaches values corresponding to diastolic arterial pressure, the arterioles will be compressed during diastole. Under these circumstances the arterioles present a very high resistance to flow and they will not be refilled during systole. The result is a cessation of blood flow."[110]

It is entirely possible that the mechanism described earlier (morphologically intact arterial channels combined with extensive, although mostly periodical, obstruction of flow in the drainage system and high tissue tension) is responsible for the intermittent high pulseless pressure observed[14,15] in the patella during sustained maximal flexion, particularly in patients with PP syndromes (compression deformation in combination with partial drainage blockage). The same mechanism may equally produce the occasional high peaks of pulseless pressure seen during some joint maneuvers in nontraumatic femoral head necrosis: intraosseous intravascular venous blockage, capsular strangulation of extraosseous veins by torsion, and compression deformation supplemented by intraarticular venous blockage during the osteoarthritic end stages. In these cases of extreme venous flow resistance and high tissue tension, the effect on capillary blood flow may be similar to that of interrupted or severely reduced arterial supply.

The structure of the bone seems to be another important factor that governs the level of intraosseous pressure. Thus, compression of the patella against the femoral condyle raised the intraosseous pressure in both the condyle and the patella. However, because of the noncompliance of the closed patellar marrow space, the pressure rise was always greater there than in the "open" marrow of the femoral condyle, where pulseless tracings were never observed. However, opening of the patellar bone marrow (osteotomy or fenestration and core decompression) always significantly reduced the intraosseous pressure there, just as osteotomy or fenestration also lowered the pressure in the osteoarthritic and osteonecrotic femoral head marrow.

Our results thus indicate that because of increased tissue tension, decreased effective transmural vessel pressure, and arteriovenous pressure difference, impairment of venous drainage from juxtachondral bone marrow always influences capillary flow. Under certain circumstances tissue tension becomes so high that the flow of blood ceases. Hemoconcentration due to increased osmotic pressure of extravascular proteins and the effects on cellular metabolism of abnormal proteins in the interstitial fluid compartment may also be important in the pathogenesis of degenerative tissue changes. In this connection it should be remembered that synovial fluid is essentially a plasma dialysate and that this is the fluid on which cartilage metabolism depends.

Differences and Similarities Between Osteoarthritis and Nontraumatic Osteonecrosis of the Femoral Head

Until the appearance of the work by Harrison et al.[2] it was generally accepted that osteoarthritis is caused by a deficiency of arterial supply to the femoral head. This concept now has few supporters. However, nontraumatic femoral head necrosis is generally accepted as an avascular necrosis, implying that the localized bone tissue death is due to interruption of arterial inflow to the affected bone marrow area.

The results of the investigations on osteonecrosis of the femoral head mentioned here, together with observations made by many other authors, make it natural to reexamine and discuss the evidence regarding the cause or causes of osteocyte death, the replacement of bone by other mesenchymal tissues, and the progression to secondary osteoarthritis.

Interruption of Arterial Supply Versus Blocking of Venous Drainage

Total interruption of arterial supply to an organ, or part of an organ, leads to infarction (total death due to anoxemia of the tissues involved). It is, however, equally true that cessation of arterial flow is accompanied by lowered tissue tension, in this case lowered pressure in the affected bone marrow. At the same time the pulsatile excursions on the pressure tracings diminish or disappear.[97] On the other hand, with intact arterial inflow, blockage of venous outflow raises the tissue tension in the area affected, and, as previously reported, the pulsatile excursions on pressure tracings tend to increase, at least as long as the rise of intraosseous tissue tension does not exceed the local diastolic arteriolar pressure.

All published works report increased and pulsatile pressure in bone marrow in intraosseous engorgement–pain syndromes, radiographically silent and manifest osteoarthritis, late-stage rheumatoid arthritis, and even the very early stage of experimental osteoarthritis. Even higher intraosseous pressures are found in early and late nontraumatic femoral head necrosis, pulsatile even inside the demarcated sequester.

These findings indicate that blockage of venous drainage is a common feature in all these disorders. They cannot, however, be taken as signs of interruption of arterial supply to the bone marrow.

Histological Evidence

Death and disintegration of large areas of subchondral bone are common in the late stages of nontraumatic osteonecrosis. However, focal and even widespread areas of bone death were also found in advanced osteoarthritis,[110] and local areas of osteocyte death have been noted by many authors. Pedersen et al.[75] found no characteristic histological pattern differentiating osteoarthritis from osteonecrosis.

In all disorders, from the earliest to the latest stages, bone and bone marrow tissues are replaced by invasion of more primitive mesenchymal tissues. These areas seem larger in osteonecrosis than in osteoarthritis, as are the areas of avascular disorganized debris. However, histologically, the character and vascularization of these invasive tissues do not differ in the two disorders.

Histological Signs of Venous Blockage

In all cases examined—osteoarthritic, rheumatoid arthritic, and osteonecrotic—the synovium showed essentially the same picture of vein and venule dilation with stasis, erythrocyte agglutinations, and fibrin thrombi of various ages. The synovium of early nontraumatic osteonecrosis has not been examined in this way. However, the evidence at hand indicates that vascular synovitis is a secondary phenomenon in osteonecrosis.

In the bone marrow the venules and veins of osteoarthritic and rheumatoid arthritic femoral heads showed the same picture of intravascular blockage, and in both these disorders and in nontraumatic osteonecrosis the tendency to vessel blockage was prominent in the well-vascularized invasive fibrous tissue. All disorders showed agglutinations and fibrin thrombi in the haversian vessels. They were even observed in cases of radiographically silent osteoarthritis. However, haversian blockage was a much more prominent feature in the late stages of nontraumatic osteonecrosis.

The general impression gained by histological observations is that in osteoarthritis and rheumatoid arthritis intravascular blockage is predominantly due to extraosseous, intraarticular causes. The intramedullary blockage is secondary, whereas vessel blockage in osteonecrosis is primarily due to intraosseous causes.

Nature of Haversian Blockage and Osteocyte Death

Whereas the intact endothelium proved that the blockage of veins and venules of soft tissues (synovium, bone marrow, and invasive primitive tissues) was obviously due to intravascular stasis, erythrocyte agglutinations, or fibrin thrombi, my histological findings indicate that the cause of haversian blockage may not be so easily explained.

In some cases MSB staining showed amorphous yellow or red thrombi (Figure 83.24) inside clearly defined haversian venules, but in the majority the blockage, stained blue (Figure 83.31), showed no signs of identifiable vascular structures. Further, in many of these cases the blue mass showed typical collagen strands. In fact, in these slides the blockage appeared to be due to fibrous tissue (also stained blue with MSB). The intravascular origin of the blockage that tended to fill the canal space was far from obvious.

From studies on thrombosis of peripheral veins, the transformation of the thrombus into fibrous tissue is a well-known observation. However, the possibility remained that the histologically observed blockage of the canals by fibrous tissue could also be a phenomenon parallel to the massive invasion of primitive tissues with low oxygen demands into the bone marrow of the femoral head characteristic of osteoarthritis and osteonecrosis. To try to solve this question Starklint et al.[92] used immunohistochemical techniques with antibodies against factor VIII and Ulex europeus lectin to visualize the endothelium of the blood vessels. As a result they suggested that obstruction to the venous outflow was due to intravascular thrombosis and perivascular fibrosis. Intravascular blockage or extravascular constriction, the fact remains that in the locations where they occur, the osteocytes of the region degenerate or die.

Fat Embolism as a Cause of Nontraumatic Femoral Head Necrosis

The possible association between fat embolism of the subchondral vessels (arterioles) of bone, especially those of the haversian canals, and osteonecrosis was suggested by Jones et al.,[111] and a synthesis of the evidence supporting this concept was published later.[85] This hypothesis is based on epidemiological, experimental, and clinical research. Because it represents a concept accepted by many students of the disorder, it is summarized here, together with some of the reports with observations and conclusions adverse to the theory. Finally, it is compared with the observations of my own research.

Epidemiological Studies

Jacobs[112] found that 89% of 269 patients with nontraumatic femoral head osteonecrosis had concomitant disorders known to be complicated by disturbed fat metabolism.

Experimental Studies

Several authors[113–117] have treated rabbits with corticosteroids and observed hyperlipemia, fatty liver, fat embolism in the vessels of the femoral head, and osteocyte death. The observation times varied between 21 and 150 days. Kenzora et al.[118] confirmed the findings of fatty liver and femoral head fat embolism but not osteocyte death (observation time 63 and 365 days). Paolaggi[115] found significant bone marrow necrosis after 3 weeks of corticosteroid administration. Increased intrafemoral head pressure was noted by Wang[119] with decreased blood flow[120] after 6 to 8 weeks. Jaffe et al.[121] found fat embolism in the subchondral capillary beds of both the femoral and humeral heads, and Gold et al.[122] noted a large number of empty lacunae during the second and third weeks, together with an accumulation of necrotic debris within the marrow spaces.

From Fat Embolism to Thrombosis

Figure 83.35 represents Jones's[85] view of the transition from fat embolism to thrombosis in the vessels of the femoral head. Oleic acid, generated by neutral embolic fat, causes a marked stripping of capillary endothelium, passive congestion, and edema. (It also produces local

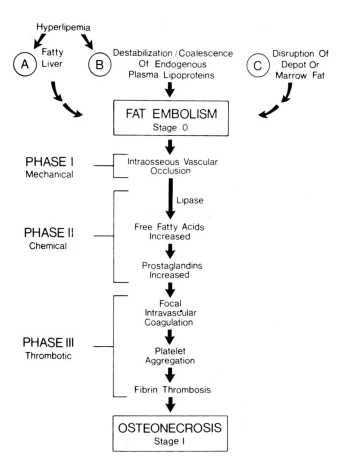

FIGURE 83.35. Three mechanisms (A, B, and C) capable of producing intraosseous fat embolism and triggering a three-phase process of focal intravascular coagulation resulting in early osteonecrosis. (From Jones.[85])

thrombosis when injected into an isolated vein segment.) Platelet aggregation and fibrin deposition occur in the vicinity of the fat.[123] However, the precise mechanism by which fat produces thrombosis is not known. It has been shown that platelet aggregation and fibrin thrombi are associated with fat emboli[125,126] and that intravascular coagulation may be precipitated by endothelial damage and fat embolism.

Opposing Views Based on Experience with Human Nontraumatic Osteonecrosis

Glimcher and Kenzora[86] compared sections of healthy femoral heads, osteoarthritic femoral heads without osteonecrosis, and femoral heads from patients with clear clinical and microscopic osteonecrosis. Using Jones's criteria and staining methods they detected fat "emboli" in the vascular spaces in almost all samples of healthy bone. However, the bone adjacent to the presumptive embolus was viable. Also, the capillary endothelial cells in which the fat was located were viable. They concluded only a negligible role for fat deposits in the pathology of osteonecrosis.

Jones[85] could demonstrate deformed fat globules that seemed to be intravascular in the subchondral haversian canals in necrotic femoral heads from alcoholic patients and patients taking high doses of corticosteroids. Nonetheless, Solomon[87] was unconvinced that the fat globules demonstrated in his patients were intravascular, and Catto[77] and Mulligan et al.[126] were not able to find them in the osteonecrotic hip and knee, respectively.

Author's Observations

My observations, as described in this chapter, neither prove nor disprove Jones's hypothesis, as set forth in Figure 83.35, although I could confirm the findings in phase III (at least as regards veins and venules). My histological observations were made on late stages of nontraumatic osteonecrosis. Staining by four different lipid-staining methods failed to show intravascular fat globules in the vessels of the haversian canals or in those of the soft tissues of the femoral head bone marrow. I also found, however, a large number of young, middle-aged, and what may have been old fibrin thrombi in the haversian canals. They may or may not have developed from early fat emboli. However, intravascular fibrin thrombi of the same location were also extremely common in the synovium of osteoarthritis (early and late), rheumatoid arthritis, and the parapatellar synovium of PP syndromes.[15] In PP syndromes haversian blockage was found, although rarely, in the subchondral bone and the trabeculae. In these locations thrombi were frequently observed in osteoarthritis and rheumatoid arthritis; all patients without signs of nontraumatic osteonecrosis or diseases presumably were connected with this disorder.

My own conclusion (based on observations recorded over the years and set forward in this chapter) is that fat embolism or abnormally high lipid contents in the blood might play a role in some types of nontraumatic femoral head necrosis. The evidence put forward by Jones is most convincing in dysbaric disease and less when it comes to osteoarthritis.[127] The failure to create an experimental model counts heavily against a general acceptance of fat embolism as the common cause of osteonecrosis. Osteoarthritis can now be produced in animals by so many methods, none of them related to disturbed fat metabolism, that it seems futile to maintain the idea that fat embolism is the cause of this type of degenerative joint disorder.

Reaction of Bone Tissue in Osteoarthritis and Osteonecrosis

The gross morphological differences between osteoarthritis of the hip joint and early and late stages of nontraumatic osteonecrosis are readily observed on radiographs and in greater detail by magnetic resonance imaging.[128] Although the overall picture of nontraumatic osteonecrosis is segmental bone death, histological examinations using isotope and tetracycline labeling have demonstrated reparative bone processes in the transitional area between the sequestered and "normal" cancellous bone.[70] Rebuilding in other areas is rare and is not marked until secondary osteoarthritis has developed, which is also when the acetabulum may be involved.

Conversely, osteoarthritis is characterized by a mixture of bone destruction and repair. Histological findings of dead bone trabeculae overlaid by new bone formation, growth of osteophytes, and a general tendency for the form of the femoral head to adapt to altered mechanical demands dominate the picture. The acetabulum is involved throughout the pathological process.

From all evidence collected I conclude that both disorders to a large degree owe their pathologic development to vascular factors. Also, this evidence indicates a common background: increased resistance to venous drainage from, and capillary flow in, the femoral joint region. The difference between osteoarthritis and nontraumatic osteonecrosis seems to be one of degree.

Reaction of Various Mesenchymal Tissues to Changes in Bone Marrow Capillary Blood Flow Conditions

Rösingh and James[129] demonstrated that complete blockage of arterial inflow to bone results in the death of osteocytes within 8 to 24 hours. Although total blockage of venous drainage has the same effect on capillary flow as a blockage of arterial inflow, in most of the clinical disorders examined here total venous blockage is of short duration (intermittent venous hypertension). In most conditions the blockage is incomplete (i.e., capillary flow is more or less retarded but has not entirely ceased). Several authors have stated that a moderately severe reduction of Po_2 in bone marrow may induce new bone formation.[2,11,130–132] Evidence of reduced oxygen tension in juxtachondral bone marrow of osteoarthritic joints was presented by Brookes and Helal[133] and Pujol et al.[134] Recently, mass spectrometry measurements have confirmed these observations in both osteoarthritis and nontraumatic femoral head necrosis.[75,135,136]

Hypoxia seems to be a stimulating factor for some mesenchymal tissue activity. Stern et al.[137] studied the effect of various oxygen tensions on the synthesis and degradation of collagen in bone. With an oxygen content of 10% to 20% in the incubation medium, synthesis exceeded collagen degradation; at 30% both processes increased and at 50% the processes were equal. These observations have been confirmed several times. Thus, although anoxia results in tissue death, experimental and clinical evidence confirms that hypoxia may actually stimulate growth of mesenchymal tissues. However, my histological evidence suggests a considerable difference in the reaction of the different tissues of the juxtachondral bone marrow.

Tissue Rivalry in Low-Oxygen Environment

Osteoarthritis, rheumatoid arthritis, and especially the later stages of nontraumatic femoral head necrosis were characterized histologically by ingrowth of masses of primitive tissues into the bone marrow. In many cases they seemed to have displaced healthy soft marrow tissue and the bone trabeculae. In the apparently intact trabeculae a common finding was blockage, perhaps by fibrin thrombi in the vessels of the haversian canals, surrounded by empty cell lacunae, especially in nontraumatic osteonecrosis. The impression gained from these histological studies was dead and dying bone giving place to extremely vital and vascularized primitive fibrous tissues, sometimes transformed into or continuing as broad areas of fibrocartilage.

The conception of the sequester of the osteonecrotic femoral head as devitalized is thus not entirely correct. Isotope scintigraphy may show the sequester as a cold-in-hot area; however, because the isotopes used for diagnostic purpose are bone seeking, this cold area only indicates a substantial local decrease in anabolic and/or catabolic bone metabolism and cannot be trusted to reflect activity in other tissues.

Revascularization of the sequestered area by vessels in the soft tissue components and the tendency to clogging of the veins and venules by erythrocyte agglutinations and thrombi are probable explanations of the high pressure and the slow but pulsatile flow. In light of the experiments by Stern et al.[137] and the recent findings of low or lowered oxygen tension in the femoral head in these disorders, the predominance of primitive mesenchymal tissues could be due to their adaptability to low oxygen tensions in the environment, a characteristic absent in the more specialized bone marrow cells including the osteocytes.

Pain Relation to Intraosseous Hypertension and Venous Distension: Role of Neuropeptides

Nerves of Joints and Their Role in Vascular Synovitis

Pain is one of the main causes of disability in patients with joint disorders. In fact, pain is the deciding factor for most surgical interventions. Pain is caused by irritation of nociceptive nervous elements in the joint structures. Although hyaline cartilage is devoid of such pain receptors, investigations by conventional histological methods (e.g., silver impregnation) have demonstrated nerves in various other joint structures.[138–141] Although it is generally agreed that fasciae, tendons, ligaments, and periosteum are richly supplied with nerves, the results obtained from the synovium have varied. Thus, Harvey[142] suggested that no pain receptors are present in the synovium, whereas Kennedy et al.[141] found this structure richly innervated. In bone tissue the bone marrow trabeculae and the haversian canals were reported to contain nerve fibers[143–145] and in certain pathologic states (e.g., osteoarthritis) the number of nerves in the femoral head seems to increase.[146]

Grönblad et al.[147,148] found nerve elements staining with neurofilament antiserum perivascularly in both healthy synovium and synovium from patients with rheumatoid arthritis and osteoarthritis. Free nerve fibers were also present in these tissues, and some of them stained with antisera to the neuropeptides Substance P is a sensory transmitter and vasodilator, increases vascular permeability and thus protein extravasation, and stimulates fibroblast proliferation; calcitonin gene–related peptide is also a potent vasodilator and a sensory transmitter. Levine et al.[149] suggested that the nervous system, and more specifically the neuropeptide substance P, might be involved in the pathophysiology of rheumatoid arthritis. They noted that the joints most affected have the highest concentration of substance P, and when substance P was infused into these joints the arthritis became more severe. Konttinen et al.[150] suggest that these neuropeptides may be involved in joint dis-

ease, possibly in both pain and inflammation. The inflammatory effect they attribute to the well-known effects of both substance P and calcitonin gene–related peptide as vasodilators and to increased vascular permeability and protein extravasation.

These new observations and suggestions are interesting, as regards both the origin of pain and synovial vascular inflammation. The illustrations given by these authors show the nerve fibers in close contact with the vessel walls. Considering the sometimes extreme vascularization of the synovial membrane of osteoarthritis (the proliferative stage), for example, where most of the vessels are dilated venules, their discoveries suggest a circulus vitiosus starting with experimental osteoarthritis with inflammatory hyperemia, going on to the stasis stages, and being perpetuated by the influence of a rising content of vasodilative neuropeptides.

In some of the disorders, notably chondromalacia (PP syndromes), osteoarthritis, rheumatoid arthritis, and the late stages of nontraumatic osteonecrosis, the normally avascular and aneural joint cartilage is invaded by vascularized fibrous tissue. This tissue can be from either (as in rheumatoid arthritis and hemophilic arthropathy) the pannus covering the surface facing the joint cavity or (as in osteoarthritis and particularly chondromalacia) the tissues of the region of the osteochondral junction. According to Badalamente and Cherney[151] the invading vessels in the basal layer of the chondromalacial cartilage are accompanied by small myelinated nerves that contain substance P and serotonin. Thus, in many of the disorders dealt with here, the normally aneural and avascular hyaline cartilage may have become innervated and partly vascularized.

Finally, when considering the origin of pain, especially in connection with loading and joint movements, it should be remembered that other joint structures such as the periosteum also show an increased number of sensory nerves in arthritic joints.

Pain and Degenerative Changes in Relation to Venous Distension and Hypertension

Pain at Rest

My investigations on patients with osteoarthritis and especially the intraosseous engorgement–pain syndrome indicate that pain at rest is more closely correlated to intraosseous venous stasis than to the degree of bone marrow pressure. A priori it must be assumed that in osteoarthritis and related disorders the tissue tension in the noncompliant semiclosed medullary space leaves very little room for venous expansion (dilation) in spite of great resistance to flow and increased intraluminar pressure. In one place, however, the difference in vessel caliber between healthy bone marrow and that of patients with osteoarthritis or intraosseous engorgement–

pain syndromes is obvious to the naked eye in the phlebographs. The caliber of the small vessels around the tip of the cannula is visibly larger in the bone marrow of the disordered joint than in the marrow of the healthy side. This constant difference in small-vessel caliber is a fairly reliable indication that high resistance to venous flow is accompanied by venous distension and intraosseous hypertension.

The connection between pain and venous distension per se is perhaps most convincingly demonstrated in patients with idiopathic dysfunction of the venous pump of the calf (cruralgia orthostatica),[50,152] as described in Chapter 82. In these women the disorder is dominated by severe bursting pain in the calf. The pain is orthostatic; that is, it is felt when the patient is standing, sitting, and walking but disappears after a period with the feet up or when a sufficiently strong compression bandage is applied to the lower leg. Phlebography shows abnormally wide deep veins of the calf but with healthy valves. The contraction pressures produced by the calf muscles during walking are abnormally low, and venous leg ulcers and skeletal changes due to high systolic pressures transmitted to the subcutaneous tissues of the ankle region through incompetent perforating veins are never seen in these patients.

Thus, in patients with incompetence or dysfunction of the venous pump of the calf it is possible to distinguish quite sharply between the effects of venous hypertension and venous distension. In ambulatory systolic intermittent hypertension of the ankle degenerative changes of mesenchymal tissues dominate (induration, leg ulcers, and skeletal changes).[153] In women with cruralgia orthostatica the abnormal orthostatic deep vein distension (with activation of pain sensors) is obviously correlated to the characteristic pain suffered by these patients.

Pain During Joint Maneuvers

In osteoarthritis, nontraumatic osteonecrosis, and PP syndromes it was observed that all joint maneuvers that are usually characterized by increased pain (rotation, flexion, and loading) were accompanied by a rise in intramedullary pressure above the already high pressure at rest. In addition to the pain released from nocireceptors in other joint structures, it would be reasonable to assume that these intermittent periods of sharply increased resistance to flow coincide with periods of accentuated distension of veins, venules, sinusoids, and capillaries of the bone marrow and that this may be another source of activation of sensory transmitters.

A common clinical observation: fenestration or core decompression, which reduces intraosseous hypertension but does not denervate any structures of the femoral joint, is generally effective not only for pain at rest but also pain on joint movements and loading.

References

1. Pridie KH. The development of osteoarthritis of the hip joint. *J Bone Joint Surg (Br)*. 1952;34:153–164.

2. Harrison WH, Schajowicz F, Trueta J. Osteoarthritis of the hip: a study of the nature and evolution of the disease. *J Bone Joint Surg (Br)*. 1953;35:598–627.

3. Meriel P, Ruffie R, Fournie A. La phlebographie de la hanche dans les coxarthroses. *Rev Rhum*. 1955;22:328–341.

4. Hulth A. Circulatory disturbances in osteoarthritis of the hip. *Acta Orthop Scand*. 1958;28:81–89.

5. Helal B. *Osteoarthritis of the Knee* [dissertation]. Liverpool, England: University of Liverpool; 1962.

6. Philips RS. Phlebography in osteoarthritis of the hip. *J Bone Joint Surg (Br)*. 1966;48:280–288.

7. Arlet J, Ficat P, Sebbag D. Interet de la mesure de la pression intra medullaire dans la massif trochanterien chez l'homme. *Rev Rhum*. 1968;35:250–256.

8. Arnoldi CC, Linderholm H, Müssbichler H. Venous engorgement and intraosseous hypertension in osteoarthritis of the hip. *J Bone Joint Surg (Br)*. 1972;54:409–421.

9. Arnoldi CC, Linderholm H. Intraosseous pressure of the calcaneus and venous pressure in the calf of healthy human subjects in the erect position. *Acta Chir Scand*. 1966;132:646–662.

10. Arnoldi CC, Linderholm H. Intracalcanean pressure in patients with different forms of dysfunction of the venous pump of the calf. *Acta Chir Scand*. 1971;137:21–27.

11. Arnoldi CC, Linderholm H, Vinnerberg Å. Skeletal and soft tissue changes in patients with intracalcanean hypertension. *Acta Chir Scand*. 1972;138:25–37.

12. Arnoldi CC, Reimann I, Mortensen S, Christensen SB. The effect of joint position on juxta-articular bone marrow pressure. *Acta Orthop Scand*. 1980;51:893–897.

13. Bünger C, Harving S, Bünger EH. Intraosseous pressure in the patella in relation to simulated joint effusion and knee position: an experimental study in puppies. *Acta Orthop Scand*. 1982;53:745–753.

14. Hejgaard N, Arnoldi CC. Osteotomy of the patella in the patello-femoral pain syndrome: the significance of intraosseous pressure during sustained knee flexion. *Int Orthop*. 1984;8:189–194.

15. Arnoldi CC. Patellar pain. *Acta Orthop Scand*. 1991;(suppl 244):1–29.

16. Arnoldi CC. Vascular aspects of degenerative joint disorders: a synthesis. *Acta Orthop Scand*. 1994;(suppl 261): 1–82.

17. Tenland T. *On Laser Doppler Flowmetry: Methods and Microvascular Applications* [dissertation]. University of Linköping, Sweden: ;1982.

18. Swiontkowski MF, Ganz R, Schlegel U, Perren SM. Laser Doppler flowmetry for clinical evaluation of femoral head osteonecrosis: preliminary experience. *Clin Orthop*. 1987;218:18–26.

19. Smits GJ, Roman RJ, Lombard JH. Evaluation of laser Doppler flowmetry as measure of tissue blood flow. *J Appl Physiol*. 1986;61:666–673.

20. Hellem S, Jacobsson LS, Nilsson GE. Microvascular response in cancellous bone to halothane-induced hypotension in pigs. *Int J Oral Maxillofac Surg*. 1983;12:178–183.

21. Basset GS, Apel DM, Wintersteen VG, Tolo VT. Measurement of femoral head microcirculation by laser Doppler flowmetry. *J Pediatr Orthop.* 1991;11:307–311.

22. Vegter J, Klopper PJ. Effect of intracapsular hyperpressure on femoral head blood flow: laser Doppler flowmetry in dogs. *Acta Orthop Scand.* 1991;62:337–340.

23. Swiontkowski MF, Tepic S, Perren SM. Laser Doppler flowmetry for bone blood flow measurements, correlation with microsphere estimates, and evaluation of the effect of intracapsular pressure on femoral head blood flow. *J Orthop Res.* 1986;4:362–371.

24. Bouteiller G, Blasco A, Vigoni F, De Camps JL. The relationships between bone blood flow and intraosseous pressure. In: Arlet J, Ficat P, Hungerford DS, eds. *Bone Circulation.* Baltimore, Md: Williams & Wilkins; 1984.

25. Wilkes CH, Visscher MB. Some physiological aspects of bone marrow pressure. *J Bone Joint Surg (Am).* 1975;57:49–63.

26. Lausten GS, Arnoldi CC. Blood perfusion uneven in femoral head necrosis. *Acta Orthop Scand.* 1993;64: 533–536.

27. Arnoldi CC, Djuurhuus JC, Heerfordt J, Karle A. Intraosseous phlebography, intraosseous pressure measurements, and ^{99m}Tc-polyphosphate scintigraphy in patients with various painful conditions in the hip and knee. *Acta Orthop Scand.* 1980;51:19–28.

28. Arnoldi CC, Reimann I. The pathomechanism of human coxarthrosis. *Acta Orthop Scand.* 1979;(suppl 181):1–47.

29. Ficat P. Idiopathic bone necrosis of the femoral head. *J Bone Joint Surg (Br).* 1985;67:3–11.

30. Bohr H, Heerfordt J. Autoradiography and histology in a case of idiopathic femoral head necrosis. *Clin Orthop.* 1977;129:209–212.

31. Christensen SB. Osteoarthrosis: changes of bone, cartilage, and synovial membrane in relation to bone scintigraphy. *Acta Orthop Scand.* 1985;(suppl 214):1–43.

32. Arnoldi CC, Reimann I, Bretlau P. The synovial membrane in human coxarthrosis: light and electron microscopic studies. *Clin Orthop.* 1980;148:213–230.

33. Brånemark P-I, Ekholm R, Goldie IF, Lindström J. Synovectomy in rheumatoid arthritis: experimental, biological, and clinical aspects. *Acta Rheum Scand.* 1967;13:161–179.

34. Dryll A, Lansaman J, Cazalis H. Light and electron microscopy study of capillaries in normal and inflammatory human synovial membrane. *J Clin Pathol.* 1977;30:556–562.

35. Goldie IF. The synovial microvascular derangement in rheumatoid arthritis and osteoarthritis. *Acta Orthop Scand.* 1970;40:751–766.

36. Eyring EJ, Murray WR. The effect of joint position on the pressure of intraarticular effusion. *J Bone Joint Surg (Am).* 1964;46:1235–1241.

37. Ropes MW, Bauer W. *Synovial Fluid Changes in Joint Disease.* New York, NY: Harvard University Press; 1953.

38. Kushner I, Somerville A. Permeability of human synovial membrane to plasma proteins: relationship to molecular size and inflammation. *Arthritis Rheum.* 1971;14:560–570.

39. Pruzanski W, Russel ML, Gordon DA, Ogryzio MA. Serum and synovial fluid proteins in rheumatoid and degenerative joint diseases. *Am J Med Sci.* 1973;265:483–490.

40. Willumsen L, Friis JA. A comparative study of the protein pattern in serum and synovial fluid. *Scand J Rheum.* 1975; 4:234–245.

41. Reimann I, Arnoldi CC, Nielsen OS. Permeability of synovial membrane to plasma proteins in human coxarthrosis. *Clin Orthop.* 1980;147:296–300.

42. Laurell C-B. Quantitative estimation of proteins by electrophoresis in agarose gel containing antibodies. *Ann Biochem.* 1966;15:45–51.

43. Burnett D, Wood SM, Bradwell AR. Estimations of the Stokes radii of serum proteins for a study of protein movement from blood to amniotic fluid. *Biochem Biophys Acta.* 1976;427:231–234.

44. Felgenhauer K. Protein size and cerebrospinal fluid composition. *Klinica Wochenschrift.* 1974;52:1158–1164.

45. Renkin EM. Multiple pathways of capillary permeability. *Circ Res.* 1977;41:735–742.

46. Arnoldi CC, Lemperg RK, Linderholm H. Immediate effect of osteotomy on the intramedullary pressure of the femoral head and neck in patients with degenerative osteoarthritis. *Acta Orthop Scand.* 1971;42:357–365.

47. Lemperg RK, Arnoldi CC. The significance of intraosseous pressure in normal and diseased states, with special reference to intraosseous engorgement–pain syndrome. *Clin Orthop.* 1978;136:143–156.

48. Ficat P, Arlet J. In: Hungerford DS, ed. *Ischemia and Necrosis of Bone.* Baltimore, Md: Williams & Wilkins; 1980.

49. Arnoldi CC, Lemperg RK, Linderholm H. Intraosseous hypertension and pain in the knee. *J Bone Joint Surg (Br).* 1975;57:360–363.

50. Arnoldi CC. Physiology and pathophysiology of the venous pump of the calf. In: Eklöf B, Gjöres JE, Thulesius O, Gergquist D, eds. *Controversies in the Management of Venous Disorders.* London: Butterworths; 1989:6–23.

51. Danielsson LG. Incidence and prognosis of coxarthrosis. *Acta Orthop Scand.* 1964;(suppl 66):21–24.

52. McDevitt C, Gilbertson E, Muir H. An experimental model of osteoarthritis: early morphological and biochemical changes. *J Bone J Surg (Br).* 1977;59:24–33.

53. Christensen SB, Reimann I, Henriksen O, Arnoldi CC. Experimental osteoarthritis in rabbits: a study of 133-xenon washout rates from the synovial cavity. *Acta Orthop Scand.* 1982;53:167–174.

54. Hulth A, Lindberg L, Telhag H. Experimental osteoarthritis in rabbits. *Acta Orthop Scand.* 1970;41:522–526.

55. Lassen NA. Muscle blood flow in normal man and in patients with intermittent claudication evaluated by simultaneous 133-Xe and 24-Na clearance. *J Clin Invest.* 1964;43:1895–1911.

56. Phelps P, Steele AD, McCarthy DJ. Significance of xenon-133 clearance rate from canine and human joints. *Arthritis Rheum.* 1972;15:361–730.

57. Kofoed H. Haemodynamics and metabolism in arthrosis: studies in the rabbit knee. *Acta Orthop Scand.* 1986;57:119–122.

58. Edwall G. *Stable and Reproducible Antimony–Antimony Oxide Electrodes* [dissertation]. University of Stockholm, Sweden: 1976.

59. Grønlund J, Kofoed H, Svalastoga E. Effect of increased knee joint pressure on oxygen tension and blood flow in

subchondral bone. *Acta Physiol Scand.* 1984;121:127–133.

60. Arnoldi CC, Reimann I, Christensen SB, Mortensen S. The effect of increased intra-articular pressure on juxtachondral bone marrow pressure. *ICRS.* 1979;7:471.

61. Bünger C, Sørensen J, Djuurhuus JC, Lucht U. Intraosseous pressures in the knee in relation to simulated joint effusion, joint position, and venous obstruction. *Scand J Rheum.* 1981;10:283–291.

62. Bünger C, Harving S, Hjermind J, Bünger EH. Relationship between intraosseous pressure and intra-articular pressure in arthritis of the knee. *Acta Orthop Scand.* 1983; 54:188–201.

63. Christensen SB. Localisation of bone-seeking agents in developing experimentally induced osteoarthritis in the knee joint of the rabbit. *Scand J Rheum.* 1983;12:343–349.

64. Reimann I, Christensen SB, Diemer NH. Observation of reversibility of glycosaminoglycan depletion in articular cartilage. *Clin Orthop.* 1982;168:258–265.

65. Finsterbush A, Friedman B. Early changes in immobilized rabbit knee joints: a light and electron microscopic study. *Clin Orthop.* 1973;92:305–312.

66. Langenskjöld A, Michelsson JE, Videmann T. Osteoarthritis of the knee in the rabbit produced by immobilisation. *Acta Orthop Scand.* 1979;50:1–13.

67. Shu-zheng H, Zhenhua X, Hansen ES, Bünger C. Microvascular morphology of bone in arthrosis: scanning electron microscopy in rabbits. *Acta Orthop Scand.* 1990; 61:196–200.

68. Merle d'Aubigne R, Postel M, Dahlen DC. Idiopathic avascular necrosis of the femoral head in adults. *J Bone Joint Surg (Br).* 1965;47:612–633.

69. Patterson RJ, Bickel WH, Dahlen DC. Idiopathic avascular necrosis of the head of the femur: a study of 52 cases. *J Bone Joint Surg (Am).* 1964;46:267–283.

70. Lausten GS, Christensen SB. Distribution of ^{99m}Tc-phosphate compounds in osteonecrotic femoral heads. *Acta Orthop Scand.* 1989;60:419–423.

71. Serre H, Simon L. L'osteonecrose primitive de la tete femorale chez l'adulte, I: aspect symptomatique. *Rev Rhum.* 1962;29:527–535.

72. Arlet J. Petrochanteric phlebography in primary necrosis of the femoral head in the initial stage (stage I). In: Zinn WM, ed. *Idiopathic Ischemic Necrosis of the Femoral Head in Adults.* Stuttgart, Germany: Georg Thieme Verlag; 1971: 152–157.

73. Hungerford DS, Zizic TM. Alcoholism associated ischemic necrosis of the femoral head: early diagnosis and treatment. *Clin Orthop.* 1978;144:144–153.

74. Hungerford DS, Lennox DW. The importance of increased intraosseous pressure in the development of osteonecrosis of the femoral head: implications for treatment. *Orthop Clin North Am.* 1985;16:635–654.

75. Pedersen NW, Kiær T, Kristensen KD, Starklint H. Intraosseous pressure, oxygenation, and histology in arthrosis and osteonecrosis of the hip. *Acta Orthop Scand.* 1989; 60:415–417.

76. Kiær T, Pedersen NW, Kristensen KD, Starklint H. Intraosseous pressure, oxygen tension in avascular necrosis, and osteoarthritis of the hip. *J Bone Joint Surg (Br).* 1990; 72:1023–1030.

77. Catto M. Pathology of aseptic bone necrosis. In: Davidson JK, ed. *Aseptic Necrosis of Bone.* Amsterdam: Excerpta Medica; 1976.

78. Welfing J. Hip lesions in decompression disease. In: Zinn WM, ed. *Idiopathic Ischemic Necrosis of the Femoral Head in Adults.* Stuttgart, Germany: Georg Thieme Verlag; 1971: 103–106.

79. Atsumi T, Kuroki Y, Yamano KA. A microangiographic study of idiopathic osteonecrosis of the femoral head. *Clin Orthop.* 1989;246:186–194.

80. Riniker P, Huggler A. Idiopathic necrosis of the femoral head: a further patho-anatomical study. In: Zinn WM, ed. *Idiopathic Ischemic Necrosis of the Femoral Head in Adults.* Stuttgart, Germany: Georg Thieme Verlag; 1971:67–73.

81. Zinn WM. Idiopathic necrosis of the femoral head in adults. In: *Modern Trends in Rheumatology.* 2nd ed. London, England: Butterworths; 1971:348–365.

82. Jacqueline F, Rutishauser E. Idiopathic necrosis of the femoral head. In: Zinn WM, ed. *Idiopathic Ischemic Necrosis of the Femoral Head in Adults.* Stuttgart, Germany: Georg Thieme Verlag; 1971:34–48.

83. Kahlstrom SC, Burton CC, Phemister DB. Aseptic necrosis of bone, I: infarction of bone in Caisson disease resulting in encapsulated and calcified areas in diaphyses and in arthritis deformans. *Surg Gynecol Obstet.* 1939;68:129–146.

84. Jones JP, Englemann EP, Jajarian JS. Systemic fat embolism after renal homotransplantation and treatment with corticosteroids. *N Engl J Med.* 1965;273:1453–1458.

85. Jones JP. Fat embolism and osteonecrosis. *Orthop Clin North Am.* 1985;16:595–633.

86. Glimcher MJ, Kenzora JE. The biology of osteonecrosis of the human femoral head and its clinical implications. *Clin Orthop.* 1979;140:273–296.

87. Solomon L. Drug-induced arthropathy and necrosis of the femoral head. *J Bone Joint Surg (Br).* 1973;55:247–261.

88. Hungerford DS. Bone marrow pressure, venography, and core decompression in ischemic necrosis of the femoral head. In: *The Hip: Proceedings of the Seventh Open Scientific Meeting of the Hip Society.* St Louis, Mo: CV Mosby; 1979: 218–237.

89. Lausten GS, Mathiesen B. Core decompression for femoral head necrosis. *Acta Orthop Scand.* 1990;61:1–5.

90. Arnoldi CC. Intraosseous pressure in juxtachondral bone during loading and joint movements [editorial]. *ARCO Newsletter.* 1990;2.

91. Proposition of a classification of bone necrosis. *ARCO Newsletter.* 1989; 1.

92. Starklint H, Lausten GS, Arnoldi CC. Microvascular obstruction in avascular necrosis: immunohistochemistry of 14 femoral heads. *Acta Orthop Scand.* 1995;66:9–12.

93. Lucht U, Djuurhuus JC, Sørensen SS. The relationship between increasing intraarticular pressure and intraosseous pressures in the juxtaarticular bone. *Acta Orthop Scand.* 1981;52:491–497.

94. Soto-Hall R, Johnson LH, Johnson RA. Variations in the intra-articular pressure of the hip joint in injury and disease: a probable factor in avascular necrosis. *J Bone Joint Surg (Am).* 1964;46:509–516.

95. Egund N, Nilsson LT, Strömquist B. Hemarthrosis after femoral neck fracture fixation. *Acta Orthop Scand.* 1988; 59:526–529.

96. Strömquist B, Nilsson LT, Egund N. Intracapsular pressures in undisplaced fractures of the femoral neck. *J Bone Joint Surg (Br)*. 1988;70:192–194.

97. Arnoldi CC, Linderholm H. Fracture of the femoral neck, I: vascular disturbances in different types of fractures, assessed by measurements of intraosseous pressure. *Clin Orthop*. 1972;84:116–127.

98. Vegter J, Lubsen CC. Fractional necrosis of the femoral epiphysis after transient increase in joint pressure: an experimental study in juvenile rabbits. *J Bone Joint Surg (Br)*. 1987;69:530–535.

99. Svalastoga E, Kiær T, Jensen PE. The effect of intracapsular pressure and extension of the hip on oxygenation of the juvenile femoral epiphysis. *J Bone Joint Surg (Br)*. 1989; 71:222–226.

100. Kristensen KD, Kiær T, Pedersen NW. Intraosseous Po_2 in femoral neck fracture: restoration of blood flow after aspiration of haemarthrosis in undisplaced fractures. *Acta Orthop Scand*. 1989;60:303–304.

101. Harper WM, Barnes MR, Gregg PJ. Femoral head blood flow in femoral neck fractures. *J Bone Joint Surg (Br)*. 1991; 73:73–75.

102. Jayson MI, Dixon AS. Intra-articular pressure in rheumatoid arthritis of the knee, III: pressure changes during joint use. *Ann Rheum Dis*. 1970;29:401–408.

103. Boersma W, van Limborgh J. Experimental investigations on the development of the ulcus cruris in the frog, I: the effects of increased mean venous pressure. II: the effects of intermittently increased venous pressure. *Folia Angiol*. 1967;9:448–454.

104. Zweifach BW. The structural basis of permeability and other functions of blood capillaries (Cold Spring Harbor Symposia). *Quant Biol*. 1940;8:216–223.

105. Burch GE, Sodeman WA. Studies in tissue pressure. *Proc Soc Exp Biol Med*. 1937;36:256–258.

106. Wells HS, Youmans JB, Miller DG. Tissue pressure as related to venous pressure, capillary filtration, and other factors. *J Clin Invest*. 1938;17:489–498.

107. Burton C, Yamada S. Relation between blood pressure and flow in the human forearm. *J Appl Physiol*. 1951;4: 329–341.

108. Ryder HW, Molle WE, Ferris EB. The influence of the collapsibility of veins on venous pressure, including a new procedure for measuring tissue pressure. *J Clin Invest*. 1944;23:333–341.

109. Nielsen HV. *Effects of Increased Tissue Pressure on Regional Blood Flow in the Lower Limb of Man* [thesis]. Copenhagen, Denmark: Lægeforeningens Forlag; 1984.

110. Wong SY, Evans RA, Needs C. The pathogenesis of osteoarthritis of the hip: evidence for primary osteocyte death. *Clin Orthop*. 1987;214:305–312.

111. Jones JP. Alcoholism, hypercortisonism, fat embolism, and osseous avascular necrosis. In: Zinn WM, ed. *Ischemic Necrosis of the Femoral Head in Adults*. Stuttgart, Germany: Georg Thieme Verlag; 1971:112–132.

112. Jacobs B. Epidemiology of traumatic and non-traumatic osteonecrosis. *Clin Orthop*. 1978;130:51–67.

113. Fisher DE, Bickel WH. Corticosteroid-induced avascular necrosis: a clinical study of seventy-seven patients. *J Bone Joint Surg (Am)*. 1971;53:859–873.

114. Cruess RL. Osteonecrosis of bone: current concepts as to etiology and pathogenesis. *Clin Orthop*. 1986;208:30–39.

115. Paolaggi JB. Early alterations of bone and marrow after high doses of steroids: results in two animal species. In: Arlet J, Ficat P, Hungerford DS, eds. *Bone Circulation*. Baltimore, Md: Williams & Wilkins; 1984:42–47.

116. Surat A. Isolation of prostaglandin E_2–like material from osteonecrosis induced by steroids and its prevention by kallikrein-inhibitor, aprotinin. An experimental study in rabbits. *Prostaglandins Leukot Med*. 1984;13:159–167.

117. Kawai T, Tamki A, Hirohata K. Steroid-induced accumulation of lipid in the osteocytes of the rabbit femoral head: a histochemical and electron microscopic study. *J Bone Joint Surg (Am)*. 1985;67:755–763.

118. Kenzora JE, Steel RE, Yosipovitch ZH, Glimcher MJ. Experimental osteonecrosis in the femoral head in adult rabbits. *Clin Orthop*. 1978;130:8–46.

119. Wang G-J. Cortisone-induced intrafemoral head pressure change and its response to a drilling decompression method. *Clin Orthop*. 1981;159:274–278.

120. Wang G-J, Rawles JG, Hubbard SL. Steroid-induced femoral head pressure changes and their response to lipid clearing agents. *Clin Orthop*. 1983;174:298–302.

121. Jaffe WL, Epstein M, Heyman N, Mankin HJ. The effect of cortisone on femoral and humeral heads in rabbits. *Clin Orthop*. 1972;82:221–228.

122. Gold EW. Corticoid-induced avascular necrosis: an experimental study in rabbits. *Clin Orthop*. 1978;135:272–280.

123. Sikorski JM. Venous thrombosis produced by the local injection of fat. *J Bone Joint Surg (Br)*. 1983;65:340–354.

124. Bradford DS, Foster RR, Nosel HL. Coagulation alterations, hypoxemia, and fat embolism in fracture patients. *Trauma*. 1970;10:307–321.

125. Philp RB. A review of blood changes associated with compression–decompression: relation to decompression sickness. *Undersea Biomedical Research*. 1974;1:117–150.

126. Mulligan WH, Briggs JD, Canavan A, Catto M. Unpublished observations. Cited by: Catto M. Pathology of aseptic bone necrosis. In: Davidson JK, ed. *Aseptic Necrosis of Bone*. Amsterdam: Excerpta Medica; 1976.

127. Jones JP Jr. Fat embolism, intravascular coagulation, and osteonecrosis. *Clin Orthop*. 1993;292:294–308.

128. Steinberg ME, Hayken GD, Steinberg DR. A new method for evaluation and staging of avascular necrosis of the femoral head. In: Arlet J, Ficat P, Hungerford DS, eds. *Bone Circulation*. Baltimore, Md: Williams & Wilkins; 1984: 398.

129. Rösingh GE, James J. Early phases of avascular necrosis of the femoral head in rabbits. *J Bone Joint Surg (Br)*. 1969; 51:165–174.

130. Pistolesi GF. Il circulo venoso profondo dell'anca nell'ártrosi. Russegna internationale del film scientifici-diduttio. Universita di Padova, Italia; 1962.

131. Abdalla ABE, Harrison RG. Observations on the reaction of tubular bone to venous stasis. *J Anat*. 1966;100: 627–638.

132. Philips RS, Bulmer JH, Hoyle G, Davies W. Venous drainage in osteoarthritis of the hip. *J Bone Joint Surg (Br)*. 1967;49:301–309.

133. Brookes M, Helal B. Primary osteoarthritis, venous engorgement, and osteogenesis. *J Bone Joint Surg (Br)*. 1968; 50:493–502.

134. Pujol M, Tran M-A, Arlet J. Premiers resultats d'une etude gasometrique de sang osseux trochanterien dans les coxopathies. *Rev Rhum.* 1973;40:515–521.

135. Kiær T, Sørensen KK, Grønlund J. Intraosseous pressures of oxygen and carbon dioxide in coxarthrosis. *Acta Orthop Scand.* 1986;57:115–121.

136. Svalastoga E. *Local Tissue Hypoxia in the Pathogenesis of Osteoarthritis* [dissertation]. Copenhagen, Denmark: Royal Veterinary and Agricultural University; 1988.

137. Stern B, Glimcher MJ, Goldhaber P. The effect of various oxygen tensions on the synthesis and degradation of bone collagen in tissue culture. *Proc Soc Exp Biol Med.* 1966;121:869–872.

138. Kellgren JH, Samuel EP. The sensitivity and innervation of the articular capsule. *J Bone Joint Surg (Br).* 1950;32:85–92.

139. Samuel EP. The autonomic and somatic innervation of the articular capsule. *Anat Rec.* 1952;113:84–92.

140. Ralston HJ III, Miller MR, Kasahara M. Nerve endings in human fasciae, tendons, ligaments, periosteum, and joint synovial membrane. *Anat Rec.* 1960;36:137–147.

141. Kennedy JC, Alexander IJ, Hayers KC. Nerve supply of the human knee and its functional importance. *Am J Sports Med.* 1982;10:329–335.

142. Harvey AR. Neurophysiology of rheumatic pain. *Clin Rheumatol.* 1987;1:1–26.

143. Milgram JW, Robinson RA. An electron microscopic demonstration of unmyelinated nerves in the haversian canals of the adult dog. *Bull Johns Hopkins Hosp.* 1965;117:63–73.

144. Cooper NS. Arthritis and the rheumatic diseases. *Journal of the American Physical Therapy Association.* 1964;44:574–589.

145. Sherman MS. The nerves of bone. *J Bone Joint Surg (Am).* 1963;45:522–528.

146. Reimann I, Christensen SB. A histological demonstration of nerves in subchondral bone. *Acta Orthop Scand.* 1977;48:345–358.

147. Grönblad M, Konttinen YT, Korkala O. Neuroanatomical basis for pain reception in joint disease. XXII Scandinavian Congress of Rheumatology, Reykjavik, Iceland. *Scand J Rheumatol.* 1988;(suppl 72):39.

148. Grönblad M, Konttinen YT, Korkala O. Neuropeptides in the synovium of patients with rheumatoid arthritis and osteoarthritis. *J Rheumatol.* 1988;15:1807–1810.

149. Levine JD, Clark R, Devor M. Intraneuronal substance P contributes to the severity of experimental arthritis. *Science.* 1984;226:547–549.

150. Konttinen YT, Grönblad M, Hukkanen E. Pain fibers in osteoarthritis: a review. *Semin Arthritis Rheum.* 1989;18:35–40.

151. Badalamente MA, Cherney SB. Periosteal and vascular innervation of the human patella in degenerative joint disease. *Semin Arthritis Rheum.* 1989;18(suppl 2):61–65.

152. Arnoldi CC, Linderholm H. Venous blood pressures at rest and during exercise in patients with idiopathic dysfunction of the venous pump of the calf. *Acta Chir Scand.* 1969;135:601–609.

153. Arnoldi CC, Linderholm H. On the pathogenesis of the venous leg ulcer. *Acta Chir Scand.* 1968;134:427–440.

84

Internal Valvuloplasty: Surgical Technique, Valve Location, Indication, Quantitative Assessment, and Long-Term Follow-Up

V. S. Sottiurai

Whether single or multiple valvuloplasty is needed to correct deep vein valve incompetence of the lower extremity is controversial. For technical expedience valvuloplasty is often performed in the proximal superficial femoral or common femoral vein.[1-6] However, Gooley and Sumner[7] and Shull et al.[8] have independently demonstrated the relationship of venous reflux and the physiologic advantage of popliteal valve over femoral valve correction. This concept was supported by Bry and associates[9] in valve transfer to the popliteal vein. In a prospective randomized study of 38 valvuloplasties performed in the proximal to mid superficial femoral valve ($n = 15$), the femoropopliteal valve at the adductor hiatus ($n = 15$), and the popliteal valve ($n = 8$), Sottiurai has demonstrated the hemodynamic advantage of the juxtapopliteal or popliteal valvulo-plasty over femoral valvuloplasty (Table 84.1). His cumulative data on valvuloplasty performed exclusively at the femoropopliteal junction ($n = 98$) and popliteal vein ($n = 33$) further emphasized the theory of the hemodynamic advantage of popliteal valve over superficial femoral or common femoral valve reconstruction (Table 84.2).

In this chapter I address (1) the hemodynamic, durability, and efficacy of popliteal vein over superficial femoral vein valvuloplasty; (2) the technique of internal valvuloplasty; (3) the value of intravenous pressure in the assessment of venous reflux and extravalvular reflux via collateral veins before, during, and after valvuloplasty; and (4) the value of using elastic stockings and a pneumatic compression pump to control superficial venous hypertension.

TABLE 84.1. Comparison of valve competence in proximal superficial versus femeropopliteal valves at adductor hiatus and popliteal open valvuloplasty.

Site	No.	Follow-up (mo)	Valve competence (initial)	Intravenous pressure improvement	Valve competence (late)	Venous ulcer
Proximal superficial femoral valve	15	10–49 (32)	12/15	13/15	8/15	2/5
Femoropopliteal valve at adductor hiatus	15	3–46 (30)	15/15	15/15	14/15	None
Popliteal valve	8	12–57 (36)	8/8	8/8	8/8	None

Mean times are in parentheses.

TABLE 84.2. Comparison of results following valvuloplasty of a valve near the adductor hiatus and in the popliteal vein.

Site	No.	Follow-up (mo)	Valve competence	
			Early	Late
Femoropopliteal valve at adductor hiatus	98	9–152 (72)	96/98 (97.9%)	73/98 (74.6%)
Popliteal valve	33	8–150 (63)	32/33 (96.9%)	26/33 (78.8%)

Diagnostic Evaluation and Patient Selection

A total of 131 limbs from 120 nonindigent patients (68 men and 52 women) with a mean age of 54 years were treated with deep vein valvuloplasty for Kistner's grades III and IV venous reflux.[10] Preoperative and postoperative descending venography and intravenous pressure measurements via the dorsal vein of the foot in a supine position, >45-degree reversed Trendelenburg's position with and without Valsalva's maneuver and during standing and ambulation were the standard protocols.

Impedance plethysmography was replaced by duplex scan in 1986. Air plethysmography (APG) was added to the diagnostic protocol in 1990 to complement photoplethysmography. Ascending and descending venographies were performed on patients who were candidates for venous reconstruction. Only patients with intractable ulcers, swelling, and pain not improved with pneumatic compression pump and compression stockings for more than 6 months were considered for valvuloplasty. Coagulopathy survey for antithrombin III, protein C, protein S, fibrinogen factor V Leiden, and plasminogen levels was part of the patient evaluation.

For the surgical techniques,[11,12] a medial thigh incision was used for superficial femoral or popliteal valve exposure. The adductor tendon was detached from the femur to allow access to the popliteal fossa. Incompetent valves located at the adductor hiatus occurred in >90% of patients. Vein segments with incompetent valves in the femoral vein, femoropopliteal vein junction, or popliteal vein were occluded with atraumatic vascular clamps. A supravalvular transverse venotomy encompassing 60% of the circumference of the vein was made with right-angle Potts scissors. A vertical venotomy originating at the midpoint of the transverse venotomy was extended into the valvular sinus using right-angle Potts scissors. Commissures and valve cusps were brought into view by retracting the venous flaps laterally using 6-O polypropylene sutures (Figure 84.1). Double-ended 7-O Prolene sutures inserted obliquely through the valve cusps and vein wall from opposite directions and tied externally at each commissure were repeated to suspend and tighten the loose valve cusps. Multiple tacking at each commissure was needed to produce tight apposition of the valve cusps (Figure 84.2). The vertical venotomy was closed with running 6-O Prolene sutures. The transverse venotomy was approximated with 6-O Prolene sutures using running stitches with frequent interruption to prevent suture-line stricture (Figure 84.3).

A strip test was used before and after valvuloplasty for qualitative assessment of valve competence. Intravenous pressures obtained via the dorsal vein of the foot in supine and 45-degree reversed Trendelenburg's positions with and without Valsalva's maneuver (>50 mm

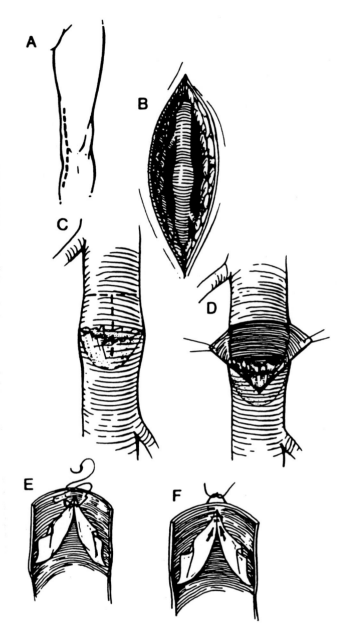

FIGURE 84.1. Vein valve exposure and valvuloplasty: **A,** Vertical skin incision at the medial aspect of the distal thigh. **B,** Femoral vein exposed through a vertical incision. **C,** Transverse and vertical venotomies as indicated by broken lines. **D,** Vein flaps retracted laterally with suture to display the valve cusps. **E,** Double-ended suture used to suspend valve cusps at the commissure. **F,** Ties placed outside of the vein to tack valve cusps to the venous wall.

Hg) were more accurate and reliable to quantitatively determine valve competence and venous reflux (Figure 84.3). Intraoperative Valsalva's maneuver was performed by changing the mechanical mode of ventilation to manual mode using an Ambu bag to increase and maintain the airway pressure gauge to more than 50 mm Hg while intravenous pressures were recorded via a foot vein with the transducer maintained at the same level. Valsalva's

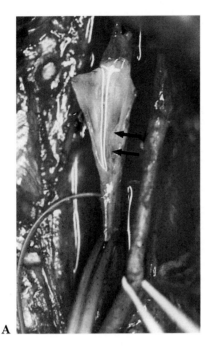
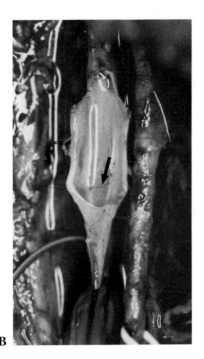
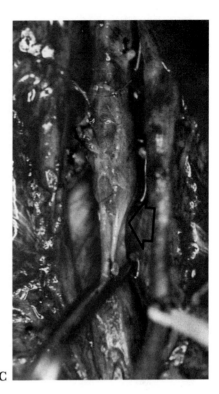

FIGURE 84.2. Femoropopliteal valvuloplasty performed on a valve near the adductor hiatus using supravalvular open technique: **A,** Transverse and vertical venotomies allow exposure of redundant valve leaflet by retracting the venous flap laterally. Note redundant valve leaflets (arrow). **B,** The edge of each valve cusp is tightly apposed after multiple tacking using 7-O polypropylene stitches (arrow). **C,** Completion of open valvuloplasty revealed a competent valve in a 45-degree reversed Trendelenburg's position with >50 mm Hg Valsalva's maneuver (arrow).

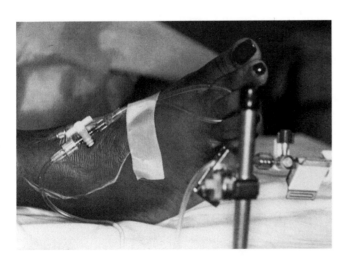

FIGURE 84.3. A 20-gauge angiocatheter was placed in a dorsal vein of the foot for intravenous pressure measurements in a supine and 45-degree reversed Trendelenburg's position intraoperatively. Preoperative and postoperative standing and ambulatory intravenous pressures were also taken with and without Valsalva's maneuver (>50 mm Hg) by placing the transducer at the level of the Intracath.

maneuver often produced venous reflux in a vein with a negative strip test (Figures 84.4 and 84.5A). Venous reflux became more pronounced when patients were placed in the reversed Trendelenburg's position in excess of 45 degrees with Valsalva's maneuver (Figure 84.5B). The diameter of the vein often enlarged by 20% to 30% while Valsalva's maneuver was being performed and even more so in the reversed Trendelenburg's position. More tacking was needed when valve reflux persisted, which was rare.[12] I do not routinely use external wrapping of the vein after valvuloplasty unless the vein is excessively thin and dilated. My initial prospective randomized comparison of external wrapping using polytetrafluoroethylene was inconclusive.

Determination of Data

No postoperative venous thrombosis or valve disruption from valvuloplasty was documented by duplex scan and descending venography. Intravenous pressure improvement after valvuloplasty was a consistent and statistical

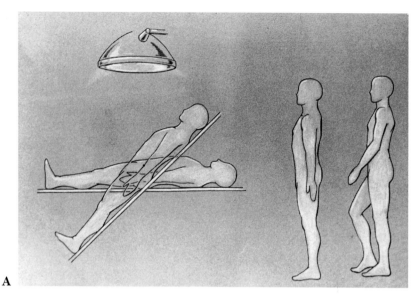

FIGURE 84.4. **A,** Various positions (supine, reversed Trendelenburg's, standing, and ambulatory) in which the recordings of intravenous pressure were taken via a foot vein with the transducer positioned at the site of angiocatheter placement. Intravenous pressures were taken with and without Valsalva's maneuver (>50 mm Hg). **B,** Changes of mean intravenous pressure before and after valvuloplasty in supine, 45-degree incline, and ambulation positions with and without Valsalva's maneuver (>50 mm Hg).

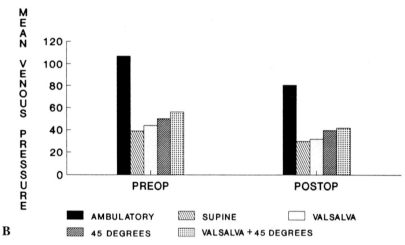

B

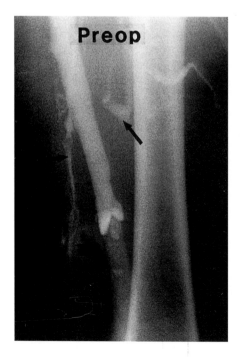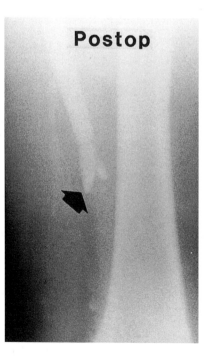

FIGURE 84.5. Prevalvuloplasty and postvalvuloplasty collateral venous reflux via collateral veins: **A,** Preoperative descending venogram shows mild collateral venous reflux (small solid arrow). Large solid arrow indicates the incompetent valve near the adductor hiatus of the femoropopliteal vein for open valvuloplasty. **B,** Descending venogram after valvuloplasty reveals that function of the preoperative incompetent femoropopliteal valve near the adductor hiatus was restored (large solid arrow). However, reflux via the collateral vein located superior to the valve that underwent valvuloplasty was markedly accentuated (small solid arrow).

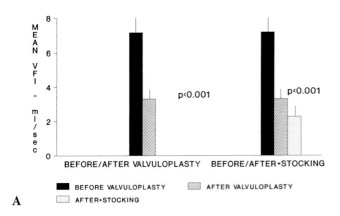

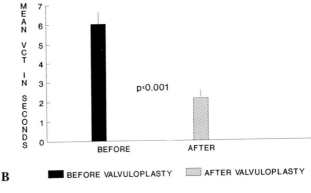

A

B

FIGURE 84.6. **A,** Comparison of venous filling indices (VFI) of air plethysmography demonstrating improvement of venous reflux following valvuloplasty and elastic stocking application. Normal VFI = <2 mL/s. **B,** Comparison of valve closure time (VCT) in duplex analysis before and after valvuloplasty. Normal valve closure time is <1 second.

observation. Similar findings were seen with APG and duplex scanning (Figure 84.6). Intraoperative Valsalva's maneuver was particularly useful in the assessment of valve competence and collateral vein reflux. Division of the collateral veins significantly reduced extravalvular reflux and reduced intravenous pressure. Valsalva's maneuver in reversed Trendelenburg's position not only demonstrated collateral reflux but also identified inade-

quate valvuloplasty (Figure 84.5). Large vein and dilated saphenous vein were the major sources of reflux. Transposition of saphenous vein or accessory femoral vein distal to the site of valvuloplasty is useful in avoiding the need for saphenous stripping (Figure 84.7).

Postoperatively, as determined by descending venography, APG, and duplex scan, 15 of 15 femoropopliteal valves were competent, 8 of 8 popliteal valves were com-

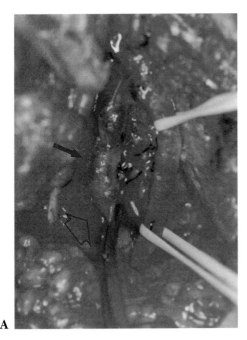

A

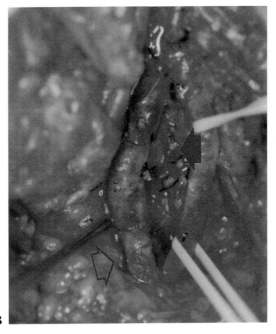

B

FIGURE 84.7. **A,** After valvuloplasty the incompetent valve became competent even with Valsalva's maneuver (>50 mm Hg) in reversed Trendelenburg's position. **B,** The adjacent large collateral vein located to the right was ligated and tied with 3-O silk (solid arrow). The inferior transected end of the vein was transposed to the femoropopliteal vein near the adductor hiatus in an end-to-side configuration (open arrow). Valvuloplasty was located cephalad to the vein transposition. **C,** Descending venograms before and after valvuloplasty and vein transposi-

tion. Preoperative: solid arrow points to incompetent valve to undergo valvuloplasty; open arrow points to incompetent valve of adjacent large collateral vein. Preoperative: solid arrow points to incompetent valve to undergo valvuloplasty; open arrow points to incompetent valve to undergo transposition. Multiple small white solid arrows indicate venous reflux below the knee. Postoperative: solid arrow points to competent valve of the vein after valvuloplasty; open arrow indicates ligated end of adjacent large collateral vein.

petent, and 12 of 15 middle superficial femoral valves were competent (Table 84.1). Late valve incompetence (mean 34-month follow-up) occurred in 8 of 15 patients who had undergone superficial femoral valvuloplasty versus 1 of 23 who had undergone femoropopliteal valvuloplasty ($P < .001$). Of the 15 limbs treated with superficial femoral valvuloplasty, 2 developed recurrent venous ulcers in comparison to 0 of 23 for femoropopliteal and popliteal valvuloplasty ($P < .05$).[13]

In a retrospective review of 131 valvuloplasties, 73 of 98 (74.5%) femoropopliteal valves were competent and 26 of 33 (78.8%) popliteal valves were competent after a mean follow-up of 72 months. Recurrent venous ulcers in this series were seen in 32 of 131 (24.4%) limbs. Valve competence and ulcer healing were comparable in valvuloplasty performed at the femoropopliteal junctions and in the popliteal veins (Table 84.2).

A correlation also exists in the recurrence of valve incompetence and ulcer redevelopment. In this study, the recurrent ulcers were managed by subfascial ligation and saphenous stripping ($n = 18$) and multiple-incision subfascial ligation and varicose vein excisions ($n = 14$). Except for women who did not work outside the home ($n = 14$) and retirees ($n = 22$), 95 (72.5%) patients returned to full employment after venous valvular reconstruction.

Discussion

Numerous techniques have been proposed to correct valve incompetence of the lower extremities. Kistner's innovation in transcommissure open valvuloplasty in 1975[4] and closed external valvuloplasty in 1990 has become the cornerstone of venous valve reconstruction of the lower extremities.[1,3,4,6] Raju in 1983 and Sottiurai in 1988 proposed supravalvuloplasty using a transverse venotomy and combined transverse and vertical venotomies, respectively.[5,11] Jessup and Lane in 1988 advocated external wrapping to restore competence to the valve without the need for a venotomy.[14] Psathakis[15] claimed success in using a fascial or synthetic sling to intermittently interrupt venous flow at the popliteal vein to regulate venous return. The opponents of venous valve repair tend to adhere to the concept that all leg ulcers can be healed with bed rest, leg elevation, and elastic stocking or Unna boot.

Perhaps the confusion of ulcer healing resides in the definitions of *healed ulcer* and *recurrent ulcer*. The term *healed ulcer* implies that no additional ulcer develops after the initial healing. Ulcers that have healed and then recur should be classified as recurrent ulcers. Subscribing to this strict and precise definition prevents confusion about ulcer healing and recognizes the successes of ulcer treatment. Similarly, a uniform parameter to deter-

mine valve competence and venous reflux is needed to assess the immediate and long-term results of valvuloplasty. Until such criteria are established, success in valvuloplasty will remain controversial and inconsistent. Our method of determining success in valvuloplasty can be enumerated as follows: (1) ulcer heals permanently; (2) valve competence is restored and confirmed by APG, duplex scan, and descending venogram; (3) intraoperative venous pressure improves with Valsalva's maneuver (>50 mm Hg) in reversed Trendelenburg's position; and (4) the postoperative descending venography shows cessation of venous reflux in the repaired valve in a 45- to 60-degree inclined position with Valsalva's maneuver.

Whether single or multiple valvuloplasty is needed to correct venous reflux has been the subject of debate. For technical expedience and easy accessibility, internal valvuloplasty is often performed in the proximal superficial femoral or common femoral vein. Multiple internal valvuloplasty is not a common practice due to uncertainty about its need, its time-consuming nature, and its technical demands. However, the technical ease of external valvuloplasty introduced by Kistner[6] has encouraged the practice of femoral and tibial valve reconstruction reported by S. Raju.[16]

Whether single valvuloplasty is adequate to prevent venous reflux and correct valve incompetence depends on the following factors: (1) site of valvuloplasty with an optimal hemodynamic effect, (2) control of collateral vein reflux, (3) durability of the repaired valve, and (4) extent of saphenous and superficial vein reflux.

Retrospective and randomized prospective comparisons of valvuloplasty for superficial femoral veins, femoropopliteal junctions, and popliteal veins suggest that valvuloplasty performed in the femoropopliteal and popliteal veins produced comparable results and has offered the following advantages over valvuloplasty in the superficial femoral and common femoral veins:

1. The femoropopliteal and popliteal valves are located close to the calf muscle pump (the important driving force of venous return from the leg).
2. The popliteal vein is anatomically and physiologically analogous to the gateway between the tibial veins and thigh veins.
3. The termination of the popliteal vein is frequently solitary with a single valve located near the adductor hiatus.
4. The popliteal vein is formed by a confluence of converging tibial veins.[17]
5. Collateral veins are more numerous adjacent to the superficial femoral and deep femoral veins than the popliteal vein.

Division of collateral veins to control extravalvular reflux can be achieved more easily at the adductor hiatus and popliteal fossa, where collateral veins are fewer in number and lie juxtaposed to the popliteal vein. In contradistinction, collateral veins that connect with the superficial femoral vein are numerous and widely distributed. Many are located beyond the limits of the operating field in the thigh (Figure 84.8B).

The durability of internal valvuloplasty has been well established by numerous studies.[11,12,16,17] After a mean follow-up of 72 months (8–152 months), valve competence after valvuloplasty in a retrospective review was seen in more than 74% of patients.[17] Conversely, there is no documented long-term study that includes follow-up data for valve competence of patients who have undergone external valvuloplasty. In our experience, valve incompetence recurred in patients who had undergone external valvuloplasty ($n = 12$) 5 to 11 months after the operation.[17]

Like collateral vein reflux, saphenous and superficial vein reflux can significantly enhance the intravenous pressure. Although saphenous vein ligation is considered an acceptable mode of treatment, I prefer (1) great

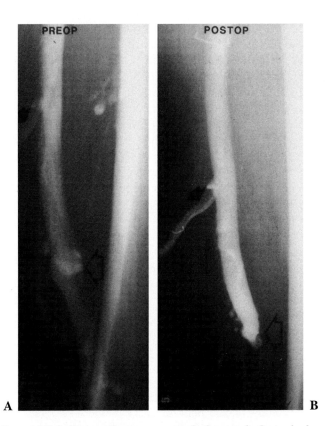

A   **B**

FIGURE 84.8. Descending venograms before and after valvuloplasty of the femoropopliteal vein junction near the adductor hiatus: **A,** Solid arrow indicates mild collateral venous reflux before correction of incompetent valve near adductor hiatus (large open arrow). **B,** Solid arrow indicates enhanced venous reflux via collateral veins above the valvuloplasty of the femoropopliteal vein near the adductor hiatus (large open arrow).

and small saphenous vein stripping and varicose cluster excision or (2) distal saphenous to femoropopliteal vein transposition and stripping of the incompetent proximal saphenous vein. Tightly fitted thigh-length elastic stockings (>45 mm Hg) can reduce the saphenous and superficial vein reflux and improve the intravenous pressure obtained via the dorsal veins of the foot or APG (Figures 84.3 and 84.6A).

Prospective randomized valvuloplasty performed in the proximal to middle superficial femoral vein, femoropopliteal vein at the adductor hiatus, and popliteal vein has demonstrated that (1) early venous reflux and valve incompetence are more prevalent in superficial femoral valvuloplasty (3 of 15) than femoropopliteal and popliteal valvuloplasty (0 of 23) ($P < .01$), (2) late recurring valve incompetence is more common in the superficial femoral valve (7 of 15) than in the valves of the femoropopliteal junction or the popliteal vein (1 of 23) ($P < .001$), (3) leg ulcers recurred more often in extremities that underwent superficial femoral valvuloplasty (2 of 15 versus 0 of 23) ($P < .05$) after a mean follow-up of 32 months (3–57 months),[18] and (4) collateral vein reflux occurred more after superficial femoral vein valvuloplasty than femoropopliteal or popliteal vein valvuloplasty. Similar results were seen in the previously mentioned study of valvuloplasty for 131 limbs performed at the femoropopliteal junction ($n = 98$) and the popliteal vein ($n = 33$).

The improved valve function and reduced venous reflux documented by APG, duplex scan, descending venography, and intravenous pressure quantitation (Tables 84.1 and 84.2 and Figures 84.4B and 84.6) after valvuloplasty of the popliteal vein or the junction of the femoropopliteal veins is in agreement with the theoretical advantage recognized by Gooley and Sumner[7] and Shull et al.[8] regarding the relation between the popliteal valve and venous reflux. The data also support the tenet that single valvuloplasty can adequately correct the venous reflux when performed (1) near the muscle pump of the leg, (2) in the solitary valve of the popliteal vein or junction of the femoral and popliteal veins, (3) with division of the adjacent collateral vein or elimination of the saphenous reflux, and (4) with transposition of large accessory superficial femoral or distal saphenous veins to the vein undergoing valvuloplasty (Figure 84.7A,B). Postoperative descending venography has demonstrated repeatedly that restoring competence to the valve at the femoropopliteal junction or popliteal vein also reduces venous reflux in the superficial femoral valves. This observation illustrates the anatomical and hemodynamic importance of the popliteal valve and its ability to influence the function of other preceding valves in the superficial femoral vein (Figure 84.9).[17,18]

On the basis of 131 valvuloplasties performed in venous valves located at the femoropopliteal junction

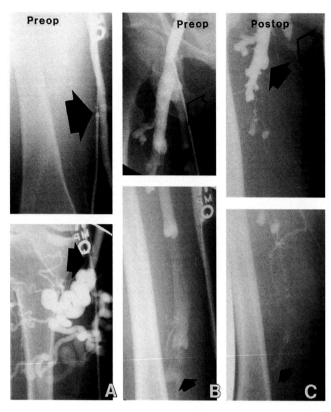

FIGURE 84.9. Descending venograms before and after valvuloplasty of the femoropopliteal junction near the adductor hiatus: **A,** Large incompetent saphenous vein with extensive varicosity below the knee (medium solid arrow). Large solid arrow points to saphenous vein in the thigh. **B,** Large open arrow points to saphenous vein with reflux at the saphenofemoral junction. Large solid arrow indicates incompetent proximal superficial femoral valve followed by a series of incompetent valves with venous reflux. Midsize solid arrow indicates valve located near adductor hiatus that has been selected for valvuloplasty. **C,** Large open arrow points to great saphenous vein ligation at the saphenofemoral junction after saphenous vein stripping. Large solid arrow indicates competence of the proximal superficial femoral valve and a series of superficial femoral valves with minimal reflux after restoring competence to the femoropopliteal valve at the adductor hiatus with valvuloplasty (midsize solid arrow).

($n = 98$) and the popliteal vein ($n = 33$), plus the supportive data derived from the prospective randomized study, a favorable conclusion of the value and adequacy of single valvuloplasty is unequivocal. Single valvuloplasty is functionally more effective when performed in valves located at the femoropopliteal junction or in the popliteal vein than in the proximal to middle femoral vein. Multilevel valvuloplasty, including the tibial valve, may be needed when valvuloplasty is not performed close to the calf muscle pump (i.e., common femoral or proximal superficial femoral valvuloplasty). The time required to perform multiple valvuloplasty outweighs the

unproven potential benefits, particularly when single valvuloplasty in the popliteal vein has already established its effectiveness. To date no long-term data favor multilevel valvuloplasty over valvuloplasty performed in the popliteal vein or at the femoropopliteal vein junction. Similarly, no long-term results are available for angioscopic-assisted single external valvuloplasty performed in the common femoral valve; a hemodynamic advantage over external valvuloplasty performed in the same site has not been established.

Conclusion

Single valvuloplasty is effective and corrects venous reflux when performed in the popliteal vein or at the femoropopliteal junction. Anatomically and physiologically, the popliteal vein functions strategically as a gateway between the confluence of the calf veins and the thigh veins. Collateral veins near the vein undergoing valvuloplasty should be ligated to reduce venous reflux. Large collateral veins or saphenous veins with incompetent valves should be transposed to the vein undergoing valvuloplasty to channel venous flow through a newly restored competent valve. A strip test performed in the pressure neutral supine position is inadequate in assessing valve competence without Valsalva's maneuver (>50 mm Hg). Intravenous pressure recorded via a foot vein is useful in determining the competence of the repaired valve and venous reflux of the collateral and saphenous veins. When patients are in reversed Trendelenburg's position with Valsalva's maneuver the accuracy in the assessment of valve competence and venous reflux is further enhanced.

Acknowledgment
I gratefully acknowledge the assistance of Shirley Lim Sue in preparation of this chapter. The study is supported by the Romi Sottiurai Foundation, MISIA, and Jobst.

References

1. Kistner RL. Transvenous repair of the incompetent femoral vein. In: Bergan JJ, Yao JST, eds. *Venous Problems.* Chicago, Ill: Year Book Medical Publishers; 1987:493–509.
2. Raju S, Fredericks R. Valve reconstruction procedures for non obstructive venous insufficiency: rationale, techniques, and results in 107 procedures with 2–8 years follow-up. *J Vasc Surg.* 1988;7:301–310.
3. Kistner RL, Ferris EB. Technique of surgical reconstruction of femoral vein valves. In: Bergan JJ, Yao JST, eds. *Operative Technique in Vascular Surgery.* New York, NY: Grune & Stratton; 1980:291–295.

4. Kistner RL. Surgical repair of the incompetent femoral vein valve. *Arch Surg.* 1975;110:1336–1342.

5. Raju S. Venous insufficiency of the lower limb and stasis ulceration. *Ann Surg.* 1983;197:688–697.

6. Kistner RL. Surgical technique of external venous valve repair. *Straub Foundation Proceeding.* 1990;55:5515–5516.

7. Gooley N, Sumner DS. Relationship of venous reflux to the site of venous valvular incompetence: implications for venous reconstructive surgery. *J Vasc Surg.* 1988;7:50–57.

8. Shull KC, Nicolaides AN, Fernandes e Fernandes JF, et al. Significance of popliteal reflux in relationship to ambulatory venous pressure and ulceration. *Arch Surg.* 1979;114:1304–1306.

9. Bry JDL, Muto PA, O'Donnell TF, Isaacson LA. The clinical and hemodynamic results after axillary-to-popliteal vein valve transplantation. *J Vasc Surg.* 1995;21:110–119.

10. Kistner RL, Ferris EB, Randhawa G, et al. A method of performing descending venography. *J Vasc Surg.* 1986;4:464–468.

11. Sottiurai VS. Technique in direct valvuloplasty. *J Vasc Surg.* 1988;8:646–648.

12. Sottiurai VS. Supravalvular incision for valve repair in primary valvular insufficiency. In: Bergan JJ, Kistner RL, eds. *Atlas of Venous Surgery.* Philadelphia, Pa: WB Saunders; 1992:135–145.

13. Sottiurai VS, Cooper M, Ross C, et al. Comparison of initial and late hemodynamics in proximal-mid and superficial femoral vein versus femoro-popliteal junction and popliteal valvuloplasty. *J Vasc Surg.* In press.

14. Jessup G, Lane RJ. Repair of incompetent venous valves: a new technique. *J Vasc Surg.* 1988;8:569–575.

15. Psathakis MN. Has the "substitute valve" at the popliteal vein solved the problem of venous insufficiency of the lower extremity? *J Cardiovasc Surg.* 1986;9:64–70.

16. Raju S. Venous reconstruction for chronic venous insufficiency of the leg. In: Ernst CB, Stanley JC, eds. *Current Therapy in Vascular Surgery,* 2nd ed. Philadelphia: B.C. Decker, Inc.: 1991:977–981.

17. Sottiurai VS. Current surgical approaches of venous hypertension and valvular reflux. *Int Angiol.* 1996;5:49–54.

18. Sottiurai VS. Is single valvuloplasty adequate? *Bull Vasc Surg.* In press.

85

Chronic Venous Insufficiency Disease: Its Etiology and Treatment

Dinker B. Rai

Venous disease is a common problem worldwide. In the United States alone more than 20 million people are estimated to suffer from the morbid effects of some kind of venous abnormality.

In the initial stages venous insufficiency can manifest as sprouting of unattractive spiderlike veins seen through the skin. It can also be associated with aching, subcutaneous ecchymosis, and occasionally external bleeding secondary to local trauma that may result in an emergency situation.

In its later stages patients present with larger veins seen as flat bluish streaks under the skin; these veins are known as reticular veins. Some of them later become tortuous and wormlike under the skin and are known as varicose veins. Most patients seek medical care at this stage .

Later on patients begin to manifest skin changes. The most common feature of these changes is the typical brownish to black pigmentation of the skin around the ankle. Approximately 10% to 15% of patients with untreated venous insufficiency develop frank ulcers of the skin on the foot and leg. The most common location of venous ulcers is the malleolar area.

It is well known that strict 24 -hour bed rest with elevation of the legs and local care help to heal most of these ulcers. Skillful application of compression bandages (the most commonly used type in the United States is the Unna boot dressing) can also heal the ulcers. However, ulcer recurrence is observed in a very high percentage of patients. The ulcers are often viewed as purely skin lesions and treated by dermatologists. Because the ulcers are chronic, however, they attract the attention of surgeons.

Trendelenburg first described the underlying etiology of chronic venous insufficiency disease (CVID) in the 1890s. His concepts were based mostly on clinical examination. Trendelenburg's theory of "private circulation" as the underlying cause is worth mentioning. On the basis of his theory, stripping and ligation of the great or

short saphenous vein became part of the surgical treatment of venous insufficiency. Stripping and ligation were once the most common surgical procedures practiced in the United States, and they remain the preferred treatment among surgeons.

Linton in the United States[5] and Boyd, Dodd, and Cockett in Europe[1,2] described the incompetency of perforating veins as the main cause of ulcer recurrence. Linton called it the *perforating burst theory*. Subfascial ligation of the incompetent perforating veins has become a routine surgical procedure.

In 1938 Homans first described several cases of what he referred to as *postphlebitic induration and ulceration*.[3] He placed the affected patients in a separate group. This classification opened a new wave of information on venous ulcers secondary to venous obstructive disease.

Also in 1938, Leriche described leg ulcers in patients who had previously been diagnosed with deep venous thrombosis (DVT). Each time a new etiology was described, a particular surgical procedure followed, and all patients with venous disease were believed to have the same underlying etiology diagnosed on the basis of clinical examination and subjected to the currently accepted surgical procedure.

Surgeons who followed Linton's school of thought treated all patients by subfascial ligation of incompetent perforating veins. Those who followed Trendelenburg's theory stripped and ligated only the veins of the saphenous system. The remaining surgeons followed Homans's theories of postphlebitic syndrome.[3] Only the few patients whose underlying etiology of the ulcer matched that of the clinician's theory benefited from the surgical treatment rendered; for the rest of the patients surgical treatment made no difference. Hence, the surgical procedures used in the past offered only marginal benefits for most of the patients who suffered from severe CVID with ulcers.

The clinical manifestation (i.e., the signs and the symptoms) of the disease is the same for all patients, but

TABLE 85.1. Noninvasive tests.

Impedence plethysmography
Phleborheography
Bidirectional Doppler
Duplex imaging
Maximum venous outflow measurement
Venous capacitance measurement
Venous reflux measurement

the underlying etiology can be quite different from one patient to another. The medical community understood this situation after interest was renewed in the study of venous valves and their function when descending and ascending phlebography were developed as diagnostic tests. More recently noninvasive procedures have markedly contributed to the understanding of the disease (Table 85.1). Today it is important to diagnose the underlying etiology in each patient and choose the treatment accordingly.

Chronic Venous Insufficiency Disease

The manifestations of venous sequelae and venous insufficiency vary in degree among patients. A few spider veins may be the initial sign. In its terminal stage venous insufficiency results in intractable ulcers with various types of skin changes in the legs that completely disable the patient. We have categorized under the diagnosis of CVID only patients who go into a terminal stage of venous insufficiency. To fit into this category the patients should have the following symptom complex:

1. Intractable nonhealing ulcer that does not respond to traditional medical management or recurs within a few weeks
2. Pain on weight bearing
3. Inability to ambulate freely; most patients limp and develop anatomical deformities of the ankle, and some are wheelchair bound or bedridden

Because all of these changes occur slowly over a long period of time, patients accept them as part of the aging process rather than manifestations of a disabling disease that markedly changes their lifestyles. Hence, most patients resist physicians' treatment plans.

In the past adjunctive surgical procedures were done in addition to the medical treatment to prevent recurrence of symptoms. Symptoms improved only marginally. Failure of treatment was due mainly to an inability to understand the exact underlying etiology of the venous disorder.

In this chapter I classify the underlying etiology found among 100 patients with CVID. Classification is based on clinical tests and then noninvasive and invasive diagnostic tests. Among all the tests a combination of descending and ascending phlebographies has been the most informative in the classification. I also describe my experience with CVID secondary to venous valvular incompetency and its treatment by reconstructive valvular surgery.

Clinical Examination

After the history and general examination the tests discussed in the following sections are performed.

Trendelenburg Test

The Trendelenburg test[12] determines the valvular competency of superficial and communicating systems. The patient is placed in the recumbent position, and the veins are emptied by raising the leg and gently stroking the varicose veins. A tourniquet is then applied at the level of the saphenofemoral junction and the patient is made to stand quickly. One of two methods may be used:

1. In the first method the tourniquet is released immediately. If the varices fill quickly from above downward by retrograde flow of blood, the saphenofemoral valve and the rest of the valves in the saphenous system are considered incompetent.
2. In the second method the tourniquet is released after 30 seconds. Gradual filling of varicose veins during this time indicates the incompetency of communicating veins, which allow the blood to flow from the deep veins to the superficial veins.

Both of the preceding findings are considered positive Trendelenburg tests. The tests can be repeated at the saphenopopliteal junction to evaluate the short saphenous vein.

Perthe's Test

Perthe's test helps to determine whether the deep veins are healthy. A tourniquet is applied at the saphenofemoral junction. The patient is advised to walk quickly for some time with the tourniquet in place. If the communicating and deep venous systems are normal and have competent valves, the superficial varicose veins shrink. If there is blockage of the deep system, varicose veins become more distended and the patient may complain of discomfort and pain. The patient then undergoes the noninvasive studies listed in Table 85.1.

Patients with infected ulcers, cellulitis, pain, and swelling are admitted to the hospital. Initial treatment involves 24-hour bed rest (with walking allowed only to the bathroom), elevation of the legs, culture from the ul-

TABLE 85.2. Invasive tests.

Radionuclide imaging
Ascending phlebography
Descending phlebography
Venous pressure studies (done with patient lying, standing, excercising)

TABLE 85.3. Signs of chronic venous insufficiency disease.

Spider veins	Hyperpigmentation
Varicose veins	Hyperkeratosis
Edema	Calcified vein*
Eczema	Thrombophlebitis
Dermatitis	Periostitis*
Cyanosis	Talipes equinus*
Hair loss	Nonhealing ulcer
Muscle wasting	

* Rare signs

TABLE 85.4. Symptoms of chronic venous insufficiency disease.

Swelling of leg
Pain on weight bearing
Inability to ambulate
Itching
Weeping skin
Hemorrhage

cer, and intravenous antibiotic administration. The immediate response to the medical treatment is remarkable. Within 24 to 48 hours swelling, pain, cellulitis, and infection subside. Ulcers become clean but never heal completely. If the patient is allowed to ambulate or sit the symptoms recur immediately. During this time the invasive studies listed in Table 85.2 are performed.

Etiology

I have studied 100 patients with CVID (Figure 85.1). They all had severe skin changes as described in Tables 85.3 and 85.4. In addition, they had two or more of the symptoms necessary to fit into the category of CVID as described earlier in this chapter (intractable ulcer, pain on weight bearing, and inability to ambulate fully). These patients were admitted to the hospital and underwent extensive laboratory tests. Final diagnosis was based on information obtained from ascending and descending phlebographies.[6]

Venous Obstructive Disease

Most patients with venous obstructive disease are found to have intraluminal occlusions (Table 85.5). In the past we believed the occlusions to be secondary to venous thrombosis. However, none of these patients indicated a history of DVT or anticoagulation treatment. Consequently, we have not grouped them under the diagnosis of postthrombotic syndrome. In three patients obstruction of the iliac vein was secondary to therapeutic ligation of the iliofemoral vein after trauma. In two patients

TABLE 85.5. Venous obstructive disease.

Inferior vena cava and iliac vein	1
Ileofemoral vein	12
Iliac vein ligation (for trauma)	3
Iatrogenic ligation (during abdominal surgery)	2
Ileocaval compression syndrome	3
Femoropopliteal vein	2
Total	23

iliac veins were ligated iatrogenically during abdominal surgery.

Venous Valve Incompetency

The total number of patients with venous valve incompetency was 56 (see Table 85.6). Of them, four patients who gave a definite history of DVT with anticoagulation treatment were classified as having postthrombotic syndrome. Some patients who had competent proximal common and superficial femoral venous valves were found to have incompetent venous valves in the popliteal vein distally. This diagnosis is made possible by selective catheterization of the superficial femoral vein and performance of descending phlebography. To achieve this it is necessary to advance the catheter beyond the femoral vein valve without damaging it (see Chapter 86).

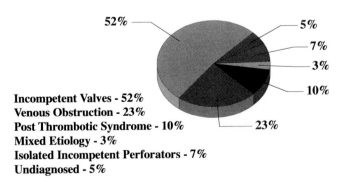

52%
5%
7%
3%
10%
23%

Incompetent Valves - 52%
Venous Obstruction - 23%
Post Thrombotic Syndrome - 10%
Mixed Etiology - 3%
Isolated Incompetent Perforators - 7%
Undiagnosed - 5%

FIGURE 85.1. Etiologies of 100 patients with chronic venous insufficiency disease.

TABLE 85.6. Venous valve incompetency.

Isolated saphenofemoral incompetency	7
Proximal femoral valve incompetency	11
Distal popliteal valve incompetency	8
Generalized valvular incompetency	30
Total	56

Postthrombotic Syndrome

Many of the obstructive venous diseases and some of the valvular incompetency diseases are probably secondary to past DVT. However, we were unable to include them under this classification because a clear-cut history was lacking. Hence, the 10 patients who had a definite history of hospitalization for DVT and long-term anticoagulation therapy are included in the category of postthrombotic syndrome. Among them four patients had generalized valvular incompetency (author's classification level IV; see Table 85.7) and were treated with venous valve transplantation.

Mixed Etiology

Patients with mixed etiology had occlusive arterial disease in addition to CVID (Figure 85.1). The presentation of the signs and symptoms of the disease was similar to that of the cases of CVID. Two patients had venous obstructive disease, and one also had valvular incompetency.

Incompetent Perforating Veins

Patients with venous obstructive disease and valvular incompetency sometimes have incompetent perforating veins (Figure 85.1). However, patients diagnosed with incompetent perforating veins after workup were found to have competent valves in the superficial and deep venous system, and none had evidence of venous obstructive disease of the large veins to account for CVID. The only underlying pathology found in these patients was incompetent perforating veins (Table 85.7, level V).

Undiagnosed

After extensive workups, we were unable to find any specific underlying etiology in five of the patients (Figure 85.1). These patients, who presented with clinical manifestations identical to those of CVID, are thus classified as undiagnosed. One of these patients had vasculitis secondary to scleroderma, but this did not explain the clinical manifestation.

TABLE 85.7. Descending phlebography: author's classification.

Level 0	Competent valves
Level I	Saphenofemoral valve incompetency
Level II	Proximal valvular incompetency (valves at common femoral level involving profunda femoris, superficial femoral, and great saphenous veins)
Level III	Distal valvular incompetency (femoral vein valves mentioned in level II are competent, but valves distal to them in popliteal vein onwards are incompetent)
Level IV	Generalized incompetency (all valves of superficial and deep system are incompetent)
Level V	Incompetent perforator vein associated with or without any of the preceding levels.

Treatment

Medical management of the patients was outlined earlier in this chapter. The surgical approach is based totally on the underlying etiology. Patients who were found to have isolated saphenofemoral incompetency underwent high ligation of the great saphenous vein and all of its tributaries followed by sclerotherapy of distal varicose veins. Those with isolated incompetent perforating veins underwent subfascial ligation of incompetent perforating veins. Those classified as having CVID of mixed etiology had both arterial and venous insufficiency. One patient had valvular incompetency, and two patients had obstructive venous disease. In these patients the primary procedure was to correct occlusive arterial disease by arterial bypass surgery, which resulted in healing of the ulcers. After correction of the arterial occlusion patients with venous obstructive disease showed increased swelling of the limb, although the ulcer healed.

Correction of the arterial insufficiency was undertaken only when the arteries proximal to the popliteal segment were occluded. Patients who had palpable popliteal pulses with tibial arterial disease and a marginal fall in ankle–brachial arterial index were not grouped in this category. However, in venous reconstruction good ankle perfusion is necessary for satisfactory results. Patients who had distal valvular incompetency and generalized valvular incompetency (classifications III and IV; see Table 85.7) underwent venous valve transplantation.

The patients who had proximal deep venous valve incompetency (classification II; see Table 85.7) underwent venous valvuloplasty. Kistner[4] first described venous valvuloplasty, and Taheri[11] first described valve transplantation. I have devised a new technique to transplant valves from the upper extremity brachial vein segment into the distal popliteal vein below the knee. The surgical techniques of venous valve transplantation and vein valvuloplasty are described in detail in the following section.

Surgical Technique

Venous Valve Transplantation

The venous valve is harvested from the brachial vein in the following manner.[7] A 5-cm vertical incision is made under 1% lidocaine anesthesia in the upper one third of the upper arm along the bicipital groove. After incision of the deep fascia the brachial vein is identified and the valve is located as a bulge in the vein. A 1.5-cm segment of vein is dissected out on either side of the valve. A strip test is performed to check the competency of the valve. A 3-cm length of vein segment with the competent valve in the middle is resected and preserved in heparinized blood. If a competent valve is not available then a search is made on the upper arm of the opposite side. Only if both brachial vein segments fail to provide a competent valve is the axillary vein valve harvested in a similar manner. The wound is closed in layers, and a medium Jackson Pratt drain is left in place. Good hemostasis during the entire procedure is critical.

The distal popliteal vein is then exposed. A 10-cm incision is made beginning at the medial epicondyle of the femur 1 cm medial to the inner margin of the tibia. The deep fascia is incised and the medial head of the gastrocnemius muscle is retracted downward and the popliteal fossa entered. The popliteal vein is identified, and a 5-cm length is carefully dissected out. The patient is administered heparin systemically. Vascular clamps are applied proximally and distally to the popliteal vein. The middle of the popliteal vein is ligated deliberately using a large hemoclip. Flat ligation of the popliteal vein is the result. The popliteal vein is not ligated using ties that cause one pointed ligation because wrinkling of the vein wall at the site of the ligation results. Flat ligation of the vein can also be done by suturing the vein wall in a transverse fashion instead of using a hemoclip. A venotomy is performed about 1.5 cm above the ligation. The length of the venotomy should correspond to the diameter of the harvested vein. The cephalic end of the harvested vein is anastomosed to the venotomy by using 6-O Prolene sutures. The proximal popliteal vein and anastomosed segment of vein are irrigated with heparinized normal saline solution. A second venotomy is then made on the popliteal vein about 1.5 cm distal to the ligation. The caudal end of the harvested vein is anastomosed to the venotomy by using the same material and technique.

Intraoperative venography is performed to evaluate the anastomosis and valve. A 21-gauge angiocatheter is introduced into the popliteal vein distal to the distal anastomosis. Contrast material is injected, and a roentgenogram is taken. Good hemostasis must be established during the procedure. The wound is closed in layers with a Jackson Pratt drain left in place. The drain should be located away from the transplanted vein segment.

Double popliteal veins are present only rarely. If the popliteal veins have incompetent valves on descending phlebography the following procedure should be used. The vein is transected as high as possible, and the proximal end is ligated. The distal end is anastomosed to the side of the main popliteal vein distal to the transplanted segment of the vein, so that the venous drainage from the leg into the thigh now goes through the transplanted segment of the brachial veins with competent valves (Figure 85.2). In many patients the accessory popliteal vein draining into the main popliteal vein just around the knee shows incompetent valves on descending phlebography. This vein can be managed by simple ligation. If the descending phlebography also shows an incompe-

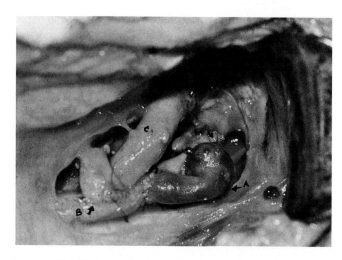

FIGURE 85.2. Venous valve transplant in a patient with incompetent double popliteal vein: **A,** Transplanted brachial vein into main popliteal vein. **B,** Accessory popliteal vein anastomosed to main popliteal vein in an end-to-side fashion distal to the transplantation. **C,** Popliteal artery.

tent great saphenous vein or short saphenous vein that vein is also ligated. During the first 24 hours after surgery 500 mL dextran 40 is administered. The drains are subsequently removed and the patient is administered 800 to 1000 units of heparin per hour for 7 days. The patient also wears compression stockings and is placed on intermittent venous compression pumps.

Femoral Vein Valvuloplasty

Femoral vein valvuloplasty is usually done under epidural or spinal anesthesia. Usually there are two to three valves in the superficial femoral veins distal to the saphenofemoral junction. Saphenofemoral valve incompetency is treated with ligation of the saphenous vein at the saphenofemoral junction with heavy silk sutures. Usually the valve in the superficial femoral vein distal to the junction of the profunda femoris vein is repaired in the following way. A midinguinal incision is made. Most of the dissection is done with cauterization. Meticulous maintenance of hemostasis is critical. The anterior femoral sheath is opened. The common femoral, profunda femoris, superficial femoral, and great saphenous veins are dissected out carefully, and control is obtained by applying rubber loops. Incompetency of the superficial femoral vein valve is established before surgery by descending phlebography. It can be further confirmed with a strip test.

Kistner originally described a vertical incision for the exposure of the valve. Raju has proposed a transverse incision. In my experience a T incision is ideal for venotomy.[10] Initially I use a transverse incision just above the valves, which can be identified externally after some ex-

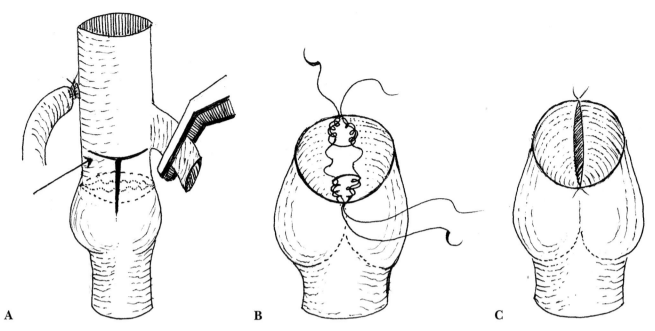

FIGURE 85.3. Internal valvuloplasty: **A,** Femoral vein. Note ligated great saphenous vein and clamped profunda femoris. Arrow points to T incision. **B,** Internal valvuloplasty technique. Note the redundant valves with wide base. **C,** Corrected valve.

perience. If the exposure is not adequate then we convert it into a T incision, as shown in Figure 85.3; 7-O Prolene stay stitches are applied. The valves may not be visible immediately to inexperienced clinicians. Usually we irrigate the area of the valve with a mild jet of heparinized normal saline solution. Then the valves can be seen floating in the normal saline. Extreme care has to be taken in handling the valves. After stroking the valve a couple of times, the approximate percentage of the length of the redundant valve margin that needs to be shortened can be estimated. Usually one fifth, or 20%, of the length is shortened on each side. A 9-O nylon suture is used (Figure 85.3). One side is treated at a time. The vein is entered from the external surface of the vein wall at the junction of the commissure and the free margin of the valve. After entering the lumen of the vein at the free margin of the upper valve cusp, a reefing suture is applied for one fifth of its length. At this stage the suture is brought into the free margin of the lower valve cusp. Reefing suture along this margin is continued, and the suture is brought out of the vein wall at approximately the same place it is entered. The two ends of the suture are then tied on the external surface of the wall of the vein. During the process the whole valve cusp free margin is shortened by one fifth of its length. A similar technique is used to shorten the opposite valve cusp margins at their junction at the opposite commissure. This results in two fifths plication of the entire valve length. Figure 85.3 shows the plicated and now competent valve that is no longer redundant.

External Vein Valvuloplasty

External vein valvuloplasty was first described by Kistner.[4] The procedure is easier than internal repair and less time-consuming because several valves can be corrected simultaneously. Figure 85.4 depicts the technique.

The site of attachment of the lateral margins of the valve cusps to the wall of the vein can be identified as a firm, thin white streak from the external surface of the vein wall. The two lines of the adjacent valves start as a wide base and approach each other at an acute angle, where they join their free margins. In nonrefluxive valves the angle where they join each other is usually less than 11 degrees. Incompetent valves show a wide commissural angle. The external repair technique aims to reduce this angle to less than 11 degrees and provide good coaptation. A 9-O nylon suture is used. After identifying the commissure, suturing is begun from the top and continued toward the base as a continuous stitch. A through-and-through stitch is applied at the upper end of the commissure. The two valve cusps, where the commissure joins its free margin, are brought together by this technique, and suturing is continued toward the base and tied on the outside. In the process the wide angle is converted into an acute angle that stops reflux. Disadvantages of the technique include that it is done without direct visualization of the valve cusp, which may result in inadequate repair of valve cusps. Raju has used this technique extensively in multiple valve reconstruction.[9]

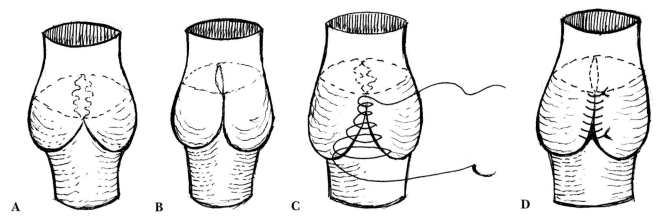

FIGURE 85.4. Technique of external valvuloplasty: **A,** Abnormal valve. Note the wide base of more than 11-degree angle. **B,** Normal valve. **C,** External valvuloplasty technique. Valve commis-sures are brought together by running suture. **D,** Corrected valve. Note that the running suture is tied externally.

Postoperative Follow-Up

All the patients were followed up with noninvasive and invasive studies. Noninvasive studies included maximum venous outflow, venous capacitance, and venous reflux studies. Studies are usually performed 3 months after the procedure and then repeated on a yearly basis.

Preoperative and postoperative venous reflux results with 90% recovery time are provided in Figure 85.5. In most of these patients postoperative 90% stable recovery time was found to be more than 9 seconds, suggesting a decrease in venous reflux following the procedure (Figure 85.6).

Postoperative invasive studies included venous pressure tests, ascending and descending phlebographies, and for some patients venous velocity studies (see Figures 85.7 and 85.8). Venous pressures were recorded with the patient lying down, standing, and exercising. Most of the patients showed a spontaneous healing of ulcers, and few needed skin grafts, as shown in Table 85.8. In the series of patients I studied, the remarkable clinical improvement seen after valvular reconstructive procedures did not reflect a similar change in postoperative ambulatory venous pressures (Table 85.9). This result has led to questions about the role of venous pressure as a test that might reflect the subtle changes that take place in the motion of venous blood in disease and in health.

After considering other alternatives to understanding the hemodynamics in health and disease, we came up

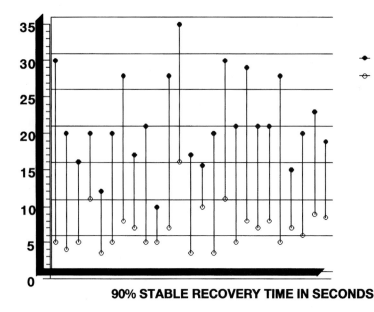

90% STABLE RECOVERY TIME IN SECONDS

◆ **Postoperative**
○ **Preoperative**

FIGURE 85.5. Study on 25 patients with venous valve transplantation.

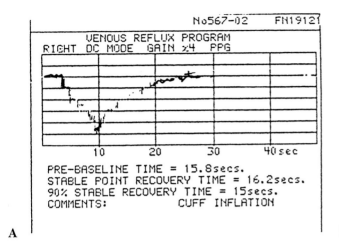

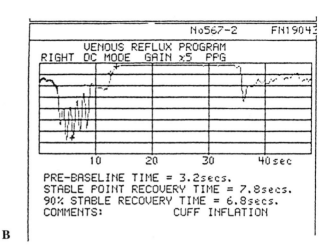

A B

FIGURE 85.6. Preoperative (**A**) and postoperative (**B**) venous reflux studies. (From Rai and Lerner.[8])

with a concept of understanding the velocity of circulation in these patients. Although the test, concept, and findings are in the preliminary stages, the test is worth mentioning in this chapter because it has the potential for future development in hemodynamics.

Venous Velocity as a Test to Understand Venous Hemodynamics

I first considered venous velocity as a test to understand venous hemodynamics in 1990. So far, we have conducted 29 studies. Of these, 20 studies were of patients with venous valve incompetency before and after surgery. Two healthy individuals provided control data.

Method

Venous velocity is measured by the following method: 20 mCi of technetium 99m in human serum albumin is injected into the femoral artery of the diseased leg. The data are acquired by gamma camera and stored and processed by computer. In each study, gamma variant graphs were obtained. The time–activity curve is generated by drawing a region of interest on the iliac vein of the same side. The expression t_1 is the transit time to reach peak activity (Figure 85.9).

Finding

In patients with valvular incompetency the highest t_1 recorded was 267 seconds in a patient before surgery. The average fall of t_1 following surgery is 88 seconds ($P = .0431$). For healthy patients t_1 is 25 seconds. In all patients preoperative and postoperative exercise venous

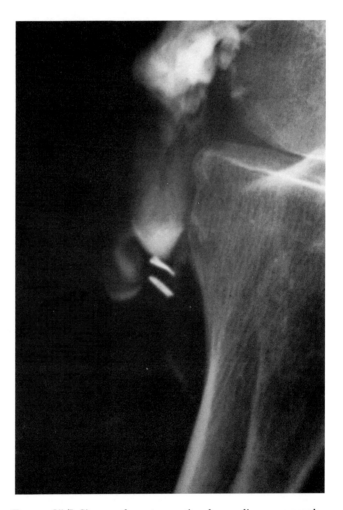

FIGURE 85.7. Six-month postoperative descending venography. Note popliteal vein ligated with hemoclips. Blind loop of popliteal vein below the proximal anastomosis is patent; transplanted vein segment is seen in front with competent valves. (From Rai and Lerner.[8])

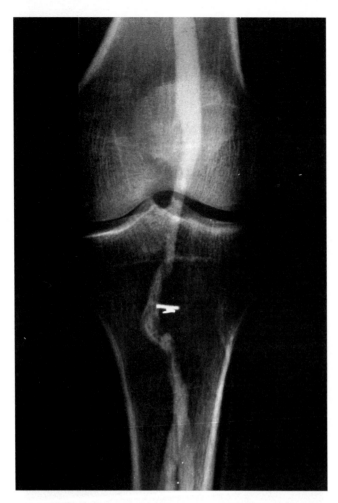

FIGURE 85.8. Ascending venography 1 year after surgery. Note transplanted segment of brachial vein that is patent and of normal caliber similar to a minibypass around the ligated popliteal vein with hemoclips. (From Rai and Lerner.[8])

TABLE 85.9. Venous pressures.*†

1.	15, 120, 120
	18, 125, 120
2.	10, 125, 88
	15, 130, 90
3.	10, 88, 78
	10, 90, 75
4.	15, 110, 110
	15, 105, 100
5.	10, 80
	10, 76
6.	12, 93, 90
	15, 95, 90
7.	10, 90, 88
	10, 90, 88
8.	15, 110, 85
	15, 110, 80
9.	10, 95
	12, 95
10.	17, 88, 92
	15, 82, 80
11.	15, 95, 85
	15, 96, 85

* Preoperative lying, standing, exercising
  Postoperative lying, standing, exercising
† Eleven patients after venous valve transplantation.

TABLE 85.8 Vein valve transplantation: author's technique

Adjunctive procedures	
High ligation of great saphenous vein	12
Ligation of accessory popliteal vein	3
Bypass of accessory popliteal vein	1
Skin graft	4
Femoral vein valvuloplasty	1*

*Done 2 yr later.

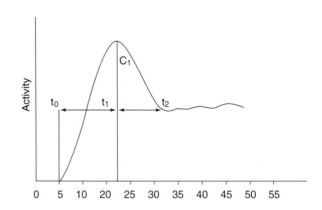

C_1—Peak activity
t_0—Time of injection
t_1—Transit time to reach peak activity
t_2—Transit time to reach plateau due to
      systemic dilution of technitium

FIGURE 85.9. Time–activity curve. C_1, peak activity; t_0, time of injection; t_1, transit time to reach peak activity; t_2, transit time to reach plateau due to systemic dilution of technetium.

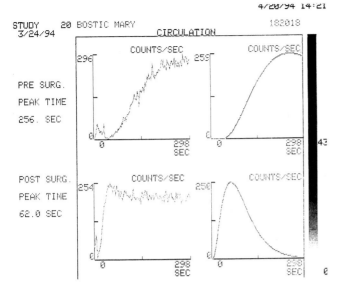

FIGURE 85.10. Preoperative and postoperative time–activity curve that reflects significant changes in postoperative venous velocity.

pressures did not vary noticeably. Hence, this significant change in velocity of the venous blood reflected in the recording of t_1 provides some new understanding on the motion of venous circulation responsible for the clinical improvement in these patients. Whether the velocity of the blood rather than the pressure of the blood is the deciding factor in tissue oxygenation and nutrition is thus a question of importance. Figure 85.10 shows preoperative and postoperative images in a patient. Although this is a preliminary study, I believe that this new concept could be a reliable test to understand the subtler aspects of hemodynamics in the future and is worth further evaluation.

Results

The patients who had venous valve incompetency as the underlying etiology were classified on the basis of descending phlebography (Table 85.7). On the basis of this classification only patients with level II valve incompetency underwent femoral vein valvuloplasty; and those with levels III and IV underwent venous valve transplantation. In each group adjunctive procedures such as high ligation of the great saphenous vein or short saphenous

TABLE 85.10. Vein valvuloplasty: nine cases of adjunctive procedures.

High ligation of great saphenous vein	8
External cuffing	3
Healed with skin graft	1
Complication: postoperative hematoma (reexplored)	1
Recurrence in 6 mo	1

TABLE 85.11. Follow-up valve transplantation: author's technique.

Number of patients	Result	Time postoperative
2	Died	10 d and 60 d
1	Ischemic disease	2 yr
1	Ischemic disease	1 yr
1	Lost to follow-up	3 yr
1	Died	3 yr

Follow-up 13 to 112 mo; average follow-up 68 mo; six patients not included in follow-up

TABLE 85.12. Author's technique for vein valve transplantation (33 patients).

Result	
Nonhealing	1
Recurrence 1 yr	0
Recurrence 2 yr	2
Recurrence 3 yr	3*
Recurrence 4 yr	1
Recurrence 5 yr	2
Complications	
Heparin-induced thrombocytopenia	1
Postoperative hematoma and reexploration	1
Death due to myocardial infarction	1*

* Developed severe ischaemic disease.

vein or management of an incompetent accessory popliteal vein were done (refer to Tables 85.8 and 85.10).

Patients who underwent vein valve transplantation were followed up for 13 to 112 months, with an average follow-up period of 68 months. Six patients who were not included in the follow-up are listed in Table 85.11. In one patient the ulcer never healed; this patient had poor ankle perfusion due to occlusive arterial disease distal to the popliteal artery that was not correctable (Table 85.12). One patient who had severe reflux in the transplanted brachial vein segment suffered recurrence 2 years later. This patient later underwent femoral vein valvuloplasty. The ulcer healed for a short time immediately after the surgery but then recurred. Patients who underwent femoral vein valvuloplasty were followed for 3 to 84 months, with an average follow-up period of 66 months. Adjunctive surgical procedures for these patients with results and complications are provided in Table 85.10.

References

1. Boyd AM. Discussion on primary treatment of varicose veins. *Proc R Soc Med.* 1948;41:633–639.
2. Dodd H, Cockett FB, eds. *The Pathology and Surgery of the Veins of the Lower Limb.* Edinburgh: Livingstone; 1956 (2nd ed, Edinburgh: Churchill Livingstone; 1976).
3. Homans J. The etiology and treatment of varicose ulcer of the leg. *Journal International Chirurgie.* 1938;3:599–606.
4. Kistner RL. Surgical repair of the incompetent femoral vein valve. *Arch Surg.* 1975;110:1336–1142.

5. Linton RR. The communicating veins of the lower leg and the operative technique for their ligation. *Ann Surg.* 1953;138:415.

6. Rai DB. Descending venography: various approaches. *Proceedings of the 12th Annual Congress of the Phlebology Society of America.* 1989:58–64.

7. Rai DB. Vein valve transplantation: a new technique. In: Montorsi M, Zennaro F, eds. *Second World Week of Professional Updating in Surgery and in Surgical and Oncological Disciplines of the University of Milan.* Bologna: Monduzzi Editore; 1990:341–343.

8. Rai DB, Lerner R. Chronic venous insufficiency disease and etiology: a new technique for vein valve transplantation. *Int Surg.* 1991;76:176–178.

9. Raju S. Multiple valve reconstruction for venous insufficiency: indications, optimal technique, and results. *Current Critical Problems in Vascular Surgery.* 1992;4:122–125.

10. Sottirai VS. Current surgical approaches to venous hypertension and valvular reflux. *Int J Angiol.* 1996;5:49–54.

11. Taheri SA, Lazar L, Elias SM, Merchand P. Vein valve transplant. *Surgery.* 1982;91:28–33.

12. Trendelenburg F. Uber die underbindunger vena saphena magna bei underschen-kelvarizen. *Bruns Beitr Klin Chir.* 1890:7:195.

86

Phlebography

Dinker B. Rai

In the evaluation of arterial disease, the arterial tree must be studied from the aorta downward. Likewise, in the evaluation of chronic venous insufficiency disease (CVID), the venous tree must be studied from the inferior vena cava (IVC) down to the ankle.

At present, the venous tree can be studied only by the combination of ascending and descending phlebography. Other noninvasive tests are available, including impedence plethysmography, phleborheography, bidirectional Doppler ultrasound, and radionuclide techniques. However, phlebography remains the standard against which the sensitivity and specificity of noninvasive tests are compared. Noninvasive tests are currently adjunctive tests that provide additional information; they do not act as substitutes for phlebography, especially when the patient is subjected to venous reconstructive procedures of the venous tree.

Ascending phlebography is a well-established test. Descending phlebography was first described in the early 1950s. Interest in descending phlebography gradually waned, but the test has regained importance in the study and treatment of CVID. However, descending phlebography is not a well-established and routinely performed test with which the radiologist is familiar.

Because no technique for descending phlebography has been uniformly accepted, performance results are not available. No details about methods of cannulation, type, volume, and injection rate of contrast have been published. The catheters and instruments used are borrowed from those in use for angiograms. None of them are specifically designed for use on the venous system or are suitable for different approaches. Thus, descending phlebography is a crudely performed procedure at this time.

Since 1986, I have performed approximately 300 ascending and descending phlebographies in an attempt to understand the technique in detail by using different approaches according to the needs of the patient. The anatomy, classification of the approach, method, and ad-

vantages and disadvantages of various methods pertaining to descending phlebography are explained in more detail in this chapter. Other types of phlebographies are well-known standardized procedures and so are mentioned only briefly here.

Ascending Phlebography

Ascending phlebography of the affected lower extremity is performed before beginning descending phlebography. The dorsal vein of the foot, ankle, or leg is used. If edema makes finding a vein difficult, any available normal vein or even varicose vein is used.

Usually a 21-gauge angiocatheter is inserted into the vein. The patient is kept in a 30- to 45-degree semierect position. The contralateral leg bears the weight of the whole body on a wooden block kept below the foot. For better opacification of the deep system a tourniquet is applied 4 to 5 cm above the site of the angiocatheter. To opacify the superficial system the tourniquet should be released. The contrast material is then injected using a 60-mL syringe. Two to three aliquots of contrast material (15 mL at a time) are necessary for the complete evaluation. The following films are obtained in sequence:

1. Calf: anteroposterior, medial and lateral rotations, one shot each
2. Knee: anteroposterior, one shot
3. Thigh: anteroposterior, one shot
4. Pelvis: anteroposterior, one shot

Additional images are taken as required. During the pelvic exposure the calf is compressed manually to allow for better filling of the iliac veins. Despite various techniques described for better opacification of the pelvic veins and IVC, evaluation of these veins in most healthy patients and almost all patients with disease is found to be inadequate. Opacification of iliac veins is better performed by descending phlebography.

A combination of 60 mg meglumine with 520 mg/mL diatrizoate or 80 mg/mL sodium diatrizoate and 600 mg/mL iothalamate meglumine are the most common contrast materials used. These are water-soluble contrast media. Tri-iodinated derivatives of benzoic acid are excreted by the kidneys. The radiopaque component of the contrast is the iodine. Frequently used anions are diatrizoate and iothalamate, and frequently used cations are sodium and methylglucamine. These substances are used in different combinations to change the viscosity, osmolality, toxicity, and renal excretion of the contrast material.

Intraosseous Venography

Intraosseous venography is used to evaluate the deep venous system not evaluated by standard methods or when venous access is not available for the injection of contrast material. Because the procedure is very painful, premedication or general anesthesia may be necessary.

A sternal puncture trocar is inserted into the bone marrow of the appropriate bone for which venous drainage must be evaluated. For example, the calcaneus is used for calf veins, the pubic bone is used for internal iliac veins and the obturator plexus, the greater trochanter is used for the iliac vein and IVC, and the proximal tibia is used for femoral veins.

Varicography

Varicography is direct phlebography of the varicose veins. It is used to determine the anatomy of these veins and connections to incompetent perforating veins. Varicography is informative and useful before the treatment of these veins with sclerotherapy or local excision. Varicose veins are made prominent by keeping the extremity in a dependent position (sitting or standing).

A 21-gauge angiocatheter is introduced into the varicose vein, and diluted contrast is injected with the patient on a tilt table in the semiupright position. After the test, care should be taken to wash the contrast material from the varicose veins by injecting normal saline and manually compressing the veins with the patient in Trendelenburg's position. Otherwise, varicose veins can be predisposed to thrombosis or local ulceration.

Descending Phlebography

Descending phlebography is also known as retrograde phlebography. In conventional ascending phlebography contrast material is injected into the vein of the distal part of the lower extremity (e.g., foot or ankle) and flows centripetally toward the heart. In descending phlebography, infradiaphragmatic IVC or any preceding distal segment of that vein is selectively catheterized by either retrograde or antegrade approach. The contrast material is injected in a retrograde fashion with the patient kept in a 75-degree semierect position. Two important results help to indicate the underlying causes of CVID:

1. In venous occlusive disease descending phlebography gives the exact anatomical details of the upper level of such occlusions (demonstrated in Figures 86.1 and 86.2).
2. In valvular incompetency disease descending phlebography helps to evaluate the valvular function at the femoral level and if necessary the function of the valves distal to it situated in the great saphenous vein, profunda femoris, superficial femoral vein, and popliteal vein (demonstrated in Figures 86.3 and 86.4).

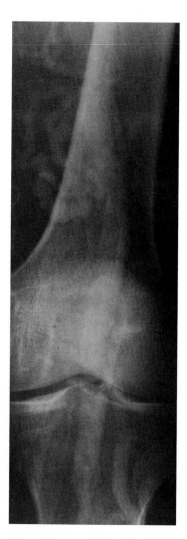

FIGURE 86.1. Ascending phlebography showing lower level of occlusion. Note the formation of collateral vessels at the site of occlusion.

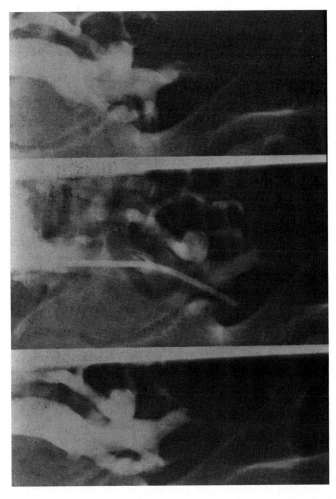

FIGURE 86.2. Descending phlebography showing upper level of venous occlusion at right distal common iliac vein. Note the anatomical details at the site of occlusion.

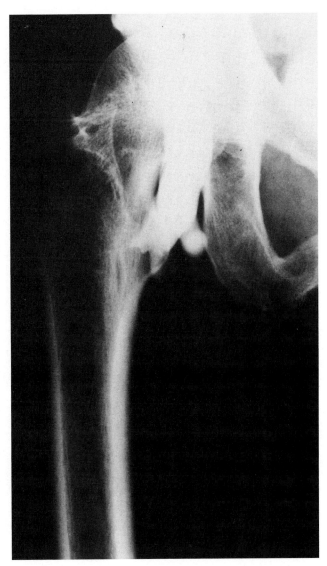

FIGURE 86.3. Normal descending phlebography showing competent valves in the great saphenous vein, profunda femoris, and superficial femoral vein.

Bauer[1] published an article in 1948 in which he described evaluation of the femoral vein by surgical exposure of the great saphenous vein and retrograde injection of aqueous iodine solution into the proximal part of the femoral vein. The foot of the operating table was lowered to an angle of 45 degrees. Bauer noticed contrast filling of the femoropopliteal vein in many patients and even of the tibial vein in some patients. He claimed this finding was due to incompetency of venous valves and retrograde flow of contrast.[2]

In 1950 Tore Sylvan[3] published an article on this subject and reported retrograde phlebography by percutaneous injection of contrast medium directly into the femoral vein. Radiologists today use the same technique when performing descending phlebography.[4] I initially used the same approach but soon realized the following shortcomings:

1. Inadequate evaluation of the venous tree is common.

2. Only the function of femoral vein valves can be evaluated.

3. The tip of the needle must be kept very close to the valve. Because it is a blind approach, such attempts result in extravasation of contrast in many patients.

4. A short catheter inserted farther into the external iliac vein to prevent extravasation results in antegrade injection with most of the contrast lost into the iliac veins and thus inadequate evaluation of the femoral vein valves.

5. Retrograde injection of contrast material into the femoral vein requires insertion of the needle into the femoral vein in retrograde fashion in the groin, which exposes the femoral vein valves to direct injury, thereby causing iatrogenic incompetency of the valves.

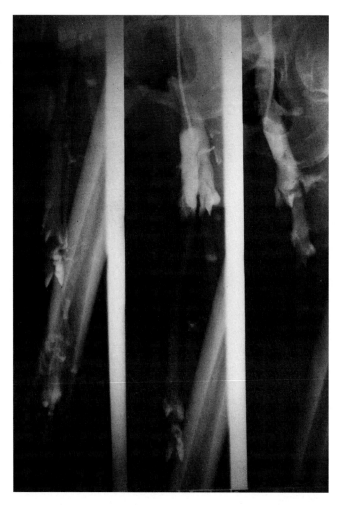

FIGURE 86.4. Descending phlebography: incompetent valves allow retrograde contrast flow into the profunda femoris, superficial femoral vein, and great saphenous vein.

The management of CVID depends on the correct understanding of underlying cause in the venous tree. The initial technique depends on chance and at most allows evaluation of femoral vein valve function only.

Obstructive venous disease escapes diagnosis with selective evaluation of the distal vein valves. Hence, in this method complete evaluation of the venous tree is not adequate. In many cases the etiology of CVID was unclear. Therefore, complete refinement of the approach and exploration of new approaches to suit the needs of different patients were necessary.

I have been performing descending phlebography since 1986. The various approaches are classified as indicated in Table 86.1. We report here the first 100 procedures and group them according to the classification in

Table 86.2. Each patient underwent ascending phlebography followed by descending phlebography and venous pressure studies with the patient lying, standing, and exercising. Each approach is described in detail in Table 86.1.

Supradiaphragmatic Approach

The materials necessary for the supradiaphragmatic approach include the following:

1. 18-gauge angiocatheter
2. 5-mL syringe
3. 7- or 8-F vessel dilator
4. 155-cm-long, 0.028-in-diameter guide wire with 1.5-mm J tip
5. 7- or 8-F, 110-cm-long venous catheter double lumen with balloon and curved tip

Pericarpal Percutaneous Method

For the pericarpal percutanous method,[5] a prominent superficial vein of the forearm is selected. The basilic vein at the cubital fossa below the elbow is the most ideal vein. The forearm and wrist of the patient are sterilized and draped. A tourniquet is applied proximally. Under local anesthesia, an 18-gauge angiocatheter is introduced into the vein. The guide wire with the J tip is introduced into the vein through the angiocatheter and carefully advanced 20 cm. Then the angiocatheter is removed and a small skin incision is made to introduce the vessel dilator, which dilates the opening. The vessel dilator is removed, and the main catheter, which is the 7- or 8-F, 110-cm-long catheter with double lumen with balloon and curved tip, is introduced. The catheter is advanced on the guide wire. Passage of the guide wire from the subclavian vein into the IVC through the right atrium of the heart is always done under fluoroscopy. Although the catheter slips into the IVC naturally more than 90% of the time, it occasionally enters the right ventricle. When it does, the guide wire begins to oscillate and curves to the left. Under such circumstances the guide wire is pulled back into the atrium and manipulated into the IVC.

Progression of the guide wire must be smooth and without resistance. Occasionally while advancing it into the IVC the guide wire can get into one of the tributaries of the IVC (e.g., the hepatic vein). In such cases immedi-

TABLE 86.1. Classification of different approaches.

Supradiaphragmatic	Pericarpal percutaneous catheterization
	Trans brachial
	Trans cervical (internal jugular and subclavian)
Infradiaphragmatic	Ipsilateral femoral
	Contralateral femoral

TABLE 86.2. Report on 100 cases.

Procedure	Number of patients
Pericarpal percutaneous catheterization	51
Transbrachial	10
Internal jugular	3
Transcervical	0
Subclavian	1
Ipsilateral femoral	32
Contralateral femoral	3
Total	100

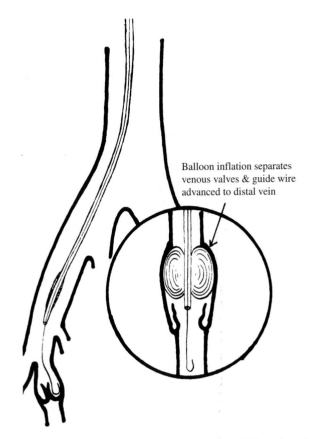

Balloon inflation separates venous valves & guide wire advanced to distal vein

FIGURE 86.5. Retrograde catheterization beyond the vein valve.

ate resistance is encountered during advancement of the guide wire. When this occurs, the guide wire is removed with the catheter in place and a phlebography is performed by injecting contrast media to delineate the anatomy. During this time balloon inflation is useful to prevent retrograde flow of the contrast material. Then the catheter is advanced into the desired external iliac vein and placed at the level of the inferior ramus of the ischium. At this stage, the x-ray table is tilted to a 75-degree upright position and the contrast material is manually injected from a 60-mL syringe. Competency of the valves and patency of the veins are studied under fluoroscopy. When the valves are incompetent the contrast flows retrograde into the veins of the thigh and leg (Figure 86.4). Contrast (15–20 mL) is injected and films are taken of the pelvic, thigh, and calf areas. Normally, 60 to 90 mL of contrast material is sufficient to complete the study.

Some patients with CVID may have competent femoral vein valves. They can have pathology in the distal segment of the vein. In such patients the catheter should be passed beyond the femoral valves, and selective catheterization of the superficial femoral vein, popliteal vein, profunda femoris, or great saphenous vein is necessary. The catheter should be advanced beyond the valves without damaging them. Three methods aid in retrograde catheterization beyond the venous valves:

1. The catheter is advanced close to the venous valve, and the catheter balloon is inflated to dilate the vein segment. This results in wide separation of the valve cusps. Then the guide wire is advanced between the cusps to the distal vein. The balloon is deflated, and the catheter is advanced on the guide wire beyond the valves (Figure 86.5).
2. The patient is asked to breathe deeply. During expiration venous blood flow increases from the femoral vein into the iliac vein and IVC, which separates the valve cusps. At the same time, the guide wire is manipulated and advanced easily between the valve cusps.
3. An assistant pumps the calf muscles. This augments venous outflow, which separates the valve cusps and helps to advance the guide wire and then the catheter.

Transbrachial Approach

In patients who have no superficial veins visible in the cubital fossa or forearm, superficial vein visibility in the arm is not likely and a deep vein in the arm is used.[6] A venous cut is made just above the medial epicondyle of the humerus. One of the venae comitantes of the brachial artery is identified, isolated, and used for catheterization. The succeeding steps of the procedure and technique are the same as described for the pericarpal percutaneous approach.

Transcervical Approach

Under local anesthesia, an 18-gauge angiocatheter is introduced blindly into the internal jugular or subclavian vein. (The technique of this procedure is similar to that for central venous pressure catheterization.) Once the angiocatheter is in the vein, venous blood is aspirated easily. Without disturbing the angiocatheter, the guide wire is introduced into the vein through the angiocatheter. Approximately 15 cm of the guide wire is advanced, and then the angiocatheter is removed. At the site of entry of the guide wire, a small skin incision is made using a knife blade. The access is dilated using the vessel dilator. The vessel dilator is removed, and the ve-

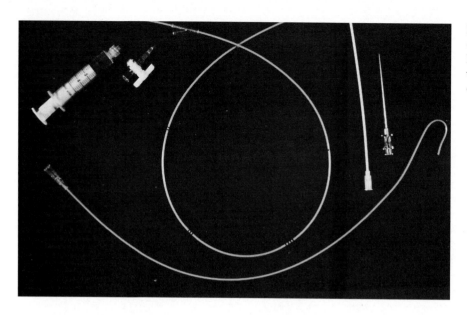

FIGURE 86.6. Catheters for a contralateral femoral approach include a 45-cm-long, 7-F catheter with 2-cm-wide J tip with 10-degree curve from the distal end.

nous catheter is introduced over the guide wire and advanced. The succeeding steps of the procedure and technique are similar to those described previously for the pericarpal percutaneous approach.

Infradiaphragmatic Approach

Contralateral Femoral Vein Catheterization

The following materials are necessary for contralateral femoral vein catheterization:

1. 18-gauge, 3-in-long needle
2. 5-mL syringe
3. 7-F vessel dilator
4. 7-F, 45-cm-long catheter with J tip (Figure 86.6)
5. 7-F, 75-cm-long venous catheter with balloon and a curved tip

Method

The contralateral groin of the affected leg is sterilized and draped. The femoral artery pulsation is felt at the midinguinal point, and the region adjacent and medial to the artery is injected with local anesthesia. The femoral vein is blindly entered with an 18-gauge needle. Once the needle enters the vein venous blood is freely aspirated. Without disturbing the needle, the guide wire is introduced into the vein through the needle. The needle is removed, and the site of entry is dilated using the vessel dilator. With the dilator in place, the guide wire is advanced through the dilator and into the contralateral common iliac vein. Keeping the guide wire in place, the dilator is removed and a venous catheter is introduced into the contralateral common iliac vein and advanced to the external iliac vein. However, it should be noted

that in most patients the guide wire has a tendency to enter the IVC. If the guide wire enters the IVC the following technique should be used. Instead of the venous catheter, a 7-F, 45-cm-long catheter with J tip should be inserted over the guide wire and advanced up to the bifurcation of the IVC. At that point the guide wire is deliberately pulled back into the catheter, and the catheter is advanced into the IVC, where it can be seen under fluoroscopy floating free in the lower part of the IVC with the tip of the J curve pointing downward (Figure 86.7).

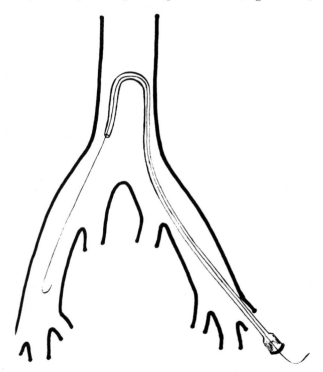

FIGURE 86.7. Contralateral transfemoral approach. Note that the J-tip catheter helps to insert the guide wire into the contralateral iliac vein.

Then the guide wire is advanced through the catheter tip in a retrograde fashion toward the bifurcation of the IVC, where it is manipulated into the contralateral iliac vein. Once the guide wire is in place, the introducer catheter is removed and the main catheter with the balloon is advanced to the desired level. Succeeding steps of the procedure are similar to those described for the pericarpal percutaneous method.

Ipsilateral Femoral Vein Approach

The following materials are necessary for the ipsilateral femoral vein approach:

1. 18-gauge, 3-in-long needle
2. 5-mL syringe
3. 7-F vessel dilator
4. 75-cm-long 0.028-in-diameter guide wire with 1.5-mm J tip
5. 7-F, 45-cm-long, three-lumen venous catheter with balloon (Figure 86.8)

Method

The ipsilateral groin is sterilized and draped. The femoral vein is entered as described previously. Once the guide wire is introduced, the access is dilated with a ve-

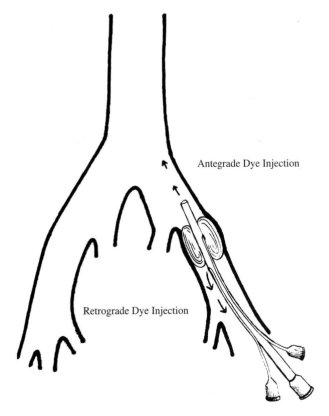

FIGURE 86.8. Ipsilateral transfemoral approach with three-lumen balloon catheter.

Antegrade Dye Injection

Retrograde Dye Injection

nous dilator. Then the dilator is removed and the venous catheter is introduced.

The venous catheter has three lumens. One is for introduction of the guide wire, one is for inflation of the balloon, and one is for injection of contrast material, which opens proximal to the balloon. Once the catheter is introduced into the femoral vein, it is deliberately pushed into the iliac vein. The balloon is partially inflated, and the catheter is pulled back gently until resistance is encountered. Resistance indicates that the balloon is close to the puncture site of the femoral vein. Then the catheter is advanced forward about 1 cm, which ensures injection of the contrast material into the femoral vein close to the femoral valve and adequately away from the puncture site of the femoral vein. This maneuver prevents extravasation of contrast material and injection of contrast material close to the femoral valves. Before the injection of the contrast the balloon is inflated. This technique results in retrograde injection of the contrast and also prevents wasting contrast by washout toward the heart.

Discussion

My colleagues and I have used the pericarpal percutaneous method most often. It is easy to perform after the first few procedures. Although it gives the maximum information with the highest satisfaction, it cannot be performed in all patients (Table 86.3).

In two patients we were unable to negotiate the catheter into the left common iliac vein for unknown reasons. We presume occasional venous webs may prevent retrograde advancement of the catheter. In one patient the procedure was discontinued because of subclavian vein obstruction. In all patients alternative approaches were used and the test completed. Most tedious of all the approaches is the contralateral femoral vein approach. We resorted to it only when the other approaches either failed or were not feasible.

In the ipsilateral femoral vein approach initial procedures were conducted by direct puncture of the femoral vein with a long, 18-gauge needle. Many of these procedures resulted in extravasation of the contrast material. Also, contrast injection was difficult with the patient in an upright position. We replaced the needle with a short catheter, but the test was never satisfactorily completed

TABLE 86.3. Contraindications of supradiaphragmatic approach.

Kyphoscoliosis
Cardiac anomalies
Venous anomalies
Superior vena cava obstruction
Subclavian and internal jugular vein obstruction

because contrast material was injected very high in the iliac vein. Hence, we devised the three-lumen catheter. Use of this catheter has perfected the technique, eliminated the chances of extravasation of contrast material, and provided optimal information. The disadvantage of this approach is that selective catheterization of the vein segments beyond the common femoral vein valves (e.g., superficial femoral vein and popliteal vein) is not possible and in some patients selective catheterization is important to complete the diagnosis. In his earlier work Kistner classified valvular incompetency into four grades on the basis of descending phlebography findings.[7] In our experience the grading does not correlate with the severity of the disease. However, it is necessary to understand the level of incompetency of the venous valves in treatment of the disease.[8] Hence, we have rated severity according to five categories:

1. *Saphenofemoral valve incompetency:* isolated incompetency of the valves at the saphenofemoral junction
2. *Proximal valvular incompetency:* only valves in the common femoral vein are incompetent (involving the profunda femoris, superficial femoral vein, and great saphenous vein)
3. *Distal valvular incompetency:* the femoral vein valves mentioned in category 2 are competent, but the valves distal to them present in the superficial femoral and popliteal veins are incompetent
4. *Generalized incompetency of the venous valves:* all of the valves present in the superficial and deep venous systems are incompetent
5. *Incompetency of perforating veins:* with or without preceding categories

The most common complaint after descending phlebography has been dizziness or weakness in the upright position (Table 86.4). These symptoms may be seen because the patient is kept fasting for the procedure and occasionally develops hypoglycemia. Hypoglycemia precipitates the mentioned symptoms when the patient is placed in a semierect position. Although most patients respond to reassurance and restoration of the horizontal

TABLE 86.4. Complications of descending phlebography.

Dizziness and weakness	10
Phlebitis	3
Allergic reactions	1

position, a few require intravenous dextrose infusions. In three of our patients local phlebitis was noticed along the basilic vein, but it responded to local care and spontaneously resolved. Local warm soaking and antiinflammatory medication should be prescribed as needed.

Surgeons who are interested in reconstructive venous surgery should work with the radiologist and perform the procedure to gain firsthand information during fluoroscopy. Experience provides a better understanding of venous anatomy and the underlying etiology of CVID. Venous diseases are far more complex in nature than arterial diseases.

References

1. Bauer G. Observation on the technique of phlebography. *Acta Radiol.* 1945;26:557–588.
2. Bauer G. The etiology of leg ulcers and their treatment by resection of popliteal vein. *Journal International de Chirurgie.* 1948;8:937.
3. Sylvan T. Percutaneous retrograde phlebography of the leg. *Acta Radiol.* 1951;36:66–80.
4. Herman RJ, Neiman HC, Yao JST, et al. Descending venography: a method of evaluation of lower extremity venous valvular function. *Radiology.* 1980;137:63–69.
5. Rai DB, Ortega C, Borzouye A, Lerner R. Descending venography: pericarpal percutaneous venous catheterization of the lower extremity. *Proceedings of the 10th Annual Congress of the Phlebology Society of America.* 1986:115–124.
6. Taheri SA, Sheehan F, Elias S. Descending venography angiology. *J Vasc Dis.* 1983;34:301.
7. Kistner RL. Transvenous repair of the incompetent femoral vein valve. In: Burgan JJ, Yao JST, eds. *Venous Problems.* Chicago, Ill: Year Book Medical; 1978:493–509.
8. Josephus LP. Deep vein valves: a venographic study in normal and post phlebitic stages. *Surgery.* 1956;29:381.

87

The Venous Valve

Travis J. Phifer

History

Hieronymus Fabricius of Aquapendente is considered to be the discoverer of the venous valve.[1] This teacher of anatomy at the University of Padua correctly described venous valves in a 24-page volume, *De Venarum Ostiolis*, published in 1603.[2] Figure 87.1 shows a typical drawing from this work.

William Harvey later made reference to Fabricius in the landmark 72-page publication *Anatomic Treatise of the Motion of the Heart and the Blood in Animals* that contains our modern concept of the circulatory system.[3] In this work Harvey described the venous valve and offered clarification as to function. To quote Harvey (cited in Gottlob,[1] page 6):

The celebrated Hieronymus Fabricius of Aquapendente, a most skilful anatomist, and venerabel old man, or, as the learned Riolan will have it, Jacobus Silvius, first gave representations of the valves in the veins, which consists of raised or loose portions of the inner membranes of these vessels, of extreme delicacy, and a sigmoid or semilunar shape. They are situated at different distances from each other, and diversely in different individuals; they are connate at the sides of the veins; they are directed upwards or towards the trunks of the veins; the two—for there are for the most part two together—contact by their edges, that if anything attempt to pass from the trunks into the branches of the veins, or from the greater vessels into the less, they completely prevent it; they are further so arranged, that the horns of those that succeed are opposite the middle of the convexity of those that precede, and so on alternately.

Embryology

The first vestiges of venous valves at the level of the saphenofemoral junction in the human embryo appear at about 3.5 months. By the end of the fifth month, however, valve development is much more complete. Venous valve development apparently occurs commensurate with the differentiation of media in the endothelial tubes. Before this time in embryologic life, endothelial tubes are devoid of a muscular layer. Kampmeir and Birch[4] actually divided development of the venous valve into five phases and provided detailed descriptions and anatomical diagrams (Figure 87.2) for each of these phases. The contribution of physical factors to development of these vestiges of the venous valve is not completely clear, with conflicting data concerning the matter provided by different scholars.[5] Vortices certainly develop around oblique obstacles in the venous lumen, as is the case with some experimental fixed valves.[6] The extremely smooth and pliant character of the normal fully developed venous valve produces very little turbulence, however, with the gossamerlike leaflets of these delicate structures floating almost passively in the blood stream and yielding easily to impulses of the current.

Macroscopic Anatomy

There are two distinct identifiable macroscopic varieties of venous valves—parietal and ostial.[7] Parietal valves occur most frequently and are generally found at sites of more proximal entry of a tributary or at the junction of two veins of nearly equal diameter. The term *free parietal valve* applies if a parietal valve occurs with no relationship to an entrance or junction. Ostial valves occur at the entry of a small vein into a larger vessel and exist in the two forms of marginal (low) and recessed (high). The best nomenclature for ostial valves, per the discussion that follows, is perhaps simply ostial valve with marginal cusps and ostial valve with recessed cusps.

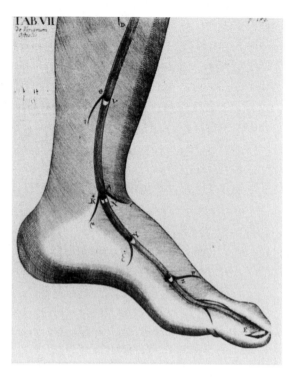

FIGURE 87.1. Valves of the distal greater saphenous vein as depicted by Hieronymus Fabricius of Aquapendente in 1603.[1]

Parietal Valves

Components of a parietal valve are the cusps, agger, cornua, and sinus.[7] In veins of less than 80- to 100-μm diameter, however, there is no valve agger. Most parietal valves are bicuspid, although rare valves occur with one to five cusps. Cusps are usually in the shape of a three quarter to half moon. These extremely thin and delicate cusps consist simply of a collagenous skeleton covered by endothelium. Sometimes a band of collagenous fibers of particular thickness, however, parallels and reinforces the free border of the cusp. Cusps connect to the vein wall by insertion onto the agger. This agger, which contains smooth muscle, is in the shape of a double horse-shoe with the convex aspect faced distally. Juncture of the aggers in the region of the valve commissure forms the cornua. The sinus is the space between the valve cusp and vein wall. The vein wall is particularly thin at the level of the sinus, which perhaps facilitates sinus expansion on hydrostatic loading.

In parietal valves, the geometric relationships of cusps to the vein wall are of some interest. In bicuspid valves, the vertical length of the cusp is often twice the diameter of the vessel.[8] On valve closure, cusps touch over a length of from one fifth to one half the venous diameter at the respective level.[9] An interesting question probably related to valvular competence is the angle optimally portended by the two valve aggers of a bicuspid valve at the level of the cornua.

Ostial Valves

Ostial valves usually consist of a single fold. The insertion of this fold occupies about two thirds of the circumference of the entry of the small vein into the larger vein.[8] If an ostial valve has two folds, they are generally of unequal length but form an oyster shell–like structure. The location of the agger of ostial valves varies between the varieties with marginal insertions and those with recessed insertions.

In the variety of ostial valve with marginal (low) insertion, the valve is directly at the circumference of the entry. The agger for the distal cusp is in the lumen of the major vessel, and the cusp hangs freely into the lumen of this vessel. There is no sinus for the distal cusp. The agger for the proximal cusp is at the site of merging of the walls of the small and large vessels. The sinus for the proximal cusp is proximal to the agger for this cusp and entirely in the wall of the major vein. The wall of the major vein is characteristically thin at the level of the sinus.

In the variety of ostial valve with recessed (high) insertion, the aggers are entirely within the entering vessel. The valve cusps generally hang out of the ostium into the lumen of the major vessel in this situation. There is a sinus for each half of the valve.

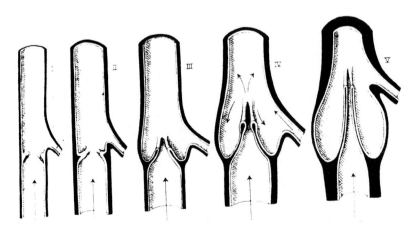

FIGURE 87.2. Embryologic development of a bicuspid venous valve as depicted by Kampmeier and Birch[4]: I–IV, between fetal months 3.5 and 5; V, at full term.

Spatial Orientation

The shape of the veins in the cross section in vivo depends on the degree of luminal filling and is generally elliptical.[9] This is particularly so at the level of a valve. The alignment of valve cusps is along the longitudinal axis of the ellipse. Valve cusps thus normally coapt in a plane parallel to the skin or the fascia surrounding the muscles. Normal cusps join smoothly, an impossible situation with any other spatial orientation of the valve mechanism.

Microscopic Anatomy

The following excerpt from the monograph *Venous Valves* by Gottlob and May[7] succinctly describes the histology of the venous valve as demonstrated by light microscopy using paraffin sections and is thus worthy of direct quotation. Figure 87.3, taken from the same source, is an excellent illustration of this verbal description.

The valvular cusps may be divided into two regions, a luminal part facing the lumen of the vessel, and a parietal part facing the wall of the vessel. Both parts are covered by a layer of unicellular endothelium. Underneath the endothelium of the luminal part there is a thin elastic layer, which is an extension of the internal elastic membrane of the vein. The elastic membrane is slightly undulated. According to Saphir and Lev (1953) extremely thin elastic fibrils may branch off occasionally and invade the adjacent collagenous layer. The surface of the luminal part is relatively smooth, whereas the parietal part is rather irregularly outlined. Crypts and crevices covered by endothelium invade the substance of the valves. These crypts are arranged in an irregular manner; occasionally they are absent. Saphir and Lev attributed the superficial irregularity of the parietal part to the absence of an elastic layer in that region. The stroma of the valve mainly consists of collagen; the valve contains few connective tissue cells. In the region of the valvular agger smooth muscle cells are found, but such cells do not invade farther into the valvular cusp.(33, 34)

In the avalvular portion of veins, endothelial cells run with their longitudinal axes parallel to the axis of the vessel. In the valve sinus, however, the endothelial arrangement is either crosswise to or in irregular alignment with the axis of the vessel. Arrangement of endothelia on the parietal aspect of the valve cusp is analogous to the valve sinus. On the luminal aspect of the valve cusp, however, endothelial alignment is predominantly along the long axis of the vessel as is the case in avalvular portions of the vein.

Electron microscopy confirms and embellishes the findings of light microscopy. Endothelial cells found on venous valves contain the organelles and cellular elements typical of endothelial cells in general. Transport vesicles and coated vesicles are common, with variable numbers of Weibel–Palade bodies. There are many intracellular filaments of intermediate size, with an occasional single cilium. Endothelial cells on the valve surface attach by closed junctions, with superficial borders of cytoplasm on both the parietal and luminal layers gathered in regular overlapping marginal folds. The distance between endothelial cells varies on both sides of the cusp, with this space ranging from a thickness of only a few collagenous fibrils or less to a thickness of either one or more bundles of fibrils or one or more cellular elements (myofibroblasts). Stroma cells are in general sparse but more frequent toward the free edge of the valve cusp. These cells are of two types, both morphologically distinct from fibroblasts and fibrocytes. Because of bundles of cytoplasmic filaments potentially corresponding to actin, some classify these connective tissue cells as myofibroblasts. Myofibroblasts and smooth muscle cells occur with comparable frequency only at the level of valvular insertion. Collagenous fibrils comprise the main portion of the fibrillar material of the valve, with the thickness of this material varying from a single layer of fibrils in thin areas to two or more bundles at wider spaces between endothelial cells.

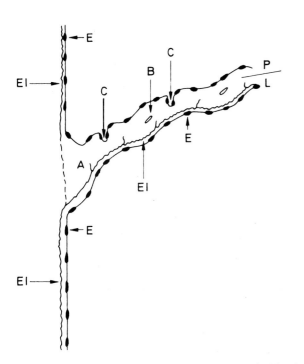

FIGURE 87.3. Scheme of venous valve structure[7]: El, elastic membrane; E, endothelial cells; A, valvular agger; C, crypts; B, connective tissue cell; P, parietal aspect; L, luminal aspect.

Occurrence and Distribution

Numerous studies of varying degrees of comprehensiveness provide interesting information with regard to occurrence and distribution of venous valves.[10] Although absent in some veins, venous valves occur throughout the animal kingdom and are not unique to the bipedal human. For example, venous valves occur in amphibians such as the frog. Venous valves also occur in birds but less frequently than in humans. In domestic animals, the distribution of venous valves approximates that of humans.

Valves occur in postcapillary veins as small as 20 to 145 μm diameter. The large capacitance veins, however, are devoid of valves. The first venous valves craniad from the heart are at the subclavian and internal jugular levels. Valves occur more frequently in the lower extremity veins; they assume a particularly important role in these veins in humans because of their relationship to hydrostatic loading and the common human affliction of chronic venous insufficiency.

A brief synopsis[10,11] regarding occurrence and distribution of valves in the lower extremity veins (Figure 87.4) is as follows:

Deep veins

1. Inferior vena cava: 0 valves
2. Common iliac vein: valves in the common iliac vein are rare, with reported absence of valves above even the saphenofemoral junction varying from 20% to 24%.
3. External iliac and common femoral vein (above saphenofemoral junction): reported occurrence of a single valve varies from 35% to 80%
4. Femoral vein (below saphenofemoral junction): 3 valves
5. Popliteal vein: 1 valve

6. Posterior tibial vein: 19 valves
7. Anterior tibial vein: 11 valves
8. Peroneal vein: 10 valves

Superficial veins

1. Long saphenous: average of 3.5 valves in the thigh and 4 valves in the calf, with about 8 in the foot; the most important superficial valve mechanism is just below the saphenofemoral junction, with the uppermost (terminal) valve an ostial valve located at the entrance into the femoral vein and a second (subterminal) valve about 5 cm distal to the proximal valve[12]
2. Short saphenous: 8 valves
3. Communicating veins of the calf: about 75% of these veins contain valves, with an average of 1 to 5 valves per vein; there are apparently no valves outside the muscular fascia, and all valves are bicuspid
4. Perforating veins of the foot: these veins have either a single valve or no valves at all; the physiological flow of blood at this level, in contrast to the perforating veins of the calf, is from deep to superficial[13]
5. Veins of the gastrocnemius and soleus muscles: variation is considerable at this level; valves are generally abundant, however, at least before age 30

Bardeleben in the late 1800s postulated a constant distance between venous valves in any individual depending on such factors as body height and limb length.[14] Although this concept is now basically considered untenable,[10] calculation of average distances between these valves is feasible and provides some constants germane to the current understanding of lower extremity venous dynamics. The average distance between valves in the deep system (22 mm) is shorter than in the superficial system (40 mm). This variation seemingly favors efficiency in blood return, because blood at this level normally flows from superficial to deep and then centrally on engagement of the deep muscle pump of the calf.

An interesting question relates to the issue of disappearance of venous valves with age.[10] Bardeleben suggested a retention rate of only 19% of original valves.[14] Rather than de novo disappearance of valves, however, pathologic processes more likely result in structural atrophy and valvular incompetence.[15–17] An exception is spontaneous regression of the ostial and free valves of fetal and infant kidneys. Regional variation is also apparently important, in that constant unidirectional flow conditions predispose a patient to the loss of functional valves and hydrostatic loading and frequent reversal of flow favor preservation of valve function. Pathologic processes potentiating valve dysfunction and atrophy include overdilation of the vein wall and perivalvular thrombus formation. With overdilation of the vein wall, valve leaflets unable to coapt not only become functionally incompetent but also change morphologically. Any distortion of the valve mech-

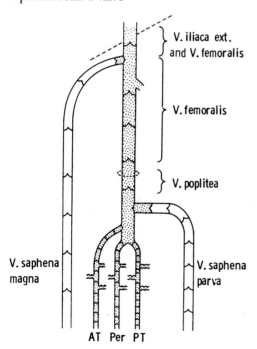

FIGURE 87.4. Valves in the venous system of the leg.[10]

FIGURE 87.5. Valve function in the veins of the calf.[18]

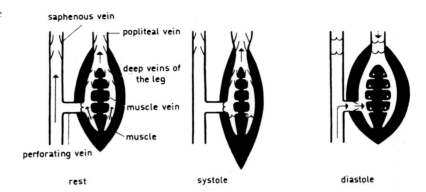

anism results in turbulence and thus predisposes a patient to thrombus formation. The formation of simple microthrombi around and in the valve sinus or on the leaflets often causes leaflet distortion after lysis and organization, perhaps related to shrinkage or synechial formation. With thrombotic occlusion of the venous lumen, irreparable damage to valves occurs even with thrombolysis and recanalization of the lumen.[18] Other than pathologic processes directly affecting the valves, occlusion of the iliac or caval veins often results in shunting of venous blood through valveless venous collaterals.[9]

Function

The primary function of the venous valve, as asserted by Harvey in his classic work in 1628,[3] is maintenance of the direction of blood flow. This occurs by both hydrodynamic and hydrostatic mechanisms.[19,20] Also, the venous valve plays a pivotal role in mechanisms related to the pathogenesis of thrombus formation in lower extremity veins.

Hydrodynamic Mechanisms

On ambulation and compression of the plantar plexus (venous insole), valves in communicating veins direct the flow of blood from deep to superficial in the foot. Blood also enters the deep veins from the foot, however, because communicating veins at this level often have no valves and are thus capable of bidirectional flow. This is in contrast to the calf (Figure 87.5), where valves in perforating veins open during muscle relaxation and close during muscle contraction and thus direct blood flow from superficial to deep. In the saphenous systems and deep veins, more proximal valves open and distal valves close in synchrony with skeletal muscle contraction during calf pump systole (with sequence reversal during diastole). This mechanism inhibits retrograde flow yet promotes antegrade flow. Similarly, increased pressure within the abdominal cavity during inspiration produces passive closure of valves in infrainguinal veins and, in association with the concomitant reduction of intrathoracic pressure (associated with depression of the diaphragm and expansion of the thoracic cage), enhances central blood return. On expiration, this sequence also reverses and blood flows into the capacitance veins of the abdomen from the lower extremities in preparation for repetition of the cycle. Bollinger[21] described this phenomenon in terms of a thoracoabdominal suction pressure pump (Figure 87.6). Finally, venous valves also function to some degree in the central return of blood by synchronization of impulses exerted by arteries on immediately adjacent accompanying veins.

FIGURE 87.6. Schematic of thoracoabdominal suction pressure pump depicting three regions of differing pressure encountered by venous blood passing from the lower extremities to the heart and showing the effect of this pump on lower extremity venous hemodynamics.[19] Solid arrows depict blood flow; open arrows depict pressure on the inferior vena cava with ventilation. VCI, inferior vena cava; VCS, superior vena cava; AD, right atrium.

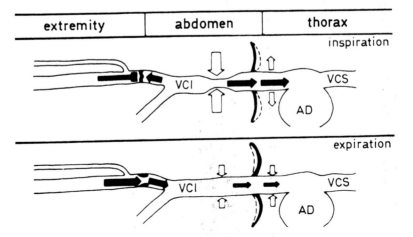

Hydrostatic Mechanisms

Even at rest, blood flow continues in the veins. On sudden changes of position, dramatic hydrostatic pressure fluxes often occur within the lower extremity veins. The maximal hydrostatic pressure exerted at any level in the erect human is the weight of the perpendicular column of blood from the point of measurement to the phlebostatic axis, as described by Winsor and Birch[22] at approximately the level of the right atrium. A sudden change in intraluminal venous pressure results in prompt valve closure. Valve closure then continues until normal antegrade filling from below the level of the closed valve eliminates the pressure gradient across the valve. When this steady state is reached, the valve opens and leaflets simply float in the luminal flow until another change in pressure occurs.

Mechanisms of Valve Failure

Failure of the venous valve with development of valvular incompetence occurs by both primary and secondary mechanisms.[23] Primary valvular incompetence probably involves a process of fibroelastic degeneration of valve tissue, with development of redundancy in the valve leaflets and stretching of the valve wall. Redundant valve leaflets described as cauliflowerlike are characteristic. Secondary valvular incompetence is commonly a postphlebitic event, however, with valve leaflets permanently damaged and encased in fibrous tissue after recannulation of thrombosed veins.[18]

Thrombus formation in lower extremity veins often begins at the level of the sinus aspect of the valve and is likely related to the unique hemodynamic characteristics of the venous valve. Vortices produced in the valve sinus during flow increase the dwell time of particles before their ultimate expulsion from a deteriorating orbit into the main luminal stream.[6] This process retards blood flow and potentiates accumulation of cellular elements, with apparent progressive desaturation of hemoglobin toward the base of the sinus.[24] Endothelial hypoxia is the likely consequence of this series of events. Endothelial hypoxia results in leukocyte adhesion[25] followed by platelet deposition and degranulation with release of substances such as thromboxane and platelet thromboplastin. Further platelet aggregation with fibrin formation and trapping of cells results in mature thrombus formation, sometimes limited to the valve sinus but at other times propagating and occluding the venous lumen. Venous thrombosis involving valve cusps causes an increase of capillary permeability at the base of the cusp. This increased permeability results in early transcapillary migration of leukocytes, followed later by capillary budding and fibroblast proliferation with collagen deposition. Ulceration and attachment of the valve cusp to the

vein wall occurs. Fibrinolytic activity eventually results in restoration of luminal patency to the thrombosed vein but with virtual destruction of the valve leaflets leaving only remnants of elastica remaining in the thickened and scarred wall of the recannulated vein.[18]

Relationship to Chronic Venous Insufficiency

Venous valvular incompetence is a common denominator to all categories of chronic venous insufficiency,[26] although valvular reflux and disordered calf muscle function also occur in limbs with little or no manifestations of venous disease.[25] The significance of valvular reflux at different levels thus remains controversial. Calf muscle pump dysfunction seems particularly likely with incompetence of communicating veins. Also, incompetence of the communicating veins seems to occur in 80% or more of patients with venous ulceration.[28] Some thus favor treating reflux in the superficial system (including the communicating veins) before considering correction of deep venous valvular incompetence. Others emphasize the importance of deep venous valvular incompetence in failure of the calf muscle pump and consider superficial venous imcompetence a secondary phenomenon, however, reporting 75% to 88% pure deep vein valvular reflux in legs with venous ulceration.[29] Regardless of this mechanism, the pathologic potential of calf muscle pump failure includes the clinical syndrome of chronic venous insufficiency manifest as a painful edematous limb with varicosities and stasis dermitis progressing to lipodermatosclerosis and eventual dermal ulceration. The dermal consequences of this syndrome are apparently related to a combination of derangements at the microcirculatory and cellular levels initiated by chronic venous hypertension and associated with altered fibrinolysis as well as leukocyte dysfunction and cytokine release.[30-33] Chronic venous insufficiency is a substantial worldwide health problem that is extremely costly not only in terms of days lost from gainful employment and in expense of medical therapy but also in terms of human morbidity and thus warrants serious consideration with regard to prevention and treatment.

Surgical Procedures

Carrel and Guthrie in 1906 reported autotransplantation of canine vein segments containing valves.[34] Almost half a century later, in 1953, Eiseman and Malette described an intussusception technique for construction of a valve in the canine inferior vena cava.[35] Kistner in 1968 introduced the technique of valvuloplasty in humans[36,37] and with Sparkuhl in 1979 described valve transposition.[38] De-Weese and Niquidula in 1960 reported venous valves autotransplantation in the canine,[39] although Taheri et al. in 1982 reported the first vein valve autotransplant in a human.[40]

Clinical Studies

Procedures currently accepted with favorable clinical data for treatment of venous valve incompetence include valvuloplasty,[37,39,41] valve transposition,[38,42] and valve autotransplantation.[40,43] Other techniques reported for correction of lower extremity deep vein valve incompetence include the intravascular procedure of creating a xenogeneic monocuspid patch[44,45] valve, as well as the extravascular procedures of placement of a popliteal sling[46] and valve banding.[47]

Valvuloplasty

The procedure for venous valve repair described by Kistner in 1968 is a direct technique of internal valvuloplasty accompanied by placement of pleating sutures at the commissures of incompetent valves such as to tighten redundant leaflets and restore valvular competence.[36,37] Minor modifications of the original technique for gaining access to the redundant cusps include a transverse venotomy advocated by Raju and Fredericks[29] and the T-shaped incision employed by Sottiurai[41] rather than the vertical incision used by Kistner. Also, Jones et al. used axial plication of the valve sinus to reduce excessive dilation and restore valve competence.[48] Kistner later described a technique of external valvuloplasty that is less precise than internal valvuloplasty but faster to perform and applicable to smaller-caliber veins.[49]

Valvuloplasty is an effective procedure for restoration and maintenance of venous valve competence. Ferris and Kistner in 1982 showed valve competence as determined by descending phlebography in the majority of 31 valves studied 13 years after valvuloplasty.[50] The exact effect of the valvuloplasty on clinical disease was more difficult to assess because of concomitant communicating vein surgery in most of these cases. Raju and Fredericks in 1968 reported results of 61 valvuloplasty procedures studied beyond 2 years, however, and showed relief of pain and swelling in 87% and 83%, respectively, with maintenance of dermal healing in 63%.[29]

Transposition

Valve transposition as described by Kistner and Sparkuhl in 1979[38] involves transfer of an incompetent venous segment to a vein with at least one competent valve, usually accomplished as an end-to-side anastomosis between the transected incompetent venous segment below a competent valve in the recipient vein.[42] Several different

anatomical arrangements are possible. Although effective in the initial improvement of calf muscle pump function,[42,50] this procedure fails to confer long-term competence with valve failure reported in as many as 50% of cases.[51]

Autotransplantation

Valve autotransplantation uses a segment of either brachial or axillary vein containing a single autogenous valve, interposing this valvular conduit at either the superficial femoral or popliteal level.[40,43] This procedure provides at least short-term correction of valvular reflux and improvement of calf muscle pump function with healing of dermal ulceration and resolution of symptoms in some patients. Raju and Fredericks showed at over 2 years improvement of pain and edema in 50% and 39%, respectively, with resolution of problems with dermal ulceration in 46%.[29] Eriksson and Almgren studied 34 autotransplanted valves using duplex scanning as well as descending phlebography, however, and showed incompetence of 16 with thrombosis of 8 at 27 months.[52] Also using duplex scanning as well as descending venography, Perrin et al. showed competence of only 6 valves in 17 autotransplants assessed at 28 months.[53] Durability of autotransplanted venous valves is thus a significant question.

Xenogeneic Monocuspid Patch

Garcia-Rinaldi et al. described a xenogeneic monocuspid patch valve. The model for this valve is the cardiac sinus of Valsalva. Computer simulation apparently aided design of the valve, which is constructed from xenogeneic patch material with a single valve leaflet in a cusp supported by a ring. Reported clinical results were excellent after placement of this device in the lower extremity of a single patient with chronic venous insufficiency; a later report of two additional patients supplemented the data.[44,45]

Banding

Hallberg reported in 1972 a technique of indirect valvuloplasty utilizing a Dacron cuff wrapped around the valve sinus to reduce sinus dilation.[54] Raju and Fredericks later used this technique as a adjunct to valve autotransplantation.[29] Jessup and Lane in 1988 introduced a similar process of valve banding, using an extravascular prosthetic wrap for reduction of valve circumference.[47] The purpose of this procedure using either technique is to improve leaflet coaptation and restore valve competence. Long-term benefit of this procedure is questionable, however, with available data limited. Of note, Raju and Fredericks reported no significant benefit in axillary vein transfers using the adjunct of a Dacron sleeve.[29]

Popliteal Sling

The popliteal sling is an extravascular approach to treatment of lower extremity venous valvular incompetence.[46] This procedure, as modified, uses a prosthetic spacer passed between the popliteal artery and vein connecting the gracilis and biceps tendons. This spacer compresses the popliteal vein during muscle pump diastole by contraction of the gracilis muscle with the foot off the ground. The originator of this procedure reported ulcer healing in all patients and relief of pain with improvement in ambulatory venous pressure in more than 85% of patients. Confirmatory multicenter studies, however, are not available. Technical nuances of this intriguing concept perhaps make reproduction of these excellent results difficult.[55]

Animal Studies

A basic prerequisite for valvuloplasty performed by any technique (internal or external, direct or indirect) is the presence of redundant but otherwise grossly normal valve leaflets (i.e., primary valvular incompetence). Valvuloplasty is generally of limited value in valves damaged by the postphlebitic process. Transposition and autotransplantation procedures require a competent valve in the recipient vein or donor segment, respectively. As many as 40% of axillary vein valves are incompetent,[29] however, with size matching another consideration in autotransplantation. Although valvuloplasty seems to confer lasting competence in the majority of cases, durability of transposed and autotransplanted valves is less certain.[56] Valve dilation possibly related to size mismatch as well as shedding of endothelium with fibrosis and degeneration perhaps related to ischemia are potential mechanisms of valve failure.[57,58] The xenogeneic monocuspid patch is basically an experimental device of unproven value. Long-term benefit of valve banding is questionable, even when the procedure is possibly limited to cases of primary valvular incompetence. Reproducibility of results is a problem with the popliteal sling. None of the aforementioned clinical procedures is thus totally satisfactory and universally applicable. A prosthetic venous valve is needed that is readily available in multiple sizes with proven safety and satisfactory function as well as established durability, easily implantable, possibly in tandem in lower extremity veins. Such a prosthesis is not yet available for clinical application, however, despite extensive investigational work with various tissues and mechanical devices.

After Carrel and Guthrie reported autotransplantation of valve-bearing vein segments in animals in 1906,[34] there was little apparent interest in venous surgery until Johns undertook studies of venous anastomotic techniques reported in 1947.[59] Eiseman and Malette in 1953 first described a technique for construction of a valve in the canine inferior vena cava.[35]

The technique described by Eiseman and Malette was a type of wall intussusception used earlier by Perl for creation of a conical valve in jejunostomies.[60] Venous valves constructed by this technique remained patent at 6 months without anticoagulation, although results of tests for competence were not clear.

Three decades later, Hill et al. reported implantation over a stainless-steel stent in the canine external jugular vein of a bicuspid flutter valve mechanism produced in both glutaraldehyde-fixed human umbilical vein as well as pellethane polymer.[61] Despite anticoagulation, thrombotic occlusion occurred in all umbilical vein units by 48 hours and in all pallethane units by 8 days.

Ackroyd in 1985 reported implantion of glutaraldehyde-preserved homogeneic valves in a canine model at the femoral level.[62] Even with adjuncts including heparinization and defibrinogenation as well as construction of an arteriovenous fistula, thrombosis of all units occurred by 6 weeks. Kaya et al. in similar canine experiments a few years later, however, noted improved patency with glutaraldehyde-fixed autografts and allografts despite valve function in only 25% of the allografts at 7 weeks.[63]

Also in 1985, Warmenhoven et al. implanted valve-shaped Silastic mandrels at various positions in dogs such as to incite production of a collagen sheath around the mandrel.[64] Subsequent removal of the mandrel and excision of the sheath and 4 to 13 weeks resulted in production of a collagen valve. Implantation of these valves at either the femoral or jugular level without anticoagulation, however, resulted in thrombosis of all units by 16 weeks.

Rosenbloom et al.[65] in 1988 described an autogenous venous valve produced from the canine external jugular vein using an elegant approach modified after the technique described earlier by Eiseman and Malette.[35] The technique involved somewhat tedious dissection of the intima from the media and adventitia of a donor vein, fashioning a nipple-type valve within the remaining cylindric intimal conduit. Hydrostatic tests indicated potential for function of these units under physiological conditions, with low opening and closing pressures in the range of 3–5 cm H_2O yet competence at pressures up to 55 cm H_2O. Although 6 of these valves interposed at the femoral level in the canine remained patent and competent at 7 days without anticoagulation, 4 of the units were incompetent because of perileaflet thrombus formation. With anticoagulation, 3 valves were both patent and competent at 13 days after implantation. Long-term data are not available.

Taheri then developed a sutureless center-hinged bicuspid mechanical valve composed of either platinum or pyrolyte carbon-covered titanium[66] and in 1988 reported results from implantation of these valves in the canine at the femoral level as well as in the inferior vena cava.[67] Marginal patency and problems such as valve migration and tilting as well as cracking of the leaflet attachment limited results of these experiments. Phifer et al. similarly reported experiments with a mechanical tilt-disc valve implanted in the canine inferior vena cava, with 9 of 12 valves patent at 2 to 4 weeks but with function limited by nonocclusive thrombus formation in the valve mechanism.[68]

In 1989, Phifer et al. demonstrated feasibility for prolonged patency of valvular biprostheses placed in the venous system, using modified xenogeneic cardiac valves interposed in the canine inferior vena cava.[69] At the time of either elective sacrifice or final study of the 22 animals in this report at intervals of 1 to 28 months, 12 valves remained patent with a plausible cause of occlusion identified in 8 of the 10 unsuccessful units. There were no pulmonary emboli demonstrated by angiography or autopsy in animals with patent valves, although nonfatal pulmonary embolization occurred in 9 of the 10 dogs with occluded valves. Despite acceptable competence upon retrograde valvulography in 6 of 8 patent valves evaluated for reflux, perileaflet thrombus formation with subsequent organization and collagen deposition limited leaflet function in these units as demonstrated at autopsy.

Spiegowski et al. autotransplanted canine venous valve cusps from the brachial to the femoral level, and in 1989 reported 100% patency and 80% competency at 10–16 weeks.[70] These valves were competent only at relatively low pressures (16 mm Hg), however, and isolated cusp placement resulted in low patency. The same investigators also autotransplanted canine valve segments. Using the usual end-to-end anastomotic technique, 80% of the units were patent with 70% competence at 4 months. Using an innovative biterminal end-to-side anastomoses, 80% were both patent as well as competent at 4 months.[71]

Also in 1989, Van den Broek described a microsurgical technique using peritoneum for creation of a monocusp valve mechanism. In autogenous implantation studies performed in a rat model, valves remained patent and free of thrombus, although few were competent.[72]

In 1990, Wilson et al. reported production of size-matched autogenous venous valves with an endothelial lining[73] using a technique of vein wall intussusception similar to that used by Eiseman and Malette in 1953[35] and Rosenbloom et al. in 1988.[65] Hydrostatic studies showed opening and closing pressures of less than 5 cm H_2O, with competence at pressures up to 250 cm H_2O. In canine implantation experiments performed without chronic anticoagulation, 6 valves remained patent with no evidence of thrombus formation and with phlebographic competence at 1 to 112 days. Long-term studies, however, are not available.

In 1993, Delaria et al. described basic criteria considered necessary for a prosthetic venous valve.[74] These investigators then used an in vivo test circuit to produce conditions analogous to hemodynamics of the venous circulation and evaluated a valvular bioprosthesis produced from glutaraldehyde-fixed bovine jugular vein designed specifically for application in the venous circulation. Results of the in vitro tests were encouraging, although in vivo data are not yet published.

The most interesting current work comes from a group of investigations evaluating cryopreserved venous valvular allografts.[75] A preliminary report showed patency (assisted with a distal arteriovenous fistula) at approximately 6 weeks in 6 of 8 implants to an incompetent femoral venous system in a canine model. These 6 valves were grossly and histologically normal, with partial correction of venous hemodynamics. Multicenter human trials are in progress.

Conclusion

Despite a substantive body of experimental work, no suitable prosthesis is yet available for replacement of the venous valve. The functional and anatomical configuration of the autogenous venous valve, as described earlier in this chapter, is deceivingly simple. Development of a durable and functional prosthesis, however, is incredibly difficult. Correction of venous valvular incompetence at this time thus depends on techniques using autogenous tissue valvuloplasty, autotransplantation, and transposition. Development of a prosthetic venous valve remains an elusive dream.

References

1. Gottlob R, May R. History. In: Gottlob R, May R, eds. *Venous Valves*. Vienna, Austria: Springer-Verlag; 1986:3–10.
2. Fabricius H ab Aquapendente. *De Venarum Ostiolis*. Padua, Italy; 1603.
3. Harvey W. Exercitatio anatomica de motu cordis et sanguinis in animalibus. 1628.
4. Kampmeier OF, Birch CLF. The origin and development of the venous valves with particular reference to the saphenous district. *Am J Anat.* 1917;38:451–499.
5. Gottlob R, May R. Embryology of venous valves. In: Gottlob R, May R, eds. *Venous Valves*. Vienna, Austria: Springer-Verlag; 1986:13–15.
6. Karino T, Motomiya M. Flow through a venous valve and its implication for thrombus formation. *Thromb Res.* 1984; 36:245–257.
7. Gottlob R, May R. Anatomy of venous valves. In: Gottlob R, May R, eds. *Venous Valves*. Vienna, Austria: Springer-Verlag; 1986:25–61.
8. Franklin KJ. Valves in veins: an historical survey. *Proceedings of the Royal Society of Medicine.* 1927;21:1.

9. Edwards A. The treatment of varicose veins: anatomical factors of ligation of the great saphenous vein. *Surg Gynecol Obstet.* 1934;59:916–928.

10. Gottlob R, May R. Occurrence and distribution of venous valves. In: Gottlob R, May R, eds. *Venous Valves.* Vienna, Austria: Springer-Verlag; 1986:16–24.

11. Ludbrook J. *Aspects of Venous Function in the Lower Limbs.* Springfield, Ill: CC Thomas; 1968.

12. Cotton LT. Varicose veins gross anatomy and development. *Br J Surg.* 1961;48:589–598.

13. Lofgren EP, Myers TT, Lofgren KA, et al. The venous valves of the foot and ankle. *Surg Gynecol Obstet.* 1968;127:289–290.

14. Bardeleben KV. Das klappendistanzgesetz. *Jenaische Z Naturwiss.* 1880;14:467.

15. Paterson JC, McLachlin J. Precipitating factors in venous thrombosis. *Surg Gynecol Obstet.* 1954;98:96–102.

16. Sevitt S. Organization of valve pocket thrombi and the anomalies of double thrombi and valve cusp involvement. *Br J Surg.* 1974;61:641–649.

17. Sevitt A. The structure and growth of valve-pocket thrombi in femoral veins. *J Clin Pathol.* 1974;27:517.

18. Edwards AE, Edwards JE. The effect of thrombophlebitis on the venous valve. *Surg Gynecol Obstet.* 1937;65:310–320.

19. Gottlob R, May R. Functions of venous valves. In: Gottlob R, May R, eds. *Venous Valves.* Vienna, Austria: Springer-Verlag; 1986:62–76.

20. Sumner DS. Applied physiology in venous disease. In: Sakaguchi S, ed. *Advances in Phlebology.* London: John Libbey; 1987:5.

21. Bollinger A. Klappenagenesie und-dysplasie der beinvenen. *Schweiz Med Wochenschr.* 1971;101:1348.

22. Winsor T, Burch GE. Phlebostotatic axis and phlebostatic level for venous pressure measurements in man. *Proc Soc Exp Biol Med.* 1945;58:165–169.

23. Kistner RL. Primary venous valve incompetence of the leg. *Am J Surg.* 1982;140:218–224.

24. Hamer JD, Malone PO, Silver JA. The Po₂ in venous valve pockets: its possible bearing on thrombogenesis. *Br J Surg.* 1981;68:166–170.

25. Schaub RG, Simmons CA, Kott MH, et al. Early events in the formation of a venous thrombus following local trauma and sepsis. *Lab Invest.* 1984;51:218–224.

26. Schanzer H, Peirce EC. A rational approach to surgery of the chronic venous stasis syndrome. *Ann Surg.* 1982;195:25–29.

27. Stacey MC, Burnand KG, Pattison M, et al. Changes in the apparently normal limb in unilateral venous ulceration. *Br J Surg.* 1987;74:936–939.

28. Negus D. Prevention and treatment of venous ulceration. *Ann R Coll Surg Engl.* 1985;67:144–148.

29. Raju S, Fredericks R. Valve reconstruction procedures for nonobstructive venous insufficiency: rationale, techniques, and results in 107 procedures with two- to eight-year follow-up. *J Vasc Surg.* 1988;7:301–310.

30. Thomas RS, Nash GB, Dormandy JA. White cell accumulation in dependent legs of patients with venous hypertension: a possible mechanism for trophic changes in the skin. *Br Med J.* 1988;296:1693–1695.

31. Pappas PJ, DeFouw DO, Venezio LM, et al. Morphomatic assessment of the dermal microcirculation in patients with chronic venous insufficiency. *J Vasc Surg.* 1997;26:784–795.

32. Burnand KG, Whimster I, Naidoo A, et al. Pericapillary fibrin in the ulcer-bearing skin of the leg: the cause of lipodermatosclerosis and venous ulceration. *Br Med J.* 1982;285:1071–1072.

33. Falanga V, Eaglstein WH. The trap hypothesis of venous ulceration. *Lancet.* 1993;341:1006–1008.

34. Carrel A, Guthrie CC. Uniterminal and biterminal venous transplantation. *Surg Gynecol Obstet.* 1906;2:266–286.

35. Eiseman B, Mallette W. An operative technique for the construction of venous valves. *Surg Gynecol Obstet.* 1953;97:731–734.

36. Kistner RL. Surgical repair of a venous valve. *Straub Clin Proc.* 1968;34:41–43.

37. Kistner RL. Surgical repair of the incompetent femoral vein valve. *Arch Surg.* 1975;110:1336–1342.

38. Kistner R, Sparkuhl MD. Surgery in acute and chronic venous disease. *Surgery.* 1979;85:31–41.

39. DeWeese JA, Niquidula F. The replacement of short sequents of veins with functional autogenous venous valves. *Surg Gynecol Obstet.* 1960;110:303–308.

40. Taheri SA, Lazar L, Elias SM, et al. Vein valve transplant. *Surgery.* 1982;91:28–33.

41. Sottiurai VS. Technique in direct venous valvuloplasty. *J Vasc Surg.* 1988;8:646–648.

42. Queral LA, Whitehouse WM, Flinn WR, et al. Surgical correction of deep venous insufficiency by valvular transposition. *Surgery.* 1980;87:688–695.

43. O'Donnell TF, Mackey WC, Shepherd AD. Clinical, hemodynamic, and anatomic follow-up of direct venous reconstruction. *Arch Surg.* 1987;122:474–482.

44. Garcia-Rinaldi R, Revuelta JM, Martinez MJ, et al. Femoral vein valve incompetence: treatment with a xenograft monocusp patch. *J Vasc Surg.* 1986;3:932–935.

45. Garcia-Rinaldi R, Revuelta JM. Experimental prosthetic vein valve [letter]. *Am J Surg.* 1990;159:186.

46. Psathakis N, Psathakis D. Rationale and efficacy of the substitute "valve" operation by technique II in deep venous insufficiency of the lower limb. *Vasc Surg.* 1986;20:211–224.

47. Jessup G, Lane RJ. Repair of incompetent venous valves: a new technique. *J Vasc Surg.* 1988;8:569–575.

48. Jones JW. Elliot F, Kerstein MD. Triangular venous valvuloplasty. *Arch Surg.* 1982;117:1250–1251.

49. Kistner R. Surgical technique of external venous valve repair. *Proc Straub Pacific Health Foundation.* 1990;55:15.

50. Ferris EB, Kistner RL. Femoral vein reconstruction in the management of chronic venous insufficiency. *Arch Surg.* 1982;117:1571–1579.

51. Wilson NM, Rutt DL, Browse NL. Repair and replacement of deep vein valves in the treatment of venous insufficiency. *Br J Surg.* 1991;78:388–394.

52. Eriksson I, Almgren B. Surgical reconstruction of incompetent deep vein valves. *Upsala J Med Sci.* 1988;93:139–143.

53. Perrin M, Hiltbrand B, Bolot JE, et al. Resultats de la chirurgie veineuse restauratrice dans les reflux de la voie veineuse profonde au niveau des nembres inferieurs. *Proc 10eme Congress Mondial Union Internationale de Phlebologie.* Strasbourg: John Libby; 1989:1085–1086.

54. Hallberg D. A method for repairing incompetent valves in deep veins. *Acta Chir Scand.* 1972;138:143–145.

55. Plate G, Brudin L, Eklof B, et al. Physiologic and therapeutic aspects in congenital vein valve aplasia of the lower limb. *Ann Surg.* 1983;198:229–233.

56. Raju S. Venous insufficiency in the lower limb and stasis ulceration. *Ann Surg.* 1983;197:688–697.

57. Nash T. Long term results of vein valve transplants placed in the popliteal vein for intractable post-phlebitic venous ulcers and pre-ulcer skin changes. *J Cardiovas Surg.* 1988; 29:712–716.

58. Raju S, Perry JT. The response of venous vascular endothelium to autotransplantation and in vitro preservation. *Surgery.* 1983;94:770–775.

59. Johns TNPA. A comparison of suture and non-suture methods for the anastomosis of veins. *Surg Gynecol Obstet.* 1947;84:939–942.

60. Perl JI. Intussuscepted conical valve formation in jejunostomies. *Surgery.* 1949;25:297–299.

61. Hill R, Schmidt S, Evancho M, et al. Development of a prosthetic venous valve. *J Biomed Mater Res.* 1985;19: 827–832.

62. Ackroyd JS. Venous valve homografts. M Chir Thesis, Cambridge University, 1985.

63. Kaya M, Grogan JB, Lentz D, et al. Glutaraldehyde-preserved venous valve transplantation in the dog. *J Surg Res.* 1988;45:294–297.

64. Warmenhoven PG, Klopper PJ, Keeman JN. Construction of valves in the venous system. A preliminary report of an experimental study in dogs. *Eur Surg Research.* 1985;17 (Suppl 1):105.

65. Rosenbloom MS, Schuler JJ, Bishara RA, et al. Early experimental experience with a surgically created, totally autogenous venous valve: a preliminary report. *J Vasc Surg.* 1988;7:642–646.

66. Taheri SA, Rigan D, Wels P, et al. Experimental prosthetic venous valve. *Am J Surg.* 1988;156:111–114.

67. Taheri SA, Shores R. Successful use of sutureless prosthetic vein valves in dogs. *Proc 10eme Congress Mondiale Union Internationale de Phlebologie.* Strasbourg: John Libby; 1989:1035–1037.

68. Phifer TJ, Price DT, Thomas MB, et al. Performance of the tilt-disc valve in the inferior vena cava: an animal study. *Vascular Surgery.* 1990;24:496–502.

69. Phifer TJ, Gerlock AJ, Grafton WD, et al. Valvular xenografts in the inferior vena cava: an animal study. *Am J Surg.* 1989;157:588–592.

80. Spiegowski M, Ziolkowski P, Przetakiewicz Z, et al. Reconstruction of the venous valves. *Proc 10eme Congress Mondial Union Internationale de Phlebologie.* Strasbourg: John Libby; 1989:1032–1034.

71. Spiegowski M, Nowecki Z, Przetakiewicz Z, et al. Transplantation of the venous segments with valves. *Proc 10eme Congress Mondial Union Internationale de Phlebologie.* Strasbourg: John Libby; 1989:1029–1031.

72. van den Broeck TAA. Experimentele chirurgie. In: *Chronische Veneuze Insufficiente en Veneuze Reconstructieve Chirurgie.* Vrije Universiteit te Amsterdam: Krips repro Meppel, 1989.

73. Wilson NM, Rutt DL, Browse NL. Venous valve replacement: a new technique. *Br J Surg.* 1990;77:A701–702.

74. DeLaria GA, Phifer T, Roy J, et al. Hemodynamic evaluation of a bioprosthetic venous prosthesis. *J Vasc Surg.* 1993;18:577–586.

75. Burkhart HM, Fath SW, Dalsing MG, et al. Experimental repair of venous valvular insufficiency using a cryopreserved venous valve allograft aided by a distal arteriovenous fistula. *J Vasc Surg.* 1997;26:817–822.

88

Superficial Venous Insufficiency: Varicosities and Management, Especially With Sclerotherapy

Joel Steinberg

The term *venous insufficiency* indicates that the ability of the superficial veins to perform their normal functions is diminished. The major function of the peripheral venous system is to act as a conduit for return of blood to the central venous system and heart. In addition, the ability of veins to dilate and accommodate relatively large volumes of blood has led to their designation as capacitance, or storage, vessels. The superficial veins of the lower limbs are redundant in that they are not necessary for normal function unless the deep venous system is sufficiently obstructed. Thus, superficial venous pathology does not usually interfere with normal circulatory function to the point of causing morbidity. Nevertheless, the superficial veins can undergo various changes that are often clinically undesirable. They can become thrombosed with consequent obstruction, inflammation, and pain. They can become abnormally dilated, with the development of various sequelae including (1) bulging from engorgement with blood and associated clinical symptoms and/or cosmetic problems; (2) incompetency, with development of venous hypertension and associated adverse sequelae; (3) spontaneous rupture of varicose veins with substantial hemorrhage; and (4) ulcer formation that may require therapeutic interventions.

To some physicians, even vascular specialists, venous problems tend to be perceived as uninteresting and undeserving of attention because of their usually low morbidity. Yet patients afflicted with superficial venous problems, whether symptomatic or cosmetic, require well-thought-out, often customized attention and care. My main emphasis in this chapter is the treatment of superficial dilated veins. Many patients initially seek medical attention because of symptoms. Others desire medical care for the cosmetic problems associated with dilated superficial veins or, to paraphrase a concept of Dr. David Duffy, they have unwanted superficial veins.[1]

In this chapter I address the spectrum of superficial venous insufficiency and emphasize major aspects of this clinical problem, including basic anatomy and physiology, pathogenesis, and treatment options. The role of sclerotherapy in treating patients with superficial venous insufficiency is discussed in detail.

Superficial Veins: Anatomy

For the clinician to properly evaluate and treat superficial veins, a fundamental knowledge of their anatomy and physiology is required.

Greater Saphenous System

The major superficial veins are depicted in Figures 88.1 and 88.2 (L. L. Tretbar, personal communication, 1996).[2] The major vessel, the greater saphenous vein (GSV), begins as the medial continuation of the dorsal arch vein, anterior to the medial malleolus, and travels medially up the limb, usually remaining quite superficial until just distal to the groin. At that point it proceeds anteriorly and deep, passing through the foramen ovale to join the deep system's superficial femoral vein, forming the saphenofemoral junction. Immediately distal to the saphenofemoral junction, the GSV contains two valves, the terminal and subterminal valves. These valves are of major clinical importance because if they leak they give rise to saphenofemoral junction incompetency.

Branches of the GSV are not clinically evident in most people. However, those with varicose veins exhibit some common patterns of branches. A knowledge of locations of frequently occurring branches provides the clinician with a convenient method of locating and naming them, especially when there is a role for treatment. The most proximal branches of the GSV lie in the area of the foramen ovale. They usually drain into the GSV immediately

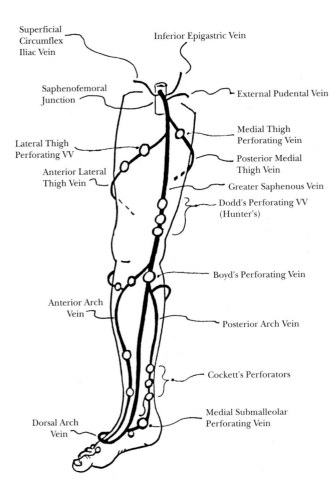

FIGURE 88.1. Anterior and medial superficial and perforating veins of the lower limbs. See text for explanation.

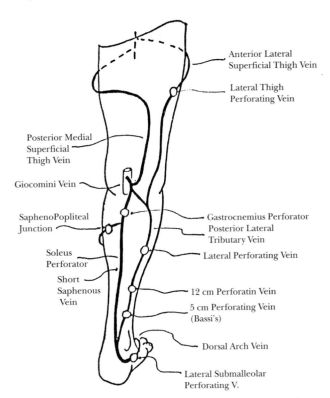

FIGURE 88.2. Posterior and lateral superficial and perforating veins of the lower limbs. See text for explanation.

distal to the saphenofemoral junction. The superficial circumflex vein extends anteriorly, and two veins extend posteriorly, the inferior epigastric vein, which ascends, and the external pudendal vein, which drains into the proximal GSV just distal to the drainage site of the inferior epigastric vein. However, as with most superficial veins, locations and drainage sites of these can vary widely. The three most proximal branches just described are of clinical significance in the presence of saphenofemoral junction incompetency. When the junction is treated surgically, exposure, identification, and ligation and division of these branches are considered standard parts of a complete saphenofemoral junction flush ligation and division procedure. If these branches are not divided, the risk of recurrence of junctional incompetency via collateral development is increased.

At the level of the thigh, two superficial branches often occur. One is the anterior lateral thigh vein, also known as the accessory saphenous vein, which ascends diagonally (upward and medially) from the lateral thigh's distal aspect, across the anterior thigh, to drain into the proximal GSV. At its distal end, the accessory

saphenous vein can extend over the popliteal area and the calf to merge with other superficial veins. The other major thigh-level branch of the GSV is the posterior medial thigh vein. Its course mirrors that of the anterior lateral thigh vein. It can course upward and medially to the anteromedial aspect of the thigh, just below the groin, where it drains into the GSV. Its distal course can sometimes extend down the posterior thigh to the popliteal fossa area. At this location, it sometimes drains into the proximal lesser, or short, saphenous vein near the saphenopopliteal junction. It then takes on the characteristics of a superficial vein that drains both proximally and distally into another superficial vein and thus anastomoses the two veins; it is then called the Giacomini vein. This vein is of potential clinical significance because if incompetent it can feed substantial hypertension into the lesser saphenous system. Occasionally, a subfascial vein may extend from the proximal lesser saphenous vein upward as the femoropopliteal vein to drain into the deep venous system in the thigh.[3]

At the level of the leg at and below the knee, the GSV may have two branches. The anterior arch vein extends as a middle instep branch of the dorsal arch vein, ascending up the anterior leg to just below the knee, where it courses medially to drain into the GSV. The posterior arch vein extends as the medial branch of the dorsal arch vein, behind the medial malleolus, rather close to the posterior tibial vein, and courses superficially up the posteromedial calf to drain into the GSV below the knee. This vein is of potential significance clinically because of associated Cockett's perforating veins that drain from it into the posterior tibial vein; if incompetent Cockett's perforators may contribute substantially to chronic venous insufficiency problems. The medial malleolus acts as a helpful anatomical landmark by which to distinguish the GSV and posterior arch vein. This distinction becomes important when performing duplex mapping in preparation for sclerotherapy if the posterior arch vein is to be closed but the GSV preserved. The GSV begins anterior to the medial malleolus; the posterior arch vein begins behind the malleolus. To define each of these veins anatomically, duplex imaging is best begun at the level of the ankle, where their different locations provide for easy identification.

Lesser Saphenous System

The lesser saphenous vein begins as the lateral continuation of the dorsal arch vein located at the instep and ascends behind the lateral malleolus up the posterior calf. It usually drains into the popliteal vein to form the saphenopopliteal junction. However, the location of lesser saphenous drainage into the deep venous system can vary from along the course of the popliteal vein to a more distal location such as the gastrocnemius vein or a more proximal location via the femoropopliteal or Giacomini veins. As noted previously, a branch of the GSV, the posterior medial thigh vein, may extend down the posterior thigh as the Giacomini vein to drain into the proximal lesser saphenous vein just distal to its junction with and drainage into the popliteal vein. An occasional major branch of the lesser saphenous vein is the posterior lateral tributary vein, which ascends up the posterior lateral aspect of the calf from the ankle to drain into the lesser saphenous vein at the popliteal fossa. Occasionally, the anterior lateral thigh vein branch of the GSV courses distally toward the back of the knee to anastomose with the proximal aspect of the posterior lateral tributary vein.

Perforating (Communicating) Veins

In addition to having a working knowledge of the common branches of the saphenous systems, it is important to be aware of the location of the common perforating veins, because, when incompetent, their treatment becomes an essential part of interrupting saphenous system reflux. The most proximal perforating vein of the lower limbs is the proximal end of the GSV. Because this segment of the GSV traverses the fascia to connect the GSV to the deep system, it fulfills criteria for the definition of a perforating vein. As already noted, it contains

two valves, the terminal and subterminal valves, that if incompetent generate backflow and venous hypertension. At the midlevel of the thigh, Hunter's perforating veins drain the GSV; at the lower third of the thigh, Dodd's perforating veins drain the GSV. Lateral thigh perforating veins may drain from the anterior lateral thigh vein. Medial thigh perforating veins may drain from the posterior medial thigh vein at the level of the medial thigh.

A few collections of perforators may occur in the leg. Boyd's perforating veins drain from the GSV below the anteromedial aspect of the knee into the trifurcation area. Cockett's perforating veins drain from the posterior arch vein, at the distal third of the leg, into the posterior tibial veins. Inferior to the medial malleolus, medial submalleolar perforating veins may drain the distal aspect of the posterior arch vein.

Several perforating veins can sometimes be found as part of the lesser saphenous system. The gastrocnemius perforating veins, if present, drain the proximal lesser saphenous vein into gastrocnemius muscle veins and then into the popliteal vein. Soleus, or midcalf, perforating veins may drain the lesser saphenous vein or branches into the soleal muscle sinusoids. A series of perforators that may be present along the course of the posterior lateral tributary vein have been named, including the lateral perforating vein, and, more distally, Bassi's perforating vein. Perforating veins are sometimes also named by their distance above the bottom of the foot (e.g., the 6-, 12-, and 18-cm perforating veins). Inferior to the lateral malleolus, the lateral submalleolar perforating vein may be present. Most superficial and perforating veins vary widely in location, if they are present at all.

Superficial Veins: Physiology

In a healthy person, a combination of muscle pump activity and one-way valves that allow for flow in the cephalad direction and through perforating veins from the superficial to the deep system maintain drainage of the lower limbs. When a person walks, contracting muscle generates pressure against the deep venous system, pushing on the blood. One-way valves mediate the upward direction of flow. Perforating and superficial veins normally contribute little to this process because of their usually small caliber.

In venous disease, two major factors are frequently involved in initiating pathological events: obstruction, usually from thrombi, and valve incompetency. These two factors are often present together and accelerate the development of pathological events. Obstruction sets up stagnation of flow, stasis, and various subsequent processes, such as rerouting of blood through the superficial system, development of incompetent valves, and venous hypertension. Valve incompetency, due to either thrombotic damage on a primary basis or other mechanisms (e.g., primary vein wall dilation, as in primary varicose veins), can also initiate venous pathology sequelae. A long column of blood created by a series of incompetent valves can exert downward pressure because of gravity. This pressure is increased when the patient stands. The column of blood, unaided by one-way valves to route blood upstream, exerts increased venous pressure in the legs that causes venous hypertension. Subsequent soft tissue changes, the clinical picture of chronic venous insufficiency, evolve.

In most cases of venous insufficiency, whether by thrombotic obstruction, valvular incompetence, a combination of the two, or other mechanisms, the veins are dilated. Indeed, primary venous wall dilation (e.g., at the saphenofemoral junction) is probably a significant factor in the development of many varicose veins.

When varicose veins and associated findings are related to prior deep venous thrombosis, the veins are called secondary varicose veins. When the deep system appears to be normal, the varicosities are referred to as primary varicose veins.

Other factors besides venous obstruction and valvular incompetency may contribute to venous insufficiency, including elevated central venous pressure from, for example, right ventricular failure, tricuspid valve regurgitation, cor pulmonale, arteriovenous anastomoses, and congenital disorders such as Klippel–Trénaunay syndrome. Additional details of events that underlie venous insufficiency are presented in the section on pathogenesis.

Dilated Vein Classification

Most insufficient superficial veins are dilated. Vein diameter often determines clinical presentation (i.e., symptoms) and is an important consideration when planning treatment, especially sclerotherapy. Vein diameter thus provides a convenient and practical means of characterizing superficial veins. Several classifications by diameter have been developed. The one presented in this chapter has been found to be simple and convenient. Dilated superficial veins of the lower limbs can be categorized into six groups (see Table 88.1).

TABLE 88.1. A classification of superficial dilated veins of the lower limbs.

Varicosed truncal veins
Great saphenous vein
Small saphenous vein
Usually bulge from the skin level
May have normal skin color, dark skin color, or skin with blue tinge
Usually greater than 5 mm in diameter

Varicosed saphenous branches or tributaries of greater and lesser saphenous systems
Color can be similar to surrounding skin, slightly darker, or with bluish tinge
Usually greater than 4 mm in diameter
Some, especially in popliteal area, may be 2–4 mm in diameter, with frank bluish color

Reticular (or "blue") veins
Pale blue color with indistinct margins
Usually 2–4 mm in diameter
Located about 1–2 mm below skin surface (do not bulge above skin level)
Often found in the thigh, especially lateral thigh
Often drain an arch of venulectasias into the deep system as the lateral subdermic venous system

Venulectasias
1–2 mm in diameter
Red or blue in color
Occasionally bulge just above the skin level
Variant
   Bullous venulectasias, also called "blue blebs," thin-walled phlebectasias
   Occur at the ankle as the corona phlebectatica
   Classified here because of their very thin walls and bulging, fragile appearance
   Diameter of 2–5 mm

Telangiectasias (spider veins)
0.1–1 mm in diameter
Blue or red in color
Rarely bulge

Telangiectatic mats
Less than 0.2 mm in diameter
Usually bright red
Typically occur as clusters, neovascularization after a skin injury or injection

The largest abnormally dilated veins are sometimes the greater (see Figure 88.3) and lesser saphenous veins, sometimes called the truncal veins. They can be 8 mm in diameter or greater. The color may be similar to surrounding skin, slightly darker, or have a bluish tint.

Dilated branches of the saphenous trunks, tributary saphenous veins (Figure 88.3), are typically greater than 4 mm in diameter and have a color similar to the surrounding skin, slightly darker, or with a bluish tinge. Some, typically found in the popliteal fossa area, may be 2 to 4 mm in diameter, often with a frank bluish color.

Reticular veins are recognized by their pale blue color with indistinct margins; they do not bulge above the level of the skin. They are usually 2 to 4 mm in diameter and may be 1 to 2 mm below the surface of the skin. They are frequently found in the lateral thigh as part of the lateral thigh system of subdermal veins[4] (see Figure 88.4). Venulectasias are 1 to 2 mm in diameter, blue or red in color, and sometimes bulge or are just below the level of the skin (see Figures 88.4 and 88.5).

So-called blue blebs can be considered a subcategory of venulectasias because they have very thin walls, much thinner than those of varicosities. When found as a clus-

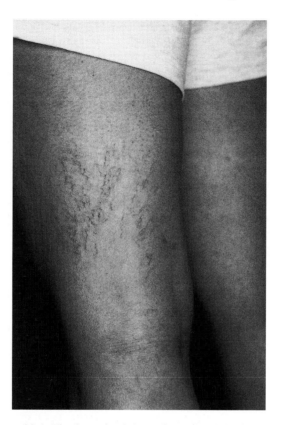

FIGURE 88.4. The lateral subdermal system of thigh veins can, as depicted in this patient, sometimes be found at the posterior thigh and elsewhere as well. Venulectasias are arranged more or less parallel to each other, in a gentle arc, and drain into the deep system by way of reticular veins. In this patient, the reticular vein, which tends to show poorly in black-and-white prints, appears as a vague shadow at the lower thigh and extends from the inferior margin of the venulectatic arch, which it usually drains, toward the knee crease.

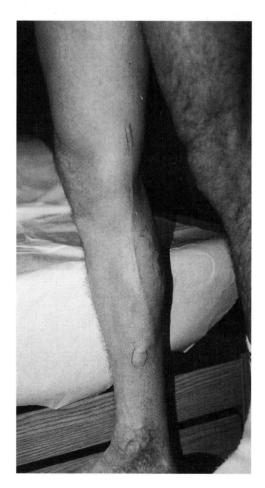

FIGURE 88.3. Greater saphenous vein.

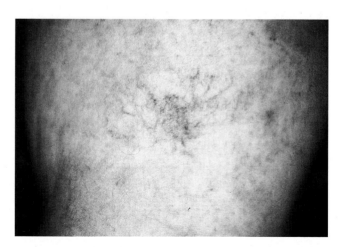

FIGURE 88.5. Venulectasias are often found as clusters or radiating in an arc.

ter at the ankle, they are given the group name *corona phlebectatica*. They have also been called *bullous venulectasias*. They are sometimes found at the level of the knee and elsewhere. They are typically 2 to 5 mm in diameter, blue, as their name implies, and have a fragile appearance because of their bulging and very thin walls (see Figure 88.6).

Telangiectasias, more simply known as spider veins, are usually 0.1 to 1 mm in diameter and sometimes reddish but more often blue to purple in color. They do not usually bulge above the level of the surrounding skin (see Figure 88.5). Telangiectatic mats are less than 0.2 mm in diameter, tend to be bright red, almost by definition occur in clusters, and are sometimes seen as postinjection sequelae via neovascularization.

Pathogenesis of Superficial Dilated Veins

Multiple investigations and observations underlie our current knowledge of dilated superficial vein pathogenesis. As noted previously, secondary varicose veins are defined as those that are secondary to deep venous pathology (i.e., obstruction and/or incompetency, factors that elevate venous pressure of the lower limbs). Historically, deep venous thrombosis and associated valve damage (postphlebitic syndrome) were considered to be the major etiology for secondary varicose veins. The development of duplex ultrasound analysis, a noninvasive test that provides both anatomical and physiological information about veins, has improved our understanding of deep venous changes in the presence of varicose and other venous pathology. Thus, many patients with secondary varicose veins are found by duplex analysis to have no evidence of prior deep venous thrombosis, such as sclerotic or thickened walls. They are suspected of having developed deep venous incompetency as a primary event. Mechanisms underlying the development of primary deep venous incompetency may relate to both primary wall dilation and valvular dysfunction from cusp changes.

In most patients, primary superficial varicose vein development probably reflects pathologic events that occur initially in the vein wall rather than the valves. Clinical observations and histological studies support this thesis. For example, the clinical finding of segmental varicosed bulging not always accompanied by reflux supports vein wall pathology as the initial source of varicose development, with reflux developing if wall dilation occurs at a valve site. If proximal valves at, for example, the saphenofemoral junction and thigh perforating veins become incompetent, the resultant reflux can in turn generate a hydrostatic force from the weight of the blood, especially with the patient standing, that creates venous hyperten-

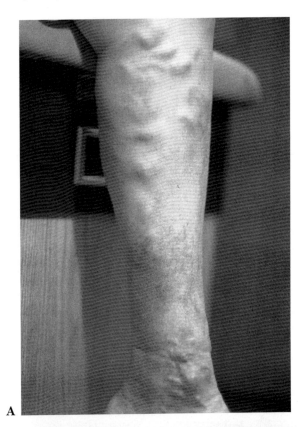

A

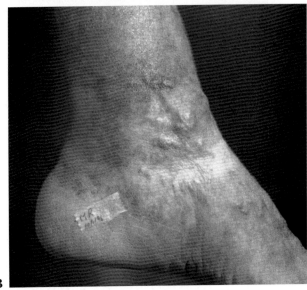

B

FIGURE 88.6. **A,** Ankle phlebectasias and greater saphenous trunk as well as branch varicosities. Venous hypertension of the ankle ectatic veins is fed by reflux from more proximal saphenous system varicosities. The ankle bullae are at risk for rupture. This problem is best addressed by interrupting proximal reflux varicosities, via, for example, sclerotherapy and ligations, to reduce venous hypertension. Thereafter, the ankle venulectasias can be sclerosed closed. **B,** Small (2- to 5-mm diameter), thin-walled, bulging, round venulectasias are often called blue blebs. When occurring as a cluster at the ankle, the group is sometimes called corona phlebectatica.

sion. Venous hypertension in turn generates the additional varicose changes distally that ultimately lead to chronic venous insufficiency syndrome.

Several studies of varicose vein wall histology have shown changes to help explain the development of dilation.[5-12] For example, cell-type selective staining of vein walls has demonstrated the presence in varicosities of fragmented rather than continuous elastin fibers, irregular rather than uniform orientation of smooth muscles, and substantial hypertrophy of noncontractile collagen fibers. An increase in collagen and fibrous content of the wall, with separation of smooth muscle cell bundles into smaller units and consequent decreased overall wall contractility, may explain the decreased tone of varicosed walls and their dilation. Also, the actual collagen content of varicose veins may be decreased compared with that of normal veins, with the bulk of the wall consisting of ground substances such as mucopolysaccharides. This noncontractile material may also underlie varicosed wall dilation. Recently, Rai and Iqbal described histopathological changes in varicose veins in the form of atrophy of the media layer.[13] These findings may explain weakened walls that underlie dilation.

Several factors probably contribute to the development of small-caliber dilated superficial veins (reticular, venulectatic, and telangiectatic veins). These factors include genetic predisposition, pregnancy, high estrogen levels, varicose veins, occult incompetent perforating veins, arteriovenous connections, injury, primary congenital disorders (e.g., Klippel–Trénaunay syndrome), and acquired diseases (e.g., lupus and human immunodeficiency virus infection).

Histological findings in small-caliber dilated veins include interfibrillar collagenous dysplasia and variable diameters of collagenous microfibrils with only a few elastic fibers but numerous oxytalan fibers (detected via peracetic acid oxidation followed by Corori's aldehyde fuchsin staining). Overall vessel diameter is enlarged and accompanied by asymmetric thickening of the wall. These findings may reflect abnormal collagen metabolism.[14]

Approach to the Patient With Superficial Venous Insufficiency

Several sequelae of superficial venous insufficiency may prompt a patient to seek medical attention. To help plan proper care, it is usually best to determine the status of the deep, superficial, and perforating systems. The history and physical examination often provide much of this information. Doppler and/or duplex studies can usually further define venous anatomy and hemodynamics so as to guide therapeutic plans. As the clinician begins to evaluate the patient, the diagnostic possibilities

should be considered so that the history taking, examination, and any necessary laboratory studies can be customized to determine the pathologic problem and, in turn, the appropriate therapeutic options.

When obtaining a history, it is helpful to keep in mind that patients with superficial venous insufficiency seek medical care for a variety of reasons. Some have innocuous findings and merely need reassurance about the benign nature of their problem. Some see their veins as unsightly and unwanted and seek cosmetic improvement. Many present with symptoms from which they desire relief. And, of course, in those with such morbid problems as ulcers and varicose bleeding, the need for treatment is obvious.

As the patient evaluation proceeds and the history leads into the examination, the accumulated information will help further refine the differential diagnoses so that laboratory studies, as may be warranted, can be selected to further define underlying pathology. For example, at one end of the pathologic spectrum, the young adult patient with undesired telangiectasias and an otherwise unremarkable examination and history may be an obvious candidate for sclerotherapy with little need for diagnostic tests. At the other extreme of the superficial venous disease spectrum, the patient who presents with varicosities and stasis hyperpigmentation with or without a clear history of deep venous thrombosis may raise a diagnostic and therapeutic challenge. For example, sclerotherapeutic closure of major superficial venous conduits of limb drainage is usually contraindicated if the deep venous system has occlusions. In such a patient, duplex analysis of the deep veins is usually warranted to determine proper and safe care. Also, in patients with deep venous incompetency, venous reflux and hypertension tend to foster development of dilated superficial veins. Thus, for the patient with both dilated superficial veins and deep venous incompetency who desires sclerotherapy, the possibility of (early) recurrences of problems with treated veins should be explained so that an informed decision can be made about treatment.

Symptoms

Varicosed and other dilated superficial veins can be associated with a variety of symptoms, including swelling, aches, pain, heaviness, burning, and itching (see Table 88.2). Symptoms often become more bothersome with prolonged standing, warm weather, high humidity, or premenstrually. The effects of gravity in increasing blood volume and engorgement of the veins with blood probably underlie these exacerbations. In many patients veins become progressively more dilated and prominent with each pregnancy to a point where they become so annoying that they interfere with normal lifestyle. Both mechanical and hormonal factors of pregnancy probably underlie these changes. When obtaining a history, it is

TABLE 88.2. Symptoms reported with superficial dilated veins.

Aching
Swelling
Heaviness, especially with prolonged standing, premenses
Cramps
Paresthesias (itching, tingling)
Pain (burning, dull, throbbing, sharp)
Tiredness
Vague discomfort

often helpful to ascertain types of symptoms, duration, exacerbating factors, and so forth. Some patients express a variety of strong negative emotional reactions to their superficial veins. This view may increase their perception of a physical problem and contribute substantially to their interest in obtaining cosmetic improvement.

Patients frequently seek evaluation of superficial veins for cosmetic reasons. Adverse sequelae from small-caliber dilated superficial, reticular, venulectatic, and telangiectatic veins are probably less frequently encountered than from the larger veins. However, these small-caliber veins can be associated with symptoms (e.g., aches, pain, and heaviness) found with varicose veins. Interestingly, individual patient perception of vein size varies, and some with only slightly bulging venulectasias may perceive these on a par with much larger veins. The impact of small-caliber dilated veins on the patient's sense of well-being should not be underestimated. In addition to dilated superficial veins themselves, several rather significant sequelae—stasis fibrosis, inflammation, varicose ulcers, and hemorrhage—can cause symptoms and prompt a patient to seek care.

Stasis Fibrosis and Associated Sequelae

Hyperpigmentation and other stasis change markers of chronic venous insufficiency are typically found above the medial malleolus, along the path of the superficial veins, in the stasis or gaiter area,[2] or on the skin of the distal leg. The normally soft tissues above the medial malleolus can become firm, even hard, in the presence of chronic varicose veins, and the underlying tissues usually become fibrotic. I call these findings *stasis fibrosis*. This term, admittedly newly coined, helps to indicate the likely pathogenic events: stasis from long-standing venous insufficiency and venous hypertension that leads to the pathologic findings of fibrotic changes of the soft tissues. Other terms that have been used to describe stasis events include *lipodermatosclerosis*[2,15] and *chronic indurated cellulitis*.[16] The clinical manifestations and means of diagnosis are the findings of semifirm to hard tissues for up to several centimeters above the ankle, at least medially, and often with a nodular or irregular texture along the distal medial leg. Some mild hyperpigmentation is usually seen in the stasis area secondary to hemosiderin deposition.

The patient may seek medical care when the stasis or gaiter area becomes tender, warm, painful, or erythematous. These complaints and findings are evidence that the tissues have become actively inflamed. In this situation, a variety of descriptive terms have been employed, including *indurated cellulitis*, *acute lipodermatosclerosis* (which emphasizes skin involvement), and *panniculitis*[2] (to indicate inflammation of subcutaneous adipose tissue radicles). If the skin is actively inflamed, terms such as *venous dermatitis*, *stasis dermatitis*,[16] *stasis eczema*, and *varicose eczema*[17] have been applied.

A likely sequence of events leading to chronic stasis fibrosis and its complications may include valve incompetency, which leads to venous hypertension, which leads to slowed venous flow and sludging, consequent adherence of leukocytes to the venule intima, consequent damage of the vein wall with loss of intima integrity, subsequent leakage of proteins into surrounding tissues, with resultant inflammation as an autoimmune process and, in turn, reactive accumulation of fibrotic tissues, including accumulation of fibrin material around the veins (the so-called fibrin cuff).

Although the various stasis changes just described are more commonly seen in the presence of chronic deep venous insufficiency, they can be found when varicose insufficiency is a prominent finding. Varicose interruptions, for example, via sclerotherapy and ligations as needed (see section on sclerotherapy), can sometimes resolve the acute inflammatory progression of stasis fibrosis, an observation that indicates the potential for varicose insufficiency to be the underlying factor in cellulitic flares.

Varicose Ulcers

Skin ulceration can develop in the presence of varicose veins. If varicose insufficiency is the major etiology, the term *varicose ulcer* is appropriately employed. The patient may complain of a sore or pain. As described in detail in a later section of this chapter, interruption and closure of feeding proximal refluxing veins with, for example, sclerotherapy can be used to block underlying varicose-generated hypertension and facilitate ulcer healing. When the clinical picture raises the possibility that both superficial and deep venous insufficiency are contributing to the ulcer's formation (e.g., in the presence of substantial hyperpigmentation), Doppler or duplex analysis can help to determine the contribution of each of these systems to the wound's development so that appropriate care can be planned.

Varicose Hemorrhage

Hemorrhage, spontaneous or traumatic, can sometimes occur from bullous venulectasias (sometimes called superficial phlebectasias, blue blebs of the corona phlebectatica, or ankle flare[18]) at the ankle or foot. Patients may present because of a bleeding episode or concern about the appearance (usually because of the blue color). The veins are often firm to palpation (i.e., under substantial pressure), when examined with the patient standing, an indicator of the underlying venous hypertension generated by proximal feeding incompetent varicose veins. As described in the next sections, sclerotherapy of the blebs and sclerotherapy combined with ligation interruption of feeding varicosities can provide an effective means of treating this problem and reducing the risk of further bleeding.

Differential Diagnosis

The presence of dilated superficial veins and lower limb symptoms cannot always be equated with a cause–effect relationship. The differential diagnoses of leg symptoms that can mimic superficial venous insufficiency are listed in Table 88.3. Some examples and suggested workup are as follows: popliteal cysts may cause knee or proximal calf pain. An ultrasound of the area usually clarifies the diagnosis. Inflammatory joint disease should also be considered. Crepitus of the knee on passive range of motion supports this consideration, as does warmth and/or swelling of the knee. If a routine knee x-ray examination does not reveal pathology, a magnetic resonance imaging scan can be instructive to demonstrate changes such as occult meniscal tears. Lumbosacral radiculopathies that cause paresthesias of the lower limbs can occur in the presence of dilated veins. A clue to the radiculopathic nature of the symptoms is their extension into the hip, buttock, and lumbar areas, whose involvement is not seen with venous symptoms. A history of arthritis, low back symptoms, a positive straight leg raise test, and/or a positive nerve conduction velocity–electromyography

TABLE 88.3. Differential diagnosis of symptoms in patient with dilated superficial veins.

Lumbosacral radiculopathies
Peripheral neuropathies
Arthritis
Synovitis
Baker's cyst
Ruptured Baker's cyst
Deep venous thrombophlebitis
Idiopathic muscle cramps
Restless leg syndrome
Ischemic claudication
Neurogenic claudication
Myalgias
Fibromyalgias
Tendinitis
Indurated cellulitis (acute lipodermatosclerosis)
Stasis eczema

test also supports radiculopathy as a factor in the patient's symptoms.

Physical Examination

A general and pertinent physical examination is warranted for the patient who presents with superficial venous insufficiency. Evidence of a systemic disorder may exclude some types of vein care. For example, the finding of slowly healing wounds in a diabetic patient or a history of brittle diabetes raises the strong possibility that stab avulsion phlebectomy would be too risky. Thus, a basic comprehensive history and physical examination in most newly presenting patients is wise. The examination room setting for evaluation of the lower limbs should include the basic tools for any physical examination. The patient should be comfortable and appropriately draped (or in suitable attire such as loose or high-cut shorts) to minimize potential embarrassment; the room should be quiet, warm, well ventilated, and well lit.

It is easiest to examine the legs with the patient standing on a platform elevated about 1 to 3 ft above the floor to allow the clinician, while sitting on a comfortable stool, good direct visualization of the lower limbs. An examination platform measuring about 2 ft square, preferably with a side rail, enables the patient to safely turn around so that all surfaces of the lower limbs can be inspected. Room overhead lighting usually does not provide for adequate inspection of the legs. Accordingly, it is quite helpful to employ a floor lamp with a gooseneck or comparably flexible method to adjust the angle of the light and sufficient power (e.g., a 75-W or higher flood bulb). To optimally examine the patient for varicose veins, he or she should stand to increase filling of the veins with blood and demonstrate bulging. The patient should stand for 30 seconds to 1 minute to facilitate filling of varicosities and proper inspection. It is often helpful to have the patient slightly bend the knee of the leg being examined while holding onto the railing for support to relax the muscles and thus facilitate evaluation of the superficial veins.

In addition to inspection, palpation of veins with the ball of the thumb or other finger along the course of varicosities and above where they can be seen may help to determine their course. Pressing in on the varicose veins also aids access for two additional and important findings. Pressing firmly may help to identify indentations or voids in the subcutaneous tissues that indicate fascial defects through which incompetent perforating veins are located. These sites have been called *points of control* by Beesley and Fegan to emphasize their contribution to varicose development by providing reflux that feeds venous hypertension.[19] However, such defects may merely represent a void or depression in subcutaneous fat occupied by a varix.[2] A digital modification of the Brodie–Trendelenburg tourniquet test (see later section) often helps to differentiate an incompetent perforating site from a subcutaneous depression.

Pressing along the path of varicosities also provides a rough estimate of the pressure they are under. Veins that are firm to palpation are usually found distally. The firmness indicates that they are under higher pressure, probably being fed by proximal sites of reflux and sources of hypertension that should be determined by physical examination and, as warranted, Doppler or duplex analysis. During sclerotherapy, high-pressure veins may require the use of higher strengths of sclerosant and firmer compression bandaging than might low-pressure veins. Palpation of varicosities also helps to identify such potentially significant findings as thrombi. Palpation should extend up as far proximally as possible, even to the junction with the deep venous system.

Some documentation of the patient's baseline varicose status is warranted, especially if procedures to obliterate the varicose veins are contemplated. Some clinicians use written descriptions in their progress notes, others use standard leg outlines and fill in the contents with hand drawings, and still others use photographs.

Auscultation over superficial veins can serve to identify bruits created by an arteriovenous anastomosis. Vein percussion can be of value as part of special tests described in the following section.

Special Tests

Several special tests can help to determine the status of varicose veins and valve competency. Familiarity with these tests, as well as their capabilities and limitations, is important so that they can be employed as needed.

The Schwartz percussion test assists in evaluating continuity of a column of blood. A proximal varicose segment is palpated, and a distal segment is tapped. If the percussion impulse is felt over the proximal segment, the distal segment probably represents a branch. The test can be reversed by palpating the distal branch while tapping the proximal segment. The ability to sense the percussion impulse distally supports the presence of incompetent valves between the segments with a connecting continuous column of blood.

The cough test helps to determine valve competency between the thorax and site of distal palpation. The saphenofemoral junction or other vein site is palpated while the patient coughs. Detection of an impulse over the palpated segment supports the presence of incompetent valves between there and the thorax.

The Brodie–Trendelenburg tourniquet test is a valuable method to help determine the location of incompetent perforating veins. With the patient in a supine posi-

tion, the leg to be examined is elevated at least 45 degrees for several seconds so that blood can drain out of the varicosities. A tourniquet is then placed at the proximal thigh just below the foramen ovale–saphenofemoral junction location. The patient stands, and the leg is inspected for 30 seconds to observe varicose filling. Appearance of varicose bulging within 30 seconds of standing indicates the presence of incompetent perforating veins distal to the saphenofemoral junction. If varicosities do not become prominent until the tourniquet is removed, the saphenofemoral junction is most likely the major source of varicose reflux.

If this initial test shows varicose bulging within 30 seconds of standing, the test can be repeated with the tourniquet placed more distal on the limb to help ascertain the level of incompetent perforating veins. Thus, the leg is elevated and the tourniquet placed immediately above the knee; the patient then stands and is inspected. If varicosities do not become obvious within 30 seconds, the incompetent perforating veins are likely located above the knee in the thigh, at the level of Hunter's perforating veins. This location can be confirmed by releasing the tourniquet, which allows rapid filling of varicosities. On the other hand, if varicosities of the calf fill rapidly on standing before the tourniquet is removed, incompetent perforating veins are likely located below the tourniquet in the calf. In this case, one can repeat the test but with the tourniquet below the knee to block reflux from potential Boyd's perforating veins at the medial knee. Delayed varicose filling supports those perforating veins as the source of reflux; rapid filling points toward the presence of incompetent perforating veins more distally.

A few caveats about the nuances of performing the Brodie–Trendelenburg tourniquet test are worth noting. Good lighting at the leg level is warranted. An adjustable floor lamp is helpful for this purpose. The clinician should examine the leg at a comfortable eye level. If the varicosities of interest are subtle to inspection, their location can be marked on the skin with a felt-tip pen or the like while the patient is standing and before the test is done, so the examiner knows where to look for varicosities on the leg when the patient stands during the test.

The Brodie–Trendelenburg tourniquet test has been modified into a digital form. For this test, the patient is placed in a supine position with the examined leg elevated. After the varicosities are allowed to drain and collapse, the examiner places a finger firmly over a site of suspected perforating vein incompetency, such as the proximal GSV (see Figure 88.7) or a previously palpated fascial defect. The patient then stands while continuous firm digital pressure is maintained over the site of interest. After 30 seconds of standing, the finger is removed. Subsequent rapid filling of a previously collapsed varicosity confirms the clinician's suspicion that an incom-

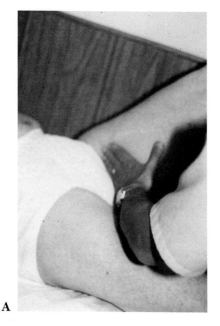
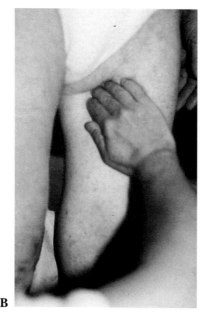
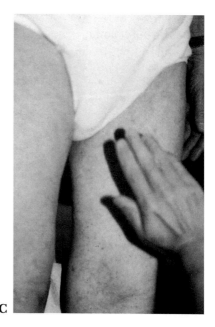

A   B   C

FIGURE 88.7. Digital modification of the Brodie–Trendelen-burg tourniquet test. The test is being used to evaluate for saphenofemoral junction competency. On the left side (A), the leg has been elevated to drain varicosities, after which the soft tissues in the region of the proximal greater saphenous vein are firmly compressed. With this compression maintained, the patient stands (B) and filling of varicosities is observed during the first 30 seconds and after compression is removed (C).

TABLE 88.4. Highlights of some noninvasive vascular laboratory tests used to evaluate superficial venous insufficiency and sclerotherapy candidates.

Venous Doppler flow analysis
When performed with the patient in supine or 10-degree Trendelenburg's position, can be used to evaluate for venous patency and reflux
With the patient standing and examined leg unweighted, can be used to evaluate venous patency and the degree of incompetency

Venous duplex analysis (preferably with color flow)
More accurate than nonimaging Doppler flow analysis (≥ 95%).
To assess for incompetency, preferably performed with the patient standing and examined leg unweighted
Optimal method to map superficial veins
Preferred method for determining presence and degree of reflux at the saphenofemoral junction, saphenopopliteal junction, and other perforating vein sites

Direct current photoplethysmography
Potential method to determine the ability of superficial vein interruption (via sclerotherapy) to improve or correct venous reflux by obstructing superficial vein regurgitation with a tourniquet and repeating the test after an initial test examination without a tourniquet; short recovery time is reflective of substantial reflux
Nonspecific monitor of skin erythematous characteristics and, if these changes from nonvenous incompetency (e.g., cellulitis) are present, may give false-positive evidence of reflux, even with the use of tourniquets
Light reflection rheography and modifications are described as not affected by skin color, pigment, or edema

Air plethysmography
Provides objective characteristics of muscle venous pump function
Can provide objective evidence of effects of various strengths of compression gradient stockings on calf muscle pump function

Segmental venous capacitance and maximal venous outflow study via volume or strain-gauge plethysmography
Infrequently performed since the advent and popularity of venous duplex analysis
Capacitance part of the study can estimate total varicose size
Maximal venous outflow is diminished with proximal deep venous obstruction to outflow from the limb

petent perforating site had been compressed by the examiner's finger, or, employing terminology coined by Beesley and Fegan, a point of control has been identified.[19] Incompetent perforating sites can then be marked for selected injections or ligations, just distal to the site, to facilitate varicose closure with sclerotherapy.

Vascular Laboratory Tests

Several vascular laboratory tests are available to help diagnose and direct care for patients with superficial venous insufficiency. Most of them are noninvasive and thus have some inherent advantages, especially safety. Most noninvasive tests can be performed with mobile equipment, which offers the added advantage of portability. The most common tests as they apply to superficial venous insufficiency, and in particular the sclerotherapy candidate, are reviewed in the following sections. This information is summarized in Table 88.4. More in-depth resources should be consulted for details of physics, techniques, and so forth.

Doppler Analysis

Doppler ultrasound flow instrumentation, either nondirectional or directional, can help determine underlying venous hemodynamics. Most equipment uses a pencil-shaped probe that contains two Doppler crystals. An emitting crystal sends out a sound wave. For superficial vessel work, an 8- to 10-MHz frequency is used, because it generates a narrow beam to vessels near the skin and thus minimizes return signal interference from other sources. A second receiving crystal detects sound waves that reflect off moving blood cells. That ultrasound signal, via electronics, is converted into an audible signal. More rapidly moving blood generates a stronger signal. In some equipment, the signal is also converted into a graphic record on a paper recorder. A potential disadvantage of Doppler technology is its inability to visualize the tested vein. Therefore it may not be able to decipher which vessel is being insonated when neighboring vessels are present. In addition, Doppler flow analysis is often unable to define partially thrombosed or obstructed veins versus nonobstructed veins. Performance and evaluation of Doppler tests require technical expertise. Nevertheless, in spite of its shortcomings, continuous wave Doppler flow analysis provides an inexpensive and practical means of evaluating venous hemodynamics, especially in the hands of an experienced person.

Continuous wave nonimaging Doppler flow analysis is helpful in analyzing the hemodynamics of both deep and superficial veins when detailed information about anatomy is not necessary and when there is a low clinical index of suspicion of partially thrombosed obstructed veins. It is thus a good screening tool to ensure patency of deep veins in otherwise clinically healthy patients who are candidates for sclerotherapy. Continuous wave nonimaging Doppler flow analysis is helpful, for example, in the swollen leg to assess venous hemodynamics as a preliminary test modality. Doppler analysis can identify occluded veins, as no flow will be detected in them. According to the literature, accuracy of continuous wave pencil-probe Doppler analysis is about 85%.

Doppler flow analysis is helpful in assessing deep and superficial venous system reflux, which is best done with the patient standing (see Figure 88.8). It readily aids in determining competency versus reflux of bulging varicose veins when a distal compression–release maneuver is performed with the patient standing. Generally, greater than half a second reflux with release of a compressed limb segment distal to the level of insonation with the Doppler probe indicates reflux of probable clinical significance. Doppler flow analysis can also be used to approximate the status of possible perforating veins. If palpation demonstrates a fascial defect along the course of a varicose vein, and/or Brodie–Trendelenburg tourniquet testing above a suspected perforating site leads to rapid filling of the vein, or other findings suggest perforating reflux, Doppler flow analysis can be helpful in confirming this suspicion. Tourniquets are applied just proximal and distal to the site of suspected perforating vein incompetency. The Doppler probe is applied over the site of suspected reflux. The distal limb segment is compressed distal to the site of the distal tourniquet. If flow is augmented with this compression, because the tourniquets exclude reflux through superficial veins, the increased Doppler signal supports the presence of incompetency of the insonated perforating vein.

Venous Duplex Analysis

Venous duplex analysis is presently the gold standard of noninvasive vascular studies. The term *duplex* is perhaps not the best one, because it does not explicitly describe the technical features of the testing equipment. However, the term has become ingrained as part of the standard phlebological and radiological vocabulary. The term *duplex* is meant to indicate that two separate modalities are used during the analysis; one is pulsed wave Doppler flow analysis, and the other is B-mode, real-time ultrasound imaging. In more advanced units, Doppler information is translated into a color signal, and the accepted standard is to adjust instrumentation so that flow toward the heart appears blue and flow toward the periphery appears red. Ultrasound imaging provides actual visualization of the tested vessel. This feature gives duplex studies some invaluable capabilities for studying venous disease. In evaluating a vein for deep venous thrombosis, the overlying duplex probe is pressed inward to compress the visualized vein. Ability to coapt the

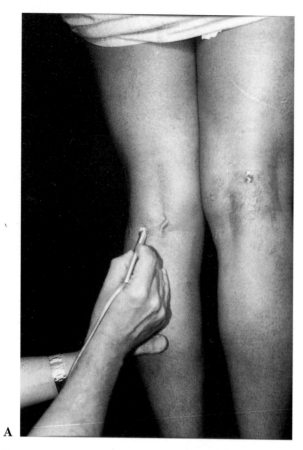

A

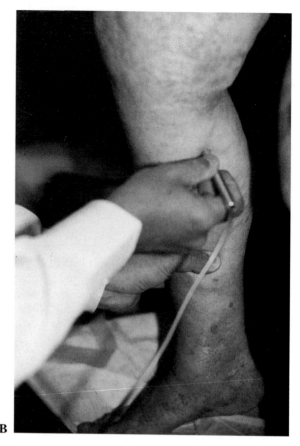

B

FIGURE 88.8. Doppler pencil probe analysis of venous flow. In experienced hands, this technique is very helpful. In **A,** the popliteal vein is analyzed. Note that the patient is standing to bring out potential reflux; the probe is lateral to the midline of the popliteal fossa, where the popliteal vessels are located; and the examiner's left hand is poised to perform a distal compression–release maneuver to determine forward and backward flow patterns. In **B,** the greater saphenous vein is being interrogated. The examiner's left hand is compressing the limb distally while the examiner listens for cephalad flow (an augmentation maneuver).

opposing vein walls so that they contact each other virtually rules out obstruction. Inability of the compression maneuver to bring the walls together usually indicates thrombosis (see Figure 88.9). Duplex analysis can also help to identify partially obstructed veins, in contrast to Doppler flow analysis, which cannot readily distinguish clear, healthy veins from partially thrombosed, nonoccluded veins. Duplex evidence of partial obstruction, as with nonocclusive or evolving thrombosis, includes an inability to completely coapt vein walls by compression of the overlying soft tissues with the ultrasound transducer, visualization of some stationary echoes in the lumen, and lack of total filling by Doppler color of the entire vein lumen. Imaging capabilities also enable detection of duplicated vessels, as can sometimes occur in the popliteal and femoral systems, that is not possible with (continuous wave) Doppler assessment.

Because duplex studies look at all soft tissue components within the beam's range, this technology can visualize not only vessels but also other tissues with potentially significant changes. For example, a popliteal or Baker's cyst in the popliteal fossa area can be readily appreciated on duplex imaging and can explain swelling that was thought to reflect venous thrombosis. Ultrasound imaging also enables the clinician to guide insertion of a needle to aspirate the cyst and provide relief of symptoms. These duplex capabilities offer major advantages over contrast venography, which only visualizes the intraluminal status of vessels.

When mapping varicosities, duplex analysis can be invaluable in visualizing superficial venous system veins that are not bulging or are otherwise not visible by inspecting the skin (e.g., subcutaneous veins) (see Figures 88.10 and 88.16). This information can be invaluable when performing sclerotherapy and ligations of, for example, the proximal GSV (see Figure 88.16), saphenofemoral junction, and saphenopopliteal junction areas. Details of this application are discussed in a later section of this chapter. Imaging has other applications for the sclerotherapist. It shows the exact site of the often variably located saphenopopliteal junction and allows direct visualization of perforating veins and assess-

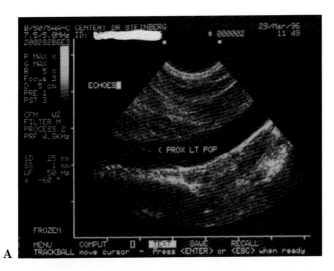

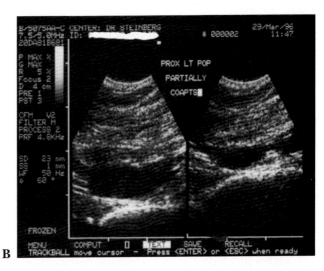

FIGURE 88.9. Venous duplex detection of thrombosis. On the left side (A) some intraluminal echoes are seen in part of the popliteal vein. On the right side (B) compression of the overlying soft tissues with the duplex probe fails to totally coapt the opposing vein walls together.

ment for reflux via pulsed wave Doppler audible signal, waveform, and color flow analyses (see Figure 88.10). This information can facilitate ultrasound-guided sclerotherapeutic injections of incompetent perforating veins.

Duplex technology has some limitations for vein imaging. The superficial femoral vein in the adductor canal may be difficult to see or compress; noncompressibility may lead to a false-positive interpretation of thrombosis. Infrapopliteal vein visualization is not always accurate. It can miss short segments of clots or not differentiate a diseased tibial–peroneal vein from a healthy one of these normally paired vessels. Very superficial veins, often of interest in diagnosing superficial venous insufficiency, may be missed if the ultrasound probe inadvertently compresses them or the technician sets the depth adjust-

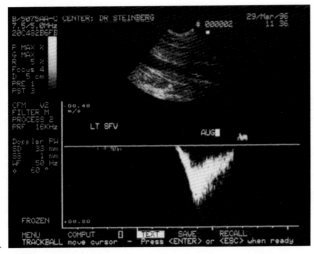

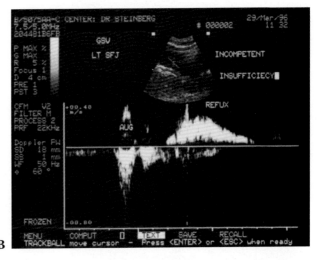

FIGURE 88.10. Use of venous duplex analysis to determine competency status of specific veins. The limb distal to the site of insonation is compressed and, in the absence of proximal obstruction, will augment flow toward the heart. On release of the compressed segment, backflow or reflux, if longer than a half second, is usually considered abnormal. The recorded waveform and audible signal indicate flow patterns. On the left side (A), the record of the left superficial femoral vein shows normal flow with distal compression toward the heart (note down-ward waveform), with minimal backward flow on release (note negligible upward tracing). On the right side (B), the left proximal greater saphenous vein, just below the bifurcation (saphenofemoral junction), demonstrates prominent reflux (note prominent and prolonged upward waveform, indicative of reflux, that develops after the leg, distal to the duplex probe, is compressed, causing antegrade flow [downward wave], and then released).

ment to look at deeper vessels. The phlebologist should keep these limitations in mind when reading studies and when instructing the technician on areas of interest.

Direct Current Coupled Photoplethysmography

Photoplethysmography (PPG) and its newer diagnostic cousin, light reflection rheography, use an infrared light source directed onto the skin and a sensor to measure reflected light. The equipment is used to assess superficial blood content of the skin as a means of determining venous insufficiency patterns and sources. To perform a test, the PPG probe is applied to the skin above the medial malleolus, typically with double-sided cellophane tape (see Figure 88.11A). The patient, in a sitting position with the tested leg freely dangling, is instructed to alternately move the foot up (dorsiflexion) and down (plantar flexion). After five such maneuvers in continuous succession, the leg is again allowed to freely dangle, and resultant waveforms, printed on a paper strip recorder, are observed. The foot exercise is designed to facilitate emptying of blood from the venous pool in the skin. The reflected light detects the amount of blood in the skin. During the exercise, there is a stepwise decrease of the PPG waveform as, with calf muscle pump

function, venous blood is pushed out of the distal leg upward (see Figure 88.11B, top strip, left). During the post-exercise rest, with normal deep and superficial venous hemodynamics, the waveform slowly returns to the baseline over at least 20 seconds (see Figure 88.11B, top strip, middle and right). In the presence of reflux the waveform returns to baseline in less than 20 seconds (see Figure 88.11B, middle strip), and in moderate to advanced reflux the baseline is reached in less than 10 seconds (see Figure 88.11B, bottom strip).

Tourniquets are then applied at various places on the lower limb, just below the groin, above or below the knee, and so forth to block superficial venous reflux. If the waveform remains abnormal with the tourniquet in place, the veins distal to that location are refluxing. If the waveform normalizes with the tourniquet in place, the pretourniquet reflux was mediated by superficial veins that, with the tourniquet in place, is blocked from supplying rapid skin filling (see Figure 88.11). This test can be used to predict the benefit of interrupting superficial veins on leg hemodynamics. If, for example, treatment of superficial veins with sclerotherapy is being considered and the study shows normalization of waveforms with a tourniquet, the patient and physician have evidence that the patient's venous insufficiency is probably due to superficial vein reflux and the contemplated treatment will substantially relieve associated symptoms.

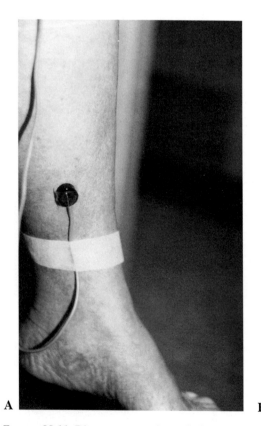

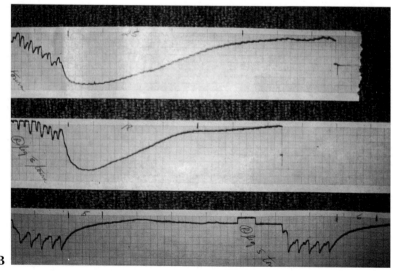

A   B

FIGURE 88.11. Direct current photoplethysmograph study of venous reflux. See text for explanation.

PPG is a relatively simple test to perform. The technician must properly position the patient and use the tourniquets appropriately. PPG has the potential to give false-positive results if the skin is discolored. These problems may be circumvented by recent modifications of the instrumentation. PPG may be particularly informative for the patient with normal or minimally discolored distal legs who complains of heaviness or other symptoms suggestive of venous insufficiency. In most patients with venous problems, Doppler or duplex analysis is more helpful in determining pathology.

Air Plethysmography

Air plethysmography is the name applied to a device, developed in the mid 1980s, to measure calf volume changes. The device uses a plastic air chamber that is placed around the leg and connected to a pressure–electricity transducer, and, in turn, to a paper strip recorder to print a generated waveform. Although named *air plethysmography*, the device is actually a specialized volume plethysmograph, which, from a physicist's point of view, is really a pressure plethysmograph. Regardless, the device can be used via various patient maneuvers to provide a functional venous volume (the increase of leg volume after the patient moves from a supine position with 45-degree leg elevation to a standing position), the time or speed over which the functional venous volume takes to develop (measured as the "venous filling time 90," or the time required to reach 90% of the venous volume), and the volume expelled from the leg with a single foot plantar flexion–dorsiflexion (tiptoe) maneuver (called the ejection volume). Other volumes and derived calculations can also be measured. The instrument was designed to measure calf venous pump function. It can be used while the patient is wearing a stocking. Thus, it has the potential to allow comparison of venous hemodynamics with and without compression stockings and between the various strengths of compression gradient or elastic stockings to determine an optimal strength.

Contrast Venography

Contrast venography is generally accepted as the gold standard for evaluating the lower limb veins. It is more commonly called venography, although technically, because duplex technology also visualizes veins, it too is a form of venography. Even the use of the term *contrast* can be disputed because the injected material that produces the image is visible to the naked eye under the conditions in which it is studied (i.e., with roentgen rays) and therefore has the characteristics to a physicist of a dye. Regardless, venography usually provides an excellent picture of the luminal characteristics of the leg veins.

Contrast venography remains the best method of analyzing infrapopliteal veins. To perform the study, a foot dorsal vein is located, needle inserted, and contrast injected. The examined leg is usually unweighted to avoid potential spurious findings such as muscle tension–induced compression of veins. Such veins may not fill with contrast; if they do not, they may be interpreted as obstructed and inappropriately treated. As part of venography, a tourniquet is usually placed around the ankle to help direct contrast into the deep system, usually the area of primary concern when this study is performed. Contrast venography can also be used to demonstrate incompetent perforating veins if contrast refluxes into the superficial system. With the advent of venous duplex and color flow technology, contrast venography is now used less frequently. It may be used when diagnosis of infrapopliteal deep venous thrombosis might be of clinical importance.

Advantages of contrast venography include its high-resolution visualization of the venous system and a long history of reliability. Its accuracy does not usually depend on technician skill as much as does duplex technology. In contrast to duplex analysis, it can provide good visualization of the iliac veins. Disadvantages include the extra cost of the study over duplex analysis, risk of allergic reaction to dye (which can be fatal), risk of contrast-induced phlebitis (which is probably a markedly overrated concern), and a usual reluctance to do repeated studies because of associated pain, cost, and potential renal insult. Spurious findings are possible. For example, if the examined leg is not relaxed and the knee is hyperextended during the study, the popliteal vein may be stretched or compressed closed, not fill with contrast, and mimic occlusion. If dye load, flow rate, or timing of imaging is not optimal, contrast appearance in proximal veins may not be sufficient, and interpretation of the study may be difficult. For example, a localized partial thrombus in the iliofemoral veins may be missed. Information from ascending venography about deep venous incompetency is usually poor, but descending venography addresses this problem. However, if proximal valves are competent, descending studies may not demonstrate reflux in more distal vein segments. Duplex analysis circumvents this potential limitation of contrast venography. Contrast studies may be quite helpful when venous valve reconstruction or transplantation is being considered and detailed anatomical information is desired.

Treatment of Superficial Venous Insufficiency

After obtaining a general and pertinent history, examination, and laboratory studies, options for treatment can be reviewed with the patient. In approaching treatment of superficial venous insufficiency, several issues should be considered, including the pathologic problem, available treatment options, and the patient's goals. In addition, concomitant medical problems should be factored in when planning therapy. For example, the aged, arthritic patient with varicosities may not be able to put on or tolerate compression gradient stockings. For the diabetic patient with a history of slow healing, vein ligation procedures may create an unacceptable risk of complications such as infection.

Because superficial venous insufficiency usually involves treatment of refluxing and/or dilated veins, options to treat these problems are addressed first. Then some selected clinical problems that may warrant customized care are discussed. Four major methods of treating dilated superficial veins—reassurance; elevation, compression, and pneumatic pumps; sclerotherapy techniques; and surgical methods—can be considered. Laser and radiofrequency devices are employed to treat some types of dilated veins. These technologies are not yet in such widespread use as is injection sclerotherapy, and their discussion is beyond the scope of this chapter.

For the patient who presents with varicose or other dilated superficial veins, it is important to explain all treatment options (Table 88.5) and some of the advantages and disadvantages relevant to that particular patient (see Table 88.6). For example, when discussing compression gradient stockings, if the patient has features that might make their use difficult or unrealistic (e.g., obesity or neuromuscular weakness) these difficulties will be explained.

TABLE 88.5. Dilated superficial veins: choices of therapy.

Reassurance, without other therapy
Compression gradient stockings or other compression bandaging
Injection sclerotherapy with ligations preceded by proximal reflux site (e.g., saphenofemoral junction) interruption (ligated and divided or ultrasound guided compression sclerotherapy) as needed
Ambulatory stab avulsion phlebectomy
Stripping

Reassurance

The most conservative means of treating varicose veins is reassurance as to their usually benign character. This "treatment" is especially applicable to the occasional patient who seeks medical input because of concerns due merely to the presence of dilated veins but has few if any symptoms. The patient's initial visit is an opportune time to acquaint him or her with other therapeutic options (e.g., stockings, sclerotherapy, and stripping) so the patient can make an informed decision about treatment selection. If the patient has no sequelae of varicose veins, the initial evaluation also affords the opportunity to explain the potential for symptoms to develop (e.g., hyperpigmentation, ulcers, and spontaneous ankle area bullous venulectasia rupture with hemorrhage) so that he or she can become aware of the possibility for future problems that might warrant reevaluation.

Elevation and Compression

Elevation is a mainstay for treating venous insufficiency. Elevation of the feet well above the hips uses gravity to

TABLE 88.6. Varicose vein treatment options: advantages and disadvantages.

Treatment	Advantages	Disadvantages
Reassure patient of benign nature of veins; otherwise, do nothing	May be all that is required for asymptomatic patients Inexpensive	Does not address symptoms or cosmetic problems
Compression gradient stockings	Compresses varicosities so they don't fill with blood, bulge, and cause symptoms	Ongoing cost Hard to get on Poorly tolerated in hot weather
Ligation and compression sclerotherapy	Usually very effective compared with stripping Low risk Relatively low cost Good cosmetic results Minimal anesthesia needed	Very technique dependent No uniform technique in general use Equivocal efficacy for saphenofemoral junction reflux
Mini-incision (stab) avulsion (ambulatory) phlebectomy	Low risk Good cosmetic results	Technique dependent Labor intensive Extensive infiltrate anesthesia required
Stripping	Usually very effective Low risk	Requires patient acceptance of procedure Incisional scars Higher costs because it is performed in operating room

circumvent venous valve incompetency and stasis by draining blood proximally out of the legs and toward the central circulation. Thus, elevation overcomes the essential problem of venous insufficiency, which is venous hypertension. Elevation is particularly helpful for patients who develop leg heaviness with prolonged standing in spite of using compression stockings. An optimal position for elevation is placing the feet at least 6 and preferably 12 in above the hips, with the knees slightly bent (to avoid uncomfortable pulling or stretching on the popliteal musculature).

Elevation is not a panacea or always practical. One cannot function in daily life with the legs constantly elevated; such practicalities as vocational and family obligations, meal preparation, and so forth limit the duration of compliance with elevation. Obesity and other medical conditions such as arthritis often limit a patient's ability to elevate his or her legs. Restlessness is another limiting factor. Nevertheless, in selected patients a course of elevation may be a very helpful initial treatment for varicose ulcers. Compliance with elevation is often best achieved in the hospital or nursing facility environment, where reinforcement and assistance with activities of daily living are provided.

Compression therapy is another mainstay for treating venous insufficiency. Most modalities consist of various ambulatory compression devices (e.g., stockings or bandages). Stockings specifically designed to treat chronic venous insufficiency are designated compression gradient stockings (see Figure 88.12). They are designed to provide a gradient of pressure that is highest at the foot and ankle and decreases proximally. If sufficiently strong, they markedly reduce bulging of varicosities, engorgement with blood, and symptoms and even facilitate ulcer healing. They are usually classified based on their strength at the ankle. Commonly available strengths are 20 to 30 mm Hg (European class I), 30 to 40 mm Hg (class II), and 40 to 50 mm Hg (class III). Open- and closed-toe designs and various lengths (below or above the knee, high thigh, or with a waist attachment) are available. Open-toe stockings permit the use of a silk sleeve to slide the stocking over the foot and heel to ease pulling them on; however, these stockings run the risk that the open forefoot portion of the stocking will ride up the instep, compress it too tightly, and block blood flow to the foot. Some companies offer different textures and linings to improve appearance, ease application of the stocking, and/or reduce irritation of the skin. The clinician can order whichever model might best suit a particular patient. Because the gradient of pressure is manufactured into compression gradient stockings and thus counteracts underlying pathogenic venous hypertension, the stockings offer a preferred method of providing bandaging or compression in patients with dilated symptomatic leg veins. Compression stockings and other compression methods probably do not facilitate substan-

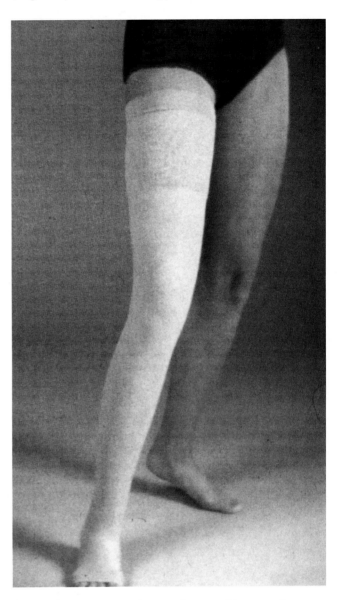

FIGURE 88.12. Compression gradient stockings, as shown on the right leg, are often helpful to treat chronic venous insufficiency. Several lengths and strengths are available. See text for further discussion.

tial regression of dilated vein size except while they are worn. However, they probably retard progression of venous insufficiency and its sequelae and indeed are a standard therapy for such cases. Mild elastic stockings (e.g., antiembolism stockings) may provide symptomatic relief of small varicose veins and those under low pressure, and they are easier to apply than 20– to 30–mm Hg and stronger stockings.

Unfortunately, stocking use may not be practical for several reasons. Stockings may last only 3 to 6 months and thus must be replaced regularly; because they are not usually covered by insurance carriers their use can create a financial burden on the patient. They can be cosmetically undesirable. Stronger stockings tend to be more difficult to put on, and in some patients, such as the elderly, arthritic, and obese, putting the stocking on can be quite difficult. Various devices are available to ease stocking application. Examples are the Miraculous Assist, Medi-Butler, Sigvaris SOS, and JuzoR Easypad and Slippie. Nevertheless, some motivation and agility are still required to use these devices.

In addition to compression gradient stockings, other compression methods are available and have met with varying popularity. Elastic bandages such as Ace's, can be helpful if applied in a compression gradient fashion (i.e., firmly around the instep, wrapped in a figure-8 pattern around the ankle—the heel rarely needs to be covered—and then firmly wrapped in a spiral pattern up the leg to below the knee using each turn to cover the upper half of the one below). The 4-in-wide, self-adherent type is most practical (see Figure 88.13). Disadvantages of elastic bandages include a need for some skill to apply them properly; their ability to generate higher compression strengths, in the ≥40 mm Hg range, is probably difficult to accomplish; elastic bandages offer no ready method of application to produce a reliable, reproducible gradient of compression. After several uses and with washing, elasticity is markedly diminished. However, the ready availability of Ace and similar bandages makes them an attractive alternative to compression gradient stockings, especially for patients with mild venous insufficiency. They are probably best used when an experienced nurse is available to apply them. Their relatively low cost also makes them practical for patients who are able to learn proper self-application of the elastic bandage (see Figure 88.13).

Additional methods of compression are available. The Coban 4-in-wide bandage has minimal elasticity, and the ability to adhere to itself reduces its slippage down the leg during ambulation. The Setopress elastic bandage has rectangles imprinted along its length. This product is designed so that when it is pulled sufficiently during application to convert the rectangles to squares, a compression of 30 mm Hg is generated. This characteristic probably helps to improve proper application of the bandage.

Inelastic but fully adjustable compression devices, such as the CircAid and CircPlus with foot–ankle wrap, offer another potential option of treatment. They are made of a series of hook and loop (Velcro) straps that are wrapped around the leg from the instep upward. Some may consider these devices unattractive. Their major advantage is that they avoid the need to pull a stocking on because the devices wrap around the leg; they are easier for some patients to apply than a stocking.

Pneumatic Pumps

Intermittent pneumatic limb compression may help treat superficial venous insufficiency by augmenting return flow and decreasing interstitial fluid pressure. It can be a useful adjunct, especially in patients who cannot use compression stockings. Several types of pumps are available. Single-compartment appliances are less expensive, but sequential pumps, especially with adjustable gradients, may be more effective.

Surgical Stripping

Surgical stripping offers a permanent means of treating varicose veins by removing them, and many patients prefer this approach. Various modifications have been developed to facilitate stripping. For example, perforate in-

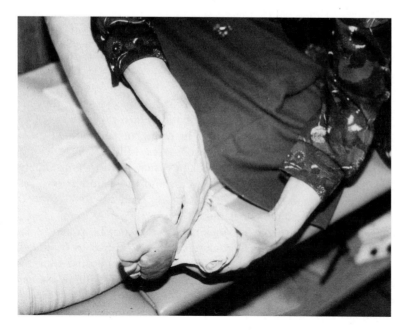

FIGURE 88.13. Use of Ace bandaging and a compression pad to reduce risk of recurrence of stasis ulcers. This patient with chronic venous insufficiency uses a pad over the area above the medial malleolus where ulcers have since healed and then applies an Ace elastic bandage in a pressure gradient fashion. In the dexterous, motivated, compliant patient, this method affords an economical method of treating chronic venous insufficiency and reducing the risk of skin breakdown.

vagination stripping facilitates saphenous trunk (greater and lesser saphenous veins) removal with minimal risk to other soft tissues.[20-22]

Patients may perceive some aspects of stripping—including the presence of residual surgical scars; the time, risk, and expense of the procedure; and the use and added risk of anesthesia—as negative. However, for the patient who wants the assuredness of vein removal with minimal risk of recurrence, surgical stripping does offer an attractive option. In particular, stripping down to below the knee offers an effective means of eradicating thigh-level sources of reflux and venous hypertension that are generated through incompetent Hunterian, Dodd, and Boyd perforating veins and the saphenofemoral junction. More distal leg- or calf-level stripping risks injury of the accompanying saphenous nerve in an area in which sclerotherapy can usually be performed quite effectively without this risk. Furthermore, because leg-level incompetent perforating veins usually do not connect with the GSV, saphenous stripping at the leg level distal to Boyd perforating veins usually does not address leg-level perforating incompetency and thus is rarely warranted. Rather, leg-level varicosities may drain via unclassified and unnamed veins, including perforating veins along their path sometimes via subtle connections to named saphenous branches. Careful examination, sometimes coupled with Doppler or duplex ultrasound mapping, can often identify proximal reflux sources so as to guide sclerotherapy injections and ligations.

The named leg-level perforating veins, the Cockett's groups, drain from the posterior arch vein. This vein courses just posterior and parallel to the GSV in the leg and drains into the GSV just below the knee. Incompetent Cockett's perforating veins can be addressed by interruption with Linton's procedure. Recently, endoscopic methods have been developed to interrupt Cockett's perforating veins without using the long incision of the traditional Linton's procedure. Endoscopic subfascial perforating interruption[23-25] utilizes a small incision to introduce the endoscope at the proximal leg, and CO_2 insufflation is used to enlarge the subfascial space to provide a larger area in which the operator can visualize the perforating veins and gain access to them with an instrument to clip them.

Sclerotherapy

Sclerotherapy offers the patient what can be considered a midway option between the aggressiveness of surgical removal and the nuisance and perhaps suboptimal value of compression stockings. Clinical factors that favor a role for sclerotherapy to treat dilated superficial veins are listed in Table 88.7. Sclerotherapy is discussed in detail in a later section of this chapter.

TABLE 88.7. Clinical factors favoring sclerotherapy to treat dilated superficial veins.

Varicose veins
Old age or disability
Presence of medical contraindications to surgery
Below-knee varicosities
Isolated varicosities (without saphenous reflux)
Recurrent varicosities
Patient preference against surgery or anesthesia
Preference for less labor-intensive treatment versus resection
Preference for lower-liability procedure versus resection

*Reticular veins**

*Venulectasias**

*Telangiectastasias**

*Sclerotherapy is probably the best treatment.

Mini-Incision Avulsion Phlebectomy (Ambulatory Stab Avulsion Phlebectomy)

In recent years, ambulatory stab avulsion phlebectomy has grown in popularity as a means to treat unwanted superficial veins.[26,27] It provides a method of removing varicose veins without large incisions. The varicosities are mapped, and the patient is placed in a supine position. The overlying skin is sterilized, and the underlying tissues are aggressively infiltrated with anesthetic (e.g., 1% lidocaine with epinephrine). Small 3-mm stab incisions are made along the path of the treated vein by either a no. 11 pointed blade or a 16-gauge needle.

The clinician extends a special hook through the incision to get under the offending vein, hooks it, and pulls it through the incision to externalize it. Both ends of the formed loop are then held with hemostats. The vein is pulled, while simultaneously pushing off adherent tissues with the use of a dissecting probe as needed, until it avulses and is removed. Sterile dressing, padding, and compression bandage are then applied and worn for perhaps 2 weeks.

This technique is usually performed in an outpatient facility, such as a short procedure unit. Some clinicians perform it in the office with suitable facilities. The procedure is somewhat labor intensive. Some malpractice carriers may categorize this procedure as surgery, which adds to the clinician's cost of providing ambulatory stab avulsion phlebectomy.

Sclerotherapy

This section deals with sclerotherapy in considerable detail. The essence of sclerotherapy is the injection of a chemical into the vein with consequent disruption of the intima and adherence of opposing walls to each other to convert the vessel from a blood-filled, visible, and often bulging vein to a thin fibrotic tissue that no longer bulges above the skin surface and is no longer discernible. This idealized goal is sometimes but not always achieved, in part because of the clinician's technique, inherent limitations of sclerotherapy, and the individual patient's pathology. The upper part of Figure 88.14 depicts the ideally sclerosed vein. But, as shown in the lower part, such problems as entrapped or residual blood in the injected vein, with eventual recanalization, can lead to treatment failure.

The origins of sclerotherapy may date back to ancient times, when varicose veins were recognized as a clinical entity. The development of the hypodermic needle in the mid 1800s provided a convenient means to inject substances into a vein. One of the first described attempts to accomplish sclerotherapy was Chassaignac's injection of a varicosity with ferric chloride.[28]

Modern methods of sclerotherapy have their origins in the work of several investigators from the mid 1930s to the 1960s. Biegeleisen[29] of New York did some of the early pioneering work in this field. In the early 1950s in Switzerland Sigg[30,31] developed techniques of injecting the entire length of a varicosity in one treatment session. Tourney[32] of France emphasized the value of interrupting proximal sources of venous reflux (e.g., the thigh perforating veins) before treating more distal veins. In the early 1960s in Ireland, Fegan[33,34] emphasized the value of injecting incompetent perforating veins, the im-

portance of postsclerotherapy continuous compression of the limb, and a role for injecting the leg with it elevated. Orbach[35–37] of Connecticut can be credited with developing the air block technique and the use of butterfly needles with catheters to facilitate insertion of needles into the leg followed by elevation for the injections. Hobbs[38,39] published reports on trials in London that demonstrated the different roles of compression sclerotherapy (CST) and surgery depending on the presence of proximal reflux.

More recently, in the late 1980s and early 1990s, other clinicians, including many Americans, developed or popularized some significant techniques to improve treatment. Katz[40] of Ohio developed and Malkoff[41] of California further advocated varicose ligation as a means to facilitate sclerotherapeutic treatment. In 1989 Knight[42] of Florida published his initial experience with use of duplex ultrasound technology to guide sclerotherapy of subcutaneous veins and the saphenofemoral junction. Several phlebologists are noteworthy not only for their research contributions but also for organizing phlebology societies. These individuals include Biegeleisen[43] of New York City and Butie[44] formerly of California. deGroot[45] of Seattle taught the fundamental principles of sclerotherapy. Goldman[46] of California has not only provided basic research but also has written prolifically about sclerotherapy and thus contributed substantially

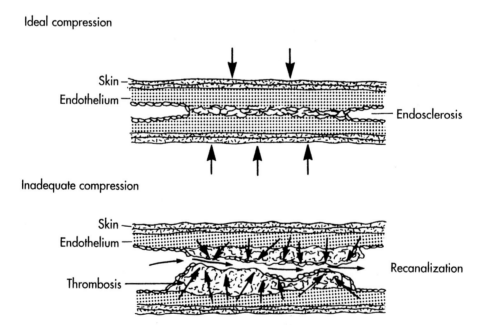

FIGURE 88.14. In the ideally sclerosed vein, injection induces the development of a thin layer of fibrosis along the endothelial surfaces of opposing vein walls (upper diagram). The result is permanently adjoined vein walls. Aggressive compression of the treated veins after injections is felt to be a key step in accomplishing this goal, by keeping the vein's opposing lumen surfaces in intimate contact to facilitate development of in-

terendothelial fibrosis. The lower diagram depicts reopening of an injected vein. This is thought to often result from the presence of thrombosed blood in the injected vein that then recanalizes. Aggressive compression of the treated veins immediately after they are injected offers a potential means to reduce this unwanted outcome of sclerotherapy. See text for further details. From Wenner L, cited in Goldman.[46]

to its popularity. Techniques of small-vein (e.g., telangiectasia) sclerotherapy have their origins in the pioneering work of Biegeleisen[47] of New York City who coined the term *microinjection* in 1934 and the more recent works of Duffy[1] of California, Goldman[46] of California, Chang[48] of Long Island, and many others.

The techniques of sclerotherapeutic treatment of superficial veins are still evolving. Several schools of therapy exist, including the so-called French and Swiss schools. There is no consensus about a best technique that the majority of sclerotherapists use. This unsettled state of the art suggests that several different techniques are comparable, or, alternatively, that some are better but their superiority has yet to be widely recognized. The techniques presented in this chapter represent the melding of input from innumerable sources, including the works of the previously mentioned investigators. In my experience the techniques described herein have provided good initial and long-term results with infrequent complications. These techniques can be labeled American, because they emphasize a particular component of the treatment in widespread acceptance in the United States, compression. Indeed, compression is so broadly recognized as an inherent part of sclerotherapy as practiced in the United States that many American phlebologists call the procedure compression sclerotherapy (CST). Thus, the remainder of this chapter deals with CST. The role of compression as part of sclerotherapy is discussed later in this chapter.

Another general observation about sclerotherapy is important to note. "Modern" CST has evolved to a much more sophisticated level than practiced by the pioneers of the 1950s and 1960s. As will be seen in the sections that follow, CST of varicose veins often incorporates the accompanying use of ultrasound duplex imaging to map veins and guide injections, as well as vein ligations. The latter technique is used to facilitate vein closure and obliterate reflux. Accordingly, this chapter deals with CST with as needed ultrasound guidance and vein ligations.

Contraindications and Precautions

A note of caution about sclerotherapy is warranted. For the overwhelming majority of patients who desire this treatment and have veins suitable for the procedure, a good outcome can be expected. However, in certain conditions, this procedure is contraindicated or unwise, such as when a patient exhibits any of the following: (1) active cellulitis of the leg (the exception is distal leg indurated cellulitis or acute lipodermatosclerosis for which sclerotherapy and ligation of offending proximal refluxing varicosities is actually a treatment of choice), (2) active thrombophlebitis of the vein segments under consideration for treatment, (3) pregnancy (although data is lacking to show that sclerotherapy during pregnancy is risky, at least two factors make this timing of treatment unwise—varicose size and pressure often decrease in the postpartum period, so that the patient symptoms that motivate injection treatment may improve after delivery and negate a need for sclerotherapy, and, in a highly litigious society, it is always tempting to blame a poor outcome of pregnancy on any event during it, even though a causal relationship cannot be determined), (4) previous side effect from the proposed sclerosant, (5) expectation of poor compliance with postsclerotherapy directions (e.g., premature removal of the compression stocking can result in thrombophlebitis; if the patient's behavior suggests a risk of noncompliance, such as those with dementia, language barrier to understanding directions, cavalier attitude toward medical care, or insistence on removing the compression stocking to shower, other therapies may be safer), (6) active cardiopulmonary or other systemic disorder with substantial potential for morbidity (e.g., diabetic patients with poor healing), and (7) infection.

Evidence that sclerotherapy presents a risk in patients who take oral contraceptives or in those with abnormal heart valves is lacking. Some conditions offer a relative risk for sclerotherapy but are infrequently seen in clinical practice. These conditions include use of anticoagulant agents and congenital hypercoagulability states.

Treatment Plan

Selection of sclerotherapy as a treatment for an individual patient usually requires consideration of several factors (see Table 88.7). Most patients who select sclerotherapy to treat their varicose veins do so because of their preference for a simpler, less involved, and less potentially risky office-based treatment compared with surgical procedures (e.g., stripping or avulsion phlebectomy). From a practical point of view, varicose sclerotherapy, including ligation (see later section), probably requires one half to one third of the time of stab avulsion phlebectomy. Thus, sclerotherapy is also attractive to the practitioner as a more efficient use of time.

With respect to reticular and smaller-caliber veins, such as venulectasias and telangiectasias, sclerotherapy is probably the best method of treatment. Several lasers are on the market and advertised to treat leg veins, but they are quite costly. Furthermore, laser treatment of a vein may require more than one treatment, and it may not disappear as rapidly as veins do when injected.

When a patient chooses sclerotherapy, with or without adjunctive surgery, a systematic plan of care should be planned, as summarized in Tables 88.8 and 88.9. Some important fundamental principles underlie these plans. First, proximal sources of reflux should usually be interrupted before or during treatment of more distal veins.

TABLE 88.8. Summary of sclerotherapy treatment sequence of events

- Obtain general and pertinent history (e.g., history of deep vein thrombosis, oral contraceptive use, diabetes, murmur, heart or lung disease, hypercoagulability).
- Perform general and pertinent physical examination (e.g., check for murmur, wheezes, pulses, do as necessary tourniquet or digital venous reflux tests).
- Obtain, as warranted, noninvasive vascular laboratory studies (e.g., duplex or Doppler analysis to determine perforating vein incompetency and location, access deep veins for patency; arterial Doppler segmental pressures and indices to assure adequate blood supply).
- Interrupt proximal junctional sources of distal venous hypertension (saphenofemoral and saphenopopliteal junctions).
- Interrupt (via sclerotherapy and ligations) large-caliber varicose veins and incompetent perforating veins.
- Sclerotherapeutically close reticular and small-caliber (venulectatic and telangiectatic) veins.

If proximal reflux sources are not obliterated initially, these usually low-pressure sources of retrograde flow and distal venous hypertension will continue to exert their hemodynamic influence of elevated pressure and increase the possibility of recurrence of previously treated more distal dilated veins. Thus, as part of a plan of sclerotherapy, proximal reflux sources are usually obliterated initially. A second important principle is to treat large-caliber dilated veins before small vessels. For example, venulectasias and telangiectasias should usually not be treated until associated varicosities are obliterated. If smaller veins are treated without first obliterating large-caliber sources of reflux and venous hypertension, the chance that smaller veins will recur is substantially increased, leading to frustration and disappointment on the part of the patient. With these fundamental principles of sclerotherapy in mind, the practitioner can plan the patient's care.

TABLE 88.9. Sclerotherapy and surgical options for treatment of dilated superficial veins.

If saphenofemoral junction is incompetent; interruption via
Flush ligation and division of junction and tributaries
or
Ultrasound-guided compression sclerotherapy
or
Proximal great saphenous vein sclerotherapy and ligation followed by sclerotherapy or mini-incision avulsion phlebectomy of remaining varicosities

If incompetent thigh perforating veins
Great saphenous vein stripping to below knee
or
Ultrasound-guided compression sclerotherapy and ligations followed by sclerotherapy or mini-incision avulsion phlebectomy of remaining varicosities

If varicose veins with competent saphenous trunk
Compression sclerotherapy, including perforator sites, with ligations
or
Mini-incision avulsion phlebectomy

If only reticular and smaller veins
Compression sclerotherapy
or
Laser therapy

Keeping in mind the sequence of events that enables CST to work is important when applying different techniques to different types and sizes of veins. These events may be summarized as follows:

1. Insert the tip of the injecting needle into the vein lumen (e.g., with reticular veins, this is accomplished by attempting to aspirate blood as the needle is advanced; when blood is aspirated, the needle tip is in the lumen).
2. Maintain the needle tip in the vein lumen during injection (for butterfly needles used on varicose veins, this is accomplished by taping the butterfly wings to the skin; for smaller veins, a steady hand is the key).
3. Provide a relatively empty vein for injection in order to minimize dilution of sclerosant by blood (for varicose vein injections, this is accomplished via the empty vein–air block method, by elevating the leg; for reticular and smaller vein injections, this is accomplished by injecting a small volume of either air or sclerosant, which pushes blood out of the vein ahead of it).
4. Remove the injecting needle.
5. Apply and maintain sufficiently strong compression on the injected vein until a semipermanent fibrotic scar develops.

Table 88.10 summarizes the sequence of events used for veins of various sizes to accomplish the described steps or goals. In the later section on techniques reference to this table will facilitate appreciation of how and why specific steps in sclerotherapy are performed. The following sequence of events is usually followed in treating dilated superficial veins: interrupt incompetent perforating veins (saphenofemoral junction, saphenopopliteal junction, and thigh and leg perforating veins), obliterate varicose veins, and treat reticular and telangiectatic veins.

Sclerosing Agents

Before describing specific injection techniques, it is important to review sclerosing agents. The sclerotherapist

TABLE 88.10 How steps in sclerotherapy are achieved for various sizes of dilated superficial veins.

Step in sclerotherapy	Type of vein		
	Telangiectasias and venulectasias	Reticular veins	Varicose veins
Insert needle tip into vein lumen and determine that the tip is in the lumen	As needle is advanced, try to inject air from the syringe hub into the vein	As needle is advanced, aspirate plunger until blood is withdrawn	As butterfly needle is inserted, observe appearance of regurgitant dark nonpulsatile blood in tubing
Maintain needle tip in vein lumen during injection	Use a steady hand	Use a steady hand	Tape butterfly needle to skin
Inject sclerosant into empty vein	As sclerosant is injected, blood is pushed out of the superficial vein	As sclerosant is injected, blood is pushed out of the superficial vein	Keep leg elevated at about 45 degrees to empty vein of blood and inject air before the sclerosant
Maintain vein closed (walls coapted together) until vein is scarred or fibrosed closed	Apply compression dressing: cotton balls and 30–40 mm Hg stocking for 1–3 d continuously	Apply compression dressing: cotton balls and 30–40 mm Hg stocking for 3–5 d continuously	Ligate refluxing and large bulging vein segments; use cotton balls and 30–40 mm Hg stocking continuously for 2 wk

should become familiar with these agents, their attributes, and their potential complications so that appropriate agents can be used. Descriptions of actual techniques include my preferences for sclerosing agents and strengths.

The currently available products frequently used for sclerotherapy can be grouped into three categories according to their major mode of action. These categories are detergents, osmotic agents, and those that act by means of chemical reactivity. Some commercial products contain more than one type of agent, and some contain additives for specific purposes. Some sclerosing solutions and products are discussed in the following sections. A more detailed description of these can be found elsewhere.[46]

Detergent Sclerosing Agents

Available detergent solutions include sodium tetradecyl sulfate, morrhuate sodium, ethanolamine oleate, and polidocanol.

Sodium Tetradecyl Sulfate

Sodium tetradecyl sulfate (STS) (available from Elkins-Sinn, Inc., Division [Cherry Hill, N.J.] of Wyeth-Ayerst Labs of Philadelphia), a synthetic surface active agent or detergent, is one of the most popular sclerotherapy agents in the United States. Chemically, STS is sodium 1-isobutyl-4-ethyloctyl sulfate. Structurally, it is a long-chain fatty acid salt of an alkali metal, with the low surface tension detergent properties of soap. Available in 1% and 3% solutions, commonly used concentrations for telangiectasias range from 0.1% to 0.5%; the latter strength is commonly used to treat varicose veins, and 1% to 3% strengths are sometimes used to treat large veins, such as the saphenofemoral junction.

Advantages include approval by the US Food and Drug Administration (FDA) for sclerotherapy. STS has enjoyed widespread use with rare significant side effects or complications overall. Most patients tolerate STS well, especially if the strength of the solution is adjusted to accommodate the size and pressure of the injected vein.

Disadvantages are several but rare. Skin necrosis occurs in perhaps 1% of patients; its incidence is most likely related to techniques and the agent's inherent potential to disrupt tissue integrity. I have very rarely seen skin ulcers and necrosis with a strength of 0.25% or less for treatment of veins 4 mm or smaller in diameter. Postsclerotherapy hyperpigmentation has been reported as a frequent problem but may be more reflective of the quality of the patient's veins and overlying skin than of the technique. Deep venous thrombosis has been reported rarely and again most likely reflects techniques rather than any unique quality of STS. An occasional patient develops an erythematous, apparently allergic local reaction of overlying skin after injection of even diluted 0.125% STS. This reaction probably in part reflects a natural mast cell and histamine release reaction to the injection. This occurrence, especially if prominent, may prompt a switch to an alternative agent to avoid potential complications.

Morrhuate Sodium

Morrhuate sodium (available from American Regent Labs of Shirley, N.Y., and Palisades Pharmaceuticals of Tenafly, N.J.) is a mixture of sodium salts of saturated and unsaturated fatty acids in cod liver oil. Each milliliter contains 50 mg of morrhuate sodium. The 5% concentrations can be diluted with normal saline solution as desired. For telangiectasias, strengths of 0.25% to 0.5% have been used with reportedly good results.

Advantages include approval by the FDA for varicose sclerotherapy, minimal postinjection local discomfort, and reports of infrequent significant side effects such as anaphylactoid-type reactions. Potential disadvantages include an extremely caustic behavior, lack of widespread use, and some rare reports of fatal anaphylactic reactions.

Ethanolamine Oleate

Ethanolamine oleate (available from Block Drug Co., Piscataway, N.J.) is a mixture of ethanolamine and oleic acid; it is available as a 5% solution that contains 50 mg of ethanolamine oleate per milliliter.

Potential advantages include only rare instances of allergic reactions and FDA approval for sclerotherapy. Potential disadvantages include a viscous nature, lack of widespread use and experience with it, and relatively weak detergent action.

Polidocanol

Polidocanol (available from Chemische Fabrik Kreussler and Co. of Weisbaden-Biebrich, Germany; Globopharm AQ of Kusnacht, Switzerland; and Laboratories Pharmaceutiques DEXO, S.A. of Nanterre, France) contains hydroxypolyethoxydodecane in water with 5% ethanol. Detergent characteristics derive from an apolar lipid-soluble, hydrophobic component, dodecyl alcohol, and a polar hydrophilic component, polyethylene glycolic ether. Concentrations advocated are 0.25% to 1% to treat telangiectasias, 1 to 3% to treat varicose veins 4 to 8 mm in diameter, and 4% to treat larger varicosities and perforating veins.

Advantages include lack of ulceration at injection sites, rare (1%) reports of adverse reactions (e.g., general urticaria, systemic pruritis, rash, anaphylaxis, brief inguinal paresthesias, and taste changes), and widespread use. The incidence of pain on injection and injection pigmentation is also reported as low compared with other detergent sclerosants. Potential disadvantages include lack of FDA approval (as of this writing) and perhaps 50% less sclerosing strength compared with other detergent agents.

Osmotic Agents

Hypertonic saline solution (HTS) and its variants are the major osmotic agents available (available from American Regent Laboratories Inc. of Shirley, N.Y.) in a strength of 23.4%. HTS is a popular agent in the United States for treating small-caliber veins, telangiectasias, and venulectasias. It has been modified in various ways in an effort to improve its efficacy and decrease potential side effects. For example, a product called Heparasal contains 20% hypertonic saline with heparin, which may prevent intraluminal thrombi and procaine, to reduce the pain of in-

jections. The value of this product has been debated. When using hypertonic saline, I routinely add 3 mL of 2% lidocaine to a 30-mL vial of 23.4% HTS and have observed a substantially decreased incidence of burning with injection from perhaps 40% to 5%–10%. In my experience, whether used alone or with lidocaine, the pain of hypertonic saline injections is usually brief, lasting less than 30 seconds. When injecting venulectasias and telangiectasias, I usually maintain a small volume of air in the hub of the needle. It is injected before the sclerosant to clear the vein of blood and ensure location of the needle tip in the vein. Others have used this technique with the rationale of avoiding dilution of HTS by blood so as to increase its efficacy.

Potential advantages of HTS include lack of allergenicity. This characteristic has been put forth as an argument against modifying virgin HTS solutions with such agents as lidocaine. However, in my experience, the addition of lidocaine rarely if ever leads to allergic reactions. HTS is approved by the FDA as an abortifacient and thus can be used legally in the United States, although it is not approved for use in sclerotherapy.

Potential disadvantages of HTS include pain on injection (see earlier comments) and hemolysis due to its nonspecific osmotic effects on all tissues. The latter effect can theoretically cause the cosmetically undesired presence of dark-colored hemolyzed erythrocytes within the injected vein lumen. However, with proper techniques, such as injection of an air bolus to clear the vein of blood before the HTS is injected, and aggressive injection of a sufficient volume of sclerosant to clear the vein of blood, and/or immediate firm compression of the vein after injection, the appearance of dark blood products in the injected vein can be minimized and usually prevented. The loss of HTS's sclerosing ability due to its dilution in the blood stream as it travels away from the injection site can be viewed as a disadvantage. However, this phenomenon can also be seen as an added safety factor for HTS, because there is less risk that it will cause undesired sclerosing effects at sites distant from the point of injection.

Variants of Hypertonic Saline

Hypertonic Glucose/Saline

A commercially available product, Sclerodex (by Omega of Montreal, Canada) contains 250 mg dextrose, 100 mg sodium chloride, and 100 mg propylene glycol per milliliter of solution. A hypertonic solution, its use has been advocated primarily for treating small-caliber veins such as telangiectasias.

One reported advantage of Sclerodex is less pain on injection due to a reduction of sodium chloride concentration; the addition of dextrose facilitates adequate sclerosing effects in spite of the lowered sodium chloride content. Another proposed advantage is rare reports of allergic reactions. Disadvantages include lack of FDA approval for use in the United States, reported mild pain on injection, rare skin necrosis, and substantially increased viscosity when mixed with blood if aspirated into the syringe to determine location of the needle tip in the vein lumen (see later comments).

I have experienced good results with the use of hypertonic saline–lidocaine mixtures, as described earlier. However, comparable successes with dilute STS, at strengths of 0.125% or 0.25% for sclerotherapy of telangiectasias and venulectasias, has made use of this mixture less common. However, occasionally, perhaps 5% of the time, I have seen immediate reactions at and adjacent to the injection site of small veins with even dilute STS in the form of cutaneous erythema and dilation of nearby veins. These responses may reflect a reaction with substantial vasodilation through interaction with mast cells and release of vasodilating substances such as histamine. An alternative agent to dilute STS with a good safety–complication profile was sought. Efficacy with hypertonic saline and the value of dextrose as an additive have been noted previously. In addition, experienced sclerotherapists such as Katz and Malkoff (personal communication, 1992) have reported the value of using 10% dextrose as the diluent for STS. I sought an alternative agent for patients intolerant to STS solutions as dilute as 0.125%. A combination of hypertonic saline and dextrose was considered. I use a solution consisting of three parts 23.4% hypertonic saline and one part 50% dextrose. To date, good results have been seen with this mixture for telangiectasias and venulectasias without complications such as burning and ulcers. The concerns that dextrose can cause excessive stickiness and difficulty in using the sclerosant have not been borne out with repeated uses. Indeed, I see the potential increased viscosity with dextrose as an advantage. The use of dextrose may help prevent, after injection of the vein, regurgitation of blood distal from the injected site back into the visible vein because of its viscosity effects on blood with resultant sludging and reduction of backflow.

Chemically Reactive Agents

Two chemically reactive agents on the market are chromated glycerin and polyiodinated iodine. Chromated glycerin is available in 72% strength (as Chromax, from Omega Laboratories of Montreal, Canada, and Giouami Pelli Pharmacia of Lusano, Switzerland). A relatively weak sclerosing agent, it is possibly the most widely used agent to treat telangiectasias, except within the United States.

Advantages of chromated glycerin include its low incidence of side effects such as skin ulcers and hyperpigmentation; perivascular injections are reported to cause only minimal problems such as temporary ecchymoses but without skin damage. Disadvantages of chromated

glycerin include lack of FDA approval for use in the United States, high viscosity, and local pain at injection sites. The latter problem can be reduced with the addition of lidocaine.

Polyiodinated iodine (PI) (available as Varigloban, from Chemiese Fabrik Kreussler and Co. of Wiesbaden-Biebrich, Germany; as Variglobin by Globopharm, of Kusnacht, Switzerland; and as Sclerodine from Omega of Montreal, Canada) is perhaps the most potent sclerosing agent. It contains diatomic iodine and sodium iodine in an aqueous solution. The product is available in strengths ranging from 2% to 12%. The active ingredient, iodine, interacts with the vessel wall proteins to provide a sclerosing effect. The remaining iodine is reduced and without sclerosing action. Reactivity of this agent only at the injection site may help mediate its safety by reducing the risk of distant adverse sequelae. Manufacturer-recommended strengths for veins of various calibers are 0.15% for telangiectasias; 2% for small-caliber, 2- to 4-mm-diameter varicose veins; 2% to 4% for 48-mm-diameter varicosities; and 6% to 12% for large-caliber varicosities such as truncal veins and the saphenofemoral junction. Some sclerotherapists have combined PI with other agents and report better efficacy. Sigg and his successor, Hoerdegen, popularized this agent; they reported very good results with negligible complications, especially for use in large varicosities including the saphenofemoral junction.

Advantages of PI include its brief localized action due to neutralization by blood components. Complications have been reported to be infrequent and minor. Disadvantages include tissue necrosis on perivenous injection, necessitating great care with technique, and, in the United States, lack of FDA approval.

Techniques

Varicose Veins

Surgery for Saphenofemoral Junction Incompetency

Following principles detailed previously, the first step in sclerotherapy is to obliterate proximal sites of reflux. In many patients, the most proximal reflux site is the saphenofemoral junction. Saphenofemoral junction incompetency can be detected by clinical examination, Brodie–Trendelenburg tourniquet test, and venous duplex or Doppler analysis. Several methods have been developed to interrupt saphenofemoral junction reflux.

The most accepted and probably most reliable technique is open surgical flush ligation and division with concurrent ligation and division of the three tributaries located in this area, the superficial circumflex iliac vein, inferior epigastric vein, and external pudendal vein. In the patient with a varicosed GSV who elects to undergo stripping, this procedure eradicates saphenofemoral junction incompetency. The details of saphenofemoral junction flush ligation and division are beyond the scope of this chapter.

Most authorities believe that both ligation and division are required to provide long-term eradication of reflux. They argue that if interruption alone is done, without division, collateral venous flow pathways will develop over the course of time around the ligations and cause redevelopment of reflux. Some experienced surgical phlebologists, such as Tretbar, have used interruption of the proximal GSV and tributaries via surgical clipping of the vessels. Good results are described. Such a method has an advantage of reducing surgical time.

Ultrasound-Guided Sclerotherapy

Ultrasound-guided sclerotherapy is a method that was first reported by Knight.[42] Some patients with saphenofemoral junction reflux may be adamantly against any surgical technique. For this and other reasons, a variety of techniques have been proposed and developed to interrupt the proximal GSV without open surgical procedures. Several phlebologists have developed sclerotherapy techniques to address saphenofemoral junction incompetency. My technique and the rationale behind some of the particulars are described in this chapter.[49]

The patient's deep and superficial venous systems are analyzed in the usual technique with venous duplex technology to rule out deep venous thrombosis. With the patient standing and the evaluated leg unweighted, the GSV is insonated with specific attention to the proximal GSV and saphenofemoral junction (Figure 88.15). Various maneuvers are used to determine presence of reflux, such as Valsalva's maneuver and manual compression and release of the lower limb musculature. Reflux of less than a half second at the junction and proximal GSV is usually considered to be within a physiologic range. Longer durations of reflux are usually considered pathologic. Especially if reflux is longer than 1 second and rather loud via Doppler flow analysis, the junction area is considered appropriate for reflux interruption.

With the patient again placed in a supine position, the proximal GSV is identified with the duplex probe at a site approximately 10 cm distal to the junction. The depth of the vein below the skin and its diameter are determined by internal duplex marker calibrations (Figure 88.16). This information is used to help guide the sclerotherapist as the injecting catheter (see later section) is advanced. The skin overlying the GSV and immediately distal to the probe is sterilized with a 10% povidine–iodine solution, and the overlying skin is anesthetized with infiltrate injections of 1% lidocaine. A 16-gauge, 2¼-in-long flexible Teflon catheter placement unit with a central hollow steel needle is then introduced (Figure 88.17) through the skin and subcutaneous tissues toward the GSV under continuous ultrasound guidance (Figure 88.12) . As the needle and catheter are seen to approach and indent the vein wall, they are then inserted deeper until the tip enters the vein lumen (Figure 88.18). This is confirmed by spontaneous backflow of blood, slowly, under low pressure, through the hollow flexible steel stylet needle (Figure 88.19) and by the ability to aspirate blood. The outer Teflon catheter is then passed further into the vein lumen, after which the central hollow needle stylet is removed. Injection of saline solution through the catheter, under ultrasound guidance, confirms its intraluminal location. The ultrasound probe is then removed.

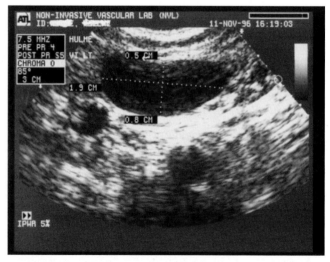

FIGURE 88.16. Use of duplex imaging to direct sclerotherapeutic injection of subcutaneous superficial system veins. The diagonal straight white line on the right side above the saphenous vein helps to indicate the path of the injection needle as it is passed through the soft tissues toward the vein.

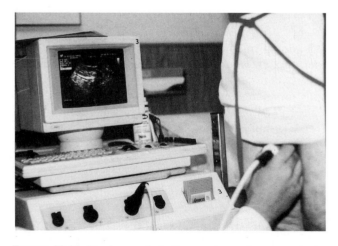

FIGURE 88.15. Duplex analysis for greater saphenous vein incompetency. Note that the patient is standing, which helps make reflux more evident.

The lower limb is elevated to approximately 35 degrees to reduce blood content in the saphenous vein via gravity. Further reduction of blood content of the vein is provided by direct firm manual compression over the proximal saphenous vein in the area at the tip of the catheter. This approach is used to minimize blood in the veins and thus dilution of sclerosant to maximize sclerosant efficacy. STS (1% to 3%) in an amount of 0.5 to 1 mL is slowly injected through the catheter into the vein. Injection of ½ mL air or normal saline further empties the catheter contents into the vein and minimizes tracking of sclerosant through subcutaneous tissues as the catheter is withdrawn. Concurrently, continuous strong compression is maintained over the injected area. The catheter is then withdrawn. Manual compression of the proximal GSV is immediately replaced by a dense, firm synthetic rubber material with beveled edges, precut to the size of the area (approximately 8 by 12 cm), and held in position with a self-adhesive elastic bandage (Coban). A class II compression gradient stocking is pulled proximally to cover this area. The patient is allowed to sit up and wrap the stocking's Velcro belt around his or her waist.

The patient returns in a week for assessment of the injected area by venous duplex analysis, which is done with the patient in a supine position. Duplex analysis may be repeated a week later, or a physical examination or pencil-probe Doppler analysis may be used to determine persisting interruption of the proximal GSV. In my experience, this technique is approximately 80% successful and may require a second injection to accomplish full interruption of the vein. This technique does not always

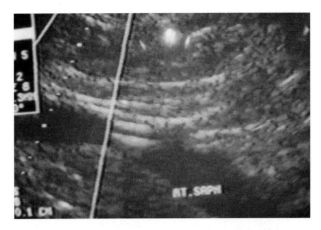

FIGURE 88.18. Visualization of a successfully inserted IV catheter placement unit under ultrasound guidance. This step is the major component of sclerosing the proximal greater saphenous vein. The parallel white lines in the vein lumen (to the left of center) confirm proper placement of the Teflon catheter in the vein. In addition, regurgitation of blood through the catheter (Figure 88.19) and visualization of a stream as saline is injected also confirm proper catheter placement before the sclerosant is injected.

result in vein wall coaptation, and sometimes a thrombus can be seen on the ultrasound image. The patient is informed before the procedure, and signs informed consent papers that explain to them the possibility of recurrence of venous reflux via recanalization. In my experience, with 3-year follow-up assessments, recurrence of reflux has been rare.

Some phlebologists have developed methods of externalizing the proximal GSV to ligate and divide it.[50] A

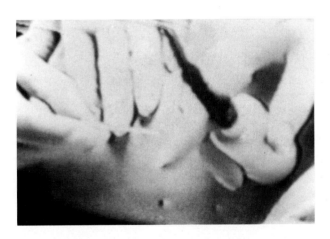

FIGURE 88.17. Duplex ultrasound is being used to guide insertion of an intravenous catheter placement unit. The technician is holding the probe over the proximal greater saphenous vein (patient's head is to the right) while the sclerotherapist inserts the "needle" assembly (the straight white object being held by the hand at the left) and uses the ultrasound image to help guide insertion depth and angle. (The fuzzy picture quality probably reflects the origin of this print, a color slide of a videotape.)

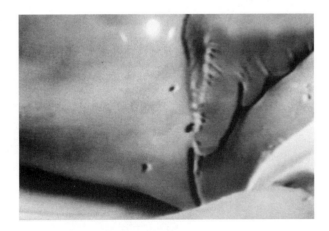

FIGURE 88.19. Successful insertion of a catheter tip into the greater saphenous vein is confirmed by spontaneous slow appearance and regurgitation of blood out of the catheter hub. In addition, ultrasound visualization of a stream of saline solution as it is injected into the catheter further confirms proper placement of the tip in the lumen and indicates that sclerosant can be safely injected. See text for details.

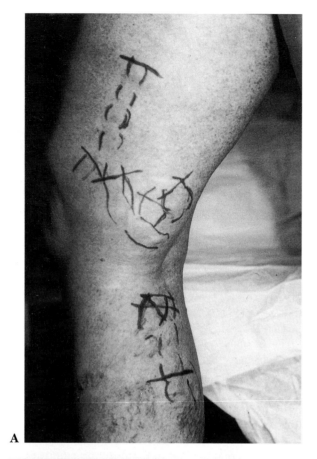

A

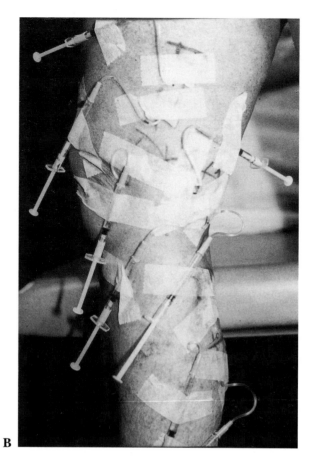

B

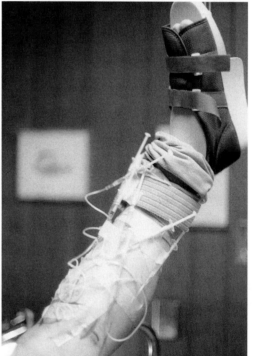

C

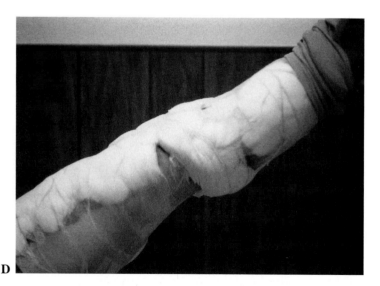

D

FIGURE 88.20. Sequence of events in varicose sclerotherapy. **A,** Varicose veins have been mapped, and sites for ligations have been marked with straight lines. **B,** Butterfly needles have been inserted into the veins and taped to the skin; the catheters have been flushed of regurgitant blood, and sclerosant-containing syringes are taped conveniently on the leg. **C,** The leg has been elevated, and injections will begin. Note that the stocking is in place, for ready application. **D,** After injections and vein ligations, cotton is placed over the mapped varicosities, held in place with tape, and the stocking will be applied.

third approach to saphenofemoral junction reflux that I sometimes use is to sclerose and ligate the most proximal aspect of the GSV that remains superficial just before it courses deeply at the proximal thigh. This location is defined by venous duplex imaging analysis. The overlying skin is marked and sterilized, a butterfly needle is inserted, the leg is elevated, sclerosant is injected, and the subcutaneous vein is ligated immediately proximal and distal to the injection site. Although the junction is not interrupted with this method, it is a simple practice and usually effective in preventing reflux.

Single-Session Ligation Compression Sclerotherapy With Empty Vein–Double Air Block Method

After proximal GSV reflux is corrected by the various methods previously described, attention is concentrated on the remaining varicosities. My procedure, described later, is summarized in Table 88.11 and depicted in Figure 88.20. As noted previously, there are as yet no established standard methods for sclerotherapy of varicosities. Many sclerotherapists imply comparably good efficacy with different techniques. However, the variability in efficacy and complication rates among some sclerotherapists may reflect deficiencies in some techniques. To make the inexperienced sclerotherapist's selection of techniques even more difficult, the long-term efficacy and complication rates with many methods have not been reported; judging them based on literature reports is thus difficult. Long-term results of methods by several pioneers (e.g., Fegan and Hobbs[38]) suggest that injection therapy is comparable in efficacy to surgical techniques.

TABLE 88.11. Single session ligation and compression sclerotherapy with empty vein–double air block method (method of Steinberg).

1. With patient standing, mark visualized and palpable veins.
2. Using duplex analysis, follow marked veins proximally and map overlying skin of subcutaneous veins, especially if refluxing.
3. Mark proximal refluxing sites and bulging veins for ligations.
4. Insert butterfly needles (e.g., $3/8$-in-long, 25-gauge needle with 3-in tubing) into varicosities at about every 3–6 cm.
5. Regurgitation of dark, nonpulsatile blood into the butterfly catheter is indicative of proper needle tip placement.
6. Place patient in a supine position and elevate patient's leg to 30–45 degrees; inject about 0.25 mL of air (first air block) to clear vein of blood.
7. Slowly inject sclerosant (e.g. 0.5 mL of 0.5% sodium tetradecyl sulfate).
8. Inject air again (second air block) to flush sclerosant out of tubing into vein to avoid tracking.
9. Remove needles.
10. Ligate veins at previously marked sites.
11. Pack cotton balls along path of treated veins, hold in place with Micropore tape, and apply 30–40 mm Hg high thigh compression gradient stocking with waist attachment.
12. Keep stocking on continuously for 2 wk.

In spite of a lack of standardization of techniques, sclerotherapy remains an extremely attractive treatment modality to patients, perhaps because of their preference to avoid surgery. The literature does suggest that the techniques of pioneers in sclerotherapy had some associated but acceptable side effects, such as postinjection thrombi. The method described in the following reflects my amalgamation of procedural details of several accomplished clinicians, including Orbach,[35] Goren,[51] Katz,[40] and Malkoff,[41] and the incorporation of several of my own techniques.[49,52] In my experience, these methods have resulted in good long-term efficacy with rare side effects and complications and can thus be comfortably recommended.

In the patient with interrupted or competent saphenofemoral junction and saphenopopliteal junction, the following sclerotherapy procedures are utilized. A class II (30–40 mm Hg) or class III (40–50 mm Hg) compression gradient stocking is placed over the foot to the ankle level. With the patient standing and the leg unweighted, varicosities to be treated are identified by inspection. The lateral borders of these veins are marked (see Figure 88.20A). In addition, palpation is used to determine vein locations, because some may not be apparent on inspection. Again, the overlying skin is marked. Palpation is performed along the course of these veins to detect fascial defects that may reflect sites of incompetent perforating veins. Incompetency can then be determined as desired with venous duplex, Doppler, or digital Brodie–Trendelenburg testing. A straight line is marked perpendicular to the long axis of the vein just below such fascial defects to indicate where the vein will be ligated. In addition, similar lines are marked over large varicose bulges for eventual ligation. The proximal course of varicosities with reflux is determined with venous duplex analysis, because proximal refluxing extensions of the varicosities may not be evident to inspection and palpation (see Figure 88.21). Again, the overlying skin is marked, and a line is also marked across the proximal refluxing subcutaneous veins to indicate location for future ligations.

The overlying skin is sterilized with 70% isopropyl alcohol. Caution must be taken to ensure that the skin markings remain clear and are not washed away by overzealous alcohol use if the skin marker is alcohol soluble.

With the patient standing on an elevated platform and the sclerotherapist comfortably sitting so that the veins to be treated are at or near eye level and under good lighting, 25-gauge, ⅜-in butterfly needles, with 3-in-long catheters, are sequentially inserted from distal to proximal sites every several centimeters along the previously marked varicosities. The needle is inserted parallel to the skin. Immediately on visualization of regurgitating dark, nonpulsatile blood, further insertion of the needle is discontinued, and the butterfly is held in place with

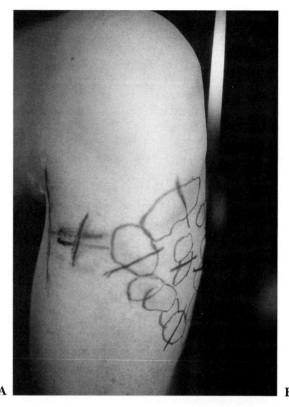

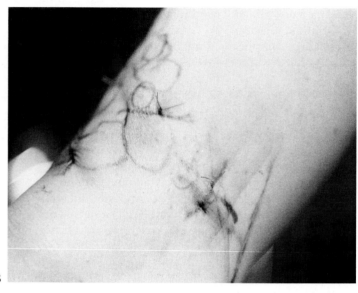

A   **B**

FIGURE 88.21. Use of venous duplex mapping to help guide sclerotherapy and placement of vein ligations. In **A,** varicose veins, indicated by the ovals, were readily found by inspection and/or palpation. Locations of the greater saphenous vein (long vertical line) and the feeding branch of it (parallel hori-zontal lines) were found by duplex mapping. Cross lines indi-cate sites for planned ligations, to interrupt reflux. In **B,** after the leg was elevated and veins injected, ligations have been placed. A compression gradient stocking will now be applied.

1-in-wide Micropore tape. The distal cap of the catheter is unscrewed, and a 1-mL syringe that contains the de-sired sclerosant, usually 0.5 mL of 0.5% STS, and 0.5 mL of air is quickly screwed onto the Luerlock fitting. Suffi-cient air is then injected through the catheter to clear it of blood. The syringe is then attached to the neighbor-ing skin with tape. This process is continued from distal to proximal sites until all vein portions to be injected have had a butterfly needle inserted (see Figure 88.20B).

The patient is instructed to sit. If the butterfly needles have been placed at or near the knee, the patient is in-structed to keep the leg under treatment unweighted with the knee straight and to use the contralateral limb to support body weight and to lower himself or herself into a sitting position at the foot end of the examination table immediately adjacent to the treatment platform. The table leg support shelf is then extended so that the nontreated leg can rest comfortably on it. The leg under treatment is elevated to approximately 45 degrees above horizontal and maintained there. Support of the ele-vated leg can be accomplished by various means. Some use a sling that extends from the patient's ankle to the top of an intravenous pole. I use an orthopedic platform shoe (e.g., Darco or comparable shoe) held onto the

foot with hook and loop fastener (Velcro) straps. A chain extending from the forefoot of the shoe is attached to a hook in the ceiling (see Figure 88.20C).

Starting distally and moving proximally, injections are begun. The individual butterfly syringe may be aspirated to observe regurgitant blood as a method of ensuring that the needle tip remains in the vein lumen. Alterna-tively, gentle pressure on the plunger with lack of resis-tance is a practical means of ensuring proper location of the needle tip intraluminally. A small volume of air (0.3–0.5 mL) is slowly injected to help clear the vein seg-ment of blood. The sclerosant is then slowly injected. Some sclerotherapists advocate maintaining mild digital pressure proximal and distal to the injection site. If the butterfly needles are not too close, this approach can be readily used. If some resistance to injection is appreci-ated, mild pressure of the middle finger on the skin overlying the needle tip often helps to create a clear path for continued injection, presumably by moving the tip lumen away from the wall.

After the sclerosant is injected, a second volume of air is slowly injected until the sclerosant in the tubing clears out of it and into the vein. I call this technique the empty vein–double air block method, in contrast to the empty vein–air block method as popularized by Orbach.[35,37] The rationale of leg elevation is to empty the vein of blood so that the injected sclerosant is not diluted and maximal benefit from the sclerosant is achieved upon injection into an empty vein. Some have, probably rightfully, argued that the vein is never totally emptied of blood. Nevertheless, injection of sclerosant with the leg elevated has been found by me and many others to be an efficacious method of accomplishing sclerosis. A French method of injecting the vein in the horizontal position, without it being emptied, is also reported to give good results. Orbach has proposed an initial injection of air before the sclerosant is injected to further clear blood from the vein in the elevated leg. I use this technique routinely. The second air block, by flushing sclerosant through the butterfly catheter into the vein with an additional volume of air, is purposely done to avoid tracking sclerosant through the subcutaneous tissue and skin as the butterfly needle is withdrawn after completion of the injection.[52] If sclerosant is tracked, there is a risk, albeit small, of inducing cutaneous ulceration, which can take some time to heal. The second air block markedly reduces this risk.

After the second air block is injected, the butterfly is removed and the next butterfly injection of sclerosant is performed sequentially from distal to proximal sites until all injections are completed. After each injection, the patient is instructed to bend the knee of the treated leg slightly and repeatedly alternate between dorsiflexion and plantar flexion at the ankle. This is purposely done to increase deep venous blood flow and flush any sclerosant that may have entered the deep system to reduce the risk of the sclerosing agent harming the deep system veins.

With the technique just described, I have yet to experience clinical evidence of either skin ulcerations or deep venous thrombosis.

After all injections are completed, the vein ligation procedures are initiated. The skin at sites previously marked for ligation is sterilized with povidine–iodine in a 10% solution. The skin and subcutaneous tissues at the sites are anesthetized with infiltrate of 1% lidocaine. Sutures are then selected for ligation from distal to proximal sites or as convenient for the clinician. Usually 4-O absorbable sutures are used with a ⅜-circle curved cutting needle. I use Polysorb sutures.

The markings on the skin that indicate the lateral borders of the varicosed segment to be ligated and the straight line across the segment are then used. The needle is inserted, relatively perpendicular to the skin, at one side of the vein, extended under the vein and across it, and brought out on the opposite side. The needle is then reinserted, at the same site from where it has just been drawn through, passed just under the skin, and is again brought out through the skin on the opposite side of the vein at the site of the initial needle insertion. The

suture is pulled firmly to pucker the skin and securely tied.

The remaining suture sites are ligated. They are covered with a sterile dressing (e.g., gentamicin ointment and a bandage) (see Figure 88.21B). Large cotton balls are then placed along the full extent of the previously marked varicosities (see Figure 88.20D). As suggested by the work of Tazelaar and Neumann,[53] cotton material has the ability to become quite firm when compressed and also conforms to the configuration of the space in which it is placed. Thus, cotton balls tend to fit quite nicely along the fascial and cutaneous gaps where varicosities are located and usually provide effective compression of the varicosities. (In my experience, material other than cotton balls, such as foam products of various densities, have not been found to provide effective compression of varicose veins and therefore are not used.) The cotton balls are placed along the entire course of the varicosities and held in place with 2- to 3-in-wide Micropore tape. In a few patients, the technique causes blistering, which can usually be minimized by not pulling the tape tightly across the cotton balls to opposing sides. The only role of the tape is to keep the cotton balls in place so they will not move as the compression gradient stocking is placed over the leg. Some sclerotherapists use Coban for this purpose. In my experience it does not work nearly as well as paper tape.

After all dressing, such as cotton balls or dense foam, is placed and stabilized, a compression gradient stocking is applied. I usually use a class II high thigh-length stocking with waist attachment. They are made by several companies. If rather high pressure varicosities are found while the patient is standing, a class III stocking is used. The stocking is applied and the patient stands and ambulates for at least 10 minutes in the treatment area. Fegan[33,34] first popularized the virtues of postinjection ambulation. Clear scientific evidence of its value is lacking, and some schools of sclerotherapy do not advocate ambulation. In my opinion, brief ambulation in the physician's presence offers some potential benefits. It ensures additional flushing of the deep system soon after injections to reduce the risk of sclerosant harm to deep veins. The physical action may help to set the compression pads in place over the underlying varicosities to ensure a secure location. And the extra time for ambulation ensures that the patient is comfortable, not experiencing discomfort from an inadvertently improperly applied stocking or overzealously tied ligation, and not experiencing such remote complications as vasovagal attack.

The patient is given instructions to follow during the ensuing weeks while the stocking is in place. These instructions include the following: the stocking is to remain in place constantly until removed by the physician. For purposes of hygiene, the top of the stocking can be lowered to just above the most proximal cotton ball and a plastic trash bag applied and held in place with 2-in-wide duct tape to provide a waterproof seal so that the patient can shower safely and comfortably without wetting the stocking. Some clinicians prefer the use of a cast cover, which is more expensive but also more convenient. The patient is instructed to continue all normal activities but to avoid activities that could inflict trauma on the leg. Accordingly, physically demanding contact sports such as tackle football should be avoided. Occupational activities that could inadvertently expose the leg to trauma should also be avoided.

The patient is seen a week after injection. With the patient in a semi-Fowler or supine position, the compression gradient stocking is pulled down to expose all cotton balls or foam padding. The padding material is gently removed to expose the injected veins, which are then inspected and palpated to determine the presence of potential complications such as suture site infections, tender thrombophlebitic areas, and entrapped blood. These various potential but rare complications are treated as warranted. If an infected suture site is found, a culture can be obtained, suture removed, and a first-generation cephalosporin used to eradicate typically offending microorganisms such as *Staphylococcus* and *Streptococcus*. In my experience, the occurrence of suture-associated infections is rare. If palpation demonstrates the presence of fullness, indicative of trapped blood, the blood can be evacuated by first sterilizing the skin, piercing it with a no. 11 blade or a 16-gauge needle, and gently kneading the skin to remove the underlying coagulum. Again, in my experience, the occurrence of this complication is rare.

The padding material and stocking are then reapplied, and the wounds are reinspected in another week. A 2-week period is usually sufficient to ensure effective sclerotherapy with negligible if any problems. Accordingly, the stocking and padding are usually removed 2 weeks after the initial treatment. The patient then stands. Treated veins are insonated with a pencil probe Doppler and the distal leg is compressed and released. If appreciable reflux of greater than 1 second is found, the vein segment is injected; ligated; cotton balls, tape, and stocking applied; and reassessed in 1 and 2 weeks. The resclerotherapy procedure is rarely required, but when warranted provides a more effective treatment with less risk of varicose recurrence. A patient's reticular and/or small-caliber veins are treated at a later time.

Reticular Vein Sclerotherapy

Reticular veins are treated with sclerotherapy via an aspiration injection method, as promulgated by Tretbar and others (Table 88.12). If the reticular veins have associated venulectasias and telangiectasias, as commonly occurs at the lateral thigh, both usually warrant treatment in the same session. Reticular veins can be quite pale and on occasion only appreciated on inspection by patients

TABLE 88.12. Reticular (blue) vein injection technique.

1. Insert angled 30-gauge needle, bevel up, into skin.
2. Aspirate as needle is advanced slightly downward toward vein.
3. When blood is seen in the hub, slowly inject sclerosant.
4. Apply compression bandage (e.g., cotton balls, tape in place, cover with class II stocking).

because of their particular angle of observation of their own veins. If such faint veins are present, the clinician may want the patient to point them out so that the clinician can visualize them at a low angle and mark the overlying skin for easy visualization of locations for injections. In addition, some reticular veins may only be evident with the patient standing; the overlying skin should thus be marked at this time. A special light source, marketed as the Venoscope, may facilitate reticular vein sclerotherapy by illuminating reticular veins not otherwise visible with ambient light inspection.

Most reticular veins are injected with the patient in a supine position. Rarely, the patient must stand for the needle to penetrate the vein wall. The overlying skin is sterilized with isopropyl alcohol. A 30-gauge disposable needle with a clear plastic hub is used; it is bent 30 degrees with the bevel up. A typical sclerosant for reticular vein injections is 0.25% or 0.125% STS. If the patient demonstrates allergy to STS, I use a 3:1 mixture of hypertonic saline and 50% dextrose, as described earlier.

The procedure is performed as follows. The needle is inserted slowly. Immediately after the tip is placed under the skin, the plunger is pulled back gently. The needle is advanced, and as soon as blood is seen in the clear plastic hub (see Figure 88.22) to verify that the needle tip is in the vein lumen, sclerosant is gently injected until the vein is seen to clear. Compression is immediately applied by pressing cotton balls on the injected vein segment and maintaining pressure while the needle is removed. Micropore tape is applied to hold the cotton in place, and a compression gradient stocking is brought up to compress the cotton ball padding. The application of compression immediately after injection and maintaining continuous compression of the vein after injection are usually reliable methods to keep the vein closed with negligible if any risk of backward refilling and discoloration. Many sclerotherapists do not apply compression stockings or other bandaging until they have completed all injections and report good results. However, others[54] who apply compression at the end of a session of injecting several veins report the common development of intravascular thrombi, temporary pigmentation, and bruising. The discoloration related to these postinjection sequelae can last weeks to months. Such posttreatment problems can usually be prevented by employing immediate compression after each vein is injected. The disadvantage of this technique is that immediate covering of an injected vein with a cotton ball and compression gra-

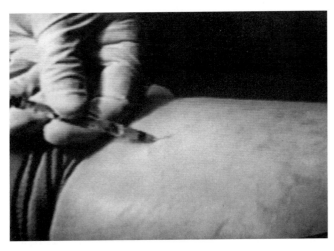

FIGURE 88.22. Sclerotherapy of reticular veins. The vein is too faint to be seen in the picture. However, the key step in confirming placement of the needle tip in the vein lumen is depicted. At the needle end of the syringe, dark blood can be seen upon an aspiration maneuver. This finding signals the ability to proceed with injection of sclerosant. Typically, as this is done, the vein can be seen to clear, as the sclerosant displaces blood in the vein lumen.

dient stocking prevents the ability to inject other veins in the same area. Accordingly, I systematically begin injections from distal to proximal sites, bringing the stocking up over the injected site after (a group of) veins are injected and cotton balls placed. This method of immediate postinjection compression is also used when injecting venulectasias and telangiectasias.

When injections are completed, the patient is instructed to walk briefly and informed how long to keep the pressure gradient stocking or other appropriate bandage in place. A uniform opinion about this time is still debated. I recommend 3 to 4 days of continuous stocking application after sclerotherapy for reticular veins. Many clinicians report good results from only a few hours or overnight stocking use. The strength of the stocking and the duration of application remain debated issues within the field of sclerotherapy. For good results the first time, patients are usually willing to tolerate the nuisance of the stocking to ensure efficacy. Most patients describe the use of the stockings as a greater nuisance than the actual injections.

Sclerotherapy of Venulectasias and Telangiectasias (Spider Veins)

After varicosities, if present, have been treated and closed, smaller-caliber veins are treated (Table 88.13). If reticular veins are infrequent and not anatomically associated with smaller veins, they can be treated, as just described, followed by treatment of the small-caliber veins.

TABLE 88.13. Telangiectasia and venulectasia injection technique.

1. Draw sclerosant into syringe, and draw air into hub.
2. Insert 30-gauge needle, bent 30 degrees, bevel up, into vein.
3. If gentle pressure on plunger clears vein, inject sclerosant (if air infiltrates tissue or bleb develops, stop).
4. Withdraw needle and knead skin.
5. Apply compression bandage (cotton balls and stocking).

Quite often, reticular veins are present in conjunction with venulectasias and telangiectasias in the form of a lateral thigh subdermal network of veins. This system was described by Albanese et al.[55] and further studied by Weiss and Weiss.[56] Typically, the venulectatic and telangiectatic veins are arranged in an arc at the midlevel of the lateral thigh, concave side down, and drain into some central reticular veins that, in turn, drain toward the knee (see Figure 88.4). Studies indicate that these veins probably drain into the deep venous system in the general area of the knee. Thus, the reticular veins serve as a conduit to drain the arch veins. When the lateral subdermal network is present, it is usually best to treat both the reticular and smaller-caliber veins together. Otherwise, if the reticular veins are not closed, they may act as an ongoing source of venous backflow that may lead to recurrence of the arch veins. If the reticular veins are of a sufficiently large caliber to form small-caliber varicosities with distinct borders, sclerotherapeutic closure and ligation, as employed for larger varicosities, can assist in ensuring effective interruption. When injecting the lateral subdermal system, the sclerosant sometimes travels from the reticular or slightly smaller components of the system into the arch branches and vice versa. Thus, with injection of a single vein component of the system, other branch veins can simultaneously be reached and treated.

For sclerotherapy of venulectasias and telangiectasias, I use a technique that reflects modifications of the methods of Biegeleisen (personal communication, 1988), Duffy (1), and Chang (personal communication, 1992). A 30-gauge disposable needle with a clear plastic hub is used. The usual sclerosing agent is STS 0.125%. If inadequate results are obtained, 0.25% STS is used. If untoward reactions are seen a 3:1 mixture of 23.4% sodium chloride and 10% dextrose is used.

The patient is placed in a supine position. A class II compression gradient high-thigh stocking with waist attachment is placed on the foot to above the ankle. Injections are begun distally and continued proximally. A 1-mL syringe containing sclerosant is used. A 30-gauge needle is attached (but is not used to draw up sclerosant, because the dense rub stopper of most injectable bottles may blunt the tip). The needle is bent 30 degrees with the bevel up (see Figures 88.23 and 88.24). A small

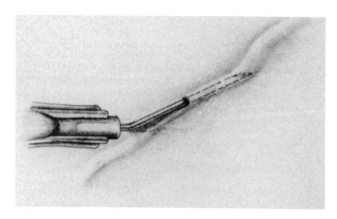

FIGURE 88.23. For sclerotherapy of venulectasias and telangiectasias, a 30-gauge needle is used. The needle is bent 30 degrees, with the bevel up to facilitate ease of insertion into the vein. From Goldman MP and Bennett RG, as cited in Goldman.[46]

The injection is continued until the vein clears, after which a compression pad is immediately applied and then the stocking. As for reticular veins, I use cotton balls and Micropore tape for sclerotherapy of telangiectasias and venulectasias. The next proximal vein is then injected in a likewise manner. On occasion, if a venulectatic vein caliber is large, I use an aspiration technique as described for reticular veins. The needle is passed under the skin, the plunger gently pulled back, and the injection is performed after blood is seen to enter the hub of the needle. After injections are completed and the stocking applied, the patient is allowed to walk briefly in the office and instructed on how long the stocking must be worn. For venulectatic or telangiectatic veins, 3 days is typically sufficient. This may be much longer than necessary; some clinicians require only a few hours of compression bandaging.

Not all clinicians use a compression bandage or stocking. Some dermatologists, after the spider veins are injected, infiltrate the surrounding skin with a sufficient degree of inert solution (e.g., saline solution) to create a local bulge. This technique appears to provide de facto compression of the vein and thus an effective means of treating it. This technique may be effective for small-caliber short veins. Special concentrated lighting (e.g., with a Venoscope) may help illuminate and visualize reticular veins to guide injections.

amount of air is maintained in the hub of the needle. The needle, with bevel up, is advanced parallel to and just under the skin along a straight line, if possible, where the vein course is relatively straight. The plunger is gently pressed, and lack of resistance and ready entry of air into the vein, with clearing of the vein, confirms proper placement of the needle tip in the vein lumen.

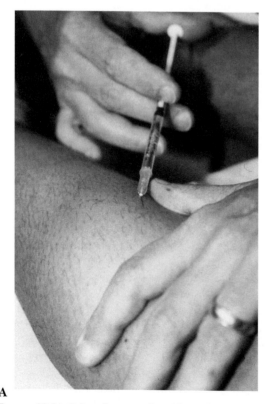

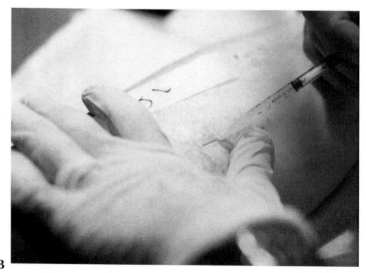

A   **B**

FIGURE 88.24. Sclerotherapy of venulectasias and telangiectasias. See text for explanation. Gloves are now and should be used during this and all sclerotherapy procedures.

Complications of CST

As with most widely accepted medical procedures, CST is usually safe but has the potential for complications. Many complications are related to technique, and some are related to the use of sclerosants and their inherent potential to damage tissue. Only a few potential complications are described here.

One of the most serious potential complications of varicose vein sclerotherapy is the inadvertent injection of an artery. Substantial sequelae, such as ischemia and even necrosis of the tissues supplied by the artery, can result. Prevention of such problems is a must. If the sclerotherapist suspects that the injecting needle is in an artery, the needle should be removed. Arterial puncture is usually easy to discern. Upon inserting a butterfly needle into the vein of a standing patient, the blood return from a vein is usually sudden initially and then usually quickly slows down or stops, with a steady, nonpulsatile pattern. The blood is dark in color. If, however, the return is pulsatile, with a bright red color, the inadvertent puncture of an artery should be presumed and the needle withdrawn. The field of anesthesiology has a very apt saying to avoid the potential pitfalls of accidentally intubating the esophagus instead of the trachea: "when in doubt, pull it out." Likewise, if the sclerotherapist suspects that an artery may have been entered, removing the needle is the safest route to follow.

Fortunately, in contrast to the deep system veins, which are usually accompanied by arteries, superficial veins rarely have adjacent arteries. Thus, injections of veins of the superficial system rarely entail risks of entering an artery. However, there are exceptions to this rule that the sclerotherapist should keep in mind. In at least three anatomical areas of the lower limbs, arteries may be in the vicinity of the superficial venous system: the infrainguinal area, where the deep external pudendal artery can lie near the saphenofemoral junction and the inferior pudendal artery courses down the anterior proximal thigh; the knee, where various arteries (e.g., genicular arteries, patellar plexus, and gastrocnemius artery) can course; and behind the medial malleolus, where the posterior arch vein branch of the GSV lies near the posterior tibial vessels. Caution when injecting in these areas is warranted. For example, if bright red, pulsatile blood return is found on entering a vessel in these areas, the needle should be removed and direct compression applied as needed to control bleeding. Also, duplex inspection of the vessel to be injected, especially in the saphenofemoral junction area, should enable determination that it is the proper vessel to be treated.

Skin necrosis has been reported, especially with STS. I deliberately use the double air block technique to treat varicose veins with CST, as described earlier, to flush sclerosant out of the syringe and needle into the veins and thus minimize tracking of sclerosant through the skin. This method has been very successful (no ulcers have yet been seen) and can thus be recommended. Also, using the lowest strength of STS that will successfully sclerose the vein for venulectasias and telangiectasias should help prevent ulcers, which may take weeks to months to heal.

Rarely, after successful clearing of venulectasias with injections and removal a few days later of compression bandages, some segments of the treated veins are found to be dark. The etiology of this result is unclear. Backflow of blood and its precipitation may occur. Reaction of the sclerosant with the vein wall may also be a factor. Regardless, this complication is an annoyance, because the patient's veins have been converted from unsightly blue veins to even more unsightly dark veins. I have found that flushing the veins with 1% lidocaine usually leads to clearing. The liquid acts as a flushing agent, and the lidocaine numbs the area so the patient does not mind this second set of injections.

On occasion, a week or so after injecting varicose veins, they are found to contain, on palpation, a soft, sometimes tender coagulum. This development probably reflects inadequate compression and/or ligation interruption of the veins. Coagula can probably be minimized by the aggressive use of ligation and soft material such as cotton balls. This compression material can conform to the shape of the subcutaneous cavity in which many varicosities lie and firmly coapt the walls. If coagula develop, removal is preferred to prevent their solidification and formation of a persisting lump. To remove them, the overlying skin is sterilized and infiltrate anesthetized, a puncture is made (e.g., with a no. 11 blade or 16-gauge needle), and the surrounding skin is kneaded to evacuate the coagulum (see Figure 88.25).

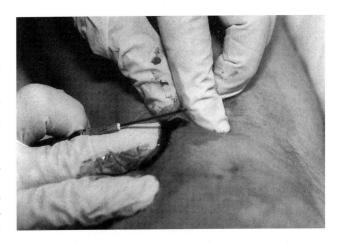

FIGURE 88.25. Extrusion of coagulum from an injected varicosity. The skin has been sterilized and numbed; a 16-gauge needle was inserted to create a path for extrusion. This potential complication of sclerotherapy can often be prevented with aggressive postinjection compression.

Several more complications have been well documented but are beyond the scope of this chapter. Refer to texts and journal articles to explore this subject further.

Complications of Superficial Venous Insufficiency and Special Applications of Sclerotherapy and Ligation

In addition to varicose veins themselves some patients may develop various secondary sequelae, such as varicose ulcers, acute indurated cellulitis (acute lipodermatosclerosis), and bullous venulectasias of the ankles. Varicose insufficiency may be the major or a contributing factor in their pathogenesis.

Varicose Ulcers

Varicose ulcers may respond to the same treatments used for deep venous stasis ulcers. Thus, constant high leg elevation that reduces venous hypertension often leads to healing. Unfortunately, patients' poor compliance with this method makes it an impractical treatment except in the controlled setting of a hospital or nursing facility. The use of topical preparations of the patient's blood (processed with a combination of natural and synthetic moisturizers and emulsifiers, including mineral oil and water) has been found in my experience and that of others to accelerate healing. Most likely, granulation-stimulating factors explain this finding. Some published studies support these observations.[57]

If patients cannot comply with leg elevation instructions, other approaches, such as serial Dome paste or Unna boot applications (I prefer zinc oxide preparations without calamine to prevent the occasional allergic reaction to the boot), can be used. They are changed every 5 to 10 days. Another alternative is the use of compression gradient stockings in the form of an ulcer kit now commercially available. The stocking length should reach above the most proximal insufficient vein. Intermittent pneumatic limb compression therapy bas also been helpful to facilitate healing. Pentoxifylline has been advocated as adjunctive therapy, in part because of its ability to decrease leukocyte adherence. This adherence may be a major factor in the development of soft tissue stasis changes. Studies have demonstrated more rapid healing of stasis ulcers with pentoxifylline[58] in doses up to 800 mg three times daily.[59]

The previously described treatment methods are not always effective or practical. Sclerotherapeutic interruption, as described in the following, can sometimes be beneficial.

Indurated Cellulitis (Acute Lipodermatosclerosis)

Examination findings in patients with acute lipodermatosclerosis include tender, often painful, and lumpy changes of the normally soft tissue in the gaiter area above the ankle, especially above the medial malleolus; skin hyperpigmentation; erythematous changes at the tender areas; and proximal venous insufficiency. Surrounding normally soft tissues are firm because of chronic stasis and secondary fibrosis (see section titled "Approach to the Patient With Superficial Venous Insufficiency"). When related to superficial venous insufficiency, varicose veins are usually apparent just proximal to the inflamed area. In addition to examination findings, Brodie–Trendelenburg tourniquet tests and venous Doppler or duplex analysis help to confirm superficial venous reflux. In such cases, varicose interruption by CST, as described in the following, may be of substantial value to facilitate treatment.

Several treatment options can be considered for acute lipodermatosclerosis. As for varicose ulcers, high leg elevation is usually helpful, but compliance limits its practicality. Use of compression gradient stockings or an intermittent pneumatic pump, preferably a sequential device, may be helpful if tolerated. Antiinflammatory agents are sometimes of benefit. The nonsteroidal type is usually preferred because it is safer than corticosteroids. Stanozolol, an anabolic steroid, has been advocated to treat acute lipodermatosclerosis. More recently, dapsone has been found to be helpful.[60] Doses can be started at 25 mg twice daily and increased to 100 mg three times daily until a clinical benefit is seen. Because of the potential for blood dyscrasias, monitoring a regular complete blood count and differential with platelet count is recommended. Again, as with varicose ulcers, if varicose insufficiency is a major factor underlying the acute lipodermatosclerosis, venous interruption may provide a more rapid, efficacious means of therapy than the aforementioned treatments.

Sclerotherapy and Ligations for Varicose Ulcers and Acute Lipodermatosclerosis

In practice, an examination and Brodie–Trendelenburg or digit modification test is initially performed to document varicose insufficiency. Then venous duplex mapping is performed with the patient sitting and legs dangling, or, if needed to better fill the varicosities with blood so they will show up, the patient stands without weight on the examined leg. Varicose mapping begins at or just above the ulcer or inflammation. Refluxing veins are identified, and the overlying skin is marked. Mapping is continued upward to the proximal sources of the refluxing veins. After mapping is completed and sites for ligation (e.g., beginning of reflux or bifurcations) are marked, the patient is treated with CST and ligation as described in previous sections of this chapter.

Usually, skin inflammation is noted to overtly decrease within a week of treatment. Varicose ulcers may often require a few weeks or longer to heal (see Figure 88.26). The gradient compression stocking, used as part of the CST treatment, is worn constantly for a minimum of 2 weeks. Thereafter, if the clinical situation warrants, as in the case of chronic stasis fibrosis and contributions from both superficial and deep venous insufficiency, long-term ambulatory use of the stocking is recommended.

Dilated Ankle Veins and Rupture

Dilated superficial veins at the ankle are frequently seen in practice (see the end of the section titled "Approach to the Patient With Superficial Venous Insufficiency"). They present as sparse to innumerable blue ectatic blebs, with a typical diameter of 1 to 4 mm, that often bulge out prominently. They are usually innocuous. However, they can occasionally rupture, either spontaneously or via trauma, and bleed profusely. Factors that predispose them to rupture include their bulging shape, which may increase their exposure to trauma; very few layers of cells between the vein lumen and the outermost skin layers

with thus a rather inherently weak wall; and high intraluminal pressure because of underlying venous hypertension from proximal venous incompetency (see Figure 88.6).

Fortunately, rupture of these veins is rare. However, when it occurs, often spontaneously, a spurt of blood may result that, because of underlying high venous pressure, can shoot out some distance. Rupture often occurs in a patient who does not expect this event and does not know how to handle it. If left untreated, the patient can suffer unnecessary blood loss and risk syncope from, for example, a vasovagal reaction. Many patients have presented to emergency units with hemorrhage from ruptured ankle veins.

However, this problem is easily treated. Should hemorrhage occur, immediate direct compression over the bleeding site will stop the bleeding and permit a clot to form. Alternatively, or in addition, the leg can be elevated high enough to drop venous pressure that feeds the hemorrhage. A compression bandage can then be applied. For long-term control or prophylaxis, sclerotherapeutic closure can be used.[18] First, proximal sources of reflux that supply venous hypertension from leg and thigh varicosities are identified, usually by examination and duplex analysis. They are then closed with

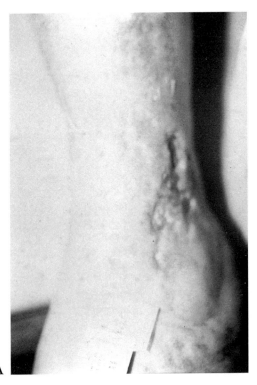
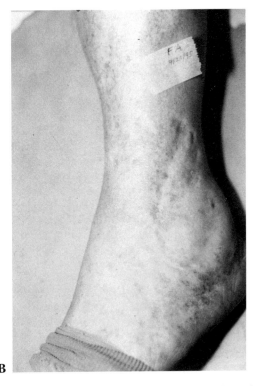

A   **B**

FIGURE 88.26. Use of sclerotherapy and ligations to treat a varicose ulcer. Although the dilated superficial veins that fed the ulcer in this patient were subtle to exam, duplex analysis demonstrated them. **A,** The ulcer before varicose interruption. Note the depth and extent. The proximal feeding veins were then interrupted by sclerotherapy and ligations. After several weeks, with adjunctive use of a compression stocking, the ulcer is just about healed (**B**). This patient was intolerant of Unna boots.

CST and ligation as described earlier in this chapter. Then the bullous venulectasias themselves are also treated with CST. The venulectasias can be injected, usually with dilute STS; a compression dressing or bandage maintained for 1 to 2 weeks allows for fibrous conversion of the injected veins.

References

1. Duffy DM. Technique for Injection Sclerotherapy of Spider and Varicose Veins [videotape]. 1991.

2. Browse NL, Burnand KG, Thomas ML, et al. *Diseases of the Veins.* London: E. Arnold; 1989:39–46.

3. Georgiev M. The femoropopliteal vein. *Dermatologic Surgery.* 1996;22:613–616.

4. Weiss RA, Weiss MA. Doppler ultrasound findings in reticular veins of the thigh subdermic lateral venous system and implications for sclerotherapy. *Journal of Dermatologic Surgery and Oncology.* 1993;19:947.

5. Svjcar J, et al. Biochemical differences in the composition of primary varicose veins. *Am Heart J.* 1964;67:572.

6. Cornu-Thenard A. The role of heredity in the varicose vein disease: a case control study. *Journal of Dermatologic Surgery and Oncology.* 1992;18:62.

7. Bouissou H, et al. Vein morphology. *Phlebology.* 1988;3 (suppl 1):1.

8. Acsady G, Lengyel I. Modifications between histomorphological and pathobiochemical changes leading to primary varicosis. In: Davy A, Stemmer R, eds. *Phlebologie 89.* Montrouge, France: John Libbey Eurotext; 1989.

9. Staubesand J, Fischer N. The ultrastructural characteristics of abnormal collagen fibrils in various organs. *Connect Tissue Res.* 1980;7:213–217.

10. Rose SS, Ahmed A. Some thoughts on the aetiology of varicose veins. *J Cardiovasc Surg.* 1986;27:534–543.

11. Clarke H, Smith SR, Vasdekis SN, et al. Role of venous elasticity in the development of varicose veins. *Br J Surg.* 1989;76:577–580.

12. Fuchs U, Petter O. Phlebosclerosis of the stem veins in varicosis. *Phlebologie und Proktologie.* 1990;19:120.

13. Rai DB, Iqbal S. Saphenofemoral incompetency and varicose veins: histopathology and management. Paper presented at: 17th Annual Congress of the Phlebology Society of America; November 1997; Coronado, Calif.

14. Wokalek H, et al. Morphology and localization of sunburst varicosities: an electron microscopic and morphometric study. *Journal of Dermatologic Surgery and Oncology.* 1989; 15:149–154.

15. Browse NL, et al. Venous ulceration. *BMJ.* 1983;286:19201.

16. Juergens JL, Spittell JA Jr, Fairbairn JF II. *Peripheral Vascular Diseases.* Philadelphia, Pa: WB Saunders; 1980.

17. Gravitational eczema. In: Rook A, et al., eds. *Textbook of Dermatology.* Melbourne, Australia: Blackwell Scientific, 1986.

18. Tretbar LL. Treatment of small bleeding varicose veins with injection sclerotherapy. *Dermatol Surg.* 1996;22:78–80.

19. Beesley WH, Fegan WG. An investigation into the localization of incompetent perforating veins. *Br J Surg.* 1970;157: 30–32.

20. Oesch A. "Pin-stripping": a novel method of atraumatic stripping. *Phlebology.* 1993;4:171–173.

21. Oesch A. PIN-stripping. *Phlebologie.* 1996;25:177–182.

22. Goren G, Yellin AE. Minimally invasive surgery for primary varicose veins: limited invaginated axial stripping and tributary (hook) stab avulsion. *Ann Vasc Surg.* 1995;9: 401–414.

23. Saharay M, Scurr JH. Minimally invasive surgery for perforator vein incompetence. *Cardiovasc Surg.* 1996;4:701–705.

24. Whiteley MS, Smith JJ, Galland RB. Tibial nerve damage during subfascial endoscopic perforator vein surgery. *Br J Surg.* 1997;84:512.

25. Iafrati MD, Welch HJ, O'Donnell TF Jr. Subfascial endoscopic perforator ligation: an analysis of early clinical outcomes and cost. *J Vasc Surg.* 1997;25:995–1001.

26. Muller R. Traitment des varices par la phlebectomie ambulatoire. *Phlebologie.* 1966;19:277.

27. Ricci S, et al. *Ambulatory Phlebectomy: A Practical Guide for Treating Varicose Veins.* St Louis, Mo: Mosby–Year Book; 1995:89–114.

28. Chassaignac E. Nouvelle Methode pour la traitment des Tumours Hoemorhoidaies. Paris: Bailliere; 1885.

29. Biegeleisen HI. *Primer of Sclerotherapy: Injection Treatment.* New York, NY: Froben Press; 1944.

30. Sigg K. The treatment of varicosities and accompanying complications. *Angiology.* 1952;3:355–379.

31. Sigg K. Treatment of varicose veins by injection-sclerotherapy: a method practiced in Switzerland. In: Hobbs JT, ed. *The Treatment of Venous Disorders: A Comprehensive Review of Current Practice in the Management of Varicose Veins and the Post-Thrombotic Syndrome.* Philadelphia, Pa: JB Lippincott; 1977:113–137.

32. Tournay R. Indications et resultats de la mothode sclerosante dans la traitement des varices. *Bulletin Medical (Paris).* 1931;45:73.

33. Fegan WG. Continuous compression technique of injecting varicose veins. *Lancet.* 1963;1:109–112.

34. Fegan WG. Treatment of varicose veins by injection-compression: a method practiced in Eire. In: Hobbs JT, ed. *The Treatment of Venous Disorders.* Philadelphia, Pa: JB Lippincott; 1977:99–112.

35. Orbach EJ. Sclerotherapy of varicose veins (utilization of an intravenous airblock). *Am J Surg.* 1944;66:362–366.

36. Orbach EJ. A new look on sclerotherapy. *Folia Angiologica Haupt and Koska.* 1977;25:181.

37. Orbach EJ. Hazards of sclerotherapy of varicose veins: their prevention and treatment of complications. *VASA.* 1979;8:170–173.

38. Hobbs JT. Surgery and sclerotherapy in the treatment of varicose veins: a random trial. *Arch Surg.* 1974;109: 793–796.

39. Hobbs JT. The management of varicose veins. *Surg Ann.* 1980;12:169–186.

40. Katz W. Circumferential ligations followed by sclerotherapy. In: *Proceedings, Western Phlebology Conference.* April 24–26, 1991; Whistler, British Columbia, Canada: 1991: 128–129.

41. Malkoff J. Injection compression sclerotherapy. Paper presented at: 15th Annual Congress of the Phlebology Society of America; May 28, 1993; New Orleans, La.

42. Knight RM, Zygmunt JA. Echosclerotherapy. Proceedings of the 12th Annual Congress of the Phlebology Society of America. 1989:37–39.

43. Beigeleisen K, Nielsen RD. Failure of angioscopically guided sclerotherapy to permanently obliterate greater saphenous varicosity. *Phlebology*. 1994;9:799.

44. Butie A. Experience with injections at the saphenofemoral junction in the United States. In: Davy A, Stemmer R, eds. *Phlebologie 89*. Montrouge, France: John Libbey Eurotext; 1989.

45. deGroot WP. Treatment of varicose veins: modern concepts and methods. *Journal of Dermatologic Surgery and Oncology*. 1989;15:191–198.

46. Goldman MP. *Sclerotherapy: Treatment of Varicose and Telangiectatic Leg Veins*. St Louis, Mo: Mosby–Year Book; 1995.

47. Beigeleisen HI. Telangiectasia associated with varicose veins: treatment by a micro-injection technique. *JAMA*. 1934;102:2092.

48. Chang J. Experiences with sclerotherapy. Paper presented at: 13th Annual Congress of the Phlebology Society of America; September 11, 1991; Cincinnati, Ohio.

49. Steinberg J. Catheter-mediated sapheno-femoral junction sclerotherapy under ultrasound guidance with an empty vein–air block method. *Journal of Dermatologic Surgery and Oncology*. 1994;20:67.

50. Vin F, et al. An ambulatory treatment of varicose veins associating surgical section and sclerotherapy of large saphenous veins (35 techniques). *Dermatol Surg*. 1996;22:65–70.

51. Goren G. Single session sclerotherapy of truncal varicosities. Paper presented at: 13th Annual Congress of the Phlebology Society of America; May 11, 1990; Chicago, Ill.

52. Steinberg J. Empty vein–double air block: a sclerotherapy technique to prevent skin necrosis. A poster presentation at: 8th Annual Congress of the North American Society of Phlebology; February 25–28, 1995; Fort Lauderdale, Fla.

53. Tazelaar RJ, Neumann HAM. Macrosclerotherapy and compression. In: Goldman MP, Bergan JJ, eds. *Ambulatory Treatment of Venous Disease*. St Louis, Mo: Mosby–Year Book; 1996:105–112.

54. Fronek HS. Sclerotherapy of reticular veins. In: Goldman MP, Bergan JJ, eds. *Ambulatory Treatment of Venous Disease*. St Louis, Mo: Mosby–Year Book; 1996:49–56.

55. Albenese AR, et al. The lateral subdermic venous system of the legs. *Vasc Surg*. 1969;3:81.

56. Weiss RA, Weiss MA. Doppler ultrasound findings in reticular veins of the thigh subdermic lateral venous system and implications for sclerotherapy. *Journal of Dermatologic Surgery and Oncology*. 1993;19:947.

57. Knighton DR, et al. Stimulation of repair in chronic, non-healing, cutaneous ulcers using platelet-derived wound healing formula. *Surg. Gynecol Obstet*. 1990;170:56–60.

58. Weltgasser H. The use of pentoxifylline ('Trental' 400) in the treatment of leg ulcers: results of a double-blind trial. *Pharmatherapeutica*. 1983;3(suppl 1):143.

59. Tretbar L. Results of FDA pentoxifylline (Trental®) study for the healing of venous ulcers. Paper presented at: 17th Annual Congress of the Phlebology Society of America; November 11, 1997; Coronado, Calif.

60. Lack EB. The use of dapsone in the treatment of lipodermatosclerosis. *Proceedings of the 12th Annual Congress of the Phlebology Society of America*. 1989:57.

Section 12
Deep Vein Thrombosis

89

Acute Vein Thrombosis

Michael Martin

The diagnosis and treatment of deep vein thrombosis (DVT) is a significant challenge to the medical profession. According to a recent study of 2500 patients who were admitted to the hospital with DVT[63] and a calculation based on the number of hospital beds available, an average number of about 30,000 patients per year are treated for acute thrombosis in Germany every year. With a total population of 80,000,000, this translates into an annual incidence of 0.04%. DVT is a disabling and dangerous disease associated with severe skin lesions and the potential for fatal pulmonary embolism. Prandoni et al.[81] followed 355 patients with DVT over eight years. Severe postthrombotic changes developed in 10% of these persons, and the cumulative incidence of recurrent venous thrombosis was recorded at 30%. Furthermore, seven groups reported on fatal pulmonary embolism during hospital stay (Table 89.1) and six groups on fatal pulmonary embolism 1.5 months to 4.8 years after discharge from the hospital (Table 89.2). Obviously, the severity of the sequelae of DVT is related to the thrombosis site. Thus, a 3-year follow-up study[25] showed that postthrombotic changes in patients with iliac thromboses were recorded at a rate of 37.9% (ulcer 17.2%), of patients with femoral vein thromboses in 47.2% (ulcer 11.1%), in patients with popliteal vein thromboses of 19.2% (ulcer 11.5%), and in patients with calf vein thromboses of 3.57% (no ulcer).

Until 1940 the only method of treatment of DVT available was bandaging and bed rest. At that time the rate of lethal embolism was as high as 18%. Bauer[8,9] was one of the first to introduce heparin as a prophylactic measure for the early stages of thrombosis. This strategy has reduced in-hospital mortality rates dramatically.

Another approach to the management of DVT is the use of thrombolytic agents. They were first studied in human volunteers by Johnson and McCarthy[45] and introduced for clinical use by Schmutzler.[92] Unlike heparin, which is given for prophylactic reasons, fibrinolytic treatment is administered to remove thrombi (i.e., therapeutic intervention) (Table 89.3). However, fibrinolytic therapy has not gained universal recognition.

In some European countries such as Germany fibrinolytic treatment is routinely used as standard therapy for DVT. However, in other countries, including the United States, fibrinolysis has not stimulated significant interest. Surgical methods still predominate and are often the only therapeutic modality used apart from heparin.

TABLE 89.1. Rates of fatal pulmonary embolism during heparin therapy of patients treated for deep vein thrombosis in the hospital.

Authors	Number of patients	Fatal pulmonary embolism	
		n	%
Bauer[9]	288	3	1.04
Coon et al.[20]	1744	10	0.57
Kakkar et al.[46]	10	1	10.0
Tsapogas et al[107]	15	—	—
Widmer et al.[115]	42	—	—
Elliot et al.[27]	25	2	8.00
Watz & Savidge[113]	17	—	—
Fagher & Lundh[28]	28	—	—
Arnesen et al.[7]	21	—	—
Biland et al.[15]	278	2	0.72
Hull et al.[42]	219	3	1.37
Martin[61]	1674	39	2.33

TABLE 89.2. Fatal pulmonary embolism after discharge from hospital.

Authors	Number of Patients	Period of follow-up investigation	Fatal pulmonary embolism	
			n	%
Widmer et al.[115]	204	4.8 ± 1.8 y	6	2.49
Hull et al.[42]	219	3 mo	4	1.83
Prandoni et al.[81]	170	51–155 d	5	2.94
Franzeck et al.[31]	58	12 y	2	2.94
Prandoni et al.[81]	170	6 mo	6	3.53
Koopman et al.[49]	404	6 mo	3	0.743

TABLE 89.3. Heparin and streptokinase treatment for deep vein thrombosis: results of six controlled studies.

Authors	Fully cleared or substantial lysis		Partially cleared or moderate lysis		Unchanged or worse	
	H	SK	H	SK	H	SK
Kakkar et al.[46]	2	6	2	1	5	2
Robertson et al.[86]	1	5	1	1	5	3
Seaman et al.[94]	1	6	14	11	10	4
Arnesen et al.[6]	2	11	3	4	16	6
Elliot et al.[27]	0	9	0	9	25	5
Watz and Savidge[113]	1	8	4	3	3	3
Total Number	7	45	24	29	64	23
Percentage	7.37	46.4	25.3	29.9	67.4	23.7

H, heparin; SK, streptokinase.

A relatively new development has been the advent of low molecular weight heparin (LMWH), which has been shown to be more than or at least as effective as unfractionated heparin (UFH) (Table 89.4).

In this chapter an overview of the causes of DVT, the methods used for its diagnosis, the possibilities for treating this condition, and the various therapeutic tools now available to the different forms of thrombosis will be described.

Causes of DVT

A recent study on the outcome of DVT treatment with heparin[61] and fibrinolytic treatment[63] has shown that immobility was the main cause of thrombosis. Thus, patients with paralysis, people traveling long distances by bus or air, and those working in unnatural postures for hours or days at a time are prone to developing venous occlusion. Other causal mechanisms relate to surgery (which in most cases is connected with immobility), tumor, pregnancy, oral contraceptive use, and blood coagulation abnormalities.

Some controversy still exists over whether the starting point of a thrombosis is located in the small veins of the calf muscles[9,46] or in the cusps of the valves of the larger vessels.[12,75] The latter view is sustained by hemodynamic flow analysis (Figure 89.1) and venographic series before and after fibrinolytic treatment of DVT (Figure 89.2).

Tumors are a well-established cause of DVT and account for 5% to 8% of cases.[72,75] Evidence of coagulation system activation in cancer patients was obtained in a first large study by Morrison,[73] but the precise mechanism responsible for tumor-related thrombus formation is still unclear.[38] There are, however, indications for the existence of a factor VII–activating tissue factor that, on contact with tumor cells, is produced by macrophages.[24] Furthermore, tumor cells can produce a procoagulant with a factor X–activating capacity.[30]

Irregularities of the coagulation system include the following:

- Low level of protein C
- Low level of protein S

TABLE 89.4. Low molecular weight heparin versus unfractionated heparin in the treatment of deep vein thrombosis.

Authors	LMWH			UFH	Score improvement LMWH/UFH	Thrombosis progression LMWH/UFH
	Substance	Daily dose		Mode of application		
Lockner et al.[58]	Fragmin	2 × 240 anti-Xa U/kg SC		INF	−/−	0/+
Albada et al.[2]	Fragmin	15,000 anti-Xa U/24 h IV		INF	−/−	−/−
Bratt et al.[18]	Fragmin	2 × 240 or 120 anti-Xa U/kg SC		INF	−/−	+/++
Collaborative European Multicenter Study [1]	Fraxiparin	2 × 225 anti-Xa U/kg SC		INF	+/−	−/−
Study 1991						
Hull et al.[42]	LMWH	1 × 175 anti-Xa U/kg SC		INF	−/−	+/++
Lopaciuk et al.[59]	Fraxiparin	2 × 225 anti-Xa U/kg SC		2 × SC	−/−	+/++
Prandoni et al.[81]	Fraxiparin	2 × 15,000 anti-Xa U/55−80 kg SC		INF	−/−	+/++
Simonneau et al.[96]	Enoxaparin	2 × 1 mg/kg SC		INF	−/−	+/++
Lindmarker et al.[57]	Fragmin	1 × 200 anti-Xa U/kg SC		INF	−/−	−/−
Koopman et al.[49]	Fraxiparin	2 × 8,200−18,400 anti-Xa U/l SC		INF	−/−	+/++
Levine et al.[55]	Enoxaparin	2 × 1 mg/kg SC		INF	−/−	+/++

LMWH, low molecular wieght heparin; UFH, unfractionated heparin; SC, subcutaneous injection; INF, continuous infusion.

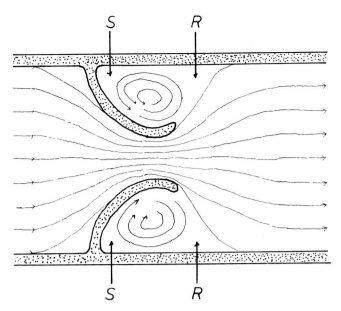

FIGURE 89.1. Flow pattern of blood in front of and behind a venous valve (see Karino and Goldsmith[47]). Whirls develop in the pockets of the valves. The reattachment point, R (situated between the whirl area and the normalized flow), and the site at the base of the valve, S, are still regions where cellular material can deposit and thrombi develop.

- Low level of antithrombin III
- Resistance of factor Va to protein C [activated protein C (APC) resistance]
- Presence of lupus anticoagulant

Table 89.5 indicates the risks for DVT associated with the mentioned coagulation abnormalities. As is evident, APC resistance (Factor V Leiden mutation) is a coagulation abnormality most frequently met in the population.[99] It is a heritable condition linked with a heterogeneous or homogeneous genetic trait.[14,85]

The normal incidence of DVT in women aged 14 to 45 is 1 to 2/10,000 per year. Pathologic APC resistance increases the risk of thrombosis 3-fold to 4-fold. Oral contraceptive use leads to another 4-fold increase of risk, and a combination of APC resistance and contraceptive medication leads to a 35-fold increase.[10]

Lupus anticoagulant is an antibody that attacks the phospholipid component of the prothrombin activator complex. This results in a lengthening of the activated partial thromboplastin time (APTT). Lupus anticoagulant may also attack prostacyclins in the vessel wall, a condition that would inhibit the capacity of prostacyclin to repulse platelets and, consequently, further the forma-

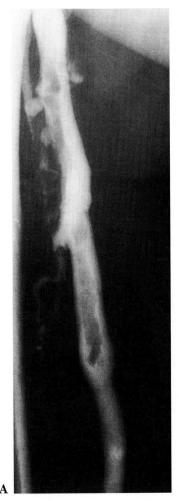
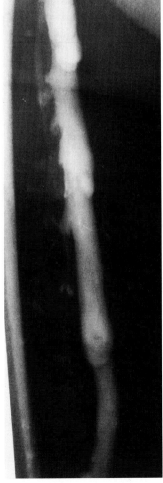

FIGURE 89.2. Demonstration of the development of a femoral thrombosis originating from a venous valve: **A,** Venogram before therapy. A tonguelike thrombus extends in a proximal direction. **B,** Dissolution of the thrombus under fibrinolytic treatment.

A

B

TABLE 89.5. Statistics on protein C, protein S, and antithrombin III deficiency; lupus anticoagulant occurrence; and activated protein C resistance.

Abnormality	Frequency	Authors
Frequency of protein C deficiency in the general population	0.2%–0.4%	Broekmans et al.[19] Miletich et al.[71]
Frequency of protein C deficiency in patients with thrombosis	3%–7%	Beck and Scharrer[11] Heijboer et al.[37]
Frequency of thrombosis with protein C deficiency	50%–60%	Bovill et al.[17] Allart et al.[3]
Frequency of protein S deficiency in the general population	—	—
Frequency of protein S deficiency in patients with thrombosis	2%	Heijboer et al.[37] Scharrer et al.[90]
Frequency of thrombosis with protein S deficiency	—	—
Frequency of antithrombin III deficiency in the general population	0.02%	Tait et al.[100]
Frequency of antithrombin III deficiency in patients with thrombosis	1%	Rosendaal et al.[87]
Frequency of thrombosis with antithrombin III deficiency	50%	Thaler & Lechner[101]
Frequency of lupus anticoagulant in the general population	—	—
Frequency of lupus anticoagulant in patients with thrombosis	—	—
Frequency of thrombosis with lupus anticoagulant	30%–50%	Verstraete & Vermylen[111]
Frequency of activated protein C resistance in the general population	3%–7%	Koster et al.[50] Rosendaal et al.[88] Svensson et al.[99]
Frequency of activated protein C resistance in patience with thrombosis	20%	Rosendaal et al.[88]
Frequency of thrombosis with activated protein C resistance	25%	Svensson et al.[99]

tion of mural thrombi.[54] Stress is another cause of thrombosis *(thrombose par effort)*. However, this mechanism is relevant almost exclusively for the subclavian vein. Patients whose occupations require them to work frequently or continuously with their arms elevated are in danger of compressing the subclavian vein between their clavicula and first rib. This in turn irritates the vessel wall, a process that can produce a thrombotic stenosis that ultimately leads to occlusion of the subclavian vessel[41] (Figure 89.3).

Clinical Investigation

Inspection

In DVT the circumference of the involved limb is greater than normal. The swelling is always one segment lower than the thrombosis site (e.g., a swollen calf is produced by a femoral vein thrombosis and a swollen thigh by an iliac vein thrombosis). In addition, the thrombosed leg presents with a bluish hue as a result of the increase in cutaneous blood flow due to the occlusion of the deep veins. Collateral vein networks are seen in the groins of patients with iliac vein thromboses and over the upper lateral chest in patients with subclavian vein thromboses.

Palpation

On compression of the calf musculature increased stiffness can be felt on the side of the thrombosis (subfascial edema). Pitting of the pretibial skin is also present (epifascial edema). Palpation of the calf musculature elicits circumscribed tenderness, which is typical of acute DVT. Swelling and discoloration are often absent in patients confined to bed, and this tenderness is then often the only sign of acute DVT.

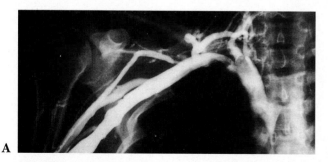

A

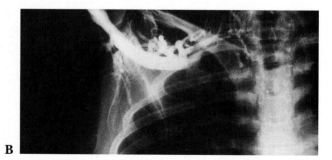

B

FIGURE 89.3. Compression of the subclavian vein by elevation of the arm: **A,** Venography with the arm in a downward position. **B,** Elevation of the arm with compression of the subclavian vein between the first rib and clavicula produces an interruption of blood flow.

Perthes' Test

Perthes' test evaluates the function of the calf muscle pump function. It can only be carried out if a certain degree of varicosis is present. The patient stands erect. A tourniquet is fastened below the knee, and the patient is asked to walk about briskly. After this exercise the varicose veins are inspected. Collapse of the veins indicates normal muscle pump function. Conversely, an absence of drainage implies blockage of the deep veins or insufficiency of a great number of perforating veins (Figure 89.4).

Linton's Test

While the patient is in an upright position, a tourniquet is fastened below the knee. The patient then lies down and raises the affected leg. Drainage of the foot veins indicates free passage, and failure of drainage indicates occlusion of the deep veins.

Phlebodynamometry

A plastic cannula is introduced into the dorsal pedis vein. Via a Y junction two catheters are connected to a pressure-measuring device and to an infusion machine (Figure 89.5). The latter guarantees proper flushing of the cannula with 1 mL saline solution per minute. With the patient standing erect the dorsalis pedis vein pressure is about 90 mm Hg. The patient is then asked to perform heel-raising exercises at a rate of one rise per second. Under normal conditions the exercise leads to a pressure drop of 50 to 60 mm Hg (Figure 89.6). In patients with deep vein occlusions or multiple incompetent perforating veins the pressure drop is less than 30 mm Hg or can even rise above the pressure at rest (Figure 89.7).

Plethysmography

Plethysmography is carried out with the patient lying on the examination table. A cuff is placed around the thigh, and a circumference-measuring device (e.g., cuff or strain gauge) is fixed around the calf. Subsequently, the leg is raised by 25 to 30 degrees and the cuff around the thigh inflated to a pressure at which the arterial blood can enter the limb but venous backflow is prevented. After a predefined period the cuff is deflated. The resultant drainage per units of time is proportional to the

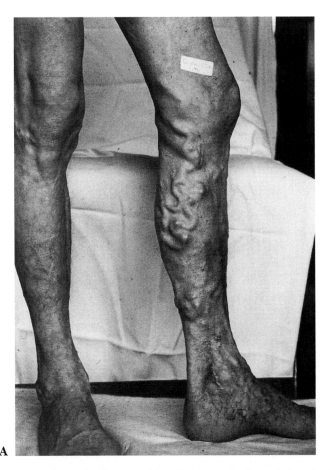

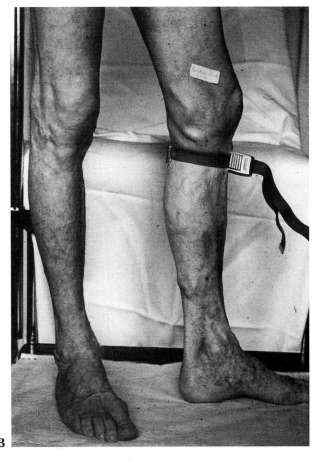

A   **B**

FIGURE 89.4. Perthes' test: **A,** After fixing a tourniquet below the knee the patient walks. **B,** During this activity the varicose veins drain and disappear. This indicates free passage through the deep vein system and the sufficiency of perforating veins.

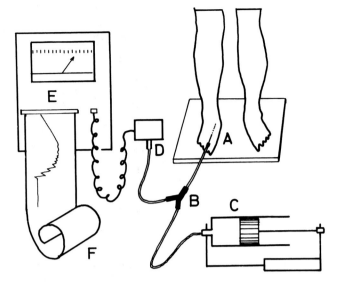

FIGURE 89.5. Schematic representation of the phlebodynamic investigation method: A cannula is fixed in the dorsal pedis vein (**A**). Three catheters are joined by a Y junction (**B**). One goes to the cannula, one to an infusion machine (**C**), and one to a pressure-measuring device (**D**) with recording facilities (**E,F**).

speed of decrease in calf circumference. In patients with DVT this return flow is significantly slower than under normal conditions. Plethysmography is a reliable means of detecting iliac and femoral vein occlusion but yields poorer results in calf vein thrombosis. In addition, there is always a danger of mobilizing thrombotic material during the measurement procedure.

Continuous Wave Doppler Sonography

A continuous wave transducer is placed in the groin over the femoral vein. The patient is asked to inhale deeply. Under normal circumstances lowering of the diaphragm increases the intraabdominal pressure and thus immediately stops flow from the leg into the iliac vein. When the patient exhales the blood resumes its flow into the iliac vein (spontaneous sound, or S sound) (Figures 89.8 and 89.9). Therefore, if an iliac thrombosis is present, either no flow or a continuous flow unaffected by breathing is recorded (the venous pressure distal to the iliac occlusion is higher than the intraabdominal pressure) (Figure 89.10). Continuous wave Doppler sonography can also be performed with the continuous wave transducer posi-

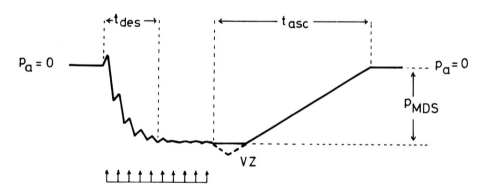

FIGURE 89.6. Normal phlebodynamic recording. P_a, pressure at rest; t_{des}, period up to maximal pressure reduction; VZ, additional pressure drop after exercise; t_{asc}, period of pressure restitution; P_{MDS}, maximal pressure drop by heel-raising exercise.

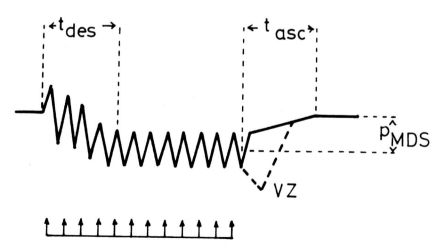

FIGURE 89.7. Pathologic phlebodynamic recording. Maximal pressure drop by heel-raising exercise (P_{MDS}) is significantly reduced, which indicates deep vein thrombosis or multiple insufficiency of the perforating veins. t_{des}, period up to maximal pressure reduction; t_{asc}, period of pressure restitution; VZ, additional pressure drop after exercise.

FIGURE 89.8. Continuous wave Doppler sonography of the iliac veins. The transducer is positioned in the groin. **A,** Flow signal of a healthy person. With inhaling the flow into the pelvic veins decelerates or stops (lowering of the diaphragm produces an abdominal pressure higher than the venous pressure of the leg). **B,** After taking a deep breath the flow signal disappears until the patient exhales again and the flow returns to its normal pattern (S sound). **C,** In a patient with iliac thrombosis a deep breath does not influence the flow pattern (lowering of the diaphragm produces an abdominal pressure that is still lower than the venous pressure of the leg with iliac thrombosis). **D,** Under normal conditions light hand pressure on the abdomen stops the venous flow. **E,** In a patient with iliac thrombosis even heavy pressure on the abdomen does not influence the flow pattern.

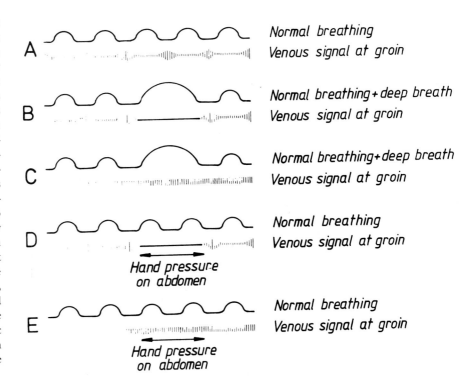

tioned in the popliteal fossa. Venous blood flow affected by breathing is indicative of free popliteal and/or femoral veins, whereas continuous flow independent of breathing points to occlusion of the popliteal and/or femoral veins.

In healthy individuals compression of the calf muscles produces an increase of flow that can be recorded in the groin by continuous wave Doppler sonography (aug-mented sound, or A sound). Usually, A sounds cannot be elicited in a leg with DVT.

Color-Coded Duplex Sonography

A two-dimensional picture is produced by placing the duplex transducer on the venous segment of interest. The color component is adjusted so that the arterial flow

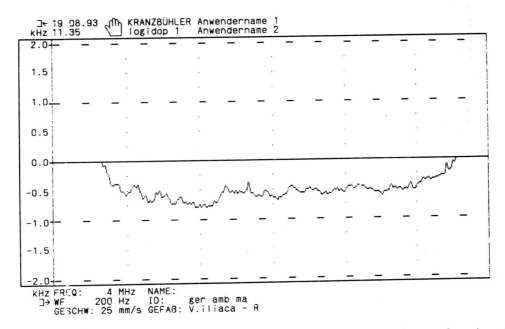

FIGURE 89.9. Original tracing of continuous wave Doppler sonography in a healthy patient. The transducer is positioned in the groin. After taking a deep breath the patient exhales forcefully, which results in flow acceleration for several seconds.

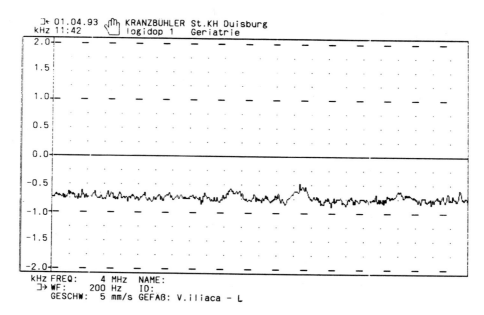

01.04.93   KRANZBUHLER St.KH Duisburg
kHz 11:42   logidop 1   Geriatrie

FIGURE 89.10. Original tracing of continuous wave Doppler sonography in a patient with iliac thrombosis. The transducer is positioned in the groin. After taking a deep breath the pa-tient exhales forcefully, but the flow into the pelvic veins remains unchanged.

is marked in red and yellow (red is normal, and yellow indicates accelerated flow) and the venous flow in blue and green (blue is normal, and green indicates accelerated flow). The speed of flow can thus be measured, possible narrowings assessed, and thrombotic depositions detected (Figure 89.11). In addition, a Doppler window can be positioned in the colored flow signal to allow spectrographic registration of flow characteristics.

Best results are achieved in the femoral and popliteal areas. The iliac vein is difficult to evaluate because of the depth at which the vessel is situated. Here, as in the continuous wave Doppler sonography investigation, the breathing-related interruption of blood flow in the groin indicates free passage into the iliac veins. Another weakness of the duplex method is its low predictability for calf vein occlusions.

Even without color, the two-dimensional image is a reliable tool for assessing whether a vessel segment is patent or occluded. The transducer must be pressed firmly onto the area of skin over the vein of interest. If the vein is not obstructed, its grayish structure will disappear (a vein with relatively low pressure becomes compressed). If, however, a thrombotic occlusion is present, compression will not lead to obliteration and the venous structure remains unchanged.

Venography

Venography is mandatory before and after any attempt at revascularization (whether by lysis or by surgery). The patient stands in the x-ray apparatus tilted backward at 45 degrees. After a tourniquet has been placed around the ankle the dorsal foot vein is punctured and a cannula is inserted. The contrast medium is injected, and x-ray films are taken in a distal to proximal progression. Femoral veins must never be punctured in the groin. Because of possible bleeding complications (e.g., inadvertent arterial puncture or puncture of the posterior wall of the vein) fibrinolytic treatment is then contraindicated.

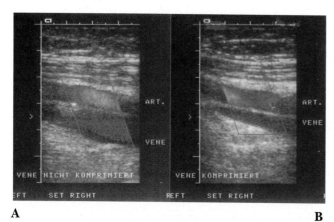

A   **B**

FIGURE 89.11. Color-coded duplex sonography in a healthy person (artery is red, and vein is blue): **A,** The transducer is not applying pressure. **B,** Pressure to the skin results in obliteration of the venous structure.

Laboratory Investigation

Risk Evaluation

Protein C, protein S, antithrombin III, lupus anticoagulant, and the action of APC are frequently altered in patients with DVT (Table 89.5). Because proteins C and S are vitamin K dependent they cannot be measured in patients who take coumarin; and because antithrombin III complexes with heparin, its level cannot be determined properly in patients who receive heparin medication.

Control of Heparin Infusion

The tests that best measure the effects of heparin on coagulation are the activated thromboplastin time (APTT) and the plasma thrombin time (TT). Conversely, UFH and LMWH administered subcutaneously are not monitored on a routine basis.

Control of Coumarin Treatment

Coumarin agents are monitored by using the prothrombin time, prothrombin time ratio, Quick's value, or international normalized ratio (INR).

Control of Fibrinolytic Therapy

Monitoring of streptokinase (SK) and urokinase (UK) treatment (ultrahigh or conventional dosage) is not recommended because in terms of bleeding complications and clinical efficacy the optimum infusion rates or plasma concentrations are unknown. Conversely, recombinant tissue plasminogen activator (rtPA) must be closely monitored because of the close relationship between dosage and bleeding complication. A relatively high rate of bleeding was reported with rtPA doses of 0.8 to 1.76 mg/kg per day, whereas an influx of 0.5 mg/kg per day was relatively safe.[116]

Therapeutic Measures

Heparin Infusion

The loading dose of heparin is 5000 IU, and the initial maintenance dose is 1200 IU/h. Thereafter, the heparin infusion influx must be adjusted on the basis of APTT or plasma thrombin time. The therapeutic target is a 2 to 2.5 times prolongation of normal.

Subcutaneously Administered Heparin

Recommended doses for UFH are injections of 5000 or 7500 IU subcutaneously in 8- or 12-hour intervals. The standardization of LMWH is still under discussion. Anti-factor Xa units and milligrams are in current use. Despite beneficial results with LMWH in acute DVT (Table 89.4), it is not yet licensed for the treatment of acute DVT in all countries. Subcutaneous injections every 12 or 24 hours are recommended (doses adjusted to body weight).

Coumarin Agents

Intracapillary thrombosis (coumarin necrosis) is a serious side effect in the initial stages of coumarin treatment. An accelerated fall of the coagulation inhibiting protein C level with procoagulant factors still at normal concentrations can produce this complication.[19,112] Coumarin should therefore always be administered along with heparin (subcutaneous or infusion). The therapeutic target of coumarin medication is Quick's value 25% to 38% (INR 2.0–3.0).[40]

Fibrinolytic Treatment

Conventional SK Infusion

Conventional SK infusion is systemic SK infusion via the brachial vein. The loading dose is 250,000 IU SK over 20 minutes. Forty percent of patients experience initial reactions during the first 10 minutes of infusion that consist of (1) facial flush, (2) dyspnea, (3) back pain, and (4) a fall in blood pressure. In most cases only one or two of these reactions occur. Early reactions are not anaphylactic in nature but the result of kinins released into the circulation under the influence of plasmin. They occur within the first 10 minutes of SK infusion, last for about 5 minutes, and do not return during the following days of infusion. Before therapy, the patients are informed of these possible and harmless side effects and asked to tell the doctor (who is always in attendance while the loading dose is infused) if they experience any of these reactions. If reactions occur, the infusion is stopped. Only when the symptoms have subsided is the infusion resumed. As mentioned previously, early reactions are produced by kinins rather than antigenic mechanisms. Cortisone medication is therefore not indicated. Early reactions are never a reason for prematurely ending SK therapy.

After the loading dose a maintenance infusion of 100,000 IU SK/h follows. From day 2 onward, heparin is added and coagulation monitored by APTT or plasma thrombin time. A 3-day infusion is usually necessary to remove all thrombotic material. SK cannot be administered for longer than 5 days. After that time antistreptokinase production sets in and makes further treatment futile.

As explained, SK infusion alone requires no laboratory control; only heparin is monitored by APTT. However, hemoglobin tests every 12 hours are recommended to detect occult bleeding.

Ultrahigh SK Short-Term Treatment

Ultrahigh SK (UHSK) short-term treatment is a systemic treatment via the brachial vein.[64] The loading dose is 250,000 IU SK over 20 minutes, and the maintenance dose is 9 million IU SK over 9 hours (1.5 million SK/h) (Figure 89.12). As in conventional SK therapy, early reactions are to be expected and are dealt with according to the directions provided earlier. In most cases two UHSK series are given on 2 subsequent days, after which the first follow-up venography is carried out. No heparin is necessary after the first series, but from the second series on heparin infusions are mandatory. Only heparin infusion is monitored by APTT; other coagulation tests are not needed. The importance of regular hemoglobin monitoring has already been mentioned.

Lysis Under the Protection of a Temporary Caval Filter

In patients who undergo fibrinolytic therapy, iliac thrombosis can be the source of fatal pulmonary embolism.[63] To prevent this complication, a temporary caval filter has proven effective (Figure 89.13). To date, most experiences are reported with the Anthéor filter.[62,97,118] One advantage of this type of filter is the brachial vein introduction, which allows effective control of possible bleeding from the puncture wound. The Anthéor filter contains two components: the port catheter and the filter catheter, the latter of which carries an expansible metal filter on one end. After positioning the port catheter in the lumen of the inferior vena cava, the branches of the filter are released into the vessel's lumen. Fibrinolytic treatment starts on the day of filter implantation, and the filter is removed the following day after cessation of treatment (Figure 89.13). Before removal, a contrast medium injection via the axial channel of the filter catheter must confirm that the filter is free of thrombotic material. If thrombotic material is caught in the filter, two options are available: (1) fibrinolytic treatment is continued to dissolve the embolus or (2) a minicatheter is introduced into the axial channel of the filter catheter. The tip of this catheter is guided directly into the embolus. The embolus is then lysed locally with UK (300,000 IU/h, infusion lasts up to 3 hours if necessary).

Conventional UK Treatment

The loading dose for conventional UK treatment is 600,000 IU over 30 minutes. No early reactions are anticipated during this period. The maintenance dose is 100,000 IU/h. Because the effects on coagulation are minimal, concomitant heparin infusion monitored on the basis of APTT is recommended. UK is a relatively weak fibrinolytic agent. Therefore, 1 to 2 weeks of continuous infusion are needed to fully dissolve leg vein thrombosis.

Ultrahigh UK Short-Term Treatment

Ultrahigh UK (UHUK) short-term treatment consists of a 6-hour infusion of 9 million IU UK.[52,66] No loading dose is given, and no early reactions are anticipated. One or more series of UHUK can be given on consecutive days. Heparin infusions are interposed between two UHUK series and after the last one.

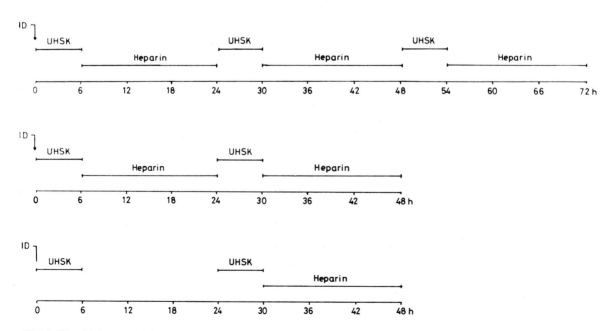

FIGURE 89.12. Ultrahigh streptokinase (UHSK) dosage scheme. Several series can be given on subsequent days. Heparin infusion is not necessary after the first UHSK series. Here fibrinogen degradation products provide for adequate anticoagulation.

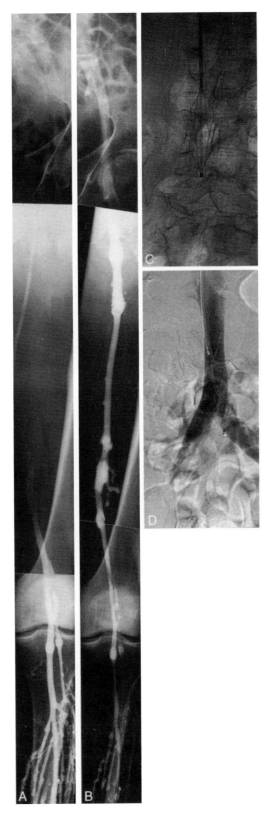

FIGURE 89.13. Removal of iliofemoral thrombosis with two series of ultrahigh streptokinase treatments under the protection of a temporary caval filter. **A,** Situation before lysis. **B,** Clearance of the vein. **C,** Caval filter positioned. **D,** Visualization of the inner filter space with contrast medium for detection of possible clots caught in the filter.

Systemic rtPA Infusion

Systemic rtPA infusion is still in an experimental phase. Only five trials have been published so far (see Table 89.6).

Locoregional Treatment

Locoregional treatment consists of SK, UK, or rtPA infusions lasting 4 to 5 hours. They are given on 1 or more days (one infusion per day) into the dorsal pedis vein of the thrombosed leg. During infusion, a tourniquet is applied around the ankle and the leg is bandaged up to the thigh (see Table 89.7).

Lysis Block Treatment

Lysis block treatment is a new form of fibrinolytic therapy for distal femoral, popliteal, and calf vein thromboses.[39,67] Strictly local lysis is achieved by placing a cuff around the thigh, inflating the cuff to a pressure of 500 mm Hg (Bier's blockade), and giving 50 mL Mepivacain 1%, 5000 IU heparin, and 40 mg rtPA as an intravenous injection into the dorsal pedis vein (Figure 89.14). Occlusion lasts for 45 minutes. During the blockade APTT and rtPA remain nearly unchanged in the systemic circulation. Only after removal of the cuff is the APTT prolonged (due to the influx of heparin) and the rtPA concentration increased. Because of the short half-life of rtPA, its concentration falls to zero within about 15 minutes after ending the blockade. This short half-life is important for patients with bleeding tendencies for whom lytic treatment might normally be contraindicated. Lysis block treatment necessitates that a patient stay only a few days in hospital, and it has also been performed on an outpatient basis.

Compression Therapy

During fibrinolytic therapy and 1 week thereafter the affected leg is bandaged from the foot up to the groin. The calf is compressed with elastic bandages (Figure 89.15) or Unna's paste dressing (Figure 89.16). An adhesive bandage compresses the thigh. Gradual pressure reduction from distal to proximal is essential in bandaging technique for both the reduction of edema and the comfort of the patient. In this context it is important that the number of bandage layers wrapped around the leg on the one hand and the pressure exerted with one layer alone on the other are interchangeable (several layers on top of one another need lesser pressure than one layer alone).[36]

If complete thrombus removal is achieved, the patient wears a thigh-high elastic stocking for another month. After this period no further compression is necessary. When no lysis was possible, however, the patient wears a thigh-high elastic stocking for 3 months. Subsequently,

TABLE 89.6. Systemic recombinant tissue-type plasminogen activator treatment for deep vein thrombosis.

Authors	Number of patients	Doses and duration of therapy		Result
Verhaeghe et al.[110]	19	First day	100 mg/8 h	Decrease of Marder score but no significant difference with heparin
		Second day	50 mg/8 h	
	6	First day	50 mg/8 h	
		Second day	50 mg/8 h	
Goldhaber et al.[33]	53	0.05 mg/kg/per h	24 h	Complete or >50% lysis in 28%–29% of patients
Marder et al.[60]	18	0.24 mg/kg/2 h	2 h	Reduction of thrombus of 3%, 13%, and 50%
		0.06 mg/kg/per h	4, 22, or 34 h	
Turpie et al.[108]	12	0.5 mg/kg/per 4 h	4 h	40% reduction of thrombus
	28	0.5 mg/kg/per 8 h	8 h	In 20% lysis more than 50%
Zimmermann et al.[116]	22	0.53–1.78 mg/kg/per d	1–10 d	Substantial recanalization in 86%
Bounameaux et al.[16]	32	0.25 mg/kg/per d	3–7 d	No substantial change in the venogram
		0.50 mg/kg/per d	3–7 d	

TABLE 89.7. Locoregional treatment of deep vein thrombosis.

Method	Authors	Regimen	Result
Peripheral local lysis	Meyer[70]	Infusion of 100,000 IU SK/20 min or 300,000 IU UK/20 min into the dorsal pedis vein with tourniquet around the ankle One series per day up to 5 SK series or 14 UK series	Complete lysis in 6/23 = 26.1%
Low-dose fibrinolytic therapy	Hagg[35]	Infusion of 20 mg rtPA or 250,000 IU UK/4 h into the dorsal pedis vein One series per day On the average 4 series	With rtPA compete lysis in 53% ($n = 32$) With UK complete lysis in 60% ($n = 10$)
Locoregional ultra-high fibrinolysis	Mumme et al.[74]	Isolated perfusion of a leg vein with 3 million IU SK under hyperthermic condition	Complete clearance in 2/5 = 40%
Local fibrinolysis	Unkel and Hajjar[109]	Infusion of 20 mg rtPA/8 h into the dorsalis pedis vein with a tourniquet around the ankle One series per day up to 3 series	Very good results in 93% ($n = 42$)
Local fibrinolytic therapy	Timmermann et al.[104]	Infusion of 250,000 IU UK/4 h or 20 mg rtPA/4 h with subsequent infusion of 25,000 IU heparin/24 h in a dorsal pedis vein with the leg bandaged One series per day Total of 3–5 series	50% complete lysis with UK 65.4% complete lysis with rtPA ($n = 62$)
Locoregional thrombolysis	Althoff and Rudofsky[4]	4-h infusion of 20 mg rtPA into the dorsalis pedis vein with the leg bandaged Heparin runs parallel (20,000 IU per day) One series per day Total of 6–8 series	Complete lysis 31%–34% Partial lysis 47%–50% No lysis 17%–21% ($n = 162$)

SK, streptokinase; UK, urokinase; rtPA, recominant tissue-type plasminogen activator.

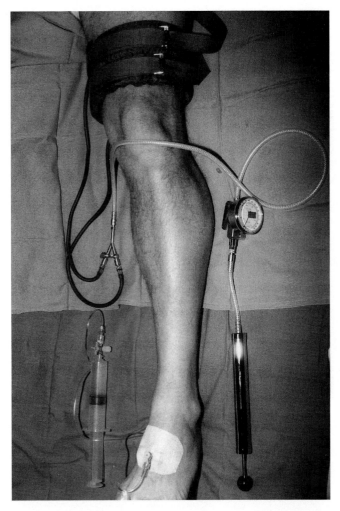

FIGURE 89.14. Lysis block treatment. The leg with thrombosis is prepared for treatment. The cuff around the thigh has been inflated to 500 mm Hg. Heparin, an anesthetic agent, and a fibrinolytic drug have been injected into the dorsal pedis vein.

the long stocking is exchanged for a knee-length elastic sock that must be worn during the day for an indefinite period of time.

Result of Treatment

Heparin Treatment

In the literal sense heparin is not a therapy for DVT. In a small percentage of patients veins blocked by thrombosis open up spontaneously, and heparin may help to further this process (Table 89.3). Otherwise heparin works in a solely prophylactic fashion and consequently differs fundamentally from fibrinolytic treatment.

Heparin infusion inhibits thrombosis progression and reduces the risk of pulmonary embolism. Bauer[9] was one of the first to show that heparin significantly lowers the

rate of fatal pulmonary embolism (in his data from 47% to 3%). IV heparin is now a generally acknowledged medication for DVT.

Presently, patients with femoropopliteal vein thrombosis are prescribed either bed rest plus heparin infusion or are permitted to stay ambulatory under an overlapping regimen of subcutaneous heparin and oral anticoagulation. During this regimen the leg is firmly bandaged. Conversely, patients with iliac vein thrombosis remain always in bed and undergo 1-week heparin infusion with subsequent coumarin treatment. One working group[78] advocates an ambulatory regimen for patients with fresh iliac vein thrombosis. However, this approach has not yet been generally accepted.

In recent years several studies have been published comparing the results of subcutaneously administered LMWH with infusions of UFH (Table 89.4). Results show that in terms of thrombosis progression subcutaneously administered LMWH was more efficient than UFH infusions. The reason for this surprising outcome is still unclear, but a longer period of bed rest for patients who receive infusions may play a role (i.e., because of thrombosis progression due to immobility).

Although heparin treatment lowers the rate of pulmonary embolism considerably, fatal embolism still occurs (Table 89.1). These embolic events depend on the thrombosis location: iliac vein thrombosis is associated with a higher incidence of embolism than femoral vein thrombosis, and femoral vein thrombosis is associated with a higher rate of embolic events than popliteal vein thrombosis.[61]

Coumarin Treatment

Only a few studies have investigated the progression of DVT with and without oral anticoagulant therapy. One of these is a prospective study on patients in whom the rate of newly formed thrombosis (events per 1000 patient months) was registered.[20] A substantial difference in thromboembolism was recorded in patients who either were or were not treated with anticoagulant agents. This difference was greatest from the first to the ninth week of observation. Later on the difference was less dramatic.

In another randomized study[53] two groups of patients with calf vein thrombosis were investigated. One group of patients received warfarin, and the other group received placebo. During the first 3 observation months 29% of patients in the placebo group revealed thrombosis progression compared with none in the warfarin group ($P < 0.01$). After 1 year 4% of patients in the warfarin group had suffered a recurrence compared with 32% in the placebo group ($P < 0.02$).

Early reports[20,95] described more thromboembolic events in patients with Quick's values over 24% than un-

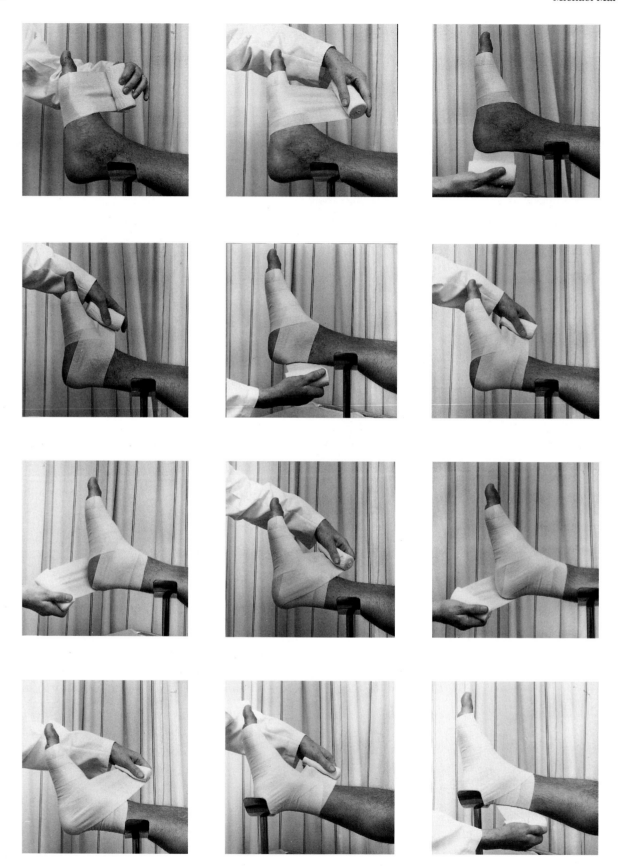

FIGURE 89.15. Bandaging a leg. For calf compression an elastic bandage and for thigh compression adhesive bandages (that are cut off after each bandage tour) are used.

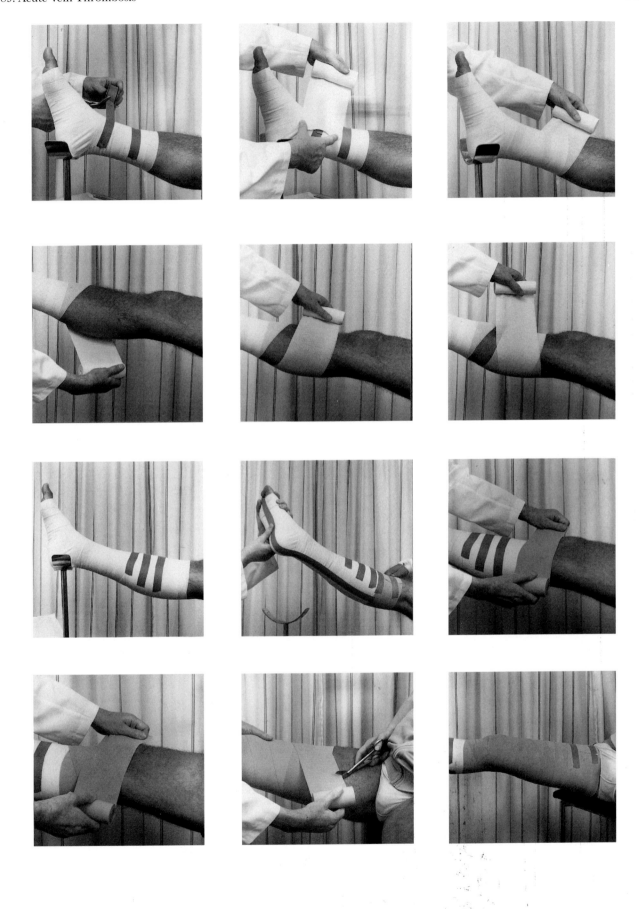

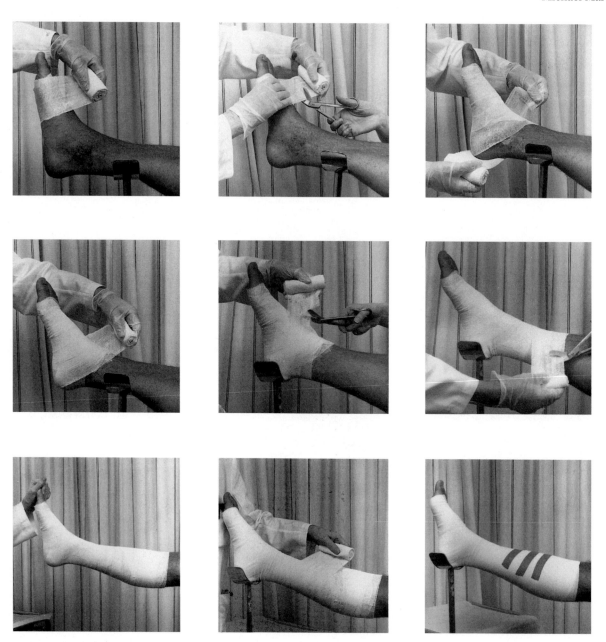

FIGURE 89.16. Applying an Unna's paste dressing. After every turn the paste bandage is cut off.

der 24%. To date, Quick's values of between 25% and 38% (INR 2.0–3.0) are regarded as sufficient for the prevention of thrombosis recurrence.[40,80]

Fibrinolytic Therapy

Conventional SK Regimen

The following data are derived from a meta-analysis of 18 trials with 850 patients (Table 89.8). Treatment consisted of SK infusions of 100,000 IU/h over 2 to 6 days. Complete clearance was seen in 42.1% ± 13.0% and partial clearance in 31.3% ± 17.8% of vessels previously occluded by thrombosis (Figure 89.17).

Ultrahigh SK Short-Term Regimen

The following data are derived from a meta-analysis of 10 trials involving 490 patients (Table 89.9). The treatment regimen consisted of infusions of 1.5 million IU SK per hour over a period of 6 hours. Up to five infusions were given. From the first or second series on, an intermittent heparin infusion was administered between the UHSK series. Complete clearance was seen in 49.6% ± 12.6%

TABLE 89.8. Fibrinolytic treatment of deep vein thrombosis: studies with a conventional streptokinase regimen.

Authors	Number of patients	Thrombosis site				Thrombosis age (d)	Group	Heparin control	Result	fPE	CB
		IL	FEM	C	SC						
Kakkar et al.[46]	10	8	1	2	—	0.5–3	Yes	Complete lysis	67%	0	0
								Partial lysis	11%		
Robertson et al.[86]	9	—	9	—	—	< 8	Yes	Complete lysis	56%	0	0
								Partial lysis	11%		
Olow et al.[76]	13	Leg veins				< 4	No	Complete lysis	55%	0	0
								Partial lysis	18%		
Mavor et al.[69]	39	39	—	—	—	1–10	No	Complete lysis	25%	0	0
								Partial lysis	60%		
Tsapogas et al.[107]	19	Leg veins				< 5	Yes	Complete lysis	53%	0	0
								Partial lysis			
Widmer et al.[115]	86	35	47	4	—	Mean 7,9	Yes	Substantial lysis	42%	2	1
								Partial lysis	25%		
Giercksky et al.[32]	11	3		8	—	< 28	No	Significant lysis	70%	0	0
Johansson et al.[43]	19	11	8	—	—	0–16	No	Complete lysis	42%	0	0
Seaman et al.[94]	37	Leg veins				< 14	Yes	Complete lysis	43%	0	1
								Partial lysis	19%		
Arnesen et al.[6]	21	Leg veins				< 5	Yes	Significant lysis	71%	0	0
Elliot et al.[27]	23	15	9	—	2	< 8	Yes	Complete lysis	39%	0	0
								Partial lysis	52%		
Rahmer et al.[83]	51	33	16	2	—	1–14	No	Complete lysis	43%	1	1
								Partial lysis	18%		
Watz and Savidge[113]	18	4	14	—	—	0–7	Yes	Complete lysis	44%	0	0
								Partial lysis	22%		
Theiss et al.[103]	23	Leg and subclavian veins				< 7	No	Complete lysis	39%	0	0
								Partial lysis	52%		
Scharrer and Hetzel[91]	198	100	72	—	26	< 21	No	Complete lysis		7	4
								Iliac	30%		
								Femoral	36%		
								Subclavian	31%		
Trübestein et al.[105]	126	Leg veins				1–6	No	Complete lysis	69%	0	2
								Partial lysis	25%		
						7–21		Complete lysis	22%		
								Partial lysis	52%		
Schulman et al.[93]	39	11	28	—	—	< 7	No	Complete lysis	33%	0	0
Ott et al.[77]	108	—	84	—	21	< 4	No	Complete lysis	31%	3	0
								Partial lysis	25%		

IL, iliac; FEM, femoropopliteal; C, calf; SC, subclavian; fPE, fatal pulmonary embolism; CB, cerebral bleeding.

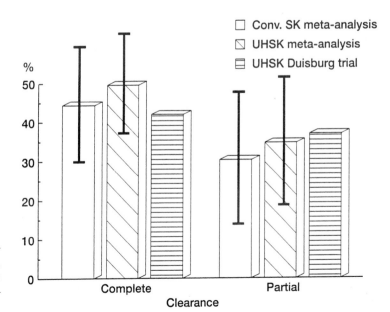

FIGURE 89.17. Meta-analysis of the results of conservative streptokinase (SK) treatment (100,000 IU/h), meta-analysis of the results of ultrahigh streptokinase (UHSK) treatment (1.5 million IU/h), and the results of the Duisburg UHSK trial.

TABLE 89.9. Fibrinolytic treatment of deep vein thrombosis: studies with short-term ultrahigh streptokinase treatment.

Authors	Number of patients	Thrombosis site				Thrombosis age (d)	Result	fPE	CB
		IL	FEM	C	SC				
Anders et al.[5]	11	8	3	—	—	2–10	Complete lysis 36% Partial lysis 46%	0	0
Koch[48]	15	2	5	8	—	—	Complete lysis 45% Partial lysis 67%	0	0
Theiss et al.[102]	21	11	9	—	2	2–14	Complete lysis 62% Partial lysis 29%	1	0
Krzywanek[52]	11	Leg veins				1–21	Complete lysis 36% Partial lysis 46%	0	0
Straub et al.[98]	20	Leg veins				1–21	Success 70%	0	0
Podlaha and Schlichting[79]	11	1	9	1	—	2–35	Complete lysis 64% Partial lysis 9%	0	0
Fahn et al.[29]	56	18	37		1	—	Complete lysis 43% Partial lysis 40%	1	1
Krüger[51]	37	5	28	3	1	3–18	Complete lysis 70% Partial lysis 22%	0	0
Trübestein et al.[106]	89	Leg veins				1–6	Complete lysis 48% Partial lysis 16 %	0	0
Martin and Fiebach[65]	219	45	149	2	23	8.74 ± 9.27	Complete lysis 42% Partial lysis 37%	4	2

IL, iliac; FEM, femoropopliteal; C, calf; SC, subclavian; fPE, fatal pulmonary embolism; CB, cerebral bleeding.

TABLE 89.10. Fibrinolytic treatment of deep vein thrombosis: studies with conventional urokinase treatment.

Authors	Number of patients	Thrombosis site				Thrombosis age	Therapeutic regime	Result	fPE	CB
		IL	FEM	C	SC					
Greul and Tilsner[34]	34	Deep veins of the leg				2–12 wk 8–14 d	37,500 IU/h	Complete lysis 32% Partial lysis 24%	0	0
Theiss et al.[103]	30	Deep veins of the leg				1 d–6 wk	21 patients pretreated with streptokinase 40,000 IU/h 4–23 d	Complete lysis 35% Partial lysis 35%	0	0
Trübestein et al.[105]	99	Deep veins of the leg				1–6 d 6–12 d 1–3 wk	80,000 IU/h	Complete lysis 42% Partial lysis 25% Complete lysis 15% Partial lysis 56%	1	0
Zimmermann et al.[117]	17	—	—	—	17	< 10 d <2 wk > 10 d	70,000–140,000 IU/h	Complete lysis 71% Partial lysis 11% Complete lysis 0%	0	0
D'Angelo and Manucci[23]	41	Deep veins of the leg				4–15 d 2 d 3 d 7 d 4 d	105,000 IU/h 175,000 IU/h 175,000 IU/h 280,000 IU/h	Substantial lysis 20% Substantial lysis 36% Substantial lysis 20% Substantial lysis 40%	0	0
Martin et al.[67]	52	52	—	—	—	2–14 d < 1 wk	100,000 IU/h	Iliac clearance 60% Iliac clearance 72%	1	1

IL, iliac; FEM, femoral; C, calf; SC, subclavian; fPE, fatal pulmonary embolism; CB, cerebral bleeding.

and partial clearance in 34.7% ± 17.8% of vessels previously occluded by thrombosis (Figure 89.17).

Data from the Duisburg experiences are derived from 219 patients. In the unselected cohort complete clearance was seen in 42% of patients and partial clearance in 37.0% (Figure 89.17). The clearance rate for femoropopliteal vein thrombosis (Figure 89.18) was 70.5%. Clearance rates were related to thrombosis age. Thus, 1- to 3-day-old occlusions were totally removed in 50.0%, 4- to 7-day-old occlusions in 48.4%, 8- to 10-day-old occlusions in 35.7%, 11- to 14-day-old occlusions in 34.1%, and over 14-day-old occlusions in 14.3%. Iliac vein occlusions were invariably combined with femoral occlusions. Iliac veins were cleared in 71.1% with or without removal of thrombi in the femoral segment and in 24.4% in which iliac as well as femoral veins became patent. As in the femoropopliteal group, clearance rates of iliac veins were related to thrombosis age. Thus 1- to 7-day-old iliac thromboses were removed in 78.1%, 8- to 14-day-old occlusions in 62.5%, and over 14-day-old occlusions in 50.0%.

Conventional UK Regimen

The results of UK infusion in six trials with a total of 273 patients are listed in Table 89.10. The average rate of complete thrombus removal was 32.5% ± 24.3% and of partial removal 35.0% ± 19.1%.

Ultrahigh UK Short-Term Lysis

Because only limited studies have been undertaken the value of UHUK is difficult to define. Krzywanek[52] reported on 14 thromboses. None could be removed by UHSK alone, but six (42.9%) were removed by subsequent UHUK treatment. In addition, 12 out of 55 (21.8%) thromboses were directly dissolved by UHUK. In another study[68] UHUK was successful in treating one of four venous occlusions.

Systemic rtPA Treatment

Six studies have been published on the results of systemic rtPA infusion (Table 89.6). From the information given, the rate of partial lysis was low and complete revascularization was seldom achieved. This observation corresponds with the results of the Phlebothrombosis–Fibrinolysis (PHLEFI) Study,[63] in which the therapeutic benefit of systemic rtPA treatment was last in comparison with other fibrinolytic regimes.

Locoregional Treatment

In recent years locoregional treatment has gained some attention. The results of six studies carried out with this method are summarized in Table 89.7.

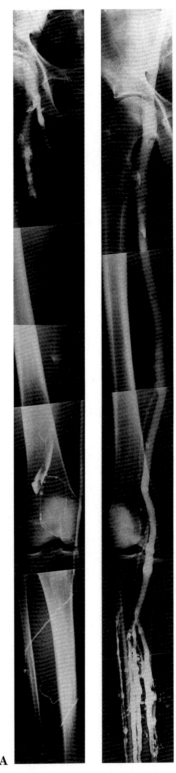

A   **B**

FIGURE 89.18. Removal of femoral and calf vein thromboses with two series of ultrahigh streptokinase (UHSK). **A,** Venography before lysis. **B,** Complete clearance 18 hours after conclusion of UHSK therapy.

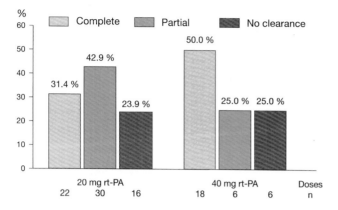

FIGURE 89.19. Result of lysis block treatment according to dosage in patients with distal femoral, popliteal, and/or calf vein thromboses.

Lysis Block Treatment

On the average 1.92 ± 0.681 series of lysis block treatment were administered. The clearance rate of distal femoral, popliteal, and calf vein thromboses depended on the rtPA doses administered. Thus, with 20 mg rtPA complete thrombosis removal was achieved in 31.4% and with 40 mg rtPA in 50.0% of patients. Partial lysis occurred in 42.9% of those receiving 20 mg rtPA and 43.8% receiving 40 mg rtPA (Figures 89.19 and 89.20).

Complications and Side Effects

Heparin Treatment

Heparin treatment lowers, but does not prevent, the occurrence of fatal pulmonary embolism. As is evident from Table 89.1, considerable discrepancies exist in the reported incidences of pulmonary embolism in patients treated with heparin.

The Phlebothrombosis–Conservative Treatment (PHLECO) Study[61] obtained data on the risk of fatal pulmonary embolism in 1674 inpatients. UFH (continuous infusion and/or subcutaneous injection) was used for treatment. The incidence of fatal pulmonary embolism was 2.33%, and iliac vein thrombosis was the principal cause of mortality (Figure 89.21). Fatal pulmonary embolism was positively correlated with female sex and high patient age.

The PHLECO Study showed only a 0.18% incidence of major bleeding in patients administered heparin. This finding corresponds with the average result of six studies compiled by Levine and Hirsh[55] with a bleeding rate of 0.46%.

Oral Anticoagulant Agents

Oral anticoagulant agents can induce life-threatening bleeding. Coon and Willis[21] reported on 263 (6.8%) major bleeds and 4 bleeding-related deaths (0.1%) in 3862 courses of anticoagulant treatment. In 11 studies with a total of 1873 patients, the average incidence of major bleeding in terms of 100 patient years was 4.18 ± 6.35, and the average mortality rate was 1.61 ± 2.62.[56]

The frequency of bleeding increases with the intensity of treatment. Accordingly, a prothrombin activity of >30% (INR <2.5) was accompanied by 0.25 major episodes per 1000 days, an activity of 10% to 29% (INR 2.5–7.0) with 1.9 episodes, and an activity of <10% (INR >7.0) with 31 episodes.[21]

Fibrinolytic Treatment

Cerebral Bleeding

Intracranial hemorrhage is one of the most dangerous complications of fibrinolytic therapy. The PHLEFI Study[63] investigated the incidence of cerebral bleeding in 1498 patients who had received various forms of fibri-

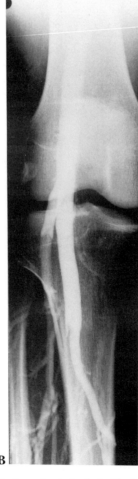

FIGURE 89.20 Removal of popliteal thrombosis by lysis block treatment (LBT). **A,** Venography prior to lysis. **B,** Dissolution of the thrombus after two series of LBT.

FIGURE 89.21. In-hospital rate of fatal pulmonary embolism of patients treated with heparin. The death rate depends on the proximal thrombosis site. (Results of the PHLECO study.[61])

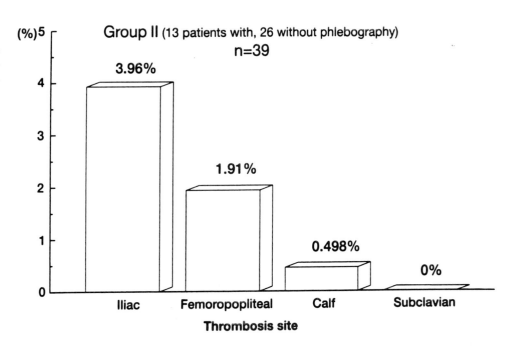

Group II (13 patients with, 26 without phlebography)
n=39

3.96%

1.91%

0.498%

0%

Iliac   Femoropopliteal   Calf   Subclavian

Thrombosis site

nolytic therapy for DVT. A total of 21 bleeds (1.4%) and 5 subsequent deaths (0.334%) were reported.

The patient's age was the most important factor for intracerebral hemorrhage. Bleeding was rare in patients under age 50 (0.355%), but the risk was considerably elevated in patients over age 50. The highest incidence of cerebral bleeding was found in patients between ages 70 and 90 (3.83%) (Figure 89.22).

Pulmonary Embolism

In the PHLEFI Study,[63] the incidence of fatal pulmonary embolism during UHSK therapy was recorded at 0.664%

and with UK at 0.870%. Iliac veins emerged as the principal source of fatal embolism (6.25% with UHSK [Figure 89.23] and 1.39% with UK treatment). Thrombosis of the right iliac vein was distinctively more dangerous than that of the left iliac vein. Femoral vein thrombosis was seldom responsible for fatal embolism (0.358% with UHSK, 0% with UK).

A temporary caval filter can prevent the occurrence of pulmonary embolism under fibrinolytic therapy.[62,97,118] This kind of prophylaxis is recommended as a supporting measure of fibrinolytic treatment for iliac vein thrombosis.

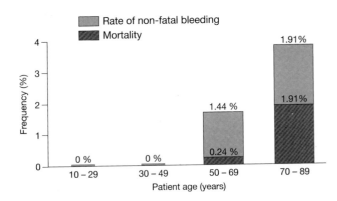

FIGURE 89.22. Cerebral bleeding rates in 807 patients treated with ultrahigh streptokinase for deep vein thrombosis. Patients under age 50 (n = 284) were safe from intracranial hemorrhage, but beyond this limit an exponential rise with age was recorded. (Results of the PHLEFI Study.[63])

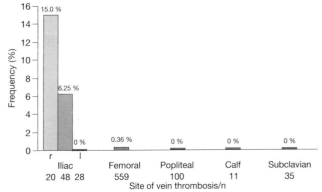

FIGURE 89.23. Fatal pulmonary embolism in 753 patients treated with ultrahigh streptokinase for deep vein thrombosis. Patients with right-sided iliac vein thrombosis were especially endangered. (Results of the PHLEFI Study.[63])

Follow-Up Studies

Fibrinolytic Treatment

After successful lytic treatment of DVT, follow-up studies were conducted by either venographic or clinical examination.

Venographic Examination

Table 89.11 lists five studies dealing with venographic follow-up investigation. The interval between lysis and reexamination was 1 month to 6 years. The overall results show that 80% of veins formerly thrombosed but cleared by fibrinolytic treatment remained open. One study group[26] looked at the venographic outcome according to the thrombosis site and investigated 8 patients with iliofemoral and 19 patients with femoral thrombosis. In the iliofemoral group 8 of 8 iliac veins and 3 of 8 femoral veins had become patent and the clearance rate of the femoral group was 19 of 19. After an average interval of 18.9 ± 6.7 months a follow-up venography was carried out. With the exception of one reocclusion in the femoral thrombosis group all veins were still open.

Clinical Examination

Johansson et al.[43] reported on 18 patients with acute DVT of the leg treated with SK. Venography performed immediately after treatment revealed complete clearance in 7 patients, remnants of thrombi in 4, and no effect in 7. Follow-up examinations 6 to 50 months later demonstrated normal venographies in 8 of the 18 patients. All of them were free from postthrombotic symptoms. By contrast, in the group with pathologic venographies, patients complained of edema and aching.

Elliot et al.[27] reported on 23 patients with DVT who were treated with SK and 25 patients with DVT who were treated with heparin. Both groups were randomized. Directly after treatment 17 of the 23 patients treated with SK presented with 80% to 100% thrombosis removal. No lysis was seen in the patients with heparin treatment. After an average follow-up period of 19 months, 22 patients in the SK group were free of postthrombotic syndromes (e.g., aching and edema) but only two of the patients in the heparin group.

Eichlisberger et al.[25] investigated 223 patients with DVT of whom 144 had received fibrinolytic and the rest heparin treatment. Venography directly after fibrinolytic therapy showed complete lysis in 25 and partial lysis in 75 patients. In 44 patients thrombus removal was not possible. Thirteen years later, a clinical follow-up investigation demonstrated that patients with complete and partial lysis displayed significantly lower rates of postthrombotic changes than patients who were treated with heparin or lysed unsuccessfully. These findings indicate that after complete thrombus removal postthrombotic complications are minimal or do not occur at all.

Coumarin Treatment

Long-term investigations have shown that 3 to 4 months of anticoagulation treatment are necessary after acute DVT to significantly reduce the incidence of further thromboembolic complications.[20,22,84,89] Because the curve for risk of thrombosis recurrence is hyperbolic (high recurrence rate within the first 2 weeks and lower rates thereafter), the administration of oral anticoagulant agents is recommended for a period of at least 3 months.

Recommendation for Treatment of Acute DVT

Patients Under Age 50

Oral anticoagulant agents for the treatment of calf vein thrombosis should be given for 3 months. Fibrinolytic therapy is contraindicated because only an insignificant percentage of patients develop postthrombotic sequelae[25,114] or pulmonary embolism.[63] Walking with the leg compressed (e.g., with a bandage or compression stocking) is essential.

Popliteal vein thrombosis is an excellent indication for lysis block treatment. This method can be recommended because it has almost no side effects, requires only a rela-

TABLE 89.11. Venographic follow-up investigation of veins previously thrombosed but subsequently cleared by fibrinolytic therapy.

Authors	Number of veins cleared by fibrinolysis	Drug	Interval between fibrinolysis and venography	Number of veins patent on inspection
Kakkar et al.[46]	7	SK	6–12 mo	4
Johansson et al.[44]	8	SK	5–50 mo	8
Olow et al.[76]	6	SK	1–10 mo	6
Arnesen et al.[7]	12	SK	6.3 y	5
Eickerling et al.[26]	27	UHSK	18.9 mo	25

UHSK, ultrahigh dose of streptokinase; SK, streptokinase.

tively short treatment period, and can probably also be performed as an outpatient procedure.

Therapy of choice for femoral vein thrombosis is UHSK short-term treatment. In patients under age 50 the incidence of side effects such as cerebral hemorrhage and fatal pulmonary embolism is extremely low.

Iliac vein thrombosis is also a good indication for UHSK treatment. However, because of a potentially high rate of fatal pulmonary embolism during UHSK infusion, a temporary caval filter should be implanted before lysis. The Anthéor filter is recommended because it can be inserted via the brachial vein, which permits easy control of possible bleedings from the puncture site.

Patients Over Age 50

Calf vein thrombosis does not require fibrinolytic therapy and is treated according to the guidelines provided for younger patients. Lysis block treatment has no major side effects (e.g., cerebral bleeding or pulmonary embolism). Therefore, elderly patients with popliteal vein thrombosis can receive this treatment without undue risk.

Because of a cerebral bleeding risk in patients over age 50, systemic lysis of femoral vein thrombosis is contraindicated. For these patients, initial subcutaneous heparin treatment with overlapping coumarin therapy is the best possible approach. During the first weeks the patients should walk with their legs bandaged or with compression stockings. Patients unable to walk remain in bed and receive heparin infusion for 1 week followed by coumarin therapy.

Some controversy exists over whether patients with acute iliac vein thrombosis should walk or remain in bed. Most clinicians recommend a 1-week bed rest during which heparin infusions and later coumarin medication are administered.

References

1. Collaborative European Multicenter Study. A randomized trial of subcutaneous low-molecular-weight heparin (CY216) compared with intravenous unfractionated heparin in the treatment of deep-vein thrombosis. *Thromb Haemost.* 1991;65:251–256.
2. Albada J, Nieuwenhuis HK, Sixma JJ. Treatment of acute venous thromboembolism with low-molecular-weight heparin (Fragmin): results of a double-blind randomized study. *Circulation.* 1989;80:935–940.
3. Allart RF, Poort SR, Rosendaal FR, Reitsma PH, Bertina RM, Briet E. Increased risk of venous thrombosis in carriers of hereditary protein C deficiency defect. *Lancet.* 1993; 341:134–138.
4. Althoff M, Rudofsky G. Die lokoregionale Thrombolyse bei tiefer Venenthrombose. *Die gelben Hefte (Behringwerke).* 1994;34:105.
5. Anders O, Lakner V, Konrad H, Ernst B. Kurzzeitlysen bei venösen Thrombosen mit ultrahoher Streptokinasedosierung. *Folia Haematologica.* 1986;113:82–87.
6. Arnesen H, Heilo A, Jakobsen E, Ly B, Skaga E. A prospective study of streptokinase and heparin in the treatment of deep vein thrombosis. *Acta Med Scand.* 1978;203:457–463.
7. Arnesen H, Hoiseth A, Ly B. Streptokinase or heparin in the treatment of deep vein thrombosis. *Acta Med Scand.* 1982;211:65–68.
8. Bauer G. Early diagnosis of venous thrombosis by means of venography and abortive treatment with heparin. *Acta Med Scand.* 1941;107:136–147.
9. Bauer G. Heparin therapy in acute deep venous thrombosis. *JAMA.* 1946;131:196–203.
10. Bauersachs R, Kuhl H, Lindhoff-Last E, Ehrly AM. Thromboserisiko bei oralen Kontrazeptiva: Stellenwert eines Thrombophilie-Screenings. *Vasa.* 1996;25:209–220.
11. Beck KH, Scharrer I. Protein C: ein Inhibitor der Blutgerinnung. *Diagnose and Labor.* 1988;38:35–42.
12. Beckering RE, Titus JL. Femoral-popliteal venous thrombosis and pulmonary embolism. *Am J Clin Pathol.* 1969;52: 530–537.
13. Bertina RN. The control of hemostasis: protein C and protein S. *Biomed Prog.* 1989;4:53–56.
14. Bertina M, Koelman BPC, Kostert T, et al. Mutation in blood coagulation factor V associated with resistance to activated protein C. *Nature.* 1994;369:64–67.
15. Biland L, Zemp E, Widmer LK. Zur Epidemiologie der venösen Thromboembolie. *Internist.* 1987;28:285–290.
16. Bounameaux H, Banga JD, Bluhmki E. Double-blind, randomized comparison of systemic continuous 0.25 versus 0.50 mg/kg/24 h of altplase over 3 to 7 days for treatment of deep venous thrombosis in heparinized patients: results of the European Thrombolysis With rt-PA in Venous Thrombosis (ETTT) Trial. *Thromb Haemost.* 1992;67: 627–630.
17. Bovill EG, Bauer KA, Dickman JD, Callas P, West B. The clinical spectrum of heterozygote protein C deficiency in a large New England kindred. *Blood.* 1989;73:712–717.
18. Bratt G, Aberg W, Johansson M. Two daily subcutaneous injections of Fragmin as compared with intravenous standard heparin in the treatment of deep venous thrombosis (DVT). *Thromb Haemost.* 1990;564:506–510.
19. Broekmans AW, Bertina RM, Loeliger EA, Hofmann V, Klingemann HG. Protein C and the development of skin necrosis during anticoagulant therapy. *Thromb Haemost.* 1983;49:244–251.
20. Coon WW, Willis PW, Mich AA. Recurrence of venous thromboembolism. *Surgery.* 1973;73:823–827.
21. Coon WW, Willis PW, Mich AA. Hemorrhagic complications of anticoagulant therapy. *Arch Intern Med.* 1974;133: 386–392.
22. Coon WW, Willis PW, Symons MJ. Assessment of anticoagulant treatment of venous thromboembolism. *Ann Surg.* 1969;170:559–568.
23. D'Angelo A, Manucci PM. Outcome of treatment of deep-vein thrombosis with urokinase: relationship to dosage, duration of therapy, age of the thrombus, and laboratory change. *Thromb Haemost.* 1984;51:236–239.
24. Dvorak HF. Abnormalities of hemostasis in malignancy. In: Colman RW, Hirsh J, Marder VJ, Salzman EW, eds. *Hemo-*

stasis and Thrombosis: Basic Principles and Clinical Practice. Philadelphia, Pa: JB Lippincott; 1987:1143–1157.

25. Eichlisberger R, Frauchiger B, Widmer MTH, Widmer LK, Jäger K. Spätfolgen der tiefen Venenthrombose: ein 13-Jahres-Follow-up von 223 Patienten. *Vasa.* 1994;23: 234–243.

26. Eickerling B, Rakus H, Martin M. Phlebographische Nachuntersuchung erfolgreich fibrinolytisch behandelter tiefer Beinvenenthrombosen. *Vasa.* 1990;19:142–148.

27. Elliot MS, Immelman EJ, Jeffery P, et al. A comparative randomized trial of heparin versus streptokinase in the treatment of acute proximal venous thrombosis: an interim report of a prospective trial. *Br J Surg.* 1979;66: 838–843.

28. Fagher B, Lundh B. Heparin treatment of deep vein thrombosis. *Acta Med Scand.* 1981;210:357–361.

29. Fahn H, Maubach P, Merl R, Senner H, Hellwig H, Wirtzfeld A. Ultrahoch dosierte Thrombolysetherapie mit Streptokinase bei peripherer Phlebothrombose. *Med Klin.* 1989;84:183–187.

30. Folkman J. How is blood vessel growth regulated in normal and neoplastic tissue? *Cancer Res.* 1986;46:467–473.

31. Franzeck UK, Schalch I, Jäger KA, Schneider E, Grimm J, Bollinger A. Prospective 12-year follow-up study of clinical and hemodynamic sequelae after deep vein thrombosis in low-risk patients (Zürich Study). *Circulation.* 1996;93: 74–79.

32. Giercksky KE, Sorlie DG, Odegaard H, Johnson JA. Fibrinolytic treatment of post-operative deep vein thrombosis. *Surg Gynecol Obstet.* 1975;141:576–578.

33. Goldhaber SZ, Meyerovitz MF, Green D, et al. Randomized controlled trial of tissue plasminogen activator in proximal deep venous thrombosis. *Am J Med.* 1990;88:235–240.

34. Greul W, Tilsner V. Thrombolysis with urokinase in arterial and venous thrombosis. In: Paoletti R, Sherry S, eds. *Thrombosis and Urokinase: Serono Symposia.* Vol 9. London: Academic Press; 1977:235–242.

35. Hagg NB. Niedrig dosierte Fibrinolysetherapie mit rt-PA bei Thrombosen des tiefen Venensystems. *Vasa.* 1991; 33 (suppl):124–125.

36. Hansson C, Swanbeck G. Regulating the pressure under compression bandages for venous leg ulcers. *Acta Derm Venereol.* 1988;68:245–249.

37. Heijboer H, Branjes DP, Buller HR, Sturk A, Ten Cate JW. Deficiency of coagulation inhibiting and fibrinolytic proteins in outpatients with deep vein thrombosis. *N Engl J Med.* 1990;323:1512–1516.

38. Heimburger N, Pâques EP, Römisch J. Coagulation and fibrinolysis in cancer. *Behring Inst Mitt.* 1992;91: 169–182.

39. Heimig T, Martin M. Lyseblocktechnik: eine neue lokale Behandlungsform für Unterschenkelvenen- und Arterienverschlüsse. *Vasa.* 1992;21:289–293.

40. Hirsh J, Fuster V. Guide to anticoagulant therapy, II: oral anticoagulants. *Circulation.* 1994;89:1469–1480.

41. Huber P, Häuptli W, Schmitt HE, Widmer LK. Die Axillar-Subclaviavenenthrombose und ihre Folgen. *Internist.* 1987;28:336–343.

42. Hull RD, Raskob GE, Pineo GF, et al. Subcutaneous low-molecular-weight heparin compared with continuous intravenous heparin in the treatment of proximal-vein thrombosis. *N Engl J Med.* 1992;326:975–983.

43. Johansson E, Ericson K, Zetterquist St. Streptokinase treatment of deep venous thrombosis of the lower extremity. *Acta Med Scand.* 1976;199:89–94.

44. Johansson L, Nylander G, Hedner U, Nilsson IM. Comparison of streptokinase with heparin: late results in the treatment of deep venous thrombosis. *Acta Med Scand.* 1979; 206:93–98.

45. Johnson AJ, McCarthy WR. The lysis of artificially induced vascular clots in man by intravenous infusion of streptokinase. *J Clin Invest.* 1959;38:1627–1643.

46. Kakkar VV, Flanc C, Howe CT, O'Shea M, Flute PT. Treatment of deep vein thrombosis: a trial of heparin, streptokinase, and arwin. *BMJ.* 1969;1:806–810.

47. Karino T, Goldsmith HL. Rheological factors in thrombosis and hemostasis. In: Bloom AL, Thomas DP, eds. *Hemostasis and Thrombosis.* Edinburgh: Churchill Livingstone; 1987.

48. Koch HU. Lysetherapie tiefer Phlebothrombosen mit ultrahoch dosierter Streptokinase gefolgt von konventionell dosierter Urokinase. *Medizinische Welt.* 1988;39:245–250.

49. Koopman MMW, Prandoni P, Piovella F, et al. Treatment of venous thrombosis with intravenous unfractionated heparin administered in the hospital as compared with subcutaneous low-molecular-weight heparin administered at home. *N Engl J Med.* 1996;334:682–687.

50. Koster T, Rosendaal FR, Ronde De H, Briet E, Vandenbroucke JP, Bertina RM. Venous thrombosis due to poor anticoagulant response to activated protein C: Leiden Thrombophilia Study. *Lancet.* 1993;342:1503–1506.

51. Krüger P. Streptokinase in ultrahoher Dosierung (UHSK): Thrombolytische Therapie tiefer venöser Thrombosen. *Herz-Gefäße.* 1989;9:2–8.

52. Krzywanek HJ. Vergleichende Untersuchungen zur intermittierenden fibrinolytischen Behandlung akuter Phlebothrombosen mit Streptokinase und Urokinase in ultrahoher Dosierung. *Innere Medizin.* 1988;14:179–184.

53. Lagerstedt CI, Olsson CG, Fagher BO, Öqvist BW. Need for long-term anticoagulant treatment in symptomatic calf-vein thrombosis. *Lancet.* 1985;325:515–518.

54. Lellouche F, Martinuzzo M, Said P, Maclouf J, Carreras LV. Imbalance of thromboxane/prostacyclin biosynthesis in patients with lupus anticoagulant. *Blood.* 1991;78: 2894–2899.

55. Levine M, Gent M, Hirsh J, et al. A comparison of low-molecular-weight heparin administered primarily at home with unfractionated heparin administered in the hospital for proximal deep-vein thrombosis. *N Engl J Med.* 1996; 334:677–681.

56. Levine MN, Hirsh J. Hemorrhagic complications of anticoagulant therapy. *Semin Thromb Hemost.* 1986;12:39–57.

57. Lindmarker P, Holmstrom M, Granqvist S, Johansson H, Lockner D. Comparison of once-daily subcutaneous Fragmin with continuous intravenous unfractionated heparin in the treatment of deep venous thrombosis. *Thromb Haemost.* 1994;72:186–190.

58. Lockner D, Bratt G, Tornebohm E, et al. Intravenous and subcutaneous administration of Fragmin in deep venous thrombosis. *Haemostasis.* 1986;16:25–29.

59. Lopaciuk S, Meissner AJ, Filipecki S, et al. Subcutaneous low-molecular-weight heparin versus subcutaneous unfractionated heparin in the treatment of deep vein thrombosis: a Polish multicenter trial. *Thromb Haemost.* 1992;68: 14–18.

60. Marder V, Brenner B, Rubin R. Comparison of dosage schedules of rt-PA in the treatment of deep vein thrombosis. *Circulation.* 1990;82:376–377.

61. Martin M. PHLECO: a multicenter study of the fate of 1647 hospital patients treated conservatively without fibrinolysis and surgery. *Clinical Investigation.* 1993;71:471–477.

62. Martin M. Systemic fibrinolytic treatment of iliofemoral vein thrombosis. *Int J Angiol.* 1996;5(suppl):38–40.

63. Martin M. Results of the PHLEFI Study (PHLEbothrombosis—Fibrinolytic Therapy): a prospective multicentre study of the fate of 1498 patients receiving fibrinolytic therapy for deep vein thrombosis. *Int J Angiol.* In press.

64. Martin M, Fiebach BJO. Short-term ultrahigh streptokinase treatment of chronic arterial occlusions and acute deep vein thrombosis. *Semin Thromb Hemost.* 1991;17: 21–38.

65. Martin M, Fiebach BJO. *Fibrinolytische Behandlung peripherer Arterien- und Venenverschlüsse.* Huber, Switzerland: Göttingen; 1994.

66. Martin M, Fiebach BJO, Feldkamp M. Ultrahohe Streptokinase-Infusionsbehandlung bei peripheren Gefäßverschlüssen. *Dtsch Med Wochenschr.* 1983;108:167–171.

67. Martin M, Heimig T, Fiebach BJO, Magnus L, Riedel C. Lysis block treatment: a new form of local thrombosis. *Angiol.* 1994;45:43–48.

68. Martin M, Riedel C, Bauer A. Ultrahohe Kurzzeitlyse mit Urokinase. *Medizinische Welt.* 1989;40:1431–1434.

69. Mavor GE, Dhall DP, Duthie JS, et al. Streptokinase therapy in deep vein thrombosis. *Br J Surg.* 1973;60:468–474.

70. Meyer J. Die periphere lokale Lyse (PLL). Eine neue zusätzliche Behandlungsmöglichkeit bei tiefer Bein- und Becken-venenthrombose. Bericht über 23 Patienten. *Z Herz-Thorax-Gefäßchirurgie.* 1990;4:151–156.

71. Miletich J, Sherman L, Broze G. Absence of thrombosis in subjects with heterocygous protein C deficiency. *N Engl J Med.* 1987;317:991–996.

72. Minar E, Ehringer H, Marosi L, et al. Akute Venenthrombose: Lokalisation, Ausdehnung, und Ätiologie mit besonderer Berück-sichtigung der Paraneoplasie. *Dtsch Med Wochenschr.* 1982;7:1303–1309.

73. Morrison M. Analysis of the blood picture in 100 cases of malignancy. *J Lab Clin Med.* 1932;17:1071.

74. Mumme A, Kemen M, Ernst R, Zumtobel V. Lokoregionäre ultrahochdosierte Fibrinolyse tiefer Beinvenen-Thrombosen. *Vasa.* 1991;33:122–121.

75. Nordström M, Lindblad B, Anderson H, et al. Deep venous thrombosis and occult malignancy: an epidemiological study. *BMJ.* 1994;308:891–894.

76. Olow B, Johansson C, Andersson J, Eklöf B. Deep venous thrombosis treated with a standard dosage of streptokinase. *Acta Chir Scand.* 1970;136:181–189.

77. Ott P, Eldrup E, Oxholm P, Vestergard A, Knudsen JB. Streptokinase therapy in routine management of deep venous thrombosis in lower extremities: a retrospective study of phlebography results and therapeutic complications. *Acta Med Scand.* 1986;219:295–300.

78. Partsch H, Oburger K, Mostbeck A, König B, Köhn H. Frequency of pulmonary embolism in ambulant patients with pelvic vein thrombosis: a prospective study. *J Vasc Surg.* 1992;16:715–722.

79. Podlaha R, Schlichting P. Erfahrungen mit Streptokinase in ultrahoher Dosierung bei der Behandlung der tiefen Beinvenenthrombosen. *Phlebologie und Proktologie.* 1988;17: 197–201.

80. Poller L, McKeran A, Thomson JM, Elstein M, Hirsh PJ, Jones JB. Fixed minidose warfarin: a new approach to prophylaxis against venous thrombosis after major surgery. *Br Med J.* 1987;295:1309–1312.

81. Prandoni P, Lensing AW, Büller HR, et al. Comparison of subcutaneous low-molecular-weight heparin with intravenous standard heparin in proximal deep-vein thrombosis. *Lancet.* 1992;339:411–415.

82. Prandoni P, Lensing AWA, Cogo A, Cuppini S, Villalta S. Carta M, Cattelan AM, Polistena P, Bernardi E, Prins MH. The long-term clinical course of acute deep venous thrombosis. *Ann Int Med.* 1996;125:1–7.

83. Rahmer H, Wahl S, Stunkat R, Hertel K. Akute tiefe Bein-und Beckenvenenthrombosen: Thrombolytische Therapie. *Diagnostik und Intensivmedizin.* 1979;4:65–67.

84. Research Committee of the British Thoracic Society. Optimum duration of anticoagulation for deep-vein thrombosis and pulmonary embolism. *Lancet.* 1992;340:873–876.

85. Ridker PM, Hennekens CH, Lindpaintner K, Stampfer MJ, Eisenberg PR, Miletich JP. Mutation in the gene coding for coagulation factor V and the risk of myocardial infarction, stroke, and venous thrombosis in apparently healthy men. *N Engl J Med.* 1995;332:912–917.

86. Robertson BR, Nilsson IM, Nylander G. Thrombolytic effect of streptokinase as evaluated by phlebography of deep venous thrombi of the leg. *Acta Chir Scand.* 1970;136: 173–180.

87. Rosendaal FR, Heidboer H. Mortality related to thrombosis in congenital antithrombin III deficiency. *Lancet.* 1991; 337:1545.

88. Rosendaal FR, Koster T, Vandenbroucke JP, Reitsma PH. High risk of thrombosis in patients homozygous for factor V Leiden (activated protein C resistance). *Blood.* 1995;85: 1504–1508.

89. Sarasin FP, Bounameaux H. Duration of anticoagulant therapy after proximal deep vein thrombosis: a decision analysis. *Thromb Haemost.* 1994;71:286–291.

90. Scharrer I, Hach-Wunderle V, Heyland H. Incidence of defective tPA release in 158 unrelated young patients with venous thrombosis in comparison to PC, PS, AT III, fibrinogen, and plasminogen deficiency. *Thromb Haemost.* 1989; 61:50–54.

91. Scharrer I, Hetzel D. Auswertung der zwischen 1962 und 1981 durchgeführten Lysetherapie an 285 Patienten. In: Trübestein G, Etzel F, eds. *Fibrinolytische Therapie.* Stuttgart, Germany: FK Schattauer; 1983:151–154.

92. Schmutzler R, Koller F. Die Thrombolysetherapie: *Ergebnisse der Inneren Medizin und Kinderheilkunde.* 1965;22: 157–210.

93. Schulman S, Lockner D, Granquist S, Bratt G, Paul C, Nyman D. A comparative randomized trial of low-dose versus high-dose streptokinase in deep vein thrombus of the thigh. *Thromb Haemost.* 1984;51:261–265.

94. Seaman AJ, Common HH, Rösch J, et al. Deep vein thrombosis treated with streptokinase or heparin: a randomized study. *Angiology.* 1976;27:549–556.

95. Sevitt S, Innes D. Prothrombin-time and Thrombotest in injured patients on prophylactic anticoagulant therapy. *Lancet.* 1964;1:124–129.

96. Simonneau G, Charbonnier B, Decousus H, et al. Subcutaneous low-molecular weight heparin compared with continuous intravenous unfractionated heparin in the treatment of proximal deep vein thrombosis. *Arch Intern Med.* 1993;153:1541–1546.

97. Stöhr G, Hey D. Anwendung eines passageren Vena-Cava-Filters bei der Lyse von Bein-/Beckenvenenthrombosen mit ultrahoher Streptokinase bzw. Urokinase. *Medizinische Welt.* 1991;42:1061–1065.

98. Straub H, Drews S, Jäger D. Die thrombolytische Therapie der Venenthrombose mit Streptokinase in konventioneller Dauerlyse oder ultrahoher Kurzlyse. *Vasa.* 1988;23(suppl):91.

99. Svensson PJ, Dahlbäck B. Resistance to activated protein C as a basis of venous thrombosis. *N Engl J Med.* 1994;330:517–522.

100. Tait RC, Walker ID, Perry DJ, Islam SI, Daly ME, McCall F, Conkie JA, Carrell RW. Prevalence of antithrombin deficiency in the healthy population. *Br J Haematol.* 1994;87:106–112.

101. Thaler E, Lechner K. Antithrombin III deficiency and thromboembolism. *Clinicum Haematologicum.* 1981;10:369–390.

102. Theiss W, Baumann G, Klein G. Fibrinolytische Behandlung tiefer Venenthrombosen mit Streptokinase in ultrahoher Dosierung. *Dtsch Med Wochenschr.* 1987;112:668–674.

103. Theiss W, Hofer E, Kriessmann A, Lutilsky L, Sauer E, Wirtzfeld A. Streptokinase-Behandlung tiefer Venenthrombosen. *Med Klin.* 1980;75:580–586.

104. Timmermann J, Rudofsky G, Hagg N, Ranft J, Ruch U. Lokale fibrinolytische Therapie (PLL) der tiefen Beinvenenthrombosen mit rt-PA. *Phlebologie.* 1992;21:205–209.

105. Trübestein G, Brecht T, Ludwig M, Brecht G, Etzel F. Fibrinolytische Therapie mit Streptokinase und Urokinase bei tiefer Venenthrombose. In: Trübestein G, Etzel F, eds. *Fibrinolytische Therapie.* Stuttgart, Germany: FK Schattauer; 1983:193–201.

106. Trübestein G, Trübestein R, Ludwig M, Christ F. Die Thrombolysetherapie der Becken- und Beinvenenthrombosen. In: Bruhn HD, ed. *Hauptvorträge und ausgewählte Vorträge auf dem 6. Kongreß der Gesellschaft für Thrombose- und Hämostaseforschung.* Stuttgart, Germany: FK Schattauer; 1990:277–286.

107. Tsapogas MJ, Peabody RA, Wu KT, Karmody AM, Devaray KT, Eckert C. Controlled study of thrombolytic therapy in deep vein thrombosis. *Surgery.* 1973;74:973–984.

108. Turpie AGG, Levine MN, Hirsh J, et al. Tissue plasminogen activator (rt-PA) vs heparin in deep vein thrombosis. *Chest.* 1990;97:172–175.

109. Unkel B, Hajjar H. Fibrinolyse mit Plasminogen-Humanaktivator (Actilyse) bei peripheren Venenthrombosen. Vortrag 8. Jahrestagung der deutschen Gesellschaft für Gefäßchirurgie. Dresden, Germany: Springer-Verlag; 1992.

110. Verhaeghe R, Besse P, Bournameaux H, Marbet GA. Multicenter pilot of the efficacy and safety of systemic rt-PA administration in the treatment of deep vein thrombosis of the lower extremities and/or pelvis. *Thromb Res.* 1989;55:5–11.

111. Verstraete M, Vermylen J. Molecular defects of the factors of coagulation and of the fibrinolytic system associated with thrombo-embolism. *Essentiala.* 1987;16:1–12.

112. Vigano S, Manucci PM, Solinas S, Botasso B, Mariani G. Decrease in protein C antigen and formation of an abnormal protein soon after starting an anticoagulant therapy. *Br J Haemost.* 1984;57:213–220.

113. Watz R, Savidge GF. Rapid thrombolysis and preservation of valvular venous function in high deep vein thrombosis. *Acta Med Scand.* 1979;205:293–298.

114. Widmer LK, Brandenberg E, Schmitt HE, et al. Zum Schicksal des Patienten mit tiefer Venenthrombose. *Dtsch Med Wochenschr.* 1985;110:993–997.

115. Widmer IK, Marder G, Schmitt HE, Ducker F, Da Silva D, Müller G. Heparin oder Thrombolyse in der Behandlung der tiefen Beinvenenthrombose. *Vasa.* 1974;3:422–432.

116. Zimmermann R, Abdulkadir G, Horn A, Harenberg J, Diehm C, Kübler W. Fibrinolytic therapy of deep vein thrombosis with continuous intravenous infusion of a recombinant tissue plasminogen activator. *Semin Thromb Hemost.* 1991;17:48–54.

117. Zimmermann R, Janssen E, Harenberg J, Kossakowski A, Diehm C, Mörl H. Ergebnis der thrombolytischen Behandlung der Achselvenenthrombose mit Urokinase. In: Trübestein G, Etzel F, eds. *Fibrinolytische Therapie.* Stuttgart, Germany: FK Schattauer; 1983:239–242.

118. Zwaan M, Kagel CH, Mierenhof N, et al. Erste Erfahrungen mit temporären Venen-Cava-Filtern. *Fortschritte auf dem Gebiete der Röntgenstrahlen und der neuen bildgebenden Verfahren.* 1995;163:171–176.

90

Pulmonary Embolism

J. Ernesto Molina

The incidence of pulmonary embolism (PE) in the United States is now estimated at over 500,000 people per year, with a 10% death rate. Published figures from the 1970s[1-3] placed the incidence at 500,000 to 600,000 cases diagnosed every year, with 50,000 deaths. The most recent figures from the 1980s and 1990s[1,4-7] do not show any difference whatsoever in incidence or death rate, in spite of prophylactic measures recommended since the mid 1960s and early 1970s in an attempt to decrease the incidence of deep vein thrombosis (DVT), and therefore of PE, in postsurgical patients. However, many surgeons still do not prescribe any prophylactic treatment for their patients.

The number of patients hospitalized with this diagnosis, according to Anderson et al.,[5] is 250,000 per year. The estimate of the National Institutes of Health Consensus Conference on thromboembolism in 1986 was 300,000 to 600,000, with a death rate of about 50,000, including both surgical and nonsurgical patients.[4] Similar figures have been published by Goldhaber.[6,7] However, fewer patients develop PE secondary to surgical interventions. As Bergqvist and Lindblad[8] indicate, the postsurgical group of PE patients constitutes only about 28% of the total number so diagnosed. Therefore, a large proportion (up to 72%) of PE patients have chronic medical disorders. The percentage attributed to multiple traumatic injuries, which constitutes another group, is no more than 10% of the total population.

Of the total number of PE patients, many have other serious conditions; PE is only coincidental or merely a contributing factor in the total picture of their illness. Therefore, surgical patients are better candidates for a prophylactic approach to prevent DVT and, as an immediate result, produce a decrease in PE.

Several prophylactic regimens have been demonstrated to prevent DVT,[9] including use of subcutaneous heparin,[10,11] low molecular weight dextran,[12] warfarin, and even antiplatelet agents[9,13] preoperatively. In addition, anesthesia methods have improved significantly,

and pneumatic intermittent compression of the lower extremities is now routine during and after surgery. Once DVT has occurred and PE develops, intravascular inferior vena cava (IVC) filters, which prevent large emboli from reaching the lung or avoid the recurrence of the problem, can be implanted; more aggressive direct treatment of the embolus with thrombolytics can also be undertaken. An even newer percutaneous surgical procedure aimed at removing the clots from the lung has been designed and implemented with various degrees of success,[14] although direct mechanical intervention to remove the embolus from the pulmonary artery on an emergency basis is rarely needed. During the past few years, new thrombolytic agents and modalities for their use have been introduced; combined with safer protocols, they have effectively helped prevent bleeding complications. The different thrombolytic methods will continue to be reviewed; as the medical community becomes more confident as to their proper use, surgical intervention (namely, embolectomy) probably can be avoided altogether in the future.

Clinical Presentation

Regardless of which category the patient belongs to (see "Categories" section), PE can present in three different ways:

Class 1: Symptoms of PE (chest pain, dyspnea, diaphoresis) with compromised but stable cardiorespiratory function. These patients are not in shock but are usually short of breath. They may or may not have experienced chest pain or rapid heart beat. Their blood pressure usually remains above 90 peak systolic, with no signs of hemodynamic deterioration.

Class I: Sudden signs of shock, with peak systolic blood pressure lower than 90 mm Hg, hypoxia, and tachypnea. Within a few minutes, the patients may suffer cardiac arrest.

Class III: Chronic PE. The patients have no obvious signs or symptoms. Nevertheless, over long periods of time—weeks or months—they start noticing shortness of breath and less ability to perform physical tasks. They experience tiredness, occasional coughing, or dyspnea. Dyspnea is often associated with a previous history of DVT in the lower extremities, usually extending above the knee.

These three groupings have helped us decide which test to perform to confirm or rule out PE and which course of action to take. To diagnose PE, the clinician must consider it a possibility in every patient who complains of shortness of breath that suggests cardiorespiratory compromise.

Etiology

The occurrence of PE is intimately related to the development of DVT. Most studies done with iodine 125–labeled fibrinogen and venography show the calf as the primary site. However, the calf's clinical relevance is limited, because calf thrombi usually produce no symptoms; they do not cause significant PE or late postphlebitic leg syndrome.[15] In up to 80% of cases, such thrombi disappear spontaneously.[16,17] Up to 25% of patients over 40 years of age undergoing major abdominal surgery develop DVT in the postoperative period.[2,8,15,17] Above-knee thrombosis is definitely associated with a high risk of PE and late postthrombotic sequelae in the leg.

In a double-blind randomized study by Lahnborg et al.,[18] ventilation perfusion (VQ) scans were obtained routinely in patients undergoing major surgery. Without any prophylaxis, the incidence of PE was 56%, but when subcutaneous heparin was used perioperatively, the incidence was reduced to 19%. Dyspnea and cyanosis of lips were noticed in only 15% of the patients; most (85%) never had any symptoms. Therefore, when symptoms are present, a very large embolus exists, and no time should be wasted in implementing immediate treatment.[17,19–21]

In a separate study, Partsch et al.[22] found that only 12.5% to 14.5% of patients with PE had symptoms. These patients had iliofemoral vein thrombosis and were being treated in an ambulatory facility.

Other studies have shown that up to 7% of patients over 40 years of age undergoing major surgery develop DVT above the knee.[9] This finding is worrisome: up to 0.9% of these patients may die of PE, as confirmed by autopsy studies.[4,9]

In a study by Murray et al.[23] of patients undergoing major orthopedic surgery (e.g., hip arthroplasty), the incidence of fatal PE was 1.5%. In cases of traumatic hip fracture, the incidence of fatal PE is known to be around 4%.[4] It is also known that fatal PE can occur even after patients are discharged from the hospital.[24,25] In studies by Huber et al.,[24] 30% of the total number of PE cases occurred within 30 days after the patients left the hospital. Other types of surgery done in the pelvis (e.g., gynecologic or urologic procedures) produce a significant incidence of DVT and PE. The magnitude of surgery also makes a difference in the incidence of these complications.

The European Consensus Statement of 1991[26] on thromboembolism showed that the incidence of PE depended on the type of surgery. The DVT rate was as high as 75% after knee arthroplasty, decreasing gradually for leg amputation, hip fracture surgery, hip arthroplasty, open prostatectomy, general abdominal surgery, gynecologic surgery, kidney transplantation, noncardiac thoracic surgery, and neurosurgery. The lowest rate was after open meniscectomy: 20% to 25%.

Risk factors are also additive. The development of DVT depends not only on the type of surgery but also on other factors such as increasing age, cancer, diabetes, or polycythemia.[9,27–29] The type of thrombus is also important; the incidence of PE in patients with free-floating thrombi in the iliac system was 26% for unilateral involvement but 42.9% with bilateral thrombi, as reported by Berry et al.[30] In 93% of patients with pulmonary embolism, the location of the thrombus was proximal (downstream) to the superficial femoral vein.

Categories

The seven types of patients prone to develop PE are described in the following sections.

Postoperative Patients

PE may follow any major operation in patients over 40 years of age. It may be the first symptom of a thromboembolic event and is most common after operations in the pelvis or abdomen or after an orthopedic procedure. However, other operations in other parts of the body are not completely free of this potential complication, including kidney or lung transplants, coronary bypasses, thoracotomies, and even thoracic organ transplants or spinal surgery.

Posttrauma Patients

PE can be associated with multiple traumas and bone fractures of the pelvis, lower extremities, or chest wall. These patients have usually been involved in serious automobile accidents or falls and have multiorgan injuries.

Patients With Chronic Debilitating Diseases

PE can occur in bed-confined patients or those with prolonged periods of immobilization. Such patients may have malignancies for which they are undergoing chemotherapy or radiation therapy, sepsis of various causes, or multiorgan failure (with renal insufficiency or diabetes). They may have experienced previous episodes of thromboembolism, usually with no recent surgery performed.

Patients With Recurrent Venous Thrombosis

Patients with recurrent venous thrombosis are fairly healthy but may be morbidly obese, old, or chronically dehydrated. They may have subclavian vein "effort" thrombosis in the subacute or chronic stage.

Women During Pregnancy or After Delivery

Women during pregnancy or after delivery may develop lower extremity venous hypertension or venous varicosities associated with edema of the lower extremities.

Young Women Who Take Birth Control Pills

PE may occur in young women in their teens, 20s, or 30s with a history of steady intake of birth control pills.

Patients With Long-Term Indwelling Central Catheters

Because of the widespread use of central catheters for chemotherapy, antibiotic therapy, renal dialysis access, or placement of transvenous pacemakers and defibrillators (among other reasons), subclavian vein, innominate, or even superior vena cava strictures or stenosis occurs quite frequently. Even after the catheters are removed, if local fibrosis of the vein has occurred and caused stenosis, then thrombosis and PE can result at that site. The process may be silent and not diagnosed until the patient has developed recurrent, multiple PE episodes without symptoms. Sometimes, by the time the patient is evaluated, pulmonary hypertension and even right-sided heart failure already exist. Intracardiac thrombus formed at the tip of central catheters may sit in the atrium or ventricle and sometimes cause massive PE.

Clinical Approach

Treatment sometimes depends on the patient's classification. No single protocol can be applied uniformly across the board to all patients.

The clinician must weigh the pros and cons of the optimal therapy in every instance but must have a clear understanding of what the options are. The most important factor is thoroughness. Failure is usually caused by inappropriate use of drugs, poor follow-up, or unclear treatment plan.

Therapeutic Options

Initially, in the early years, heparin was the drug of choice, and it is still used at many centers. It is adminis-

tered to prevent further formation of thrombus and to help the normally present thrombolysins in the body dissolve the clot already formed and lodged in the lungs. Heparin is not effective at dissolving clots; moreover, the natural lytic process undertaken by the normal enzymes in the circulation is a limited and very slow process that requires several days to significantly reduce the size of clots. At the same time, heparin also acts to prevent further clot formation in the lower veins of the body where the embolus originated.

A second option, much more effective and faster, is the use of thrombolytic agents. Their adoption has been rather slow because of the feared risk of causing bleeding, particularly in patients who have undergone recent surgical procedures. These agents act directly on the thrombus by inducing lysis. Depending on the age of the clot, it could completely dissolve in less than 48 hours, leaving the patient with perfectly clear and open pulmonary arteries.

Most objections to thrombolytic agents derive from the risk of bleeding, particularly in the central nervous system. However, this risk seems to depend on the manner in which thrombolytics are administered. On the one hand, therefore, lies the thrombolytic therapy option. Embolectomy, on the other hand, is a direct surgical approach aimed at removing the embolus from the pulmonary circulation. It is always a major intervention entailing thoracotomy and extracorporeal circulation. A less formidable operation using a steerable instrument inserted by way of the femoral vein, with a suction mechanism to aspirate the clots from the main pulmonary trunks, has been proposed by Greenfield et al. since the early 1970s.[14,31] However, even recent reports on the surgical results of pulmonary embolectomy using either technique show a very high mortality rate.[32-37] Careful analysis of these patients shows that they could probably have been treated with thrombolytic agents much more safely. The only candidates for embolectomy are patients in whom thrombolytic agents are contraindicated. It is therefore important that physicians become familiar with thrombolytic therapy, which seems to offer better results than any other methods previously or currently attempted.

Thrombolytic Therapy

Because PE is a sudden event that often leads to cardiac arrest and death, the ideal therapy is aimed at dissolving the clot rapidly, reopening the pulmonary vasculature, stabilizing the hemodynamics of the patient, and curing him or her within a very short period.

All reports in the 1960s and 1970s definitely proved that thrombolytic therapy was superior to heparin treatment[38-42] and also more effective than pulmonary embolectomy. The patients subjected to embolectomy usually were in more critical condition, which prompted the surgical intervention.

Several thrombolytic agents have been used throughout the past 20 years. Streptokinase was approved for use in the United States in 1977, followed by urokinase in 1978.

The advantages of thrombolytic therapy are several: rapid lysis of the clot (in less than 48 hours), reestablishment of pulmonary tissue perfusion, and improvement and increase in the pulmonary capillary blood volume. These changes occur rather rapidly, reducing the mortality caused by hemodynamic embarrassment. Thrombolytic therapy also rapidly reverses the right-sided heart failure produced by the embolus; by clearing all the small pulmonary artery branches, it reduces the incidence of later development of pulmonary hypertension.

Because of the continuing discovery of newer thrombolytic agents, comparison of their effectiveness and safety has prompted numerous publications, focusing mostly on safety, cost, acceleration of activity, and side effects.

Studies by Miller et al.,[38] Sharma et al.,[39] Dalen et al.,[42] Tow et al.,[40] and others have shown that thrombolytic therapy for PE is superior to treatment by heparin alone. Urokinase was superior to streptokinase in several trials involving not only PE[43,44] but also arterial thromboembolic phenomena and myocardial infarction.[45-47] More recently, the recombinant tissue-type plasminogen activator (rtPA) used in treating myocardial infarction has been successfully used also in PE.[48,49] Newer thrombolytic agents such as alteplase are being tested effectively,[50,51] but no results showing the advantages or disadvantages of these drugs over urokinase are available yet.

Comparison of Thrombolytic Agents

All thrombolytic agents act directly or indirectly as plasminogen activators. Plasminogen is the proteolytic enzyme of plasma that binds to fibrin to produce a thrombus. Thrombolytic agents break the equilibrium of the plasminogen–plasmin enzyme system.

Streptokinase is an indirect activator of plasminogen. Urokinase, however, is a direct activator; its thrombolytic action depends largely on increased activity expressing the presence of fibrin.

Streptokinase, a protein from the group C streptococci, is antigenic, may lead to a severe anaphylactic reaction, and also tends to be pyrogenic. It has been used as a fixed dose infused over 20 to 30 minutes.[43,44,46,52]

Urokinase is a human product obtained from fetal kidney tissue and therefore is not antigenic or pyrogenic. Consequently, it can be injected several times if need be without causing sensitization of the patient.

The half-life of streptokinase is 10 to 12 minutes, and the half-life of urokinase is 11 to 16 minutes. Clinical studies have favored urokinase over streptokinase whether given as a single dose or by continuous infusion over a 24-hour period.

rtPAs have also been used as a fixed dose to treat PE. These very fast acting thrombolytic agents have been and still are used extensively in myocardial infarction trials. Use of acylated plasminogen–streptokinase–activator complex has not been reported in PE studies, but it is expected to work similarly to streptokinase.

Choosing a Thrombolytic Agent

Deciding which thrombolytic agent to use depends on several factors. As explained in the previous chapter, urokinase seems to be superior to streptokinase in several aspects; for example, significant cerebral hemorrhage has been reported with streptokinase more often than with urokinase. This finding may relate to the general thrombolytic stage level, which is greatest with streptokinase and acylated plasminogen–streptokinase–activator complex using a fixed dose; it is only at an intermediate level with urokinase.

Another factor to be considered is cost. We compared the cost of the three available thrombolytic agents now in use in the United States to determine which is the most economical and convenient but also effective and safe. We compared a single dose of each drug: 250,000 U/vial of streptokinase, 250,000 U/vial of urokinase, and 50 mg/vial of rtPA. The cost of one vial of streptokinase was assigned one unit ($12.31); the comparable cost of urokinase would amount to 18 units ($221.10) and of rtPA, 95 units ($1166.00). The most economical was streptokinase. However, it was the least safe. Therefore, at the University of Minnesota, urokinase is preferred over the other agents. Our thrombolytic protocols were developed not only for PE but also for venous thrombosis at any level. Our protocol for PE uses only urokinase as the agent of choice.

In a study by Verstraete et al.,[49] rtPA was given in a single dose of 50 mg as a bolus to stabilize or reverse the hemodynamic embarrassment caused by massive PE. However, they did not use continuous infusion to pursue total lysis of the clot. Actually, some patients required a second dose, which was also given as a bolus. In their experience, this injection caused a drastic drop in the fibrinogen level—a drop not observed when urokinase is infused continuously in the pulmonary artery trunk.[21]

Furthermore, if a single bolus of a fixed dose of thrombolytics is given, there is practically no need to take laboratory tests during the thrombolytic infusion because no dosage adjustments are provided. The same method was used with other trials using streptokinase and urokinase before 1990.[32,38] Bleeding complications or rapid drop in fibrinogen level is not seen when urokinase is used according to our protocol (as described in this chapter): we carefully monitor the fibrinogen levels, and as soon as they reach a critical, preset level, we stop the urokinase infusion; we do not restart it until the fibrinogen comes back to the proper level. In our experience with continuous infusion of urokinase for PE, iliofemoral vein thrombosis, or subclavian vein thrombosis, no bleeding complications have occurred as long as the protocol was followed as outlined.

Postoperative Patients

Many studies have been done of patients undergoing surgery to prevent DVT, all aimed at decreasing the incidence of PE. Yet the treatment of PE once it occurs has not changed significantly over the past 30 years.

Even after thrombolytic therapy became available, one of the contraindications that was considered absolute by previous investigators[44,48,50,51] was recent surgery (within the previous 2 weeks). However, most postoperative right-sided thromboembolic events occur within 2 weeks of major surgery. Theoretically, the benefits of thrombolytic therapy would not have any significance for postsurgical patients, according to those investigators. This policy, however, changed recently. In the early 1990s, a therapeutic plan using urokinase in recently postsurgical patients was set forth and implemented.[16] It was safe and effective, even in the early postoperative stage.

Protocol for Acute Postoperative Pulmonary Embolism

Class 1

For patients with stable hemodynamic parameters who are not acutely compromised, the following protocol is implemented:

1. Pulmonary arteriogram is done by invasive radiology, and the diagnosis is firmly established or completely ruled out.
2. If the embolus is visualized, occupies a large percentage (over 40% of the diameter) of the pulmonary artery branch, and is mostly localized to one of the lungs (usually the right pulmonary artery branch), the angiographic catheter is placed in the branch involved or positioned in the main trunk of the pulmonary artery. Measurements of the pulmonary artery pressures are taken at this point.
3. Baseline coagulation studies are carried out before the urokinase is administered to the patient, including prothrombin time, thrombin time, partial thromboplastin time, and fibrinogen level. Usually, fibrinogen levels in people with venous thrombosis are very high, varying from 0.4 to 0.8 μmol/L. Dur-

ing therapy, the fibrinogen levels should be monitored every 6 hours along with the other coagulation parameters. Hemoglobin value and hematocrit should be determined every 12 hours.

4. As soon as the diagnosis is confirmed, a bolus of urokinase is injected by way of the angiographic catheter at a dose of 2200 U per kilogram of patient's weight. Then a continuous infusion pump of urokinase solution set at a rate of 2200 U/kg per hour is connected. Heparin therapy (already started before the angiogram) is administered at the rate of 500 U/h peripherally (usually in the opposite arm). The patient is monitored in the intensive care unit during continuous infusion of urokinase, until total lysis of the clot is obtained. A pulmonary arteriogram is repeated at 12 or 24 hours. Depending on the degree of clot resolution, the decision is made to continue with urokinase infusion after the first 12 hours. Usually, complete lysis is obtained in less than 30 hours of infusion. When resolution of the clot has occurred, urokinase administration is stopped, the pulmonary catheter is removed, and the intravenous heparin dose is increased to 1000 U/h and from then on is adjusted after either the prothrombin time or thrombin time, monitoring results until further therapy is decided on. Implanting an IVC filter may be necessary; however, staying with anticoagulation therapy until the patient is discharged may be preferable.
5. As therapy with urokinase progresses, the fibrinogen level will drop, and two possibilities must be considered: (1) If the patient has had surgery within 2 weeks, the fibrinogen level should not be allowed to drift below 0.2 μmol/L; otherwise, bleeding will be a significant risk. (2) If the patient has not had any recent surgery, the fibrinogen levels are allowed to drift down to 0.15 μmol/L. On average, it takes between 48 and 72 hours for the fibrinogen to reach such a level with the stated dose of urokinase administered by continuous infusion.
6. Venous Doppler ultrasound is obtained after pulmonary emboli have cleared but while the patient is still being given heparin. Venograms may be necessary if ultrasound is insufficient to find the source of the embolism. A bidimensional echocardiogram may be needed occasionally if a cardiac source of thrombus is suggested.
7. At this point, further therapy depends on the findings of the venogram or ultrasound studies.
8. Long-term anticoagulation is necessary for only 3 months if all the venous system is clear or if a definite source of embolism is found and treated—for example, partial vein obstruction (stenosis) that requires surgical intervention or percutaneous trans-

venous balloon angioplasty with or without implanting a stent. Most of the time, the source of the embolism can be determined. If PE recurs, or if conditions are found that make recurrence likely, an IVC filter is definitely implanted.

9. If the IVC or iliac veins cannot be studied or visualized by ultrasound, venography should be obtained to assess thrombosis, stricture, or extrinsic compression.

10. The patient may need an IVC filter implant at this time if free-floating thrombi exist in the iliac veins, if an embolus occurs again during lytic therapy, or if the risk of recurrence is too dangerous (because of, for example, a previous pneumonectomy, unresolvable venous strictures in the large veins of the lower body, or malignant tumors directly invading the vein wall).

Thrombolytic therapy for PE in any hospital should be organized in a manner that is safe for all patients. A written protocol must be available in all the intensive care units and the emergency room; it must be given to the house staff at teaching hospitals. At the University of Minnesota, a small pocketbook with the standard written protocol for the use of lytic agents is given to all house staff and nursing personnel. It is also readily available in the intensive care units, the pharmacy, and the surgery office. It is very important that all personnel be familiar with this protocol to avoid serious complications or undertreatment.

Class 2

Patients who show sudden signs of shock and imminent signs of cardiac arrest are given a urokinase bolus of 2200 U per kilogram of patient's weight, intravenously, preferably by way of a centrally placed catheter. Resuscitative measures are implemented with the use of inotropic agents or fluids until the patient stabilizes hemodynamically. Cardiac massage may be needed. As soon as the patient is stable, the steps for class 1 are followed.

Class 3

Patients with chronic recurrent PE and pulmonary hypertension should be prophylactically treated with an IVC filter to prevent recurrence. They should be evaluated for a possible pulmonary thromboendarterectomy procedure if no other solution or effective therapy is found.

We showed the effectiveness and safety of treating PE with intrapulmonary urokinase infusion in 1992[21] in 13 initial patients. Our current number has increased to 30 patients, and the results have remained the same. None of the patients have died of PE, even massive types of PE.

In fact, two patients required cardiac massage and resuscitation at the time of the massive embolic event, but they recovered with the use of concomitant inotropic agents and gradually improved after receiving the bolus injection of urokinase by way of a central catheter.

We contend that thrombolytic therapy is the treatment of choice for PE of any severity in postoperative patients, no matter how recent the surgical procedure, as long as the outlined protocol is followed as described.

Posttrauma Patients

Patients suffering from severe trauma (e.g., after automobile accidents or falls), with fractured pelvic or lower extremity bones, are at high risk for PE. They tend to develop extensive pelvic venous thrombosis and a hypercoagulable state.

Their treatment differs substantially from that provided for other PE patients. Trauma patients usually have extensive injuries, frequently including a ruptured spleen or liver, and sometimes involving the great vessels. It is advisable to prophylactically implant an IVC filter (as suggested by several investigators) to prevent a fatal outcome after any surgery for life-threatening conditions.

The use of thrombolytic agents, or even heparin, leads to certain bleeding complications. If PE occurs, trauma patients cannot be treated with thrombolytic agents or even with anticoagulants. The risk of death is real.

Traumatized regions that would most likely lead to PE are the pelvis, spinal cord, and head. In a study by Winchell et al.[53] involving 9721 patients with trauma, 36 suffered PE (0.4%). The highest risk for PE was for patients with head and spinal cord injury, followed by the combination of head and long bone fractures. The third highest risk was a combination of pelvic and long bone fractures, followed closely by multiple long bone fractures. Rogers et al.[54] strongly recommended placement of an IVC filter in severely injured trauma patients. In many situations, it is the only measure that will prevent a fatal outcome after surgery to repair injuries in other parts of the body.

Multiple trauma is probably one of the few contraindications to the use of thrombolytic therapy among the wide spectrum of PE patients. All patients with a severity score greater than 15 should have a prophylactic IVC filter implanted.[55,56] This category of patients should not be treated with thrombolytic therapy under any circumstances.

Patients With Chronic Debilitating Diseases

The vast majority of PE patients have chronic debilitating diseases. Because they have not had recent surgery or trauma, they are perfect candidates for our protocol;

we use urokinase as a continuous infusion either in the pulmonary artery trunk or by way of a central catheter in the right atrium. The fibrinogen levels can be allowed to drop to 0.15 μmol/L without risking any bleeding. As long as no contraindications exist, thrombolytic agents are the treatment of choice in this category.

Because these patients are chronically prone to develop venous thrombosis in the future, it is sometimes beneficial to prescribe maintenance doses of antiplatelet aggregation agents such as aspirin or dipyridamole orally (in addition to warfarin) on a temporary or permanent basis after the PE is resolved. Many of these patients are candidates for implant of an IVC filter because of their chronic conditions and the likelihood of recurrent thrombosis and further embolization.

The outlook for long-term survival should be carefully evaluated, particularly for patients suffering advanced degrees of malignancy and multiorgan failure. Thus, some chronically ill patients may not be candidates for thrombolytic therapy.

Patients With Recurrent Venous Thrombosis

PE patients with recurrent DVT or other conditions that chronically affect their otherwise relatively good health are definitely candidates for thrombolytic therapy. The source of the embolism should be identified and treated directly to prevent recurrence, particularly for patients with so-called effort thrombosis of the subclavian vein (if they have not been treated properly and significant stenosis has remained in the subclavian vein).

The incidence of PE in this category is high[57–60]: 11% in our own series[61] and as high as 16.6% in the literature.[58] Such patients should have the stenotic subclavian vein operated on and widened[61,62] to prevent recurrent thrombosis.

PE patients with recurrent iliofemoral vein thrombosis who have not had their veins reopened (by balloon angioplasty, with or without stenting, thus reestablishing adequate flow) are candidates for implant of an IVC filter. If embolism occurs in these patients, they should also be treated with thrombolytic therapy.

Women During Pregnancy or After Delivery

Although rare, PE may occur in women either during pregnancy or shortly after delivery. Our experience is limited in this area. However, we have treated patients with iliofemoral vein thrombosis during pregnancy with thrombolytics[63] without any problems; following our protocol, we did not allow the fibrinogen level to decrease below 0.2 μmol/L. One patient with PE 3 days after delivery was also treated successfully with our protocol, again keeping the fibrinogen levels at the preset safety margin of 0.2 μmol/L.

Young Women Who Take Birth Control Pills

The use of estrogen by young women is widely known to be a causative factor of venous thrombosis and PE. Because of the extensive use of birth control pills even by patients in their teens, more DVT and PE in this population are being diagnosed in patients without any previous history of trauma or phlebitis. The first signs of thromboembolic phenomena could be PE.

At the University of Minnesota, we have seen two patients (aged 14 and 23) who developed massive PE from the use of birth control pills. The first patient survived thanks to our thrombolytic therapy protocol; she was also diagnosed with iliofemoral vein thrombosis. The second patient sat for more than 12 hours on a transatlantic flight and suffered a fatal PE 24 hours after she had deplaned.

PE in this category is definitely best treated with our protocol (continuous urokinase, 2200 U per kilogram of patient's weight per hour by way of a pulmonary catheter).

Patients With Indwelling Central Catheters

Patients with long-term placement of subclavian catheters for dialysis or chemotherapy or implanted pacemakers or transvenous defibrillators[64] who develop subclavian stricture are at risk for PE. They should be studied if significant stenosis remains in the upper veins.

Summary of Indications for Lytic Therapy in PE

The use of thrombolytic therapy for PE is recommended in all patients in categories 1, 3, 4, 5, 6, and 7. The only exception is category 2; administration of thrombolytic agents in posttrauma patients invariably leads to serious bleeding complications of lethal proportion.

The attitude of the physician treating patients with PE is of drastic importance today. As soon as the diagnosis of PE is made, the physician should contemplate thrombolytic therapy as a first-line approach. Only if contraindications exist should other options be considered.

Monitoring Thrombolysis

Because our protocol entails continuous infusion of urokinase instead of a fixed dose, the amount of lysis must be controlled and bleeding prevented, particularly in recent surgical patients. The protocols in the initial urokinase trials caused significant problems with bleeding because of the very high fixed dose of 4400 U/kg implemented at that time. Some of the bleeding that has been reported with the use of rtPA and streptokinase also may be caused by the manner of administration.

Monitoring throughout the period of urokinase continuous infusion is very important; at the same time, it is practical and easy to do. The tests to monitor the effectiveness and safety of urokinase as well as the anticoagulation levels obtained are partial thromboplastin time, thrombin time, prothrombin time, or International Normalized Ratio (INR), and fibrinogen. These are the only tests that are useful. Any other, more sophisticated tests would take too long in the laboratory and would be impractical for patients who need readjustments every few hours.

Before fibrinolytic therapy is implemented, a routine coagulation battery of tests must be obtained. The four tests mentioned earlier are to be used during the entire course of treatment because the results can usually be reported from the coagulation laboratory within a half hour. The most important test to assess fibrinolytic activity is the level of fibrinogen. Patients with hypercoagulable states, such as those with PE, DVT, or venous thrombosis in any location, usually have very high fibrinogen levels. We have observed up to 0.8 μmol/L in the initial assessment (normal value is 0.3 μmol/L).

Once therapy is under way, the fibrinogen level will drop but should not be allowed to drift below a value preset as follows: if the patient had surgery within the past 2 weeks, the fibrinogen level should not be allowed to drop below 0.20 μmol/L to prevent bleeding. If the patient has not had any recent surgery, or none within the previous 6 weeks, then the level may be allowed to drift further down to 0.15 μmol/L. Fibrinogen levels are requested every 6 hours throughout the period of therapy; if they reach the preset level of safety, then the infusion is stopped for 4 to 6 hours (usually 6 hours) and reinitiated when the fibrinogen value again returns above the preset level.

After completion of fibrinolytic therapy (which never lasts more than 30 hours), the patient remains on heparin as indicated in Table 90.1. The administration of heparin is monitored with either prothrombin time or

thrombin time at 1:4 dilution. These tests should also be checked every 6 hours. Because the patients are eventually switched to warfarin therapy, they should have INR measurements daily. In our experience, as previous publications show,[21] resolution of the pulmonary embolus has never taken more than 30 hours. Therefore, it is achieved even before the levels of fibrinogen reach a critical point.

In patients with iliofemoral vein thrombosis or subclavian vein thrombosis, with prolonged periods of infusion, we have observed that it takes between 48 and 72 hours on average for the fibrinogen to reach the preset levels.[65,66] Because our PE protocol was originally designed for patients who had recently undergone surgery (within 2 weeks) and because it has worked safely with no bleeding complications, it is very safe for patients who have not had any recent surgery.

As a corollary, therefore, we believe our protocol can be implemented for any PE patient, with great effectiveness and very minimal or nonexistent risk of bleeding. The only category for which this protocol does not apply is posttrauma patients (or individuals with other contraindications, discussed in the next section).

Contraindications for Use of Thrombolytics

Some of the classic contraindications given by previous investigators are relative and must be evaluated individually, but absolute contraindications for use of thrombolytics include the following:

1. Recent percutaneous biopsy of internal organs (e.g., kidney, liver, or lung)
2. Recent needle puncture of vessels inaccessible to manual compression (i.e., abdominal aorta or subclavian–axillary artery)
3. Lumbar puncture if done within the previous 5 days, chest tube insertion, hemothorax, and insertion of intraperitoneal catheters
4. Recent active bleeding in the gastrointestinal or genitourinary tracts
5. Known potentially serious bleeding conditions (e.g., cerebrovascular accidents, brain surgery within previous 2 months, intracranial malignancy, uncontrollable arterial hypertension, severe liver disease, renal failure, uncontrolled coagulation defects, or postpartum period within 3 days after cessation of bleeding)
6. Other miscellaneous conditions such as cavitary tuberculosis (very rare), recent trauma with internal injuries, cardiovascular resuscitation with rib fractures, and bacterial endocarditis

TABLE 90.1. Pulmonary embolism protocol for urokinase administration.

↓
Pulmonary arteriogram
Heparin 500 U/h
↓
Urokinase bolus in PA, 2200 U/kg
↓
Urokinase in PA, 2200 U/kg per hour (in ICU)
Systemic heparin 500 U/h
↓
Repeat arteriogram
↓
Stop urokinase
Heparin ↑ 1000 U/h

PA, pumonary artery; ICU, intensive care unit.

Recent surgery per se is not a contraindication; rather, each particular situation should be carefully evaluated individually. In our series,[21] we have used urokinase as early as 3 days after an operation. If urokinase is contraindicated and the patient has IVC, iliac, or iliofemoral thrombosis, then implantation of an IVC filter is probably indicated.

References

1. Lillienfeld DE, Chan E, Ehland J, Godbold JH, Landrigan PJ, Marsh G. Mortality from pulmonary embolism in the United States: 1962–1984. *Chest.* 1990;98:1067–1072.

2. Prevention of fatal postoperative pulmonary embolism by low doses of heparin: an international multicentre trial. *Lancet.* 1975;2:45–51.

3. Dalen JE, Alpert JS. Natural history of pulmonary embolism. *Prog Cardiovasc Dis.* 1975;17:259–270.

4. Prevention of venous thrombosis and pulmonary embolism. NIH Consensus Development. *JAMA.* 1986;256: 744–749.

5. Anderson FA Jr, Wheeler HB, Goldberg RJ, et al. A population-based perspective of the hospital incidence and case-facility rates of venous thrombosis and pulmonary embolism. The Worcester DVT Study. *Arch Intern Med.* 1991; 151:933–938.

6. Goldhaber SZ. Pulmonary embolism death rates. *Am Heart J.* 1988;115:1342–1346.

7. Goldhaber SZ. Thrombolytic therapy for pulmonary embolism. *Semin Vasc Surg.* 1992;5:69–75.

8. Bergqvist D, Lindblad B. A 30-year survey of pulmonary embolism verified at autopsy: an analysis of 1274 surgical patients. *Br J Surg.* 1985;72:105–108.

9. Clagett GP, Reisch JS. Prevention of venous thromboembolism in general surgical patients. Results of meta-analysis. *Ann Surg.* 1988;208:227–240.

10. Kakkar V, Cohen AT, Edmonson RA, et al. Low molecular weight versus standard heparin for prevention of venous thromboembolism after major abdominal surgery. *Lancet.* 1993;341:259–265.

11. Nurmohamed MT, Verhaeghe R, Haass S, et al. A comparative trial of a low molecular weight heparin (enoxaparin) versus standard heparin for the prophylaxis of postoperative deep vein thrombosis in general surgery. *Am J Surg.* 1995;169:567–571.

12. Atik M, Harkess JW, Wichman H. Prevention of fatal pulmonary embolism. *Surg Gynecol Obstet.* 1970;130:403–413.

13. Harris WH, Salzman EW, Athanasoulis Ca, Waltman AC, DeSanctis RW. Aspirin prophylaxis of venous thromboembolism after total hip replacement. *N Engl J Med.* 1977;297:1246–1249.

14. Greenfield LJ, Bruce TA, Nichols NB. Transvenous pulmonary embolectomy by catheter device. *Ann Surg.* 1971; 174:881–886.

15. Lindhagen A, Bergqvist D, Hallböök T. Deep vein insufficiency after postoperative thrombosis diagnosed with I-125 labeled fibrinogen uptake test. *Br J Surg.* 1984;71:511–515.

16. Ramaswami G, Nicolaides AN. The natural history of deep vein thrombosis. In: Bergqvist D, Comerota AJ, Nicolaides AN, Scurr JH, eds. *Prevention of Venous Thromboembolism.* London: Med-Orion; 1994:109–114.

17. Bergentz SE. What is new in the prophylaxis and treatment of venous thromboembolism? *World J Surg.* 1996;20: 1141–1148.

18. Lahnborg G, Berström K, Friman L, Lagergren H. Effect of low-dose heparin on incidence of postoperative pulmonary embolism detected by photoscanning. *Lancet.* 1974;1:329–331.

19. Miller GAH, Hall RJC, Paneth M. Pulmonary embolectomy, heparin, and streptokinase: their place in the treatment of acute massive pulmonary embolism. *Am Heart J.* 1977;93:568–574.

20. Sasahara AA, Sharma GVRK, Parisi AF, et al. Pulmonary embolism, pulmonary microcirculation, and thrombolytic therapy. *Angiology.* 1982;33:368–374.

21. Molina JE, Hunter DW, Yedlicka JW, Cerra FB. Thrombolytic therapy for postoperative pulmonary embolism. *Am J Surg.* 1992;163:375–381.

22. Partsch H, Kechavarz B, Mostbeck A, Köhn H, Lipp C. Frequency of pulmonary embolism in patients who have iliofemoral deep vein thrombosis and are treated with once or twice daily low-molecular weight heparin. *J Vasc Surg.* 1996;24:774–782.

23. Murray DW, Carr AJ, Bulstrode CJK. Pharmacological prophylaxis in total hip replacement [editorial]. *J Bone Joint Surg.* 1995;77:3–5.

24. Huber O, Bounameaux H, Borst F, Rohner A. Postoperative pulmonary embolism after hospital discharge: an underestimated risk. *Arch Surg.* 1992;127:310–313.

25. Kroshus TJ, Kshettry V, Hertz MI, Bolman RM III. Deep venous thrombosis and pulmonary embolism after lung transplantation. *J Thorac Cardiovasc Surg.* 1995;110: 540–544.

26. Nicolaides AN. Prevention of thromboembolism: European Consensus Statement (1991). In: Bergqvist D, Comerota AJ, Nicolaides AN, Scurr J, eds. *Prevention of Venous Thromboembolism.* London: Med-Orion; 1994:443–452.

27. Thomas DP. Treatment of pulmonary embolic disease. *N Engl J Med.* 1965;273:885–892.

28. Bauer G. Thrombosis, early diagnosis, and abortive treatment with heparin. *Lancet.* 1946;1:447–454.

29. Barritt DW, Jordan SC. Anticoagulant drugs in treatment of pulmonary embolism. *Lancet.* 1960;1:1309–1312.

30. Berry RE, George JE, Shaver WA. Free-floating deep venous thrombosis. *Ann Surg.* 1990;211:719–723.

31. Greenfield, LJ, Bruce TA, Nichols NB. Transvenous pulmonary embolectomy by catheter device. *Ann Surg.* 1971; 174:881–886.

32. Sautter RD, Myers WO, Wenzel FJ. Implications of the urokinase study concerning the surgical treatment of pulmonary embolism. *J Thorac Cardiovasc Surg.* 1972;63: 54–59.

33. Schmid C, Zietlow S, Wagner TOF, Laas J, Borst HG. Fulminant pulmonary embolism: symptoms, diagnostics, operative technique, and results. *Ann Thorac Surg.* 1991;52: 1102–1107.

34. Soyer R, Brunet AP, Redonnet M, Borg JY, Hubscher C, Letac B. Follow-up of surgically treated patients with massive pulmonary embolism with reference to 12 operated patients. *Thorac Cardiovasc Surg.* 1982;30:103–108.

35. Berger RL Pulmonary embolectomy with preoperative circulatory support. *Ann Thorac Surg.* 1973;16:217–227.

36. Reul GJ, Beall AC. Emergency pulmonary embolectomy for massive pulmonary embolism. *Circulation.* 1974;50 (suppl II):II236–II241.

37. Meyer G. Tamisier D, Sors H, et al. Pulmonary embolectomy: a 20-year experience at one center. *Ann Thorac Surg.* 1991;51:232–236.

38. Miller GAH, Sutton GC, Kerr IH, Gibson RV, Honey M. Comparison of streptokinase and heparin in treatment of isolated acute massive pulmonary embolism. *BMJ.* 1971;2: 681–684.

39. Sharma GVRK, Burleson VA, Sasahara AA. Effect of thrombolytic therapy on pulmonary-capillary blood volume in the patients with pulmonary embolism. *N Engl J Med.* 1980;303:842–845.

40. Tow DE, Wagner HN Jr, Holmes RA. Urokinase in pulmonary embolism. *N Engl J Med.* 1967;277:1161–1167.

41. Sasahara AA, Canilla JE, Belko JS, Morse RL, Criss AJ. Urokinase therapy in clinical pulmonary embolism. *N Engl J Med.* 1967;277:1168–1173.

42. Dalen JE, Haffajee CI, Alpert JS, Howe JP III, Ockene IS, Paraskos JA. Pulmonary embolism, pulmonary hemorrhage, and pulmonary infarction. *N Engl J Med.* 1977;296: 1431–1435.

43. Marder VJ, Sherry S. Thrombolytic therapy: current status (1). *N Engl J Med.* 1988;318:1512–1520.

44. Sasahara AA, Ho DD, Sharma GVRK. When and how to use fibrinolytic agents. *Drug Therapy.* 1979;4:67–84.

45. Belkin M, Belkin B, Buckman CA, Straub JJ, Lowe R. Intra-arterial fibrinolytic therapy. *Arch Surg.* 1986;121:769–773.

46. Van Breda A, Graor RA, Katzen BT, Risius B, Gillings D. Relative cost-effectiveness of urokinase versus streptokinase in the treatment of peripheral vascular disease. *J Vasc Interv Radiol.* 1991;2:77–87.

47. Tennant SN, Dixon J, Venable TC, et al. Intracoronary thrombolysis in patients with acute myocardial infarction: comparison of the efficacy of urokinase with streptokinase. *Circulation.* 1983;69:756–760.

48. Goldhaber SZ, Kessler CM, Heit JA, et al. Recombinant tissue-type plasminogen activator versus a novel dosing regimen of urokinase in acute pulmonary embolism: a randomized controlled multicenter trial. *J Am Coll Cardiol.* 1992;20:24–30.

49. Verstraete M, Miller AH, Bounameaux H, et al. Intravenous and intrapulmonary recombinant tissue-type plasminogen activator in the treatment of acute massive pulmonary embolism. *Circulation.* 1988;77:353–360.

50. Goldhaber SZ, Agnelli G, Levine MN. Reduced dose bolus alteplase vs conventional alteplase infusion for pulmonary embolism thrombolysis: an international multicenter randomized trial. *Chest.* 1994;106:718–724.

51. Sors H, Pacouret G, Azarian R, Meyer G, Charbonier B, Simonneau G. Hemodynamic effects of bolus vs. 2 hour infusion of alteplase in acute massive pulmonary embolism: a randomized controlled multicenter trial. *Chest.* 1994; 106:712–717.

52. Neuhaus KL, Wurm K, Köstering H, Tebbe U, Nebel H, Kreuzer H. Lokale Streptokinasebehandlung bei akuter lungenembolie mit shock. *Dtsch Med Wochenschr.* 1980;105: 1392–1395.

53. Winchell RJ, Hoyt DB, Walsh JC, Simons RK, Eastman AB. Risk factors associated with pulmonary embolism despite routine prophylaxis: implications for improved protection. *J Trauma.* 1994;37:600–606.

54. Rogers FB, Shackford SR, Wilson J, Ricci MA, Morris CS. Prophylactic vena cava filter insertion in severely injured trauma patients: indications and preliminary results. *J Trauma.* 1993;35:637–641.

55. Greenfield LJ, Michna BA. Twelve-year clinical experience with Greenfield vena cava filter. *Surgery.* 1988;104: 706–712.

56. Hunter JA, DeLaria GA. Hunter vena cava balloon: rationale and results. *J Vasc Surg.* 1984;1:491–497.

57. Aufses AH Jr. Venous thrombosis of the upper extremity complicated by pulmonary embolus. *Surgery.* 31954;5: 957–961.

58. Adams JT, McErog RK, DeWeese JA. Primary deep vein thrombosis of upper extremity. *Arch Surg.* 1965;91:29–42.

59. Barnett T, Levitt LM. "Effort" thrombosis of the axillary vein with pulmonary embolism. *JAMA.* 1951;146: 1412–1413.

60. Abruahma AF, Sadler DL, Robinson PA. Axillary subclavian vein thrombosis: changing patterns of etiology, diagnostic and therapeutic modalities. *Am Surg.* 1991;57: 101–107.

61. Molina JE. Surgery for effort thrombosis of the subclavian vein. *J Thorac Cardiovasc Surg.* 1992;103:341–346.

62. Molina JE. Need for emergency treatment in subclavian vein effort thrombosis. *J Am Coll Surg.* 1995;181:414–420.

63. La Valleur J, Molina E, Williams PP, Rolnick SJ. Use of urokinase in pregnancy. *Postgraduate Med.* 1996;99: 269–273.

64. Vanherwegham J-L, Yassine T, Goldman M, et al. Subclavian vein thrombosis: a frequent complication of subclavian vein cannulation for hemodialysis. *Clin Nephrol.* 1986;26:235–238.

65. Molina JE, Hunter DW, Yedlicka JW. Thrombolytic therapy for iliofemoral venous thrombosis. *Vasc Surg.* 1992;26: 630–637.

66. Bjarnason H, Kruse JR, Asinger DA, et al. Iliofemoral deep venous thrombosis: safety and efficacy outcome during five years of catheter-directed thrombolytic therapy. *J Vasc Intervent Radiol.* 1997;8:405–418.

91

Venous Thrombectomy

Gunnar Plate

The first attempts at surgical removal of deep venous thromboses were performed during the beginning of this century.[49,50,77] Larger series were presented during the late 1950s and early 1960s by Mahorner et al.,[54] Haller and Abrams,[34] Bradham and Buxton,[6] De-Weese,[17] and Fontaine and Tuchmann.[27] These communications demonstrated that fatal pulmonary embolism and venous gangrene were prevented by venous thrombectomy, and the authors assumed that the late postthrombotic sequelae were also prevented. The enthusiasm for venous thrombectomy was turned into skepticism and abandonment when Lansing and Davis in 1968[48] presented their long-term follow-up of the series reported by Haller and Abrams, demonstrating that late sequelae and valvular incompetence had developed in the majority of the patients. Karp and Wylie,[41] Mavor and Galloway,[58] and Brunner and Wirth[9] explained the poor long-term results by demonstrating that rethrombosis occurs frequently after venous thrombectomy. To avoid this complication, attempts at refining the surgical technique have continued at some institutions. Fogarty et al.[26] introduced the balloon catheter, which makes venous thrombectomy easier, safer, and more effective. It should be stressed that the patients of the crucial series reported by Lansing and Davis[48] were operated on without balloon catheters, which to some extent explains the disappointing results. Mavor and Galloway[58] have clearly demonstrated that complete vein clearance is mandatory for continued venous patency. For this purpose, Kiely[42] proposed exploration of the veins below the knee, whereas Egeblad et al.[21] and Mansfield et al.[56] stressed the importance of intraoperative phlebography. Postoperative local infusion of heparin or thrombolytic agents directly into the vein after thrombectomy has been advocated by some authors[19,31,58,73] as a means of reducing the incidence of early rethrombosis. Based on experimental work by Kunlin[47] and Bryant et al.,[10] a temporary arteriovenous fistula has also been used as protection against postoperative rethrombosis.[8,45,55]

Some recent communications[3,14,31,37,43,72,73] have demonstrated encouraging early results using variations of these new techniques for thrombectomy of iliofemoral thrombosis. All these communications lack comparison with a control group treated with conventional anticoagulation treatment, and the long-term results have not been well elucidated. In addition, the objective interpretation of the results is in many instances compromised by an insufficient number of late phlebographic examinations.

Pathophysiology

The etiology of extensive iliofemoral thromboses is basically the same as in most deep venous thromboses.[67] Compression of the left iliac vein by the overriding iliac artery may cause intraluminal fibrosis and narrowing, the so-called May–Turner syndrome,[59] explaining the marked left-sided predominance of iliofemoral thromboses. Severe cases of phlegmasia cerulea dolens are often associated with malignant disease causing venous compression as well as increased thrombogenicity.[15,51] Upper extremity thromboses are often caused by venous compression or indwelling catheters.[30,35,52,60]

The main hazards of extensive deep venous thromboses are life-threatening pulmonary embolism, limb loss from venous gangrene, and development of late sequelae. The risk for pulmonary embolism is mainly related to the location of the thrombus; the larger the vein, the greater the risk. Around 40% to 50% of patients with iliofemoral venous thrombosis have scintigraphic signs of pulmonary embolism, which in most instances is asymptomatic and of minor importance.[71] The risk for embolism seems to be less in upper extremity thrombosis but may be frequent in patients with thrombosis caused by indwelling catheters.[30,35,52,60] Venous gangrene is extremely rare in the upper extremity, but develops occasionally in extensive lower extremity thrombosis. This complication is related to an increased pressure in the muscle compartments, causing reduced tissue perfusion.[75] The incidence of late postthrombotic sequelae is difficult to establish because this syndrome deteriorates progressively with time. Still, it seems quite clear that these sequelae are more frequent with more extensive initial thrombosis.[53,64,86] Development of leg ulceration is closely related to destruction of the femoropopliteal vein valves,[79] and leg pain during exercise (venous claudication) is the result of persistent outflow obstruction caused by occluded iliac veins.[82] In patients with iliac vein obstruction combined with incompetent femoropopliteal veins, major venous hypertension and severe sequelae frequently develop.[40,53,64,86] The incidence of postthrombotic sequelae after upper extremity thrombosis is not well known. Some authors claim that chronic symptoms are extremely rare, whereas others have demonstrated postthrombotic sequelae in around 20% to 50% of patients.[30,35,52]

Clinical Features and Their Basis

The clinical presentation of extensive deep venous thromboses is usually quite obvious, with sudden onset of massive swelling and pain of the involved extremity. Physical examination reveals distended superficial veins with leg edema and tenderness. In descending thromboses starting in the pelvic area, leg swelling may be preceded by several days of diffuse pain and tenderness in and above the groin region. The swelling is obviously due to reduced venous outflow causing venous hypertension. The pain may be due to an inflammation of the vein wall (phlebitis). Patients with postoperative thrombosis often have less inflammation and less pain.[80] Severe pain may be due to a secondary compartment syndrome that develops if the venous and intracompartmental pressures exceed the perfusion pressure.[75] This condition is related to the clinical feature of phlegmasia cerulea dolens. The two well-known conditions, phlegmasia alba dolens and phlegmasia cerulea dolens, are by definition related to the actual color of the involved extremity.[29] Because the color of the limb may vary with time and elevation of the extremity, there is no clear-cut delineation between the two conditions. Still, the blue variant is more severe, with secondary affection of peripheral perfusion that increases the risk for development of venous gangrene.[29,74] Phlegmasia alba dolens and phlegmasia cerulea dolens may be misinterpreted as being caused by primary arterial obstruction. The typical swelling of the entire extremity should alert the physician to a primary venous disorder.

A carefully obtained history is crucial for the selection of therapy. Previous episodes of deep venous thrombosis make thrombectomy less likely to be of benefit to the patient. Determination of the likely age of the thrombus is

also of utmost importance. Endothelial damage and tissue ingrowth make thrombectomy or thrombolysis less successful after 5 to 7 days. Therefore, any symptom indicating when the thrombotic process started must be scrutinized. The onset of limb swelling is usually noted by the patient, but it is not uncommon that the thrombosis initially causes pain only in the pelvic area. This pain is often misjudged by the patient as well as by the physician. Symptoms of pulmonary embolism may also precede limb swelling, indicating that the thrombus is older than initially expected.

Diagnostic Tests

Diagnostic tests are first used to confirm or exclude the presence of thrombosis in the deep venous system. This is usually sufficient if only anticoagulation therapy is intended. If thrombolysis or thrombectomy is intended, information about the likely age and extension of the thrombosis is also of utmost importance. Various noninvasive tests may be used to confirm the diagnosis of deep

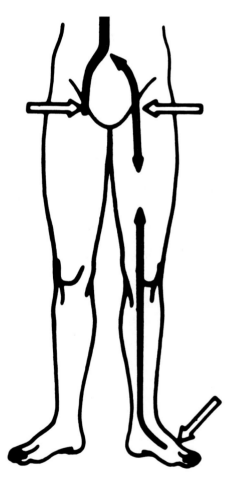

FIGURE 91.1. Technique of three-point phlebography performed in clinically suggested acute iliofemoral venous thrombosis. (From Plate et al.,[69] by permission.)

venous thrombosis. Duplex ultrasound is most reliable in femoropopliteal thromboses but is sometimes insufficient in demonstrating iliac vein thromboses. Contrast phlebography is in most cases mandatory to delineate the cephalad extension of the thrombus and to tailor the surgical procedure for the individual patient. We have found the so-called three-point phlebography to be a safe and useful procedure (Figure 91.1). The initial ascending phlebogram of the affected leg (step 1) usually confirms the presence of an extensive deep venous thrombosis, although the cranial extension of the thrombus is sometimes not visualized. This is accomplished with contrast injection into the ipsilateral common femoral vein (step 2), but injection into the contralateral femoral vein (step 3) is often required to exclude thrombus progression into the vena cava. No patient should be operated on with venous thrombectomy from the groin alone unless thrombosis of the inferior vena cava has been excluded.

Patients with iliofemoral thrombosis secondary to chronic venous obstruction are less amenable to thrombectomy alone, especially if the obstruction is caused by a neoplasm. Computerized tomography of the abdomen and pelvis is most useful for identification of such conditions before surgery. The role of nuclear magnetic resonance imaging in the diagnostic process needs further evaluation. Ventilation/perfusion scintigraphy may be used for detection of pulmonary embolism before surgery.

Medical Treatment

In addition to venous thrombectomy, two modes of treatment are available today: anticoagulation and induced thrombolysis. The main objectives of all regimens are to reestablish and preserve venous patency and to preserve valvular function, thereby avoiding major complications such as pulmonary embolism, venous gangrene, and late postthrombotic sequelae.

Anticoagulation Treatment

Anticoagulation treatment does not by itself reestablish venous patency but is in most cases successful in preventing progression and dislodgment (embolization) of the thrombus.[71] The individual's own fibrinolytic system may produce some thrombolysis, which in combination with subsequent recanalization and development of collaterals will provide sufficient venous outflow in most less-severe cases.[7,87] Therefore, anticoagulation is still the most common treatment of deep venous thromboses confined to the calf veins and the femoropopliteal segment. In patients with extensive thrombosis, these mechanisms are often insufficient, and valvular incompetence with severe venous reflux often develops with

time.[1,46,58,64] Thus, although the early clinical outcome in most cases is satisfactory with anticoagulation treatment alone, the incidence of late sequelae is not.[7,24,40,63,72] Because the postthrombotic sequelae develop over several decades, the same doctor is not likely to see the patient both at the time of the acute event and when the patient returns with late sequelae several years later. Therefore, many physicians have a falsely optimistic conception of the beneficial long-term effects with anticoagulation treatment alone. Still, in patients with a limited life expectancy, this treatment is sufficient to provide acceptable short-term results even for extensive thromboses.

As soon as a diagnosis of extensive deep venous thrombosis has been established, adequate anticoagulation treatment should be instituted. This is accomplished by a bolus intravenous injection of 5000 IU of heparin followed by a continuous heparin infusion of about 500 IU/h, adjusted to a two to three times prolongation of the activated partial thromboplastin time. Although low molecular weight heparins are commonly used for treatment of deep venous thrombosis, their efficacy has not yet been sufficiently studied for extensive iliofemoral thrombosis. The patient is allowed to ambulate with compression support on the first day after admission. Oral anticoagulation therapy is instituted and continued for at least 6 months. All patients should be encouraged to use compressive stockings if leg swelling develops in the future.

Induced Thrombolysis

Several reports have demonstrated rapid dissolution of deep venous thrombi with early restoration of venous patency.[4,13,24] Venous clearance is often incomplete, however, and rethrombosis after discontinuation of the thrombolysis is common in patients with extensive thrombosis.[13,18,81,83] After iliofemoropopliteal thromboses, venous patency and valvular competence are preserved in only a minority of the patients treated.[2,4,13,24] Venous gangrene and fatal emboli are infrequent with thrombolysis,[24] but some authors have reported slightly more fatal pulmonary emboli with thrombolytic than with anticoagulant treatment.[4,16] The long-term outcome after thrombolytic therapy has not been satisfactorily analyzed. Late sequelae seem to develop less frequently than with anticoagulant treatment alone, but this has been demonstrated mostly for less extensive thromboses localized to the femoropopliteal veins.[5,40,86] Following iliofemoral thrombosis, more than 60% of the patients develop postthrombotic sequelae with thrombolytic treatment.[24,86] In addition, there is a significant risk for hemorrhagic complications, which prohibits such treatment during pregnancy, in the puerperium, after trauma, surgery, and cerebrovascular accidents, and in patients with hemorrhagic diathesis, severe hypertension, liver disease, kidney disease, and gastroduodenal ulcers. These are all conditions in which deep venous thromboses are common. More effective and safer drugs are now available, but their effect has not yet been sufficiently evaluated, and the costs are substantial for the doses required for lysis of extensive deep venous thromboses. Therefore, the value of thrombolytic treatment in routine practice is still doubtful.

Local catheter infusion of thrombolytic agents directly into the thrombus has recently been employed at several institutions with promising early results.[14,78] This may in the future become the treatment of choice, perhaps in combination with surgery under certain circumstances. The experience is still not sufficient to provide any clear-cut conclusions regarding the long-term results of this treatment.

Surgical Treatment

The operative mortality rate has been extremely low in several series.[23,39,43,70] Scintigraphic pulmonary emboli have not occurred more frequently than with medical treatment.[71] Because thrombectomy usually is the most expeditious method of removing thrombi from the deep venous system, development of venous gangrene is most effectively prevented. In addition, venous thrombectomy is often successful in restoring iliac vein patency when thrombolytic therapy has failed.[14,81]

The long-term benefit of surgery has not been convincingly proven. At 5-year follow-up in the only prospective, randomized study of surgery for iliofemoral thrombosis,[72] the clinical and physiological results were slightly better after venous thrombectomy with an arteriovenous fistula than with anticoagulation treatment alone (Table 91.1). Whether this means that the postthrombotic sequelae are clearly prevented is still unresolved, however.

Indications

The main indications for venous thrombectomy are as follows:

1. Phlegmasia cerulea dolens or phlegmasia alba dolens
2. Other iliofemoral thrombosis if the thrombus is fresh (less than 5 to 7 days) and the patient is young and healthy

Careful patient selection is of utmost importance in achieving good results. The success of surgery depends to a great extent on the age of the thrombus. After 5 to 7 days, organization of the thrombus and valvular destruction make complete venous clearance impossible, and rethrombosis and valvular incompetence are likely to develop after thrombectomy.

Thromboses limited to the iliac veins are usually easy to remove surgically with good long-term results,[28,84] but

TABLE 91.1. Long-term results after iliofemoral venous thrombectomy: clinical and physiological 5-year results in 22 patients treated with anticoagulation (medical group) and 19 patients treated with venous thrombectomy combined with a temporary arteriovenous fistula and anticoagulation treatment (surgical group).

	Medical group	Surgical group
Leg swelling	77%	63%
Leg ulcer	14%	5%
Iliac vein occlusion	50%	21%
Venous reflux	89%	50%
Venous hypertension	89%	50%

these patients also do fairly well with conservative treatment alone. Complete clearance of the deep venous system is possible in more than a third of patients with thrombosis involving the entire extremity with excellent long-term outcome.[39,72] Even if the late results after thrombectomy of extensive thrombosis are not as good as with proximal thrombosis, these patients also do worse after conservative treatment.[7,46,53] Therefore, the extension of the thrombus per se does not affect the decision for or against surgery. Deep venous thromboses limited to the femoropopliteal segment have occasionally been operated on, but the usefulness of surgery has not been established in these cases.

Iliofemoral thromboses that develop during pregnancy must be managed in close cooperation with an obstetrician. During early pregnancy, thrombectomy combined with an arteriovenous fistula may be performed safely. During late pregnancy, venous thrombectomy may be combined with simultaneous cesarean delivery. Because these patients are usually young, they are likely to develop late sequelae if venous outflow obstruction persists and if the peripheral vein valves are destroyed. Pregnant women and women taking oral contraceptives are presently the two categories of patients most commonly subjected to venous thrombectomy.[84]

Preparations

Routine laboratory tests including anticoagulation studies and blood grouping and cross-matching should be initiated in cooperation with the radiologist and the anesthetist to decrease the risk for thrombus propagation or embolization during the time required for diagnostic procedures and preparations for surgery. These patients have a significant amount of fluid in their swollen legs and are often hypovolemic. This volume deficit must be corrected by intravenous administration of crystalloid or colloid solutions before surgery. Prophylactic antibiotics are administered to reduce the risk of wound infection.[11] The operation may be performed under local or regional anesthesia, but general intubation anesthesia is preferred. This method allows for application of a positive end-expiratory pressure of 10 to 15 cm of water during manipulation of the thrombus in the iliac or caval veins, which may reduce the risk of pulmonary embolism. Autotransfusion is recommended because these patients may lose a significant amount of blood during clearance of thrombus material from the deep veins.

Operative Technique

The long saphenous vein, the common femoral vein, and the superficial femoral artery are exposed with minimal perivascular dissection and meticulous hemostasis. A transverse or longitudinal venotomy is performed in the common femoral vein while controlling bleeding with digital compression or application of soft clamps (e.g., Fogarty clamps). A venous balloon catheter (Fogarty, no. 8 to 10) is introduced into the vena cava, the balloon is inflated with contrast material, and intraoperative fluoroscopy is used to verify the position of the catheter. Repeated thrombectomies are performed until no further thrombus material is retrieved from the iliac veins (Figure 91.2). Occasionally, the catheter may pass into the ascending lumbar vein, which may rupture if the balloon is inflated. There is also a risk that thrombus material at the caval bifurcation may become dislodged from the vena cava during return of an inflated balloon from the ascending lumbar vein (Figure 91.3). Occasionally, it is difficult to pass the catheter from the left iliac vein into the vena cava because of compression from the overlying artery and intraluminal fibrosis (venous spur). This problem can sometimes be overcome by bending the tip of the catheter before the attempted passage into the vena cava.

The peripheral veins are cleared with simultaneous occlusion of the cephalad common femoral vein to prevent embolization. If the thrombosis is fairly fresh, the peripheral thrombi are easily milked out of the deep venous system by vigorous manual compression from the foot toward the groin (Figure 91.4) or by application of an Esmarch bandage. This has to be repeated several times and may cause significant blood loss, which must be compensated for. Some thrombus material may be retrieved by careful introduction of a balloon catheter in a retrograde fashion into the deep and superficial femoral veins. This passage is compromised by the vein valves, which may be passed after careful inflation of the balloon to dilate the valvular region.

The venotomy is closed with interrupted or continuous 6-O polypropylene sutures. Finally, clearance of the iliac segment is checked by intraoperative phlebography or angioscopy.[56,76,85] An arteriovenous fistula is created by performing an end-to-side anastomosis between the divided long saphenous vein and the superficial femoral artery. The fistula is fashioned as a loop close to the skin and wrapped with a Teflon patch to facilitate later clo-

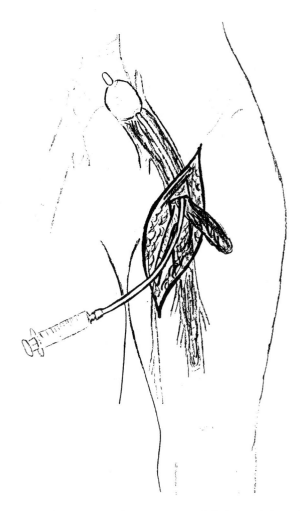

FIGURE 91.2. Venous thrombectomy of iliofemoral thrombosis. From Plate,[65] by permission.

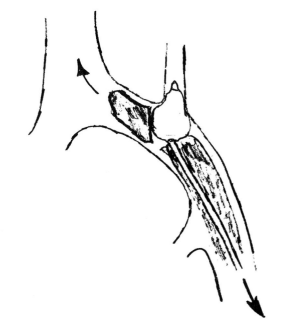

FIGURE 91.3. Dislodgment of thrombus material during balloon catheter thrombectomy.

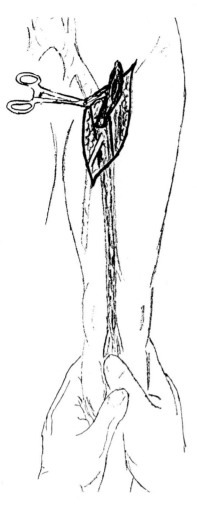

FIGURE 91.4. Peripheral vein clearance by use of manual compression. From Plate,[65] by permission.

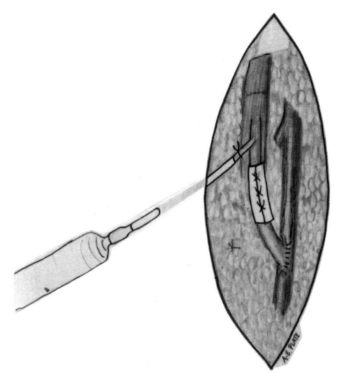

FIGURE 91.5. Constructed arteriovenous fistula with Teflon patch and infant-feeding catheter in side branch. From Plate et al.,[66] by permission.

sure. An infant-feeding catheter may be introduced through a side branch and used for intraoperative and postoperative phlebography (Figure 91.5). Suction drainage is brought out through a separate stab incision, and the wound is closed in layers, care being taken to avoid kinking of the fistula.

Technical Problems

Many surgeons have hesitated to perform venous thrombectomy because of the fear of creating pulmonary emboli. Some have used additional balloon catheters introduced by way of the same venotomy or the contralateral groin veins with the balloon inflated cephalad of the thrombus during thrombectomy. We have not used this technique because it has proved to be unnecessary if the thrombus is confined to the iliofemoral vein.[71]

If the thrombosis extends into the vena cava, the risk of pulmonary embolism is increased and other measures are required. In elderly patients with proved pulmonary

embolism it is often preferable to start the procedure by inserting a filter into the inferior vena cava cephalad of the thrombus. This is easily performed percutaneously or by surgical exposure of the right internal jugular vein. Various devices are available for this purpose.[32] This may be the only procedure required in some patients. In most young patients, it is better to remove the caval thrombus to preserve venous outflow from both lower limbs.[62] The inferior vena cava is exposed using a right-sided, transverse subcostal incision with extraperitoneal dissection. Bleeding from the vein is controlled by application of soft clamps. A longitudinal venotomy is performed, and the vein edges are separated with stay sutures during careful removal of the thrombus by milking, suction, and use of venous balloon catheters. The venotomy is closed with continuous or interrupted 5-O polypropylene stitches. It is often advantageous to perform the caval exploration at the same time as thrombectomy from the groin to secure complete venous patency before the cavotomy is closed (Figure 91.6). In patients with only minimal protrusion of the thrombus into the vena cava, it is not always necessary to perform a cavotomy; embolization is prevented by temporary application of a caval clip during thrombectomy from the groin.

Left-sided iliofemoral thromboses are often caused by compression from the overlying right common iliac artery with secondary intraluminal fibrosis, a so-called venous spur.[12,38] In these cases, complete venous clear-

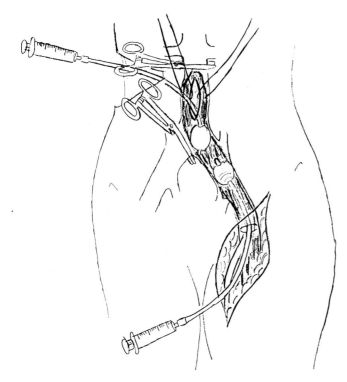

FIGURE 91.6. Simultaneous direct removal of thrombus from the vena cava and venous thrombectomy from the groin. From Plate,[65] by permission.

ance is difficult, the risk for rethrombosis is greatly increased, and the long-term results are more dubious. Some surgeons use ring strippers, balloon dilatation, and stents to overcome such venous spurs.[13,38,85] Others suggest direct exposure and reconstruction of the caval inflow.[82] The value of such aggressive measures has not been convincingly proved.[68] Therefore, we have relied on iliofemoral thrombectomy in combination with an arteriovenous fistula to keep most of the iliac vein patent and to promote development of collateral flow.

In ascending thrombosis when the peripheral thrombus is older, clearance of the peripheral veins may be difficult. Gruss[33] has suggested exploration of the popliteal and/or tibial veins with construction of a peripheral fistula to allow clearance and maintenance of femoropopliteal venous patency in such cases. Intraoperative administration of thrombolytic agents has also been used in some institutions.[61] The benefit with these additional procedures is not obvious, because the vein valves are likely already destroyed in the case of an old thrombus. On the contrary, ligation of the superficial femoral vein has been proposed to prevent pulmonary embolism and late venous reflux. Although still controversial, it seems as if this procedure is fairly well tolerated if the deep femoral vein is patent and competent.[57] This may be difficult to assess in the acute situation, however.

In severe cases of phlegmasia cerulea dolens it is of utmost importance to achieve a rapid decompression of the muscle compartments below the knee. Except for immediate and successful thrombectomy, this is best accomplished by fasciotomy of all muscle compartments of the calf. In less severe cases, the need for fasciotomy may be assessed by measurement of intracompartmental pressures, the critical level being about 30 mm Hg.[75]

Venous thrombectomy is seldom indicated in upper extremity thrombosis but may be beneficial in some patients with severe arm swelling.[30,35,52] It is performed by exposing the axillary vein and using a venous balloon catheter. The value of an arteriovenous fistula or other adjunctive procedures has not been elucidated. The presence of venous compression may indicate a need for resection of the first rib or a cervical rib.

Postoperative Management

Full anticoagulation therapy should be resumed as soon as possible (meticulous operative hemostasis is therefore crucial). Oral anticoagulation administration is started

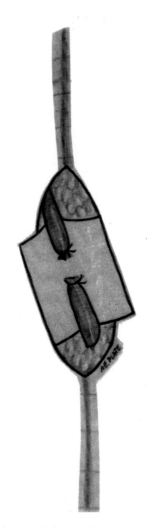

FIGURE 91.7. Closure of the arteriovenous fistula. From Plate et al.,[66] by permission.

on the first postoperative day and continued for at least 6 months. Heparin administration is continued for at least 5 days and until therapeutic oral anticoagulation has been achieved. The patient is allowed to ambulate on the first postoperative day. Compressive stocking support should be used for several months and as long as leg swelling persists. The patient may in most cases be discharged from the hospital 1 week after the operation.

The arteriovenous fistula could be closed after 6 to 8 weeks when healing of the venous endothelium has occurred.[23] In pregnant women, the fistula is maintained until several weeks after delivery. Fistula closure is a simple procedure using local anesthesia and a short skin incision over the maximum thrill created by the fistula (Figure 91.7), which is easily identified by the Teflon patch and then divided and ligated. An intraoperative phlebogram may be obtained to check iliac vein patency. This operation is performed as an outpatient procedure. Other techniques for fistula closure have been described elsewhere.[20,25]

Summary

The most important measures in performing a safe and successful venous thrombectomy are as follows:

- Careful patient selection
- Identification and control of thrombus in the vena cava
- Complete clearance of central and peripheral veins
- Effective prevention of rethrombosis

Most likely, the technique of surgical thrombectomy could be further improved by the following:

- More aggressive clearance of the peripheral veins with placement of the fistula at a more peripheral level to improve the preservation of valvular function
- Combination of thrombectomy with infusion of thrombolytic agents to provide more effective vein clearance
- Use of intravascular devices to overcome vein compression

References

1. Åkesson H, Brudin L, Dahlström JA, Eklöf B, Ohlin P, Plate G. Venous function assessed during a 5 year period after acute iliofemoral venous thrombosis treated with anticoagulation. *Eur J Vasc Surg.* 1990;4:43–48.
2. Albrechtsson U, Andersson J, Einarsson E, Eklöf B, Norgren L. Streptokinase treatment of deep vein thrombosis and the postthrombotic syndrome. Follow-up evaluation of venous function in the post-thrombotic legs. *Arch Surg.* 1981;116:33–37.
3. Andriopoulos A, Wirsing P, Bötticher R. Results of iliofemoral venous thrombectomy after acute thrombosis. Report on 165 cases. *J Cardiovasc Surg.* 1982;23:123–124.
4. Arnesen H, Heilo A, Jacobsen E, Ly B, Skaga E. A prospective study of streptokinase and heparin in the treatment of deep vein thrombosis. *Acta Med Scand.* 1978;203:457–463.
5. Arnesen H, Höiseth A, Ly B. Streptokinase or heparin in the treatment of deep vein thrombosis. *Acta Med Scand.* 1981;211:65–68.
6. Bradham RR, Buxton JT. Thrombectomy for acute iliofemoral venous thrombosis. *Surg Gynecol Obstet.* 1964; 119:1271–1275.
7. Browse NL, Clemenson C, Lea Thomas M. Is the postphlebitic leg always postphlebitic? Relation between phlebographic appearances of deep-vein thrombosis and late sequelae. *BMJ.* 1980;281:1167–1170.
8. Brunner U. Die femoroiliakale Thrombose als evolutive Venenobstruktion: Probleme in chirurgischer Sicht. *Vasa.* 1974;3:22–26.
9. Brunner U, Wirth W. Spätresultate nach Thrombektomie bei Iliofemoralvenenthrombose im klinisch-radiologischen Vergleich. *Schweiz Med Wochenschr.* 1971;101: 1327–1334.
10. Bryant MF, Lazenby WD, Howard JM. Experimental replacement of short segments of veins. *Arch Surg.* 1958;76: 289–293.
11. Christensson J, Einarsson E, Eklöf B. Infection complications after thrombectomy in deep venous thrombosis. *Acta Chir Scand.* 1977;143:431–434.
12. Cockett FB, Lea Thomas M, Negus D. Iliac vein compression. Its relation to iliofemoral thrombosis and the postthrombotic syndrome. *BMJ.* 1967;2:14–19.
13. Comerota AJ, Aldridge SC. Thrombolytic therapy for deep venous thrombosis, a clinical review. *Can J Surg.* 1993;36: 359–364.
14. Comerota AJ, Aldridge SC, Cohen G, Ball DS, Pliskin M, White JV. A strategy of aggressive regional therapy for acute iliofemoral venous thrombosis with contemporary venous thrombectomy or catheter-directed thrombolysis. *J Vasc Surg.* 1994;20:244–254.
15. Coon WW. Epidemiology of venous thromboembolism. *Ann Surg.* 1977;186:149–164.
16. Denck H. Operative therapie (Thrombektomie, Schirmfilter, Cavaligatur). *Langenbecks Arch Chir.* 1977;345:381–388.
17. DeWeese JA. Thrombectomy for acute iliofemoral venous thrombosis. *J Cardiovasc Surg.* 1964;5:703–712.
18. Dhall DP, Dawson AA, Mavor GE. Problems of resistant thrombolysis and early recurrent thrombosis in streptokinase therapy. *Surg Gynecol Obstet.* 1978;146:15–20.
19. Edwards WH, Sawyers JL, Foster JH. Iliofemoral venous thrombosis: reappraisal of thrombectomy. *Ann Surg.* 1970; 171:961–970.
20. Edwards WS. A-V fistula after venous reconstruction. A simplified method of producing and obliterating the shunt. *Ann Surg.* 1982;196:669–671.
21. Egeblad K, Bojsen-Möller J, Jacobsen B. Kirurgisk behandling av dyb venös trombose. *Nord Med.* 1970;83:438–443.
22. Einarsson E, Albrechtsson U, Eklöf B, Norgren L. Follow up evaluation of venous morphologic factors and function after thrombectomy and temporary arteriovenous fistula

in thrombosis of iliofemoral vein. *Surg Gynecol Obstet.* 1986; 163:111–116.

23. Einarsson E, Eklöf B, Kuenzig M, et al. Scanning electron-microscopy and Evans blue staining for assessing endothelial trauma and reconstruction after venous treatment. *Scan Electron Microsc.* 1984;1:273–278.

24. Elliot MS, Immelman EJ, Jeffery P, et al. A comparative randomized trial of heparin versus streptokinase in the treatment of acute proximal venous thrombosis: an interim report of a prospective trial. *Br J Surg.* 1979;66: 838–843.

25. Endrys J, Eklöf B, Neglén P, Zyka I, Peregrin J. Percutaneous balloon closure of temporary femoral arteriovenous fistula after venous thrombectomy. *Acta Chir Scand.* 1985; 151:607–611.

26. Fogarty TJ, Dennis D, Krippachne WW. Surgical management of iliofemoral venous thrombosis. *Am J Surg.* 1966; 112:211–217.

27. Fontaine R, Tuchmann L. The role of thrombectomy in deep venous thromboses. *J Cardiovasc Surg.* 1964;5: 298–312.

28. Gänger KH, Nachbur BH, Ris HB, Zurbrügg H. Surgical thrombectomy versus conservative treatment for deep venous thrombosis: functional comparison of long-term results. *Eur J Vasc Surg.* 1989;3:529–538.

29. Gloviczki P, Hollier LH, Cherry KJ, Pairolero PC, Gale SS, Schirger A. Phlegmasia cerulea dolens: the continuing morbidity. *Int Angiol.* 1982;1:127–134.

30. Gloviczki P, Kazmier FJ, Hollier LH. Axillary-subclavian venous occlusion: the morbidity of a nonlethal disease. *J Vasc Surg.* 1986;4:333–337.

31. Goto H, Wada T, Matsumoto A, Matsumoto H, Soma T. Iliofemoral venous thrombectomy. *J Cardiovasc Surg.* 1980; 21:341–346.

32. Greenfield LJ, DeLucia A Endovascular therapy of venous thromboembolic disease. *Surg Clin North Am.* 1992;72: 964–989.

33. Gruss JD. Venous reconstruction, I. *Phlebology.* 1988;3: 7–18.

34. Haller JA, Abrams BL. Use of thrombectomy in the treatment of acute iliofemoral venous thrombosis in forty-five patients. *Ann Surg.* 1963;158:561–569.

35. Horattas MC, Wright DJ, Fenton AH, et al. Changing concepts of deep venous thrombosis of the upper extremity. Report of a series and review of the literature. *Surgery.* 1988;104:561–567.

36. Horsch S, Zehle A., Eisenhardt HJ, Landes T, Pichlmaier H. Chirurgische Behandlung der akuten Bein- und Beckenvenenthrombose. *Med Klin.* 1979;74:101–108.

37. Hutschenreiter S, Vollmar J, Loeprecht H, Abendschein A, Rödl W. Rekonstruktive Eingriffe am Venensystem-Spätergebnisse unter kritscher Bewertung funktioneller und gefässmorphologischer Kriterien. *Chirurg.* 1979;50: 555–563.

38. Jakob H, Maass D, Schmiedt W, Schild H, Oelert H. Treatment of major venous obstruction with an expandable endoluminal spiral prosthesis. *J Cardiovasc Surg.* 1989;30: 112–117.

39. Juhan CM, Alimi YS, Barthelemy PS, Fabre DF, Riviere CS. Late results of iliofemoral venous thrombectomy. *J Vasc Surg.* 1997;25:417–422.

40. Kakkar VV, Lawrence D. Hemodynamic and clinical assessment after therapy for acute deep vein thrombosis. *Am J Surg.* 1985;150:54–63.

41. Karp RB, Wylie EJ. Recurrent thrombosis after iliofemoral venous thrombectomy. *Surg Forum.* 1966;17:147.

42. Kiely PE. A new venous thrombectomy technique. *Br J Surg.* 1973;60:850–852.

43. Kistner RL, Sparkuhl MD. Surgery in acute and chronic venous disease. *Surgery.* 1979;85:31–43.

44. Kitainik E, Quiros RS. Thrombectomy and caval interruption. *J Cardiovasc Surg.* 1972;13:440–445.

45. Köpf RI, Stahlknecht CD. Temporäre Arterialisation der Venenstrombahn nach operativer Thrombektomie. *Bruns Beitr Klin Chir.* 1973;220:719–724.

46. Kriessman A, Rupp N. Natürlicher Verlauf der venösen Drainage-Insuffizienz bei Becken- und tiefer Beinvenenthrombose. *Vasa.* 1977;6:124–127.

47. Kunlin JL. Le rétablissement de la circulation veineuse par greffe en cas d'oblitération traumatique ou thrombophlébitique. Greffe de 18 cm entre la veine saphéne interne et la veine iliaque externe. Thrombose aprés trois semaines de perméabilité. *Mem Acad Chir (Paris).* 1953;79: 109–110.

48. Lansing AM, Davis WM. Five-year follow-up study of iliofemoral venous thrombectomy. *Ann Surg.* 1968;168: 620–628.

49. Läwen A. Ueber Thrombektomie bei Venenthrombose und Arteriospasmus. *Zentralbl Chir.* 1937;64:961–968.

50. Leriche R. Traitement chirurgical des suites éloignées des phlébites et des grands oedémes non medicaux des membres inférieurs. *Bull Mem Soc Nat Chir.* 1927;53:187–195.

51. Lieberman JS, Borrero J, Urdaneta E, Wright IS. Thrombophlebitis and cancer. *JAMA.* 1961;177:72–75.

52. Lindblad B, Bergqvist D. Aggressive or conservative treatment in subclavian vein thrombosis. In: Eklöf B, Gjöres JE, Thulesius O, Bergqvist D, eds. *Controversies in the Management of Venous Disorders.* London: Butterworths; 1989: 141–158.

53. Lindner DJ, Edwards JM, Phinney ES, Taylor LM, Porter JM. Long-term hemodynamic and clinical sequelae of lower extremity deep vein thrombosis. *J Vasc Surg.* 1986; 4:436–442.

54. Mahorner H, Castleberry JW, Coleman WO. Attempts to restore function in major veins which are the site of massive thrombosis. *Ann Surg.* 1957;146:510–522.

55. Maillard J-N, Gillot C. Artérialisation du segment veineux thrombectomise dans le traitement chirurgical tarif d´une thrombose de la veine cave inférieure. *Presse Med.* 1970; 78:2417–2419.

56. Mansfield AO, Carmichael JHE, Parry EW. Thrombectomy employing continuous radiological control. *Br J Surg.* 1971;58:119–123.

57. Masuda EM, Kistner RL, Ferris EB. Long-term effect of superficial femoral vein ligation: thirteen-year follow-up. *J Vasc Surg.* 1992;16:741–749.

58. Mavor GE, Galloway JMD. Iliofemoral venous thrombosis. *Br J Surg.* 1969;56: 43–59.

59. May R, Thurner J. Ein Gefässporn in der v. iliaca com. sin als wahrscheinliche Ursache der überwiegend linksseiti-

gen Beckenvenenthrombose. *Z Kreislaufforsch.* 1956;45: 912–922.

60. Monreal M, Lafoz E, Rutz J, Valls R, Alastrue A. Upper-extremity deep venous thrombosis and pulmonary embolism: a prospective study. *Chest.* 1991;99:280–283.

61. Nachbur B, Wiesman A. Können die Behandlungsergebnisse bei tiefer Thrombophlebitis verbessert werden durch Kombination von chirurgischer Thrombektomie und regionale Fibrinolyse? *Helv Chir Acta.* 1977;44:791–796.

62. Neglén P, Nazzal MMS, Al-Hassan HK, Christenson JT, Eklöf B. Surgical removal of an inferior vena cava thrombus. *Eur J Surg.* 1992;6:78–82.

63. O'Donnell TF, Browse NL, Burnand KG, Lea Thomas M. The socioeconomic effects of an iliofemoral venous thrombosis. *J Surg Res.* 1977;22:483–488.

64. Partsch H. Funktionelle Resultate nach tiefer Venenthrombose des Oberschenkels und des Beckens in Abhängigkeit det Therapieform. *Vasa.* 1987;20(suppl): 90–94.

65. Plate G. Surgical treatment of acute deep venous thrombosis. In: Waerstad A, Westbye O, Beerman B, Strandberg K, eds. *Workshop: Treatment of Venous Thrombosis and Pulmonary Embolism.* Oslo, Norway: Falch Hurtigtrykk; 1995:141–162.

66. Plate G, Albrechtsson U, Einarsson E, Eklöf B. Technical problems in thrombectomy with a temporary arteriovenous fistula in the treatment of acute iliofemoral vein thrombosis. In: May R, Weber J, eds. *Pelvic and Abdominal Veins.* Amsterdam: Excerpta Medica; 1981:224–230.

67. Plate G, Einarsson E, Eklöf B. Etiologic spectrum in acute iliofemoral venous thrombosis. *Int Angiol.* 1986;5:59–62.

68. Plate G, Einarsson E, Eklöf B, Jensen R, Ohlin P. Iliac vein obstruction associated with acute iliofemoral venous thrombosis. Results of early reconstruction using polytetrafluoroethylene grafts. *Acta Chir Scand.* 1985;151: 607–611.

69. Plate G, Einarsson E, Ohlin P, Jensen R, Qvarfordt P, Eklöf B. Thrombectomy with temporary arteriovenous fistula: the treatment of choice in acute iliofemoral venous thrombosis. *J Vasc Surg.* 1984;1:867–876.

70. Plate G, Eklöf B, Norgren L, Ohlin P, Dahlström JA. Venous thrombectomy for iliofemoral vein thrombosis: 10-year results of a prospective randomized study. *Eur J Vasc Endovasc Surg.* 1997;14:367–374.

71. Plate G, Ohlin P, Eklöf B. Pulmonary embolism in acute iliofemoral venous thrombosis. *Br J Surg.* 1985;72:912–916.

72. Plate G, Åkesson H, Einarsson E, Ohlin P, Eklöf B. Long-term results of venous thrombectomy combined with a temporary arterio-venous fistula. *Eur J Vasc Surg.* 1990; 4:483–489.

73. Poilleux J, Chermet J, Bigot J-M, Deliere T. Les thromboses veineuses ilio-femorales recentes. *Ann Chir.* 1975; 29: 713–719.

74. Provan JL, Rumble EJ. Re-evaluation of thrombectomy in the management of iliofemoral venous thrombosis. *Can J Surg.* 1979;22:378–381.

75. Qvarfordt P, Eklöf B, Ohlin P. Intramuscular pressure in the lower leg in deep vein thrombosis and phlegmasia cerulea dolens. *Ann Surg.* 1983;197:450–453.

76. Risberg B, Konrad P, Örtenwall P, Smith L. Venous endoscopy in thrombectomy of the iliac vein using the choledochoscope. *Eur J Vasc Surg.* 1990;4:297–300.

77. Schnitzler J. Ueber die chirurgische Behandlung der Varicen nebst Bemerkungen zur postopertiven Phlebitis. *Wien Med Wochenschr.* 1911;61:241–245.

78. Semba CP, Dake MD. Iliofemoral deep venous thrombosis: Aggressive therapy with catheter-directed thrombolysis. *Radiology.* 1994;191:487–494.

79. Shull KC, Nicolaides AN, Fernandes e Fernandes J. Significance of popliteal reflux in relation to ambulatory venous pressure and ulceration. *Arch Surg.* 1979;114:1304–1306.

80. Solis MM, Ravel TJ, Nix ML, et al. Is anticoagulation indicated for asymptomatic postoperative calf vein thrombosis? *J Vasc Surg.* 1992;16:414–419.

81. Stiegler H, Hiller E, Arbogast H, Heim G, Schildberg FW. Thrombektomie nach erfolgloser Lysetherapie tiefer Bein-Becken venenthrombosen: ein sinnvolles verfahren? *Vasa.* 1992;21:280–288.

82. Taheri SA, Nowakowski P, Pendergast D, Cullen J, Pisano S, Boman L. Iliocaval compression syndrome. *Phlebology.* 1987;2:173–179.

83. Thiess W, Wirtzfield A, Fink U, Maubach P. The success rate of fibrinolytic therapy in fresh and old thrombosis of the iliac and femoral veins. *Angiology.* 1983;34: 61–69.

84. Törngren S, Bremme K, Hjertberg R, Swedenborg J. Late results of thrombectomy for ilio-femoral venous thrombosis. *Phlebology.* 1991;6:249–254.

85. Vollmar J, Loeprecht H, Hutschenreiter S. Rekonstruktive Eingriffe am Venensystem. *Chirurg.* 1978;49:296–302.

86. Watz R, Savidge GF. Rapid thrombolysis and preservation of valvular venous function in high deep vein thrombosis. *Acta Med Scand.* 1979;205:293–298.

87. Widmer LK, Brandenberg E, Widmer M-T, et al. Late sequelae of deep venous thrombosis. *Int Angiol.* 1982;1: 31–37.

92

Principles in Hemostasis

Gernold Wozniak

Basic Considerations

Since 1905, when Morowitz[1] first initiated clotting research and summarized his classical scheme, scientific interest in hemostasis has increased enormously. In 1955 Deutsch[2] wrote a renowned book titled *Blood Coagulation Factors* and began his preface as follows:

In the last two decades, coagulation research has gone through a speedy development. Biochemical working methods and ways of thinking have found input and have extensively suppressed pure clinical and pathophysiological points of view. This development has not only led to discovering a larger number of coagulation factors, but it has also enabled gain of the pure form of many of these factors and to characterize them so well in their physical and chemical attributes that their existence is ascertained, whereas 20 years ago, it seemed that this could only be made evident in fibrinogen. The opinions about the theory of the coagulation process have also gone through corresponding changes. But now the development seems to have come to a conclusion. (v)

Today, more than 40 years later, it seems only natural to write similar statements, but developments in recent years have taught us that *coagulation* means far more than generally assumed. Aside from the latest knowledge about proteins, proteases, and enzymes, such as protein C,[3-7] protein S,[5,8-10] heparin cofactor II,[11,12] and tissue-type plasminogen activator (tPA),[13-15] the knowledge about manifold cross-linking of the coagulation cascade with other cascadelike systems, such as the kallikrein system,[16-19] the complement system,[16,20-23] and the fibrinolysis system,[18,24] has increased enormously.[21,22,25,26] Scientific and clinical discovery about these relevant facts and clarification about relationships between corpuscular blood parts, plasmatic components, and the endothelial system[18,20,25,27,28] make hemostasis an exceptional interdisciplinary field of science, research, and therapy.

The occurrence of heparin-associated thrombocytopenia (HAT) with clinically relevant venous thrombosis or arterial thromboembolism,[29-34] lupus anticoagulants (LAs), anticardiolipin antibodies[35-39] (which are related to women of childbearing age with distinct tendencies toward miscarriage[40,41]), prognostically valuable hemostatic changes in patients with septic diseases or polytrauma,[42-45] and the numerous cell-bound or systemic hemostatic findings in various forms of carcinoma in oncology[46-52] elucidate the interdisciplinary importance of hemostasis. In this chapter I present the physiological bases of hemostasis, the causes of venous thrombosis and the hypercoagulable state, and the essential mechanisms and facts of therapeutic fibrinolysis.

Physiology of Hemostasis

The essential task of hemostasis is to maintain the integrity of blood circulation. In cooperation with thrombocytes and the vessel wall via the first (vasoconstriction and platelet aggregation) and second phases (development of fibrin clot) of hemostasis, the coagulation system (Figure 92.1) prevents loss of blood after injury of a blood vessel or of the endothelium. The fibrinolytic system, which also cooperates with endothelial and thrombotic factors, provides balance so that excessive thrombus formation, which could otherwise clot the vessel lumen and thus impair blood supply to the organs, is inhibited. In addition to the factors of the clotting and fibrinolysis systems, a series of other inhibitors also influence the balance of both systems. A close correlation exists between vessel content and vessel wall in all of these processes. These correlations have to be understood as a permanent dynamic occurrence in which factors of other cascade systems (Figure 92.2) participate as either inhibitors or accelerators,[16-20,22] because many results support the theory that coagulation and fibrinolytic proteins, including their inhibitors, are continuously converted.[28]

Apart from the synthesis of quantitatively sufficient and qualitatively functional hemostasis and adequate vascular perfusion, an intact clearance function of the reticuloendothelial system for the activated proteins and their split products is required for physiological hemostasis balance.[28] The reduction of clotting ability under a critical limit leads to hypocoagulability and thus to possible hemorrhagic diathesis. Multiplication and activation of the coagulation factors with limited clearance may lead to local or disseminated hypercoagulability.

Vessel Wall

Vasoconstriction not only provides some control of bleeding, but initiation of coagulation is influenced by the accumulation of thrombocytes in impaired circulation. Because of the complexity of vasoconstriction, it is not yet clear which mediators and reactions maintain the function; however, various vasoactive substances, such as

serotonin and thromboxane A_2 (TXA_2), which are generated and released from thrombocytes, play a significant role.[53,54] TXA_2 is itself a stimulus for further adhesion and aggregation of thrombocytes. The endothelium is also able to produce vasoconstrictive substances such as endothelin.[55] Other smaller peptides such as bradykinin, which can develop through contact activation via factor XII and kallikrein, cause increased contractility of smooth muscle cells and even alter vascular permeability.[18,19,56–59] A fragment split off during the conversion of fibrinogen to fibrin is fibrinopeptide B, which is also able to induce contraction in the smooth vascular muscle cells.[60]

The intact endothelium has the task of relaxing the vessel and providing as antithrombogenic a vascular inner space as possible (Figure 92.3). Some of the dilating substances produced in endothelium are prostacyclin and the endothelial-derived relaxing factor. Therefore, by indirectly reducing thrombocyte adhesion, prostacyclin is also an antithrombotic working substance but with only local effect. Prostacyclin's biological half-life is only

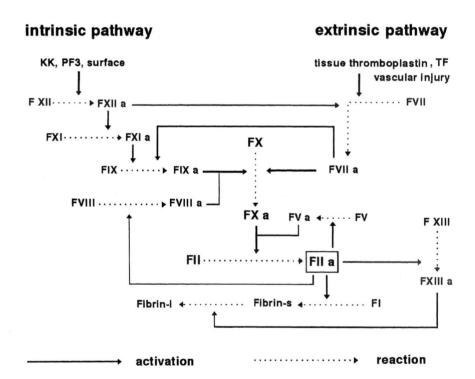

FIGURE 92.1. Coagulation pathway.

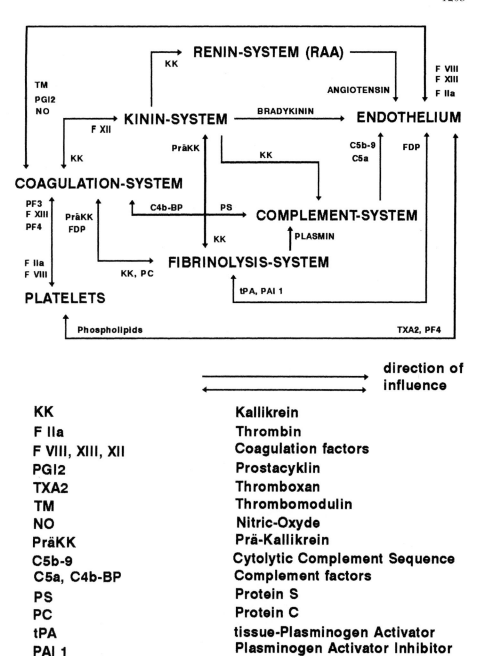

FIGURE 92.2. Cross-linking between different mediator and hemostatic systems.

KK	Kallikrein
F IIa	Thrombin
F VIII, XIII, XII	Coagulation factors
PGI2	Prostacyklin
TXA2	Thromboxan
TM	Thrombomodulin
NO	Nitric-Oxyde
PräKK	Prä-Kallikrein
C5b-9	Cytolytic Complement Sequence
C5a, C4b-BP	Complement factors
PS	Protein S
PC	Protein C
tPA	tissue-Plasminogen Activator
PAI 1	Plasminogen Activator Inhibitor
FDP	Fibrin (ogen) Degradation Products

a few seconds, as is that of TXA$_2$.[61] The negative-loaded endothelial surface and heparin sulfates and thrombomodulin also offer important antithrombogenic protective mechanisms.[17,62] Thrombomodulin is found on all endothelial cell surfaces except those in the microcirculation of the brain.[62] The amount of thrombomodulin is subjected to some up-regulation and down-regulation, which is responsible for thrombophilic coagulation in some diseases. Apart from protein C activation, thrombin loses its thrombogenic potency after linking with thrombomodulin.[3,4,8]

Thrombogenic factors, such as von Willebrand's factor, plasminogen activator inhibitor 1 (PAI-1), and platelet activating factor, are also formed in the endothelial cells,[63] but the endothelium also supplies an essentially fibrinolytic substance with the tPA.

Similar to a vascular or endothelial injury, exposure of endothelium to endotoxins, interleukin 1, or tumor necrosis factor results in multiple tissue factor activity and hence to quicker thrombin generation and reduction of thrombomodulin function.[64] Because tumor necrosis factor and interleukin 1 are both mediators of inflammation, there is a close correlation via the endothelium between inflammatory mechanisms and coagulation.[65]

The quantity and quality of endothelial mechanisms, which directly or indirectly participate in hemostasis

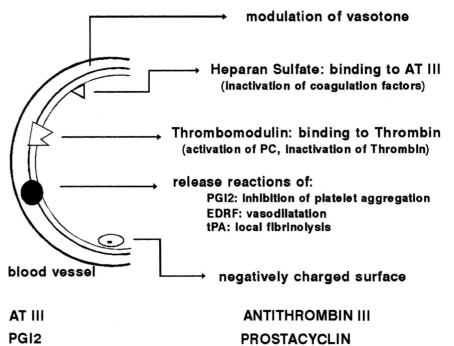

modulation of vasotone

Heparan Sulfate: binding to AT III
(inactivation of coagulation factors)

Thrombomodulin: binding to Thrombin
(activation of PC, inactivation of Thrombin)

release reactions of:
PGI2: inhibition of platelet aggregation
EDRF: vasodilatation
tPA: local fibrinolysis

blood vessel

negatively charged surface

FIGURE 92.3. Antithrombotic properties of intact endothelium.

AT III	ANTITHROMBIN III
PGI2	PROSTACYCLIN
EDRF	ENDOTHELIAL DERIVED RELAXING FACTOR
tPA	TISSUE-PLASMINOGEN ACTIVATOR

processes, depend considerably on localization of endothelial cells. Therefore, capillary endothelium secretes about 100-fold more tPA than venous endothelium, but both endothelial cells produce a comparable level of thrombomodulin activity.[66]

Platelet

Thrombocytes derive from the cytoplasm of the megakaryocytes, have a length diameter of 2 to 4 μm, a cross diameter of about 1 μm, and a life span of 7 to 11 days in circulating blood. These anuclear cells circulate as free-floating cells and do not adhere to normal vascular endothelium or to each other. Cytoplasm from dormant thrombocytes is surrounded by glycocalix, which show variable invagination in cytoplasm. These invaginations are referred to as a surface-connected open canalicular system and play a role in the uptake and conversion of substances from plasma.[28,62] Actin filaments and a circumferential band of microtubules may be necessary for stabilizing the dormant thrombocytes. Various subcellular storage granules, such as α-granules and β-granules (dense bodies) are seen under electronic microscope. Among other substances, α-granules store β-thromboglobulin, platelet factor 4, platelet-derived growth factor, von Willebrand's factor, factor V, fibrinogen, and thrombospondin.

The dense bodies contain metabolically inactive adenosine diphosphate, adenosine triphosphate, calcium, and serotonin.[62]

The so-called dense tubular system, which consists of a membrane system of channels and bubbles, is also found. This membrane system, with its similarity to the sarcoplasmic reticulum of the muscle, is a site for calcium storage and TXA_2 synthesis.[28] Regardless of the means of activation, platelets provide a procoagulant surface on which blood coagulation is accelerated. Platelets also inhibit the anticoagulant activity of heparin by secreting platelet factor 4 and serve as donors for the phospholipids required for plasma coagulation.[53]

On the whole, platelets have different ways of influencing coagulation. The essential task of thrombocytes is to form a hemostatic plug at either the vascular or endothelial injury site and to supply phospholipids, which are critical for plasmatic coagulation. After stimulation platelets are capable of the following functional and morphological changes: adhesion, shape change, aggregation, and release reaction. Within seconds of injury, platelets accumulate at the site of vascular damage and begin to adhere to subendothelial or perivascular connective tissue that has become exposed to circulating blood.[62] This phenomenon of platelet adhesion is the initial step in the formation of a hemostatic plug.[67] Besides subendothelial structures, thrombocyte activation and adhesion can also be caused by thrombin, immune complexes, adenosine diphosphate, adrenaline, noradrenaline, serotonin, vasopressin, and turbulent (shear forces) blood flow.[28,62,68] Laminin, fibronectin, microfibrils, and collagen, which is the major component to which platelets adhere, all belong to the subendothelial structures.[62]

The exact mechanism of platelet adhesion is not yet fully understood, but investigations on patients with hereditary bleeding disorders and platelet adhesion problems (e.g., von Willebrand's disease and Bernard–Soulier syndrome) have provided some clarity. Current information suggests that platelets bind to collagen through von Willebrand's factor and a specific receptor on the platelet surface (glycoprotein Ib) (Table 92.1). von Willebrand's factor binds to the collagen structure in the first stage, and thrombocytes bind to the formed surface complex in the second stage. After adhesion, thrombocytes become spherical rather than disk shaped and develop pseudopodia. Reversible shape change is followed by an irreversible release reaction after sufficient activation in which various substances such as adenosine diphosphate, platelet factor 4, von Willebrand's factor, platelet-derived growth factor, serotonin, and TXA$_2$ are actively discharged from the platelets. The release reaction is caused by contraction of the circumferential band of microtubules. The cell membrane remains fully intact, because stored substances are released after fusion of the granule membrane to the membrane of the surface-connected open canalicular system. The release of adenosine diphosphate causes further adhesion of platelets to each other and thus aggregation of thrombocytes, which increases the hemostatic plug.

Prostaglandins play a special role in thrombocytic release reaction and aggregation. Among other substances, collagen leads to activation of phospholipases in the thrombocytic membrane that release arachidonic acid via hydrolysis of phospholipids. Cyclooxygenase then forms prostaglandin endoperoxides that, after further reactions, also produce TXA$_2$ and greatly influence

aggregation of the platelets.[62,68-70] Fibrinogen is also responsible for further aggregation and stabilization, because thrombocytes exhibit a receptor for fibrinogen (glycoproteins IIb/IIIa) that connects them to each other (Table 92.1). However, with the different functional and morphological changes, these stages always run simultaneously to fulfill their hemostatic task. In addition to formation of a hemostatic plug, thrombocytes supply phospholipids, which are essential for coagulation. Platelet factor 3 is only supplied on the surface of activated thrombocytes and induces not only intrinsic activation via contact factors (e.g., factor XII, prekallikrein, and high molecular weight kininogen) but also the activation of prothrombin to thrombin by activated factor X (Xa). Local conversion from prothrombin to thrombin through surface receptors for factors Va and Xa is increased enormously so that, apart from the hemostatic plug, plasmatic coagulation contributes to further elimination of vascular injury.[62] The thrombocyte-connected activated factor X (Xa) is additionally protected by this binding from inactivation through antithrombin III (AT III).

Plasmatic Coagulation

Vasoconstriction and thrombocyte aggregation are the first steps in a complex series of functions that ultimately results in temporary formation of stable fibrin. The first thrombocytic formation of a hemostatic plug is followed after activation by conversion from prothrombin to thrombin, which does not normally circulate freely in blood. Thrombin (factor IIa) causes activation of factors V, VIII, and XIII and is also responsible for splitting fibrinogen and thus for the formation of fibrin monomers (Figure 92.1). A stable fibrin network, insoluble in uric or monochloracetic acid, is formed with the help of the activated factor XIII (XIIIa) and calcium through cross-linking of fibrin polymers. The coagulation factors (Table 92.2), which for the most part participate in these activation procedures, are serine proteinases that carry the amino acid serine in their catalytic centers.[53,62] The six serine proteinases (factors II, VII, IX, X, XI, and XII) are inactive zymogens in blood and are activated and become effective during the coagulation cascade (IIa, VIIa, IXa, Xa, XIa, and XIIa). The Roman numerals do not signify the time sequence in the coagulation procedure but rather were chosen with reference to their discovery.[62] Factors V and VIII are not enzymes but cofactors that accelerate the specific reaction procedures. Factor III is the specification of the tissue thromboplastin; factor IV signifies calcium ions. Most reactions of the coagulation factors take place on the surfaces of phospholipids.

The plasmatic activation from prothrombin to thrombin can be initiated via either the intrinsic or extrinsic

TABLE 92.1. Platelet glycoproteins and their function.

Glycoproteins	Function
GP Ia	In complex with GP IIa receptor for collagen
GP Ib	Receptor for antibodies, thrombin and von Willebrand's factor
GP Ic	Receptor for fibronectin
GP IIa	In complex with GP Ia receptor for collagen
GP IIb	In complex with GP IIIa receptor for fibrinogen, von Willebrand's factor, and fibronectin
GP IIIa	In complex with GP IIb receptor for fibronectin and vitronectin
GP IV	Receptor for thrombospondin
GP IX	In complex with GP Ib

Table 92.2 Characteristics of coagulation factors.

Name (synonym)	Specification	Molecular Weight (d)	Half-life (h)	Plasma concentration
Procoagulants				
II (prothrombin)	Single-chain serine proteinase; vitamin K dependent	72,500	41–72	100 µg/mL
VII (proconvertin)	Single-chain glycoprotein; vitamin K dependent	48,000	2–5	0.5 µg/mL
IX (plasma thromboplastin component)	Single-chain glycoprotein; vitamin K dependent	57,100	18–30	5 µg/mL
X (Stuart–Power)	Two-chain serine proteinase; vitamin K dependent	54,800	20–42	10 µg/mL
I (fibrinogen)	Glycoprotein	340,000	96–120	300 µg/mL
V (proaccelerin)	Single-chain nonenzymatic cofactor	350,000	12–15	200 µg/mL
Tissue factor	Single-chain glycoprotein	37,000	Unknown	Unknown
VIII	Complexing to von Willebrand's factor	320,000	10–18	0.1 µg/mL
XIII (fibrin stabilizing factor)	Zymogen, transglutaminase	320,000	100–120	15 µg/mL
High molecular weight kininogen Fitz-Gerald-F	Single-chain cofactor, contact phase	110,000	Unknown	70 µg/mL
Prekallikrein (Fletcher)	Single-chain serine proteinase, contact phase	85,000	Unknown	50 µg/mL
XI (plasma thromboplastin antecedent)	Two identical sulfide-linked chains, contact phase	160,000	10–20	6 µg/mL
XII (Hageman)	Single-chain serine proteinase, contact phase	84,000	50–70	30 µg/mL
Inhibitors				
Tissue factor pathway inhibitor	Inhibits Xa and VIIa/tissue factor catalytic activity	33,000	Unknown	60–80 µg/mL
Protein C	Two-chain serine proteinase; vitamin K dependent	62,000	6–8	2–6 µg/mL
Protein S	Single-chain cofactor for activated protein C; vitamin K dependent	75,000	55–65	25 µg/mL
Thrombomodulin	Endothelial cell surface receptor for thrombin; activation of protein C	450,000	Unknown	Unknown
Antithrombin III (Heparin cofactor I)	Single-chain glycoprotein; 1:1 complexed with thrombin, IXa, Xa, XIa and XIIa	65,000	50–72	18–30 µg/mL
Heparin cofactor II	1:1 complexed with thrombin	65,000	35–50	30–67 µg/mL

pathway. Exposure of injured tissue in circulating blood leads to activation of the extrinsic pathway. The term *extrinsic* derives from the fact that tissue thromboplastin itself does not originate from circulating blood. After activation, thrombocyte phospholipids (e.g., platelet factor 3) can be exposed on the surface, which also starts the intrinsic pathway. The specification *intrinsic* derives from the fact that all of the factors required for this procedure are present in circulating blood. Strictly speaking, though, this distinction is only relevant under the didactic aspect, because on the one hand tissue factor can also be produced in circulating blood by monocytes,[62] and on the other hand different activation interactions between the so-called intrinsic and extrinsic systems are well known.

A functional difference exists between both activation pathways. Activation of the extrinsic pathway leads to the formation of a few thrombin within seconds. The intrinsic pathway is slower (taking minutes) but with more effective formation of thrombin.[16,17,53] These functional differences are diagnostically useful but have lost clinical relevance through evidence that the activated factor XII

(intrinsic) can activate factor VII (extrinsic) and also that activated factor VII (extrinsic) can lead to activation of factor IX (intrinsic).[16,17,24,53] These two mutual possibilities of activation mean that initiation of a reaction in the intrinsic pathway always signifies activation of the extrinsic pathway and vice versa.

The intrinsic and extrinsic pathways lead to activation of factor X (Xa). In this reaction, in which calcium and phospholipids are also required, the activated factor VIII (VIIIa) takes over the role of cofactor. Activation of factor X (Xa) triggers off the joint final pathway of coagulation, in which prothrombin is again activated to thrombin in the presence of calcium and phospholipids (platelet surface). Factor V is a cofactor in this reaction. The developed thrombin subsequently detaches itself from the platelet surface and takes on various hemostatic tasks.[17,19,24–26]

The most important task of thrombin is converting fibrinogen (factor I) to fibrin. Fibrinogen has a molecular weight of 340,000 d, is synthesized in the liver, and has a half-life of nearly 4 days. Factor I is a dimer in which both chains consist of three different peptide sequences and are held together by disulfide links. In the first step, thrombin splits one peptide each from the A α-chain and the B β-chain (fibrinopeptides A and B). This splitting forms a fibrin monomer. In the second step, fibrin polymers are formed, but they are soluble in uric acid. Finally, fibrin polymers cross-bind to insoluble fibrin due to the fibrin-stabilizing factor XIII under the influence of calcium.[71,72]

Physiologically, the coagulation system is confronted by a series of antagonistic mechanisms.[3,8,11,16,24] Clearance of activated coagulation factor and split products through the reticuloendothelial system and proteolytic reduction of fibrin through fibrinolysis and a series of plasma inhibitors prevent unlimited coagulation. Among all the different inhibitors of coagulation, AT III is surely

the most relevant because this glycoprotein inhibits all serine proteinases[6,53] (Figure 92.4).

AT III belongs to the α_2-globulins and is generated mainly in the liver. Inhibition is caused by formation of an inactive complex, related to covalent formation between the inhibitor and the serine proteinase. The binding speed is collectively slow, but it can be increased manifold through heparin administration.[62] Inhibitory binding of thrombin is especially relevant and is also the quickest binding. The molecular relationship between AT III and the sum of the coagulation factor are calibrated under normal conditions, so that even a slight fall of AT III level under the usual value can promote development of thromboembolic complications.[6,8,16,24,53] Protein C is a further relevant inhibitor of the coagulation

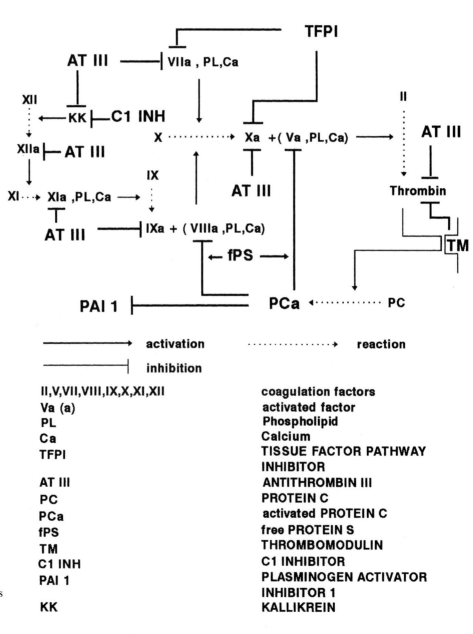

FIGURE 92.4. Coagulation inhibitors and their function.

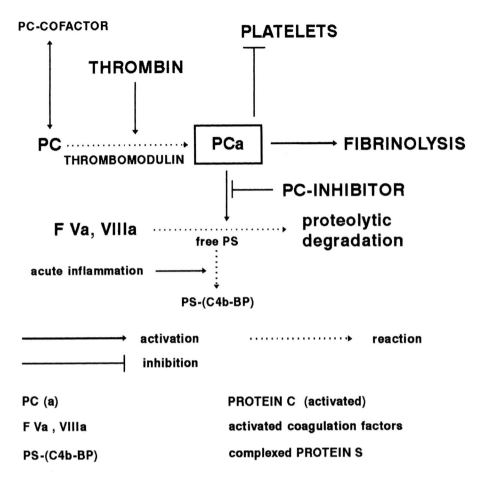

FIGURE 92.5. Protein C pathway.

system, which, in contrast to AT III, has to be activated first. Thrombin is the only physiological activator linked to an endothelium-fixed thrombomodulin (Figure 92.5). In inactive form, this two-chain serine proteinase is developed in a vitamin K–dependent reaction in the liver, and it is the most important inhibitor of activated factors V (Va) and VIII (VIIIa).[3,4,6,8] In addition, activated protein C (PCa) has a stimulating influence on fibrinolysis by inhibiting PAI-1 and also seems to have a slightly inhibitory function during thrombocyte activation. However, at least one cofactor is required for development of the inhibitory capacity. Single-chain protein S is also developed in a vitamin K–dependent reaction in the liver and is a cofactor. About 40% of protein S is free and thus effective as a cofactor, and the remaining 60% is normally linked with a complement factor (C4 binding protein) and ineffective. The relationship between linked and free protein S is subject to various influences,[9–11,73] so that a procoagulant status also results by reducing the free portion of protein S.

However, according to reports from Dahlbäck,[5] it has to be assumed that another cofactor exists, because patients who lack protein C still suffer constant hypercoagulability in spite of treatment with protein C. Heparin cofactor II, tissue factor pathway inhibitor, C1 esterase

inhibitor, and the α_2-macroglobulin are other inhibitors.[16,24,25]

Venous Thrombosis and the Hypercoagulable State

Thrombophilia

Thrombophilia increases the risk of thrombosis or embolism due to inherited or acquired disorders of either hemostasis or fibrinolysis. Prevalence of thrombophilia is estimated at about 1 in 2000 and is five times higher than the prevalence of hemophilia.[74] Unrelated to any causal factor, thrombophilia and thus hypercoagulable status always occur either in increased presence of coagulation activators combined with decreased presence of inhibitors or in situations with decreased presence of fibrinolytic activators combined with increased fibrinolytic inhibitors. Unlike inherited disorders of hemostasis, in which patients are mostly young and thrombosis localization with strong recidivism is present, the acquired disorders of hemostasis are not limited to any age and causal factors can be clarified in many cases because certain risks can be exposed.

Screening for thrombophilia includes measurement of the coagulation inhibitors (i.e., AT III, heparin cofactor II, protein C, and protein S) and determination of several participating factors of fibrinolysis, such as plasminogen, histidin-rich glycoprotein, fibrinogen, factor XII, tPA, urokinase type plasminogen activator, and PAI. Furthermore, LA and reduced activated protein C cofactor levels should be measured.[74] Because no reliable prospective investigations have yet been undertaken, reports about the causes of single occurrences of thrombophilia are not exact, but it seems that in a thrombosis collective with young patients deficiencies of AT III, protein C, protein S, and factor XII happen more often, with a prevalence of 2% to 15%.[75,76] Deficiencies of heparin cofactor II, plasminogen, fibrinogen, and histidin-rich glycoprotein are more rare, with a prevalence of less than 2%.[77] Also, there are not enough reliable reports about defects of fibrinolysis[25,78] and LA[39,42,79,80] and lack of activated protein C cofactor.[5] However, a superficial look through the literature suggests that these defects occur more frequently than assumed.[74]

AT III deficiency was described as the first thrombophilia factor by Egeberg in 1965.[81] Clinical correlation consists of venous and arterial thrombosis, and manifestation is more frequent in the venous vascular region. AT III essentially inhibits activated factor X (Xa), thrombin formation, and also thrombin effect and must be sufficiently available so that heparin can become more efficacious. The two types of defects are distinguished by molecular and functional aspects. Type I defects show differences in heparin binding; type II defects include the various forms of molecular defects of AT III.[74] AT III deficiency is usually transmitted in an autosomal dominant manner. Mutations that alter the heparin-binding domains in the protein molecule seem to be less afflicted with the risk of thrombosis. Furthermore, because both inherited and acquired deficiencies are possible, actual clinical circumstances have to be considered in AT III testing. AT III levels can be lowered in systemic heparinization of patients during the third trimester of pregnancy or with acute deep vein thrombosis. However, levels can rise during therapy with vitamin K antagonists. Also, AT III deficiency can occur because of reduced synthesis in patients with liver cirrhosis due to augmented consumption of disseminated intravascular coagulation or greater loss (e.g., in nephrotic syndrome). According to investigations by Pabinger,[8] pregnant women with AT III deficiency have an extremely high risk of thrombosis. Furthermore, administration of oral contraceptives increases the risk of thrombosis in women with AT III deficiencies.[8] There is a strong similarity between AT III and heparin cofactor II, which is formed in the liver and is also a thrombin inhibitor. However, the affinity of heparin cofactor II to heparin is far less distinct compared with that of AT III. Likewise, deficiency can generate enhanced thromboemboli.

In 1981 Griffin[3] first described the association between protein C deficiency and multiple thromboses. Protein C is synthesized in the liver if vitamin K is present and is activated in plasma through the endothelial thrombin–thrombomodulin complex.[3,4,6,82] Activated protein C inactivates coagulation factors Va and VIIIa in the presence of protein S, calcium ions, and phospholipids and thus inhibits thrombin formation. Inhibition of factors Va and VIIIa is especially important, because these factors are not subject to the effect of AT III so that clotting inhibition is additive and synergistic. In addition to this anticoagulant effect, protein C can activate fibrinolysis by inhibiting PAI-1, and protein C is thought to exercise a certain inhibitory effect on thrombocyte adhesion.[6,74] By forming the thrombin–thrombomodulin complex required for protein C activation, bound thrombin loses its procoagulant effect, so that the described complex also inhibits clotting.[5,8,74,82] In contrast, a decrease of endothelium-fixed thrombomodulin involved in the protein C pathway means a procoagulant threat to patients associated with an increased risk of thrombosis.[6,12,28] A down-regulation of endothelial thrombomodulin expression can be observed in different diseases, such as malaria and generalized sepsis. Protein C deficiency is also divided into two types. The immunological activity and biological activity are low in the frequently occurring classic type I protein C deficiency; immunological activity is normal but the biological activity is low in type II. Familiar protein C deficiency is transmitted in an autosomal dominant manner and recessively inherited. Newborns with homozygous protein C deficiency who have survived to birth develop purpura fulminans, which has a high mortality rate.[83] Similar to manifested disseminated intravascular coagulation, laboratory findings of homozygous protein C deficiency show an antigen level of less than 1% of normal values.[83,84]

The biological activity of the heterozygous deficiency is decreased to 50% of normal values. These patients demonstrate an increased risk of thromboembolic complications but are rarely symptomatic until their early 20s, with more individuals experiencing thrombotic events as they reach age 50.[83] Approximately 75% of patients up to that age have experienced one or more thrombotic events. The first event develops spontaneously in almost 70% of patients. The most common thrombotic manifestation involves the deep leg veins, the iliofemoral veins, and the mesenteric veins. More than 60% of patients develop recurrent venous thrombosis, and there are signs of past lung embolism in almost 40%.[85] The investigations of the Dutch group on first manifestation showed an especially high frequency of superficial thrombophlebitis in the leg veins and cerebral venous thrombosis in several protein C–deficient patients.[86] The protein C levels in newborns are about 20% to 40% of adult standard values and even lower in premature infants.[87]

Acquired protein C deficiency occurs in several clinical disorders (e.g., liver disease, disseminated intravascular coagulation, and adult respiratory distress syndrome), postoperatively, and in association with various drug treatments.[6,83,87] Unlike AT III, the antigenic concentrations of vitamin K–dependent plasma proteins, including protein C, were often elevated in patients with nephrotic syndrome.[83] Therapy with L-asparaginase particularly led to a clear decrease of protein C levels.[88] Whether oral contraceptive use is a risk factor is controversial. Overall, however, the threat of thromboembolic complications with contraceptive use seems less than that of women with AT III deficiency.[74] Because protein C and protein S depend on vitamin K for synthesis, every medication that influences vitamin K metabolism also leads to a change in protein C and protein S formation. The biological activity during coumarin treatment is markedly reduced, corresponding to Quick's value, and thus protein C and protein S determination is irrelevant during appropriate treatment with vitamin K antagonists. Vitamin K–dependent carboxylation cannot ensue in vitamin K–dependent coagulation factor (factors II, VII, IX, and X) during coumarin treatment; consequently, the so-called proteins induced by vitamin K absence develop and are released as nonfunctional precursors in the circulation.[28,74]

Several other medications, due to their biochemical construction, are able to inhibit vitamin K–epoxide reductase and also intervene in vitamin K metabolism. These medications consist of the β-lactamase antibiotics with an N-methyltetrathiazole side chain. My investigations of a large group of patients with temporary protein C and protein S deficiency showed an apparent coincidence of deficiency status and earlier long-term therapy with antibiotics.[6,82] These considerations are also supported by the results of Uchida,[89] but they are partially based on animal studies. Patients in intensive care units over a long period who are fed parenterally and treated extensively with antibiotics and sedatives are prone to temporary protein C and protein S deficiency due to a shortage of vitamin K storage unless vitamin K is administered. Shortage of vitamin K storage involves not only the vitamin K–dependent coagulation inhibitors but also the vitamin K–dependent coagulation factors. However, reduction of protein C levels can be measured initially, because protein C has a distinctly shorter half-life than the remaining vitamin K–dependent coagulation factors (Table 92.2).

Due to these varying half-lives of the procoagulant factors (II, VII, IX, and X) and the anticoagulant inhibitors (proteins C and S), a special problem arises in the application of vitamin K antagonists if protein C deficiency has not been diagnosed. These patients are especially threatened by the occurrence of coumarin-induced skin necrosis (Figures 92.6 and 92.7). Because of the shorter half-life, treatment with vitamin K antagonists lessens the activity of protein C at first so that during the first days of treatment there is an imbalance in favor of the procoagulant side. The more distinguished protein C deficiency is present before therapy with vitamin K antagonists begins, the longer the imbalance and thus the greater the danger to patients. If these patients are not sufficiently heparinized, microthromboses that initially are undetected can develop during the first days of administration of vitamin K antagonists. The most common sites for these microthromboses are the extremities and especially the mechanically stressed regions of the body (those covered with bandages). However, some authors have also reported manifestations in the breast, genital region, inner organs, and brain.[4,6,10,74,83]

Bleeding in the previously microthrombosed area begins when sufficient anticoagulation is obtained and the activity of the other coagulation factors is reduced. Necrosis, appearing as a hemorrhagic area at first, is then visible. Depending on how pronounced microthrombosis is, a slight superficial or a deep defect can occur that can lead to necrotic impairment of musculature.[6] If such coumarin-induced skin necrosis occurs, prophylactic therapy is no longer possible, but local surgical treatment may be helpful. To prevent necrosis, protein C deficiency should be excluded and heparinization continued. Sufficient treatment with heparin is mandatory in the initial period of coumarin treatment. Several medications (e.g., Stanozolol and Danazol) have been reported to substantially raise the protein C levels in heterozygous patients with type I protein C deficiency.[90]

As mentioned previously, the presence of protein S as a cofactor is required so that PCa can develop its inhibitory capacity. Protein S also depends on vitamin K for synthesis in the liver, endothelium, and megakaryocytes. Only the freely circulating part in plasma (40%) is suitable as a cofactor. The other 60% remains inactive for the protein C pathway because of reversible binding to the C4 binding protein. Both parts are subjected in ratio to numerous influences, among others to a rise in C4 binding protein levels in sepsis, by activating the complement system, followed by multiple binding of free protein S, which leads to reduction of cofactor activity.[6,10,16,17,20,83]

Arterial thrombosis is especially common with protein S deficiency, and central arterial thrombosis and infarction have been repeatedly described as clinical correlates.[9–11,73,74] Protein S deficiency is divided into three types. Criteria for classification are behaviors of total protein S and free protein S and their activity.[74]

Dahlbäck[5] recently described another cofactor of protein C. His article deals with the reduced reaction of activated protein C (activated protein C resistance). This defect, with a relatively high prevalence, is supposedly the cause of almost 30% of cases of thrombophilia of unknown origin.

FIGURE 92.6. Coumarin-induced skin necrosis (first day of appearance on proximal thigh).

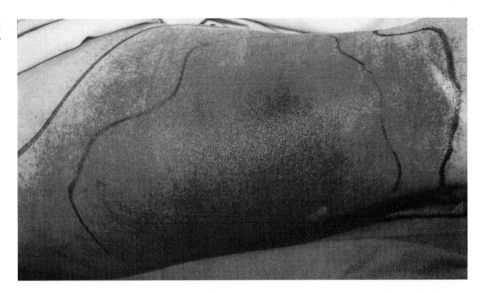

As well as the endothelium with thrombomodulin takes over relevant anticoagulant task, it occupies a key role in fibrinolysis. Different activators and inhibitors regulate fibrinolysis activity (Figure 92.8), which concludes in a conversion from plasminogen to plasmin. This conversion is endogenously possible via three activators: tPA, prourokinase, and the contact factors (e.g., factor XII, prekallikrein, and high molecular weight kininogen). There are fewer activators and more inhibitors during a procoagulant disturbance of regulation. Rare causes of thrombophilia are plasminogen deficiency and abnormal plasminogen molecules[91]; both are inherited in a mostly autosomal dominant manner and manifest themselves from clinically mild to very severe thrombotic events.[74] The increased level of histidin-rich glycoprotein that inhibits fibrinolysis by binding to plasminogen and dysfibrinogenemia, whose prothrombotic behavior is explained by the resistance of abnormal fibrin molecules to tPA, is rare.[74]

In comparison to previously described rare defects, factor XII deficiency[92,93] and the tPA release disorders occur far more frequently.[94] tPA release disorder is reported to have an incidence of 15% to 30% in the juvenile population with thrombotic events. The two types of disorder depend on the reaction of tPA antigen, tPA activity, and PAI level.[94] Reduced tPA antigen and tPA activity levels are measured in one group with normal PAI values, and the other group shows normal tPA antigen levels, reduced tPA activity, and increased PAI values.

Although factor XII deficiency with its prolonged partial thromboplastin time can be striking, it does not primarily lead to hemorrhagic diathesis as assumed. Instead, patients such as John Hageman (Table 92.2) suffer from thrombophilic coagulation, because initiation of fibrinolysis, depending on contact factors, does not ensue with sufficient power but coagulation activity is nearly normal via factor XI.[92,93]

Factor XII, the Hageman factor, is a serine proteinase that can be activated by either contact with negative-loaded surfaces or enzymatic splitting. Activated factor XII (XIIa) can activate both the intrinsic coagulation system and fibrinolysis and is also able to generate

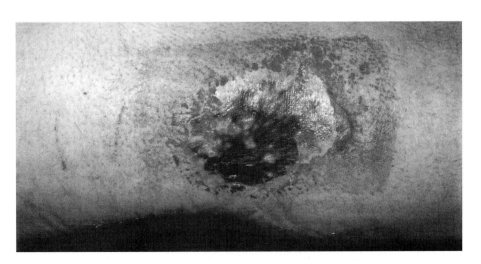

FIGURE 92.7. Same patient as in Figure 92.6 14 days after appearance of skin necrosis.

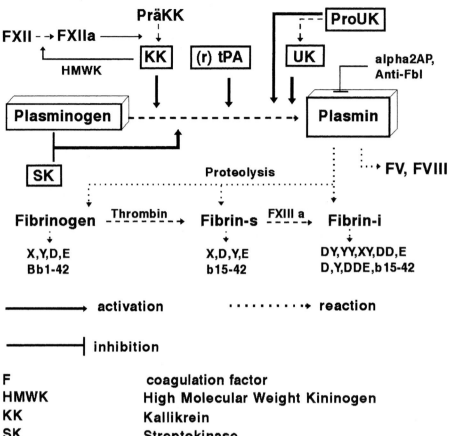

FIGURE 92.8. Fibrinolytic scheme.

kallikrein via a proteolytic process.[92] After initial activation of factor XII, the self-activation and amplifier loop maintain the procoagulant clotting status over a longer period. This self-activation ensues from kallikrein, which is developed from prekallikrein, and which transports inactive zymogen (factor XII) to active serine proteinase (factor XIIa).[92–94] As in other serine proteinases, factor XII deficiency appears as a quantitative cross-reacting material negative or as a qualitative cross-reacting material positive deficiency. Since the description by Saito[95] of the first qualitative factor XII deficiency, many others have reported on different dysfunctional factor XII variations.[96]

Factor XII deficiency is inherited in an autosomal recessive manner. Patients with factor XII deficiency inherited heterozygously are seldom conspicuous due to prolonged partial thromboplastin time and therefore can easily remain undiagnosed.[92] However, despite receiving 50% factor XII activity, the patients with factor XII deficiency also have tendencies to venous thrombosis (Figures 92.9 and 92.10), as shown in studies by me and my colleagues.[6] Various working groups have reported about different meanings of factor XII deficiency, but this variation is due only to the different groups of patients.[97,98] On the whole, the incidence of factor XII deficiency in patients with recurrent venous thrombosis is reported to be between 8% and 10%.[92] However, the incidence of factor XII deficiency is supposedly higher in patients who have thromboembolism or myocardial infarction. Halbmayer[98] reported that the incidence in these patients is 20%. On the other hand, some reports, including that of Goodnough et al.,[97] that deal with the incidence of venous and thromboembolic events in patients with diagnosed factor XII deficiency show that

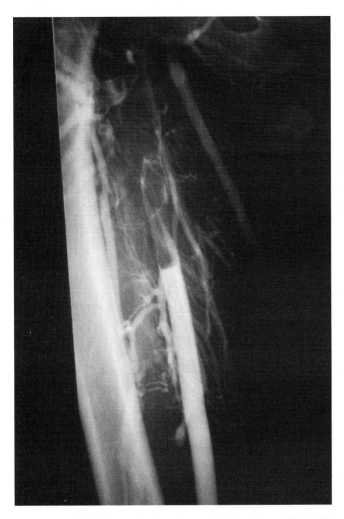

FIGURE 92.9. Phlebography in a 9-year-old boy (factor XII deficiency) with descending deep vein thrombosis from the vena cava to the superficial femoral vein.

8.3% of these patients had venous thrombosis and 8.3% myocardial infarction. According to an investigation of 300 healthy patients, it can be assumed that the frequency of factor XII deficiency lies between 1.5% and 3% in a healthy population.

Lupus Anticoagulants (LA)

LAs are autoantibodies of immunoglobulin M or G classification that work against negative-loaded phospholipids and protein–phospholipid complexes[41,79] and block their function by binding coagulation factors onto these phospholipids. Formation of prothrombin activator complexes is obstructed, as are protein C activation, prostacyclin synthesis and release, and the effect of plasminogen activator. Contrary to corresponding laboratory results, patients with markedly prolonged partial thromboplastin times tend toward venous or thromboembolic events.[35,36,38] Investigations by Lechner[36] proved that 30% of the patients with ascertained LA presence have had at least one thrombotic event. Two thirds of these patients suffered from venous thrombosis

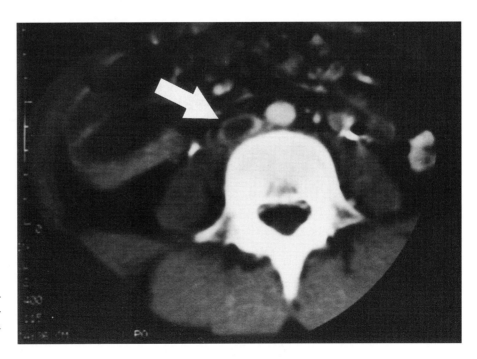

FIGURE 92.10. Computed tomography image in the patient from Figure 92.9 with thrombus in the vena cava (arrow).

and one third from arterial thrombosis, especially cerebral thrombosis. Women with habitual spontaneous abortions in the second and third trimesters of pregnancy often have LAs.[36] A possible pathophysiological connection can be explained by the imbalance between prostacyclin and thromboxane B_2. Similar to preeclampsia, a reduced prostacyclin concentration was seen in female patients with LAs.[35,80]

The incidence of LAs is reported to be between 10% and 48% in women who have had habitual spontaneous abortions.[35] Classically, these LAs appear in patients with systemic lupus erythematosus,[39,80] but they are also evident in patients with other autoimmune diseases. These LAs appear in approximately one third of all systemic lupus erythematosus patients according to Love and Santoro.[39] However, LAs have also been seen in other diseases, after various pharmacotherapy regimens (e.g., chlorpromazine, procainamide, and hydantoin),[99] and in healthy patients without recognizable cause. Many patients with evidence of LAs do not require special therapy, but immunosuppressive therapy should be considered if thrombocytopenia and severe prothrombin deficiency occur simultaneously. Thrombocytopenia and prothrombin deficiency often correlate with the presence of LAs.[36] Therapy with prednisolone should be considered with pregnant women with detectable LAs to diminish the threat of spontaneous abortion. However, heparin treatment may be just as efficacious.

Heparin-Associated Thrombocytopenia (HAT)

The incidence of HAT is reported to be between 1% and 2% in all patients who have been therapeutically heparinized over a period of 5 days.[12,30,31,34] However, HAT can also appear in patients after a single administration of low molecular weight heparin.[12] HAT is the most frequent form of drug-induced thrombocytopenia, whereby the antibodies bind via Fc receptors, contrary to other drug-dependent thrombocytopenias.[99] HAT is generally regarded as an immunological process in which highly sulfated oligosaccharides and a releasable platelet protein (usually platelet factor 4) form a multimolecular neoantigen complex to which patients become immune.[31,34,100] The created antibodies then lead to platelet activation in a further or new presence of heparin[101,102] or other sulfated oligosaccharides.[31,103] However, endothelium seems to be activated via heparin sulfate–platelet factor 4 complexes and consequently is involved in the development of HAT.[33] The decreased platelet count is clinically noticeable and becomes evident about 8 days (4–14 days) after first exposure to heparin or 1 to 3 days after repeated exposure.

The severity of thrombocyte degradation does not always cause further clinical symptoms. Because the number of thrombocytes apparently seldom drops to mini-

mal values, most of the patients are primarily threatened by the massive platelet activation and after thromboembolic events.[12,29,30] Arterial thrombosis is found in two thirds of patients with HAT, yet recurrent venous thrombosis is also a manifestation of HAT.[12] A special problem results from occlusions in the microcirculation, which often lead to partial or complete amputation of extremities later in the course of the illness.[12] Care must be taken to immediately stop heparin exposure if HAT is suspected. In most cases, the platelet count then returns to normal within a few days. However, if anticoagulant therapy is mandatory, Orgaran, a low molecular weight heparin of a different chemical composition that cross-reacts with heparin antibodies in only 20% (in vitro), can be given.[12] Oral anticoagulation therapy should either be started or continued. In some hospitals HAT patients are treated with hirudin after positive cross-reaction of Orgaran, but there are no reports yet about indications for hirudin, which is still being tested. According to encouraging reports from Greinacher,[29] high-dose intravenous immunoglobulin G administration seems to effectively inhibit platelet activation in HAT patients. This therapy can also be used during pregnancy and provides good results until the circulation is completely free of heparin.

Basics of Drug Thrombolysis

Despite an early observation that blood does not always clot,[104] interest in stopping blood coagulation first began at the end of the nineteenth century. The term *fibrinolysis*, first used by Dastre,[105] derives from this period. The fundamental theory of dynamic balance between coagulation and fibrinolysis was developed in 1905 by Morawitz and Nolf.[1] Between 1958 and 1962 Astrup[106] and Fearnley[107] improved and added to this theory with new facts but without altering the fundamental idea.

When Tillet and Garner[108] reported about the fibrinolytic capacity of hemolysing streptococci in 1933, and Christensen and MacLeod[109] succeeded in clarifying streptococcal fibrinolysis, the principle of fibrinolysis moved to the scientific foreground. Later on, several reports further clarified the molecular levels of enzymatic courses of fibrinolysis and their regulation.

Fibrinolysis is a proteolytic enzymatic process of dissolving fibrin. In the human vascular system this means first localizing thrombotic events and subsequently dissolving the local clot formation to prevent unlimited thrombus generation and vascular occlusion. The most important enzyme of the fibrinolysis system is serine proteinase plasmin. Its most obvious and important task is to split fibrin through proteolysis. If there is a high concentration of plasmin, fibrinogen is also proteolytically degraded. However, other factors of blood coagulation (factors V and VIII) depend on degradation by plasmin,[110,111] so that hyperplasmia is marked by loss of fibrinogen, by a flooding of fibrin and fibrinogen split products, and by decreased activity of factors V and VIII. Laboratory and clinical findings show extensive incoagulability of blood.[13,24,112,113] The more powerful and more prolonged these effects are in therapeutic treatment with thrombolytic drugs, the less heparinization that accompanies thrombolytic treatment is necessary (Table 92.3) and the greater the risk of bleeding.

To prevent such uncontrollable fibrinolysis, different inhibitors are available (e.g., PAI, α_2-antiplasmin, α_2-macroglobulin, and C1 esterase inhibitor) to induce plasmin proteolysis or inactivation by binding,[13,112] so that no distinct fibrinolytic activities of plasmin can be detected in healthy resting patients.[13,17,28] Physiologically, free circulating plasmin is neutralized within a few seconds ($t_{1/2} = 0.1$ second) by the most important inhibitor, α_2-antiplasmin.[13] The capacity of plasmin formation is controlled by a 20-fold inhibitor potential.[113] Apart from directly neutralizing plasmin, α_2-antiplasmin seems to control fibrinolysis directly at the thrombus site.[13] One mechanism of this control results from the calcium-dependent and covalent fibrin net through thrombocytic (intracellular) or plasmatic (extracellular) factor XIII that, as a transglutaminase, also binds α_2-antiplasmin to stable fibrin, so that circulating plasmin, transported on a thrombus, is also immediately neutralized by the presence of α_2-antiplasmin.[71] Unlike plasmatic factor XIII, which is composed of two A and two B chains, the thrombocytic factor XIII as dimer consists of two identical A chains.[72] This difference and thus other binding behaviors of fibrin with α_2-antiplasmin seem to be one reason that platelet-rich thrombi are less soluble due to fibrin-specific thrombolytic drugs; a larger dose is thus necessary for lysis.[71,72]

However, apart from the direct plasmin inhibitors, plasminogen activator inhibitors (PAI-1 and PAI-2) also regulate plasmin formation earlier on, and these inhibitors are in turn exposed to a complex regulation of enhancement and neutralization. Hence, the fibrinolysis inhibiting effect of PAI-1 is also attenuated by protein C.[6,11,16,112] In all, the fibrinolysis system shows a distinct similarity in its proteolytic processes to the cascadelike functioning coagulation system and has cross-links with the coagulation, endothelium, and complement systems (Figure 92.11).[16–20,22–24,26,82]

Thrombolytic Drugs (Plasminogen Activators)

As an active serine proteinase, plasmin generates from the inactive preliminary stage of plasminogen through a limited proteolytic process that is induced and maintained by circulating plasminogen activators.[112] Besides the endogenous tPA and the prourokinase (single-chain urokinase-PA) that are formed endogenously and under physiological conditions cause only a local fibrinolysis, pure plasminogen activators can also be used to imitate endogenous fibrinolysis or to enhance the effects.[13] Endogenous plasminogen activators from organs beyond the blood system are called extrinsic activators to distinguish them from intrinsic activators, the so-called contact factors of blood coagulation (e.g., factor XII, prekallikrein, and high molecular weight kininogen) that develop in blood (Figure 92.1). In contrast to extrinsic activators (e.g., tPA and prourokinase), which demonstrate a multiple increase of their proteolytic activity only in the presence of fibrin (Table 92.3) and therefore display a small although dose-dependent effect, the exogenous activators (e.g., streptokinase, urokinase, and acylated plasminogen–streptokinase–activator complex) are only slightly fibrin specific. Their therapeutic application is therefore marked by the occur-

TABLE 92.3. Characteristics of fibrinolytic drugs.[13]

	Streptokinase	APSAC	Urokinase	rtPA	Prourokinase
Molecualr weight (d)	47,000	137,000	54,000	70,000	54,000
Type of activation	Indirect	Direct	Direct	Direct	Direct
Plasma half-life	20 min	100 min	10–15 min	4–7 min	8 min
Fibrin caused increasing activity	-	+	++	++++	+++ ?
Quickness of thrombolysis	++	+++	+	++++	+++
Systemic effects	++++	++++	++	+	+++
Continuous infusion of heparin	No	No	Yes	Yes	Yes
Risk of bleeding	Low	Low	Low	Low	Low
Management of therapy	Poor	Very poor	Good	Good	Good
Allergic reaction	Yes	Yes	No	No	No
Decreasing of blood pressure (therapy)	Yes	Yes	No	No	No

APSAC, acetylized plasminogen activator complex; rtPA, recombinant tissue-type plasminogen activator.

-       no effect
+   effect/influence little
++++   effect/influence strong

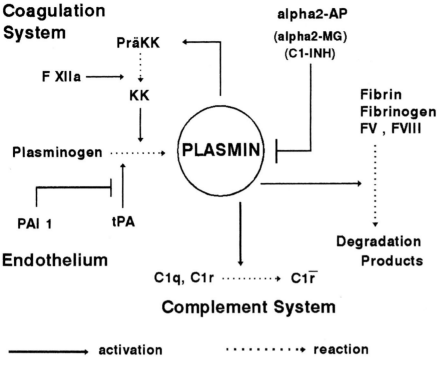

FIGURE 92.11. Cross-linkings in plasmin generation.

F	coagulation factor
AT III	Antithrombin III
KK	Kallikrein
PAI 1	Plasminogen-Activator-Inhibitor 1
tPA	tissue-Plasminogen-Activator
alpha2-AP	alpha2-Antiplasmin
alpha2-MG	alpha2-Macroglobulin
C1-INH	C1-Inhibitor
C1q, C1r	complement factors
PräKK	Prekallikrein

rence of a systemic fibrinogenolysis and fibrinolysis with corresponding systemic effects, such as generalized bleeding tendency.

Fibrin-Unselective Thrombolytics (Exogene Activators)

Acylated Plasminogen–Streptokinase–Activator Complex

Acylated plasminogen activator complexes are a further development of streptokinase, whereby the active center is reversibly esterized and thus primarily inactivated. A slow and almost uncontrollable loss of an acetyl group first arises in blood and at the thrombus site, followed later by development of enzymatic activity.[114,115] Subjected to this slow hydrolytic loss of the acetyl

group, there is a plasma half-life of about 100 minutes. Despite fibrin affinity, clinical application of acylated plasminogen–streptokinase–activator complex shows a similar influence on the coagulation system as the application of streptokinase. Likewise, the streptokinase portion can also lead to development of antibodies.[13]

Urokinase

Urokinase can be found in human urine. It is a matter of a physiological two-chain glycoprotein that, after activation of prourokinase, splits into at least two enzymatically active and pharmacologically and clinically similar effective parts. With regards to transformation of plasminogen, the high molecular weight urokinase with a molecular weight of 55,000 d seems to be more potent than the low molecular weight urokinase with a molecular weight of 33,000 d. Urokinase has a high affinity to plasminogen and leads to direct activation of plasminogen to plasmin. Urokinase can be administered repeatedly and does not lead to formation of antibodies.

Streptokinase

Streptokinase is a nonphysiological thrombolytic drug and a catalytic metabolic product of the β-hemolytic streptococci of Lancefield group C. Streptokinase is not fibrin selective and does not itself have any proteolytic activity, but it demonstrates a high affinity for plasminogen. Activation of plasminogen to plasmin occurs in two stages. First of all, an equimolecular complex develops between streptokinase and plasminogen. This complex transforms circulating plasminogen to plasmin through proteolysis. Because development of effective activator complexes depends on circulating plasminogen, too high of a dosage may lead to insufficient circulating plasminogen for plasmin transformation after forming the activator complexes; the therapy is thus ineffective. Consequently, the appropriate dose would mean sufficient formation of the activator complex without consuming the total circulating plasminogen. The half-life of streptokinase depends on the presence of specific streptokinase antibodies that can arise during administration or that are present due to streptokinase treatment in the past. Thus, repeated administration after a short time is contraindicated.

Fibrin-Selective Thrombolytics (Extrinsic Activators)

Prourokinase

Prourokinase is a glycoprotein that is transformed to urokinase by hydrolysis of peptide bindings. This substance has not yet been approved for widespread clinical use on patients. Based on animal experimental investigations and administration in some patients, prourokinase has a half-life of about 4 to 8 minutes, so that, similar to tPA, it seems that long-term use is required to achieve a therapeutic concentration.[116] Plasma clearance is essentially influenced by liver metabolism.

Tissue Plasminogen Activator

In a recombinant form, fibrin-selective tPA is biotechnically produced as recombinant tissue-type plasminogen activator (rtPA) and is available for clinical use. Native tPA is a glycoprotein from 527 amino acids and is synthesized in the vascular endothelium. tPA is a two-chain glycoprotein and consists of a C-terminal light chain, which contains the active center, and an N-terminal heavy chain, which exhibits the domain structure responsible for the specific binding of fibrin. tPA is a less effective enzyme in plasma. The therapeutic effect of plasminogen activation is primarily increased in the presence of fibrin in a tertiary complex (i.e., fibrin, tPA, and plasminogen). Formation of this tertiary complex is responsible for fibrin selectivity, because only plasminogen is changed to plasmin via tPA, which is bound to fibrin at the complex. This fibrin selectivity is in turn the cause of the minor systemic effect on the coagulation system. Because the rate of hypofibrinogenemia and amount of ensuing split products is small, generalized clot inhibition or bleeding tendency does not arise. This low intrinsic anticoagulant capacity, however, makes accompanying and therapeutically effective heparinization necessary to prevent appositional thrombus generation during therapy or rethrombosis after fibrinolysis.[13,28,112,113] tPA's short half-life enables good control, but continuous application is required to maintain a long-lasting effect on the plasma concentration. Elimination is essentially influenced by liver clearance.

Patient Selection and Laboratory Control Factors

In all cases, before carrying out fibrinolysis, alternative therapies such as operative venous thrombectomy, arterial embolectomy, arterial reconstruction, or purely conservative treatment must be considered, because arterial or venous fibrinolysis is not suitable for every patient. Fibrinolysis is rarely successful, especially in the venous vascular region, if an obstructive outflow (e.g., hematoma, tumor, or vein spur) (Figures 92.12 and 92.13), which can be surgically or interventionally treated, is responsible for generation of thrombosis.[117] Additionally, fibrinolysis naturally means a risk for the patient in terms of failure or arising side effects. Contraindications (Table 92.4) for fibrinolytic treatment essentially derive from the spectrum of side effects, which differ among thrombolytic drugs. However, the most important and significant side effect for all thrombolytic drugs is heavy bleeding; its incidence depends greatly on lysis pattern and thus duration of lysis.[78,118] The incidence of fatal hemorrhage, mostly due to meningeal bleeding, is about 1%.[119] Short-term lysis with streptokinase has an incidence of fatal meningeal hemorrhage of less than 0.5%.[119] Various authors have reported that bleeding complications in general arise in patients undergoing long-term lysis (3–6 days) with streptokinase, with an incidence between 4% and 10%.[120] The incidence with use of urokinase over a period of 5 to 10 days is between 1% and 1.2%.[78] The incidence of general bleeding complications with tPA administration is reported to be up to 40%, mostly at the puncture site.[75] In comparison to streptokinase, the number of treatments with rtPA is too small to determine the incidence of severe bleeding complications.

Apart from the obligatory phlebography control, fibrinolysis therapy also requires certain laboratory tests before and especially during lysis. A latent or manifested hemorrhagic diathesis has to be excluded before starting lysis. If hemorrhagic diathesis is not suspected clinically, a rough but sufficient method of investigation consists of the hemoglobin test, thrombocyte count, global test of coagulation (Quick's value), partial thromboplastin test, thrombin time, and evaluation of fibrinogen and AT III levels.[78] In special cases, a thromboelastogram can provide some information about the hemostatic status.

Determination of thrombin time and fibrinogen plasma level plays a significant role during lysis therapy. If possible, fibrinogen content should not drop below 100%. After extremely prolonged thrombin time at the beginning of lysis due to flooding with fibrin or fibrinogen split products, attempts should be made to prolong thrombin time up to three times the normal value.[78] Determination of partial thromboplastin time, which reacts sensitively on split products, is less helpful during fibrinolysis, because it is influenced by fibrinogen plasma level and the amount of factors V and VII, which can also be subjected to proteolysis. If fibrinolysis is combined with heparin (e.g., as necessary from the beginning onward during tPA treatment), the reptilase time might need to be determined to evaluate the altered coagulation status due solely to split products. Heparin therapy has no influence on reptilase time. Changes of these parameters reflect fibrinolytic effect of the thrombolytic drug during lysis through flooding of split products; they

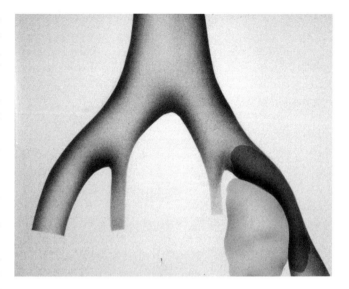

FIGURE 92.12. Extravascular venous compression.

TABLE 92.4. Contraindications to fibrinolysis.[78]

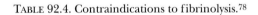

Absolute
Current bleeding, bleeding short time ago
Hemorrhagic diathesis
Hypertension (diastolic pressure above 105 mm Hg)
Streptosepticemia
Bacterial endocarditis
Stroke, short time ago (6 mo after stroke for recombinant tissue-type
    plasminogen activator)
Antistreptokinase titer above 300 IU/mL blood (for streptokinase)
Within 7 d of operation (14 d for recombinant tissue-type
    plasminogen activator)
Carcinoma in digestive system or bronchial carcinoma
Ulcerative colitis or gastroduodenal ulcer
Glomerulonephritis, pancreatitis
Diabetes mellitus that affects eye area
Mitral valvular defect with atrial fibrillation
8 wk after neurosurgical operations
4 wk after opthalmologic operations
Aneurysms

Relative
Treatment with streptokinase within last 3 mo
Severe hepatopathy
Current pulmonary tuberculosis
Old age (over 70 years)
Within first 16 wk of pregnancy
Puncture of great vessels, biopsy

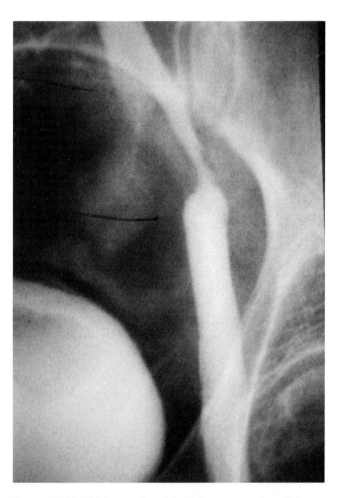

FIGURE 92.13. Phlebography with distinct narrowing of the external iliac vein (tumor).

FIGURE 92.14. Development of activation markers.

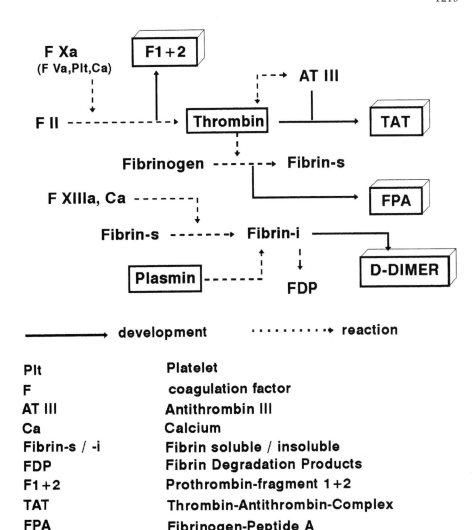

Plt   Platelet
F   coagulation factor
AT III   Antithrombin III
Ca   Calcium
Fibrin-s / -i   Fibrin soluble / insoluble
FDP   Fibrin Degradation Products
F1+2   Prothrombin-fragment 1+2
TAT   Thrombin-Antithrombin-Complex
FPA   Fibrinogen-Peptide A
D-Dimer   Fibrin Degradation Product

do not, however, allow determination or predictive evaluation of successful lysis. Measurement of so-called activation markers (thrombin–antithrombin complex, prothrombin fragment 1+2, fibrinopeptide A, D-dimer) (Figure 92.14) have also increasingly established themselves as measures for evaluating the hemostasis status before therapy.[82,113,121,122] The necessity for the broad use of these measurements has not yet been proven in any study, so the tests are still restricted to specific situations.

Some investigations dealing with the therapy of deep vein thrombosis with tPA, which due to its fibrin selectivity rarely leads to systemic changes of the hemostatic balance, showed that the actual coagulation status of patients before regional thrombolysis greatly influences the success of lysis.[113] These investigations were based on the estimation of markers of activation (prothrombin fragment 1+ 2, D-dimer), forming a quotient (coagulation–lysis index). Lower quotients correlated significantly with better rates of recanalization.[123]

Further Developments

Various disciplines have tried to associate the favorable attributes of different plasminogen activators to obtain as high a thrombolytic efficacy rate and as low an incidence of side effects and systemic influence as possible. Thus, by combining rtPA with streptokinase, a high capacity of thrombolysis is connected with hemorheological properties of streptokinase to reocclusion prophylaxis. Due to their synergistic effect and resulting low dose, the combination of prourokinase with rtPA is likewise sensible.[13] Unforeseeable possibilities are presented by the genetic development of hybrid molecules and mutants, which show highly selective efficacy. For a long time now, special attention has been focused on the hybrids and mutants of rtPA.[14,124,125] Some of these mutants are already being studied in clinical trials.[15] The combined therapeutic application of such a selective fibrinolytic drug with stronger potency and a useful systemic effect with improved selective antithrombotic drugs, also in development, would reduce the number of reocclusions.[126]

References

1. Morawitz P. Die Chemie der Blutgerinnung. *Ergeb Physiologie, Biochemie, Biophysik, und Psychophysik.* 1905;4:307–422.

2. Deutsch E. *Blutgerinnungsfaktoren.* Vienna: Franz Deuticke; 1955.

3. Griffin JH, Evatt B, Zimmerman TS, Kleiss AJ, Wideman C. Deficiency of protein C in congenital thrombotic disease. *J Clin Invest.* 1981;68:1370–1373.

4. Broekmans AW, Veltkamp JJ, Bertina RM. Congenital protein C deficiency and venous thromboembolism: a study in three Dutch families. *N Engl J Med.* 1983;309:340–344.

5. Dahlbäck B, Carlsson M, Svensson J. Familial thrombophilia due to a previously unrecognized mechanism characterized by poor anticoagulant response to activated protein C: prediction of a cofactor to activated protein C. *Proc Natl Acad Sci U S A.* 1993;90:1004–1008.

6. Wozniak G, Montag H, Alemany J. Incidence of disorders of hemostasis in patients with deep vein thrombosis. *Int J Angiol.* 1995;4:99–102.

7. Conlan MG, Folsom AR, Finch A, Davis CE, Sorlie P, Wu KK. Correlation of plasma protein C levels with cardiovascular risk factors in middle-aged adults: the Atherosclerosis Risk in Communities (ARIC) Study. *Thromb Haemost.* 1993;70:762–767.

8. Pabinger I, Schneider B, and GTH Study Group on Natural Inhibitors. Thrombotic risk of women with hereditary antithrombin III-, protein C-, and protein S-deficiency taking oral contraceptive medication. *Thromb Haemost.* 1994; 71:548–552.

9. Comp PC, Nixon RR, Cooper MR, Esmon CT. Familial protein S deficiency is associated with recurrent thrombosis. *J Clin Invest.* 1984;74:2082–2088.

10. Engesser L, Broekmans AW, Briet E, Brommer EJP, Bertina RM. Hereditary protein S deficiency: clinical manifestation. *Ann Intern Med.* 1987;106:677–682.

11. Nielsen HK. Pathophysiology of venous thromboembolism. *Semin Thromb Hemost.* 1991;17(suppl 3):250–253.

12. Hathaway WE, Goodnight SH. *Disorders of Hemostasis and Thrombosis.* New York, NY: McGraw-Hill; 1993.

13. Seifried E. Das Fibrinolysesystem und seine Aktivatoren. In: Hach-Wunderle V, Neuhaus K, eds. *Thrombolyse und Antikoagulation in der Kardiologie.* Berlin: Springer-Verlag; 1994:3–22.

14. Krause J. Catabolism of tissue-type plasminogen activator (tPA): its variants, mutants, and hybrids. *Fibrinolysis.* 1988; 2:133–142.

15. Martin U, von Möllendorf E, Akpan W, Kientsch-Engel R, Kaufmann B, Neugebauer G. Pharmacokinetic and hemostatic properties of the recombinant plasminogen activator BM06.022 in healthy volunteers. *Thromb Haemost.* 1991;66:569–574.

16. Müller-Berghaus G. Wechselwirkung zwischen Komplement, Kallikrein-Kinin-System und Hämostasesystem. In: Tilsner V, Matthias FR, eds. *Immunologie und Blutgerinnung.* Basel, Switzerland: Editiones Roche; 1990:27–46.

17. Bennett B, Booth NA, Ogston D. Potential interactions between complement, coagulation, fibrinolysis, kinin-forming, and other enzyme systems. In: Bloom AL, Thomas DP, eds. *Haemostasis and Thrombosis.* Edinburgh: Churchill Livingstone; 1987:267–282.

18. Egberg N, Gallimore M, Green K, Jakobsen J, Vesterquist O, Wiman B. Effects of plasma kallikrein and bradykinin infusions into pigs on plasma fibrinolytic variables and urinary excretion of thromboxane and prostacyclin metabolites. *Fibrinolysis.* 1988;2:101–106.

19. Kaplan AP, Silverberg M. The coagulation-kinin pathway of human plasma. *Blood.* 1987;70:1–15.

20. Blajchman MA, Özge-Anwar AH. The role of the complement system in hemostasis. In: Brown E, ed. *Progress in Hematology.* Vol 14. New York, NY: Grune & Stratton; 1986: 149–161.

21. Seifert PS, Hugo F, Hansson GK, Bhakdi S. Prelesional complement activation in experimental atherosclerosis: terminal C5b–9 complement deposition coincides with cholesterol accumulation in the aortic intima of hypercholesterolemic rabbits. *Lab Invest.* 1989;60:747–754.

22. Sundsmo JS, Fair DS. Relationship among the complement, kinin, coagulation, and fibrinolytic systems. *Seminar Immunopathology.* 1983;6:231–258.

23. van Deventer SJH, Buller HR, ten Cate JW, Aarden LA, Hack CE, Sturk A. Experimental endotoxemia in humans: analysis of cytokine release and coagulation, fibrinolytic, and complement pathways. *Blood.* 1990;76:2520–2526.

24. Müller-Berghaus G. Physiologie der Blutgerinnung und Fibrinolyse. In: Müller-Eckhardt C, ed. *Transfusionsmedizin.* Berlin: Springer-Verlag; 1988:53–78.

25. Müller-Berghaus G. Pathophysiologic and biochemical events in disseminated intravascular coagulation: dysregulation of procoagulant and anticoagulant pathways. *Semin Thromb Hemost.* 1989;15:58–87.

26. Preissner KT. The role of vitronectin as multifunctional regulator in the hemostatic and immune systems. *Blut.* 1989;59:419–431.

27. Petersen LC, Bjorn SE, Nordfang O. Effect of leucocyte proteinases on tissue factor pathway inhibitor. *Thromb Haemost.* 1992;67:537–541.

28. Matthias FR. *Blutgerinnungsstörungen.* Berlin: Springer-Verlag; 1985.

29. Greinacher A, Liebenhoff U, Kiefel V, Presek P, Müller-Eckardt C. Heparin-associated thrombocytopenia: the effects of various intravenous IgG preparations on antibody mediated platelet activation—a possible new indication for high dose i.v. IgG. *Thromb Haemost.* 1994;71: 641–645.

30. Warkentin TE, Kelton JG. Heparin-induced thrombocytopenia. *Progress in Hemostasis and Thrombosis.* 1991;10: 1–34.

31. Greinacher A, Michels I, Liebenhoff U, Presek P, Müller-Eckhardt C. Heparin-associated thrombocytopenia: immune complexes are attached to the platelet membrane by the negative charge of highly sulfated oligosaccharide. *Br J Haematol.* 1993;84:711–716.

32. Greinacher A, Michels I, Müller-Eckhardt C. Heparin-associated thrombocytopenia: the antibody is not heparin specific. *Thromb Haemost.* 1992;67:545–549.

33. Cines DB, Tomaski A, Tannenbaum S. Immune endothelial-cell injury in heparin-associated thrombocytopenia. *N Engl J Med.* 1987;316:581–589.

34. Greinacher A, Pötzsch B, Amiral J, Dummel V, Eichner A, Müller-Eckhardt C. Heparin-associated thrombocytopenia: isolation of the antibody and characterization of a multimolecular PF4-heparin complex as the major antigen. *Thromb Haemost.* 1994;71:247–251.

35. Triplett DA. Lupus-Antikoagulantien: Klinische Aspekte und Laborbefunde. *Diagnose und Labor.* 1993;43:154–161.

36. Lechner K, Jäger U, Kapiotis S, Pabinger I. Lupus-Antikoagulantien. In: Tilsner V, Matthias FR, eds. *Immunologie und Blutgerinnung.* Basel, Switzerland: Editiones Roche; 1990: 153–160.

37. Galli M, Comfurius P, Maassen C, et al. Anticardiolipin antibodies (ACA) directed not to cardiolipin but to a plasma protein cofactor. *Lancet.* 1990;335:1544–1547.

38. Gastineau DA, Kazmier FJ, Nichols WL, Bowie EJW. Lupus anticoagulant: an analysis of the clinical and laboratory features of 219 cases. *Am J Hematol.* 1985;19:265–275.

39. Love PE, Santoro SA. Antiphospholipid antibodies: anticardiolipin and the lupus anticoagulant in systemic lupus erythematosus (SLE) and in non-SLE disorders. *Ann Intern Med.* 1990;112:682–698.

40. de Boer K, Büller HR, ten Cate JW, Levi M. Deep vein thrombosis in obstetric patients: diagnosis and risk factors. *Thromb Haemost.* 1992;67:4–7.

41. Unander AM, Norberg R, Hahn L, Arfors L. Anticardiolipin antibodies and complement in ninety-nine women with habitual abortion. *Am J Obstet Gynecol.* 1987;156: 114–119.

42. Matthias FR, Leithäuser B, Reitz D. Sepsis und Blutgerinnung: diagnostisches procedere. *Diagnose und Labor.* 1993; 43:162–168.

43. Leithäuser B, Matthias FR, Voss R. Sepsis und Hämostasesystem. In: Tilsner V, Matthias FR, eds. *Blutgerinnung und Intensivmedizin.* Basel, Switzerland: Editiones Roche; 1991: 61–65.

44. Corrigan JJ, Ray WL, May N. Changes in the blood coagulation associated with septicemia. *N Engl J Med.* 1986;279: 851–856.

45. Voss R, Matthias FR, Borkowski G, Reitz D. Activation and inhibition of fibrinolysis in septic patients in an intensive care unit. *Br J Haematol.* 1990;75:99–105.

46. van Wersch JWJ, Tjwa MKT. Coagulation/fibrinolysis balance and lung cancer. *Haemostasis.* 1991;21:117–123.

47. Dvorak HF. Thrombosis and cancer. *Hum Pathol.* 1987; 18:275–284.

48. Chew E, Wallace AC. Demonstration of fibrin in early stages of experimental metastases. *Cancer Res.* 1976;36: 1904–1909.

49. Evers JL, Patel J, Madeja JM, et al. Plasminogen activator activity and composition on human breast cancer. *Cancer Res.* 1983;42:219–226.

50. Duffy MJ, O'Grady P, Devaney D, O'Siorain L, Fennelly JJ, Lynen HJ. Urokinase-plasminogen activator, a marker for aggressive breast carcinomas. *Cancer.* 1988;62:531–533.

51. Mussoni L, Acero R, Conforti MG, Riganti M, Mantovani A, Donatie MB. Enhanced expression of plasminogen activator (PA) activity by tumor-associated macrophages (TAM). *Thromb Haemost.* 1985;54:162–164.

52. Wojtukiewicz MZ, Zacharski LR, Memolo VA, et al. Abnormal regulation of coagulation/fibrinolysis in small cell carcinoma of the lung. *Cancer.* 1990;65:481–485.

53. Hiller E, Riess H. *Hämorrhagische Diathese und Thrombose.* Stuttgart, Germany: Wissenschaftliche Verlags Gesellschaft; 1988.

54. Haverback BJ, Dutcher TF, Shore PA, et al. Serotonin changes in platelets and brain induced by small daily doses of reserpine: lack of effect of depletion of platelet serotonin on hemostatic mechanisms. *N Engl J Med.* 1975; 256:343–345.

55. Yanagisawa M, Kurihara H, Kimura S, et al. A novel potent vasoconstrictor peptide produced by vascular endothelial cells. *Nature.* 1988;332:411–415.

56. Ratnoff OD, Saito H. Surface-mediated reactions. *Current Topics Hematology.* 1979;2:1–57.

57. Cochrane CG. Exposure of blood to foreign surfaces: what are the consequences? In: Dudziak R, Reuter HD, Kirchhoff PG, Schumann F, eds. *Proteolyse und Proteinaseninhibition in der Herz- und Gefäßchirurgie.* Stuttgart, Germany: Schattauer; 1985:5–16.

58. Neuhof H. Acute respiratory distress syndrome: the pathogenetic role of the "classical" cascade systems and the arachidonic acid metabolism. *Intensive Care News.* 1983;2: 5–9.

59. Wachtfogel YT, Kucich U, James HL, et al. Human plasma kallikrein releases neutrophil elastase during blood coagulation. *J Clin Invest.* 1983;72:1672–1677.

60. Colman RW, Osbahr AJ. New vasoconstrictor, bovine peptide-B, released during blood coagulation. *Nature.* 1967;214:1040–1041.

61. Neuhof H. Zur Rolle der Mediatoren bei der Sepsis. *Intensivmedizin.* 1989;26(suppl 1):3–9.

62. Saito H. Normal hemostatic mechanisms. In: Ratnoff OD, Forbes CD, eds. *Disorders of Hemostasis.* Philadelphia, Pa: WB Saunders; 1991:18–47.

63. Prescott SM, Zimmermann GA, McIntyre TM. Human endothelial cells in culture produce platelet activating factor (1-alkyl-2-acetyl-sn-glycero-3-phosphocholine) when stimulated with thrombin. *Proc Natl Acad Sci U S A.* 1984; 81:3534–3538.

64. Stern D, Nawroth P, Handley D, et al. An endothelial cell dependent pathway of coagulation. *Proc Natl Acad Sci U S A.* 1985;82:2523–2527.

65. Esmon CT. The regulation of natural anticoagulant pathways. *Science.* 1987;235:1348–1352.

66. Speiser W, Anders E, Preissner KT, et al. Differences in coagulant and fibrinolytic activities of cultured human endothelial cells derived from omental tissue microvessels and umbilical veins. *Blood.* 1987;69:964–967.

67. Sixma JJ. Platelet adhesion in health and disease. In: Verstraete M, Vermylen J, Lijnen HR, eds. *Thrombosis and Haemostasis 1987.* Leuven, Belgium: Leuven University Press; 1987:127–146.

68. Crawford N, Scrutton MC. Biochemistry of the blood platelets. In: Bloom AL, Thomas DP, eds. *Haemostasis and Thrombosis.* 2nd ed. Edinburgh: Churchill Livingstone; 1987: 47–77.

69. Klein J. *Immunologie.* Weinheim, Germany: VCH Verlagsgesellschaft; 1991.

70. Dapper F, Neppl H, Wozniak G, Strube I, Neuhof H. EKZ: Humorale Systeme und Mediatoren. In: Preuße CJ, Schulte HD, eds. *Extrakorporale Zirkulation Heute*. Darmstadt, Germany: Steinkopff Verlag; 1991:31–36.

71. Sakata Y, Aoki M. Crosslinking of alpha₂-plasmin inhibitor to fibrin by fibrin-stabilizing factor. *J Clin Invest*. 1980; 65:290–297.

72. McDonagh J. Biochemistry of fibrin-stabilizing factor (XIII). In: McDonagh J, Seitz R, Egbring R, eds. *Factor XIII*. Stuttgart, Germany: Schattauer Verlag; 1993:2–8.

73. Pabinger I, Kyrle PA, Heistinger M, Eichinger S, Wittmann E, Lechner K. The risk of thromboembolism in asymptomatic patients with protein C and protein S deficiency: a prospective cohort study. *Thromb Haemost*. 1994;71: 441–445.

74. Scharrer I. Bekannte Ursachen der Thrombophilie. In: Tilsner V, Matthias FR, eds. *Thrombophilie und Antikoagulation*. Basel, Switzerland: Editiones Roche; 1993:7–21.

75. Gladson CL, Scharrer I, Hach V, Beck KH, Griffin JH. The frequency of type I heterozygous protein S and protein C deficiency in 141 unrelated young patients with venous thrombosis. *Thromb Haemost*. 1988;59:18–22.

76. Scharrer I, Hach-Wunderle V. Prävalenz und klinische Bedeutung der hereditären Thrombophilie. *Innere Medizin*. 1988;15:5.

77. Hach-Wunderle V, Scharrer I. Prävalenz des hereditären Mangels an Antithrombin III, Protein C, und Protein S. *Dtsch Med Wochenschr*. 1993;118:187–190.

78. Jaenecke J. *Antikoagulanzien- und Fibrinolysetherapie*. Stuttgart, Germany: Georg Thieme Verlag; 1991.

79. Thiagarajan P, Shapiro SS, De Marco L. Monoclonal immunoglobin M lambda coagulation inhibitor with phospholipid specificity. *J Clin Invest*. 1980;66:397.

80. Triplett DA, Brandt JT, Musgrave KA, Orr CA. The relationship between lupus anticoagulants and antibodies to phospholipid. *JAMA*. 1988;259:550–554.

81. Egeberg O. Inherited antithrombin deficiency causing thrombophilia. *Thrombosis Diethesis Haemorrhagia*. 1965;13: 516.

82. Wozniak G, Altmeyer W, Montag H, Alemany J. Thrombophilie: Gerinnungs-Screening in Diagnostik und Therapiekontrolle. *Diagnose und Labor*. 1992;2:120–124.

83. Bauer KA, Rosenberg RD. The hypercoagulable state. In: Ratnoff OD, Forbes CD, eds. *Disorders of Hemostasis*. Philadelphia, Pa: WB Saunders; 1991:267–291.

84. Branson HE, Katz J, Marble R, Griffin JH. Inherited protein C deficiency and coumarin-responsive chronic relapsing purpura fulminans in a newborn infant. *Lancet*. 1983; 2:1165–1168.

85. Broekmans AW, Bertina RM. Protein C. In: Poller L, ed. *Recent Advances in Blood Coagulation*. Vol 4. New York, NY: Churchill Livingstone; 1985:117–137.

86. Wintzen AR, Broekmans AW, Bertina RM, et al. Cerebral hemorrhagic infarction in young patients with hereditary protein C deficiency: evidence for "spontaneous" cerebral venous thrombosis. *BMJ*. 1985;290:350–352.

87. Karpatkin M, Mannucci P, Bhogal M, et al. Low protein C in the neonatal period. *Br J Haematol*. 1986;62:137–142.

88. Pui CH, Chesney CM, Bergum PW, et al. Lack of pathogenetic role of proteins C and S in thrombosis associated with asparaginase-prednisone-vincristine therapy for leukaemia. *Br J Haematol*. 1986;64:283–290.

89. Uchida K. Influence of antibiotics on vitamin K metabolism. *Ann Hematol*. 1992;64(suppl):53.

90. Gonzalez R, Alberca I, Sala N, Vicente V. Protein C deficiency: response to danazol and DDAVP. *Thromb Haemost*. 1985;53:320-322.

91. Hach-Wunderle V, Scharrer I, Lottenberg R. Congenital deficiency of plasminogen and its relationship to venous thrombosis. *Thromb Haemost*. 1988;59:277–280.

92. Halbmayer WM, Mannhalter CH, Fischer M. Faktor XII-Mangel und Thrombophilie. *Hämostaseologie*. 1993;13: 157–160.

93. Halbmayer WM, Haushofer A, Schön R, et al. The prevalence of moderate and severe F XII (Hageman factor) deficiency among the normal population: evaluation of the incidence of F XII deficiency among 300 healthy blood donors. *Thromb Haemost*. 1994;71:68–72.

94. Juhan-Vague I, Valadier J, Alessi M, et al. Deficient t-PA release and elevated PA inhibitor levels in patients with spontaneous or recurrent deep venous thrombosis. *Thromb Haemost*. 1987;57:67.

95. Saito H, Scott JG, Movat HZ, Scialla SJ. Molecular heterogeneity of Hageman trait (f XII deficiency): evidence that two of 49 subjects are cross-reacting material positive (CRM+). *J Lab Clin Med*. 1979;94:256–265.

96. Wuillemin WA, Huber I, Furlan M, Lämmle B. Functional characterization of an abnormal factor XII molecule (F XII Bern). *Blood*. 1991;78:997–1004.

97. Goodnough LT, Saito H, Ratnoff OD. Thrombosis or myocardial infarction in congenital clotting factors abnormalities and chronic thrombocytopenias: a report of 21 patients and a review of 50 previously reported cases. *Medicine*. 1983;62:248–255.

98. Halbmayer W-M, Mannhalter C, Feichtinger C, Rubi K, Fischer M. The prevalence of factor XII deficiency in 103 orally anticoagulated outpatients suffering from recurrent venous and/or arterial thromboembolism. *Thromb Haemost*. 1992;68:285–290.

99. Christie DJ, Mullen PC, Aster RH. Fab-mediated binding of drug-dependent antibodies to platelets in quinidine and quinidine-induced thrombocytopenia. *J Clin Invest*. 1985;75:310–314.

100. Amiral J, Bridey F, Reyfus M, et al. Platelet factor 4 complexed to heparin is the target for antibodies generated in heparin-induced thrombocytopenia. *Thromb Haemost*. 1992;68:95–96.

101. Kelton JG, Sheridan D, Santos A, et al. Heparin-induced thrombocytopenia: laboratory studies. *Blood*. 1988;72: 925–930.

102. Chong BH, Fawaz I, Chesterman CN, Berndt MC. Heparin-induced thrombocytopenia: mechanism of interaction of the heparin-dependent antibody with platelets. *Br J Haematol*. 1989;73:235–240.

103. Anderson GP. Insights into heparin-induced thrombocytopenia. *Br J Haematol*. 1992;80:504–508.

104. Morgagni JB. The Seats and Causes of Diseases Investigated by Anatomy. 3rd ed. London; 1796.

105. Dastre A. Fibrinolyse dans le sang. *Archiv Physiology Normale Pathology*. 1893;5:661–663.

106. Astrup T. The hemostatic balance. *Thrombosis et Diathesis Haemorrhagia.* 1958;2:347–357.

107. Fearnley GR. A concept of natural fibrinolysis. *Lancet.* 1961;992–993.

108. Tillett WS, Garner RL. The fibrinolytic activity of hemolytic streptococci. *J Exp Med.* 1933;58:485–491.

109. Christensen LR, MacLeod CM. A proteolytic enzyme of serum: characterization, activation, and reaction with inhibitors. *J Gen Physiol.* 1945;28:559–565.

110. Kirby EP, Martin N, Marder VJ. Degradation of bovine factor VIII by plasmin and trypsin. *Blood.* 1974;43:629–640.

111. Pasquini R, Hershgold EJ. Effects of plasmin on human factor VIII (AHF). *Blood.* 1973;41:105–111.

112. Sherry S. *Fibrinolysis, Thrombosis, and Hemostasis.* Philadelphia, Pa: Lea & Febiger; 1992.

113. Wozniak G, Montag H, Alemany J. Correlation between results of regional thrombolysis with rtPA in patients with deep vein thrombosis and the coagulation status before therapy: predictive value of the F1+2/D-dimer-index. In: *Proceedings of the European Congress of the International Union of Phlebology, Budapest 1993.* Essex, England: Multi-Science Publishing; 1993:424–434.

114. Paques EP, Heimburger N. Das fibrinolytische System. *Hämostaseologie.* 1986;6:139–147.

115. Smith RAG, Dupe RJ, English PD, Green J. Fibrinolysis with acyl enzymes: a new approach to thrombolytic therapy. *Nature.* 1981;290:505–508.

116. Van de Werf F, Nobuhara N, Collen D. Coronary thrombolysis with human single-chain, urokinase-type plasminogen activator (pro-urokinase) in patients with acute myocardial infarction. *Ann Intern Med.* 1986;104:345–348.

117. Alemany J, Montag H, Wozniak G. Rezidivthrombosen nach chirurgischer Thrombektomie ilio-femoraler Thrombosen. *Archiv Angiologie.* 1993;24:147–150.

118. Martin M, Fiebach BJO. *Fibrinolytische Behandlung peripherer Arterien- und Venenverschlüsse.* Bern, Switzerland: Verlag Hans Huber; 1994.

119. Straub H. *Fibrinolytische Therapie.* Stuttgart, Germany: Schattauer Verlag; 1983.

120. ISAM Study Group. A prospective trail of intravenous streptokinase in acute myocardial infarction: mortality, morbidity, and infarct size at 21 days. *N Engl J Med.* 1986; 314:1465–1471.

121. Carter CJ, Doyle DL, Dawson N, Fowler S, Devine DV. Investigations into the clinical utility of latex D-dimer in the diagnosis of deep vein thrombosis. *Thromb Haemost.* 1993; 69:8–11.

122. Bauer KA, Rosenberg RD. The pathophysiology of the prethrombotic state in humans: insights gained from studies using markers of hemostatic system activation. *Blood.* 1987;70:343–345.

123. Wozniak G, Dapper F, Alemany J. Prädiktive Bedeutung des aktuellen Gerinnungsstatus für die semi-lokale rtPA-Lyse der Unterschenkelvenenthrombose. *Schweiz Med Wochenschr.* 1995;125(suppl 66):11.

124. Pannekoek H, de Vries C, van Zonneveld AJ. Mutants of human tissue-type plasminogen activator (tPA): structural aspects and functional properties. *Fibrinolysis.* 1988;2: 123–132.

125. Jackson CV, Crowe VG, Craft TJ, et al. Thrombolytic activity of a new plasminogen activator, LY210825, compared to recombinant tissue-type plasminogen activator in a canine model of coronary artery thrombosis. *Circulation.* 1990;82:930–940.

126. Phaneuf MD, Ozaki CK, Johnstone MT, Loza J-P, Quist WC, LoGerfo FW. Covalent linkage of streptokinase to recombinant hirudin: a novel thrombolytic agent with antithrombotic properties. *Thromb Haemost.* 1994;71: 481–487.

Section 13
Chronic Lymphedema

93

Chronic Lymphedema

Robert Lerner

Chronic lymphedema is a major health problem that plagues millions of people all over the world. In underdeveloped countries, filarial infestation is the major cause. In industrialized countries, the majority of cases result from cancer treatments, that is, lymph node dissections and/or radiation therapy. Chemotherapy is probably not a significant contributing factor.

The approximate numbers of lymphedema cases, based on a World Health Organization report,[1] are listed in Table 93.1. From this listing it is obvious that lymphedema is a major health problem.

Lymphedema is defined as the protein-rich edema that occurs when the lymph load (volume) exceeds lymph transport capacity in any body segment. As more and more protein and other macromolecules accumulate in the interstitial spaces, colloid-osmotic pressure rises and edema worsens. The presence of stagnant protein in the interstitium incites a low-grade chronic inflammation that leads to connective tissue proliferation, fibrosis, induration, skin thickening, skin erythema, and, in long-standing cases, hyperkeratotic papilloma formation and other changes typical of elephantiasis.

Because of the presence of stagnant, protein-rich fluid in the tissue spaces, patients with lymphedema are prone to have repeated episodes of infection: cellulitis, erysipelas, and lymphangitis. Lymphedema also results in increased lymphatic pressure, dilation of lymph vessels, valvular incompetence, and, as a result, additional lymph stasis.

Földi et al.[2] described three lymphedema stages, which are listed in Table 93.2. In early lymphedema, the edema

TABLE 93.1. Incidence of lymphedema.

Parasites	90 million
Breast cancer	20 million
Primary	2–3 million
Chronic venous insufficiency	300 million

TABLE 93.2. Three stages of lymphedema.

Stage I
Reversible lymphedema
    Accumulation of protein-rich edematous fluid

Stage II
Spontaneously irreversible lymphedema
    Protein-rich edematous fluid
    Connective and scar tissue

Stage III
Lymphostatic elephantiasis
    Protein-rich edematous fluid
    Connective and scar tissue
    Hardening of dermal tissues
    Papillomas of the skin

is soft and pitting; therapy is rapid, easy, and usually successful in returning the limb to normal size. In later stages, the skin and subcutaneous tissues are fibrotic, and pitting cannot be elicited. In these later stages, treatment requires more time and effort, and the results are generally less favorable. Because of this difference, clinicians are urged to advise appropriate therapy as early as possible in the course of the disease.

Types of Lymphedema

Primary Lymphedema

Primary lymphedema occurs because of the imperfect development of the lymph-vascular system in utero. It can be familial or sporadic. The exact incidence of primary lymphedema is unknown because patients frequently receive no treatment for the condition and it is not reportable.

Histologically, biopsy specimens may reveal aplasia, hypoplasia, or hyperplasia of the lymph vasculature, any of which can result in chronic extremity lymphedema. Primary lymphedema develops mostly in women. It is some-

TABLE 93.3. Types of primary lymphedema.

I. Congenital (present at birth)
II. Precocious (begins at puberty)
III. Tardive (begins after age 35)

TABLE 93.5. Lymphedema defense mechanisms.

Naturally occurring lymphovenous anastomoses
Active macrophage/phagocytic resorption mechanism
Abundant collateral circulation
Active (versus sedentary) lifestyle
Patent connections between superficial and deep drainage systems

times accompanied by a fibrotic, enlarged lymph node or cluster of lymph nodes in the groin, as described by Kinmonth,[3] the excision of which results in further damage to lymph transport capacity and worsening of the lymphedema.

Primary lymphedema usually appears without obvious cause or after a minor traumatic event occurring at different stages of life. These stages are listed in Table 93.3.

About 80% of all cases of primary lymphedema are of the lymphedema praecox variety, usually starting at puberty or in teenage years.

Secondary Lymphedema

Secondary lymphedema is more common than primary lymphedema. It occurs as a result of a wide variety of causes, which are listed in Table 93.4.

Most secondary lymphedemas are the result of parasites in underdeveloped countries and of breast cancer treatments in industrialized nations. Because of the millions of patients who must endure the burden of lymphedema after breast cancer, there is currently great impetus to remove fewer and fewer axillary nodes or to even forego axillary dissection in certain cases. Radiation therapists also avoid axillary irradiation whenever possible.

Whether primary or secondary, chronic lymphedema is incurable, despite the many previous heroic attempts to restore the injured or inadequate lymph vessels. It is also progressive over time. The rate of progression varies with temperature, humidity, body build, activities, number of infectious complications, and so forth. Treatment is very challenging and time-consuming, causing many clinicians to ignore the problem completely or, if they do treat the lymphedema, to prescribe ineffective or inappropriate measures. In addition, because lymphology is not yet a fully recognized medical specialty, patients are usually left with no treatment at all or must seek help

from physicians with little expertise or experience in the field.

In the case of arm lymphedema after axillary surgery or radiation therapy (or both), the edema is often more distressing to the patient than the mastectomy or lumpectomy because the edematous upper extremity cannot easily be disguised and because the patient must deal with lymphedema and its complications for life.

In the lower extremities, lymphedema is even more distressing because patients must deal with a variety of special problems, such as a different shoe size for each foot, difficulty walking, excessive fatigue from heavy lower extremities, back pain, diminished agility, and sedentary lifestyle. Lymphedema begins soon after axillary treatment in some cases; in others, it begins years later. The difference lies in the degree of damage caused by the treatment and by the potency of the patient's defense mechanisms; the latter are listed in Table 93.5.

It appears certain that obesity, excessive postoperative wound drainage, and infections are associated with increased lymphedema occurrence.[4,5] Swelling of the ipsilateral upper extremity after axillary treatment (surgery and/or radiation therapy) occurs very frequently. The exact numbers have been studied for nearly a century, and too much time has been wasted in the past just to learn that upper extremity lymphedema is very common. According to the National Cancer Institute, it occurs in 50% to 70% of patients after axillary treatment[6] but is severe in only about 10%. Many other studies have confirmed this overall figure,[7,8] although studies that evaluate patients soon after their treatment indicate a lesser incidence.[9-11] Whenever the percentage of lymphedema is cited, it is important to state how long after the axillary treatment it occurred, because lymphedema can develop 20 or even 30 years after treatment. Some of the previously cited studies are listed in Table 93.6.

In all studies reviewed, lymphedema is more prevalent in patients who have had both axillary surgery and radia-

TABLE 93.4. Causes of secondary lymphedemas.

Surgery
Radiation therapy
Trauma
Filariasis
Cancer
Self-induced
Infectious
Iatrogenic

TABLE 93.6. Lymphedema incidence after axillary treatment.

Britton and Nelson[7]	7%–63%
Hughes and Patel[8]	41%–70%
National Cancer Institute[6]	50%–70%
Johns Hopkins[42]	16%
Memorial Hospital[43]	16%
Royal Marsden[44]	26%
Ivens et al.[11]	18%

tion therapy. Even when the radiation is given only to the breast, as is usually done after lumpectomy, there is enough radiation delivered to the axilla to place the patient into the highest risk category for lymphedema.[12]

Parasitic Lymphedema

Parasitic lymphedema is very common in tropical areas of the world. It is caused by the microfilariae of *Wuchereria bancrofti* and *Brugia malayi,* which can be transmitted to humans by many different mosquito species. When these microfilariae reach the lymph vessels, they develop into adult worms. The resulting inflammation and fibrosis cause increasing lymphatic obstruction. The infection may cause chills, fever, and general malaise. These symptoms may also be associated with lymphangitis, lymphadenitis, and so forth. Elephantiasis is the result of repeated infections over many years.

Ivermectin and diethylcarbamazine are of value in patients with microfilariae in the blood. The lymphedema is treated by complete or complex decongestive physiotherapy (CDP), if available.

Lymphedema and Reflux

Lymph flow is always centripetal except in cases of reflux. Reflux is the result of lymph valve insufficiency, allowing the lymph or chyle to flow the wrong way. Complications of lymphatic reflux are numerous: lymph-filled cysts (of the penis, scrotum, or labia), skin papillomas, lymph-cutaneous fistulas, chylous-joint reflux, chyluria, chylous ascites, chylous pericarditis, and others. Reflux is a surgically treatable disease if the refluxing segment and fistulous tracts can be located and resected. These operations should be undertaken after careful study of the anatomical situation and only by surgeons with experience in this field.

Pure Lymphedema and Combination Forms

Most patients with lymphedema have pure lymphedema. Lymphedema sometimes appears in combination with morbid obesity, lipedema, or rheumatoid arthritis or in patients with long-standing chronic venous insufficiency.

In chronic venous insufficiency, most of the interstitial fluid is unable to return to the heart by way of the obstructed iliofemoral veins. As a result, the volume of fluid transported by the lower extremity lymphatics increases to compensate for the venous occlusion. This safety-valve function of the lymph vessels continues until, at some point, the lymphatic valvular mechanism be-

comes insufficient, the lymph vessels become insufficient, reflux occurs, swelling of the limb increases, and venous ulcers develop.

Lipedema is a condition affecting only women and usually only the pelvic girdle and lower extremities. It is a bilateral, symmetrical swelling of the lower extremities extending from the pelvic brim to the ankles. Histologically, its hallmark is a great increase in the subcutaneous fat layer but only in the areas just mentioned. The patient may be normal in weight or even thin in the upper half of the body, but grossly obese from the pelvic brim down. Patients with lipedema occasionally have a similar fat-storage problem in the arms, but this is much less common. If the arms are involved, these areas show large amounts of subcutaneous fat, loose skin, and thin forearms.

Lipedema and lymphedema frequently coexist as the lymph vessels in lipedema are coiled, the prelymphatic canals and initial lymph vessels are abnormal, lymph transport velocity is decreased, and the lymphedema eventually involves both lower extremities and the feet. Lipedematous limbs are tender and bruise easily because the subcutaneous veins have no support as they course through the layers of loose, subcutaneous fat.

Diagnosis and Differential Diagnosis

Lymphedema after node dissection or radiation therapy is to be expected. In patients treated for breast cancer who develop lymphedema, the usual tests to rule out recurrence of tumor should be carried out. Lymphangiography, venography, and lymphoscintigraphy are unnecessary in such cases and may further damage the remaining lymph vasculature. Similarly, venous sonography is not indicated because axillary vein thrombosis is a diagnosis that is easily made clinically and such thrombosis does not cause lymphedema. Axillary vein obstruction or narrowing, moreover, does not require surgical correction.

In patients with other types of cancer, care should be taken to rule out recurrence. If none is found, the lymphedema should be treated as early as possible.

In patients with primary lower extremity lymphedema, the swelling usually starts in the ankle and foot for no obvious reason or after minor trauma. In some cases it begins after an infection, inguinal hernia repair, or a biopsy of an inguinal lymph node. Often it begins after an airplane trip or following great physical exertion. It usually begins in one ankle.

If primary lymphedema is suggested, the clinician should rule out pelvic, anal, and external genital cancer before treating the lymphedema. Venous sonography is usually not necessary but certainly should be done in patients with varicose veins and whenever femoral vein thrombosis is possible. Because most of the patients are teenage girls, the latter diagnosis is not usually considered.

Lymphoscintigraphy (radioisotope lymphography) should always be done if the diagnosis of lymphedema is in question or if there are other congenital anomalies or complicating factors such as angiodysplasias, hemangiomas, lymphangiomas, or bone malformations. Lymphoscintigraphy is by far the most valuable and least invasive diagnostic test that can be done in these circumstances. It is minimally invasive and does not damage the visualized lymph vessels.

Prevention

Upper Extremity

Several recent studies have shown that without dissection or irradiation of clinically negative axillae, there was only a 2% to 5% failure rate,[13-15] even though about one third of such axillae contain metastatic cancer.[16,17] In patients with breast cancer, axillary dissection should probably not be done in the very elderly, in patients with in situ or very early or very tiny breast cancers, in patients with serious, life-threatening medical conditions, or in patients with small areas of intraductal carcinoma. The indications for level I, II, or III axillary dissection are still being debated in the surgical community.

There is no doubt, however, that a clinically negative axilla or a completely dissected axilla should not be subjected to postoperative radiation therapy. Some physicians[18] also advocate the avoidance of postoperative exercises for 2 weeks to lessen the incidence of lymphedema.

After axillary treatment, however, there is broad consensus that the patient should avoid trauma to the ipsilateral upper extremity; avoid venipunctures, blood pressure measurements, heat of all types, and insect bites; and avoid constricting clothes and bra straps. In addition, all vigorous exercises should be done only when the arm is supported by a compression sleeve or lymphedema bandage.

Lower Extremity

Many cases of lower extremity lymphedema can be avoided. In the child with a fibrotic inguinal lymphadenopathy, the physician should avoid excisional biopsy and rely whenever possible on fine-needle aspiration biopsy. If there is a family history of lower extremity lymphedema, biopsy should not be done. Vein stripping operations should rarely be done because many lymphedema cases begin after these procedures. Inguinal

and femoral hernia operations should be done through small incisions that parallel Langer's lines. Popliteal cysts should be aspirated and bandaged whenever possible because excision is sometimes associated with postoperative lymphedema. In patients with melanoma, groin dissection should not be done for early, superficial lesions. The technique of sentinel node biopsy should be more widespread because this method often avoids a full groin dissection. When a groin dissection is done, postoperative seromas should be kept to a minimum by compression bandaging and adequate drainage of the wound.

Treatment

Over the past century, three basic treatment methods have evolved from a huge number that were tried and mostly abandoned. Lymphedema has never been cured by any method. The best that medicine can offer the patient with lymphedema is to improve appearance, improve function, and prevent further progression of the swelling.

The three methods currently in use include the following:

1. Surgery of some kind
2. CDP
3. Pneumatic compression pump therapy

Surgeons have tried many innovative procedures to restore the damaged lymph circulation, bridge (or bypass) the obstructed segment, or debulk the swollen limb. Restoration operations include lymphangioplasties using silk threads,[19] nylon tubes,[20] small veins,[21] and others. Bridging procedures include the Goldsmith operation (omentopexy),[22] the Standard operation,[23] lymphovenous anastomoses done by microsurgeons,[24] Thompson's operation,[25] Kondoleon's procedure,[26] the enteromesenteric bridge procedure,[27] and others. Debulking or resective procedures include Homans's operation,[28] Sistrunk's operation,[29] Charles's procedure,[30] and so forth.

None of the operations just mentioned can be recommended for patients with lymphedema because they are major procedures associated with frequent complications, poor cosmetic results, scarring of the limbs, and varying degrees of success in controlling the progression of the lymphedema. Even the microsurgical procedures introduced in the 1960s and 1970s are being done less and less often these days because of lack of long-term success.

Surgeons sometimes recommend operations because "conservative therapy" has failed. As Földi et al. point out,[31] "conservative therapy of lymphedema is in disarray or chaotic." Before an operation, one must carefully define who did the conservative therapy and what methods were used. In the United States, for example, patients with lymphedema are often referred for physical therapy that is given by therapists with the most rudimentary knowledge of lymphedema and its treatment.

CDP was practiced in Berlin in 1892 by von Winiwarter.[32] It flourished in various clinics from time to time afterward but was largely unused until Földi popularized the method in the 1970s.[33-35] Since then, he has been the greatest force worldwide in explaining the pathophysiology of lymphedema and the singular value of CDP for its control. In a recent publication, he wrote,

had the clinical outcome as shown in many articles treated by operation occurred in Germany where combined physiotherapy is the preferred method of treating peripheral lymphedema, the results would be considered cosmetically and functionally unacceptable. . . . Nonetheless, by means of combined physiotherapy, a manipulative form of treatment free of noticeable side effects, lymphedema of the extremities even in the most advanced stages can be remedied with remarkable consistency.[36]

CDP (complex or complete decongestive physiotherapy) is a two-phase method of treating patients with lymphedema. Phase I is carried out by specially trained therapists who work under the supervision of a physician with great experience and expertise in lymphedema. Treatments are given once or twice daily, 5 days a week, for this treatment period. The patient and family are taught everything that must be done in phase II, the maintenance phase, that is then carried out by patient and family at home. Follow-up visits are usually done every 6 months thereafter to assess the patient's progress, measure the volume of the limb, fit a new compression garment, and so on. Because lymphedema is chronic and incurable, CDP effectively transfers the day-to-day care of the patient from physician and clinic to patient and family. This feature is an important cost-saving mechanism that should be noted by physicians and the health care industry.

In addition, as the swollen limb is decompressed and emptied of stagnant protein-rich fluid, the patient is much less likely to develop cellulitis and lymphangitis, the most common complications of lymphedema.

CDP has four major components:

1. Meticulous skin and nail care. This includes eradication of infections and application twice daily of a low-pH skin lotion to reduce the number of skin microorganisms.
2. Manual lymph drainage, a lymphatic massage technique that decongests the trunk first, the proximal swollen limb next, and the distal parts of the limb last.
3. Immediately after the manual lymph drainage, multilayered compression bandaging of the involved limb using minimally elastic bandages. This prevents any evacuated fluid from returning and also increases di-

minished skin and tissue pressure, avoids any new lymph formation, and promotes resorption of interstitial fluid.
4. Remedial exercises carried out under supervision and only when the patient is wearing the nonyielding bandages just described. These exercises force the muscles and joints to further propel any stagnant lymph and interstitial fluid proximally, increasing volume and force of flow. Repeated treatments establish additional collateral circulation and restore the limb to normal or near normal.

If phase I is done in the early stages of lymphedema, the swelling disappears and the limb returns to normal size and shape. If treatment is done in stage II or III, CDP reduces the swelling but cannot return the limb to normal. For these advanced cases, home maintenance, which the patient has learned, will continue to improve the lymphedema, and a normal appearance may be achieved over a period of a few years.

CDP is extremely effective and cost-effective. Practically no risks or side effects are associated with CDP. Treatments are painless and relaxing. Well-trained therapists, great attention to detail, and experienced physicians are necessary for successful practice of CDP.

Posttreatment maintenance consists of wearing a surgical-grade elastic sleeve or stocking by day, compression bandaging of the limb at night, and remedial exercises every morning before removing the bandages. If a family member has learned manual lymph drainage, this technique is sometimes added. Before-and-after photographs of typical patients treated by CDP are shown in Figures 93.1 through 93.4.

Pneumatic compression pump therapy was introduced in the early 1970s. These devices are made so that the patient can insert the swollen limb into a large sleeve that contains multiple chambers attached by hoses to a compression pump. Compressed air is forced into one chamber at a time in the distal to proximal direction. As the chamber expands, it forces fluid from the most distal area to the next adjacent area; the first chamber then deflates, the second chamber is inflated, and so forth. In this manner, excess fluid is "milked" from the swollen extremity in the distal to proximal direction. Compression pumps are made by many different manufacturers. The patient usually buys or leases one. They have the great advantage of being available at home and of not requiring a therapist in their application or usage.

They have many disadvantages as well. The affected limb that has been decongested usually swells once the motor is turned off and the patient resumes normal activity. Use of a pneumatic pump disregards the fact that the ipsilateral trunk quadrant is also congested or lymphedematous, so the pump is essentially forcing fluid from a congested limb to a congested trunk. The pump

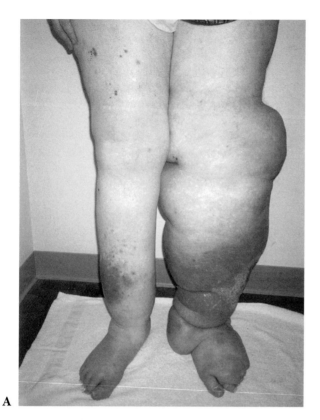 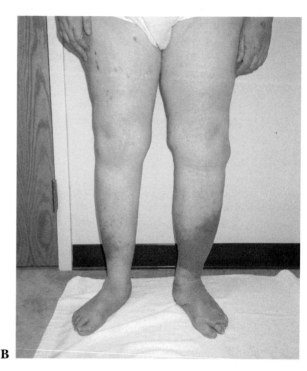

FIGURE 93.1. **A,** Primary lymphedema praecox of both lower extremities in a 48-year-old man with chronic infection, before CDP. **B,** Same patient after one course of CDP lasting 6 weeks.

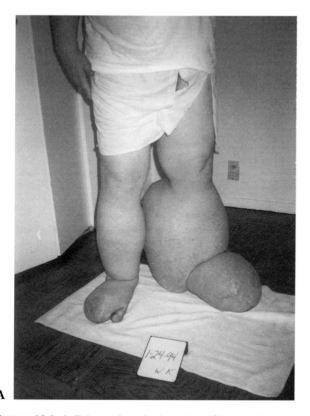 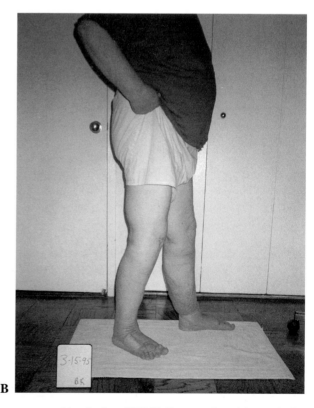

FIGURE 93.2. **A,** Primary lymphedema in a 67-year-old man. Both lower extremities, before CDP. **B,** Same patient 14 months later, after intensive CDP.

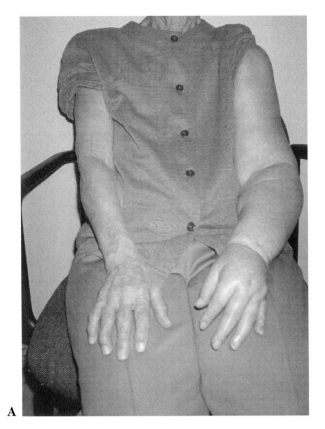

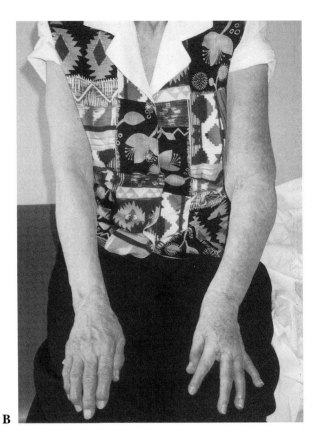

A

B

FIGURE 93.3. **A,** Secondary, postmastectomy lymphedema, before CDP therapy. **B,** Same patient after 20-day course of CDP.

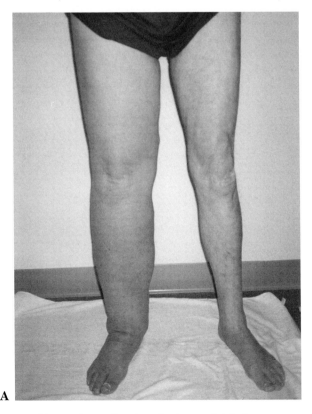

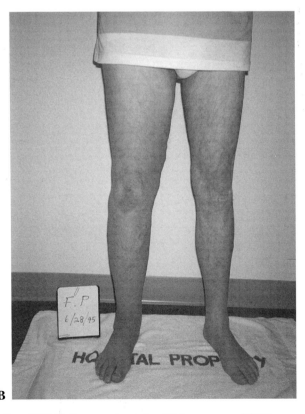

A

B

FIGURE 93.4. **A,** Secondary lymphedema of right lower extremity, before CDP. **B,** Same patient after 20-day course of CDP.

has no value in stages II and III lymphedema because it has no effect on fibrous connective or scar tissue. The external genitalia sometimes swell as a result of pump therapy when the lymphedema involves a lower extremity. Pneumatic pumps may also traumatize residual, functioning lymph vessels, much as blood pressure cuffs may do.

Physicians faced with a patient who has lymphedema often tell the patient that "nothing can be done" or the patient "must learn to live with it." Other physicians are quick to recommend pneumatic pumps because they are aware that the surgical results are not optimal, they do not have access to a CDP clinic or are unaware of the excellent results of CDP, and they feel it is their duty to recommend something. Because pumps are available in most developed countries, they are widely prescribed. Patients often use them for a period of months or years and then stop because of disillusionment or frustration.

Földi has written, "To squeeze edema fluid towards the groin or axilla of a lymphedematous limb, especially if the regional lymph nodes have been removed or are diseased, defies an understanding of basic anatomy and physiology."[36](pp1-2)

Adjuvant Therapy

Elevation

Physicians often tell their patients to elevate the arm or sleep with the arm or leg elevated. This is good advice but only in stage I lymphedema. It is also impractical for a patient with lymphedema of the arm to move about during the day with the arm elevated. Similarly, even if a patient goes to sleep with the swollen arm on two pillows, it is doubtful that the arm will be in that position when the patient awakes the next morning.

Elastic Support Garments

Elastic support garments are very important after any treatment for lymphedema, whether surgery, CDP, or pneumatic pump therapy. It is essential for the elastic support garment to be measured after the swollen limb has been decompressed because of considerations of comfort and appearance. It is most distressing for a patient to wear an elastic garment on a swollen limb. The garment never fits properly; it cuts in here and there and is very uncomfortable. In most such cases, the patient stops wearing the garment.

Elastic garments must also be measured and fitted by professionals with expertise in this area and not by a clerk who happens to be on duty in a surgical supply store. The physician who prescribes the garment should specify the compression class, the length of the garment desired, and, if possible, the type of fabric. Fabrics should be durable, seamless, comfortable, and nonallergenic.

Medications

The medications most often prescribed for lymphedema are diuretics. They are sometimes of value in the initial stages of CDP. Long-term use is probably harmful for patients with lymphedema because it results in an increase in intercellular colloid-osmotic pressure that attracts edema fluid and may also cause electrolyte imbalances. Diuretics are of value in patients who have body cavity effusions or protein-losing enteropathy.[37]

Antibiotics must of course be given to lymphedema patients with cellulitis or erysipelas. If these infections are not aborted by CDP, prophylactic antibiotics should be considered. For fungal infections, the patient should be treated vigorously and promptly with antimycotic medications. To treat patients with blood-borne filariasis, ivermectin or diethylcarbamazine is recommended. The skin of such patients should be cleansed with a mild disinfectant and topical antibacterial–antifungal cream should be applied.[37](p116)

Benzopyrones have been recommended as an adjunct to CDP for some years.[38-40] They are available as oral preparations, a topical cream, and a dusting powder. These substances are thought to stimulate macrophage activity and extralymphatic tissue protein absorption. Coumarin, a commonly recommended oral benzopyrone, sometimes produces a toxic, idiosyncratic hepatitis. The exact role of the benzopyrones and their value in treating lymphedema are still unknown. The drugs still lack US Food and Drug Administration approval in the United States. The great excitement caused by the idea of an oral tablet that can improve lymphedema has not yet led most clinicians or the executive committee of the International Society of Lymphology to recommend these drugs.[37] When they are used, Casley-Smith has recommended that they be used in conjunction with CDP.[41]

Summary

Because cure of lymphedema has never been achieved, physicians and others should concentrate on prevention. Many cases can be prevented.

A candid discussion between patient and physician before cancer treatment is in order. Physicians must stress everything that can be done to prevent the problem. The patient should be made aware of the chances of getting lymphedema and the problems associated with the condition. CDP must become more readily available. Physicians must explain to their patients that lymphedema is a lifelong condition but that it can be controlled and its progression stopped by CDP. They should also tell their patients that pneumatic pumps are helpful only in stage I lymphedema and ineffective in later stages.

Most importantly, physicians must observe their patients carefully, recognize lymphedema promptly, and refer the patient for treatment as early as possible. If this is not done, we will continue to see patients whose lymphedema has been neglected and whose lifestyles have been diminished by a treatable, nonlethal, and often debilitating condition.

References

1. *Worldwide Incidence of Lymphedema.* WHO Technical Report. Series 702. Geneva, Switzerland: World Health Organization; 1984.
2. Földi E, Földi M, Weissleder H. Conservative treatment of lymphoedema of the limbs. *Angiology.* 1985;36:171–180.
3. Kinmonth JB. *The Lymphatics.* London: Edward Arnold; 1972.
4. Földi M, Kubik S. *Lehrbuch der Lymphologie.* Stuttgart, Germany: Gustav Fischer Verlag; 1989.
5. Földi E, Földi M, Clodius L. The lymphedema chaos: a lancet. *Ann Plast Surg.* 1989;22:505–515.
6. *The Breast Cancer Digest: A Guide to Medical Care, Emotional Support, Educational Programs, and Resources.* 2nd ed. Bethesda, Md: Office of Cancer Communications, National Cancer Institute. 1984.
7. Britton RC, Nelson PA. Causes and treatment of lymphedema of the arm: report of 114 cases. *JAMA.* 1962; 180:95–98.
8. Hughes JH, Patel AR. Swelling of the arm following radical mastectomy. *Br J Surg.* 1966;53:4–9.
9. Lin PP, Allison DC, Wainstock J, et al. Impact of axillary lymph node dissection on the therapy of breast cancer patients. *J Clin Oncol.* 1993;11:1536–1540.
10. Werner RS, McCormick B, Petrek JA, et al. Arm edema in conservatively managed breast cancer: obesity is a major factor. *Radiology.* 1991;180:177–179.
11. Ivens D, Hoe AL, Podd CR, et al. Assessment of morbidity from complete axillary dissection. *Br J Cancer.* 1992;66:136–139.
12. Petrek JA, Lerner R. *Diseases of the Breast.* Philadelphia, Pa: Lippincott-Raven; 1996.
13. Recht A, Pierce SM, Abner L, et al. Regional nodal failure after conservative surgery and radiotherapy for early-stage breast carcinoma. *J Clin Oncol.* 1991;9:988–991.
14. Halverson KJ, Taylor ME, Perez CA, et al. Regional nodal management and patterns of failure following conservative surgery and radiation therapy for stage I and II breast cancer. *Int J Radiat Oncol Biol Phys.* 1993;26:593–595.
15. Sarrazin D, LeM Arriagada R, et al. Ten year results of a randomized trial comparing a conservative treatment to mastectomy in early breast cancer. *Radiother Oncol.* 1989; 14:177–184.
16. Kinne DW. Primary treatment of breast cancer: surgery. In: Harris JR, Helman S, Henderson IC, et al., eds. *Diseases of the Breast.* 2nd ed. Philadelphia, Pa: JB Lippincott; 1991; 347–373.
17. Haagensen CD. *Diseases of the Breast.* 3rd ed. Philadelphia, Pa: WB Saunders; 1986.
18. Lerner R. Breast surgery without lymphedema. In: Cluzan RV, Pecking AP, Lokiec FM, eds. *Progress in Lymphology XIII.* Amsterdam: Elsevier Science Publishers; 1991:405–406.
19. Handley WS. A new method for the relief of the brawny breast cancer and for similar conditions of lymphatic oedema. *Lancet.* 1908;1:1783–1785.
20. Degni M. New technique of drainage of the subcutaneous tissue of the limbs with nylon net for treatment of lymphedema. *Rev Bras Cardiovasc.* 1974;10:1–8.
21. Campisi C. The autologous vein grafts in reconstructive microsurgery for lymph stasis. In: Olszewski WL, ed. *Lymph Stasis: Pathophysiology and Treatment.* Boca Raton, Fl: CRC Press; 1991:553–573.
22. Goldsmith HS. Long-term evaluation of omental transposition for chronic lymphedema. *Ann Surg.* 1974;180:847–849.
23. Standard S. Lymphedema of the arm following radical mastectomy for carcinoma of the breast: new operation for its control. *Ann Surg.* 1942;116:816–820.
24. Nielubowicz J, Olszewski W. Surgical lymphaticovenous shunts in patients with secondary lymphedema. *Br J Surg.* 1968;55:440–442.
25. Thompson N. Buried dermal flap operation for chronic lymphedema of the extremities. *Plast Reconstr Surg.* 1970; 45:541–546.
26. Kondoleon E. Operative Behandlung der elephantiastischen Oedema. *Zentralbl Chir.* 1912;39:1022.
27. Hurst P, Stewart G, Kinmonth JB, Browse NL. Longterm results of the enteromesenteric bridge operation in the treatment of primary lymphedema. *Br J Surg.* 1985;72:272–278.
28. Homans J. Lymphedema of the limbs. *Arch Surg.* 1940;40:232–235.
29. Sistrunk WE. Further experiences with the Kondoleon operation for elephantiasis. *JAMA.* 1918;71:800–806.
30. Latham A, English TC, eds. *A System of Treatment.* London: Churchill, 1912.
31. Földi M. Treatment of lymphedema [editorial]. *Lymphology.* 1994;27:1–5.
32. Von Winiwarter A. *Die Elephantiasis, Deutsche Chirurgie.* Stuttgart, Germany: Enke; 1892.
33. Földi E, Földi M, Clodius L. The lymphedema chaos: a lancet. *Ann Plast Surg.* 1989;22:505–515.
34. Földi M. *Lymphology.* 1995;28:3. Review of: *Modern Treatment for Lymphoedema,* Casley-Smith JR, Casley-Smith JR.
35. Földi E, Földi M, Weissleder H. Conservative treatment of lymphedema. *Angiology.* 1985;36:171–179.
36. Földi , M. Treatment of lymphedema [editorial]. *Lymphology.* 1994;27:1–5.
37. The diagnosis and treatment of peripheral lymphedema: consensus document of the International Society of Lymphology Executive Committee. *Lymphology.* 1995;28:113–117.
38. Jamal S, Casley-Smith JR, Casley-Smith JR. The effects of 5,6 benzo-[a]-pyrone (coumarin) and DEC on filaritic lymphoedema and elephantiasis in India. Preliminary results. *Ann Trop Med Parasitol.* 1989;83:287–290.
39. Piller NB, Morgan RG, Casley-Smith JR. A double blind, cross-over trial of benzopyrones in the treatment of lymphedema of the arms and legs. *Br J Plast Surg.* 1988;41:20–27.

40. Piller NB. Pharmacological treatment of lymph stasis. In: Olszewski WL, ed. *Lymph Stasis: Pathophysiology, Diagnosis, and Treatment.* Boca Raton, Fl: CRC Press; 1991:501–523.

41. Casley-Smith J. Treatment of lymphedema of the arms and legs with 5,6 benzopyrone. *N Engl J Med.* 1993;329: 1158–1163.

42. Lin PP, Allison DC, Wainstock J, et al. Impact of axillary lymph node dissection on the therapy of breast cancer patients. *J Clin Oncol.* 1993;11:1536–1539.

43. Werner RS, McCormick B, Petrek JA, et al. Arm edema in conservatively managed breast cancer: obesity is a major predictive factor. *Radiology.* 1991;180:177–180.

44. Kissen MW, della Rovere QG, Easton D, et al. Risk of lymphedema following the treatment of breast cancer. *Br J Surg.* 1986;7:580–582.

Section 14
Vascular Malformations and Hemangiomas

94

Vascular Malformations and Hemangiomas

Stefan Belov

The primary defect in vascular formation, which is a direct result of disturbances in the embryonal development, is "Vitium vasorum primae formationis" (congenital vascular defect, i.e., vascular malformation).[1] In comparison with anomalies in origin, number, distribution, or course of the vessels that do not provoke changes in hemodynamics, the vascular malformations (VMs) are congenital organic vascular diseases that cause disturbances in blood and lymph circulation and tissue metabolism.

The literature is rich in publications of the clinical pictures of peripheral vascular malformations. Each author names the syndrome observed by him or her, for example, Klippel–Trénaunay syndrome, Weber's syndrome, and so forth.[1]

Recently experts on VMs have established the inexpediency of the use of eponyms in nosography of VM. In light of modern thinking and of his great personal experience Malan is convinced that "the Klippel-Trenaunay-Parkes Weber eponym is meaningless and should be abandoned."[2] Moreover, after the detailed study of VM morphology Leu[3] and van der Stricht[4] concluded that the use of proper names to designate congenital vascular pathology is "highly confusing" and should be replaced with descriptive nosography including clinical picture, kind of VM, and systemic alterations.

Similar to the abuse of eponyms, many classifications of VM exist as well. However, some of them are collections of different kinds of congenital vascular pathology and phakomatoses, hamartoses, and name syndromes that are difficult to use in daily practice.

Another type of systematization is the hemodynamic classification of Mulliken,[5] based on radiologic or ultrasonic characteristics of the blood flow within the malformations. This classification divides VM into the main groups of slow flow and fast flow, to which the complex-combined malformations with the name syndromes are added.

Including different kinds of VMs in the indicated main groups is regretfully very difficult or even impossible. On the one hand, VMs are most often polyangiopathies, and, on the other hand, the blood flow disturbances in different parts of the affected organ caused by polyangiopathies have precise characteristics. Thus, classification of arterial malformations (e.g., aneurysm or coarctation) as fast flow is very strange, because these vascular defects significantly reduce the peripheral blood supply.

VMs with reduction of deep venous truncuses often cause opening of the Sucquet–Hoyer's channels to ensure a satellite shunt circulation centrally to the communications, which was confirmed both experimentally and clinically in congenital and acquired disturbances of deep venous drainage. Definition of this primary venous malformation as slow flow or fast flow is very difficult.

The principal classification of arteriovenous (A-V) defects as fast flow is also difficult, because the parameters of the entire peripheral blood circulation in one and the same affected limb vary depending on the localization of A-V communications. As demonstrated in studying the pathophysiology of hemodynamics, centrally from the communications the blood circulation manifests fast flow, whereas peripherally from the communications it registers slow flow as a result of the steal phenomenon. Concerning the advisability of including the name syndromes in the classification, we have already indicated the stand of Malan,[2] Leu,[3] and van der Stricht.[4]

Because of these difficulties in the systematization of VM Bourde[6] maintains that one simple, coherent, and intelligible classification that excludes confusing nomenclatures is necessary. Leu[3] himself believes that a pathoanatomical classification of vascular defects is the best basis for current management. Based on classic categories and contemporary knowledge of the morphology of VM, I proposed at the 7th Meeting of the International Workshop on Vascular Malformations in

Hamburg in 1988 the pathoanatomical classification, which was named Hamburg Classification (Table 94.1).[1,7,8] As seen in the table the five main species of vascular defects have two basic morphological forms: truncular and extratruncular. Attribution to one of these forms is embryologically defined, depending on the part of the primary vascular system from which the malformation has originated.

Truncular defects are dysembryoplasia of differentiated vessels and can be in the form of aplasia, hypoplasia or obstruction, dilatation, A-V communication, and combined vascular defect with or without shunt. Extratruncular defects derive from remnants of the primitive capillary network. They can have the following pathoanatomical features: infiltrative form, showing invasion in the neighboring muscles, tendons, and sometimes bones, and limited form, demonstrating expansive growth.

The discussions regarding some new terms in the Hamburg Classification demand their additional explanation.[9] This concerns first the terms *truncular* and *extratruncular vascular malformations*. These basic conceptions are clear from a pathoanatomical point of view, are embryologically explained, and have proven practical value, because they define the indications and possibilities of therapeutic tactics: surgery, vaso-occlusive angiotherapy, nonsurgical treatment, or combined management.

Therefore nothing imposes the substitution of these intelligible terms by the theoretical conceptions *mature* and *primitive* or by the unclearly defined terms *macrofistulas* and *microfistulas* in A-V shunting malformations. The last terms often lead to confusion in practice, as well as in scientific discussions. The statements that truncular macrofistulas, whose diameters in peripheral vascular malformations are not larger than 1 to 2 mm, are visualized angiographically and cause hyperdynamic circulation but extratruncular microfistulas are not visualized and have minor hemodynamic impact are incorrect. The visualization of A-V communications, which is rarely direct, is demonstrated by indirect arteriographic signs depending not on the size of the A-V fistulas but on the he-

modynamic significance of the shunt effect. Regarding the hemodynamic impact of congenital A-V communications I cite Malan.[2] According to this Nestor in VM, the shunt effect is characterized not by the size of individual A-V fistulas but "is defined by the total section area of the communication between the arterial and the venous system" (31). Other important parameters, according to Malan,[2] are "the geometry concerns the shape, number, and distribution of the A-V fistulae and the location, which is important especially in terms of the size of the supplying artery or arteries." All this is well demonstrated in Figure 94.1, which shows the indirect arteriographic symptoms of A-V shunt caused by an extratruncular microfistulous area infiltrating the shoulder region and having generated considerable shunt effect and ischemia of the arm as a result of the hemodynamic steal phenomenon.

Lastly, the conceptions *infiltrating form* and *limited form* of VM should not be equated with the terms *diffuse* and *localized*.[9] The terms *infiltrated form* and *limited form* are basic morphological conceptions for extratruncular VMs and indicate not the dimension of VMs but the character of their growth. The infiltrating form showing invasion in neighboring tissues (e.g., muscles, bones, glands, and parenchymatous organs) was observed until recently only in malignant formations. This form could be localized, infiltrating the extratruncular area (Figure 94.1), or diffuse, infiltrating the entire extremity or a part of it (Figure 94.2). The infiltrating VMs are the most difficult therapeutic problem and are treated with embolization or most often with combined management, including surgery and vaso-occlusive angiotherapy. The limited form, on the other hand, demonstrates expansive growth (Figure 94.3), which alleviates significantly its treatment.

The issues discussed so far confirm the contention that creating terminology and classification in science is very difficult. The congenital vascular defects are so different from acquired vascular diseases and are so various that they often surprise even the most experienced re-

TABLE 94.1. Classification of congenital vascular defects according to their species and anatomopathological forms.

Species	Forms	
	Truncular	Extratruncular
Predominantly arterial defects	Aplasia or obstruction	Infiltrating
	Dilatation	Limited
Predominantly venous defects	Aplasia or obstruction	Infiltrating
	Dilatation	Limited
Predominantly lymphatic defects	Aplasia or obstruction	Infiltrating
	Dilatation	Limited
Predominantly arteriovenous shunting defects	Deep arteriovenous fistulas	Infiltrating
	Superficial arteriovenous fistulas	Limited
Combined vascular defects	Arterial and venous without shunt	Infiltrating hemolymphatic
	Hemolymphatic with or without shunt	Limited hemolymphatic

Hamburg Classification. From Belov 1988.

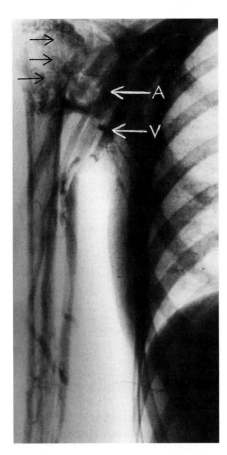

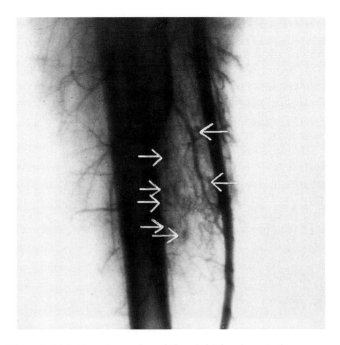

FIGURE 94.2. Arteriography of the right leg in arteriovenous (A-V) malformation causing congenital angio-osteohypertrophy (length discrepancy 6 cm). Discrete signs of A-V shunt: multiple "snowflake" spots in the thigh (arrows) indicating diffuse extratruncular infiltrating A-V fistulas.

FIGURE 94.1. Arteriography of the right arm in arteriovenous (A-V) malformation causing congenital angio-osteohypertrophy (length discrepancy 5 cm). Indirect signs of A-V shunt: extratruncular area of tortuous communicating arterial and venous branches infiltrating the shoulder region (arrows) and causing a significant A-V shunt demonstrated by simultaneous opacification of axillary arteries (A) and veins (V) and slight opacification of the distal arterial segment with peripheral ischemia. Reprinted with permission from Belov.[10]

geons, radiologists, and pediatric surgeons, whose subjects of diagnostics and management are all juxtacardial, visceral, and peripheral VMs of the extremities,[11–19] and also of plastic surgeons, who along with radiologists treat the VMs localized in the specific regions of the face, head, and neck.[20,21]

The capillary malformations are not included in the classification because, according to Azzolini,[21] they "are

searcher. This explains their late inclusion in the textbooks of angiology. Naturally, every classification can be a subject of criticism, but it is a necessary systematization of knowledge intended for use in practice, as well as for scientific analyses. Classification should combine scientific authority with practical applicability and should be founded on significant practical efficiency because experience is the best teacher.

The Hamburg Classification, based on pathoanatomical analysis of 932 patients with VM over a period of 30 years, is comprehensive yet simple.[7,8] In most patients the pathoanatomy was verified through the comparison of clinical manifestations and noninvasive investigations with angiographic pictures, operative findings, and histological examinations. Use of the Hamburg Classification is convenient in formulating precise clinicopathoanatomical diagnoses and planning the causal and combined treatment in the daily practice of vascular sur-

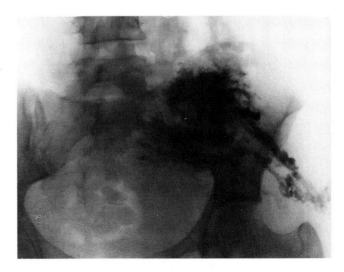

FIGURE 94.3. Phlebography of an extratruncular malformation in the abdominal wall: a limited extratruncular venous malformation is opacified.

of small significance from the hemodynamic and evolutionary points of view, being comparable with a mildly pathological capillary network" (266). Useful in practice will be not to classify the different cutaneous hemangiomas together with the cutaneous angiodysplasias (e.g., birthmarks and port-wine stains) that are not connected with the systemic blood and lymph circulation, taking into consideration Mulliken's[5] description of the well-defined differences in their pathoanatomy and evolution. Such systematization will serve many specialists including dermatologists, plastic surgeons, and pediatricians, whose subjects are the specific methods for treatment of these kinds of congenital vascular pathologies.[5,22-24]

References

1. Belov S. Classification, terminology, and nosology of congenital vascular defects. In: Belov S, Loose DA, Weber J, eds. *Vascular Malformations*. Reinbek, Germany: Einhorn-Presse; 1989:25–30.
2. Malan E. *Vascular Malformations (Angiodysplasias)*. Milan, Italy: Carlo Erba; 1974:17–31.
3. Leu HJ. Pathomorphology of vascular malformations: analysis of 310 cases. *International Angiology*. 1990;9:147–155.
4. van der Stricht J. Les syndromes "Type" Klippel et Trenaunay. *Phlebologie*. 1992;45:483–487.
5. Mulliken JB. Cutaneous vascular anomalies. *Semin Vasc Surg*. 1993;6:204–218.
6. Bourde C. Les angiodysplasies. *Artères et Veines*. 1990;9:401–402.
7. Belov S. Classification of congenital vascular defects. *International Angiology*. 1990;9:141–146.
8. Belov S. Anatomopathological classification of congenital vascular defects. *Semin Vasc Surg*. 1993;6:219–224.
9. Rutherford RB. Classification of peripheral congenital vascular malformations. In: Ernst C, Stanley J, eds. *Current Therapy in Vascular Surgery*. 3rd ed. St Louis, Mo: Mosby; 1995:834–838.
10. Belov S. Grundsätze der chirurgischen Behandlung angevorener Gefässfehler. In Belov S, Loose DA, and Müller E, eds. *Angeborene Gefässfehler*. Reinbek, Germany: Einhorn-Presse; 1985.
11. Loose DA, Wang Z. The surgical treatment of predominantly venous defects. *International Angiology*. 1990;9:189–196.
12. Loose DA, Wang Z. Surgical treatment of predominantly arterial defects. *International Angiology*. 1990;9:183–188.
13. Loose DA. Surgical treatment of predominantly venous defects. *Semin Vasc Surg*. 1993;6:252–259.
14. Loose DA. Angiodysplasien. In: Alexander K, ed. *Gefässkrankheiten*. Munich, Germany: Urban & Schwarzenberg; 1994:599–600.
15. Mattassi R. Differential diagnosis in congenital vascular-bone syndromes. *Semin Vasc Surg*. 1993;6:233–244.
16. Mattassi R. Diagnosis and treatment of venous malformations of the lower limbs. In: Wang Z-B, Becker H-M, Mishima Y, Chang JB, eds. *Vascular Surgery: Proceedings of the International Conference on Vascular Surgery*. Beijing, China: International Academic Publishers; 1993:397–404.
17. Weber JH. Vaso-occlusive angiotherapy (VAT) in congenital vascular malformations. *Semin Vasc Surg*. 1993;6:279–296.
18. Tasnadi G. Clinical investigations in epidemiology of congenital vascular defects. In: Balas P, ed. Progress in Angiology, 1991. Proceedings of the 7th European Congress of the International Union of Angiology and 3rd Mediterranean Congress of Angiology. Torino, Italy: Edizioni Minerva Medica; 1992:391–394.
19. Tasnadi G. Epidemiology and etiology of congenital vascular malformations. *Semin Vasc Surg*. 1993;6:200–203.
20. Petrovici V. Surgical treatment of congenital arteriovenous malformations in the scalp and ear. In: Belov S, Loose DA, Weber J, eds. *Vascular Malformations*. Reinbek, Germany: Einhorn-Presse; 1989:235–239.
21. Azzolini A, Azzolini C. Treatment of congenital vascular malformations of the face. *Semin Vasc Surg*. 1993;6:266–278.
22. Landthaler M, Hoherleutner U. Laser treatment of congenital vascular malformations. *International Angiology*. 1990;9:208–213.
23. Kimmig W. Laser therapy of congenital vascular malformations. In: Belov S, Loose DA, Weber J, eds. *Vascular Malformations*. Reinbek, Germany: Einhorn-Presse; 1989:195–196.
24. Ehringhaus C. Corticosteroid treatment of infantile cutaneous hemangiomas. In: Belov S, Loose DA, Weber J. eds. *Vascular Malformations*. Reinbek, Germany: Einhorn-Presse; 1989:197–199.

95

Vascular Malformations and Hemangiomas: Pathophysiology

Stefan Belov

The pathophysiology of the hemodynamics in peripheral vascular malformations (PVMs) depends on their pathoanatomy and especially on the presence of direct arteriovenous (AV) communications. Hemodynamic disturbances are basically of two types: parasitic shunt circulation and reduced circulation.

Parasitic shunt circulation is observed in predominantly AV malformations (for the most part, multiple truncular and extratruncular AV communications), in cases of deep venous reduction and AV fistulas toward the superficial embryonal vein, and in combined hemolymphatic defects associated with an AV shunt. The existence of AV communications toward compensatory veins in patients with impassible deep veins is explained by the activation of the normally existing channels for derivation of Sucquet–Hoyer to assist the venous drainage. This finding was discovered in patients with aplasia of deep venous trunci,[1-4] and the opening of AV shunts was confirmed also in acquired venous congestion after deep venous thrombosis.[5-9] Moreover, Lamy and Bourde[10] in 1957 for the first time proposed the opening of AV communications as a result of intrauterine obliterating thrombosis. The best proof of the connection between restricted venous drainage and the development of short circuits is provided by the experiments of Soltész,[11] Brookes and Sigh,[12] and Solti et al.,[9] who after ligatures of the femoral veins in animals have angiographically, hemodynamically, and histologically established the opening of AV communications, which ensure a satellite circulation. Solti et al.[13] discovered that lymphedema also leads to AV shunting, which explains the finding of AV fistulas in hemolymphatic defects.

Typical signs of peripheral parasitic circulation at different degrees and levels of the affected extremity (Figure 95.1)[14] include the following:

- A large blood flow volume and high venous oxygen saturation centrally to the shunt (arterialization of the venous blood)
- Low peripheral arterial pressure and venostasis as a result of the steal phenomenon
- Compensatory increased local blood pressure around the fistular area to ensure a peripheral blood supply
- Low oxygen tension of the capillary blood in the metaphyses of tubular bones, causing hypoxia of the osteoblasts in zones of bone growth because blood shunting through the AV communications does not serve a metabolic function[15]

Reduced circulation is observed in PVMs without shunt: predominantly venous defects, such as hypoplasia venous obstruction or diffuse phlebectasias, and rarely predominantly arterial defects, such as hypoplasia or obstruction and combined arterial and venous hypoplasia.[15-23]

Parameters of peripheral reduced circulation in the diseased extremity[15] are as follows:

- Decreased blood flow volume in the limb as a consequence of restricted arterial supply and poor venous drainage
- Delayed blood flow
- Diffuse ischemia
- Diffuse venostasis

One of the important pathophysiological problems in PVMs is the pathogenesis of bone pathology, which causes osteohypertrophy, with lengthening of the affected limb, or osteohypotrophy, with shortening of the affected limb.

Several theories exist for the explanation of bone hypertrophy. The oldest is the theory of *panhistia*, according to which just one teratogenic agent causes diffuse mesodermal malformations, including vascular and bone pathology.[24,25] This theory was rejected by authors

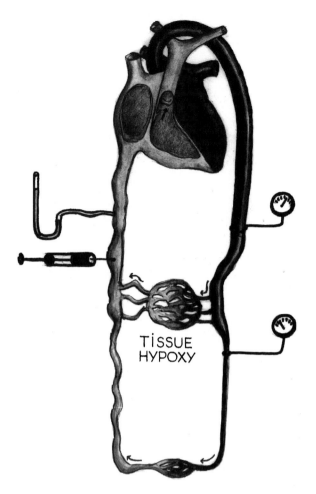

TISSUE HYPOXY

FIGURE 95.1. Scheme of peripheral blood circulation in AV communications. Increased "fast flow" blood perfusion centrally to the shunt and reduced "slow flow" circulation distally to the AV communications, causing peripheral ischemia and venostasis. Compensatory increased blood pressure and tissue hypoxia occur in zones of the fistular area. (Adapted from Malan.[14])

who considered that the hemodynamic disturbances in PVMs are the pathogenic cause for the osteohypertrophy.[10,26-28] Moreover, Malan and Puglionisi[27,28] indicated that in patients examined by them, the bone pathology had been of hyperplastic and not of dysplastic type.

Another theory connected bone hypertrophy with the *venous stasis* caused by vascular malformation.[10,29-31] Actually, it has been well known since the time of Ambroise Paré that venostasis influences the increase of ossification and helps the consolidation of fractures. However, this influence is insufficient to be the sole cause of the hyperostosis. Proof of this is provided by the experiments of Dickinson[32] and the many patients with predominantly venous malformations (segmental deep venous hypoplasia, diffuse phlebectasias) in whom the congenital venostasis causes the opposite effect—

namely, osteohypotrophy and shortening of the extremity.[16-21]

Other authors consider that the basic pathogenic factor of osteohypertrophy is the increased arterial bone supply in AV shunting circulation.[33-35] The theory of *arterial hyperemia,* however, is also rejected. In the first place, in parasitic circulation, increased blood supply is only a compensatory mechanism for the improvement of peripheral circulation.[28] In the second place, it is well known that the blood volume shunted through AV communications does not participate in tissue metabolism. Present-day angiology proves the hemodynamic genesis of congenital angioosteohypertrophy, although differences of opinion among individual authors exist about the pathogenic role of the various parameters of disturbed peripheral blood circulation.[10,28,36-50]

Several excellent experimental works studying the role of hemodynamic and metabolic disturbances in parasitic shunt circulation give the best possibility for understanding the pathogenesis of bone pathology in PVMs. The biochemical studies of Cartier[51] established that a permanent enzymatic connection exists between the specific activity of the osteoblasts in relation to calcification and their respiratory activity. Thus, the reduction of respiration of the osteoblasts leads to accumulation of the phosphorus ester and accelerates the mineralization of the bones. This *primum movens* was demonstrated by Cartier with experimentally provoked osteopetrosis by inhibiting the respiration of the osteoblasts.

Very important is the polarographic study of Ingebrigsten et al.,[52] which concerns blood circulation in femoral AV fistulas in animals. The basic pathophysiological effect established by these authors is the decrease of oxygen tension in the fistular metaphyses in comparison with the sound legs. The experimental investigations of Vanderhoeft et al.[53] made it clear that an increase in blood pressure around the epiphysial cartilage in AV communications provoked lengthening of the tubular bones.

The pathogenic role of circulatory hypoxia of osteoblasts and of increased blood pressure in zones of bone growth was brilliantly proved by the experimental works of Hauss.[54] These two factors occupy, respectively, third and sixth place among 19 noxae studied by Hauss that cause "unspecific mesenchymal reaction of proliferation."

Comparison of the clinical and experimental investigations demonstrates that the indicated parameters of *parasitic circulation* and the *hypoxia of osteoblasts* in the zones of bone growth are included in a chain in pathogenesis of angioosteohypertrophy with lengthening of tubular bones. This gave the reason to the author to define the described bone pathology as "circulatory-hypoxic hyperostosis" (Figure 95.2).[15,55]

Examinations showed that the genesis of congenital angioosteohypotrophy can be hemodynamically or me-

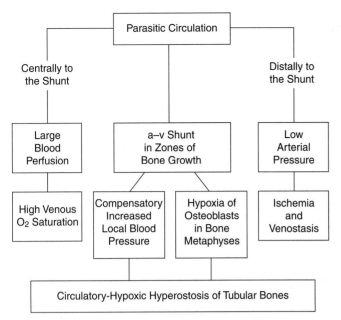

FIGURE 95.2. Pathogenesis of congenital circulatory-hypoxic hyperostosis.

chanically vascularly conditioned. The hemodynamic pathogenesis appears in cases of congenital reduced circulation due to the enumerated peripheral vascular defects. A mechanical vascular cause is apparent in patients with large, deep extratruncular vascular formations pressing the metaphyses of tubular bones in childhood (Figure 95.3).[15,55]

The evaluation of late postoperative results showed correction or considerable decrease of lower limb length discrepancy after vascular surgery performed between

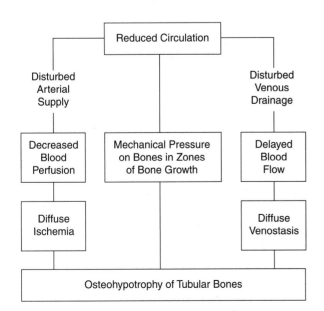

FIGURE 95.3. Pathogenesis of congenital angioosteohypotrophy.

ages 5 and 12 years.[55] It is impressive that these results were achieved after normalization of hemodynamics in childhood, mainly by functional radical operations to remove congenital vascular defects. These results are the best confirmation of the hemodynamic pathogenesis of bone pathology in PVMs.[55-59]

In general, it must be emphasized that PVMs differ significantly from acquired vascular pathology in morphology and pathophysiology. Serious circulatory and metabolic disturbances cause the protean and severe clinical pictures and possible complications. The specifics of pathoanatomy, hemodynamics, and pathogenesis, defining the diagnostic and treatment methods for congenital vascular defects, demanded the training by physicians in postgraduate courses and the inclusion of PVMs in textbooks as the newest part of angiology.

References

1. Belov S. Congenital agenesia of the deep veins of the lower extremities: surgical treatment. *J Cardiovasc Surg (Torino)*. 1972;13:594–598.
2. Loose DA. Surgical strategy in congenital venous defects. In: Belov S, Loose DA, Weber J, eds. *Vascular Malformations*, Reinbek, Germany: Einhorn-Presse Verlag; 1989:163–180.
3. Mattassi R. Individual indications for surgical and combined treatment in so-called inoperable cases of congenital vascular defects. In: Balas P, ed. *Progress in Angiology 1991. Proceedings of the 7th European Congress of the International Union of Angiology and 3rd Mediterranean Congress of Angiology*. Torino, Italy: Minerva Medica; 1992:383–386.
4. Rudofsky G, Brosig H-J, Ehinger W, Vogt K, Nobbe F, Vollmar J. Klinische und hämodynamische Untersuchungsbefunde beim Gliedmassenriesenwuchs (Typ Klippel-Trenaunay, Typ FP Weber). In: Vollmar JE, Nobbe FP, eds. *Arteriovenöse Fisteln—Dilatierende Arteriopathien (Aneurysmen)*. Stuttgart, Germany: Thieme; 1976:82–86.
5. Acsady G, Solti F, Frank J, Turbok E. The development of extremital arteriovenous shunts after deep venous thrombosis. In: Maurer PC, Becker HM, Heidrich H et al., eds. *What Is New in Angiology. Proceedings of the 14th World Congress of the International Union of Angiology*. Munich, Germany: W. Zuckschwerdt Verlag; 1986:457–459.
6. Fontaine R, Le Gal Y, Fontaine JL. Zur Klinik der arteriovenösen Anastomosen. In: *Aktuelle Probleme in der Angiologie*. Vol 2. Bern, Switzerland: Huber; 1968:92.
7. Haimovici M. Abnormal arteriovenous shunts associated with chronic venous insufficiency. *J Cardiovasc Surg (Torino)*. 1976;17:473.
8. Soltész L, Solti F, Gloviczki P, Szlavi L, Entz L. Limb circulation in varicosity of various types. *Acta Med Acad Sci Hung*. 1982;39:63–67.
9. Solti F, Soltész L, Ungvari Gy, Szlavi L, Gloviczki P. Limb circulation after deep venous thrombosis. *Acta Chir Acad Sci Hung*. 1982;23:145–152.
10. Lamy I, Bourde C. Urgences vasculaires des membres. Paris: Masson; 1957.
11. Soltész L. Contributions to clinical and experimental studies of the hypertrophy of the extremities in congenital ar-

teriovenous fistulae. *J Cardiovasc Surg (Torino).* 1965; (suppl):260.

12. Brookes M, Sigh M. Venous shunt in bone after ligation of the femoral vein. *Surg Gynecol Obstet.* 1972;135:85.

13. Solti F, Ungvari GY, Balint A, Nagy P. The regulation of the limb circulation in lymphoedema. *Angiologia.* 1971;8: 117–127.

14. Malan E. Hemodynamic phenomena in congenital arteriovenous fistulae. In: Malan E, ed. *Vascular Malformations.* Milan, Italy: Carlo Erba, 1974.

15. Belov S. Hemodynamic pathogenesis of vascular-bone syndromes in congenital vascular defects. *Int Angiol.* 1990;9: 155–162.

16. Belov S, Loose DA, Müller E. *Angeborene Gefässfehler.* Reinbek, Germany: Einhorn-Presse Verlag; 1985:230–245.

17. Belov S, Loose DA, Müller E. *Malformazioni Vascolari Congenite.* Milan, Italy: Linea Carlo Erba; 1992:207–221.

18. Belov S, Loose DA, Müller E. Defeitos vasculares congênitos. *Rev Bras Angiol Cir Vasc.* 1988;18:159–173.

19. Belov S. Diagnostik angeborener Gefässfehler. In: Loose DA, ed. *Aktuelle Aspekte der peripheren arteriallen Verschlusskrankheit.* Reinbek, Germany: Einhorn-Presse Verlag; 1988: 7–35.

20. Belov S. Gefässfehlers des Armes. In: Loose DA, ed. *Der schmerzhafte Arm aus angiologischer Sicht.* Reinbek, Germany: Einhorn-Presse Verlag; 1988:49–55.

21. Loose DA, Wang Z. The surgical treatment of predominantly venous defects. *Int Angiol.* 1990;9:189–196.

22. Moskalenko YD. *Acquired Aneurysms, Arteriovenous Fistulae and Congenital Vascular Defects* [dissertation]. Moscow: Inst. Cardio-Vascular Surg. Academy of Medical Sciences SSSR; 1970.

23. Volkolakov JV, Tkhor SM. *Reconstructive Surgery of the Blood Vessels in Children.* Leningrad: Medicina; 1979.

24. Klippel M, Trenaunay J. Du noevus variqueux et osteo-hypertrophique. *Arch Gén Méd.* 1900;3:641–672.

25. Vollmar J, Vogt K. Angiodysplasie und Skeletsystem. *Der Chirurg.* 1976;47:205–213.

26. Jouve A, Bourdoncle E, Bourde C. Fistules artério-veineuses congénitales des membres et syndrome de Klippel-Trenaunay. *Semin Hôp Paris.* 1952;28:2674.

27. Malan E, Puglionisi A. Congenital angiodysplasias of the extremities, note I: generalities and classification; venous dysplasias. *J Cardiovasc Surg (Torino).* 1964;5:87–130.

28. Malan E, Puglionisi A. Congenital angiodysplasias of the extremities, note II: arterial, arterial and venous, and hemolymphatic dysplasias. *J Cardiovasc Surg (Torino).* 1965;6: 255–345.

29. Servelle M. Stase veineuse et croissance osseuse. *Bull Acad Natl Méd.* 1948;132:471–474.

30. Servelle M. *Les Affections Veineuses.* Paris: Masson; 1978.

31. Servelle M. Klippel and Trenaunay's syndrome. *Ann Surg.* 1985;201:365–373.

32. Dickinson P. Venous stasis and bone growth. *Exp Med Surg.* 1953;11:49–53.

33. Vollmar J. *Rekonstruktive Chirurgie der Arterien.* Stuttgart, Germany: Thieme; 1967.

34. Holman E. *Abnormal Arteriovenous Communications.* Springfield, Ill: Charles C. Thomas; 1968.

35. Sumner D. Hemodynamics and pathophysiology of arteriovenous fistulas. In: Rutherford RB, ed. *Vascular Surgery.* Vol 8. 3rd ed. Philadelphia, Pa: WB Saunders Company; 1989.

36. Belov S. *Congenital Angiodysplasias and Their Surgical Treatment.* Sofia, Bulgaria: Med i Fizk; 1971:61–68.

37. Belov S. *Vascular Malformations: Diagnostics and Surgical Treatment.* Sofia, Bulgaria: Med i Fizk; 1982:163–172.

38. Fontaine R. Spezielle therapeutische Aspekte gewisser arteriovenöser Missbildungen. In: Schobinger RA, ed. *Periphere Angiodysplasien.* Bern, Switzerland: Huber; 1977: 197–206.

39. Franz D. Klinische und experimentelle Beiträge betreffend das Aneurysma arterio-venosum. *Arch Klin Chir.* 1905;75:572.

40. Janes JM, Jennings WK. Effect of induced arteriovenous fistula on leg length: 10 year observations. *Proc Staff Meetings Mayo Clin.* 1961;36:1–11.

41. Janes JM, Musgrove JE. Effect of arteriovenous fistula on growth of bone: an experimental study. *Surg Clin North Am.* 1950;30:1191–1200.

42. Kinmonth JB, Negus D. Arterio-venous fistulae in the management of lower limb discrepancy. *J Cardiovasc Surg (Torino).* 1974;15:447–453.

43. Kiz̆aev VI. *Traumatic Hemangiomas of Lower Extremities.* Moscow: Vopr Klin Khir; 1955.

44. Koskinen EVS, Tala P, Siltanen P. The effect of massive arteriovenous fistula on hemodynamics and bone growth. *Clin Orthop.* 1967;50:305.

45. Leu HJ. Zur Morphologie der arteriovenösen Anestomosen bei kongenitalen Angiodysplasien. *Morphol Med.* 1982;2:99–107.

46. Loose DA. The combined surgical therapy in congenital A-V shunting malformations. In: Belov S, Loose DA, Weber J, eds. *Vascular Malformations.* Reinbek, Germany: Einhorn-Presse Verlag; 1989:213–226.

47. Mattassi R, Colombo R, Boccalon L, Vaghi M, D'Angelo F, Tacconi A. Experiences in the surgical treatment of congenital vascular malformations: changes in diagnosis and surgical tactics in the view of new experiences. In: Belov S, Loose DA, Weber J, eds. *Vascular Malformations.* Reinbek, Germany: Einhorn-Presse Verlag; 1989:202–206.

48. Mattassi R. Surgical treatment of congenital arteriovenous defects. *Int Angiol.* 1990;9:196–202.

49. Mattassi R. Differential diagnosis in congenital vascular-bone syndromes. *Semin Vasc Surg.* 1993;6:233–244.

50. Soltész L, Temesvari A, Vas G. Über angeborene arteriovenöse Fisteln. *Zentralbl Chir.* 1955;80:1665–1677.

51. Cartier P. Biochimie des troubles de l'ossification. In: Polonowsky M, ed. *Pathologie Chimique.* Paris: Masson; 1952:1462–1473.

52. Ingebrigsten R, Krog J, Lerand S. Circulation distal to experimental arterio-venous fistulas of the extremities: a polarographic study. *Acta Chir Scand.* 1963;125:308–317.

53. Vanderhoeft PJ, Kelly PJ, Janes JM, Peterson LFA. Growth and structure of bone distal to an arterio-venous fistula. *J Bone Joint Surg [Br].* 1963;45:582.

54. Hauss WH. Transport und Stoffwechsel im Bindegewebe. In: Klüken N, ed. *Aktuelle Angiologie,* Folia Angiologica

Suppl. Vol 2. Berlin, Germany: Verlag Haupt & Koska; 1973:174–191.

55. Belov S. Correction of lower limb length discrepancy in congenital vascular-bone diseases by vascular surgery performed during childhood. *Semin Vasc Surg.* 1993;6: 245–251.

56. Belov S. Spätergebnisse der chirurgischen Behandlung von 100 Kranken mit kongenitalen Angiodysplasien. *Zentralbl Chir.* 1974;99:935–945.

57. Belov S. Late results of surgical treatment of congenital vascular defects. In: Maurer PC, Becker HM, Heidrich H et al., eds. *What Is New in Angiology? Proceedings of the 14th World Congress of the International Union of Angiology.* Munich, Germany: Zuckschwerdt Verlag; 1986:249–250.

58. Loose DA, Belov S. Chirurgische Terapiemöglichkeiten bei angeborenen peripheren Gefässdysplasien. In: Loose DA, ed. *Aktuelles aus Angiologie und Gefässchirurgie.* Reinbek, Germany: Einhorn-Presse Verlag; 1985:55–85.

59. Belov S, Loose DA, Mattassi R, Špatenka J, Tasnadi G, Wang Z. Therapeutic strategy, surgical tactics, and operative techniques in congenital vascular defects (multicentre study). In: Strano A, Novo S, eds. *Advances in Vascular Pathology 1989. Proceedings of the 15th World Congress of the International Union of Angiology.* Amsterdam, The Netherlands: Excerpta Medica; 1989:1355–1360.

96

Vascular Malformations and Hemangiomas: Clinical Features and Their Basis

Dirk A. Loose

Diagnosis

Usually, the diagnosis of vascular malformations and hemangiomas is clinical. In most instances, a precise history and assessment of symptoms, together with a very careful physical examination of the patient, yield a diagnosis sufficiently precise for a prognosis and indication of necessary investigations.

In neonates or very young children, clinical assessment may be difficult, and, quite often, it may be impossible to offer any prognosis at this stage. Here, it is very important for the physician to refrain from making an overconfident prognosis. Initially the physician should examine the child at monthly intervals to determine within the first year whether the lesion is a hemangioma, which is likely to regress, or a malformation, which does not regress at all. They may spread, enlarge, or be problematic without any obvious change in size. Arteriovenous (AV) fistulas, edema, sepsis, lymphatic leakage, and deep structures caused by vascular malformations all cause problems. Such early investigations are necessary for early treatment, between the ages of 3 and 7 years.[3] With vascular malformations in an older child or adult, in most instances, it is possible to predict the future of the lesion at the time of the first clinical examination. There are, however, some additional problems when assessing late vascular malformations. One of these

problems is that the wide range of the differential diagnosis expands. For example, anomalies of leg veins may resemble postthrombotic syndrome, and length discrepancy of the legs may appear without the presence of any vascular lesion.[1]

Practically no angiologic disease appears in such clinical variety as congenital vascular defects (CVDs), down to different combinations of CVDs in one specific case. The clinical appearance of CVDs depends on their being well marked according to the following component parts:

Anatomic region (Table 96.1)
    Central
    Visceral
    Peripheral
    Associated
Localization (Table 96.2)
    Species
    Anatomicopathological form
    Extent

Not only the clinical but also the symptomatic features depend on these factors. Contrary to hemangiomas, spontaneous regression of CVDs has not been observed. Moreover, it is not rare that nonsymptomatic forms eventually become symptomatic in adolescence or adulthood.

TABLE 96.1. Anatomic regions of congenital vascular defects.

Central CVDs	Visceral CVDs	Peripheral CVDs	Associated CVDs
Systemic circulation	Brain	Head	Central and visceral vessels
Pulmonary circulation	Thoracic organs	Neck	Central and peripheral vessels
Communication between aorta and pulmonary artery	Abdominal organs and urogenital system	Trunk	Visceral and peripheral vessels
Multiple	Multiple	Multiple	Central, visceral and peripheral vessels

CVDs, congenital vascular defects.

TABLE 96.2. Classification of congenital vascular defects according to their species and anatomic form: Hamburg Classification 1988.

Species	Anatomical forms	
	Truncal	Extratruncal
Predominantly arterial defects	Aplasia or obstruction	Infiltrating
	Dilatation	Limited
Predominantly venous defects	Aplasia or obstruction	Infiltrating
	Dilatation	Limited
Predominantly lymphatic defects	Aplasia or obstruction	Infiltrating
	Dilatation	Limited
Predominantly arteriovenous shunting defects	Deep arteriovenous fistulas	Infiltrating
	Superficial AV fistulas	Limited
Combined vascular defects	Arterial and venous, (without arteriovenous shunt)	—
	Hemolymphatic (with or without arteriovenous shunt)	Infiltrating hemolymphatic
		Limited hemolymphatic

Presenting Symptoms

The presenting symptoms depend on the hemodynamic influence of the affected region or on the central or venous circulation. It is difficult to predict whether, after a stable period, the CVD will cause circulatory insufficiencies. Thus, it is important to judge whether the CVD is only a minor cosmetic problem or whether it will create symptoms in the near future. In the former case it usually suffices to check the child who has a CVD at yearly intervals. Problems may well arise.

Unfortunately, in our experience, many patients with vascular malformations present late. One reason is the so-called "Pontius to Pilatus syndrome," that is, time wasted searching for the appropriate treatment center. A second reason is that the malformation remains stable, only developing a complication at a late stage such as in adolescence or adulthood. The vascular malformation can cause bleeding, lymphatic leakage, variable discomfort, or even aggravating outright pain. Also, infection or thrombosis can occur. Especially in AV lesions, pain distant from the lesion can occur, either from the pressure on nerves or from a steal phenomenon, resulting in ischemic pain, ulceration, or gangrene.

Long-time silent AV malformations may suddenly progress after puberty, pregnancy, or even the beginning of oral contraceptive hormonal therapy. Pregnancy can activate not only AV malformations but also venous and hemolymphatic lesions, which are known for a capacity to expand during pregnancy, presumably under the influence of some nonspecific humoral agent. The increased blood volume and other hemodynamic changes associated with pregnancy may also precipitate these changes.

The most frequent clinical findings in 210 patients with predominantly venous CVD and 80 patients with predominantly AV CVD are demonstrated in Table 96.3. Venectasias were the most frequent signs in predominantly venous as well as predominantly AV cases. Second

in frequency were nevi and circumscribed tissue augmentation. A further, very important finding in the clinical features of CVDs was the length discrepancy of the extremities.

Predominantly arterial defects are very seldom seen. In a 30-year-old man, arteriography revealed such a defect. A vascular defect was suggested by the marked length discrepancy and coldness of the affected leg. Arteriography demonstrated hypoplasia of the external iliac artery to the femoral branch. The arteriographic morphology of an elongation of the artery in young patients can indicate dysplastic changes of the vessel wall. After reconstruction of the pelvic artery, the patient had no further problems.

The most frequent CVDs are predominantly venous defects, which account for about 60% of the cases. A 20-year-old man had varied findings of extensive areas of nevus flammeus (port-wine stain) and patterns of hyperkeratotic vascular staining, combined with venectasias and skeletal overgrowth (Figure 96.1). Angiographic re-

TABLE 96.3. Frequency of clinical findings in patients with predominantly venous congenital vascular defects and with predominantly arteriovenous congenital vascular defects.

Total number of patients	210	80
Findings	Venous	Arteriovenous
Diffuse varicosity	(21%)	(10%)
Limited varicosity	(39%)	(27%)
Cutaneous nevi	(28%)	(19%)
Limited mass	(17%)	(25%)
Ulcer	(2%)	(6%)
Limb enlargement (swollen leg)	(4%)	(14%)
Bleeding	—	(2%)
Hyperthermia	—	(8%)
Edema	(9%)	(4%)
Pain	(4%)	(8%)
Length discrepancy		
Shortening	20	10
Lengthening	25	18

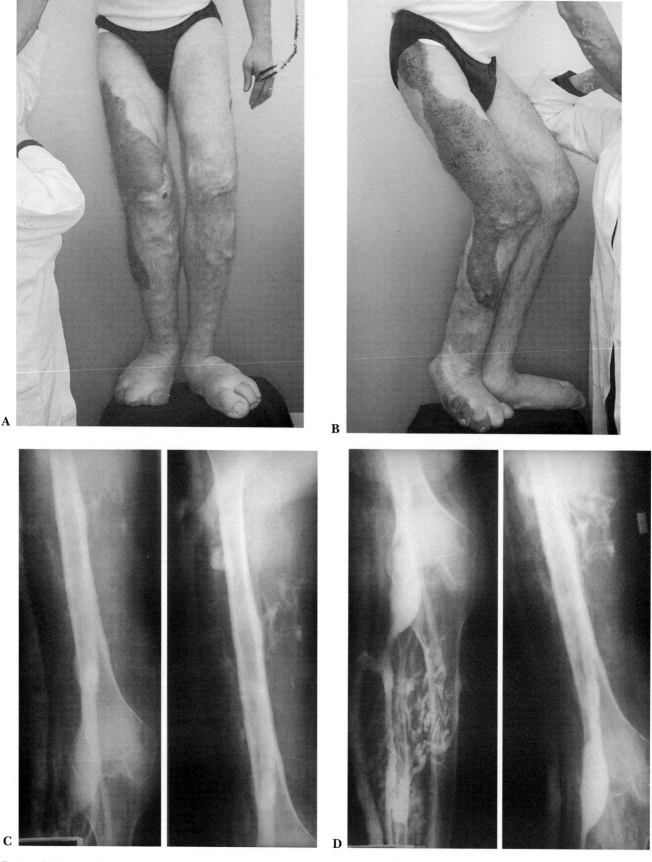

FIGURE 96.1. **A** and **B,** Severe, predominantly venous congenital defect with bone overgrowth in both legs and extended areas of nevus flammeus (port-wine stain). **C** and **D,** Phlebogram of the right leg demonstrating venectasias (marginal vein) and malformed veins infiltrating the calf muscles.

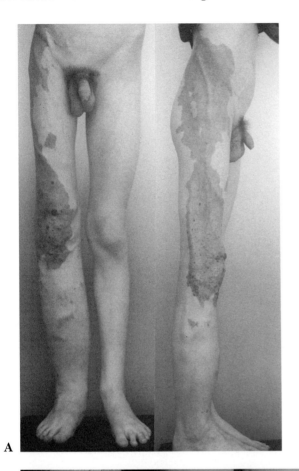

A

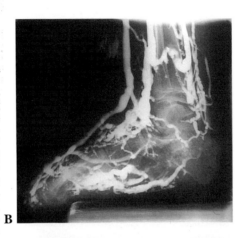

FIGURE 96.2. **A,** Clinical appearance of congenital vascular defect of the right leg in a 15-year-old boy. Nevus flammeus, angiokeratosis, venectasias (marginal vein), swelling, and length discrepancy are present. **B,** Phlebogram of the right foot in lateral projection demonstrating dilated, malformed veins. **C,** Phlebogram demonstrating venectasias, a marginal vein, and malformed veins infiltrating the muscles of the thigh. **D,** Phlebogram showing the drainage by way of the circumflex femoral vein and gluteal veins.

B

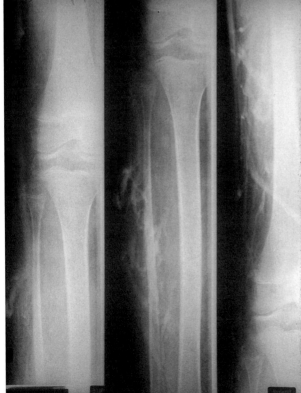

C

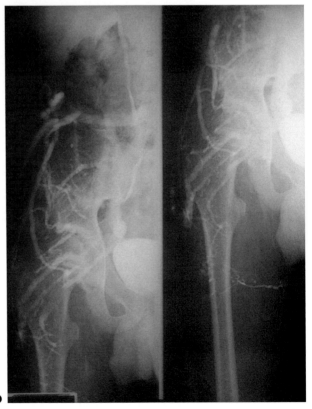

D

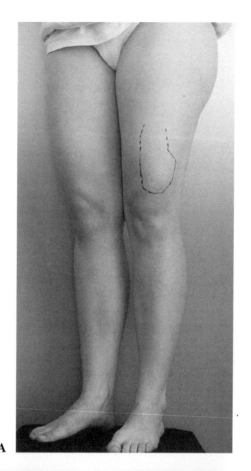

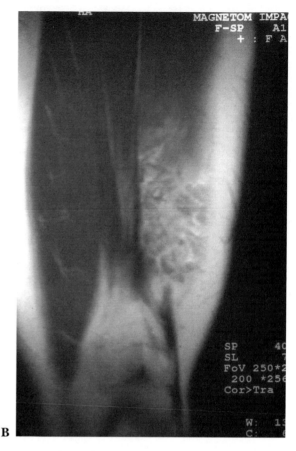

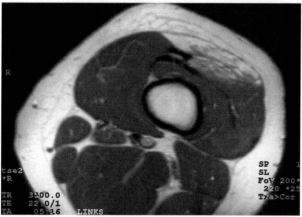

FIGURE 96.3. **A,** Clinical appearance of a 20-year-old woman with pain in her left suprapatellar region. (The painful region is marked.) **B and C,** Magnetic resonance images of the region of interest of the left thigh disclosing an extratruncal infiltrating form of a predominantly venous defect, located subfascially.

sults revealed pathologic findings in the arterial circulation, whereas phlebography detected extensive areas of malformed veins, truncal dilatations, and extratruncal infiltrating forms (Figure 96.1C, D). In the right leg there was a dilated, valveless, typical marginal vein (Figure 96.1C). In the left leg there was a similar, but less extensive, clinical feature.

Comparable clinical findings were present in a 15-year-old boy, who was scheduled for amputation in a Ukrainian hospital. He sought a second opinion as to whether the amputation could be avoided. Again, the clinical findings included multivascular defects: nevus flammeus (port-wine stain), venectasias, angiokeratosis,

length discrepancy, and swelling (Figure 96.2). Arteriography showed no pathologic finding. Phlebography revealed an extensive marginal vein as well as areas of malformed veins infiltrating the muscles (Figure 96.2B–D). The venous drainage was through the circumflex femoral vein and the gluteal veins (Figure 96.2D).

During the initial examination of a patient suspected of having a vascular malformation, most cases can roughly be categorized within the "Hamburg classification"[2] (Table 96.2). The anatomic form, in most instances, can be detected precisely after arteriography and phlebography. That is why we adhere to the recommendation of Malan[4] and Bollinger,[3] who agreed in conformity, "The

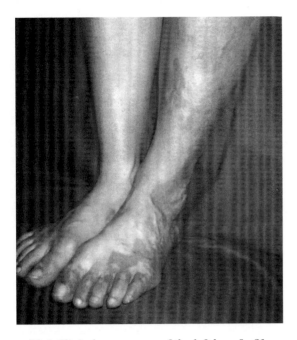

FIGURE 96.4. Clinical appearance of the left leg of a 21-year-old woman demonstrating nevus flammeus (port-wine stains), length discrepancy, venectasias, and distinct swelling. Angiographically no evidence of congenital vascular defect was found, and the diagnosis was varicosis of the great saphenous vein and side branches.

ghosts of Klippel, Trénaunay, and Weber which hover over a virtual thicket of clinical manifestations should be exorcised in favor of case-by-case analysis based on clear results."

The clinical feature of predominantly venous CVDs can be difficult to detect if they are located subfascially. A 20-year-old woman, for example, had pain in her left suprapatellar region that was quite circumscribed (Figure 96.3A). Neither by phlebography nor by arteriography could the character of the lesion be determined. At last, magnetic resonance imaging was able to settle the question; the reason for the discomfort and pain was an extratruncal, subfascially located, infiltrating, predominantly venous malformation (Figure 96.3B, C).

In a 21-year-old woman, different clinical findings pointed to the diagnosis of vascular malformations; that is, she had nevus flammeus (port-wine stain), venectasias, and length discrepancy of the legs (Figure 96.4A). However, the functional tests, as well as the angiographic findings, excluded any CVDs but revealed a varicosis with insufficient perforating veins.

A 4-year-old girl had gigantism of the left leg and foot. She also had a lipoma of the abdominal wall (Figure 96.5 A, B). No venectasias were found. Neither phlebography

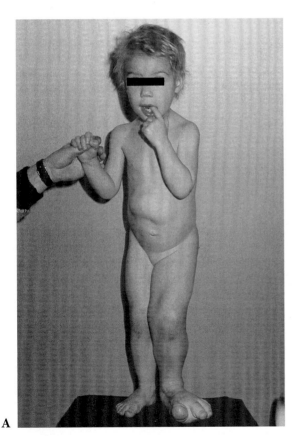

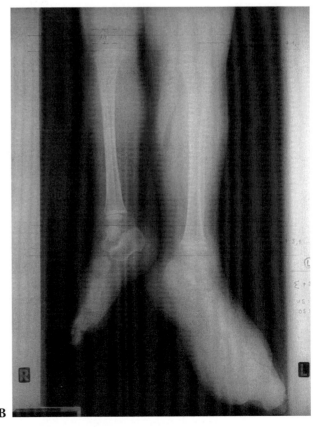

A   B

FIGURE 96.5. **A,** Four-year-old girl with enlarged left leg and abdominal lipoma. **B,** Radiography demonstrating the extent of the length discrepancy of the leg.

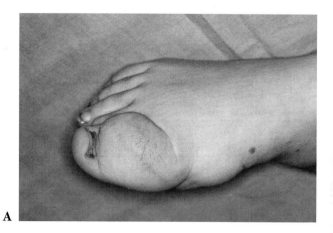 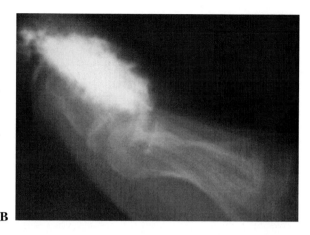

FIGURE 96.6. **A,** Clinical view of the first toe of the right foot with soft tissue "tumor." **B,** Lymphography by direct puncture revealing numerous lymphatic cysts.

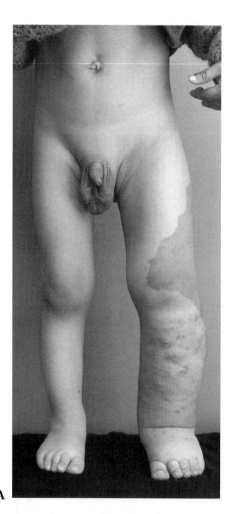 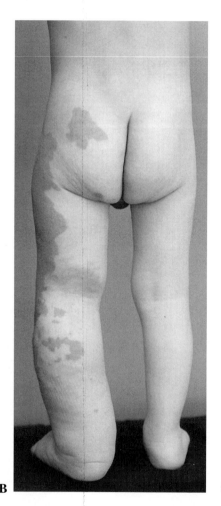 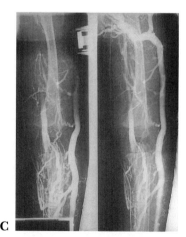

FIGURE 96.7. **A** and **B,** Clinical view of a 4-year-old boy demonstrating nevus flammeus (port-wine stain), swelling (lymphedema), length discrepancy, and "varicosity." **C,** Phlebogram of the left leg demonstrates a valveless marginal vein and hy-poplasia of the principal veins, indicating that the swelling of the left leg is caused partially by venous insufficiency and partially by lymphostasis.

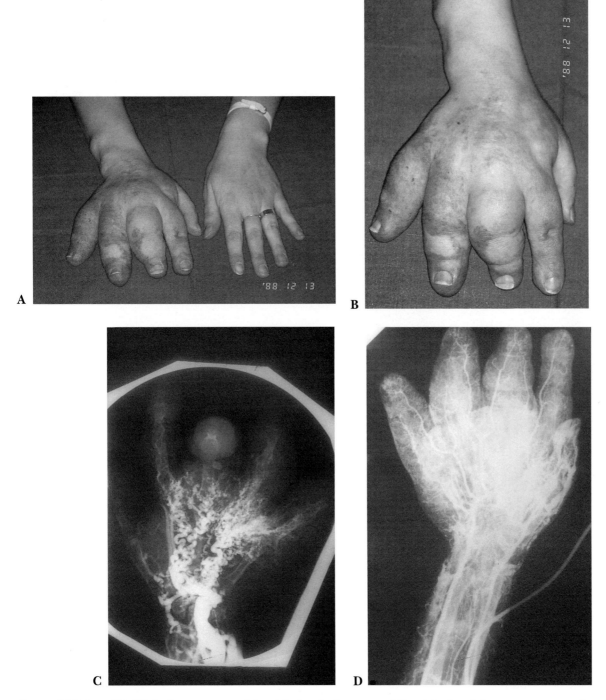

FIGURE 96.8. **A** and **B,** Clinical appearance of the right hand of a 22-year-old woman with swelling of the second to the fifth finger, including the metacarpus. Both nevus flammeus (portwine stain) and localized venectasias are present. **C,** Phlebo-gram of the right hand demonstrates extensive venectasias in the hand and finger areas. **D,** Arteriography of the right hand reveals numerous AV fistulas.

nor arteriography showed any cause for the gigantism of the leg. In this case, orthopedic surgery was required to reduce the length discrepancy.

Predominantly lymphatic CVDs are very rare compared with the venous ones. The clinical features in a 5-year-old girl suggested a lymphatic defect because there was a localized, infiltrating, soft mass in the right

first toe (Figure 96.6A). Phlebography did not reveal the character of the lesion, whereas by direct puncture and injection of a contrast agent (Figure 96.6B) a localized cystic appearance of the underlying tissue was detected. The malformed lymphatic tissue was totally extirpated by surgery, and the histologic findings proved the predominantly lymphatic nature of the malformation.

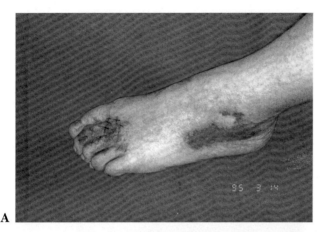

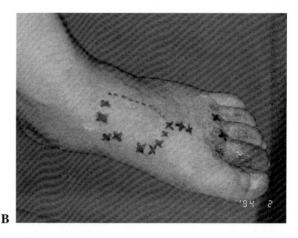

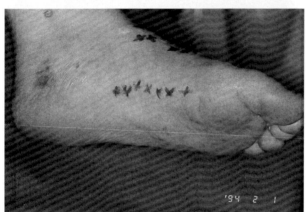

FIGURE 96.9. **A,** Clinical aspect of the left foot with preulceration due to ischemia caused by peripheral AV fistulas. **B** and **C,** Ultrasonic Doppler mapping of the AV fistulas of the left foot. Every identified AV fistula is marked by an X.

Quite often, predominantly venous CVDs are combined with lymphatic defects. That is why, as in the case of a 4-year-old boy, mixed clinical features are present: nevus flammeus (port-wine stain), length discrepancy, venectasias, swelling, and lymphedema (Figure 96.7A, B). Phlebography demonstrated a distinct marginal vein and a hypoplastic, subfascial principal vein system (Figure 96.7C). Arteriography did not show any pathologic findings.

Many problems arise when such combined CVDs are present in the hand and forearm region. Here, it is advised that the diagnosis and treatment be directed cooperatively by not only the vascular surgeon but also the hand surgeon. In a 22-year-old woman, for example, there was a distinct swelling and disfiguration of the second to the fifth finger of the right hand and of the midhand region. Venectasias and nevus flammeus (port-wine stain) were present. The fingertips showed a bluish color, and the patient described discomfort and pain in the right hand, although functionally she had no serious handicap (Figure 96.8A, B). Arteriography and phlebography (Figure 96.8C, D) revealed a combined vascular defect with hemolymphatic malformations and venectasias as well as very small AV fistulas (Figure 96.8C).

Specific Symptoms of Congenital Arteriovenous Defects

The clinical appearance of predominantly AV defects may vary in cutaneous malformation from a simple pink stain to a mass of pulsatile vessels. The patients' symptoms are varied. In our cases the main symptoms were as follows:

Pain in the affected area or distally
Heaviness of the affected limb
Uncomfortable pulsation in the lesion
Heaviness in the area of the lesion
Severe local hyperhidrosis
Local hypertrichosis
Local hyperthermia
A thrill in the lesion
Functional impairment of the affected limb
Trophic changes in the skin
Intermittent hemorrhage from ischemic ulceration

Such ischemic ulcerations provoke severe pain, and the underlying lesion can be diagnosed by invasive techniques such as arteriography and phlebography. A 22-year-old woman had severe pain of her left foot, which demonstrated dystrophic changes of the skin, hyperthermia, hyperhidrosis, and swelling (Figure 96.9A). Ultrasonic Doppler mapping demonstrated the main localization of the AV fistula areas (Figure 26.9B, C). Arteriography precisely documented all AV fistula regions.

The extreme variety of the findings sometimes does not admit a diagnosis at first sight. That is why, especially during the first clinical examination, the recommendation of Malan[4] and Bollinger[3] should be remembered, when they advise: "The nouns have to be abandoned in favor of a precise, morphologic functional description of each special case."

Literature

1. Belov S, Loose DA, Müller E. *Angeborene Gefäßfehler.* Reinbek, Germany: Einhorn-Presse Verlag; 1985.
2. Belov S, Loose DA, Weber J, eds. *Vascular Malformations.* Reinbek, Germany: Einhorn-Presse Verlag; 1989.
3. Bollinger A. *Funktionelle Angiologie, Lehrbuch und Atlas.* Stuttgart, Germany: Georg Thieme. 1979:244–258.
4. Malan E. *Vascular Malformations (Angiodysplasias).* Milan, Italy: Carlo Erba; 1974.
5. Tasnádi G. Postnatal development of the lower extremities in some forms of vascular malformations. Paper presented at: 9th International Workshop for the Study of Vascular Anomalies; July 1–3, 1992; Denver, Colo.

97

Vascular Malformations and Hemangiomas: Diagnostic Tests and Nonsurgical Treatment

Dirk A. Loose

Vascular malformations are complex lesions with a variety of manifestations and findings depending on the dominant lesion—arterial, venous, lymphatic, arteriovenous, or combined. To fully evaluate these lesions, it is necessary to first define the predominant type of lesion and second define the precise anatomic location. To obtain this information, a combination of direct imaging and noninvasive hemodynamic testing is necessary. A multimodality approach can provide a precise diagnosis of congenital vascular malformation by combining information from a variety of sources.

Several radiologic techniques exist where contrast media are not necessary to localize and demonstrate the morphologic structural characteristics of the malformation. X-ray examination of the extremities can demonstrate the length discrepancy in centimeters and also show macroscopic morphological changes of the bones and also of phleboliths in the soft tissues.

Computed tomography (Table 97.1) and magnetic resonance imaging provide anatomic detail not possible with either arteriography or noninvasive testing. These imaging modalities accurately define the involvement of adjacent musculoskeletal elements (see Figure 97.1). Computed tomography and magnetic resonance imaging, however, do not provide information about arterial or venous hemodynamics. Computed tomography angiography and magnetic resonance angiography are emerging technologies that may provide this information in future.

The duplex scan is used to estimate the total limb blood flow and to define the characteristics of the lesions. This technique provides both anatomic and hemodynamic evaluation of peripheral arteries and veins. The duplex scan provides important information in patients with suspected arteriovenous malformations in the affected extremity; the major arteries (e.g., axillary, femoral, or subclavian artery) are visualized and the diameter determined. The diameter of the artery on the side of the vascular malformation is often larger than that of the contralateral extremity because of adaptive enlargement with increased blood flow. In addition, the arterial waveform documents a loss of resistance with increased velocity.

If the arterial blood flow is not different on the affected side, the venous system is studied more carefully. Major venous lesions often result in incomplete deep venous systems (hypoplasia or aplasia) with large lateral veins and aneurysm formation. Such careful characterization of the deep venous system is useful. Segmental limb blood pressures are useful only when shunting through fistulas is sufficient to decrease distal arterial blood pressure.

Very useful is the Doppler analysis of the waveform proximal to the fistulas that documents increased forward flow and loss of backflow due to diminished resistance. In the artery distal to the fistulas, backflow is continuous throughout the cardiac circle. Also, the veins with fistulas exhibit continuous blood flow and pulsatility. With discrete arteriovenous communication, it may be possible to occlude the arteriovenous communication by pressure and ablate the venous pulsatility. In patients with primary venous and lymphatic malformations, limb arterial hemodynamics are not altered.

Electrocardiography demonstrates the diastolic load of the right side of the heart in marked peripheral left–right shunt. The electronic oscillography is able to register multiple oscillations in the region of the extremity with the vascular malformation, especially when arteriovenous fistulas and/or aneurysms are present.

Electronic volumetry can precisely document the differences of the volumes of the extremities in patients with congenital vascular malformations. Dermal thermography is a simple technique to document the dermal temperature. An elevated dermal temperature of the whole extremity, for example, is an important finding that indicates a diffuse form of arteriovenous malformation.

The impedance plethysmography demonstrates, by comparing the extremities, a relative decrease of the

TABLE 97.1. Anatomic regions of congenital vascular defects.

	Arterial malformation	Venous malformation	Lymphatic malformation
Computed tomography	Enhanced vascular mass Enlarged arteries and veins	Enhanced vascular mass Enlarged draining veins	Mass plus or minus enhancement No enlarged vessels
Magnetic resonance imaging	Flow voids in mass and draining vessels	Signal brightness T_1: Fat greater than malformation in muscle (fat is the brightest tissue in the field) T_2: Malformation greater than fat (malformation is the brightest tissue in the field)	Signal brightness Same as venous malformation
Ultrasound	Resistance index: 0 Increased flow velocity and volume flow	Resistance index: normal Dilated veins	Resistance index: normal Normal flow

blood volume when the arterial or venous circulation is reduced and a relative increase of the blood volume of the extremities when parasitic circulation is present (e.g., in arteriovenous malformations).

The transcutaneous oxygen partial pressure measurement determines the local circulatory hypoxia. In this technique measurements from normal areas of the body are compared with those from the affected extremity. Such a quantitative result can be obtained concerning the microcirculation and the rate of circulatory tissue hypoxia. The duplex scan with color flow Doppler echocardiography provides a precise diagnosis of the shunt loading of the heart.

No single test is able to supply all of the information necessary to accurately assess the pathoanatomy and pathophysiology of major vascular malformations. Arteriography and phlebography remain essential before a therapeutic strategy can be determined. Other invasive techniques such as blood oxygen saturation analysis, phlebodynamometry, and cardiac scintigraphy are also useful.

Nonsurgical Treatment

Nonsurgical treatment of congenital vascular malformations is indicated when surgical therapy is impossible or must be delayed for an unknown period.

Subjective complaints in patients with central and visceral malformations can be decreased and sometimes complications can be avoided with administration of certain medications. When symptoms are first manifest and the hemodynamic disturbances are not marked distinctly, pharmacotherapy can provide temporary improvement of the patient's condition.

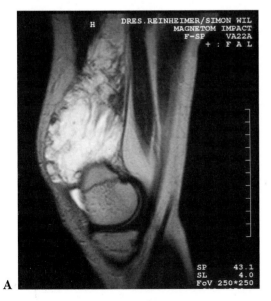

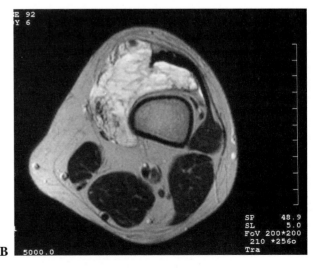

FIGURE 97.1. **A,** Magnetic resonance imaging scan of the left distal thigh region demonstrating extensive involvement of the quadriceps muscle by predominantly venous malformation. **B,** Magnetic resonance imaging cross section of the distal part of the left thigh demonstrating nearly complete involvement of the distal part of the quadriceps muscle.

Compression bandages or compression stockings are indicated when an extremity tends to develop edema due to a congenital vascular defect. Quite often the subjective complaints can also be relieved with use of compression bandages.[1] Sclerotherapy may be indicated in patients with limited, localized vascular defects as additional treatment or if extensive superficial malformations must be reduced before surgery.[2-5]

Systemic treatment with corticosteroids is indicated only in selected infants with hemangiomas that are rapidly growing; that seriously distort facial features; that cause recurrent bleeding, ulceration, or infection; or that interfere with normal physiological functions (e.g., breathing, hearing, eating, or seeing). Other situations that justify a trial of steroids are large hemangiomas and multicentric hemangiomas that cause bleeding (secondary to thrombocytopenia) and/or high-output cardiac failure.[6,7] Predominantly venous malformations do not respond to this kind of treatment.[8]

Congenital treatment of flat, superficial, predominantly venous malformations of the skin, without any other vascular defect, was performed successfully with cryotherapy.[9] Laser treatment of superficial, limited, localized, predominantly venous malformations may be used with some success. New laser technologies may prove useful in treating congenital vascular malformations.[10-12]

Transcatheter embolization of congenital vascular malformations is generally the treatment of choice when the malformation cannot be easily excised. This additional treatment has rapidly improved, and selective catheterization of small feeding vessels has become routine. Whether to use this technique should be determined by an interdisciplinary team under the guidance of a vascular surgeon.

Embolic materials have progressed from autologous muscle clots, muscles, and absorbable gelatin sponges to polyvinyl, alcohol, liquid silicon, acrylic tissue adhesives, and Ethibloc. These newer agents, which penetrate and obliterate the nidus of the malformation, have significantly improved management of patients with arteriovenous vascular malformations. Many lesions feared to be untreatable due to the extent or anatomic position are now controlled, if not cured, by embolization therapy or by the combined treatment of transcatheter embolization and surgery.

References

1. Paes EH, Vollmar JF. Aneurysmal transformation in congenital venous angiodysplasias in lower extremities. *International Angiology*. 1990;9:90–96.
2. Hunter DW, Amplatz K. Sclerotherapy of peripheral AVMs and hemangiomas through a retrograde transvenous approach. In: Belov S, Loose DA, Weber J, eds. *Vascular Malformation: Periodica Angiologica*. Vol 16. Reinbek, Germany: Einhorn-Presse; 1989:279.
3. van der Stricht J. The sclerosing therapy in congenital vascular defects. *International Angiology*. 1990;9:224–227.
4. Mulliken JB. Vascular malformations of the head and neck. In: Mulliken JB, Young AE, eds. *Vascular Birthmarks, Hemangiomas, and Malformations*. Philadelphia, Pa: WB Saunders; 1988:323.
5. Riché M-C, Merland J-J. Embolization of vascular malformations. In: Mulliken JB, Young AE, eds. *Vascular Birthmarks, Hemangiomas, and Malformations*. Philadelphia, Pa: WB Saunders; 1988:436–440.
6. Mulliken JB. Treatment of hemangiomas. In: Mulliken JB, Young AE, eds. *Vascular Birthmarks, Hemangiomas and Malformations*. Philadelphia, Pa: WB Saunders; 1988:88–90.
7. Ehringhaus C. Corticosteroid treatment in infantile cutaneous hemangiomas. In: Belov S, Loose DA, Weber J, eds. *Vascular Malformation: Periodica Angiologica*. Vol 16. Reinbek, Germany: Einhorn-Presse; 1989:197–199.
8. Belov S, Loose DA. Surgical treatment of congenital vascular defects. *International Angiology*. 1990;9:175–182.
9. Djawari D, Cremer HJ. Frühtherapie der kutanen Hämangiome mit der Kontaktkryochirurgie. *Padiat Prax*. 1994;47:633–650.
10. Philipp C, Berlien H-P, Poetke M, Waldschmidt J. Ten Years of laser treatment of congenital vascular disorders: techniques and results. SPIE proceedings 2327. Medical Applications of Laser. 1994.
11. Kimmig W. Laser therapy of cutaneous congenital vascular malformations. In: Belov S, Loose DA, Weber J, eds. *Vascular Malformation: Periodica Angiologica*. Vol 16. Reinbek, Germany: Einhorn-Presse; 1989:195–196.
12. Landthaler M, Hohenleutner U. Laser treatment of congenital vascular malformations. *International Angiology*. 1990;9:208–213.

98

Radiological Diagnostic Strategies and Interventional Radiology

J. Weber

Until now, the classification of congenital vascular defects has meant a serious problem for the adequate and well-timed therapy of the diseased patients.[6,25,28,31,70,64]

Many of the disciplines involved are still following their own definitions,[23,44,52,56] each transmitting historical syndromes, such as Klippel and Trénaunay's from 1900[18] and F. P. Weber's from 1907,[55] that were defined at that time only according to clinical signs.[51]

Recently it has become more and more evident that there are two completely different types of vascular abnormalities, namely, *hemangiomas* on the one hand and *vascular malformations* (or angiodysplasias) on the other.[30,31]

After a long and controversial discussion,[3,4,6,7] the goal for the 1988 *Hamburg classification*[7] of congenital vascular malformations (CVMs) seems to be more and more accepted in the literature (Table 98.1).[42,49] It means a *descriptive* definition of the individual manifestations of the CVM, including clinical signs, angiographic findings, soft tissue and bone involvement, and, even more, the functional disorders (arteriovenous [AV] fistulas, valveless veins, etc.[7,64,69]) that are components or consequences of the congenital defect.

The aspects of classification must be pointed out before discussing morphologic findings, documented by *imaging modalities* (Doppler ultrasound, duplex ultrasound, computed tomography, magnetic resonance imaging, angiography) and *functional tests* (blood pressure measurements, plethysmography, Doppler ultrasound, duplex ultrasound, angiography) (Table 98.2).[41,42]

In my view, the decision for using more or less invasive diagnostic modalities depends on the experience of specialists, leading to an adequate selection of methods offered to the patient according to the actual clinical signs and the prospective development of symptoms to be expected in the future.[70]

Radiological Diagnostic Strategies

Rutherford[41,42] presented diagrams on the diagnostic approach and vasosurgical management of the CVM in 1989, based on his recent experiences as a surgeon.

In my experience—considering surgical, interventional radiological, and combined forms of therapy—the "decision tree" of diagnostic tests depends mainly on the angiographic findings, which define the vascular lesion to be predominantly venous versus AV, showing low flow respectively to the high flow in the demonstrated AV fistulas (Table 98.3).[67,70]

TABLE 98.1. Classification of the congenital vascular defects according to their species and anatomical form.

Species	Anatomical form	
Predominantly arterial defects	Truncular forms ———————	aplasia or obstruction dilatation
	Angiomatous form	
Predominantly venous defects	Truncular forms ———————	aplasia or obstruction dilatation
	Infiltrating form	
	Angiomatous form	
Predominantly AV shunting defects	Truncular forms ————————	deep AV fistulae
	Infiltrating form	superficial AV fistulas
	Angiomatous form	
Combined vascular defects	Truncular forms ————————	arterial and venous
	Hemolymphatic	hemolymphatic
	angiomatous form	

TABLE 98.2 Imaging modalities and functional tests for diagnosis and classification of congenital vascular malformations.

I. Functional tests Doppler/duplex ultrasound Pressure measurement Plethysmography	*II. Noninvasive imaging* Duplex scan Ultrasound (B-mode) Computed tomography Magnetic resonance imaging
Localization of arteriovenous fistulas, definition of low-flow and high-flow arteriovenous malformations; venous reflux, chronic venous insufficiency	Flow direction of arteries and veins, infiltrative forms, subfascial and epifascial manifestation, muscular involvement, cystic degeneration, calcification
III. Phlebography Ascending leg phlebography Varicography Serial venography	*IV. Arteriography* Arterial overview Selective arteriography Subselective arteriography Balloon occlusion arteriography
Pathoanatomy of deep and suprafascial veins, venous valves, reflux, phlebectasias, persistent embryonal or marginal vein.	Axial arterial anatomy, identification and localization of arteriovenous fistulas, exact definition of low-flow and high-flow lesions, collaterals, cartography of feeding vessels for vaso-occlusive therapy (transcatheter embolization)
V. Lymphography Direct or indirect (seldom needed)	

Functional Tests

The functional tests ought to give qualitative and quantitative information about the hemodynamic parameters, such as arterial and venous pressure, blood flow and shunting volume, pump function, venous reflux, and chronic venous insufficiency.[35,67,70]

Magnetic Resonance Imaging

Magnetic resonance imaging offers additional important information on the attachment of diseased vascular structures and surrounding soft tissue based on the transverse cut scanning of the areas of interest and the characteristics of signal intensity of blood vessels locally. Especially in the periphery of diseased extremities, the exact localization and relationship to subcutaneous and intramuscular structures can be demonstrated much more clearly compared with angiography and even more so compared with computed tomography imaging—and without radiation exposure. This is also important for infants and adolescent patients who have CVMs.[49,70]

However, the detailed differentiation of arteries, veins, and shunting vessels by magnetic resonance imaging is limited because of the variety of controverse flow-directed signals, limiting also the quality of the digital reconstruction of vascular structures. This makes it evident that MRI cannot substitute entirely for angiography.

Angiography

Clear and detailed demonstration of the individual vascular pathoanatomy is the key for classification and therapeutic considerations in all types of CVM. This is seldom needed in hemangiomas, being required mainly for definition of the nutritive arterialization in huge tumor-like lesions, or in critical areas of localization such as the craniofacial space.[49] Nevertheless, functional aspects revealed by angiography should be studied very carefully:

- *Arteriography* can demonstrate the degree of high-flow and low-flow lesions, collateralization, and steal effects due to the AV-shunting vascular areas.
- *Phlebography* shows primary and secondary signs of the CVM under orthostatic conditions, such as valveless

TABLE 98.3. Diagnostic approach to congenital vascular malformations.

Clinical symptoms	Plain film	Functional tests	Phlebography	Arteriography	Magnetic resonance imaging
Extremity difference in length	+++				
Predominantly venous defect	(+)	Doppler, duplex, pressure measurements, plethysmography	+++	(+)	(+)
Low-flow arteriovenous malformations	++	Doppler, duplex	(+)	+++	(+)
High-flow arteriovenous malformations	++	Doppler, duplex	(+)	+++	(+)
Infiltrative forms (arterial and venous)					+++

+: indicated; (+) in special cases
++: highly indicated
+++: obligatorious

decompensation or reflux due to reduction and dysfunction of venous valves of the limb. It also shows collateral circulation resulting from varicose degeneration or primary congenital phlebectasias.

- *Lymphography* can also demonstrate reflux ("dermal backflow") and lymphedema. Lymphatic cysts are relatively rare. They can be documented by direct fine-needle puncture and contrast enhancement.

Phlebography

Phlebography in my view is obligatory in the majority of peripheral CVMs and should be carried out before arteriography. The method is less invasive. It can be easily performed on an outpatient basis. And it can be combined with direct peripheral blood pressure measurements, giving additional and directly correlated information about the degree of chronic venous insufficiency, which occurs very early in the presence of AV fistulas and persisting large embryonal or marginal veins (Figure 98.1).[54,67,70]

Phlebography should be performed even in young children who show direct or indirect clinical signs of phlebectasias, such as swelling of the leg and difference in length of the limb, to prevent progressive functional decompensation on the venous side (which is much more common compared with AV shunting problems in

the AV malformations [AVMs] and more or less incurable by active therapy after a while).

Phlebography clearly shows axial abnormalities and variations of the deep venous system of the limb[65,67] and its correlation to superficial subcutaneous dysplastic collecting veins (e.g., saphenous and persistent marginal veins, phlebectasias). Phlebographic demonstration thereby leads to an adequate surgical resection and ligation in predominantly venous and combined AV low-flow lesions.[5,23,24]

Phlebography also frequently shows indirect signs of AV shunting of blood flow and its dominant localization, guiding the way to its subsequent direct demonstration and classification by arteriography.[20,70] Phlebography in the end demonstrates congenital disorders in the pelvic and abdominal area, such as aplasia, dysplasia, duplication, and so forth, at the level of the iliofemoral, iliocaval, and inferior caval space.[57,59]

Technique

The technique of phlebography ought to be mainly adapted to the clinical pathology, indicating and guiding the surgical approach to the varicose syndrome within the CVM, including ascending leg phlebography and varicography.

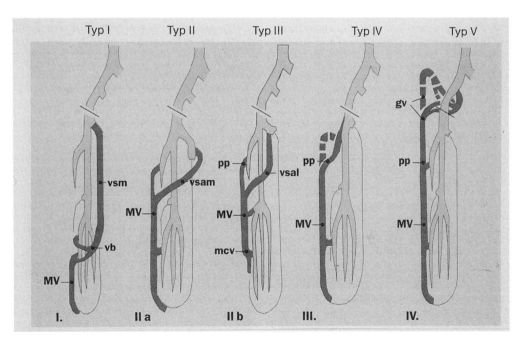

FIGURE 98.1. Persistent marginal vein: types of drainage. **A,** Persistent lower leg, long saphenous drainage. **B,** Persistent lower and upper leg drainage into the deep femoral and accessory posterior saphenous veins. **C,** Persistent lower and upper leg drainage into the deep femoral and accessory anterior saphenous veins. **D,** Persistent lower and upper leg drainage into the deep femoral and lateral circumflex veins. **E,** Persistent lower and upper leg drainage into the inferior/superior glutaean veins. Abbreviations: MV = marginal vein; gv = glutaean veins; mcv = mid crural veins; pp = deep femoral perforator veins; vb = arcuad veins; vsm = long saphenous vein; vsal = accessorial lateral saphenous vein; vsam = accessorial medial saphenous vein. From Weber.[72]

Ascending leg phlebography. With the patient standing in a half-erect position on a tilted table, phlebography is performed by taking films under fluoroscopy and by means of Valsalva's maneuver as a functional angiography, showing valves, reflux at the level of the deep veins, perforators, and saphenous orifices as well as collateral flow and venostasis.

Varicography. As an additional method, varicography by direct puncture is indicated to demonstrate localized varicosities, superficial phlebectasias, and the upper and lower points of connection of persisting marginal veins with the deep venous system.

If there is a discrepancy in length at the level of the lower extremities, I take plain films of both legs with the patient in a standing position at the tilted table before phlebography. At a distance of about 150 cm between the x-ray tube and the plain film, there is only a little magnification to be calculated. Differences in lengths at one side can be clearly measured and correlated.[70] This is important mainly as long as the epiphyseal closure of the stems has not yet taken place, as in children and other growing young patients. By therapeutic reduction of the unilateral vascular problems (AV shunting and venostasis), the difference in length can be reduced or even balanced in many patients without further orthopedic aid.

Arteriography

Arteriography can be omitted in individual patients who show no direct or indirect clinical and phlebographic signs indicating AV fistulas.[19,41,42,46,49,67,70] As an invasive method (being mostly performed on children under full anesthesia[43]), arteriography should be indicated only if there is a strong clinical demand for active surgical and/or interventional treatment.[41,46] This also means that the angiographic pattern of the lesion and its functional character ought to demonstrate the actual state of pathoanatomy and pathophysiology,[29] considering the evolution of AV-shunting high-flow lesions during growth, puberty, pregnancy, and so forth.[21,25–27,31,61,69]

As for the angiographic technique, indirect transvenous demonstration of the arterial pattern of the AVMs is obsolete in my eyes. The direct opacification of the feeding arteries and the AV fistulas themselves is necessary for adequate therapeutic planning, including the decision as to which type of active intervention is needed.

Technically it can be very difficult to realize a qualified documentation under high-flow conditions of the vascular lesion.[46] A flow-directed balloon-tipped catheter (Swan–Ganz type[46]) may improve the opacification of the afferent vessels (balloon occlusion arteriography[68]). Road-mapping by digital subtraction arteriography and a detailed cartography of the area of interest may guide one directly to the center of the network of AV fistulas to be resected or embolized.[32]

When planning the interventional approach by transcatheter embolization, arteriography should be performed as a separate diagnostic procedure.[71,73] The large amount of contrast medium needed for diagnostic purposes will limit the angiographic control of a subsequent therapeutic vaso-occlusion if both procedures are carried out within one session. Separate diagnostic and therapeutic angiography also allows interdisciplinary discussion and decision making to find the best individual therapeutic solution for the patient, by offering surgical and/or interventional therapy.[23,24,71]

A separate diagnostic approach by arteriography also enables a detailed and selected check of all feeding arteries and collaterals. One can calculate the risks of therapy according to the amount of embolization volume and materials needed to occlude the AV fistulas safely, without damaging adjacent structures to be spared from vaso-occlusion.[61,62,69,71]

Also, it makes good sense for the diagnostic and therapeutic arteriographic procedures to be carried out in one hand, so as to avoid errors and to improve the radiologist's morphologic and functional knowledge about the lesion to be treated. As a matter of fact, there is a high rate of repeated diagnostic arteriography in patients with AVMs because of inadequate documentation according to the previously discussed criteria. In particular, poor technical quality of the angiograms, such as subtraction artifacts and reduction of film sequences documented during the phases of disturbed AV circulation, may lead to misinterpretation.

It is very important in low-flow lesions to demonstrate small direct and even indirect signs of AV fistulas by filming the local sequence of arterial, late arterial, AV, and venous phases of the vascular area being involved. The enlargement of small side branches of the injected arteries, early venous filling, and pooling of the contrast medium may guide the examiner to the identification of microshunts, draining frequently into suprafascial phlebectasias also in the predominantly venous vascular defects. Surgery in these cases can treat the hypodynamic AV fistulas by resecting phlebectasias that show "arterialized veins" at the site of incision.[7,22]

Interventional Radiology

The interventional radiological approach to CVMs is generally limited to the high-flow lesions that show arteriographically hyperdynamic AV shunting by means of enlarged feeding vessels to be catheterized.

Indications and Tactics

Vaso-occlusion by transcatheter embolization can be considered as a method by itself in selected cases.[1,2,29,32,40,47,68,69] If it is a part of a combined treatment, the radiological approach should be carried out before surgery, for several reasons.[24]

Many patients show high-flow AV fistulas with enlarged afferent arterial side-branches at the level of the lower extremities localized to the areas of joints (hip, knee, ankle, and foot). These vascular areas can frequently be treated by transcatheter embolization, whereas many hypodynamic microfistulas, situated in between (and mostly leading to outside subcutaneous venous drainage), can be resected much more safely and effectively by the vascular surgeon.

Primary transcatheter vaso-occlusion of the bigger AV fistulas enables subsequent surgical resection of the small fistulas and phlebectasias with reduced risk of local bleeding and loss of blood volume (and thus reduced need of blood transfusion).[23,24]

Contraindications to transcatheter embolization must be discussed by balancing the advantages and disadvantages of the method, focusing on the risk of complications and the long-term perspective of a permanent vaso-occlusion, also causing local ischemia and perhaps permanent functional defects. Contraindications should be discussed in terms of the possibilities and the limits of alternative therapeutic procedures, mainly surgery.[33] Contraindications may also be caused by preceding therapeutic activities, such as surgical ligation, skeletonization, and resection of feeding arteries without having removed the AV fistulas themselves.[53] The same negative results can be caused by inadequate transcatheter embolization that has occluded the afferent vessels without blocking the AV shunting fistulas,[12] pushing collateralization of the lesion and inducing local progressive ischemia at the same time.

Embolization Materials

Many embolizing substances have been recommended in the literature (Table 98.4).[9,14,15,34,66] However, capillary embolization[17] cannot be realized by using materials such as detachable balloons,[38] coils,[13] and macroparticles,[10,12] which can only occlude the afferent vessels. Likewise, resorbable particulate substances mostly do not cause permanent vaso-occlusion in high-flow lesions.[17,33,62,66]

Fluid and semifluid materials, in comparison, are suitable for the direct occlusion of small and very small AV fistulas, blocking the complex network of the mostly infiltrative type of lesion by cutting the connections to other feeders that are involved (Figure 98.2).[2,15,17,66,74]

However, the different characteristics such as viscosity (i.e., injectability), enhancement (for fluoroscopic control), and reactivity against the intimal vascular wall (for solidity and permanence of vaso-occlusion) must be calculated.[17,33,66] They also depend on the localization of the lesion (acral as opposed to parenchymal vessels), the size of the afferent arteries, and the caliber of the fistulas themselves.[8,9]

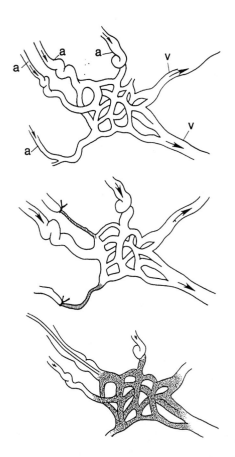

FIGURE 98.2. Vaso-occlusion of the center of AV-fistulas. Ideally, embolization of an AV malformation should aim at the core of the lesion rather than the feeding arteries. **A,** Schematic drawing of AV malformation. a = artery; v = vein. **B,** Surgical ligation or proximal occlusion of feeding arteries is not effective because collaterals take over. **C,** When core of lesion is obliterated, occlusion is effective. From Weber.[64]

TABLE 98.4. Vaso-occlusive materials suitable for embolization of arteriovenous malformations.

Particulate materials	
Silicon spheres	+
Polyvinyl alcohol (Ivalon)	+
Dura and fascia lata	+
Mechanical devices	
Steel coils (Gianturco type)	++
Steel "spiders"	++
Detachable balloons	++
Fluid and semifluid materials	
Absolute alcohol (ethanol)	++
Iso-butyl-cyanoacrylate (acrylate)	+++
Amino acids (prolamine)	+++

+ indicated; ++ highly indicated; +++ optimal

Acrylate. Acrylate (iso-butyl-cyanoacrylate) as a fluid agent can be offered by thin and coaxial catheters. It polymerizes immediately on contact with blood,[11] causing, however, irregular blockade of arteries and major AV shunting of the substance to the venous side.[17] The material generally works like a glue.

Absolute alcohol. Absolute alcohol (ethanol) also can be injected easily by tiny catheters into very small arteries.[74,75] Vaso-occlusion by hyperosmotic intimal damage and subsequent local thrombosis is effective, with permanent results under the longtime blocked ("wedge") position of the application catheter and only in smaller vessels. Injection can also be protected by means of balloon-tipped catheters in bigger afferent arteries during the time of solidification of local clots that are induced by alcohol injection and as an additional protective measure against reflux.[8,62,74,75]

Prolamine. Prolamine actually is the ideal substance in my opinion for vaso-occlusion of high-flow AV fistulas.[33,60,62] The semifluid alcoholic solution of biocompatible amino acids precipitates—comparable with acrylates—in direct contact with blood. However, solidification occurs much more slowly and can be balanced—if wanted—by adding iodized oil.[17,33] When diluted with this lymphographic contrast medium, prolamine can also be applied in smaller vessels, using coaxial catheters. In bigger arteries, however, balloon-tipped catheters may prevent reflux and help to protect the solidification of the vascular spout.

In large AV fistulas and in very big afferent arteries, I combine prolamine injection with the application of Gianturco coils,[13] creating a "frame" to incorporate the precipitating material thereafter, thereby blocking a branching artery centrally to protect it from reflux (Figure 98.3).[60,62,66]

Sclerotherapy. Sclerotherapy may be a special therapeutic approach for patients in whom the direct surgical or interventional access is not (or is no longer) available.[16] Instead of direct arterial catheterization and subsequent vaso-occlusion, local retrograde venous sclerotherapy may be helpful in reducing phlebectasias and local swelling of the adjacent soft tissue structures.

In low-flow lesions these therapeutic effects may be long lasting; in high-flow lesions, however, the results appear to be relatively poor and diminish after a short time of improvement, limited by progressive venous collateralization.[68]

Recently I have made my first attempts toward sclerosing intraosseous AV fistulas by direct needle puncture under temporary exsanguination, using the Esmarch technique. With a very small amount of sclerosant needed and in a high concentration (polydocanol, 3% to 4%), locally good results can be gained by direct occlusion of the fistulas and the efferent phlebectatic veins locally.

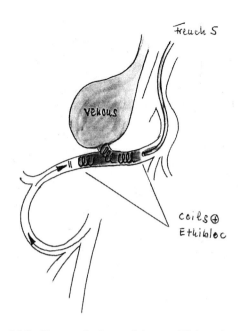

FIGURE 98.3. Vaso-occlusion of large AV-shunting fistulas. Frame of detached Gianturco coils, blocking prograde and retrograde collateral arterial flow. Solid occlusion by Prolamine incorporated thereafter. From Weber.[64]

Catheter Materials

Many different catheter systems, including those with various calibers and configurations of the catheter tip and flow-directed smooth Tracker-type, coaxial, and balloon-tipped devices, are commercially available.[8,33] Also, different smooth guide wires help to direct the catheter's approach to the desired peripheral and selective position.[33] Working with a locking delivery device, the exchange of catheters can be performed easily and much more safely.

Complications and Side Effects

Complications of transcatheter embolization depend on many factors. First, the management of catheters, guide wires, and so forth is part of the standard angiographic technique.[1,36] The delivery of the embolizing substances, however, may cause special complications, depending on the type of material to be used and its injectability. Complications can be reduced by the skilled ability of the experienced angiographer.[8,9,33]

Reflux of the embolizing substances may also be reduced by optimal fluoroscopic control of opacified materials.[57,60] A nonoptimal position of mechanical devices (coils) can be corrected or removed under fluoroscopy as well.[58]

Necroses of the adjacent tissues, of nerves, and of the skin have been mainly reported after ethanol injection.[39,50,73] After arterial embolization, Novak[34] generally calculated an overall complication rate of 3.8% and mortality rate of 0.9%. However, the risks of severe complications may be even higher in different areas (pelvic, 5.0%; neuroradiological, 6.7%).[34]

Because few patients have undergone embolization as treatment of AVMs, there are no statistically significant data available in the literature so far. Side effects and discomforts are considered to be unavoidable with a complete and permanent therapeutic vaso-occlusion by transcatheter embolization. They are part of the "postembolization syndrome" (or postinfarction syndrome)[35,63]:

- Pain
- Mild fever
- Leukocytosis
- Local edema

These, and others, are clinical signs of a locally induced ischemia, which generally leads to thrombosis, infarction, and corresponding inflammatory soft tissue reaction of the surrounding tissues. The degree of these symptoms mainly depends on the extension of infarction and the solidity of the vaso-occlusion that was produced.[63,68,69]

In the majority of patients with AVMs, transcatheter embolotherapy (as well as surgical therapy) means more or less palliation, seldom curative treatment. To achieve the best results available while causing only minor complications, a step-by-step treatment is mandatory.[1,24,39,71,73] Transcatheter embolization of about three afferent main vessels at a maximum within one session means protection of adjacent structures, especially saving the skin and the nutrition of nerves passing nearby.[39,71]

Because of the invasiveness of the procedure, the potential risks of complications, and the severe pain syndrome, which frequently requires patient care and monitoring in the intensive care unit over the first few days, guidance of the patient is very important.[43,69] It is also indispensable to inform the patients (or the parents of the diseased children) about the character of the vascular defect and the strategy of separate and repeated diagnostic and therapeutic approaches. Otherwise, it seems nearly impossible to win their confidence and to guide them over a long, perhaps lifelong period of recurrent interventions and continuing conservative treatment in between (e.g., with elastic stockings, orthopedic aid). A detailed explanation should also include information about the pain syndrome and other side effects of the vaso-occlusive therapy.

Embolotherapy of AVMs demands good interdisciplinary teamwork of the specialists involved, mainly between the interventional radiologist and the vascular surgeon. Likewise, cooperation with the anesthesiologist is mandatory. Most patients should be treated while fully anesthetized. Peridural anesthesia in addition offers much comfort during the first 1 to 3 days of the postembolization syndrome.[43]

Orthopedists can help in the osteodysplastic syndrome by surgically increasing or reducing the difference in length of the involved lower extremity on the diseased side.[7,23,24] Reconstructive surgery enables us to improve on the first surgical results for cosmetic and functional reasons, if needed.[37]

Conclusions

Clinical signs, the natural history, and all available noninvasive and invasive diagnostic investigations ought to lead to an optimal classification of the individual congenital vascular defect. Angiographic examinations (phlebography first, then arteriography in the majority of cases, with lymphography in selected patients) are obligatory in patients with CVMs to find an adequate therapeutic access to the lesion. Magnetic resonance imaging can help both surgical planning and interventional embolotherapy by showing the correlation of adjacent soft tissue structures.

Transcatheter embolization should be limited to the active treatment of hyperdynamic AVMs (high-flow lesions) only and can be indicated as a therapeutic procedure on its own or before surgical resection as a part of the combined treatment. A careful selection of suitable catheter devices and of embolization materials, directed occlusion of the AV fistulas, and creation of permanent vaso-occlusion are imperative for attaining long-lasting clinical results and reducing risks and complications.

Good clinical experience, diagnostic knowledge, and skilled angiographic training are as important as the interdisciplinary teamwork among specialists who are familiar with all aspects of congenital vascular defects. From the patient's viewpoint, therapeutic aid during the period of postembolization syndrome is mandatory. Guidance of the patient ought to include good information, optimal management of the invasive therapy, and long-term observations and follow-up studies.

References

1. Allison DJ, Kennedy A. Embolization technique in arteriovenous malformations. In: Belov S, Loose DA, Weber J, eds. *Vascular Malformations.* Vol 16. Reinbek, Germany: Einhorn-Presse Verlag; 1989.
2. Athanasoulis CA. Transcatheter arterial occlusion for arteriovenous fistulas and malformations of the trunk, pelvis, and extremity. In: Athanasoulis CA, Pfister RC, Greene

RE, Roberson GH, eds. *Interventional Radiology*. Philadelphia, Pa: WB Saunders; 1982.

3. Belov S. Chirurgische Behandlung der kongenitalen Angiodysplasien. *Zentralbl Chir.* 1967;192:1595.

4. Belov S. Congenital angiodysplasias and their surgical treatment. *Medicina i Fizkultura.* Sofia; 1971.

5. Belov S. Surgical treatment of congenital predominantly venous defects. In: Belov S, Loose DA, Weber J, eds. *Vascular Malformations.* Vol 16. Reinbek, Germany: Einhorn-Presse Verlag; 1989.

6. Belov S, Loose DA, Müller E, eds. *Angeborene Gefäßfehler.* Vol 10. Reinbek, Germany: Einhorn-Presse Verlag; 1985.

7. Belov S, Loose DA, Weber J, eds. *Vascular Malformations.* Vol 16. Reinbek, Germany: Einhorn-Presse Verlag; 1989.

8. Berenstein A, Kricheff II. Catheter and material selection for transarterial embolization. Technical considerations: catheters. *Radiology.* 1979;132:619.

9. Berenstein A, Kricheff II. Catheter and material selection for transarterial embolization. Technical considerations: materials. *Radiology.* 1979;132:631.

10. Brooks B. The treatment of traumatic arteriovenous fistulas. *South Med J.* 1930;23:100.

11. Cromwell LD, Kerber CW. Modification of cyano-acrylate for therapeutic embolization: preliminary experience. *AJR Am J Roentgenol.* 1979;132:799.

12. van Dongen RJAM. Therapie der angeborenen arteriovenösen Angiodysplasien unter besonderer Berücksichtigung der operativen Embolisation. *Angiology.* 1993;5:169.

13. Gianturco G, Anderson JH, Wallace S. Mechanical devices for arterial occlusion. *Am J Roentgenol Radium Ther Nucl Med.* 1975;124:428.

14. Grace DM, Pitt DF, Gold RE. Vascular embolization and occlusion by angiographic technique as an aid or alternative to operation. *Surg Gynecol Obstet.* 1976;142:469.

15. Greenfield AJ. Transcatheter vessel occlusion: methods and materials. In: Athanasoulis CA, Pfister RC, Greene RE, Roberson GH, eds. *Interventional Radiology*. Philadelphia, Pa: WB Saunders; 1982.

16. Hunter DW, Amplatz K. Sclerotherapy of peripheral AVMs and hemangiomas through a retrograde transvenous approach. In: Belov S, Loose DA, Weber J, eds. *Vascular Malformations.* Vol 16. Reinbek, Germany: Einhorn-Presse Verlag; 1989

17. Kauffmann G, Wimmer B, Bischoff W, et al. Experimentelle Grundlagen für therapeutische Gefäßverschlüsse mit Angiographiekathetern. *Radiologe.* 1977;17:489.

18. Klippel M, Trénaunay P. Du naevus variqueux ostéohypertrophique. *Arch Gen Med.* 1900;3:641.

19. Lea Thomas M, Andress MR. Angiography in venous dysplasias of the limb. *AJR Am J Roentgenol Radium Ther Nucl Med.* 1971;113:722.

20. Lea Thomas M, Macfie GB. Phlebography in the Klippel-Trénaunay syndrome. *Acta Radiol.* 1974;15:43.

21. Leu HJ. Pathoanatomy of congenital vascular malformations. In: Belov S, Loose DA, Weber J, eds. *Vascular Malformations.* Vol 16. Reinbek, Germany: Einhorn-Presse Verlag; 1989.

22. Loose DA. Surgical strategy in congenital venous defects. In: Belov S, Loose DA, Weber J, eds. *Vascular Malformations.* Vol 16. Reinbek, Germany: Einhorn-Presse Verlag; 1989.

23. Loose DA. The combined surgical therapy in congenital av-shunting malformations. In: Belov S, Loose DA, Weber J, eds. *Vascular Malformations.* Vol 16. Reinbek, Germany: Einhorn-Presse Verlag; 1989.

24. Loose DA, Weber J. Indications and tactics for combined treatment of congenital vascular defects. In: *Progress in Angiology 1991.* Torino, Italy: Minerva Medica; 1991.

25. Malan E. *Vascular Malformations (Angiodysplasias).* Milan, Italy: Carlo Erba Foundation; 1974.

26. Malan E. Surgical problems in the treatment of congenital arteriovenous fistulae. *J Cardiovasc Surg.* 1965;6:251.

27. Malan E, Puglionisi A. Congenital angiodysplasias of the extremities. *J Cardiovasc Surg.* 1965;6:255.

28. May R, Nißl R. Beitrag zur Klassifizierung der "gemischten kongenitalen Angiodysplasien." *Fortschr Röntgenstr.* 1970; 113:170.

29. Merland JJ, Chiras J, Riche MC. Embolization of lesions in the limbs. In: Veiga-Pirex JA, Martins da Silva M, Oliva L, eds. *Intervention Radiology.* Amsterdam: Excerpta Medica Foundation; 1980.

31. Mulliken JB. Cutaneous vascular anomalies. *Semin Vasc Surg.* 1993;6:204.

30. Mulliken JB, Young AE, eds. *Vascular Birthmarks: Hemangiomas and Malformations.* Philadelphia, Pa: WB Saunders; 1988.

32. Natali J, Merland JJ. Superselective arteriography and therapeutic embolization for vascular malformations (angiodysplasias). *J Cardiovasc Surg.* 1976;17:465.

33. Novak D. Embolization materials. In: Dondelinger RF, Rossi P, Kurdziel JC, Wallace S, eds. *Interventional Radiology.* New York, NY: Thieme; 1990.

34. Novak D. Complications of arterial embolization. In: Dondelinger RF, Rossi P, Kurdziel JC, Wallace S, eds. *Interventional Radiology.* New York, NY: Thieme; 1990.

35. Novak D, Weber J, Wieners H, Zabel G. New liquid and semi-liquid embolizing substances for tumour-embolization. *Ann Radiol.* 1984;24:4.

36. Partsch H. Non-invasive investigations, measurement of shunt-volume, and indirect lymphography in vascular malformations of the limbs. In: Belov S, Loose DA, Weber J, eds. *Vascular Malformations.* Vol 16. Reinbek, Germany: Einhorn-Presse Verlag; 1989.

37. Petrovici P. Surgical treatment of congenital arteriovenous malformation in the scalp and ear. In: Belov S, Loose DA, Weber J, eds. *Vascular Malformations.* Vol. 16. Reinbek, Germany: Einhorn-Presse Verlag; 1986.

38. Rankin RN, McKenzie FN, Ahmad D. Embolization of arteriovenous fistulas and aneurysms with detachable balloons. *Can J Surg.* 1983;26:317.

39. Riche MC, Reizine D, Melni JP, Merland JJ. Les complications et les pièges de l'embolisation des membres. *Ann Radiol.* 1984;27:287.

40. Roche A. Peripheral arteriovenous malformations. In: Dondelinger RF, Rossi P, Kurdziel JC, Wallace S, eds. *Interventional Radiology.* New York, NY: Thieme; 1990.

41. Rutherford RB. New approaches to the diagnosis of congenital vascular malformations. In: Belov S, Loose DA, Weber J, eds. *Vascular Malformations.* Vol 16. Reinbek, Germany: Einhorn-Presse Verlag; 1989.

42. Rutherford RB. Congenital vascular malformations: diagnostic evaluation. *Semin Vasc Surg.* 1993;6:225.

43. Schilke PM. Special methods of anaesthesia for vascular surgery and interventional radiology. In: Belov S, Loose DA, Weber J, eds. *Vascular Malformations.* Vol 16. Reinbek, Germany: Einhorn-Presse Verlag; 1989.

44. Schobinger RA. *Periphere Angiodysplasien.* Bern, Switzerland: Huber; 1977.

45. Servelle M, Tringuecoste P. Des angiomes veineux. *Arch Mal Coeur.* 1948;47:436.

46. Sörensen R. Congenital arteriovenous malformations: diagnostic approach. In: Belov S, Loose DA, Weber J, eds. *Vascular Malformations.* Vol 16. Reinbek, Germany: Einhorn-Presse Verlag; 1989.

47. Stanley RJ, Cubillo E. Nonsurgical treatment of arteriovenous malformations of the trunk and limbs by transcatheter embolization. *Radiology.* 1975;115:609.

48. Swan HJ, Ganz W, Forrester J, et al. Catheterization of the heart in man with use of a flow-directed balloon-tipped catheter. *N Engl J Med.* 1970;283:447.

49. Trout HH, Feinberg RL. Vascular anomalies and acquired arteriovenous fistulas. In: Dean RH, Yao JST, Brewster DC, eds. *Current Diagnosis and Treatment in Vascular Surgery.* Norwalk, Conn: Appleton & Lange; 1995.

50. Twomey BP, Wilkins RA, Mee AD. Skin necrosis: a complication of alcohol infarction of a hypernephroma. *Cardiovasc Intervent Radiol.* 1985;8:202.

51. Vollmar JF. Zur Geschichte und Terminologie der Syndrome nach F. P. Weber und Klippel-Trénaunay. In: Vollmar JF, Nobbe FP. *Arteriovenöse Fisteln—dilatierende Arteriopathien (Aneurysmen).* Stuttgart, Germany: Thieme; 1976.

52. Vollmar JF, Nobbe FP. *Arterio-venöse Fisteln—dilatierende Arteriopathien (Aneurysmen).* Stuttgart, Germany: Thieme; 1976.

53. Vollmar JF, Stalker CG. The surgical treatment of congenital arterio-venous fistulas in the extremities. *J Cardiovasc Surg.* 1976;17:340.

54. Vollmar JF, Voss E. Vena marginalis lateralis persistens— die vergessene Vene der Angiologen. *Vasa.* 1979;8:192.

55. Weber FP. Angioma formation in connection with hypertrophy of limbs and hemihypertrophy. *Br J Dermatol.* 1907;19:231.

56. Weber J. Der umschriebene Riesenwuchs, Typ Parkes-Weber. *Fortschr Röntgenstr.* 1970;113:734.

57. Weber J. Entwicklungsstörung der Vena cava inferior und der Beckenvenen. Untersuchungen zur Hämodynamik im venösen Niederdrucksystem. *Fortschr Röntgenstr.* 1974;121: 273.

58. Weber J. A complication with the Gianturco coil and its non-surgical management. *Cardiovasc Intervent Radiol.* 1980;3:156.

59. Weber J. Congenital abnormalities of the inner pelvic veins and the iliocaval junction. In: May R, Weber J, eds. *Pelvic and Abdominal Veins.* Amsterdam,: Excerpta Medica Foundation; 1981.

60. Weber J. Experimental renal embolization using contrast-labeled Ethibloc and follow-up observations by computed tomography. In: Oliva L, Veiga Pires JH, eds. *Intervention Radiology 2.* Amsterdam: Excerpta Medica Foundation; 1982.

61. Weber J. Embolisationstherapie arteriovenöser Mißbildungen. *Radiol Diagn (Berl).* 1987;28:513.

62. Weber J. Embolizing materials and catheter techniques for angiotherapeutic management of the AVM. In: Belov S, Loose DA, Weber J, eds. *Vascular Malformations.* Vol 16. Reinbek, Germany: Einhorn-Presse Verlag; 1989.

63. Weber J. The post-infarction and pain syndrome following catheter embolization and its treatment. In: Belov S, Loose DA, Weber J, eds. *Vascular Malformations.* Vol 16. Reinbek, Germany: Einhorn-Presse Verlag; 1989.

64. Weber J. Kongenitale Angiodysplasien (Gefäßmal-formationen). In: Weber J, May R, eds. *Funktionelle Phlebologie.* Stuttgart, Germany: Thieme, 1990.

65. Weber J. Kongenitale Achsen- und Verlaufs-anomalien. In: Weber J, May R. *Funktionelle Phlebologie.* Stuttgart, Germany: Thieme; 1990.

66. Weber J. Technique and results of therapeutic catheter embolization of congenital vascular defects. *Int Angiol.* 1990;9:214.

67. Weber J. Kongenitale Angiodysplasien. In: Weber J, May R, eds. *Funktionelle Phlebologie.* Stuttgart, Germany: Thieme; 1990.

68. Weber J. Invasive radiological diagnostic of congenital vascular malformations (CVM). *Int Angiol.* 1990;9:168.

69. Weber J. Vaso-occlusive angiotherapy in congenital vascular malformations. In: Loose DA, ed. *Semin Vasc Surg.* 1993;6:279.

70. Weber J, Ritter H. Diagnostic management of the venous and lymphatic components of av-malformations (AVM). In: Belov S, Loose DA, Weber J, eds. *Vascular Malformations.* Vol 16. Reinbek, Germany: Einhorn-Presse Verlag; 1989.

71. Weber J, Ritter H. Strategies for the radiological angiotherapy of hyperdynamic av-malformations. In: Belov S, Loose DA, Weber J, eds. *Vascular Malformations.* Vol 16. Reinbek, Germany: Einhorn-Presse Verlag; 1989.

72. Weber J. Invasive diagnostik angeborener gefässfehler. In: Loose DA, Weber J. *Angeborene Gefässmissbildungen.* Nordlanddruck, Luenebung; 1997.

73. Wojtowycz M. *Handbook of Interventional Radiology and Angiography.* St Louis, Mo: Mosby–Year Book; 1995.

74. Yakes WF, Haas DK, Parker SH, et al. Symptomatic vascular malformations: ethanol embolotherapy. *Radiology.* 1994; 170:1059.

75. Yakes WT. Extremity venous malformations. Diagnosis and management. *Semin Intervent Radiol.* 1994;11:332.

99

Arteriovenous Malformations of the Upper Limb

S. Sulaiman Shoab and J. H. Scurr

The term *arteriovenous malformations* (AVMs) usually refers to congenital defects. About 10% of these malformations involve the upper extremities. AVMs are pathologically a diverse group of lesions. They are, in general, much more difficult to cure than the acquired arteriovenous fistulas (AVFs). This has led to less than appropriate management in many instances. Clinically, AVMs of the limbs are taken to include simple and cavernous hemangiomas, microarteriovenous and macroarteriovenous fistulas, venous angiomas, and mixed congenital vascular malformations (Figure 99.1). They range in size from tiny glomus tumors to massive AVFs.[2] New growths of the vascular elements, on the other hand, are acquired lesions. These are identifiable by their cellular or gross appearance. They are not AVMs, by definition. Experience with AVMs is limited to specialized centers, and many studies referred to are case reports.

Pathology and Pathophysiology

AVMs occur because of focal defects in vascular development in utero. This happens between the 4th and 10th weeks of development. A focal persistence of primitive vascular elements is suggested as a mechanism for these lesions (Figure 99.2). There is a possible connection between abnormal neural and vascular development. Venous lesions may have their origin in some form of vascular obstruction in utero.[3] The peripheral vascular system is laid out in its adult form at a very early stage in life. Although no hereditary pattern has been noted, it has been reported that defects in the TIE1 and TIE2 receptors for vascular endothelial growth factor lead to cavernous angioma formation.[4] The defect lies in the smooth muscle coat of the vascular wall, which is lacking. Recognition of this defect has made future gene therapy a realistic possibility in these pathologies.

Anatomically, AVMs are divided into *capillary, venous, lymphovenous,* and *arteriovenous* types. Functionally, AVMs are often classified as *microfistulous* and *macrofistulous.* This latter classification is based on angiographic appearance (see later discussion). A high venous PO$_2$ is found in most of these lesions. Arteriovenous fistulization occurs to some degree in most AVMs. The arteries break up into a number of branches, which in turn communicate with a connecting bunch of radiating veins. The terms *cirsoid aneurysm, pulsatile nevus, racemose aneurysm, diffuse arterial ectasia,* and *congenital AVF* have been applied to the macrofistulous variety. Microfistulous AVMs are difficult to distinguish from angiomas, and 70% of microfistulous AVMs contain areas of angioma in any case.[5] Cavernous angiomas are by definition venous and have no arterial connections. Lymphatic malformations are not discussed here, although they may exist in a combined form, mostly as lymphovenous anomalies.

Extension into deeper layers including muscles and bone is frequent. In some cases the accompanying deep veins are either defective or absent. In these cases venous hypertension and its sequelae may be seen.

Congenital vascular–bone syndromes are an example of AVM. Establishing the precise hemodynamic pathogenesis of the vascular defects in congenital vascular–bone syndromes is very important in determining the principles of their surgical treatment. It offers the possibility of the correct choice of operative tactics and techniques in these severe vascular diseases, which in many cases lead to disability and cardiovascular insufficiency.[6] If accompanied by bone overgrowth, the condition is known as the Klippel–Trénaunay syndrome. Congenital AVFs can exist in a hand and extend to involve the whole limb and shoulder (pelvis in lower limb) region (Figure 99.3). An accompanying increase in the size of the limb constitutes the Parker–Weber syndrome.

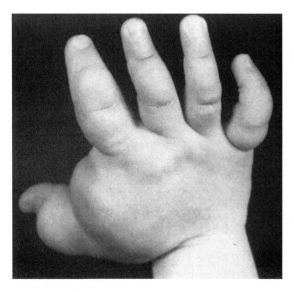

FIGURE 99.1. AVM of the hand. (From Riles and Rosen,[1] with permission.)

Hemangiomas

Strictly speaking, hemangiomas are a distinct entity. They share with AVMs the properties of growth in response to trauma, menarche, antiovulatory medication, and pregnancy and can be potentially serious because of their size or location. The suffix *-oma* should be reserved for lesions that grow by cellular proliferation. During the proliferative phase, these lesions have a high mast cell count, which returns to normal levels once involution is complete. These changes are in contradistinction to AVMs. Although AVMs usually first appear after childhood, hemangiomas are thought to be congenital. Women are affected two to three times more frequently.

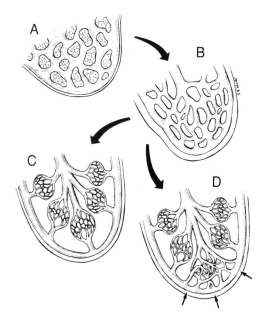

FIGURE 99.2. Persistence of primitive vasculature as a mechanism for AVM. From Riles and Rosen,[1] with permission.)

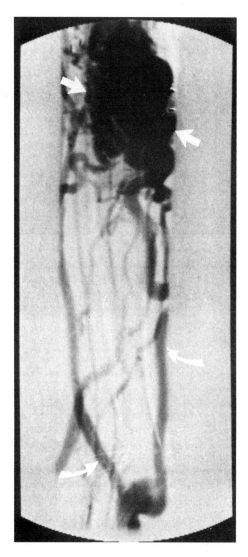

FIGURE 99.3. Arteriogram of an AVM of the forearm showing a classic appearance of the abnormal blood vessels. (From Cohen, Weinreb, and Redman,[14] with permission.)

Hemangiomas can involve skeletal muscle, heart, liver, bone, or the central nervous system. Medical attention is sought because of cosmesis, ulceration of overlying skin, or rapid increase in size. Most remain quiescent until they encounter a stimulatory factor. On physical examination, the mass is not pulsatile and no bruit is audible. Because of the high resistance, cardiac involvement due to arteriovenous shunting is most unusual.

Clinical Presentations and Complications

With regard to clinical presentation of hemangiomas, the best-known birthmark is the *port-wine stain*. This is characteristically pink at birth, changing to purple as the child grows. These lesions may be associated with deeper venous, venolymphatic, or true arterial malformations. The latter can, of course, be present without any skin involvement. Café-au-lait spots are sometimes observed.

Presentation

Venous malformations in the palm, interdigital web spaces, forearm, or dorsum of a digit or hand may remain unnoticed for quite some time. They usually become evident as they fill up when the hand is dependent. Similarly, arterial malformations may be present at birth but be asymptomatic and remain undetected for many years. Once they are brought to attention, the diagnosis is often evident clinically. In a typical case there is discoloration of the overlying skin, hyperhidrosis may occur, obvious pulsation may be present, and a "machinery murmur" may be auscultated. Increase in pulse rate is seen with significant shunting. The pulse rate is seen to decrease on occluding the feeding artery (Nicoladoni–Branham sign). Detectable cardiomegaly may occur. Pigmentation of the skin may occur distal to the lesion because of venous hypertension. Cavernous angiomatosis can occur extensively over the limb (although the lower limb is more commonly affected). Skin involvement shows as a dark purple, irregular, compressible swelling.

In one series of peripheral AVMs, the abnormality was localized in the upper limb in 32 patients and in the lower extremity in 49 patients. Signs, symptoms, treatment modalities, and long-term results were found to vary over a relatively broad spectrum. In the upper extremity, pain was the most frequent presenting symptom.[7] Painful subungual, glomus tumor–like lesions are an unusual presentation. Hemangiomalike skin lesions of the trunk and nodular lesions of the finger joints are sometimes associated with them, and prominent arteriovenous shunting may be present. The etiology of all these abnormalities is thought to be extensive proliferation of glomus cells.[8]

In another series of 32 patients,[9] the presenting symptoms were pain ($n = 9$), swelling ($n = 6$), varices ($n = 6$), none ($n = 4$), and hypertrophy ($n = 2$). In the same group the clinical signs reported were swelling ($n = 11$), vascular nevus ($n = 4$), hypertrophy ($n = 4$), subcutaneous tumor ($n = 3$), varices ($n = 2$), tenderness ($n = 1$), and "indifferent" ($n = 7$).

Rarely, a Kaposi's sarcoma may be mistaken for an AVM. Angiographic findings can be misleading, and careful histopathological analysis of such lesions is advocated so that the correct treatment may be carried out.[10]

Complications

Enlargement of AVMs usually parallels the growth of the patient. Sudden enlargement may occur after changes in the systemic blood pressure or hormonal status or in response to trauma. The exact mode of these aggravating factors is not known. Profuse hemorrhage can occur from these lesions, and high-output cardiac failure has been reported. Large hemangiomas are known to cause platelet trapping and may lead to clinically significant thrombocytopenia (Kasabach–Merritt syndrome).

Cardiac complications with AVMs are not frequently seen. They are even less common with upper limb lesions, in which case they are almost always associated with above-elbow lesions. The hyperdynamic circulation in pregnancy can significantly alter blood flow through these lesions. Worsening symptomatology during pregnancy may demand early delivery. Persistent debilitating symptoms may resolve partially after delivery.[11] Cases have been described of young women with progression of a macrofistulous AVM during pregnancy resulting in severe symptoms and necessitating cesarean delivery. There is often a dramatic postpartum recovery in these cases.[11] However, it is difficult to advise patients with AVMs about the effects of a pregnancy because many of them are known to carry normal pregnancies to full term.

Hemangiomas in infants may require relatively extensive surgery because of ensuing complications. After complete resection of the hemangioma, extensive defects of the skin and subcutaneous tissue may have to be replaced with flaps.[7]

Direct involvement of nerves may occur. Leakage of blood may cause locoregional pressure symptoms. In one reported case, a 15-year-old boy with a long-standing history of congenital AVM in his left arm was seen with an acute posterior interosseous nerve palsy. Exploration showed this to be caused by bleeding from a congenital AVM in the radial tunnel. Decompression and evacuation of the hematoma resulted in full recovery.[12]

Investigations

The diagnosis is often obvious clinically. Unless treatment is being planned, an extensive diagnostic workup is not indicated. This is especially true in children.

- Doppler examination can confirm the strong pulsation in the superficial tissues.
- Duplex examination can reveal abnormal flow patterns in major vessels, venous insufficiency, or thrombosis. It can demonstrate AVFs readily but is of somewhat limited value in operative decision making. It could be used as the only test in patients for whom no active treatment is being planned.
- Dynamic computed tomography can be a useful diagnostic modality. It identifies the location and often demarcates the muscle group involved. Deeper lesions show up as mottled masses. Intravenous contrast

medium (given by bolus or infusion) produces variable enhancements. Cellular lesions with relatively lesser vascularity may not enhance well. The extent of these lesions may be underestimated. In addition, usually only transverse sections are obtained with computed tomography because longitudinal scans are not easy to obtain.

- Magnetic resonance imaging (MRI) can reveal the true extent of the lesion and its relation to the surrounding structures. It also avoids the use of contrast media and has become a most useful part of the workup.
- Plain radiographs show a soft tissue mass. Bony changes may be revealed if present. Phleboliths may be seen in venous lesions.
- Ascending phlebography is a useful technique, especially in venous angiomas. It can also be used where other modalities are either unavailable or cannot be used. Venous dilatation, sinusoids, and isolated venous abnormalities show up well with this technique.
- Other tests include plethysmography, temperature probe recordings, radionuclide scans, and blood gas estimations.
- Contrast angiography remains the gold standard to confirm the fistula and show the feeding arteries.

In differentiating the various forms of AVM, Doppler waveform analysis, labeled microsphere studies, arteriography, closed-space phlebography, and contrast-enhanced computed tomography scans have all been advocated. Each test may have significant limitations in various scenarios.

Angiography

Angiography is recommended before an operation or embolization to locate the feeding and draining vessels and delineate the anatomy of the lesion. Selective catheterization may be used for optimal imaging. Microfistulous AVMs may not show up clearly. Arteriography does not define the fascial planes or specify the musculo-osseous groups involved. In some cases the entire limb may appear filled with contrast material. Angiography may be extremely difficult in infants and young children.

The classification described by Mullikan is very useful[13]:

- AVMs show a high flow, enlarged feeding arteries, and rapid arteriovenous shunting.
- Capillary lesions have low flow, appear as a dense capillary blush, and show a normal or slightly early venous return.
- Venous malformations, on the other hand, have dilated, tortuous, slow-filling veins with no arteriovenous shunting. The arterial supply is normal, and these are low-flow lesions.

These distinctions are important for therapeutic considerations.

Magnetic Resonance Imaging

MRI provides a noninvasive assessment of the anatomical extent of the flow patterns and cellularity of AVMs. This benefit is offset by the lack of availability of MRI and its cost in many places. MRI allows differentiation between muscle, bone, and blood vessels based on signal characteristics. This allows accurate demarcation of the extent of "invasion" of surrounding tissues by the AVM (Figure 99.4). The MRI appearance is that of dilated, tortuous vessels. Vessels appear as low-signal tubular or rounded structures. This is caused by the rapidly flowing blood, which produces the "flow-void" phenomenon.[14]

MRI can quantify blood from the signal intensity depending on (1) proton density, (2) speed of proton relaxation after the excitation pulse (T_1 and T_2), and (3) the blood flow (proton flux). High-flow feeding arteries and draining veins appear as "black holes." Intravascular thromboses can be identified, and the age of extravasated blood can even be determined in many instances.

AVMs were evaluated by MRI in eight patients, four with AVM in the upper and four with AVM in the lower extremity. Before MRI, seven patients had arteriography, five had phlebography, and five had Doppler waveform analysis. MRI showed a highly cellular network with little arteriovenous flow in five patients. In four of them, arteriography and phlebography confirmed the presence of a predominantly venous or microfistulous anomaly. In the other three patients, MRI demonstrated high-flow arterial and venous channels, and these patients were confirmed by arteriography to have macrofistulous AVMs.

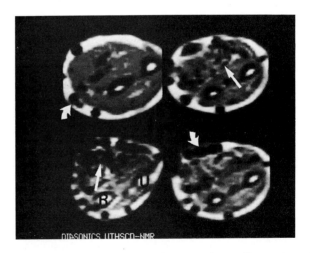

FIGURE 99.4. MRI study of low-flow vascular malformation of forearm. More clear delineation of lesion and its relationship to surrounding tissue planes. (From Cohen, Weinreb, and Redman,[14] with permission.)

In all eight patients, MRI revealed the anatomic location and the longitudinal and transverse extent of the vascular malformations as well as their relationships with contiguous muscle groups, bones, and vessels. It was concluded that AVMs of the limbs can be characterized accurately with MRI, and the anatomic extent, degree of cellularity, and flow characteristics can be readily gauged. Because MRI provides the same basic information supplied by angiography and the noninvasive laboratory tests and assesses anatomic extent and cellularity, it serves well as the primary diagnostic test for suggested AVM, particularly in infants and children, in whom other tests have additional limitations.[15]

MRI as a Primary Decision-Making Tool

Because of the ability of MRI to show the localized or diffuse nature of the AVM as well as its flow characteristics, an algorithm based on these properties has been suggested.[15]

- In patients with *low-flow discrete* lesions, surgical excision can be performed on the basis of the MRI.
- In high-flow discrete lesions, however, arteriography is essential to delineate the main vessels involved. Either surgical excision or embolization may then be employed.
- Surgical results may be poor with diffuse low-flow lesions, and they may be observed without arteriography.
- Diffuse high-flow lesions need further tests to quantitate the arteriovenous shunting and to allow accurate embolization if needed.

Hand

The use of surface coils and high-resolution capabilities has allowed MRI to be used with accuracy in the hand. In a study of 12 patients with a variety of suggested pathological conditions, high-resolution MRI of the hands and wrists was obtained at 1.5 T using a prototype surface coil. Lesions studied included ganglions, rheumatoid arthritis, carpal fractures, carpal tunnel syndrome, and AVMs. In the cases studied, MRI provided potentially relevant information in nearly all instances. It was possible to obtain surgical, pathological, and radiographic correlations.[16]

MRI affords delineation of soft tissue structure that is unmatched by other imaging methods, including computed tomography. It offers sufficient valuable clinical information in certain conditions to justify its expense outside the research setting.[14,16] Detection of a large AVM by MRI may obviate the need for an angiogram. MRI may also be used as a tool for follow-up.

Although the actual scanning time with MRI can average between 20 and 25 minutes, the time spent in the suite could be about 60 minutes. Longer times may be required if views in many different planes are required. The expense of the equipment is an important consideration.[16]

Miscellaneous

New aspects of thermography as a noninvasive diagnostic method for arteriovenous anastomoses in the extremities make it a tool of some use in selected instances.[17] Recurrence of AVMs is inevitable unless the total malformation is resected. Bony involvement in some of these malformations contributes to a quick recurrence when limited resection is undertaken. Although arteriography is one of the procedures of choice in delineating vascular and soft tissue involvement with the malformation, it does not outline osseous involvement. Xeroradiography is an adjunctive diagnostic procedure that provides information about bony involvement, which may assist in planning the total resection of the malformation.[18]

Treatment

General guidelines for surgical treatment are as follows:

1. Very large proximal lesions do well after percutaneous embolization.
2. Peripheral localized lesions may be treated with embolization, excision, or a combination of the two. Very often, however, local excision suffices in these cases.
3. Operative embolization is rarely required. For some larger lesions the emphasis is on "intermittent" treatment, possibly with alternating embolization (percutaneous/intralesional, sclerotherapy, laser therapy) and resection.[19] Coordinated management involving the vascular surgeon and the vascular interventional radiologist must be sought. Surgical treatment can be very complex, and merely tying off the feeding vessels almost never cures the lesion. In fact, this is to be avoided to prevent development of myriad collaterals and for other considerations discussed elsewhere.

Hemangiomas

Hemangiomas can be treated expectantly. Cosmetic cover on the upper limb is hardly ever necessary, unlike lesions on the face. Compression garments may help. Most hemangiomas do not recur. Excision should, however, be as complete as possible for these potentially curable lesions. Some hemangiomas are aggressive locally; this is especially true of lesions that invade the skeletal muscle. In one series, 18% recurred once and 7% recurred more than once.[20]

Conservative Management

Strong elastic support compresses the lesion and can contain further enlargement. Periodic elevation of the limb encourages venous return and will counter venous hypertension if this is present. The smaller "angiomas" can be treated expectantly, by lasers, or with sclerotherapy. Sclerotherapy can significantly reduce the size of the lesion. Sclerotherapy, however, is to be avoided if possible. Oral steroid treatment can cause regression of many of these lesions. It must be used judiciously.

Surgical Treatment

Surgical treatment is indicated for complications of AVMs. These include uncontrollable hemorrhage, uncontrolled pain, distal extremity ischemia, and congestive heart failure. Congenital AVMs of the hand may be hemodynamically significant in the neonate. Progressive cardiac decompensation is an indication for surgical intervention.[21] Primary surgical treatment is reserved for smaller, surgically accessible, symptomatic lesions. Relative indications may include discrepancies of limb length, functional impairment, or cosmetic deformity. Combined treatment is used in many instances, as discussed elsewhere.

Surgical treatment could be a considerable undertaking. Some older series show disappointing results. Szilagyi et al. in 1965 reported surgical "success" in 10 of 48 cases. In a later series they reported a favorable outcome in 10 of 18 patients.[5,22] Other contemporary reports showed similar results. More precise preoperative anatomical localization and appreciation of the pathological and hemodynamic nature of these lesions (together with better selection of patients) has led to better success rates.

Considerable skill is required because the lesions often cross anatomical boundaries and require meticulous sharp dissection. The overlying skin can easily be devascularized and subsequently necrose. Other complications include operative damage to surrounding nerves, scar formation limiting mobility of tendons, and damage to ligaments. It is important to perform an adequate excision the first time to avoid having to reenter areas of scarring. Recurrence of a lesion is due not to formation of new channels but rather to redirection of flow into preexisting "dormant" channels. Persistent leakage, ulceration, and wound breakdown are other complications sometimes seen.

In some cases surgical excision with coverage by a vascularized flap is possible. The possibility of the operation's leading to amputation or disfigurement must be discussed with the patient. The anatomical location of some lesions may make attempts at complete removal hazardous to life or function. This has to be counterbalanced against the real risk of recurrence.

Technical Aspects

The operative area should be widely prepared and draped. Tourniquets are usually required and should be used carefully. Autotransfusion is a useful technique in patients with larger lesions because these may bleed profusely. A large blood loss may necessitate transfusion of blood components. Many of these patients are hypervolemic, and up to 3 to 4 units of blood may be deposited before surgery for operative replacement.[23] Large venous "lakes" must be excised or obliterated to avoid postoperative hemorrhage. Proper drainage of the wound is of the utmost importance because hematoma is one of the most frequently seen complications. Closure may require grafting or flap reconstruction on occasion, and the help of a plastic surgeon may have to be sought. Delayed primary closure must be resorted to on occasion.

Partial resection is not ideal. Sometimes it may be resorted to in the emergency situation with bleeding or ulcerated lesions.

Transluminal Occlusion by Embolization

Transluminal occlusion by embolization is a very useful technique in the hands of experienced vascular radiologists. Its use may be more limited in AVMs of the upper extremity, however. This is especially true of the more distal lesions. Careful planning is extremely important because, generally, obliteration of the main arterial pedicle is not advisable. The goal of embolotherapy is to reduce abnormal shunting by occluding communicating vessels with embolic material. Use of nonopaque agents requires addition of a dye. Careful monitoring during the procedure is mandatory. Repeated embolization over several sittings is required in many cases.

It is important to conserve the main feeding vessels to provide a portal for the previously mentioned procedures. This is especially relevant because repeated procedures are often required. Unless the lesion is to be completely excised, the main feeding vessels must be neither ligated nor embolized.

In one study, five patients with a single AVF and one patient with numerous AVFs were studied. Three patients had undergone surgery for treatment of their AVFs, one patient had undergone isobutyl-2-cyanoacrylate embolization, and two patients had undergone no prior therapy. The AVFs recurred in the three patients who had undergone surgery and in the patient who had undergone isobutyl-2-cyanoacrylate embolization. All patients underwent ethanol embolization of their AVFs. Angiograms obtained immediately after embolization documented closure of all AVFs. At follow-up, none of the embolized lesions had recurred. The authors concluded that ethanol embolotherapy can cure these problematic lesions. Extreme caution, however, must be employed with the use of intravascular ethanol because off-target embolization may result in tissue devitalization. In this study, two patients developed a small focal area of skin necrosis that fortunately did not require skin grafting and healed with conservative management.[24]

The complications of embolization include damage to nontarget tissues as a result of inadvertently misplaced injection; emboli may pass into the venous circulation in addition. Rarely, severe infection may ensue at the site of embolization. The postembolization syndrome comprises malaise, pyrexia, and leukocytosis along with pain at the site of embolization. This does not last beyond 48 hours in most instances. Pseudoaneurysms can form at the site of arterial access but are rare and relatively easily treated. Surgical débridement may be necessary when there is extensive tissue necrosis after embolization.

Materials Used for Embolization

The choice of material depends on the indication and the nature of the AVM. Preoperative embolization is used for diminishing operative blood loss and is directed toward the center of the lesion. Small particulate material such as gelatin sponge or polyvinyl alcohol (Ivalon, 50–1000 µm) is often used. In situations in which the actual arteriovenous fistulization is minimal, a more proximal occlusion may have to be performed. Liquid sclerosants (dehydrated alcohol, cyanoacrylate [acrylic adhesive], and sodium tetradecyl sulfate) are very powerful and may cause damage to nontarget tissues. These latter agents are mostly used for treatment of venous lesions by direct injection. Coils and other larger devices cause blockage of feeding vessels and are to be avoided, as already discussed.

Combined Treatment

Combined treatment has become a very useful management approach in most sizable lesions. (In the viscera, nearly all AVMs require this approach.) Refinements in interventional radiological treatment may have relegated surgical management to a secondary place in many instances. Preoperative embolization reduces bleeding and the bulk of the lesion. This is usually performed the day before surgery to avoid the inflammatory reaction and neovascularization that may follow. Postoperative embolization is useful when uncontrolled postoperative hemorrhage is encountered. A complementary approach may be useful in patients who exhibit severe hemorrhage from proximal lesions.[25] Intraoperative injection of sclerosants may be used for residual, unresectable vascular remnants.

The transfemoral route is most often used for both initial angiography and embolization. Cutdown into the axillary or brachial artery is less commonly used. At times,

puncture into vessels immediately adjacent to the lesion is the only practical route.

A combination of treatments was evaluated in a series of 81 patients.[19] In 32 patients the abnormality was localized in the upper extremity, and in 49 patients it was localized in the lower extremity. Signs, symptoms, treatment modalities, and long-term results were tabulated. In the upper extremity, pain was the most frequent presenting symptom. Three types of malformation were distinguished: purely venous malformations, venous malformations with microshunts, and malformations with macroshunts. The treatments of choice were excision of varices and superficial nevi, combined treatment of embolization and excision, and selective embolization without resection for the first, second, and third groups, respectively. The treatment was most successful in cases of malformation with macrofistulas in the shoulder region or with only a localized lesion that could be excised.

In the same series, conservative treatment in purely venous malformations prevented progression, whereas combined treatment was successful in patients with a proximal AVM or a small excisable lesion. The purely venous abnormality can be successfully treated with conservative measures, the AVM with macroshunts in the pelvis and shoulder region should be embolized, and circumscript lesions can be excised, with or without embolization, depending on the character of the lesion.[19]

Miscellaneous

When the patient is a child, it is important to reassure the parents about the basic facts regarding these lesions; namely, they are not neoplasms, they are rarely genetically transmitted, and they often do not require any treatment.

Inequality in limb length must be monitored. Surgical correction (epiphysiodesis while the bone is still growing or bone shortening in adult life) is sometimes needed. Sympathectomy is useful in severe, uncontrollable causalagia that is sometimes caused by AVM of the upper extremity.[26] In venous hypertension due to deep vein defects, the defective segment can be bypassed. The defective vein can also be implanted into a nearby normal segment of vein. Alternatively, an interposition graft may be used. Hemangiomas may respond to steroid therapy.

Intolerable symptoms in lesions that are not treatable may require more radical measures. Amputation of the limb must be the very last resort. Even this may be difficult in the more proximal AVM. In some large AVMs, cardiac bypass with hypothermia has been used. Vascular access (for the purpose of embolization) may have to be created surgically in patients in whom the major feeding vessel has been occluded surgically or by embolization.[27] In Klippel–Trénaunay syndrome it is important to establish the anatomy of venous drainage before embarking on any vein-stripping operations.

Vascular soft tissue tumors of the extremities (e.g., hemangiopericytomas) are not strictly AVMs. However, principles very similar to those outlined in this chapter can be applied to these lesions as well. Smaller particulate material must be used for embolization. It is important to preserve a large access vessel for repeated embolotherapy sessions.

People in whom multiple treatment sessions with reconstruction are being planned will benefit from multidisciplinary conferences. Nursing and other ancillary care personnel should be involved.

References

1. Riles TS, Rosen RJ. Arteriovenous malformations. In: Strandness E, Breda AV, eds. *Vascular Diseases*. New York: Churchill Livingstone; 1994:1115–1120.

2. McClinton MA. Tumors and aneurysms of the upper extremity. *Hand Clin*. 1993; 9:151–169.

3. Servelle M. Agenesis d'une des veines principales du membre inferieur. *Coeur Med Interne*. 1965:4:53.

4. Folkman J, D'Amora P. Blood vessel formation: what is its molecular basis? *Cell*. 1996;87:1153–1155.

5. Szilagyi S, Elliot JP, DeRusso FJ, Smith RF. Peripheral congenital arteriovenous fistulas. *Surgery*. 1965;57:61–81.

6. Belov S. Haemodynamic pathogenesis of vascular-bone syndromes in congenital vascular defects. *Int Angiol*. 1990; 9:155–161.

7. Nakada K, Kawada T, Fujioka T, et al. Hemangioma of the upper arm associated with massive hemorrhage in a neonate. *Surg Today*. 1993;23:273–276.

8. Nakamura K. Multiple glomus tumors associated with arteriovenous fistulas and with nodular lesions of the finger joints. *Plast Reconstr Surg*. 1992;90:675–683.

9. Kromhout JG, v d Horst C, Peeters F, Gerhard M AD. The combined treatment of congenital vascular defects. *Int Angiol*. 1990;9:203–207.

10. Witt JD, Jupiter JB. Kaposi's sarcoma in the hand seen as an arteriovenous malformation. *J Hand Surg [Am]*. 1991; 16:607–609.

11. Elliott JA, Rankin RN, Inwood MJ, Milne JK. An arteriovenous malformation in pregnancy: a case report and review of the literature. *Am J Obstet Gynecol*. 1985;152:85–88.

12. Regan PJ, Roberts JO, Bailey BN. Acute posterior interosseous nerve palsy caused by bleeding from an arteriovenous malformation. *J Hand Surg [Am]*. 1991;16: 272–273.

13. Mullikan JB. Classification of vascular birthmarks. In: Grainger RG, Allison DJ, eds. *Vascular Birthmarks, Haemangiomas, and Malformations*. Philadelphia, Pa: WB Saunders; 1988:24–37.

14. Cohen JM, Weinreb JC, Redman HC. Magnetic resonance imaging of a congenital arteriovenous malformation of the forearm. *Surgery*. 1986;99:623–625.

15. Pearce WH, Rutherford RB, Whitehill TA, Davis K. Nuclear magnetic resonance imaging: its diagnostic value in patients with congenital vascular malformations of the limbs. *J Vasc Surg*. 1988;8:64–70.

16. Weiss KL, Beltran J, Lubbers LM. High-field MRI surface-coil imaging of the hand and wrist, II: pathologic correlations and clinical relevance. *Radiology*. 1986;160:147–152.

17. Bergqvist D, Bornmyr S. New aspects on thermography as a non-invasive diagnostic method for arterio-venous anastomoses in the extremities. *Vasa*. 1986;15:241–244.

18. Cabbabe EB. Xeroradiography as an aid in planning resection of arteriovenous malformation of the upper extremities. *J Hand Surg [Am]*. 1985;10:670–674.

19. Kromhout JG, v d Horst C, Peeters F, Gerhard M. The combined treatment of congenital vascular defects. *Int Angiol*. 1990;9:203–207.

20. Allen PW, Enzinger PM. Haemangiomas of skeletal muscle. An analysis of 80 cases. *Cancer*. 1972;29:8–22.

21. Moye SJ, Billmire DA. Congenital arteriovenous malformation of the finger resulting in cardiac decompensation: a case report. *J Hand Surg [Am]*. 1992;17:887–891.

22. Szilagyi DE, Smith RF, Elliot JP, Hageman JH. Congenital arteriovenous anomalies of the limbs. *Arch Surg*. 1976; 111:423–429.

23. Ernst CB, Reddy DJ. Surgical treatment of acquired and congenital arteriovenous fistulae. In: Jamieson CW, Yao JT, eds. *Vascular Surgery*. 5th ed. London: Chapman & Hall Medical; 1995:426–433.

24. Yakes W, Luethke JM, Merland JJ, et al. Ethanol embolization of arteriovenous fistulas: a primary mode of therapy. *J Vasc Interv Radiol*. 1990;1:89–96.

25. Jackson JE, Allison DJ. Combined therapeutic embolization and surgery. In: Jamieson CW, Yao JT, eds. *Vascular Surgery*. 5th ed. London: Chapman & Hall Medical; 1995:435–450.

26. Stolzel U, Schiffter R, Sorensen R, et al. Sympathektomie bei Kausalgieschmerz durch arteriovenose Malformationen der oberen extremitat. *Med Klin*. 1988;3:470–472.

27. Vaughan M, Henessey O, Jamieson C, Hemingway AP, Allison DJ. The preoperative embolization of vascular malformations. *Br J Radiol*. 1985;58:717–720.

100

Combined Treatment of Vascular Malformations: Indications, Methods, and Techniques

Dirk A. Loose

The treatment of congenital, predominantly arteriovenous (AV) malformations is a task that can only be performed to the highest standard in a multidisciplinary group guided by a vascular surgeon.[1,2] The treatment of congenital vascular malformations is one of the most difficult tasks in vascular surgery.[3,4] The occurrence of severe hemorrhage, endangering the patient's life during the operation, is kept in mind during every one of the surgeon's movements. Moreover, according to Fontaine,[5] the vascular surgeon constantly is placed between Scylla and Charybdis, that is, between excessively radical surgery, which may lead to severe postoperative ischemia, and excessive caution, which may result in a relapse. That is why, for a long time, treatment was mainly conservative and symptomatic. With the development of modern nonsurgical and surgical techniques, combined treatment was created,[6-14] and today it is the latest therapeutic concept in modern vascular surgery.

Choice of Combined Treatment

In more than 2500 patients with congenital vascular defects, vascular surgeons of six different countries[15] have created and proved the efficacy of therapeutic strategies, surgical tactics, and operative techniques for congenital vascular malformations.

Vascular malformations rarely affect just one type of vessel; usually it is a question of polyangiopathies. Depending on the predominant type of malformed vessel, the congenital vascular defects are as follows:

Predominantly arterial defects
Predominantly venous defects
Predominantly lymphatic defects
Predominantly AV shunting defects
Combined vascular defects

In predominantly AV shunting defects, the treatment of choice is combined therapy. It consists not only of operative embolization of the vascular malformation by way of its feeding arteries, with skeletonization and—if possible—excision,[16,17] but also of surgical and nonsurgical methods. It does not consist of alternative or competitive techniques; rather, the nonsurgical and the surgical forms of treatment are complementary.[13,14,18-22,24] Combined treatment is the latest therapeutic concept in modern vascular surgery.

The nonsurgical forms of treatment are as follows:

Laser therapy
Cortisol therapy
Sclerotherapy
Embolization therapy

The indications for nonsurgical treatment include the following:

Laser therapy: superficial cutaneous and combined cutaneous–subcutaneous, localized, small vascular defects (see Chapter 97)
Corticosteroid therapy: infantile, immature, superficial hemangiomas (extratruncal forms) (see Chapter 97)
Sclerotherapy: additional treatment for superficial malformed veins (see Chapters 97 and 98)
Embolization therapy: dependent on the morphological form and site of the malformation (see Chapters 97, 98, and 99)

Before the combined treatment starts, the type of therapy must be planned. One of the main questions is whether a predominantly embolization therapy or a predominantly surgical therapy should be performed. Although each individual case has its own indications for embolization or surgical therapy, there are some principal guidelines.

TABLE 100.1. Recommended application of combined treatment relative to location of lesion (upper extremity)

Location of lesion	Type of combined treatment	
	Predominantly surgery	Embolization
Shoulder		X
Upper arm	X	
Elbow	X	X
Forearm to wrist	X	(X)
Hand distal to wrist joint	X	

It is important to know the risks of combined treatment depending on the site of the vascular defect (Table 100.1). In the upper extremity, embolization therapy generally should not extend distally beyond the wrist joint. Otherwise, severe peripheral spasms and/or digital necrosis can occur. For the lower extremity (Table 100.2), embolization therapy generally should not extend distally beyond the proximal shank region. Should it be necessary to perform a treatment distal to these borderlines, then surgery is the method of choice in most cases. However, my colleagues and I saw a few patients with diffuse, infiltrating AV lesions in the foot for which surgery could be precisely combined with embolization therapy.

TABLE 100.2. Recommended application of combined treatment relative to location of lesion (lower extremity)

Location of lesion	Type of combined treatment	
	Predominantly surgery	Embolization
Buttocks		X
Upper thigh	X	
Knee	X	X
Proximal calf		X
Distal calf	X	
Ankle	X	
Foot	X*	

*Dependent on pathoanatomic form.

TABLE 100.3. Recommended application of combined treatment relative to pathoanatomic form for predominantly arteriovenous shunting defects

Pathoanatomic form	Type of combined treatment	
	Surgery	Embolization
Truncal forms		
Deep arteriovenous fistulas	X	
Superficial arteriovenous fistulas	X	
Extratruncal forms		
Diffuse, infiltrating	X	X
Localized	X	X

Concerning the pathoanatomical forms of the predominantly AV shunting defects, our experience has resulted in recommended choices of treatment (Table 100.3). For truncal forms with deep AV fistulas, surgery is predominantly indicated. For truncal forms with superficial AV fistulas, surgery is indicated when the AV communications must be removed together with segments of dilated afferent veins. The main candidates for combined treatment are the extratruncal forms, which are either infiltrating or limited. In both cases, combined surgical and nonsurgical treatment is indicated. The course of each treatment is determined by the special hemodynamic requirements of each individual.

Results of Combined Treatment

A typical example of combined treatment is the following case: an 18-year-old girl from Lithuania had increasing pain, swelling, and pronounced length discrepancy of her left leg, as well as worsening back pain. A severe, predominantly AV malformation was diagnosed, and she was operated on in her hometown, Vilnius. There, the surgical tactic of reducing the hemodynamic activity of the AV shunts was followed, and skeletonization of the superficial femoral artery (Vollmar's method 1[23]) was performed. No improvement was seen, however, and the patient was transferred to our institution. Our clinical findings included a pronounced length discrepancy of the left leg, which was more than 4 cm longer (Figure 100.1) and a distinct swelling of the left thigh region, where a huge scar (25 cm) was detected. Angiography revealed numerous hemodynamically active AV fistulas in the whole thigh region down to the knee joint (Figure 100.2). The therapeutic strategy was to reduce the inflow into the afferent malformed arteries by means of embolization therapy and surgery. This combined therapy began with two sessions of transcatheter embolization of several AV fistulas in the thigh region, the knee joint, and the shank region (Figure 100.3). After 2 weeks, when the postinfarction pain syndrome secondary to catheter embolization was gone, the surgical treatment could be performed. Before the surgery, the AV fistulas still existing in the region of the huge scar were revealed by means of ultrasonic Doppler tests and marked (Figure 100.4). In addition, the plastic surgery strategy for treatment of the scar was decided (see Figure 100.4). Loose's method II[25] was the surgical technique performed to reduce the hemodynamic activity of the vascular defect (Figure 100.5A). A large number of AV fistulas could be closed after ultrasonic Doppler mapping during surgery (Figure 100.5B). The postoperative clinical findings showed satisfactory results; further steps in the combined treatment still have to be performed.

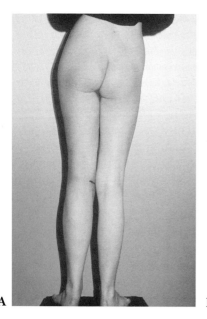
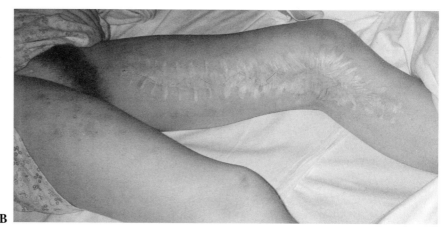

FIGURE 100.1. **A,** Clinical findings in an 18-year-old girl with left-sided length discrepancy and swelling of the whole left leg. The diagnosis was congenital, predominantly arteriovenous malformation. **B,** Huge scar after skeletonization of superficial femoral artery, before the patient was transferred to our hospital. Distinct swelling of the left thigh region is shown.

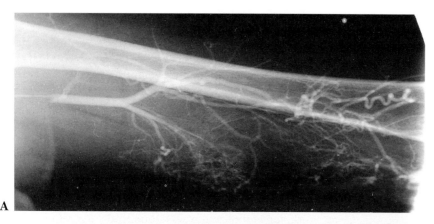

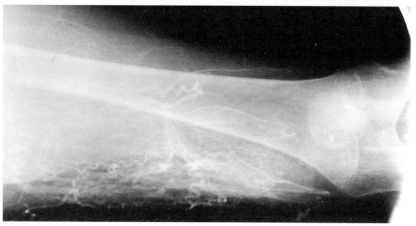

FIGURE 100.2. **A,** Selective arteriography of the deep femoral artery demonstrates numerous hemodynamically active arteriovenous fistulas. **B,** The fistulas are distributed in the whole thigh region down to the knee joint.

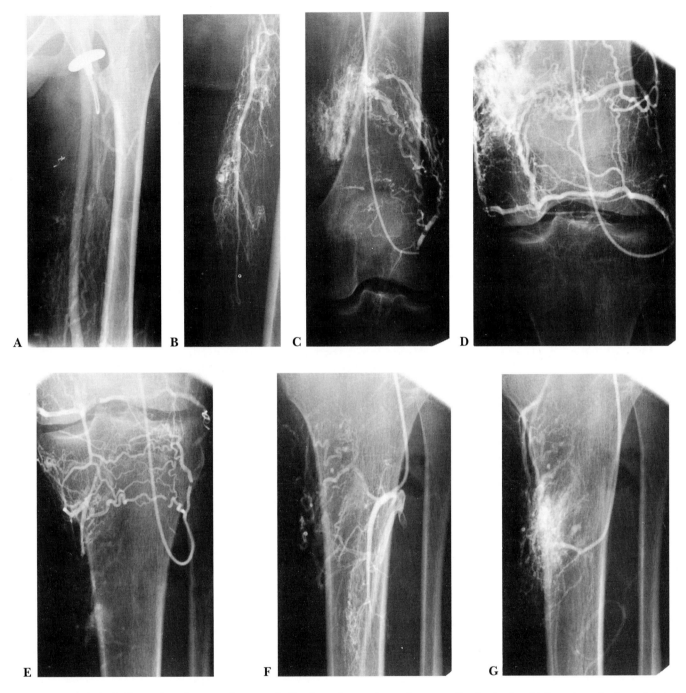

FIGURE 100.3. **A–G,** Examples of transcatheter embolization of several arteriovenous fistulas in the thigh region, the knee joint, and the shank region.

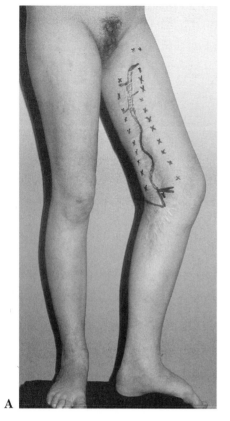
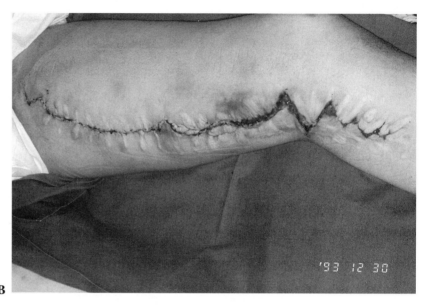

FIGURE 100.4. **A,** The left thigh region. The excision line of the huge scar is marked on the skin, as are the remaining arteriovenous fistulas, as revealed by ultrasonic Doppler. **B,** The planned partial excision of the huge scar by means of a Z-plasty technique is marked in the knee joint region.

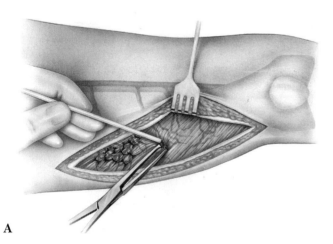
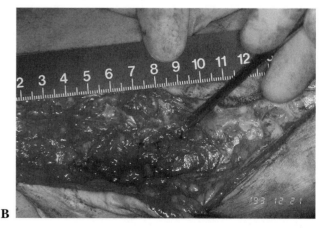

FIGURE 100.5. **A,** Sketch of the surgical technique (Loose's method II[25]) used to reduce the hemodynamic activity of the vascular defect: ultrasonic mapping of arteriovenous fistulas is carried out during surgery; the fistulas are closed by over-and-over stitches. **B,** View of the left thigh during surgery using Loose's method II.[25]

Discussion

Congenital vascular defects are not as rare as sometimes presumed. Inadequate treatment can aggravate the patient's complaints, especially the circulatory disturbance of the affected region. For this reason, a special, usually interdisciplinary treatment of such findings is mandatory. When AV communications are present, combined treatment with both surgical and nonsurgical techniques must be considered. Which specific technique should be performed? Clinical, functional, and hemodynamic parameters have to be evaluated so that the correct combination of therapeutic steps can be chosen. Usually, several steps of treatment are necessary.

References

1. Belov S, Loose DA. Surgical treatment of congenital vascular defects. *International Angiology.* 1990;9:175–182.
2. Mattassi R. Surgical treatment of congenital arteriovenous defects. *International Angiology.* 1990;9:196–202.
3. Malan E. Considerazioni sulle fistole artero-venose congenite degli arti. *Boll Soc Riem Chir 5.* 1954;24:297.
4. Malan E. *Vascular Malformations (Angiodysplasias).* Milan, Italy: Carlo Erba; 1974:17.
5. Fontaine R. Spezielle therapeutische Aspekte gewisser arteriovenöser Mißbildungen. In: Schobinger RA, ed. *Periphere Angiodysplasien.* Bern, Switzerland: Huber-Verlag; 1977:197–206.
6. Loose DA. Combined treatment of congenital vascular defects: indications and tactics. *Semin Vasc Surg.* 1993;6:260–265.
7. Loose DA. Special problems in surgery of angiodysplasias with AV communications. Communication during the 5th meeting of the International Workshop for the Study of Vascular Anomalies: Haemangiomas and Vascular Malformations in the Field of Plastic Surgery; May 25–26, 1984; Milan, Italy: Fondazione Carlo Erba.
8. Loose DA. Treatment of predominantly AVMs of legs and congenital vascular bone syndrome. Paper presented at: 9th International Workshop for the Study of Vascular Anomalies; July 1–3, 1992; Denver, Colo.
9. Loose DA. New concepts in the treatment of congenital vascular defects. In: *Proceedings of the 18th World Congress of the International College of Surgeons, Cairo, Egypt, November 16–21, 1992.* Bologna, Italy: Monduzzi Editore; 1992:477–482.
10. Loose DA, Müller E. Problems in surgery of congenital vascular malformations with arteriovenous shunts. In: de Castro Silva M, ed. *Atualizacao em Angiologia.* Belo Horizonte, Brazil: Brazilian Society of Angiology; 1978:121–141.
11. Loose DA, Belov S, Jupitz M, Weber J. Possible surgical therapies for congenital peripheral angiodysplasia. Paper presented at: 6th International Workshop for the Study of Vascular Anomalies; June 6, 1986; Boston, Mass.
12. Belov S. Surgical treatment of congenital predominantly arteriovenous shunting defects. In: Belov S, Loose DA, Weber J, eds. *Vascular Malformations: Periodica Angiologica.* Vol 16. Reinbek, Germany: Einhorn Presse; 1989:229–234.
13. Loose DA. The combined surgical therapy in congenital AV-shunting malformations. In: Belov S, Loose DA, Weber J, eds. *Vascular Malformations: Periodica Angiologica.* Vol 16. Reinbek, Germany: Einhorn Presse; 1989:213–225.
14. Loose DA. Active multidisciplinary treatment in congenital vascular defects. Communication at the London Meeting on Congenital Vascular Malformations; September 25, 1992; London.
15. Belov S, Loose DA, Mattassi R, Spatenka J, Tasnádi G, Wang Z. Therapeutical strategy, surgical tactics, and operative techniques in congenital vascular defects (multicentre study). In: Strano A, Novo S, eds. *Advances in Vascular Pathology.* Amsterdam: Excerpta Medica; 1989:1355–1360.
16. Kromhout JG, van der Horst C, Peeters F, Gerhard M. The combined treatment of congenital vascular defects. *International Angiology.* 1990;9:203–207.
17. Van Dongen RJAM. Therapie der angeborenen arteriovenösen Angiodysplasien unter besonderer Berücksichtigung der operativen Embolisation. *Angio.* 1983;5:169–179.
18. Allison DJ, Kennedy A. Embolization techniques in arteriovenous malformations. In: Belov S, Loose DA, Weber J, eds. *Vascular Malformations: Periodica Angiologica.* Vol 16. Reinbek, Germany: Einhorn Presse; 1989:261–269.
19. Weber J. Techniques and results of therapeutic catheter embolization of congenital vascular defects. *International Angiology.* 1990;9:214–223.
20. Weber J. Embolisations therapie arteriovenöser Mißbildungen. *Radiologische Diagnostik (Berlin).* 1987;28:513–516.
21. Weber J. Vaso-occlusive angiotherapy (VAT) in congenital vascular malformations. *Semin Vasc Surg.* 1993;4:279–296.
22. Loose DA, Weber J. Indications and tactics for a combined treatment of congenital vascular defects. In: Balas P, ed. *Progress in Angiology 1991.* Torino, Italy: Edizioni Minerva Medica; 1992:373–378.
23. Vollmar, J. *Rekonstruktive Chirurgie der Arterien.* Stuttgart: Thieme; 1996:169–173.
24. Loose, DA, Funck, J: Angeborene Venenfehler: diagnostische und therapeutische Möglichkeiten. *Akt. Chir.* 1995;30: 329–340.
25. Loose DA. Systematik, radiologische Diagnostik und Therapie vaskulärer Fehlbildungen. In: Hohenleutner U, Landthaler M: *Operative Dermatologie im kindes und Jugendalter.* Berlin: Blackwell Wissenschafts-Verlag. 1997.

101

Vascular Malformations and Hemangiomas: Surgical Treatment

Stefan Belov

Surgical treatment is indicated for the five main types of peripheral vascular malformations, which cause vascular insufficiency, cardiac overload, and limb-length discrepancy, disfiguration, and dysfunction, and can lead to complications such as recurrent hemorrhages, trophic ulcers, and gangrene. Therapeutic strategy should follow the principles of early, active, causal, functionally radical, individual, multidisciplinary, surgical, and combined treatment by stages, including vascular surgery, interventional radiology, and nonsurgical methods, when necessary combined with plastic surgery and orthopedic procedures.[1,2]

The oldest and most common therapeutic principle formulated by Hippocrates is "Sublata causa tollitur morbus" ("when the cause is removed, the illness is removed"). Regrettably, the morphology, extent, and localization of peripheral vascular malformations in many cases do not permit the application of this principle. Therefore, four types of surgical tactics and techniques are applied.

Reconstructive Operations (Revascularization)

The first operations to be discussed are the reconstructive operations[1,2]:

1. Resection of the segment with congenital vascular stenosis, aneurysmal dilatation, or large arteriovenous (AV) communication and reconstruction of vascular integrity by vascular suture or implantation of an autologous venous graft (i.e., a vascular prosthesis)
2. Bypass operation
3. Patch-plastic
4. Membranotomy (i.e., resection of an obstructive membrane in the vascular lumen)

Reconstructive operations are rarely possible in peripheral vascular malformations because of the diffuse nature of vascular defects. Operative techniques are similar to those applied in acquired vascular pathology. Postoperative results are usually good because of removal of the malformation and restitution of the affected vessels.

Operations to Remove Vascular Defects (Devascularization)

The second type of surgical tactics and techniques consists of operations for removal of vascular defects.

Removal of Truncular Vascular Defects

Removal of truncular vascular defects includes the following[3-6]:

1. Resection of dysplastic phlebectasias
2. Resection of deep AV communications
3. Resection of superficial AV communications together with efferent veins

Operative technique in resection of truncular dysplastic phlebectasias demands multiple, most often atypical incisions along the affected vessels and possibly radical resection of dilated veins and venous convolutes (Figure 101.1).

The operative approach in truncular, deep AV communications consists of typical incisions toward the main vessels. The AV fistulas are carefully dissected and resected consecutively along the vessels (Figure 101.2A).

The superficial truncular AV communications are reached by atypical incisions along the superficial, dilated efferent veins at the places where clinical, angiographic, and hemodynamic AV communications are discovered. They are resected, together with segments of the efferent phlebectasias (Figure 101.2B,C).

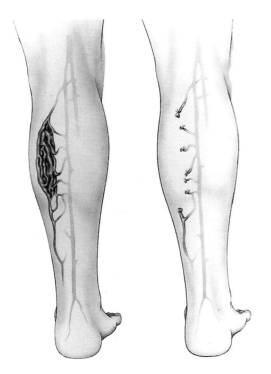

FIGURE 101.1. Resection of truncular dysplastic phlebectasias. (Reprinted with permission from Belov S. Surgical treatment of congenital predominantly venous defects. In: Belov S, Loose DA, Weber J, eds. *Vascular Malformations.* Reinbek, Germany: Einhorn-Presse; 1989.)

The success of operative treatment in multiple truncular AV communications depends on their precise localization. Because this sometimes proves to be quite difficult, a systematic search is necessary. It was pointed out that the hemodynamic significance of congenital AV fistulas is defined by the size of the total cross-sectional area of the AV communications. Thus, multiple AV fistulas of a small caliber could nevertheless provoke hemodynamic disturbances and circulatory hypoxic hyperostosis. With their radical elimination in childhood, the parasitic circulation is eliminated and elongation of the tubular bones is discontinued, thus correcting the limb-length discrepancy (Figure 101.3).[7]

Removal of Extratruncular Vascular Defects

Removal of extratruncular vascular defects includes the following[8,9]:

1. Extirpation of extratruncular limited vascular malformation
2. Radical extirpation of extratruncular infiltrating vascular malformation together with tissues and organs (demolitive surgery) (Malan's method I)

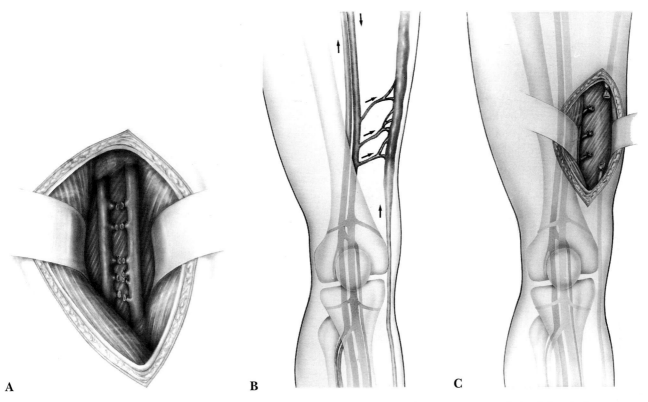

A   B   C

FIGURE 101.2. Resection of truncular arteriovenous (AV) communications. **A,** Dissection and resection of deep, truncular AV fistulas. **B,** Multiple superficial truncular AV fistulas. **C,** Resection of AV fistulas together with segments of efferent veins.

(Reprinted with permission from Belov S. Surgical treatment of congenital predominantly arteriovenous shunting defects. In: Belov S, Loose DA, Weber J, eds. *Vascular Malformations.* Reinbek, Germany: Einhorn-Presse; 1989.

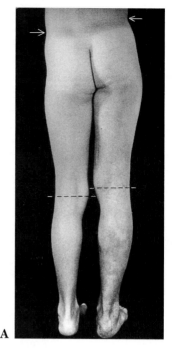

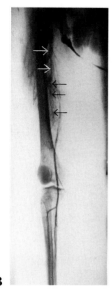

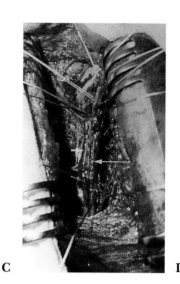

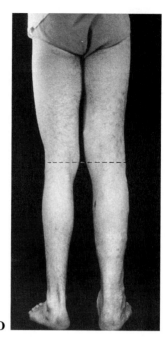

A   B   C   D

FIGURE 101.3. **A,** A boy aged 10 with congenital angio-osteohypertrophy of the right leg, with a 5-cm length discrepancy (dotted lines), diffuse telangiectatic nevi, superficial dilated veins, pelvic tilting to the sound leg (arrows), and compensatory lumbar scoliosis. **B,** Arteriography shows early opacification of deep femoral veins (white arrows) and "snowflake spots" (black arrows), indicating multiple deep and superficial arteriovenous (AV) fistulas in the thigh. **C,** Operative technique involves resection of direct AV communications between the femoral artery and vein in Hunter's channel, having a diameter of 1 to 2 mm. **D,** Postoperative appearance 10 years after the operation, showing correction of the lower limb–length discrepancy (dotted line). (Reprinted with permission from Belov S. Grundsätze der chirurgischen Behandlung angeborener Gefässfehler. In: Belov S, Loose DA, Müller E, eds. *Angeborene Gefässfehler.* Reinbek, Germany: Einhorn-Presse; 1985.)

The surgical approach in extratruncular venous and AV malformations is best attained by flap incisions. Dissection of the vascular malformation (VM) is in many cases very difficult or even impossible, because of infiltrative growth in encompassing tissues and fragility of the dysplastic vessels, and is often accompanied by abundant hemorrhage. In such cases a radical extirpation of the extratruncular VM together with muscles and bone segments can be performed (Malan's method I).[8,9] This technique is in accordance with Malan's opinion that the criteria of surgical treatment in VM are not different from those applied in cancer surgery. One must be extremely radical, even when this produces considerable mutilation.[8]

The operations to remove vascular defects are most often applied in peripheral VM. Postoperative results after early and functionally radical operations are usually good. Correction of the lower limb-length discrepancy, as mentioned previously, can be achieved after vascular surgery in childhood.[10–14] Recovery of form and function is also possible after meticulously executed operation in parts of extremities where embolization is dangerous and surgery is difficult.

Operations to Reduce the Arteriovenous Shunt

The third type of surgical tactics and techniques is not radical but consists of anatomically appropriate and physiologically grounded operations to reduce the arteriovenous shunt.

Operations to reduce AV shunt include the following[8,15]:

1. Arterial deafferentation (Malan's method II)
2. Skeletonization of principal vessels (Vollmar's method I)
3. Ligature by stages of two principal arteries distal to the elbow or the knee (Vollmar's method II)

Arterial deafferentation (Malan's method II)[8] consists of isolating the principal arteries of the limb and tying all branches that supply the shunt region. The skeletonization of principal vessels (Vollmar's method I)[15] consists of ligatures of all branches of both principal artery and vein and aims to reduce the parasitic circulation. These two operative methods were applied in anatomically inaccessible, extratruncular, diffuse infiltrating AV fistulas.

Experience showed that exclusion only of arterial supply of the shunt region is not enough, and the result of skeletonization of both artery and vein is only a temporary reduction of parasitic circulation. Consequently, both operative techniques have been replaced successfully with transcatheter embolization of the diffuse extratruncular AV communications.

The ligature method, involving partial resection of two principal arteries, is performed in two stages distally from elbow or knee (Vollmar's method II).[15] The method was proposed in areas of infiltrating AVM in distal parts of extremities where surgery is difficult and hazardous. A better and more lasting effect is reached by the combination of preoperative embolization with additional partial resection of the fistulous area.

Unconventional Surgical Methods

The fourth type of therapeutic tactics and techniques include the so-called unconventional operative methods applied in conventionally inoperable forms of VM. These inoperable forms are the extratruncular vascular defects that infiltrate the neighboring tissues and organs, destroying their form and function and making their dissection and resection difficult, hazardous, or even impossible. Another form is the frequent reduction of vascular truncuses (mainly aplasia or hypoplasia of long segments of deep veins), disturbing greatly the venous drainage and the complete hemodynamics of the affected limb, when reconstructive surgery is impossible.

The results of new scientific research on morphology, pathophysiology, and pathogenesis of VM, as well as the further development of operative techniques, enabled the creation of the unconventional surgical methods in VM considered inoperable.[2–4,16–21]

Unconventional surgical methods include the following:

1. Sparing resection of extratruncular vascular area (Belov's method III)
2. Segmental resection of infiltrating vascular area (Belov's method IV)
3. Ultrasound examination with Doppler mapping intraoperatively and stitching ligatures of infiltrating AV fistulas (Loose's method II)
4. Skeletonization of embryonal vein (Belov's method I)
5. Restoration of deep venous drainage by rerouting the venous flow through its normal way (Belov's method II)
6. Resection of marginal vein (Loose's method I)

In an AV or venous area located in an anatomically critical region, a sparing resection of the VM is possible (Belov's method III)[4,16,17] (Figure 101.4). The surgical technique consists of step-by-step, meticulous resection of the extratruncular vascular area using small hemostatic clamps and piercing stitches, retaining the principle

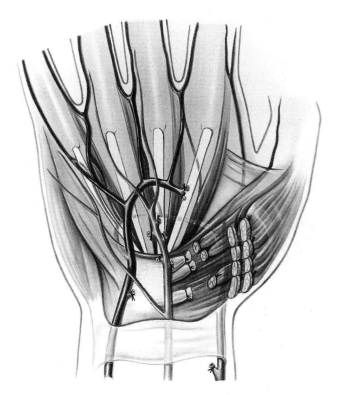

FIGURE 101.4. Sparing resection of extratruncal vascular malformation (Belov's method III). The arteriovenous area is economically resected, together with tissues. Reprinted with permission from Belov.[4]

"as radical as possible, as conservative as necessary"[2] (Figure 101.5).

In extratruncular VMs that cannot be dissected from the involved adjacent tissues and anatomical structures, segmental resection of the infiltrating vascular area is indicated (Belov's method IV).[2,16,17] The surgical technique consists of exposure and clipping of the dysplastic vascular formation by atraumatic Satinsky clamps and segmental resection of vascular area, saving important anatomical structures (Figure 101.6). A running mattress suture in the manner of Blalock[2] is performed just below the instruments, followed by a second hemostatic over-and-over suture along the line of resection (Figure 101.7).

The technique of ultrasound examination with Doppler mapping intraoperatively and stitching ligatures of AV fistulas (Loose's method II)[20] is performed successfully in peripheral, inaccessible and nonresectable, multiple, extratruncular infiltrating AV fistulas, impossible to treat by embolization (Figure 101.8).

The operative technique for skeletonization of the embryonal vein (Belov's method I)[2,3,17,18] consists of dissection and resection of the superficial AV fistulas by numerous incisions, leaving the single persistent embryonal vein intact (Figure 101.9). This operative method is indicated in patients with aplasia of a long segment of

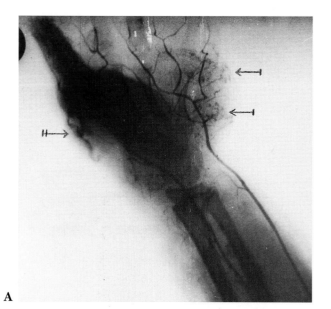

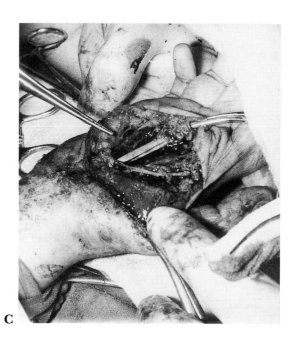

FIGURE 101.5. **A,** Arteriography[14] shows arteriovenous malformation infiltrating palm and fingers of the right hand. The arrows indicate the neatly contrasted pattern of reticular and snowflake arteriovenous fistulae. **B,** Operative technique of resection of the extratruncular vascular area together with tissues, using hemostatic clamps. **C,** Condition after sparing resection of the arteriovenous area; tendons and arterial and nerve branches are preserved.

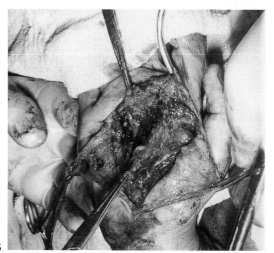

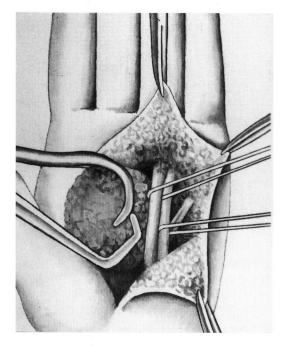

FIGURE 101.6. Segmental resection of extratruncular vascular malformation (Belov's method IV). Two atraumatic Satinsky clamps are placed prior to segmental resection of the infiltrating vascular area. (Reprinted with permission from Belov S. Surgical treatment of congenital vascular defects. In: Chang JB, ed. *Modern Vascular Surgery*. New York, NY: Springer-Verlag; 1994.)

FIGURE 101.7 **A,** Man aged 20 with considerable disfiguration and dysfunction of the left hand, including pain, swelling, and reduced efficiency. Operative scar from unsuccessful intervention is visible. **B,** Angiography with direct punction reveals extratruncular arteriovenous malformation infiltrating the palm and the third and fourth fingers of the left hand. **C,** Operative technique for segmental resection of the vascular malformation using Satinsky clamps, saving important anatomical structures. **D,** Postoperative appearance; form and function of hand are restored.

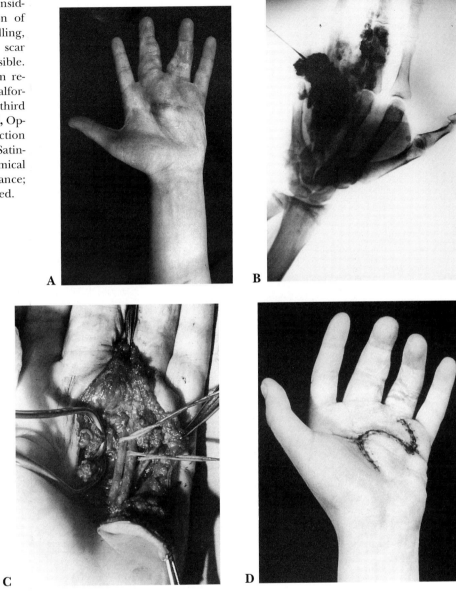

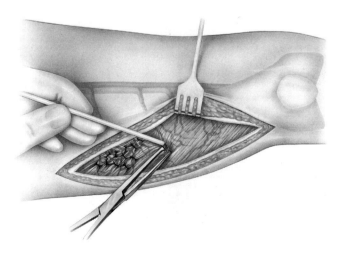

FIGURE 101.8. Ultrasound examination with Doppler mapping intraoperatively and stitching ligatures of arteriovenous fistulas (Loose's method II). Reprinted with permission from Loose.[20]

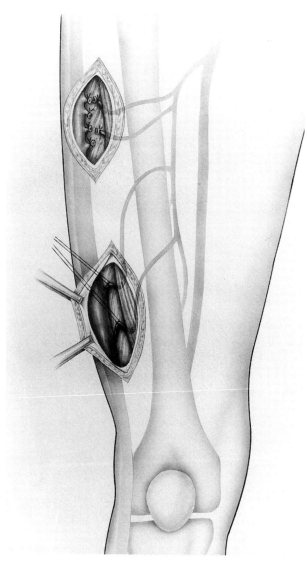

FIGURE 101.9. Skeletonization of embryonal vein (Belov's method I). Resection of the arteriovenous fistulas by numerous incisions, leaving the single persistent vein intact. (Reprinted with permission from Belov S. Surgical treatment of congenital predominantly venous defects. In: Belov S, Loose DA, Weber J, eds. *Vascular Malformations.* Reinbek, Germany: Einhorn-Presse; 1989.)

the deep venous trunks and sometimes also of the normal superficial veins, combined with multiple small AV fistulas toward the compensatory embryonal vein. As mentioned, the pathogenic connection between decompensated deep venous flow and the opening of AV communications toward the embryonal vein, most probably as an intermediary satellite circulation, is indisputably proved by experimental studies and by examinations of numerous patients with congenital deep venous reduc-

tion or with acquired postthrombotic occlusion of the deep veins. Usually the vascular reconstruction in these cases is very difficult and uncertain, because of the diffuse vascular pathology. The hemodynamic and angiographic data led to the idea of removing the parasitic circulation and reducing the venous stasis in affected extremities by way of skeletonization of the embryonal vein (Figure 101.10).[2,3,18]

The operative technique to restore deep venous drainage by rerouting the venous flow through its normal way (Belov's method II)[2,3,17,19] consists of careful resection, often in several stages, of the highly dilated superficial veins so as to reroute the venous flow by way of the hypoplastic principal deep veins (Figure 101.11).

An operation is indicated when phlebography reveals hypoplasia of a long segment of the deep veins and superficial dysplastic phlebectasias. The motivation for this operative method is the possibility of restoring deep venous drainage by removal of the superficial phlebectasias. In this manner, the basic venous flow is rerouted through its normal way (i.e., the principal deep veins) in which the lumens gradually dilate to a normal size (Figure 101.12).[2,3,19]

A special technique is required for resection of the marginal veins in deep venous hypoplasia (Loose's method I) (Figure 101.13).[21]

The unconventional operations achieved a significant improvement of the described local hemodynamic disturbances, and a decrease in the unpleasant symptoms in these patients, who until recently were considered inoperable.

The modern surgical management of peripheral VM proves that the old, simple practice of arterial ligature, removing only limited VMs (i.e., localized phlebectasias or single AV fistulas) by amputation must be abandoned. Treatment should conform to the indicated strategy, surgical tactics, and operative methods as therapeutic guidelines, but the surgical technique in each case must be individualized and often unconventional, in accordance with the polymorphism and hemodynamic peculiarities of the vascular defect in each patient.

Current surgical management in the framework of multidisciplinary surgical and combined treatment should be performed in treatment centers for vascular malformations, directed by specialists in this congenital vascular pathology, preferably by a vascular surgeon and radiologist with broad knowledge of the indications, possibilities, and limits of the different therapeutic methods. Experience shows that good will, patience, and specialized knowledge, combined with operative proficiency and therapeutic creativity, can produce good results in this difficult and challenging field in angiology.

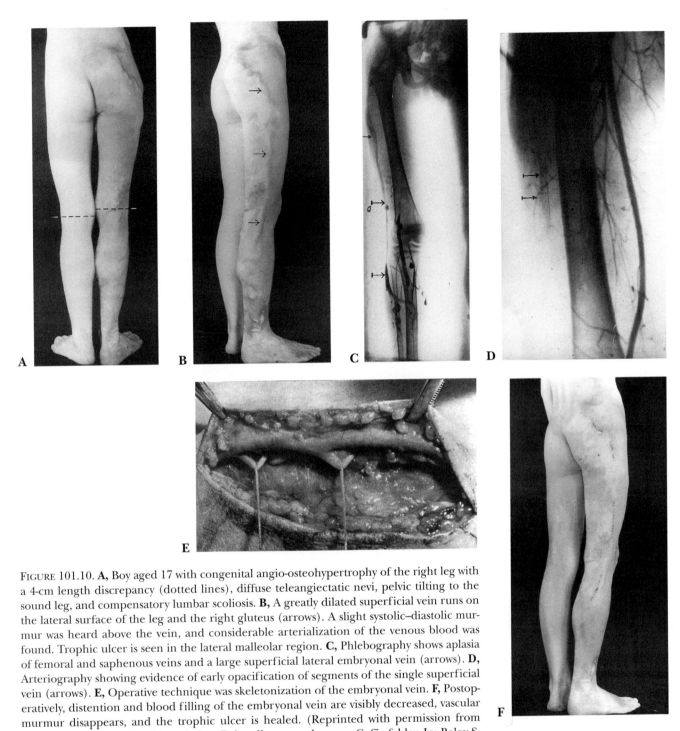

FIGURE 101.10. **A,** Boy aged 17 with congenital angio-osteohypertrophy of the right leg with a 4-cm length discrepancy (dotted lines), diffuse teleangiectatic nevi, pelvic tilting to the sound leg, and compensatory lumbar scoliosis. **B,** A greatly dilated superficial vein runs on the lateral surface of the leg and the right gluteus (arrows). A slight systolic–diastolic murmur was heard above the vein, and considerable arterialization of the venous blood was found. Trophic ulcer is seen in the lateral malleolar region. **C,** Phlebography shows aplasia of femoral and saphenous veins and a large superficial lateral embryonal vein (arrows). **D,** Arteriography showing evidence of early opacification of segments of the single superficial vein (arrows). **E,** Operative technique was skeletonization of the embryonal vein. **F,** Postoperatively, distention and blood filling of the embryonal vein are visibly decreased, vascular murmur disappears, and the trophic ulcer is healed. (Reprinted with permission from Belov S. Grundästze der chirurgischen Behandlung angeborener Gefässfehler. In: Belov S, Loose DA, Müller E, eds. *Angeborene Gefässfehler.* Reinbek, Germany: Einhorn-Presse; 1985.)

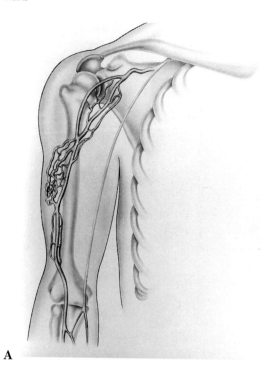

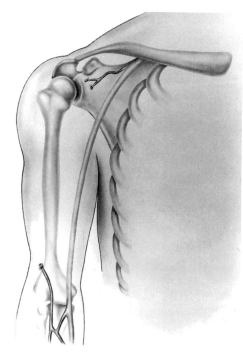

A

B

FIGURE 101.11. Restoration of deep venous drainage by rerouting the venous flow through its normal way (Belov's method II). **A,** Hypoplasia of deep veins in the right arm and superficial dysplastic phlebectasias. **B,** Resection of the highly dilated superficial veins to reroute the venous flow by way of deep principal veins. (Reprinted with permission from Belov S. Surgical treatment of congenital predominantly venous defects. In: Belov S, Loose DA, Weber J, eds. *Vascular Malformations.* Reinbek, Germany: Einhorn-Presse; 1989.)

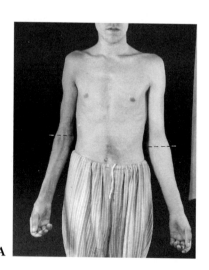

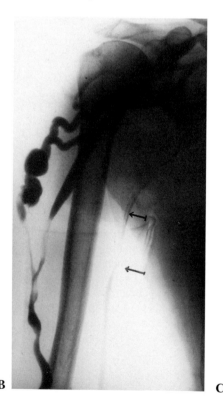

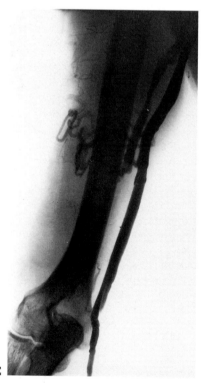

A

B

C

FIGURE 101.12. **A,** Man aged 24 with congenital angio-osteohypotrophy of the right arm with a 2.5-cm length discrepancy (dotted lines) and diffuse phlebectasias along the whole extremity. **B,** Phlebography reveals hypoplasia of the brachial vein (arrows) and superficial dilated, tortuous veins. **C,** Postoperative phlebography shows the brachial vein to be well opacified and with a normal lumen, which ensures the basic venous drainage in the arm.

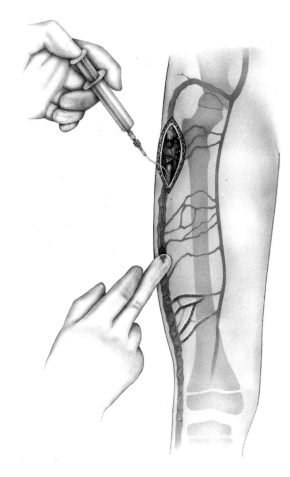

FIGURE 101.13. Resection of marginal vein (Loose's method 2). Reprinted with permission from Loose.[21]

References

1. Belov S, Loose DA. Surgical treatment of congenital vascular defects. *Int Angiol.* 1990;9:175–182.
2. Belov S. Surgical treatment of congenital vascular defects. In: Chang JB, ed. *Modern Vascular Surgery.* New York, NY: Springer-Verlag; 1994:383–397.
3. Belov S. Surgical treatment of congenital predominantly venous defects. In: Belov S, Loose DA, Weber J, eds. *Vascular Malformations.* Reinbek, Germany: Einhorn-Presse; 1989:158–162.
4. Belov S. Surgical treatment of congenital predominantly arteriovenous shunting defects. In: Belov S, Loose DA, Weber J, eds. *Vascular Malformations.* Reinbek, Germany: Einhorn-Presse; 1989:229–234.
5. Loose DA. Surgical treatment of predominantly venous defects. *Semin Vasc Surg.* 1993;6:252–259.
6. Loose DA, Wang Z-G. Surgical treatment of predominantly arterial defects. *Int Angiol.* 1990;9:183–188.
7. Belov S. Grundsätze der chirurgischen Behandlung angeborener Gefässfehler. In: Belov S, Loose DA, Müller E, eds. *Angeborene Gefässfehler.* Reinbek, Germany: Einhorn-Presse; 1985:63–101.
8. Malan E, ed. *Vascular Malformations (Angiodysplasias).* Milan, Italy: Carlo Erba Foundation; 1974;6:104–109.
9. Belov S. Chirurgische Behandlung der kongenitalen Angiodysplasien. *Zentralbl Chir.* 1967;92:1595–1609.
10. Belov S. Correction of lower limbs length discrepancy in congenital vascular-bone diseases by vascular surgery performed during childhood. *Semin Vasc Surg.* 1993;6:245–251.
11. Belov S. Spätergebnisse der chirurgischen Behandlung von 100 Kranken mit kongenitalen Angiodysplasien. *Zentralbl Chir.* 1974;99:935–945.
12. Belov S. Late results of surgical treatment of congenital vascular defects. In: Maurer PC, Becker HM, Heidrich H, Hoffmann G, Kriessmann A, Müller-Wiefel H, Prätorius K., eds. *What Is New in Angiology? Trends and Controversies. Proceedings of the 14th World Congress of the International Union of Angiology, July 6–11, 1986, Munich, West Germany.* Munich: Zuckschwerdt Verlag; 1986:249–250.
13. Loose DA, Belov S. Chirurgische Terapiemöglichkeiten bei angeborenen peripheren Gefässdysplasien. In: Loose DA, ed. *Aktuelles aus Angiologie, Gefässchirurgie, Chirurgie.* Reinbek, Germany: Einhorn-Presse; 1985:55–85.
14. Belov S, Loose DA, Mattassi R, Spatenka J, Tasnadi G, Wang Z-G. Therapeutical strategy, surgical tactics, and operative techniques in congenital vascular defects (multicentre study). In: Strano A, Novo S, eds. *Advances in Vascular Pathology 1989. Proceedings of the 15th World Congress of the International Union of Angiology, Rome, 17–22 September 1989.* Amsterdam: Excerpta Medica; 1989:1355–1360.
15. Vollmar J, Vogt K. Angiodysplasie und Skeletsystem. *Chirurg.* 1976;47:205–213.
16. Belov S. Operative–technical peculiarities in operations of congenital vascular defects. In: Balas P, ed. Progress in Angiology 1991. Proceedings of the 7th European Congress of the International Union of Angiology and 3rd Mediterranean Congress of Angiology. Turin, Italy: Minerva Medica; 1992:379–382.
17. Mattassi R. Diagnosis and treatment of venous malformations of the lower limbs. In: Wang Z-G, Becker HM, Mishima Y, Chang JB, eds. *Vascular Surgery. Proceedings of the International Conference on Vascular Surgery.* Vol 1. Beijing, China: International Academic Publishers; 1993:397–404.
18. Belov S. Congenital agenesia of the deep veins of the lower extremities: surgical treatment. *J Cardiovasc Surg.* 1972;13:594–598.
19. Belov S. *Vascular Malformations: Diagnostics and Surgical Treatment.* Sofia, Bulgaria: Med i Fizk; 1982:98–102.
20. Loose DA. Systematik, radiologische Diagnostik und Therapie vasculärer Fehlbildungen. In: Hohenleutner, Landthaler, eds. *Fortschritte der operativen und onkologischen Dermatologie.* Vol 12. Berlin, Germany: Blackwell; 1997:79–94.
21. Loose DA, Funk I. Angeborene Venenfehler—Diagnostische und Therapeutische Möglichkeiten. *Akt Chir.* 1995;30: 329.

102

Vascular Tumors (Hemangiomas) in Childhood

Hansjörg Cremer

Definition

Until recently the definition for *vascular anomalies* given by the International Society for the Study of Vascular Anomalies encompassed hemangiomas and vascular malformations. But the term *hemangioma* represented a very nonhomogenic group of vascular disorders. It included on the one hand those very common, strictly located hemangiomas that often were not yet visible at birth, became apparent during the first weeks of life, and grew initially for several weeks until they mostly regressed spontaneously within years. But there were also other—admittedly very rare—types of hemangiomas that differed vastly from this group of common hemangiomas. Consequently, in 1996 at its last general meeting in Rome, the International Society for the Study of Vascular Anomalies replaced the term *hemangioma* with the term *vascular tumor*.

The new definition of vascular anomalies is that they encompass vascular tumors and vascular malformations. Thereby a definition that contained virtually all vascular disorders that did not belong to the category of malformations was created. However, this vague definition makes the understanding of these vascular disorders somewhat difficult for those who are not familiar with this subject.

In 1982 Mulliken and Glowacki[19] classified the main groups of hemangiomas as superficial, deep, or mixed hemangiomas and distinguished between a proliferative and a regressive phase. I call this group localized classical hemangiomas (LCHs). But this classification by Mulliken and Glowacki did not include the disseminated forms and other rare then unknown or hardly known vascular disorders that differed fundamentally from the LCHs with respect to their clinical outcome and their histology. Even the subgroup superficial hemangiomas is by no means uniform and needs to be divided into further subgroups.

Therefore I found it necessary to create a clearer classification system that allows for a more comprehensive understanding of the numerous different types of vascular tumors, following a clinical approach. Clearer classification is also necessary if we wish to compare therapeutic results, because otherwise incongruous forms may be compared.

Suggestion for a New Classification of Vascular Tumors

1 Localized classical hemangiomas
  1.1 Superficial LCHs
    1.1.1 Singular elevated LCHs with regular circumference
    1.1.2 Precursor lesions (pale maculae, or white hemangiomas)
    1.1.3 Flat, diffusely erythematous patches with irregular circumference
    1.1.4 Packed clusters of small erythematous papules
    1.1.5 Telangiectatic patches with or without a pale halo
  1.2 Deep LCHs
  1.3 Mixed LCHs (other important components such as type, size, velocity of growth, localization, complications, and so on, as discussed later, also have to be taken into account)
2 Hemangiomatosis
  2.1 Disseminated neonatal hemangiomatosis
    2.1.1 With skin and visceral involvement
    2.1.2 Without skin involvement but with visceral involvement
  2.2 Benign neonatal hemangiomatosis (with only skin involvement)

3 Special forms of hemangiomas
  3.1 Extended (superficial, mixed, or deep) hemangiomas in the craniofacial area that involve at least one half of the head
    3.1.1 With associated visceral involvement
    3.1.2 Without visceral involvement
  3.2 Eruptive angiomas
  3.3 Tumorlike congenital hemangiomas of the newborn, fully developed at birth
    3.3.1 With rapid spontaneous regression
    3.3.2 With incomplete regression
    3.3.3 Without regression
4 Hemangiomas combined with malformations of other organs
  4.1 Lumbosacral hemangiomas combined with tethered cord syndrome, malformations in the urogenital or sacral area, or lipomeningomyelocele
  4.2 Extended hemangiomas in the facial area combined with posterior fossa malformations
  4.3 Other combined forms
5 Other congenital vascular tumors
  5.1 Kasabach–Merritt syndrome
  5.2 Tufted angioma
  5.3 Hemangiopericytoma
  5.4 Kaposiform hemangioendothelioma

Localized Classical Hemangiomas (Group 1)

Because LCHs are by far the most frequent vascular tumors, they are discussed in great detail.

Frequency of the LCH Groups

The percentages given refer to an evaluation of 1130 vascular anomalies (1000 LCHs) that I saw at the Pediatric Hospital in Heilbronn between 1991 and 1996 and that I have classified according to my recommendations. Approximately 85% of all LCHs are superficial, 13% are mixed LCHs, and only about 2% are deep LCHs.

Pathogenesis of LCHs

The vasculature is initially organized in a single plane. Subsequently two planes of vessels develop parallel to the epidermis. After the seventh week of gestation, two planes of vessels that differ in diameter and structure from the walls of the vessels are identifiable. The superficial plane of the cutaneous vasculature is the equivalent of the subpapillary plexus in adult skin. The deep vascular plexus is probably the forerunner of the vasculature in the lower reticular dermis of the adult.[9] By the fifth month of fetal life the vessel walls have differentiated and permit identification of arterioles and venules.

Postnatal Changes

Newborns possess a disorderly dermal capillary network with numerous anastomoses and only a few papillary loops.[20] The major cutaneous vascular pattern is already formed, but the microvasculature, particularly in the subpapillary dermis, continues to change. This reorganization is an ongoing process for the first several months of life. By the fourth postnatal month a stable cutaneous vascular pattern is established. The epidermis is supplied by many papillary loops, including hair follicles and sweat glands. These vessels do not form well-defined horizontal plexuses but cross the dermis at varying angles.[24]

Role of Angiogenesis for the Pathogenesis of Hemangiomas

Angiogenesis is somehow connected with the development of hemangiomas. The proliferative phase in infants coincides with the period of continued organization of the dermal vascular network in postnatal life. Perturbation of this physiological process could conceivably result in the formation of abnormal collections of dermal vessels (incipient hemangiomas) responsive to angiogenic promoters and inhibitors in the tissue.[9]

Predisposing Factors for the Development of LCHs

Approximately 10% to 12% of children develop LCHs during their first year of life. Prematurity seems to be a predisposing factor. The more premature the child, the greater the risk of development of a LCH.[1]

Female Predominance

Girls are more frequently affected (my results: 538:237 = 2.3:1). Particularly in superficial LCHs, I have noticed an even stronger female predominance (438:173 = 3.1:1) but less dominance in mixed and deep LCHs (100:64 = 1.6:1).

Clinical Examples of LCHs

Superficial LCHs (Group 1.1 and Subgroups 1.1.1 Through 1.1.5)

Group 1.1 superficial LCHs must be further divided into five subgroups, each differing completely in appearance. By far the most common subgroup is 1.1.1, or singular elevated LCHs with regular circumference (Figure 102.1). This group represents approximately 85% of all LCHs and about 95% of the superficial LCHs.

Subgroup 1.1.2 lesions (i.e., precursor lesions, or white hemangiomas) (Figure 102.2) can often be seen at birth.[13] From these precursor lesions flat hemangiomas

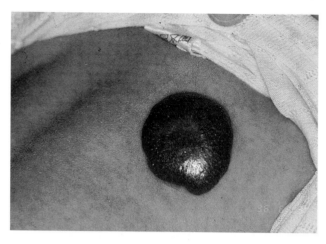

FIGURE 102.1. Singular elevated LCHs with regular circumference on an infant.

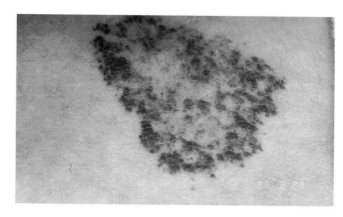

FIGURE 102.4. A flat hemangioma has developed from a white hemangioma.

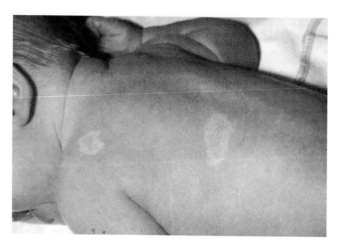

FIGURE 102.2. Precursor lesions (white hemangiomas) on a newborn.

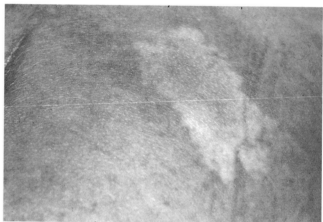

FIGURE 102.5. Nevus anemicus on a young infant.

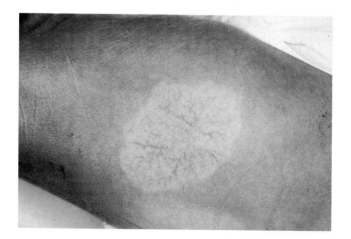

FIGURE 102.3. A close-up view of white hemangiomas.

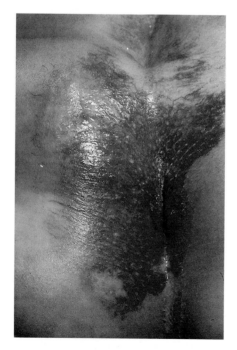

FIGURE 102.6. Flat, diffusely erythematous patches with irregular circumference in the anal area.

may develop (Figures 102.3 and 102.4). White hemangiomas must be distinguished from nevus anemicus, which is caused by a momentary vasoconstriction (Figure 102.5).

Subgroup 1.1.3 lesions—flat, diffusely erythematous patches with irregular circumference—can be quite extensive (Figures 102.6 and 102.7). Some tend to grow, and others quickly regress. Subgroup 1.1.4 lesions—packed clusters of small erythematous papules (Figure 102.8)—can originate from ill-defined bluish areas (Figures 102.9 and 102.10). Subgroup 1.1.5 lesions are telangiectatic patches with threadlike telangiectasias that can be seen with (Figures 102.11 and 102.12) or without a pale halo (Figures 102.13 and 102.14). The subgroups 1.1.2 through 1.1.5 are rare; they represent only about 5% of all superficial LCHs.

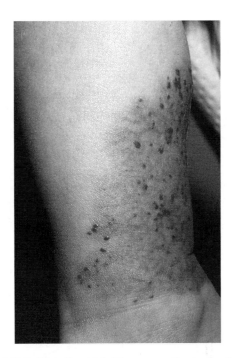

FIGURE 102.9. Ill-defined bluish area on the back of the right leg of a 2-week-old infant.

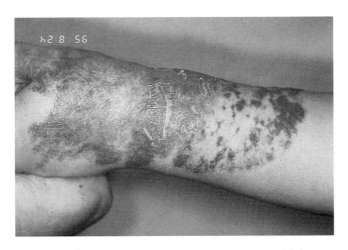

FIGURE 102.7. Flat, diffusely erythematous patches with irregular circumference on the left arm of a 5-month-old infant.

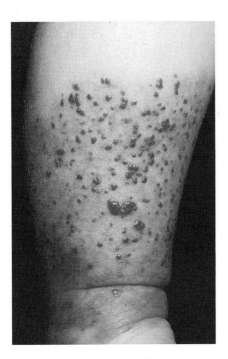

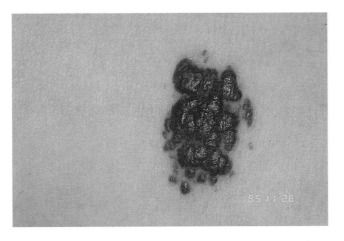

FIGURE 102.8. Packed clusters of small erythematous papules.

FIGURE 102.10. Packed clusters of small erythematous papules have originated from the ill-defined bluish area on a 7-week-old infant (same infant as in Figure 102.9).

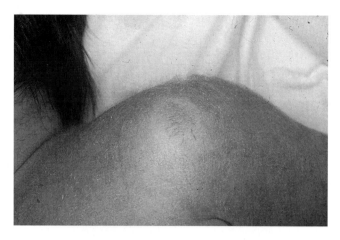

FIGURE 102.11. Telangiectatic patches with threadlike telangiectasias with a pale halo on the shoulder of a 2-week-old infant.

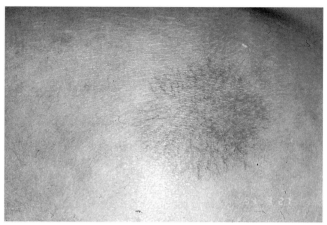

FIGURE 102.14. Telangiectatic patches with threadlike telangiectasias without a pale halo on the forehead of a 3-week-old infant.

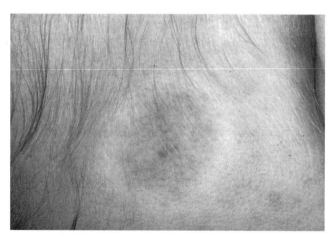

FIGURE 102.12. Telangiectatic patches with threadlike telangiectasias without a pale halo on the neck of a 6-week-old infant.

Deep Hemangiomas (Group 1.2)

Deep hemangiomas (Figure 102.15) are often difficult to distinguish from vascular malformations. They are sometimes combined with lymphangiomas.

Mixed Hemangiomas (Group 1.3)

In mixed hemangiomas (Figure 102.16) the deep component is not always apparent in the early stages.

First Appearance of LCHs

About 10% to 12% of children develop LCHs during their first year of life. About 30% are already present at birth; most appear within the first weeks of life, and 99% appear within the first year. Approximately 85% can be recognized by the end of the first month, and only 5% appear after the third month of life.

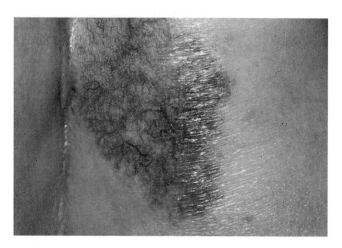

FIGURE 102.13. Telangiectatic patches with threadlike telangiectasias without a pale halo on the rim of the anus of a 4-month-old infant.

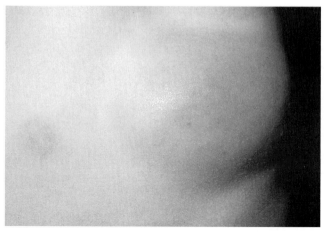

FIGURE 102.15. Deep hemangioma under the left axilla.

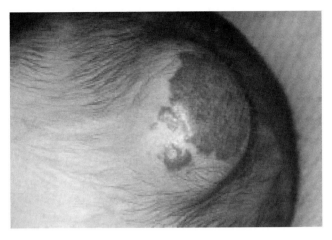

FIGURE 102.16. Mixed hemangioma on the scalp.

Growth and Regression of LCHs

Growth

About 70% of all LCHs grow more or less rapidly for a few months. LCHs in the facial area sometimes show excessive growth (Figure 102.17). Early diagnosis of these hemangiomas is essential because they can be treated ei-

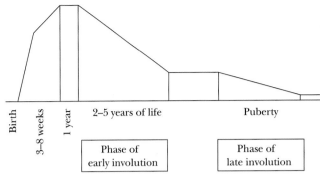

FIGURE 102.18. Growth and regression of hemangiomas over a period of years.

ther by contact cryosurgery or by pulsed dye laser in their initial stages.

In superficial LCHs spontaneous involution usually begins in the second half of the first year of life (Figure 102.18). Over a period of years about 70% of all LCHs regress completely, 10% show no sign of regression, and 20% regress partially (Figure 102.19).

Regression

The hemangioma gradually flattens and the bright red color (Figure 102.20) is replaced by a grayish color (Figure 102.21). Usually a more or less distinct scar remains of the largest size of the hemangioma (Figure 102.22). Disfiguring scars sometimes remain (Figure 102.23). Deep and mixed LCHs often take a long time to regress. Some hemangiomas—especially those located on the lips—do not regress at all.

Size of LCHs

LCHs are small (<1 cm^2), middle sized (1–5 cm^2), or large (>5 cm^2). The final size of a LCH is influenced by

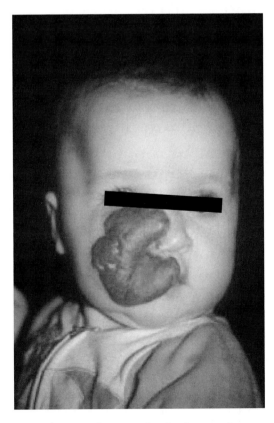

FIGURE 102.17. Excessive growth of a hemangioma on a 7-month-old infant; the hemangioma appeared shortly after birth as only a slight discoloring of the cheek.

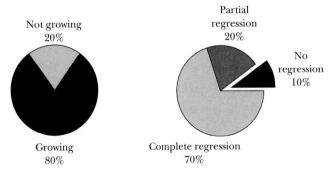

FIGURE 102.19. Natural history of LCHs.

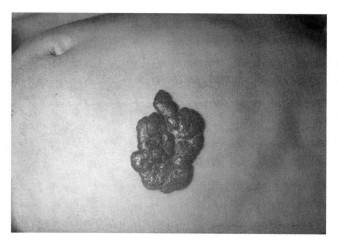

FIGURE 102.20. Elevated, bright red hemangioma on a 3-month-old infant.

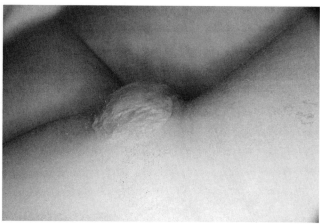

FIGURE 102.23. Completely regressed hemangioma that has left a flabby scar.

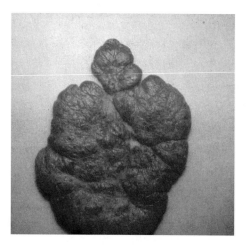

FIGURE 102.21. Same child as in Figure 102.20 at 1 year of age; hemangioma shows signs of regression.

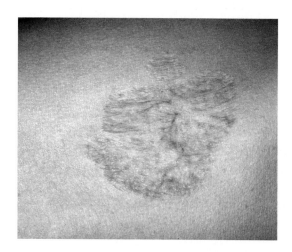

FIGURE 102.22. Same child as in Figure 102.20 at 12 years of age; hemangioma has completely regressed, but a scar the size of the hemangioma at its greatest extension remains.

the speed and the duration of growth. Because the duration of growth is nearly always limited to only a few months, the speed of growth becomes the decisive factor for determining the final size. Of all the superficial LCHs I have seen, about 55% were small, about 40% were middle sized, and less than 5% were large.

Number of LCHs

Most LCHs occur singly (70%); in 20% two LCHs occur, and in only about 10% of all cases are three or more hemangiomas seen.

Localization of LCHs

Besides the size, the localization of LCHs plays an important role in the degree of severity. Of the 1000 LCHs I observed, 51% were located in the head area, 3% on the neck, 27% on the trunk, 4% in the anogenital region, 6% on the upper extremities, and 9% on the lower extremities (Figure 102.24).

Hemangiomas Located in Problem Zones

For cosmetic reasons LCHs in the facial area are especially problematic for the child and also his or her parents (Figure 102.25).

Hemangiomas in the Eye Area

Obstruction of vision by hemangiomas (Figure 102.26) quickly leads to functional blindness. All hemangiomas in this area must be considered emergencies. Immediate therapy can prevent visual obstruction. If contact cryosurgery or laser therapy is not possible, steroids or

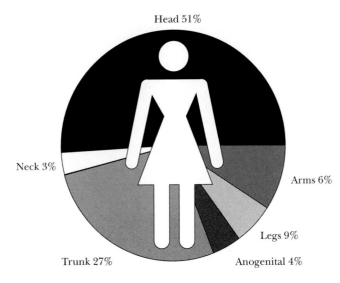

FIGURE 102.24. Localization of LCHs ($n = 1050$) seen at the Pediatric Hospital Heilbronn (Sept. 1991–June 1996).

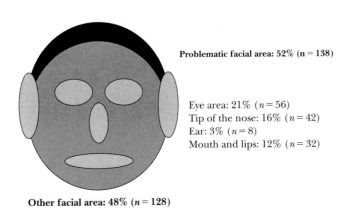

Problematic facial area: 52% (n = 138)

Eye area: 21% ($n = 56$)
Tip of the nose: 16% ($n = 42$)
Ear: 3% ($n = 8$)
Mouth and lips: 12% ($n = 32$)

Other facial area: 48% ($n = 128$)

FIGURE 102.25. Distribution of 266 LCHs in the facial area.

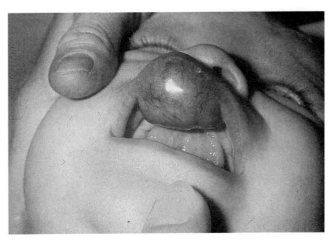

FIGURE 102.27. Large hemangioma on the lips that does not regress.

interferon alfa-2a can be administered. Surgical intervention is only rarely indicated.

Hemangiomas in the Mouth Area

Hemangiomas on lips often do not regress (Figure 102.27).

Hemangiomas on the Tip of the Nose

Hemangiomas on the tip of the nose—also called Cyrano nose—are very disfiguring (Figure 102.28). Even if they regress, islands of fatty tissue often remain (Figure 102.29).

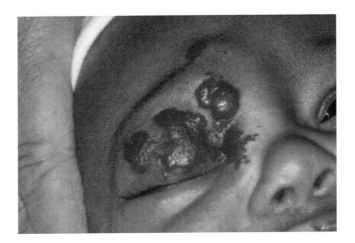

FIGURE 102.26. Obstruction of vision by a hemangioma.

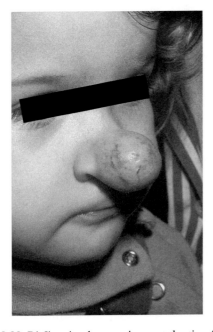

FIGURE 102.28. Disfiguring hemangioma at the tip of the nose.

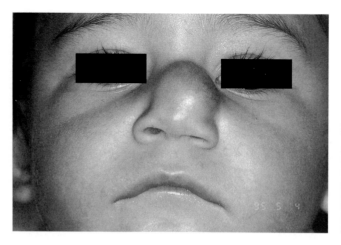

FIGURE 102.29. Remaining fatty tissue after regression of a nasal hemangioma.

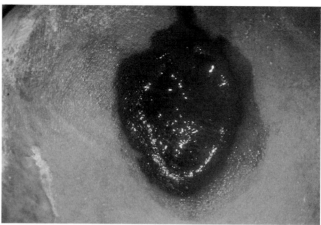

FIGURE 102.31. Ulcerated hemangioma on the buttock of a 5-month-old infant.

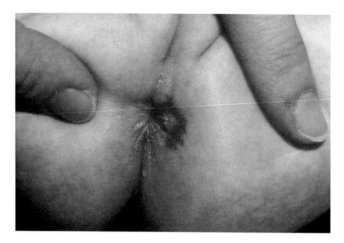

FIGURE 102.30. Ulcerated hemangiomas in the anogenital region.

Hemangiomas in the Anogenital Region

Hemangiomas in the anogenital region tend to ulcerate (Figure 102.30).

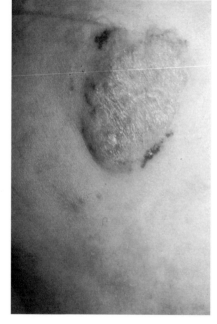

FIGURE 102.32. Same infant as in Figure 102.31, 7 weeks after contact cryosurgery.

Complications of LCHs

Ulceration and Necrosis

The most frequent complications of LCHs are ulceration and necrosis. The danger of secondary infection is always present in patients with ulceration or necrosis. The ulcerations are often very painful. My colleagues and I have observed good results by treating ulcerated hemangiomas with contact cryosurgery (Figures 102.31 and 102.32); others have reported similarly good results by using argon laser and the pulsed dye laser.[18] Conservative local therapy consists of applying antiseptic lotions or antibiotic ointments. Nonadhesive biosynthetic dressings (as used in the local treatment of burns) are very helpful. Zinc oxide ointment can also be used.

Infection

Infections can occur in ulcerated hemangiomas. In rare cases systemic infections can cause life-threatening complications in patients with hemangiomas. I once observed necrotizing fasciitis, caused by toxin-producing streptococcus, in an extended superficial hemangioma. The patient could be saved only by immediate and ex-

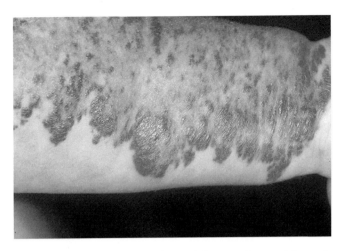

FIGURE 102.33. Extended elevated hemangioma with early signs of regression in a 7-week-old infant.

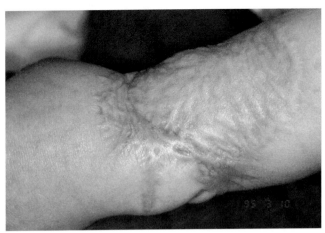

FIGURE 102.36. Same child as in Figure 102.35, 8 months after surgery.

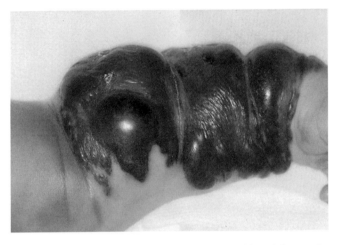

FIGURE 102.34. Same infant as in Figure 102.33 at 3.5 months of age; the hemangioma worsened severely, and within hours the infant suffered shock.

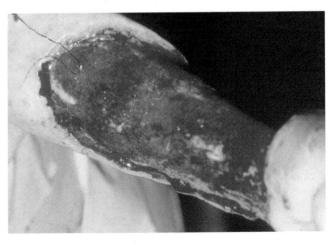

FIGURE 102.35. Same infant as in Figure 102.34 on the same day; the patient underwent emergency surgery to remove the whole affected area.

tensive excision of the affected area (Figures 102.33, 102.34, 102.35, and 102.36).

Bleeding

Parents often fear severe bleeding from a hemangioma. Fortunately bleeding occurs only rarely. Parents should be provided with simple guidelines on what to do if bleeding occurs (simple compression is usually sufficient). Disseminated intravascular coagulation does not occur in LCHs[8]; it only occurs in Kasabach–Merritt syndrome, which is not classified as a LCH.

Obstruction

In some rare cases obstruction (e.g., of the trachea or eye) can result.

Diagnostic Technique

Superficial LCHs are diagnosed clinically. Usually lengthy examinations are not required. In deep and mixed LCHs the use of magnetic resonance imaging Doppler echography sound is very helpful. Sometimes it may be difficult to distinguish between vascular malformations and deep LCHs. If embolization is planned, angiography is necessary.

Therapy of LCHs

Choice of Therapy

The choice of therapy in LCHs depends on their classification (Figures 102.37 and 102.38). Superficial LCHs of subgroup 1.1.1 (singular elevated hemangiomas with

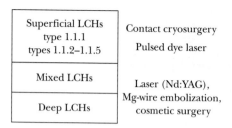

Superficial LCHs type 1.1.1 types 1.1.2–1.1.5	Contact cryosurgery Pulsed dye laser
Mixed LCHs	Laser (Nd:YAG), Mg-wire embolization, cosmetic surgery
Deep LCHs	

FIGURE 102.37. Choice of therapy of LCHs depends on their classification.

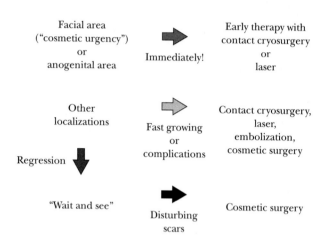

FIGURE 102.38. Recommended therapy for LCHs.

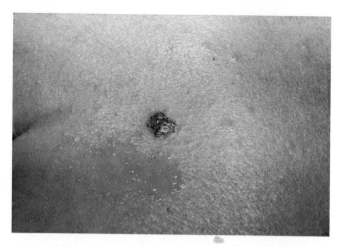

FIGURE 102.39. Small hemangioma before treatment on a 5-month-old infant.

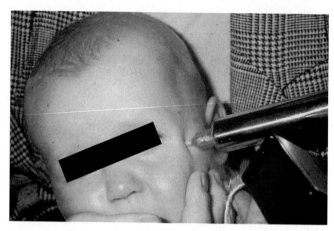

FIGURE 102.40. Contact cryosurgery on the same infant as in Figure 102.39.

regular circumference) are best treated by contact cryosurgery.[5] Pulsed dye laser is recommended for subgroups 1.1.2 through 1.1.5. Most deep hemangiomas (group 1.2) can be treated with laser, but additional surgical intervention—in some cases combined with embolization—is also often necessary. In mixed hemangiomas (group 1.3) the superficial part can be treated with contact cryosurgery or pulsed dye laser.

Timing of Therapy

If LCHs are located in a critical area such as the face or the anogenital region, early treatment (the earlier the better) often spares the patient and the parents much trouble. In these cases treatment should be performed while the angioma is still small or as soon as the hemangioma becomes visible.[5] In other less critical areas hemangiomas should be treated when they begin to grow more quickly. No therapy is necessary when hemangiomas show signs of regression.

Various Therapeutic Methods

Contact Cryosurgical Treatment

Superficial hemangiomas are best treated by contact cryosurgery. In contact cryosurgery a metal stick, cooled

by liquid nitrogen of $-195°C$, is placed on the hemangioma with controlled pressure for 10 seconds (Figures 102.39, 102.40, and 102.41). The best results are obtained if therapy starts very early while the hemangiomas are still small (Figures 102.42, 102.43, 102.44, and 102.45). Ulcerated hemangiomas also respond favorably to contact cryosurgery (Figures 102.31 and 102.32), as do hemangiomas on the lips (Figures 102.46 and 102.47) and on the tip of the nose (Figures 102.48 and 102.49).

Contact cryosurgery is useful in cases that require only limited penetration. I do not recommend using a spray. Contact cryosurgery—especially when used in the early stages of growing hemangiomas—does not cause scarring. In most cases general anesthesia is not necessary. A local anesthetic ointment can be used.

Contact cryosurgery works as follows: during the process of deep-freezing of a hemangioma, crystallization occurs in cells with high water content, such as the endothelial cells of blood vessels. As a result the cells are destroyed. Epidermal keratinocytes contain much less

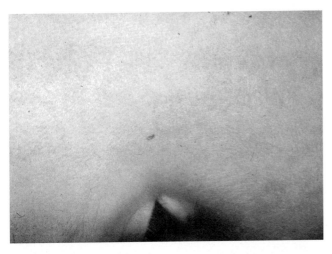

FIGURE 102.41. After 2 months, the hemangioma has completely regressed without scarring (same infant as in Figure 102.40).

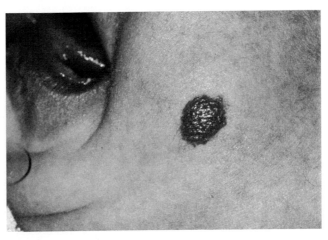

FIGURE 102.44. Growing hemangioma on the left cheek of a 4-week-old infant.

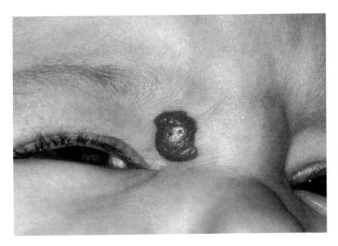

FIGURE 102.42. Growing hemangioma near the eye of a 3-month-old infant.

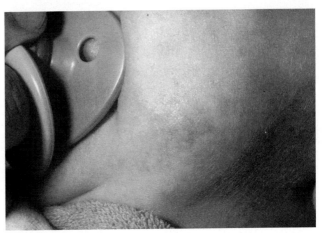

FIGURE 102.45. Same infant as in Figure 102.44, 4 weeks after contact cryosurgery.

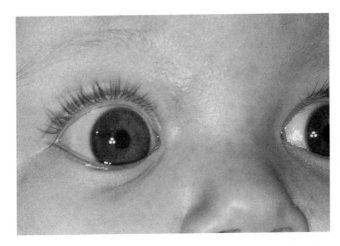

FIGURE 102.43. Same infant as in Figure 102.42, 4 weeks after contact cryosurgery.

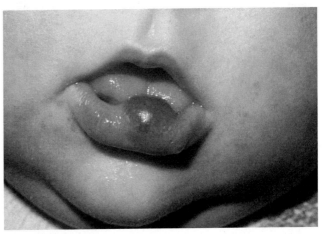

FIGURE 102.46. Growing hemangioma on the lip of a 3-month-old infant.

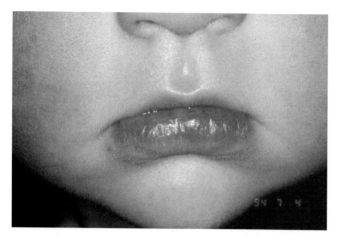

FIGURE 102.47. Same child as in Figure 102.46, 6 weeks later, after contact cryosurgery.

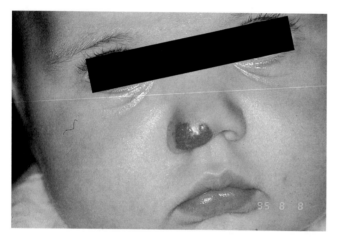

FIGURE 102.48. Growing hemangioma on the tip of the nose of a 7-month-old infant.

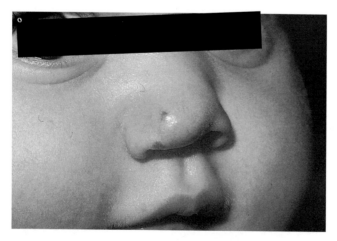

FIGURE 102.49. Same infant as in Figure 102.48, 5 weeks after contact cryosurgery.

water and are therefore much less vulnerable to the process of deep-freezing.

Laser Therapy

Mixed and deep hemangiomas should be treated by laser therapy. The choice of the type of laser used (e.g., argon laser or neodymium:yttrium–aluminum–garnet laser) depends on the size and extension of the hemangiomas. Here too the best results are obtained by early therapy. Good results are obtained by using ice cubes for cooling. Flat, extended hemangiomas are probably best treated with pulsed dye laser.

Cosmetic Surgery

Cosmetic surgery is sometimes preferable in treating deep, well-localized LCHs, but it requires great skill and experience. Disfiguring scars should be corrected by cosmetic surgery.

Embolization

Embolization, mostly in combination with surgery, has been used in deep-lying LCHs that are inaccessible by other methods. It should be reserved for hemangiomas that require immediate treatment and should be performed only by very experienced teams.

Corticosteroids

Vascular tumors in children with life-threatening symptoms or LCHs in the eye area with obstruction of eyesight not accessible by other methods have been treated successfully with corticosteroids (3–5 mg/kg prednisone per day). However, only about 30% respond well. Intralesional corticosteroids are of doubtful value.[4]

Interferon Alfa-2a

Researchers first noticed that recombinant human interferon alfa-2a inhibited tumor growth in patients with Kaposi's sarcoma, which presents with vascular tumors.[11] Interferon alfa-2a has also been effective in treating hemangiomatosis of children[26,28] and Kasabach–Merritt syndrome.[23] However, this therapy can cause neurotoxic side effects.[2] Hemangiomas in children with life-threatening symptoms and hemangiomas in the eye area with obstruction of eyesight have also been successfully treated with interferon alfa-2a therapy.[6]

Angiogenesis Inhibitors

New approaches have resulted from research on angiogenic factors. Therapeutic consequences may be drawn from the recognition of angiogenesis inhibitors.[25]

Neonatal Hemangiomatosis (Group 2)

Disseminated Neonatal Hemangiomatosis With Visceral Involvement (Group 2.1)

Disseminated neonatal hemangiomatosis with visceral involvement affects both the skin (with numerous 0.2- to 2-cm reddish-blue, sharply defined elevated hemangiomas) and the viscera. The liver is usually involved, but other organs (e.g., eyes, lung, and central nervous system) can also be affected. The prognosis is poor. Patients often suffer from progressive high-output congestive heart failure.[6] In suspected cases, ultrasound, computed tomography, or magnetic resonance imaging is helpful for diagnosis.

Therapy

In some patients with disseminated neonatal hemangiomatosis the administration of prednisone (3–5 mg/kg per day) has been effective.[4,12] Interferon alfa-2a (3,000,000 U/m² per day) has been used with varying success.[10,21,27,28]

Benign Neonatal Hemangiomatosis (Group 2.2)

The benign neonatal hemangiomatosis (Figure 102.50) in which only the skin is involved should not be included in the category of disseminated neonatal hemangiomatosis because of the good prognosis. At birth affected infants have numerous hemangiomas that resemble eruptive angiomas. Because the hemangiomas usually regress spontaneously within a few months, no therapy is necessary.

Special Forms of Hemangiomas (Group 3)

Extended Hemangiomas in the Craniofacial Area (Group 3.1)

Extended hemangiomas, which can affect one half of the head or more, with or without associated visceral involvement, are rare (Figure 102.51).[9] They are problematic cases that are difficult to treat. Laser therapy may be effective in the early stages; in later stages corticosteroids and/or interferon alfa-2a may be used successfully.

Eruptive Angioma (Group 3.2)

Eruptive angiomas are quite common in children. They are often located on the face (Figure 102.52) but can also appear on the trunk (Figure 102.53). Eruptive angiomas can occur at any age and tend to bleed. Pathologically, an eruptive angioma is a neoformation of endothelial cells caused by minor violations of superficial vessels, such as by scratching. Eruptive angiomas may erode and heal spontaneously, but they should usually be removed by curettage (with local anesthesia), laser therapy, or contact cryosurgery. Eruptive angiomas can also originate from port-wine stains (Figure 102.54).

Tumorlike Congenital Hemangiomas of the Newborn (Group 3.3)

The existence of tumorlike congenital hemangiomas of the newborn was first brought to my notice in 1994.[17] There are three different forms of these hemangiomas. In all three forms the hemangiomas are already full size at birth. They are generally surrounded by a pale halo.

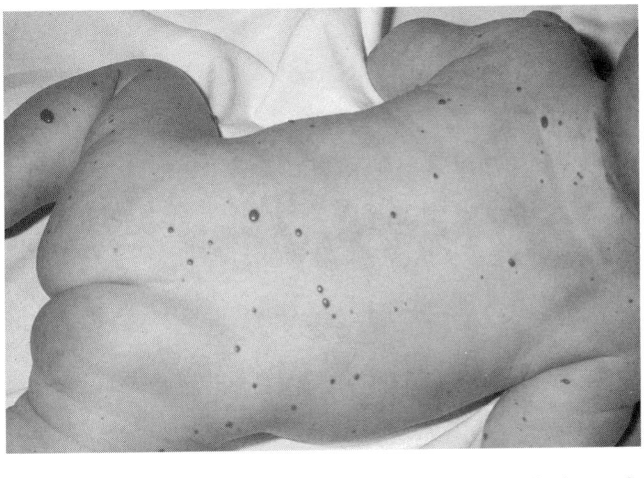

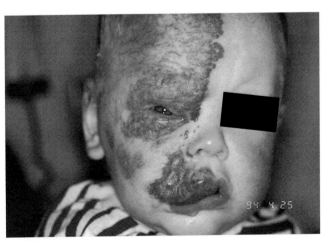

FIGURE 102.50. Benign neonatal hemangiomatosis in a 2-month-old infant.

FIGURE 102.51. Extended hemangioma in a 7-month-old infant in the craniofacial area without associated visceral involvement.

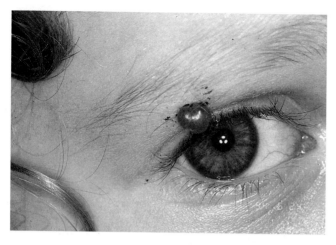

FIGURE 102.52. Eruptive hemangioma on the upper lid.

In the subgroup 3.3.1, tumorlike congenital hemangiomas of the newborn with rapid spontaneous regression (Figures 102.55, 102.56, 102.57, and 102.58), the tumor starts to regress soon after birth. Regression is usually completed after 1 to 2 years, sometimes leaving atrophic scars or loose skin. In the subgroup 3.3.2, tumorlike congenital hemangiomas of the newborn with incomplete regression,[7] the tumor also starts to regress quickly but then stops regressing after about 1 year (Figures 102.59 and 102.60). Subgroup 3.3.3, tumorlike congenital hemangiomas without regression (Figure 102.61 and 102.62), usually show the histological pattern of tufted angiomas.[7]

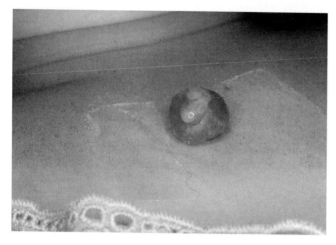

FIGURE 102.53. Large eruptive hemangioma on the chest of an 8-year-old child.

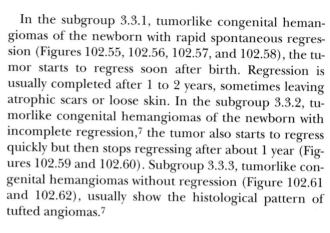

FIGURE 102.55. Huge, solid bluish tumor on the right cheek of a 10-day-old infant.

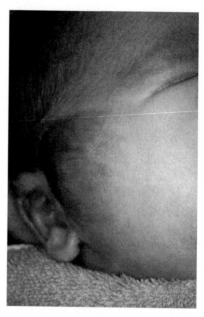

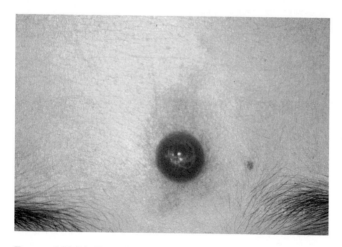

FIGURE 102.54. Eruptive hemangioma on a 10-year-old child; the hemangioma originated from a port-wine stain.

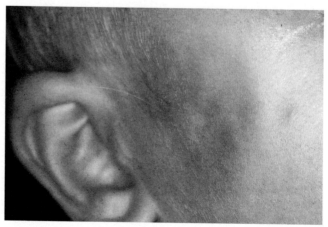

FIGURE 102.56. Same child as in Figure 102.55 at 2 years of age; the tumor has completely regressed.

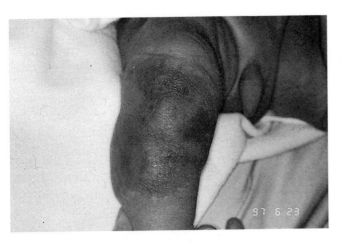

FIGURE 102.57. Huge, solid bluish tumor surrounded by a pale halo on the right leg of a 3-day-old infant.

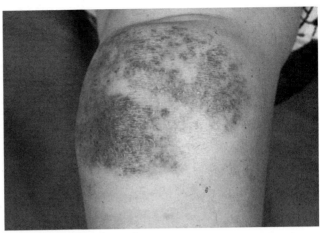

FIGURE 102.60. Same infant as in Figure 102.59 at 2 years of age; the tumor has only partially regressed.

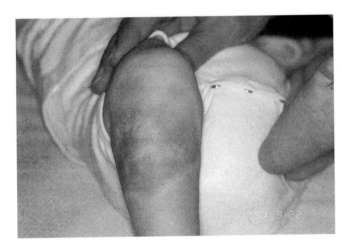

FIGURE 102.58. Same infant as in Figure 102.57 at 3 months of age; the tumor has regressed.

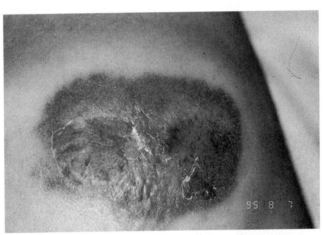

FIGURE 102.61. Solid bluish tumor surrounded by a pale halo on the right arm of a 2-month-old infant.

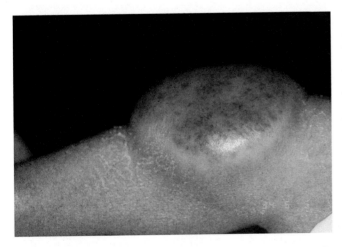

FIGURE 102.59. Huge, solid bluish tumor surrounded by a pale halo on the right knee of a 3-week-old infant.

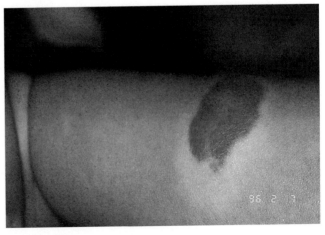

FIGURE 102.62. Same child as in Figure 102.61 at 1 year of age; the tumor shows no sign of regression.

Tumorlike congenital hemangiomas of subgroup 3.3.3 are probably identical to noninvoluting congenital hemangiomas.[26] Clinically some of these hemangiomas appear as solid, elevated, violet tumors with ecstatic veins and a white halo; others are of a grayish color with multiple ectasias or are flat with a violet coloring.[3] Knowing that these special forms of hemangiomas often heal without treatment can spare affected children unnecessary aggressive therapy.

Hemangiomas Combined With Malformations of Other Organs (Group 4)

In hemangiomas combined with malformations of other organs, extended hemangiomas are associated with congenital anomalies of other organs. Lumbosacral hemangiomas can be associated with tethered cord syndrome (Figure 102.63), malformations in the urogenital or sacral area, or lipomeningomyelocele.[11] Extended hemangiomas in the facial area can be combined with posterior fossa malformations such as Dandy–Walker syndrome and cerebellar malformations.[23] Other very rare forms of hemangiomas associated with organic malformations have also been noted.[9]

Other Congenital Vascular Tumors (Group 5)

Congenital vascular tumors not otherwise classified resemble LCHs but differ considerably histologically and in their clinical course.

Kasabach–Merritt Syndrome (Group 5.1)

Kasabach–Merritt syndrome (Figure 102.64) shows histologically the pattern of a tufted angioma or a kaposiform hemangioendothelioma.[8] Unlike LCHs there is no female predominance. Typical of the clinical course of Kasabach–Merritt syndrome is the development of disseminated intravascular coagulation with severe thrombocytopenia and a tendency to bleeding that is often critical. Corticosteroids[22] and/or interferon alfa-2a,[15] surgery, and radiation have been used successfully to treat Kasabach–Merritt syndrome. Despite this success, the prognosis is poor. Some cases have regressed spontaneously after several years.

Tufted Angioma (Group 5.2)

Tufted angiomas[29] are rare. The term *tufted angioma* is derived from the histological pattern. Clinically they vary considerably. Some are present at birth,[7] and others appear after a few years (acquired forms) (Figures 102.65 and 102.66). They are often located in the area of the upper trunk and on the neck. They tend to spread slowly, but there is no malignancy. As mentioned earlier, some of the tumorlike congenital hemangiomas of the newborn and also the Kasabach–Merritt syndrome show the pattern of tufted angiomas histologically.

Hemangiopericytoma (Group 5.3)

Hemangiopericytoma is a very rare tumor derived from the wall of smooth muscle cells that surround the wall of small blood vessels. Coarse, reddish-brown lumps a few centimeters in diameter often occur within the first year of life.[14] In about 20% of cases they become malignant. Superficial tumors are mostly benign. Because they tend

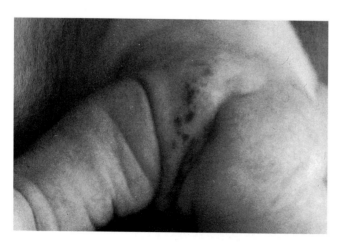

FIGURE 102.63. Lumbosacral hemangioma, tethered cord syndrome, and right-sided renal aplasia in a 2-week-old infant.

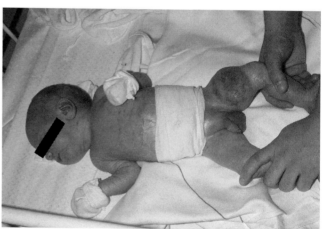

FIGURE 102.64. Kasabach–Merritt syndrome in a 1-week-old infant.

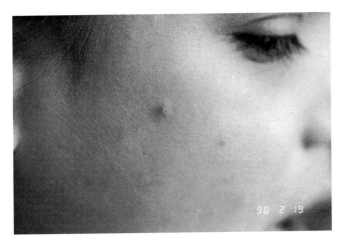

FIGURE 102.65. Tufted angioma in a 6-year-old child.

to become malignant, hemangiopericytomas should be excised thoroughly.

Kaposiform Hemangioendothelioma (Subgroup 5.4)

Kaposiform hemangioendothelioma, a very rare disease, is not clearly defined.[16] In spite of being invasive, it is a benign tumor. Morphologically it is difficult to distinguish between the benign infantile form and the malignant adult form. Clinically and histologically the hemangioendothelium lies between hemangioma and hemangiosarcoma. Hemangioendotheliomas develop fast-growing reddish-blue to bluish-violet cutaneous and subcutaneous infiltrating plaques and lumps with ecchymosis, necrosis, and ulcerations. The main location is the trunk. They seem to be closely related to the tufted angioma—as in the case of Kasabach–Merritt syndrome.[8]

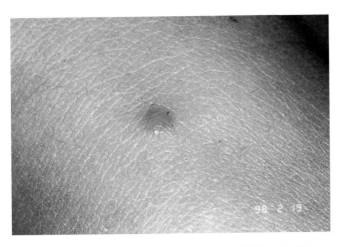

FIGURE 102.66. Close-up view of the same child as in Figure 102.65.

Vascular Malformations Resembling Hemangiomas

Some vascular anomalies, such as glomangiomas, blue rubber bleb nevus syndrome, Gorham–Stout syndrome, angiokeratomas, and verrucous angiomas, which may resemble hemangiomas, are actually vascular malformations and are therefore not included in this chapter.

References

1. Amir J, Krikler R, Metzker A, et al. Strawberry hemangioma in preterm infants. *Pediatr Dermatol.* 1986;3: 331–332.
2. Barlow C, Priebe CJ, Mulliken JB, Barnes P. Neurotoxicity in the treatment of hemangiomas with interferon alpha 2a. Paper presented at: ISSVA 11th International Workshop on Vascular Anomalies; June 23–26, 1996; Rome.
3. Boon LM, Enjolras O, Mulliken JB. Congenital hemangioma: evidence of accelerated involution. *J Pediatr.* 1996; 128:329–335.
4. Clemmensen O. A case of multiple neonatal hemangiomatosis successfully treated by systemic corticosteroids. *Dermatologica.* 1979;159:485–499.
5. Cremer HJ, Djawari D. Frühtherapie der kutanen Hämangiome mit der Kontaktkryochirurgie pädiat. *Pädiatrische Praxis.* 1994; 47:633–650.
6. Enjolras O, Riche MC, Merland JJ, Escandej P. Management of alarming hemangiomas in infancy: a review of 25 cases. *Pediatrics.* 1990;85:491–498.
7. Enjolras O, Wassef M, Dompmartin A, Labreze C, Josset P. Congenital tufted angiomas. Paper presented at: ISSVA 12th International Workshop on Vascular Anomalies; June 27–28, 1998; Berlin.
8. Enjolras O, Wassef M, Mazoyer E, Frieden IJ, Rieu PN, Drouet L, Taieb A, Stalder JF, Escande JP. Infants with Kasabach-Merritt syndrome do not have "true" hemangiomas. *J Pediatr.* 1997;130:631–640.
9. Esterly NB. Current Problems in Dermatology: Cutaneous Hemangiomas, Vascular Stains and Malformations, and Associated Syndromes. St. Louis, MO: Mosby; 1995: 65–108.
10. Ezekowitz RAB, Mulliken JB, Folkman J. Interferon alfa-2a therapy for life-threatening hemangiomas of infancy. *N Engl J Med.* 1992;326:1456–1463.
11. Goldberg NS, Herbert AA, Esterly NB. Sacral hemangiomas and multiple congenital anomalies. *Arch Dermatol.* 1986;122:684–687.
12. Gozal D, Saad N, Boder D, et al. Diffuse neonatal hemangiomatosis: successful management with high dose corticosteroid. *Eur J Pediatr.* 1990;149:321–324.
13. Hidano A, Nakajima S. Earliest features of the strawberry mark in the newborn. *Br J Dermatol.* 1972;83:138–144.
14. Kaufman SL, Stout AP. Hemangiopericytoma in children. *Cancer.* 1960;13:695–710.
15. Klein C, Hauser M, Hadorn HB. Interferon alpha-2a therapy of consumptive coagulopathy in Kasabach-Merritt syndrome. *Eur J Pediatr.* 1992;151:919.

16. Kobayashi H, Furukawa M, Fukai K, et al. Cellular angioma of infancy with dermal melanocytosis. *Int J Dermatol.* 1988;27:40–42.

17. Martinez-Perez D, Mulliken JB. All hemangiomas do not look like strawberries. Paper presented at: ISSVA 10th International Workshop on Vascular Anomalies; June 15, 1994; Budapest.

18. Morelli JG, Tan OT, Weston WL. Treatment of ulcerated hemangiomas with the pulsed tunable dye laser. *Am J Dis Child.* 1991;145:1062–1064.

19. Mulliken JB, Glowacki J. Hemangiomas and vascular malformations in infants and children: a classification based on endothelial characteristics. *Plast Reconstr Surg.* 1982; 69:412–420.

20. Norman M, Herin P, Fagrell B, et al. Capillary blood cell velocity in full-term infants as determined by video-photometric microscopy. *Pediatr Res.* 1988;23:585–588.

21. Orchard PJ, Smith CM, Woods WG, Day DL, Dehner LP, Shapiro R. Treatment of haemangioendotheliomas with alpha interferon [letter]. *Lancet.* 1989;8662:565–567.

22. Ozoylu S, Irhen C, Gurgey A. High dose intravenous methylprednisolone for Kasabach-Merritt syndrome. *Eur J Pediatr.* 1989;148:403–405.

23. Reese V, Frieden IJ, Paller AS, et al. Association of facial hemangiomas with Dandy-Walker and other posterior fossa malformations. *J Pediatr.* 1993;122:379–384.

24. Ryan TJ. Cutaneous circulation. In: Goldsmith LA, ed. *Biochemistry and Physiology of the Skin.* Vol. 2. New York: Oxford University Press; 1983:817–877.

25. Schweigerer L, Fotsis T. Angiogenesis and angiogenesis inhibitors in paediatric diseases. *Eur J Pediatr.* 1992;151: 472–476.

26. Wassef M, Boon L, Kozakewich HPW, Enjolras O, Burrows PE, Mulliken JB. Non-involuting congenital hemangioma. Paper presented at: ISSVA 12th International Workshop on Vascular Anomalies; June 27–28, 1998; Berlin.

27. White CW, Sondheimer HM, Edmond C, Crouch PH, Wilson H, Fan LL. Treatment of pulmonary haemangiomatosis with recombinant interferon alfa-2a. *N Engl J Med.* 1989;380:1197–1225.

28. White CW, Wolf STJ, Korones DN, Sondheimer HM, Tosi MF, Yu A. Treatment of childhood angiomatous diseases with recombinant interferon alfa-2a. *J Pediatr.* 1991;118: 59–66.

29. Wilson JE, Orkin M. "Tufted angioma" (angioblastoma): a benign progressive angioma, not to be confused with Kaposi's sarcomas. *J Am Acad Dermatol.* 1989;20:214–225.

Section 15
Tissue Plasminogen Activator: Biological Perspective for Surgeons

103

Tissue Plasminogen Activator: Biological and Physiological Relevance for Vascular Surgeons

Robert Chang, Khurrum Kamal, and Bauer E. Sumpio

Over the past few years, enormous strides have been made in the development and use of thrombolytic therapy for occlusive vascular disease. Insight into the endogenous properties of thrombolytic agents, such as tissue-type plasminogen activator (tPA), has enabled researchers to begin exploring the efficacy of treatment for patients after myocardial infarction or cerebrovascular accident. Preliminary work has shown that tPA and other agents such as streptokinase and urokinase are effective in improving clinical outcome in both animal and human trials. Thrombolytic therapy is already an effective treatment for pulmonary embolism and deep venous thrombosis.

The efficacy of tPA results from its central role in endogenous fibrinolysis. tPA is one of the many substances responsible for the relative nonthrombogenicity of the vascular system in vivo. The exquisite balance between the procoagulant factors and the production of fibrin is counteracted by clotting inhibitors and the fibrinolytic system, which produces plasmin. The main protectants of thrombosis in vivo include tPA, plasmin, heparin, thrombomodulin, and antithrombin III. These substances are necessary to regulate the coagulation process, which responds to even the slightest arterial insults. Clearly, elucidation of the complex regulatory factors of this system as it pertains to fibrinolysis and thrombus dissolution would show much benefit for patients with vascular disease. Much of the current effort focuses on the molecular signaling of the dynamic vascular system as it responds to changes in pressure, flow, and volume.

The cellular and fluid milieu of the blood vessel wall in vivo is a complex interactive system in which the endothelial lining assumes a major role in hemostasis (Figure 103.1). In addition to circulating vasoactive substances, blood cellular elements secrete agents that can modulate local cell and tissue function. The relative nonthrombogenicity of the endothelium in vivo results from several properties of endothelial cells (ECs), in-

cluding their ability to synthesize and secrete anticoagulant molecules such as prostacyclin and heparinlike molecules and the expression of thrombomodulin on cell surfaces. In addition, ECs participate in fibrinolysis by secreting enzymes with fibrinolytic activity, including urokinase and tPA. Vascular diseases such as neointimal hyperplasia and venous thrombosis represent major disturbances in hemostasis. Impaired fibrinolysis and its association with recurrent venous thrombosis involves defective tPA secretion. tPA is the essential endogenous participant in the fibrinolytic pathway that converts inactive plasminogen into the active plasmin. In addition to its role in fibrinolysis, tPA has also been implicated in the progression of cancer metastasis and regulation of the ovulatory cycle.

New molecular biology and genetic research techniques have significantly increased our understanding of the structure and function of tPA and its role in vascular pathosis. In this chapter we address the numerous forces and substances responsible in regulating tPA secretion and activity. We examine the possible mechanisms regulating the role of tPA in fibrinolysis. The discussion is limited to the extrinsic regulatory factors and includes an overview of the well-elucidated plasminogen activator inhibitor and antiplasmin regulatory pathways only.

Biochemistry of tPA

tPA is a highly specific serine protease that converts the zymogen plasminogen into active plasmin (Figure 103.2). When activated, plasmin attacks fibrin and disrupts the covalent nature of the fibrin clot to form soluble degradation products.[1] Two types of plasminogen activators have been identified: one found in mammalian urine and the other found in tissues (tPA). The major plasminogen activator found in the blood and implicated in the fibrinolytic situation occurring in vascular

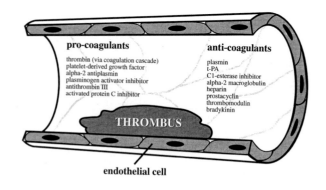

FIGURE 103.1. Contributions to in vivo homeostasis of relative nonthrombogenicity. t-PA, tissue-type plasminogen activator.

disease has been found to be secreted primarily by ECs.[2] The first satisfactory purification of human tPA was from human uterine tissue,[3] and by 1981, several laboratories had purified enough tPA from melanoma cell lines to satisfactorily study its biological and chemical properties.[4–6]

Mature tPA is a single-chain glycoprotein (Figure 103.3A). It is about 70 kD and composed of a single polypeptide chain of 527 amino acids.[7] The amino terminal contains three regions: one corresponds to the fibronectin finger domain,[8–10] the second resembles a growth factor domain,[10–12] and the third contains two looped kringle regions.[13]

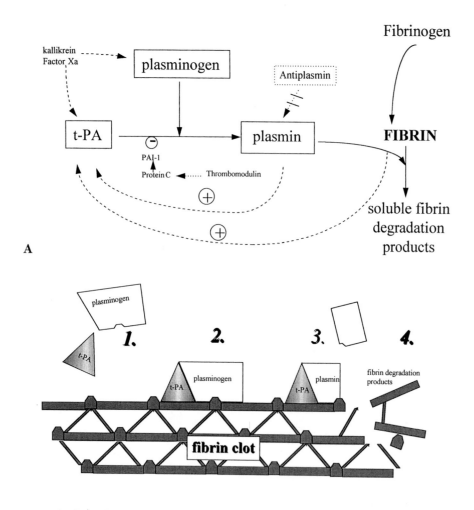

FIGURE 103.2. **A,** Fibrinolytic pathway. t-PA, tissue-type plasminogen activator; PAI-1, plasminogen activator inhibitor 1. **B,** Plasminogen activation: **1,** t-PA released into circulation. **2,** Binding of t-PA in close proximity with plasminogen on fibrin surface. **3,** Cleavage and activation of plasmin. **4,** Degradation of fibrin clot.

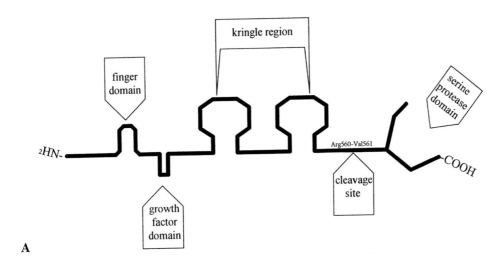

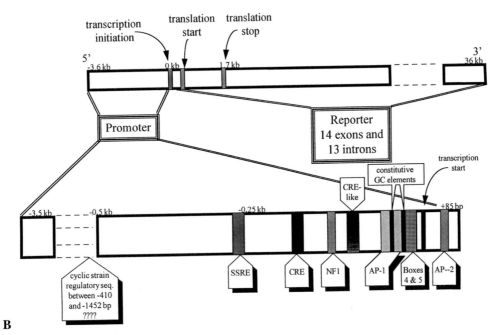

FIGURE 103.3. **A,** Peptide structure of tissue-type plasminogen activator. **B,** Tissue-type plasminogen activator gene. CRE, cyclic adenosine monophosphate response element; G, gua-nine; C, cytosine; SSRE, shear stress response element; NF1, neurofibromatosis 1; AP, activator protein.

The tPA protein contains an NH_2 terminal extension of three additional amino acids (Gly-Ala-Arg).[14] It has 17 disulfide bonds and an additional free cysteine at position 83. The NH_2 terminal region is composed of several domains. Some of the domains are homologous to domains in other proteins such as fibronectin and human epidermal growth factor and also to other serine proteases. These distinct domains in tPA appear to be involved in binding to fibrin, binding to endothelial receptors, and the specificity of tPA with fibrin.[15] The structures involved in binding tPA to the fibrin mass have been shown to be localized within the heavy (A) chain.[16,17]

Deletional peptide mutant investigation has shown that tPA binding to fibrin is mediated by the finger domain and the second kringle region.[18,19] A tPA variant lacking both the finger domain and the growth factor regions, but still containing the kringle regions, can still have enzymatic activity, but it binds poorly to fibrin.[20,21] The structures responsible for enzymatic function are located in the light chain (B chain), because an isolated B chain tPA protein construct is active.[16,17] Plasmin, plasma kallikrein, or factor Xa can activate tPA by cleaving the Arg 278–Ile 279 peptide bond to yield a two-chain enzyme with two chains (A and B) that are held together by disulfide bonds. It has been shown that both single- and double-chain forms exhibit similar catalytic efficiency.[22]

The exact peptide regions necessary for proteolytic activity of the tPA moiety are unclear at this time; studies report conflicting and confusing information. As well as can be determined, the various kringle domains in the heavy chain have been implicated in the functional activity of tPA. The light chain is thought to contain the catalytic site for the serine protease. A possible hindrance in the elucidation of this mechanism might be that deletion or mutation studies of the tPA molecule complicate the picture by changing the existing tertiary conformational arrangements that result in aberrant activity.[15] It is known that both single- and double-chain tPA activate plasminogen by cleaving the Arg 560–Val 561 peptide bond of the zymogen. This creates a heavy and a light chain, with the latter possessing a trypsinlike active site.[23,24]

Physiology

The deposited fibrin present in both normal and pathologic vascular states is the end result of the coagulation cascade that begins with the stimulation of thrombin (Figure 103.3B). tPA is less effective in the absence of fibrin because the presence of fibrin strikingly enhances the activation rate of plasminogen.[25,26] Fibrin provides the surface for optimal reaction between tPA and plasminogen. Degradation of fibrin reveals further binding sites for tPA, thus enhancing the fibrinolytic activity.[27] It is also believed that the fibrin–tPA complex formation renders tPA relatively inaccessible to plasminogen activator inhibitor, thereby enhancing fibrinolysis.[28]

Endothelial cells can also modulate hemostatic and thrombotic events at the cell surface by providing specific binding sites for the activation of plasminogen.[29] Binding of tPA to ECs results in a threefold to fourfold increase of its apparent catalytic efficiency for plasminogen activation.[29] Endothelial cells most likely provide the tPA molecule with additional protection from inhibition by circulating antifibrinolytic agents.[30] This may explain why plasminogen activation does not freely take place in circulation and why fibrinolysis is mainly limited to the clot. The possibility has been raised of two distinct binding sites for tPA on cultured human umbilical vein ECs.[31] By varying the expression of these cell surface receptors, the EC can control the longevity and efficiency of the tPA molecule. Decreased expression of these low-affinity binding sites in the vessel wall is thought to contribute to the development of thrombi in vascular disease states.

Platelets also seem to play a role in fibrinolysis. Miles and Plow[32] have reported that platelets can bind plasminogen and that this bound plasminogen is more sensitive to activation by tPA. In this case, platelets illustrate a common cellular paradox because they initiate the coagulation cascade while also modulating the resultant fibrinolytic pathway. Further evidence affirms this interplay between cellular components. Lipoproteins that disrupt certain cell surface binding sites inhibit tPA at the transcriptional level and at the translational level.[33] A molecular mechanism may link the resulting impairment of fibrinolysis with the initiation of atherosclerosis.

Regulation of tPA

Saksela[34] has characterized the dependence of tPA production on hormonal and developmental control in vivo. Studies with rat ovarian cells exemplify the diversity and complexity of the regulatory mechanism in different systems. Gonadotropins, epidermal growth factor, and vasoactive intestinal peptide have all been shown to affect tPA activity. Interleukin 1 is also known to preferentially stimulate tPA production in human articular chondrocytes.[35]

Recent investigation has revealed more specific sites of regulation as well as proposed modes of action. Regulation of tPA can occur at several different points. Messenger RNA (mRNA) levels may be influenced by transcriptional activity, posttranscriptional alterations may change the mRNA degradative instructions, or tPA protein stability properties may be altered.

After completion of transcription, tPA mRNA and its resulting protein product are additionally influenced by hemostatic forces and agents. Exact mechanisms are not well enumerated, but the second messenger pathways have been implicated (Figure 103.4).

Endogenous substances and known vasoactive agents in the blood play a crucial role in tPA release. Thrombin stimulates release of tPA and plasminogen activator inhibitor 1 (PAI-1).[36,37] Hinsbergh and coworkers[38] observed an increase in tPA production in human microvascular cells with administration of thrombin, which is thought to be mediated by a protein kinase C (PKC) pathway. Administration of thrombin results in an increase in tPA mRNA levels, thus suggesting that thrombin is a transcriptional regulator.[39] Histamine also stimulates secretion of tPA protein but not PAI-1.[37] Histamine may have an additive effect on phorbol monoacetate (PMA) activation of tPA, whereas histamine and thrombin exhibit no synergistic effect.[40]

tPA activity and mRNA levels are increased in HeLa cells and ECs exposed to tumor-promoting phorbol esters.[41] Numerous studies of tPA regulation have been done with administration of phorbol ester, a known stimulator of the PKC pathway, to examine this second messenger's effect on tPA secretion. This response is potentiated fivefold with simultaneous administration of cyclic adenosine monophosphate (cAMP). This was not seen

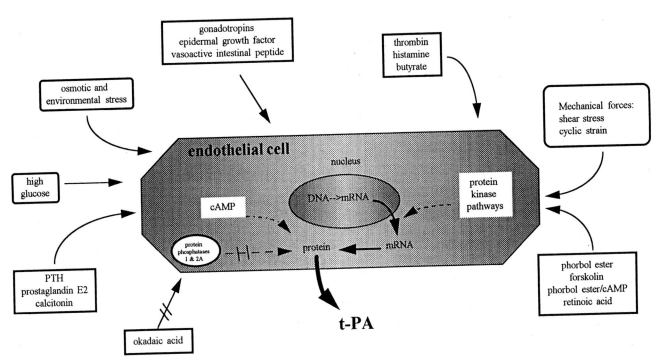

FIGURE 103.4. Modulators of tissue-type plasminogen activator (t PA) activity. cAMP, cyclic adenosine monophosphate; mRNA, messenger ribonucleic acid; PTH, parathyroid hormone.

with cAMP alone but in conjunction with phorbol ester.[42] In 1989 Levin and colleagues[43] reported that changes in mRNA levels in response to PMA and PMA/forskolin precede and determine tPA antigen secretion. They noted that this response was modulated by a cAMP-sensitive pathway. Additional investigation with PMA led to the conclusion that both factors interacted using the PKC–tyrosine kinase and cAMP–dependent signal transduction pathway.[44] Epidermal growth factor has also been shown to have a stimulatory effect on transcription.[44]

The biology of the activation of tPA appears to be largely mediated through various second messenger systems that control many aspects of regulation. Allan and associates[1] observed cAMP mediation of parathyroid hormone, prostaglandin E_2, and calcitonin in increasing tPA activity. In addition, they noted a cAMP-independent regulatory mechanism with a vitamin D derivative. Increases of tPA mRNA levels mediated by PMA are known to depend on ongoing protein synthesis. This may be due to a cyclic regulatory effect in this system.[45]

Peraldi and colleagues[2] noted that kidney mesangial cells were inhibited by PKA, in contrast with ECs, which showed no change in baseline tPA levels. These changes were concluded to be posttranscriptional, through inhibition of protein synthesis or activation of protein degradation.

Glucocorticoids also up-regulate tPA production, which suggests a possible glucocorticoid receptor–mediated pathway of activation.[46] Under high blood glucose conditions, up-regulation of tPA protein has been observed. A posttranslational mechanism has been proposed for the impaired fibrinolysis seen in some patients with diabetes.[47] Butyrate treatment of ECs induces significant increases in tPA mRNA levels and in tPA production without influencing the level of PAI-1. A four-carbon moiety was found to maximally stimulate activity in cultured human ECs.[48] Other agents in the second messenger pathway have also been shown to affect tPA synthesis. Okadaic acid, an inhibitor of protein phosphatases 1 and 2A, is a significant suppressor of tPA mRNA levels. This suggests an active role for phosphatases in tPA transcription.[49]

Cell structure and morphology are also critical in tPA synthesis. Disruption of the cellular microtubule system by colchicine, nocodazole, and tubulozole partly blocked the PMA-induced stimulation of tPA mRNA levels, suggesting the importance of the relationship between cytoskeletal arrangement and tPA gene expression.[50]

Physiological Regulation

In addition to chemical effectors, vascular ECs are subjected to numerous mechanical forces in vivo. The modulation of cellular processes by mechanical force is a widely accepted concept, and recent studies have delineated important factors. Two such forces, shear stress and cyclic strain, have previously been shown to exert wide-ranging effects on the arterial environment in vitro and in vivo. Shear stress is a function of the tangential force of blood flow on the arterial wall, and cyclic strain is a pressure force exerted on the endothelium and vessel layers by the distension and relaxation of systole and diastole.

In vivo canine studies have shown that fluid flow alters the alignment and morphology of intact endothelium.[51] Aortic ECs alter their orientation relative to the direction and flow pattern of circulation in experimental conditions. These cells also exhibit a more elongated and elliptical shape when exposed to increasing hemodynamic force (i.e., a larger vessel in vivo). Other in vivo studies have investigated the effects of exercise and venous occlusion on steady-state levels of tPA. Increased rates of exercise and cases of venous occlusion were separately observed to increase tPA secretion.[52-55] The dependence of tPA activity on hemodynamic forces has been known for some time.[56-61] The relative flow seems to affect the rate of tPA complex formation, and it may be involved in regulation of the intrinsic inhibitor system.

In 1989 Diamond and coworkers[62] showed that shear stress stimulated tPA secretion in cultured ECs. Later, Diamond and associates[63] observed that tPA mRNA levels increased in cells exposed to laminar shear stress. Control cells were maintained in stationary culture, and the experimental group was exposed to 25 dyn/cm² shear stress for 24 hours. The tPA mRNA levels increased 10-fold compared with controls, whereas the secreted tPA levels increased 3-fold compared with the stationary cells. These results suggested a transcriptional and posttranscriptional mechanism for modulation by shear stress.[63]

A shear stress response element in the platelet-derived growth factor gene promoter has been identified.[64] A series of nested deletion mutants of the gene promoter, coupled to the chloramphenicol acetyl transferase reporter gene, were transfected into bovine aortic endothelial cells and exposed to 10 dyn/cm² shear stress for 4 hours. After the mutant cells that showed a shear stress–related increase were isolated, further analysis pinpointed the exact location of this shear stress–responsive area. Interestingly, the shear stress response element is also found in the tPA promoter, located −284 base pairs (bp) upstream from the transcription initiation site. Whether this binding site can selectively up-regulate tPA levels in response to in vitro shear stress remains to be determined.

In vivo measurements in patients and animals and in vitro models replicating the major geometric features of blood vessels indicate a 5% to 6% wall excursion at peak systole under normal physiologic conditions that can be as high as 10% under hypertensive conditions.[65,66] Our laboratory has investigated the response to cyclic strain in cultured ECs. Previous work has shown that stretched ECs can selectively stimulate tPA production.[67] Endothelial cells harvested from human saphenous veins were seeded on flexible collagen membranes and grown to confluence. In cells exposed to −20 kPa of vacuum, which deformed the membranes to 24% maximum strain at a frequency of 60 cycles/min (0.5 seconds of elongation alternating with 0.5 seconds of relaxation), there was a threefold to fivefold increase of tPA secretion after exposure at 3 and 5 days. Endothelial cells exposed to this regimen secreted approximately 1.7-fold higher levels of tPA compared with the stationary cells.

In recent studies, tPA promoter elements were examined for their potential significance in cyclic strain regulation.[68] Bovine aortic ECs were transfected with promoter variants that were coupled to the CAT reporter gene. Deletional mutants of lengths −1452, −410, −196, and −105 bp were constructed. Transfected cells were seeded on flexible collagen membranes and were maintained in conditioned media in a 37°C incubator. All cells were stretched using −20 kPa vacuum (10% average strain) at 60 cycles/min for up to 48 hours. A significant drop-off in activity was noted in the stretched −410 bp promoter construct cells compared with the −1452 bp cells, thus raising the possibility of a strain-dependent regulatory element located in the region between −410 and −1452 bp.

In similar studies, the cAMP responsive element and AP-2 sites of the promoter were mutated and transfected into bovine aortic endothelial cells to observe their possible involvement in strain regulation. Both mutant forms showed significant decreases in stretched cells compared with the wild-type promoter constructs, with the cAMP responsive element mutant showing the most significant decrease. Although these sites are important for cyclic strain regulation, they did not prove to be necessary or sufficient for tPA synthesis.

In addition, transfection with a promoter construct containing a defective shear stress response element segment showed no significant decrease in activity when exposed to cyclic strain. It appears that this element is responsive to shear stress only and is not influenced by mechanical deformation.

The mechanism for cyclic strain regulation is not currently known. We have previously shown that cyclic strain increases inositol triphosphate and diacylglycerol levels in ECs and that phosphatidylcholine hydrolysis by phospholipase D can contribute to the sustained diacylglycerol formation in ECs subjected to cyclic strain.[69,70] The sustained elevation in diacylglycerol can potentially stimulate PKC expression that has been implicated in increased tPA activity. These results suggest that tPA production can be regulated by changes in the pulsatile flow. The most likely mechanism appears to be the PKC/cAMP pathway, which has been shown to be activated by other biological influences.

In addition to the effects from mechanical forces, environmental stress has also been shown to influence tPA activity. Levin and coworkers[71] reported an increase in tPA production in cells exposed to a hyperosmotic environment. Endothelial cells that were incubated in hyperosmotic media showed a dose-dependent decrease in cell volume, and a 1.9-fold and 3.7-fold induction of tPA secretion at 425 and 485 mOsm/kg H_2O, respectively. The measurements were taken within 24 hours of incubation. The compounds used to manipulate the osmolality (mannitol, raffinose, sorbitol, or NaCl) did not affect the dose-dependent increase of tPA. Levin and coworkers[71] postulated that this increase uses a different signal pathway, because inositol triphosphate and diacylglycerol levels were unchanged in the hyperosmotic cells.[71] Because plasmin, the cleavage product of tPA, functions nonspecifically, the environmental effects on tPA may play a crucial role in protein degradation and the induction of pathophysiologic processes.

Clinical Implications and Future Perspectives

Impairment of fibrinolysis, from deficient synthesis or release of tPA from the vessel wall or increased levels of PAI-1, is associated with a tendency to thrombosis. Excessive fibrinolysis due to increased tPA levels may cause bleeding complications. Lifelong hemorrhagic disorders of this type have been described.[72,73]

The importance of the EC on clot dissolution in vivo seems clear. The fibrin specificity of tPA has led to its use in antithrombotic therapy. With the development of recombinant DNA techniques, tPA has become one of the first drugs utilized in treatment of stroke and myocardial infarction dysfunction.[1] In fact, retroviral-induced overexpression has been suggested to be a useful therapy in thromboocclusive failure of implanted vascular devices and mechanically denuded vessels.[74]

Administration of tPA has recently been shown to improve clinical outcome as of 3 months after a stroke. Studies suggest that doses of less than 0.95 mg of tPA per kilogram of body weight are relatively safe and resulted in early neurological improvement in a significant proportion of patients observed. Regardless of the subtype of stroke diagnosed, tPA treatment within 3 hours of cerebrovascular accident resulted in a more favorable outcome compared with no treatment.[75]

Work remains to be done to determine the precise mechanisms and the exact areas of regulation for the role of tPA in fibrinolysis. tPA modulation has been implicated in the relative nonthrombogenicity of vessels in vivo. Because many transcription factors and their effector sites on the gene promoter are common among various products in the endothelium, the elucidation of transcriptional mechanics is eagerly sought after for more relevant understanding of the hemostatic scenario and the long-term benefit for treatment of vascular disease.

References

1. Medcalf R, Ruegg M, Schleuning W. A DNA motif related to the cAMP-responsive element and an exon-located activator protein-2 binding site in the human tissue-type plasminogen activator gene promoter cooperate in basal expression and convey activation by phorbol ester and cAMP. *J Biol Chem.* 1990;265:14618–14626.
2. Levin E, Loskutoff D. Cultured bovine endothelial cells produce both urokinase and tissue-type plasminogen activators. *J Cell Biol.* 1982;94:631–639.
3. Rijken D, Wijngaards G, Jong MZ-D, Welbergen, J. Purification and partial characterization of plasminogen activator from human uterine tissue. *Biochim Biophys Acta.* 1979;580:140–144.
4. Rijken D, Collen D. Purification and characterization of the plasminogen activator secreted by human melanoma cells in culture. *J Biol Chem.* 1981;256:7035–7039.
5. Collen D, Rijken D, Damme JV, Billiau A. Purification of human tissue-type plasminogen activator in centigram quantities from human melanoma cell culture fluid and its conditioning for use in vivo. *Thromb Haemost.* 1982;48:294–298.
6. Kruithof E, Schleuning W, Bachmann F. Human tissue-type plasminogen activator. Production in continuous serum-free cell culture and rapid purification. *Biochem J.* 1985;226:631–635.
7. Pennica D, Holmes WE, Kohr WJ, et al. Cloning and expression of human tissue-type plasminogen activator cDNA in E. coli. *Nature.* 1983;301:214–221.
8. Skorstengaard K, Thorgersen H, Petersen T. Complete primary structure of the collagen-binding domain of bovine fibronectin. *Eur J Biochem.* 1984;140:235–243.
9. Petersen T, Thorgersen H, Skorstengaard K, et al. Partial primary structure of bovine plasma fibronectin: three types of internal homology. *Proc Natl Acad Sci U S A.* 1983;80:137–141.
10. Banyai L, Varadi A, Patthy L. Common evolutionary origin of the fibrin-binding structures of fibronectin and tissue-type plasminogen activator. *FEBS Lett.* 1983;1635:37–41.
11. Savage C, Inagami T, Cohen S. The primary structure of epidermal growth factor. *J Biol Chem.* 1972;247:7612–7621.
12. Gregory H, Preston B. The primary structure of human urogastrone. *Int J Pept Protein Res.* 1977;9:107–118.
13. Magnusson S, Peterson T, Sottrup-Jensen L, Claeys H. Complete structure of prothrombin: isolation, structure, and reactivity of ten carboxylated glutamic acid residues and regulation of prothrombin activation by thrombin. In: Reich E, Rifkin D, Shaw E, eds. *Proteases and Biological Control.* Cold Spring Harbor, NY: Cold Spring Harbor Laboratory; 1975:123–149.
14. Jornvall H, Pohl G, Bergsdorf N, Wallen P. Differential proteolysis and evidence for a residue exchange in tissue

plasminogen activator suggest possible association between two types of protein microheterogeneity. *FEBS Lett.* 1983;156:47.

15. Collen D, Lijnen H, Verstraete M. Fibrinolytic system and its disorders. In: Handin R, Lux S, Stossel T. *Blood: Principles and Practice of Hematology.* Philadelphia, Pa: JB Lippincott; 1995:1261–1288.

16. Holvoet P, Lijnen H, Collen D. Characterization of functional domains in human tissue-type plasminogen activator with the use of monoclonal antibodies. *Eur J Biochem.* 1986;158:173–180.

17. Rijken D, Groeneveld E. Isolation and functional characterization of the heavy and light chains of human tissue-type plasminogen activator. *J Biol Chem.* 1986;261: 3098–3105.

18. Verheijen J, Caspers M, Chang G, et al. Involvement of finger domain and kringle 2 domain of tissue-type plasminogen activator in fibrin binding and stimulation of activity by fibrin. *EMBO J.* 1986;5:3525–3529.

19. Zonneveld AV, Veerman H, Pannekoek H. Autonomous functions of structural domains on human tissue-type plasminogen activator. *Proc Natl Acad Sci U S A.* 1986;83: 4670–4678.

20. Kalyan N, Lee S, Wilhelm J, et al. Structure-function analysis with tissue-type plasminogen activator. Effect of deletion of NH_2-terminal domains on its biochemical and biological properties. *J Biol Chem.* 1988;263:3971–3980.

21. Larsen G, Henson K, Blue Y. Variants of human tissue-type plasminogen activator: fibrin binding, fibrinolytic, and fibrinogenolytic characterization of genetic variants lacking the fibronectin finger-like and/or the epidermal growth factor domains. *J Biol Chem.* 1988;263:1023–1032.

22. Rijken D, Hoylaerts M, Collen D. Fibrinolytic properties of one-chain and two chain human extrinsic (tissue-type) plasminogen activator. *J Biol Chem.* 1982;257:2920–2927.

23. Robbins K, Summaria L, Hsieh B, Shah R. The peptide chains of human plasmin: mechanism of activation of human plasminogen to plasmin. *J Biol Chem.* 1967;242: 2333–2339.

24. Groskopf W, Summaria L, Robbins K. Studies on the active center of human plasmin: partial amino acid sequence of a peptide containing the active center serine residue. *J Biol Chem.* 1969;244:3590–3597.

25. Hoylaerts M, Rijken D, Lijnen H, Collen D. Kinetics of the activation of plasminogen by human tissue plasminogen activator: role of fibrin. *J Biol Chem.* 1982;257:2912–2918.

26. Camiolo S, Thorsen S, Astrup T. Fibrinogenolysis and fibrinolysis with tissue plasminogen activator, urokinase, streptokinase-activated human globulin, and plasmin. *Proc Soc Exp Biol Med.* 1971;138:277–287.

27. Nieuwenhuizen W, Voskuilen M, Vermond A, et al. The influence of fibrin(ogen) fragments on the kinetic parameters of the tissue-type plasminogen-activator-mediated activation of different forms of plasminogen. *Eur J Biochem.* 1988;174:163–171.

28. Wun T, Capuano A. Initiation and regulation of fibrinolysis in human plasma at the plasminogen activator level. *Blood.* 1987;69:1354–1362.

29. Hajjar K, Hamel N, Harpel P, Nachman R. Binding of tissue plasminogen activator to cultured human endothelial cells. *J Clin Invest.* 1987;80:1712–1719.

30. Speiser W, Anders E, Binder B, Muller-Berghaus G. Clot lysis mediated by cultured human microvascular endothelial cells. *Thromb Haemost.* 1988;60:463–467.

31. Barnathan E, Kuo A, Keyl HVD, et al. Tissue-type plasminogen activator binding to human endothelial cells: evidence for two distinct binding sites. *J Biol Chem.* 1988; 263:7792–7801.

32. Miles L, Plow E. Binding and activation of plasminogen on the platelet surface. *J Biol Chem.* 1985;260:4303–4310.

33. Levin E, Miles L, Fless G, et al. Lipoproteins inhibit the secretion of tissue plasminogen activator from human endothelial cells. *Arteriosci Thromb.* 1994; 14:438–442.

34. Saksela O. Plasminogen activation and regulation of pericellular proteolysis. *Biochim Biophys Acta.* 1985;823:35–65.

35. Bunning R, Crawford A, Richardson H, et al. Interleukin 1 preferentially stimulates the production of tissue-type plasminogen activator by human articular chondrocytes. *Biochim Biophys Acta.* 1987;924:473–478.

36. Gelehrter T, Sznycer-Laszuk R. Thrombin induction of plasminogen activator–inhibitor in cultured endothelial cells. *J Clin Invest.* 1986;77:165–171.

37. Hanss M, Collen D. Secretion of tissue-type plasminogen activator and plasminogen activator inhibitor by cultured human endothelial cells: modulation by thrombin, endotoxin, and histamine. *J Lab Clin Med.* 1987;109:97–108.

38. Van Hinsbergh VW, Binnema D, Scheffer M, et al. Production of plasminogen activators and inhibitor by serially propagated endothelial cells from adult human blood vessels. *Arteriosclerosis.* 1987;7:389–400.

39. Villamediana L, Rondeau E, He C, et al. Thrombin regulates components of the fibrinolytic system in human mesangial cells. *Kidney Int.* 1990;38:956–961.

40. Levin E, Santell L. Thrombin- and histamine-induced signal transduction in human endothelial cells. Stimulation and agonist-dependent desensitization of protein phosphorylation. *J Biol Chem.* 1991;266:174–181.

41. Wigler M, Weinstein I. Tumour promoter induces plasminogen activator. *Nature.* 1976;259:232–233.

42. Levin E, Santell L. Stimulation and desensitization of tissue plasminogen activator release from human endothelial cells. *J Biol Chem.* 1988;263:9360–9365.

43. Levin E, Marotti K, Santell L. Protein kinase C and the stimulation of tissue plasminogen activator release from human endothelial cells. Dependence on the elevation of messenger RNA. *J Biol Chem.* 1989;264:16030–16036.

44. Medcalf R, Schleuning W. Regulation of human tissue-type plasminogen activator gene transcription by epidermal growth factor and 3′,5′-cyclic adenosine monophosphate. *Mol Endocrinol.* 1991;5:1773–1779.

45. Waller E, Schleuning W. Isolation and characterization of the human tissue-type plasminogen activator structural gene including its 5′ flanking region. *J Biol Chem.* 1985; 260:6354–6360.

46. Medcalf RL, Van den Berg E, Schleuning WD. Glucocorticoid-modulated gene expression of tissue- and urinary-type plasminogen activator and plasminogen activator inhibitor 1 and 2. *J Cell Biol.* 1988;106:971–978.

47. Maiello M, Boeri D, Podesta F, et al. Increased expression of tissue plasminogen activator and its inhibitor and reduced fibrinolytic potential of human endothelial cells cultured in elevated glucose. *Diabetes.* 1992;41:1009–1015.

48. Kooistra T, van den Berg J, Tons A, Platenburg G, Rijken DC, van den Berg E. Butyrate stimulates tissue-type plasminogen-activator synthesis in cultured human endothelial cells. *Biochem J.* 1987;247:605–612.

49. Medcalf R. Cell- and gene specific interactions between signal transduction pathways revealed by okadaic acid. Studies on the plasminogen activating system. *J Biol Chem.* 1992;267:12220–12226.

50. Santell L, Marotti K, Bartfeld N, et al. Disruption of microtubules inhibits the stimulation of tissue plasminogen activator expression and promotes plasminogen activator inhibitor type 1 expression in human endothelial cells. *Exp Cell Res.* 1992;201:358–365.

51. Flaherty J, Pierce J, Ferrans V, et al. Endothelial nuclear patterns in the canine arterial tree with particular reference to hemodynamic events. *Circ Res.* 1971; 30:23–33.

52. Biggs R, Macfarlane R, Pilling J. Observations on fibrinolysis. Experimental production by exercise or adrenaline. *Lancet.* 1947;1:402–404.

53. Clarke R, Orandi A, Cliffton E. Induction of fibrinolysis by venous obstruction. *Angiology.* 1960;11:367–370.

54. Holemans R. Increase in fibrinolytic activity by venous occlusion. *J Appl Physiol.* 1963;18:1123–1129.

55. Wiman B, Mellbring G, Ranby M. Plasminogen activator release during venous stasis and exercise as determined by a new specific assay. *Clin Chim Acta.* 1983;127:279–288.

56. Wiman B, Chmielewska J, Ranby M. Inactivation of tissue plasminogen activator in plasma. *J Biol Chem.* 1984;259: 3644–3647.

57. Verheijen J, Chang G, Kluft C. Evidence for the occurrence of a fast-acting inhibitor for tissue-type plasminogen activator in human plasma. *Thromb Haemost.* 1984;51: 392–395.

58. Thorsen S, Philips M. Isolation of tissue-type plasminogen activator-inhibitor complexes from human plasma. Evidence for a rapid plasminogen activator inhibitor. *Biochim Biophys Acta.* 1984;802:111–118.

59. Kruithof E, Tran-Thang C, Ransijn A, Bachman F. Demonstration of a fast-acting inhibitor of plasminogen activators in human plasma. *Blood.* 1984;64:907–913.

60. Fearnley G, Tweed J. Evidence of an active fibrinolytic enzyme in the plasma of normal people with observations on inhibition associated with the presence of calcium. *Clin Sci.* 1953;12:81–89.

61. Fearnley G, Lackner R. The fibrinolytic activity of normal blood. *Br J Haemotol.* 1955;1:189–198.

62. Diamond S, Eskin S, McIntire L. Fluid flow stimulates tissue plasminogen activator secretion by cultured human endothelial cells. *Science.* 1989;243:1483–1485.

63. Diamond S, Sharefkin J, Dieffenbach C, et al. Tissue plasminogen activator messenger RNA levels increase in cultured human endothelial cells exposed to laminar shear stress. *J Cell Physiol.* 1990;143:364–371.

64. Resnick N, Collins T, Atkinson W, Bonthron DT, Dewey CF Jr, Gimbrone MA Jr. Platelet-derived growth factor B chain promoter contains a *cis*-acting fluid shear stress-responsive element. *Proc Natl Acad Sci U S A.* 1993;90:4591–4595.

65. Steinman D, Ethier C. The effect of wall distensibility on flow in a 2D end-to-side anastomosis. *J Biomech Eng.* 1994; 96:234–239.

66. Patel DJ, Greenfield JC Jr, Austen WG, Morrow AG, Fry DL. Pressure-flow relationships in the ascending aorta and femoral artery of man. *J Appl Physiol.* 1965;20:459–463.

67. Iba T, Shin T, Sonoda T, Rosales O, Sumpio B. Stimulation of endothelial secretion of tissue-type plasminogen activator by repetitive stretch. *J Surg Res.* 1991;50:457–460.

68. Sumpio BE, Chang R, Xu W, Wang X, Du W. Regulation of tissue plasminogen activator in bovine endothelial cells exposed to cyclic strain: the functional significance of the CRE, AP-2, and SSRE sites. *Am J Physiol.* 1997;42: C1441–C1448.

69. Rosales O, Sumpio B. Changes in cyclic strain increase inositol triphosphate and diacylglycerol in endothelial cells. *Am J Physiol.* 1992;262:C956–C962.

70. Evans L, Frenkel L, Brophy CM, et al. Activation of diacylglycerol in cultured endothelial cells exposed to cyclic strain. *Am J Physiol.* 1997;41:C650–C659.

71. Levin E, Santell L, Saljooque F. Hyperosmotic stress stimulates tissue plasminogen activator expression by a PKC-independent pathway. *Am J Physiol.* 1993;265:C387–C396.

72. Booth NA, Bennett B, Wijngaards G, Grieve JH. A new lifelong hemorrhagic disorder due to excess plasminogen activator. *Blood.* 1983;61:267–275.

73. Aznar J, Estelles A, Vila V, Reganon E, Espana F, Villa P. Inherited fibrinolytic disorder due to an enhanced plasminogen activator level. *Thromb Haemost.* 1984;52: 196–200.

74. Dichek D, Anderson J, Kelly A, et al. Enhanced in vivo antithrombotic effects of endothelial cells expressing recombinant plasminogen activators transduced with retroviral vectors. *Circulation.* 1996;93:301–309.

75. National Institute of Neurological Disorders and Stroke rt-PA Stroke Study Group. Tissue plasminogen activator for acute ischemic stroke. *N Engl J Med.* 1995;333:1581–1587.

Index

Index